FOR INSTRUCTORS

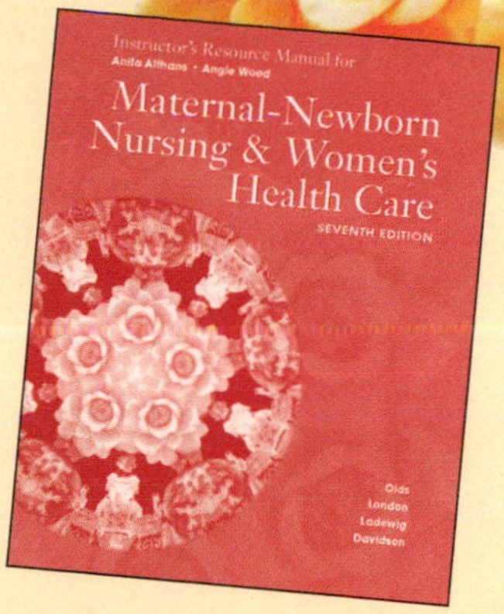

Instructor's Resource Manual

ISBN: 0131122762

This manual contains a wealth of material to help faculty plan and manage the maternity nursing course. It includes chapter overviews, detailed lecture suggestions and outlines, learning objectives, a complete test bank, answers to the textbook critical thinking exercises, teaching tips, and more for each chapter. The IRM also guides faculty how to assign and use the text-specific Companion Website, www.prenhall.com/olds, and the free Student CD-ROM that accompany the textbook.

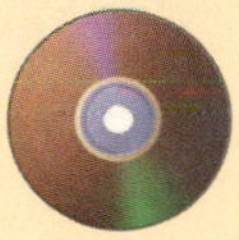

Instructor's Resource CD-ROM

ISBN: 0131100114

This cross-platform CD-ROM provides text and illustrations in PowerPoint from the new Seventh Edition of this textbook for use in classroom lectures. It also contains an electronic test bank, answers to the textbook critical thinking exercises, and animations and video clips from the Student CD-ROM. This supplement is available to faculty free upon adoption of the textbook.

Companion Website Syllabus Manager

www.prenhall.com/olds

Faculty adopting this textbook have ***free*** access to the online **Syllabus Manager** feature of the Companion Website, www.prenhall.com/olds. Syllabus Manager offers a whole host of features that facilitate the students' use of the Companion Website, and allows faculty to post syllabi and course information online for their students. For more information or a demonstration of Syllabus Manager, please contact a Prentice Hall Sales Representative.

Companion Website

Online Course Management Systems

Also available are online companions available for schools using course management systems. The online course management solutions feature interactive assessment modules, electronic test bank, PowerPoint images and text slides, animations and video clips, and more. For more information about adopting an online course management system to accompany **Maternal-Newborn Nursing & Women's Health Care**, please contact your Prentice Hall Health Sales Representative or go to the appropriate website below:

Bb Blackboard www.blackboard.com

WebCT

http://cms.prenhall.com/webct/index.html
http://cms.prenhall.com/blackboard/index.html
http://cms.prenhall.com/coursecompass/

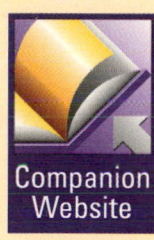

Brief Contents

Maternal-Newborn Nursing & Women's Health Care

SEVENTH EDITION

Sally B. Olds, MS, RNC, SANE
Professor Emerita
Beth-El College of Nursing
Colorado Springs, Colorado

Marcia L. London, PhDc, RNC, NNP
Senior Clinical Instructor
Beth-El College of Nursing and Health Sciences
University of Colorado
Colorado Springs, Colorado

Patricia A. Wieland Ladewig, PhD, RN
Professor and Academic Dean
School for Health Care Professions
Regis University
Denver, Colorado

Michele R. Davidson, PhD, CNM, RN
Assistant Professor of Nursing and Women's Studies
George Mason University
Fairfax, Virginia
Staff Midwife Women's Healthcare Associates of Loudoun
Lansdowne, Virginia

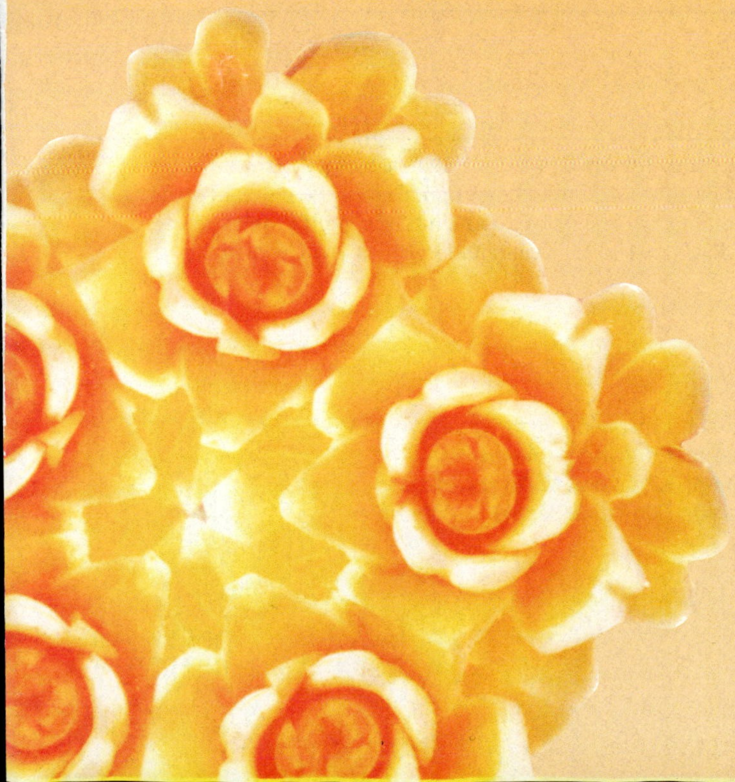

PEARSON
Prentice Hall

Upper Saddle River, New Jersey 07458

Library of Congress Cataloging-in-Publication Data

Maternal-newborn nursing and women's healthcare / Sally B. Olds . . . [et al.].— 7th ed.
p. cm.
Previous ed. published under the title: Maternal-newborn nursing.
Includes bibliographical references and index.
ISBN 0-13-099009-4
1. Maternity nursing—Handbooks, manuals, etc. I. Olds, Sally B., (date) II. Olds, Sally B., (date) Maternal-newborn nursing.

RG951.O4327 2004
610.73'678—dc21 2002192996

Publisher: Julie Levin Alexander
Assistant to the Publisher: Regina Bruno
Editor-in-Chief: Maura Connor
Executive Development Editor: Marilyn Meserve
Development Editor: Laura Bonazzoli
Media Development Editor: John J. Jordan
Assistant Editors: Yesenia Kopperman & Sladjana Repic
Permissions Coordinator: Amy Puchino
Director of Production & Manufacturing: Bruce Johnson
Managing Production Editor: Patrick Walsh
Production Liasion: Danielle Newhouse
Production Editor: Amy Hackett, Carlisle Communications
Manufacturing Manager: Ilene Sanford
Design Director: Cheryl Asherman
Senior Design Coordinator: Maria Guglielmo
Interior Designer: Christine Cantera
Cover Designers: Cheryl Asherman & Mary Siener
Cover and Interior Illustrations: *Passport to Paris* by Judith Paul and Tom Durden/Images Kaleidoscopes, as seen in *Kaleidoscope Artistry* by Cozy Baker
Electronic Art Creation: Precision Graphics
Manager of New Media Production : Amy Peltier
New Media Project Manager: Stephen Hartner
New Media Production : Eclectic Multimedia
Marketing Manager: Nicole Benson
Marketing Coordinator: Janet Ryerson
Channel Marketing Manager: Rachele Strober
Composition: Carlisle, Inc.
Cover Printer: Lehigh Press
Printer/Binder: RR Donnelley & Sons

Notice: Care has been taken to confirm the accuracy of information presented in this book. The authors, editors, and the publisher, however, cannot accept any responsibility for errors or omissions or for consequences from application of the information in this book and make no warranty, express or implied, with respect to its contents.

The authors and publisher have exerted every effort to ensure that drug selections and dosages set forth in this text are in accord with current recommendations and practice at time of publication. However, in view of ongoing research, changes in government regulations, and the constant flow of information relating to drug therapy and drug reactions, the reader is urged to check the package inserts of all drugs for any change in indications of dosage and for added warnings and precautions. This is particularly important when the recommended agent is a new and/or infrequently employed drug.

All photographs/illustrations not credited on page or below the piece, were photographed/rendered on assignment and are property of Pearson Education/ Prentice Hall Health.

Pearson Education LTD.
Pearson Education Australia PTY. Limited
Pearson Education Singapore. Pte. Ltd
Pearson Education North Asia Ltd
Pearson Education Canada, Ltd.
Pearson Educación de Mexico, S.A. de C.V.
Pearson Education—Japan
Pearson Education Malaysia, Pte. Ltd
Pearson Education. Upper Saddle River, NJ

PEARSON
Prentice Hall

10 9 8 7 6 5 4 3
ISBN 0-13-099009-4

Dedication

The future of maternal-newborn nursing rests in the hands of today's nursing students. And so we dedicate this text to all nursing students—future professional nurses.

May you have the vision to see possibilities and opportunities;
The compassion to identify the needs and desires of childbearing families;
The knowledge and skill necessary to provide effective care;
The wisdom to recognize what needs to be changed;
The courage to implement these changes effectively;
And the firm commitment to remain men and women for others.

For truly, you are our hope and the hope of childbearing families everywhere.

Then too, as always, we dedicate this text to our families with love.
To Joe Olds, Scott, Roy, Allison, and Dave
To David London, Craig, and Matthew
To Tim Ladewig, Ryan, Amanda, and Erik
To Nathan Davidson, Hayden, and Chloe

Contents

Appendices

Preface

Most often, pregnancy and childbirth are times of great joy, a celebration of life, and a promise of the future. But, they may also be times of deepest sorrow as families deal with illness, complications, and loss. Nurses play a central role in all aspects of the childbearing experience, from the earliest days of pregnancy, through the moments of birth, and during the early days of parenthood. Often the quality of the nursing care that a family receives profoundly influences their perceptions of the entire experience—for better or for worse. However, the changes occurring in the healthcare delivery system are altering the way we practice nursing and have staggering implications for nurses everywhere, even nurses caring for childbearing women and their families.

Now, more than ever, nurses must be flexible, creative, and open to change. They must be able to think critically and problem solve effectively. They must be able to meet the teaching needs of their clients so that their clients can, in turn, better meet their own healthcare needs. They must be open to an increasingly multicultural population. They must understand and use the technology available in their chosen area of practice. Most crucially, they must never lose sight of the importance of excellent nursing care in improving the quality of people's lives.

The underlying philosophy of ***Maternal-Newborn Nursing & Women's Health Care*** remains unchanged. We believe that pregnancy and birth are normal life processes and that family members are co-participants in care. We believe that women's healthcare is an important aspect of nursing. We remain committed to providing a text that is accurate and readable; a text that helps students develop the skills and abilities they need now and in the future in an ever-changing healthcare environment.

Underlying Themes and Contemporary Trends

The cover on this edition of the text depicts a kaleidoscope. The kaleidoscope theme is an important one for us because through the magic of a kaleidoscope, its images—like life itself—change from moment to moment. Like pregnancy, "kaleidoscopes are a universal celebration. . . . Each kaleidoscope is a little world unto itself where one can hear silent music, feel wondrous joy, count the interlacing stars, find peace and calm, experience oneness. . . ."[1] We hope to help capture for you the magic that childbearing families experience and the deep satisfaction that maternal-newborn nurses feel in their practice.

Fostering Evidence-Based Practice. Seasoned nurses, like health professionals in all disciplines, are increasingly aware of the importance of using reliable information as the basis for planning and providing effective care. This approach, referred to as *evidence-based practice*, draws on information from a variety of sources, including nursing research. To help nurses become more comfortable in using evidence-based practice, we include a brief discussion of the concepts in Chapter 1 and then, throughout the text, we provide a series of **Evidence-Based Practice** boxes relating research evidence to women's health and maternal-newborn nursing. We also include a series of **Research in Practice** boxes that provide strong examples of relevant clinically focused research.

Commitment to Diversity. As nurses and as educators, we recognize the importance of honoring diversity and of providing culturally competent care. Thus, we continually strive to make our text ever more inclusive. As part of this effort, we added a new, important chapter—Chapter 2, *Care of the Family in a Culturally Diverse Society.* This chapter provides the theoretical basis for the consideration of cultural factors that influence a family's expectations of their healthcare providers and their experience with the healthcare system. We then elaborate upon this information throughout the text in a boxed feature entitled **Developing Cultural Competence.** In addition, we have worked hard to ensure that our photos, illustrations, charts, and case scenarios are inclusive in their appearance and in the information they provide. Furthermore, this edition includes a new feature, **Global Perspectives,** which looks at childbirth practices and women's health issues around the world. As our society becomes more global in nature, nurses need to cultivate their awareness of these issues since they ultimately do affect how we deliver healthcare in this country.

Women's Healthcare. In this edition, content related to women's health has been expanded dramatically with the addition of several new chapters, including a separate chapter on family planning and a new chapter on commonly occurring infections. In addition, another new chapter addresses common gynecologic problems. Moreover, because of the text's focus on community-based care, gynecologic cancers are addressed briefly in the text and then can be found in greater detail on our Companion Web Site at www.prenhall.com/olds.

Addressing Complementary and Alternative Therapies. In recent years interest has grown in the use of complementary and alternative therapies as a credible component of holistic care. To help nurses become familiar with this content, we include a new chapter on these therapies—Chapter 3, *Complementary and Alternative Therapies.* Throughout the text, we expand upon this content by providing a boxed feature that highlights specific therapies. We think that both practicing nurses and students will find this information especially relevant in today's clinical environment.

[1]From Kaleidoscope Artistry by Cozy Baker (2002) C & T Publishing, Lafayette, CA

Organization: A Nursing Care Management Framework

While some books cover the role of the medical community in childbirth as a separate topic, our book gives an overview of all aspects of the childbearing process with a specific emphasis on nursing care throughout pregnancy, labor and birth, and the postpartal period. A new heading, **Nursing Care Management,** delineates the important care management role of the nurse within the organizing framework of the nursing process. Numerous special features reinforce the nursing care management role. The **Assessment Guides** incorporate expected findings, possible alterations, and causes, as well as guidelines for interventions. The **Clinical Pathways** help nurses organize care and evaluate its effectiveness. **Procedures** describe interventions specific to maternal-newborn nursing care in an illustrated, step-by-step fashion. These procedures can also be found on the Student CD-ROM in a printable format. The **Clinical Tips** are among our favorite features. These tips, or "pearls of wisdom," are gleaned from our own clinical practice or that of colleagues and are addressed directly to the students. They are designed to help students practice more effectively by offering tried-and-true approaches.

Community-Based Nursing Care. By its very nature, maternal-newborn nursing is community-based nursing. Only a brief portion of the entire pregnancy and birth is spent in a birthing center or hospital. Moreover, because of changes in practice, even women with high-risk pregnancies are receiving more care in their homes and in the community and spending less time in hospital settings. Similarly, most aspects of women's healthcare are addressed in ambulatory settings.

The provision of nursing care in community-based settings is a driving force in healthcare today and, consequently, is a dominant theme throughout this edition. We have addressed this topic in several ways. **Community-Based Nursing Care** is a heading used throughout the text to assist students in identifying specific aspects of this content. Because we consider **Home Care** to be one form of community-based care, it is often a separate heading under Community-Based Nursing Care. Even more important, Chapter 36, *Home Care of the Postpartal Family*, provides a thorough explanation of home care as an important aspect of care for childbearing families.

Emphasis on Client and Family Teaching. Client and family teaching is a crucial responsibility of the maternal-newborn nurse, one we continue to emphasize strongly and highlight in this seventh edition. Again, our focus is on the teaching that nurses do at all stages of pregnancy and the childbearing process including the important postpartal teaching that is done before and immediately after families are discharged.

In several places a more detailed discussion of client/family teaching is summarized in a **Client Teaching** box, such as the one on sexual activity during pregnancy. These teaching guides help students plan and organize their client teaching. The tear-out **Client/Family Teaching Cards** are also handy tools for the student to use while studying or for quick reference in the clinical setting. Furthermore, a foldout, full-color **Fetal Development Chart** depicts maternal/fetal development month by month and provides specific teaching guidelines for each stage of pregnancy. Students can use this chart as another tool for study or as a quick clinical reference.

Notable Learning Aids

Instructors and students alike continue to praise the abundance of in-text learning aids included in our books. With this edition, we once again create a book that is both easy to learn from and easy to use as a reference. Each chapter opens with a **Family Vignette,** a story from our clinical experience or those of colleagues. The vignette helps set the tone for the chapter. Learning **Objectives** and a list of **Key Terms** follow the vignette, offering students a quick glance at the topics covered in the chapter. A **Glossary** of terms that are commonly used in the field of maternal-newborn nursing can be found at the back of the book. The textbook glossary includes phonetic pronunciations of those terms that are most difficult to pronounce, while a comprehensive Audio Glossary can be found on the Student CD-ROM or the Companion Web Site. Throughout the chapters, we incorporate **Quotes** from women and family members. These quotes make a specific point and help students reflect on the humanity of the women and families for whom they care. Additionally, photographs, quotes, and vignettes from nurses, clients, and students bring a personal perspective to the text by presenting real-life situations. Where appropriate, we include **Drug Guides** for those medications commonly used in maternal-newborn nursing. These charts guide students in correctly administering medications. Each chapter ends with a section titled **Focus Your Study,** which summarizes important concepts, as well as a list of References.

New MediaLink Applications. At the beginning of each chapter, the **MediaLink** box identifies chapter-specific topics, animations, videos, NCLEX review questions, tools, and other interactive exercises that appear on the accompanying Student CD-ROM and the Companion Web Site. Special **MediaLink** icons appear in the margins throughout the chapter to refer students to those topics and activities available on the media supplements. At the end of each chapter, **EXPLORE MediaLink** sections encourage students to use the CD-ROM and the Companion Web Site to apply what they have learned from the text in case studies, to practice NCLEX questions, and to use additional resources. The purpose of the MediaLink feature is to further enhance the student experience, build upon knowledge gained from the textbook, prepare students for the NCLEX, and foster critical thinking.

Supplements that Inspire Success for the Student and the Instructor

- **Clinical Handbook.** This handbook serves as a portable, quick reference to maternal-newborn nursing care for students. Covering pregnancy through the postpartum and newborn stages, this handbook allows students to take the information they learn from class into any clinical setting.

- **Student Workbook.** This popular workbook incorporates strategies for students to focus their study and increase comprehension of concepts of nursing care. It contains a variety of activities, MediaLinks referring students to the Student CD-ROM and Companion Web Site, and more.
- **Student CD-ROM.** Packaged *free* with the textbook, this CD-ROM provides an interactive study program that allows students to practice answering NCLEX-style questions with rationales for right and wrong answers. It also contains animated tutorials of difficult topics, such as fetal heart circulation, and videos of labor, vaginal birth, and cesarean birth.
- **Companion Web Site—www.prenhall.com/olds.** This free online study guide is designed to help students apply the concepts presented in the book. Each chapter-specific module features objectives, additional NCLEX review questions, chapter outlines for lecture notes, case studies, care plan activities, critical thinking activities, WebLinks, audio glossary, and more. Instructors adopting this textbook have free access to the online Syllabus Manager feature of the Companion Web Site. Syllabus Manager offers a whole host of features that facilitate the students' use of the Companion Web Site, and allows faculty to post syllabi and course information online for their students. For more information or a demonstration of Syllabus Manager, please contact your Prentice Hall sales representative.
- **Instructor's Resource Manual.** This manual contains a wealth of material to help faculty plan and manage the maternity nursing course. It includes chapter overviews, detailed lecture suggestions and outlines, learning objectives, a complete test bank, answers to the textbook critical thinking exercises, teaching tips, and more for each chapter. It also guides faculty how to assign and use the text-specific Companion Web Site, www.prenhall.com/olds, and the free Student CD-ROM that accompany the textbook.
- **Instructor's Resource CD-ROM.** This cross-platform CD-ROM prepares instructors for the classroom and clinical. It provides illustrations and text slides in PowerPoint for use in classroom lectures. It also contains an electronic test bank, answers to the textbook critical thinking exercises, animations and video clips from the Student CD-ROM, an electronic version of the Instructor's Resource Manual, and other instructional aids.
- **Online Course Management Systems.** For schools using Blackboard, WebCt, or CourseCompass, Prentice Hall offers online course management solutions to enhance your course. These *free* solutions feature interactive assessment modules, electronic test bank, gradebook functions, PowerPoint images and text slides, animations and video clips, and more. For more information about adopting an online course management system to accompany ***Maternal-Newborn Nursing & Women's Health Care***, please contact your Prentice Hall Health sales representative or visit the appropriate Web site below:

  http://cms.prenhall.com/webct/index.html

  http://cms.prenhall.com/blackboard/index.html

  http://cms.prenhall.com/coursecompass

A Note to Students

We believe that working with childbearing families gives you the opportunity to experience the essence of nursing at its best. You can play a vital role in helping families learn what they need to know in order to be as independent as possible. You can improve and refine your assessment skills as you work with essentially healthy women and infants, as well as those with complications. And, you can also use the other nursing skills you have learned in a variety of acute and community-based care settings.

We love this field, and we know that many of you will as well. Some of you, on the other hand, may find that this area of nursing is not your first interest, and that's OK, too. We would have a real problem if every nurse loved the same area!

We do hope that you will use this opportunity to grow in professional ability and to appreciate the importance of all you do as nurses—not just the technical and organizational tasks, although they are undoubtedly crucial, but also the caring you bring to the role of nurse. When you hold the hand of a laboring woman or help an adolescent plan a way to tell her parents of her pregnancy; when you provide accepting care to a woman with AIDS or gently stroke the skin of a preterm infant; when you rejoice with a delighted father or console a grieving one; you are practicing the heart of nursing.

Caring in an optimal environment is not difficult, but caring in today's practice setting is more of a challenge. Finding a way to maintain a caring environment when you are overworked and stretched by fiscal constraints and a lack of adequate staffing requires great dedication, creativity, and personal resolve. We attempt to help you translate caring into practice in this textbook through the tone of the book, the photos and illustrations, the personal quotes, and the content itself with its emphasis on holistic care.

As you work to transfer what you learn into practice, please take care of yourselves as well. Providing excellent nursing care is infinitely rewarding and can be energizing, but it is also draining both physically and emotionally. Make time to play, rest, exercise, be with loved ones, and participate in things that rejuvenate you.

We think that nurses are very special people, and we are proud to be counted among them. Good luck with your studies! We wish you well.

Sally B. Olds
Marcia L. London
Patricia W. Ladewig
Michele R. Davidson

Acknowledgments

Our goal with every revision is to incorporate the latest research and information from the literature of nursing and related fields to make our text as relevant and useful as possible. This would not be possible without the support and encouragement of our colleagues in nursing. The comments and suggestions we have received from nurse educators and practitioners around the country have helped us keep this text accurate and up-to-date. Whenever a nurse takes the time to write or to speak to one of us at a professional gathering, we recognize again the intense commitment of nurses to excellence in practice. And so we thank our colleagues.

We are grateful, too, to our students, past, present, and future. They stimulate us with their interest; they reinvigorate us with their enthusiasm; they challenge us with their questions to make each edition of this text clear and understandable. We learn so much from them.

In publishing, as in healthcare, quality assurance is an essential part of the process. That is the dimension our reviewers have added. Some reviewers assist us by validating the accuracy of the content, some by their attention to detail, and some by challenging us to examine our ways of thinking and to develop a new awareness about a given topic. Thus, we extend our sincere thanks to all those who reviewed the manuscript for this book. Their names and affiliations are listed on the following pages.

We are also grateful to the contributors to the seventh edition of *Maternal-Newborn Nursing & Women's Health Care.* Their knowledge of clinical practice and current literature in their areas of expertise helps make the chapters relevant and accurate. They, too, are listed on the following pages.

The success of a project of this scope requires the skills and dedication of many people. We would personally like to thank the following people:

Our editor, Maura Connor, deserves our deepest thanks. She is always there for us, ensuring that we have the support and resources we need to produce an exceptional text, one designed to support students and foster the profession of nursing. Maura's energy and enthusiasm are contagious. When we come together as a team, the synergy is incredible and we are the better because of her commitment to the project. She is our close friend and staunch ally.

Julie Alexander, our publisher, has played an important role in the development of our text. Her leadership of Prentice Hall Health has resulted in the growth of a company committed to excellence, to technology, and to student support. She is a visionary in publishing.

Laura Bonazzoli, our developmental editor, is a dear friend and a creative genius. She is a Renaissance woman, widely read and able to challenge us when our vision becomes myopic. Moreover, her organizational skills and eye for detail help us produce a tighter, more readable text. We would be lost without her.

Special thanks to Assistant Editor, Sladjana Repic, who handled the overall manuscript for both the book and the media supplements. She was fast and efficient in responding to needs and concerns and unfailingly calm and helpful. Sladjana, it is a pleasure to work with you.

We are also grateful to Yesenia Kopperman, former Assistant Editor, who handled the production of the text supplements. She did a marvelous job of pulling the pieces together into a coherent whole.

Thanks, too, to Marilyn Meserve, executive managing editor, who stepped in to coordinate the process during Maura's maternity leave, and to Danielle Newhouse, production editor, who handled the in-house production issues. You both have been wonderful to work with, and we appreciate your support.

And, finally, we extend our deepest appreciation to two amazing Amys! Amy Hackett of Carlisle Publisher Services handled the myriad of responsibilities inherent in the production of a manuscript of this size. Throughout the process, she remained gracious, helpful, and focused. She solved every problem, excused every error, and brought us a finished text on schedule. She is quite a woman. Amy Puchino handled all the permissions for the text. What an accomplishment. She is a master at tracking down sources, at expediting permissions, at following leads. We would be totally lost without her. Amy, you are amazing!

During these times of uncertainty in the healthcare environment, we are sustained by our passion for nursing and our vision of what childbirth means. Time and again, we have seen the difference a skilled nurse can make in the lives of people in need. We, like you, are committed to helping all nurses recognize and take pride in that fact. Thank you for your letters, your comments, and your suggestions. We are renewed by your support.

Sally B. Olds
Marcia L. London
Patricia W. Ladewig
Michele R. Davidson

Reviewers

We are grateful to all the nurses, both clinicians and educators, who reviewed the manuscript of this textbook. Their insights, suggestions, and eye for detail helped us prepare a more relevant and useful textbook, one that will prepare caring and competent nurses in the field of maternal-newborn and women's health nursing.

Cindy Anderson, MS, WHNP
Clinical Associate Professor
University of North Dakota
Grand Forks, North Dakota

Karen Bess, RN, MSN
Assistant Professor
Jewish Hospital College of Nursing & Allied Health
St. Louis, Missouri

Sara E. Bishop, RNC, MSHP
Assistant Professor of Nursing
Midwestern State University
Wichita Falls, Texas

Suzanne Hetzel Campbell, PhD, APRN, WHNP
Assistant Professor
Fairfield University
Fairfield, Connecticut

Nancy Wilson Darland, RNC, MSN, CNS
Professor
Louisiana Tech University
Ruston, Louisiana

Judith N. Halle, PhD, RNC
Associate Professor/Director, Perinatal Research & Education Project
West Virginia Wesleyan College
Buckhannon, West Virginia

Janice G. Harris, MSN, RNC
Associate Professor
Columbus State University
Columbus, Georgia

Linda E. Jensen, RN, MN, PhD
Assistant Professor
University of Nebraska Medical Center
Kearney, Nebraska

Maryanne F. Lachat, RNC, PhD
Associate Professor
Georgetown University
Washington, DC

Betty Spencer Lemon, MSN, RNC, CNN, CNS, ALSO
Assistant Professor
The University of Toledo
Toledo, Ohio

Christine H. Milhollan, RNC, BS
Clinical Manager, Mother-Baby Unit
Memorial Hospital
Colorado Springs, Colorado

Karen B. Moody, RNC, PhD
Assistant Professor
Southeastern Louisiana University
Baton Rouge, Louisiana

Sarah Rhoads, MNSc, WHNP, APN-C, RN-C
Clinical Assistant Professor
University of Arkansas for Medical Sciences
Little Rock, Arkansas

Kathy Roberts, RN, MSN
Assistant Professor
Lamar University
Beaumont, Texas

Karen A. Stevens, MSN, PhD
Associate Professor
Bowie State University
Bowie, Maryland

Stephanie N. Wyatt, MNSc, APN
Clinical Instructor
University of Arkansas Medical Sciences
Little Rock, Arkansas

Contributors

We are grateful to the contributors to the seventh edition of *Maternal-Newborn Nursing & Women's Health Care.* Their knowledge of clinical practice and current literature in their areas of expertise helps make the chapters relevant and accurate.

Laura Bonazzoli, MFA
Medical Writer
Camden, Maine
Chapter 3

Adele C. Brandmark, FNP, MSN
Planned Parenthood of Metro Washington Area
Falls Church, Virginia
Chapter 35

Margie Brandquist, CNM, MSN
Women's Healthcare Associates of Loudoun
Landesdowne, Virginia
Chapter 23

Nancy Brenner, RNC, BSN
Presbyterian/St. Luke's Medical Center
Denver, Colorado
Chapter 28

Linda Chapman, RN, DNSc
Samuel Merritt College
Oakland, California
Chapter 26

Wendy Dotson, CNM, MSN
Women's Healthcare Associates of Loudoun
Landesdowne, Virginia
Chapters 3 and 23

Kimberly K. Eby, PhD
George Mason University
Fairfax, Virginia
Chapter 9

Victoria A. Flanagan, RN, MS
Dartmouth-Hitchcock Medical Center
Lebanon, New Hampshire
Chapter 19

Kathleen K. Furniss, RNC, MSN
Women's Health Initiative, UMDNJ
Newark, New Jersey
Chapters 4 and 5

Carol Ann Harrigan RNC, MSN, NNP
Desert Samaritan Medical Center
Level III NICU
Mesa, Arizona
Chapter 32

Janet Houser, PhD, RN
Regis University
Denver, Colorado
Research in Practice boxes

Lisa Jensen, CNM, FNP, MS
Midwifery and Family Health Nurse
Practitioner Programs
Stony Brook University
Stony Brook, New York
Chapter 21

Peter Johnson, CNM, PhD
Stony Brook University
Stony Brook, New York
Chapter 21

Denise Jurow, CNM, MSN
Nurse Midwifery Program
Stony Brook University
Stony Brook, New York
Chapter 21

Cheryl Pope Kish RNC, MSN, EdD, WHNP
Georgia College & State University
School of Health Sciences
Milledgeville, Georgia
Chapter 37

Linda J. Kobokovich, PhD, RN
Dartmouth-Hitchcock Medical Center
Lebanon, New Hampshire
Chapter 17

Deborah Cooper McGee, RNC, MSN, PNNP, RDMS
Obstetrix Medical Group of Colorado
Denver, Colorado
Chapter 20

Roxann M. Moran, BSN, MEd, CMT
Private Practice
Leesburg, Virginia
Chapter 3

Julie Nadeau, RN, MSN
University of the Incarnate Word
San Antonio, Texas
Chapter 36

Lisa R. Pawloski, PhD
George Mason University
Fairfax, Virginia
Chapter 2

Lisa Smith-Pedersen APRN, MSN, CNNP
Northwestern State University of Louisiana
Louisiana State University Medical Center
Shreveport, Louisiana
Chapters 10, 33, and 34

Candace Polzella, RD, MSS
University of Vermont
Burlington, Vermont
Chapter 18

Carol Roehrs, PhD, RN
University of Northern Colorado
Greeley, Colorado
Chapter 14

Lisa Sams, RNC, MSN
Clinical Linkages
Arlington, Virginia
Chapter 26

Candice Tolve Schoeneberger, RNC, PhD
Regis University
Denver, Colorado
Chapter 16

Kathleen R. Stevens, RN, EdD, FAAN
Academic Center for Evidence-based Practice
The University of Texas Health Science Center at San Antonio
San Antonio, Texas
Evidence-Based Practice boxes

Monica Taylor, RN, MEd, LCCE
The Toledo Hospital
Toledo, Ohio
Chapter 29

Rebecca A. Walter, MA
George Mason University
Fairfax, Virginia
Chapter 8

Karen Zimmerman, RN, MSN, PNNP
Rocky Mountain Women's Care
Denver, Colorado
Chapters 6 and 7

Supplement and Media Contributors

We are grateful to the following educators who contributed their teaching expertise to the student and instructor supplements accompanying *Maternal-Newborn Nursing & Women's Health Care.* Their contributions provide applications that help prepare students for NCLEX-RN while also developing their clinical judgment skills.

Ellise D. Adams, CNM, MSN, CD(DONA), ICCE
Nursing Faculty, Calhoun Community College
Decatur, Alabama
Student CD-ROM and Companion Web Site

Anita Althans, MSN
Assistant Professor, Our Lady of Holy Cross College
New Orleans, Louisiana
Instructor's Resource Manual and Instructor's Resource CD-ROM

Ann L. Bianchi, RN, MSN, ICCE, ICD
Nursing Faculty, Calhoun Community College
Decatur, Alabama
Student CD-ROM and Companion Web Site

Carol Boswell, RN, EdD
Associate Professor, Texas Tech University Health Sciences Center
School of Nursing
Odessa, Texas
Companion Web Site

Katharine West, MPH, MSN, RN, CNS
Azusa Pacific University
Azusa, California
Companion Web Site

Angie F. Wood, PhD
Professor, Carson-Newman College
Jefferson City, Tennessee
Instructor's Resource Manual and Instructor's Resource CD-ROM

About the Authors

Sally B. Olds

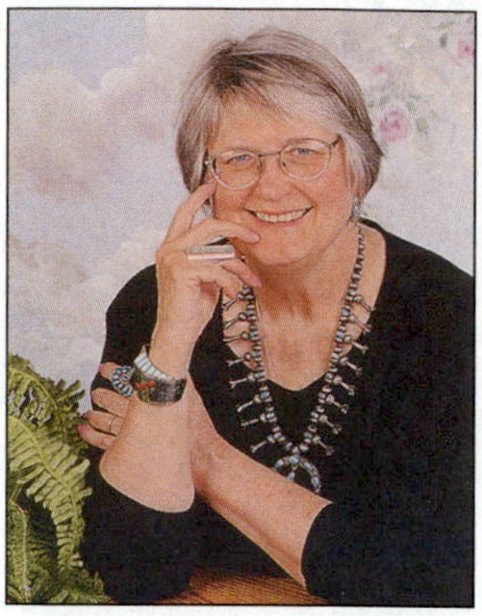

Sally B. Olds provided hands-on maternal-newborn nursing care and mentored students and colleagues for more than 30 years. She received her BSN from the University of Kansas and her MS in nursing from the University of Colorado. Completing her master's degree provided Mrs. Olds with the opportunity to achieve one of her life's goals—teaching nursing students. She began teaching at the Beth-El School of Nursing and Health Science in 1975, eventually becoming the chair of the Department of Holistic Nursing, and was instrumental in developing the Clinical Nursing Specialist Program in Holistic Health for the master's program. Her teaching philosophy has been to nurture and support students as they learn, to focus on the positive aspects of learning, and to teach students the importance of respecting the client and family for whom they provide care. Mrs. Olds taught at Beth-El for over 22 years before retiring in 1997, and was named professor emerita. She became a sexual assault nurse examiner (SANE), working one-on-one with sexual assault survivors in 1996, and she continues her involvement with issues affecting women and children. Since her retirement, Mrs. Olds has had more time to spend with her husband and two grown children, and her Old English sheepdog.

Marcia L. London

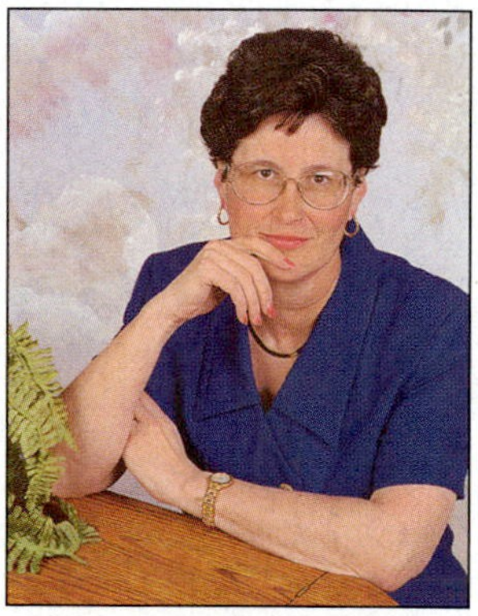

Marcia L. London has been able to combine her two greatest passions—being both a nurse caring for children and families and a teacher for almost 29 years. She received her BSN and school nurse certificate from Plattsburgh State University in Plattsburgh, New York. After graduation, she worked as a pediatric nurse at Saint Luke's Hospital in New York City, and then moved to Pittsburgh where she began her teaching career. Mrs. London accepted a faculty position at Pittsburgh's Children's Hospital Affiliate program and received her MSN in pediatrics from University of Pittsburgh in Pennsylvania. Mrs. London began teaching at Beth-El School of Nursing and Health Science in 1974 after opening the first intensive care nursery at Memorial Hospital of Colorado Springs. She has served in many faculty positions at Beth-El, including assistant director of the School of Nursing. Mrs. London obtained her post-master's neonatal nurse practitioner certificate in 1983, and subsequently developed the neonatal nurse practitioner certificate and the master's programs at Beth-El. She is active nationally in neonatal nursing and was involved in the development of the Neonatal Nurse Practitioner Educational Program guidelines. Mrs. London is currently completing her PhD in higher education administration and adult studies at University of Denver in Colorado. She feels fortunate to be involved in the education of her future colleagues. Her teaching philosophy is that with support, students can achieve more than they may initially believe they are capable of achieving. Mrs. London and her husband have two sons and two dogs (Samantha and Betsy—daughters by proxy). Her son Matthew is studying computer animation in college and her son Craig is combining college and computers. Both are more than willing to give mom helpful hints.

Patricia A. Wieland Ladewig

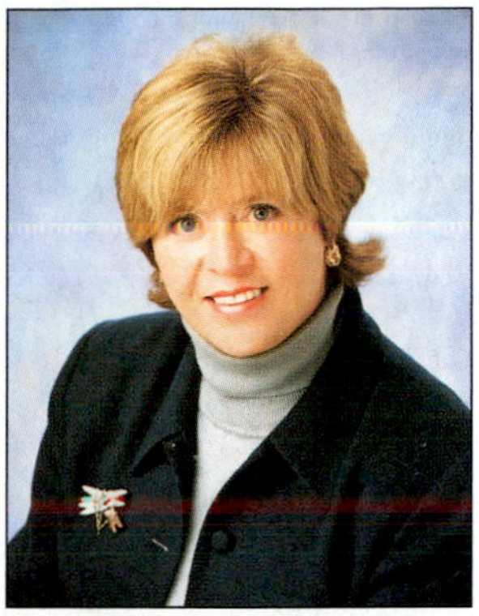

Patricia A. Wieland Ladewig received her BSN from the College of Saint Teresa in Winona, Minnesota. After graduation, she worked as a pediatric nurse before joining the Air Force. After completing her tour of duty, Dr. Ladewig relocated to Florida where she accepted a faculty position at Florida State University. There she discovered teaching as her calling. Over the years, she taught at several schools of nursing while earning her MSN in maternal-newborn nursing from Catholic University of America in Washington, DC, and her PhD in higher education administration from the University of Denver in Colorado. In addition, she became a women's health nurse practitioner and maintained a part-time clinical practice. In 1988 Dr. Ladewig became the first director of the nursing program at Regis College in Denver, and in 1991, when the college became Regis University, she became dean of the School for Health Care Professions. Under her guidance, the Department of Nursing has added a graduate program and the School for Health Care Professions has added two departments: the Department of Physical Therapy and the Department of Health Services Administration and Management. Dr. Ladewig feels that teaching others to be excellent, caring nurses gives her the best of all worlds because it keeps her in touch with the profession she loves and enables her to help shape the future of nursing professionals. When not at work or writing textbooks, Pat and her husband, Tim, enjoy skiing, climbing Colorado's 14'ers (14,000 foot mountains—she has climbed 15 to date), and traveling. They are parents of two sons, Erik, a graduate of Regis and an avid snowboarder, and Ryan, who has a master's degree in computer science and works in Web design. The newest member of the Ladewig clan is Ryan's wife, Amanda, who is also a nurse! She works on a telemetry unit at a Denver hospital.

Michele R. Davidson

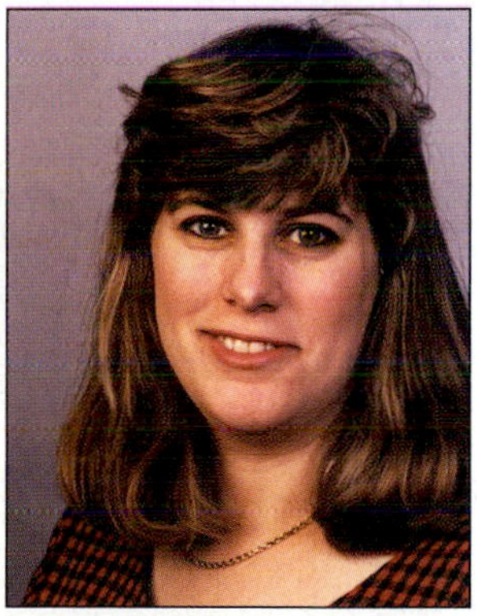

Michele R. Davidson received an ADN from Marymount University in 1990 and upon graduation began working in postpartum and the newborn nursery in a women's specialty hospital in Washington, DC. Because of her interest in educating expectant and new families, she began an education and consulting service providing childbirth education classes, lactation consultant services, and newborn care courses. Her role as a nurse entrepreneur enabled her to work with families from various cultures and countries throughout the world. During this time she also worked as a reproductive endocrinology/infertility nurse while she obtained a BSN from George Mason University. Dr. Davidson then attended Case Western Reserve University where she earned her MSN and a certificate in nurse midwifery. She worked as a certified nurse midwife at Columbia Hospital for Women in Washington, DC, while completing her PhD in nursing administration and health care policy from George Mason University. During her PhD program, she discovered her love for writing and routinely publishes clinical and research articles in various nursing journals and magazines. Dr. Davidson began teaching at George Mason University in 1999 after the birth of her son, Hayden. She is a member of the American College of Nurse Midwives Certification Council, the body that writes the national certification examination for certified nurse midwives. Dr. Davidson has maintained a part-time clinical position as a nurse-midwife at Women's Healthcare Associates of Loudoun since the birth of her daughter, Chloe, because she strongly believes that active clinical practice is essential to provide nursing students with updated clinical and critical thinking skills. In addition to teaching in the undergraduate nursing program, Dr. Davidson has developed an immersion clinical experience on a remote island in the Chesapeake Bay where she teaches community health to students who reside in that community. In 2003, she founded the Smith Island Foundation, a nonprofit organization in which she serves as the executive director. In her free time, Michele enjoys spending time with her mom, gardening, reading, and camping with her nurse practitioner husband, Nathan, their two preschoolers, Hayden and Chloe, and their dog, Katie.

A Guide to

Maternal-Newborn Nursing & Women's Health Care

SEVENTH EDITION

This textbook contains numerous learning tools to help increase your understanding of key concepts and guide you in applying maternal-newborn women's health nursing care.

Vignettes
Each chapter begins with a personal vignette that helps set the tone for the chapter.

Objectives
Learning objectives introduce students to the topics covered in each chapter.

MediaLink
MediaLink introduces each chapter of the text and lists additional content, animations, videos, NCLEX Review, and other interactive exercises and tools that appear on the accompanying Student CD-ROM and the Companion Website. Throughout the chapter, the MediaLink tab in the margin refers the student to specific animations, additional content, resources or activities contained on the Student CD-ROM or the Companion Website **www.prenhall.com/olds** that accompany this textbook.

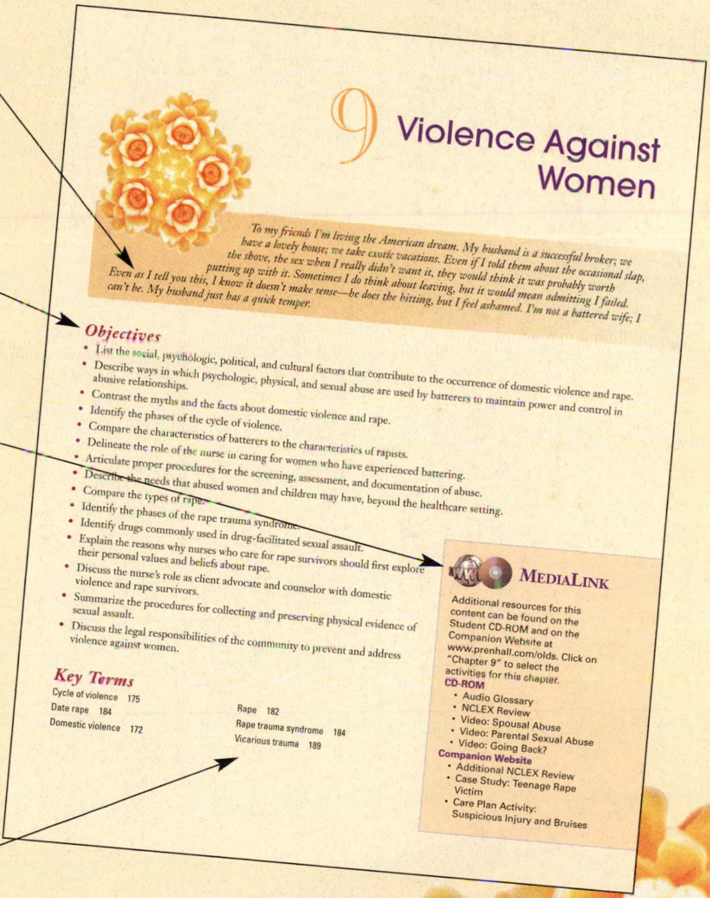

9 Violence Against Women

To my friends I'm living the American dream. My husband is a successful broker; we have a lovely house; we take exotic vacations. Even if I told them about the occasional slap, the shove, the sex when I really didn't want it, they would think it was probably worth putting up with it. Sometimes I do think about leaving, but it would mean admitting I failed. Even as I tell you this, I know it doesn't make sense—he does the hitting, but I feel ashamed. I'm not a battered wife; I can't be. My husband just has a quick temper.

Objectives

- List the social, psychologic, political, and cultural factors that contribute to the occurrence of domestic violence and rape.
- Describe ways in which psychologic, physical, and sexual abuse are used by batterers to maintain power and control in abusive relationships.
- Contrast the myths and the facts about domestic violence and rape.
- Identify the phases of the cycle of violence.
- Compare the characteristics of batterers to the characteristics of rapists.
- Delineate the role of the nurse in caring for women who have experienced battering.
- Articulate proper procedures for the screening, assessment, and documentation of abuse.
- Describe the needs that abused women and children may have, beyond the healthcare setting.
- Compare the types of rape.
- Identify the phases of the rape trauma syndrome.
- Identify drugs commonly used in drug-facilitated sexual assault.
- Explain the reasons why nurses who care for rape survivors should first explore their personal values and beliefs about rape.
- Discuss the nurse's role as client advocate and counselor with domestic violence and rape survivors.
- Summarize the procedures for collecting and preserving physical evidence of sexual assault.
- Discuss the legal responsibilities of the community to prevent and address violence against women.

Key Terms

Cycle of violence 175
Date rape 184
Domestic violence 172
Rape 182
Rape trauma syndrome 184
Vicarious trauma 189

MEDIALINK

Additional resources for this content can be found on the Student CD-ROM and on the Companion Website at www.prenhall.com/olds. Click on "Chapter 9" to select the activities for this chapter.

CD-ROM
- Audio Glossary
- NCLEX Review
- Video: Spousal Abuse
- Video: Parental Sexual Abuse
- Video: Going Back?

Companion Website
- Additional NCLEX Review
- Case Study: Teenage Rape Victim
- Care Plan Activity: Suspicious Injury and Bruises

Key Terms
Key terms introduce each chapter, with page numbers showing where each term first appears in the chapter, in bold type.

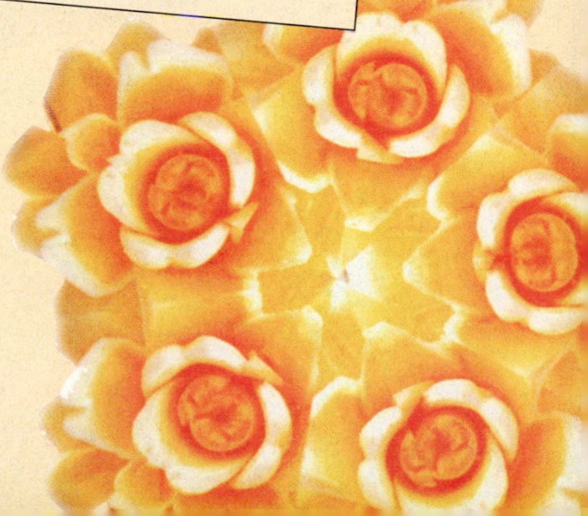

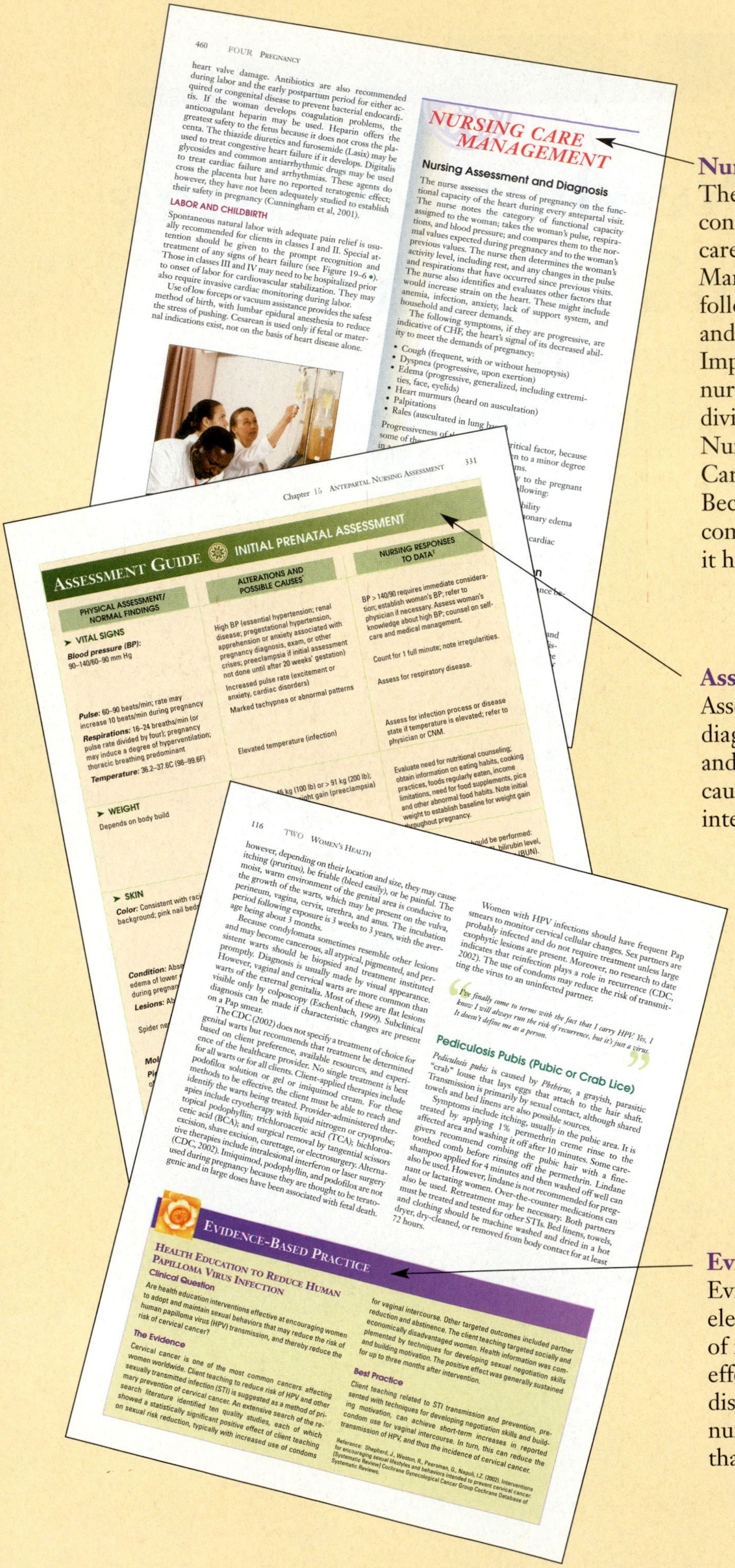

Nursing Care Management

The nursing process is presented in a consistent manner throughout the nursing care chapters. The heading Nursing Care Management highlights nursing actions, followed by sections on Nursing Assessment and Diagnosis, Nursing Plan and Implementation, and Evaluation. Since not all nursing care occurs in the hospital, the authors divide care into the sections Hospital-based Nursing Care and Community-based Nursing Care, which is highlighted by a special icon. Because home care is considered a form of community-based care, students will often find it highlighted in this section.

Assessment Guides

Assessment Guides assist students with diagnoses by incorporating physical assessment and normal findings, alterations and possible causes, as well as guidelines for nursing interventions.

Evidence-Based Practice

Evidence-based practice is an important element to help students understand the use of reliable information to plan and provide effective nursing care. These boxes provide discussions of clinical situations, typical nursing practice, and the current research that supports or fails to support that practice.

Complementary and Alternative Therapies
In addition to an entire chapter introducing the student to complementary and alternative therapies, these boxes inform students about therapies their clients might be using or therapies the nurse might safely suggest. In all cases, research is cited for safe practice of these therapies.

Client Teaching
These effective guides provide students with a teaching plan to use when educating the client and family about any aspect of self-care or a special health care issues.

Family Quotations
These quotations from clients help students reflect upon the humanity of the women and families for whom they care—from women's issues, to pregnancy, labor and the birth experience.

Developing Cultural Competence
These boxes expose students to cultural factors that influence a family's expectations of and responses to their health care provider and their experiences with the health care system.

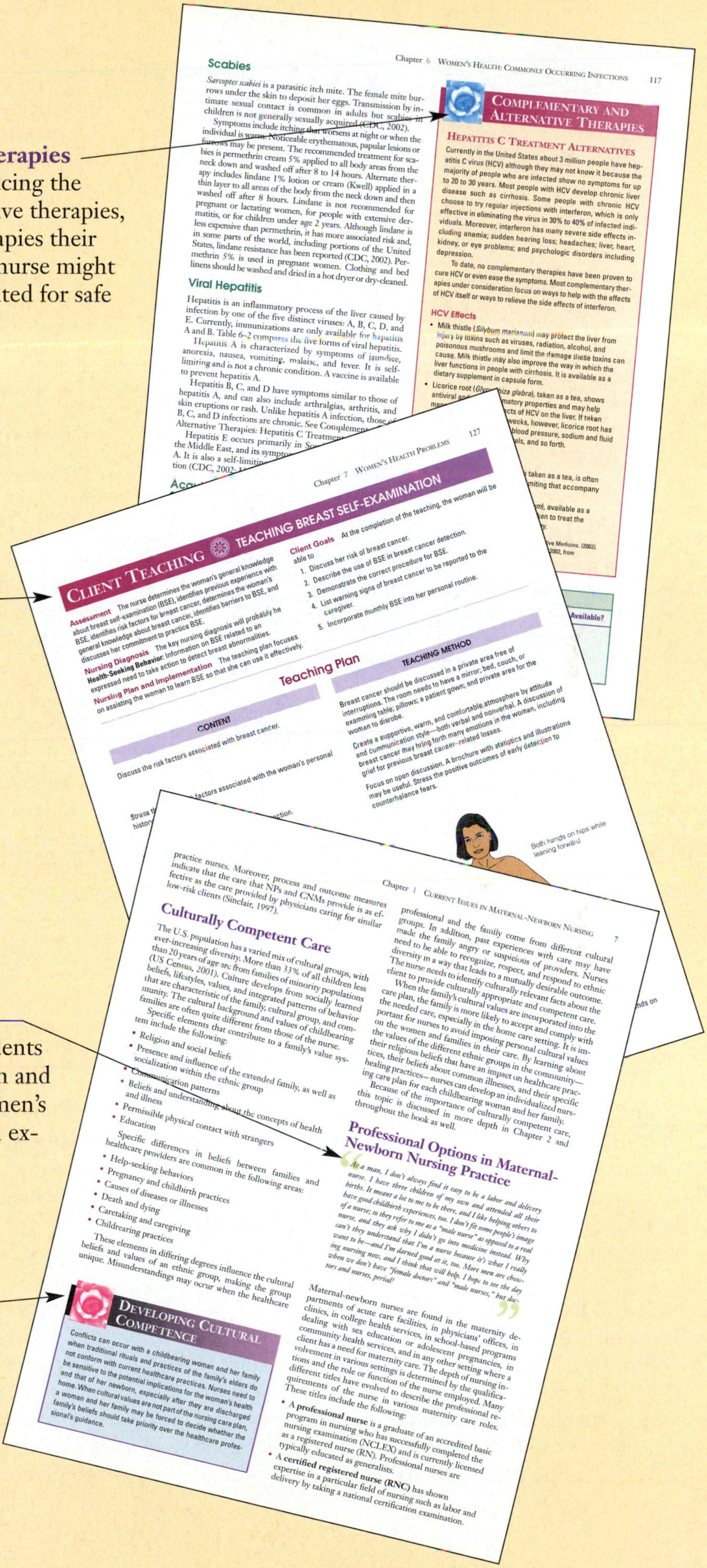

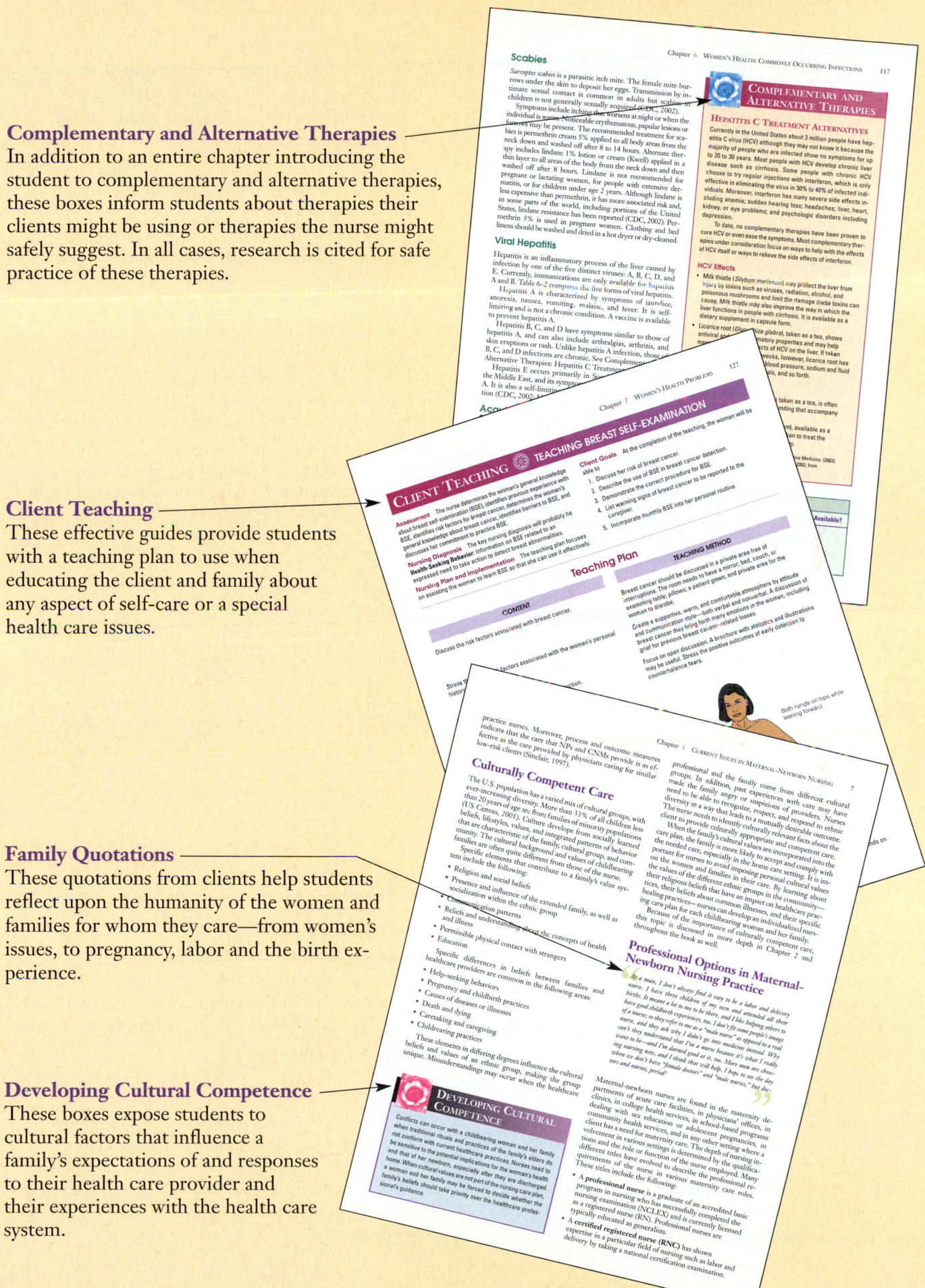

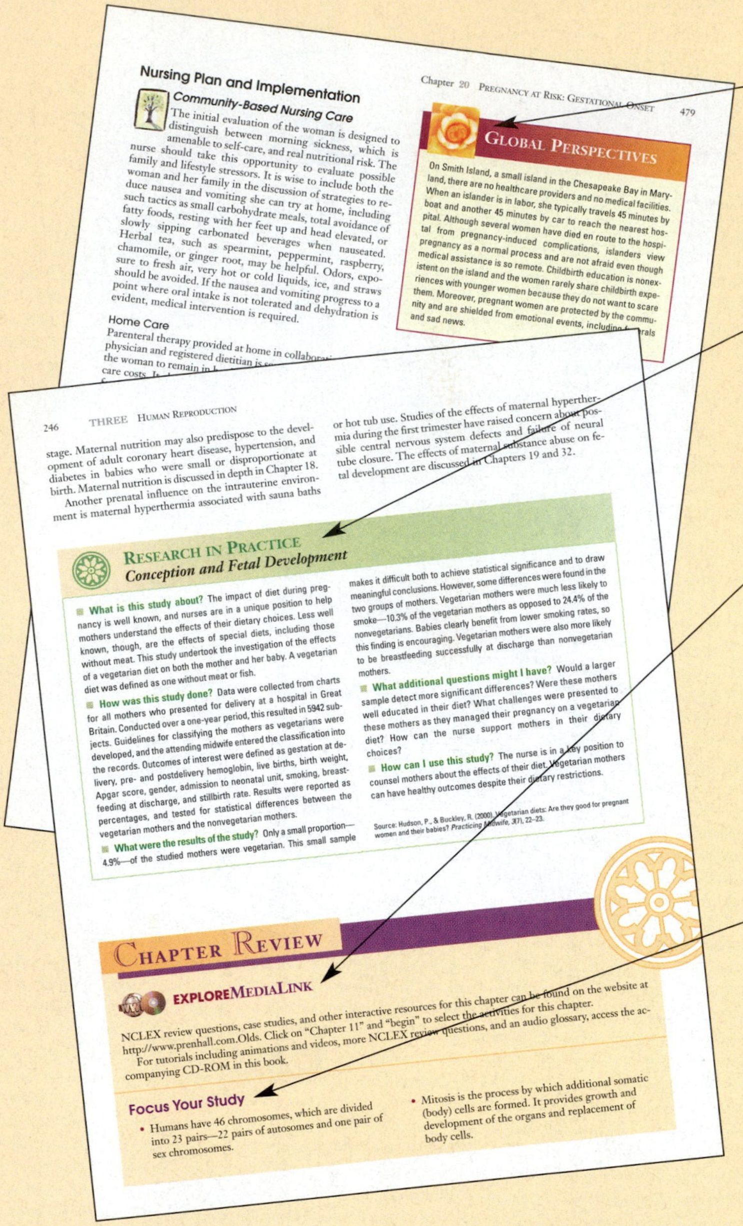

Global Perspectives
This new feature looks at the values and practices of other communities around the world with regard to pregnancy, childbirth, and women's health.

Research in Practice
These exemplars provide strong examples of relevant, clinically focused nursing research.

EXPLORE MediaLink
Found at the end of each chapter, EXPLORE MediaLink encourages students to use the CD-ROM and the Companion Website to apply what they have learned from the text in case studies, practice NCLEX questions, and to use additional resources.

Focus Your Study
At the end of each chapter, students will find a bulleted summary of chapter highlights. Students who review these concepts before reading the chapter will find this helpful in focusing their attention. Chapter highlights are also an appropriate tool to quickly review the chapter content.

ADDITIONAL MEDIA RESOURCES

Animation and Video Tutorials
On the Student CD-ROM, the student will find animations illustrating difficult concepts, such as fetal heart circulation, and video clips showing nursing care during labor, vaginal birth, cesarean birth, and postpartum and newborn care.

NCLEX Reviews
Both the Student CD-ROM and the free Companion Website offer the student an abundance of NCLEX review questions for each chapter of the book. The questions provide comprehensive rationales, as well as identify how the questions correlate to the NCLEX test plan.

Care Plan Activities
Each clinical chapter on the Companion Website provides the student with a case scenario and asks the student to develop a care plan for the client. Students can email these care plans to instructors as homework assignments.

Case Studies
For each chapter on the Companion Website, the student can review a client scenario and answer several critical thinking questions related to that client's care. Students can email the responses to the case studies to instructors as homework assignments.

Special Features

Assessment Guides

Client Teaching

Clinical Pathways

Complementary and Alternative Therapies

Critical Thinking in Practice

Developing Cultural Competence

Drug Guides

Evidence-Based Practice

Global Perspectives

Procedures

Research in Practice

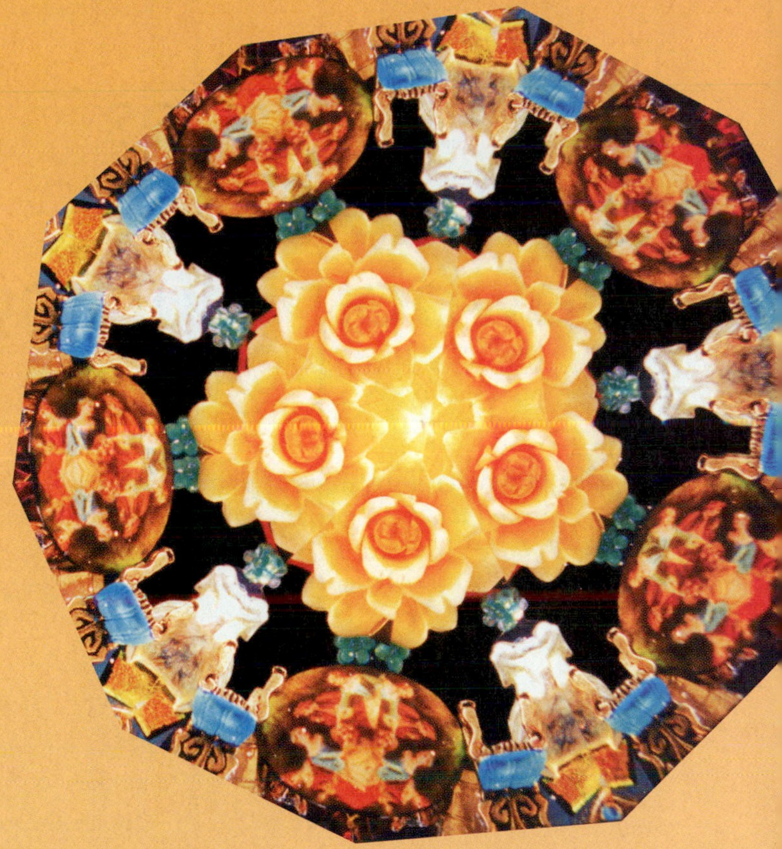

ONE

Contemporary Maternal-Newborn Nursing

Current Issues in Maternal-Newborn Nursing

1

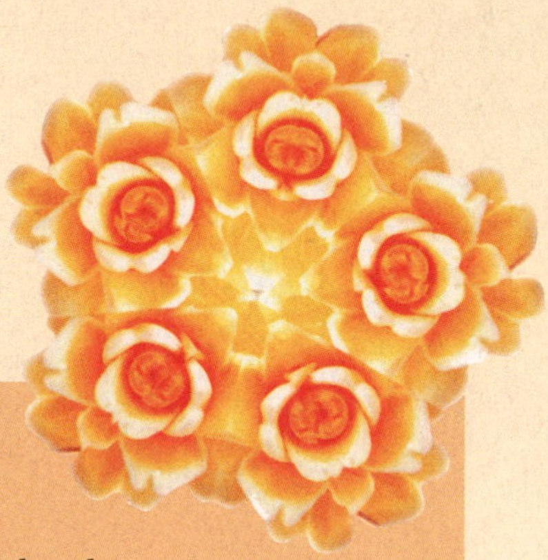

Our daughter just told us that she is 3 months pregnant with our first grandchild. As a labor and delivery nurse for 25 years, I've helped with hundreds of births, but it still seems magical to me, especially now. I'm excited for her and a little worried because I know all the risks as well as the joys. She is so happy; when I am with her I just want to laugh out loud. I already know I love being a grandmother, even though I really am too young!

Objectives

- Relate the concept of the expert nurse to nurses caring for childbearing families.
- Discuss the impact of the self-care movement on contemporary childbirth.
- Compare the nursing roles available to the maternal-newborn nurse.
- Identify specific factors that contribute to a family's value system.
- Delineate significant legal and ethical issues that influence the practice of nursing for childbearing families.
- Evaluate the potential impact of some of the special situations in contemporary maternity care.
- Contrast descriptive and inferential statistics.
- Relate the availability of statistical data to the formulation of further research questions.
- Delineate the benefits of evidence-based nursing practice to the client, the institution, and the profession of nursing.

Key Terms

Assisted reproductive technology (ART) 15
Birth rate 17
Certified nurse-midwife (CNM) 8
Certified registered nurse (RNC) 7
Client 5
Clinical nurse specialist (CNS) 8
Evidence-based practice 21
Infant mortality rate 18
Informed consent 11
Intrauterine fetal surgery 14
Maternal mortality rate 20
Nurse practitioner (NP) 8
Professional nurse 7
Therapeutic insemination (TI) 14

MediaLink

Additional resources for this content can be found on the Student CD-ROM and on the Companion Website at www.prenhall.com/olds. Click on "Chapter 1" to select the activities for this chapter.

CD-ROM
- Audio Glossary
- NCLEX Review

Companion Website
- Additional NCLEX Review
- Case Study: Cord Blood Banking
- Care Plan Activity: Request for Second Trimester Abortion

The practice of most nurses is filled with special moments, shared experiences, times in which they know they have practiced the essence of nursing and, in doing so, have touched a life. What is the essence of nursing? Simply stated, nurses care for people, care about people, and use their expertise to help people help themselves.

> *I like working with students. I enjoy the enthusiasm they bring, the questions they ask, the ways they cause me to examine my practice. I love being a nurse. I am passionate about the importance of what I do, and I feel the need to seize every chance to influence those who will be practicing beside me someday. Last week was a perfect example. I had a nursing student working with me in one of our birthing rooms. It was her first day caring for a laboring woman, and she was scared and excited at the same time. We were taking care of a healthy woman who had two boys at home and really wanted a girl.*
>
> *As labor progressed, the student and I worked closely together monitoring contractions, teaching the woman and her husband, doing what we could to ease her discomfort. Sometimes the student would ask how I knew when to do something, a vaginal exam, for example, and I'd have to think beyond "I just do" to give her some clues. At the birth the student stayed close to the mother, coaching and helping with breathing. The student was excited but felt she had an important role to play, and she handled it beautifully. At the moment of birth the student and the dad were leaning forward watching as the baby just slipped into the world. There wasn't a sound until the student said in a voice filled with awe, "Oh, it's a girl!" Then we all laughed and hugged each other. What a day—using my expertise to help others and helping a future nurse recognize the importance of what we do!*

All nurses who provide care and support to childbearing women and their families can make a difference. But how does this happen? How do nurses develop expertise and become skilled, caring practitioners?

In her classic work, Benner (1984) suggested that as nurses develop their skills in making clinical judgments and intervening appropriately, they progress through five levels of competence. Beginning as a novice, the nurse progresses to advanced beginner and then to competent, proficient, and finally, expert nurse.

In the preceding situation, the student was clearly a novice. Lacking experience, the novice relies on rules to guide actions. As nurses gain experience, they begin to draw on that experience to view situations more holistically, becoming increasingly aware of subtle cues that indicate physiologic and psychologic changes. Expert nurses, like the nurse in the preceding situation, have a clear vision of what is possible in a given situation. This holistic perspective is based on a wealth of knowledge bred of experience and enables nurses to act "intuitively" to provide effective care. In reality nurses' intuition reflects their internalization of information. When faced with a clinical situation, nurses draw almost subconsciously on their stored knowledge and judgment.

This intuitive perception is integral to the "art of nursing," especially in areas such as maternal-newborn nursing, where change occurs quickly and families look to the nurse for help and guidance. Labor nurses become attuned to a woman's progress or lack of progress; nursery nurses detect subtle changes in their infant charges; antepartal and postpartal nurses become adept at assessing and teaching. Similarly, nurses who are cross-trained as labor, delivery, recovery, and postpartum (LDRP) nurses become skilled at caring for childbearing families during all phases of childbirth. Thus skilled nursing practice depends on a solid base of knowledge and clinical expertise delivered in a caring, holistic manner.

Empowerment is an important concept for nurses and clients today. Empowerment may be viewed as both a process and an outcome. As an internal process, empowerment results as individuals develop ever-increasing awareness of competence, mastery, and control over their own lives. An empowered self develops as a consequence of five processes—control, competence, credibility, confidence, and comfort. For nurses, these attributes often evolve as they mature in the profession (Moores, 1997).

Control develops as nurses learn to handle their own emotions and to master clinical situations by making and acting on client care decisions. Control issues are often difficult for advanced beginners, who can demonstrate only marginally acceptable performance (Benner, 1984) and they may look to expert nurses for guidance. As nurses provide good nursing care and develop a knowledge base, they gain competence. From this competence flows credibility as others begin to trust and believe in them. Nurses in turn become self-reliant, gaining confidence in their judgment, which is critical to feelings of empowerment. Finally a sense of comfort develops and nurses feel able to predict probable outcomes (Moores, 1997).

Empowered nurses are better able to approach client care situations effectively with full knowledge that they are ethically, legally, and morally accountable for their actions. Empowered nurses are able to interact as equals with other healthcare providers and collaborate with them to resolve problems and accomplish goals (Moores, 1997). When empowered nurses practice proactively, they anticipate problems before they develop and avoid undesirable client outcomes (Hagedorn, Gardner, Laux, et al, 1997). Empowered nurses share responsibility and accountability with each childbearing family, thereby helping the family become self-determining (Figure 1–1 ●).

> *My first pregnancy ended in spontaneous abortion at 8 weeks, so this time I decided not to tell anyone I was pregnant until I was 3 months along. We had just told both families the news the preceding day when it happened again. I began bleeding heavily, and we rushed to the ER. Here I was, a maternal-newborn nursing instructor, and I couldn't seem to handle a pregnancy. I was in the bathroom when I passed the fetus into the Johnny cap. My poor baby—so small, maybe 3 or 4 inches long. I began to sob uncontrollably as I rang for the nurse. I told her what happened, and she helped me to bed. My husband sat with his arm around me as I*

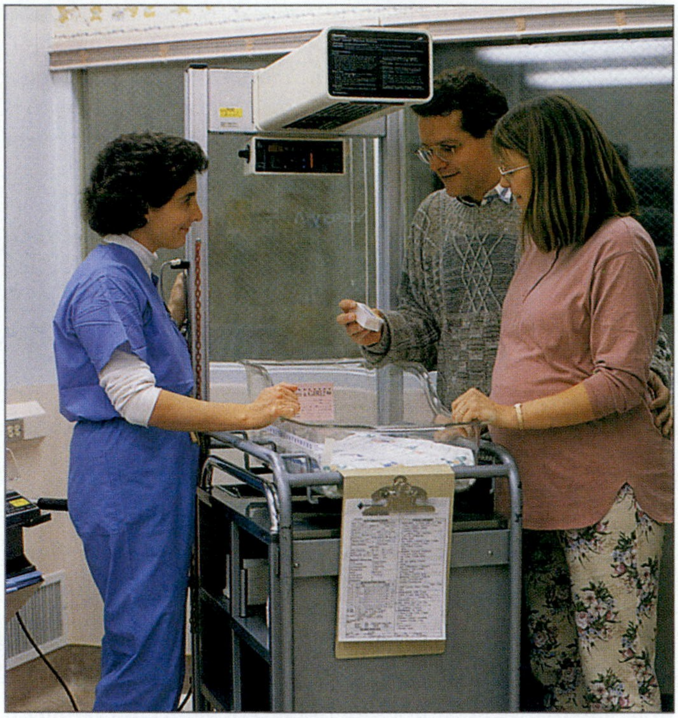

Figure 1–1 • Individualized education for childbearing couples is one of the prime responsibilities of the maternal-newborn nurse.

cried while the nurse took our baby out. A few minutes later, she came back and said, "I saw on your record that you are Catholic. Would you like me to baptize your baby?" I said, "Oh, yes, please," and she left. I've never forgotten how that made me feel. She saw me as a total person. I'm still teaching, and now I have two children. Whenever I teach high-risk pregnancy, I tell that story to the students. I want them to know what a difference a nurse can make."

We believe that many nurses who work with childbearing families are experts: They are sensitive, intuitive, knowledgeable, critical thinkers. They are technically skilled, empowered professionals who can collaborate effectively with others and advocate for those individuals and families who need their support. Such nurses do make a difference in the quality of care that childbearing families receive.

Contemporary Childbirth

The scope of practice of maternal and newborn nurses has changed dramatically in the past 25 years. Today's maternal-newborn nurses have far broader responsibilities and focus more on the specific goals of the individual childbearing woman and her family.

Not only has maternal-newborn nursing changed, so has the whole experience of childbirth. No longer do laboring women leave their partners and family at the labor room door while they work to give birth without the family's loving presence; no longer are newborns routinely whisked away for a prescribed period, to reappear magically for feedings every 4 hours and then return to the safe atmosphere of a central nursery; no longer are young siblings treated like walking sources of infection that threaten every infant. Today fathers are active participants in the birth experience. Families and friends are also often included. Siblings are encouraged to visit and meet their newest family member and may even attend the birth. Today the concept of "family-centered childbirth" is accepted and encouraged.

In addition, new definitions of family are evolving as discussed in Chapter 2. For example, the family of the single mother may include her mother, sister, another relative, a close friend, or the father of the child. Many cultures also recognize the importance of extended families, where several family members often provide care and support.

The family can generally make choices about many aspects of the childbirth experience, including the place of birth (hospital, free-standing birthing center, or home birth); the primary caregiver (physician, certified nurse-midwife, or even certified midwife); and birth-related experiences (methods of childbirth preparation, use of analgesia and anesthesia, and position for labor and birth, for example).

As recently as the early 1990s, women who gave birth vaginally remained in the hospital for approximately 3 days. This provided ample time for nurses to assess the family's knowledge and skill and complete essential teaching. By the mid-1990s, in an effort to control costs, hospitals were routinely discharging new mothers within 12 to 24 hours or less following birth. For women with supportive families, thorough prenatal preparation, and adequate resources for necessary follow-up care, this practice did not necessarily pose a problem. However, because early discharge severely limits the time available for client teaching, women with little knowledge, experience, or support were at greater risk of being inadequately prepared to care for themselves and their newborn infants.

Fortunately, the negative impact of this practice gained recognition nationwide. As a result, Congress passed the Newborns' and Mothers' Health Protection Act of 1996, which took effect in January 1998. This act provides for a postpartum stay of up to 48 hours following vaginal birth and up to 96 hours following cesarean birth at the discretion of the mother and her healthcare provider. However, it does not contain a provision for home care follow-up if a new mother chooses to leave the birthing facility earlier than the length of stay mandated by the act. Some states have developed home care provisions that strengthen the federal legislation.

It seems likely that home follow-up nursing care will continue to gain acceptance because it is a cost-effective approach with favorable long-term family outcomes. In addition, families can access a variety of community resources, from local programs focusing on specific topics such as parenting or postpartal exercise to the widely recognized support provided by national organizations such as La Leche League.

For families with access to the Internet, a wealth of information and advice is available. For example, the Department of Health and Human Services' Office on Women's Health offers a wide variety of educational resources designed to help promote women's health and well-being. This source provides information on a variety of topics such as "Pick Your Health," a yearlong campaign focused on assisting women to take practical, simple steps to improve their health and the "HHS Blueprint for Action on Breastfeeding," which is designed to promote breastfeeding, and includes Web links to a variety of organizations and consumer publications. Additional information about women's health resources can be found at the Web site of the Office on Women's Health: www.4woman.gov/owh/index.htm.

Interest in complementary and alternative medicine (CAM) practices is growing nationwide and will have an impact on the care of childbearing families. In response to this trend, the National Institutes of Health now has an Office of Alternative Medicine. Nurses caring for childbearing families need to recognize that a significant percentage of Americans are using some form of unconventional or alternative practice although they may not share this information with their healthcare provider. Thus it is important for nurses to communicate a willingness to work with the client to recognize and respect these alternative approaches. To assist nurses caring for these childbearing families we have included a new chapter—Chapter 3—on complementary and alternative therapies.

Many women elect to have their pregnancy and birth managed by a certified nurse-midwife (CNM), a registered nurse who is also prepared as a midwife. A few women choose to receive care from a certified midwife or even a lay midwife. The preparation and role of the CNM is described on page 8. Training as a lay midwife typically follows an apprenticeship or internship model, with a more senior midwife teaching a younger one. Today, however, a cadre of professional midwives is developing. These midwives complete a direct-entry midwifery education program and may take a certification exam to become a *certified midwife (CM)*. Accreditation for both CNMs and CMs is offered through the American College of Nurse-Midwives (American College of Nurse-Midwives, 2002).

Some women choose to give birth at home although healthcare professionals do not generally recommend this approach. The concern of the healthcare professional is that, in the event of an unanticipated complication that threatens the well-being of the mother or her infant, delay in obtaining emergency assistance might result. Some CNMs do attend home births; other home births are attended by CMs or by lay midwives.

The Self-Care Movement

The self-care movement began to emerge in the late 1960s as consumers sought to understand technology and take an interest in their own health and basic self-care skills. More and more people have begun to exercise, control their diet, monitor their psychologic and physiologic status, and in some cases even do their own diagnostic tests. They thus assume many primary care functions. Furthermore, today's healthcare consumers are requiring greater information and accountability from their healthcare providers. These consumers recognize that knowledge, indeed, is power.

Practicing self-care—assuming responsibility for one's own health—often requires assertiveness and taking an active role in seeking necessary information. Nurses can foster self-care by providing information readily and by acknowledging people's right to ask questions and become actively involved in their own care.

Maternal-newborn care offers a special opportunity to promote active participation in healthcare because it is essentially health focused; in most cases, clients are well when they enter the system. The consumer movement that has already influenced childbirth encourages people to speak up for preferences in dealing with healthcare providers.

Self-care has gained an even broader appeal in recent years because research suggests that it can significantly reduce healthcare costs. We believe that self-care will be a vital part of healthcare for years to come. Obviously, self-care is not always realistic or appropriate, especially in acute emergencies, but in many situations it is appropriate. With this in mind, throughout this book we have attempted to suggest ways in which nurses might offer health education that would enable the childbearing family to meet their own healthcare needs. We see this as one of nursing's most important functions and one that nurses are especially well qualified to perform.

Because of our support of self-care, we have used the term *client* rather than patient when referring to the childbearing woman. The term **client** implies an active, rather than a passive, role. The client seeks assistance from professionals who have special skills and knowledge that the client does not. The healthcare professional offers information and suggestions for a plan of action regarding the client's particular situation. The client can choose not to accept the professional's advice. Furthermore, the healthcare professional cannot proceed with the plan of action without the client's consent. In this relationship, clients assume responsibility for their decisions.

The nursing profession has been at the forefront in recognizing that people who are able to do so should take an active role in their own healthcare, and the term *client* best fits this concept. Nurses must understand that it is their professional expertise and skill that the client is seeking. Any attempt to make decisions for the client is inappropriate.

The Healthcare Environment

Healthcare issues are at the top of policy and legislative agendas. Cost, access, and quality of healthcare have become the "bywords" of the times. In 1960, healthcare costs in the United States accounted for approximately 5% of the gross domestic product (GDP). In 2000, however, despite efforts to contain healthcare costs, healthcare expenditures accounted for 13.2% of the GDP. Currently the United States spends a greater portion of the GDP on health than any other major industrialized nation worldwide (Pastor, Makuc, Reuben et al, 2002). Healthcare reform is in part a reaction to a cost problem out of control. The real question is whether the United States can develop solutions that are not

MediaLink
Office of Women's Health

simply reactive incremental changes, but that truly address the cost issue and other fundamental problems in the system.

In addition to high cost, lack of access to appropriate healthcare services is a second serious problem in the existing system. Currently about 41.2 million people in the United States, or 14.6% of the population, have no health insurance (US Census Bureau, 2002). Estimates suggest that an even greater number are underinsured. Among women of childbearing age (15 to 44 years), one in six, or about 11 million women, is uninsured. This group accounts for 30% of uninsured Americans. Significantly, Native American, Hispanic, African American, and Asian women are more likely to be uninsured than Caucasian women in this age group (Thorpe, 2001).

The United States spends more per capita than any other country in the world on healthcare; nevertheless, compared with other industrialized nations, the United States has higher infant mortality rates, similar life expectancy, and less access to care. Many people who have insurance fear changing or losing jobs because they may lose healthcare benefits and access to insurance. They may be denied insurance in the future because of preexisting conditions. The increase in serious, debilitating illnesses such as AIDS and tuberculosis and in chronic illnesses such as diabetes and hypertension makes this problem of "job lock" and lack of transferability of insurance benefits even more significant. For some uninsured people, the only access to the healthcare system is an emergency department. This inappropriate use of expensive services for basic primary care is both an access and a cost problem.

Demographic and environmental changes are increasing the need for services. Most significantly, as the overall population ages, the number of elderly and chronically ill continues to rise. Children and female heads of households also require a large share of health services. In the United States, 16.2% of children under age 18 live in poverty. This is the lowest poverty rate for children since 1979 but is still above the lows of the late 1960s and 1970s, which were about 14%. In 2000 the poverty rate for female-headed households was at an all-time low—24.7%. Experts attribute these decreases to the economic recovery that occurred in the 1990s (Dalaker, 2001). However, these numbers appear to be changing again in response to the economic declines that have marked the country recently. Perhaps most significantly, the United States has the highest child poverty rate of the 19 most developed countries in the world, well above rates in countries such as Canada, Great Britain, France, and Sweden (Madrick, 2002). The issue of women and poverty is explored in more detail in Chapter 8.

Currently about 62.6% of people in the United States are covered by employment-based health insurance (US Census Bureau, 2002). Many of these people are enrolled in some type of managed care organization because, in an effort to curtail costs, many employers have moved from fee-for-service coverage to some form of managed care. Thus managed care is now the dominant form of healthcare delivery in the United States. The move toward managed care has sparked concerns about the quality of healthcare. Because a fee-for-service model allows the consumer to register dissatisfaction by choosing to seek care elsewhere, quality is a high priority among fee-for-service providers. A managed care model, in contrast, limits consumer choice and, in turn, potentially affects quality. Establishing managed care's effects on quality poses a problem because in the US system, quality indicators such as outcomes of care usually have not been well determined. An outcome-based system is essential if there is to be comprehensive healthcare reform.

Changing the current system requires a new way of thinking and providing services. Primary healthcare services should be the base on which all other secondary and tertiary services are built. Today in the United States the opposite is still the case. The system emphasizes high-technology care rather than prevention. However, morbidity and mortality from disease are reduced significantly when people use preventive health services. There are some areas of improvement. For example, between 1990 and 2000, the percentage of pregnant women who received prenatal care increased from 76% to 83%. Similarly, between 1987 and 2000, the percentage of women age 40 and over who had had a mammogram in the preceding 2 years more than doubled, increasing from 29% to 70% (Pastor et al, 2002).

Providing all segments of the population with access to primary healthcare should be the chief criterion for meaningful reform of the US healthcare system. This includes a focus on health promotion, prevention, and individual responsibility for one's own health. In this model, secondary healthcare services would use a smaller proportion of the healthcare dollar.

The current emphasis on healthcare reform has yielded an unexpected benefit: Many healthcare providers and consumers have become more aware of the vitally important role nurses play in providing excellent care to clients and families. The emerging shift in the US healthcare system presents a significant opportunity for the nursing profession. However, this opportunity for responding to and creating change in nursing and healthcare delivery requires a new way of thinking. Nurses must clearly articulate their role in the changing environment. They must define and differentiate practice roles and the educational preparation required for those new roles, especially in community-based nursing practice and advanced practice roles such as nurse practitioners (NPs) and CNMs. Nurses must delineate roles of caregiver and care manager. Nurses must also assume greater roles in promoting health and preventing disease. In reality, in many settings nurses assume the primary responsibility for preventive healthcare services and screening programs.

Healthcare reform is influencing women's health and maternal-newborn nursing. Several factors, including demographic changes, the nationally recognized need to improve access to care, public demand for more effective healthcare options, new research findings, and women's preferences for healthcare, are contributing to changes in the field. Changes are predicted in clinical procedures, provider roles, care settings, and financing of care. As access to healthcare and the need to control costs increase, so will the need for, and utilization of, nurses in advanced practice roles. It is estimated that 80% to 90% of primary and preventive care services can be appropriately and cost-effectively provided by advanced practice nurses. Moreover, process and outcome measures indicate that the care that NPs and CNMs provide is as effective as the care provided by physicians caring for similar low-risk clients (Sinclair, 1997).

Culturally Competent Care

The U.S. population has a varied mix of cultural groups, with ever-increasing diversity. More than 33% of all children less than 20 years of age are from families of minority populations (US Census, 2001). Culture develops from socially learned beliefs, lifestyles, values, and integrated patterns of behavior that are characteristic of the family, cultural group, and community. The cultural background and values of childbearing families are often quite different from those of the nurse.

Specific elements that contribute to a family's value system include the following:

- Religion and social beliefs
- Presence and influence of the extended family, as well as socialization within the ethnic group
- Communication patterns
- Beliefs and understanding about the concepts of health and illness
- Permissible physical contact with strangers
- Education

Specific differences in beliefs between families and healthcare providers are common in the following areas:

- Help-seeking behaviors
- Pregnancy and childbirth practices
- Causes of diseases or illnesses
- Death and dying
- Caretaking and caregiving
- Childrearing practices

These elements in differing degrees influence the cultural beliefs and values of an ethnic group, making the group unique. Misunderstandings may occur when the healthcare professional and the family come from different cultural groups. In addition, past experiences with care may have made the family angry or suspicious of providers. Nurses need to be able to recognize, respect, and respond to ethnic diversity in a way that leads to a mutually desirable outcome. The nurse needs to identify culturally relevant facts about the client to provide culturally appropriate and competent care.

When the family's cultural values are incorporated into the care plan, the family is more likely to accept and comply with the needed care, especially in the home care setting. It is important for nurses to avoid imposing personal cultural values on the women and families in their care. By learning about the values of the different ethnic groups in the community—their religious beliefs that have an impact on healthcare practices, their beliefs about common illnesses, and their specific healing practices—nurses can develop an individualized nursing care plan for each childbearing woman and her family.

Because of the importance of culturally competent care, this topic is discussed in more depth in Chapter 2 and throughout the book as well.

DEVELOPING CULTURAL COMPETENCE

Conflicts can occur with a childbearing woman and her family when traditional rituals and practices of the family's elders do not conform with current healthcare practices. Nurses need to be sensitive to the potential implications for the woman's health and that of her newborn, especially after they are discharged home. When cultural values are not part of the nursing care plan, a woman and her family may be forced to decide whether the family's beliefs should take priority over the healthcare professional's guidance.

Professional Options in Maternal-Newborn Nursing Practice

> *As a man, I don't always find it easy to be a labor and delivery nurse. I have three children of my own and attended all their births. It meant a lot to me to be there, and I like helping others to have good childbirth experiences, too. I don't fit some people's image of a nurse; so they refer to me as a "male nurse" as opposed to a real nurse, and they ask why I didn't go into medicine instead. Why can't they understand that I'm a nurse because it's what I really want to be—and I'm darned good at it, too. More men are choosing nursing now, and I think that will help. I hope to see the day when we don't have "female doctors" and "male nurses," but doctors and nurses, period!*

Maternal-newborn nurses are found in the maternity departments of acute care facilities, in physicians' offices, in clinics, in college health services, in school-based programs dealing with sex education or adolescent pregnancies, in community health services, and in any other setting where a client has a need for maternity care. The depth of nursing involvement in various settings is determined by the qualifications and the role or function of the nurse employed. Many different titles have evolved to describe the professional requirements of the nurse in various maternity care roles. These titles include the following:

- A **professional nurse** is a graduate of an accredited basic program in nursing who has successfully completed the nursing examination (NCLEX) and is currently licensed as a registered nurse (RN). Professional nurses are typically educated as generalists.
- A **certified registered nurse (RNC)** has shown expertise in a particular field of nursing such as labor and delivery by taking a national certification examination.

- A **nurse practitioner (NP)** is a professional nurse who has received specialized education in either a master's degree program or a continuing education program and thus can function in an expanded role. Nurse practitioners often provide ambulatory care services to the expectant family (women's health nurse practitioner, family nurse practitioner); some NPs also function in acute care settings (neonatal nurse practitioner, perinatal nurse practitioner). NPs focus on physical and psychosocial assessment, including health history, physical examination, and certain diagnostic tests and procedures. The nurse practitioner makes clinical judgments and begins appropriate treatments, seeking physician consultation when necessary. The emerging emphasis on community-based care has greatly increased opportunities for NPs.
- A **clinical nurse specialist (CNS)** is a professional nurse with a master's degree who has additional specialized knowledge and competence in a specific clinical area. CNSs assume a leadership role within their specialty and work to improve client care both directly and indirectly.
- A **certified nurse-midwife (CNM)** is educated in the two disciplines of nursing and midwifery and is certified by the American College of Nurse-Midwives (ACNM). The certified nurse-midwife is prepared to manage independently the care of women at low risk for complications during pregnancy and birth and the care of normal newborns (Figure 1–2 •). In 2001 the American College of Obstetricians and Gynecologists (ACOG) and the ACNM issued a joint statement describing the independent, collaborative, and interdependent responsibilities of both groups, namely obstetricians/gynecologists and certified nurse-midwives/certified midwives. This agreement affirms that the "quality of care is enhanced by the interdependent practice of the obstetrician/gynecologist and the certified nurse-midwife/certified midwife working in a relationship of mutual respect, trust and professional responsibility." This agreement does not require the physical presence of an OB/GYN physician but does include the use of mutually agreed upon written medical guidelines/protocols.

  Typically CNMs care for women with low to average risk pregnancies. Research indicates that women with high-risk pregnancies can also benefit from CNM care if the CNM has unlimited access to physician consultation (Davidson, 2002).

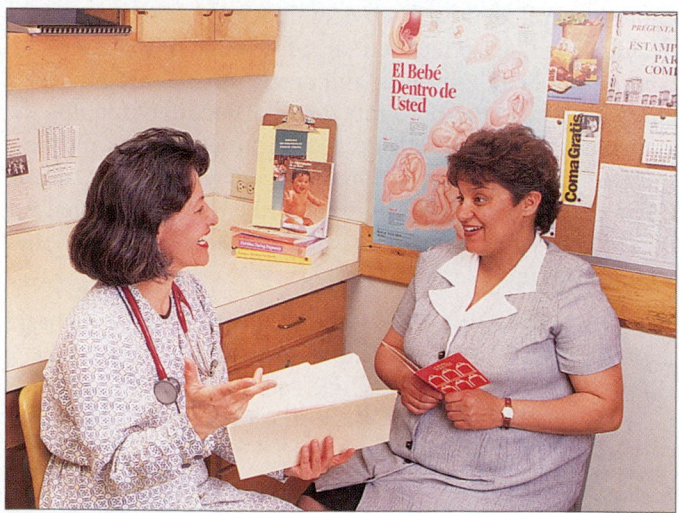

Figure 1–2 • A certified nurse-midwife confers with her client.

The term *advanced practice nurse* is used to describe nurses who, by education and practice, function in an expanded nursing role. The term, often used in a legal sense in state nurse practice acts, most frequently applies to NPs, CNSs, CRNAs (certified registered nurse anesthetists), and CNMs. As NPs assume a more prominent role in providing care, the distinctions between the roles of the nurse practitioner and the clinical nurse specialist are beginning to blur and these roles may ultimately merge.

Collaborative Practice

Managed care has led to a rethinking of care delivery. One approach that is becoming increasingly popular is collaborative practice. Collaborative practice is a comprehensive model of healthcare that uses a multidisciplinary team of health professionals to provide cost-effective, high-quality care. In maternal-newborn settings, the team generally includes CNMs and NPs in practice with physicians (often obstetricians or family practice physicians) and may include other health professionals, such as lactation consultants, social workers, or CNSs (Figure 1–3 •).

Successful teams have certain characteristics (Simpson & Knox, 2001):

- They have established consensus about their mission and vision, their goals, and their objectives and strategies.
- They recognize, respect, and value the unique contributions of each team member.
- They share a sense of mutual accountability—the team, not an individual, is responsible for success or failure.

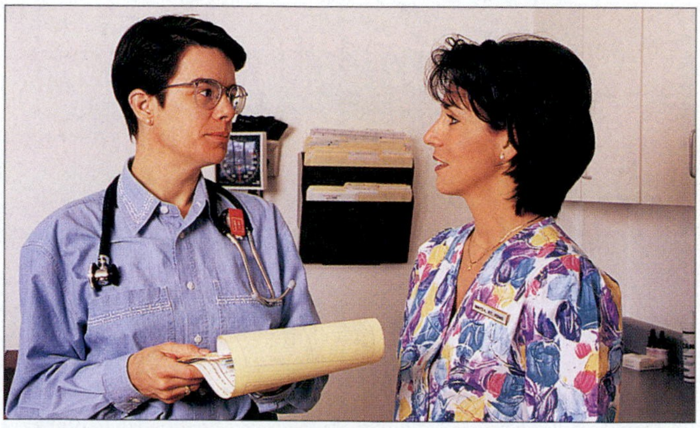

Figure 1–3 • A collaborative relationship between nurse and physician contributes to excellent client care.

- They are part of an organization that has strong, well-delineated performance standards and expectations.
- They have established effective communication.

In a successful team, each individual has autonomy but functions within a clearly defined scope of practice. In such a collaborative approach, no single profession "owns the client." Rather, the team seeks to empower clients and families and include them as partners in their care and in decision making.

Challenges of Contemporary Nursing Practice

The stresses inherent in the growing demand for nurses, coupled with the aging of the nursing workforce (the average age of practicing nurses is 43), the emphasis on cost containment as healthcare costs once again begin to escalate, regulatory and quality pressures, and organizational downsizing are constant challenges for nurses and, indeed, for all healthcare professionals. Many nurses enjoy caring for pregnant women, childbearing families, and newborns, so areas where maternal-newborn nurses practice have not felt the impact as much as other practice settings. Nevertheless, the impact of the nursing shortage is still apparent, as are efforts to curtail costs, especially by limiting staffing.

Nurses are beginning to explore ways to change education and practice. Colleges and universities are partnering with healthcare organizations to develop innovative educational opportunities. Nurses are working hard to stress the uniqueness of nursing practice and to present the rewarding side of the profession, not simply the challenges that nurses face. Healthcare providers are beginning to consider long-term solutions rather than settle for "quick fixes" to major challenges.

Beginning in fall 2001, leaders from 60+ nursing organizations came together to complete an in-depth strategic planning process, which led to the development of a comprehensive plan, *Nursing's Agenda for the Future*. This plan focuses on 10 major areas or domains including economic values, leadership and planning, work environment, delivery systems and nursing models, public relations and communication, legislation/regulation/policy, professional/nursing culture, recruitment/retention, education, and diversity (American Nurses Association, 2002). A steering committee of 19 nursing organizations, including the Association of Women's Health, Obstetric, and Neonatal Nurses (AWHONN), is guiding implementation of the plan. Nursing leaders next hope to put forth a call to stakeholders outside the profession seeking support for the plan to help ensure that high-quality nursing care is available.

> *I love being a neonatal intensive care nursery nurse. It is important work—caring for the innocents, helping families deal with the worry, and sometimes the heartbreak. I do get scared though when we are understaffed or have a float nurse who doesn't know much about the subtle changes that indicate that trouble is approaching. My friend who is a clinical instructor told me that nursing enrollments are up, in part because of the economy but also because the events of September 11th have caused people to rethink their priorities. I am so glad something positive is coming out of that tragedy. I hope it continues to influence people's choices about what matters.*

Community-Based Nursing Care

Many advocates of a new direction for healthcare support the increasing emphasis on primary care. Primary care includes a focus on health promotion, illness prevention, and individual responsibility for one's own health. These services are best provided in community-based settings. Third-party payers and managed care organizations are beginning to recognize the importance of primary care in containing costs and maintaining health. Community-based health services providing primary care and some secondary care will be available in schools, workplaces, homes, churches, clinics, transitional care programs, and other ambulatory settings.

The growth and diversity of managed care plans offer both opportunities and challenges for women's healthcare. The potential exists for managed care organizations to work with consumers to provide a model for coordinated and comprehensive well-woman care that includes improved screening and preventive services. One challenge managed care organizations will face is how to relate to essential community providers of care—organizations such as family planning clinics or women's health centers—that offer a unique service or serve groups of women with special needs (adolescents, disabled women, ethnic or racial minorities). Community-based care remains an essential element of healthcare for uninsured and underinsured individuals as well as for those individuals who benefit from programs such as Medicare or state-sponsored health-related programs. Some of these programs, such as those offered through public health departments, are broad based; others, such as parenting classes for adolescents, are geared to the needs of a specific population.

Community-based care is also part of a trend initiated by consumers, who are asking for a "seamless" system of family-centered, comprehensive, coordinated healthcare, health education, and social services. This seamless system requires coordination as clients move from primary care services to acute care facilities and then back into the community. The shortened length of hospital stays further mandates the need for coordination of services. Nurses can assume this care management role and perform an important service for individuals and families.

Maternal-newborn nurses are especially sensitive to these changes in healthcare delivery because the vast majority of healthcare provided to childbearing families takes place outside hospitals in clinics, offices, and community-based organizations. In addition, maternal-newborn nurses offer specialized services such as childbirth preparation classes or postpartal exercise classes. In essence, we are already experts at providing community-based nursing care. However, it is important that we remain knowledgeable about current practices and trends and open to new approaches to meet the needs of women and children.

HOME CARE

The provision of healthcare in the home is emerging as an especially important dimension of community-based nursing care. The shortened length of hospital stays has resulted in the discharge of individuals who still require support, assistance, and teaching. Home care can help fill this gap. Conversely, home care also enables individuals to remain at home with conditions that formerly would have required hospitalization.

Nurses are the major providers of home care services. Home care nurses perform direct nursing care and also supervise unlicensed assistive personnel who provide less skilled levels of service. In a home setting, nurses can use their skills in assessment, therapeutics, communication, teaching, problem solving, and organization to meet the needs of childbearing families. They also play a major role in coordinating services from other providers, such as physical therapists or lactation consultants.

Postpartum and newborn home visits are becoming a recognized way of ensuring that childbearing families make a satisfactory transition from the hospital or birthing center to the home. We see this trend as positive and hope that this method of meeting the needs of childbearing families becomes standard practice. Chapter 36 discusses home care in more detail and provides guidance about making a home visit. In addition, throughout the text we have provided information on how home care can meet the needs of women with health problems such as diabetes or preterm labor, which put them at risk during pregnancy. We believe that home care offers nurses the opportunity to function in an autonomous role and make a significant difference for individuals and families.

Legal and Ethical Considerations

Professional nursing practice requires full understanding of practice standards, institutional or agency policies, and local, state, and federal laws. Professional practice also requires an understanding of the ethical implications of those standards, policies, and laws that impact care, care providers, and care recipients. Every professional nurse is responsible for obtaining and maintaining current information regarding ethics and laws related to nursing practice and healthcare.

Scope of Practice

State nurse practice acts protect the public by broadly defining the legal *scope of practice* within which every nurse must function and by excluding untrained or unlicensed individuals from practicing nursing. Although some state practice acts continue to limit nursing practice to the traditional responsibilities of providing client care related to health maintenance and disease prevention, most state practice acts cover expanded practice roles that include collaboration with other professionals in planning and providing care, diagnostic and prescriptive privilege, and the delegation of client care tasks to other specified licensed and unlicensed personnel. Specified care activities for certified nurse-midwives and women's health, perinatal, or neonatal nurse practitioners may include diagnosis and prenatal management of uncomplicated pregnancies (CNMs may also manage births) and prescribing and dispensing medications using protocols in specified circumstances. A nurse must function within the scope of practice or risk being accused of practicing medicine without a license.

Correctly interpreting and understanding state practice acts enables the nurse to provide safe care within the limits of nursing practice. State boards of nursing may provide official interpretation of practice acts when the limits are not clear. On occasion hospital policy may conflict with a state's nurse practice act. It is important to recognize that hospital or agency policy may restrict the scope of practice specified in a state practice act, but such policy cannot legally expand the scope of practice beyond the limits stated in the practice act.

Nurse practice acts are subject to change. One component of professional nursing practice is the responsibility of each nurse to remain up-to-date regarding scope of practice and even to participate actively in promoting appropriate changes.

Nursing Negligence

Negligence is defined as omitting or committing an act that a reasonably prudent person would not omit or commit under the same or similar circumstances. Negligence consists of four elements:

1. There was a duty to provide care.
2. The duty was breached.
3. Injury occurred.
4. The breach of duty caused the injury (proximate cause).

Duty may be breached by omission—failing to give a medication, failing to assess properly, failing to notify a physician of a change in a laboring woman's condition, and so on. Duty may also be breached by commission—giving the wrong medication, placing an infant in the wrong crib, and so on. The injury that results may be physical or mental (pain and suffering). In determining whether nursing negligence occurred, the care that was given is compared to the standard of care. If the standard was not met, negligence occurred.

Standards of Nursing Care

Standards of care establish minimum criteria for competent, proficient delivery of nursing care. Such standards are designed to protect the public and are used to judge the quality of care provided. Legal interpretation of actions within standards of care is based on what a reasonably prudent nurse with similar education and experience would do in similar circumstances.

SOURCES OF CARE STANDARDS

Written standards of care are provided by a number of different sources. The American Nurses Association (ANA) has published standards of professional practice since 1950. In 1973, the ANA Congress for Nursing Practice began to write generic standards for all nurses in all settings. In addition, the ANA Divisions of Practice have published standards that include nursing practice for maternal-child health. The Council of Perinatal Nurses has published standards for perinatal nursing. Other specialty organizations, such as the Association of Women's Health, Obstetric, and Neonatal Nurses (AWHONN), the Association of Operating Room Nurses (AORN), and the National Association of Neonatal Nurses (NANN), have developed standards of specialty practice. Agency policies, procedures, and protocols also provide appropriate guidelines for care standards. The Joint Commission on Accreditation of Healthcare Organizations (JCAHO), a private, nongovernmental agency that audits the operation of hospitals and healthcare facilities, has also contributed to the development of nursing standards.

Agency policies, procedures, and protocols also provide appropriate guidelines for care standards. For example, *clinical practice guidelines* and clinical pathways are comprehensive interdisciplinary care plans for a specific condition that describe the sequence and timing of interventions that should result in expected client outcomes. Clinical practice guidelines or clinical pathways are adopted within a healthcare setting to reduce variation in care management, to limit costs of care, and to evaluate the effectiveness of care (Melnyk, Fineout-Overholt, Stone, et al, 2000).

Some standards carry the force of law; others, although not legally based, still carry important legal significance. Any nurse who fails to meet appropriate standards of care invites allegations of negligence or malpractice. (*Malpractice* is negligent action of a professional person.) However, any nurse who practices within the guidelines established by agency, local, or national standards is assured that clients are provided with competent nursing care, which, in turn, diminishes the potential for litigation.

ETHICAL COMPONENTS OF CARE STANDARDS

Standards of care are based on a legal model rather than on ethics. However, they incorporate important ethical components that extend the narrow legal interpretation of the term *standard.* Although there is a great deal of interplay between the two disciplines, each has a different perspective.

Law is based primarily on a rights model that establishes rules of conduct to define relationships among individuals. Law may also define relationships to impersonal entities like formal organizations, agencies, or hospitals.

Ethics, in contrast, is based on a responsibility or duty model that considers a wider range of factors than the rights model of law. Ethics incorporates factors such as risks, benefits, other relationships, concerns, and the needs and abilities of persons affected by and affecting decisions.

Law and ethics are interrelated; they share a similar decision process and standards. Both disciplines incorporate fact-finding, conflict negotiation, prioritization of related issues and values, and the application of resolutions of particular cases in decision making. Professional nurses must consider the ethical implications of legal decisions and the legal implications of ethical decisions.

Understanding the distinctions among medical or healthcare decisions, legal decisions, and ethical decisions is important. Consider the case in which parents from a culture unfamiliar to the nurse refuse surgery for their newborn based on a deeply held spiritual belief that intentional cutting of a body will result in spiritual death. Such a decision to forgo surgery may be viewed as negligent in the eyes of the law, unwise and inappropriate from a medical perspective, yet fully justifiable ethically. Similarly, legally sanctioned maintenance of life support for a severely damaged newborn with little hope for meaningful existence may remain a medically viable alternative, but to many it is not ethically justifiable. Recognizing the type of decision to be made often helps measure the worth and outcome of a decision more appropriately.

Clients' Rights

Law and ethics impact all of nursing practice, and several topics have specific implications for maternal-child nursing practice. Clients' rights encompass such topics as informed consent, privacy, and confidentiality.

INFORMED CONSENT

Informed consent is a legal concept designed to allow clients to make intelligent decisions regarding their own healthcare. Informed consent means that a client, or a legally designated decision maker, has granted permission for a specific treatment or procedure based on full information about that specific treatment or procedure as it relates to that client under the specific circumstances of the permission. While this policy is usually enforced for such major procedures as surgery or regional anesthesia, it pertains to any nursing, medical, or surgical intervention. To touch a person without consent (except in an emergency) constitutes battery.

Several elements must be addressed to ensure that the client has given informed consent. The information must be clearly and concisely presented in a manner understandable to the client and must include risks and benefits, the probability of success, and significant treatment alternatives. The client also needs to be told the consequences of receiving no treatment or procedure. Finally, the client must be told of the right to refuse a specific treatment or procedure. Each client should be told that refusing the specified treatment or procedure does not result in the withdrawal of all support or care.

The individual who is ultimately responsible for the treatment or procedure should provide the information necessary to obtain informed consent. In most instances, this is a physician. In such cases, the nurse's role may be to witness the client's signature giving consent. A nurse who knows the client and the procedure may certainly help the physician obtain the client's consent by clarifying the information the physician provides. It is also part of the nurse's role to determine that the client understands the information prior to making a decision. Anxiety, fear, pain, and medications that alter consciousness may influence an individual's ability to give informed consent. An oral consent is legal but written consent is easier to defend in a court of law.

Society grants parents the authority and responsibility to give consent for their minor children. Parents are presumed to possess what a child lacks in maturity, experience, and capacity for judgment in life's difficult decisions. Although the age of majority is 18 years in most states, variations in certain states require that nurses be aware of the law in the state where they practice. Children under 18 or 21 years of age, depending on state law, can legally give informed consent in the following circumstances:

- When they are minor parents of the infant or child client
- When they are *emancipated minors* (self-supporting adolescents under 18 years of age, not subject to parental control)
- When they are adolescents between 16 and 18 years of age seeking birth control, mental health counseling, or substance abuse treatment (Dickey & Deatrick, 2000)

Mature minors (14- and 15-year-old adolescents who are able to understand treatment risks) can give consent for treatment or refuse treatment in some states.

Special problems can occur in maternity nursing when a minor gives birth. It is possible, depending upon state law, that a minor may be able to consent to treatment for her infant but not for herself. In some states, however, a pregnant teenager is considered an emancipated minor and may therefore give consent for herself as well.

Additionally, some states require a married woman to obtain the consent of her spouse when a procedure involves sterilization or threatens the life of a fetus. Although childbearing women sign a general consent form on admission to an agency, separate informed consent is often required for surgery, cesarean birth, the administration of anesthesia, tubal ligation, or participation in research.

Refusal of a treatment, medication, or procedure after appropriate information also requires that a client sign a form to release the physician and agency from liability. Jehovah's Witnesses' refusal of blood transfusion or Rh immune globulin is an example of such refusal.

Nurses are responsible for educating clients about any nursing care provided. Before each nursing intervention, the maternal-child nurse lets the individual and/or family know what to expect, thus ensuring cooperation and obtaining consent. Afterward, the nurse documents the teaching and the learning outcomes in the person's record. The importance of clear, concise, and complete nursing records cannot be overemphasized. These records are evidence that the nurse obtained consent, performed prescribed treatments, reported important observations to the appropriate staff, and adhered to acceptable standards of care.

RIGHT TO PRIVACY

The *right to privacy* is the right of a person to keep his or her person and property free from public scrutiny. Maternity nurses need to remember that this includes avoiding unnecessary exposure of the childbearing woman's body. In the context of healthcare, the right to privacy dictates that only those responsible for a client's care should examine the client or discuss the client's case.

Most states have recognized the right to privacy through statutory or common law, and some states have written that right into their constitution. The ANA, National League for Nursing (NLN), and JCAHO have adopted professional standards protecting clients' privacy. Healthcare agencies should also have written policies dealing with client privacy. The new Health Insurance Portability and Accountability Act of 1996 (HIPAA), which was fully implemented in 2002, also has a provision to guarantee the security and privacy of health information.

Laws, standards, and policies about privacy specify that information about clients' treatment, condition, and prognosis can be shared only by the health professionals responsible for their care. Authorization for the release of any client information should be obtained from competent clients or their surrogate decision maker. Although it may be legal to reveal vital statistics such as name, age, occupation, and prognosis, such information is often withheld because of ethical considerations. The client should be consulted regarding what information may be released and to whom. When a client is a celebrity or is considered newsworthy, inquiries may be best handled by the public relations department of the agency.

CONFIDENTIALITY

Given the highly personal and intimate information requested of clients, the need for maintaining confidentiality is extremely crucial for the development of trust in the relationship between client and provider. Privileged communications exist between client and physician, client and attorney, husband and wife, and clergy and those who seek their counsel. In some states laws of privilege also protect nurses. Nurses should become well informed regarding privileged communication laws in their state.

A client may waive the right to confidentiality of medical records by action or words. For example, if a childbearing woman sues a physician, hospital, or other care provider, she waives the right to confidentiality of the medical record because the record becomes a source of evidence. Clients commonly consent to disclose information to insurance companies or to their employers. Computerization of medical records has created a greater concern for the integrity of records and the potential invasion of privacy.

In some instances, the public good takes precedence over an individual's right to privacy. For example, state laws require that care providers report gunshot wounds, child abuse, elder abuse, and some communicable diseases.

The Federal Patient Self-Determination Act requires all healthcare institutions that are reimbursed by Medicare or Medicaid to provide all hospitalized individuals with written information about their rights, which include expressing a preference for treatment options and making *advance directives* (writing a living will or authorizing a durable power of attorney for healthcare decisions on the individual's behalf). This often comes as a surprise to young women and couples of childbearing age who may have no experience of hospitals. However, with an advance directive in place, a childbearing woman can be certain that, even if she becomes incompetent, she can retain her autonomy about healthcare decisions (Rittley & Porter, 2001). Nurses often discuss these issues with clients and their families and can help them explore their beliefs and values about treatment options and dying.

Ethical Decision Making

Healthcare and bioethical literature are filled with examples of ethical decision-making models and frameworks. Decision-making models help nurses and other care providers confront seemingly unresolvable conflicts among the rights, duties, theories, principles, values, and individuals impacted by the ethical dilemmas of practice. There are six critical components of ethical decision making; they are very similar to the components of the nursing process.

1. Establish a means of determining who is involved in the dilemma, who is involved in the decision, and who will be affected by the outcome of the decision. This data-gathering step allows the nurse to identify and define the issue and determine who owns the problem, the information, the decision, and the consequences of it.
2. Establish a mechanism for obtaining all the information relevant to the conflict, including data related to diagnosis, prognosis, treatment options, available healthcare, and psychosocial, spiritual, financial, and other appropriate resources.
3. Formulate a plan to outline all potential options and the consequences of each option. Be sure that opposing viewpoints are presented and considered. Set individual values aside during this phase in order to encourage divergent views.
4. In the conflict resolution process that follows, review driving and restraining forces, assess risks and benefits, and assess the likelihood of a successful outcome with each option. At this stage, be sure that the moral values of everyone involved are addressed. In addition, review peripheral issues—such as the possible impact on other individuals or systems related to the decision, changes in client condition, pertinent laws, or new information—within the context of general and individual moral principles.
5. Select and act on a plan to resolve the conflict. Before acting on the resolution, determine who is ultimately responsible for the decision, who is most impacted by the outcome, and whether consensus is required.
6. Evaluate the resolution, its consequences, and the decision process itself. This step is critically important to avoid making similar decisions in isolation.

Ethical decisions in maternal-child nursing are often complicated by moral obligations to more than one client. Straightforward solutions to the ethical dilemmas nurses encounter in caring for childbearing families are often, quite simply, not available. By using a formal decision-making structure, nurses may, however, increase the likelihood of addressing multiple needs in complex care situations in an ethically appropriate and legal manner.

Special Ethical Situations in Maternity Care

Maternity care is fraught with unique circumstances in which an ethical dilemma may arise. These include situations of maternal-fetal conflict, issues related to termination of pregnancy, embryonic and fetal research, reproductive assistance, and cord blood banking. Additionally, the use of data from the Human Genome Project may give rise to ethical challenges.

Maternal-Fetal Conflict

Until fairly recently, the fetus was viewed legally as a nonperson. Mother and fetus were viewed as one complex client—the pregnant woman—of which the fetus was an essential part. However, advances in technology have permitted the physician to treat the fetus and monitor fetal development. The fetus is increasingly viewed as a client separate from the mother, although treatment of the fetus necessarily involves the mother. Thus the medical emphasis has shifted from one of unity to one of duality (Hornstra, 1999). This focus on the fetus intensified in 2002 when President George W. Bush announced that "unborn children" would qualify for government healthcare benefits. The move was designed to promote prenatal care, but it represented the first time that any U.S. federal policy had defined childhood as starting at conception.

Most women are strongly motivated to protect the health and well-being of their fetus. In some instances, however, women have refused interventions on behalf of the fetus, and forced interventions have occurred. These include forced cesarean birth, coercion of mothers who practice high-risk behaviors such as substance abuse to enter treatment, and, perhaps most controversial, mandating experimental in utero therapy or surgery in an attempt to correct a specific birth defect. These interventions infringe on the autonomy of the mother. They may also be detrimental to the baby if, as a result, maternal bonding is hindered, the mother is afraid to seek prenatal care, or the mother is herself harmed by the actions taken (Hornstra, 1999).

Attempts have also been made to criminalize the behavior of women who fail to follow a physician's advice or who engage in behaviors (such as substance abuse) that are considered harmful to the fetus. This raises two thorny questions: (1) What practices should be monitored? and (2) Who will determine when the behaviors pose such a risk to the fetus that the courts should intervene?

The American College of Obstetricians and Gynecologists (ACOG) Committee on Ethics (1999) and the American Academy of Pediatrics (AAP) Committee on Bioethics (1999) both affirm the fundamental right of pregnant women to make informed, uncoerced decisions about medical interventions. ACOG and AAP also recognize that cases of maternal-fetal conflict involve two clients, both of whom deserve respect and treatment. Such cases are best resolved by using internal hospital mechanisms including counseling, the intervention of specialists, and consultation with an institutional ethics committee. Court intervention should be considered a last resort, appropriate only in extraordinary circumstances.

Abortion

Since the 1973 Supreme Court decision in *Roe v. Wade*, abortion has been legal in the United States. It can be performed until the period of viability, after which abortion is permissible only when the life or health of the mother is threatened. Before viability, the mother's rights are paramount; after viability, the rights of the fetus take precedence.

Personal beliefs, cultural norms, life experiences, and religious convictions shape people's attitudes about abortion. Ethicists have thoughtfully and thoroughly argued positions supporting both sides of the question. Nevertheless, few issues spark the intensity of response seen when the issue of abortion is raised.

At present, decisions regarding abortion are made by a woman and her physician. Nurses (and other caregivers) have the right to refuse to assist with the procedure if abortion is contrary to their moral and ethical beliefs. However, if a nurse works in an institution where abortions may be performed, the nurse may be dismissed for refusing. To avoid being placed in a situation contrary to their values and beliefs, nurses should determine the philosophy and practices of an institution before going to work there. A nurse who refuses to participate in an abortion because of moral or ethical beliefs does have a responsibility to ensure that someone with similar qualifications is able to provide appropriate care for the client. Clients may never be abandoned, regardless of the nurse's beliefs.

MediaLink CARE PLAN: SECOND TRIMESTER ABORTION

Fetal Research

Research with fetal tissue has been responsible for remarkable advances in the care and treatment of fetuses with health problems and advances in the treatment of progressive, debilitating adult diseases such as Parkinson disease, Alzheimer disease, and DiGeorge syndrome. Therapeutic research with living fetuses has been instrumental in the treatment of Rh-sensitized infants, the evaluation of lung maturity using the lecithin/sphingomyelin ratio, and the treatment of pulmonary immaturity in the newborn. Because it is aimed at treating a fetal condition, therapeutic fetal research raises fewer ethical questions than does nontherapeutic fetal research. To be approved, nontherapeutic research requires that the risk to the fetus be minimal, that the knowledge to be gained be important, and that the information be unobtainable by any other means. Control over research standards and attention to state and federal regulations remain foci of debate regarding fetal research.

Intrauterine fetal surgery, which began in 1981 and developed through therapeutic research, is a therapy for anatomic lesions that can be corrected surgically and are incompatible with life if not treated. Intrauterine fetal surgery involves opening the uterus during the second trimester (prior to viability), treating the fetal lesion, and replacing the fetus in the uterus. The risks to the fetus are substantial, and the mother is committed to cesarean births for this and subsequent pregnancies because the upper, active segment of the uterus is incised during the surgery. The parents must be informed of the experimental nature of the treatment, the risks of the surgery, the commitment to cesarean birth, and alternatives to the treatment.

As with other aspects of maternity care, the pregnant woman's autonomy must be respected. The procedure does involve health risks to the woman, and she retains the right to refuse any surgical procedure. In 2001, ACOG issued a news release calling fetal surgery "experimental." Speaking specifically about fetal surgery for open neural tube defects, ACOG reported that long-term neurologic outcomes have not yet been demonstrated and the surgery exposes the mother to the risks of anesthesia, hemorrhage, preterm labor, and uterine rupture and also poses additional risk to the fetus. Healthcare providers must be careful that their zeal for new technology does not lead them to focus unilaterally on the fetus at the expense of the mother.

Reproductive Assistance

The number and sophistication of reproductive assistance techniques continue to grow. Infertile couples now have available a wide range of reproductive options from therapeutic insemination to in vitro fertilization and beyond. The ethical dimensions of such techniques are discussed here. The techniques themselves are identified and described in detail in Chapter 12.

Therapeutic insemination (TI) is accomplished by depositing into a woman sperm obtained from her husband, partner, or other donor. Some women who are single are choosing TI as a childbearing option. No states prohibit therapeutic insemination using a husband's sperm because there is no question of the child's legitimacy. Legal problems may occur with TI using donor sperm, however. Because the child is the biologic child of the mother, legal concerns center on the donor. A donor must sign a form waiving all parental rights. The donor must also furnish accurate health information, particularly regarding genetic traits or diseases. Donor sperm must be tested for HIV. Husbands often are requested to sign a form to agree to the insemination and to assume parental responsibility for the child. Some men legally adopt the child so there is no question of parental rights and responsibilities. Several states have enacted legislation regarding paternity of the child conceived by insemination with donor sperm.

A variety of procedures such as testicular sperm aspiration (TESA) have been developed to address severe male factor infertility. Although these procedures have been quite promising, they do raise questions about the increased risk of genetic defects related to bypassing of certain aspects of the process of natural selection. In the United States there are no established barriers to the use of these procedures.

Assisted reproductive technology (ART) is the term used to describe any fertility treatment in which both the egg and sperm are handled. Treatments in which only the sperm are handled (e.g., therapeutic insemination) or in which a woman takes medication to stimulate egg production without subsequent egg retrieval are not included in the definition of ART. In vitro fertilization and embryo transfer (IVF-ET), a therapy offered to selected infertile couples, is perhaps the best known ART technique. Some effort has been made legislatively to address consumer concerns about ART. In the United States, the Federal Fertility Clinic Success Rate and Certification Act of 1992 (FCSRCA) addresses issues related to laboratory quality and the standardized reporting of pregnancy success rates associated with ART programs. The act requires all clinics performing ART in the United States to report their success rates annually to the Centers for Disease Control and Prevention (CDC). However, it does not contain provisions to deal with the unethical practices that may occur, nor does it address false reporting of success rates. To help ensure data accuracy, a validation process, which includes site visits to a portion of reporting clinics, is completed.

The success rates of the ART procedures vary significantly by maternal age. Specifically, in 1999, 24.8% of all ART procedures that used fresh, nondonor eggs or embryos resulted in a live birth. However, the success rate was 32.2% for women under age 35 and only 18.5% for women ages 38 to 40 (CDC, 2001).

Of the pregnancies that result from ART, about 37% include more than one fetus (29% twins, 8% triplets or greater). Multiple pregnancy occurs because the use of ovulation-inducing medications typically triggers the release of multiple eggs, which, when fertilized, produce multiple embryos that are then implanted. Multiple pregnancy increases the likelihood of miscarriage, preterm birth, and neonatal morbidity and mortality. It also increases the mother's risk of cesarean birth and of complications such as hypertensive diseases of pregnancy, gestational diabetes, and hemorrhage. To help prevent a high-level multiple pregnancy, the American Society for Reproductive Medicine has issued guidelines to limit the number of embryos transferred. This practice raises ethical considerations about the handling of the unused embryos. When a multiple pregnancy does occur, the physician may suggest that the woman abort some of the embryos—nonselective embryo reduction—to give the remaining embryos a better chance for survival. Clearly, this procedure raises ethical concerns about the sacrifice of some so that the remainder can survive (ACOG, 2002).

Surrogate childbearing is another approach to addressing the issue of infertility. Surrogate childbearing occurs when a woman agrees to become pregnant for another woman or for a couple who are usually childless. Depending on the infertile woman's or couple's needs, the surrogate may be therapeutically inseminated with the male partner's sperm or a donor's sperm, or she may even receive a gamete transfer. If fertilization occurs, the woman carries the fetus to term and then releases the infant to the couple after birth.

These methods of resolving infertility raise many ethical questions, including the problem of religious objections to artificial conception, the question of who will assume financial and moral responsibility for a child born with a congenital defect, the issue of candidate selection, and the threat of genetic engineering. Other ethical questions include the following:

- What should be done with surplus fertilized oocytes?
- To whom do frozen embryos belong—parents together or separately? The hospital or infertility clinic?
- Who is liable if a woman or her offspring contracts HIV disease from donated sperm?
- Should children be told the method of their conception?

> *Our son was born after artificial insemination. Nick, my husband, was sterile because of radiation therapy so his cousin was the donor for us. I thought that might be awkward but the whole family was so excited that there was a way to help us after Nick's battle with cancer that it has been OK. Every time we look at Vincent Joseph (he is named for his grandfathers) and see him smile, we know that we would do it again in an instant.*

Embryonic Stem Cell Research

Human stem cells can be found in embryonic tissue and in the primordial germ cells of a fetus. Research has demonstrated that in tissue cultures these cells can be made to differentiate into other types of cells such as blood, nerve, or heart cells, which might then be used to treat problems such as diabetes, Parkinson and Alzheimer diseases, spinal cord injury, or metabolic disorders. The availability of specialized tissue or even organs grown from stem cells might also decrease society's dependence on donated organs for organ transplants (Ryan, 2000).

In 2001, President George W. Bush decided to permit federal funding of embryonic stem cell research, but only on the 64 existing cell lines identified by the National Institutes of Health (NIH). The president also announced the creation of a President's Council on Bioethics, which is to oversee all federally funded embryonic stem cell research and study the range of ethical issues found in the biomedical and behavioral sciences. Later that year the National Academy of Sciences released a new report on the subject. In the report the academy stated that public funding should be provided for further stem cell research and that, ultimately, new embryonic stem cell lines will have to be developed (American Association for the Advancement of Science, 2002).

The ethical questions and dilemmas associated with embryonic stem cell research are staggering and complex. The following are two of the most pressing, initial issues to be considered (Roche & Grodin, 2000):

- What moral status should be attached to the human embryo? How should an embryo be viewed? With full status as a person? As a cluster of undifferentiated cells with no moral status? As having status somewhere in between, that is beyond mere cells and deserving of special respect?
- What sources of embryonic tissue are acceptable for research? Is it ever ethical to create embryos solely for stem cell research? Is there justification for using embryos remaining after fertility treatments?

Equally significant, advancements in stem cell research play a major role in the rapidly approaching convergence of reproductive and genetic technologies with all of their related ethical dilemmas.

MediaLink CASE STUDY: CORD BLOOD BANKING

Cord Blood Banking

Cord blood, which is taken from a newborn's umbilical cord by the physician or nurse-midwife assisting with the birth, may play a role in combating leukemia, certain other cancers, and other immune and blood system disorders. Cord blood, like bone marrow, contains regenerative stem cells, which are able to replace diseased cells in the affected individual. The value of bone marrow transplants has long been recognized, and a national registry of potential bone marrow donors has been established. The process of collecting bone marrow is expensive and uncomfortable, however, and the National Marrow Donor Registry often has difficulty finding a matching bone marrow donor.

Cord blood has some advantages over bone marrow:

- Collecting cord blood is less invasive and involves no risk to mother or infant.
- Large-scale cord blood banking would increase the availability of stem cells for minority groups, who are seriously underrepresented in bone marrow registries.
- Cord blood is less likely than bone marrow to trigger a potentially fatal rejection response.
- Cord blood works with a less-than-perfect match.
- Cord blood is available for use more rapidly than bone marrow.

Although the use of cord blood is an option that is gaining interest, cord blood also has its limitations (Crooks, Lill, Feig, et al, 1997): For example:

- A limited number of cells are available to be transplanted.
- There is little definitive information about effectiveness based on recipient size.
- There is an increased likelihood of leukemic relapse.
- Transplantation cannot be repeated.

Cord blood banks that process and store cord blood have now been established in the United States. Families can elect to register their infant's cord blood privately. The blood is collected at birth and the family assumes all costs for analyzing, preparing, and storing the blood. The blood is quickly available for use by the donor, a sibling, or the mother. (During pregnancy, mother and infant seem to become immunologically tolerant of each other.) This option is especially useful in families with a history of cancer or genetic blood disease. Alternatively, families may elect to donate the cord blood to an established registry for use by others. Currently, however, this option is not widely available.

Ethical issues associated with cord blood banking include the following (Smith & Thomson, 2000):

- Who owns the blood? The donor? The parents? Private blood banks? Society?
- How will informed consent be obtained and by whom?
- How will confidentiality be ensured? Family members need to understand that, if they choose to donate, the mother will be asked to provide a blood sample and a detailed history about her health and infectious disease status.
- How will obligations to notify the family and donor be addressed if testing of the blood reveals infectious diseases or genetic disorders? Should there be any ongoing assessment of donors so that if health problems develop, recipients can be notified?
- How can the harvested blood be distributed fairly, so that it is available to individuals from all races, ethnic groups, and income levels?

The Human Genome Project

The *Human Genome Project (HGP)* is an international, multidisciplinary effort begun in 1990 to explore and map human genetic material. In the United States, the Human Genome Project is a coordinated, 15-year national research program to identify all human genetic material—the genome—by developing a human genetic map of all chromosomes, by improving existing genetic maps, and by determining the complete sequence of human DNA. Jointly sponsored by the US Department of Energy and the NIH, the project is also designed to develop new technologies and techniques to support the effort. In addition, the HGP is charged with analyzing the legal, ethical, and social implications resulting from the availability of genetic information about individuals; developing public policy options to deal with the complex issues that will arise; and identifying advanced ways of sharing the information that emerges with researchers, scientists, physicians, and others so that the data may quickly be used for the public good (National Center for Human Genome Research, 2001). As part of the effort, the HGP has also established research training programs for pre- and postdoctoral fellows.

The implications of the effort are staggering. In June of 2000, the scientific community was excited by the announcement that a rough draft of the human genome had been finished a year ahead of schedule. This draft sequence provides information about 90% of the human genome. On April 14, 2003, a date that coincides with the 50th anniversary of the discovery of the DNA double helix by Watson and Crick, researchers announced that 99% of the human genetic code had been identified. (Ault, 2003). This effort, the work of scientists from 18 countries, was completed 2½ years ahead of schedule and forms the basis for future genomic research.

As more genetic information becomes available, questions regarding the use and protection of such information arise. Gene manipulation and gene therapy, once limited to science fiction novels, now present a reality that adds to the complex ethical questions of the use and control of technology. Other emerging issues include the question of payment for genetic testing; appropriate counseling following testing; confidentiality; qualifications of individuals engaged in testing, counseling, and interventions; mandated testing; and the right to refuse genetic information.

Implications for Nursing Practice

The complex ethical issues facing maternal-newborn nurses have many social, cultural, legal, and professional ramifications. Nurses, like all healthcare professionals, need to learn to anticipate ethical dilemmas, clarify their own positions and values related to the issues, understand the legal implications of the issues, and develop appropriate strategies for ethical decision making. To accomplish these tasks, they may read about bioethical issues, participate in discussion groups, or attend courses and workshops on ethical topics pertinent to their areas of practice. Most nurses develop solid skills in logical thinking and critical analysis. These skills, coupled with theoretical knowledge about ethical decision making, can serve nurses well in dealing with the many ethical dilemmas found in healthcare.

Statistical Data and Maternal-Infant Care

Increasingly nurses are recognizing the value and usefulness of statistics. Health-related statistics provide an objective basis for projecting client needs, planning use of resources, and determining the effectiveness of treatment.

There are two major types of statistics: *descriptive* and *inferential. Descriptive statistics* describe or summarize a set of data. They report the facts—what is—in a concise and easily retrievable way. How the data are compiled and presented is determined by the question being asked. An example of a descriptive statistic is the birth rate in the United States. Although no conclusion may be drawn from these statistics about why some phenomenon has occurred, they can identify certain trends and high-risk "target groups" and generate possible research questions.

Inferential statistics allow the investigator to draw conclusions or inferences about what is happening between two or more variables in a population and to suggest or refute causal relationships between them. For example, descriptive statistics reveal that the infant mortality rate in the United States has declined over the past decade. Exactly why that trend has occurred cannot be answered by simply looking at these data, however. More data and inferential statistics using smaller samples of the population of pregnant women are needed to determine whether this finding is due to earlier prenatal care, improved maternal nutrition, use of electronic fetal monitoring during labor, and/or any number of factors potentially associated with maternal-fetal survival.

Descriptive statistics are the starting point for the formation of research questions. Inferential statistics answer specific questions and generate theories to explain relationships between variables. Theory applied in nursing practice can help change the specific variables that may cause or contribute to certain health problems.

This section discusses descriptive statistics that are particularly important to maternal-newborn healthcare. Inferences that may be drawn from these descriptive statistics are addressed as possible research questions that may help identify relevant variables.

Birth Rate

Birth rate refers to the number of live births per 1000 people. In 2001, the US birth rate was 14.5. Table 1–1 • provides valuable information about births in the United States in 2000 and 2001. In 2001 the number of births was 4,040,121, down slightly from 2000. The number of births to white (non-Hispanic) and black women decreased 1% to 3%, while births to Native American and Asian/Pacific Islander women remained essentially unchanged. Births to Hispanic women increased by 4%. Teenage birth rates decreased for all race and ethnic groups, while birth rates for women ages 30 to 44 increased (Martin, Park, & Sutton, 2002).

Table 1–2 • provides interesting information about selected demographic and health characteristics. Although the proportion of births to unmarried mothers increased slightly in 2001 (to 33.4% as compared to 33.2% in 2000), that percentage has changed very little since 1994. It typically ranges between 32.2% and 33.4%. Unfortunately the cesarean birth rate rose from 22.9% of all births in 2000 to 24.4% in 2001, an increase of 7%. On a more positive note, the percentage of women beginning prenatal care in the first trimester rose slightly from 83.2% to 83.4% (Martin et al, 2002).

Birth rates also vary dramatically from country to country. Table 1-3 • identifies the birth rates for selected countries.

- Is there an association between birth rates and changing societal values?
- Do the differences in birth rates between various age groups reflect education? Changed attitudes toward motherhood?
- Do the differences in birth rates among various countries reflect cultural differences? Do they represent availability of contraceptive information? Are there other factors at work?

Table 1–1 • BIRTHS AND BIRTH RATES BY AGE, RACE, AND ORIGIN OF MOTHER: UNITED STATES, FINAL 2000 AND PRELIMINARY 2001

[Data for 2001 are based on a continuous file of records received from the States. Figures for 2001 are based on weighted data rounded to the nearest individual, so categories may not add to totals. Rates per 1000 women in specified age and racial group]

	2001		2000	
Age and Race/Hispanic Origin	**Number**	**Rate**	**Number**	**Rate**
All races				
Total[1]	**4,040,121**	**67.2**	**4,058,814**	**67.5**
10–14 years	7,791	0.8	8,519	0.9
15–19 years	447,367	45.9	468,990	48.5
15–17 years	145,646	25.3	157,209	27.4
18–19 years	301,721	75.8	311,781	79.2
20–24 years	1,024,933	110.2	1,017,806	112.3
25–29 years	1,062,590	121.8	1,087,547	121.4
30–34 years	946,598	95.6	929,278	94.1
35–39 years	452,960	41.4	452,057	40.4
40–44 years	92,805	8.1	90,013	7.9
45–54 years[2]	5,076	0.5	4,604	0.5
White, non-Hispanic	**2,336,033**	**58.0**	**2,362,968**	**58.5**
Black	**604,834**	**69.3**	**622,598**	**71.7**
Native American	**41,809**	**70.7**	**41,668**	**71.4**
Asian/Pacific Islands	**200,493**	**69.4**	**200,543**	**70.7**
Hispanic	**849,800**	**107.4**	**815,868**	**105.9**

[1]The total number includes births to women of all ages, 10–54 years. The rate shown for all ages is the fertility rate, which is defined as the total number of births, regardless of age of mother, per 1000 women aged 15–44 years.

[2]The number of births shown is the total for women aged 45–54 years. The birth rate is computed by relating the number of births to women aged 45–54 years to women aged 45–49 years, because most of the births in this group are to women aged 45–49.

[3]Race and Hispanic origin are reported separately on the birth certificate. Data for persons of Hispanic origin are also included in the data for each race group, according to the mother's reported race.

[4]Includes births to Aleuts and Eskimos.

[5]Includes all persons of Hispanic origin of any race.

Note: Rates for some population groups, particularly Hispanic and Asian or Pacific Islander, may be overstated.

Source: *National Vital Statistics Report*, Vol 50, No 10, June 6, 2002.

Infant Mortality

The **infant mortality rate** is the number of deaths of infants under 1 year of age per 1000 live births in a given population. In 2000 the US infant mortality rate was 6.9 (Table 1–4 •). However, the infant mortality rate varied widely by race of the mother from 5.6 for infants of Hispanic mothers to 13.6 for infants of black mothers (Mathews, Menacker, & MacDorman, 2002). *Neonatal mortality* is the number of deaths of infants less than 28 days of age per 1000 live births. *Perinatal mortality* includes both neonatal deaths and fetal deaths per 1000 live births. (*Fetal death* is death in utero at 20 weeks or more gestation.)

In 2000, infant mortality rates were highest for the babies of adolescent mothers and lowest for women in their late 20s and early 30s. They were also high for women in their forties and older. In general, infant mortality rates also decreased with increasing maternal educational levels. On the other hand, the infant mortality rate for babies of unmarried mothers was more than 83% higher than the mortality rate for infants of women who were married. In addition, the infant mortality rate in 2000 was higher for the infants of mothers who smoked than for the infants of nonsmokers (Mathews et al, 2002). Figure 1-4 • depicts the leading causes of death for infants in the United States in 2000.

The US infant mortality rate has continued to be of concern because the United States has fallen to 22nd place among industrialized nations in infant mortality rankings. Healthcare professionals, policy makers, and the public have continued to stress the need in the United States for better prenatal care, coordination of health services, and the provision of comprehensive maternal-child services.

Table 1–3 identifies infant mortality rates for selected countries. As the data indicate, the range is dramatic among the countries listed. Unfortunately, information about birth rates and mortality rates is limited for some countries because of a lack of organized reporting mechanisms.

The information prompts questions about access to healthcare during pregnancy and following birth, standards of living, nutrition, sociocultural factors, and more. Additional

Table 1–2 • TOTAL BIRTHS AND PERCENT OF BIRTHS WITH SELECTED DEMOGRAPHIC AND HEALTH CHARACTERISTICS BY RACE AND ORIGIN OF MOTHER: UNITED STATES, FINAL 2000 AND PRELIMINARY 2001

[Figures for 2001 are based on weighted data rounded to the nearest individual]

	All Races[1]		White, Total[2]		Non-Hispanic White		Black[2]		Hispanic[3]	
Characteristic	2001	2000	2001	2000	2001	2000	2001	2000	2001	2000
					Number					
Births	4,040,121	4,058,814	3,192,985	3,194,005	2,336,033	2,362,968	604,834	622,598	849,800	815,868
					Percent					
Births to unmarried mothers	33.4	33.2	27.6	27.1	22.5	22.1	68.3	68.5	42.4	42.7
Low birth weight[4]	7.6	7.6	6.7	6.5	6.7	6.6	12.9	13.0	6.5	6.4
Very low birth weight[5]	1.43	1.43	1.15	1.14	1.16	1.13	3.02	3.06	1.13	1.14
Total cesarean delivery rate[6]	24.4	22.9	24.2	22.8	24.5	23.1	25.8	24.3	23.5	22.1
Primary cesarean rate[7]	16.9	16.1	16.7	15.9	17.2	16.4	18.2	17.3	15.2	14.5
VBAC rate[8]	16.5	20.6	16.4	20.4	16.9	21.1	16.8	20.5	14.8	18.5
Prenatal care beginning in first trimester	83.4	83.2	85.2	85.0	88.5	88.5	74.5	74.3	75.7	74.4
Prenatal care beginning in third trimester or no care	3.8	3.9	3.2	3.3	2.3	2.3	6.6	6.7	5.9	6.3

[1]Includes races other than white and black.

[2]Race and Hispanic origin are reported separately on the birth certificate. Data for persons of Hispanic origin are included in the data for each race group according to the mother's reported race.

[3]Includes all persons of Hispanic origin of any race.

[4]Birth weight of less than 2500 grams (5 lb 8 oz).

[5]Birth weight of less than 1500 grams (3 lb 4 oz).

[6]Total births by cesarean as percent of all births.

[7]Number of primary cesareans per 100 live births to women who have not had a previous cesarean.

[8]Number of vaginal births after previous cesarean delivery per 100 live births to women with a previous cesarean delivery.

Source: *National Vital Statistics Report*, Vol 50, No 10, June 6, 2002.

Table 1–3 • LIVE BIRTH RATES AND INFANT MORTALITY RATES FOR SELECTED COUNTRIES

Country	Birth Rate	Infant Mortality Rate
Afghanistan	41.4	147.0
Argentina	18.4	17.8
Australia	12.9	7.2
Bangladesh	25.3	70.0
Cambodia	33.2	65.4
Canada	11.2	5.0
China	16.0	28.1
Egypt	24.9	60.5
Germany	9.2	4.7
Ghana	29.0	56.5
India	24.3	63.2
Iraq	34.6	60.0
Japan	10.0	3.9
Latvia	8.0	15.3
Mexico	22.8	25.4
Peru	23.9	39.4
Russia	9.4	20.1
Sweden	9.9	3.5
United Kingdom	11.5	5.5
United States	14.5	6.9

Source: *World Almanac and Book of Facts 2002.* New York: World Almanac Books.

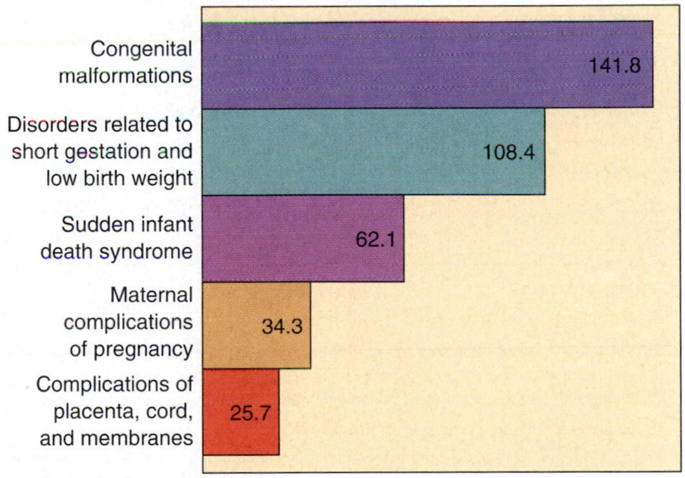

Figure 1–4 • Leading causes of death for infants in the United States, 2000.

Source: Mathews, T.J., Menacker, F., & MacDorman, M.F. (2002). Infant mortality statistics for the 2000 period. Linked birth/infant death data set. *National Vital Statistics Report, 50*(12), 1–27.

Table 1–4 • INFANT, NEONATAL, AND POSTNEONATAL DEATHS AND MORTALITY RATES BY ORIGIN OF MOTHER: UNITED STATES, 2000.

Hispanic Origin and Race of Mother	Live Births	Number of Deaths			Mortality Rate per 1000 Live Births		
		Infant	Neonatal	Postneonatal	Infant	Neonatal	Postneonatal
All origins[1]	4,058,882	27,960	18,733	9,227	6.9	4.6	2.3
Total Hispanic	815,883	4,564	3,078	1,486	5.6	3.8	1.8
Non-Hispanic white	2,362,982	13,461	8,924	4,537	5.7	3.8	1.9
Non-Hispanic black	604,367	8,212	5,552	2,660	13.6	9.2	4.4
Not stated	42,969	480	368	112	...	...	...

. . . Category not applicable.

[1]Origin of mother not stated included in "All origins" but not distributed among origins.

Note: Neonatal is less than 28 days and postneonatal is 28 days to under 1 year.

Source: *National Vital Statistics Report*, Vol 50, No 12, August 28, 2002.

Table 1–5 • MATERNAL MORTALITY FOR COMPLICATIONS OF PREGNANCY, CHILDBIRTH, AND THE PUERPERIUM, ACCORDING TO RACE AND AGE: UNITED STATES, SELECTED YEARS 1950–1999

[Data are based on the National Vital Statistics System]

Race, Hispanic Origin, and Age	1950[1]	1960[1]	1970	1980	1990	1995	1996	1997	1998	1999[2]
					Number of deaths					
All persons	2,960	1,579	803	334	343	277	294	327	281	391
White	1,873	936	445	193	177	129	159	179	158	214
Black	1,041	624	342	127	153	133	121	125	104	154
American Indian or Alaska Native	—	—	—	3	4	1	6	2	2	5
Asian or Pacific Islander	—	—	—	11	9	14	8	21	17	18
Hispanic[3]	—	—	—	—	47	43	39	57	42	67
White, non-Hispanic[3]	—	—	—	—	125	84	114	121	116	149
All persons					Deaths per 100,000 live births					
All ages, age adjusted	73.7	32.1	21.5	9.4	7.6	6.3	6.4	7.6	6.1	8.3
All ages, crude	83.3	37.1	21.5	9.2	8.2	7.1	7.6	8.4	7.1	9.9
Under 20 years	70.7	22.7	18.9	7.6	7.5	3.9	*	5.7	*	6.6
20–24 years	47.6	20.7	13.0	5.8	6.1	5.7	5.0	6.6	5.0	6.2
25–29 years	63.5	29.8	17.0	7.7	6.0	6.0	6.6	7.9	6.7	8.2
30–34 years	107.7	50.3	31.6	13.6	9.5	7.3	7.6	8.3	7.5	10.1
35 years and over[4]	222.0	104.3	81.9	36.3	20.7	15.9	19.0	16.1	14.5	23.0

—Data not available.

*Based on fewer than 20 deaths.

[1]Includes deaths of persons who were not residents of the 50 States and the District of Columbia.

[2]Starting with 1999 data, changes have been made in the classification and coding of maternal deaths under ICD—10. The large increase in the number of maternal deaths between 1998 and 1999 is due to changes associated with ICD—10. See Appendix II, *International Classification of Diseases (ICD)*, and Rate: Death and related rates.

[3]Excludes data from States lacking an Hispanic-origin item on their death and birth certificates. See Appendix 1, National Vital Statistics System.

[4]Rates computed by relating deaths of women 35 years and over to live births to women 35–49 years.

Sources: National Center for Health Statistics. Health, United States, 2002. Hyattsville, MD.

factors affecting the infant mortality rate may be identified by considering the following research questions:

- Does infant mortality correlate with a specific maternal age?
- What are the leading causes of infant mortality in each country?
- Is there a difference in mortality rates among racial groups? If so, is it associated with the availability of prenatal care? With educational level of the mother or father?

Maternal Mortality

The **maternal mortality rate** is the number of deaths from any cause during the pregnancy cycle (including the 42-day postpartal period) per 100,000 live births. In 1999, 391 women died of maternal causes as compared to 281 in 1998 and 327 in 1997. Prior to 1996, the maternal mortality rate in the United States had decreased steadily in the last 40 years or more (Table 1–5 •). Factors influencing the decrease in maternal mortality include the increased use of hospitals and specialized healthcare personnel by antepartal, intrapartal, and postpartal maternity clients; the establishment of care centers for high-risk mothers and infants; the prevention and control of infection with antibiotics and improved techniques; the availability of blood and blood products for transfusions; and the lowered rates of anesthesia-related deaths.

Additional factors to consider may be identified by asking the following research questions:

- Is there a correlation between maternal mortality and age?
- Is there a correlation with availability of healthcare? Economic status?

Implications for Nursing Practice

Nurses can use statistics in a number of ways. For example, statistical data may be used to

- Determine populations at risk.
- Assess the relationship between specific factors.
- Help establish databases for specific client populations.
- Determine the levels of care needed by particular client populations.
- Evaluate the success of specific nursing interventions.
- Determine priorities in caseloads.
- Estimate staffing and equipment needs of hospital units and clinics.

Statistical information is available through many sources, including professional literature; state and city health departments; vital statistics sections of private, county, state, and federal agencies; special programs or agencies (family-planning and similar agencies); and demographic profiles of specific geographic areas. Most of these sources are accessible via the Internet. Nurses who use this information will be better prepared to promote the health needs of maternal-newborn clients and their families.

Evidence-Based Practice in Maternal-Child Nursing

Evidence-based practice—that is, nursing care in which all interventions are supported by current, valid research evidence—is emerging as a force in healthcare. It provides a useful approach to problem solving/decision making and to self-directed, client-centered, lifelong learning. Evidence-based practice builds on the actions necessary to transform research findings into clinical practice by also considering other forms of evidence that can be useful in making clinical practice decisions (Goode & Piedalue, 1999). These other forms of evidence may include, for example, statistical data, quality improvement measurements, risk management measures, and information from support services such as infection control.

As practicing clinicians, nurses need to meet two basic competencies related to evidence-based practice. Specifically, nurses need to

1. Recognize which clinical practices are supported by good evidence, which practices have conflicting findings as to their effect on client outcomes, and which practices have no evidence to support their use.
2. Use data in their clinical work.

Rote memorizing and practicing from habit and opinion are passé, part of the industrial age. Unfortunately, some agencies and clinical units where nurses practice still operate in the old style, which often generates conflict for nurses who recognize the need for more responsible clinical practice. In truth, market pressures are forcing nurses and other healthcare providers to evaluate routines in order to improve efficiencies and provide better outcomes for clients.

Nurses need to know what data are being tracked where they work and how care practices and outcomes are improved as a result of quality improvement initiatives. However, there is more to evidence-based practice than simply knowing what is being tracked and how the results are being used. Competent, effective nurses learn to question the very basis of their clinical work.

Throughout this text we have provided *snapshots* of evidence-based practice related to childbearing women, children, and families such as the one on page 86. We believe that these snapshots will help you understand the concept more clearly. We also expect that these examples may challenge you to question the usefulness of some of the routine care you observe in clinical practice. That is the impact of evidence-based practice—it moves clinicians beyond practices of habit and opinion to practices based on reliable, valid, current science.

Nursing Research

Research is vital to expanding the science of nursing, fostering evidence-based practice, and improving client care. Research also plays an important role in advancing the profession of nursing. For example, nursing research can help determine the psychosocial and physical risks and benefits of both nursing and medical interventions.

The gap between research and practice is being narrowed by the publication of research findings in popular nursing journals, the establishment of departments of nursing research in hospitals, and collaborative research efforts by nurse researchers and clinical practitioners. Interdisciplinary research between nurses and other healthcare professionals is also becoming more common. This ever-increasing recognition of the value of nursing research is important because well-done research supports the goals of evidence-based practice. Most chapters of this text, therefore, include Research in Practice boxes such as the one shown here.

RESEARCH IN PRACTICE
Ethical Decision-Making Regarding Terminating a Pregnancy

What is this study about? Prenatal diagnosis has resulted in the early detection of fetal abnormalities, but an identified abnormality creates the dilemma of decision making about selective termination of the pregnancy. These diagnoses are often unavailable until after the 14th week of pregnancy, when curettage is no longer possible as a method of termination and induction of labor becomes necessary. This procedure may fall within the responsibility of a midwife, and may result in ethical conflicts for the care provider. The purpose of this study was to investigate how midwives view the termination of pregnancy due to a fetal abnormality and to clarify ethical issues related to this situation.

How was this study done? Thirteen midwives participated in this qualitative study. All of the subjects were working in the delivery unit of a university clinic. Data were collected by interviews, which lasted between 40 and 90 minutes. The interviews were transcribed and evaluated using content analysis.

What were the results of the study? The midwives universally described a heavy emotional burden in the situation of abnormality-related termination of pregnancy. They reported feelings of sadness, anger, helplessness, and contradictory feelings. A strong sense of uneasiness about their role identity—essentially a shift from midwife to abortionist—was reported. They were particularly disturbed about being confronted with a situation that they could not change. On the other hand, most of the midwives described the procedure itself as part of their professional duties and scope of competencies. All of these midwives chose to support the principle of the woman's right to self-determination. They did, however, express their uneasiness about the termination as a loss of life. There was universal agreement that this procedure was among the most emotionally stressful activities for them in their professional capacity.

What additional questions might I have? Would the midwives feel differently if they helped parents in the decision-making process prior to the termination? Did these midwives feel that their internal conflicts affected their care processes? If so, in what way?

How can I use this study? Nurses are often in situations that create ethical conflicts for them. Determining a personal decision-making framework can help nurses reconcile their professional identity in the face of ethical conflicts.

Source: Cignacco, E. (2002). Between professional duty and ethical confusion: Midwives and selective termination of pregnancy. *Nursing Ethics, 9*(2), 179–192.

Clinical Pathways

One result of nursing research into the nursing process has been the creation of clinical pathways. *Clinical pathways* specify essential nursing activities and provide basic guidelines about expected outcomes at specified time intervals. These guidelines are research based and enable the nurse to determine whether a client's responses meet expected norms at any given time. In the text, we have provided sample clinical pathways for a woman experiencing a normal vaginal birth and a cesarean birth. We have also provided sample clinical pathways for the normal newborn, for a woman in the postpartal period, and for women or newborns with selected conditions or problems.

Evidence-Based Practice: An Example

In using evidence-based practice, nurses draw on a variety of tools such as statistical data, nursing research and other research, standards of care, statistics, and critical analysis skills. These tools can exist separately, but in practice they overlap and build upon each other. An example of just one possible situation is presented in the following case study.

> Two birthing unit nurses express concerns to each other about the seemingly high number of adolescents who have been giving birth in their unit. At the next staff meeting, they voice their concerns and raise questions about whether the number of teenage mothers seen in their unit is higher than normal. After the discussion, the nurses decide they need to formulate a plan to gather more information. Each nurse volunteers to pursue a particular aspect of the plan of action. Their plan includes contacting the local public health department for local and national statistics on this age group; looking at the availability of healthcare for adolescents in their community; investigating the particular health problems of pregnant teenagers and risks to their infants; checking the availability of prenatal education groups for adolescents; finding out whether their community has school health programs and what the program content is; looking at national statistics identifying when adolescents seek prenatal care; talking with local certified nurse-midwives, physicians, and prenatal clinic personnel to see if the national statistics apply to their community; collecting information about current legislative issues affecting adolescent healthcare; seeking further information about the needs of adolescents during pregnancy and birth by doing a library search; and looking for continuing education programs dealing with the pregnant adolescent client.
>
> At subsequent staff meetings, nurses share information and investigate other areas as the need is identified. How they evaluate the data and apply them will depend on the requirements of their maternal-newborn unit and the unique needs of their community. Possible outcomes may include developing a research study, volunteering in local adolescent clinics, developing and teaching prenatal classes for adolescents, volunteering to teach in community school health programs, organizing a continuing education program on the adolescent mother for community hospitals, and forming a network within their professional nursing organization to stay informed about legislative issues pertaining to adolescents.

As the example illustrates, the application of tools of evidence-based practice assists the nurse in analyzing data and planning a course of action.

Chapter Review

EXPLOREMediaLink

NCLEX review questions, case studies, and other interactive resources for this chapter can be found on the Web site at http://www.prenhall.com/olds. Click on "Chapter 1" to select the activities for this chapter.

For tutorials including animations and videos, more NCLEX review questions, and an audio glossary, access the accompanying CD-ROM in this book.

Focus Your Study

- Many nurses working with childbearing families are expert practitioners who are able to serve as role models for nurses who have not yet attained the same level of competence.
- Contemporary childbirth is family centered, offers choices about birth, and recognizes the needs of siblings and other family members.
- The self-care movement, which emerged in the late 1960s, emphasizes personal health goals, a holistic approach, and preventive care.
- The US healthcare system is facing a variety of challenges including the high cost of healthcare and the need for cost containment while retaining quality; the large numbers of uninsured and underinsured people; high infant mortality rates as compared to other industrialized nations; and a high incidence of poverty, especially among children and women-headed households.
- The nurse who provides culturally competent care recognizes the importance of the childbearing family's value system, acknowledges that differences occur among people, and seeks to respect and respond to ethnic diversity in a way that leads to mutually desirable outcomes.
- A nurse must practice within the scope of practice or be open to the accusation of practicing medicine without a license. The standard of care against which individual nursing practice is compared is that of a reasonably prudent nurse.
- Nursing standards provide information and guidelines for nurses in their own practice, in developing policies and protocols in healthcare settings, and in directing the development of quality nursing care.
- Informed consent—based on knowledge of a procedure and its benefits, risks, and alternatives—must be secured prior to providing treatment.
- State constitutions, statutes, and common law protect the right to privacy.
- Maternal-fetal conflict may arise when the fetus is viewed as a person of equal rights to those of the mother's and external agents attempt to force the mother to accept a therapy she wishes to refuse, or similarly attempt to restrict a mother's actions to support the well-being of the fetus.
- Abortion can be performed until the age of viability. Caregivers have the right to refuse to perform an abortion or assist with the procedure.
- A variety of procedures are available to help infertile couples achieve a pregnancy. However, some of these procedures provoke serious ethical dilemmas.
- Embryonic stem cell research using human stem cells obtained from a human embryo is marked by controversy. On the one hand, it raises the possibility of treatment for a variety of major diseases such as diabetes, Parkinson disease, and Alzheimer disease. On the other hand, ethicists question the ethical implications of using embryonic tissue—especially tissue obtained specifically for stem cell research.
- Cord blood banking provides the opportunity to make stem cells available to treat a variety of cancers and blood system disorders. Its growing popularity has revealed several ethical issues, such as: Who owns the blood? How will informed consent be obtained and by whom? How will confidentiality be ensured? How can the harvested blood be distributed fairly, so that it is available to individuals from all races, ethnic groups, and income levels? And so forth.
- Descriptive statistics describe or summarize a set of data. Inferential statistics allow the investigator to draw conclusions about what is happening between two or more variables in a population.

- Evidence-based practice—that is, nursing care in which all interventions are supported by current, valid research evidence—is emerging as a positive force in healthcare.
- Nursing research plays a vital role in adding to the nursing knowledge base, expanding clinical practice, and expanding nursing theory.

References

American Academy of Pediatrics, Committee on Bioethics. (1999). Fetal therapy—Ethical considerations (RE9817). *Pediatrics, 103*(5), 1061–1063.

American Association for the Advancement of Science. (2002). *Stem cell research.* (Policy Brief). Washington, DC: Author.

American College of Nurse-Midwives. (2002). *Program types.* Retrieved August 19, 2002, from http://www.midwife.org

American College of Obstetricians and Gynecologists. (2001). *Joint statement of practice relationships between obstetrician-gynecologists and certified nurse-midwives/certified midwives* (ACOG Statement of Policy). Washington, DC: Author.

American College of Obstetricians and Gynecologists. (2001, February 28). *ACOG calls fetal surgery experimental.* ACOG press release retrieved April 27, 2002, from http://www.acog.com/from_home/publications/press_releases/nr02-28-01-1.html

American College of Obstetricians and Gynecologists. (2002). *Nonselective embryo reduction: Ethical guidance for the obstetrician-gynecologist* (Committee Opinion). Washington, DC: Author.

American College of Obstetricians and Gynecologists, Committee on Ethics. (1999). *Patient choice and the maternal-fetal relationship* (Opinion No. 214). Washington, DC: Author.

American Nurses Association. (2002). Nursing profession unveils strategic plan to ensure safe, quality patient care and address root causes of growing shortage. Press release, April 4, 2002. Retrieved October 3, 2002 from http://nursingworld.org/pressrel/2002/pr0404.htm

Ault, A. (2003). Completion of human genome first step toward comprehensive genetic medicine. Retrieved May 8, 2003 from www.mcdscape.com/viewarticle/452355?mpid=12569 & Weblogicsession=PrcMy8.

Benner, P. (1984). *From novice to expert.* Menlo Park, CA: Addison-Wesley.

Centers for Disease Control and Prevention. (2001). *1999 assisted reproductive technology success rates.* Retrieved July 16, 2002 from http://www.cdc.gov/needphp/drh/ART99

Crooks, G. M., Lill, M., Feig, S., & Parkman, R. (1997). Cord blood—new source of stem cells for transplants. *Contemporary OB/GYN, 42*(8), 114–126.

Dalaker, J. (2001). *Poverty in the United States: 2000* (US Census Bureau, Current Population Reports, Series P60-214). Washington, DC: US Government Printing Office.

Davidson, M. R. (2002). Outcomes of high-risk women cared for by nurse-midwives. *Journal of Midwifery and Women's Health, 47*(1), 46–49.

Department of Commerce. (1997). Vital statistics. In *Statistical abstract of the United States, 1997* (117th ed., pp. 70–108). Washington, DC: Author.

Dickey, S. B., & Deatrick, J. (2000). Autonomy and decision making for health promotion in adolescence. *Pediatric Nursing, 26*(5), 461–467.

Dower, C. N., & Miller, J. E. (1999). *Taskforce on midwifery. Charting a course for the 21st century: The future of midwifery.* San Francisco: Pew Health Professions Commission and the University of California–San Francisco Center for the Health Professions.

Fetal surgery: Past, present, and future work in this frontier [Symposium; Special issue]. (1994, April 15). *Contemporary OB/GYN, 39*(S), 59–66.

Goode, C., & Piedalue, F. (1999). Evidence-based clinical practice. *Journal of Nursing Administration, 29,* 15–21.

Gorman, C. (1994, August). Brave new embryos. *Time, 144*(9), 60–61.

Hagedorn, M. I. E., Gardner, S. L., Laux, M. G., & Gardner, G. L. (1997). A model for professional nursing practice. In S. L. Gardner & M. I. E. Hagedorn (Eds.), *Legal aspects of maternal-child nursing practice* (pp. 67–94). Menlo Park, CA: Addison Wesley Longman.

Hornstra, D. (1999). A realistic approach to maternal-fetal conflict. *Neonatal Intensive Care, 12*(2), 24–31.

Macklin, R., & White, G. B. (1997). Assisted reproductive technologies, ads, and ethics: Philosophical, ethical, and clinical perspectives on the use of advertising in reproductive medicine. A conference held by the National Advisory Board on Ethics in Reproduction [Executive summary]. *Women's Health Issues,* 7(3), 127–131.

Madrick, J. (2002, June 13). A rise in child poverty rates is at risk in U.S. *The New York Times,* Retrieved June 18, 2002 from www.nytimes.com

Mahowald, M. B. (1997). An overview of the Human Genome Project and its implications for women. *Women's Health Issues,* 7(4), 206–208.

Martin, J. A., Park, M. M., & Sutton, P. D. (2002). Births: Preliminary data for 2001. *National Vital Statistics Report, 50*(10), 1–20.

Mathews, T. J., Menacker, F., & MacDorman, M.F. (2002). Infant mortality statistics for the 2000 period. Linked birth/infant death data set. *National Vital Statistics Report, 50*(12), 1–27.

Melnyk, B. M., Fineout-Overholt, E., Stone, P., & Ackerman, M. (2000). Evidence-based practice: The past, the present, and recommendations for the millennium. *Pediatric Nursing, 26*(1), 77–80.

Moores, P. (1997). Empowering women in the practice setting. In S. L. Gardner & M. I. E. Hagedorn (Eds.), *Legal aspects of maternal-child nursing practice* (pp. 9–23). Menlo Park, CA: Addison Wesley Longman.

National Center for Human Genome Research. (2001). *U.S. human genome project 5-year research goals 1998–2003.* Retrieved October 7, 2002 from http://www.ornl.gov/TechResources/Human_Genome/home.html

Pastor, P. N., Makuc, D. M., Reuben, C., & Xia, H. (2002). *Health, United States, 2002.* Hyattsville, MD: National Center for Health Statistics with chartbook on trend in the health of Americans.

Peters, K. D., Kochanek, K. D., & Murphy, S. L. (1998, November 10). Deaths: Final data for 1996. *National Vital Statistics Reports, 47*(9), 1–82.

Plotnick, J., & Presler, B. (1996). Rugged individualism and compassion: The foundation of public policy. *American Journal of Maternal Child Nursing, 21*(1), 20–33.

Rittley, D., & Porter, J. (2001). Exploring advanced directives in the OB setting. *AWHONN Lifelines, 5*(5), 10–12.

Roche, P. A., & Grodin, M. A. (2000). The ethical challenge of stem cell research. *Women's Health Issues, 10*(3), 136–139.

Ryan, K. J. (2000). The politics and ethics of human embryo and stem cell research. *Women's Health Issues, 10*(3), 105–110.

Sackett, D., Richardson, W., Rosenberg, W., & Haynes, R. B. (1997). *Evidence based medicine: How to practice and teach EBM.* New York: Churchill-Livingstone.

Simpson, K. R., & Knox, G. E. (2001). Perinatal teamwork: Turning rhetoric into reality. *AWHONN Lifelines, 5*(5), 56–59.

Sinclair, B. P. (1997). Advanced practice nurses in integrated healthcare systems. *Journal of Obstetric, Gynecologic, & Neonatal Nursing, 26*(2), 217–223.

Smith, F. O., & Thomson, B. G. (2000). Umbilical cord blood collection, banking, and transplantation: Current status and issues relevant to perinatal caregivers. *Birth,* 27(2), 127–135.

Thorpe, K. (2001). *The distribution of health insurance coverage among pregnant women, 1999.* White Plains, NY: March of Dimes.

Thorp, J. M., Jr., Bowes, W. A., & Cefalo, R. C. (1997). Medical and legal considerations of court-ordered OB intervention. *Contemporary Obstetrics and Gynecology, 42*(6), 41–48.

US Census Bureau (2001). Population estimates for children by age and race. Population Estimates Program, Population Division. Washington, DC: Author.

US Census Bureau. (2002). *Health insurance in America: Numbers of Americans with and without health insurance rise, Census Bureau reports.* Press release retrieved October 21, 2002, from http://www.census.gov/Press-Release/www/2002/cb02-127.html

Ventura, S. J., Martin, J. A., Curtin, S. C., & Mathews, T. J. (1998, June 30). Report of final natality statistics, 1996. *Monthly Vital Statistics Report, 46*(11S), 1–99.

Weisman, C. S. (1996). Proceedings of women's health and managed care: Balancing cost, access, and quality [Meeting report]. *Women's Health Issues, 6*(1), 1–38.

Care of the Family in a Culturally Diverse Society

2

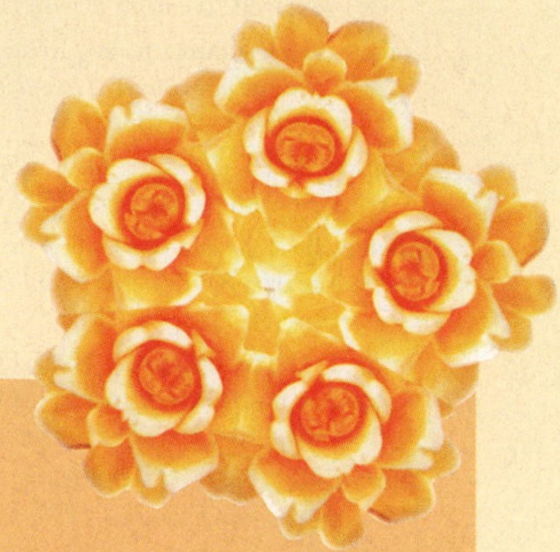

I can't imagine going through pregnancy, birth or those initial few weeks after my daughter was born without my family. My brother called regularly throughout my pregnancy to check on me. Dad gave me pep talks on eating right and taking care of myself. My husband and my mom were both with me during my labor and my unexpected cesarean birth. After Rosario was born, my husband accompanied our new daughter to the nursery and mom stayed with me, talking and holding my hand. What a difference a family can make.

Objectives

- Explore factors that influence the values, decision making, and roles within the family unit.
- Summarize employment, marital, and economic trends affecting the contemporary family.
- Distinguish among several different types of families.
- Identify major developmental tasks to be completed by the childbearing family.
- Delineate the advantages of using a family assessment tool.
- Discuss the impact of culture in caring for the childbearing family.
- Identify prevalent cultural norms related to childbearing and childrearing.
- Summarize the importance of cultural competency in providing nursing care.
- Discuss the use of a cultural assessment tool as a means of providing culturally sensitive nursing care.
- Identify the key considerations in providing spiritually sensitive nursing care.

Key Terms

Acculturation 35
Assimilation 35
Cultural competency 40
Culture 35
Ethnicity 35
Ethnocentrism 40
Family 27
Family assessment 34
Family development 31
Family power 27
Family roles 27
Family values 27
Religion 43
Spirituality 43
Taboos 39

MEDIALINK

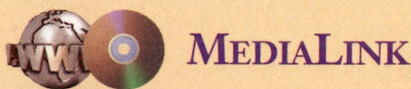

Additional resources for this content can be found on the Student CD-ROM and on the Companion Website at www.prenhall.com/olds. Click on "Chapter 2" to select the activities for this chapter.

CD-ROM
- Audio Glossary
- NCLEX Review

Companion Website
- Additional NCLEX Review
- Case Study: Family Assessment
- Care Plan Activity: Midcycle Pain in Perimenopausal Woman

Although a woman may arrive for her healthcare appointment physically alone, in another sense, she is always accompanied by her family. Her parents, partner, spouse, or in-laws may accompany her in the form of internalized messages about her body, contraception, sex, or childbearing, or in the form of their expectations for her behavior. In addition, her family's culture and religious beliefs will influence her healthcare practices, decisions, and needs. Thus, a nurse may provide expert teaching about condom use to an adolescent, but the teaching may not be put into practice because the client's partner objects. Or a nurse may encourage a pregnant client to increase her consumption of cow's milk, but a religious proscription against consuming animal products may prohibit this behavior. The goal of effective, holistic nursing care requires nurses to recognize that their clients' values, behaviors, decisions, and needs do not exist in a vacuum; instead, nurses must actively seek to learn about and care for the entire childbearing family.

In this chapter, we provide a perspective on the childbearing family in a culturally diverse society. We begin by discussing family values, power, and roles, as well as key social changes affecting the contemporary family. We then identify a variety of different family types the nurse is likely to encounter, and explore the developmental tasks of these varied families. Since families cannot be considered in isolation from their culture, we introduce several concepts essential to culturally competent nursing care. We close the chapter with a brief look at the influence of a family's religious beliefs on health outcomes, and identify key considerations in providing spiritually sensitive nursing care.

Defining Family

A number of definitions of families can be found in the literature. For example, a nurse researcher defines **family** as "two or more persons who are joined together by bonds of sharing and emotional closeness and who identify themselves as being part of a family" (Friedman, 1998, p. 9). The US Census Bureau defines *family* in more traditional terms as individuals joined together by marriage, blood, adoption, or residence in the same household.

Family Values

Families have values that guide their behavior and interactions within society and their own family units. In a classic study of families in crisis, **family values** are defined as a "system of ideas, attitudes, and beliefs about the worth of an entity or concept that consciously or unconsciously bind together the members of the family in a common culture" (Parad & Caplan, 1965, p. 55). These values are greatly influenced by external factors including cultural background, social norms, education, environmental influences, socioeconomic status, and beliefs held by peers, coworkers, political and community leaders, and other individuals outside of the family unit. Because of the influence of these external factors, a family's values may change significantly over the years.

Family Power and Decision Making

Within each family, there is an individual or group who possesses **family power;** that is, the potential or actual ability to change the behavior of other family members (Olson & Cromwell, 1975, p. 143). This individual or group may affect how a client responds to a healthcare provider, a diagnosis, treatments, or health teaching. Research has shown that many families make health-related decisions only with the aid of other family members. For example, in the Korean culture, in which elders are highly respected and play a key role in family matters, family power may rest with the grandfather. If the son wanted to make a health-related change in the family's diet, for example, he would first seek the advice and approval of his grandfather. Similarly, many Chinese identify themselves in relation to other members of the family and believe that personal independence is not as important. Thus, a Chinese client may avoid taking action regarding a health matter unless a family leader gives permission (Purnell & Paulanka, 1998).

In many traditional families, the father figure is the decision maker. In traditional Cuban culture, for example, the father may be aggressive and dominant and is critical to all family decisions (Purnell & Paulanka, 1998). In contrast, the mother typically remains at home, passive and dependent. However, Cubans in the United States have become much more egalitarian because women are usually the first ones able to find jobs and contribute to their families (Purnell & Paulanka, 1998). Thus, among Cubans who have assimilated, one may find equal decision-making power.

Filipino families also consider the father to be the major decision maker in most cases. However, the mother has an equal say with the father about issues of health, welfare, and money (Purnell & Paulanka, 1998).

In many immigrant families, the child is first to learn the new language and may be used as an interpreter in healthcare settings. In families in which the father is considered the power holder, this situation can cause problems if the family perceives that the healthcare provider is relating only to the child. They may feel that their child is being placed in a superior position, which may be unacceptable to them (Murray & Zentner, 2001).

Family Roles

Family roles are "homogeneous sets of behaviors that are normatively defined and expected of an occupant of a given social position. Roles are based on role expectations or prescriptions defining what individuals in a particular situation should do in order to meet their own or another's expectations of them" (Nye & Gecas, 1976, p. 7).

Roles vary depending on age, position within the family, conflict within the family, stressors, cultural backgrounds, health status of family members, and demographic trends. However, within each family, roles commonly encountered include breadwinner, homemaker, nurturer, social planner, and peacemaker. Although roles are sometimes perceived to be gender specific, they are more accurately assigned to the family member who performs that specific function. In the majority of US households in the 1950s, a male was the sole breadwinner and a female performed all homemaker functions. In contemporary society, these roles are often shared. For example, both parents may be employed and may participate equally in the care of the children. Segregated roles are more evident in certain cultures where roles are defined more sharply based on gender.

Any one individual within a family may have two or more roles. In nuclear families, roles are typically paired and consist of father-husband, wife-mother, son-brother, and so forth. In extended families the number of paired roles increases, whereas in single-parent families the numbers are less.

Increasingly important in the contemporary US family is the role of the grandparent. High adolescent pregnancy rates have created a sizable population of young grandparents (as young as the 30s), and increased life expectancy rates have created a sizable population of great-grandparents. Grandparents vary in how they express their role. Role functions may include: (1) witness who is simply present for the grandchildren, (2) protector who provides care and ensures safety when needed, (3) peacemaker who helps resolve conflicts between parents and children, and (4) active participant who maintains involvement in family life in the past, present, and future.

Grandparents can offer a great deal to children and provide substantial support and advice to parents (Figure 2–1 •). Often grandparents are able to spend more quality time with grandchildren than they did with their own children. Many grandparents are retired and use this opportunity to build lasting bonds with grandchildren. Although extended families are often geographically separated, many grandparents have identified alternative means to stay connected with grandchildren when frequent visits are not possible. These alternatives include phone calls, e-mails, and letters, as well as sharing journals, photos, and videotapes.

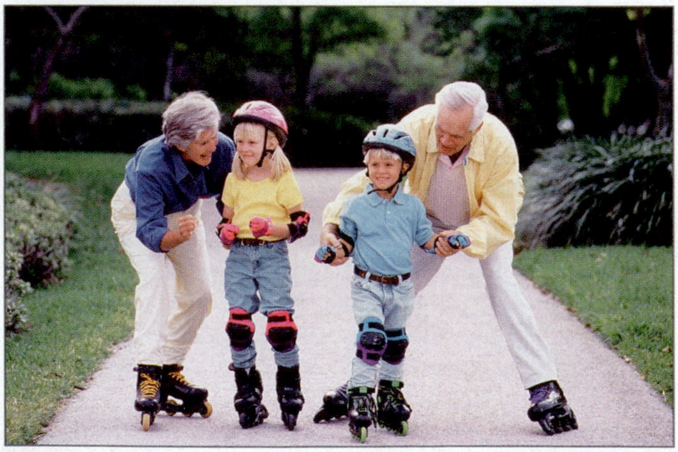

Figure 2–1 • Grandparents can offer nurturing and guidance to their grandchildren, not to mention lots of fun.
SOURCE: Paul Barton/CORBIS.

> *I call my grandchildren every day! I know what they did in school, what sports and hobbies they are involved in, and what special moments have occurred throughout their day. My grandchildren also take turns visiting me, one at a time. They know whose turn is next and what special things they will get to do at "Mimi's" house. My grandson knows he will get to go for ice cream, stay up late watching television, and eat popcorn in bed. My granddaughter knows that we will go to her favorite playground and stomp through the woods in back of the house, looking for "treasures." And of course I send them lots of cards, and they send me photographs and drawings they have made. I'm having lots of fun being a long-distance granny!*

Changes Affecting the Contemporary Family

The contemporary family has changed dramatically from the family unit of the 1950s, which typically consisted of a working father and a stay-at-home mother who cared for the children and ran the family home (Figure 2–2 •). Today, this model makes up only 7% of all US households (US Census Bureau, 1999). Affecting the contemporary family are employment trends, changes in marriage rates, and economic trends.

EMPLOYMENT TRENDS

Employment trends have changed with the shift from a male-dominated workforce to a mixed male-female workforce. In 1999, 25% of women earned more than their spouses (Fullerton, 1999a). Today, the majority of households consist of dual-earner families in which both the mother and father have employment outside of the home. Dual-earner families may have different needs than traditional families. For example, when a child becomes ill in a dual-earner family, the parents

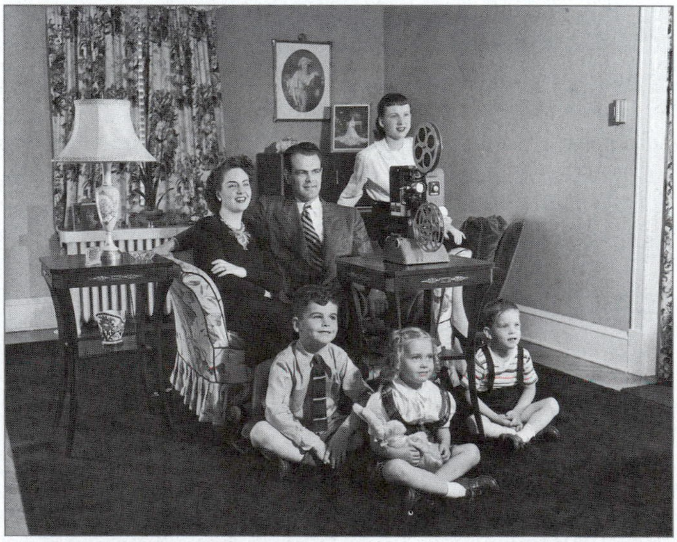

Figure 2–2 • The traditional family of the mid-20th century consisted of a father who worked outside of the home, a mother who performed all homemaking and childrearing functions, and one or more children.
SOURCE: Getty Images, Inc.–Hulton Archive Photos.

must decide who will take off work to care for the child. In traditional families, the mother would care for the child and work stresses from illness-related absences would not be a concern.

CHANGES IN MARRIAGE RATES

Since World War II, there has been a consistent decline in marriage rates. As recently as 1970, nearly 90% of white children were being raised in a two-parent household. By 1998, this number had dropped to 74%. Similar trends occurred in Hispanic families with a decline from 78% to 64%. African American children have historically had the lowest numbers of two-parent households. In 1970, 60% of African American children lived in a two-parent household; this number fell to 36% by 1998 (Teachman & Paasch, 1999b).

Along with the high proportion of single-parent families, there is also a higher proportion of never-married individuals in the United States than ever before, and those who do marry tend to do so at a later age than in the past. A combination of factors has led to delayed childbearing (see Chapter 8). There is also a growing trend for women to remain childless. In 1980, 10% of women ages 40 to 44 were childless compared to 19% in 1998 (US Census Bureau, 1999b). American women spend fewer childbearing years in marriage, which increases the likelihood of nonmarital childbearing.

Other trends in the United States include increasing acceptance of single women giving birth. In 1950, 3% of births were to unmarried women. Today, approximately one third of births are to unmarried women (Teachman, 2000). While this trend is increasing in the United States, in some cultures, an unmarried woman giving birth is viewed negatively. We discuss cultural views on birth outside of marriage later in this chapter.

ECONOMIC TRENDS

Changes in income levels have directly affected families. The household income of most American families increased by over 17% between 1970 and 1997. Families that experienced the most economic growth had two wage earners and higher educational preparation. More recently, the terrorist attacks of September 11, 2001, continued revelations of corporate wrongdoing, and the threat of global conflict have led to a downturn in the stock market and a rise in unemployment. The 2001 annual census revealed a downturn in median family income that may negatively impact the health and well-being of American families.

Types of Families

Various types of families—both traditional and nontraditional—exist in contemporary society.

Nuclear Family

The *nuclear family* consists of a husband provider, a wife who stays home, and children (see Figure 2–2). Although the nuclear family was once the norm in the United States, it is no longer the most common type of family.

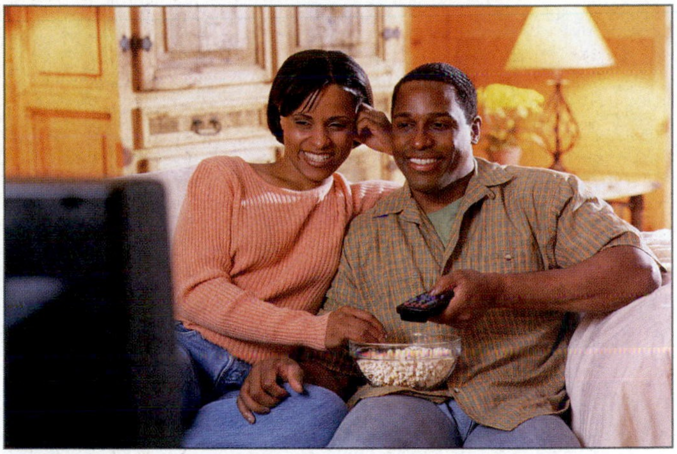

Figure 2–3 • Today, 5% of married couples voluntarily choose to remain childless.
SOURCE: Michael Keller/CORBIS.

Dual-Career/Dual-Earner Family

The *dual-career/dual-earner family* is now considered the norm in modern society. Today, two thirds of all two-parent families have both parents working. While many women work outside the home because of financial necessity, other women work either full- or part-time out of personal choice. Dual-career/dual-earner families have specific challenges. Because both parents are working, child care, household chores, and spending time with other family members are priorities that need to be addressed.

Childless Family

A growing trend exists for couples to remain childless (Figure 2–3 •). While as many as 10% of couples experience infertility problems, 5% of married couples are voluntarily without children. This trend is continuing to grow with the increased opportunities available to women in the workplace, delayed marriage, and wider acceptance of women choosing not to become mothers.

Extended Family

Extended families consist of a couple who shares household responsibilities, chores, and expenses with parents, siblings, or other relatives. Multigenerational family living arrangements are more common in non-US cultures and in working-class families. Children are reared by parents and other relatives. Extended families are also common when an elderly or ill relative requires care by the younger family members.

Extended Kin Network Family

An *extended kin network family* is a specific form of an extended family in which two nuclear families of primary or unmarried kin live in close proximity to each other. The family shares a social support network, chores, goods, and services. This type of family model is common in the Latino community (Figure 2–4 •).

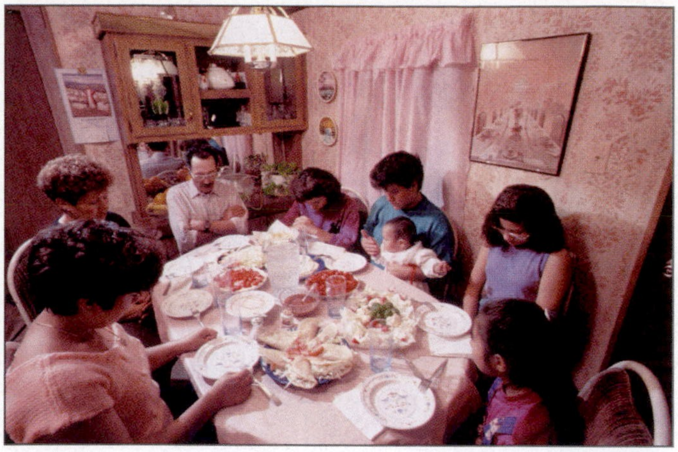

Figure 2–4 • In an extended kin network family, two nuclear families live in close proximity to each other and share responsibilities and resources.
SOURCE: Getty Images, Inc.

Single-Parent Family

Single-parent families are headed by only one parent (Figure 2–5 •). Although rare in the past, by the year 2000 there were 12 million such families in the United States, almost one third of all families. Since 1970 there has been a 14% increase in single-mother families and a 4% increase in single-father families.

In the traditional single-parent family the head of the household is widowed, divorced, abandoned, or separated. In the nontraditional single-parent family the head of the household, most often the mother, was never married. Single-parent families often face difficulties because the sole parent may lack social and emotional support, need assistance with childrearing issues, and face financial strain. Mothers who have never married tend to have more financial difficulties than those who are divorced (Fields & Casper, 2001).

Stepparent Family

With divorce rates exceeding 50% and rates of remarriage for women at 72%, *stepfamilies* have become increasingly common (Friedman, 1998). Stepfamilies include a biologic parent with children, and a new spouse who may or may not have children. These families are also known as *remarried families*, *reconstituted families*, or *blended families*. It is estimated that 75% of all divorced individuals eventually remarry. Sixty-five percent of these remarriages involve children from a prior marriage. (Stepfamily Association of America, 2000).

Stepfamily models have both strengths and weaknesses. Although marriage is often a new opportunity for success in a marital relationship for the parents, the relationship between stepparents and stepchildren can be strained. Stresses can include discipline issues, adjustment problems, role ambiguity, strain with the other biologic parent, and communication issues. While stepfamilies may have fewer financial issues and may actually offer the child a new support person and role model, open communication is imperative to ensure a smooth transition.

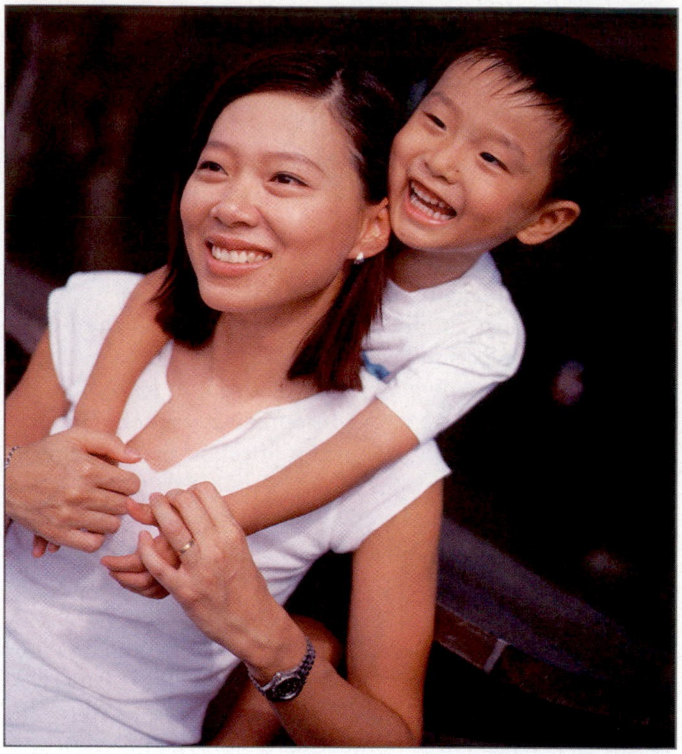

Figure 2–5 • Single-parent families account for nearly one third of all US families.
SOURCE: Joyce Choo/CORBIS.

Binuclear Family

A *binuclear family* is a postdivorced family in which the biologic children are members of two nuclear households, both that of the father and that of the mother. The children alternate between the two homes, typically spending a week with the father and a week with the mother. This is also called *co-parenting*, and involves joint custody. Legally, *joint custody* refers to situations in which both parents have equal responsibility and legal rights, regardless of where the children live. Although this type of family represents a small number as yet, there has been an increase in this type of household as fathers assume a more active role in parenting. The increased recognition of the importance of having both a maternal and paternal presence has encouraged more parents to actively raise their children together, regardless of their relationship with each other. The benefits of a binuclear family include the ability to have both the mother and father involved in the child's upbringing, a model for effective communication (in a successful family model), and additional support and role models from extended family members.

Nonmarital Heterosexual Cohabitating Family

A *nonmarital heterosexual cohabitating family* is a heterosexual couple who may or may not have children and live together

Clinical Tip *It is important to establish which parent has legal custody, current visitation policies, and other legal variables (restraining orders, supervised visitation, etc.) when communicating information to parents about their children. Certain legal issues may prohibit the nurse from sharing some information with the noncustodial parent.*

outside of marriage. This may include never-married individuals, as well as divorced or widowed persons. Unmarried cohabitating couples made up 3.7% of all US households in 2000. There are 3.8 million families classified as cohabitating, but it is estimated that this number is underreported (Fields & Casper, 2001).

While some individuals may choose this model for personal reasons, others may do so for financial reasons or to seek companionship. For example, a widow may fear losing her pension if she remarries, or an individual who owns significant assets may fear losing these assets to a spouse, especially if residing in a community-property state.

Gay and Lesbian Families

Gay and *lesbian families* include those in which two or more people who share a same-sex orientation live together (with or without children), as well as families consisting of a gay or lesbian single parent rearing a child (Figure 2–6 •). The number of gay and lesbian families is underreported. Although data are not collected on the census regarding this family status, the *Current Population Report* by the US Census Bureau estimates there are 1.6 families in this category. Of the families, 865,000 are male couples and 809,000 are female couples (US Census Bureau, 1998). Same-sex couples make up 3% of all couples, including married and cohabitating couples. The number of children who reside in gay or lesbian households is not known.

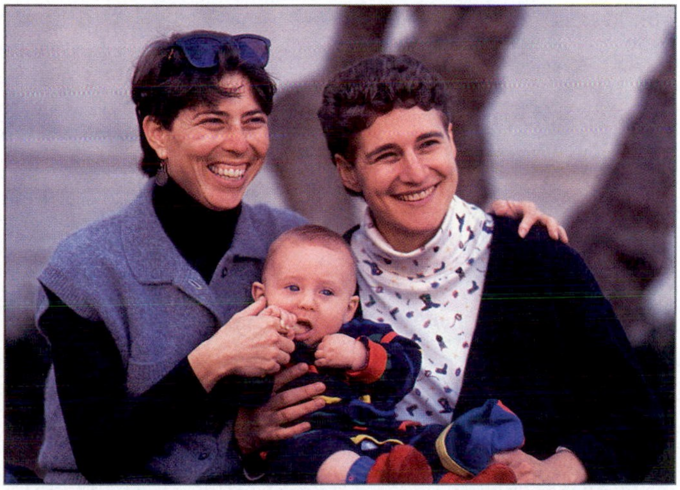

Figure 2–6 • Some gay and lesbian couples choose to adopt children in need of loving homes.
SOURCE: Dana White/PhotoEdit.

Small studies have evaluated children raised by gay and lesbian couples and have found that they show no significant differences from children raised in other types of families. These children get along with their parents and peers the same as children raised in heterosexual households. Children raised in gay or lesbian families may face unique issues in interacting with peers and in revealing their parents' sexual orientation. In cases where the biologic parents divorced or separated because of one parent's newfound sexual orientation, children may be particularly vulnerable during the adjustment phase (Wald, 1999).

Contemporary Family Development Frameworks

Family development refers to the dynamics or changes that families experience over time. It includes relationships, communication patterns, roles, and changes in interactions. Although each family is unique, the members must go through a set of fairly predictable changes. The amount of time in each stage and the duration between stages vary within each family unit.

Multiple family models and frameworks have been proposed over the years to facilitate an understanding of the complexities of family development. These developmental frameworks observe a family's progression over time by identifying specific stages in family life. Contemporary models, primarily based on the developmental framework by Duvall (1977), have embraced the trends and changes of contemporary society and family life. Duvall developed an eight-stage family life cycle that describes the developmental process that each family encounters. This model is based on a nuclear family (Table 2–1 •). The oldest child serves as a marker for the family's developmental stage except in the last two stages when the children are no longer present. Couples with more than one child may be in overlapping stages with developmental advances occurring simultaneously.

Model of the Childbearing Family

Multiple tasks exist for the childbearing family. The couple must first arrange the home to meet the needs of the newborn. This entails preparing for the infant by providing a safe environment, a safe clean place to sleep, and appropriate clothing and supplies.

At the time of birth of the first child, the childbearing family will engage in behaviors aimed at identifying responsibility and accountability for the newborn. Couples are rapidly faced with the realization that infants require 24-hour care. While fathers are taking a more active role in childrearing, the mother is frequently the primary care provider, especially if she is breastfeeding. Although a breast pump can be used and milk can be given by bottle, the breastfeeding mother still assumes the majority of the feeding responsibilities. The father may assume other household tasks or other baby care activities, such as changing, bathing, and

Table 2-1 • THE EIGHT-STAGE FAMILY LIFE CYCLE

Stage I	Beginning families	Marriage between partners, identification as partners, establishing goals for future, interaction and building relationships with kin.
Stage II	Childbearing families	Birth of first child, new role as parents, integrating new family member into existing family.
Stage III	Families with preschool children	Establishing family network, socialization of children, reinforcing independence in children when separating from parents.
Stage IV	Families with school-age children	Facilitating peer relationships while maintaining family dynamics, adjusting to outside influences.
Stage V	Families with teenagers	Increase in children's independence and autonomy; parents' concerns shift to aging parents, careers, and marital relationship.
Stage VI	Families launching young adults	Readjustment of marital relationship; parents and children establish separate identities outside the family unit.
Stage VII	Middle-aged parents	Renewed marital relationship, new outside interests, fewer family responsibilities, new roles as grandparents and as in-laws, increased concern for aging parents, death, and disability of older generation.
Stage VIII	Retirement and old age	End of career, shift to retirement, maintain functioning during the aging process, maintain marital relationship, adjust to potential loss of spouse, friends, and siblings, prepare for eventual death.

Source: Adapted from Duvall, Elizabeth M. *Marriage and Family Development,* 5th ed. Published by Allyn and Bacon, Boston, MA. Copyright © 1977 by Pearson Education. Adapted by permission of the publisher; and Friedman, M.M. (1998). *Family Nursing: Research, Theory, and Practice* (4th ed., p. 113). Reprinted by permission of Pearson Education, Upper Saddle River, NJ.

putting the infant down to sleep. During the early stages, new roles will be identified as couples strive to establish a daily routine that includes the new family member.

Another task of the childbearing family is reestablishing a satisfying sexual relationship. Nurses can play an active role in teaching couples about normal changes during this period of family life. For example, in the postpartum period, sexual activity typically declines or ceases. The parents are transitioning to new roles, especially the mother. Fatigue is common. Women may also feel discomfort due to the birth and may fear pain with resumption of sexual intercourse. Reduced desire and vaginal dryness due to low estrogen levels are especially common in breastfeeding women. Counseling can provide the couple with reassurance that these changes are a common part of this developmental stage.

Couples need to communicate effectively and share thoughts and feelings as they adjust to their new roles. Fathers may feel isolated or "left out" as the mother embraces her new role. New mothers may feel overwhelmed with the responsibility of caring for an infant when alone. Even dual-career families typically have a transition period in which the mother is at home caring for the newborn and the father is working. For some women who previously worked full-time, being at home may cause feelings of isolation.

"*I thought I would love being at home with my beautiful new son. It wasn't that I didn't love him and want to be with him, I just felt like I was losing part of myself. I wasn't me anymore, and I missed talking with other adults and working. I felt tremendously guilty when I returned to work at 3 months; however, it made my time with him so much more special and I regained my self-confidence and felt like a real person again.*"

As the new family adapts to their changing roles and responsibilities, the role of other family members also emerges. Some extended families take an active role, whereas others may be more passive. Family members frequently provide guidance, advice, and assistance with child care. Both sets of grandparents may have strong beliefs about childrearing and may attempt to promote their own beliefs and rituals. Couples must effectively communicate with each other and other family members to avoid conflict. Although both families may want their traditions followed in terms of childrearing, the couple may wish to develop new traditions and rituals within their own family unit.

Along with changes in family relationships, the childbearing family may also experience changes in personal relationships and outside activities. After the birth of an infant, couples are typically more involved with their home life, may stay home more often, and may engage in different activities. Many women, especially women who formerly worked outside of the home, may feel like they have less in common with previous coworkers or friends who do not have children. This may lead to new friendships with other families who have more in common with the new family unit.

"*Allie and I met in high school, and from then on, we were inseparable. Even after I got married, we stayed close, going out to lunch or shopping together every couple of weeks, and talking on the phone every few days. When she found out I was pregnant, she threw a surprise shower for me, but as my due date approached, we started to drift apart. Since my daughter's birth, we've gotten together just once. Allie says she feels excluded and that all I ever talk about is the baby. I guess she's right—my daughter is the center of my world now, so it's hard to talk about anything else. I haven't seen Allie for several months now. It makes me sad when I think about it.* ”

Childbearing families face multiple changes and challenges as they embark into new parenthood. The nurse can assist the childbearing family by providing teaching about family-planning issues, infant care and appropriate development, and safety concerns. The nurse can also offer guidance to the couple as they transition into parenthood by identifying interventions that can assist in meeting the emotional and physical needs of caring for a newborn. The nurse can provide support by actively listening as the couple expresses their feelings related to current role transition and changes in personal and family relationships. Resources can be provided to the new parents that will enable them to establish new relationships within their community.

Model Incorporating the Unattached Young Adult

Other models have been created to encompass the changes in contemporary families. For instance, Carter and McGoldrick (1989) modified the Duvall (1977) model to include the unattached young adult. This stage begins when the young adult leaves the family home and becomes financially independent, and lasts throughout young adulthood as long as the individual remains unmarried. Developmental tasks in this stage include differentiating self from the family unit, developing intimate peer relationships, and establishing a career and financial independence.

Since the median age at first marriage continues to rise, it is important to include the unattached young adult in family models. In 1970 the median age at first marriage was 23.2 years for men and 20.8 years for women. By 2000 the median age had increased to 26.8 and 25.1 years, respectively (Fields & Casper, 2001). Because of this increased age at first marriage, it is less common for adolescents to go directly from their parental home to a marital relationship. However, there is also a trend for young adults to reside with their parents well into their 20s. This is especially true for young men. In 2000, 56% (7.5 million) of men and 43% of women aged 18 to 24 lived at home with a parent or parents (Fields & Casper, 2001). It was fairly uncommon for young adults in the 18 to 24-year-old age group to live alone (4%).

Model Incorporating Divorce and Remarriage

Carter and McGoldrick (1989) devised another developmental model to describe issues encountered in undergoing divorce and in postdivorce (Table 2–2 •). Both emotional and developmental issues are encountered as families dissolve during the divorce process. Family members not only mourn the loss of a two-parent family, they also must adjust to a single-parent family model. Child visitation, financial issues, guilt, and attachment difficulties all play a major role in the changing family dynamics. Remarriage, which is becoming increasingly common, is another transitional stage in which family members must adjust to new roles and expectations (Table 2–3 •).

Table 2-2 • STAGES IN DIVORCE AND POSTDIVORCE

Stage	Issues
Divorce	
I. Decision to divorce	Accepting responsibility/part of responsibility for failed marriage.
II. Planning the breakup	Collaboratively working to resolve marital issues: financial, child care/custody. Communicating dissolution of marriage to relatives and friends.
III. Separation	Adapting to loss of previously established family unit, reorganizing relationships with spouse and children, restructuring finances, adapting to living apart, addressing issues related to attachment to spouse, maintaining bonds with extended family and spouse's extended family.
IV. Divorce	Grieving related to loss of prior family unit, accepting that the marriage is over, retrieving positive aspects of marriage (hopes, memories, dreams, expectations), overcoming negative feelings (anger, guilt, hurt, disappointment), maintaining relationships with extended family members.
Postdivorce	
I. Single parent (custodial)	Dealing with issues related to visitation and custody, rebuilding social relationships. Ensuring financial stability.
II. Single parent (noncustodial)	Continuing parenting role, identifying new means to relate to children, facilitating relationship between ex-spouse and children, providing support with childrearing decisions, providing financial support to ex-spouse for children, establishing new social relationships.

Source: From Betty Carter and Monica McGoldrick (Eds). *The Changing Family Life Cycle: A Framework for Family Therapy,* 2nd ed., p. 22. Published by Allyn and Bacon, Boston, MA. Copyright © 1989 by Pearson Education. Reprinted by permission of the publisher.

Model of the Lesbian or Gay Family

Lesbian or gay families face unique challenges in completing their developmental tasks. For example, they are frequently faced with discrimination and disapproval from mainstream society. For this reason, many gay or lesbian families opt to keep their sexual orientation a secret. In most states, they do not have the option of legal marriage and therefore do not have many of the benefits of marriage that heterosexual couples have such as insurance benefits, rights to property, custody issues, and family leave benefits associated with family illness or childbirth (Wald, 1999). Chapter 8 provides an overview of obstacles faced by lesbians.

Table 2-3 • STAGES IN REMARRIAGE

Stage	Issues
I. Establishing a new relationship	Resolve feelings from divorce, determine new marriage is desired, evaluate emotional readiness for new family, commit to new family.
II. Planning new marriage and family	Deal with personal fears and fears of new spouse and children, establish openness and open communication, determine financial obligations and coparenting roles with former spouses, plan for adjustment to new roles for parents and children, set new boundaries, resolve loyalty conflicts, maintain relationships with extended family members of ex-spouses, foster relationships between extended family and new spouse.
III. Remarriage and reconstitution of family	Include new spouse into family unit, dissolve previous attachment to former spouse and image of the "ideal family," restructure family system to include stepparent role, incorporate both families into a system to support children, foster all family relationships with extended family (including ex-spouses), share special memories to enhance family bonding and integration.

Source: Adapted from Betty Carter and Monica McGoldrick (Eds). *The Changing Family Life Cycle: A Framework for Family Therapy,* 2nd ed., p. 24. Published by Allyn and Bacon, Boston, MA. Copyright © 1989 by Pearson Education; and Friedman, M. (1992). Family Nursing: Theory and Practice (3rd ed., pp. 82–105). Norwalk, CT: Appleton & Lange.].

Slater (1995) developed a model specific to the stages of family life for lesbian and gay families (Table 2–4 •). The model identifies five stages in the development of the gay or lesbian family and addresses different issues and tasks in each stage.

Family Assessment

The nurse's understanding of the family structure helps provide insight into the family's support systems and needs. A **family assessment** is a collection of data regarding the family's current level of functioning, support systems, sociocultural information, environmental information, type of family, family structure, and needs.

In order to obtain an accurate and concise family assessment, the nurse needs to establish a trusting relationship with the woman and her family. Data is best collected in a comfortable, private environment, free from interruptions. The nurse can use therapeutic communication skills, such as active listening, reflection, and silence, to encourage the woman and family to verbalize information. Basic information should include

- Name, age, sex , and family relationship of all family members residing in the household.
- Cultural associations, including cultural norms and customs related to childbearing, childrearing, and infant feeding (discussed shortly).

Table 2-4 • LESBIAN AND GAY FAMILY STAGES

Stage	Issues
I. Formation of couple	Establish themselves as a couple versus individuals, combine two lives together, develop trust, reveal details about self, respond empathetically to partner to encourage further risk taking in relationship, tell others about their relationship.
II. Ongoing couplehood	Move from a physical passionate relationship to a stable relationship that includes passion and dailiness, manage differences between partners and handle conflict, increase sense of security and belonging as a couple.
III. Middle years	Progress into a long-term relationship with commitment, continue sense of security, make efforts to keep relationship fresh and new, rework rewards and disappointments.
IV. Generativity	Create a legacy beyond their own self-identity that will endure.

Source: Adapted with permission of The Free Press, a division of Simon & Schuster Adult Publishing Group, from *The Lesbian Family Life Cycle* by Suzanne Slater. Copyright © 1995; and Friedman, M.M. (1998). *Family Nursing: Research, Theory, and Practice* (4th ed., p. 143). Reprinted by permission of Pearson Education, Upper Saddle River, NJ.

- Religious affiliations, including specific religious beliefs and practices related to childbearing.
- Support network, including extended family, friends, and religious and community associations.
- Family type, structure, roles, and values.
- Communication patterns, including language barriers.

Health History

The health of individual family members can have a great impact on the health, well-being, and functioning of the family as a whole. The nurse should gather data about acute and chronic illnesses, genetic conditions, history of family violence, and mental health. A personal history beginning with pregnancies, pregnancy losses, infant health concerns, or deaths is also obtained. The nurse completes a comprehensive review of current health practices and health promotion behaviors to assess the family's ability to prevent accidents and chronic health conditions, and performs a brief nutritional assessment. Families with nutritional excesses or deficits are provided with nutritional education to reduce the risk of nutrition-related illnesses.

The health history should also assess current exercise and activity patterns, sleep patterns, occupational exposures, use of prescription and nonprescription drugs, alcohol consumption, smoking, and use of illegal drugs.

Environmental Considerations

A family's home environment can be assessed through home visits. Although not always possible, multiple home visits will yield more information than a single visit. A home visit enables the nurse to observe the family directly in their own environment and personal space. It also provides a more realistic view of family relationships, roles, parenting styles, and family needs. Often, the first visit serves as an introduction for the nurse to lay the foundation for a therapeutic relationship.

Observations should include the availability of personal space for all family members, including a place to sleep. The home should have basic necessities for daily living such as safe drinking water, a working waste-disposal system, electricity, and heat. The nurse can ensure that adequate cooking facilities, including a stove and refrigerator, are available for safe meal preparation. The availability of a phone is important so family members have access to healthcare providers and emergency services as needed.

The childbearing family should have resources available for the new baby including a safe place to sleep, appropriate clothing, blankets, hygienic equipment, and age-appropriate resources for other children.

The home should also be inspected for potential hazards. Childproofing the home is a topic generally covered during the home visit. A safe place to bathe the infant should be identified. Parents should be taught never to leave the infant unattended during bathing and never to leave the infant in a location where a fall can occur. Environmental hazards such as open stairs, uncovered electrical outlets, fragile items that could harm the infant or other children if the items were broken, and unattended electrical appliances need to be discussed. Many new childbearing families may not recognize the potential environmental dangers and will benefit from a brief review.

During the home visit, the nurse can also assess the neighborhood in which the family lives. Observations should include availability of resources (drug store, grocery store, closest medical facility, child care resources, and schools), characteristics of the neighborhood (safety issues, proximity of public transportation), and community resources (new mothers' groups, breastfeeding support groups, and availability of infant development/first aid classes).

Upon completion of the home visit(s), the nurse can make recommendations and identify community resources and sources of support for the new family. Families can also be counseled on the availability of social services, such as the Special Supplemental Food Program for Women, Infants, and Children (WIC), and financial support programs. Parents without health insurance coverage should be encouraged to apply for Medicaid coverage for their infant. Community health programs, such as local health department immunization clinics, should also be discussed.

Family Assessment Tool

Multiple tools are available to assist the nurse in collecting data regarding the family. The Friedman Family Assessment tool is a comprehensive assessment of family functioning and other essential family data (Figure 2–7 •). It can be used during the home visit to obtain pertinent information and provide a framework for the nurse when planning and implementing interventions for the family.

Cultural Influences Affecting the Family

When caring for families, it is critical to consider the influence of culture, which may affect how a family reacts and responds to health-related issues. Cultural beliefs that may seem strange to a person born and raised in Ohio might have significant meaning for an immigrant from West Africa. Developing knowledge about cultural beliefs and traditions can increase the nurse's appreciation of diversity, prevent violation of cultural norms, and most important, improve the family's healthcare experience.

Within the United States there is tremendous cultural diversity. The 2000 census reported that 12.5 % of Americans are Hispanic or Latino, 12.3% are of African descent, 3.6% are of Asian descent, and 0.9% are American Indian or Alaska Native. Thus it is important for nurses to have an understanding of how culture can influence family care.

Cultural Concepts

Culture can be defined as the beliefs, values, attitudes, and practices that are accepted by a population, a community, or an individual. Culture is learned and not ingrained in our genetic material, yet it can be passed on from generation to generation by means of *enculturation.* When a group is isolated, whether geographically or economically, culture is often reinforced.

Ethnicity is a social identity that is associated with shared behaviors and patterns. These include family structure, religious affiliation, language, dress, eating habits, and health behaviors. Many Americans define ethnicity by physical characteristics such as skin color. However, many individuals consider themselves "biracial" or identify themselves with a specific ethnic group not because of skin color but because of a shared ideology or attitude. Many Americans are blends of ethnic backgrounds and it is often difficult to assign a specific ethnic identity to someone (Murray & Zentner, 2001). Although some beliefs and cultural practices are common among certain ethnic groups, one must be careful to avoid stereotyping individuals. It is important not to assume that because individuals identify themselves as a specific ethnicity they must practice a certain custom.

Within the United States, cultures have in the past been forced to blend. When people from one culture are transported to another place with new cultural norms, many adapt to these new behaviors. This process by which people adapt to a new cultural norm is called **acculturation.** Moreover, when a group completely changes their cultural identity to become part of the majority culture, **assimilation** occurs.

MEDIALINK CASE STUDY: FAMILY ASSESSMENT

Acculturation

Many immigrants acculturate, and sometimes the acculturation process has an effect on the family's health. Acculturation is frequently associated with improved health status and health behaviors; however, this does not suggest that the

Meeting of Physical, Emotional, and Spiritual Needs of Members
- Ability to provide food and shelter
  - Space management as regards living, sleeping, recreation, privacy
  - Crowding if over 1.5 persons per room
  - Territoriality or control of each member over lifespace
  - Access to laundry, grocery, recreation facilities
  - Sanitation including disposal methods, source of water supply, control of rodents and insects
  - Storage and refrigeration
  - Available food supply
  - Food preparation, including preserving and cooking methods, (stove, hotplate, oven)
  - Use of food stamps and donated foods as well as eligibility for food stamps
  - Education of each member as to food composition, balanced menus, special preparations or diets if required for a specific member
- Access to health care
  - Regularity of health care
  - Continuity of caregivers
  - Closeness of facility and means of access such as car, bus, cab
  - Access to helpful neighbors
  - Access to phone
- Family health
  - Longevity
  - Major or chronic illnesses
  - Familial or hereditary illnesses such as rheumatic fever, gout, allergy, tuberculosis, renal disease, diabetes mellitus, cancer, emotional illness, epilepsy, migraine, other nervous disorders, hypertension, blood diseases, obesity, frequent accidents, drug intake, pica
  - Emotional or stress-related illnesses
  - Pollutants that members are chronically exposed to such as air, water, soil, noise, or chemicals that are unsafe
- Neighborhood pride and loyalty
- Job access, energy output, shift changes
- Sensitivity, warmth, understanding between family members
  - Demonstration of emotion
  - Enjoyment of sexual relations
    - Male: Impotence, premature or retarded ejaculation, hypersexuality
    - Female: Frigidity (inability to achieve orgasm), enjoyment of sexual relations, feelings of disgust, shame, self-devaluation; fear of injury, painful coitus
    - Menstrual history, including onset, duration, flow, missed periods and life situation at the time, pain, euphoria, depression, other difficulties
- Sharing of religious beliefs, values, doubts
  - Formal membership in church and organizations
  - Ethical framework and honesty
  - Adaptability, response to reality
  - Satisfaction with life
  - Self-esteem

Childrearing Practices and Discipline
- Mutual responsibility
  - Joint parenting
  - Mutual respect for decision making
  - Means of discipline and consistency
- Respect for individuality
- Fostering of self-discipline
- Attitudes toward education, reading, scholarly pursuit
- Attitudes toward imaginative play
- Attitudes toward involvement in sports
- Promotion of gender stereotypes

Communication
- Expression of a wide range of emotion and feeling
- Expression of ideas, concepts, beliefs, values, interests
- Openness
- Verbal expression and sensitive listening
- Consensual decision making

Support, Security, Encouragement
- Balance in activity
- Humor
- Dependency and dominance patterns
- Life support groups of each member
- Social relationship of couple: go out together or separately; change since marriage mutually satisfying; effect of sociability patterns on children

Growth-Producing Relationships and Experiences Within and Without the Family
- Creative play activities
- Planned growth experiences
- Focus of life and activity of each member
- Friendships

Responsible Community Relationships
- Organizations, including involvement, membership, active participation
- Knowledge of and friendship with neighbors

Growing with and Through Children
- Hope and plans for children
- Emulation of own parents and its influence on relationship with children
- Relationship patterns: authoritarian, patriarchal, matriarchal
- Necessity to relive (make up for) own childhood through children

Unity, Loyalty, and Cooperation
Positive interacting of members toward each other

Self-Help and Acceptance of Outside Help in Family Crisis

Figure 2–7 • The Family Assessment tool.
SOURCE: Murray, R. B. & Zentner, J. P. (2001). *Health promotion strategies through the lifespan* (7th ed.). Upper Saddle River, NJ: Prentice Hall, p. 200, Figure 4–2 Family Assessment Tool.

American lifestyle is somehow more healthful. Instead, it seems that many factors contribute to the improved health status of acculturated immigrants. Primary among these are socioeconomic factors. Many immigrants are financially better off in the United States than they were in their country of origin, particularly those who have immigrated from developing nations. Several studies have examined the impact that improved socioeconomic status has among immigrants and have revealed improved health. For example, children adopted from the former Soviet Union have better health and nutritional status than children who still live there. One study by Cousins et al (1992) showed that Mexican American women who were more acculturated were more likely to have regular Pap smear and mammogram screenings; however, the study also showed that this association did not occur when socioeconomic status was factored into the analysis. Other factors that are thought to improve the health of immigrants to the United States include improved medical care, nutrient dense foods, and overall improved environment.

Sometimes health declines with acculturation. For example, obesity is a problem that is growing rapidly within the United States and particularly among immigrant populations. Kalhan, Puthawala, Agarwal, et al (2001) found that South Asians who immigrate to the United States have a greater chance of developing central obesity as well as elevated cholesterol levels and insulin resistance. A study done by Cairney and Ostbye (1999) in Canada reported that the prevalence of excess weight increases with time since immigration in both men and women.

Some studies have also shown that there is very little difference in health status related to the level of acculturation within an ethnic group if strong traditional ties remain within a culture. Parsons, Goodson, Williams, et al (1999) compared the diets of children from first-generation and second-generation Pakistani immigrants and found no significant differences. The research suggested that there was such a strong cohesiveness within the Pakistani community that the level of acculturation regarding diet was minimal.

Impact of Culture on Family Structure

Traditional family structure within the United States usually consists of a nuclear family with an extended family living separately. However, many immigrants to the United States live together with and rely on a network of grandparents and even aunts, uncles, and cousins. For example, Cuban families are often multigenerational and consider grandmothers to be part of the nuclear family. Further, godparents (or *compadrazgos*) are often considered part of the family even if they are not related by blood (Purnell & Paulanka, 1998).

Many Islamic families from West Africa practice polygamy. Although they do not often freely admit this when in the United States, sometimes women live in households with their co-wives. Sometimes the co-wives work well together and get along, and in some cases they do not. Often children view each co-wife as their own mother.

Clinical Tip *When caring for a family in which grandparents play a key role in family decision making, the nurse should include the grandparents in the decision-making and teaching sessions, since their views are highly respected within the family unit.*

Research in Practice
Cultural Considerations in Planning Health Promotion Programs

What is this study about? Creating health promotion programs without considering cultural influences can lead to ineffective programs. This study was conducted to develop an understanding of the emotional context of adolescent pregnancy in a Latin-American country. The goal was to improve health promotion efforts aimed at the prevention of adolescent pregnancy.

How was this study done? This qualitative study was conducted in Colombia, South America. A purposive sample was solicited from antenatal clinics in and around Medellin, Columbia, and 21 adolescents ranging in age from 13 to 19 years consented to participate. The subjects were interviewed using an open-ended guide. The interviews lasted 30 to 60 minutes and were transcribed verbatim for analysis. Analysis was conducted concurrently with data collection and involved three stages: first, categories of meaning were named; second, the categories were linked analytically; and finally, the categories and their links were validated. The study design and analysis were based on symbolic interactionism, which emphasizes the importance of meaning in understanding social behavior.

What were the results of the study? This study found that the reasons Latin-American adolescents become sexually active and risk pregnancy are complex and emotional. These respondents placed their sexual behavior in the context of a genuine love affair, in which ideas of romantic love guided the girl's behavior. This experience of love was strongly influenced by gender identity, following their notions of the rules of feminine behavior. The girls used these gender rules as a resource to guide their interactions with their boyfriends. In this context, to engage in sexual activity was a key part of the task of being a "girlfriend." The context of sexual relations did not appear abruptly but emerged as the relationship matured. Often associated with a special moment–an anniversary or reunion after an absence–entering into a sexual relationship was not focused on reproduction but rather establishing intimacy. These events were seen as important but as natural events in the framework of the relationship. For these girls, sex was inextricably linked with their romantic view of the relationship. Since the boyfriend was seen as "the one," sexual relationships were legitimized. These girls did not fit the stereotypical view of the promiscuous teen who becomes pregnant, but rather a romantic youth who conforms to an idealized gender role.

What additional questions might I have? How do the boys feel about these ideas? This study focused exclusively on the adolescent girl. Understanding the cultural influences of the boy in the relationship might inform health promotion programs more effectively.

■ **How can I use this study?** In order to provide effective health promotion services, the nurse must take into account the cultural and contextual influences that guide behavior. Programs aimed at reducing the teen pregnancy rate in this culture must take into account these notions of romantic love and gender behavior if they are to be effective.

Source: De La Cuesta, C. (2001). Taking love seriously: The context of adolescent pregnancy in Columbia. *Journal of Transcultural Nursing, 12,* 180–192.

Cultural Influences on Childbearing and Childrearing

A family's culture may influence its beliefs about and practices surrounding many aspects of childbearing and childrearing, including beliefs about the importance of children, beliefs and attitudes about pregnancy, health practices, and infant feeding behaviors.

BELIEFS REGARDING THE IMPORTANCE OF CHILDREN

Children are generally valued all over the world, not only for the joy they bring, but also because they ensure continuation of the family and cultural values. This valuing of children may manifest in different ways, however. Families in the United States and many Western countries commonly only have one or two children, often out of a desire to provide the children with the best home and education they can afford, and to spend as much free time with them as possible. Many fear that additional children would too greatly dilute their financial and emotional resources. In contrast, in many cultures throughout the world, it is common to have as many children as possible. In Mali, West Africa, for example, the average woman has about seven children in her lifetime.

An understanding of the meaning of children in a culture may explain reactions of joy or shame to pregnancy. Pregnancy is a joyful event in a culture that values children. In some cultures, a woman who gives birth achieves higher status, especially if the newborn is male. The latter is especially true in traditional Chinese culture and some Middle Eastern cultures. Similarly, in the western United States, people of the Mormon faith view motherhood as the most important aspect of a woman's life, comparable with the male role of priesthood (Faust, 2000). In Mexican American society and among many other Hispanic groups, having children is evidence of the male's virility and is a sign of manliness, or *machismo,* a desired trait.

In cultures that value children only when they are born to a legally married couple, however, pregnancy is a shameful event if it occurs outside of marriage. In Ireland, for example, it is the norm to ignore the pregnancy of an unmarried woman throughout most of her gestation (Hyde, 1998). This behavior significantly increases the stress levels experienced by pregnant women who are not married. Pregnancy outside of marriage may even be dangerous. In many Muslim countries, an unmarried pregnant woman may seek a clandestine abortion because the consequences of carrying an illegitimate child can be social ostracism or even death—in some cases, even when the pregnancy has resulted from rape.

There are also many culturally influenced beliefs related to contraception. Many Muslims from the Middle East do not practice contraception because children are highly valued and it is believed that the traditional role of the woman is to bear children. Further, many Muslim clients will not seek prenatal care because of their feeling of fatalism, the idea that the future is in the hands of God, thus there is little need to prepare for the future.

In a culture in which children are highly valued, a woman's self-esteem may be related to her childbearing ability. In such cultures, women may even be made to feel that it is their fault if they are unable to bear children. Such women may go to great lengths to preserve their fertility. For example, Greek women may refuse gynecologic examinations because they fear that the exam will diminish their fertility (Purnell & Paulanka, 1998).

BELIEFS AND ATTITUDES ABOUT PREGNANCY

Beliefs and attitudes about pregnancy may also be culturally influenced, and may influence a woman's health behaviors. Thus certain health behaviors can be expected if a culture views pregnancy as a sickness, whereas other behaviors can be expected if pregnancy is viewed as a natural occurrence. Prenatal care may not be a priority for women who view pregnancy as a natural occurrence. For example, in India pregnancy is not considered an illness but a normal physiologic event, so a traditional Indian woman may seek healthcare only in the event of a problem (Choudhry, 1997). On the other hand, healthcare throughout Southeast Asia tends to be crisis oriented, with symptom relief as the goal (D'Avanzo, 1992).

Attitudes about pregnancy do vary somewhat among cultures. Americans of African descent, for example, usually consider pregnancy as a state of wellness. Mexican Americans generally view pregnancy as a natural and desirable condition, and most Native American groups consider pregnancy a normal process. Although pregnancy is perceived as a natural occurrence in many cultures, it may also be viewed as a time of increased vulnerability. Individuals with European/Western ideas might expect the woman to be away from work before and right after childbirth. In Orthodox Judaism, it is a man's responsibility to procreate, but it is a woman's right, not her obligation, to do so. This is because, according to Orthodox Jewish law, the health of the mother, both physically and mentally, is of primary concern, and she should never be obliged to do something that threatens her life (Bodo & Gibson, 1999a).

Individuals of many cultures take certain protective precautions based on their beliefs. For example, many women of Malawi, Africa, avoid preparing clothes for the infant during the prenatal period because they believe that this action will lead to the birth of a stillborn infant (Gennaro, Kamwendo, Mbweza, et al, 1998). Similarly, many Southeast Asian women fear that they will have a complicated labor and birth if they sit in a doorway or on a step. Thus they tend to avoid areas near doors in waiting rooms and examining rooms (Mattson, 1995). For many Vietnamese women, lifting the arms above the head is believed to increase the risk of preterm birth. Vietnamese women are also discouraged from sitting or lying down for lengthy periods because doing so might allow the baby to become too large (Bodo & Gibson, 1999b).

In the Mexican American culture, the concept of *mal aire*, or bad air, is sometimes related to evil spirits. It is thought that air, especially night air, may enter the body and cause illness. Preventive measures, such as keeping the windows closed or covering the head, are used. Some Latinos may place a raisin on the cord stump of a newborn to prevent drafts from entering the baby's body (Murray & Zentner, 2001).

For many Southeast Asians, the wind (or *vata*) is a potentially negative force that can disturb the body's internal harmony when a person is in a vulnerable state, such as during and after childbirth or during surgery (Mattson, 1995). The natural forces thought to be more desirable during pregnancy include the earth, for groundedness, and water, for fluidity. Thus, in addition to avoiding wind and drafts, the pregnant woman is encouraged to eat creamy, oily, and other heavy foods, retire early and sleep until dawn, avoid stimulants and stress, and drink plenty of water.

Taboos refer to behaviors or things that are avoided. Many cultures, including those found in the United States, have taboos centered around the unborn baby that are meant to ensure that the baby will survive. Many of these beliefs stem from the fear of injuring an unborn child or the worry that a baby might die. In developing countries, mortality rates among infants and young children are extremely high; thus, certain traditions have centered around preventing early death. For example, it is common among Muslims to avoid naming babies until after birth and to ensure that the first words a baby hears are from God (Purnell & Paulanka, 1998). In the western part of Mali, babies' faces are covered in mud and they are called ugly names to ward off evil spirits. Taboos also emanate from the fear that a pregnant woman has evil powers. For this reason, pregnant women are sometimes prohibited from taking part in certain activities with other people.

Many cultures ascribe to the *equilibrium model of health*, which is based on the concept of balance between light and dark, heat and cold. As described in the next chapter, Far Eastern philosophical belief systems focus on the notion of yin and yang. Yin represents the female, passive principle—darkness, cold, and wetness. Yang is the masculine, active principle—light, heat, and dryness. When the two are combined, they are all that can be.

The hot-cold classification is also seen in cultures in Latin America, the Near East, and Southeast Asia. The dimensions and meanings of this classification vary, however, and require further investigation. Spanish priests brought the concept of "hot" and "cold" to Mexico, where it was combined with ancient Aztec beliefs. Consequently, some Mexican Americans may consider illness to be an excess of either hot or cold (Spector, 2000). To restore health, imbalances are often corrected by the proper use of foods, medications, or herbs. These substances are also classified as hot or cold. For example, an illness attributed to an excess of coldness will be treated only with hot foods or medications. The classification of foods is not always consistent, but it does conform to a general structure of traditional knowledge. Certain foods, spices, herbs, and medications are perceived to cool or heat the body. These perceptions do not necessarily correspond to the actual temperature; some hot dishes are said to have a cooling quality.

Southeast Asians believe it is important to keep the woman "warm" after the birth because blood, which is considered "hot," has been lost, and the woman is at risk of becoming "cold." Therefore, they avoid cold drinks and foods following birth (Mattson, 1995). In addition, many women in India consider pregnancy a hot period and eat cool foods to counterbalance the hot state (Choudhry, 1997).The concepts of hot and cold are not as important in Native American or African American beliefs. There are some similarities, however, in all of these groups because of the emphasis on a balance in nature.

> **Clinical Tip** *When caring for a woman of Asian descent, ask her if she would prefer hot water or ice water at her bedside. This can help ensure that proper oral hydration is maintained and cultural beliefs are supported.*

HEALTH PRACTICES DURING PREGNANCY

Health practices during pregnancy are influenced by numerous factors, such as the prevalence of traditional home remedies and folk beliefs, the importance of indigenous healers, and the influence of professional healthcare workers. In an urban setting the age of the family members, length of time in the city, marital status, and strength of the family may affect these patterns. Socioeconomic status is also important because modern medical services are more accessible to those who can afford them.

An awareness of alternative health sources is crucial for health professionals because these practices affect health outcomes. For example, many members of the Mexican American community utilize the *partera*, a lay midwife, as a healer who gives advice and treats illnesses during pregnancy as well as being in attendance during labor and birth (Spector, 2000).

Indigenous healers are also important in some cultures. In the Mexican American culture the healer is called a *curandero* or *curandera*. In some Native American tribes the medicine man may fulfill the healing role. Herbalists are often found in Asian cultures; and faith healers, root doctors, and spiritualists are sometimes consulted in the African American culture.

CULTURAL NORMS REGARDING INFANT FEEDING PRACTICES

Culture can greatly affect new mothers' as well as experienced mothers' choices in feeding decisions. For example, in the Hispanic culture, women often believe that newborns need to be supplemented with infant formula before the milk comes in. Although colostrum provides vital antibodies for the infant, many Hispanic women refuse to nurse until their milk supply is established. It is important for the nurse to understand cultural norms and make recommendations that complement these norms, rather than conflict with them. In the preceding example, the nurse may advise the woman to first nurse her newborn at the breast and then offer the infant formula.

The majority of research on formula-feeding behavior has been conducted among Hispanic mothers and African American mothers. One common practice in these cultural groups is the addition of foods to the formula bottle, usually after 2 to 3 months, but for some, as early as 2 weeks into a baby's life. The kinds of food added vary from nonnutritive, high-calorie substances like sugar to adult foods like rice, beans, cereal, potatoes, yams, and eggs. Once the food is added, the nipple is often enlarged so that the baby can consume the food creating a potential choking hazard.

Such supplementation may be done for a variety of reasons. Hispanic mothers report that it is important to add these foods to the formula to help the baby grow to be large. In Latin American culture, many people believe that "the bigger the baby, the better," so parents supplement the breast or formula hoping for a big and healthy baby. Unfortunately, the parents are usually unaware of the fact that the addition of these foods can hurt the growth and health of the infant. Indeed, if a mother does not feed her child in the culturally accepted way, she may appear to be unfit or irresponsible in the community.

A second reason why foods are added to formulas lies in the belief that the addition of traditional foods at a very young age will prepare children to accept and enjoy their traditional foods when they are older. Food is an extremely important component of many Hispanic cultures; it ties people together and is usually the centerpiece of religious events and holidays. This relates to the third reason why foods are added to formula. During the holidays, it is considered important that everyone eat the same thing and participate equally; thus, infants are often included by being given the same foods the adults are eating.

African American mothers have also reported adding foods like cereal, potatoes, evaporated milk, or even extra scoops of powdered formula to thicken the formula. As with Hispanic families, the addition of these foods is thought to be necessary to help the child grow to be big and healthy, but more immediately, it is thought that this thickened formula will better satisfy a baby, so that he or she will sleep better through the night and allow the mother to do so as well. Thin formulas are associated with making a baby cry at night.

Overfeeding is a common cultural behavior as well. Hispanic mothers are reported to often overfeed their infants. Some mothers have reported to feed a child until he or she spits up. That is the indication that a child is eating in a healthful manner. Puerto Rican mothers believe overfeeding to be a protective care behavior that keeps a child healthy, well fed, and safe from illness or harm.

Many immigrants choose formula-feeding over breastfeeding. While this choice may be partly due to their busy lives, it also can be due to cultural beliefs, particularly among immigrants from developing countries, where the ability to formula-feed is a status symbol because it is so expensive. In Mali, for example, a can of formula can cost the equivalent of $2, while the average individual only earns $200 per year. In the United States, formulas are more affordable and available to the poor; however, when additional cultural practices come into play, such as overfeeding and adding extra formula, the subsidized formulas can run out quickly, and mothers may choose to substitute cow's milk, use canned evaporated or condensed milk, dilute the formula, or purchase unsafe formulas on the "black market." Obviously, these choices have dangerous health implications for the infant.

A nurse may educate a mother in her native language about appropriate infant feeding practices, but the influences from her family and their cultural beliefs may have a greater impact than the health teaching on her feeding behavior. Understanding parents' beliefs and traditions can help nurses to educate families more effectively about healthful feeding behaviors.

Cultural Diversity in Family Nursing Care

Cultural attitudes, behaviors, and beliefs that are related to health can greatly affect how a client will respond to and comply with health advice. Thus it is critical that nurses develop a holistic understanding of their clients' needs. Healthcare providers are often unaware of the cultural characteristics they themselves demonstrate. Without cultural awareness, caregivers tend to project their own cultural responses onto foreign-born clients; clients from different socioeconomic, religious, or educational groups; or clients from different regions of the country. This leads caregivers to assume that clients are demonstrating a specific behavior for the same reason that they themselves would. Moreover, healthcare providers frequently fail to recognize that medicine has its own culture, which has been dominated historically by traditional, middle-class values and beliefs (American College of Obstetricians and Gynecologists [ACOG], 1998).

Ethnocentrism is the conviction that the values and beliefs of one's own cultural group are the best ones or the only acceptable ones. It is characterized by an inability or unwillingness to understand the beliefs or world view of another group or culture. To a certain extent, most people are guilty of ethnocentrism, at least some of the time. Thus the nurse who values stoicism during labor may be uncomfortable with the more vocal response of a Latin American woman. Another nurse may be disconcerted by the Southeast Asian woman who believes that pain is something to be endured rather than alleviated and is very intent on maintaining self-control in labor (Mattson, 1995).

Healthcare providers sometimes believe that if members of other cultures do not share Western values, they should adopt them. This is especially difficult for a nurse caring for childbearing families if the nurse is a firm believer in the equality of the sexes and feminism. The nurse may find it difficult to remain silent if a woman from a Middle Eastern culture defers to her husband in decision making. It is important to remember that pressure to defy cultural values and beliefs can be stressful and anxiety provoking for these women.

To address issues of cultural diversity in the provision of healthcare, emphasis is being placed on developing **cultural competency**—that is, the skills and knowledge necessary to appreciate, understand, and work with individuals from different cultures. It requires self-awareness, awareness and understanding of cultural differences, and the ability to adapt clinical skills and practices as necessary (Beckman & Dysart, 2000).

The nurse can begin developing cultural competence by becoming knowledgeable about the cultural practices of local groups. For example, is it considered courteous to avoid eye contact? Should last names be used in conversation as a sign of respect? Is a female healthcare provider necessary? Do communication and language barriers exist? If so, how can they be addressed?

Mattson & Smith (2000) have suggested that care providers conduct a "cultural assessment" to glean information about health practices based on the client's beliefs, values, and customs. This kind of assessment might include questions such as:

1. Who in the family must be consulted before decisions are made about a person's care?
2. Does the client see primarily in the present or does he or she have a futuristic time orientation?
3. What type of health provider is most appropriate for the client?
4. Does the client have beliefs or traditions that may impact the care plan?

Several cultural assessment tools are in use to assist the nurse in obtaining cultural information. Giger & Davidhizar (1995) developed a transcultural assessment tool that identifies the cultural background, communication patterns, issues related to personal space, social organization, time, roles within the environment, biologic variations, and a nursing assessment (Figure 2–8 •).

It is imperative when caring for families that nurses provide culturally sensitive care that supports cultural differences. The nurse who respects cultural diversity is an asset to the childbearing family as they adjust to their new role. Establishing a trusting relationship enables the nurse to assist the family in meeting educational needs.

A Transcultural Assessment Model

CULTURALLY UNIQUE INDIVIDUAL

1. Place of birth
2. Cultural definition
   What is . . .
3. Race
   What is . . .
4. Length of time in country

COMMUNICATION

1. Voice quality
   A. Strong, resonant
   B. Soft
   C. Average
   D. Shrill
2. Pronunciation and enunciation
   A. Clear
   B. Slurred
   C. Dialect
3. Use of silence
   A. Infrequent
   B. Often
   C. Length
      (1) Brief
      (2) Moderate
      (3) Long
      (4) Not observed
4. Use of nonverbal
   A. Hand movement
   B. Eye movement
   C. Moves entire body
   D. Kinesics (gestures, expressions, or stances)
5. Touch
   A. Startles or withdraws when touched
   B. Accepts touch without difficulty
   C. Touches others without difficulty
6. Ask these and similar questions:
   A. How do you get your point across to others?
   B. Do you like communicating with friends, family, and acquaintances?
   C. When asked a question, do you usually respond (in words or body movements, or both)?
   D. If you have something important to discuss with your family, how would you approach them?

SPACE

1. Degree of comfort
   A. Moves when space invaded
   B. Does not move when invaded
2. Distance in conversations
   A. 0 to 18 inches
   B. 18 inches to 3 feet
   C. 3 feet or more
3. Definition of space
   A. Describe degree of comfort with closeness when talking with or standing near others
   B. How do objects (e.g., furniture) in the environment affect your sense of space?
4. Ask these and similar questions:
   A. When you talk with family members, how close do you stand?
   B. When you communicate with co-workers and other acquaintances, how close do you stand?
   C. If a stranger touches you, how do you react or feel?
   D. If a loved one touches you, how do you react or feel?
   E. Are you comfortable with the distance between us now?

SOCIAL ORGANIZATION

1. Normal state of health
   A. Poor
   B. Fair
   C. Good
   D. Excellent

Figure 2–8 • Cultural assessment tool. *(continued on next page)*

2. Ask these and similar questions:
   A. How do you define social activities?
   B. What are some activities that you enjoy?
   C. What are your hobbies, or what do you do when you have free time?
   D. Do you believe in a Supreme Being?
   E. How do you worship that Supreme Being?
   F. What is your function (what do you do) in your family unit/system?
   G. What is your role in your family unit/system (father, mother, child, advisor)?
   H. When you were a child, what or who influenced you most?
   I. What is/was your relationship with your siblings and parents?
   J. What does work mean to you?
   K. Describe your past, present, and future jobs.
   L. What are your political views?
   M. How have your political views influenced your attitude toward health and illness?

TIME

1. Orientation to time
   A. Past-oriented
   B. Present-oriented
   C. Future-oriented
2. View of time
   A. Social time
   B. Clock-oriented
3. Physiochemical reaction to time
   A. Sleeps at least 8 hours a night
   B. Goes to sleep and wakes on a consistent schedule
   C. Understands the importance of taking medication and other treatments on schedule
4. Ask these and similar questions:
   A. What kind of timepiece do you wear daily?
   B. If you have an appointment at 2 PM, what time is acceptable to arrive?
   C. If a nurse tells you that you will receive a medication in "about a half hour," realistically, how much time will you allow before calling the nurses' station?

ENVIRONMENTAL CONTROL

1. Locus-of-control
   A. Internal locus-of-control (believes that the power to affect change lies within)
   B. External locus-of-control (believes that fate, luck, and chance have a great deal to do with how things turn out)
2. Value orientation
   A. Believes in supernatural forces
   B. Relies on magic, witchcraft, and prayer to affect change
   C. Does not believe in supernatural forces
   D. Does not rely on magic, witchcraft, or prayer to affect change
3. Ask these and similar questions:
   A. How often do you have visitors at your home?
   B. Is it acceptable to you for visitors to drop in unexpectedly?
   C. Name some ways your parents or other persons treated your illnesses when you were a child.
   D. Have you or someone else in your immediate surroundings ever used a home remedy that made you sick?
   E. What home remedies have you used that worked? Will you use them in the future?
   F. What is your definition of "good health"?
   G. What is your definition of illness or "poor health"?

BIOLOGIC VARIATIONS

1. Conduct a complete physical assessment noting:
   A. Body structure
   B. Skin color
   C. Unusual skin discolorations
   D. Hair color and distribution
   E. Other visible physical characteristics (e.g., keloids, chloasma)
2. Ask these and similar questions:
   A. What diseases or illnesses are common in your family?
   B. Describe your family's typical behavior when a family member is ill.
   C. How do you respond when you are angry?
   D. Who (or what) usually helps you to cope during a difficult time?
   E. What foods do you and your family like to eat?
   F. Have your ever had any unusual cravings for:
      (1) White or red clay dirt?
      (2) Laundry starch?
   G. When you were a child what types of foods did you eat?
   H. What foods are family favorites or are considered traditional?

NURSING ASSESSMENT

1. Note whether the client has become culturally assimilated or observes own cultural practices.
2. Incorporate data into plan of nursing care:
   A. Encourage the client to discuss cultural differences; people from diverse cultures who hold different worldviews can enlighten nurses.
   B. Make efforts to accept and understand methods of communication.
   C. Respect the individual's personal need for space.
   D. Respect the rights of clients to honor and worship the Supreme Being of their choice.
   E. Identify a clerical or spiritual person to contact.
   F. Determine whether spiritual practices have implications for health, life, and well-being (e.g., Jehovah's Witnesses may refuse blood and blood derivatives; an Orthodox Jew may eat only Kosher food high in sodium and may not drink milk when meat is served).
   G. Identify hobbies, especially when devising interventions for short or extended convalescence or for rehabilitation.
   H. Honor time and value orientations and differences in these areas. Allay anxiety and apprehension if adherence to time is necessary.
   I. Provide privacy according to personal need and health status of the client (Note: the perception and reaction to pain may be culturally related).
   J. Note cultural health practices
      (1) Identify and encourage efficacious practices.
      (2) Identify and discourage dysfunctional practices.
      (3) Identify and determine whether neutral practices will have a long-term ill effect.
   K. Note food preferences
      (1) Make as many adjustments in diet as health status and long-term benefits will allow and that dietary department can provide.
      (2) Note dietary practices that may have serious implications for the client.

Figure 2–8 • Cultural assessment tool. *(continued)*
SOURCE: Reprinted from Giger, J.N. and Davidhizar, R.E.: Transcultural Nursing: Assessment and Intervention. © 1991, with permission from Elsevier Science.

In planning care, the nurse considers the extent to which the woman's personal values, beliefs, and customs are in accord with those of the woman's identified cultural group, the nurse providing care, and the healthcare agency. If discrepancies exist, the nurse then considers whether the woman's system is supportive, neutral, or harmful in relation to possible interventions. If the woman's system is supportive or neutral, it can be incorporated into the plan. For example, individual food practices or methods of pain expression may differ from those of the nurse or agency but would not necessarily interfere with the nursing plan.

In contrast, certain cultural practices might pose a threat to the health of the childbearing woman. For example, some Filipino women will not take any medication during pregnancy. The primary care practitioner may consider a certain medication essential to the woman's well-being. In this case, the woman's cultural belief may be detrimental to her own health. The nurse and client must carefully discuss the reasons for her refusal. After discussing and understanding the reasons, the nurse faces three possible outcomes: (1) identifying ways to persuade the woman to accept the proposed medication, (2) accepting the woman's decision to refuse the medication if she is not willing to adapt her belief system, or (3) explaining alternative therapies that might be acceptable to the woman in light of her cultural beliefs.

The nurse can also provide community resources. An in-depth knowledge of culturally diverse resources available will assist the nurse in providing resources for clients. Multiple resources can also be found on the Internet (Table 2–5 •). The nurse should assess each family's ability to use and access computers before providing them with a list of Internet-related resources. Whenever possible, written information should be provided in the individual's primary language. Women with language barriers should be given both written and verbal information with the assistance of an interpreter. The nurse's role in caring for families with diverse backgrounds requires sensitivity, therapeutic communication skills, and awareness of community-based resources available for culturally diverse populations.

Impact of Religion and Spirituality

The goal of truly holistic care of the childbearing family requires that the nurse understand the influence that religion and spirituality may have on their childbearing experience.

Diverse Meanings of Religion and Spirituality

The terms *religion* and *spirituality* mean very different things to different people. Although many people think of **religion** as an institutionalized system that shares a common set of beliefs and practices, others define it more simply as a belief in a transcendent power. The latter definition approaches most people's understanding of **spirituality** as a concern with the spirit or soul.

Philosophers and mystics have debated the meaning of religion for millennia, but within the last 200 years, technologic advances and the ascendance of rationalism and postmodernism have led many influential thinkers to condemn religion as mere wishful thinking. For example, in 1844, philosopher Karl Marx famously decried religion as "the opium of the people," (Marx, 1971), and in 1932, in his *New Introductory Lectures on Psychoanalysis*, psychologist Sigmund Freud stated: "Religion is an illusion. . . an attempt to get control over the sensory world, in which we are placed, by means of the wish-world. . . " (Freud, 1965). More recently, however, religious teachers as diverse as the Buddhist monk Thich Nhat Hanh, Benedictine monk Brother David Steindl-Rast, and the mystic J. Krishnamurti have offered new visions of a religious life grounded in day-to-day experience. For Hanh (1995), "Religious life is life." According to Krishnamurti (1989), "To be religious is to be sensitive to reality."

Range of Religious Beliefs

These diverse meanings and approaches to religion and spirituality are reflected in the diversity of religious beliefs encountered in contemporary childbearing families. Some may belong to large institutionalized religious organizations, while others may feel deeply religious yet have no formal affiliation or practice. Many clients are *agnostic*, or doubtful about the existence of a transcendent being, or truly *atheist*, meaning that they believe there is no higher power. Internationally and in the United States, Christianity is the largest organized religious group, with over 2 billion members worldwide accounting for approximately 33% of the world's population. Another 22% of people worldwide are Islamic, and 15% are Hindu. Whatever their religious affiliation, Americans are overwhelmingly religious: fully 95% state that they believe in a higher power (Reeves, 2000).

A childbearing family's religious beliefs, affiliation, and practices can influence deeply their experience and attitudes toward healthcare, childbearing, and childrearing. Members of certain religious groups such as Christian Scientists may attempt to avoid all medical interventions, whereas others such as Jehovah's Witnesses may refuse specific interventions, such as blood transfusions. Roman Catholics may refuse contraception. Many religions promote childbearing as a sacred right and responsibility, and some prescribe childrearing practices as well. In most cases, the woman and her family gain comfort from acknowledgment of and respect for their religious beliefs and practices in the healthcare setting. However, the agnostic or atheist family may be offended if care providers assume that references to God or a higher power will be comforting.

Table 2-5 • CULTURAL RESOURCES

Networks: Health-Related Organizations

National Black Child Development Institute
1023 Fifteenth Street, NW
Suite 600
Washington, DC 20005
(202) 387-1281

National Center for the Advancement of Blacks in the Health Professions
(NCABHP)
P.O. Box 21121
Detroit, MI 48221
(313) 345-4480

American Indian Health Care Association
1550 Larimer Street
Suite 225
Denver, CO 80202
(303) 607-1048

National Indian Health Board
1385 South Colorado Blvd.
Suite A-708
Denver, CO 80222
(303) 759-3075

Asian American Health Forum
116 New Montgomery Street
Suite 531
San Francisco, CA 94105
(415) 541-0866

Asian Pacific Center on Aging
1511 Third Avenue
Seattle, WA 98101
(206) 624-1221

Association of Asian Pacific Community Health Organizations
(AAPCHO)
1212 Broadway, Suite 730
Oakland, CA 94612
(510) 272-9536

Hispanic Health Council
9648 Cedar Street
Hartford, CT 06106
(203) 527-0856

National Coalition of Hispanic Health and Human Services Organizations (COSSMHO)
1501 Sixteenth Street, NW
Washington, DC 20036
(202) 387-5100

American Public Health Association
African American, Asian, Hispanic, and Native American Caucus
1015 Fifteenth Street, NW
Washington, DC 20005
(202) 789-5600

National Council for International Health
1701 K Street, NW
Suite 600
Washington, DC 20006
(202) 833-5903

National Multicultural Institute
3000 Connecticut Avenue, NW
Suite 438
Washington, DC 20008
(202) 483-0700

Cross-Cultural Health Care Program
1200 Twelfth Avenue S
Seattle, WA 98144
(206) 621-4161
http://www.xculture.org/

The Center for Cross-Cultural Health
1313 SE Fifth Street, Suite 100B
Minneapolis, MN 55414
(612) 379-3573
http://www.crosshealth.com/

Web sites

Ethnomed
This site provides health information for a variety of ethnic groups.
http://ethnomed.org/

Culture Clues

Culture Clues are tip sheets for clinicians designed to increase awareness about concepts and preferences of patients from the diverse cultures served by the University of Washington Medical Center. Currently there are five cultures represented, with additional ones in progress.
http://depts.washington.edu/pfes/cultureclues.html

Transcultural and Multicultural Health Links
This site provides general resources for a variety of ethnic and special population groups.
http://www.iun.edu/~libemb/trannurs/trannurs.htm

Provision of Spiritually Sensitive Nursing Care

For all these reasons, nurses are increasingly committed to providing spiritually sensitive nursing care to childbearing families. On admission to the clinic or labor setting, a religious or spiritual history is now included when assessing the childbearing family. Many clients specify a religious affiliation on admission to an acute care facility, but more specific information is also needed. The assessment can include questions about current spiritual beliefs and practices that will affect the mother and baby during the hospital stay, or preferences for religious rituals during labor and birth.

Whenever possible, the nurse and other healthcare providers should attempt to accommodate religious rituals and practices requested by the childbearing family. Most such requests, such as for certain music, foods, or keeping a statue or picture by the bed, can be accommodated without causing danger; however, some, such as lighting candles, could present a risk in an acute care setting. In these circumstances, the family should be given a clear explanation of why the particular action cannot safely be carried out. In addition, nurses can provide clients with resources to meet their religious needs, such as consultation with on-staff chaplains. In settings where chaplains are not readily available, the nurse should be familiar with community resources in the area and offer referral as needed. In circumstances of spiritual distress, such as with severe fetal deformity or loss of a newborn, the family may prefer to meet with their personal religious adviser, and the nurse can arrange for that visit.

Considering the diversity of religious beliefs, it is not unusual for nurses to encounter childbearing families whose beliefs conflict with their own. This is not problematic as long as the nurse avoids attempts to influence the client's decision making. For example, a nurse who does not believe in baptism should avoid revealing this belief to a Catholic client seeking baptism for her stillborn infant. Nurses should also examine their religious beliefs related to genetic screening procedures, use of assisted reproductive technology to achieve pregnancy, use of technology to support life in a severely compromised newborn, abortion, and even less dramatic issues such as methods of contraception, circumcision, and infant feeding. In many institutions, nurses can ask to be reassigned to a different client if their religious beliefs are in conflict; however, if other personnel are not available, it is the nurse's responsibility to provide sensitive, appropriate, and nonjudgmental care to that client.

CHAPTER REVIEW

EXPLOREMEDIALINK

NCLEX review questions, case studies, and other interactive resources for this chapter can be found on the Web site at http://www.prenhall.com/olds. Click on "Chapter 2" to select the activities for this chapter.

For tutorials including animations and videos, more NCLEX review questions, and an audio glossary, access the accompanying CD-ROM in this book.

Focus Your Study

- Family values, power, and roles are important to consider when attempting to provide holistic healthcare to contemporary families.
- Multiple trends have influenced changes in the traditional family, including employment trends, changes in marital status patterns, and economic trends.
- Nuclear families consist of a mother, father, and children.
- Dual-career/dual-earner families make up the majority of contemporary families in the United States.
- Childless families are a growing trend in American culture.
- Extended family members can play an active role in family life, decision making, and family roles.
- Single-parent families account for almost a third of all US families, and stepparent and binuclear families are increasingly common.
- The developmental framework looks at a family over time as it progresses through predictable stages within the life cycle.
- A family assessment provides an in-depth tool to collect pertinent family life information that can assist the nurse in planning care.
- Culture plays a significant part in a family's development, roles, and observance of traditions, customs, and taboos.

- Cultural norms influence a family's beliefs about the importance of children, pregnancy, health practices, and infant feeding.
- A cultural assessment can assist the nurse in identifying cultural norms and providing culturally appropriate nursing care.
- A religious history is included when assessing contemporary families. Whenever possible, the nurse accommodates the family's religious-based preferences for care.

References

American College of Obstetricians and Gynecologists (ACOG). (1998). *Cultural competency in healthcare* (ACOG Committee Opinion 201). Washington, DC: Author.

Beckman, C. R. B., & Dysart, D. (2000). The challenge of multicultural medical care. *Contemporary OB/GYN, 45*(12), 12–33.

Bodo, K., & Gibson, N. (1999a). Childbirth customs in Orthodox Jewish traditions. *Canadian Family Physician, 45*, 682–686.

Bodo, K., & Gibson, N. (1999b). Childbirth customs in Vietnamese traditions. *Canadian Family Physician, 45*, 690–697.

Cairney, J., & Ostbye, T. (1999). Time since immigration and excess body weight. *Canadian Journal of Public Health, 90*(2), 120–124.

Carter, E. A., & McGoldrick, M. (Eds.). (1989). *The changing family life cycle: A framework for family therapists* (2nd ed.). New York: Gardner Press.

Cherlin, A. J. (2001). *Public & private families* (2nd ed.). Boston: McGraw-Hill.

Choudhry, U. K. (1997). Traditional practices of women from India: Pregnancy, childbirth, and newborn care. *Journal of Obstetric, Gynecologic, & Neonatal Nursing, 26*(5), 533–539.

Cousins, J. H., Rubovits, D. S., Dunn, J. K., Reeves, R. S., Ramirez, A. G., & Foreyt, J. P. (1992). Family versus individually oriented intervention for weight loss in Mexican American women. *Public Health Reports, 107*(5), 549–555.

D'Avanzo, C. E. (1992). Bridging the cultural gap with Southeast Asians. *American Journal of Maternal Child Nursing, 17*(4), 204–208.

Duvall, E. M. (1977). *Marriage and family development* (5th ed.). New York: Harper Row.

Elder, G. H. (2001). Family influence on physical health during the middle years: The case of onset of hypertension. *Journal of Marriage and Family, 63*, 527–539.

Faust, J. E. (2000). *Womanhood: The highest place of honor.* Salt Lake City, UT: The Church of Jesus Christ Latter-day Saints.

Fields, J., & Casper, L. M. (2001, June). *America's families and living arrangements: Population characteristics.* Washington, DC: US Census Bureau.

Freud, S. (1965). *New introductory lectures on psychoanalysis* (lecture 35). New York: W. W. Norton & Company. (Original work published 1932)

Friedman, M. M. (1998). *Family nursing: Research, theory & practice* (4th ed.). Stamford, CT: Appleton & Lange.

Frisch, N. C., & Frisch, N. E. (1998). *Psychiatric mental health nursing.* Boston: Delmar.

Fullerton, H. N. (1999, November). Labor force projections to 2008: Steady growth, changing composition. *Monthly Labor Review, 122*, 19–32.

Gennaro, S., Kamwendo, L. A., Mbweza, E., & Kershbaumer, R. (1998). Childbearing in Malawi, Africa. *Journal of Obstetric, Gynecologic, and Neonatal Nursing, 27*(2), 191–196.

Giger, J. N., & Davidhizar, R. E. (1995). *Transcultural nursing: assessment and interventions.* (2nd ed.). St Louis: Mosby.

Hanh, T. N. (1995). *Living Buddha, living Christ.* New York: Riverhead Books.

Higgins, B. (2000). Puerto Rican cultural beliefs: Influence of infant feeding practices in western New York. *Journal of Transcultural Nursing, 11*(1), 19–30.

Hyde, A. (1998, September). From mutual pretense awareness to open awareness: Single pregnant women's public encounters in an Irish context. *Qualitative Health Research, 8*(5), 634–643.

Kalhan, R., Puthawala, K., Agarwal, S., Amini, S. B., & Kalhan, S. C. (2001). Altered lipid profile, leptin, insulin, and anthropometry in offspring of South Asian immigrants in the United States. *Metabolism: Clinical and Experimental, 50*(10), 1197–1202.

Krishnamurti, J. (1989). *Think on these things.* New York: Harper Perennial.

Marx, K. (1971). *Critique of the Hegelian Philosophy of Right.* Cambridge, England: Cambridge University Press. (Original work published 1844)

Mattson, S. (1995). Culturally sensitive perinatal care for Southeast Asians. *Journal of Obstetric, Gynecologic, and Neonatal Nursing, 24*(4), 335–341.

Mattson, S., & Smith, J. E. (2000). *Core curriculum for maternal-newborn nursing* (2nd ed.). Philadelphia: Saunders.

Mui, A. C., Choi, N. G., & Monk, A. (1998). Long-term care and ethnicity. Westport, CT: Auburn House.

Murray, R. B., & Zentner, J. P. (2001). *Health promotion strategies through the lifespan* (7th ed.). Upper Saddle River, NJ: Prentice-Hall.

Nye, F. I., & Gecas, V. (1976). The role concept: Review and delineation. In F. I. Nye (Ed.), *Structure and analysis of the family.* Beverly Hills, CA: Sage.

Olson, D. H., & Cromwell, R. E. (1975). Methodological issues in family power. In R.E. Cromwell & D. H. Olson (Eds.), *Power in families.* New York: Sage.

Parad, H. J., & Caplan, G. (1965). A framework for studying families in crisis. In H. J. Parad (Ed.), *Crisis intervention: Selected readings.* New York: Family Services of America.

Parsons, S., Goodson, J. H., Williams, S. A., & Cade, J. E. (1999). Are there intergenerational differences in diets of young children born to first and second-generation Pakistani Muslims in Bradford, West Yorkshire, UK? *Journal of Human Nutrition and Dietetics, 12*(2), 113–122.

Purnell, L. D., & Paulanka, B. J. (1998). *Transcultural healthcare: A culturally competent approach.* Philadelphia: F.A. Davis.

Reeves, T. C. (2000). *Twentieth century America: A brief history* (p. 284). New York: Oxford University Press.

Roberts, R. (1990). *Developing culturally competent programs for families of children with special needs.* Washington, DC: Georgetown University Child Development Center, Maternal and Child Health Bureau.

Slater, S. (1995). *The lesbian family life cycle.* New York: Free Press.

Spector, R. E. (2000). *Cultural diversity in health and illness* (2nd ed.). Norwalk, CT: Appleton & Lange.

Stepfamily Association of America. (2000). *Stepfamily factsheet.* Lincoln, NE: Author. Retrieved on December 5, 2002, from the world wide web at www.saafamilies.org

Teachman, J. (2000). The changing demography of America's families. *Journal of Marriage and the Family, 62*(4); 1234–1246.

Teachman, J. & Paasch, K. (1999). The social and economic context of increasing demographic diversity of families. In Demo, D., Allen, K. & Fine, M. (Eds.) *Handbook of Family Diversity.* New York: Oxford University Press, 32–58.

US Census Bureau. (1998). *Current population reports. Table 8: Marital status and living arrangements.* Washington, DC: US Census Bureau.

US Census Bureau. (1999a). *Marriage and family: Nuclear meltdown.* Retrieved August 9, 2001, from http://www.ameristat.org/marfam/tradfam.htm

US Census Bureau. (1999b). *Fertility: Having children later or not at all.* Retrieved August 9, 2001, from http://www.ameristat.org/fertility/HavingChildrenlaterNot.html

Wald, M. S. (1999). *Same-sex couples: Marriage, families, and children.* Stanford CA: Stanford Law School.

Complementary and Alternative Therapies

3

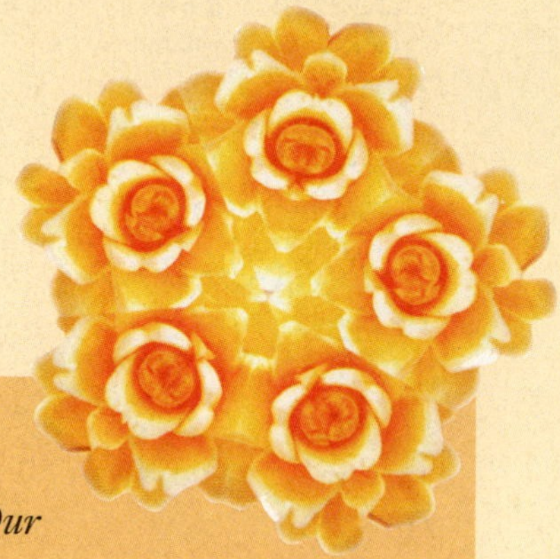

As part of a continuing education course on body-based therapies for nurses, I was giving a back massage to one of my classmates. At one point, I felt a buzz of energy shoot up my hands and arms. At that exact moment, the other student said, "Wow!" Our instructor just laughed and said, "Oh, you're just exchanging friendly energy." That experience changed forever my views as a nurse and educator. I like the fact that nursing is based in science, but I remain open to the mysteries of the human body, mind, and spirit.

Objectives

- Distinguish between *complementary* and *alternative therapies.*
- Identify several factors that have contributed to the rise in popularity of complementary and alternative therapies in the United States and Canada.
- Describe the role of the National Center for Complementary and Alternative Medicine.
- Explain the role of complementary and alternative therapies in promoting wellness, disease prevention, and holistic healing.
- Delineate the risks of using complementary and alternative therapies.
- Compare the basic principles and components of naturopathy, homeopathy, traditional Chinese medicine, and ayurvedic medicine.
- Describe the use of biofeedback, hypnosis, meditation, prayer, visualization, and guided imagery in promoting the well-being of childbearing families.
- Contrast the different body-based therapies, including chiropractic, craniosacral therapy, the Alexander technique, Feldenkreis, massage, reflexology, hatha yoga, and regular physical exercise.
- Explain the advantages and disadvantages to childbearing women of therapies involving ingestion of substances such as foods, dietary supplements, herbs, flower essences, and homeopathic remedies.
- Distinguish between acupressure and acupuncture.
- Distinguish between Reiki and therapeutic touch.
- Discuss complementary therapies appropriate for the nurse to use with childbearing families.

Key Terms

Acupressure 62
Acupuncture 62
Alternative therapy 49
Aromatherapy 61
Ayurveda 55
Biofeedback 56
Chiropractic 57
Complementary therapy 49
Guided imagery 57
Hatha yoga 59
Homeopathy 54
Hypnosis 56
Massage therapy 58
Naturopathy 54

MediaLink

Additional resources for this content can be found on the Student CD-ROM and on the Companion Website at www.prenhall.com/olds. Click on "Chapter 3" to select the activities for this chapter.

CD-ROM
- Audio Glossary
- NCLEX Review

Companion Website
- Additional NCLEX Review
- Case Study: Complementary Therapies
- Care Plan Activity: Use of CAM in High-Risk Adolescent Pregnancy

Overview of Fetal Development by Gestational Age in Weeks

Age	Length & Weight	Neurological and Musculoskeletal Systems	Cardiovascular and Respiratory Systems	Gastrointestinal and Genitourinary Systems	Endocrine, Integumentary and Immune Systems, Eye/Ear
2–3	2 mm crown-to-rump (C-R)	Groove forms along middle back; neural tube forms from closure of groove	Blood circulation begins; tubular heart begins to form in 3rd week; nasal pits form	Liver begins to function; kidneys begin to form	***Endo:*** thyroid tissue forms ***Eyes:*** optic cup and lens pit formed; pigment in eyes ***Ears:*** auditory pit closes
4	4-6 mm C-R; 0.4 grams	Anterior neural tube closes to form brain; posterior closure forms spinal cord; limb buds noted	Tubular heart beats (28 days); primitive RBCs circulate	Oral cavity forms; primitive jaws present; esophagus and trachea begin to divide; stomach forms; esophagus and intestine become tubular; pancreatic/liver ducts forming	***Eyes:*** primitive eye is present ***Ears:*** primitive ear is present
6–7	**6 wks:** 12 mm C-R **7 wks:** 18 mm C-R	**6 wks:** Brain became differentiated with cranial nerves present at week 5; bone rudiments present; primitive skeleton forming; muscle mass begins to develop; skull and jaw ossification begins	**6 wks:** Heart chambers present (atrial division at 5 weeks); blood cell groups identifiable; trachea, bronchi, lung buds present **7 wks:** Fetal heartbeats detectable; diaphragm separates abdominal/thoracic cavities	**6 wks:** Oral/nasal cavities and upper lip formed; liver starts to form RBCs; embryonic sex glands appear **7 wks:** Tongue separates; palate folds; stomach in final form; bladder and urethra separate from rectum; sex glands become testes or ovaries	**6 wks:** ***Ear:*** formation of external, middle, and inner ear continues **7 wks:** ***Eyes:*** optic nerve formed, eyelids present, lens thickens
8	2.5-3 cm C-R; 2 grams	Digits formed; skeletal cells differentiate further; ossification begins in cartilaginous bones; muscle development in head, trunk, and limbs allows some movement	Development of heart and fetal circulation complete	Lip fusion complete; rotation in mid-gut; anal membrane has perforated; external male and female genitalia appear similar until end of 9th week	***Ear:*** external, middle and inner ear assuming final forms
10	5-6 cm crown-to-heel (C-H); 14 grams	Neurons appear at caudal end of spinal cord; brain has basic divisions; nail growth begins in fingers/toes	By 9th week RBCs produced in the liver	Lips separate from jaw; palate folds fuse; developing intestines are enclosed in abdomen; bladder sac formed; testosterone physical characteristics at 8-12 wks (males)	***Endo:*** Islets of Langerhans differentiated ***Eyes:*** lids fused closed
12	8 cm C-R; 11.5 cm C-H; 45 g	Clear outline of miniature bones (12-20 wks); process of ossification established; involuntary muscles in viscera appear	Lungs acquire definitive shape	Mouth palate completed; muscles in gut appear; bile secretion begins; liver produces most of RBCs	***Skin:*** delicate, pink ***Endo:*** thyroid secretes hormones; insulin present in pancreas ***Immune:*** lymphoid tissue in thymus gland
16	13.5 cm C-R; 15 cm C-H; 200 g	Teeth begin to form hard tissue for central incisors	Fetal heart tones audible with feto scope at 16-20 weeks	Hard and soft palate differentiating; gastric and intestinal glands developing; intestines start to collect meconium; kidneys assume shape and organization; able to note sex	***Skin:*** scalp hair appears; body has lanugo; visible blood vessels beneath transparent skin; sweat glands developing ***Eyes, ears, nose:*** formed
20	25 cm C-H; 435 g (6% fat)	Spinal cord myelination begins; teeth begin to form hard tissue for canine and first molar (lateral incisors at 18 wks); lower limbs have final relative proportions	Fetal heart tones audible; primitive respiratory-like movements begin; iron is stored in the blood; bone marrow important	Fetus sucks and swallows amniotic fluid; peristalsis begins	***Skin:*** lanugo covers entire body; brown fat and vernix caseosa begin to form ***Endo:*** iron is stored; bone marrow functioning, fetal antibodies detectable ***Immune:*** fetal IgG levels detectable
24	28 cm C-H; 780 g	Brain appears mature; teeth begin to form 2nd molars	Resp. movements occur (24-40 wks), nostrils reopen, alveoli appear and begin to produce surfactant, gas exchange possible	Testes descend into inguinal ring (males)	***Skin:*** reddish and wrinkled ***Immune:*** IgG at mature levels ***Eyes:*** structurally complete
28–32	**28 wks**: 35 cm C-H; 1200-1250 g **32 wks**: 38-43 cm C-H; 2000 g	**28 wks:** Nervous system begins regulation of some bodily processes **32 wks:** More reflexes present	Viability is reached at 26-27 weeks; if born now, intensive care is needed to support respirations	Testes descend into inguinal canal and upper scrotum (males)	**28 wks:** ***Eyes:*** eyelids open ***Skin:*** adipose tissue begins to accumulate; eyebrows and eyelashes develop
36–40	**36 wks**: 42-48 cm C-H; 2500-2750 g **40 wks**: 48-52 cm C-H; 3200+ g (16% fat)	**36 wks:** Ossification centers present in distal femur	**38 wks:** Lecithin-spingomyelin (L/S) ratio approaches 2:1 (less risk of respiratory distress from inadequate surfactant if born)	**36 wks:** small scrotum with few rugae (males), final descent of testes into upper scrotum (36-40 wks), labia majora/minora equally prominent (females) **40 wks:** rugous scrotum (males); labia majora well-developed and cover the smaller labia minora and clitoris (females)	**36 wks:** ***Skin:*** pale, lanugo disappearing, hair fuzzy/wooly, few sole creases, increased vernix caseosa (36-40 wks) ***Ears:*** lobes soft with little cartilage **40 wks:** ***Skin:*** smooth, pink; vernix in skinfolds, silky hair, lanugo on shoulders and upper back, nails extend to tips of digits, creases cover sole ***Ears:*** lobes firmer, increased cartilage

 BA999030 ISBN 0-536-80700-0

PEARSON Custom Publishing

Prentice Hall's *Nursing Notes*

MATERNAL-NEWBORN NURSING

Newborn Vital Signs

Pulse

120–160 bpm

During sleep as low as 100 bpm; if crying, up to 180 bpm

Apical pulse counted for 1 full minute

Respirations

30–60 respirations/minute

Predominantly diaphragmatic but synchronous with abdominal movements

Respirations are counted for 1 full minute

Blood Pressure

80–60/45–40 mm Hg at birth

100/50 mm Hg at day 10

Temperature

Normal range: 36.5–37.5C (97.7–99.4F)

Axillary: 36.4–37.2C (97.5–99F)

Skin: 36–36.5C (96.8–97.7F)

Rectal: 36.6–37.2C (97.8–99F)

Newborn Measurements

Weight

Average: 3405 g (7 lb, 8 oz)

Range: 2500–4000 g (5 lb, 8 oz–8 lb, 13 oz)

Weight is influenced by racial origin and maternal age and size.

Physiologic weight loss: 5%–10% for term newborns, up to 15% for preterm newborns

Growth: 198 g (7 oz) per week for first 6 months

Length

Average: 50 cm (20 in)

Range: 48–52 cm (18–22 in)

Growth: 2.5 cm (1 in) per month for first 6 months

Head Circumference

32–37 cm (12.5–14.5 in)

Approximately 2 cm larger than chest circumference

Chest Circumference

Average: 32 cm (12.5 in)

Range: 30–35 cm (12–14 in)

Complications/Side Effects of Oral contraceptives

A Abdominal Pain (severe)
C Chest Pain (severe)
H Headaches
E Eye Problems
S Severe Leg Pain (calf or thigh)

Note: Chest pain also includes complication of shortness of breath and coughing up blood. Eye problems include complications such as blurred vision, flashing lights, and blindness.

Estrogen Effects

- Alterations in lipid metabolism
- Breast tenderness, engorgement, increased breast size
- Cerebrovascular accident
- Changes in carbohydrate metabolism
- Chloasma
- Fluid retention; cyclic weight gain
- Headache
- Hepatic adenomas
- Hypertension
- Leukorrhea, cervical erosion, ectopia
- Nausea
- Nervousness, irritability
- Telangiectasia
- Thrombophlebitis, pulmonary embolism

Progestin Effects

- Acne, oily skin
- Breast tenderness; increased breast size
- Decreased libido
- Decreased high-density lipoprotein (HDL) cholesterol levels
- Depression
- Fatigue
- Hirsutism
- Increased appetite; weight gain
- Increased low-density lipoprotein (LDL) cholesterol levels
- Oligomenorrhea, amenorrhea
- Pruritus
- Sebaceous cysts

Key Maternal Newborn Laboratory Values

Test	Non-pregnant Values	Pregnant Values	Neonatal Values
Hematocrit (%)	37–47	32–42	51–56
Hemoglobin (g/dL)	12–16	10–14	16.5 (cord blood)
Platelets (mm^3)	150,000–350,000	≠ 3 days after birth	150,000–400,000
Partial thromboplastin time (seconds)	22–34	Slight Ø in pregnancy and again in labor	≠ slightly for 1st 3 months
Fibrinogen (mg/dL)	175–400	Up to 600	——
Serum glucose (mg/dL)	70–80 (fasting) 60–110 (2-hr PP)	65 (fasting) < 140 (2-hr PP)	40–80
White blood cells (mm^3)	4,500–10,000	5,000–15,000	18,000
Sodium (mEq/L)	135–145	135–145	135–147
Potassium (mEq/L)	3.5–5.1	3.5–5.1	4–6
Chloride (mEq/L)	100–108	100–108	90–114
Bicarbonate (mEq/L)	22–26	22–26	20–26 (lower if premature)
Calcium (mg/dL)	8.5–10.5	Falls 10% by term	7.4–14

The Apgar Score

Sign	0	1	2
Heart rate	Absent	Less than 100/min	Greater than 100/min
Respiratory effort	Absent	Slow, irregular	Regular or crying
Reflex irritability	No response	Grimace, frown	Cry, cough
Muscle tone	Limp	Some motion, some flexion of extremities, some resistance to extension of extremities	Active, spontaneous flexion, good tone
Color	Cyanotic or pale	Body pink, extremities cyanotic	Completely pink

Episiotomy/Wound Assessment

The REEDA scale helps the nurse remember to consider each of the following:

R Redness
E Edema
E Ecchymosis
D Discharge
A Approximation of skin edges

ISBN 0-536-80700-0
90000
9 780536 807007
PEARSON
Prentice Hall

Roxann Moran
209 Primrose Ct. S.W.
Leesburg, VA 20175

Key Terms

Reflexology 58
Reiki 63
Therapeutic touch 63
Traditional Chinese medicine 54
Visualization 56

Until the latter part of the 20th century in the United States, it was rare for European American childbearing families to consult anyone except their obstetrician for advice about their pregnancy, birth, and postpartum. Though such clients are still encountered today, perinatal nurses are more likely to care for childbearing families who integrate other types of practitioners and therapies with traditional Western medicine. Families choosing complementary and alternative therapies may include those whose health practices are rooted in their cultural heritage, as well as European Americans who have explored one or more of the vast number of non-Western healing approaches available today. The nurse may even encounter families who consider alternative approaches superior to the diagnostics and treatments that conventional Western medicine offers, and who enter a clinic or hospital environment only reluctantly.

Since the use of complementary and alternative therapies has become so widespread, all nurses need to have at least a fundamental understanding of their benefits and risks, and guidelines for their safe use. The chapter begins with an overview of the evolution of complementary and alternative therapies. A brief description of the most common therapies currently used by childbearing families is also provided.

Evolution of Complementary and Alternative Therapies

A **complementary therapy** may be defined as an adjunct to conventional medical treatment that has been through rigorous scientific testing, which shows that it has some reliability. Although complementary therapies were entirely absent from clinics and hospitals until the last few decades, they are now often used together with conventional medical care. For example, both acupuncture and chiropractic are now commonly used in conjunction with pharmaceuticals and other conventional treatments for a variety of injuries and illnesses, and most health insurance plans cover at least a portion of the cost of such therapies.

In contrast, an **alternative therapy** is usually considered a substance or procedure that has not undergone rigorous scientific testing in this country, although it might have been thoroughly tested in other countries. Thus, alternative therapies are not usually available in conventional clinics and hospitals, and their costs are not typically covered under most health insurance policies. For example, research studies indicating the benefits of magnet therapy in treating some chronic conditions such as carpal tunnel syndrome have been conducted in India, Japan, and Russia; however, researchers in the United States are only beginning to study the effects of magnet therapy. Thus, this therapy is still considered experimental and would be classified as an alternative therapy.

The very terms *complementary* and *alternative* suggest the contemporary view that herbs, homeopathy, chiropractic, and other such healing techniques are peripheral to conventional Western medicine, which is the "primary" treatment. How did we come to hold this view? And what has contributed to the resurgence in complementary and alternative therapies in the last few decades?

Historical Perspective

Five hundred years ago, a Native American woman drinking hot water steeped with chamomile to settle her stomach would never have described her beverage as a complementary or alternative therapy. She was merely following a custom handed down to her by her ancestors and practiced widely in her tribe. If her symptoms continued, she would likely have consulted a medicine woman or medicine man, who might have performed a healing ritual using other herbs, stones, chanting, and/or communion with the "animal spirits" or ancestors who had passed on. Such forms of self- and community-based treatment, though varying somewhat from one culture to another, are thought to have been the norm around the world for thousands of years.

Many therapies that are today considered complementary or alternative grew out of indigenous cultures' use of the herbs, spices, flowers, fruits, and other plants and natural materials available in the region, and reflected their health concerns. For example, it has been proposed that one rationale for the highly spiced cuisine of India is that the spices used, in addition to being widely available, have an antimicrobial effect. This would have been important for a hot region of the world where food could not be preserved without fear of spoilage. In contrast, people in colder regions of the world, such as northern Europe, developed techniques such as salting, drying, and freezing foods during long winters to preserve them from microbial decay.

Many other complementary and alternative therapies developed from cultures' spiritual beliefs. Thousands of years ago, most cultures held the belief that illnesses and injuries—as well as therapies to heal them—were spiritually based. For example, peoples from ancient China, India, and the Americas shared the belief that all animals, plants, and even minerals contain a spiritual "essence," a vibrational life force that could be employed in healing. European peoples once believed that disease was caused by supernatural forces either to punish human beings or to teach them spiritual lessons. Others, such as the people of ancient India, believed that illness demonstrated a lack of alignment of the mind and body with God. For Patanjali, who wrote the *Yoga Sutras* in the third century BCE, a healthy body was a precondition for spiritual wholeness. In some cultures, spiritual healers performed rituals to exorcise the evil spirit from the diseased body.

Around 400 BCE, Hippocrates became the first practitioner in the West known to challenge the idea that illnesses and injuries have spiritual causes and remedies. His school of medicine investigated impurities in the individual's food, water, and environment as causes of disease, and attempted to base healing practices in the known laws of nature. Students began to investigate systematically the healing properties of local plants and other substances, and to develop standards of practice.

Over the next millennium, indigenous peoples worldwide continued to hand down the knowledge of healing plants and practices. Shamans, alchemists, and midwives were highly respected members of their communities and were relied upon for their cures. However, between the 13th and 17th centuries in Europe, Church-led inquisitions sought out and killed indigenous healers, typically burning them as "witches." At the same time, the new philosophy of rationalism became popular, and community leaders began to demand empirical evidence for healing practices. During the 17th century, the scientific method gained ascendancy, single-celled organisms were discovered, and the first experiments challenging the idea of spontaneous generation of life were conducted.

From the 18th to the 19th centuries, several scientific achievements further advanced the supremacy of empirically based medical techniques. High-powered microscopes were developed that could allow detection of microorganisms such as bacteria. In 1796, the English physician Edward Jenner developed the first effective vaccine, which used material from cowpox lesions to stimulate immunity to smallpox. In the mid-1800s, the French scientist Louis Pasteur conducted experiments that led to the formulation of the *germ theory of disease*; that is, the theory that microbes can cause human disease. In the 1860s, the English surgeon Joseph Lister introduced aseptic techniques using phenol and dramatically reduced the mortality rate following surgery. His techniques were widely adopted by other surgeons and led to increased acceptance of surgery as a viable treatment. By 1875, the German scientist Robert Koch had established postulates to prove whether a certain organism was pathogenic and what disease it caused. Thus, people learned that infectious disease, which was the leading cause of death at that time, was not due to spiritual flaws.

At the same time, European colonization of countries in Asia, Africa, Australia, and the Americas brought European medical practices as well. Indigenous healers and their therapies, such as the ayurvedic system of India and the nature-based therapies of Africa, were prohibited by the colonial powers and replaced with Western procedures and pharmaceuticals. In the United States, the American Medical Association (AMA) grew in prominence, replacing female midwives with male obstetricians, and homeopathic physicians (estimated to comprise about 50% of US physicians in the mid-19th century) with medical doctors who had graduated from AMA-approved schools of medicine.

In the early 20th century, several factors combined to ensure a virtual monopoly of conventional medicine in the United States. First, antimicrobial drugs and vaccines were developed that dramatically reduced morbidity and mortality due to infectious disease. Second, pharmaceutical companies began dominating medicine by heavily subsidizing US medical schools, giving rewards and subsidies to physicians who used their drugs, and lobbying US legislators for statutes and regulations favorable to their industry. Third, two world wars led to advances in both pharmaceuticals and surgical techniques that helped convince legislators of the superiority of the AMA's approach to healthcare.

Resurgence of Complementary and Alternative Therapies

Complementary and alternative therapies never entirely died out in the United States. Even in the 1950s, some people were able to eke out a living as chiropractors or herbalists. The social upheavals and "back to the land" movements of the 1960s and 1970s led to a renewed interest in the therapies of indigenous cultures and an increased interest in massage, sound, and crystals as healing therapies. Still, even in the 1980s, such therapies were not mainstream.

The dramatic increase in complementary and alternative therapies in the final decade of the 20th century was probably the result of a combination of several factors:

- Increased consumer awareness of the limitations of conventional Western medicine
- Increased international travel
- Increased media attention
- Advent of the Internet

America's love affair with conventional Western medicine began to cool in the latter part of the 20th century as costs increased, healthcare began to be seen as more technologic and less "human," and access to healthcare professionals' time became strictly limited. Childbearing families in particular began to seek more "natural" birth experiences, without anesthesia, in homelike settings attended by female certified nurse-midwives. Americans began to recognize that many health problems, such as cancer, diabetes, heart disease, autoimmune diseases, and others, could not be cured simply by swallowing a pill or "going under the knife." Such disorders came to be seen as complex, involving lifestyle factors, cultural factors, emotional elements, and—many people believed—spiritual aspects that were ignored by conventional approaches. Increasingly, people with such diseases turned to the complementary and alternative healing community.

As Americans began to engage more widely in international work, study, and travel, their exposure to other healing systems and practices increased. Indeed, several American physicians, disillusioned by the limitations of conventional Western medicine, traveled to Asia and other regions to study alternative therapies.

At the same time, the US media was beginning to pay attention to the complementary and alternative movement. The publication of Bill Moyers's *Healing and the Mind* in 1993, with its accompanying public television series, brought credibility to complementary and alternative therapies because all of Moyers's interviewees were respected scientists or physicians. For the same reason, the dramatic success of books on complementary therapies by Dr. Deepak Chopra, Dr. Andrew Weill, Dr. Joan Borysenko, and many others helped move complementary and alternative therapies into the forefront of public attention. Respected mainstream newspapers and national magazines began regularly to report on research and developments in complementary and alternative therapies, and television commercials began advertising nutritional supplements, homeopathic remedies, and other alternative products and services.

But perhaps the most explosive element in the resurgence of complementary and alternative therapies in the 1990s was the development of the Internet. With a computer and modem, information on alternative products and services was now just a few mouse clicks away. For example, a paper presented at a conference in Germany on the health benefits of reflexology might become available to Internet users worldwide the next day. The Internet increased not only information, but also communication among people with similar health concerns. A pregnant woman who had just begun to experience first trimester nausea could join a chat group debating the advantages and disadvantages of various remedies. Infertile couples could share a technique claiming to increase fertility that they had learned on a trip to Asia, or describe a fertility ritual they had learned from their Mexican grandmother. Suddenly, it became easy for people to integrate complementary and alternative therapies into their own unique approach to their healthcare concerns.

Growing Integration with Conventional Western Medicine

In this new century, it seems clear that the future of American healthcare will see an ever-increasing integration between conventional medicine and complementary therapies. Some obvious examples of this new integration in perinatal settings include the acceptance of certain herbal teas for antepartal discomforts; the use of massage, Reiki, or therapeutic touch during the first stage of labor; the use of music during childbirth; and the increased emphasis on skin-to-skin mother-to-baby bonding in the immediate postpartum period.

Further evidence of this increased integration was the establishment in 1992 of the Office of Alternative Medicine (OAM) at the National Institutes of Health. The OAM was mandated by Congress to promote research into complementary and alternative therapies and dissemination of information to consumers. In 1998 the OAM was incorporated into a new National Center for Complementary and Alternative Medicine (NCCAM) with an expanded mission and increased funding. Many studies of complementary and alternative therapies are currently under way at the NCCAM, which can be accessed via the Internet at the following site: http://nccam.nih.gov.

Benefits and Risks of Complementary and Alternative Therapies

Complementary and alternative therapies undisputedly have many benefits for the childbearing family and other healthcare consumers. However, many of these remedies have associated risks that must be considered thoughtfully before a decision is made to use them.

Benefits

Many complementary and alternative therapies emphasize prevention and wellness, and place a higher value on holistic healing than on physical cure. In addition, many are noninvasive and have few side effects, and many are more affordable and available than conventional therapies.

EMPHASIS ON PREVENTION AND WELLNESS

The therapies of conventional Western medicine—pharmaceuticals and surgery—are typically prescribed after a disease has already manifested in symptoms. These therapies are of course entirely appropriate—and may be lifesaving—in certain circumstances; for example, epinephrine for an acute asthma attack or appendectomy for appendicitis. However, they are limited in effectiveness for subacute conditions.

In contrast, most complementary and alternative therapeutic systems emphasize maintenance of wellness and prevention of illness. For example, a woman consulting a medical doctor for fatigue might be tested for iron deficiency anemia. If the lab test came back negative, the woman might be advised simply to try to get more sleep, and the physician might prescribe a sedative to help achieve a full night's rest. In contrast, a woman consulting a practitioner of naturopathy, homeopathy, traditional Chinese medicine, or ayurveda (these systems are described shortly) would likely be asked dozens of questions about every aspect of her life, including her childhood, relationships, work habits, diet, lifestyle, stressors, and even how she feels about sunny days versus rain. These questions would attempt to unearth the underlying cause of even the most subtle complaints, and to prescribe remedies in several domains (acupuncture, homeopathic treatments, herbs, nutritional modifications, lifestyle modifications, massage, color therapy, and so forth) early enough in the process of breakdown to restore wellness before true disease manifests.

MEDIALINK NATIONAL CENTER FOR COMPLEMENTARY AND ALTERNATIVE MEDICINE

EMPHASIS ON HEALING VERSUS CURE

The complementary therapeutic systems attempt to assess, diagnose, and treat the whole person. For example, the homeopathic physician and author Dr. Andrew Lockie and his associate Dr. Nicola Geddes (2000) have identified a breadth of concerns of the holistic healer that might seem

Table 3-1 • CONCERNS OF THE HOLISTIC HEALER

The holistic healer may be concerned with the following aspects of the client's life:

- Exercise, breathing, and posture
- Self-care, including dental care
- Nutrition, hydration, use of dietary supplements, and method of food preparation
- Digestion and elimination
- Sleep/wake cycles
- Stress and emotional responses
- Purity of air, food, water, and environment
- Use of alcohol, tobacco, caffeine, and other substances
- Employment and unemployment
- Hobbies, sports, and other recreational activities
- Home life and relationships
- Spirituality
- Type and age of bed and bedding
- Types of clothing, cosmetics, and personal care products used
- Pets
- Exposure to and use of sound and music
- Reactions to weather and seasons
- Electromagnetic phenomena and exposure to radiation
- Exposure to sunlight and artificial light
- Travel
- Personality and temperament
- Fears (e.g., of heights, of death, etc.)

Source: Compiled from data in Lockie, P., & Geddes, N. (2000). *Complete guide to homeopathy: The principles and practice of treatment.* New York: DK Publishing.

astonishing—and even irrelevant—to someone familiar with only conventional approaches (Table 3-1 •).

This holistic approach extends to the goal of therapy as well; that is, the goal of many complementary therapies is not curing an illness but rather healing the client's psyche, spirit, body, and even community. The physician and author Dr. Rachel Naomi Remen describes healing as "a process we're all involved in all the time." She states that healing includes education, the leading forth of wholeness in people. "Sometimes people heal physically, and they don't heal emotionally, or mentally, or spiritually. And sometimes people heal emotionally, and they don't heal physically. . . . People can heal and live, and people can heal and die" (Moyers, 1993, p. 344).

NONINVASIVE

In part because of this emphasis on healing versus cure, many of the therapeutic techniques offered by complementary systems are noninvasive and potentially enriching on many levels. For example, imagery is often used to help cancer patients enhance their immune function, but also to help increase their optimism and gain new access to feelings of love and nurturance that may have been buried by fear of their diagnosis. Meditation, hypnosis, and biofeedback are other mind-based therapies that are entirely noninvasive and can affect the client on several levels. Massage and the other body-based therapies noninvasively promote healing of both the physical body and the client's psyche. Music, light, colors, magnets, gems, and fragrances are also noninvasive, and likely achieve their effects by subtly influencing the neurochemistry, circulation, memories, and/or emotions of the client. Indeed, only a very few of the complementary therapies are invasive: these include acupuncture, certain techniques used in ayurveda, foods and dietary supplements, herbs, homeopathic remedies, and flower essences, the latter two of which are highly diluted substances.

COST AND ACCESS

Complementary and alternative therapies may be less expensive and more readily available than conventional remedies. For example, most homeopathic remedies cost less than $10 for a vial of 100 pellets or tablets. Flower essences, essential oils, herbs, and dietary supplements also tend to be far less expensive than most conventional pharmaceuticals. In fact, some complementary and alternative therapies—including meditation, prayer, visualization, self-massage, dietary modifications, regular physical exercise, music therapy, and color therapy—are free.

Visits to complementary healers are usually somewhat less expensive than visits to medical doctors; however, most insurance carriers do not cover complementary therapies unless the primary care physician has prescribed them. On the other hand, in some cases it is far easier to access complementary healers than conventional physicians—and at little or no expense to the consumer. Many neighborhood pharmacies and even grocery stores now have on staff herbalists, nutritionists, and others trained in a wide range of complementary therapies. No appointment is necessary to consult with them and no fee is charged. The same is true for complementary healers who have Web sites: by searching the Internet, it is possible for a childbearing family to glean tips on everything from relieving first-trimester nausea, to managing pain during childbirth without drugs, to preventing plugged ducts during breastfeeding.

Risks

These benefits of complementary and alternative therapies notwithstanding, it is critical that all consumers—and especially childbearing families—be aware of their not-insignificant risks. These include lack of standardization, lack of regulation and research substantiating safety and effectiveness, inadequate training and certification of some healers, and financial and health risks of unproven methods.

LACK OF STANDARDIZATION

Pharmaceuticals prescribed by a Western physician or nurse practitioner have been approved by the Food and Drug Administration (FDA). All preparations of an FDA-approved pharmaceutical, whether a brand-name drug or a generic version, have to contain identical quantities of certain precisely regulated, purified substances. In contrast, herbs, dietary supplements, and other non-FDA-approved ingested remedies may vary dramatically from one manufacturer to another. For example, preparations of herbs may use the flowers, leaves, or stems, all of which vary in potency, and preparations may contain various concentrations of the actual herb versus carrier materials. Additionally, some manufacturers use such harsh chemicals to process herbs that their healthful properties are reduced or lost. Some herbs lose their potency over time with different types of storage, whereas others vary in strength according to the soil in which they were grown or the season in which they were harvested. This lack of standardization means that one preparation may be highly potent while another is ineffective.

LACK OF REGULATION AND RESEARCH

Complementary and alternative remedies are largely unregulated, and their claims may not be backed by valid, reliable research. Approval by the FDA guarantees that a drug has been subjected to—and passed—a rigorous process requiring, in most cases, development under strictly controlled conditions, precise molecular delineation of all components, and double-blind research studies substantiating the safety and effectiveness of the drug for the purpose under investigation. For this reason, when a childbearing client is told that a certain drug will safely induce labor, or when a breastfeeding mother is told that a drug will relieve her breast tenderness without harming her infant, she can accept these statements with confidence.

In contrast, the claims to effectiveness and safety of some complementary therapies may be largely unsubstantiated, resting on flawed or inadequate research, testimonials, tradition, or merely the healer's say-so. Thus, the consumer choosing these therapies often has little valid and reliable evidence that they will work effectively and safely.

The current inadequacy of research into complementary and alternative therapies is often due to lack of funding. When drug manufacturers commit millions of dollars to research and development of new pharmaceuticals, they do so knowing that, if they succeed in developing a safe and effective drug, their financial gain will more than cover their investment. In contrast, no one profits financially from consumers who use meditation, prayer, visualization, dietary modifications, exercise, water therapy, music, or sunlight. Even the profits from essential oils, flower remedies, herbs, and the body-based therapies are minimal compared to the costs of research studies to substantiate their use. Fortunately the NCCAM is beginning to fund research into several of these therapies.

Research into complementary and alternative therapies is also hindered by the very nature of these therapies. It is comparatively easy to provide a control group with either the drug being studied or a placebo and then to measure reduction in symptoms, but how does one design a reliable, valid study of therapies that attempt to maintain wellness or prevent illness, that value healing rather than cure, that claim to work on subtle, vibrational levels, or that admit to the necessity of a therapeutic relationship with the healer? Currently there is so little understanding of the cultural, psychologic, emotional, and spiritual aspects of healing that investigators trained in quantitative research methodologies may be unprepared even to design studies of complementary and alternative therapies. On the other hand, it is interesting to note that several qualitative nursing research studies over the past decade have studied complementary and alternative therapies with some success.

INADEQUATE TRAINING AND CERTIFICATION

Many complementary therapies do have rigorous training and testing requirements that applicants must fulfill before they receive certification as practitioners. For example, naturopathic, homeopathic, and chiropractic physicians usually complete a typical undergraduate premedical program before enrolling in a 4-year graduate school in their specialty. Acupuncturists, certified massage therapists, Reiki practitioners, sound healers, and many other complementary therapists must complete a course of study at an approved school, achieve a certain number of hours of practice, and pass an exam before they are certified.

In contrast, many titles are unregulated. For example, many states do not require that people calling themselves "counselors," "nutritionists," "healers," "intuitives," or "consultants" have any particular education or license. Thus, consumers who purchase the services of such therapists must beware.

FINANCIAL AND HEALTH RISKS OF UNPROVEN METHODS

As noted earlier, complementary and alternative remedies and techniques may cost considerably less than conventional pharmaceuticals and procedures. However, consumers may make a considerable investment in unproven methods and products that do not, in the end, improve their well-being, prevent illness, or promote healing.

Although few complementary and alternative therapies actually harm consumers directly, consumers' health may indeed suffer if their belief in the therapy or healer causes them to delay or forgo conventional medical treatments. Tragically, each year in the United States, cases of fetal demise occur among childbearing families who choose to use unlicensed birth attendants in home settings.

Types of Complementary and Alternative Therapies

The following review of complementary and alternative therapies is meant as an introduction. The list is not exhaustive, and the descriptions are exceedingly brief. For more information, consult the Web sites listed in Table 3-2 ●.

The categories under which particular therapies are discussed here are somewhat arbitrary. For example, homeopathy is categorized as a complementary therapeutic system, but it could also be considered an energy therapy. Therapeutic touch and Reiki are both energy based and body based. Massage is a sense therapy in that it approaches the client through touch, yet it is classified with the body-based therapies. In truth, the holistic nature of these therapies means that they affect the client in many different ways.

MEDIALINK RESOURCES FOR COMPLEMENTARY AND ALTERNATIVE THERAPIES

Table 3–2 • SOURCES OF INFORMATION ON COMPLEMENTARY AND ALTERNATIVE THERAPIES

CAM Modality	Organization	Web Site
Acupressure	Acupressure Institute	www.acupressure.com
Acupuncture	National Acupuncture Oriental Medical Alliance	www.acuall.org
Acupuncture and Oriental medicine	National Certification Commission for Acupuncture and Oriental Medicine	www.nccaom.org
Alexander technique	North American Society of Teachers of the Alexander Technique	www.alexandertech.org
Aromatherapy	National Association for Holistic Aromatherapy	www.naha.org
Biofeedback	Association for Applied Psychophysiology and Biofeedback	www.aaph.org
Chiropractic	American Chiropractic Association	www.amerchiro.org
Craniosacral therapy	Cranio-sacral therapy (Upledger)	www.Upledger.com
Feldenkrais	Feldenkrais Guild of North America	www.feldenkrais.com
Herbs	American Botanical Council	www.herbalgram.org
Homeopathy	National Center for Homeopathy	www.homeopathic.org
Massage therapy	National Certification Board for Therapeutic Massage and Bodywork	www.ncbtmb.com
Massage therapy	American Massage Therapy Association	www.amtamassage.org
Meditation	Meditation Institute of Noetic Sciences	www.noetic.org
Reflexology	Reflexology Association of America	www.reflexology-usa.org
Sound	Sound Healers Association	www.healingsound.com
Therapeutic touch	Therapeutic Touch Nurse Healers Professional Association	www.therapeutic-touch.org

Note: The authors do not officially endorse any of these Web sites.

Complementary Therapeutic Systems

The complementary therapeutic systems described here are complex and multidimensional, incorporating several different techniques into a holistic approach to wellness, prevention, and healing.

HOMEOPATHY

Homeopathy is best understood in contrast to conventional Western medicine, which is also called *allopathic medicine.* The term *allopathy* is derived from the Greek words *allos* meaning different and *pathos* meaning suffering. Thus, allopathic medicine, which has been dominant in the United States for over 100 years, uses remedies that produce effects differing from—or in opposition to—those of the disease being treated. Thus, conventional health care practitioners may prescribe an antiinflammatory to reduce swelling or a sedative to relieve insomnia.

In contrast, the term **homeopathy** is derived from the Greek word *homos* meaning the same. Thus, it is often described as a healing system that uses like to cure like; that is, homeopathic remedies are minute dilutions of substances that, if ingested in larger amounts, would produce effects *similar* to the symptoms of the disorder being treated. For example, *Cantharis vesicatoria* is a species of beetle (commonly called Spanish fly) whose poison causes, among other things, burning urinary tract pain and a continous urge to urinate (Lockie & Geddes, 2000). Homeopathic *Cantharis* is a minute dilution of this toxin, and is thus a remedy of choice for women suffering from cystitis.

Founded by the German physician Samuel Hahnemann in the late 18th century, homeopathy traces its roots to Hippocrates, who was the first physician known to have observed the principle of like curing like. Homeopathic remedies are believed to achieve their effects by stimulating the client's immune system to mount a response against the diluted substance. Thus, it is the individual's own body, rather than the ingested remedy, that opposes the symptoms. Indeed, homeopathic physicians advise that an initial worsening of symptoms indicates that the correct remedy has been given.

It is important to note that, although homeopaths do rely on certain standard remedies such as *Cantharis* for cystitis, they believe that physical symptoms manifest disturbances on far deeper levels. Thus, they work to peel away ever-more subtle layers of disturbance, beginning with the obvious physical symptoms and moving deeper to those that may have originated in the client's childhood. Thereby, homeopaths work to effect holistic healing.

NATUROPATHY

Naturopathy is commonly referred to as *natural medicine.* It is more precisely defined as a healing system that employs various natural means of preventing and treating human disease. Many naturopathic physicians are eclectic, employing a variety of therapies in their practice. These might include clinical nutrition, botanical medicine, homeopathy, acupuncture, hydrotherapy, physiotherapy, and counseling for lifestyle modification (Murray & Pizzorno, 2001). For example, a naturopath might counsel a woman with vaginitis to eliminate from her diet all refined foods, to reduce her intake of sugars and fats, to consume lactobacillus-culture yogurt, to take B-complex vitamins and other supplements, to cleanse with a calendula preparation, and to avoid sexual intercourse.

TRADITIONAL CHINESE MEDICINE

Traditional Chinese medicine (TCM) developed more than 3000 years ago in the Chinese culture and then gradually spread with modifications to other Asian countries in-

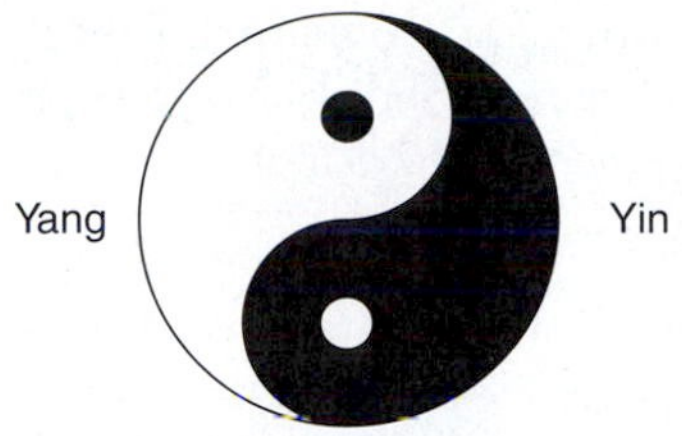

Figure 3–1 ● Traditional Chinese symbol of the opposing forces of *yin* and *yang* in perfect balance, representing integration and wholeness.

cluding Japan, Vietnam, Tibet, and Korea. Its goal is to promote health and well-being, so the underlying focus of TCM is prevention although diagnosis and treatment of disease also play an important role.

TCM seeks to ensure the balance of energy, which is called *chi* or *qi* (pronounced "chee"). Chi is the invisible flow of energy in the body that maintains health and energy and enables the body to carry out its physiologic functions. Chi flows along certain pathways or meridians, which are discussed on p. 62 under acupuncture and acupressure.

Another important concept in TCM (mentioned briefly in Chapter 2) is that of *yin* and *yang*, opposing internal and external forces that, together, represent the whole (Figure 3-1 ●). Yin is the female force—passive, cool, wet, and close to the earth. Yang is the masculine force—aggressive, hot, dry, and celestial. Yin and yang cannot exist independently because they are complementary and both are essential. Certain foods, behaviors, and environmental factors are believed to increase yin, while others increase yang. Well-being occurs when these two opposing forces are in balance, and illness can result if this balance is disturbed over a period of time.

TCM includes the following therapeutic techniques:

- Acupuncture (described shortly)
- Herbal therapy (*Note:* It is sometimes difficult to locate a skilled Chinese herbalist because there are relatively few practitioners of Chinese herbology in the United States [Bratman, 1998].)
- Nutrition
- Acupressure (Chinese massage) (described shortly)
- *Moxibustion*, which involves the application of heat from a small piece of burning herb called *moxa* (*Artemisia vulgaris*, commonly called "mugwort"). In the direct method, the herb is burned either on an acupuncture needle tip or on another substance that is then placed over the designated acupoint. The heat from the burning herbal stick, when applied to the appropriate acupoint, is believed to regulate the flow of chi. In the indirect method, which is more commonly used, smoldering moxa sticks are held near the skin (Shealy, 1999).
- *Qigong* (pronounced "chee-goong"), which is a self-discipline that involves the use of breathing, meditation, self-massage, and movement. Typically practiced daily, the movements are nontiring and are designed to stimulate the flow of chi (Figure 3-2 ●).

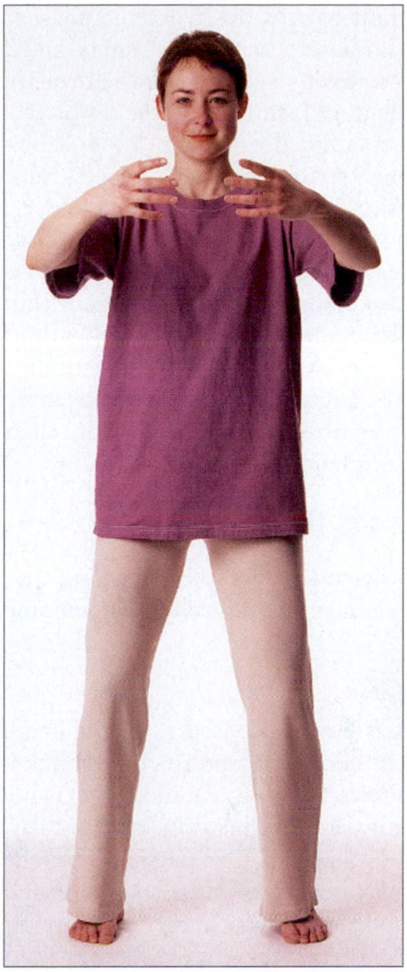

Figure 3–2 ● Pregnant woman practices the movements of *Qigong*.
SOURCE: Guy Ryecart/Dorling Kindersley Media Library.

- T'ai chi (pronounced "ty chee"), which is a form of martial art. It originally focused on physical fitness and self-defense, but is currently used more as a health discipline. T'ai chi resembles a cross between slow-motion dancing and shadow boxing and is helpful in improving balance in older adults. It is also used for hypertension, arthritis, and osteoporosis (Fontaine, 2000).

AYURVEDA

The classical system of Hindu medicine is known as **ayurveda** (Crawford, 1996). The term *ayurveda* is derived from the Sanskrit words *ayus* meaning life, health, and vitality, and *veda* meaning science or knowledge. Thus, ayurveda is the knowledge of how to live a vital, healthful life. Ayurvedic physicians believe that the five elements of ether, wind, fire, water, and earth take form in the body as three tendencies, called *doshas:* vata, pitta, and kapha. Each person's constitution is believed to reflect some combination of these three doshas. For example, vata reflects the elements of ether and wind; thus, a person in whom vata is dominant may be flighty, ungrounded, and anxious, with dry skin, eyes, and respiratory membranes. The primary element in kapha is water, and so it is not surprising that pregnancy is considered a kapha condition.

An important part of the ayurvedic physician's job is to balance the doshas to achieve harmony and holism. The physician does this by suppressing the dosha that is dominating the client and stimulating the dosha that is sluggish. For example, a fatigued woman in whom kapha is too dominant may be prescribed hot foods, spices, warm colors, energizing music, pungent aromas, and other therapies to stimulate her internal fire (pitta) and burn away some of her internal water (kapha). This is a simplistic example of a highly complex system, but the important thing to bear in mind about ayurveda is that, like homeopathy, naturopathy, and TCM, it approaches the client holistically, through the diet, the senses, breathing, posture, sleep patterns, and even through examination and alteration of the client's work life, home routine, relationships, and spirituality.

Mind-Based Therapies

This section discusses therapies engaging the mind in activities such as imagination, reflection, communication, or relaxation.

BIOFEEDBACK

Biofeedback is a method used to help individuals learn to control their physiologic responses based on the concept that the mind controls the body. An individual is hooked up to a system of highly sensitive instruments that relay information about the body back to that person. The effectiveness of biofeedback has been proven in countless studies and it is now considered a conventional therapy more than a complementary one. For example, biofeedback may focus on temperature or thermal feedback, especially in treating certain vascular diseases or in promoting relaxation. It may focus on galvanic skin response, which measures sweat gland activity in the fingers or palms, in helping people learn to deal with stress or excessive perspiration. It may use electromyography (EMG) to provide feedback about muscle tension to help in the treatment of muscle spasm, tension headache, and pain reduction. It may use electroencephalography (EEG) to gain information about brain wave activity to help with insomnia, pain management, and substance abuse.

Currently biofeedback has more than 150 applications for disease prevention and the restoration of health, including stress-related disorders such as insomnia, anxiety, headaches, hypertension, and asthma; gastrointestinal disorders such as ulcers and irritable bowel syndrome; temporomandibular joint syndrome; and hyperactivity in children (*Nurse's Handbook*, 1999).

HYPNOSIS

Hypnosis, whether guided by a trained hypnotherapist or induced through self-hypnosis, is a state of great mental and physical relaxation during which a person is very open to suggestions. Because hypnosis cannot make people do something against their will, hypnosis will not work unless an individual is really interested in changing. Studies have shown that some people are able to anesthetize themselves using hypnosis, and higher levels of endorphins, the body's natural painkiller, have been reported following hypnotherapy (Shealy, 1999). Pregnant women who receive hypnosis before childbirth have reported shorter, less painful labors and births (*Nurse's Handbook*, 1999).

MEDITATION AND PRAYER

Many people think of meditation as sitting quietly with the legs crossed and eyes closed, repeating a *mantra* or counting one's breaths in order to still the mind and bring peace. In contrast, the great spiritual teacher J. Krishnamurti (1895–1986) defined *meditation* far more simply, as something one can do every day at any moment. For Krishnamurti (2000), "Meditation is to perceive the truth each second. . . When the mind has seen the fallacy of [accumulated knowledge] completely, then it is in a constant state of 'not knowing.' Such a mind can then receive that which is not measurable and which only comes into being from moment to moment." When clients allow their family values, education, social conditioning, knowledge, desires, expectations, and all other "accumulations" to fade away, and listen receptively in a state of not knowing, they experience an emptiness that is itself transformative and healing (Figure 3-3 •).

Whereas meditation is often likened to listening, *prayer* is an act of silently or vocally addressing a deity such as Allah, Jesus, Shiva, or the Great Spirit, or for clients outside of a particular religious tradition, simply "talking to the Universe." The effect of prayer on healing has been studied and documented and more research is under way.

Nurses need to be cognizant of the spiritual needs of the people for whom they care because religion is so often a part of people's lives. Thus nurses, and all healthcare workers, need to be respectful of an individual's belief system and choices about issues of doctrine. Healthcare professionals also must avoid pushing religion onto people or attempting to convert clients to a particular faith.

VISUALIZATION AND GUIDED IMAGERY

Visualization, a complementary therapy, has been used since ancient times. In visualization a person goes into a relaxed state and focuses on or "visualizes" soothing or positive scenes such as a beach or a mountain glade. Visualization

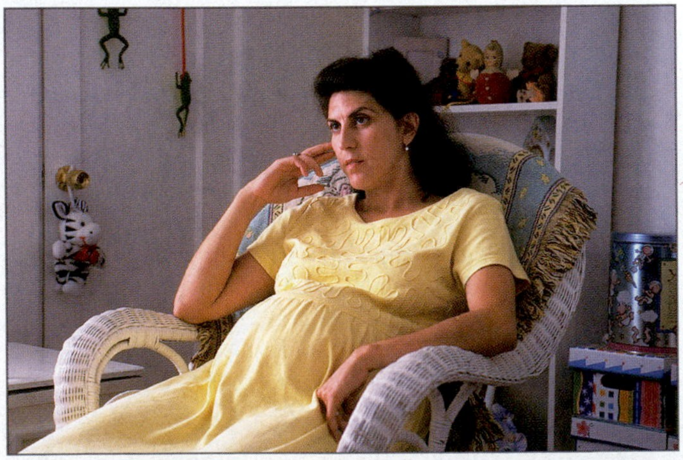

Figure 3–3 • Meditation does not have to be practiced in a particular place, time, or pose, but can be incorporated into each day.
SOURCE: Michael Newman/PhotoEdit.

helps reduce stress and encourage relaxation. For example, a therapist may work with a woman before childbirth to help her create positive images of labor.

Guided imagery is a state of intense, focused concentration used to create compelling mental images. It is sometimes considered a form of hypnosis. Guided imagery is useful in imagining a desired effect such as weight loss or in mentally rehearsing a new procedure or activity. Skill in using guided imagery improves with practice so people who wish to use it should set aside 5 to 20 minutes of quiet time once or twice daily and practice creating images that are personal and meaningful.

Body-Based Therapies

Therapies requiring practitioner manipulation of the body are discussed here, along with hydrotherapy, hatha yoga, and regular physical exercise.

CHIROPRACTIC THERAPY

Chiropractic, the third largest independent health profession in the United States (behind medicine and dentistry), is based on concepts of manipulation. It was developed by Daniel David Palmer, a self-taught American healer, in the late 19th century. Palmer believed that many diseases and illnesses were the result of abnormal nerve transmissions (subluxation) caused by misalignment of the spine. He postulated that spinal manipulation could correct these vertebral misalignments. In 1898 he founded the Palmer Chiropractic Institute in Iowa and began training others in his approach. For many years, chiropractic was viewed with scorn by traditional medical doctors, who refused to refer clients to chiropractors. In the early 1990s, however, a Supreme Court ruling against the American Medical Association (AMA) required medical doctors to cooperate with the chiropractic profession (Bratman, 1998).

Currently chiropractors are licensed in all 50 states and are regulated by state boards. Chiropractors continue to focus on the close relationship between structure and function but also stress the importance of proper nutrition and regular exercise to good health. Chiropractic is widely available, and popular demand has earned it a higher level of insurance coverage than most other alternative therapies.

A number of studies have shown chiropractic to be effective in treating problems such as lower back pain. Some women find chiropractic effective in managing the backache and physical stress resulting from spinal realignment secondary to increased body weight and changing body contours during pregnancy (Cole, 1998).

Clients who are considering chiropractic therapy should consider the following recommendations (Mayo Clinic, 2001):

- They should ask their primary caregiver for referral to the appropriate professional, which may be a chiropractor, physical therapist, or osteopathic physician.
- If they seek chiropractic care without referral, they should choose someone who has completed a training program at a school accredited by the Council on Chiropractic Education.
- They should see only chiropractors who are willing to give them a written treatment plan, who send a written report to the primary physician or care provider, and who allow the care provider to observe the chiropractic treatment, if desired.
- They should avoid chiropractors who order frequent x-rays and who ask them to extend treatment indefinitely.
- They should avoid chiropractors that consider spinal manipulation a cure for "anything that ails you." No research supports this notion.

CRANIOSACRAL THERAPY

Craniosacral therapy, developed by Dr. John Upledger in the 1970s, is a variation of cranial osteopathy, which is the belief that the bones of the skull do not fuse completely during childhood and that rhythmic impulses can be detected. The craniosacral therapist uses light touch—generally no more than the weight of a nickel—to test for restrictions in the craniosacral system. This is done by holding a client's head and other designated parts of the body and focusing on monitoring the subtle rhythm of the cerebrospinal fluid as it flows through the system. According to Upledger (1998), the therapist's light, hands-on approach assists the hydraulic forces inherent in the craniosacral system to improve the body's internal environment and strengthen its ability to heal itself.

ALEXANDER TECHNIQUE

The focus of the *Alexander technique* is on proper alignment of the head, neck, and trunk. This movement education technique was developed by F.M. Alexander, an Australian actor, in the late 1900s. Before his death, Alexander set up schools to teach his technique to others. A certified Alexander instructor has extensive training in the approach. The Alexander technique is used by many schools of music and acting worldwide, but is becoming more commonly used by people in other professions to improve their posture, alignment, and ease of movement.

After completing an assessment, an Alexander instructor uses touch, instructions (verbal cuing), and activities to guide clients into the correct use of their bodies. In the beginning the instructor monitors the student but after a time the student begins to self-monitor posture and movements. Individuals who employ the technique tend to suffer less from repetitive strain injuries and are more relaxed during performances than those who do not (Shealy, 1999).

The Alexander technique, though not in itself a therapy, has been proven to help problems related to poor posture, other musculoskeletal complaints, and even certain respiratory and digestive problems. Secondarily, it is useful in reducing both physical and mental stress. Consequently it is often recommended for stress-related disorders.

FELDENKRAIS

The *Feldenkrais method*, another movement-oriented therapy, was developed by the Russian-born physicist, educator, and judo expert, Moshe Feldenkrais. It is based on the belief that health is improved by establishing new connections between the brain and body through movement re-education. The

Feldenkrais practitioner uses verbal instruction and hands-on assistance to help clients become aware of their movements and to develop alternate ways of moving that improve posture, flexibility, and range of motion, as well as physical performance and well-being. The movements also help relieve certain forms of discomfort such as backache, muscle tension, shoulder pain, and jaw pain. Feldenkrais did not view his approach as a medical therapy but rather a training method (*Nurse's Handbook*, 1999).

MASSAGE THERAPY

Massage has been used for centuries as a form of therapy. **Massage therapy** involves the manipulation of the soft tissues of the body to reduce stress and tension, increase circulation, diminish pain, and promote a sense of well-being. Different techniques have been developed, including for example, Swedish massage, shiatsu massage, Rolfing, trigger point massage, Thai massage, and sports massage. Most forms of massage use approaches such as pressing, kneading, gliding, circular motion, tapping, and vibrational strokes.

Certification and/or licensure for massage therapists varies from state to state although most states require at least 500 hours of training. Massage therapists who have passed the written examination given by the National Certification Board for Therapeutic Massage and Bodywork (NCBTMB) are nationally certified. Continuing education is then required for recertification.

Certain massage therapists specialize in massage for women during pregnancy (Figure 3-4 •). Massage is often helpful as women adapt to the discomforts of their changing bodies. In addition, certified nurse-midwives often use perineal massage prior to labor to stretch the muscles of the perineum around the vaginal opening and thereby prevent tearing of the tissues during childbirth. During labor, massage of the back and buttocks by the nurse, labor coach, or doula can help the woman relax and may help decrease her discomfort.

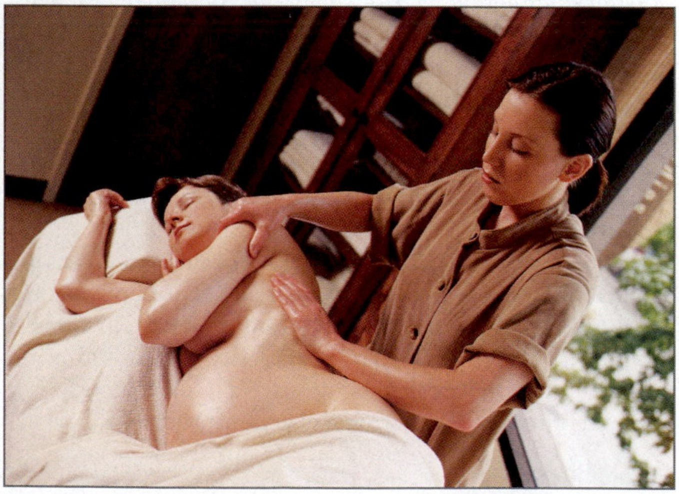

Figure 3–4 • Pregnant woman receiving massage. Massage is often useful in helping a pregnant woman cope with the discomforts of pregnancy.
SOURCE: Steve Mason/Getty Images, Inc.

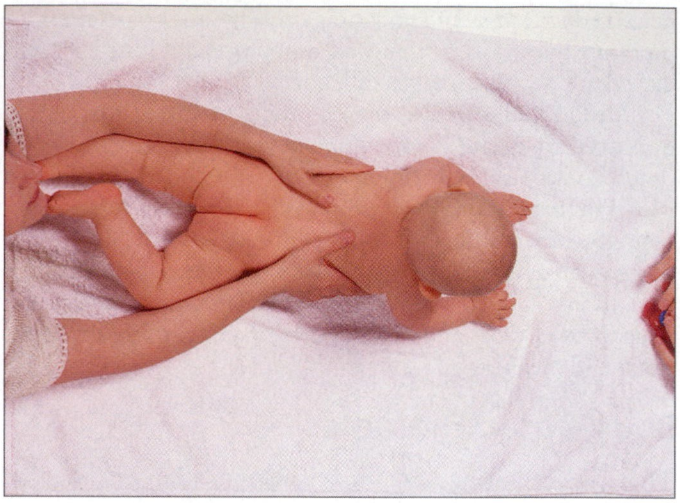

Figure 3–5 • Infant massage.
SOURCE: Jules Selmes/Dorling Kindersley Media Library.

Infant massage has become increasingly popular in the United States (Figure 3-5 •). The calm, soothing strokes of baby massage can help soothe an infant and minimize crying. In addition, research has demonstrated that massage can boost an infant's immune system, relieve colic, lower stress levels, and promote sleep (Maxwell-Hudson, 1999).

REFLEXOLOGY

Reflexology is a form of massage that involves the application of pressure to designated points or reflexes on the client's feet, hands, or ears using the thumb and fingers. Eunice Ingham, a physical therapist, mapped the specific reflex zones and is credited with spreading the practice of reflexology.

Reflexology most often involves manipulation of the feet. Practitioners believe that distinct areas of the feet correspond to particular organs or body systems. The stimulation of the appropriate region is intended to eliminate energy blockages thought to produce pain or disease. Organs on the right side of the body are represented on the right foot and organs on the left side are represented on the left foot (Figure 3-6 •). Although they are used less frequently, the hands and ears have also been mapped.

HYDROTHERAPY

Hydrotherapy is the term used to describe therapy that makes use of hot or cold moisture in any form. Hydrotherapy is used to relax muscles, promote rest, decrease pain, reduce swelling, promote healing, cleanse wounds and burns, reduce fever, lessen cramps, and improve well-being. The major types of hydrotherapy include the following:

- *Compresses* (ice packs, hot water packs, towels or dressings soaked in hot or cold water and rung out). Compresses are applied locally and are often alternated between hot and cold compresses. They are especially effective in improving circulation to a given area thereby reducing swelling and promoting healing. They are also helpful in reducing pain or achiness in a given area.

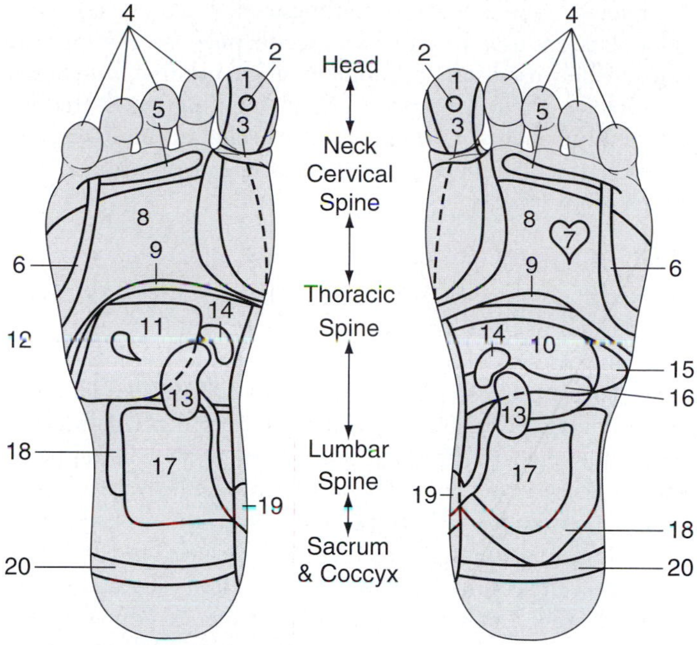

Figure 3–6 • Foot reflexology points.
SOURCE: Fontaine, K.L. *Healing practices,* 2000, p. 208. Reprinted by permission of Pearson Education, Upper Saddle River, NJ.

- *Baths* (local, such as a foot bath or sitz bath, or full immersion bath). Baths serve many of the same functions as compresses but also are effective in cleansing. Full immersion baths are often used in treating extensive burns and in rehabilitation.
- *Sweat baths* (steam bath or sauna). Sweat baths are used to open pores and induce sweating because sweating is a type of detoxification that is helpful in promoting the elimination of toxins, drugs, and salts from the body. Because high heat has been associated with neural tube defects, pregnant women should not do steam baths or saunas, especially in the first trimester (Fontaine, 2000).

HATHA YOGA

When they hear the word *yoga,* most people think of people in leotards moving through a series of postures, such as the cat stretch or the salute to the sun. In reality, the term *yoga* comes from the Sanskrit word for union, and implies a path toward union with God. **Hatha yoga** is the physical branch of yoga, and in the United States, it is commonly practiced for wellness, illness prevention, and healing. In hatha yoga, the client moves through a series of gentle stretches and postures (called *asanas*), coordinated with deep, rhythmic breathing techniques that promote oxygenation of all body tissues.

Certain yoga positions are especially beneficial during pregnancy and can be practiced safely by most women. These techniques coordinate breathing with movement while increasing strength and suppleness, providing valuable preparation for childbirth. In many communities, yoga teachers offer classes specifically designed for pregnant women (Figure 3-7 •).

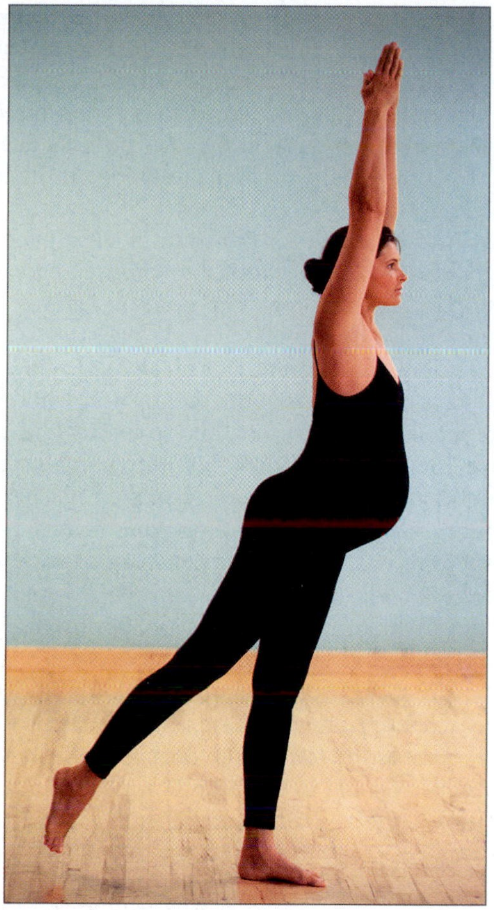

Figure 3–7 • Pregnant woman doing a hatha yoga stretch.
SOURCE: Ryan McVay/Getty Images, Inc.

REGULAR PHYSICAL EXERCISE

As more and more people are recognizing, regular physical exercise plays an important role in maintaining health and fitness. Exercise is important in maintaining muscle tone and strength, controlling weight, promoting cardiovascular health, improving digestion and elimination, reducing stress, promoting sleep, preventing a variety of chronic health problems, and providing an overall sense of fitness and well-being. In addition, exercise programs are an important component of ongoing therapy for a variety of health conditions such as arthritis, diabetes, and osteoporosis. Exercise is also crucial as part of recovery from heart attacks, fractures, orthopedic surgery, and stroke.

For further discussion of exercise during pregnancy, please refer to Chapter 16.

Nutritional and Herbal Therapies

The nutritional and herbal therapies include the use of particular foods as remedies, the use of vitamins, minerals, and other supplements, and the use of herbs.

DIETARY THERAPIES

It has long been recognized that certain foods have properties that are necessary for health, for healing, and for well-being. For example, caregivers have long known that people who are weak and easily fatigued often benefit from a diet rich in iron. Sailors learned to avoid the havoc caused by scurvy by including foods rich in vitamin C such as citrus fruits. However, the value of a nutritious diet in maintaining health is becoming more widely recognized and concerns are growing about the quality of some of the food products available today.

As part of their quest for optimum health, people make choices about their diets: whether to choose vegetarianism, a high-protein, low-carbohydrate diet, or a more balanced combination based on the Food Guide Pyramid; whether to consume alcohol in moderation or no alcohol at all; whether to include processed foods in the diet or not; whether to incorporate regular fasting or not, and so forth. The literature offers a wealth of information about nutrition and diet therapy. Some of this information is grounded in data and research; other relies more on tradition and hearsay.

Diet therapy is also an important part of treatment for many health conditions such as coronary artery disease, gout, kidney stones, gallbladder disease, Crohn disease, anemia, diverticulitis, and so forth. The importance of good nutrition for pregnant women and for infants and children cannot be overemphasized. Please refer to Chapter 18 for a discussion of nutrition for women during pregnancy and the postpartum period and to Chapter 31 for a discussion of infant nutrition.

USE OF SUPPLEMENTS

A *dietary supplement* is any product (excluding tobacco) intended to supplement the diet. It may be available for ingestion in the form of a powder, capsule, geltab, liquid, extract, and so forth, and it contains one or more of the following ingredients: a mineral, vitamin, herb, amino acid, other botanical supplements, or extracts and ingredients of animal and plant origin. Dietary supplements are not presented as conventional food products and they are not intended to be the sole item of a meal or of the diet (National Institutes of Health, 2001).

Dietary supplements, sometimes called natural food supplements, are used to achieve a specific purpose. Perhaps the most widely used form of supplement is a multivitamin tablet or capsule. Table 3-3 • provides information on selected dietary supplements. Women who are pregnant should discuss the use of supplements with their caregiver or with a registered dietician.

HERBAL THERAPIES

Herbal therapy or herbal medicine has been used since ancient times to treat illnesses and ailments. In fact, the oldest surviving prescription for garlic use was found on a clay tablet that dates from 3000 BCE (Fontaine, 2000). Like vitamins and minerals, herbs are a form of dietary supplement, but they are often used to treat the symptoms of specific ailments rather than simply to enhance overall health (Mayo Clinic, 2002). Certain herbs have become better known because of specific claims. For example, many people have used St. John's wort over the counter to help treat mild to moderate depression. However, a recent study indicates that St. John's wort is no more effective than a placebo in dealing with major depression of moderate severity (Davidson et al, 2002). Further study about its effectiveness for mild depression is needed. Other well-known herbal remedies include, for example, ginger, rosemary, ginseng, ginkgo, chamomile, oil of evening primrose, echinacea, garlic, lemon balm, and black cohosh.

Currently about 1500 botanical substances are sold in the United States as dietary supplements or as part of traditional ethnic medications. However, herbal formulations are not subject to Food and Drug Administration (FDA) premarket testing for safety and effectiveness (National Toxicology Program, 2002). Thus, these products can be sold over the counter with only little control. The FDA does have the authority to pull a product off the market if it is proven to be dangerous. Consequently most of what is known about herbs comes from Europe, where they have been studied for some time. Herbal products from Germany, France, England, and Australia are

Table 3–3 • NATURAL FOOD SUPPLEMENTS

Supplement	Benefit
Alfalfa	Rich in minerals and vitamins
Aloe vera	Used for digestive complaints; can also be used as a skin moisturizer
Bee by-products* (bee pollen, honey, Royal bee jelly)	Contains minerals, proteins, and vitamins
Brewer's yeast	Amino acids, B vitamins, and minerals
Coenzyme A	Helps to produce the energy the body needs
Coenzyme Q10	Helps with fat and energy metabolism
Colostrum (cow's)	Helps boost the immune system
Fish oil	Protects the heart and blood vessels
Garlic	Acts as an immune system stimulant; also a natural antibiotic
Green papaya	Enzymes, minerals, and vitamins
Kelp (type of seaweed)	Rich in vitamins (especially B vitamins) and minerals
Wheat germ	Source of vitamin E and most B vitamins, minerals

*Bee pollen should not be used by children, or by pregnant or lactating women (Gastel, 2000).
Source: Adapted from Balch and Balch, 2000; Graedon and Graedon, 2001; Gastelu, 2000; Hobbs and Keville, 1998

Developing Cultural Competence

The World Health Organization estimates that 80% of the Earth's population depends on plants to treat common ailments. Herbalism is an essential part of ayurvedic (Indian), traditional Asian, Native American, and naturopathic medicines. Many homeopathic remedies are also developed from herbs (Balch and Balch, 2000).

reasonably safe because in these countries herbs are regulated as if they were drugs (Graedon & Graedon, 2001).

The use of herbs during pregnancy is an especially important consideration for nurses working with childbearing families. Pregnant women interested in using herbs are best advised to follow basic principles (Belew, 1999):

1. Avoid the use of any herbs, even tonic herbs, during the first trimester, whenever possible.
2. Avoid highly concentrated extracts because the risk of side effects tends to be higher than with whole plant extracts.

In addition, pregnant women need to avoid certain categories of herbs such as abortifacient (abortion-inducing) herbs, herbs that induce menstruation, nervous system stimulants, stimulant laxatives, and so forth. Lists identifying common herbs that women are advised to avoid or use with caution during pregnancy and lactation are available. In summary, pregnant and breastfeeding women should consult with their healthcare provider before taking any herbs, even as teas.

Sense Therapies

Most practitioners who use the sense therapies are trained in several. For example, to boost immunity, one healer might prescribe a varied menu of aromas, colors, and sounds.

AROMATHERAPY

Aromatherapy is the use of certain essential oils, derived from plants, whose odor or aroma is believed to have a therapeutic effect. The essential oils may be obtained from a plant's leaves, flowers, roots, or wood (Cole, 1998). The chemicals contained in the oils are absorbed into the body to produce an effect. Thus essential oils are typically diluted in a carrier oil such as sweet almond oil, olive oil, or vegetable oil before they are applied to the skin. Essential oils can also be inhaled (a few drops in warm water) or added to bath water. Essential oils are used for many purposes such as the following (Fontaine, 2000):

- Aid in restful sleep
- Help reduce stress
- Mood regulation—some oils are sedating, others are stimulating
- Reduce weight
- Enhance the immune system
- Help a person refresh and recharge himself or herself
- Refresh a room

Aromatherapy has been used since ancient time but it is gaining great popularity in Europe and the United States. A variety of essential oils are available such as eucalyptus or peppermint from plant leaves, lavender and rose from plant flowers, cinnamon from plant bark, lemon or mandarin from plant fruit, orange plant blossoms, garlic bulbs, and sandalwood from plant wood. Oils with similar effects such as lavender and bergamot, which are calming, may also be blended to enhance their effectiveness. Oils with opposing effects should not be blended.

Opinion varies about the use of essential oils during pregnancy because certain oils may pose a risk to the woman or her fetus. A pregnant woman who is considering aromatherapy should first discuss it with a health care provider who is knowledgeable about aromatherapy or a skilled aromatherapist (Fontaine, 2000).

COLOR AND LIGHT THERAPIES

Chromotherapy or *color therapy* is designed to use colors to help restore the body to harmony. Color therapists believe that, because all matter is a form of energy, the application of energy to the body in the form of light will have effects, for good or for ill. Because light can be split into colors, it is possible to deliver this energy at very precise levels and in easily controlled doses. After an assessment is completed by the color therapist, the individual is exposed to a light source that contains the colors the therapist believes are needed to restore energy balance (Shealy, 1999).

Although sunlight has been used for healing purposes since ancient times, Western scientists have only recently begun to explore how exposure to light affects human functioning (*Nurse's Handbook*, 1999). *Light therapy* has become accepted treatment for jaundice in newborns (Chapter 33). Light therapy is also used in treating individuals with seasonal affective disorder.

MUSIC AND SOUND THERAPIES

Sound therapy is based on the premise that when the body is exposed to the correct sound frequency (including some very low and very high frequencies that humans cannot normally hear) the body restores itself. Thus sounds from Tibetan and crystal bowls, vibrating tuning forks, *mantras* (such as "Om"), and handheld machines that transmit sound waves through the skin are used to promote healing. It is suggested that certain sounds have a healing influence on the body because they influence the geometric patterns and organization of cells and living systems (Gerber, 2001). A simple application of sound therapy is to encourage a woman in childbirth to moan on as low a pitch as possible during contractions. This opens the jaw, throat, and chest, and many women report that it promotes feelings of relaxation and power. In contrast, high-pitched squealing or screaming tightens the body and may promote feelings of fear.

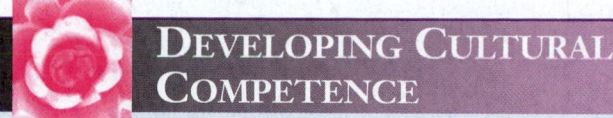

Music therapy can be considered a form of sound therapy. Music has been used during pregnancy and labor and birth to help soothe women and decrease their anxiety by stimulating endorphin release. Similarly, research involving low birth weight premature and newborn infants revealed that those infants who were played hour-long tapes of lullabies and children's songs lost 50% less weight and spent an average of 5 fewer days in the hospital (Gaynor, 1999).

Energy Therapies

The energy therapies work at the most subtle level of the body to enhance immunity, reduce allergy, improve circulation, and improve neural integration. Although acupressure and acupuncture are familiar to most healthcare professionals, many of the energy therapies are very new, and some are not widely available.

ACUPRESSURE AND ACUPUNCTURE

Both acupressure and acupuncture were originally part of traditional Chinese medicine. These practices are based on the traditional Eastern belief that the body's life energy, chi, which was discussed previously, flows along certain pathways known as meridians. The meridians—14 in number—connect all parts of the body. Each meridian is associated with a different organ system or function for which it is named such as the stomach, spleen, heart, kidney, and the like. The central meridian is associated with the brain, and the governing meridian is associated with the spine (Fontaine, 2000). The places where these meridians pass close to the skin's surface are called acupuncture points or pressure points. Applying pressure or stimulation to specific pressure points chosen based on symptoms and the specific meridian involved, can promote wellness, relieve pain, and even cure certain illnesses.

Acupressure (sometimes called Chinese massage) uses pressure from the fingers and thumbs to stimulate pressure points. Acupressure is easy to learn and is often used for self-treatment of tension-related ailments such as headaches, muscle aches, and tension due to stress. Pregnant women often use acupressure wristbands to help relieve the nausea of early pregnancy.

Acupuncture, considered the stronger technique, uses very fine (hairlike) stainless steel needles to stimulate specific acupuncture points depending on the client's medical assessment and condition. A treatment typically involves the placement of 6 to 12 needles. Acupuncture has become more widely available in most countries since the 1970s when China became more open to the West. It is particularly common in France, Canada, and New Zealand (Shealy, 1999). Acupuncture has been used in China and Europe for pain management and for vaginal births or for surgical procedures. In the United States acupuncture is becoming more popular, with over 40 schools and colleges of acupuncture now offering training in the practice. Currently states have different requirements for regulating acupuncturists. Nurses can recommend that women considering the use of acupuncture check with local, state, and national health organizations

RESEARCH IN PRACTICE
Efficacy of Complementary Approaches to First-Trimester Nausea and Vomiting

What is this study about? From 50% to 80% of all pregnant women experience nausea and vomiting in the first trimester of pregnancy, and for some women these symptoms can have a profound impact on their general sense of well-being. Women may try numerous strategies to alleviate their symptoms. Nearly half (49%) of women of childbearing age admit using complementary therapies, and a significant proportion of women may try these therapies during pregnancy. Some studies indicate that acupressure or acupuncture pericardium 6 (needle insertion on the forearm) may have an antiemetic effect, but no well-controlled trials document this effect. This study had as its goal the determination of the effect of acupuncture and pericardium acupuncture on nausea, dry retching, and vomiting in early pregnancy.

How was this study done? This single-blind randomized controlled trial was conducted in Australia and involved 593 women less than 14 weeks' pregnant with symptoms of nausea or vomiting. The women were randomly assigned to one of four groups: traditional acupuncture; pericardium 6 (p6) acupuncture; sham acupuncture; and no acupuncture (control). Participation in the trial was for 4 weeks, with women in the acupuncture groups treated twice during the first week and then weekly for the remainder of the trial. The primary outcomes were nausea, dry retching, and vomiting at days 7, 14, 21, and 26 measured by the Rhodes Index of Nausea and Vomiting Form 2, a Likert scale.

What were the results of the study? Women who received acupuncture reported less frequent and shorter periods of nausea compared with women in the control group throughout the trial, and fewer incidents of dry retching from the second week of the trial. Women who received the specific pericardium acupuncture experienced less nausea from the second week of the trial, and fewer episodes of dry retching from the third week of the trial, than did women in the control group. Women in the sham acupuncture group experienced less nausea and dry retching from the third week compared with women in the no acupuncture group. No differences in vomiting were found at any point in the trial.

What additional questions might I have? Why did the acupuncture reduce nausea but not vomiting? Is the placebo effect enhanced when nausea, dry retching, and vomiting are present for longer periods of time? Was the placebo effect a result of social support in the clinical trial? Would more frequent treatments improve the results?

How can I use this study? These results can be used to counsel mothers who may be considering nonpharmacologic and complementary treatments for nausea and vomiting associated with early pregnancy. While it appears that acupuncture may reduce the incidence of nausea and dry retching, the treatment does not show beneficial effects of this treatment in reducing vomiting.

Source: Smith, C., Crowther, C., & Beilby, J. (2002). Acupuncture to treat nausea and vomiting in early pregnancy: A randomized controlled trial. *Birth, 29*(1), 1–9.

for qualified acupuncturists. Accreditation is also available by either the National Commission on the Certification of Acupuncturists or, for physicians, the American Academy of Medical Acupuncture.

NAMBUDRIPAD'S ALLERGY ELIMINATION TECHNIQUES

An acupuncturist, chiropractor, and kinesiologist, Dr. Devi Nambudripad developed Nambudripad's allergy elimination techniques (NAET) initially to treat her own food allergies. She soon came to believe, however, that most illnesses are caused by undiagnosed blockages within the energy pathways (meridians) of the body, and that these blockages are in turn inappropriate reactions to substances. NAET attempts to identify and remove the blockages noninvasively, through a combination of muscle-response testing, energy-based desensitization, chiropractic adjustment, acupuncture or acupressure, and nutritional therapies.

MAGNETIC THERAPY

Like the earth itself, all the body's cells act as magnetic fields radiating energy outward and ultimately becoming part of other magnetic fields. Within the body electrical energy is apparent in electrocardiogram (ECG) and electroencephalogram (EEG) tracings, for example, which provide data about the magnetic fields of the heart and brain. As with other magnetic fields, the energy level is highest at its core and dissipates with distance. For humans this energy field is called "aura" and surrounds the body from head to foot. *Magnetic therapy* is believed to work by increasing blood flow and circulation to infected areas. This increased blood flow, in turn, helps relieve swelling and inflammation.

Magnetic therapy gained popularity in the mid-20th century. In Japan in the late 1950s, scientists documented a new syndrome of insomnia, low energy, aches, and pains in workers who spent extended periods of time in metal buildings shielded from the natural magnetic force of the earth. Symptoms were relieved when magnetic fields were applied externally to the bodies of affected individuals. Similarly, early Russian cosmonauts who spent a year or more in space lost over three fourths of their bone density. This was corrected when the space crafts were redesigned to provide strong artificial magnetic fields on board. Moreover, physicians who specialize in sports medicine and orthopedics have advocated the use of magnets since 1993. They report that an athlete's risk of injury is decreased and performance is enhanced when the muscles and joints are warmed up using magnets (Fontaine, 2000). Magnetic therapy is used for diagnosis and treatment of movement disorders (electromyography). It is also used for pain relief (transcutaneous electrical nerve stimulation [TENS]) and to treat insomnia and hypertension (low energy emission therapy).

Magnetic therapy is most effective when it is combined with other treatment methods. It should not be used as the only therapy for a given condition (Null, 1998). Magnets should not be used during pregnancy, especially over the abdominal area (Balch & Balch, 2000).

REIKI

Reiki, a Tibetan-Japanese technique, is a form of hand-mediated therapy designed to promote healing, reduce stress, and encourage relaxation. Reiki practitioners place their hands on or above specific problem areas and transfer energy from themselves to their clients to restore the balance of the client's energy fields (Fontaine, 2000).

THERAPEUTIC TOUCH

Therapeutic touch is a complementary therapy designed to interface with conventional medical care. It was developed in the early 1970s by Dr. Delores Krieger, a nursing professor at New York University, and Dora Kunz, a clairvoyant healer. Therapeutic Touch is grounded in the belief that people are a system of energy with a self-healing potential. The Therapeutic Touch practitioner, often a nurse, can modulate his or her energy field with that of the client's, directing it in a specific way to promote well-being and healing. Proponents of Therapeutic Touch believe that a strong desire to help the recipient is essential as is a conscious use of self to act as a link between the universal life energy and the other person (Fontaine, 2000).

Krieger asserted that healing is an innate human potential and believed that people could be trained to do healing. Her research has demonstrated that the Therapeutic Touch interaction could increase hemoglobin levels in people in the same way that chlorophyll content could be increased in healer-treated plants. This finding was one of the first that allowed quantitative biochemical measurements in humans to detect the effects of healing energy (Gerber, 2001).

Therapeutic Touch is not difficult to learn nor does it require a lengthy training process. In fact, family members have been taught to use Therapeutic Touch, to help their loved ones. There are more specific requirements including standards and scope of practice and a credentialing process for heath care workers. Table 3-4 • provides some basic facts about Therapeutic Touch, while Table 3-5 • provides a brief description of the elements of the procedure for Therapeutic Touch.

Like many other conventional and complementary therapies, therapeutic touch should be applied cautiously to pregnant women and newborns by trained providers (Figure 3-8 •).

Table 3-4 • FACTS ABOUT THERAPEUTIC TOUCH (TT)
Therapeutic touch is taught in more than 100 colleges and universities worldwide and has been taught to more than 40,000 health care providers.
The North American Nursing Diagnosis Association (NANDA) recognizes "energy field disturbance" as a nursing diagnosis, and professional organizations such as the American Nurses Association and the National League for Nursing have supported TT as a nursing intervention.
TT is used as a complementary therapy for virtually all medical and nursing diagnoses as well as for surgical procedures.
TT is best known for its ability to relieve pain and anxiety.
Source: *Nurse's handbook of alternative and complementary therapies.* Springhouse, PA: Springhouse Corporation. (1999.)

Table 3-5 • THERAPEUTIC TOUCH (TT) PROCEDURES

- The nurse should have the individual's consent to do Therapeutic Touch.
- The individual who is receiving Therapeutic Touch (who is clothed) can sit on a chair or lie on a bed or massage table.
- The nurse begins by "centering" himself or herself (a calm, focused, meditative state).
- The nurse makes an assessment of the person's energy field. While maintaining a state of sustained centering, the nurse slowly moves his/her hands about 2 to 4 inches (5 to 10 cm) over the person's body, moving in a direction from head to toe, feeling for vibrations, cold and heat, or blockages
- The nurse, using his/her hands and centered intention, seeks to facilitate the rebalancing of the client's energy field, through the actions of clearing (sometimes called "unruffling") and the direction of a universal energy.

MEDIALINK CARE PLAN: HIGH-RISK ADOLESCENT PREGNANCY

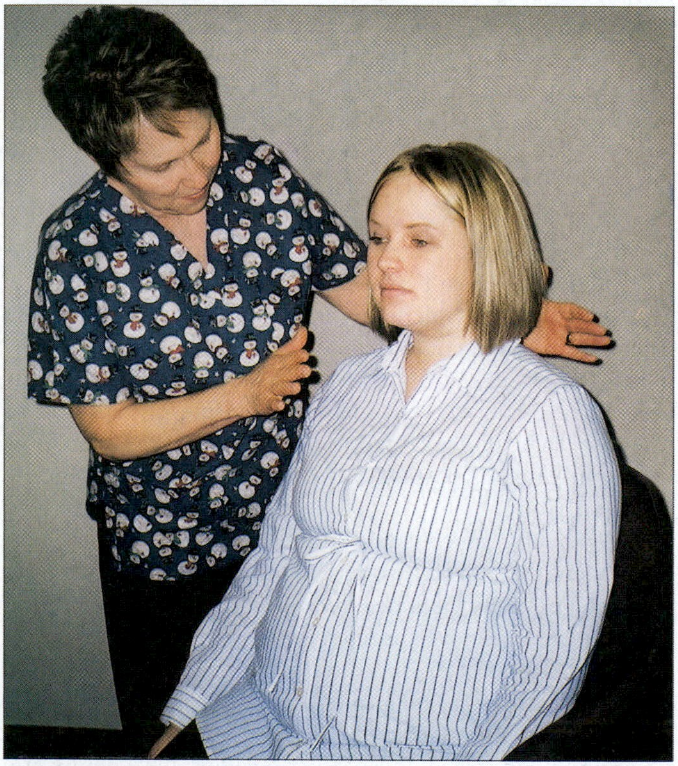

Figure 3–8 • During pregnancy, Therapeutic Touch is often helpful in easing pain and reducing anxiety.
SOURCE: Nurse Healers—Professional Associates International, The official organization for Therapeutic Touch. www.therapeutic_touch.org

Nursing Care of the Childbearing Family Using Complementary Therapies

Currently, the people most likely to use complementary and alternative medicine (CAM) are middle-aged and affluent. (See figure 3-9 •). By race, the greatest percentage are Native American, followed by Caucasian. Many people with chronic illnesses are opting to try alternative therapies. Significantly, 80% of the people who use CAM also use conventional medicine. However, 70% do not discuss their use of CAM with their traditional caregiver (Murphy, Kronenberg, & Wade, 1999).

As knowledge of alternative therapies grows, the number and type of people using one or more of them will probably increase as well. Thus, it is likely that the majority of childbearing families are using some form of alternative therapy even though they do not share that information.

Assessing a Client's Use of Complementary Therapies

The reality that women may use CAM and not reveal it raises some concern. Certain CAM modalities such as biofeedback, acupuncture, aromatherapy, massage, and prayer are not likely to cause adverse effects during pregnancy. However, the possibility exists that there might be interactions between herbal therapies and other medications prescribed by the caregiver. Similarly, complications might develop from the use of vitamin supplements immediately before or after surgery (Olson, 2001).

Nurses who create a climate of respect and openness tend to be more effective in gathering information about a woman's use of complementary or alternative therapies. The following recommendations may be useful to nurses in taking a history (Cady, 2002; Vincler & Nicol, 1997):

- Ask questions that are direct and nonjudgmental in seeking information about the client's use of CAM.
- Ask questions about specific therapies including the use of herbal therapy and homeopathy. Because many people consider herbs to be natural substances and because they are often sold as dietary supplements, clients may not think to mention them.
- Avoid making negative or disparaging comments about CAM. Such comments send the message that CAM is not desirable and may discourage people from disclosing their use of CAM therapies.

All nurses practicing today need to have at least an awareness of complementary and alternative therapies and of other systems of medicine that influence CAM. These systems include, for example, traditional Chinese medicine, ayurveda, chiropractic, naturopathy, and homeopathy. The National Institutes of Health (NIH) Web site (Table 3-2) is an excellent resource for health care providers and for childbearing women and their families.

Incorporating Complementary Therapies into Maternal-Newborn Nursing Care

Because the practice of nursing is holistic in nature, many nurses are open to and supportive of the use of complementary and alternative therapies. However, nurses in the United States need to know whether the nurse practice act in their state specifically addresses CAM therapies because some states do while others do not. For example, in Louisiana RNs may initiate and use complementary thera-

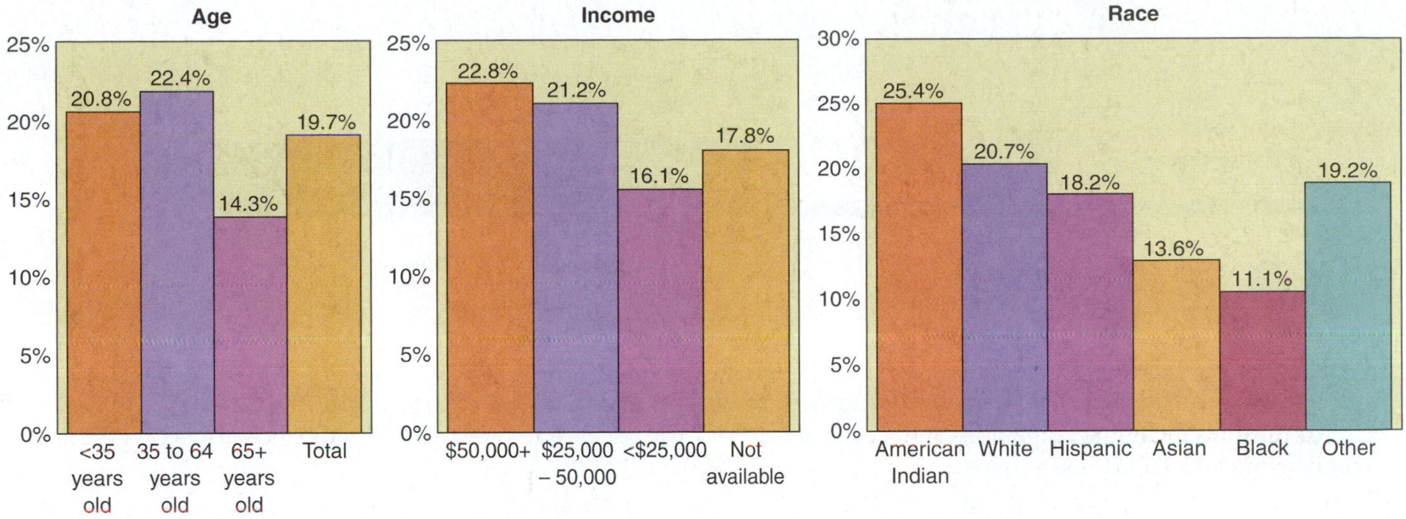

Figure 3–9 • Alternative medicine use by age, income and race.
SOURCE: Medstat.

pies for clients who seek the therapies as part of the nursing plan of care to meet goals such as relief of pain, comfort, reduction of stress, relaxation, improved coping mechanisms, and increased sense of well-being, if the individual has given informed consent. Written policies are required in all practice settings that permit the RN to perform such modalities (Cady, 2002). Nurses also need to be knowledgeable about any legal requirements that govern their use of CAM.

In working with childbearing families, or indeed with any clients, nurses who use CAM therapies should choose those methods that are within the scope of nursing practice in their state and not limited by the licensure of other providers (such as massage therapists). Nurses are also best advised to use CAM therapies that are considered somewhat mainstream and that are supported by evidence about their safety and effectiveness (Gaydos, 2001). For example, nurses working with a pregnant woman might use acupressure wristbands for the treatment of nausea. Other therapies nurses often employ include progressive relaxation, exercise and movement, therapeutic touch, visualization and guided imagery, prayer, meditation, music therapy, massage, storytelling, aromatherapy, and journaling.

Nurses who use complementary modalities should document their use within the context of nursing practice. This is most effective when the modality is identified as an intervention to address a specific nursing diagnosis or identified client need (Frisch, 2001). Thus, music therapy might be used for a laboring woman to address the identified nursing diagnosis of pain. Other modalities that might be used include progressive relaxation, massage, aromatherapy, and visualization.

Many certified nurse-midwives incorporate complementary and alternative therapies into their clinical practice with childbearing families. Research suggests that CNMs who prescribe CAM do so for the following reasons: nausea and vomiting, labor stimulation, perineal discomfort, lactation disorders, postpartum depression, preterm labor, postpartum hemorrhage, and labor analgesia. The methods most frequently used included herbal therapy, massage therapy, chiropractic, acupressure, and mind-body interventions. To a lesser degree they also recommend aromatherapy, homeopathy, spiritual healing, acupuncture, and bioelectric or magnetic applications (Allaire, Moos, & Wells, 2000).

Research on CAM sparks great interest in the public and momentum is increasing to design and carry out well-developed research on alternative modalities. Nurses have a role in conducting and supporting research of this type. Because of the variety of CAM therapies in use, research is needed in a host of areas.

The results of research sometimes support the use of a given modality; at other times they raise questions about the use of modalities that have enjoyed great popularity. For example, as discussed previously, many people have used the herbal remedy St. John's wort (*Hypericum perforatum*) to treat depression. However, recent research suggests that St. John's wort is no more effective than a placebo in treating major depression of moderate severity (Davidson, J.R.T., et al, 2002). On the other hand, research has demonstrated the effectiveness of moxibustion (described earlier) in treating breech presentation. Moxibustion has been used in China for centuries to treat pregnant women with a breech presentation. The goal is to get the fetus to turn so that birth occurs in a vertex (headfirst) position. Cardini & Weixin (1998) conducted a study with 260 women pregnant for the first time. The randomized control group received no intervention while the treatment group received moxibustion therapy. At the end of the treatment period, the moxibustion therapy group had had a significantly higher percentage of fetuses convert to a vertex presentation than the control group.

The results of research on CAM can be found in professional journals and at the NIH Web site. As the evidence supporting the use of certain interventions grows, nurses and other health care providers are incorporating the results as part of their evidence-based practice.

MediaLink CASE STUDY: COMPLEMENTARY THERAPIES

CHAPTER REVIEW

EXPLOREMEDIALINK

NCLEX review questions, case studies, and other interactive resources for this chapter can be found on the Web site at http://www.prenhall.com/olds. Click on "Chapter 3" to select the activities for this chapter.

For tutorials including animations and videos, more NCLEX review questions, and an audio glossary, access the accompanying CD-ROM in this book.

Focus Your Study

- A complementary therapy is an adjunct to conventional medical treatment that has been through rigorous scientific testing, which shows that it has some reliability.
- An alternative therapy is usually considered a substance or procedure that has not undergone rigorous scientific testing in this country, although it might have been thoroughly tested in other countries.
- The National Center for Complementary and Alternative Medicine (NCCAM) promotes research into complementary and alternative therapies and disseminates the information to consumers.
- CAM therapies have several benefits. Many of them emphasize prevention and wellness, place a higher value on holistic healing than on physical cure, are noninvasive, and have few side effects. In addition, many are more affordable and available than conventional therapies.
- Risks include lack of standardization, lack of regulation and research substantiating safety and effectiveness, inadequate training and certification of some healers, and financial and health risks of unproven methods.
- The term *homeopathy* is derived from the Greek word *homos* meaning the same. It is a healing system that uses like to cure like; that is, homeopathic remedies are minute dilutions of substances that, if ingested in larger amounts, would produce effects *similar* to the symptoms of the disorder being treated.
- Traditional Chinese medicine (TCM) seeks to ensure the balance of energy, called *chi or qi.* Techniques of TCM include acupuncture, moxibustion, herbal therapy, nutrition, acupressure, Qigong, and t'ai chi.
- Ayurveda is the classical system of Hindu medicine. It promotes balance of the three primary forces thought to influence human health and well-being.
- Biofeedback is a method used to help individuals learn to control their physiologic responses based on the concept that the mind controls the body.
- Hypnosis, whether guided by a trained hypnotherapist or induced through self-hypnosis, is a state of great mental and physical relaxation during which a person is very open to suggestions.
- Guided imagery is a state of intense, focused concentration used to create compelling mental images.
- Chiropractic, a profession practiced by licensed chiropractors, is based on concepts of manipulation, especially spinal manipulation.
- The focus of the *Alexander technique* is on proper alignment of the head, neck, and trunk. The *Feldenkrais method*, another movement-oriented therapy, is based on the belief that health is improved by establishing new connections between the brain and body through movement reeducation.
- Massage therapy involves the manipulation of the soft tissues of the body to reduce stress and tension, increase circulation, diminish pain, and promote a sense of well-being. Reflexology is a specific form of massage that involves the application of pressure to designated points or reflexes on the client's feet, hands, or ears using the thumb and fingers.
- Hydrotherapy is any therapy that makes use of hot or cold moisture in any form to relax muscles, promote rest, decrease pain, reduce swelling, promote healing, cleanse wounds and burns, reduce fever, lessen cramps, and improve well-being.

- Hatha yoga, the physical branch of yoga, is commonly practiced to improve health and well-being, to prevent illness, and to promote healing.
- A *dietary supplement* is any product (excluding tobacco) intended to supplement the diet. It contains one or more of the following ingredients: a mineral, vitamin, herb, amino acid, other botanical supplements, or extracts and ingredients of animal and plant origin.
- Herbs, a form of dietary supplement, are used to treat the symptoms of specific ailments or to enhance overall health. Pregnant women should avoid the use of all herbs during the first trimester. During the second and third trimesters, and during breastfeeding, they should avoid highly concentrated extracts, and should inform their primary care provider about any herbs they plan to take.
- Acupressure (sometimes called Chinese massage) uses pressure from the fingers and thumbs to stimulate pressure points. Acupuncture, considered the stronger technique, uses very fine (hairlike) stainless steel needles to stimulate specific acupuncture points depending on the client's medical assessment and condition.
- Therapeutic touch is based on the belief that people are a system of energy with a self-healing potential. The therapeutic touch practitioner, often a nurse, can unite his or her energy field with that of the client's, directing it in a specific way to promote well-being and healing.
- Many nurses are open to and supportive of complementary and alternative therapies. Nurses who incorporate such therapies into the practice must be certain that they are practicing within the framework of their nurse practice act and with the informed consent of their clients.

References

Allaire, A. D., Moos, M. K., & Wells, S. R. (2000). Complementary and alternative medicine in pregnancy: A survey of North Carolina certified nurse-midwives. *Obstetrics and Gynecology, 95*(1), 19–23.

Balch, P. A., & Balch, J. F. (2000). *Prescription for nutritional healing* (3rd ed). New York: Penguin Putnam.

Belew, C. (1999). Herbs and the childbearing woman: Guidelines for midwives. *Journal of Nurse-Midwifery, 44*(3), 231–246.

Bratman, S. (1998). *The alternative medicines ratings guide.* Rocklin, CA: Prima Health.

Cady, R. (2002). Are there legal issues of concern for nurses when patients use complimentary [sic] and alternative medicine? *The American Journal of Maternal/Child Nursing, 27*(2), 119.

Cardini, F., & Weixin, H. (1998). Moxibustion for correction of breech presentation: A randomized, controlled trial. *Journal of the American Medical Association, 280,* 1580–1584.

Cole, R. L. (1998). *The gentle greeting.* Naperville, IL: Sourcebooks.

Crawford, C. (1996). Ayurveda: The science of long life in contemporary perspective. In A. Sheikh & K. Sheikh (Eds.), *Healing East and West.* New York: John Wiley & Sons.

Davidson, J. R. T. Kishore, M. G., Fairbank, J. A., Krishnan, K. R. R., Califf, R. M., & Binanay, C. et al. (2002). Effect of *Hypericum perforatum* (St. John's wort) in major depressive disorder: A randomized, controlled trial. *Journal of the American Medical Association, 287,* 1807–1814.

Fontaine, K. L. (2000). *Healing practices:Alternative therapies for nursing.* Upper Saddle River, NJ: Prentice-Hall Health.

Frisch, N. C. (2001). Nursing as a context for alternative/complementary modalities. *Online Journal of Issues in Nursing, 6*(2). Retrieved June 19, 2001 from http://www. nursingworld.org.ojin/topic15/tpc15_2.htm

Gastelu, D. (2000). *The complete nutritional supplement buyer's guide.* New York: Three Rivers Press.

Gaydos, H. L. (2001). *Complementary and alternative therapies in nursing education: Trends and issues.* Retrieved June 19, 2001 from http://www. nursingworld.org.ojin/topic15/tpc15_5.htm

Gaynor, M. L. (1999). *Sounds of healing.* New York: Broadway Books.

Gerber, R. (2001). *Vibrational medicine* (3rd ed). Rochester, VT: Bear & Company.

Graedon, J., & Graedon, T. (2001). *The people's pharmacy guide to home and herbal remedies.* New York: St. Martin's Griffin.

Hobbs, C. L., & Keville, K. (1998). *Women's herbs, women's health.* Loveland, CO: Interweave Press, Inc.

Krishnamurti, J. (2000). *To be human.* Edited by David Skitt. Boston: Shambhala.

Lockie, A., & Geddes, N. (2000). *Complete guide to homeopathy: The principles and practice of treatment homeopathy.* New York: DK Publishing.

Maxwell-Hudson, C. (1999). *Massage.* New York: DK Publishing.

Mayo Clinic. (2001). *Chiropractic treatment.* Retrieved September 2, 2002, from http://www.mayoclinic.com

Mayo Clinic. (2002). *Using herbal supplements wisely.* Retrieved September 2, 2002, from http://www.mayoclinic.com

Moyers, Bill D. (1993). *Healing and the mind.* New York: Doubleday.

Murphy, P. A., Kronenberg, F., & Wade, C. (1999). Complementary and alternative medicine in women's health. Developing a research agenda. *Journal of Nurse-Midwifery, 44,* 192–204.

Murray, M., & Pizzorno, J. (2001). *Encyclopedia of natural medicine.* Rocklin, CA: Prima Publishing.

National Institutes of Health (NIH), Office of Dietary Supplements. (2001). *What are dietary supplements.* Retrieved September 2, 2002, from http://ods.od.nih.gov/whatare/whatare.html

National Toxicology Program. (2002). Herbal medicines. *NTP Factsheets—Year 2002.* Retrieved September 2, 2002, from http:// ntp-server.niehs.noh.gov/htdocs/liason/factsheets/HerbMedFacts. html

Null, G. (1998). *Healing with magnets.* New York: Carroll & Graf, Pub.

Nurse's handbook of alternative and complementary therapies. (1999). Springhouse, PA: Springhouse Corporation.

Olson, G. L. (2001). When your pregnant patient uses alternative medicine. *Contemporary OB/GYN, 46*(9), 45–58.

Shealy, N. (Consulting Ed.). (1999). *The complete illustrated encyclopedia of alternative healing therapies.* Boston: Elements Books Limited.

Upledger Institute. (1998). *Discover craniosacral therapy* [Pamphlet]. Palm Beach Gardens, FL: author.

Vincler, L., & Nicol, M. (1997). When ignorance isn't bliss: What healthcare practitioners and facilities should know about complimentary [sic] and alternative medicine. *American Health Lawyers Association, Journal of Health Law, 30*(3), 160.

TWO

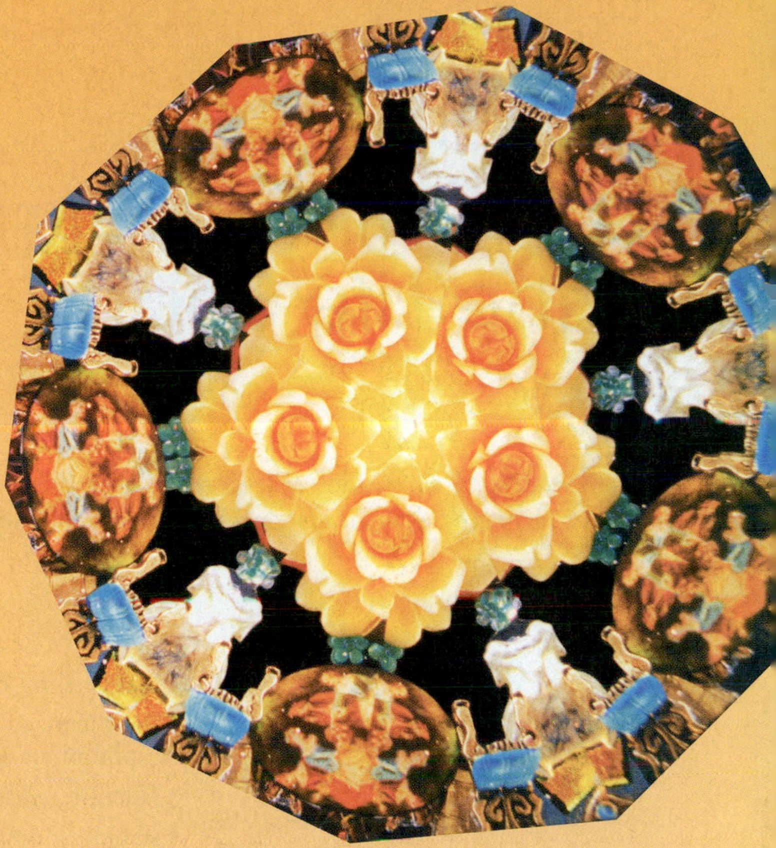

Women's Health

Women's Health Across the Life Span 4

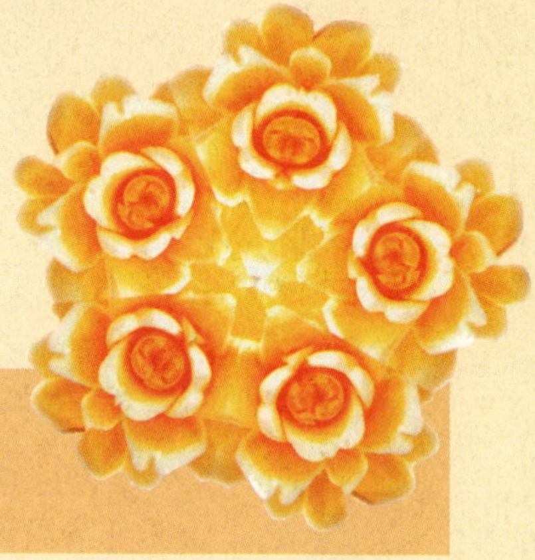

Mom was great about preparing me for my first period. I knew why I had periods and how to handle them. She NEVER called it "the curse" or made a big deal out of it, so I was surprised when friends were so negative. To me, periods were a sign of womanhood.

Objectives

- Discuss the key points a nurse should consider in taking a sexual history.
- Summarize information that women may need in order to implement appropriate self-care measures for dealing with menstruation.
- Identify causes of amenorrhea.
- Contrast dysmenorrhea and premenstrual syndrome.
- Delineate the physical and psychologic aspects of menopause.
- Explain the relationship between menopause and osteoporosis.
- Identify medical and complementary therapies to alleviate the discomforts of menopause.

Key Terms

Amenorrhea 75
Climacteric 77
Dysmenorrhea 75
Hormone replacement therapy (HRT) 82
Menopause 77
Osteoporosis 81
Perimenopause 77
Premenstrual syndrome (PMS) 76

MediaLink

Additional resources for this content can be found on the Student CD-ROM and on the Companion Website at www.prenhall.com/olds. Click on "Chapter 4" to select the activities for this chapter.

CD-ROM
- Audio Glossary
- NCLEX Review

Companion Website
- Additional NCLEX Review
- Case Study: Premenstrual Girl
- Care Plan Activity: Bone Injuries in Postmenopausal Woman

A woman's health care needs change throughout her lifetime. As a young girl she requires health teaching about menstruation, sexuality, and personal responsibility. As a teen she needs information about reproductive choices and safe sexual activity. During this time she should also be introduced to the importance of health care practices, such as breast self-examination and regular Pap smears. The mature woman may need to be reminded of these self-care issues and prepared for physical changes that accompany childbirth and aging. By educating women about their bodies, their health care choices, and their rights and responsibilities, nurses can help women be knowledgeable consumers who assume responsibility for the health care they receive.

This chapter, the first of six chapters devoted to women's health, focuses primarily on wellness care. Chapter 5 then considers issues related to family planning. Chapter 6 focuses on infections women may encounter, and Chapter 7 addresses some of the common gynecologic issues and conditions a woman may face. Chapter 8 explores some of the major social issues women face, and Chapter 9 focuses on violence against women.

Community-Based Nursing Care

Women's health refers to a holistic view of women and their health-related needs within the context of their everyday lives. It is based on the awareness that a woman's physical, mental, and social status are interdependent and determine her state of health or illness. The woman's perception of her situation, her assessment of her needs, her values, and her beliefs are valid, important factors to be incorporated into any health care intervention.

Clinical Tip *Remember that a woman's views frequently influence the health care of her entire family because women typically coordinate the family's health care needs.*

Nurses can provide health teaching and information about self-care practices in schools, during routine examinations in a clinic or office, at senior centers, at meetings of volunteer organizations, through classes offered by the local health department or community college, or in the home. Nurses can also help women with various forms of disability to address their unique health care needs and optimize their state of wellness. This community-based focus is the key to providing effective nursing care to women of all ages.

In reality, the vast majority of women's health care is provided outside of acute care settings. Nurses oriented to community-based care are especially effective in recognizing the autonomy of each individual and in dealing with clients holistically. This approach is important in addressing not only physical problems but also major health issues such as violence against women, which may go undetected unless care providers ask women specifically about violence and are alert for signs of it. See Developing Cultural Competence.

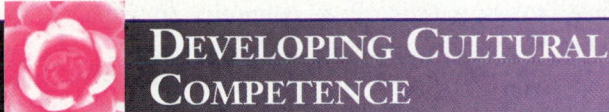

DEVELOPING CULTURAL COMPETENCE

In the course of your work as a nurse, you are bound to encounter people different from yourself. Even with the best of intentions, you may say or do something your client or the client's family finds offensive or inappropriate. If you ask someone something and get a funny look, ask what's on the person's mind. The answer may surprise you. It often leads to more honest reporting of information and a feeling of being listened to and respected. When people feel emotionally safe, cultural and other perceived differences shrink. This helps a therapeutic relationship to develop between the person you are serving and you, yourself, as the caregiver.

The Nurse's Role in Addressing Issues of Women's Wellness and Sexuality

Women expect the nurses who care for them to be knowledgeable not only about gynecologic health, but about a wide variety of health topics. Thus it is important that nurses expand their knowledge about the issues healthy women and their families may face. These include, for example, a general knowledge of normal growth and development; recommended screening procedures for both women and men, and the ages at which these procedures are indicated; signs and symptoms of substance abuse including alcoholism; health issues that well men face; signs of emotional stress and depression; community resources; and a variety of other topics. By keeping abreast of issues well families may face, the nurse becomes a more complete resource and acts to promote overall health.

On occasion, most women experience concern and even anxiety about some aspect of menstruation, contraception, sexual activity, and/or menopause. Societal standards and pressures can cause girls and adolescents to evaluate and compare with others their experiences with menstruation, sexual attractiveness, and beliefs and values about engaging in sexual activity. Young adults may be more concerned about the reproductive and health implications of sexual intercourse. The desire to achieve or avoid pregnancy and the fear of sexually transmitted infections, especially HIV/AIDS and herpes, cause many women to modify their sexual practices and activities. While older women share many of these same concerns, they may also experience anxiety about the onset of menopausal changes and wonder how these changes will affect their sexuality. Furthermore, throughout the lifespan, women may have concerns, problems, and questions about sex roles, sexual orientation, behaviors, inhibitions, morality, and related areas such as family planning. Women frequently voice these concerns to the nurse in a clinic or ambulatory setting. Thus the nurse may need to assume the role of counselor on sexual and reproductive matters.

Nurses who assume this role must be secure about their own sexuality. They must also develop an awareness of their own feelings, values, and attitudes about sexuality so that they can be more sensitive and objective when they encounter the values and beliefs of others. Nurses also need to know about the structures and functions of female and male reproductive systems. In addition, they should have accurate, up-to-date information about topics related to menstruation, sexuality, sexual practices, menopause, and common gynecologic problems.

Staying up-to-date on issues of sexuality and women's health requires constant vigilance: regular journal review, attendance at reputable conferences, library and Internet searches, and diligent perusal of women's health literature are essential activities. Continuing education for the practicing nurse and appropriate courses in undergraduate and graduate nursing education programs can also help nurses achieve and maintain the requisite knowledge. These courses can teach nurses about sexual values, attitudes, alternative lifestyles, cultural factors, and misconceptions and myths about sex and reproduction, as well as the developmental changes women experience across the lifespan.

Taking a Sexual History

Nurses today are often responsible for taking a woman's initial history, including her gynecologic and sexual history. To be effective in this role, the nurse must have good communication skills and should conduct the interview in a quiet, private place free of distractions. The sexual history is one part of a lengthier health history and covers personal and intimate topics.

> ***Clinical Tip*** *When taking a history, start your interview with less intimate areas, such as medical and surgical history, and then proceed to the sexual history toward the end of the history-taking session. This approach helps the woman develop a comfort level with you before disclosing personal information.*

Opening the sexual history discussion with a brief explanation of the purpose of such questions is often helpful. For example, the nurse might say, "As your nurse I'm interested in all aspects of your well-being. Often women have concerns or questions about sexual matters, especially when they are pregnant (or starting to be sexually active). I will be asking you some questions about your sexual history as part of your general health history."

It may be helpful to use direct eye contact as much as possible unless the nurse knows it is culturally unacceptable to the woman. The nurse should do little, if any, writing during the interview, especially if the woman seems ill at ease or is discussing very personal issues. Open-ended questions are often useful in eliciting information. For example, "What, if anything, would you change about your sex life?" will elicit more information than "Are you happy with your sex life now?" The nurse should also clarify terminology and proceed from easier topics to those that are more difficult to discuss. Throughout the interview, the nurse should be alert to the client's body language and nonverbal cues. It is essential that the nurse listen, react in a nonjudgmental manner, and use teachable moments to educate women about their bodies. It is also important that the nurse not assume the client is heterosexual. Some clients are open about discussing a lesbian relationship. Others are more reserved until they develop rapport and a sense of trust in the caregiver.

After completing the sexual history, the nurse assesses the information obtained. If there is a problem that requires further medical tests and assessments, the nurse refers the woman to a nurse practitioner, certified nurse-midwife, physician, or counselor as necessary. In many instances the nurse alone will be able to develop a nursing diagnosis and then plan and implement an appropriate intervention. For example, if the nurse determines that a woman who is interested in conceiving a child does not have a clear understanding of when she ovulates, the nurse may formulate the nursing diagnosis ***Deficient Knowledge*** related to lack of information about the timing of ovulation. The nurse can then evaluate the woman's knowledge through discussion and review and work with the woman to provide necessary information. The nurse might also suggest that the woman keep a menstrual calendar and monitor basal body temperatures to identify the time of ovulation.

The nurse must be realistic in making assessments and planning interventions. It requires insight and skill to recognize when a woman's problem requires interventions that are beyond a nurse's preparation and ability. In such cases, the nurse must make appropriate referrals.

> *"As a nurse practitioner I know that taking a thorough sexual and gynecologic history is essential if I am going to provide good care but I am constantly amazed when women, usually older women, tell me that I am the first person to ever ask about their sexuality. What a shame it is that for so long sexuality was ignored. It is such an intrinsic part of health."*

Menstruation

Girls today begin to learn about puberty and menstruation at a surprisingly young age. Unfortunately, the source of their "education" is sometimes their peers and sometimes the media; thus the information is frequently incomplete, inaccurate, and sensationalized. Nurses who work with girls and adolescents recognize this and are working hard to provide accurate health teaching and to correct misinformation about *menarche* (the onset of menses) and the menstrual cycle.

Cultural, religious, and personal attitudes about menstruation are part of the menstrual experience and often reflect negative attitudes toward women. In the past, many myths surrounded menstruation. Women were often isolated or restricted to the company of other women during their monthly

GLOBAL PERSPECTIVES

In India, menstruation is an event of embarrassment that should be hidden and not discussed. Most women do not use sanitary napkins because of financial reasons or because of lack of adequate disposal facilities. Instead, old rags and strips of clothing are used. Once used, these rags are washed for reuse and are often dried in unclean areas, such as under cots or other clothing to hide them. Because of the cultural taboos regarding menses, women are not able to dry these strips of cloth in the sun. These conditions lead to bacterial growth, which commonly causes reproductive tract infections. It is estimated that 70% to 80% of Indian women contract a reproductive tract infection in this manner.

flow because they were considered "unclean." Currently in the Western world there are fewer customs associated with menstruation, although many women hide the fact of menstruation entirely. Sexual intercourse during menstruation is a common practice and is not generally contraindicated. For most couples, the decision is one of personal preference. (The physiology of menstruation is discussed in Chapter 10.)

Counseling the Premenstrual Girl about Menarche

The average age of menarche is about 12 years for girls in the United States, although many begin their periods at an earlier age. For about 2 years before menarche, a girl experiences a series of physical changes as her body develops. Many girls find it embarrassing or stressful to discuss these changes and the menstrual experience, both because of the many taboos associated with the subject and because of their immaturity. However, the most critical factor in successful adaptation to menarche is the preteen's or adolescent's level of preparedness. Information should be given to premenstrual girls over time, rather than all at once. This allows them to absorb information and develop questions. The following basic information is helpful for young clients:

- **Cycle length.** Cycle length is determined from the first day of one menses to the first day of the next menses. Initially, cycle length is about 29 days, but the normal length may vary from 21 to 35 days. As a woman matures, cycle length often shortens to a median of 25+ days just before menopause. Cycle length often varies by a day or two from one cycle to the next, although greater normal variations may also occur.
- **Amount of flow.** The average flow is approximately 25 to 60 mL per period. Usually women characterize the amount of flow in terms of the number of pads or tampons used. Flow often is heavier at first and lighter toward the end of the period.
- **Length of menses.** Menses usually lasts from 2 to 8 days, although the length may vary.

The nurse should make it clear that variations in age at menarche, length of cycle, and duration of menses are normal because girls are likely to be concerned if their experience varies from that of their peers. It also is helpful to acknowledge the negative aspects of menstruation (messiness and embarrassment) while stressing its positive role as a symbol of maturity and womanhood.

CRITICAL THINKING IN PRACTICE

Rita Dupona is a 16-year-old, vivacious teenager who comes to the clinic because of irregular menses. She is captain of the cheerleading squad at the local high school and believes that her periods are "really messed up" and interfering with her cheering activities. She wants to get her periods regulated and asks for birth control pills.

As you take Rita's menstrual history, you find that her menarche was at age 12 and that her periods occur every 24 to 34 days. She usually has cramps, and the flow, which she describes as heavy, lasts 4 to 5 days. She uses an average of five tampons per day. What should you advise Rita about her menstrual cycle?

Answers can be found in Appendix I.

Educational Topics

The nurse's primary role is to provide accurate information and assist in clarifying misconceptions, so that girls will develop positive self-images and progress smoothly through this phase of maturation.

PADS AND TAMPONS

Since early times women have made pads and tampons from cloth or rags, which required washing but were reusable. Some women made them from gauze or cotton balls. Commercial tampons were introduced in the 1930s.

Today adhesive-stripped minipads and maxipads and flushable tampons are readily available. However, the deodorants and increased absorbency that manufacturers have added to both sanitary napkins and tampons may prove harmful. The chemical used to deodorize can create a rash on the vulva and damage the tender mucous lining of the vagina. Excessive or inappropriate use of tampons can produce dryness or even small sores or ulcers in the vagina.

MEDIALINK CASE STUDY: PREMENSTRUAL GIRL

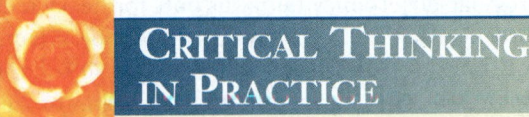

When taking a menstrual history, the nurse should attempt to determine the amount of bleeding each month. The woman can be asked what type of pad or tampon she uses, how frequently she changes, and how much blood has been absorbed. Women should be advised to change pads frequently, every 3 to 6 hours when awake, regardless of the amount of blood that is absorbed. If a woman reports she supersaturates a maxipad every 1 to 2 hours for a couple of days, she may be experiencing a gynecologic problem that needs attention to decrease the risk of anemia.

Because the use of superabsorbent tampons has been linked to the development of toxic shock syndrome (TSS) (Chapter 7), women should avoid using them. They should use regular-absorbency tampons only for heavy menstrual flow (during the first 2 or 3 days of the period), not during the whole period, and change them every 3 to 6 hours. Because *Staphylococcus aureus*, the causative organism of TSS, is frequently found on the hands, a woman should wash her hands before inserting a fresh tampon, use only tampons that have an intact protective wrapper, and avoid touching the tip of the tampon when unwrapping it or before insertion.

In the absence of a heavy menstrual flow, tampons absorb moisture, leaving the vaginal walls dry and subject to injury. The absorbency of regular tampons varies. If the tampon is hard to pull out or shreds when removed, or if the vagina becomes dry, the tampon is probably too absorbent. If a woman is worried about accidental spotting, she can check the diagrams on the packages of regular tampons. Those that expand in width are better able to prevent leakage without being too absorbent.

A woman may want to use tampons only during the day and switch to pads at night to avoid vaginal irritation. She should avoid using tampons on the last spotty days of the period and should never use them for midcycle spotting or leukorrhea. If a woman experiences vaginal irritation, itching, or soreness or notices an unusual odor while using tampons, she should stop using them or change brands or absorbencies.

The choice of sanitary protection must meet the individual's needs and feel comfortable, whether it be pads or tampons. Cultural factors may play a role in this decision for a woman. See the accompanying Global Perspectives.

VAGINAL SPRAYS AND DOUCHING

Vaginal sprays are unnecessary and can cause itching, burning, vaginal discharge, rashes, and other problems. Health care providers do not generally recommend that women use them.

> **GLOBAL PERSPECTIVES**
>
> Among Arab people, a girl's virginity is highly valued. As a result, unmarried Arab women do not use tampons during menstruation for fear of breaking the hymen. They use only sanitary pads or napkins (Al-Oballi Kridli, 2002).

If a woman chooses to use a spray, she needs to know that these sprays are for external use only and should never be applied to irritated or itching skin or used with sanitary napkins.

Although douching is sometimes used to treat vaginal infections, douching as a hygiene practice is unnecessary because the vagina cleanses itself, and caregivers advise against it. Douching washes away the natural mucus and upsets the vaginal ecology, which can make the vagina more susceptible to infection. Douching with one of the perfumed or flavored douches can cause an allergic reaction, and too frequent use of an undiluted or strong douche solution can induce severe irritation, even tissue damage. Propelling water up the vagina may also erode the antibacterial cervical plug and force bacteria and germs from the vagina into the uterus. It is essential that women avoid douching during menstruation because the cervix is dilated to permit the downward flow of menstrual fluids from the uterine lining. Douching may force tissue back up into the uterine cavity, which could contribute to endometriosis. Douching is also contraindicated during pregnancy.

CLEANSING THE PERINEUM

The mucous secretions that continually bathe the vagina are completely odor free while they are in the vagina; only when they mingle with perspiration and become exposed to the air does odor develop. Keeping one's skin clean and free of bacteria with plain soap and water is the most effective method of controlling odor. A soapy finger or soft washcloth should be used to wash gently between the labial folds. Bathing is as important (if not more so) during menses as at any other time. A long leisurely soak in a warm tub will promote menstrual blood flow and relieve cramps by relaxing the muscles.

Keeping the vulva fresh throughout the day means keeping it dry and clean. A woman can assure herself of adequate ventilation by wearing cotton panties and clothes loose enough to allow air to circulate. After using the toilet, a woman should always wipe herself from front to back and, if necessary, follow up with a moistened paper towel or toilet paper.

The most important thing to remember is that if an unusual odor persists despite these efforts, a visit to one's health care provider is indicated. Certain conditions, such as vaginitis, produce a foul-smelling discharge.

Associated Menstrual Conditions

A variety of menstrual irregularities has been identified. Several of them are discussed in Chapter 7 in the section on dysfunctional uterine bleeding. Others are addressed in the following sections.

The following terms are used to describe variations in uterine bleeding:

- **Hypomenorrhea**—short duration of menstrual flow or, in other words, regular uterine bleeding but in decreased amounts
- **Hypermenorrhea**—an abnormally long menstrual flow
- **Oligomenorrhea**—bleeding, often irregular, occurring at intervals greater than 40 days

- **Polymenorrhea**—bleeding, either regular or irregular, occurring at intervals of less than 22 days
- **Menorrhagia**—bleeding that is excessive in amount and duration, which occurs at regular intervals
- **Metrorrhagia**—bleeding, usually of a normal amount, occurring at irregular intervals
- **Menometrorrhagia**—bleeding that is excessive in amount and duration, which occurs at either regular or irregular intervals
- **Intermenstrual bleeding**—bleeding occurring between regular menstrual cycles

AMENORRHEA

Amenorrhea, the absence of menses, is classified as primary or secondary. Primary amenorrhea is said to occur if menstruation has not been established by 16 years of age. Secondary amenorrhea is said to occur when an established menses (of longer than 3 months) ceases. In reality, the distinction between the two types of amenorrhea is of little value because the causes often overlap. Typically, the causes of amenorrhea are categorized into one of four groups:

1. *Hypothalamic dysfunction.* Several types of hypothalamic disorders can occur. Some are very rare disorders and may be related to a failure of the central structures of the hypothalamus to develop properly. Other disorders may be caused by a tumor. More common forms of hypothalamic dysfunction are triggered by systemic stress related to marked weight loss (anorexia, bulimia, fad dieting), excessive exercise (associated with long-distance runners, dancers, and other athletes with a low body fat ratio), and severe or prolonged stress.
2. *Pituitary dysfunction.* Pituitary disease and pituitary tumors, such as a pituitary adenoma, can cause changes in the many hormones the pituitary manufactures. A variety of medications, including several used to treat anxiety and other psychiatric disorders, can induce a mild increase in prolactin levels, resulting in amenorrhea. Amenorrhea may also be related to low prolactin levels resulting from pituitary failure. Sheehan's syndrome, head trauma, and cancer are also serious causes of hypopituitarism.
3. *Ovarian failure.* Some forms of ovarian failure are caused by genetic disorders often related to the sex chromosomes, and are not treatable. Turner syndrome (see Chapter 12) is one of the most common genetic disorders. Other causes of ovarian failure include exposure to radiation, chemotherapy, viral infection, and surgical removal of the ovary.
4. *Anatomic abnormalities.* This category includes a variety of structural disorders such as congenital absence of the uterus, ovaries, or vagina; congenital obstruction; or imperforate hymen.

Diagnosis begins with a thorough history and careful physical examination. For women who have had periods, this evaluation begins with a pregnancy test. For a woman who has never menstruated, the pelvic examination is a crucial assessment tool in determining that she has a normal vagina, uterus, and ovaries. Regardless of type of amenorrhea, based on initial findings, further, more specific tests are usually done. For example, magnetic resonance imaging (MRI) to rule out a tumor may be indicated for a woman who has amenorrhea combined with neurologic symptoms. To evaluate pituitary function, a serum prolactin level is often obtained as a screening test. Then other pituitary hormones can be evaluated if necessary. Similarly, elevated serum follicle-stimulating hormone (FSH) levels indicate ovarian failure.

Treatment is dictated by the causative factors. Some conditions, such as imperforate hymen, are easily corrected. Other causes are not treatable. The nurse can explain that once the underlying condition has been corrected—for example, when the client gains sufficient body weight—menses will resume. Female athletes and women who participate in strenuous exercise routines may be advised to increase their caloric intake or reduce their exercise levels for a month or two to see whether a normal cycle resumes. If it does not, medical referral is indicated.

DYSMENORRHEA

Dysmenorrhea, or painful menstruation, occurs at, or a day before, the onset of menstruation and disappears by the end of menses. Dysmenorrhea is classified as primary or secondary.

Primary dysmenorrhea is defined as cramps without underlying disease. Prostaglandins F_2 and $F_2\alpha$, which are produced by the uterus in higher concentrations during menses, are the primary cause. They increase uterine contractility and decrease uterine artery blood flow, causing ischemia. The end result is the painful sensation of cramps. Dysmenorrhea typically disappears after a first pregnancy and does not occur if cycles are anovulatory.

Treatment of primary dysmenorrhea includes oral contraceptives (which block ovulation); nonsteroidal anti-inflammatory drugs (NSAIDs) (such as ibuprofen, aspirin, and naproxen), which act as prostaglandin inhibitors; and self-care measures such as regular exercise, rest, heat, and good nutrition. Biofeedback has also been used with some success.

Secondary dysmenorrhea is associated with pathology of the reproductive tract and usually appears after menstruation has been established. Conditions that most frequently cause secondary dysmenorrhea include endometriosis; residual pelvic inflammatory disease (PID); anatomic anomalies, such as cervical stenosis, imperforate hymen, or uterine displacement; ovarian cysts; or the presence of an intrauterine device (IUD). Because primary and secondary dysmenorrhea may coexist, accurate differential diagnosis is essential for appropriate treatment.

Dysmenorrhea sometimes occurs in women who are also experiencing menometrorrhagia. In such cases, a careful examination is necessary to determine what is causing both symptoms. Testing may include transvaginal ultrasound, hysterosalpingography, and hysteroscopy. If the exam shows an endocervical polyp or cervical stenosis, treatment is surgical.

For women with severe dysmenorrhea that fails to respond to treatment, a hysterectomy may be the treatment of choice if childbearing is not an issue. If childbearing is desired, a presacral neurectomy may be necessary.

Self-Care Measures for Dysmenorrhea

Some nutritionists suggest that vitamins B and E help relieve the discomforts associated with menstruation. Vitamin B_6 may help relieve the premenstrual bloating and irritability some women experience. Vitamin E, a mild prostaglandin inhibitor, may help decrease menstrual discomfort. Avoiding salt can decrease discomfort from fluid retention.

Heat is soothing and promotes increased blood flow. Any source of warmth, from sipping herbal tea to soaking in a hot tub or using a heating pad, may be helpful during painful periods. Massage can also soothe aching back muscles and promote relaxation and blood flow.

Daily exercise can ease existing menstrual discomfort and help prevent cramps and other menstrual complaints. Aerobic exercise—jogging, cycling, aerobic dancing, swimming, and fast-paced walking—is especially helpful (see Figure 4–1 •). Persistent discomfort should be medically evaluated.

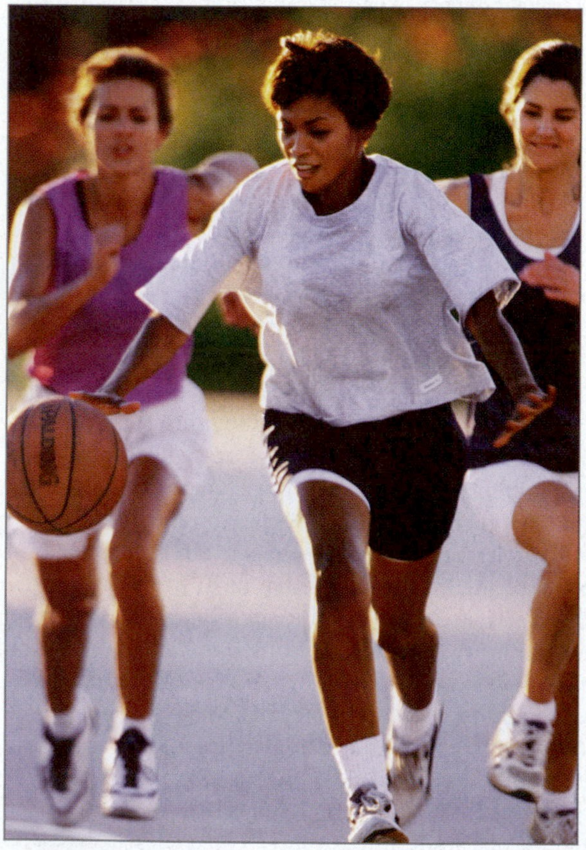

Figure 4–1 • Regular exercise is an important part of therapy for dysmenorrhea.
SOURCE: Tim Pannell-CORBIS.

PREMENSTRUAL SYNDROME

Premenstrual syndrome (PMS) refers to a symptom complex associated with the luteal phase of the menstrual cycle (2 weeks prior to onset of menses). Estimates suggest that up to 80% of women experience physical or emotional changes premenstrually, but only 20% to 40% of these women have problems as a consequence. An even smaller number—2.5% to 5%—feel that the changes jeopardize their work, home life, and relationships (Hudson, 2002).

The symptoms of PMS must, by definition, occur between ovulation and the onset of menses. They repeat at the same stage of each menstrual cycle and include some or all of the following:

- **Psychologic:** irritability, lethargy, depression, low morale, anxiety, sleep disorders, crying spells, and hostility
- **Neurologic:** classic migraine, vertigo, syncope
- **Respiratory:** rhinitis, hoarseness, occasionally asthma
- **Gastrointestinal:** nausea, vomiting, constipation, abdominal bloating, craving for sweets
- **Urinary:** retention and oliguria
- **Dermatologic:** acne
- **Mammary:** swelling and tenderness

Most women experience only some of these symptoms. The symptoms usually are most pronounced 2 or 3 days before the onset of menstruation and subside as menstrual flow begins, with or without treatment. *Premenstrual dysphoric disorder (PMDD)* is a diagnosis that may be applied to a subgroup of women with PMS whose symptoms are primarily mood related and severe enough to interfere markedly with occupational and social functioning (Endicott, Bardack, Grady-Weliky, et al, 2000).

The exact cause of PMS is unknown, although a variety of theories have been put forth to explain it. These include, for example, hormone imbalance, nutritional deficiency, prostaglandin excess, and endorphin deficiency. Researchers currently speculate that PMS is related to serotonin because serotonin levels in women with PMS fall after ovulation (Hudson, 2002).

Diagnosis is generally made after having the woman keep a menstrual calendar for 2 months on which she carefully records daily symptoms, rating them on a scale of 0 to 4, with 0 used for no symptoms and 4 used for severe, debilitating symptoms. The information provided by the diary should be very helpful. In some cases, the diary may reveal that a woman has psychologic symptoms that are present throughout her cycle but intensify premenstrually. Such women may have a dual diagnosis such as PMDD and depression or an anxiety disorder, and psychiatric consultation is indicated (Dell, Moskowitz, & Sondheimer, 2001).

Except in very severe cases, treatment focuses, at least initially, on lifestyle changes and natural approaches. These are discussed in the following section. In addition to vitamin supplements, pharmacologic treatments for PMS include diuretics, calcium supplementation, and prostaglandin inhibitors. All have been effective in some women and not in others. For women who are not planning a pregnancy, low-dose oral contraceptives, which suppress ovulation, are often an effective solution.

Serotonin agents such as fluoxetine hydrochloride (Prozac) and sertraline hydrochloride (Zoloft) can be used to help alleviate symptoms of PMDD. Previously progesterone had been used to treat PMS but it is no longer recommended. Research suggests that it is no more effective than a placebo and it may actually increase symptoms in some women (Dell et al, 2001).

NURSING CARE MANAGEMENT

The nurse can help the woman identify specific symptoms and develop healthy behavior. After assessment, the nurse may advise the woman to restrict her intake of foods containing methylxanthines, such as chocolate, cola, and coffee. It is advisable for the woman to restrict her intake of alcohol, nicotine, red meat, animal fats, and foods containing salt and sugar. Concurrently, she should increase her intake of complex carbohydrates (such as whole grains, brown rice, oatmeal), protein, fruits, vegetables, and vegetable oils; and increase the frequency of meals. A multiple vitamin and mineral supplement may also be helpful.

Supplementation with B complex vitamins, especially B_6, may decrease anxiety and depression. Vitamin E supplements may help reduce breast tenderness. Research indicates that supplementation with 1200 mg calcium carbonate is often effective in relieving several symptoms of PMS including negative mood, food cravings, water retention, and pain (Hudson, 2002).

A program of aerobic exercises such as fast walking, jogging, or aerobic dancing is generally beneficial. In fact, women who exercise regularly tend to have fewer, less severe symptoms.

An empathic relationship with a health care professional to whom the woman feels free to voice concerns is highly beneficial. The nurse can also encourage the woman to keep a journal to help identify life events associated with PMS. Stress reduction education, self-care groups, and self-help literature can also help women gain control over their bodies.

Health Maintenance for Well Women

Health care providers are becoming increasingly aware of the value of health maintenance and disease prevention, as are many consumers of health care services. Women can make lifestyle choices that promote health and well-being. These choices involve a variety of factors including:

- Eating a nutritious, balanced diet
- Maintaining normal weight for height (no fad dieting)
- Performing regular aerobic exercise and weight training several times a week
- Getting adequate sleep
- Avoiding smoking and/or stopping smoking
- Consuming alcohol in moderation
- Managing stress effectively
- Developing enjoyable hobbies and leisure activities
- Developing an inner life in some form through religion, spirituality, personal reflection, yoga, and so forth
- Fostering bonds of support and affection with family and friends
- Obtaining regular health screenings and assessments
- Ensuring that immunizations are up to date

Health screening recommendations vary by age. Table 4–1• from the National Women's Health Information Center (2002) identifies general screening and immunization guidelines for low-risk women based on their age. Nurses can share this information with well women so that they can be aware of indicated screening procedures.

Menopause

Menopause, the time when menses cease, is a time of transition for a woman, marking the end of her reproductive abilities. While it usually occurs between 45 and 52 years of age, the current median age of menopause in the United States is 51.3 years. Although not all of the physiologic mechanisms initiating menopause are precisely understood, it is known that the onset occurs when estrogen levels become so low that menstruation stops. In addition, most researchers agree that the age of onset is influenced by such factors as the woman's overall health, nutrition, lifestyle, culture, and genetic makeup.

Climacteric, or *change of life* (often used synonymously with *menopause*), refers to the host of psychologic and physical alterations that occur around the time of menopause. These aspects are discussed separately.

Perimenopause

Perimenopause refers to the period of time prior to menopause during which the woman moves from normal ovulatory cycles to cessation of menses. Perimenopause typically lasts from 2 to 8 years. It is characterized by decreasing ovarian function, unstable endocrine physiology, and highly variable, unpredictable hormone profiles.

In the United States, the number of women entering their perimenopausal years (40 to 49) has never been higher. This is due to the aging of the post-world war II baby boomers.

Table 4–1 • GENERAL SCREENING AND IMMUNIZATION GUIDELINES FOR WOMEN

Please note: These charts are guidelines only. Your health care provider will personalize the timing of each test and immunization to best meet your health care needs.

Screening Tests	Ages 18–39	Ages 40–49	Ages 50–64	Ages 65+
General health				
Full checkup, including weight and height.	Discuss with your health care provider.	Discuss with your health care provider.	Discuss with your health care provider.	Discuss with your health care provider.
Thyroid test (TSH).	Starting at age 35, then every 5 years.	Every 5 years.	Every 5 years.	Every 5 years.
Heart health				
Blood pressure test.	Starting at age 21 then once every 1–2 years if normal.	Every 1–2 years.	Every 1–2 years.	Every 1–2 years.
Cholesterol test.	Starting at age 20 then every 5 years.	Every 5 years.	Every 5 years.	Every 5 years.
Bone health				
Bone mineral density test.		Discuss with your health care provider.	Discuss with your health care provider.	Discuss with your health care provider.
Diabetes				
Blood sugar test.		Starting at age 45, then every 3 years.	Every 3 years.	Every 3 years.
Breast health				
Breast exam.	Yearly by a health care provider; monthly self-breast exam.	Yearly by a health care provider; monthly self-breast exam.	Yearly by a health care provider; monthly self-breast exam.	Yearly by a health care provider; monthly self-breast exam.
Mammogram (x-ray of breast).		Every 1–2 years. Discuss with your health care provider.	Yearly.	Yearly.
Reproductive health				
Pap test & pelvic exam.	Every 1–3 years after 3 consecutive normal tests. Discuss with your health care provider.	Every 1–3 years after 3 consecutive normal tests. Discuss with your health care provider.	Every 1–3 years after 3 consecutive normal tests. Discuss with your health care provider.	Every 1–3 years after 3 consecutive normal tests. Discuss with your health care provider.
Chlamydia test.	If sexually active, yearly until age 25.	If you are at high risk for chlamydia or other sexually transmitted diseases (STDs) you may need this test. See STD section below.	If you are at high risk for chlamydia or other sexually transmitted diseases (STDs) you may need this test. See STD section below.	If you are at high risk for chlamydia or other sexually transmitted diseases (STDs) you may need this test. See STD section below.
Sexually transmitted diseases (STDs) tests.	If you have multiple sexual partners; or a partner with multiple sexual partners; or a partner with an STD or sexual contact with STDs; or a personal history of STDs.	If you have multiple sexual partners; or a partner with multiple sexual partners; or a partner with an STD or sexual contact with STDs; or a personal history of STDs.	If you have multiple sexual partners; or a partner with multiple sexual partners; or a partner with an STD or sexual contact with STDs; or a personal history of STDs.	If you have multiple sexual partners; or a partner with multiple sexual partners; or a partner with an STD or sexual contact with STDs; or a personal history of STDs.
Colorectal health				
Colonoscopy.			Every 5–10 years.	Every 5–10 years.
Double contrast barium enema (DCBE).			Every 5–10 years. (Only if not having colonoscopy every 10 years.)	Every 5–10 years. (Only if not having colonoscopy every 10 years.)
Flexible sigmoidoscopy.			Every 5 years.	Every 5 years.
Rectal exam.	Discuss with your health care provider.	Discuss with your health care provider.	Every 5–10 years at time of each screening (sigmoidoscopy, colonoscopy, or DCBE).	Every 5–10 years at time of each screening (sigmoidoscopy, colonoscopy, or DCBE).
Fecal occult blood test.			Yearly.	Yearly.
Eye and ear health				
Vision exam with eye care provider.	Once initially between age 20 and 39.	Every 2–4 years.	Every 2–4 years.	Every 2–4 years.
Hearing test (discuss with your health care provider).	Starting at age 18, then every 10 years.	Every 10 years.	Discuss with your health care provider.	Discuss with your health care provider.
Skin health				
Mole exam.	Monthly mole self-exam; starting at age 20, by a health care provider every 3 years.	Monthly mole self-exam; by a health care provider every year.	Monthly mole self-exam; by a health care provider every year.	Monthly mole self-exam; by a health care provider every. year
Oral health				
Dental (oral exam).	One to two times every year.	One to two times every year.	One to two times every year	One to two times every year.

Table 4–1 • CONTINUED

Screening Tests	Ages 18–39	Ages 40%–49	Ages 50–64	Ages 65+
Mental health screening	Discuss with your health care provider.	Discuss with your health care provider.	Discuss with your health care provider.	Discuss with your health care provider.
Immunizations				
Influenza vaccine.	Discuss with your health care provider.	Discuss with your health care provider.	Discuss with your health care provider.	Discuss with your health care provider.
Pneumococcal vaccine.				One time only.
Tetanus-diphtheria booster vaccine.	Every 10 years.	Every 10 years.	Every 10 years.	Every 10 years.

Source: The National Women's Health Information Center, (2002) Office of Women's Health, Department of Health and Human Services, Washington, DC.

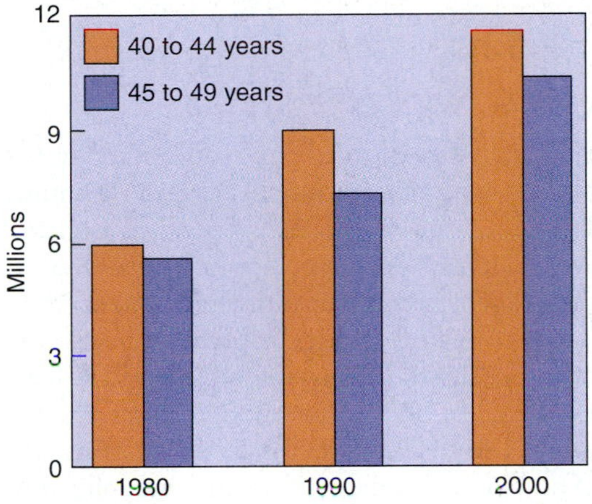

Figure 4–2 • Number of US women ages 40 to 49 years, 1980 to 2000.
SOURCE: US Census Bureau, 2001.

Currently nearly 22 million women are in the perimenopausal years. (Figure 4–2 •).

Symptoms of perimenopause may be nonexistent or bothersome. PMS, hot flashes, irregular periods, insomnia, and mood changes may be problematic. Other concerns include anovulatory dysfunctional uterine bleeding, vasomotor instability, loss of bone density, and gynecologic cancers.

Contraception remains a major concern for many perimenopausal women. In reality, although a growing number of women are choosing to delay childbearing, just over half (51%) of pregnancies for women ages 40 and higher are unplanned. Among these unplanned pregnancies, 60% are ended by induced abortion. Moreover, childbearing women ages 40 and over have a risk of death six times higher (42 per 100,000 live births) than that of women ages 25 to 29 (7 per 100,000 live births) (The Contraception Report [TCR], 2001).

In the United States, female sterilization is, in general, the most commonly used method of contraception. However, combined oral contraceptives (COCs) are gaining popularity as a contraceptive option for this time in a woman's reproductive life. COCs are considered by many to be an optimal approach to this transition, even when contraception is not a concern. Healthy nonsmokers benefit from effective contraception; regulation of menses; treatment of anovulatory bleeding; relief of symptoms of estrogen deficiency and variability such as hot flashes, sleep disturbances, menorrhagia, and vaginal dryness; and a decreased risk of endometrial and ovarian cancer. They may also experience less acne and hirsutism (abnormal hair growth, often on the face and neck), decreased osteopenia, and possible reduction in colorectal cancer incidence (Kaunitz, 2001). Other contraceptive options for perimenopausal women include the contraceptive patch, the vaginal ring, Lunelle (a monthly contraceptive injection) IUDs, progestin-only methods of contraception, and barrier methods of contraception such as male and female condoms, diaphragm, cervical cap, and spermicides (TCR, 2001). (See Chapter 5 for a discussion of these methods.)

Women describing problems that suggest perimenopause should be referred to their care provider. If oral contraceptives are not an option, other alternatives are available. Exercise, calcium and vitamin D, and other medications may be effective.

Psychologic Aspects

A woman's psychologic adaptation to menopause and the climacteric is multifactorial. She is influenced by her own expectations and knowledge, physical well-being, family views, marital stability, and sociocultural expectations. As the number of women reaching menopause increases, especially as the women of the "baby boom" generation begin to enter this phase of life, the negative emotional connotations people sometimes attach to menopause are diminishing dramatically. Menopause is no longer seen as an ending but as a time of transition.

Preliminary research suggests that three major themes often reflect the experience of menopause. These themes include the following (Damato & Winner, 2002):

- **Expectations and realization.** Women are often confused about the symptoms of menopause and fail to recognize subtle symptoms. Some women are unprepared for the fact that periods often become longer, heavier, and more frequent prior to ceasing. Others fail to recognize symptoms such as hot flashes and night sweats even though they anticipate them. Women may experience

GLOBAL PERSPECTIVES

In the United States, youth and beauty are embraced and the aging process is viewed negatively. This is not the case in all cultures.

In the Philippines, menopause is viewed as a positive and liberating event. Here, as women age, they are more respected and admired for their years of gained experiences. Older women gain status and importance as they age and are widely embraced by the younger generations within their family.

Comments from a Filipino nursing student.

emotional fluctuations—mood swings, which they may equate to "an emotional roller coaster."

- **Sorting things out.** Women may seek to explain the interrelatedness of the menopause transition and hormonal changes they experience and the impact of concurrent life events. Many women deal with issues related to aging parents, children leaving home, and the birth of grandchildren at this point in their lives. Women who have experienced PMS or postpartum depression may struggle with depression during menopause. At this point some women wrestle with the issue of whether to begin hormone replacement therapy or let the changes of menopause occur without intervention.
- **A new life phase.** For many women, menopause is a transition, one that is viewed positively. These women experience a sense of contentment about being beyond their childbearing years. They see menopause as marking a new beginning, a time to look forward, a time of freedom to do as they choose. These women also feel a newfound sense of confidence.

Despair, fatigue, and irritability are issues for some menopausal women but a hormonal link has not been conclusively proven. For many, the increased incidence of depression may be linked to menopausal symptoms and not to menopause itself. In addition, psychosocial and cultural factors appear to account for more variation in depression than menopause. In truth, the research variable that is most predictive of subsequent depression is a history of previous depression. Other potential causes of depression at this time include hypothyroidism, the use of some antihypertensive medications, and the stressful life events that often occur during midlife (Choi, 2001).

It is important to help women understand the changes that come with menopause and to deal with their feelings during this period. Moreover, caregivers need to be alert for signs that distinguish between the mood swings that are related to hormonal changes and true clinical depression (Choi, 2001).

In reality the average woman in the United States will live one third of her life after menopause. The changing perceptions of menopause and beyond are enabling menopausal women to cope more effectively and to view menopause as a time of personal growth.

> *My personal response to menopause has surprised me a little. Suddenly 52 doesn't really seem old. I look at pictures of my mother in her early fifties and she seems so much older. I imagine each generation looks back and thinks the same thing. I do wish I had known at 22 what I know now, but I still see myself as learning and growing. Now I am being more selective about my goals for the future—maybe I'll try writing a novel, or I'll take a gourmet cooking class. One thing I am committed to—I intend to do my very best to live each day as it comes and enjoy it to the hilt!*

Physical Aspects

CHANGES IN THE REPRODUCTIVE SYSTEM

The physical characteristics of menopause are linked to the shift from a cyclic to a noncyclic hormonal pattern. Beginning 2 to 8 years before menopause, women experience episodes of anovulation, reduced fertility, decreased or increased flow, irregular frequency of menses, and then ultimately, amenorrhea. Generally ovulation ceases 1 to 2 years before menopause, but individual variations exist. FSH levels rise, and ovarian follicles cease to produce estrogen. The uterine endometrium and myometrium atrophy, as do the cervical glands. The uterine cavity constricts. The fallopian tubes and ovaries atrophy. The vaginal mucosa becomes smooth and thin, and the rugae disappear, leading to loss of elasticity. As a result, intercourse can be painful, but this may be overcome by using a water-soluble lubricating gel. Dryness of the mucous membrane can lead to burning and itching. The vaginal pH level increases as the number of Döderlein's bacilli decreases. This change in the vaginal ecology can lead to an atrophic vaginitis and increase the woman's risk of vaginal infections.

Postmenopausal women can remain orgasmic, and some report that sexual interest and activity increase as the need for contraception disappears and personal growth and awareness increase. Other women report a decrease in libido following menopause, which may be related to lower testosterone levels.

Research suggests that other factors such as general health, a woman's feelings for her partner, her partner's health, any performance difficulties in the partner, psychologic issues, stress at work, and interpersonal stress also have an impact on sexual functioning. Moreover, a woman's attitudes about sex and her enjoyment of it in her younger years may influence her attitudes and enjoyment during her later years. Physiologic changes such as night sweats may cause a woman to feel irritable and tired with diminished sexual desire (Kingsberg, 2001).

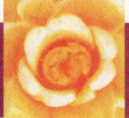

In a woman's later years, atrophic changes occur in the ovaries, vagina, vulva, and urethra and in the trigonal area of the bladder. Vulvar atrophy occurs late, and the pubic hair thins, turns gray or white, and may ultimately disappear. The labia shrink and lose their heightened pigmentation. Pelvic fascia and muscles atrophy, resulting in decreased pelvic support. Kegel exercises and regular sexual activity help prevent this change. The breasts become pendulous and decrease in size and firmness.

VASOMOTOR CHANGES

As many as 75% of menopausal women experience a vasomotor disturbance commonly known as a *hot flash*, which makes it the most commonly reported menopausal symptom (Loprinzi, Barton, Rhodes, et al, 2001). Hot flashes are typically described as a feeling of heat arising from the chest and spreading to the neck and face. The hot flashes are often accompanied by sleep disturbances triggered by profuse sweating (*night sweats*) in which a woman awakens with drenched night clothes and bedding. These episodes may occur as often as 20 to 30 times a day and generally last 3 to 5 minutes or less. Some women also experience dizzy spells, palpitations, and weakness. Many women find their own most effective ways to deal with the hot flashes. Some report that dressing in layers, using a fan, avoiding alcoholic beverages, or drinking a cool liquid helps relieve distress. Still others seek relief through hormone replacement therapy, or complementary therapies such as herbs.

CHANGES IN THE MUSCULOSKELETAL SYSTEM AND SKIN

Long-range physical changes may include **osteoporosis,** a decrease in bone strength related to diminished bone density and bone quality. This change is thought to be associated with lowered estrogen and androgen levels. Osteoporosis puts an individual at increased risk for fractures of the hip, forearm, and vertebrae. Osteoporosis is more common in women who are middle-aged or older. Research indicates that one out of every two US women and one out of every eight US men will suffer an osteoporosis-related fracture at some time (Dore, 2002). Risk factors associated with osteoporosis are identified in Table 4–2 ●.

Loss of protein from the skin and supportive tissues, especially when combined with long-term sun damage or smoking, causes wrinkling. Postmenopausal women frequently gain weight, which may be due to excessive caloric intake or to lower caloric need with the same level of intake.

Table 4–2 ● RISK FACTORS FOR OSTEOPOROSIS

- Middle-aged and elderly women
- European American or Asian ethnic origin
- Small-boned and thin body type
- Low body weight (< 127 lb)
- Family history of osteoporosis
- Lack of regular weight-bearing exercise
- Nulliparity
- Early onset of menopause
- Consistently low intake of calcium
- Cigarette smoking
- Moderate to heavy alcohol intake
- Use of certain medications such as anticonvulsants, corticosteroids, or lithium

CHANGES IN THE CARDIOVASCULAR SYSTEM

An important long-range physical change of menopause is a shift in lipid and lipoprotein levels. Estrogen has a protective mechanism that fosters elevated levels of high-density lipoprotein (HDL) and lower low-density lipoprotein (LDL). When estrogen levels fall with menopause, this protective mechanism ceases, potentially placing a woman at increased risk for coronary heart disease, hypertension, and strokes.

Although coronary heart disease (CHD) is often viewed as a "man's disease," it is the number one killer of women in both the United States and the United Kingdom. Data indicate that 42% of women who suffer a heart attack die within 1 year as compared to 24% of men. Similarly, CHD is the primary cause of death of women in the United Kingdom. In fact, mortality rates for CHD in women are higher in the United Kingdom than in any other European country or other developed country including the United States (Schifrin, 2001). Risk factors for CHD are identified in Table 4–3 ●.

CHANGES IN COGNITIVE FUNCTION

Gradually, with age, cognitive function (learning, memory, concentration, and planning ability) declines. This change is also influenced by lifestyle, genetics, and social status. In the United States, Alzheimer's disease (AD) is the most commonly occurring form of dementia (clinically apparent cognitive decline). For women over age 65 years, the prevalence of AD increases about 5% each year. It reaches 50% in women over age 85 (Naftolin, 2002).

The incidence of AD has increased, in part, because of the increase in average life span. High cholesterol levels and hypertension may increase the risk of AD as may decreased estrogen levels and possibly decreased folate levels. Preliminary research studies with mice suggest a possible link between low folic acid levels and AD (Krumen, Kumaravel, Lohani, et al, 2002). At present there are no therapies available that consistently reduce symptoms or slow the progress of the disease. Acetylcholinesterase inhibitors are the only medications approved by the Food and Drug Administration (FDA) to treat cognitive dysfunction. Some evidence does suggest that estrogen replacement therapy or hormone replacement therapy may delay the onset of AD and may also help prevent mild to moderate cognitive changes, but this finding is open to debate (Naftolin, 2002).

Table 4–3 ● RISK FACTORS FOR CHD IN WOMEN

- Family history of heart disease
- Advancing age—over 55 or postmenopausal
- Overweight and obesity
- Cigarette smoking and/or tobacco use
- Sedentary lifestyle
- Hypertension
- Diabetes
- Elevated cholesterol
- Race (highest incidence in African American women)

Premature Menopause

Some women experience menopause prematurely, either because of premature ovarian failure due to anorexia or other unknown causes, or because of oophorectomy (removal of the ovaries) or chemotherapy to treat cancer. Whatever the cause, premature menopause is traumatic and women are seldom prepared physically or psychologically to deal with the changes involved. Health care providers and nurses need to be very sensitive to women's needs at this difficult time and also need to be alert to cues that may necessitate early testing for menopause. Premature ovarian failure for any reason is devastating to a woman and needs to be identified early and treated effectively.

Medical Therapy

HORMONE REPLACEMENT THERAPY (HRT)

Hormone replacement therapy (HRT), usually involving estrogen for women without a uterus and estrogen and a progestin for women with a uterus, can be helpful in stopping or decreasing many of the symptoms of menopause. The progestin is added because when estrogen is given alone, it can produce endometrial hyperplasia and increase the risk of endometrial cancer.

Estrogen replacement using HRT is most commonly prescribed to stop hot flashes and night sweats, to reverse atrophic vaginal changes, and to prevent osteoporosis. HRT is also helpful in relieving many of the urogenital and vaginal symptoms older women experience, including vaginal dryness, dyspareunia, dysuria, urinary urgency, frequent urination, and recurrent urinary tract infections (Archer & Utian, 2001). It may also offer protection against colon cancer and AD. Currently, long-term studies are under way to determine whether estrogen can play a role in preventing or slowing the development of dementia (McKeon, 2002).

Formerly, long-term HRT was advocated for most women because of its apparent benefits. This approach changed in 2002, however, with the report that a portion of the Women's Health Initiative (WHI), a large-scale randomized study of women receiving HRT, was being stopped prematurely. The portion of the study being stopped focused on women taking a combination of estrogen and progesterone long term (more than 5 years) because evidence collected indicated that these women had a slightly increased risk of having a heart attack or stroke, of developing blood clots, and of developing invasive breast cancer. The study also revealed a slight decrease in the risk of colorectal cancer and hip fracture. However, the overall risks outweighed the benefits (Writing Group for the Women's Health Initiative Investigators, 2002). The study did not evaluate quality of life issues related to estrogen loss such as hot flashes, vaginal dryness, and cognitive issues.

Until recently, HRT was thought to provide protection against cardiovascular disease, the number one cause of death for women over age 50. However, a second study, the Heart and Estrogen/Progestin Replacement Follow-up Study (HERS II) indicated that HRT does not decrease the risk of heart attack. Moreover, women taking HRT experienced adverse effects including gallbladder disease and blood clots in the legs and lungs (Grady, Herrington, Bittner, et al, 2002).

In light of the findings from the WHI and HERS II studies, the North American Menopause Society convened an advisory panel to develop recommendations about the clinical management of postmenopausal hormone therapy. Among their recommendations they suggested the following (2002):

- The treatment of menopausal symptoms such as hot flashes and urogenital symptoms is the primary indication for HRT and estrogen therapy (ET).
- Progestin is only prescribed to protect the endometrium from unopposed estrogen. Thus women with a uterus who are taking estrogen should also have a prescription for adequate progestin coverage (HRT). Women without a uterus who are taking estrogen (ET) should *not* have a progestin prescribed.
- No estrogen therapy regimen (ET or HRT) should be used to prevent coronary heart disease. Alternative prevention regimens should be used instead (weight control, regular exercise, no smoking, healthy diet, etc).
- HRT and ET have been used for the prevention of osteoporosis. However, because of the associated risks, alternative approaches to preventing and treating osteoporosis should be considered.
- HRT and ET use should be limited to the shortest duration feasible in light of treatment goals, benefits, and risks for an individual woman.
- Lower-than-standard doses of HRT and ET should be considered for symptom relief.
- Alternate routes of administration of HRT may provide advantages, but at present the long-term risk benefit ratio has not been shown.
- Therapy decisions should be made individually based on each woman's symptoms and identified risks. Women should be informed of the known risks.

At present, HRT is still recognized as the most effective therapy for women who experience severe menopausal symptoms. For women taking short-term (1 to 4 years) HRT therapy to relieve symptoms, the benefits are likely to outweigh the risks (National Association of Nurse Practitioners in Women's Health, 2002). For women who are taking HRT, opinion varies on the number of days that progesterone (Provera) should be included. Typically, estrogen is given the first 25 days of the month with 10 mg Provera added during the last 12 days of the estrogen administration (days 14 to 25). With this regimen, 80% to 90% of women will experience monthly withdrawal bleeding. An alternative approach involves the daily administration of 0.625 mg estrogen with 2.5 mg Provera, which can be taken as two separate medications or in a combination pill, Prempro. This regimen is associated with less vaginal bleeding and is sufficient to prevent endometrial hyperplasia and osteoporosis. Although most women prefer to take estrogen orally, some choose the transdermal estrogen skin patch. Still others opt for monthly injections. Estrogen is available in a vaginal cream and is used primarily for urogenital symptoms. For women experiencing decreased libido, combination estrogen-testosterone preparations are available.

Before starting HRT, the woman should undergo a thorough history; physical examination including Pap smear; measurement of cholesterol, lipids, and liver enzyme levels; and baseline mammogram. An initial endometrial biopsy is no longer routinely recommended for all women beginning HRT; however, biopsy is indicated for women with an increased risk of endometrial cancer and if excessive, unexpected, or prolonged vaginal bleeding occurs. Caregivers who prescribe HRT should teach their clients to report immediately any signs of complications such as headaches, visual changes, signs of thrombophlebitis, or signs of myocardial infarction that are common in women (see later discussion).

PREVENTION AND TREATMENT OF OSTEOPOROSIS

Osteoporosis is rapidly becoming a significant health risk for older adults (Table 4–2). According to a report published by the National Osteoporosis Foundation (NOF) (2002), more than 10 million people in the United States have osteoporosis. Of this number, over 80% are women. If women who are at risk are added, this number increases to almost 30 million women in 2002 and could reach 35 million by 2010. These numbers are especially worrisome because osteoporosis is a largely preventable disease.

Bone mineral density (BMD) testing is useful in identifying individuals who are at risk for osteoporosis. A variety of guidelines are available for BMD testing. The American College of Obstetricians and Gynecologists (ACOG) (2002) recommends BMD testing for the following:

- All postmenopausal women aged 65 or older
- All postmenopausal women who have had a fracture
- Postmenopausal women under age 65 with one or more risk factors including Caucasian race, a history of a fracture as an adult, impaired eyesight in spite of adequate correction, and a history of alcoholism

BMD testing may also be indicated for pre- or postmenopausal women with certain medical conditions such as eating disorders, leukemia, rheumatoid arthritis, and multiple sclerosis, and for those women on certain medications such as corticosteroids or anticonvulsants.

This quick, painless test assesses whether a woman has normal bone mass or has decreased bone density (osteoporosis) or increased bone porosity or softening (osteomalacia). Optimum screening is done using a central dual-energy x-ray absorptiometry (DEXA) scan to measure bone density at the hip and lumbar spine. Increasingly, however, clinics complete a preliminary screening using smaller, more convenient BMD machines that measure BMD at peripheral sites such as the heel, forearm, or finger (Mastroianni, Ravnikar, & Wooten, 2001). Figure 4–3 • shows a sample bone density testing result.

The woman's height should be measured at each visit, because a loss of height is often an early sign that vertebrae are being compressed because of reduced bone mass. A variety of conditions, including malabsorption syndrome, cancer, cirrhosis of the liver, chronic use of cortisone, and rheumatoid arthritis, can cause secondary arthritis, which resembles osteoporosis. If these secondary causes are ruled out, treatment for osteoporosis is instituted.

Prevention of osteoporosis is a primary goal of care. Women are advised to maintain an adequate calcium intake. The Institute of Medicine recommends that women over age 50 have a daily calcium intake of 1200 mg. Most women require supplements to achieve this level. Calcium supplementation is most efficient when single doses do not exceed 500 mg and when taken with a meal. Vitamin D supplements may also be indicated.

Women are also advised to participate regularly in weight-bearing exercise, to consume only modest quantities of alcohol and caffeine, and to stop smoking. This is especially important because alcohol and smoking have a negative effect on the rate of bone resorption.

The effectiveness of estrogen in preventing osteoporosis is well documented. Women with no contraindications to estrogen who are showing evidence of bone loss are good candidates for HRT. For women who are unable or unwilling to take estrogen, other medications available to treat or help prevent osteoporosis include the following (Dore, 2002):

1. *Bisphosphonates* are calcium regulators that act by inhibiting bone resorption and increasing bone mass. The two most common, alendronate (Fosamax) and risedronate (Actonel), are both taken upon arising in the morning on an empty stomach with a large glass of water. The woman should sit upright or stand for about 30 minutes after taking the medication and before eating. New bisphosphonates may offer women alternatives that eliminate the undesirable gastrointestinal side effects. For example, in 2002, an intravenous bisphosphonate, zoledronic acid (Zometa), was approved by the FDA for use in the treatment of metastatic bone cancer. However, some clinicians are using it to treat osteoporosis. The drug, administered IV once a year, seems to achieve the same results in treating osteoporosis as other bisphosphonates taken daily or weekly without the troublesome side effects (Reid, Brown, Burckhardt, et al, 2002).
2. *Selective estrogen receptor modulators (SERMs)* have estrogen-like properties. The SERM approved for osteoporosis treatment, raloxifene (Evista), acts like estrogen by protecting against osteoporosis but does not stimulate uterine or breast tissue. Raloxifene does not relieve other menopausal symptoms, and may increase hot flashes, so it is indicated in asymptomatic women who want preventive therapy for osteoporosis.

MEDIALINK CARE PLAN: BONE INJURIES

Bedford Imaging Center
Bedford, MA 01730

Name:	**Doe, Jane**	Sex:	Female	Height:	66.5in
Patient ID:	Case A004	Ethnicity:	White	Weight:	165.0lb
Age:	66	Date of Birth:	09/02/1933	Menopause Age:	53

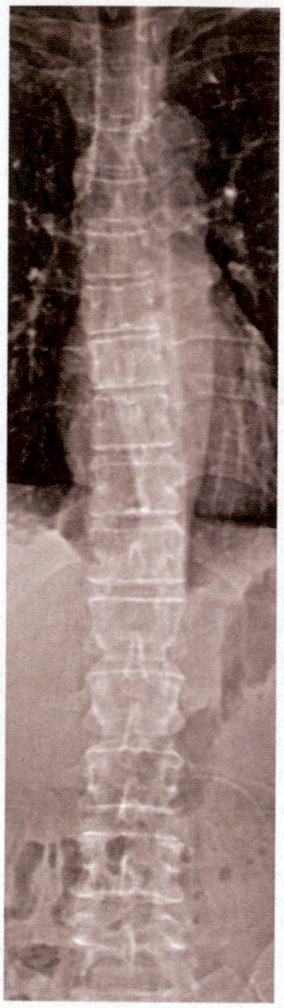

Scan Date: May 01, 2000
Scan ID: A0501000Q
Scan Type: f SE R/L Lateral Image

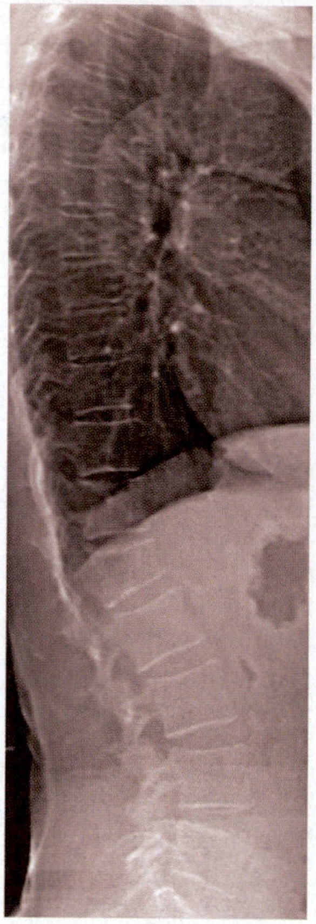

Scan Date: May 01, 2000
Scan ID: A0501000O
Scan Type: f SE AP Image

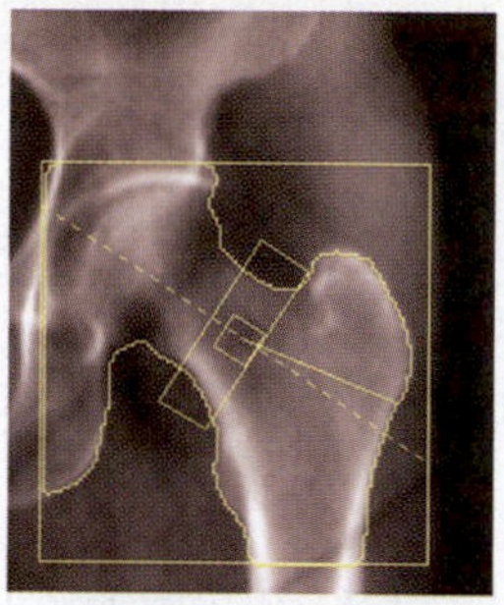

Scan Date: May 01, 2000
Scan ID: A0501000M

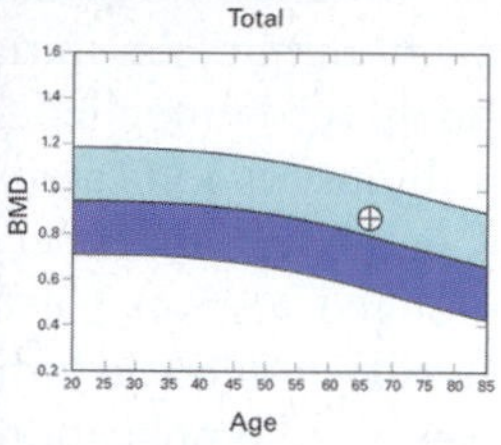

Scan Type: f Left Hip

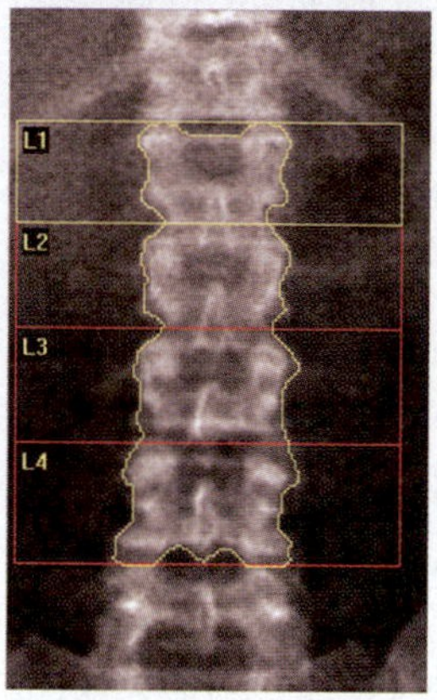

Scan Date: May 01, 2000
Scan ID: A0501000K

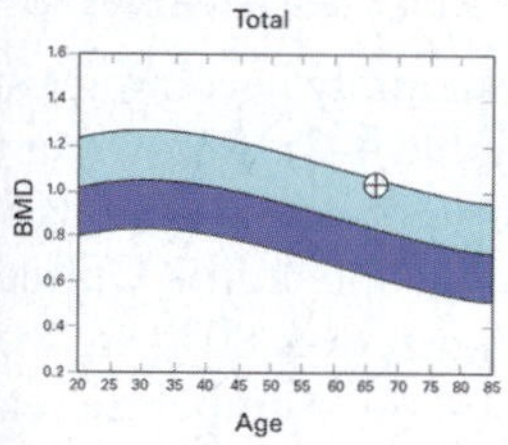

Scan Type: f Lumbar Spine

Results:

	BMD (g/cm²)	T-Score	PR (%)	Z-Score	AM (%)
Left Hip (Neck)	0.773	-0.7	91	0.9	115
Left Hip (Total)	0.870	-0.6	92	0.7	111
Spine (Total)	1.027	-0.2	98	1.7	122

Total BMD CV 1.0%

Summary:

	Classification
Left Hip BMD (Neck)	Normal
Left Hip BMD (Total)	Normal
Spine BMD (Total)	Normal
Vertebral Evaluation:	Severe Wedge Deformity at L2

A spine fracture indicates 5X risk for subsequent spine fracture and 2X risk for subsequent hip fracture.

World Health Organization criteria for BMD interpretation classify patients as Normal (T-score above -1.0), Osteopenic (T-score between -1.0 and -2.5) or Osteoporotic (T-score at or below -2.5).

HOLOGIC®
OSTEOPOROSIS ASSESSMENT

Figure 4–3 • For osteoporosis assessment, published studies demonstrate that up to 30% of clients needing treatment are missed using BMD results of the spine and hip alone. The standard of care for assessing osteoporotic fracture risk is combining BMD results with imaging of the thoracic-lumbar spine. The osteoporotic assessment examination presented here shows a 66-year-old postmenopausal woman who has not received hormone replacement therapy because of a personal history of breast cancer. Although her bone mineral density (BMD) results are within normal limits, she does have an identifiable vertebral fracture at L2. This fracture places her at increased risk for future vertebral fractures and therefore in need of treatment for osteoporosis.

SOURCE: Scan provided courtesy of Hologic, Inc., Osteoporosis Assessment Division, Bedford, MA.

3. *Salmon calcitonin* is a calcium regulator that may inhibit bone loss and is approved for use to treat osteoporosis in women who are 5 years postmenopause. Administered as a nasal spray, its value is less clear than that of the other medications listed.

Fluoride supplementation had been used effectively to treat osteoporosis. However, excessive levels can actually impair bone rebuilding, so it is no longer commonly used. New treatments are currently being investigated including parathyroid hormone (PTH) therapy.

The NOF provides a wealth of information about osteoporosis diagnosis and management. It is found at http://www.nof.org.

PREVENTION OF CORONARY HEART DISEASE

Prevention is the key to dealing with CHD. Prevention begins with lifestyle choices and with lifestyle modifications as necessary. This includes maintaining ideal body weight, exercising regularly, eating a nutritious diet, avoiding smoking, managing stress effectively, obtaining regular health care screenings as indicated, and developing a strong social support system (Table 4–3).

Unless there are contraindications, menopausal women are generally advised to begin daily low-dose aspirin therapy. In addition, women should be familiar with the signs of myocardial infarction (heart attack) that women typically experience. These include pain in the neck, back, or epigastric region; loss of appetite; shortness of breath; nausea or vomiting; and weakness in the shoulder, arms, and chest. Research indicates that women are more likely than men to delay seeking treatment. They are also more likely to die from the attack (Arslanian-Engoren, 2002). Thus it is important for nurses to stress the need to seek immediate treatment if symptoms develop.

Complementary and Alternative Therapies

Many women do not wish to take HRT or have a medical contraindication to it. A variety of therapeutic modalities has been proposed as alternative or complementary treatment or prevention measures for the discomforts and ailments of the perimenopausal and postmenopausal years. These include nutrition and nutrition supplements, such as a diet rich in calcium and vitamins E, D, and B complex.

Phytoestrogens, substances with estrogen properties found in a number of foods and herbs, may be helpful. Examples of foods rich in phytoestrogens include carrots, yams, and soy products. About 10% of women have tried herbal remedies such as dong quai and black cohosh, which have been used in traditional Chinese medicine for years but have not yet been well studied (Nachtigall, 2000). Conversely, menopausal women should avoid foods that may trigger symptoms, including caffeine, alcohol, and spicy foods.

Weight-bearing exercise, including such activities as walking, jogging, tennis, and running, is a means of increasing bone mass and potentiating the effect of estrogen on bone mass. Exercise also improves cholesterol profiles and contributes to overall health. Pelvic floor, or Kegel, exercises can help maintain vaginal muscle tone and increase blood circulation to the perineal area. Vaginal lubricants and adequate foreplay can be helpful in maintaining a satisfactory sexual experience.

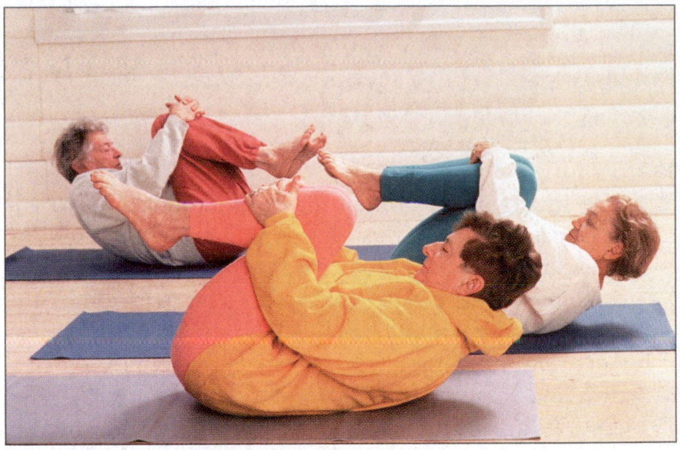

Figure 4–4 • Regular exercise is important, especially for postmenopausal women.
SOURCE: Ariel Skelley-CORBIS.

Relaxation techniques, including yoga, meditation, deep breathing, visualization, massage, use of affirmations, and biofeedback, may provide a sense of well-being. See Figure 4–4 •. Herbal remedies—ginseng, for example—can help relieve the symptoms of hot flashes, headaches, fatigue, lack of concentration, decreased libido, and irregular menses. Additional herbal remedies are dong quai, black cohosh, damiana, goldenseal, motherwort, licorice root, red raspberry leaves, sarsaparilla, and yerba buena. Other helpful therapies include homeopathy and acupuncture (Morelli & Naquin, 2002). See Complementary and Alternative Therapies.

COMPLEMENTARY AND ALTERNATIVE THERAPIES

PHYTOESTROGENS

Phytoestrogens are naturally occurring plant sterols that have an estrogen-like effect. Herbs that contain phytoestrogen include ginseng, agnus castus, beth root, black cohosh, dong quai, fenugreek, licorice, red sage, sarsaparilla, and wild Mexican yam. The phytoestrogens found in these herbs are much weaker than endogenous estrogen, but their biologic activity is equivalent to that of estradiol when the herbs are taken in large amounts. Phytoestrogens are also found in soy products such as tofu. Currently the herbs and soy are receiving considerable study of their effectiveness as more and more women elect to use alternative approachs to treat their menopausal symptoms.

Source: Ansbacher, R. (2001). Herbal medicine. *The Female Patient, 26*(1), 36–40.

NURSING CARE MANAGEMENT

Some menopausal women may need counseling to adjust successfully to this developmental phase of life. Others have no difficulty with this life transition. Reaction to menopause is determined to a large extent by the kind of life the woman has lived, by the security she has in her feminine identity, and by her feelings of self-worth and self-esteem.

Nurses and other health care professionals may be able to help the menopausal woman achieve high-level functioning at this time in her life. Of paramount importance is the nurse's ability to understand and provide support for the woman's views and feelings. Whether the woman expresses relief and delight or tearfulness and fear, the nurse needs to use an empathetic approach in counseling, health teaching, or providing physical care.

Women may discuss areas of deep concern including a history of sexual abuse, current distress, or life dilemmas. Nurses should have appropriate referrals to domestic violence hotlines and to professional therapists who work with women. Women may also be dealing simultaneously with chronically ill parents, divorce or the death of a spouse, troubled or handicapped children, children leaving home, job stressors, and/or generalized fear and anxiety. Nurses can be of assistance with referrals to support groups and counselors who are specific to each woman's need. Although this is a challenge, it is the responsibility of the nurse caring for women to be prepared to meet their needs.

MEDIALINK MENOPAUSE ONLINE

Clinical Tip *Women respond differently to the experience of menopause, so it is important to avoid generalizations. However, in working with menopausal women—and indeed, any women—touch, listening, and caring, as nursing measures, may enhance your self-actualization and that of your client.*

Nurses should explore the question of the woman's comfort during sexual intercourse. In counseling, the nurse may say, "After menopause many women notice that their vagina seems drier, and sex of any kind can be uncomfortable. Have you noticed any changes?" This gives the woman information and may open discussion. The nurse can then go on to explain that the woman can address dryness and shrinking of the vagina by using a water-soluble lubricant to help provide relief. Use of estrogen, orally or in vaginal creams, may also be indicated. Increased frequency of sexual activity will maintain some elasticity in the vagina. When assessing the menopausal woman, the nurse needs to address the question of sexual activity openly but tactfully, because the woman may have been socialized to be reticent in discussing sex. Heterosexual women who do not wish to become pregnant should be counseled to use a method of contraception for one year after their last menstrual period. They should also be advised to report any

EVIDENCE-BASED PRACTICE

EMOTIONAL WELL-BEING DURING MIDLIFE

Clinical Question

What measures are effective in promoting emotional well-being in women ages 40 to 60 years old?

The Evidence

Clinical experts from the Association of Women's Health, Obstetric, and Neonatal Nurses (A WHONN) developed these evidence-based clinical practice guidelines. The panel developed recommendations to promote the emotional well-being of women during midlife, or about ages 40 to 60 years. Quantitative and qualitative evidence was gathered and rated to address the emotional well-being and behavioral health status of women in midlife as evidenced by perceptions of health, well-being, and quality of life; positive and negative moods; levels of self-esteem; somatization; self-care strategies; coping mechanisms; presence or absence of depressive disorders, anxiety, or behavioral health problems. Each clinical practice recommendation presented in the guideline is supported by a referenced rationale.

Best Practice

The recommendations fall into six categories: (1) assessment of life transitions, (2) assessment of emotional vulnerability, (3) assessment of self-care strategies, (4) health promotion, (5) health maintenance, and (6) health restoration.

Specific examples of *health promotion recommendations* and evidence ratings are presented below:

- Provide information and education about menopause (Evidence Rating: III).
- Encourage routine diagnostic testing, such as Pap tests and mammograms (Evidence Rating: III).
- Encourage discussion of relationship issues that may influence emotional well-being (Evidence Rating: III).

Reference: Association of Women's Health, Obstetric and Neonatal Nurses (AWHONN). (2001). *Evidence-based clinical practice guideline; Promotion of emotional well-being during midlife.* Washington (DC): Author.

bleeding after one year of amenorrhea because this may indicate a problem and requires evaluation.

The crucial need of women in the perimenopausal period of life is for adequate information about the changes taking place in their bodies and their lives and support in adjusting to the changes that occur. Supplying that information and providing support as needed present both a challenge and an opportunity for nurses.

Additional information about the most current approaches to the management of menopause and the postmenopausal period can be found at the Web site of the North American Menopause Society. It is found at http://www.menopause.org.

CHAPTER REVIEW

EXPLOREMEDIALINK

NCLEX review questions, case studies, and other interactive resources for this chapter can be found on the Web site at http://www.prenhall.com/olds. Click on "Chapter 4" to select the activities for this chapter.

For tutorials including animations and videos, more NCLEX review questions, and an audio glossary, access the accompanying CD-ROM in this book.

Focus Your Study

- Nurses should provide girls and women with clear information about menstrual issues, such as the use of pads and tampons (including warnings regarding deodorant and absorbency); vaginal spray and douching practices; and self-care comfort measures during menstruation, such as maintaining good nutrition, exercising, and applying heat and massage.
- Dysmenorrhea usually begins at, or a day before, the onset of menses and disappears by the end. Hormone therapy (eg, combined oral contraceptives), nonsteroidal anti-inflammatory drugs, or prostaglandin inhibitors can alleviate dysmenorrhea. Self-care measures include improving nutrition, exercising, applying heat, and getting extra rest.
- Premenstrual syndrome occurs most often in women over 30. The most pronounced symptoms occur 2 to 3 days before onset of menstruation and subside as menstruation starts, with or without treatment. Medical management usually includes progesterone agonists, prostaglandin inhibitors, and calcium supplementation. Self-care measures include improving nutrition (taking vitamin B complex and E supplements and avoiding methylxanthines, which are found, for example, in chocolate and caffeine), undertaking a program of aerobic exercise, and participating in self-care support groups.
- During her adult years, a healthy woman should make healthful lifestyle choices such as avoiding smoking and exercising regularly. She should also participate in regular health screenings following a recommended schedule.
- Menopause is a physiologic, maturational change in a woman's life. Physiologic changes include the cessation of menses and a decrease in circulating hormones. Hormonal changes sometimes bring unsettling emotional responses. The more common physiologic symptoms are "hot flashes," palpitations, dizziness, and increased perspiration at night. The woman's anatomy also undergoes changes, such as atrophy of the vagina, reduction in size and pigmentation of the labia, and myometrial atrophy. Osteoporosis becomes an increasing concern.
- Osteoporosis is becoming a significant health problem in the United States. Prevention is the preferred approach to addressing the issue. This includes adequate calcium intake, regular weight-bearing exercise, and HRT. For women who have already developed osteoporosis, medications are available as a treatment option.
- Coronary heart disease is the number one killer of women in the United States. Prevention is the goal of therapy.
- Current management of menopause centers around hormone replacement therapy, complementary therapies, and client health care education. Decisions regarding the use of HRT should be made individually based on each woman's symptoms and risks, and women should be advised of the known risks.

References

Al-Oballi Kridli, S. (2002). Health beliefs and practices among Arab women. *MCN, American Journal of Maternal-Child Nursing, 27*(3), 178–182.

American College of Obstetricians and Gynecologists (ACOG). (2002). *Bone density screening for osteoporosis* (Committee Opinion). Washington, DC: Author.

Archer, D. F. & Utian, W. H. (2001). Decisions in prescribing HRT. *Contemporary OB/GYN, 46*(8), 86–97.

Arslanian-Engoren, C. (2002). Recognizing heart disease:Helping women seek treatment faster. *AWHONN Lifelines, 5*(2), 114–122.

Choi, M. W. (2001). Menopause and mood: Are they connected? *The Female Patient, 26*(8), 62–63.

Damato, E. G., & Winner, C. W. (2002). Cytomegalovirus infection: Perinatal implications. *Journal of Obstetric, Gynecologic, and Neonatal Nursing, 31* (1), 86–92.

Dell, D. L., Moskowitz, D., & Sondheimer, S. J. (2001). PMS and PMDD: Identification and treatment. *Contemporary OB/GYN, 46*(4), 15–30.

Dore, R. K. (2002 March). Osteoporosis: Fractures and key risk factors. *The Female Patient*, (Suppl. 27), 5–12.

Endicott, J., Bardack, L., Grady-Weliky, T. A., Ling, F. W., & Schmidt, P. J. (2000). An update on premenstrual dysphoric disorder. *The Female Patient, 25*(2), 45–56.

George, S. A. (2002). The menopause experience: A woman's perspective. *Journal of Obstetric, Gynecologic, and Neonatal Nursing, 31(1), 77–85.*

Grady, D., Herrington, D., Bittner, V., Blumenthal, R., Davidson, M., Hlathy, M., et al. (2002). Cardiovascular disease outcomes during 6–8 years of hormone therapy. Heart and Estrogen/Progestin Replacement Study Follow-up (HERS II). *Journal of the American Medical Association, 288*, 49–57.

Hudson, T. (2002). Premenstrual syndrome, Part 1. *The Female Patient, 27*(5), 47–49.

Kaunitz, A. (2001). Prescribing oral contraceptives for menopause. *Women's Health in Primary Care*, 4(9), 579–590.

Kingsberg, S. (2001). Menopause and sexual functioning. *The Female Patient, 26*(6), 35–36.

Krumen, I., Kumaravel, T. S., Lohani, A., Pederson, W. A., Cutler, R. G., Krumen, Y., et al. (2002). Folic acid deficiency and homocysteine impair DNA repair in hippocampal neurons and sensitize them to amyloid toxicity in experimental models of Alzheimer's disease. *Journal of Neuroscience, 22*(5), 1752–1762.

Loprinzi, C. L., Barton, D. L., Rhodes,D. J., et al. (2001). Newer antidepressants for hot flashes. *Contemporary OB/GYN, 46*(11), 61–70.

Mastroianni, L., Ravnikar, V. A., & Wooten, W. (2001). Assessing and maintaining bone health in the postmenopausal woman. *Contemporary OB/GYN, 46*(10), 44–60.

McKeon, V. A. (2002). Exploring HRT: Gauging the benefits, risks, and unknowns of hormone replacement therapy. *AWHONN Lifelines, 6* (1), 24–31.

Moline, M. L., & Zendell, S. M. (2000, March). Evaluating and managing premenstrual syndrome. *Medscape Women's Health, 5*(2), 1–3.

Morelli, V., & Naquin, C. (2002). Alternative therapies for traditional disease states: Menopause. *American Family Physician, 66* (1), 129–134.

Nachtigall, L. E. (2000, June). Assessing alternative approaches to menopause. *Contemporary OB/GYN*, (Suppl.) *45*, 3–10.

Naftolin, F. (2002). Cognitive function and menopause. *The Female Patient, 27*(2), 46–47.

National Association of Nurse Practitioners in Women's Health. (2002). Hormone replacement therapy: From the National Association of Nurse Practitioners in Women's Health. *Topics in Advanced Practice Nursing eJournal, 2*(3). Retrieved July 31, 2002, from www.medscape.com/viewarticle/439106_print

National Osteoporosis Foundation (NOF). (2002). *America's bone health: The state of osteoporosis and low bone mass in our nation.* Washington, DC: Author. Retrieved October 13, 2002 from http://www.nof.org

North American Menopause Society (NAMS). (2002). *Amended report from the NAMS Advisory Panel on postmenopausal hormone therapy.* Presented at the NAMS annual meeting on October 3, 2002, and amended and revised on October 6, 2002. Retrieved October 13, 2002, from www.menopause.org

Reid, I. R., Brown, J. P., Burckhardt, P., Horowitz, Z., Richardson, P., Trecksel, U., et al. (2002, February 28). Introvenous zolehydronic acid in postmenopausal women with low bone mineral density. *New England Journal of Medicine, 346*, 653–661.

Schifrin, E. (2001). An overview of women's health issues in the United States and the United Kingdom. *Women's Health Issues, 11*(4), 261–281.

The Contraception Report (TCR). (2001). Contraception for women in perimenopause. *The Contraception Report, 12*(1), 4–12.

Writing Group for the Women's Health Initiative Investigators. (2002). Risks and benefits of estrogen plus progestin in healthy postmenopausal women: Principal results from the Women's Health Initiative randomized controlled trial. *Journal of the American Medical Association, 288*, 321–333.

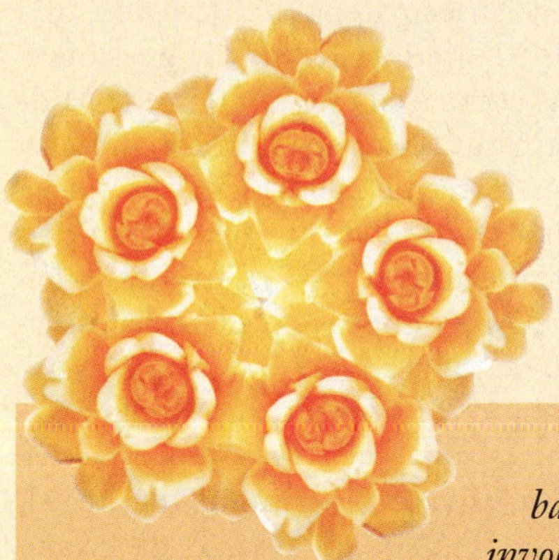

5 Women's Health: Family Planning

I was 15 when I fell in love with Joe, a 17-year-old handsome senior on our high school basketball team. My friends were so envious. We didn't plan on becoming sexually involved. It just happened. I knew I should use some method of birth control, but I didn't know where to go. I couldn't talk to my mother. She wouldn't understand. Joe tried condoms, but he didn't like the way they felt. Several months went by and nothing happened. Then one month my period was late. I was SCARED. It really hit me that a pregnancy would be so hard to handle. I was only a sophomore. My best friend took me to see her nurse practitioner. My pregnancy test was negative. The nurse practitioner encouraged me to talk. She taught me about my body and how to protect myself. She helped me build my self-esteem. I realize now that I'm not ready to be in a sexual relationship yet.

Objectives

- Describe the reasons why women and couples choose to use contraception.
- Discuss approaches to natural family planning.
- List the types of spermicides currently available.
- Compare the barrier methods of contraception with regard to correct use and advantages and disadvantages.
- Summarize the key points women who use combined oral contraceptives should know including the correct procedure for taking pills, common side effects, warning signs, and noncontraceptive benefits.
- Compare other hormonal methods of birth control including Depo-Provera, Lunelle, NuvaRing, Ortho Evra, and the minipill.
- Identify the appropriate time frame for initiating emergency postcoital contraception.
- Delineate the advantages and disadvantages of the IUD as a method of contraception.
- Contrast the two forms of sterilization—tubal ligation and vasectomy—with regard to risk, effectiveness, advantages, and disadvantages.
- Compare medical and surgical approaches to pregnancy termination.

Key Terms

Cervical cap 97
Coitus interruptus 93
Combined oral contraceptives (COCs) 99
Condom 94
Depo-Provera 101
Diaphragm 95
Fertility awareness methods 91
Intrauterine device (IUD) 98
Postcoital contraception 102
Spermicides 93
Sterilization 102
Subdermal implants (Norplant) 101
Tubal ligation 103
Vasectomy 102

MediaLink

Additional resources for this content can be found on the Student CD-ROM and on the Companion Website at www.prenhall.com/olds. Click on "Chapter 5" to select the activities for this chapter.

CD-ROM

- Audio Glossary
- NCLEX Review
- Oral Contraceptive Animation

Companion Website

- Additional NCLEX Review
- Case Study: Family Planning
- Care Plan Activity: Fertility Awareness

Family planning refers to actions an individual or a couple take to avoid a pregnancy, to space future pregnancies for a specific reason, or to gain control over the number of children conceived. Thus at a given time a woman may choose one method of contraception and at a later time, may elect to use a different approach. For example, birth control pills are an excellent method of contraception for women who are healthy and have no contraindications. A married woman in a stable sexual relationship may choose to use an intrauterine device (IUD), while a woman who has no desire for further children may elect to have a tubal ligation. While women have several contraceptive options available, currently, contraceptive approaches for men are limited to condoms and vasectomy. This chapter focuses on methods of contraception that are currently available including the advantages and disadvantages of each.

Overview of Family Planning

Demographics

Currently, about 60 million women in the United States are of childbearing age (15 to 44 years). Of these women, 64% practice contraception while 31% do not need a method of contraception because they are not sexually active, have never had intercourse, are pregnant, are postpartum, are sterile for noncontraceptive reasons, or are trying to become pregnant. Therefore, only 5% of women—approximately 3 million—between the ages of 15 and 44 who need contraception are not using it. These women account for about half (1.5 million) of the 3 million unintended pregnancies that occur annually; the remaining 1.5 million unintended pregnancies result from contraceptive failure, typically because of incorrect or inconsistent use (Alan Guttmacher Institute, 2000).

Family planning is an important component of women's health. Worldwide, women who are able to plan the number of pregnancies they have and the interval between pregnancies benefit in several ways (Alan Guttmacher Institute, 2002):

- They enjoy improved health.
- They have lower rates of induced, sometimes unsafe, abortions.
- They have fewer unwanted pregnancies and births.
- They have the opportunity to get more education and to find jobs, which enhance their economic and social status and improve the well-being of their families.

Maternal mortality remains a major health challenge in developing countries. Annually about 515,000 women die because of pregnancy or childbirth, and 98% of these women are from developing countries. As described in Chapter 1, maternal deaths are a particular problem in portions of Africa. Specifically, women in sub-Saharan Africa (Eritrea, Ethiopia, Central African Republic, Rwanda, and Mozambique) have a 1 in 13 lifetime risk of dying from a pregnancy-related cause as compared to 1 in 50 in the Middle East, North Africa, and South Asia, and 1 in 160 in Latin America (Alan Guttmacher Institute, 2002).

Most of the causes of maternal mortality are treatable or preventable with adequate healthcare. Thus, it is essential that maternal healthcare services improve if maternal mortality and morbidity are to be reduced.

In the United States, about 3 in 4 women of childbearing age receive family-planning and other reproductive healthcare services from a private practitioner or health maintenance organization (HMO) (Frost & Darroch, 2002). The remaining 1 in 4—more than 16 million women—need subsidized family-planning services. The largest funding source for this subsidy comes from the joint federal-state Medicaid program. Research suggests that this is money well spent. For every $1 spent on family-planning services, an average of $3 is saved in pregnancy-related care and care of newborns. Moreover, without these publically supported services, there would be 40% more abortions each year, and Medicaid expenditures would increase by $1.2 billion annually (Alan Guttmacher Institute, 2001).

Choosing a Method of Contraception

The decision to use a method of contraception may be made individually by a woman (or, in the case of condoms or vasectomy, by a man) or jointly by a couple. Research indicates that attitudes about contraceptive methods vary considerably. Of the contraceptive methods available, women had the highest percentages of favorable opinions about combined oral contraceptives (COCs), the male condom, vasectomy, and tubal ligation. Although 78% of women favored COCs, no other methods received a favorable rating from more than two thirds of women. Furthermore, only 26% viewed the diaphragm favorably, citing concerns about effectiveness, inconvenience, and interference with intercourse. Even fewer had favorable opinions about implants, spermicides, the IUD, injectables, the female condom, and the cervical cap (Frost & Darroch, 2002). Thus, it seems that public education about family-planning options is an important consideration for healthcare providers.

Decisions about contraception should be made voluntarily, with full knowledge of advantages, disadvantages, effectiveness, side effects, contraindications, and long-term effects. Many outside factors influence this choice, including cultural practices, religious beliefs, personality, cost, effectiveness, availability, misinformation, practicality of method, and self-esteem. Different methods of contraception may be appropriate at different times in a couple's life (Table 5–1 •). In choosing a specific method, consistency of use outweighs the absolute reliability of the given method.

RESEARCH IN PRACTICE
Association of Acculturation Level and Outcomes of Healthcare

What is this study about? For many Hispanic immigrant women, the first contact with the US healthcare system is likely a visit for reproductive healthcare. There is significant research associating acculturation status and outcomes of healthcare. The stresses associated with acculturation to an immigrant life can increase the risk of poor health and low quality of life. Several studies have indicated that adherence to traditional values as well as social support networks may serve as buffers to the stressors of immigration and may encourage positive outcomes. There is insufficient literature to determine if this relationship extends to family-planning beliefs and outcomes. The purpose of this study was to describe family-planning patterns of Hispanic women and determine if these patterns are related to acculturation level.

How was this study done? This descriptive, correlational study was completed using a convenience sample of 376 Hispanic women who accessed prenatal clinics in a teaching hospital in the Southwest. The Acculturation Rating Scale for Mexican Americans—II (ARSMA II) was used to assess acculturation. Data were collected from the medical record regarding family-planning compliance at 2 weeks, 3 months, and 1 year postbirth. Measures of association and linear regression were used to determine significant associations in the data.

What were the results of the study? Nearly 75% of the women in the study returned for at least one postpartum or family-planning visit within one year after birth. Number of pregnancies, generation in the United States, and acculturation were all significantly related to family-planning visits in the first year after a birth. Having more prenatal visits before the birth was positively correlated with return for family-planning visits. Most of the women preferred reversible family-planning methods; only 9% of the women in the study chose tubal ligation as a family-planning method.

What additional questions might I have? Is it possible the mothers who did not return used other family-planning resources available to them? Were factors omitted because of the retrospective nature of the study?

How can I use this study? Nurses working in maternal-child health settings are in a unique position to affect health choices made by Hispanic women. An assessment of acculturation level, combined with knowledge of the obstetric history of the Hispanic woman, can help guide the nurses' counseling regarding family-planning choices. The importance of prenatal visits in informing mothers and influencing family-planning choices is reinforced by this study.

Source: Jones, M. E., Bond, M. L., Gardner, S. H., & Hernandez, M. C. (2002). A call to action: Acculturation level and family-planning patterns of Hispanic immigrant women. *American Journal of Maternal Child Nursing, 27*(1), 26–33.

Table 5–1 • FACTORS TO CONSIDER IN CHOOSING A METHOD OF CONTRACEPTION

Effectiveness of method in preventing pregnancy	Personal preferences, biases
Safety of the method:	Lifestyle:
Are there inherent risks?	How frequently does client have intercourse?
Does it offer protection against STIs or other conditions?	Does she have multiple partners?
Client's age and future childbearing plans	Does she have ready access to medical care in the event of complications?
Any contraindications in client's health history	Is cost a factor?
Religious or moral factors influencing choice	Partner's support and willingness to cooperate
	Personal motivation to use method

Fertility Awareness Methods

Fertility awareness methods, also known as *natural family planning,* are based on an understanding of the changes that occur throughout a woman's ovulatory cycle. All these methods require periods of abstinence and recording of certain events throughout the cycle; cooperation of the partners is important.

On the one hand, fertility awareness methods are free, safe, and acceptable to many whose religious beliefs prohibit other methods; they provide an increased awareness of the body; they involve no artificial substances or devices; they encourage a couple to communicate about sexual activity and family planning; and they are useful in helping a couple plan a pregnancy.

On the other hand, these methods require extensive initial counseling to be used effectively; they may interfere with sexual spontaneity; they require the couple to maintain records for several cycles before beginning to use them; they may be difficult or impossible for certain groups of women to use including those with irregular cycles, women who are breastfeeding, and perimenopausal women; and, although theoretically they should be very reliable, in practice they may not be as reliable in preventing pregnancy as other methods.

Calendar Method

The *calendar,* or *rhythm,* method is based on the assumptions that ovulation tends to occur 14 days (plus or minus 2 days) before the start of the next menstrual period, that sperm are viable for up to 5 days, and that the ovum is viable for about 24 hours. To use this method, the woman must record her menstrual cycles for 6 to 8 months to identify the shortest and longest cycles. The first day of menstruation is the first day of the cycle. The fertile phase is calculated from 18 days before the end of the shortest recorded cycle through 11 days from the end of the longest recorded cycle . For example, if a woman's cycle lasts from 24 to 28 days, the fertile phase would be calculated as day 6 through day 17. Once this information is obtained, the woman can identify the fertile

MEDIALINK CARE PLAN: FERTILITY AWARENESS

and infertile phases of her cycle. For effective use of this method, she must abstain from intercourse during the fertile phase. The calendar method is the *least reliable* of the fertility awareness methods and has largely been replaced by approaches based on observable data.

Basal Body Temperature Method

The *basal body temperature (BBT)* method to detect ovulation requires that a woman take her BBT every morning upon awakening (before any activity) and record the readings on a temperature graph. To do this, she uses a BBT thermometer, which shows tenths of a degree rather than the two tenths shown on standard thermometers. After 3 to 4 months of recording temperatures, a woman with regular cycles should be able to predict when ovulation will occur. The method is based on the fact that the temperature sometimes drops just before ovulation and almost always rises and remains elevated for several days after. The temperature rise occurs in response to the increased progesterone levels that occur in the second half of the cycle. Figure 5–1 • shows a sample BBT chart. To avoid conception, the couple abstains from intercourse on the day of the temperature rise and for 3 days after. Because the temperature rise does not occur until after ovulation, a woman who had intercourse just before the rise is at risk of pregnancy. To decrease this risk, some couples abstain from intercourse for several days before the anticipated time of ovulation and then for 3 days after. Some care providers encourage both partners to check BBT daily and keep graphs. By comparing the two charts, temperature variation related to room temperature rather than physiologic changes can be evaluated.

Cervical Mucus Method

The *cervical mucus method*, sometimes called the *ovulation method* or the *Billings method*, involves the assessment of cervical mucus changes that occur during the menstrual cycle. The amount and character of cervical mucus change because of the influence of estrogen and progesterone. During the follicular phase of the cycle (from the end of menses until just prior to ovulation), cervical mucus is thin and scanty, and may even be entirely absent. At the time of ovulation, the mucus (estrogen-dominant mucus) is clearer, more stretchable (a quality called *spinnbarkheit*), and more permeable to sperm. It also shows a characteristic fern pattern when placed on a glass slide and allowed to dry.

During the luteal phase (following ovulation through the time just prior to the onset of menses), cervical mucus is thick and sticky (progesterone-dominant mucus) and forms a network that traps sperm, making their passage difficult.

Prior to using the cervical mucus method, the woman abstains from intercourse for one entire menstrual cycle, during which she assesses her cervical mucus daily for amount, feeling of slipperiness or wetness, color, clearness, and spinnbarkheit. Abstinence is important during this time not only so that the woman avoids pregnancy, but also because the presence of ejaculate in the vagina in the hours following intercourse could interfere with the woman's assessment of her cervical mucus.

When using this method, the woman assumes that the peak day of wetness and clear, stretchable mucus is the day of ovulation. However, she abstains from intercourse from the time she *first* notices that the mucus is becoming clear, more elastic, and slippery until 4 days *after* the peak wet mucus (ovulation) day. Because this method evaluates the effects of hormonal changes, women with irregular cycles can use it. Women who feel uncomfortable testing their mucus should be encouraged to use another method.

Symptothermal Method

The *symptothermal method* consists of various assessments made and recorded by the couple. These include information regarding cycle length, coitus, cervical mucus changes, and secondary signs such as increased libido, abdominal bloating, mittelschmerz (midcycle abdominal pain), and

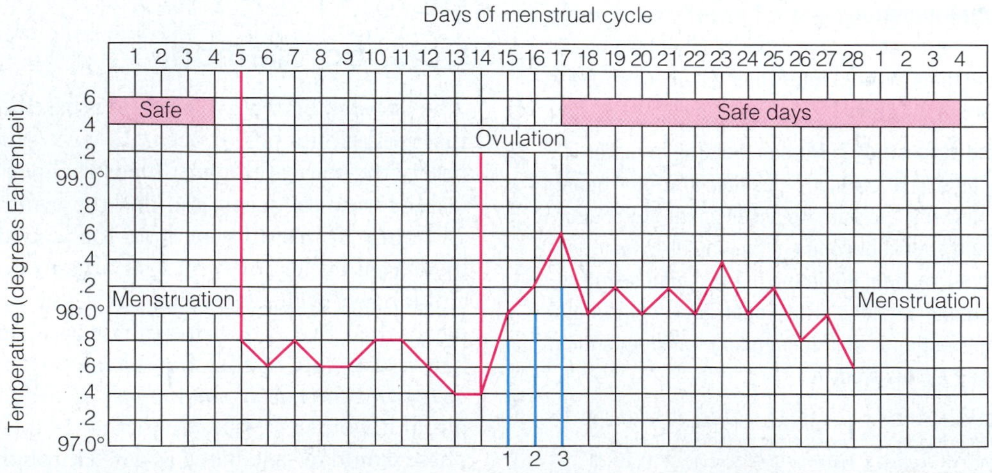

Figure 5–1 • Sample basal body temperature chart.

BBT. Through the various assessments, the couple learns to recognize signs that indicate ovulation. This combined approach tends to improve the effectiveness of fertility awareness as a method of birth control and is best taught by an expert in the method (Barron & Daly, 2001).

Situational Contraceptives

Certain practices such as coitus interruptus (withdrawal) and douching are considered situational contraceptives because they are activities an individual uses in a given situation to avoid pregnancy without benefit of clinical guidance or medical care. Abstinence, a lifestyle choice, is also considered a situational contraceptive.

Abstinence

Abstinence can be considered a method of contraception and, partly because of changing values and the increased risk of infection with intercourse, it is gaining increased acceptance among people of all ages, but especially among adolescents and young adults. In the past several years, the popular media has featured several stories about film stars, sports heroes, and other personalities who are choosing abstinence, and support groups and Web sites for abstinent teens and adults have become popular. As a result of these and other factors, more and more young people are embracing abstinence and making a commitment to delay sexual intercourse until marriage. Some have even signed pledges to that effect.

In addition, abstinence may be culturally dictated. For example, abstinence is the norm in some cultures for women during the postpartum period.

Coitus Interruptus

Coitus interruptus, or withdrawal, is one of the oldest and least reliable methods of contraception. This method requires that the male withdraw from the female's vagina when he feels that ejaculation is impending. He then ejaculates away from the external genitalia of the woman. Failure tends to occur for two reasons:

- This method demands great self-control on the part of the man, who must withdraw just as he feels the urge for deeper penetration with impending orgasm.
- Some preejaculatory fluid, which can contain sperm, may escape from the penis during the excitement phase prior to ejaculation. Because the quantity of sperm in this preejaculatory fluid is increased after a recent ejaculation, this is especially significant for couples who engage in repeated episodes of orgasm within a short period of time.

Couples who use this method should be aware of emergency postcoital contraceptive options should the man fail to withdraw in time.

Douching

Douching after intercourse is an ineffective method of contraception and is *not* recommended. Moreover, it may actually facilitate conception by pushing sperm farther up the birth canal.

Spermicides

Spermicides, available as creams, jellies, foams, vaginal film, and suppositories, are inserted into the vagina before intercourse. They destroy sperm or neutralize vaginal secretions and thereby immobilize sperm. Spermicides that effervesce in a moist environment offer more rapid protection, and coitus may take place immediately after they are inserted. Suppositories may require up to 30 minutes to dissolve and will not offer protection until they do so. The nurse instructs the woman to insert these spermicide preparations high in the vagina and maintain a supine position.

Spermicides are minimally effective when used alone, but their effectiveness increases in conjunction with a barrier method of contraception such as the diaphragm, cervical cap, contraceptive sponge, and male and female condoms. The major advantages of spermicides are their wide availability and low toxicity.

In the past, nonoxynol-9 (N-9), the main ingredient in many spermicides, was thought to offer a modest level of protection against several sexually transmitted infections. However, recent research suggests that N-9 does not offer protection against the organisms that cause gonorrhea and chlamydia, or against human immunodeficiency virus (HIV), the organism that causes HIV/AIDS (Centers for Disease Control and Prevention [CDC], 2002). Moreover, N-9 may actually increase a woman's risk of HIV infection because it has a negative effect on the integrity of vaginal cells, making them more susceptible to invasion by organisms such as HIV (Sobrero, 2002).

Barrier Methods of Contraception

Barrier methods of contraception prevent the transport of sperm to the ovum, immobilize sperm, or are lethal against them. Barrier methods are often used in conjunction with spermicides, which some authorities consider a form of chemical barrier.

Barrier methods are clearly related to an individual's sexual behavior. Each act of intercourse demands that one or both partners consciously decide whether to use a barrier contraceptive and then take action. Thus these methods require motivation on the part of the user and cooperation from the partner. They may also be used less consistently than non-coitus-related methods of contraception. However, they are also very safe methods and they do offer a level of protection against some sexually transmitted infections.

Barrier methods of contraception are a good choice for women who

- Have a contraindication to using a specific method such as COCs, the IUD, subdermal implants, and the like.

MEDIALINK CONTRACEPTION ONLINE

- Are opposed to taking systemic medications or chemicals such as COCs, monthly injections, and so forth.
- Are in early postpartum or are lactating.
- Need a backup method of contraception for a period of time such as when beginning COCs, after an IUD has been inserted, or when a male partner has just had a vasectomy.
- Have intercourse rarely or sporadically.
- Are perimenopausal but smoke and thus are not good candidates for COCs.

Before inserting any female barrier contraceptive, a woman should wash her hands with soap and water to prevent the introduction of organisms. Women who use vaginal barrier methods should avoid using oil-based products such as mineral oil or baby oil and vaginal medications such as Monistat cream (for yeast infection) and estrogen creams because they can have a negative effect on latex.

In general, female barrier methods are more effective when used with a male condom. However, a male condom should not be used with a female condom. Women who use barrier methods should be alert for signs of toxic shock syndrome such as high fever, sore throat, vomiting and/or diarrhea, faintness, weakness, muscle aches, and a rash (see Chapter 7).

Male Condom

The male **condom** offers a viable means of contraception when used consistently and properly (Figure 5–2 •). Acceptance has been increasing as a growing number of men are assuming responsibility for regulation of fertility. The condom is applied to the erect penis, rolled from the tip to the end of the shaft, before vulvar or vaginal contact. Most condoms have a reservoir tip to allow for collection of ejaculate. When using a condom without a reservoir end, a small space must be left at the end to collect the ejaculate, so that the condom does not break at the time of ejaculation. If the condom or vagina is dry, water-soluble lubricants, such as K-Y jelly or Astroglide, should be used to prevent irritation and possible condom breakage. Care must be taken in removing the condom after intercourse. For optimal effectiveness, the man should withdraw his penis from the vagina while it is still erect and hold the condom rim to prevent spillage. If after ejaculation the penis becomes flaccid while still in the vagina, the man should hold onto the edge of the condom while withdrawing to avoid spilling the semen and to prevent the condom from slipping off.

The effectiveness of male condoms is largely determined by their use. The condom is small, lightweight, disposable, and inexpensive. It has no side effects, requires no medical examination or supervision, and offers visual evidence of effectiveness. Most condoms are made of latex. Thus, their use is contraindicated if the male or his partner has a latex allergy. Polyurethane and silicone rubber condoms are also manufactured and recommended for individuals allergic to latex. Condoms are available with ribbed or smooth sides, tapered or straight-sided, lubricated or unlubricated, with or without spermicide. They come in a variety of colors, sizes, and flavors. "Natural skins" (lambs' intestines) are still available but declining in popularity. They are used primarily by individuals with latex allergies. All condoms except natural skin condoms offer protection against both pregnancy and sexually transmitted infections (STIs). Concurrent use of a vaginal spermicide does increase the overall effectiveness of skin condoms.

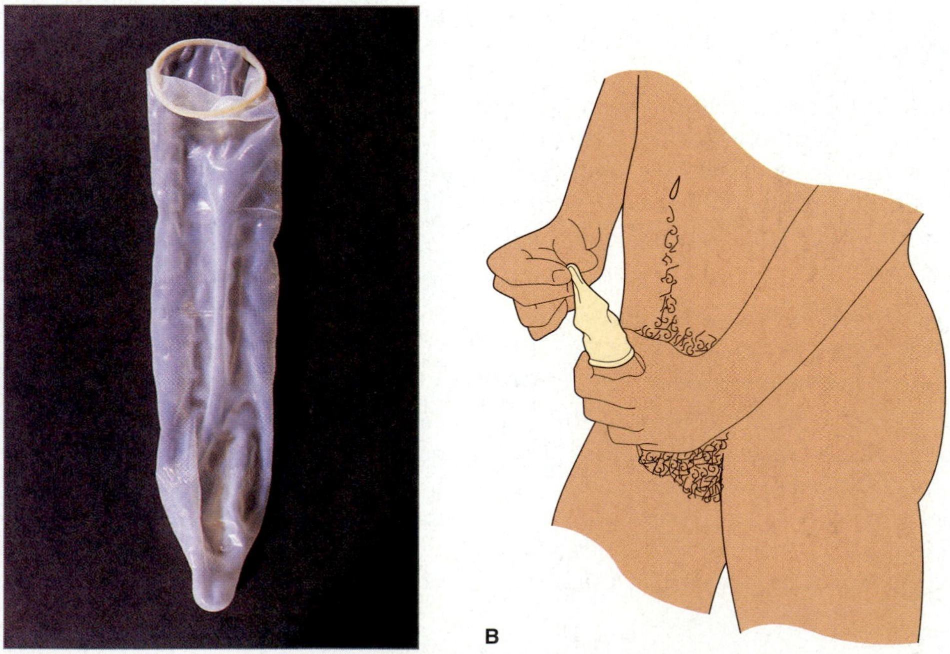

A B

Figure 5–2 • *A,* An unrolled condom with reservoir tip. *B,* Correct use.

EVIDENCE-BASED PRACTICE

CONDOM USE AND HIV TRANSMISSION

Clinical Question

How effective is the protection that condoms provide for preventing heterosexual transmission of HIV?

The Evidence

Thirteen studies of persons that reported always using condoms showed an overall effectiveness (proportionate reduction in HIV seroconversion with condom use) of approximately 80%.

Best Practice

Recommendations for the prevention of sexually transmitted HIV include consistent and correct use of condoms. Consistent use is defined as using a condom for all acts of penetrative vaginal intercourse. Consistent use of condoms during heterosexual intercourse results in 80% reduction in HIV incidence. This estimate refers to the male condom and not specifically to the latex condom. Condom use does not eliminate the risk of HIV transmission. Effectiveness is similar to, although lower than, that for contraception. The use of condoms is recommended for individuals who have multiple partners, who have a primary partner who is infected, or whose partner's serostatus is unknown.

References: Centers for Disease Control and Prevention. (1993). Update: Barrier protection against HIV infection and other sexually transmitted diseases. *Morbidity and Mortality Weekly Report,* 42, 589–591,597.

Surgeon General. (1993). Condom use for prevention of sexual transmission of HIV infection. *Journal of the American Medical Association, 269,* 2840.

Weller, S., & Davis, K. (2002). *Condom effectiveness in reducing heterosexual HIV transmission.* Cochrane HIV/AIDS Group, Cochrane Database of Systematic Reviews.

The male condom is becoming increasingly popular because of the protection it offers from infections. The protection condoms provide is especially useful for adolescent females because their developing cervical tissue increases their risk of contracting an STI (Jenkins & Raine, 2000). For women, regardless of age, an STI increases the risk of pelvic inflammatory disease (PID) and resultant infertility. Many women are beginning to insist that their sexual partners use condoms, and many women carry condoms with them.

Misplacement, risk of breakage, perineal or vaginal irritation, and dulled sensation are possible disadvantages of male condoms. Condoms should not be stored in hot conditions because heat accelerates their deterioration making them more susceptible to breaking. Thus, men should avoid placing them in their car glove box or in their wallets in a rear pants pocket.

Female Condom

The *Reality female condom* (Figure 5–3 •) is a thin polyurethane sheath with a flexible ring at each end. The inner ring, at the closed end of the condom, serves as the means of insertion and fits over the cervix like a diaphragm. The second ring remains outside the vagina and covers a portion of the woman's perineum. It also covers the base of the man's penis during intercourse. A woman needs to be careful not to twist the sheath when she inserts the condom because twisting makes male penetration impossible.

Available over the counter and designed for one-time use, the condom may be inserted up to 8 hours before intercourse. The inner sheath is prelubricated but does not contain spermicide and is not designed to be used with a male condom. Data on its effectiveness against pregnancy are still limited, although the female condom is slightly less reliable than the diaphragm, male condom, vaginal sponge, and cervical cap (Sobrero, 2002). Because it also covers a portion of the vulva it probably provides better protection against some of the pathogens that cause STIs than other methods. High cost, noisiness during intercourse, and the cumbersome feel of the device make acceptability a problem for some couples.

Diaphragm

The **diaphragm** is a barrier method that consists of a steel band that forms a ring and is covered with rubber so that, when the diaphragm is inserted, the ring lodges high in the vagina with the rubber covering the cervix. It is used with spermicidal cream or jelly and offers a good level of protection from conception. Invented in Germany in 1881 by Dr. Wilhem Mensinga, it was introduced into the United States in the early 1900s. The diaphragm was the first effective method of contraception available to women and was the mainstay of contraception for women until the development of the IUD and oral contraceptives (Sobrero, 2002).

Three types of diaphragm are available—the flat spring, the coil spring, and the arcing spring. Each type has its own advantages, and the type of coil makes the different diaphragms better suited to some women than to others. A woman must be fitted with a diaphragm and given instructions by trained personnel. The diaphragm should be rechecked for correct size after each childbirth and whenever a woman has gained or lost 10 to 15 pounds or more.

The diaphragm must be inserted before intercourse, with approximately one teaspoonful (or 1.5 inches from the tube) of spermicidal jelly placed around its rim and in the cup

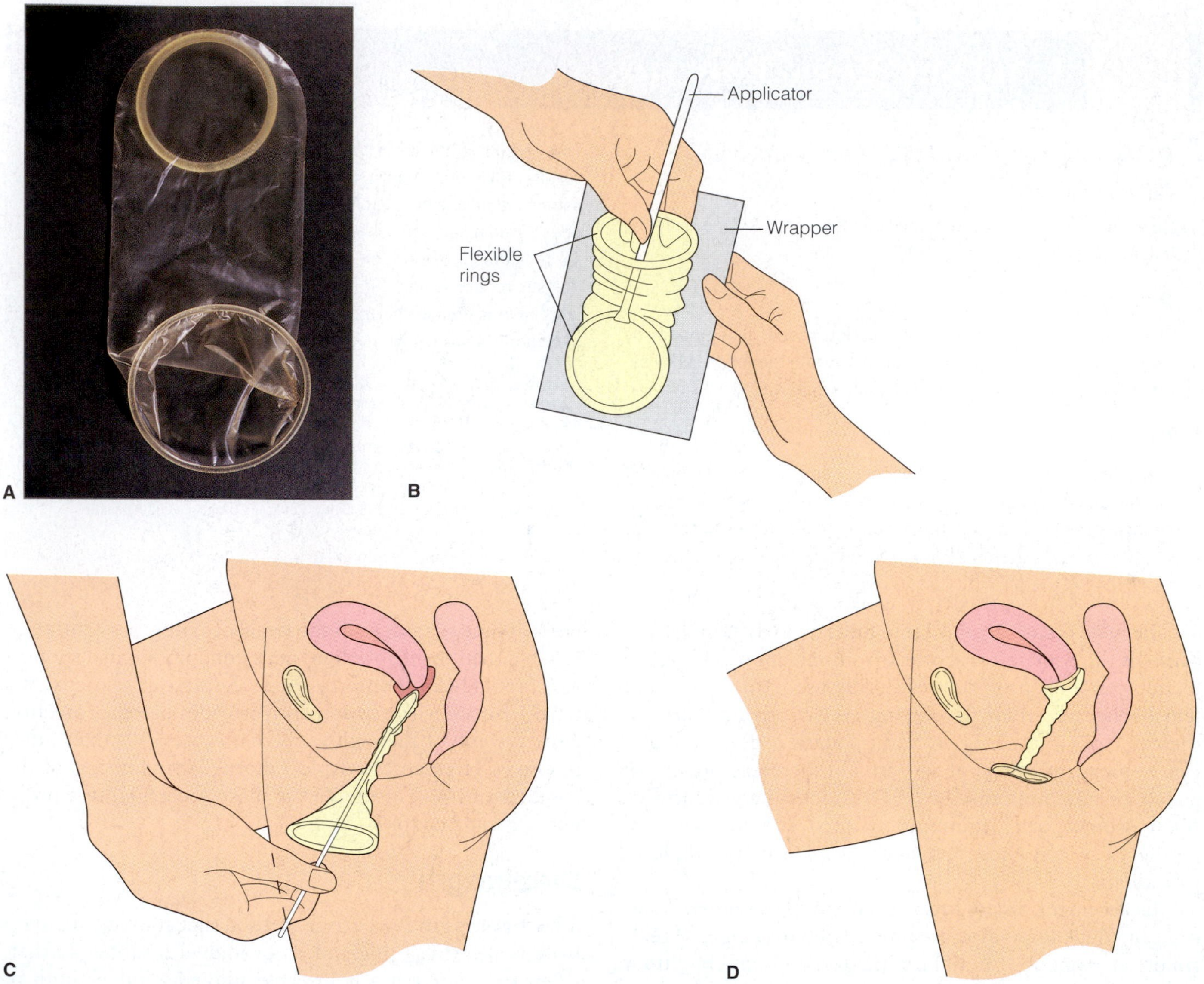

Figure 5–3 • *A,* The female condom. To insert the condom: *B,* Remove condom and applicator from wrapper by pulling up on the ring. *C,* Insert condom slowly by gently pushing the applicator toward the small of the back. *D,* When properly inserted, the outer ring should rest on the folds of skin around the vaginal opening, and the inner ring (closed end) should fit loosely against the cervix.

SOURCE: From *Our Sexuality* 5th edition by Crooks / Baur. © 1993. Reprinted with permission of Wadsworth, a division of Thomson Learning: www.thomsonrights.com. Fax 800 730-2215.

(Figure 5–4 •). This chemical barrier supplements the mechanical barrier of the diaphragm. The diaphragm is inserted through the vagina and covers the cervix. The last step in insertion is to push the edge of the diaphragm under the pubic symphysis, which may result in a "popping" sensation. When fitted properly and correctly in place, the diaphragm should not cause discomfort to the woman or her partner. Correct placement of the diaphragm can be checked by touching the cervix with a fingertip through the cup. The cervix feels like a small rounded structure and has a consistency similar to that of the tip of the nose. The center of the diaphragm should be located over the cervix.

If more than 4 hours elapse between insertion of the diaphragm and intercourse, additional spermicidal jelly should be inserted into the vagina. It is necessary to leave the diaphragm in place for at least 6 hours after coitus. If intercourse is desired again within the 6 hours, another type of contraception must be used or additional spermicidal jelly placed in the vagina with an applicator, taking care not to disturb the placement of the diaphragm. The diaphragm should not remain in the vagina for more than 24 hours.

Periodically the diaphragm should be held up to the light or filled with water and inspected for tears or holes. If properly maintained, it can last for several years, so it is a cost-effective method of contraception. The diaphragm should be washed and dried well after each use and then stored in a clean dry container. Talcum powder should not be used with a diaphragm because it contributes to the deterioration of the rubber.

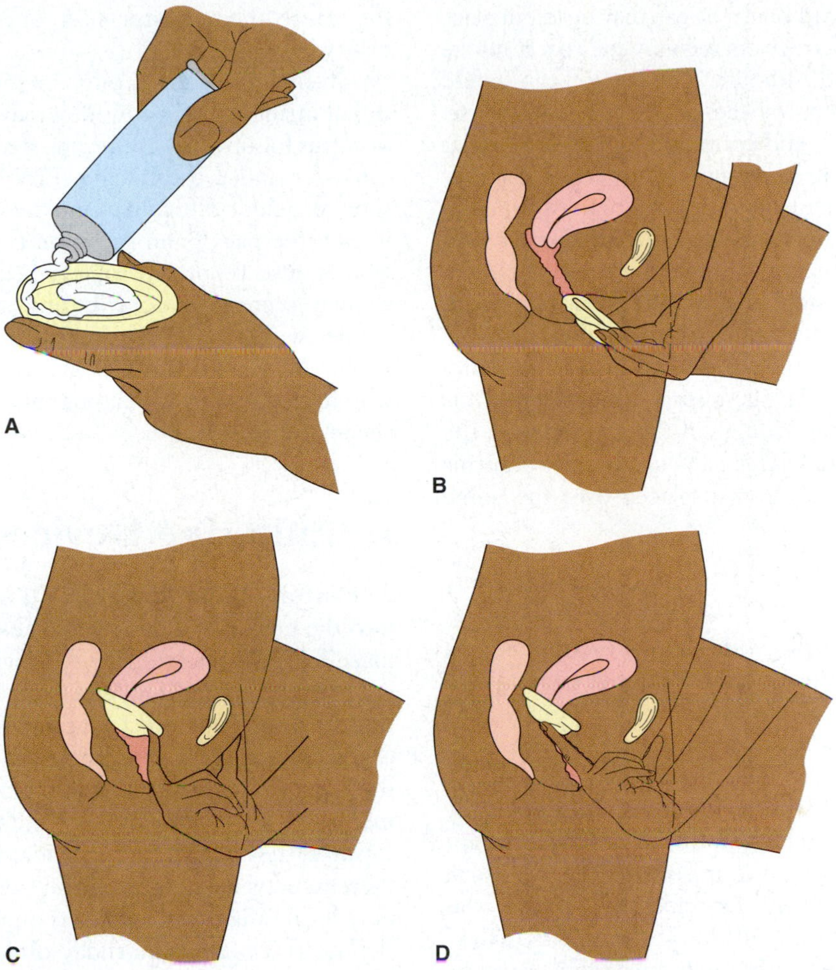

Figure 5–4 • Inserting the diaphragm. *A,* Apply jelly to the rim and center of the diaphragm. *B,* Insert the diaphragm. *C,* Push the rim of the diaphragm under the pubic symphysis. *D,* Check placement of the diaphragm. The cervix should be felt through the diaphragm.

Some couples feel that the use of a diaphragm interferes with the spontaneity of intercourse. The nurse can suggest that the partner insert the diaphragm as part of foreplay or the woman may choose to insert it herself prior to intercourse. Diaphragm use reduces the incidence of cervical gonorrhea, PID, and tubal infertility. This protection may be due in part to the simultaneous use of a spermicide (Greydanus, Patel, & Rimsza, 2001).

Women who object to touching their genitals to insert the diaphragm, check its placement, and remove it may find this method unsatisfactory. Women who are very obese or who have short fingers may find the diaphragm difficult to insert. It is not recommended for women with a history of urinary tract infection (UTI), because pressure from the diaphragm on the urethra may interfere with complete bladder emptying and lead to recurrent UTIs. They should be given information about other methods of contraception. As mentioned previously, women with a history of toxic shock syndrome should not use diaphragms or any of the barrier methods because they are left in place for prolonged periods. For the same reason, the diaphragm should not be used during a menstrual period or if a woman has abnormal vaginal discharge.

Cervical Cap

The **cervical cap** (Figure 5–5 •) is a cup-shaped device, used with spermicidal cream or jelly, that fits snugly over the cervix and is held in place by suction and by positive abdominal pressure. Effectiveness rates and method of insertion are similar to

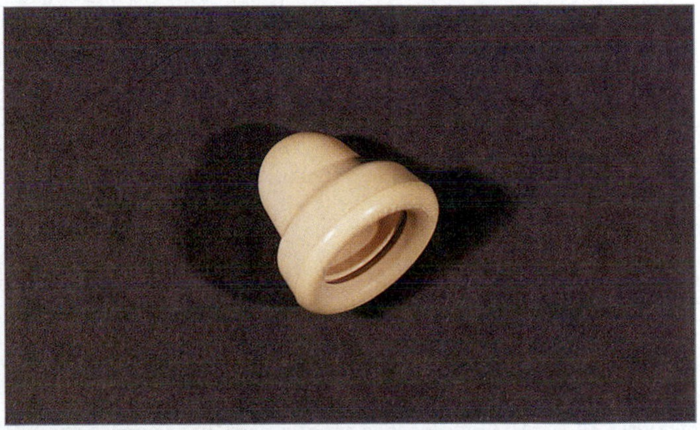

Figure 5–5 • A cervical cap.

those for the diaphragm. Although the cap may be left in place for up to 48 hours, most caregivers recommend that it not be left in place for more than 24 hours. The cervical cap should be inserted without rushing, ahead of possible intercourse. Advantages, disadvantages, and contraindications are similar to those associated with the diaphragm. The cervical cap may be more difficult to fit because of limited size options although makers of cervical caps are increasing the number of sizes available. It also tends to be more difficult for some women to insert and remove. Some women complain about unpleasant odor and discoloration of the cap, especially as the cap ages.

A new form of cervical cap—the FemCap—is currently under review. This cap looks like a small sailor's cap and is made of soft silicone. The "dome" of the cap fits over the cervix while the soft "brim" flares out slightly and conforms to the shape of the vagina. A strap placed over the dome permits easier removal.

Vaginal Sponge

The *vaginal sponge*, available without a prescription, is a pillow-shaped, soft, absorbent synthetic sponge containing a spermicide. It is made with a concave or cupped area on one side, which is designed to fit over the cervix. It also has a loop to permit easy removal. The sponge acts as a contraceptive by releasing the spermicide nonoxynol-9 gradually over a 24-hour period. Production of the only sponge approved by the Food and Drug Administrate (FDA) for use in the United States, the Today contraceptive sponge, was halted in 1994 because of manufacturing problems. However, it was reintroduced recently and is once again available.

The sponge is moistened thoroughly with water prior to use to activate the spermicide, and is then inserted into the vagina so that the cupped side fits snugly against the cervical os (Figure 5–6 •). This decreases the chances of the sponge being dislodged during intercourse. The sponge may be worn for up to 24 hours. It should be left in place for at least 6 hours after intercourse and then removed and discarded.

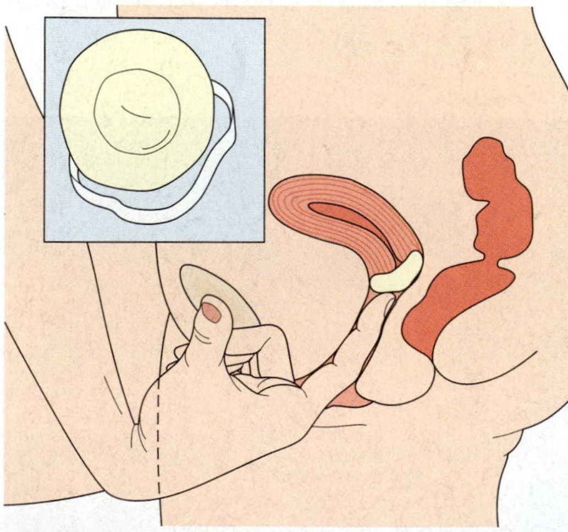

Figure 5–6 • The contraceptive sponge is moistened well with water and inserted into the vagina with the concave portion positioned over the cervix.

Advantages of the sponge include the following: professional fitting is not required; it may be used for multiple acts of coitus for up to 24 hours; one size fits all; and it acts as both a barrier and a spermicide. Problems associated with the sponge include difficulty removing it; cost (approximately $6 for a three-pack); and irritation or allergic reactions. Some women also report a problem because the sponge absorbs vaginal secretions contributing to vaginal dryness. For women without children the failure rate is comparable to that of the diaphragm and cervical cap. It is higher for women who have borne children, possibly because of changes in the shape of the cervix.

Intrauterine Devices

The **intrauterine device (IUD)** is designed to be inserted into the uterus by a qualified healthcare provider and left in place for an extended period, providing continuous contraceptive protection. The exact mechanism of IUD action is not clearly understood. Traditionally the IUD was believed to act by preventing the implantation of a fertilized ovum. Thus the IUD was considered an abortifacient or abortion-causing method. This belief is not accurate. IUDs truly are contraceptives; they trigger a spermicidal-type reaction in the body, thereby preventing fertilization. The IUD is also known to have local inflammatory effects on the endometrium.

The IUDs available today offer excellent contraceptive protection and, contrary to common myth, do not increase the risk of ectopic pregnancy or cause PID. In reality, infections in IUD users are probably related more to the woman's lifestyle than to the presence of the IUD. Unfortunately, although they are widely used throughout the world, IUDs currently account for less than 2% of contraceptive use in the United States (Chez & Strathman, 1999). Advantages of the IUD include high rate of effectiveness, continuous contraceptive protection, no coitus-related activity, and relative inexpensiveness over time. Because it is metabolically neutral, the IUD does not interact with medications. Thus it is an excellent form of contraception for women with existing medical problems. Possible adverse reactions to the IUD include discomfort to the wearer, increased bleeding during menses, increased risk of pelvic infection for about 3 weeks following insertion, perforation of the uterus during insertion, intermenstrual bleeding, dysmenorrhea, and expulsion of the device.

Two IUDs are currently available. The Copper T380A (ParaGard) is a highly effective IUD that can be left in place for up to 10 years. Copper covers parts of the stem and arms of the device. The levonorgestrel-releasing intrauterine system (LNG-IUS) (Mirena) (Figure 5–7 •) is a small, T-shaped frame with a reservoir that releases levonorgestrel gradually, is comparable in effectiveness to the Copper T, and may be left in place for up to 5 years (Zinger & Thomas, 2001). After 3 months of use of LNG-IUS, bleeding and

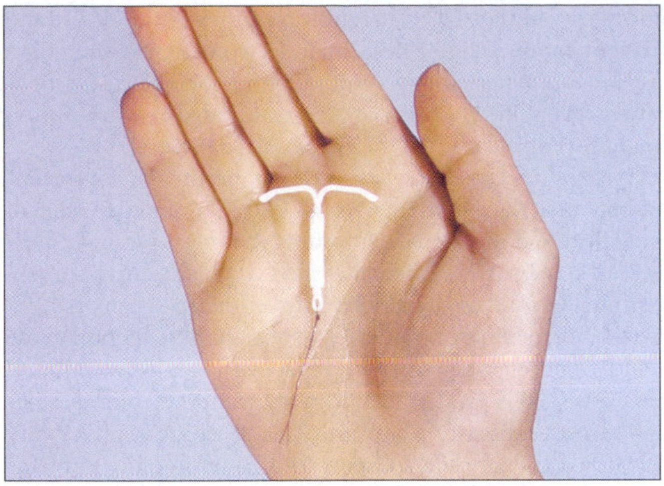

Figure 5–7 • The Mirena Intrauterine System, which releases levonorgestrel gradually, may be left in place for up to 5 years.
NOTE: Courtesy of Berlex Laboratories.

length of menstrual cycles are reduced. In fact 14% to 20% of women have amenorrhea, which they often welcome once they are advised that the absence of menses is safe and not an indication of pregnancy (Grimes & Jones, 2001).

The IUD is recommended only for women who have at least one child, have no history of PID, and are in a stable, mutually monogamous relationship, because they have the lowest risk of contracting an STI. It is not recommended for women with multiple sexual contacts, because they are at risk for STIs.

The IUD is inserted into the uterus with its string or tail protruding through the cervix into the vagina. It may be inserted during a menstrual period or during the 4- to 6-week postpartum check. After insertion, the clinician instructs the woman to check for the presence of the string once a week for the first month and then after each menses. She does this by inserting her index finger or middle finger into her vagina to feel the string. She is told that she may have some cramping or bleeding intermittently for 2 to 6 weeks and that her first few menses may be irregular. Follow-up examination is suggested 4 to 8 weeks after insertion.

Women with IUDs should contact their healthcare providers if they are exposed to an STI or if they develop the following warning signs: late period, abnormal spotting or bleeding, dyspareunia (pain with intercourse), abdominal pain, abnormal discharge, signs of infection (fever, chills, malaise), or missing string. If a woman becomes pregnant with an IUD in place, the device should be removed as soon as possible to prevent infection.

Hormonal Contraceptives

Hormonal contraceptives are available in a variety of forms. They may be progesterone-only hormones, most often using a synthetic form of progesterone called progestin, or a combination of estrogen and progesterone.

Combination Estrogen-Progestin Approaches

The use of a combination of the hormones estrogen and progesterone is a highly successful, very safe birth control method. Hormonal contraceptives work by inhibiting the release of an ovum, by creating an atrophic endometrium, and by maintaining a thick cervical mucus that slows sperm transport and inhibits the process that allows sperm to penetrate the ovum. There are several forms available, including combined oral contraceptives (COCs), transdermal patches, vaginal rings, injections, and implants.

COMBINED ORAL CONTRACEPTIVES

Combined oral contraceptives (COCs)—commonly called birth control pills or "the pill"—are a combination of a synthetic estrogen and a progestin. COCs are one of the most popular contraceptive options available to women in the United States because they are safe, highly effective, and rapidly reversible. COCs are taken daily for 21 days, following one of two methods:

1. *Day-one start.* The woman begins taking the pill on the first day of her menstrual cycle. This method prevents ovulation in the first cycle, so no backup method of contraception is needed.
2. *Sunday start.* The woman begins taking the pill on the Sunday after the first day of the menstrual cycle and ending on a Saturday. In most cases menses will occur 1 to 4 days after the last pill is taken. The Sunday start is common because it tends to prevent periods on weekends. However, a backup method of contraception is necessary during the first month of use.

With either method, 7 days after taking her last pill, the woman restarts the next cycle of pills. Thus the woman always begins the pill on the same day. Some companies offer a 28-day pack with seven "blank" pills so that the woman never stops taking a pill. The pill should be taken at approximately the same time each day—usually on arising or before retiring in the evening.

Irregular pill taking is one of the major causes of breakthrough bleeding, a side effect that leads many women to discontinue COCs. Also, although they are highly effective when taken correctly, improper use of the pill accounts for almost a third of unintended pregnancies in the United States each year (Zieman, 2001).

Birth control pills have been available for almost 40 years. In the United States, the estrogen component of the pill is either ethinyl estradiol (EE) or mestranol. Of the two, EE is by far the more commonly used estrogen and is the only estrogen used in low dose (under 50 µg) formulations. Initially, COCs contained high levels of estrogen, which were linked with increased risk for myocardial infarction (MI), thromboembolic disorders (blood clots), and stroke. Lowering the estrogen dose in the formulation eliminated the increased risk for MI and stroke and reduced the risk for thromboembolic disease. Based on this understanding, over the years the estrogen component of COCs has been decreased by 80%, from the original dose of 150 μg/day to the lowest dose currently available—20 μg/day (Ramos, Stanczyk, & Roy, 2002).

Currently nine different formulations of progestins are available. These progestins vary with respect to their biologic activity including their inhibition of ovulation. Synthetic progestins can have androgenic, antiandrogenic, estrogenic, and antiestrogenic effects. These effects are responsible for the varying progestin-related side effects.

COCs are among the most studied medications available. The current generation of low-dose pills is very safe and would be even safer if smokers over age 35 did not take COCs. In fact, research indicates that taking birth control pills is safer than being pregnant (Borgelt-Hansen, 2001). However, in an effort to reduce side effects such as bloating, breast tenderness, weight gain, and acne, regimens have been developed that use very low doses of estrogen (20 or 25 μg) and progestins that are less androgenic in effect. These very-low-dose pills may result in less contraceptive effectiveness and in weaker cycle control. In addition, researchers do not know as yet whether these low-dose pills will provide the same noncontraceptive benefits (see later discussion) as the pills that contain 30 to 35 μg of EE (Kaunitz, 2001b).

Side effects are generally identifiable as estrogen related or progestin related. Thus it is possible to modify some side effects by choosing a different oral contraceptive preparation. The side effects associated with COCs are identified in Table 5–2 •.

MEDIALINK ORAL CONTRACEPTIVE ANIMATION

Absolute contraindications to the use of oral contraceptives include pregnancy, previous history of thrombophlebitis or thromboembolic disease, acute or chronic liver disease of cholestatic type with abnormal function, presence of estrogen-dependent carcinomas, undiagnosed uterine bleeding, heavy smoking, gallbladder disease, hypertension, diabetes, and hyperlipidemia. Women with the following relative contraindications may initiate COC use; however, they require close and frequent monitoring. These include women with migraine headaches, epilepsy, depression, oligomenorrhea, and amenorrhea. Women who choose this method of contraception should be fully advised of the potential side effects.

Table 5–2 • SIDE EFFECTS ASSOCIATED WITH ORAL CONTRACEPTIVES

Estrogen Effects	Progestin Effects
Alterations in lipid metabolism	Acne, oily skin
Breast tenderness, engorgement; increased breast size	Breast tenderness; increased breast size
Cerebrovascular accident	Decreased libido
Changes in carbohydrate metabolism	Decreased high-density lipoprotein (HDL) cholesterol levels
Chloasma	Depression
Fluid retention; cyclic weight gain	Fatigue
Headache	Hirsutism
Hepatic adenomas	Increased appetite; weight gain
Hypertension	Increased low-density lipoprotein (LDL) cholesterol levels
Leukorrhea, cervical erosion, ectopia	Oligomenorrhea, amenorrhea
Nausea	Pruritus
Nervousness, irritability	Sebaceous cysts
Telangiectasia	
Thromboembolic complications—thrombophlebitis, pulmonary embolism	

Oral contraceptives have several important noncontraceptive benefits. Many women who use COCs experience relief of uncomfortable menstrual symptoms. Cramps diminish, flow decreases, and the cycle becomes more regular. Mittelschmerz is eliminated, and the incidence of functional ovarian cysts decreases. More important, there is a substantial reduction in the incidence of ectopic pregnancy, PID, ovarian cancer, endometrial cancer, colorectal cancer, iron deficiency anemia, and benign breast disease. Currently, oral contraceptives are considered a wonderful solution to the physiologic problems some women experience during the perimenopause and can be used by nonsmoking women until they transition to hormone replacement therapy at menopause (Borgelt-Hansen, 2001). Because of an increased risk of MI (heart attack), women over age 35 who smoke should not take oral contraceptives.

The woman using oral contraceptives should contact her healthcare provider if she becomes depressed, develops a breast lump, becomes jaundiced, or experiences any of the following warning signs: severe abdominal pain, severe chest pain or shortness of breath, severe headaches, dizziness, changes in vision (vision loss or blurring), speech problems, or severe leg pain.

Another oral contraceptive is the seldom-used progesterone-only pill, also called the *minipill.* It is used primarily by nursing mothers and by women who have a contraindication to the estrogen component of the combination preparation, such as history of thrombophlebitis or hypertension, but are strongly motivated to use this form of contraception. The major problems with this preparation are amenorrhea or irregular spotting and bleeding patterns. In addition, it is less effective than COCs.

TRANSDERMAL HORMONAL CONTRACEPTION

Combined hormonal contraception can now be provided transdermally using a weekly *contraceptive skin patch* called Ortho Evra. Roughly the size of a silver dollar, but square, this patch is applied weekly for 3 weeks on one of four sites: the woman's abdomen, buttocks, upper outer arm, or trunk (excluding the breasts). During the fourth week, no patch is applied and menses typically occurs. The patch is highly effective in women who weigh less than 198 pounds (Zieman, 2001). Patch users follow the same options for starting as users of oral contraception—Sunday start or day-one start.

The patch is as safe and effective as COCs and has a better rate of user compliance. Generally, women who are candidates for COCs are candidates for the patch unless they are obese (weight greater than 198 pounds) or have skin disorders that may result in reactions at the site of application.

VAGINAL CONTRACEPTIVE RING

NuvaRing vaginal contraceptive ring (manufactured by Organon), another form of low-dose, sustained-release com-

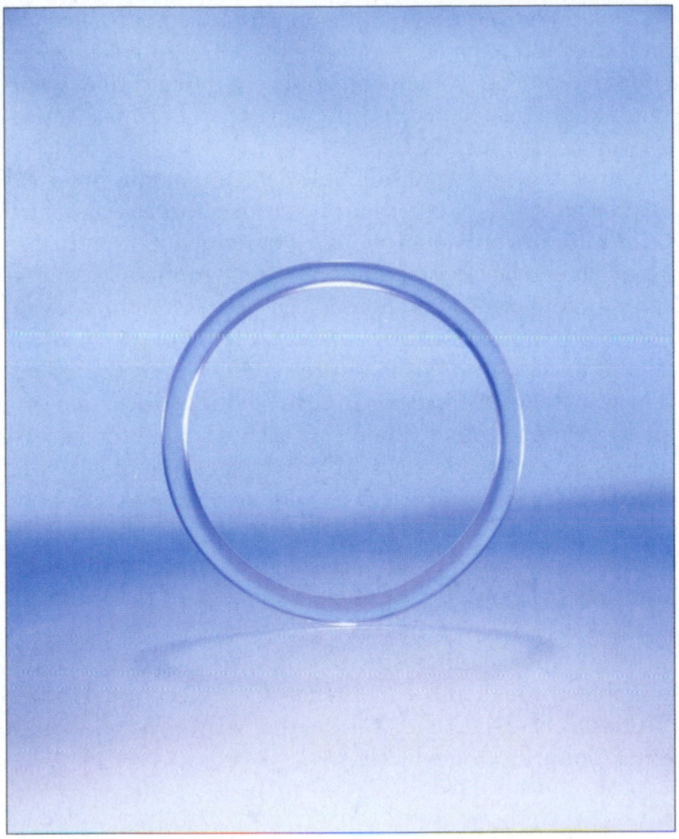

Figure 5–8 • The NuvaRing vaginal contraceptive ring.
SOURCE: Courtesy of Orgonon, Inc.

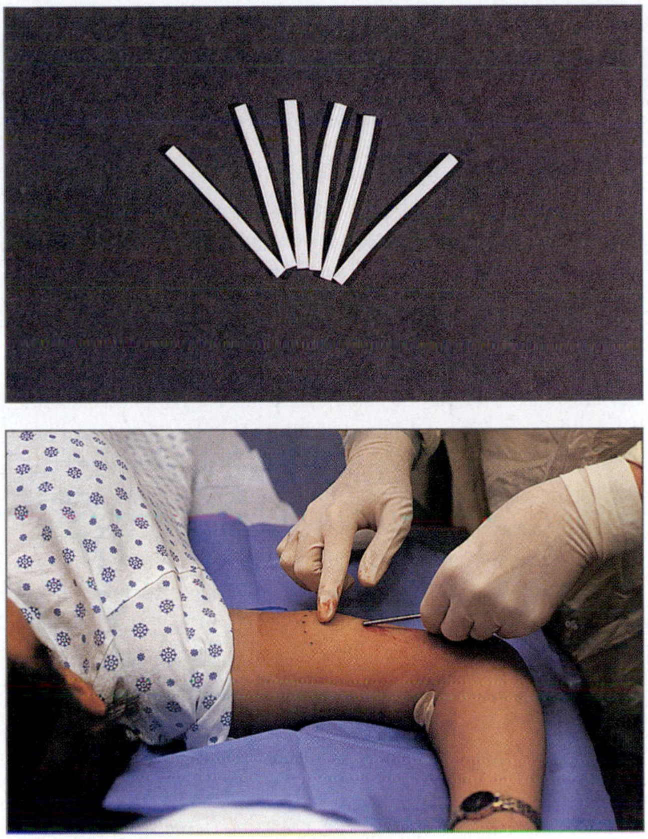

Figure 5–9 • The Norplant system.

bined hormonal contraceptive, is a flexible, soft vaginal ring that is inserted monthly (Figure 5–8 •). The ring is left in place for 21 days and then removed for 7 days (Borgelt-Hansen, 2001). One size ring fits virtually all women. Women with marked vaginal prolapse should be cautioned to check for expulsion of the ring during early use.

INJECTABLE COMBINATION CONTRACEPTIVE

Lunelle, a combination of medroxyprogesterone acetate and estradiol cypionate (MPA/E_2C), is administered every 28 to 30 days (not to exceed 33 days) as an intramuscular (IM) injection. Women using Lunelle have regular menstrual bleeding patterns and rapid return to fertility when the medication is stopped. Its contraindications and side effects are the same as those of oral contraceptives.

Long-Acting Progestin Contraceptives

With the exception of the progesterone-only oral contraceptive (the minipill), which was discussed previously, the two most common progesterone-only contraceptives are subdermal implants (Norplant) and depot-medroxyprogesterone acetate (DMPA).

SUBDERMAL IMPLANTS (NORPLANT)

Subdermal implants (Norplant) consist of Silastic capsules containing levonorgestrel, a progestin, which are implanted in the woman's arm. They are effective for up to 5 years (Figure 5–9 •). Typically, six rods are inserted, although the manufacturer is currently developing Norplant II, which uses only two rods.

Norplant prevents ovulation in most women. It also stimulates the production of thick cervical mucus, which inhibits sperm penetration. Norplant provides effective continuous contraception that is removed from the act of coitus. Possible side effects include spotting, irregular bleeding or amenorrhea, an increased incidence of ovarian cysts, weight gain, headaches, fluid retention, acne, hair loss, mood changes, and depression. Women should be advised that the implant may be visible, especially in very slender users, and that it requires a minor surgical procedure to insert and remove the implants.

DEPOT-MEDROXYPROGESTERONE ACETATE (DMPA) (DEPO-PROVERA)

Depot-medroxyprogesterone acetate (DMPA) (**Depo-Provera**), another long-acting progestin, provides highly effective birth control for 3 months when administered as a single IM injection of 150 mg. DMPA, which acts primarily by suppressing ovulation, is safe, convenient, private, and relatively inexpensive. It also separates birth control from the act of coitus. It can safely be given to nursing mothers because it contains no estrogen. DMPA provides levels of progesterone high enough to block the luteinizing hormone (LH) surge, thereby suppressing ovulation. It also thickens the cervical mucus to block sperm penetration. Side effects include menstrual irregularities, headache,

CRITICAL THINKING IN PRACTICE

Monique Hermann, age 37, was divorced 3 years ago. Her only son, now 19, is away at college. Recently, with some trepidation, Monique began dating, and she is now enjoying an active social life. She is being seen today for advice about contraception, which had not been an issue during her marriage because her husband had had a vasectomy. She reports that she is a little nervous about becoming sexually active because until this point her husband had been her only sexual partner. She is very attracted to two different men but does not prefer one over the other at this point. She states that she wants a reliable method that would permit her to have intercourse at any time without having to take action beforehand because she thinks that would be embarrassing for her. Similarly she is not interested in the patch, which is visible, nor in Norplant because she is slender and the rods might show. She is not willing to consider a tubal ligation. She is a nonsmoker who drinks occasionally. She has no known contraindications to any available methods. Which methods of contraception might be appropriate for Monique?

Answer found in Appendix I.

weight gain, breast tenderness, and depression. Return of fertility may be delayed for an average of 9 months (Kaunitz, 2001a).

MEDIALINK EMERGENCY CONTRACEPTION

Emergency Postcoital Contraception

Emergency **postcoital contraception** is indicated when a woman is worried about pregnancy because of unprotected intercourse, rape, or possible contraceptive failure (eg, broken condom, slipped diaphragm, missed oral contraceptives, or too long a time between DMPA injections). Research indicates that emergency contraception taken within 72 hours can reduce the risk of pregnancy after a single act of unprotected intercourse by 75% to 89% (Stone, Westley, & Cullins, 2002).

Two product kits, Preven, a combined hormonal approach (levonorgestrel and ethinyl estradiol) and Plan B, a progestin-only approach (levonorgestrel), are now FDA approved for emergency contraception. Though sometimes called the "morning-after pill," the phrase is misleading because the woman actually takes two pills as soon after intercourse as possible and two more 12 hours later. Prior to the development of these two kits, Ovral, a high-estrogen oral contraceptive, was often used for emergency contraception. The Plan B regimen is more effective than other emergency contraceptives and has a much lower incidence of associated nausea and vomiting (Grimes, Hanson, & Sondheimer, 2001).

This regimen must be initiated within 72 hours after unprotected intercourse. Emergency contraceptive pills are safe for almost all women. The only contraindication is a diagnosed pregnancy because the pills are ineffective (Stone, Wesley, & Cullins, 2002).

Currently there is considerable debate about the best ways to improve access to emergency contraception. It is essential that healthcare providers counsel women about the availability of emergency contraception during routine screenings and appointments. This approach ensures that women are familiar with the method before an emergency occurs. It is also helpful to have printed literature on emergency contraception available in the waiting area. In addition, discussion currently centers around other approaches to improve access such as making the kits available over the counter, allowing distribution by pharmacists, and permitting telephone screening with a prescription phoned in to a pharmacy. A nonhormonal method of postcoital contraception is also available. It involves the insertion of a copper IUD within a week of pregnancy exposure.

Information about postcoital emergency contraception is available through the Emergency Contraception Hotline (1-888-NOT-2-LATE), and on the World Wide Web at http://opr.princeton.edu/ec/.

Operative Sterilization

Operative **sterilization** is an inclusive term that refers to surgical procedures that permanently prevent pregnancy. In the man, sterilization is achieved through a procedure called *vasectomy*. In the woman, sterilization is done by *tubal ligation*.

Before sterilization is performed on either partner, the clinician provides a thorough explanation of the procedure to both. Each needs to understand that sterilization is not a decision to be taken lightly or entered into at times of psychologic stress, such as separation or divorce. Even though both male and female procedures are theoretically reversible, the permanency of the procedure should be stressed and understood.

Vasectomy

Male sterilization is achieved through a relatively minor procedure called a **vasectomy.** This involves surgically severing the vas deferens in both sides of the scrotum. It takes about 4 to 6 weeks and 6 to 36 ejaculations to clear the remaining sperm from the vas deferens. During that period, the couple is advised to use another method of birth control and to bring in two or three semen samples for a sperm count. When the sperm count is negative the couple can safely have unprotected sex. The man is rechecked at 6 and 12 months to ensure that fertility has not been restored by recanalization. Side effects of a vasectomy include pain, infection, hematoma, sperm granulomas, and spontaneous reanastomosis (reconnecting).

Vasectomies can sometimes be reversed by using microsurgery techniques. Restored fertility, as measured by subsequent pregnancy, ranges from 30% to 85%.

Tubal Ligation

Voluntary female sterilization is accomplished by **tubal ligation.** Four procedures are common in the United States:

- Tubal sterilization at the time of laparotomy for a cesarean birth or other abdominal surgery
- Postpartum minilaparotomy soon after a vaginal birth
- Interval sterilization (done at a time unrelated to a pregnancy)
- Laparoscopy

Tubal ligation may be done at any time. However, the postpartal period is an ideal time to perform a tubal ligation because the uterus is enlarged and the tubes are easy to locate. During these procedures the tubes are ligated, clipped, electrocoagulated, banded, or plugged. This interrupts the patency of the fallopian tube, thus preventing the ovum and the sperm from meeting.

Complications of female sterilization procedures include coagulation burns on the bowel, bowel perforation, pain, infection, hemorrhage, and adverse anesthesia effects. Reversal of a tubal ligation depends on the type of procedure performed. With microsurgical techniques, a pregnancy rate of 44% to 81% is possible (DeLeon & Peters, 2000).

Male Contraception

The vasectomy and the condom, discussed previously, are currently the only forms of male contraception available in the United States. Developing reversible methods of contraception for men is a challenge because healthy men produce sperm continuously whereas women produce eggs cyclically. It is easier to devise a reversible method that interrupts a cyclic process than it is to find ways to interrupt continuous fertility.

Hormonal contraception for men has yet to be developed, although studies are under way using weekly injections of testosterone enanthate (TE), a synthetic hormone that significantly inhibits sperm production in most men. A combination injection of TE and DMPA, the progestin found in Depo-Provera, is also under way. If it is successful, injections may only be needed monthly. Study is also under way on the feasibility of using subdermal implants containing gonadotropin-releasing hormone and an androgen.

"I think I'm like a lot of women. During my life I've used a variety of contraceptive methods. I took the pill back when doses were higher; I used foam alone and had a baby, then used spermicidal cream and condoms more successfully. I never wanted a tubal, and my husband refuses to consider a vasectomy, so the IUD was a perfect alternative for us. I am 47 and I like something I don't have to think about every time we want to make love. Maybe someday there will be more contraceptives for men—it seems only fair—but I'm glad that at least I've had some choices."

NURSING CARE MANAGEMENT

In most cases, the nurse who provides information and guidance about contraceptive methods works with the woman, because most contraceptive methods are female oriented. Because a man can purchase condoms without seeing a healthcare provider, only in the case of vasectomy does a man require counseling and interaction with a nurse. However, men should be encouraged to participate in contraceptive services. The nurse can play an important role in helping a woman or couple choose a method of contraception that is acceptable to both partners.

In addition to completing a history and assessing for any contraindications to specific methods, the nurse can spend time with a woman learning about her lifestyle, personal attitudes about particular contraceptive methods, religious and cultural beliefs, personal biases, and plans for future childbearing in order to help the woman select a particular contraceptive method. See Developing Cultural Competence.

Once the woman chooses a method, the nurse can help the woman learn to use it effectively. Client Teaching: Using a Method of Contraception provides guidelines for helping women use a method of contraception effectively.

The nurse also reviews any possible side effects and warning signs related to the method chosen and counsels the woman about what action to take if she suspects she is pregnant. In many cases, the nurse is involved in telephone counseling of women who call with questions and concerns about contraception. Thus it is vital that the nurse be knowledgeable about this topic and have resources available to find answers to less common questions.

MEDIALINK CASE STUDY: FAMILY PLANNING

Clinical Tip *Have informational handouts available for the various methods of contraception. Describe correct use, side effects, warning signs, and important tips for effective use. Women can then refer to the sheets at home. Be sure to include the office or clinic phone number.*

Developing Cultural Competence

Attitudes about birth control may be influenced by cultural factors. While it is impossible to attribute one attitude to an entire group of people, the following general information may be helpful as a starting point in working with women from a particular ethnic group (Cefalo & Dominguez, 2002):

- Among women from China the IUD is the most popular form of birth control although sterilization is common.
- Oral contraceptives are the most common form of birth control among African Americans.
- Birth control is an issue that causes mixed emotions for some African Americans. Those who wish to avoid pregnancy or space children see contraception as a blessing; however, some view contraception as a form of genocide.
- While many African Americans are opposed to abortion because of religious or cultural beliefs, the high rates of teen pregnancy have decreased opposition to abortion somewhat.
- Among many Hispanic women, abstinence and rhythm are the only acceptable forms of contraception and abortion is seen as morally wrong. Prolonged breastfeeding may be used to protect against pregnancy.
- Among many American Indians and Native Alaskans, large families are valued and, traditionally, birth control is not used.

Clinical Interruption of Pregnancy

Abortion, the termination of a pregnancy, was legalized in the United States in 1973. However, the associated controversy over moral and legal issues continues. This controversy is as readily apparent in the medical and nursing professions as in other groups.

Many women are strongly opposed to abortion for religious, ethical, or personal reasons. Other women feel that abortion provides a legally available alternative to a pregnancy. A number of physical and psychosocial factors influence a woman's decision to seek an abortion. The presence of a disease or health state that jeopardizes the mother's life and serious, life-threatening fetal problems are frequently suggested as indications for abortion. In other instances, the timing or circumstance of the pregnancy creates an inordinate stress on the woman, prompting her to choose an abortion. Some of these situations may involve contraceptive failure, rape, or incest. Usually the decision is best made by the woman or couple involved. A woman whose life is threatened by the pregnancy may choose to continue the pregnancy, whereas one with no obvious threat may choose abortion.

Globally, the legal status of abortion varies greatly. It ranges from complete prohibition to abortion at a pregnant woman's request. Among the 6 billion people who inhabit the Earth, national attitudes and laws about abortion can be classified into three broad categories (Henshaw, 2002):

- About one fourth of the world's people live in countries where abortion is absolutely forbidden or where it is only allowed to save the life of a pregnant woman. These include most Muslim countries of Asia, the majority of African countries, about two thirds of the Latin American countries, and one European country—Ireland.
- About one tenth live in a country where abortion is allowed to protect a woman's physical health or her mental health, and where social factors such as unmarried status, substandard housing, and inadequate income can be considered. Major countries in this group include Japan, Great Britain, and India.
- About two fifths of world countries permit abortion on request, generally without specifying a reason, although this is sometimes limited to the first trimester. Abortions for medical reasons are often allowed beyond the limits specified for an elective abortion. Countries in this category are a varied group and include the People's Republic of China, Austria, Denmark, Cuba, France, Italy, Sweden, Denmark, the United States, and most of the formerly socialist republics of Central and Eastern Europe.

Worldwide, abortion rates decline when women have access to modern methods of contraception, whether a country has legalized abortion or not.

Medical Interruption of Pregnancy

Medical abortion, now available in the United States, provides an effective alternative to surgical abortion for many women with unintended pregnancies. *Mifepristone* (Mifeprex), originally called RU 486, may be used to induce abortion medically during the first 7 weeks of pregnancy (up to 49 days following the first day of the LMP). In the United Kingdom, it can be used up to 63 days following the last menstrual period (Davtyan, 2001). Mifepristone blocks the action of progesterone, thereby altering the endometrium. After the length of the woman's gestation is confirmed, she takes a dose of mifepristone in her caregiver's office. Two days later she returns to her caregiver and takes a dose of the prostaglandin misoprostol, which induces contractions that expel the embryo/fetus. About 12 days after taking the misoprostol, the woman is seen a third time to confirm that the abortion was successful.

Surgical Interruption of Pregnancy

Surgical abortion in the first trimester is technically easier and safer than abortion in the second trimester. It may be performed by dilation and curettage (D & C), minisuction, or vacuum curettage. The major risks include perforation of the uterus, laceration of the cervix, systemic reaction to the anesthetic agent, hemorrhage, and infection. Second trimester abortion may be done using dilation and extraction (D & E), hypertonic saline, systemic prostaglandins, and intrauterine prostaglandins.

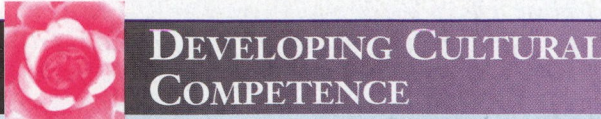

CLIENT TEACHING USING A METHOD OF CONTRACEPTION

Assessment The nurse determines the woman's general knowledge about contraceptive methods, identifies the methods the woman has used previously (if any), identifies contraindications or risk factors for any methods, discusses the woman's personal preferences and biases about various methods, and discusses her commitment (and her partner's commitment if appropriate) to a chosen method.

Nursing Diagnosis The key nursing diagnosis will probably be **Health-Seeking Behaviors:** Information on contraception related to an expressed desire to practice family planning.

Nursing Plan and Implementation The teaching plan focuses on confirming that a chosen method of contraception is a good choice for the woman. The nurse then helps the woman learn the method so that she can use it effectively.

Client Goals At the completion of the teaching, the woman will be able to

1. Confirm for herself that the chosen method of contraception is appropriate for her.
2. List the advantages, disadvantages, and risks of the chosen method.
3. Describe (or demonstrate) the correct procedure for using the chosen method.
4. Cite warning signs that should be reported to the caregiver.

Teaching Plan

CONTENT	TEACHING METHOD
Discuss the factors that a woman should consider in choosing a method of contraception (Table 5–1). Stress that the different methods may be appropriate at different times in the woman's life. Review the woman's reasons for selecting a particular method and confirm any contraindications to specific methods.	Contraception is a personal decision, so the discussion should take place in a private area free of interruptions. Create a supportive, warm, and comfortable atmosphere by attitude and communication style—both verbal and nonverbal. Provide accurate information in an open, nonjudgmental way.
Discuss the advantages, disadvantages, and risks of the chosen method.	Focus on open discussion. It may help to have written information about the method chosen. If a signed permit is required (as with sterilization or IUD insertion), the physician should also discuss the advantages, disadvantages, and risks.
Describe the correct procedure for using a method. Go through step by step. Periodically stop and have the woman review the information. If a technique is to be learned (as with inserting a diaphragm or charting basal body temperature), demonstrate and then have the woman do a return demonstration as appropriate. (*Note:* If certain aspects are beyond the nurse's level of expertise, the nurse can review the content and confirm that the woman has the opportunity to do a return demonstration. For example, an office nurse who does not do cervical cap fittings may cover information on its use, have the woman try inserting the cap herself, and then have the placement checked by the nurse practitioner or physician.)	Learning is best accomplished when material is broken down into smaller steps. Have a model or chart available to enable the woman to visualize what is being described. Have a sample of the chosen method available: a package of oral contraceptives, an open IUD, or a symptothermal chart.
Provide information on what the woman should do if unusual circumstances arise (she forgets a pill or misses a morning temperature). Stress warning signs that require immediate action on the part of the woman and explain why these signs indicate a risk. Carefully delineate the actions the woman should take.	Provide a written handout identifying the warning signs of her chosen method and listing the actions a woman should take. The handout should also cover actions the woman should take if an unusual situation develops. For example, what should she do if she vomits or has diarrhea while taking oral contraceptives? Arrange to talk with the woman again soon, either on the phone or at a return visit, to determine if she has any questions about the method and to ensure that no problems have arisen.

Evaluation

Evaluate the woman's learning by asking her to describe the method she has chosen, its contraindications and warning signs, and the procedure for using it correctly. In some cases, a return demonstration is useful.

NURSING CARE MANAGEMENT

Client selection is an important factor in medical abortion. Pregnancy needs to be verified early, by 5 weeks' gestation if possible. The woman needs to understand clearly that medical abortion takes time and follow-up is important. Moreover, women need accurate information about the cramping, bleeding, and pain that occur so that they are prepared to deal both with the discomfort and with the sight of the blood and possible uterine contents (Goss, 2002).

In general, important aspects of nursing care for a woman who chooses to have an abortion include providing information about the methods of abortion and associated risks; counseling regarding available alternatives to abortion and their implications; encouraging the woman to verbalize her feelings; providing support before, during, and after the procedure; monitoring vital signs, intake, and output; providing for physical comfort and privacy throughout the procedure; and teaching the client self-care, the importance of the postabortion checkup, and contraception review.

CHAPTER REVIEW

EXPLOREMEDIALINK

NCLEX review questions, case studies, and other interactive resources for this chapter can be found on the Web site at http://www.prenhall.com/olds. Click on "Chapter 5" to select the activities for this chapter.

For tutorials including animations and videos, more NCLEX review questions, and an audio glossary, access the accompanying CD-ROM in this book.

Focus Your Study

- Fertility awareness methods are "natural," noninvasive methods of contraception often used by people whose religious beliefs prevent them from using other methods.
- Situational contraceptives such as coitus interruptus (withdrawal) and douching are activities an individual uses in a given situation to avoid pregnancy without benefit of clinical guidance or medical care. Abstinence is also considered a situational contraceptive.
- Barrier contraceptives such as the diaphragm, cervical cap, and condom act by blocking the transport of sperm. These methods are often used in conjunction with a spermicide.
- Spermicides are far less effective in preventing pregnancy when they are not used with a barrier method.
- The IUD is a mechanical contraceptive. Although its exact method of action is not clearly understood, research suggests it acts by immobilizing sperm or by impeding the progress of sperm from the cervix to the fallopian tubes. In addition, the IUD does have a local inflammatory effect.
- Combined oral contraceptives (the "pill") are combinations of estrogen and progesterone. When taken correctly, they are one of the most effective reversible methods of fertility control.
- Hormonal options are now available through injections (Lunelle and Depo-Provera), patches (Ortho Evra), implants (Norplant), and vaginal rings (NuvaRing). These advances have broadened the range of contraceptive options available.
- Permanent sterilization is accomplished by tubal ligation for women and vasectomy for men. Although theoretically reversible, clients are advised that the method should be considered irreversible.
- The termination of pregnancy through abortion may now be achieved through either medical or surgical means.

References

Alan Guttmacher Institute. (2000). *Contraceptive use (Facts in Brief)*. New York: Author.

Alan Guttmacher Institute. (2001). *Contraceptive services (Facts in Brief)*. New York: Author.

Alan Guttmacher Institute. (2002). *Women and society: Benefits when childbearing is planned (Issues in Brief)*. New York: Author.

Barron, M., & Daly, K. (2001). Expert in fertility appreciation: The Creighton model practitioner. *Journal of Obstetric, Gynecologic, and Neonatal Nursing, 30*(4), 386–391.

Borgelt-Hansen, L. (2001). Oral contraceptives: An update on health benefits and risks. *Journal of the American Pharmaceutical Association, 41*(6), 875–886.

Cefalo, R. C., & Dominguez, L. (2002). *Culture, women, and healthcare: A multicultural approach to patients.* A continuing education monograph. New York: Medical Education Collaborative and Creative 4 Media, Inc.

Centers for Disease Control and Prevention (CDC). (2002, May 10). Nonoxynol-9 spermicide contraceptive use—United States, 1999. *Mortality and Morbidity Weekly Reports, 51*(18), 389–392.

Chez, R. A., & Strathman, I. (1999). Contraception and sterilization. In J. R., Scott, P. J. DiSaia, C. B. Hammond, & W. N. Spellacy (Eds.), *Danforth's obstetrics and gynecology* (8th ed., pp. 553–566). Philadelphia: Lippincott Williams & Wilkins.

Davtyan, C. A. (2001). Mifepristone: A practical review. *The Female Patient, 26*(12), 45–50.

DeLeon, F. D., & Peters, A. J. (2000). Reversal of female sterilization. In J. J. Sciarra (Ed.), *Gynecology and obstetrics 2002* (Vol. 6, chap. 46, pp. 1–6). Philadelphia: Lippincott Williams & Wilkins.

Frost, J. J., & Darroch, J. E. (2002). Contraceptive use and unintended pregnancy. In J. J. Sciarra (Ed.), *Gynecology and obstetrics 2002*, (Vol. 6, chap. 11). Philadelphia: Lippincott Williams & Wilkins.

Goss, G. L. (2002). Pregnancy termination: Understanding and supporting women who undergo medical abortion. *AWHONN Lifelines, 6*(1), 46–50.

Greydanus, D. E., Patel, D. R., & Rimsza, M. E. (2001). Contraception in the adolescent: an update. *Pediatrics, 107* (3), 562–573.

Grimes, D. A., Hanson, V., & Sondheimer, S. (2001). New approaches to emergency contraception. *Contemporary OB/GYN, 46*(6), 89–99.

Grimes, D. A., & Jones, K.P. (2001). *A clinician's guide to levonorgestrel intrauterine contraception.* A brochure cosponsored by the Association of Reproductive Health Professionals and the Ithaca Center for Postgraduate Medical Education. Retrieved February 26, 2002 from www.arhp.org/levonorgestrel/levonorgestrel_brochure.htm

Henshaw, S.K. (2002). Induced abortion: Epidemiologic aspects. In J. J. Sciarra (Ed.), *Gynecology and obstetrics* (2002). (Vol. 6, chap. 115, pp. 1–11). Philadelphia: Lippincott Williams & Wilkins.

Jenkins, R. R., & Raine, T. (2000). Helping adolescents prevent unintended pregnancy. *Contemporary Pediatrics* 17 (5), 75–99.

Kaunitz, A. (2001a). Injectable long-acting contraceptives. *Clinical Obstetrics and Gynecology, 44*(1), 73–91.

Kaunitz, A. M. (2001b). Reduced-dose oral contraceptives. *The Female Patient, 26*(9), 27–36.

Pollack, A. E., & Barone, M. A. (2000). Reversing vasectomy. In J. J. Sciarra (Ed.), *Gynecology and obstetrics* (2000). (Vol. 6, chap. 48, pp. 1–5). Philadelphia: Lippincott Williams & Wilkins.

Ramos, D. E., Stanczyk, F. Z., & Roy, S. (2002). Metabolic and endocrinologic effects of steroidal contraception. In J.J. Sciarri (Ed.), *Gynecology and obstetrics 2002* (Vol. 6, chap. 24). Philadelphia: Lippincott Williams & Wilkins.

Rosenberg, M. J., Meyers, A., & Roy, V. (1999). Efficacy, cycle control, and side effects of low- and lower-dose oral contraceptives: A randomized trial of 20 micrograms and 35 micrograms estrogen preparations. *Contraception, 60*(6), 321–329.

Sobrero, A. J. (2002). Use and effectiveness of barrier and spermicidal contraceptive methods. In J. J. Sciarri (Ed.), *Gynecology and obstetrics 2002* (Vol. 6, chap. 17). Philadelphia: Lippincott Williams & Wilkins.

Stone, M. H., Westley, E., & Cullins, V. E. (2002). Emergency contraception: America's best kept secret. *Contemporary OB/GYN, 47*(3), 106–116.

Wallach, M., & Grimes, D. A. (2000). *Modern oral contraception: Update from the Contraception Report.* Totowa, NJ: Emron.

Zieman, M. (2001). Transdermal contraception. *The Female Patient, 26*(12), 22–25.

Zinger, M., & Thomas, M. A. (2001). Using the levonorgestrel IUS. *Contemporary OB/GYN, 46*(5), 35–48.

Women's Health: Commonly Occurring Infections

6

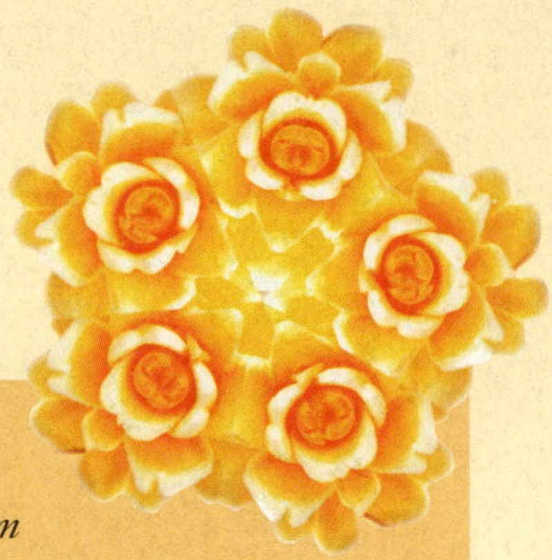

I guess I was what you would call a wild kid. I took way too many chances, even sexually, and eventually I got herpes. Now I am 32, with two kids, and married to a great man who loves me. He has never had herpes but we are very careful because I don't want him infected because of me. How much simpler life would be if I didn't carry that virus. Too bad that we can't change the past.

Objectives

- Compare vulvovaginal candidiasis and bacterial vaginosis.
- Describe the common sexually transmitted infections (STIs).
- Summarize the health teaching that a nurse needs to provide to a woman with an STI.
- Relate the implications of pelvic inflammatory disease (PID) for future fertility to its pathologic origin, signs and symptoms, and treatment.
- Contrast cystitis and pyelonephritis.
- Compare the different types of viral hepatitis.

Key Terms

Bacterial vaginosis 109
Chlamydial infection 113
Condylomata acuminata 115
Gonorrhea 114
Herpes genitalis 114
Pelvic inflammatory disease (PID) 119
Sexually transmitted infection (STI) 112
Syphilis 115
Trichomoniasis 113
Urinary tract infection (UTI) 120
Vulvovaginal candidiasis (VVC) 110

MediaLink

Additional resources for this content can be found on the Student CD-ROM and on the Companion Website at www.prenhall.com/olds. Click on "Chapter 6" to select the activities for this chapter.

CD-ROM
- Audio Glossary
- NCLEX Review

Companion Website
- Additional NCLEX Review
- Case Study: Pediculosis Pubis
- Care Plan Activity: Gynecologic Infection

Many women seek healthcare because of infections of one sort or another including those that are sexually transmitted. The nurse caring for a woman with an infection can be most helpful by providing accurate, sensitive, and supportive healthcare and health information. Additionally, the nurse is uniquely able to provide nonjudgmental health promotion, education, and counseling, in order to impact the woman's future health behaviors positively. To meet the woman's needs, the nurse needs to have up-to-date information about a variety of infections, including how they are spread, diagnosed, and treated, and their long-term implications.

This chapter focuses on several types of infections, with an emphasis on sexually transmitted infections. It is designed to provide current information to help nurses provide more effective healthcare for women and their families.

Care of the Woman with a Vaginal Infection

Vaginitis is the most common reason women seek gynecologic care. Symptoms of vaginitis, or vulvovaginitis, may include increased vaginal discharge, vulvar irritation and pruritus, external dysuria, or a foul odor. Women with vaginitis may have either infectious abnormal organisms, or an abundance or overgrowth of normal flora, such as *Candida* or *Gardnerella vaginalis* (Eschenbach, 1999).

Bacterial Vaginosis

Bacterial vaginosis (BV) is the most prevalent form of vaginal infection in the United States. BV is more prevalent in sexually active women; however, the debate continues as to whether or not BV is a sexually transmitted disease as it has also been detected in virginal women. Treatment of the male sexual partner has not been effective in preventing the recurrence of BV (Centers for Disease Control and Prevention [CDC], 2002).

Previously referred to as nonspecific vaginitis, or *Gardnerella* vaginitis, it is an alteration of normal vaginal bacterial flora resulting in the loss of hydrogen-producing lactobacilli and an overgrowth of predominantly anaerobic bacteria. Anaerobic bacteria can be found in less than 1% of the flora of normal women. In women with BV the concentration of anaerobes is 10- to 1000-fold above the norm. Lactobacilli are virtually absent (Eschenbach, 1999). The causes leading to overgrowth are not clear; however, sexual intercourse and trauma from douching are sometimes identified as contributing factors. The *Gardnerella vaginalis* and *Mycoplasma hominis* organisms have been found in the vast majority of cases, along with an increased concentration of anaerobic bacteria.

The infected woman often notices an excessive amount of thin, watery, white or gray vaginal discharge, with a foul odor sometimes described as "fishy." The characteristic "clue cells" are seen on a wet-mount preparation, and leukocytes are conspicuously absent (Figure 6–1 •). The addition of a 10% potassium hydroxide (KOH) solution to the vaginal secretions, called the "whiff" test, releases a strong, fishy, aminelike odor. The vaginal pH is usually greater than 4.5 (normal vaginal pH should be between 3.8 and 4.2). Women with BV have an increased risk of pelvic inflammatory disease (PID), abnormal cervical cytology, postoperative cuff infections after hysterectomy, and postabortion PID. The pregnant woman with BV is at risk for preterm labor, chorioamnionitis, and postcesarean endometritis (Scott & Hasik, 2001).

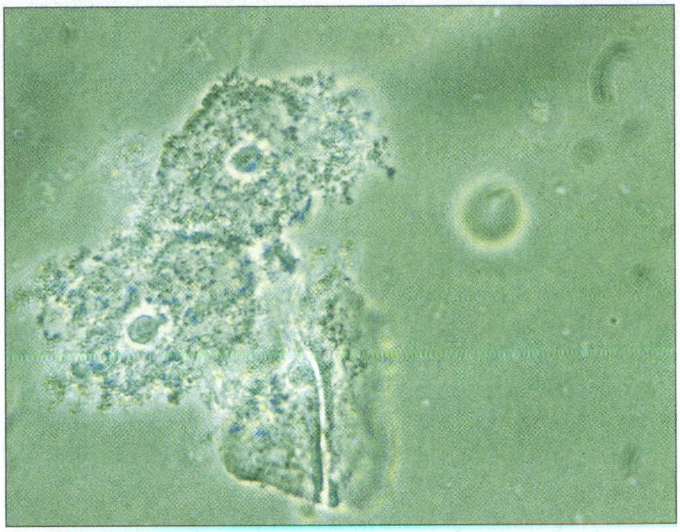

Figure 6–1 • The characteristic "clue cells" seen in bacterial vaginosis.

The nonpregnant woman who is symptomatic is generally treated with metronidazole (Flagyl) 500 mg orally twice a day for 7 days (see Drug Guide: Metronidazole) or one full applicator of metronidazole gel, 0.75% intravaginally, once daily for 5 days. Both these routes are equally effective. Alternatively the woman can be treated with 2% clindamycin (Cleocin) vaginal cream, one full applicator at bedtime for 7 days. This treatment is slightly less effective (CDC, 2002). Follow-up visits are not necessary unless symptoms recur.

For many years, metronidazole was regarded as a potential teratogen, especially in the first trimester, and its use was generally avoided, especially in early pregnancy. Recently, the CDC (2002) reported that multiple studies have not demonstrated a consistent relationship between metronidazole use during pregnancy and teratogenic effects on the newborn. Thus, currently the recommended treatment during pregnancy is metronidazole 250 mg orally three times a day or clindamycin 300 mg orally twice daily. Both should be taken for 7 days. The CDC also indicates that existing research does not support the use of intravaginal creams to treat BV during pregnancy. Some providers recommend screening of all pregnant women for BV; others recommend screening only those pregnant women at increased risk for preterm birth. In either case, if a pregnant woman is found to be positive for BV she should be treated.

MediaLink Centers for Disease Control

DRUG GUIDE METRONIDAZOLE (FLAGYL)

• Overview of Action

Metronidazole is an antiprotozoal and antibacterial agent. It possesses direct trichomonacidal and amebicidal activity against *T vaginalis* and *E histolytica.* Metronidazole is active in vitro against most obligate anaerobes but does not appear to possess any clinically relevant activity against facultative anaerobes or obligate aerobes. It is used in the treatment of various infections caused by organisms that are sensitive to this drug. It is used predominantly to treat the following infections in women: *T vaginalis,* bacterial vaginosis, endometritis, endomyometritis, tubo-ovarian abscess, and postsurgical vaginal cuff infection.

• Route, Dosage, Frequency

Trichomoniasis—1 day treatment 2 g orally in a single dose, 7-day treatment: 500 mg orally twice a day for 7 consecutive days (CDC, 2002).

Amebiasis—Adults: 750 mg orally three times a day for 5–10 days; children: 35–50 mg/kg/24 hours orally divided into three doses for 10 days.

Bacterial vaginosis—500 mg orally twice a day for 7 consecutive days or one full applicator of metronidazole gel 0.75 % intravaginally, once daily for 5 days (CDC, 2002).

• Contraindications

Blood dyscrasias

Breastfeeding women (drug secreted in breast milk)

Impaired kidney or liver function

Active CNS disease

• Side Effects

Convulsive seizures
Peripheral neuropathy
Weakness
Insomnia
Nausea/Vomiting
Headache
Anorexia
Diarrhea
Epigastric distress
Abdominal cramping
Constipation
Metallic taste in mouth
Dizziness
Vertigo
Uncoordination
Ataxia
Confusion
Irritability
Cystitis
Dysuria
Reversible neutropenia and thrombocytopenia
Flattening of the T wave on ECG
Polyuria
Incontinence
Pelvic pressure
Proliferation of *Candida* in the vagina and mouth
Joint pains
Decreased libido
Dryness in the mouth, vulva, and vagina
Dyspareunia
Depression

• Nursing Considerations

1. Inform woman about potential side effects.
2. Stress the importance of contraceptive compliance during course of treatment.
3. Obtain baseline renal and liver function tests as ordered.
4. Teach woman about the signs, symptoms, and treatment of vulvovaginal candidiasis.
5. Counsel the woman to avoid alcoholic beverages while taking the medication.
6. If the woman is taking oral contraceptives, a backup nonhormonal contraceptive method is recommended during treatment.
7. Take thorough history to rule out the woman's exposure to this medication within the last 6 weeks.
8. Teach woman to monitor the signs and symptoms of her infection.
9. Encourage cooperation with the entire course of treatment.

Vulvovaginal Candidiasis

Vulvovaginal candidiasis (VVC) is also called moniliasis or yeast infection. In the United States, 13 million cases are diagnosed annually, and it now ranks second in incidence to BV (Sinofsky, 1999). It is estimated that in their lifetime, 75% of women will have at least one episode of VVC while 40% to 45% of women will have two or more episodes (CDC, 2002). *Candida albicans* is responsible for 85% to 90% of vaginal yeast infections. Non-*albicans* species of *Candida* can also cause vulvovaginal symptoms, such as *C glabrata*, *C tropicalis*, and *C krusei*, and they are becoming more prevalent. There is evidence that some of these strains are developing resistance to therapies such as fluconazole. Predisposing factors to yeast infections include glycosuria, use of oral contraceptives, use of antibiotics, pregnancy, diabetes mellitus, and the use of immunosuppressants.

The woman with VVC often complains of thick, curdy vaginal discharge, severe itching, dysuria, and dyspareunia. A male sexual partner may experience a rash or excoriation of the skin of the penis, and possibly pruritus. The male may be symptomatic and the female asymptomatic.

On physical examination, the woman's labia may be swollen and excoriated if pruritus has been severe. A speculum examination usually reveals thick, white, tenacious, cottage cheese-like patches adhering to the vaginal mucosa. The diagnosis is made by observing mycelia or pseudohyphae upon direct microscopy in a 10% KOH preparation (Figure 6–2 •). A Gram stain or culture positive for the fungus is a more accurate way of diagnosing the causative or-

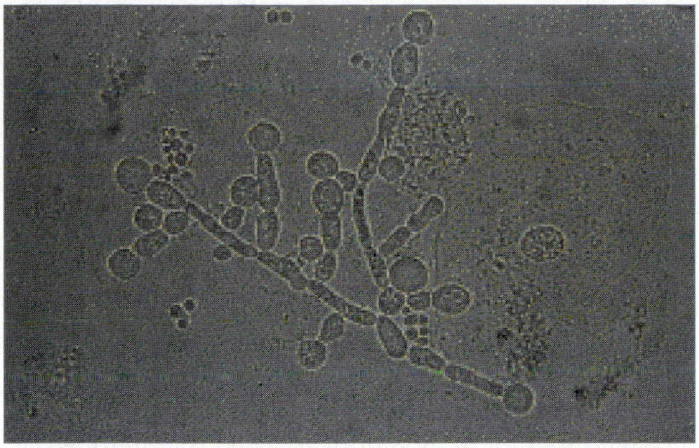

Figure 6–2 • Hyphae and spores of *Candida albicans.*

ganism. The pH of the vagina remains 4.5 or less (the normal pH of the vagina is about 3.8 to 4.25).

Local vaginal treatment with intravaginal butoconazole, clotrimazole, miconazole, nystatin, terconazole, or tioconazole cream, tablets, or suppositories is recommended. Single dose and short-course approaches (3 days) are effective for 80% to 90% of women with uncomplicated VVC. Oral fluconazole, 150 mg in a single dose, is also effective for mild VVC (CDC, 2002). Women with severe symptoms who are treated with oral fluconazole may need a repeat dose in 4 days (Mead, 2001). If the vulva is also infected, the cream is applied topically. In recurrent or resistant infections, or in cases of known non-*albicans* strains, vaginal application of boric acid or nystatin therapy works best (Eschenbach, 1999). Some of these medications are available over the counter. They are indicated for women with a history of yeast infections who clearly recognize the symptoms.

Treatment of the male partner is generally not indicated although it may be recommended for partners of women who have recurrent infection. For men who have candidal balanitis (inflammation of the glans penis) treatment with a topical antifungal medication is indicated (CDC, 2002).

Recurrent VVC, defined as four or more episodes of symptomatic VVC in one year, affects less than 5% of women (CDC, 2002). If a woman experiences frequent recurrences of monilial vaginitis, she should be tested for an elevated blood glucose level to determine whether a diabetic or prediabetic condition is present. Women at high risk for sexually transmitted infections should also be tested for HIV infection. In the absence of other risk factors, recurrent VVC treatment should include confirmation of the organism by culture, then an intensive regimen of oral and local agents for 7 to 14 days, followed by maintenance antifungal therapy using ketoconazole or itraconazole 100 mg by mouth daily, clotrimazole suppository once weekly, or fluconazole by mouth once weekly for 6 months. Women who take ketoconazole for long-term therapy should be monitored for liver toxicity (CDC, 2002).

Pregnant women with VVC should be treated only with topical azole preparations applied for 7 days (CDC, 2002). Infection at the time of birth may cause thrush (a *candidal* infection of the mouth) in the newborn.

NURSING CARE MANAGEMENT

Nursing Assessment and Diagnosis

The nurse caring for the woman should suspect VVC if the woman complains of intense vulvar itching and a curdy, white discharge. Because HIV-positive women and pregnant women with diabetes mellitus are especially susceptible to this infection, the nurse should be alert for symptoms in these women. In some areas nurses are trained to do speculum examinations and wet-mount preparations and can confirm the diagnosis themselves. In most cases, however, the nurse who suspects a vaginal infection reports it to the woman's healthcare provider.

Nursing diagnoses that might apply to the woman with VVC include the following:

- ***Risk for Impaired Skin Integrity*** related to scratching secondary to discomfort of the infection
- ***Health-Seeking Behaviors:*** Information about yeast infection related to an expressed desire to know about ways of preventing the development of VVC

Nursing Plan and Implementation

If the woman is experiencing discomfort because of pruritus, the nurse can recommend gentle bathing of the vulva with a weak sodium bicarbonate solution. If a topical treatment is being used, the woman will need to bathe the area before applying the medication.

The nurse also discusses with the woman the factors that contribute to the development of VVC and suggests ways to prevent recurrences, such as wearing cotton underwear, and avoiding douching and vaginal powders or sprays that may irritate the vulva. Women taking antibiotics should be advised about the possibility of developing VVC and encouraged to seek treatment early if symptoms develop. Some women report that adding yogurt to the diet or using activated culture of plain yogurt as a vaginal douche helps prevent recurrence by maintaining high levels of lactobacillus.

Evaluation

Expected outcomes of nursing care include the following:

- The woman's symptoms are relieved, and the infection is cured.
- The woman is able to identify self-care measures to prevent further episodes of VVC.

Care of the Woman with a Sexually Transmitted Infection

The occurrence of **sexually transmitted infection (STI)**, or sexually transmitted disease (STD), has increased over the past few decades. In fact, vaginitis and STIs are the most common reasons for outpatient, community-based treatment of women. More than one STI can occur at the same time. All symptomatic women should be tested for other infections. Table 6–1 • provides a summary of VVC and BV as well as the common STIs.

Prevention of Sexually Transmitted Infections

Effective prevention and control of STIs is based on the following concepts (CDC, 2002):

1. Education and counseling for people at risk on ways to practice safer sexual behavior
2. Identification of infected, asymptomatic individuals and of people with symptoms of STI who are not likely to seek diagnostic and treatment services
3. Effective diagnosis and treatment of people with an STI
4. Evaluation, treatment, counseling, and education for individuals who are the sex partners of people with an STI
5. Preexposure vaccination of individuals at risk for vaccine-preventable STIs

Individuals are at lowest risk for an STI if they abstain from sexual intercourse (whether vaginal, anal, or oral sex) and if they are in a long-term, monogamous relationship with a partner who is free of infection. Ideally, before entering a new sexual relationship, both partners should be tested for STIs, including HIV infection. If a person decides to have sex without knowing the partner's infection status, a new condom should be used before each act of intercourse (CDC, 2002).

Nurses can play an important role in educating and counseling individuals who have an STI, who are at risk for one, or who are the partners of an infected individual. Information should be tailored to individual needs and specific risk factors. It can include details about actions a person can take to avoid exposure to an STI or to avoid transmitting one. Nurses need to be nonjudgmental and respectful and draw on their counseling skills in sharing information.

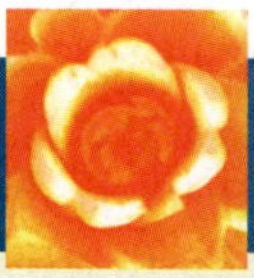

CRITICAL THINKING IN PRACTICE

Ella Matlosz is a 21-year-old, single woman, G0P0, who comes to the office today complaining of excessive, odorous vaginal discharge. She uses an IUD for contraception and has several sex partners. She states that she douches with a medicated douche after intercourse. What should you tell Ella about feminine hygiene? What would you tell Ella about the relationship between contraceptives and sexually transmitted infections?

Answers can be found in Appendix I .

Table 6–1 • SUMMARY OF SEXUALLY TRANSMITTED INFECTIONS*

			Treatment	
Disease	**Organism**	**Diagnosis**	**Nonpregnant**	**Pregnant**
Vulvovaginal candidiasis (VVC)	*Candida albicans*	Wet-mount hyphae	Topically applied azole drugs	Topically applied azole drugs
Bacterial vaginosis (BV)	*Gardnerella vaginalis* and *Mycoplasma hominis*	Wet-mount clue cells	Metronidazole	Metronidazole or clindamycin
Trichomoniasis	*Trichomonas vaginalis*	Wet-mount trichomonads	Metronidazole	Metronidazole
Syphilis	*Treponema pallidum*	Dark-field examination VDRL, RPR, or MHA-TP	Benzathine Penicillin G	Benzathine Penicillin G
Herpes genitalis	Herpes simplex virus	Herpes culture or titer	Acyclovir	Acyolovir
Chlamydia	*Chlamydia trachomatis*	Chlamydia culture	Doxycycline or azithromycin*	Erythromycin or amoxicillin
Gonorrhea	*Neisseria gonorrhoeae*	Gonorrhea culture	Cefixine, ciprofloxacin, ofloxacin, or levofloxacin plus doxycycline or azithromycin	Ceftriaxone or cefixime with erythromycin or amoxicillin
Acquired immunodeficiency syndrome	Human immunodeficiency virus	ELISA test and Western blot	Varies	Varies
Genital warts	Human papilloma virus	Virapap, biopsy, Pap smear, colposcopy	Cryotherapy, TCA, BCA, Podophyllum, podofilox, excision	Cryotherapy Trichloroacetic acid
Pediculosis pubis	*Phthirus*	Microscopic identification of lice or nits	Permethrin 1% creme rinse or lindane 1% shampoo	Permethrin 1% creme rinse
Scabies	*Sarcoptes scabiei*	Confirmation of symptoms or scraping of furrows	Lindane 1% lotion or permethrin 5% cream	Crotamiton 10% lotion or permethrin 5% cream

*Note: VVC and BV are included for comparison even though they are not spread primarily by sexual contact.

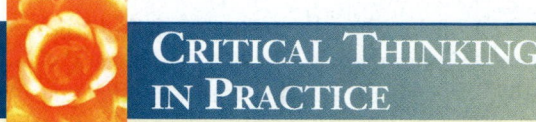

Trichomoniasis

Trichomoniasis is a sexually transmitted infection caused by *Trichomonas vaginalis*, a microscopic motile protozoan that thrives in an alkaline environment. The single-celled parasite, called a trichomonad, is an anaerobe that has the ability to generate hydrogen, which combines with oxygen to create an anaerobic environment. Most infections are acquired through sexual intimacy. Transmission by shared bath facilities, wet towels, or wet swimsuits may also be possible.

Often women with trichomoniasis are asymptomatic or have only mild symptoms. More pronounced symptoms of trichomoniasis may include a yellow-green, frothy, odorous discharge and vulvar itching. The woman may also complain of dysuria and dyspareunia. Occasionally, subepithelial hemorrhages on the cervix (strawberry-like red spots) can be seen with the naked eye; smaller areas of hemorrhage are generally visible with a colposcope. Microscopy visualization of mobile trichomonads and increased leukocytes, a vaginal pH of 4.5 or higher, and a positive whiff test are diagnostic of *T vaginalis* (Figure 6–3 •). Pregnant women with trichomoniasis may be at increased risk for premature rupture of membranes, preterm birth, and low birth weight. Pregnant women who are symptomatic should be treated with a single 2-g dose of metronidazole orally to relieve their symptoms (CDC, 2002).

Recommended treatment for trichomoniasis is metronidazole (Flagyl) administered in a single 2-g dose or, alternatively, metronidazole 500 mg twice daily for 7 days for both male and female sexual partners (CDC, 2002). Partners should avoid intercourse until both are cured (therapy is completed and both are symptom free). The woman and her partner should be cautioned to avoid alcohol while taking metronidazole; the combination has an effect similar to that of alcohol and disulfiram (Antabuse)—abdominal pain, nausea, flushing, or tremors.

Chlamydial Infection

Chlamydial infection, caused by *Chlamydia trachomatis*, is the most common bacterial STI in the United States. It occurs most frequently in sexually active adolescents and young adults. The organism is an intracellular bacterium with several different immunotypes. Immunotypes of chlamydia are responsible for lymphogranuloma venereum and trachoma, which is the world's leading cause of preventable blindness.

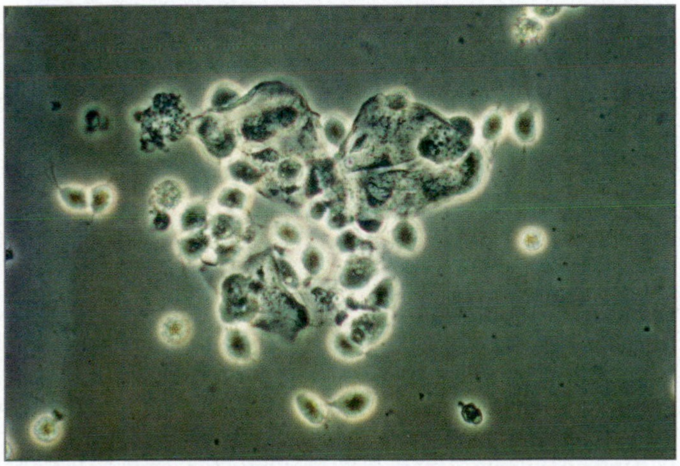

Figure 6–3 • Microscopic appearance of *Trichomonas vaginalis.*
SOURCE: Centers for Disease Control and Prevention (CDC).

Chlamydia is a major cause of nongonococcal urethritis (NGU) in men. In women it can cause infections similar to those that occur with gonorrhea. However, asymptomatic infection is common in both men and women. In women, chlamydia can infect the fallopian tubes, cervix, urethra, and Bartholin's glands. Severe sequelae can result from untreated chlamydial infection, including PID, infertility, and ectopic pregnancy. In men, chlamydial infection may result in epididymitis and infertility. In the United States, newborn exposure to chlamydia in the birth canal of the mother is the most common cause of ophthalmia neonatorum (CDC, 2002). This chlamydial conjunctivitis responds to erythromycin ophthalmic ointment but not to silver nitrate eye prophylaxis. The newborn may also develop chlamydial pneumonia.

Symptoms of chlamydia include a thin or mucopurulent discharge, cervical ectopia, friable cervix (bleeds easily), burning and frequency of urination, and lower abdominal pain. However, up to 70% of women are asymptomatic (Walsh & Irwin, 2002). The gold standard diagnostic test for chlamydia has been a culture of cervical cells. More recently, antigen detection, DNA probe assays, and polymerase chain reaction tests have become widely available. Diagnosis is frequently made after treatment of a male partner for NGU or in a symptomatic woman with a negative gonorrhea culture.

The recommended treatment is a single dose of azithromycin 1 g orally or doxycycline 100 mg by mouth twice a day for 7 days. Doxycycline costs less than azithromycin and has been used for a longer period. However, azithromycin administered at the clinic or office visit is an excellent choice for people who do not comply well with treatment or who are erratic about completing a course of medication. Sexual partners should also be treated and the couple should abstain from intercourse for 7 days after taking the single-dose treatment or for the entire 7 days of the doxycycline therapy (CDC, 2002). Doxycycline is contraindicated during pregnancy, but preliminary data on azithromycin, a category B drug, suggests that it is safe and effective, and many caregivers prescribe it. Currently the CDC (2002) recommends that pregnant women be treated with erythromycin or amoxicillin, although neither is highly effective. Thus, when these drugs are used for pregnant women, a repeat culture as a test of cure is recommended 3 weeks after completion of the prescribed medication. Because so many males and females who have chlamydia are asymptomatic, the CDC and medical specialty organizations such as the American College of Obstetricians and Gynecologists (ACOG) recommend screening as the primary method of decreasing the incidence of chlamydia. Specifically, annual screening is recommended for the following groups (CDC, 2002; Walsh & Irwin, 2002):

- All sexually active adolescent females and women ages 20 to 25 even if they are asymptomatic.
- Women over age 25 who are at risk for chlamydia (history of STIs, multiple sexual partners, new sexual partner, inconsistent use of barrier contraceptives).

- ACOG also recommends screening for high-risk pregnant women at their first prenatal visit, during the third trimester of pregnancy, or both. Some practitioners routinely screen all pregnant women.

Screening using a nucleic amplification test can be done on endocervical, urethral, or urine specimens. The urine tests are an attractive alternative for women who are not comfortable with pelvic exams or in clinics where access to gynecologic examination facilities are limited or lacking (Walsh & Irwin, 2002).

Gonorrhea

Gonorrhea is an infection caused by the bacterium *Neisseria gonorrhoeae.* The CDC (2002) estimates that 600,000 new cases of gonorrhea occur annually in the United States. Most men seek treatment for gonorrhea early because of symptoms but many women with the infection are asymptomatic until complications such as PID occur.

If a pregnant woman becomes infected after the third month of gestation, the mucous plug in the cervix will prevent the infection from ascending, and it will remain localized in the urethra, cervix, and Bartholin's glands until the membranes rupture. Then it can spread upward. A newborn exposed to a gonococcal-infected birth canal is at risk of developing ophthalmia neonatorum. Eye prophylaxis for all newborns is provided to prevent this complication.

About 50% of women with gonorrhea are asymptomatic. Thus it is accepted practice to screen for this infection by doing a cervical culture during the initial prenatal examination. For women at high risk, the culture may be repeated during the last month of pregnancy. Cultures of the urethra, throat, and rectum may also be required for diagnosis, depending on the body orifices used for intercourse.

The most common symptoms of gonorrheal infection, when they occur, include a purulent, greenish-yellow vaginal discharge, dysuria, and urinary frequency. Some women also develop inflammation and swelling of the vulva. The cervix may appear swollen and eroded and may secrete a foul-smelling discharge in which gonococci are present. Bilateral lower abdominal or pelvic pain may also occur.

Treatment for nonpregnant women consists of antibiotic therapy with cefixime, ciprofloxacin, ofloxacin, or levofloxacin orally (or ceftriaxone administered intramuscularly) plus doxycycline or azithromycin administered orally if chlamydia has not been ruled out. This combined approach provides dual treatment for gonorrhea and chlamydia because the two infections frequently occur together (CDC, 2002). Additional treatment may be required if the cultures remain positive 7 to 14 days after completion of treatment. All sexual partners must also be treated, or the woman may become reinfected. Pregnant women should be treated with a recommended cephalosporin, usually ceftriaxone intramuscularly or cefixime orally. This is combined with erythromycin or amoxicillin to address the risk of co-infection with chlamydia (CDC, 2002). Some practitioners use azithromycin to treat pregnant women for co-infection.

Women should be informed of the need for reculture to verify cure and the need for abstinence or condom use until cure is confirmed. Both sexual partners should be treated if either has a positive test for gonorrhea. Women should also be informed of signs that the infection is worsening (sharp abdominal pain, fever, or chills) and encouraged to seek further care if any of these develop.

Herpes Genitalis

The herpes simplex virus (HSV) causes herpes infections, which are recurrent, lifelong infections. Two serotypes of HSV cause human infections: HSV-1 and HSV-2. HSV-2 causes most cases of recurrent genital herpes. The clinical symptoms and treatment of both types are the same. At least 50 million people in the United States have been diagnosed with genital HSV-2 infection—**herpes genitalis.** Even so, most people infected with genital herpes have not been diagnosed because they have mild or unrecognized infections but shed the virus intermittently (CDC, 2002). Estimates suggest that between 60% and 85% of women with HSV-2 exposure have never had a recognized genital infection (Eschenbach, 1999).

The primary episode (first outbreak) of herpes genitalis is characterized by the development of single or multiple blisterlike vesicles, which usually occur in the genital area and sometimes affect the vaginal walls, cervix, urethra, and anus. The vesicles may appear within a few hours to 20 days after exposure and rupture spontaneously to form very painful, open, ulcerated lesions. Inflammation and pain secondary to the presence of herpes lesions can cause difficult urination and urinary retention. Enlargement of the inguinal lymph nodes may be present. Flulike symptoms and genital pruritus or tingling also may be noticed. Primary episodes usually last the longest and are the most severe. Lesions heal spontaneously in 2 to 4 weeks.

After the lesions heal, the virus enters a dormant phase, residing in the nerve ganglia of the affected area. Some individuals never have a recurrence, whereas others have regular recurrences. Recurrences are usually less severe than the initial episode and seem to be triggered by emotional stress, menstruation, ovulation, pregnancy, frequent or vigorous intercourse, poor health status or a generally run-down physical condition, tight clothing, or overheating. Diagnosis is made on the basis of the clinical appearance of the lesions, Pap smear or culture of the lesions, polymerase chain reaction (PCR) identification, and, occasionally, blood testing for antibodies, although this approach is controversial.

No known cure for herpes exists; however, medications are available to provide relief from pain and prevent complications from secondary infection. The recommended treatment of the first clinical episode of genital herpes is oral acyclovir, valacyclovir, or famciclovir. These same medications, in somewhat different dosages, are also recommended for recurrent herpes infection and for daily suppressive therapy for people who have frequent recurrences. Therapy should be started during the prodromal period (time prior to the onset of lesions) for the greatest benefit. The safety of acyclovir, valacyclovir, and famciclovir in pregnancy has not been established. However, because there is more documented information on acyclovir during pregnancy, it may be administered orally to pregnant women with first episode genital herpes or severe recurrent herpes. Its use in the third trimester may reduce the frequency of cesarean births by decreasing the incidence of recurrences at term (CDC, 2002). Self-care suggestions include cleansing with povidone-iodine (Betadine) solution to prevent secondary infection and with Burow's solution to relieve discomfort. Use of vitamin C or lysine is frequently suggested to prevent recurrence, although studies have not documented the effectiveness of these supplements. Sometimes 2% lidocaine (Xylocaine) is used to decrease intense pain at the site of the lesions. Keeping the genital area clean and dry, wearing loose clothing, taking sitz baths, and wearing cotton underwear or none at all will promote healing. Primary or recurrent lesions will heal without treatment.

If herpes is present in the genital tract of a woman during childbirth, it can have a devastating, even fatal, effect on the newborn. See Chapter 20 for more detail.

Syphilis

Syphilis is a chronic infection caused by the spirochete *Treponema pallidum.* Syphilis can be acquired congenitally through transplacental inoculation and can result from maternal exposure to infected exudate during sexual contact or from contact with open wounds or infected blood. The incubation period varies from 10 to 90 days, and even though no symptoms or lesions are noted during this time, the woman's blood contains spirochetes and is infectious.

Syphilis is divided into early and late stages. During the early stage (primary), a chancre (painless ulcer) appears at the site where the *Treponema pallidum* organism entered the body. Symptoms include slight fever, loss of weight, and malaise. The chancre persists for about 4 weeks and then disappears. In 6 weeks to 6 months, secondary symptoms appear. Skin eruptions called condylomata lata, which resemble wartlike plaques and are highly infectious, may appear on the vulva. Other secondary symptoms are acute arthritis, enlargement of the liver and spleen, nontender enlarged lymph nodes, iritis, and a chronic sore throat with hoarseness. Transplacentally transmitted syphilis is as high as 95% in the primary and secondary stages, but decreases to 10% in the late latent phase. Congenital syphilis may cause intrauterine growth restriction, preterm birth, and stillbirth.

As a result of the disease's impact on the fetus in utero, serologic testing of every pregnant woman is recommended; some state laws require it. Testing is done at the initial prenatal screening and repeated in the third trimester. Blood studies may be negative if blood is drawn too early in the pregnancy.

During the early primary stage, the diagnosis is made by dark-field microscopic examination of the chancre for spirochetes. Blood tests such as VDRL (Venereal Disease Research Laboratories), RPR (Rapid Plasma Reagin), or the more specific FTA-ABS (fluorescent treponemal antibody absorption test) are commonly done.

For pregnant and nonpregnant women with syphilis of less than a year's duration (early latent syphilis), the CDC (2002) recommends 2.4 million units of benzathine penicillin G intramuscularly in a single dose. If syphilis is of long duration (more than 1 year) or of unknown duration, 2.4 million units of benzathine penicillin G is given intramuscularly once a week for 3 weeks. If a woman is allergic to penicillin, and nonpregnant, doxycycline or tetracycline can be given. Clients who are allergic to penicillin whose cooperation with treatment and follow-up is questionable should be desensitized to penicillin and then treated with it. Similarly, the pregnant woman with syphilis who is allergic to penicillin should be desensitized and then treated (CDC, 2002). Maternal serologic testing may remain positive for 8 months, and the newborn may have a positive test for 3 months.

Human Papilloma Virus/Condylomata Acuminata

Condylomata acuminata, also called genital or venereal warts, is a common sexually transmitted infection caused by the human papilloma virus (HPV). Conservative estimates suggest that in the United States approximately 20 million people have productive HPV infection (ie, acute shedding of HPV). Because of the increased evidence of a link between HPV and cervical cancer, the condition is receiving increasing attention. Over 100 HPV types have been identified; of these, about 40 types can infect the genital tract (Richwald & Skaer, 2001). Most HPV infections are unrecognized, asymptomatic, or subclinical. HPV types 6 and 11 most commonly cause visible genital warts but they are rarely associated with anogenital cancers. Five specific types of HPV strains (16, 18, 31, 33, and 35) are associated with high-grade cervical dysplasia and cervical cancer; they are also found occasionally in visible genital warts. Clients with visible genital warts can be infected concurrently with different HPV types (CDC, 2002).

Often a woman seeks medical care after noticing single or multiple soft, grayish pink, cauliflower-like lesions in her genital area (Figure 6–4 •). These warts are often asymptomatic;

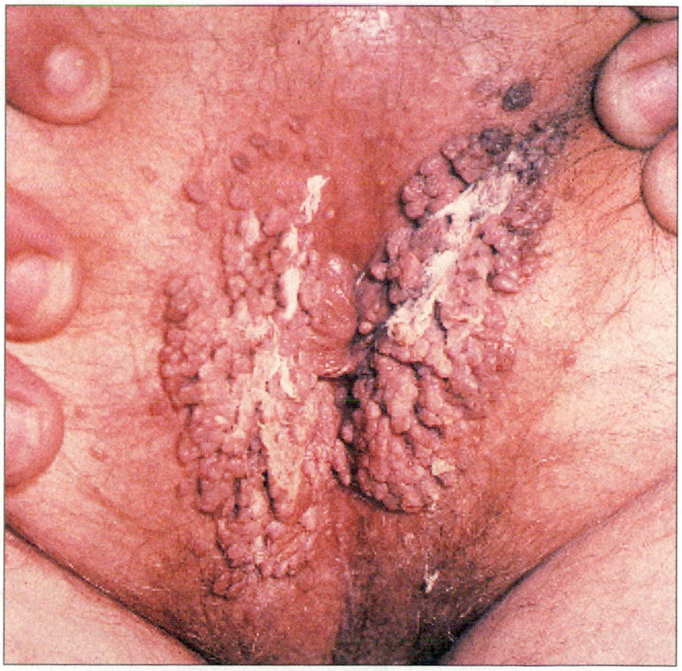

Figure 6–4 • Condylomata acuminata on the vulva.
SOURCE: Copyright Kenneth Greer/Visuals Unlimited.

however, depending on their location and size, they may cause itching (pruritus), be friable (bleed easily), or be painful. The moist, warm environment of the genital area is conducive to the growth of the warts, which may be present on the vulva, perineum, vagina, cervix, urethra, and anus. The incubation period following exposure is 3 weeks to 3 years, with the average being about 3 months.

Because condylomata sometimes resemble other lesions and may become cancerous, all atypical, pigmented, and persistent warts should be biopsied and treatment instituted promptly. Diagnosis is usually made by visual appearance. However, vaginal and cervical warts are more common than warts of the external genitalia. Most of these are flat lesions visible only by colposcopy (Eschenbach, 1999). Subclinical diagnosis can be made if characteristic changes are present on a Pap smear.

The CDC (2002) does not specify a treatment of choice for genital warts but recommends that treatment be determined based on client preference, available resources, and experience of the healthcare provider. No single treatment is best for all warts or for all clients. Client-applied therapies include podofilox solution or gel or imiquimod cream. For these methods to be effective, the client must be able to reach and identify the warts being treated. Provider-administered therapies include cryotherapy with liquid nitrogen or cryoprobe; topical podophyllin; trichloroacetic acid (TCA); bichloroacetic acid (BCA); and surgical removal by tangential scissors excision, shave excision, curettage, or electrosurgery. Alternative therapies include intralesional interferon or laser surgery (CDC, 2002). Imiquimod, podophyllin, and podofilox are not used during pregnancy because they are thought to be teratogenic and in large doses have been associated with fetal death.

Women with HPV infections should have frequent Pap smears to monitor cervical cellular changes. Sex partners are probably infected and do not require treatment unless large exophytic lesions are present. Moreover, no research to date indicates that reinfection plays a role in recurrence (CDC, 2002). The use of condoms may reduce the risk of transmitting the virus to an uninfected partner.

> *I've finally come to terms with the fact that I carry HPV. Yes, I know I will always run the risk of recurrence, but it's just a virus. It doesn't define me as a person.*

Pediculosis Pubis (Pubic or Crab Lice)

Pediculosis pubis is caused by *Phthirus*, a grayish, parasitic "crab" louse that lays eggs that attach to the hair shaft. Transmission is primarily by sexual contact, although shared towels and bed linens are also possible sources.

Symptoms include itching, usually in the pubic area. It is treated by applying 1% permethrin creme rinse to the affected area and washing it off after 10 minutes. Some caregivers recommend combing the pubic hair with a fine-toothed comb before rinsing off the permethrin. Lindane shampoo applied for 4 minutes and then washed off well can also be used. However, lindane is not recommended for pregnant or lactating women. Over-the-counter medications can also be used. Retreatment may be necessary. Both partners must be treated and tested for other STIs. Bed linens, towels, and clothing should be machine washed and dried in a hot dryer, dry-cleaned, or removed from body contact for at least 72 hours.

EVIDENCE-BASED PRACTICE

HEALTH EDUCATION TO REDUCE HUMAN PAPILLOMA VIRUS INFECTION

Clinical Question

Are health education interventions effective at encouraging women to adopt and maintain sexual behaviors that may reduce the risk of human papilloma virus (HPV) transmission, and thereby reduce the risk of cervical cancer?

The Evidence

Cervical cancer is one of the most common cancers affecting women worldwide. Client teaching to reduce risk of HPV and other sexually transmitted infections (STI) is suggested as a method of primary prevention of cervical cancer. An extensive search of the research literature identified ten quality studies, each of which showed a statistically significant positive effect of client teaching on sexual risk reduction, typically with increased use of condoms for vaginal intercourse. Other targeted outcomes included partner reduction and abstinence. The client teaching targeted socially and economically disadvantaged women. Health information was complemented by techniques for developing sexual negotiation skills and building motivation. The positive effect was generally sustained for up to three months after intervention.

Best Practice

Client teaching related to STI transmission and prevention, presented with techniques for developing negotiation skills and building motivation, can achieve short-term increases in reported condom use for vaginal intercourse. In turn, this can reduce the transmission of HPV, and thus the incidence of cervical cancer.

Reference: Shepherd, J., Weston, R., Peersman, G., Napuli, I.Z. (2002). Interventions for encouraging sexual lifestyles and behaviors intended to prevent cervical cancer. [Systematic Review] Cochrane Gynecological Cancer Group Cochrane Database of Systematic Reviews.

Scabies

Sarcoptes scabiei is a parasitic itch mite. The female mite burrows under the skin to deposit her eggs. Transmission by intimate sexual contact is common in adults but scabies in children is not generally sexually acquired (CDC, 2002).

Symptoms include itching that worsens at night or when the individual is warm. Noticeable erythematous, papular lesions or furrows may be present. The recommended treatment for scabies is permethrin cream 5% applied to all body areas from the neck down and washed off after 8 to 14 hours. Alternate therapy includes lindane 1% lotion or cream (Kwell) applied in a thin layer to all areas of the body from the neck down and then washed off after 8 hours. Lindane is not recommended for pregnant or lactating women, for people with extensive dermatitis, or for children under age 2 years. Although lindane is less expensive than permethrin, it has more associated risk and, in some parts of the world, including portions of the United States, lindane resistance has been reported (CDC, 2002). Permethrin 5% is used in pregnant women. Clothing and bed linens should be washed and dried in a hot dryer or dry-cleaned.

Viral Hepatitis

Hepatitis is an inflammatory process of the liver caused by infection by one of the five distinct viruses: A, B, C, D, and E. Currently, immunizations are only available for hepatitis A and B. Table 6–2 • compares the five forms of viral hepatitis.

Hepatitis A is characterized by symptoms of jaundice, anorexia, nausea, vomiting, malaise, and fever. It is self-limiting and is not a chronic condition. A vaccine is available to prevent hepatitis A.

Hepatitis B, C, and D have symptoms similar to those of hepatitis A, and can also include arthralgias, arthritis, and skin eruptions or rash. Unlike hepatitis A infection, those of B, C, and D infections are chronic. See Complementary and Alternative Therapies: Hepatitis C Treatment Alternatives.

Hepatitis E occurs primarily in South Central Asia and the Middle East, and its symptoms are like those of hepatitis A. It is also a self-limiting disease and not a chronic condition (CDC, 2002; Uphold & Graham, 1998).

Acquired Immunodeficiency Syndrome (AIDS)

Acquired immunodeficiency syndrome (AIDS) is a fatal disorder caused by the human immunodeficiency virus (HIV), which may be transmitted sexually. A medical-surgical text will

COMPLEMENTARY AND ALTERNATIVE THERAPIES

HEPATITIS C TREATMENT ALTERNATIVES

Currently in the United States about 3 million people have hepatitis C virus (HCV) although they may not know it because the majority of people who are infected show no symptoms for up to 20 to 30 years. Most people with HCV develop chronic liver disease such as cirrhosis. Some people with chronic HCV choose to try regular injections with interferon, which is only effective in eliminating the virus in 30% to 40% of infected individuals. Moreover, interferon has many severe side effects including anemia; sudden hearing loss; headaches; liver, heart, kidney, or eye problems; and psychologic disorders including depression.

To date, no complementary therapies have been proven to cure HCV or even ease the symptoms. Most complementary therapies under consideration focus on ways to help with the effects of HCV itself or ways to relieve the side effects of interferon.

HCV Effects

- Milk thistle (*Silybum marianum*) may protect the liver from injury by toxins such as viruses, radiation, alcohol, and poisonous mushrooms and limit the damage these toxins can cause. Milk thistle may also improve the way in which the liver functions in people with cirrhosis. It is available as a dietary supplement in capsule form.
- Licorice root (*Glycyrrhiza glabra*), taken as a tea, shows antiviral and anti-inflammatory properties and may help manage some of the effects of HCV on the liver. If taken regularly for more than 6 weeks, however, licorice root has been associated with high blood pressure, sodium and fluid retention, low potassium levels, and so forth.

Interferon Effects

- Ginger (*Zingiber officinale*), often taken as a tea, is frequently used to relieve the nausea and vomiting that accompany interferon therapy.
- St. John's wort (*Hypericum perforatum*), available as a capsule and as a tea, is sometimes taken to treat the depression caused by interferon therapy.

Source: National Center for Complementary and Alternative Medicine. (2002). *Hepatitis C: Treatment alternatives.* Retrieved October 20, 2002, from http://nccam.nih.gov

Table 6–2 • TYPES OF VIRAL HEPATITIS

Form	Primary Route of Transmission	Incubation Period	Chronic Infection	Immunization Available?
Hepatitis A	Fecal-oral, contaminated food/water	15–50 days	No	Yes
Hepatitis B	Blood/body fluids	45–160 days	Yes	Yes
Hepatitis C	Blood/blood products	14–180 days	Yes	No
Hepatitis D	Blood/body fluids	45–160 days	Yes	No
Hepatitis E	Fecal-oral	15–60 days	No	No

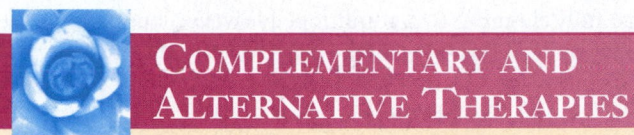

more fully describe this condition. However, because the diagnosis of HIV/AIDS or the presence of the HIV antibody has implications for a fetus if the woman is pregnant, HIV/AIDS is discussed in greater detail in Chapter 19.

NURSING CARE MANAGEMENT

Nursing Assessment and Diagnosis

The nurse working with women must become adept at taking a thorough history and identifying women at risk for sexually transmitted infections. Risk factors include multiple sexual partners; a partner's involvement with other partners; high-risk sexual behaviors, such as intercourse without barrier contraception or anal intercourse; partners with high-risk behaviors; and young age at onset of sexual activity. The nurse should be alert for signs and symptoms of STI and be familiar with diagnostic procedures if it is suspected.

While each STI has certain distinctive characteristics, the following complaints suggest the possibility of infection and warrant further investigation:

- Presence of a "sore" or lesion on the vulva
- Increased vaginal discharge or malodorous vaginal discharge
- Burning with urination
- Dyspareunia
- Bleeding after intercourse
- Pelvic pain

In many instances the woman is asymptomatic but may report symptoms in her partner, especially painful urination or urethral discharge. It is often helpful to ask the woman whether her partner is experiencing any symptoms.

Nursing diagnoses that may apply to a woman with an STI include the following:

- ***Altered Family Processes*** related to the effects of a diagnosis of sexually transmitted infection on the couple's relationship
- ***Health-Seeking Behaviors:*** Information on preventing STIs related to an expressed desire to avoid infection

MEDIALINK CARE PLAN: GYNECOLOGIC INFECTION

Nursing Plan and Implementation

In a supportive, nonjudgmental way, the nurse provides the woman who has a sexually transmitted infection with information about the infection, methods of transmission, implications for pregnancy or future fertility, and importance of thorough treatment. If treatment of her partner is indicated, the woman must understand that it is necessary to prevent a cycle of reinfection. She should also understand the need to abstain from sexual activity, if necessary, during treatment.

RESEARCH IN PRACTICE
Factors Associated with Reinfection with a Sexually Transmitted Infection

What is this study about? A key element in programs that aim to reduce the transmission of sexually transmitted infections is the identification and further prevention of infection in core groups, or groups of individuals at increased risk for reinfection. Core group members tend to exhibit high-risk sexual behavior; interventions targeting these groups have been shown to have a significant impact on infection incidence. This study investigated the demographic and behavior characteristics most frequently associated with reinfection with a sexually transmitted infection.

How was this study done? This retrospective cohort study involved review of records of 17,466 subjects who presented at one of three London, England, STD clinics with an acute sexually transmitted infection. Of these, 14% reattended for treatment of a sexually transmitted infection within one year. Demographic and diagnostic data were retrieved from subject records, while attending physicians collected behavior characteristics. Data were statistically analyzed to investigate the relationship between the rate of acute reinfection and a range of demographic and behavioral characteristics.

What were the results of the study? Of the clients with an acute sexually transmitted infection, sexual orientation and diagnosis were key predictors of reinfection. Reinfection was notably higher for subjects who presented initially with gonorrhea, nonspecific genital infection, or multiple sexually transmitted infections. Reinfection was lowest for subjects presenting initially with genital warts and herpes. Reinfection was lower for women than for men; however, younger women (ages 12 to 15 years) had the highest reinfection rate of any age group for women. Reinfection was also associated with history of previous sexually transmitted infection and for those with multiple partner changes. Ethnically, the black Caribbean population had the highest reinfection rate.

What additional questions might I have? Was the clinic a free clinic? Did it have a different socioeconomic distribution of clients than might be seen at a private clinic or physician's office? Are the rates similar for the sexually transmitted infections that may present no symptoms (eg, HIV)?

How can I use this study? Reducing the spread of sexually transmitted infections means identifying those who are at greatest risk of increasing the spread. The nurse can use these predictors to identify those individuals who are at risk for repeat sexually transmitted infections. Education, counseling, and other preventive efforts may reduce both the reinfection rate of individuals and the spread of sexually transmitted infections.

Source: Hughes, G., Brady, A., Catchpole, M., Fenton, K., Rogers, P., Kinghorn, G., et al. (2001). Characteristics of those who repeatedly acquire sexually transmitted infections: A retrospective cohort study of attendees at three urban sexually transmitted disease clinics in England. *Sexually Transmitted Diseases, 28*(7), 379–386.

Some STIs, such as trichomoniasis or chlamydia, may cause a woman concern but, once diagnosed, are rather simply treated. Other STIs may also be fairly simple to treat medically but may carry a stigma and be emotionally devastating for the woman. Thus the nurse should stress prevention with all women and encourage them to require partners, especially new partners, to use a condom.

The sensitive nurse can be especially helpful in encouraging the woman to explore her feelings about the diagnosis. She may experience anger or feel "betrayed" by a partner; she may feel guilt or see her diagnosis as a form of "punishment"; or she may feel concern about the long-term implications for future childbearing or ongoing intimate relationships. She may experience a myriad of emotions that she never expected. Opportunities to discuss her feelings in a nonjudgmental environment can be especially helpful. The nurse can offer suggestions about support groups, if indicated, and assist the woman in planning for her future with regard to sexual activity.

More subtly, the nurse's attitude of acceptance and matter-of-factness conveys to the woman that she is still an acceptable person who happens to have an infection. Table 6–3 • provides a summary of basic information the nurse should share with women who have an STI. STIs that can have an impact on pregnancy or the fetus/newborn are discussed in Chapter 20.

Evaluation

Expected outcomes of nursing care include the following:

- The infection is identified and cured, if possible. If not, supportive therapy is provided.
- The woman and her partner can describe the infection, its method of transmission, its implications, and the therapy.
- The woman copes successfully with the impact of the diagnosis on her self-concept.

Table 6–3 • PREVENTING STIs AND THEIR CONSEQUENCES

The risk of contracting an STI increases with the number of sexual partners. Because of the extended time between infection with HIV and evidence of infection, intercourse with an individual exposes a female or male to all the other sexual partners of that individual for the past 5 or more years. Because of this risk, it is important to take the following actions:

- Plan ahead and develop strategies to refuse sex (especially important for adolescents who may be less confident about saying "no" to casual sexual encounters), as abstinence is the best method of preventing STIs.
- Limit the number of sexual contacts and practice mutual monogamy.
- The condom is the best contraceptive method currently available (other than abstinence) for protection from STIs. Use one for every act of vaginal and anal intercourse. Other contraceptives such as the diaphragm, cervical cap, and spermicides also offer some protection against STIs.
- Plan strategies for negotiating condom use with a partner.
- Reduce high-risk behaviors. Use of recreational drugs and alcohol can increase sexual risk taking.
- Refrain from oral sex if your partner has active sores in mouth, vagina, or anus or on penis.
- Seek care as soon as you notice symptoms and make sure your partner gets treatment if indicated. Absence of symptoms or disappearance of symptoms does not mean that treatment is unnecessary if you suspect an STI. Take all prescribed medications completely.
- The presence of a genital infection may lead to an abnormal Pap smear. Women with certain infections should have more frequent Pap tests according to a schedule recommended by their caregiver. Ask your health care provider if you need more frequent Paps.

Care of the Woman with Pelvic Inflammatory Disease

Pelvic inflammatory disease (PID) occurs in approximately 1% of women between ages 15 and 39, although sexually active young women between 15 and 24 have the highest infection rate. An estimated 1 million cases are diagnosed annually, resulting in 200,000 hospitalizations (Scott & Hasik, 2001). The disease is more common in women who have had multiple sexual partners, a history of PID, early onset of sexual activity, a recent gynecologic procedure, or an intrauterine device (IUD). It usually produces a tubal infection (salpingitis) that may or may not be accompanied by a pelvic abscess. However, perhaps the greatest problem of PID is postinfection tubal damage, which is closely associated with infertility.

PID is defined as a clinical syndrome of inflammatory disorders of the upper female genital tract which includes any combination of endometritis, salpingitis, tubo-ovarian abscess, pelvic abscess, and pelvic peritonitis (CDC, 2002).The organisms most frequently identified with PID include *Chlamydia trachomatis* and *Neisseria gonorrhoeae* with a co-infection rate (both organisms are present) of 60%. Bacterial vaginosis may facilitate the ascending spread of pathogens. Often PID is the result of polymicrobial infection, involving other aerobic and anaerobic organisms that are often part of the normal vaginal flora (Scott & Hasik, 2001).

Symptoms of PID include bilateral sharp, cramping pain in the lower quadrants, fever greater than 101°F, chills, mucopurulent cervical or vaginal discharge, irregular bleeding, cervical motion tenderness during intercourse, malaise, nausea, and vomiting. However, it is also possible to be asymptomatic and have normal laboratory values.

Diagnosis consists of a clinical examination to define symptoms. Laboratory tests include vaginal, cervical, and possibly rectal cultures for *N gonorrhoeae* and *C trachomatis* as well as blood tests including a complete blood count (CBC) with differential, and RPR or VDRL to test for syphilis. A woman with PID often has an elevated C-reactive protein and elevated sedimentation rate. Microscopic examination of the vaginal secretions may reveal white blood cells. Physical examination usually reveals direct abdominal tenderness with palpation, and on bimanual examination, adnexal tenderness, and cervical and uterine tenderness with movement (Chandelier sign). A palpable mass is evaluated with ultrasonography. In confounding cases, laparoscopy may be used to confirm the diagnosis and to enable the examiner to obtain cultures from the fimbriated ends of the fallopian tubes.

Currently, there is no evidence comparing parenteral versus oral treatment, and outpatient treatment is an option.

The decision to hospitalize a woman is based on clinical judgment. The woman should be hospitalized if the diagnosis is uncertain, ectopic pregnancy or appendicitis is suspected, the woman is severely ill (nausea, vomiting, high fever, dehydration), there has been little response to oral therapy after 48 to 72 hours, the client is an adolescent, or the woman is unable to return for follow-up care. Treatment includes intravenous (IV) fluids, pain medication, and administration of IV antibiotics. Intravenous cefotetan or cefoxitin, plus doxycycline, is one treatment regimen. Another is clindamycin plus gentamicin (CDC, 2002). Ambulatory or outpatient treatment includes ofloxacin orally, twice daily, plus oral metronidazole twice daily, both for 14 days. This combination is highly effective in treating both gonorrhea and chlamydia, as well as BV. A different regimen would include intramuscular injection of ceftriaxone or cefoxitin, plus doxycycline, plus metronidazole (Scott & Hasik, 2001). Other supportive measures that may be helpful include increased oral fluids (up to 2 liters per day), continued bed rest or pelvic rest, acetaminophen for fever, and naproxen sodium for relief of pain. Follow-up visits are important within 48 to 72 hours, sooner if symptoms worsen. The sexual partner should also be treated. If the woman has an IUD, it is generally removed 24 to 48 hours after antibiotic therapy is started.

NURSING CARE MANAGEMENT

Nursing Assessment and Diagnosis

The nurse is alert to factors in a woman's history that put her at risk for PID. Even though fewer types of IUDs are available, many women still have them, and the nurse should question the woman about possible symptoms, such as aching pain in the lower abdomen, foul-smelling discharge, malaise, and the like. The woman who is acutely ill has obvious symptoms, but a low-grade infection is more difficult to detect.

Nursing diagnoses that may apply to a woman with PID include the following:

- ***Acute Pain*** related to peritoneal irritation
- ***Deficient Knowledge*** related to a lack of information about the possible effects of PID on fertility

Nursing Plan and Implementation

The nurse plays a vital role in helping to prevent or detect PID. Accordingly, the nurse spends time discussing risk factors related to this infection. The woman who uses an IUD for contraception and has multiple sexual partners needs to understand clearly the risk she faces. The nurse should strongly recommend that the IUD be removed and another method of contraception used. The nurse discusses signs and symptoms of PID with women at high risk and stresses the importance of early detection.

The woman who develops PID needs to understand the importance of completing her antibiotic treatment and of returning for follow-up evaluation. She should also understand that one outcome of the infection may be decreased fertility.

Evaluation

Expected outcomes of nursing care include the following:

- The woman describes her condition, her therapy, and the possible long-term implications of PID on her fertility.
- The woman completes her course of therapy and the PID is cured.

Care of the Woman with a Urinary Tract Infection

Urinary tract infection (UTI) is defined as significant bacteriuria in the presence of symptoms. Approximately 50% to 70% of women will experience a UTI in their lifetime and 20% to 30% will have a recurrent UTI (Dwyer & O'Reilly, 2002). A UTI may be life threatening or a mere inconvenience. Bacteria usually enter the sterile environment of the urinary tract by way of the urethra. The organisms are capable of migrating against the downward flow of urine. The shortness of the female urethra facilitates the passage of bacteria into the bladder. Other conditions that are associated with bacterial entry are relative incompetence of the urinary sphincter, frequent enuresis (bed-wetting) before adolescence, pregnancy, and urinary catheterization. Wiping from back to front after urination may transfer bacteria from the anorectal area to the urethra.

Voluntarily suppressing the desire to urinate is also a predisposing factor. Retention overdistends the bladder and can lead to an infection. There also seems to be a relationship between recurring UTI and sexual intercourse. General poor health or lowered resistance to infection can increase a woman's susceptibility to UTI. Factors that may inhibit bacterial growth include a low pH (5.5 or less) resulting in more acidic urine, high urea concentration, and the presence of organic acids from food such as fruits and proteins. *Asymptomatic bacteriuria (ASB)* refers to bacteria in the urine actively multiplying without accompanying clinical symptoms. It occurs in about 2% to 9% of UTIs (Dwyer & O'Reilly, 2002). This becomes especially significant if the woman is pregnant because about 20% to 30% of pregnant women with untreated ASB will develop pyelonephritis (DelRio & Pressman, 1999). ASB is almost always caused by one organism. If more than one type of bacteria are cultured, the possibility of urine-culture contamination must be considered. The most common cause of ASB is *Escherichia coli*. Other commonly found causative organisms include *Klebsiella* and *Proteus*, and less commonly, *Pseudomonas* and *Staphylococcus* species.

A woman who has had a UTI is susceptible to recurrent infection. Although the role of ASB in pregnancy complication remains controversial, the majority of evidence supports the view that bacteriuria does not, as an isolated factor, lead to low birth weight or prematurity. However, ASB is associated with low birth weight, preterm birth, hypertension, preeclampsia, maternal anemia and symptomatic UTI (Thorsen & Poole, 2002).

UTIs are more frequently encountered in pregnant women in part because of dramatic physiologic changes. Muscle tone and activity of the ureters decrease, resulting in reduced passage of urine through the urinary system. The bladder experiences decreased tone, increased capacity, and incomplete emptying. Urinary pH is elevated along with glycogen levels. All of these changes contribute to the increased risk for urinary tract disorders. All pregnant women should be screened for ASB throughout pregnancy to prevent ascending renal infections. Women at increased risk for bacteriuria, such as women with a history of UTIs, sickle cell trait, diabetes, renal calculi, chronic renal disease, or significant hypertension, should be screened every 6 to 12 weeks via clean-catch urine sample for ASB. Treatment in pregnant women includes amoxicillin, nitrofurantoin, cephalexin, trimethoprim-sulfamethoxazole, and sulfisoxazole.

Lower Urinary Tract Infection (Cystitis and Urethritis)

Because UTIs ascend, it is important to recognize and diagnose a lower UTI early to avoid the sequelae associated with upper UTI. One common lower UTI is cystitis, or infection of the urinary bladder. Several factors place a woman at increased risk for cystitis, including sexual intercourse, the use of a diaphragm and a spermicide, delayed postcoital micturition, pregnancy, and a history of a recent UTI.

E coli is present in 80% of women with UTIs. *Staphylococcus saprophyticus*, *Klebsiella*, *Proteus*, *Enterobacter*, and *Pseudomonas* are also causative pathogens. Infections without bacteriuria may indicate urethritis and are usually caused by *C trachomatis*, *N gonorrhoeae*, and herpes simplex.

When cystitis develops, the classic initial symptoms are often acute and include dysuria, specifically at the end of urination, as well as urgency and frequency. Suprapubic or low back pain may also occur. Cystitis is usually accompanied by a low-grade fever (38.3°C, or 101°F, or lower), and hematuria is occasionally seen. Urine specimens often contain an abnormal number of leukocytes and bacteria and may contain protein. Urethritis symptoms usually have a gradual onset and are associated with a cervicitis or vulvovaginal herpetic lesion.

The diagnosis can be made with a urine culture. Bacteriuria dipstick screening tests are quick office screening tests; however, they have high false-positive and false-negative rates. Prior to treatment the diagnosis should be confirmed by clinical evaluation and urine culture and sensitivity results. The treatment depends on the causative pathogen. Oral trimethoprim-sulfamethoxazole, fluoroquinolones, and fomycin tromethamine are frequently used in single-dose, 3-day, and 7-day regimens.

Upper Urinary Tract Infection (Pyelonephritis)

Pyelonephritis (inflammatory disease of the kidneys) is less common but more serious than cystitis and is often preceded by lower UTI. It is more common during the latter part of pregnancy or early postpartum and poses a serious threat to maternal and fetal well-being. Women with pyelonephritis during pregnancy are at significantly increased risk of preterm labor, preterm birth, development of adult respiratory distress syndrome and septicemia, and in some instances intrauterine growth restriction (Samuels & Colombo, 2002). Acute pyelonephritis has a sudden onset with chills, high temperature of 39.6°C to 40.6°C (103°F to 105°F), and costovertebral angle tenderness or flank pain, which may be unilateral or bilateral. The right side is almost always involved if the woman is pregnant because the large bulk of intestines to the left pushes the uterus to the right, putting pressure on the right ureter and kidney. Nausea, vomiting, and general malaise may ensue. With accompanying cystitis, the woman may experience frequency, urgency, and burning with urination.

Edema of the renal parenchyma or ureteritis with blockage and swelling of the ureter may lead to temporary suppression of urinary output. This is accompanied by severe colicky (spastic, intense) pain, vomiting, dehydration, and ileus of the large bowel. The woman with acute pyelonephritis will generally have increased diastolic blood pressure, positive fluorescent antibody titer (FA-test), low creatinine clearance, significant bacteremia in urine culture, pyuria, and presence of white blood cell casts.

Often the woman is hospitalized and started on IV antibiotics. Therapy also includes IV hydration, urinary analgesics such as Pyridium, pain management, and medication to manage fever. In the case of obstructive pyelonephritis, a blood culture is necessary. The woman is kept on bed rest. If signs of urinary obstruction occur or continue, the ureter may be catheterized to establish adequate drainage.

Initial IV treatment options include ampicillin plus gentamicin, ceftriaxone, trimethoprim-sulfamethoxazole, aztreonam, and cefazolin. With appropriate drug therapy, the woman's temperature should return to normal. The pain subsides, and the urine shows no bacteria within 2 to 3 days. Follow-up urinary cultures are needed to determine that the infection has been eliminated completely.

NURSING CARE MANAGEMENT

Nursing Assessment and Diagnosis

During the woman's visit, the nurse obtains a medical history, including a sexual history, to determine whether she is at risk for UTI. Additionally, the nurse notes any complaints from the woman of painful urination or other urinary difficulties, and systemic complaints such as fever, chills, nausea, vomiting, or back pain. If the nurse is concerned, a clean-catch urine sample is obtained to evaluate for the presence of bacteriuria.

Nursing diagnoses that may apply to the woman with a UTI include the following:

- ***Acute Pain*** related to dysuria, systemic discomforts, or back pain secondary to lower or upper urinary tract infection
- ***Health-Seeking Behaviors:*** Information about preventing UTIs related to an expressed desire to avoid recurrence
- ***Fear*** related to the possible long-term effects of the disease

Nursing Plan and Implementation

Most bacteria enter through the urethra after having spread from the anal area. Therefore, the nurse should make sure the woman is aware of good hygiene practices and provide information on other ways to avoid UTI. (See Figure 6–5 • and Table 6–4 •.) Additionally, the nurse provides the woman with information to help her recognize the signs and symptoms of a UTI to facilitate early identification and treatment of future infections. The nurse should also reinforce instructions and answer any additional questions the woman may have regarding the prescribed antibiotic, the type and amount of liquid to ingest, and the reasons for these treatments. UTI usually respond quickly to treatment, but follow-up clinical evaluation and urine cultures are important.

Evaluation

Expected outcomes of nursing care include the following:

- The woman implements self-care measures to help prevent recurrent UTI as part of her personal routine.
- The woman completes her prescribed course of antibiotic therapy.
- The woman can identify signs of recurrent UTI, or signs and symptoms of worsening urinary symptoms that would require follow-up care.
- The woman's infection is cured.

Clinical Tip *To avoid contamination of a clean-catch urine in a woman with a suspected UTI, you might try having her place a cotton ball or gauze square just inside her vagina. After she obtains the urine specimen and closes the container, she then removes the cotton or gauze and discards it in the trash receptacle.*

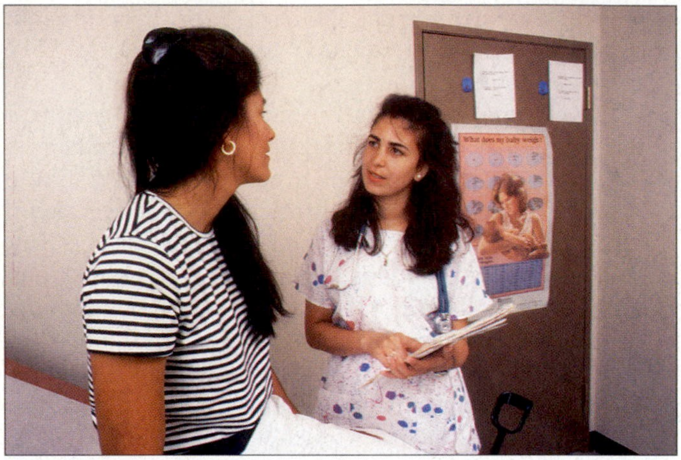

Figure 6–5 • The nurse counsels the woman about measures for preventing urinary tract infection.
SOURCE: © Michael Newman/Photo Edit—All rights reserved.

Table 6–4 • MEASURES FOR PREVENTING CYSTITIS

If you use a diaphragm for contraception, try changing methods or using another size diaphragm.
Avoid bladder irritants, such as alcohol, caffeine products, and carbonated beverages.
Increase fluid intake, especially water, to a minimum of six to eight glasses per day.
Make regular urination a habit; avoid long waits.
Practice good genital hygiene, including wiping from front to back after urination and bowel movements.
Be aware that vigorous or frequent sexual activity may contribute to urinary tract infection.
Urinate before and after intercourse to empty the bladder and cleanse the urethra.
Complete medication regimens even if symptoms decrease.
Do not use medication left over from previous infections.
Drink cranberry juice to acidify the urine. This has been found to relieve symptoms in some cases.

CHAPTER REVIEW

EXPLOREMEDIALINK

NCLEX review questions, case studies, and other interactive resources for this chapter can be found on the Web site at http://www.prenhall.com/olds. Click on "Chapter 6" to select the activities for this chapter.

For tutorials including animations and videos, more NCLEX review questions, and an audio glossary, access the accompanying CD-ROM in this book.

Focus Your Study

- Vulvovaginal candidiasis (moniliasis), a vaginal infection most often caused by *Candida albicans*, is most common in women who use oral contraceptives, are taking antibiotics, are currently pregnant, or have diabetes mellitus. It is generally treated with intravaginal miconazole or clotrimazole suppositories or fluconazole orally.
- Bacterial vaginosis (*Gardnerella vaginalis* vaginitis), a common vaginal infection, is diagnosed by its characteristic fishy odor and by the presence of "clue" cells on a vaginal smear. It is treated with metronidazole.
- Chlamydial infection is difficult to detect in a woman but may result in PID and infertility. It is treated with antibiotic therapy.
- Gonorrhea, a common sexually transmitted infection, may be asymptomatic in women initially but may cause PID if not diagnosed early. The treatment of choice is ceftriaxone and doxycycline or azithromycin.
- Herpes genitalis, caused by the herpes simplex virus, is a recurrent infection with no known cure. Acyclovir (Zovirax) may reduce the symptoms.
- Syphilis, caused by *Treponema pallidum*, is a sexually transmitted infection that is treatable if diagnosed. The characteristic lesion is the chancre. Syphilis can also be transmitted in utero to the fetus of an infected woman. The treatment of choice is penicillin.
- Condylomata acuminata (venereal warts) are transmitted by the human papilloma virus (HPV). Treatment is indicated, because research has identified seven strains of HPV linked with high-grade abnormal cervical changes. The treatment chosen depends on the size and location of the warts.
- Pelvic inflammatory disease may be life threatening and may lead to infertility. The organisms that cause PID most frequently include *C trachomatis* and *N gonorrhoeae*.
- Women with an abnormal finding on a pelvic examination will need careful explanation of the finding and techniques of diagnosis and emotional support during the diagnostic period.
- The classic symptoms of a lower UTI are dysuria, urgency, frequency, and sometimes hematuria. Oral sulfonamides are the treatment of choice except in middle to late pregnancy.
- An upper UTI is a serious infection that can permanently damage the kidneys if untreated. Generally the woman is acutely ill and may require supportive therapy as well as antibiotics.

References

Centers for Disease Control and Prevention (CDC). (2002). Sexually transmitted diseases treatment guidelines 2002. *Morbidity and Mortality Weekly Report, 51*(RR-6), 1–84.

DelRio, S., & Pressman, E. (1999). Renal, hepatic and gastrointestinal disease and systemic lupus erythematosus in pregnancy. In *Johns Hopkins Manual of Gynecology and Obstetrics.* Philadelphia: Lippincott Williams and Wilkins.

Dwyer, P., & O'Reilly, J. (2002). Recurrent urinary tract infection in the female. *Current Opinion in Obstetrics and Gynecology, 14*(5), 537–543.

Eschenbach, D. A. (1999). Pelvic infections and sexually transmitted diseases. In J. R. Scott, P. J. DiSaia, C. B. Hammond, & W. N. Spellacy (Eds.), *Danforth's obstetrics and gynecology* (8th ed., pp. 579–600). Philadelphia: Lippincott Williams & Wilkins.

Mead, P. B. (Moderator). (2001). Symposium: What's new in vaginitis diagnosis and treatment? *Contemporary OB/GYN, 46*(11), 14–42.

Richwald, G. A., & Skaer, T. L. (2001). External genital warts. *The Female Patient, 26*(11), 50–56.

Samuels, P., & Colombo, D. F. (2002). Renal disease. In S. G. Gabbe, J. R. Niebyl, & J. L. Simpson (Eds.). *Obstetrics: Normal and problem pregnancies,* (4th ed., pp. 1065–1080). New York: Churchill-Livingstone.

Scott, L. D., & Hasik, K. J. (2001). The similarities and differences of endometritis and pelvic inflammatory disease. *Journal of Obstetric, Gynecologic, and Neonatal Nursing, 30*(3), 332–341.

Sinofsky, F. E. (1999). Vulvovaginal candidiasis: Topical versus oral therapy. *The Female Patient, 24*(5), 35–42.

Thorsen, M., & Poole, J. (2002). Renal disease in pregnancy. *Journal of perinatal and neonatal nursing, 15* (4), 13–26.

Uphold, C. R., & Graham, M. V. (1998). *Clinical guidelines in family practice* (3rd ed.). Gainesville, FL: Barmarrae Books.

Walsh, C. M., & Irwin, K. L. (2002). Combating the silent chlamydia epidemic. *Contemporary OB/GYN, 47*(4), 90–98.

7 Women's Health Problems

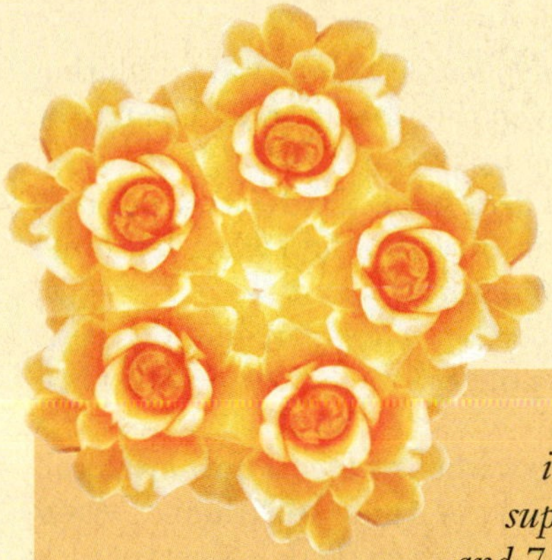

Two years ago a friend lost his wife to toxic shock syndrome. None of us knew much about it, and we were stunned by how quickly she deteriorated. Within days she was on life support until the family made the decision to stop it. My friend is now raising his 2-year old and 7-year old alone. He has made it his mission to tell women about the risks of toxic shock syndrome and the precautions they should take to avoid it.

Objectives

- Contrast the common benign and malignant breast disorders.
- Briefly describe the emotional reactions a woman may experience in regard to a diagnosis of breast cancer.
- Discuss the signs and symptoms, medical therapy, and implications for fertility of endometriosis.
- Discuss abnormal uterine bleeding and abdominal masses.
- Identify the implications of an abnormal finding during a pelvic examination.
- Summarize behaviors that help to minimize recurrence of some of the common lesions of the vulva.
- Discuss the importance of annual Pap smear evaluation, the implication of an abnormal finding, and appropriate follow-up.
- Briefly discuss the role that human papilloma virus plays in abnormal Pap smears.
- Delineate the psychosocial responses a woman may experience when facing any of the common gynecologic procedures.

Key Terms

Breast self-examination (BSE) 126
Colposcopy 144
Cystocele 147
Dysfunctional uterine bleeding (DUB) 145
Dyspareunia 134
Endometriosis 134
Fibrocystic breast changes 130
Galactorrhea 130
Hysterectomy 149
Mammogram 126
Pap smear 141
Toxic shock syndrome (TSS) 135

MEDIALINK

Additional resources for this content can be found on the Student CD-ROM and on the Companion Website at www.prenhall.com/olds. Click on "Chapter 7" to select the activities for this chapter.

CD-ROM
- Audio Glossary
- NCLEX Review

Companion Website
- Additional NCLEX Review
- Case Study: Toxic Shock Syndrome
- Care Plan Activity: Irregular Bleeding in Perimenopausal Woman
- Module: Common Gynecologic Cancers

Throughout her lifetime, a woman is likely to face a variety of gynecologic or urinary problems. Some may be minor, whereas others have the potential to be quite serious, provoking a wide array of physical and psychologic responses. This chapter provides information about selected gynecologic problems that a woman may encounter during her lifetime with an emphasis on problems commonly addressed in community-based settings. Some of the issues are addressed in detail, and other topics are discussed more briefly. The chapter concludes with a brief description of common gynecologic surgical procedures. For a detailed discussion of gynecologic cancers, for more detailed information on any of the subjects covered in this chapter, or for more in-depth discussion of gynecologic procedures, please consult a specialized text.

Care of the Woman with a Disorder of the Breast

Throughout her lifetime, a woman may experience a variety of breast disorders. Some, like mastitis, which is discussed in Chapter 37, are acute disorders, whereas others, such as fibrocystic breast disease, are chronic . This section begins with breast screening techniques and then deals with some of the common breast disorders a woman may experience.

Screening Techniques for the Breasts

Despite their limitations, breast examination and mammography remain the most effective screening techniques available for the breasts.

BREAST EXAMINATION

Like the uterus, the breast undergoes regular cyclic changes in response to hormonal stimulation. Each month, in rhythm with the cycle of ovulation, the breasts become engorged with fluid in anticipation of pregnancy, and the woman may experience sensations of tenderness, lumpiness, or pain. If conception does not occur, the accumulated fluid drains away via the lymphatic network. *Mastodynia* (premenstrual swelling and tenderness of the breasts) is common. It usually lasts for 3 to 4 days before the onset of menses, but the symptoms may persist throughout the month.

After menopause, connective breast tissue atrophies and is replaced by adipose tissue. The breasts lose elasticity and may droop and become pendulous. The recurring breast engorgement associated with ovulation ceases. If hormone replacement therapy (HRT) is used to counteract other symptoms of menopause, breast engorgement may resume.

Monthly **breast self-examination (BSE)** is a good method for detecting breast masses early. A woman who knows the texture and feel of her own breasts is far more likely to detect changes that develop. Thus it is important for a woman to develop the habit of doing routine BSE. Women at high risk for breast cancer are especially encouraged to be attentive to the importance of early detection through routine BSE. The American Cancer Society (ACS) (2002) recommends that women begin performing monthly BSE at age 20.

In the course of a routine physical examination or during an initial visit to the caregiver, the woman should be taught BSE technique and its importance as a monthly practice. The effectiveness of BSE is determined by the woman's ability to perform the procedure correctly. (See Client Teaching: Teaching Breast Self-Examination.)

BSE should be performed on a regular monthly basis about 1 week after the onset of each menstrual period, when the breasts are typically not tender or swollen. Breast self-examination is most effective when it uses a dual approach incorporating both inspection and palpation. After menopause, BSE should be performed on the same day each month (chosen by the woman for ease of remembrance).

Clinical breast examination (CBE) by a trained healthcare provider, such as a physician, nurse practitioner, or nurse-midwife, is an essential element of a routine gynecologic examination. Experience in differentiating among benign, suspicious, and worrisome breast changes enables the caregiver to reassure the woman if the findings are normal or move forward with additional diagnostic procedures or referral if the findings are suspicious or worrisome. The ACS (2002) recommends CBE every 3 years for women age 20 to 39 with no abnormal findings or history of breast-related problems and CBE annually for women age 40 and older. In clinical practice, however, many caregivers advocate annual CBE for all women over age 20.

MAMMOGRAPHY

A **mammogram** is a soft-tissue x-ray image of the breast taken without the injection of a contrast medium. It can detect lesions in the breast before they can be felt and has gained wide acceptance as an effective screening tool for breast cancer. Research indicates that mammography detects about 90% of breast cancers in women who are symptom free, although it is slightly more accurate in postmenopausal women, as compared to premenopausal women (ACS, 2002). Currently the ACS (2002) guidelines recommend that all women age 40 and over have an annual mammogram and, as discussed previously, an annual clinical breast examination. The National Cancer Institute (NCI) recommends mammograms every 1 to 2 years for women age 40 and older. The NCI also recommends that women at high risk for breast cancer should "seek expert medical advice about whether they should begin screening before age 40 and the frequency of screening" (NCI, 2002). If a woman has a history of breast cancer in a close relative (ie, mother, sister) and the cancer was diagnosed before the relative was age 40, many clinicians advocate that the client begin mammograms at that same age.

Negative consequences of mammography do exist. Thirty percent of women age 40 to 49 are likely to have a false-positive result requiring biopsy. Moreover, mammograms miss more than 25% of invasive breast cancers in women in this age group (Love, 2000). Furthermore, in some women, especially women who are quite elderly, the cancer tissue

Client Teaching: Breast Self-Examination

Assessment The nurse determines the woman's general knowledge about breast self-examination (BSE), identifies previous experience with BSE, identifies risk factors for breast cancer, determines the woman's general knowledge about breast cancer, identifies barriers to BSE, and discusses her commitment to practice BSE.

Nursing Diagnosis The key nursing diagnosis will probably be **Health-Seeking Behavior:** Information on BSE related to an expressed need to take action to detect breast abnormalities.

Nursing Plan and Implementation The teaching plan focuses on assisting the woman to learn BSE so that she can use it effectively.

Client Goals At the completion of the teaching, the woman will be able to

1. Discuss her risk of breast cancer.
2. Describe the use of BSE in breast cancer detection.
3. Demonstrate the correct procedure for BSE.
4. List warning signs of breast cancer to be reported to the caregiver.
5. Incorporate monthly BSE into her personal routine.

Teaching Plan

CONTENT	TEACHING METHOD
Discuss the risk factors associated with breast cancer.	Breast cancer should be discussed in a private area free of interruptions. The room needs to have a mirror; bed, couch, or examining table; pillows; a patient gown; and private area for the woman to disrobe.
Stress the unique risk factors associated with the woman's personal history and lifestyle.	Create a supportive, warm, and comfortable atmosphere by attitude and communication style—both verbal and nonverbal. A discussion of breast cancer may bring forth many emotions in the woman, including grief for previous breast cancer-related losses.
Discuss the use of BSE in breast cancer detection.	Focus on open discussion. A brochure with statistics and illustrations may be useful. Stress the positive outcomes of early detection to counterbalance fears.

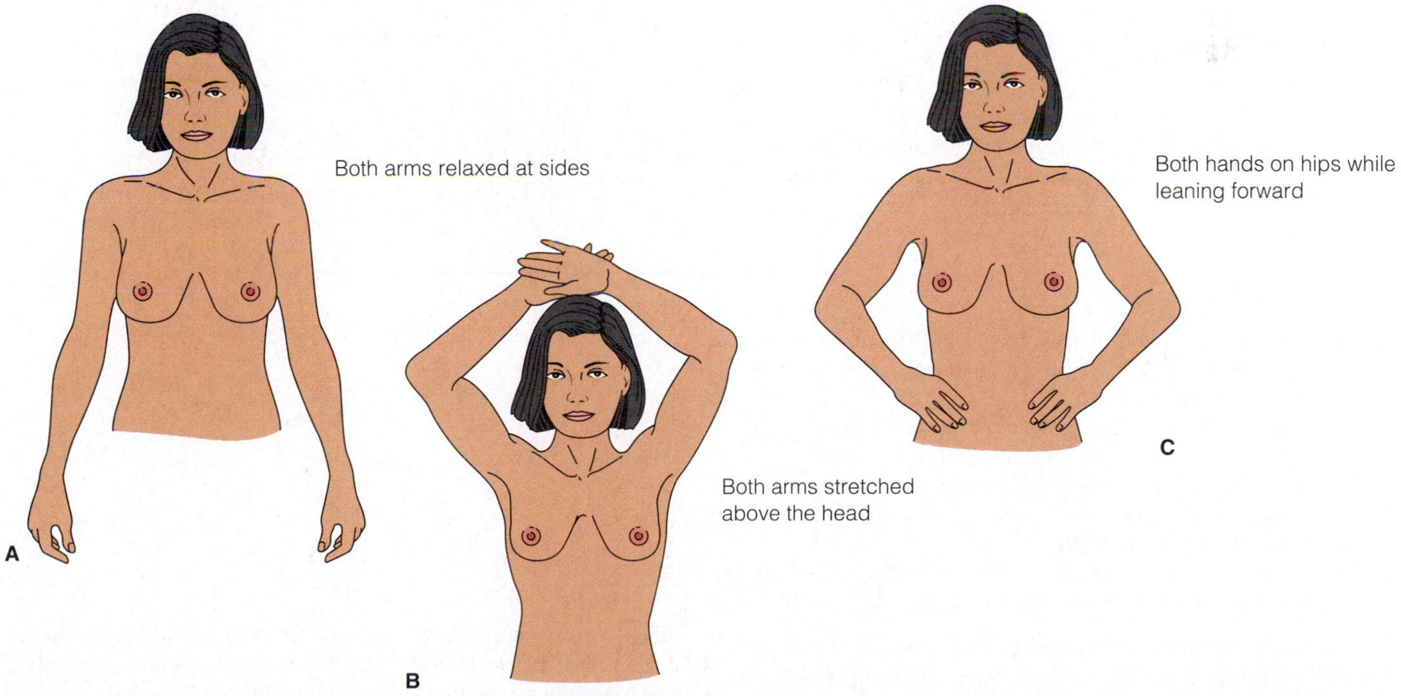

Figure 7-1 • Positions for inspection of the breasts. *A*, Both arms relaxed at sides. *B*, Both arms stretched above the head. *C*, Both hands on hips while leaning forward. *(continued on next page)*

CLIENT TEACHING BREAST SELF-EXAMINATION *(continued)*

Describe and demonstrate the correct procedure for BSE.

A. Instruct the woman to inspect her breasts by standing or sitting in front of a mirror. She needs to inspect her breasts in three positions: with both arms relaxed down at her sides, both arms stretched straight over her head, and both hands placed on her hips while leaning forward (Figure 7–1 •).

B. Advise the woman to look at her breasts individually and in comparison with one another. Note and record the following characteristics for each position:

Size and Symmetry of the Breasts

1. Breasts may vary, but the variations should remain constant during rest or movement—note abnormal contours.
2. Some size difference between the breasts is normal.

Shape and Direction of the Breasts

1. The shape of the breasts can be rounded or pendulous with some variation between breasts.
2. The breasts should be pointing slightly laterally.

Color, Thickening, Edema, and Venous Patterns

1. Check for redness or inflammation.
2. A blue hue with a marked venous pattern that is focal or unilateral may indicate an area of increased blood supply due to tumor. Symmetric venous patterns are normal.
3. Skin edema observed as thickened skin with enlarged pores ("orange peel") may indicate blocked lymphatic drainage due to tumor.

Surface of the Breasts

1. Skin dimpling, puckering, or retraction (pulling) when the woman presses her hands together or against her hips suggests malignancy.
2. Striae (stretch marks) red at onset and whitish with age are normal.

Nipple Size and Shape, Direction, Rashes, Ulcerations, and Discharge

1. Long-standing nipple inversion is normal, but an inverted nipple previously capable of erection is suspicious. Note any deviation, flattening, or broadening of the nipples.
2. Check for rashes, ulcerations, or discharge.

C. Instruct the woman to palpate (feel) her breasts as follows:

1. Lie down. Put one hand behind your head. With the other hand, fingers flattened, gently feel your breast. Press lightly (Figure 7–2, *A* •). Now examine the breast.
2. Figure 7–2, *B* shows you how to check each breast. Begin as you see in *B* and follow the arrows, feeling gently for a lump or thickening. Remember to feel all parts of each breast.
3. Now repeat the same procedure sitting up, with the hand still behind your head (Figure 7–2, *C*).
4. Squeeze the nipple between your thumb and forefinger. Look for any discharge—clear or bloody (Figure 7–2, *D*).

D. Take the woman's hand and help her to identify her "normal lumps" (eg, mammary ridge, ribs, and nodularity in the upper outer quadrants).

E. After she examines her breasts and identifies her normal lumps, instruct her to palpate her breasts once more to identify any areas that she may have questions about. If questions arise, the nurse should palpate the area and attempt to identify whether it is normal.

Learning is best accomplished when material is broken down into smaller steps and presented with multiple approaches. Prior to asking the woman to perform BSE, use a model or a chart to demonstrate the procedure. Then have the woman perform BSE. Be very supportive and give a lot of positive feedback because some women may be embarrassed. Demonstrate a nonjudgmental, accepting attitude.

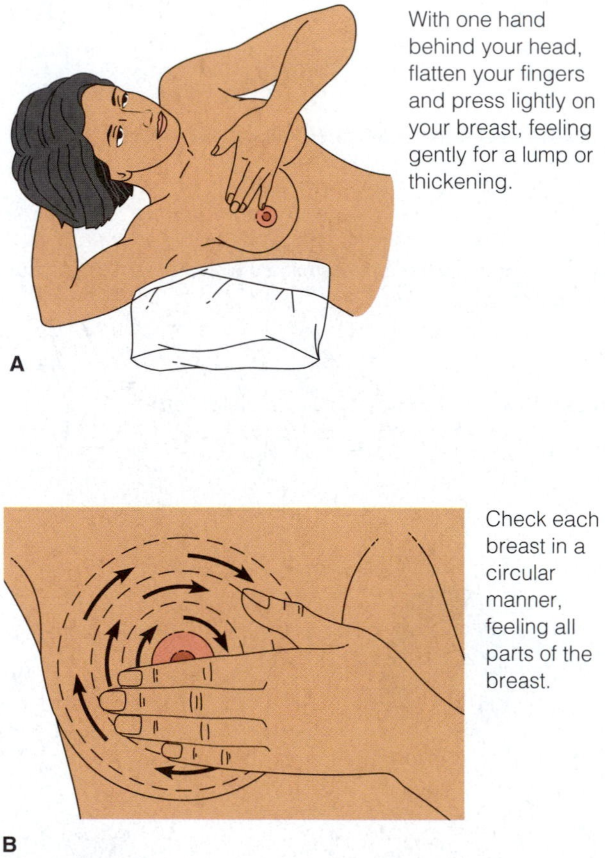

With one hand behind your head, flatten your fingers and press lightly on your breast, feeling gently for a lump or thickening.
A
Check each breast in a circular manner, feeling all parts of the breast.
B

Figure 7–2 • Procedure for breast self-examination.

Demonstrate "normal lumps" on the woman herself while guiding her hand and identifying the area. This will increase confidence that she will recognize an abnormal finding. Checking, her immediately afterward will positively reinforce her and diminish the fear associated with BSE.

Client Teaching — BREAST SELF-EXAMINATION *(continued)*

F. If a breast model is available, instruct the woman to palpate it and identify the lumps.

G. Provide information on the warning signs of breast cancer and what she should do if she identifies any of these signs during BSE.

TIMING

Instruct the woman to perform BSE on a monthly basis. Be specific based on whether she is premenopausal, pregnant, postmenopausal, or postmenopausal receiving hormone replacement therapy.

EVALUATION

Evaluate the woman's learning through discussion and return demonstration. Learning has occurred if the woman performs BSE correctly and can identify timing, normal and abnormal findings, and follow-up activities.

Provide a written handout on the warning signs of breast cancer. The handout should also cover actions that the woman should take if a warning sign is discovered. Stress the positive effects of early detection.

Provide the woman with a reminder symbol for monthly BSE. The American Cancer Society provides such items to hang in the shower, place on a refrigerator, and so forth. Praise her commitment to do monthly BSE. Give the woman a follow-up telephone number (eg, American Cancer Society) to use if she needs additional information or has questions.

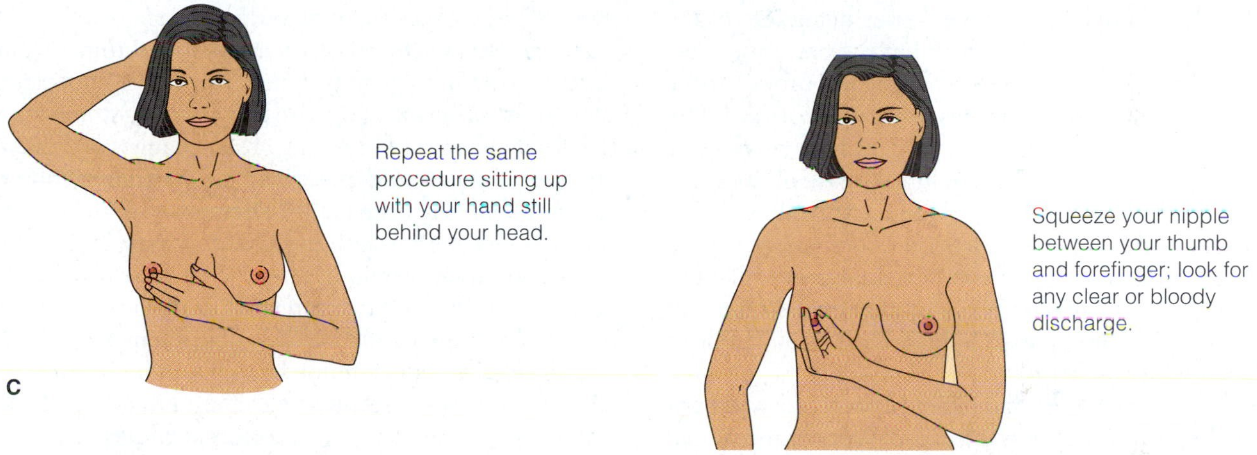
Repeat the same procedure sitting up with your hand still behind your head.
C
Squeeze your nipple between your thumb and forefinger; look for any clear or bloody discharge.

Figure 7–2 • Procedure for breast self-examination.
Source: American Cancer Society, (1973). *Breast self-examination and the nurse* (No. 3408 PB): New York: Author.

type may be so slow-growing that it would not cause morbidity or mortality within the woman's lifetime.

Breast sensitivity seems to vary from woman to woman and may be a factor in a woman's reluctance to have a mammogram. To help prevent any discomfort, the nurse can suggest that this x-ray study be scheduled when their breasts are least sensitive, which is about 2 weeks after the onset of menses. In some cases, the woman can obtain relief by reducing caffeine intake from 5 to 7 days prior to the test. In most cases, a mammogram causes feelings of compression but not pain (see Figure 7–3 •). All women should be instructed to refrain from applying lotions, powders, deodorant, or other cosmetic substances to the torso on the day of the exam because the substances may appear as questionable areas on the mammogram and may interfere with accurate interpretation. The risk of radiation exposure with mammograms is low but it does

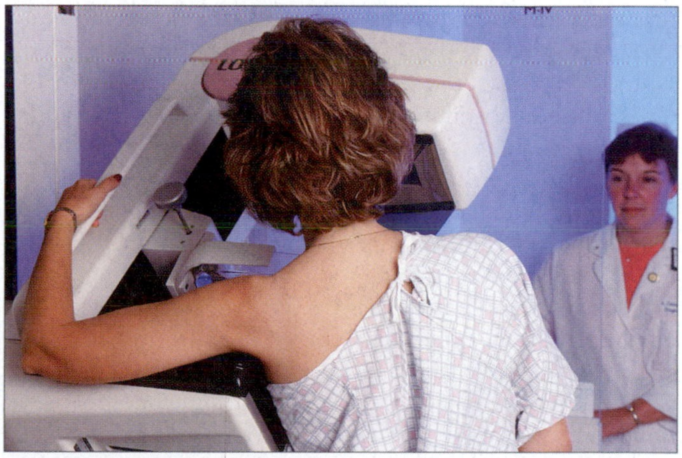

Figure 7–3 • Recommended position for mammogram.
SOURCE: Philip Bailey/CORBIS.

become more significant depending on the age of the woman at her initial mammogram and the number of mammograms she has (Love, 2000).

Benign Breast Conditions

Fibrocystic breast changes, the most common of the benign breast conditions, is most prevalent in women 20 to 50 years of age. It is rare in postmenopausal women who are not taking hormone replacement therapy. Fortunately, fibrocystic breast changes alone are not a risk factor for breast cancer. However, women who have a positive family history for breast cancer and who exhibit atypical cellular changes on biopsy do have an 11-fold increased risk for developing breast cancer (Fiorica, 1999). Fibrocystic changes may produce an asymptomatic mass, but more often are accompanied by pain or tenderness and sometimes nipple discharge. Fluctuation in size and rapid appearance or disappearance of breast masses are common. Bilateral, cyclic breast pain is the most common symptom, and the nodularities may be unilateral or bilateral, often in the upper outer quadrants of the breasts. The pathogenesis is unclear, but the presence of estrogen or an imbalance between estrogen and progesterone seems to be necessary for symptoms to occur (Fiorica, 1999).

The woman often reports pain, tenderness, and swelling that is cyclic, worsening in the late luteal phase of the menstrual cycle (just before menses), and improving about 1 to 2 days into the menstrual cycle. Physical examination may reveal only mild signs of irregularity, or the breasts may feel dense, with areas of irregularity and nodularity. Women often refer to this as "lumpiness." Some women may also have expressible nipple discharge.

If the woman has a large, fluid-filled cyst, she may experience a localized painful area as the capsule containing the accumulated fluid distends coincident with her cycle. However, if small cysts form, the woman may experience not a solitary tender lump but a diffuse tenderness. Several characteristics help differentiate a cyst from a cancerous lesion. Cysts tend to be mobile and tender and do not cause skin retraction (pulling) in the surrounding tissue, whereas cancerous lesions tend to be fixed and painless and may cause skin retraction.

Mammography, sonography, palpation, and fine-needle aspiration are used to confirm fibrocystic breast changes. Often, fine-needle aspiration provides treatment as well as relief from the tenderness or pain. Palpable cysts are often treated conservatively with medical management; however, all discrete three-dimensional masses should have a tissue sample sent for biopsy (Fiorica, 1999). Women with mild symptoms may benefit from restricting sodium intake and taking a mild diuretic during the week before the onset of menses. This counteracts fluid retention, relieves pressure in the breast, and helps decrease the pain. In other cases, a mild analgesic is necessary. Other treatment approaches include the use of thiamine and vitamin E. However, several studies have failed to demonstrate a direct benefit from these therapies (Morrow, 2000). Oral contraceptives may help alleviate symptoms, but unfortunately, maximum results may not occur until after at least a year of use. Moreover, symptoms tend to recur when the oral contraceptives are discontinued.

In severe cases, the hormone inhibitor danazol is often helpful although it can cause several undesirable side effects including masculinization. When danazol is discontinued, symptoms tend to recur in about two thirds of women. Women who do not respond to other treatment approaches may be given a trial of bromocriptine, a prolactin inhibitor. Bromocriptine improves symptoms in about three quarters of women but has many side effects, such as nausea and vomiting, alopecia (hair loss), dizziness, edema and weight gain, and headache, that cause women to discontinue its use. The antiestrogen medication tamoxifen may be used although this is an "off-label" use because tamoxifen has not been approved by the FDA for this purpose. Tamoxifen relieves symptoms in about 70% of women and has fewer side effects, but it can cause proliferation of endometrial tissue, increasing the risk of endometrial cancer, so women taking it should be monitored closely (Eskin & Sepilian, 2001). Women of childbearing age should be advised that tamoxifen has been associated with birth defects.

Some researchers suggest that methylxanthines (found in caffeine products, such as coffee, tea, colas, chocolate, and some medications) and the use of tobacco may contribute to the development of fibrocystic breast changes and that limiting use of these substances will help decrease fibrocystic changes. Other research fails to demonstrate a clear association between methylxanthines and fibrocystic breast changes. Studies in Great Britain have found treatment with evening primrose oil for breast pain related to fibrocystic changes to be effective in about 40% to 60% of women (Morrow, 2000).

Fibroadenoma is a common benign tumor affecting 10% of all women. It is the second most common benign breast lesion (Eskin & Sepilian, 2001). Fibroadenoma is most commonly seen in women in their teens and into their early thirties. It has not been significantly associated with breast cancer. Fibroadenomas are freely movable, solid tumors that are well defined, sharply delineated, and rounded, with a rubbery texture. They are asymptomatic and nontender.

If there are any disquieting features to the appearance of a lump, ultrasound, fine-needle biopsy, or excision of the mass may be indicated. Caution is exercised when deciding upon biopsy because excision of the mass in a young girl may interfere with normal breast development. Watchful observation, including monthly breast self-examination and annual clinical breast examination, is the most appropriate treatment. Surgery is often deferred, but is indicated if the mass becomes painful or continues to enlarge, if there are suspicious findings on ultrasound or cytology, or if the client needs definitive reassurance that only a biopsy can provide (Fiorica, 1999). Surgical removal of the fibroadenoma, when advisable, concludes its treatment.

The term for nipple discharge not associated with lactation (production of milk for breastfeeding) is **galactorrhea.** It is a common breast problem and has been reported in 10% to 15% of women with benign breast disease and in 2.5% to 3% of women with breast cancer (Morrow, 2000). Galactorrhea may be physiologic (as in the case with fibrocystic changes), drug induced, idiopathic, or pathologic. Physiologic discharge, usually associated with benign conditions, is characterized by clear, milky, straw-colored, or greenish fluid obtained by manual compression. Pathologic discharge, sometimes associated with malignancy, is spontaneous, unilateral, and often bloody or serosanguineous. Most providers recommend cytologic evaluation of all nipple discharge, regardless of its character; however, the absence of malignant cells does not exclude cancer, and a positive result does not distinguish in situ cancer from invasive cancer (Fiorica, 1999; Morrow, 2000).

Intraductal papillomas are tumors growing in the terminal portion of a duct or, sometimes, throughout the duct system within a section of the breast. Symptoms may include a unilateral mass or a spontaneous, and often bloody, nipple discharge. They are typically benign but have the potential to become malignant when the discharge is unilateral from a single duct, when the discharge occurs in a postmenopausal woman, or when a palpable mass is present (Fiorica, 1999).

The majority of papillomas present as solitary nodules. These small ball-like lesions may be detected on mammography but often are nonpalpable. The presence of a papilloma is often frightening to the woman, because her primary symptom is a discharge from the nipple that may be serosanguineous or brownish green due to old blood. The location of the papilloma within the duct system and its pattern of growth determine whether nipple discharge will be present. Some providers might recommend galactography or a ductogram (injecting radiopaque dye into the discharging duct and then performing mammography) for better visualization. However, the lesion must be excised and histologically examined because of the difficulty in differentiating a benign papilloma from a papillary carcinoma. Treatment for benign intraductal papilloma is excision with follow-up care.

Duct ectasia (comedomastitis), an inflammation of the ducts behind the nipple, commonly occurs during or near the onset of menopause and is not associated with malignancy. The condition typically occurs in women who have borne and nursed children. It is characterized by a thick, sticky nipple discharge of various colors and by burning pain, pruritus, and inflammation. Nipple retraction may also be noted, especially in postmenopausal women. Treatment is conservative, with drug therapy aimed at symptomatic relief. The major central ducts of the breast occasionally have to be excised.

Table 7–1 • provides a comparison of the most frequently seen benign breast disorders.

Malignant Breast Disease

The lifetime risk of breast cancer in the United States is 1 out of 8. The risk increases with age. Excluding skin cancer, breast cancer accounts for one third of female cancers. Annually approximately 15% of female cancer deaths, or 40,200 deaths, are due to breast cancer; 192,200 new cases of invasive breast cancer are diagnosed every year. Only lung cancer causes more cancer deaths in women (ACS, 2002). In women between the ages of 44 and 50 years, breast cancer is the leading cause of death in the United States (ACS, 2000).

Table 7–1 • SUMMARY OF BENIGN BREAST DISORDERS

Condition	Age	Pain	Cancer Risk	Nipple Discharge	Location	Consistency and Mobility	Diagnosis and Treatment
Fibrocystic breast changes	30–50	Yes	Yes with proliferative disease and atypical hyperplasia	Varies: none at all or may be clear, milky, straw-colored, or green	Upper outer quadrant	Multiple lumps occurring bilaterally, influenced by menstrual cycle, nodular	Needle aspiration, Pap smear of nipple discharge, observation, biopsy if unresolved mass exists or mammographic changes, sonography
Fibroadenoma	15–25, median age 20	No	No	No, but milky discharge in pregnancy	Nipple or upper outer quadrant along the lateral side	Solid, well defined, sharply delineated, rounded, rubbery, mobile	Mammography, observation, surgical excision
Intraductal papilloma	Menopausal 50–60	Yes on palpation	Yes with multiple papillomas	Yes: serous, bloody, or brownish green	No specific location	Nonpalpable or small, ball-like, poorly delineated	Pap smear of nipple discharge, mammography, ductogram, surgical excision
Duct ectasia	45–55	Yes: burning and itching around the nipple	No	Yes in perimenopausal women: thick, sticky, green, greenish brown, or bloodstained	Mass behind or around the nipple	Poorly circumscribed, inflammation, nipple retraction, axillary lymphadenopathy	Pap smear of breast discharge, mammography, drug therapy for symptoms, surgical excision, observation

PREDISPOSING FACTORS

Factors that predispose a woman to breast cancer include the following:

- Age. Incidence increases steadily with age, especially after 50. In fact, over 75% of new cases of breast cancer are diagnosed in women over age 50 (ACS, 2002).
- Female gender.
- History of previous breast cancer.
- Family history of mother , sister, or daughter with breast cancer. The risk increases if two or more relatives develop breast cancer or if the relative developed breast cancer premenopausally or in both breasts.
- Hormone replacement therapy for extended periods (more than 5 years) (Writing Group for the Women's Health Initiative, 2002).
- Being overweight after menopause.
- Alcohol consumption. The equivalent of two drinks per day, regardless of type of alcoholic beverage, increases the risk of breast cancer by 25%; moreover, this risk increases with the amount of alcohol consumed (ACS, 2002).
- No history of pregnancy or first pregnancy after age 30.
- Never breastfeeding a child.
- Longer reproductive phase (early menarche [before age 12] and late menopause [after age 55]).
- History of high-dose radiation to the chest.
- Upper socioeconomic class.
- Geographic location. High-incidence areas: North America; northern Europe; in the United States, urban areas and the Northeast. Low-risk areas: Asia; Africa; in the United States, rural areas and the Southeast.

However, when risk factors are evaluated, all together or alone, they account for only 21% of breast cancer risk among women 55 years and older. Therefore, all women are assumed to be at risk for breast cancer, especially those over 35 years of age (Fiorica, 1999).

Developing Cultural Competence

After age 40, white women are more likely to be diagnosed with breast cancer than black women, but black women with breast cancer have lower 5-year survival rates (72% versus 87%). About half of this difference is related to the fact that breast cancer in African American women tends to be diagnosed later and the tumors diagnosed tend to be more aggressive forms that are less responsive to treatment (American Cancer Society, 2002).

DIAGNOSIS

A malignant neoplasm may originate either in a duct or in the epithelium of the breast lobes. About 50% of breast cancers originate in the upper outer quadrant and spread or metastasize to the axillary lymph nodes. Common sites of distant metastasis are the lymph nodes, lungs, liver, brain, and bone.

As previously discussed, a cancerous lump may be discovered by the woman herself, by the clinician who palpates or observes an abnormality, or by mammogram. A painless mass or lump is the most important physical symptom of breast cancer, although up to 10% of women have breast pain but no palpable mass (ACS, 2002). Early detection greatly improves the treatment options available and increases women's long-term survival rates.

Worrisome findings that point to a higher risk of breast cancer include dimpling of the breast tissue, recent or acute nipple inversion, change in breast size or shape, increase of size in breast mass, skin erosion or ulceration, or presence of axillary lump. Routine mammography screening detects masses 2 to 3 years prior to clinical appearance. Other diagnostic modalities include fine-needle biopsy, ultrasonography, thermography, and magnetic resonance imaging (MRI). Biopsy is essential for a diagnosis. Once the diagnosis is made and lymph node involvement evaluated, clinical staging of the disease is determined and a treatment plan that coincides with the stage is initiated.

CLINICAL THERAPY

Once breast cancer is diagnosed, the woman and her physician make treatment decisions together. The decision is based on a consideration of the following factors:

- Stage of cancer
- Optimal treatment for that stage
- Woman's age
- Personal preferences
- Risks and benefits of each treatment protocol

Most women diagnosed with breast cancer have some form of surgery. The primary goal of the surgery is to remove the cancer from the breast and the lymph nodes, if they are involved. Surgical treatment may consist of *simple or total mastectomy*, which involves removal of the entire breast. A *modified radical mastectomy* involves the removal of the breast and the axillary lymph nodes but does not include removal of any of the pectoral muscles of the chest wall. Women who undergo mastectomy are generally given the option of having breast reconstruction surgery. This surgery may be done at the time of the mastectomy or delayed until the prescribed chemotherapy and/or radiation is completed. *Lumpectomy*, or the removal of the cancerous tissue plus a rim of normal tissue, is a breast-sparing approach that is often used for women with stages I or II breast cancer. It is almost always followed by several weeks of radiation therapy to destroy any remaining cancerous cells.

Adjunctive therapy for breast cancer includes chemotherapy, radiation, and hormone therapy. Chemotherapy typically involves a combination of drugs known to combat breast cancer. As indicated previously, radiation is often used to destroy remaining cells following surgery but it may also be used to reduce the size of a cancerous tumor before surgery. Hormone therapy is based on the knowledge that the hormone estrogen, which is produced by the ovaries, stimulates certain types of breast cancer. Women who have a form of breast cancer that tests positive for estrogen receptors can be given the antiestrogen drug tamoxifen. Tamoxifen therapy has produced a 26% annual reduction in breast cancer recurrence and a 14% annual reduction in deaths (ACS, 2002).

Research is also under way evaluating the effectiveness of tamoxifen as a preventive measure to reduce the incidence of breast cancer in women at high risk for the disease. In addition, a second-generation antiestrogen drug called raloxifene is under study. Raloxifene, a selective estrogen receptor modulator (SERM), is used to prevent osteoporosis. However, it was shown to be even more effective than tamoxifen in decreasing the risk of breast cancer in postmenopausal women who were taking it for osteoporosis. Other research focuses on the use of monoclonal antibodies such as Herceptin, which works against a protein found in breast tumors. Preliminary findings offer hope for women with metastatic breast cancer (cancer that has spread beyond the breast) (ACS, 2002).

Some women prefer a combined approach to treatment that draws on both allopathic and complementary medicine. These women elect to use complementary therapies, such as herbal remedies, therapeutic touch, acupuncture, aromatherapy, and massage, in combination with medical treatments.

When a woman is confronted with a breast cancer diagnosis, she must decide which therapy is worth what personal risk for her. Although prompt treatment is indicated, a second opinion is encouraged. Care of the woman with breast cancer involves a multidisciplinary approach, including a primary care provider, radiotherapist, surgeon, medical oncologist, and nursing specialists.

PSYCHOLOGIC ADJUSTMENT

The emotional feelings a woman experiences can range from fear of the loss of a body part, to fear of the ill effects of treatments, to fear of death. The nurse should encourage the woman to discuss her feelings and concerns, informing her of all procedures, their pros and cons, and alternative options.

The course of adjustment confronting the woman with cancer has been described in four phases: shock, reaction, recovery, and reorientation. In the *shock* phase, women make statements such as "Everything is unreal" or "I can't understand why this is happening to me." Shock generally extends from the discovery of the lump through the process of diagnosis.

Reaction occurs in conjunction with the initiation of treatment. As treatment begins, the woman is compelled to face what has occurred and begins to take in what has happened. Coping mechanisms become evident during this phase. Reaction coincides with the length of treatment. For many women, radiation treatment or chemotherapy prolongs this period to months. Treatment reinforces the diagnosis of cancer and the immediate consequences of the disease. Denial of breast loss, if a mastectomy is done, and the reality of the illness is common during the periods of diagnosis and treatment. Denial protects the woman, making therapy tolerable.

Recovery begins during convalescence following the completion of medical treatment. Anxiety about her illness diminishes and the woman looks to the future once more. She turns outward and gradually resumes her former activities. Conversely, depression and social isolation occur if the woman is unable to negotiate the recovery phase successfully.

A woman's family and friends significantly influence her recovery. Women often perceive their partners as their primary source of support. Both members of a couple must adjust to the woman's condition and its implications as well as to the effect of therapy on their sexual intimacy. Difficulties with psychosocial adjustment to breast cancer tend to be similar for women and their partners except in the area of role adjustments, where women have more difficulties. Many hospitals and community agencies sponsor suppport groups for women with breast cancer. Online support groups are also available and are of particular value to women in rural areas and in areas that lack adequate community support. In addition, the ACS sponsors support groups for cancer survivors and their families. They also have a highly successful program, Reach to Recovery, for women following surgery.

Reorientation follows recovery and is unending. It is accomplished when the woman can acknowledge that breast cancer is part of her life; yet living, for her, has returned to or perhaps exceeded its former fullness and meaning.

For additional information on breast cancer, refer to a medical-surgical text. Table 7–2 • provides a resource guide about organizations that support breast cancer research and education.

> *The physician also felt the lump and thickening and now I'm waiting to have my mammogram. My thoughts and feelings since I first felt the lump have been like a roller coaster. I'm 46 and I'm wondering if this is it. Am I dying? Now? I am afraid as I have not been afraid since one of our children was very ill.*

Table 7–2 • BREAST CANCER RESOURCES

Organizations	Web Sites
National Cancer Institute (NCI) Cancer Information Service (CIS) 800-4-CANCER (800-422-6237)	http://cancernet.nci.nih.gov (produced jointly by the International Cancer Information Center, NCI, and the Office of Cancer Communication)
National Alliance of Breast Cancer Organizations (NABCO) 212-719-0154	http://oncolink.upenn.edu/ (University of Pennsylvania)
American Cancer Society (ACS) 800-227-2345	http://www.access.digex.net/~mkragen/index.html (sponsored by the National Coalition for Cancer Survivorship, a not-for-profit organization)
Susan G. Komen Breast Cancer Foundation 800-I'M AWARE (800-462-9273)	
Y-ME 800-221-2141 (9 to 5 PM CST) or 312-986-8228 (24 hours)	

NURSING CARE MANAGEMENT

Nursing care of the woman with breast cancer is multidimensional. It involves meeting the educational, psychosexual, and physical needs of the woman and, to a certain extent, those of her family. In meeting these needs, the nurse functions as a caregiver, counselor, educator, liaison, and advocate. Nurses need to support women in their efforts to provide self-care. This increases their self-esteem and sense of control. Nursing care changes as the woman progresses from the period of diagnosis to the recovery period.

Nursing Assessment and Diagnosis

During the period of diagnosis of any breast disease, the woman may be extremely anxious. The nurse can use therapeutic communication to assess the significance the woman places on her breasts; her current emotional status, coping mechanisms used during periods of stress, and knowledge and beliefs about cancer; and other variables that may influence her coping and adjustment.

Assessment is an ongoing process. Sufficient data must be obtained to provide the nurse and other members of the healthcare team with increasing insight into the woman's physical, mental, emotional, and social situation.

Nursing diagnoses that may apply to a woman with a disorder of the breast include the following:

- ***Health-Seeking Behaviors:*** Information about diagnostic procedures for suspected breast cancer related to an expressed wish for information
- ***Anxiety*** related to threat to body image or her life

Nursing Plan and Implementation

During the prediagnosis period, the nurse should provide emotional support, clarify misconceptions, encourage the woman to express her anxiety, and urge her to ask many questions. Once a diagnosis has been made, the nurse should ensure that the woman clearly understands her condition, its association to breast malignancy, and treatment options. The nurse can also locate appropriate resources in the community and encourage the woman to make use of them as she deals with this difficult time. The woman and her partner or support person should discuss the treatment alternatives with her healthcare provider. Nursing advocacy involves supporting the woman's right to make the best treatment decision for her. With the assistance of the nurse, the woman can explore her fears, clarify her values, and identify the treatment options that would be personally acceptable. The nurse can provide psychologic support for the woman with a troublesome diagnosis, supply her with client education materials, and refer her to professional support groups.

For women who must undergo surgery, nursing care focuses on necessary perioperative interventions. Refer to a medical-surgical nursing textbook for detailed information on these aspects of nursing care.

Evaluation

Expected outcomes of nursing care include the following:

- The woman is able to discuss her fears, concerns, and questions during the period of diagnosis.
- The diagnosis is made quickly and accurately, and treatment initiated, if indicated.

Care of the Woman with Endometriosis

Endometriosis is a condition characterized by the presence of endometrial tissue outside the uterine cavity. The exact prevalence of endometriosis is unknown but it is estimated to be between 7% and 10% of women of reproductive age in the United States (Schenken, 1999). Endometriosis has been found almost everywhere in the body, including the vagina, lungs, cervix, central nervous system, and gastrointestinal tract. The most common location, however, is the pelvis. This tissue responds to the hormonal changes of the menstrual cycle and bleeds in a cyclic fashion. The bleeding results in inflammation, scarring of the peritoneum, and formation of adhesions.

Endometriosis may occur at any age after puberty, although it is most commonly diagnosed in women between ages 20 and 45 and is rare in postmenopausal women. The exact cause of endometriosis is unknown. Proposed causative factors include retrograde menstrual flow of the endometrium, physiologic disruption following gynecologic surgery or cesarean birth, hereditary tendency, and a possible immunologic defect (Hsu, 2001). Endometriosis is thought to be an autoimmune condition. It is associated with an increased risk of breast cancer, ovarian cancer, melanoma, and non-Hodgkin's lymphoma as well as hypothyroidism, fibromyalgia, chronic fatigue syndrome, autoimmune diseases, allergies and asthma (Sinaii, Cleary, Ballweg, et al, 2002). It has also been linked to dioxin exposure (dioxin is a toxic byproduct of industrial processes that involve chlorine or incineration of chlorine containing substances such as certain plastics) (Eskenazi, et al, 2002).

Although endometriosis can be asymptomatic, the most common symptom of endometriosis is pelvic pain, which is often dull or cramping although it can be debilitating. Usually the pain is related to menstruation and is thought to be dysmenorrhea by the affected woman. **Dyspareunia** (painful intercourse) and abnormal uterine bleeding are other common signs. The condition is often diagnosed when the woman seeks evaluation for infertility. Bimanual examination may reveal a fixed, tender, retroverted uterus and palpable nodules in the cul-de-sac. Diagnosis is confirmed by laparoscopy.

Treatment may be medical, surgical, or a combination of the two. During the laparoscopic examination, the physician may surgically resect any visible implants of endometrial tissue, taking care to avoid damaging any organs. Laser vaporization can be used for all but the deepest implants. This allows for more exact removal of tissue, less damage of adjacent tissue, and decreased bleeding. If the woman is experiencing severe dyspareunia or dysmenorrhea, the surgeon may perform a presacral neurectomy. In advanced cases in which childbearing is not an issue, treatment may be a hysterectomy with bilateral salpingo-oophorectomy (removal of the uterus, fallopian tubes, and ovaries). If the woman does not desire pregnancy at the present time, she may be started on oral contraceptives. In women with minimal disease and symptoms, treatment includes observation, analgesics, and nonsteroidal anti-inflammatory drugs (NSAIDs). The woman who desires pregnancy and has been unsuccessful in her attempts to conceive is often treated for a designated period of time with a medication that suppresses estrogen synthesis. This causes an atrophy of endometrial implants. Medications commonly used to treat endometriosis include oral contraceptives, progestins, antiprogestins, and gonadotropin-releasing hormones (GnRH).

Combined oral contraceptives (COCs) create a "pseudopregnancy" state that leads to decreased menstrual bleeding and possible amenorrhea. Treatment with COCs is cost effective and can relieve dysmenorrhea and pelvic pain.

Progestins such as medroxyprogesterone acetate (MPA) exert an antiendometriotic effect and ultimate atrophy. The medication is administered intramuscularly every 3 months and the effectiveness of the treatment evaluated every 3 to 6 months. Side effects may include nausea, weight gain, fluid retention, and breakthrough bleeding.

Danazol is an antiprogesterone treatment that is sometimes used to treat endometriosis. It suppresses GnRH and has high androgen and low estrogen effects that do not support the growth of the endometrium. It suppresses ovulation and causes amenorrhea. In effect, danazol and the other GnRH analogs (discussed next) induce a "pseudomenopausal" state. Danazol does have some significant side effects, including hirsutism, vaginal bleeding, acne, oily skin, weight gain, reduced libido, voice changes and hoarseness, clitoral enlargement, and decreased breast size.

GnRH agonists, such as nafarelin acetate (given as a metered nasal spray twice daily) and leuprolide acetate (Lupron, given once a month as an intramuscular injection), are gaining popularity because many women tolerate them better than danazol and their results in treating endometriosis are comparable. GnRH agonists suppress the menstrual cycle through estrogen antagonism. This may result in the hypoestrogen side effects of hot flashes, vaginal dryness, headache, breast reduction, and loss of bone density (Schenken, 1999).

NURSING CARE MANAGEMENT

Nursing Assessment and Diagnosis

The nurse should be aware of the common symptoms of endometriosis and elicit an accurate history if a woman mentions these symptoms. If a woman is being treated for endometriosis, the nurse should assess the woman's understanding of the condition, its implications, and the treatment alternatives.

Nursing diagnoses that may apply to a woman with endometriosis include the following:

- ***Acute Pain*** related to peritoneal irritation secondary to endometriosis
- ***Ineffective Individual Coping*** related to depression secondary to infertility

Nursing Plan and Implementation

The nurse can be available to explain the condition, its symptoms, treatment alternatives, and prognosis. The nurse can help the woman evaluate treatment options and make appropriate choices. If the woman begins taking medication, the nurse can review the dosage, schedule, possible side effects, and any warning signs. Women are often advised to avoid delaying pregnancy because of the risk of infertility. The woman may wish to discuss the implications of this decision on her life choices, relationship with her partner, and personal preferences. The nurse can be a nonjudgmental listener and help the woman consider her options. In addition, the nurse can refer the woman to the Endometriosis Association. This group, founded in 1980, offers women support and education. It can be accessed on the Web at www.endometriosis.org.

Evaluation

Expected outcomes of nursing care include the following:

- The woman is able to discuss her condition, its implications for fertility, and her treatment options.
- After considering the alternatives, the woman chooses appropriate treatment options.

Care of the Woman with Toxic Shock Syndrome

Although **toxic shock syndrome (TSS)** has been reported in children, postmenopausal women, and men, it is primarily a disease of women in their reproductive years, especially women at or near menses or during the postpartum period. In most cases, the causative organism is a strain of *Staphylococcus aureus.* The use of superabsorbent tampons has been widely related to an increased incidence of TSS. However, occluding the cervical os with a contraceptive device such as a diaphragm or cervical cap, especially if it is left in place for more than 48 hours, may also increase the risk of TSS.

Early diagnosis and treatment are important in preventing a fatal outcome. The most common signs of TSS include fever (often greater than 38.9C, or 102F); rash on the trunk initially followed by desquamation of the skin, especially the palms and soles, which usually occurs 1 to 2 weeks after the onset of symptoms; hypotension; and dizziness. Systemic symptoms often include vomiting, watery diarrhea, severe myalgia, and inflamed mucous membranes (oropharyngeal, conjunctival, or vaginal). Disorders of the central nervous system, including alterations in consciousness, disorientation, and coma, may also occur. Evidence of renal, hepatic, and hematologic involvement can be seen in abnormal laboratory findings, which reveal elevated blood urea nitrogen (BUN), creatinine, aspartate aminotransferase (AST), alanine aminotransferase (ALT), and total bilirubin, while platelets are often less than 100,000/mm^3.

Women with TSS are generally hospitalized and given supportive therapy, including intravenous (IV) fluids to maintain blood pressure. Severe cases may require renal dialysis, administration of vasopressors, and intubation. Penicillinase-resistant antibiotics, while of limited value during the acute phase, do help reduce the risk of recurrence from 30% to 50% (Eschenbach, 1999).

NURSING CARE MANAGEMENT

Nurses play a major role in helping to educate women about ways to prevent the development of TSS. Women should understand the importance of avoiding prolonged use of tampons. They should change tampons every 3 to 6 hours and avoid using superabsorbent tampons. Some women may choose to use other products, such as sanitary pads or minipads. The woman who chooses to continue using tampons may reduce her risk by alternating them with pads and avoiding overnight use of tampons.

Postpartal women should avoid the use of tampons for 6 to 8 weeks after childbirth. Women with a history of TSS should be advised of the risk of recurrence and should never use tampons. Women who use diaphragms or cervical caps should not leave them in place for prolonged periods and should not use them during the postpartum period or when they are menstruating.

Nurses can also help make women aware of the signs and symptoms of TSS so that they can seek treatment promptly if symptoms occur.

Care of the Woman During a Pelvic Examination

Women have a pelvic examination performed for a variety of reasons ranging from health maintenance to disease diagnosis. Many women perceive the pelvic exam as an uncomfortable and embarrassing procedure. These negative feelings may cause women to delay having yearly gynecologic examinations and this avoidance may pose a threat to life and health.

A woman's first pelvic examination is especially important because a positive experience can help allay anxiety and make subsequent pelvics less threatening. Because the initial pelvic examination is typically done when a young woman is a teenager, nurses need to be sensitive to a teen's attitudes and concerns. Teens are often shy about revealing their bodies and may feel very embarrassed by the procedure. Nurses also need to be alert for atypical responses that might indicate a history of sexual abuse.

To make the pelvic exam less threatening, and hopefully improve the woman's health-seeking behavior, it is important to create a trusting atmosphere and incorporate practices that help the woman maintain a sense of control. Additionally, it is important for the nurse to assist in facilitating a nonjudgmental and safe environment in which the woman can be honest in response to the medical providers' inquiries. Some healthcare providers are performing what is called an educational pelvic exam. During this type of exam the woman becomes an active participant and has an opportunity to learn about her body, voice her concerns, and share decisions regarding her care.

The educational exam includes offering the woman a mirror to watch the procedure, pointing out anatomic parts to her, and positioning and draping her to allow eye-to-eye contact with the practitioner. The woman is encouraged to participate by asking questions and giving feedback. The nurse can assist the woman by encouraging her to relax with specific advice such as "Keep your bottom flat against the table" and "Wiggle your toes if you find yourself beginning to tense your muscles."

Nurse practitioners, certified nurse-midwives, and physicians all perform pelvic examinations. Nurses assist the practitioner and the woman during the examination. Procedure 7–1 provides information on assisting with a pelvic examination.

The pelvic examination consists of three segments: inspection of the vulva; inspection of the vagina and the cervix via a speculum examination; and palpation of the cervix, uterus, and ovaries via a bimanual examination. Often a Papanicolaou smear is obtained during the speculum examination. The Pap smear is discussed in the section on abnormal Pap smear results, which begins on page 141.

Vulvar Self-Examination

During the pelvic examination many caregivers also provide education about self-examination of the vulva. This procedure, like self-examination of the breasts (discussed previously), permits early detection of abnormalities, thereby

Procedure 7–1 Assisting with a Pelvic Examination

Preparation

1. Ensure that the room is sufficiently warm by checking room temperature and adjusting thermostat if necessary. If overhead heat lamps are available, turn them on.
2. Explain the procedure to the woman. If she has never had a pelvic examination, show her the equipment to be used as part of the explanation.
   Rationale: Explaining the procedure helps reduce anxiety and increase cooperation.
3. Ask the woman to empty her bladder and to remove clothing below the waist.
   Rationale: An empty bladder promotes comfort during the internal examination.
4. Have padding on the stirrups. If stirrups are not padded, the woman may prefer to leave her shoes on during the procedure.
   Rationale: Stirrups are usually padded to ease the pressure of the feet against the metal and to decrease the discomfort associated with the touch of the cold stirrups. If they are not padded, however, wearing shoes accomplishes the same purpose.
5. Give the woman a disposable drape or sheet to use during the exam. Ask her to sit at the end of the examining table with the drape opened across her lap.
6. Position the woman in the lithotomy position with her thighs flexed and abducted. Place her feet in the stirrups. Her buttocks should extend slightly beyond the edge of the examining table.
7. Drape the woman with the sheet, leaving a flap so that the perineum can be exposed.
   Rationale: This position provides the exposure necessary to conduct the examination effectively. The drape helps preserve the woman's sense of dignity and privacy.

Equipment and Supplies

- Vaginal specula of various sizes, warmed with water or on heating pad prior to insertion
- Sterile gloves
- Water-soluble lubricant
- Materials for Pap smear or *ThinPrep* Pap test and cultures
- Good light source

Note: Lubricant may alter the results of tests and cultures and is not used during the speculum examination. Its use is reserved for the bimanual examination.

Procedure: Sterile Gloves

1. The examiner dons gloves for the procedure. Explain each part of the procedure as the certified nurse-midwife, nurse practitioner, or physician performs it. Let the woman know that the examiner begins with an inspection of the external genitalia. The speculum is then inserted to allow visualization of the cervix and vaginal walls and to obtain specimens for testing. After the speculum is withdrawn the examiner performs a bimanual examination of the internal organs using the fingers of one hand inserted in the woman's vagina while the other hand presses over the woman's uterus and ovaries. The final step of the procedure is generally a rectal examination.
2. Ask the woman to breathe slowly and regularly and to use any method she finds effective in helping her to remain relaxed.
3. Let her know when the examiner is ready to insert the speculum and ask her to bear down.
   Rationale: Relaxation helps decrease muscle tension. Bearing down helps open the vaginal orifice and relaxes the perineal muscles.
4. After the speculum is withdrawn, lubricate the examiner's fingers prior to the bimanual examination.
   Rationale: Lubrication decreases friction and eases insertion of the examiner's fingers.

Clinical Tip

With the examiner's consent (obtained beforehand), offer the woman a hand mirror so that she can watch all or part of the examination. This practice removes the "mystery" from the procedure and enables the woman to become familiar with the appearance of her body.

(continued on next page)

Procedure 7–1 Assisting with a Pelvic Examination *(continued)*

5. After the examiner has completed the examination and moved away from the woman, move to the end of the examination table and face the woman. Cover her with the drape. Apply gentle pressure to her knees and encourage her to move toward the head of the table. Assist her to remove her feet from the stirrups, then offer your hand to her and assist her to sit up.
   Rationale: Assistance is important because the lithotomy position is an awkward one and many women, but especially those women who are pregnant, obese, or older, may find it difficult to get out of the stirrups.
6. Provide her with tissues to wipe the lubricant from her perineum.
   Rationale: Vaginal secretions and lubricant may be discharged from the vagina when the woman sits upright.
7. Provide the woman with privacy while she dresses. Be sure that she is not dizzy and that she is standing or sitting safely before leaving the room.
   Rationale: Lying supine may cause postural hypotension.

maximizing the possibility of cure and the use of conservative treatment approaches.

Self-examination of the vulva is simple to perform. The woman is advised to assume a sitting position on a bed or a chair. In good light she holds a mirror in one hand and uses the other hand to expose the tissues of her perineum while she carefully inspects and palpates the area. Pregnant or obese women may find it easier to inspect this area in a standing position with one foot elevated on a low stool. Figure 7–4 • shows the correct procedure for vulvar self-examination.

Initially, the woman inspects the entire perineum for symmetry, discharge, and lesions. She then gently pushes back the hood of the clitoris to inspect this area. Next she separates the labia to examine the inner tissues. The woman gently palpates the vulva using the flat part of one or two fingers. Then, using her thumb and index finger, the woman palpates the lateral aspects of the genitalia along the length of the vulva, noting any tenderness, masses, or lesions. Lastly, the woman examines the vaginal opening, compressing the tissues between the index and middle fingers. The tissues should be soft, moist, nontender, and elastic. Any abnormalities should be reported to the woman's healthcare provider.

This exam should be performed monthly, at the same time as the breast self-exam, in all sexually active asymptomatic women or women over the age of 18. Women with a history of vulvar lesions or women with adverse symptoms should inspect their vulva more frequently.

Care of the Woman with Vulvitis

The term *vulvitis* refers to an inflammation of the vulva or external female genitalia. Sometimes vulvar irritation is the result of nonpathologic factors such as the following:

- Frequent douching or use of over-the-counter douches
- Feminine deodorant spray
- Detergents, harsh soaps, or bubble bath
- Colored or perfumed toilet paper
- Contraceptive creams, foams, or suppositories
- Condoms, possibly related to a latex or nonoxynol-9 sensitivity
- Dye, such as found in new clothing
- Synthetic clothing, such as nylon pantyhose, underwear, or synthetic slacks, that may trap moisture
- Tight clothing, such as jeans
- Some repetitive motion exercise, such as running or biking
- Frequent shaving of perineum
- Frequent intercourse or intercourse without adequate lubrication
- Deodorant menstrual pads or tampons, or frequent use of menstrual pads or tampons
- Estrogen deprivation due to menopause, surgical menopause, or medication-induced menopause (such as chemotherapy)

Other times, external genital irritation may be the result of inflammation or infection of the vagina or cervix. The irritation results when increased vaginal or cervical secretions flow distally and create inflammation of the vulvar tissues. This condition is called *vulvovaginitis.*

Often it is difficult to differentiate, by symptoms alone, vulvitis from vaginitis. The nurse needs to understand that vulvitis can occur as a distinct entity from vaginitis, and the previously mentioned practices may be significant contributing factors to both.

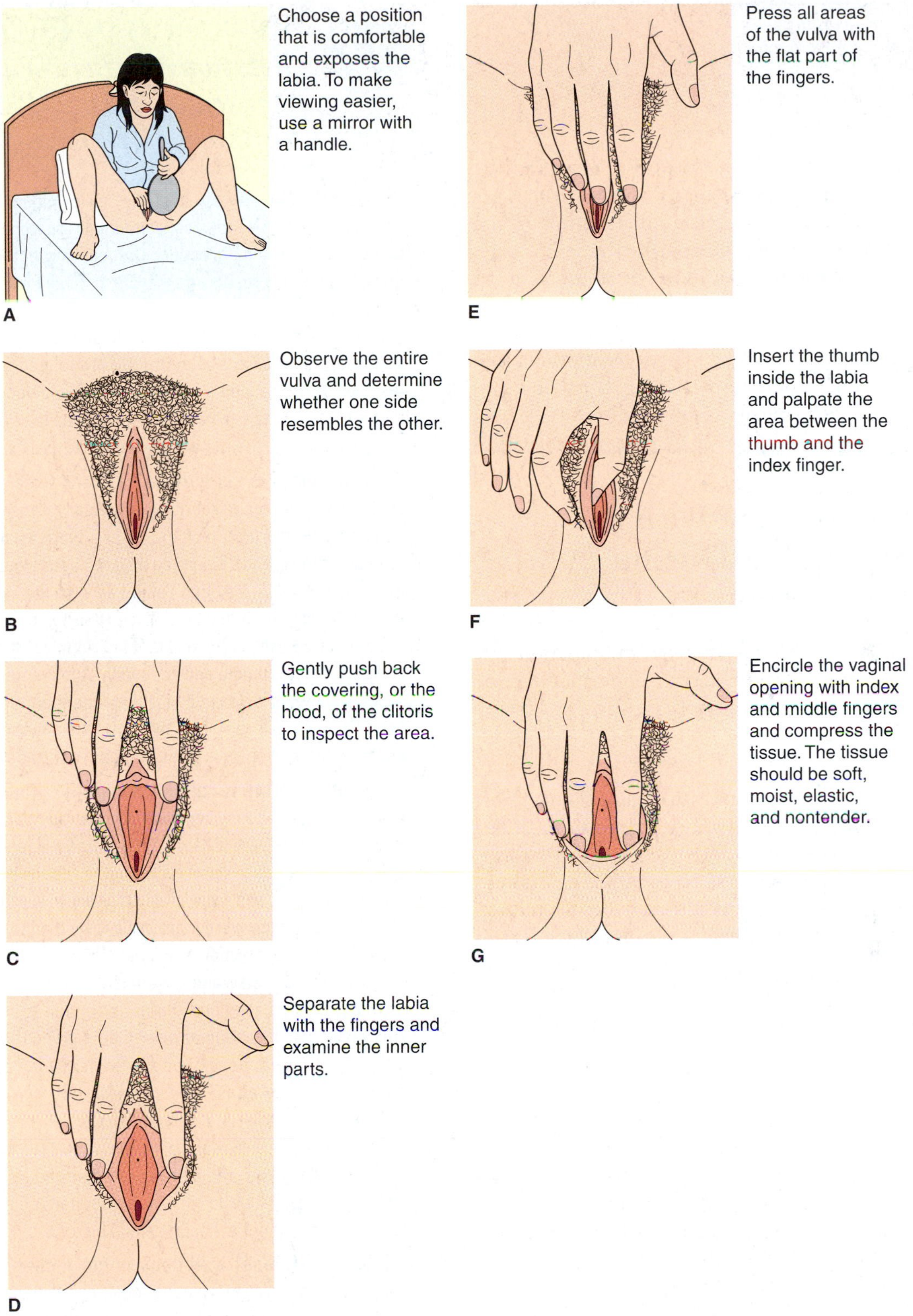

A
Choose a position that is comfortable and exposes the labia. To make viewing easier, use a mirror with a handle.
B
Observe the entire vulva and determine whether one side resembles the other.
C
Gently push back the covering, or the hood, of the clitoris to inspect the area.
D
Separate the labia with the fingers and examine the inner parts.
E
Press all areas of the vulva with the flat part of the fingers.
F
Insert the thumb inside the labia and palpate the area between the thumb and the index finger.
G
Encircle the vaginal opening with index and middle fingers and compress the tissue. The tissue should be soft, moist, elastic, and nontender.

Figure 7–4 • Steps to follow to perform vulvar self-examination.

NURSING CARE MANAGEMENT

The nurse gathers data from the woman to help differentiate behaviors that may cause isolated vulvitis from those that may cause vaginal and cervical inflammation. Once the assessment of vulvitis has been made, the nurse plays a crucial role in providing education about contributing factors that may have led to the development of vulvitis. In addition, educating the woman about behaviors to avoid, strategies or therapies to improve symptoms, and signs of a worsening condition that require further evaluation are all part of the nurse's responsibilities.

Care of the Woman with an Abnormal Finding During Pelvic Examination

An abnormal finding resulting from pelvic examination may involve tissues of the vulva or cervix, abnormal uterine bleeding, or ovarian or uterine masses.

Vulvar Lesion

The skin of the vulva is subject to diseases and changes, just as skin elsewhere on the body. Because cancer of the vulva may be present in a variety of different types of lesions it is important that the external genitalia be examined carefully at the time of pelvic examination. A common benign condition of the vulva, atrophic vaginitis, which is caused by a lack of estrogen stimulation to the vulva and vagina, is discussed in Chapter 4.

BARTHOLIN'S GLAND CYST

Infection of the Bartholin's gland resulting in inflammation of the gland itself is a common vulvovaginal lesion. The infection can be caused by a number of different organisms, the most common of which are gonorrhea and staphylococcus. Symptoms include unilateral pain and swelling of the Bartholin's gland, ranging from mild to moderate discomfort to severe pain. Treatment involves incision and drainage of the abscess, culture and sensitivity of the discharge, and appropriate antibiotic therapy (DiSaia, 1999).

VITILIGO OF THE VULVA

Vitiligo is a fairly common finding on the vulva. It is a depigmentation of the skin resulting in white patchy areas because of the absence of melanin. Vitiligo may appear anytime after puberty and anywhere on the body, but it is never associated with a systemic disorder. However, it can cause significant disfiguring cosmetic changes, particularly in dark-skinned individuals (DiSaia, 1999).

RESEARCH IN PRACTICE
Relationship Between Sexual Abuse and Risk of Pelvic Inflammatory Disease

What is this study about? Pelvic inflammatory disease (PID) can result in serious consequences for women, particularly when delayed treatment occurs. Chronic pain, ectopic pregnancy, and infertility may result, and may be more severe when delays in diagnosis prevent early treatment. Determining the characteristics of women who are at risk for PID is essential to early detection. Many factors have been strongly associated with PID, among them sexual abuse and a history of sexual violence. The purpose of this study was to evaluate the relationship between a history of sexual abuse and the risk of PID among minority women.

How was this study done? Women were eligible for this study if they had a current nonviral sexually transmitted infection confirmed by laboratory testing. Subjects were recruited from public health clinics, and 612 agreed to participate. About two thirds of the subjects were Mexican American and the remainder were African American. Of these, 32% self-reported prior sexual abuse. Descriptive statistics revealed that individuals in the sample were generally of low income and education. Ages ranged from 14 to 45 years. Data were collected initially through targeted physical examination and self-report for history of sexual abuse. Data were analyzed for relationships using standard statistical techniques.

What were the results of the study? The women with a history of sexual abuse reported a higher incidence of risk factors associated with PID, including early age of first sexual episode, more sexual partners, higher recurrence of sexually transmitted infection, and delayed health-seeking behaviors. The abused women were more likely to be diagnosed with a sexually transmitted infection after seeking treatment for symptoms, whereas nonabused women were more likely to discover a sexually transmitted infection during a routine gynecologic visit. This result may be associated with the finding that women with a history of sexual abuse had fewer visits for Pap smears and routine care. The abused women also had more severe genitourinary symptoms and abdominal pain on presentation to a healthcare provider. Results of the physical exams indicated that abused women had a higher rate of abnormal physical exams and were more likely to have a presumptive diagnosis of PID than women without a similar sexual history.

What additional questions might I have? Would these characteristics apply to women in other populations—nonminority women, women in higher economic categories, or women who are more educated? Since this study was based on self-report, could the actual magnitude of the relationship be underestimated?

How can I use this study? An assessment for history of sexual abuse is essential to the identification and early treatment of PID. The nurse is in a key position to establish rapport with women and ascertain if these risk factors may be present.

Source: Champion, J., Piper, J., Shain, R., Perdue, S., & Newton, E. (2001). Minority women with sexually transmitted diseases: Sexual abuse and risk for pelvic inflammatory disease. *Research in Nursing and Health, 24*(1), 38–43.

LICHEN SCLEROSUS

Lichen sclerosus is a benign disorder of the vulva that can occur at any age, but is more common in girls less than 10 years old and in postmenopausal women. The initial symptoms are bluish white papules that coalesce and become white plaques. The skin becomes thin, and small fissures or ulcerations may develop. Children and adults often experience pruritus, and sexually active women may have pain during intercourse related to shrinkage of the labial tissues. Diagnosis is made by clinical exam and confirmed by biopsy. Treatment includes high-dose topical steroid cream twice daily for 2 to 3 weeks, then decreased to once or twice weekly thereafter. In postmenopausal women there has been some benefit to topical progesterone or testosterone use, but women may experience undesired side effects like hair growth, acne, or clitoral enlargement (DiSaia, 1999).

VULVAR VESTIBULITIS

Women with *vestibulitis* experience local irritation and inflammation of the vulvar vestibule, pain with vaginal penetration (tampons or intercourse), burning and itching, and sometimes urinary frequency or dysuria. The cause of this disorder is poorly understood, but there is an association with excessive use of topical steroids, recurrent candidal infection, overuse of irritant soaps or deodorants, and sometimes a history of sexual abuse. No definitive treatment exists so therapies are directed at comfort measures to relieve symptoms. Therapies include sitz baths, topical steroid cream or 2% lidocaine gel, oral calcium supplements, oral corticosteroids, oral fluconazole, oral tricyclic antidepressants, biofeedback techniques, and in severe cases surgical intervention (DiSaia, 1999).

MALIGNANT TUMORS OF THE VULVA

Cancer of the vulva can occur at any age, but is more common in postmenopausal women, usually older than 70 years of age. The woman may present with pruritus, a lump, or a flat lesion, or may be relatively asymptomatic. Some risk factors include chronic vulvitis, vulvar dermatoses, history of sexually transmitted infections (STIs), and history of cervical cancer. Clinical appearances can vary greatly. Some lesions are scaly with a red background, some are flat and almost totally white or red, and others are irregularly pigmented and may be flat or raised. For these reasons, it is necessary to biopsy many vulvar lesions to confirm or rule out malignancy. Vulvar malignancies are classified as vulvar intraepithelial neoplasia (VIN), Paget's disease, and invasive cancer (DiSaia, 1999). Treatment usually involves some type of surgical procedure to remove the lesions and often the tissue surrounding the lesion, but the extent varies greatly depending on findings and degree of the lesion.

Cervicitis

Acute inflammation of the cervix is usually the result of infection from *Neisseria gonorrhoeae* or *Chlamydia trachomatis*. It may be caused by other organisms such as *Candida*, *Gardnerella vaginalis*, *Trichomonas*, herpes, staphylococci, or enterococci. Other causes may include use of intravaginal feminine hygiene products, frequent tampon use, frequent intercourse, or presence of a foreign body (such as an intrauterine device [IUD], contraceptive sponge, diaphragm, or tampon). Chronic cervicitis is believed to be present in up to 95% of women who have had vaginal birth, but it is usually asymptomatic.

Symptoms often include a yellowish white vaginal discharge or copious purulent discharge that is sometimes malodorous, depending on the etiology. Dyspareunia is a common complaint, with postcoital bleeding, and occasional irregular vaginal bleeding. Sometimes there is a sense of pelvic heaviness, and urinary symptoms such as urgency, frequency, and burning (Bristow & Karlan, 1999). Diagnosis and evaluation consists of a clinical pelvic examination, wet-mount smear, cultures, and a Pap smear. Treatment depends on the identified problem. It may include antibiotics to treat positive cultures (see chapter 6), cryotherapy to treat some lesions of the cervix, removal of foreign bodies, and in some instances treatment of nonspecific inflammation with local medication (metronidazole gel or clindamycin cream).

Abnormal Pap Smear Results

Women tend to expect a normal Pap smear report but various abnormal findings are common. Notification of an abnormal result may cause significant anxiety in the woman. Therefore, results should be provided in a caring manner, with an accurate explanation of the findings, reassurance that early detection of a problem allows early intervention, and information regarding expected further evaluation, treatment, and follow-up. The woman should be encouraged to ask questions and to voice her concerns.

PAP SMEAR

The purpose of the Papanicolaou smear (**Pap smear**) is to screen for the presence of cellular abnormalities by obtaining a sample containing cells from the cervix and the endocervical canal. Precancerous and cancerous conditions, as well as atypical findings and inflammatory changes, can be identified by microscopic examination. Estimates suggest that, annually in the United States, about 50 million women have a Pap smear done. Of these women, approximately 7% (3.5 million) are diagnosed with an abnormal finding that requires follow-up (Wright, Cox, Massad, et al, 2002).

Traditionally the test has been performed by preparing a Pap smear slide. However, the smear was often difficult to read because of obscuring factors such as blood, mucus, overlapping cells, and so forth. More recently, another test—the ThinPrep Pap smear—was approved by the Food and Drug Administration (FDA). In this test, no slide is prepared; instead, the cervical cells are transferred directly to a vial of preservative fluid, thereby preserving the entire specimen. The specimen is sent to a laboratory where a special processor prepares a slide.

Both ThinPrep Pap smears and dry slide Pap smears are acceptable methods of cervical cancer screening. ThinPreps offer the option of human papilloma virus testing if an abnormal result is obtained. ThinPreps may provide less debris and fewer cells for evaluation but they also result in more false-positive findings. Some care providers have preferences about the test to use. In some cases, insurance plans only cover the ThinPrep smear, which is more expensive, for women with a history that places them at high risk.

The Pap smear is a screening tool. A definitive diagnosis is made by studying tissue samples obtained by biopsies.

> **Clinical Tip** *Pap Smear Preparation*
> *Whenever you teach about pelvic examination and Pap smear, be certain that the woman understands that she should not douche for at least 24 hours beforehand. Douching can interfere with the accuracy of the Pap smear. For best test results, also advise women to avoid intercourse and the use of other female hygiene products and spermicidal agents immediately before a specimen is obtained. Specimens should not be obtained during menstruation or when visible cervicitis exists.*

Currently, both the American Cancer Society (ACS) (2002) and the American College of Obstetricians and Gynecologists (ACOG) recommend that all women begin having Pap smears when they reach the age of 18 or when they become sexually active, whichever comes first. ACOG recommends annual Pap smears thereafter. Alternatively, the ACS states that, following three consecutive negative Pap smears, the Pap smear may sometimes be done less frequently at the discretion of the caregiver. Less frequent Pap smears might be suggested, for example, for a woman with no history of STI or gynecologic cancer who is in a stable, monogamous relationship with a partner who is also monogamous and infection free. Some caregivers are reluctant to extend the time between Pap smears, however, because they worry that women may delay the test beyond the recommended time frames.

The Bethesda System

The Bethesda System is a standardized method of reporting cytologic Pap smear findings. This system was initially introduced in 1989 by the National Cancer Institute (NCI) to establish a uniform format and classification of terminology, and to facilitate uniformity of diagnosis and treatment. The system was revised in 1991 and again in 2001. It is the most widely used method of reporting Pap smear results (Bethesda 2001 Workshop, 2001) (see Table 7–3).

CERVICAL ABNORMALITIES

Cervical cancer is the sixth most common cancer in women in the United States, after breast, lung, colorectum, endometrium, and ovary (Bristow & Karlan, 1999). However, 50 years ago cervical cancer was the leading type of cancer in women. Since the use of Pap smear screening, in the United States and other countries that have a system of Pap smear screening, the incidence of and mortality due to cervical cancer have decreased dramatically. Worldwide, however, cervical cancer remains the most common cancer among women (Bristow & Karlan, 1999).

Cervical cancer is considered a preventable disease because it is slow-growing, has a lengthy preinvasive state, has inexpensive and available screening programs, and has effective treatment approaches for preinvasive lesions. Unfortunately, several subgroups of women in the United States have never been screened or are not screened at regular intervals. One half of women with newly diagnosed cervical cancer have never had a Pap smear, and 10% have not had a Pap smear in greater than 5 years (Bristow & Karlan, 1999).

Factors that place a woman at high risk for cervical cancer include:

- Coitus at an early age (first intercourse before 16 years of age increases the risk of cervical cancer twofold)
- History of multiple sexual partners
- Sex partner with a history of numerous sexual partners
- Exposure to sexually transmitted infections
- History of human papilloma virus (HPV) infection
- History of immunosuppressive therapy (chemotherapy) or immunocompromised state (HIV)
- Long-term oral contraceptive use (> 5 years)
- Smoking
- Antenatal exposure to diethylstilbestrol (DES)
- History of dysplasia

In the past 10 to 15 years a growing body of evidence has developed linking HPV infection with cervical dysplasia and carcinoma. As discussed in Chapter 6, over 100 different types of HPV have been identified; 40 of these types are known to infect the genital tract (Richwald & Skaer, 2001). To date, five specific types of HPV strains (16, 18, 31, 33, and 35) have been associated with high-grade cervical dysplasia and cervical cancer (Centers for Disease Control and Prevention [CDC], 2002).

The exact role of HPV in the development of cervical dysplasia is not completely understood, but it is believed that HPV-infected cells remove specific genes that regulate cell growth, leading to proliferation and neoplastic transformation of normal cells (Bristow & Karlan, 1999).

The 2001 Bethesda System (TBS) identifies three categories for premalignant squamous cell lesions: atypical squamous cells (ASC), low-grade squamous intraepithelial lesion (LSIL), and high-grade squamous intraepithelial lesion (HSIL), as well as squamous cell carcinoma (Table 7–3 •). The focus of the Pap smear is on the detection of high-grade cervical disease, especially *cervical intraepithelial neoplasia* (CIN). CIN refers to a lesion that may progress to invasive carcinoma (cancer). It is synonymous with the term *dysplasia*. To further support this objective, the ASC category is subdivided into two qualifiers that recognize the importance of detecting HSIL:

- Atypical squamous cells of undetermined significance (ASC-US)
- Atypical squamous cells—cannot exclude HSIL (ASC-H)

Table 7-3 • THE BETHESDA SYSTEM FOR CLASSIFYING PAP SMEARS

Specimen Type:

Indicate conventional smear (Pap smear) vs. liquid based vs. other

Specimen Adequacy

Satisfactory for evaluation *(describe presence or absence of endocervical/transformation zone component and any other quality indicators, eg, partially obscuring blood inflammation, etc)*

Unsatisfactory for evaluation... *(specify reason)*

Specimen rejected/not processed *(specify reason)*

Specimen processed and examined, but unsatisfactory for evaluation of epithelial abnormality because of (specify reason)

General Categorization (optional)

Negative for intraepithelial lesion or malignancy.

Epithelial cell abnormality. See Interpretation/result *(specify 'squamous' or 'glandular' as appropriate)*

Other: See Interpretation result *(eg, endometrial cells in a woman ≥ 40 years of age).*

Automated Review

If case examined by automated device, specify device and result.

Ancillary Testing

Provide a brief description of the test methods and report the result so that it is easily understood by the clinician.

Interpretation/Result

Negative for intraepithelial lesion or malignancy
(when there is no cellular evidence of neoplasia, state this in the General Categorization above and/or in the Interpretation/Result section of the report, whether or not there are organisms or other nonneoplastic findings)

ORGANISMS:

Trichomonas vaginalis

Fungal organisms morphologically consistent with *Candida* spp.

Shift in flora suggestive of bacterial vaginosis.

Bacteria morphologically consistent with *Actinomyces* spp.

Cellular changes associated with herpes simplex virus.

OTHER NONNEOPLASTIC FINDINGS (*Optional to report list not inclusive*).

Reactive cellular changes associated with

—inflammation (Includes typical repair)

—radiation

—intrauterine contraceptive device (IUD)

Glandular cells status posthysterectomy

Atrophy

Other
Endometrial cells (in a woman ≥ 40 years of age) (Specify if negative for squamous intraepithelial lesion)

Epithelial cell abnormalities

SQUAMOUS CELL

Atypical squamous cells

—of undetermined significance (ASC-US)

—cannot exclude HSIL (ASC-H)

Low-grade squamous intraepithelial lesion (LSIL)

—encompassing HPV/mild dysplasia/CIN-1

High-grade squamous intraepithelial lesion (HSIL)

—encompassing: moderate and severe dysplasia CIS/CIN-2 and CIN-3

—with features suspicious for invasion (*if invasion is suspected*)

Squamous cell carcinoma

GLANDULAR CELL

Atypical

—endocervical cells *(NOS or specify in comments)*

—endometrial cells *(NOS or specify in comments)*

—glandular cells *(NOS or specify in comments)*

Atypical

—endocervical cells, favor neoplastic

—glandular cells, favor neoplastic

Endocervical adenocarcinoma in situ

Adenocarcinoma

—endocervical

—endometrial

—extrauterine

—not otherwise specified (NOS)

Other malignant neoplasms (specify)

Educational Notes and Suggestions (optional)

Suggestions should be concise and consistent with clinical follow-up guidelines published by professional organizations (references to relevant publications may be included).

Source: Courtesy of National Cancer Institute.

The ASC-US category acknowledges equivocal results. This is considered essential because a large number of women with CIN are identified during a work-up for an equivocal finding (Solomon, Davey, Kurman, et al, 2002).

EVALUATION OF ABNORMAL CYTOLOGY

Evaluation of an abnormal Pap smear finding varies. If the results of a Pap smear indicate the presence of an infection other than HIV, the woman should be reassessed with a repeat Pap after receiving appropriate treatment for the infection (CDC, 2002).

The following points summarize the primary guidelines developed by the Bethesda 2001 Consensus Conference for managing ASC-US, ASC-H, LSIL, and HSIL (Richart, 2002; Wright, et al, 2002):

- Women with ASC-US can be treated in one of three ways: (a) immediate referral for colposcopy; (b) repeat the Pap at 4- to 6-month intervals until two negative results are obtained with referral for colposcopy if the repeat Pap shows ASC or higher; or (c) testing for HPV infection with referral for colposcopy if the testing reveals a high-risk strain of HPV. If the HPV testing is negative, the woman should have a repeat Pap in 12 months.
- Women with ASC-H are at greater risk for CIN than women with ASC-US and should be referred directly for colposcopy.

- Women with either LSIL or HSIL are also referred directly to colposcopy. (Previously LSIL was managed with repeat Paps but this approach is no longer recommended because of the risk of CIN, the likelihood that the repeat Pap would continue to be abnormal, and the risk that women would not return for follow-up multiple times.)

Based on the results of the colposcopy, of endocervical curettage of the tissue, and of biopsy if performed, further treatment may be indicated or follow-up with repeat Pap smears may be recommended. These tests are discussed next.

Colposcopy, the direct, detailed visualization and examination of the cervix, is done in most gynecologic offices. A speculum is placed in the vagina and the cervix is isolated. A 3% acetic acid solution applied on the cervix causes the abnormal epithelial cells to take on a characteristic white appearance. The colposcope, with its bright light and various color filters, provides a 6 to 40 times magnification of the cervical tissues. Lesions or other abnormalities are identified and documented, and directed biopsies can be obtained at this time, if indicated. Sometimes, the biopsy itself can be therapeutic as well as diagnostic if the entire lesion can be removed.

Endocervical curettage (ECC) may also be done at this time to evaluate for extension into the cervical canal. This involves a scraping of the endocervix from the internal os to the external os to obtain endocervical cells for cytology. Histologic evaluation of tissue biopsies and ECC samples is necessary for a definitive diagnosis.

The woman may experience moderate to severe cramplike pains during and after the biopsy and/or ECC. To help alleviate this discomfort, nurses can advise women to premedicate with 600 mg ibuprofen about 30 minutes prior to the procedure. A small amount of bleeding, initially bright red and then becoming darker, is normal for up to 2 weeks. Bleeding as heavy as a menstrual period is not normal and should be reported to the woman's care provider.

SURGICAL TREATMENT FOR ABNORMAL CYTOLOGY

Premalignant (precancerous) and malignant (cancerous) lesions are often treated with surgical procedures, varying from simple biopsy of the cervix to radical surgery of the pelvic organs, depending on the diagnosis and extent of the disease. A diagnosis of cancer can only be made after a pathologic evaluation of tissue obtained via biopsy. The goals of management are to exclude the presence of invasive cancer, to determine the extent and distribution of noninvasive cancer, and to provide appropriate treatment (Bristow & Karlan, 1999).

The treatment of cervical cancer depends on the stage of the disease, which is determined by the extent of its spread to other tissues or structures. Surgical treatment of cervical cancer may include a total abdominal hysterectomy (TAH), bilateral salpingo-oophorectomy (BSO), and bilateral lymphadenectomy. It may also include radiation therapy and chemotherapy.

Conization

A *conization* of the cervix (also known as a "cone") is generally performed when the entire lesion cannot be visualized by colposcopic examination or when there is a positive ECC sampling. In this procedure, a cone-shaped section of cervical tissue is excised. The width and depth of the tissue removed varies depending on the extent of the lesion. A large amount of normal tissue is removed, as well as the abnormal tissue, and this procedure can often be diagnostic as well as therapeutic if the entire lesion is excised. Conization is usually done as an outpatient procedure, under local or general anesthesia. Immediate postoperative risks include infection and hemorrhage; long-term risks include spontaneous abortion, incompetent cervix, or preterm labor with future pregnancies. A prolonged or profuse menstrual period may occur in two or three cycles following the procedure. Conization is used less frequently today because of the availability of loop electrosurgical excision procedure, which is discussed next.

Loop Electrosurgical Excision Procedure

Loop electrosurgical excision procedure (LEEP) can be used to treat cervical, vaginal, and vulvar intraepithelial neoplasia. When an abnormal Pap smear and a colposcopic evaluation indicate a premalignant lesion, a small electrically hot wire loop can be used to excise the entire lesion, squamocolumnar junction, and transformation zone. The cutting effect is created by a steam envelope that develops between the wire loop and the water-laden tissue. This procedure can be performed on an outpatient basis, often in the gynecologic office, under local anesthesia. Complications following LEEP are usually minimal, and it is virtually painless and bloodless (Bristow & Karlan, 1999). With the advent of LEEP many physicians have stopped performing cryosurgery and laser surgery. The woman may expect some slight bleeding, and possibly a malodorous dark brown discharge for 1 to 2 weeks after the procedure. The woman needs to know that moderate to heavy bleeding would be abnormal and should be reported to her care provider.

Cryosurgery

Cryosurgery is used to treat women with a small ectocervical lesion who have a negative ECC and no endocervical gland involvement. A double freezing method is advocated, using nitrous oxide or carbon dioxide to freeze the tissue below −20C to −30C, resulting in tissue destruction and necrosis. The freezing can also destroy normal tissue (Bristow & Karlan, 1999). The procedure is usually performed about 1 week after the last menstrual period and can easily be done in a gynecologic office or clinic without anesthesia. The woman may experience some mild cramping and should be told to expect a thin, watery, persistent, and sometimes heavy vaginal discharge for up to several weeks. She should avoid the use of tampons and avoid sexual intercourse while the discharge is present to minimize further damage to the cervix.

Laser Therapy

The carbon dioxide (CO_2) laser is used to treat cervical, vaginal, and vulvar intraepithelial lesions. The laser is used when all boundaries of the lesion are visible on colposcopy and when the ECC is negative. The invisible, highly concentrated beam is absorbed by water in the tissues, elevating the temperature in the tissues to above 100C. The targeted tissue "boils" and the exploded cells are vaporized, leaving the normal tissue intact (Bristow & Karlan, 1999). Laser treatment can be done in outpatient or office settings without anesthesia. The woman may experience mild cramping and a slight discharge for 5 to 7 days; however, bleeding is minimal. She should avoid tampon use, intercourse, and douching for 2 weeks; complete healing may take up to 12 weeks. In many clinical settings, laser therapy has become less common with the advent and effective use of LEEP.

Abnormal Uterine Bleeding

During the many years of a woman's reproductive period, she is likely to experience some form of abnormal uterine bleeding. It may occur as spotting between periods, missing several cycles followed by a heavy bleed, or menses that occur every 2 to 3 months. Heavy, unpredictable menstrual periods can cause a woman to experience fatigue, anemia, and embarrassment. Abnormal bleeding may be a symptom that accompanies infertility.

Abnormal uterine bleeding (AUB) is a common gynecologic problem. Estimates suggest that it may account for more than 20% of visits to women's healthcare providers (Williams & Parsons, 2002). AUB, with or without ovulation, that is caused by organic problems is generally classified as either a systemic or reproductive disorder. Systemic diseases that cause AUB include thyroid dysfunction, coagulation disorders, and cirrhosis. AUB may also result from trauma including accidental injury, sexual abuse, or intercourse-related trauma. Reproductive tract diseases that cause bleeding problems include the following (Oriel & Schrager, 1999):

- Pregnancy-related event, such as threatened, missed, or incomplete abortion, ectopic pregnancy, or gestational trophoblastic disease
- Endometrial, cervical, or ovarian cancer
- Uterine lesions, such as submucous fibroids, endometrial polyps, or adenomyosis
- Cervical lesions, such as polyps, cervicitis, herpes, or chlamydia

Evaluation of AUB begins with a thorough history and physical examination including a careful pelvic exam and Pap smear. Based on the information gained, specific laboratory tests may be indicated. Based on the woman's age and findings, other tests that may be indicated include transvaginal ultrasound, hysteroscopy, and endometrial biopsy (Williams & Parsons, 2002).

In the perimenopausal woman and the postmenopausal woman with abnormal uterine bleeding it is important to consider and evaluate the possibility of uterine pathology early in the investigation to rule out endometrial carcinoma. This is done with an endometrial biopsy. Most cases of endometrial cancer occur in postmenopausal women, although about 30% occur in women under 40 years of age (Brown & Cloutier, 2000).

Dysfunctional uterine bleeding (DUB) is characterized by anovulatory cycles with abnormal uterine bleeding that does not have a demonstrable organic cause. Oligomenorrhea, polymenorrhea, menorrhagia, metrorrhagia, menometrorrhagia, and intermenstrual bleeding are all forms of DUB (see Chapter 4). DUB can occur at any age but is most common at either end of the reproductive age span. Adolescents account for 20% of DUB cases due to hypothalamic immaturity after menarche. Perimenopausal women account for 50% of cases due to waning ovarian function. The remaining cases occur among women of reproductive age, generally as a result of polycystic ovary syndrome, hyperprolactinemia, or hypothalamic dysfunction.

The diagnosis is made by excluding organic causes, specifically pregnancy, uterine or ovarian pathology, medications, or systemic disease. Laboratory evaluation should include a Pap smear, thyroid function studies, pregnancy test, and possible endometrial biopsy. Additional tests may include ultrasonography, hysteroscopy, adrenal studies, liver function studies, or coagulation studies. The goals of treatment are to control bleeding, prevent or treat anemia, prevent endometrial hyperplasia or cancer, and restore quality of life. Pharmacologic treatment for DUB varies depending on the woman's desire for pregnancy and whether she is premenopausal, perimenopausal, or postmenopausal. The premenopausal and perimenopausal woman not actively trying to conceive can be treated with an oral contraceptive, which will help regulate cycles while also providing contraception. Another option is medroxyprogesterone 10 mg daily for 10 days to regulate cycles. In the woman desiring pregnancy, clomiphene (Serophene) 50 to 100 mg can be taken daily for 5 days on days 5 to 9 of her cycle to induce ovulation. The postmenopausal woman may benefit from cyclic hormone replacement therapy (HRT) to allow for withdrawal bleeding, or continuous-combined HRT to stabilize the endometrium (Oriel & Schrager, 1999).

MediaLink
Care Plan: Irregular Bleeding

Ovarian Masses

Between 70% and 80% of ovarian masses are benign. More than 50% are functional cysts (cysts that develop from ovarian follicles, from the corpus luteum, or from the theca luteum) occurring most commonly in women 20 to 40 years of age. Functional cysts are rare in women who take oral contraceptives.

Ovarian cysts usually represent physiologic variations in the menstrual cycle. Nearly all perimenopausal women have ovarian cysts, and about 15% of postmenopausal women have them. Dermoid cysts (cystic teratomas) comprise 10% of all benign ovarian masses. Cartilage, bone, teeth, skin, or hair can be observed in these cysts. Endometriomas, or "chocolate cysts," are another common type of ovarian mass.

No relationship exists between benign ovarian masses and ovarian cancer. Unfortunately, at present, no adequate techniques exist for ovarian cancer screening. Some risk factors for ovarian cancer include increased age (mean age is 59), history of treatment with fertility drugs, and early menarche or late menopause. Asbestos and talc exposure may be causative agents. Some estimates reveal a genetic link in 10% to 15% of cases. In women with a known risk factor, a CA-125 (a circulating tumor marker) level of 30 U/mL or greater may indicate an increased risk (Brown & Cloutier, 2000). In reality, ovarian cancer is the most fatal of all cancers in women because it is difficult to diagnose and often has spread throughout the pelvis before it is detected. Symptoms are often vague and nonspecific, and may include abdominal swelling and heaviness or bloating, pelvic pressure, mild constipation, and increased abdominal girth.

A woman with an ovarian mass may be asymptomatic; the mass may be noted on a routine pelvic examination. She may experience a sensation of fullness or cramping in the lower abdomen (often unilateral), dyspareunia, irregular bleeding, or delayed menstruation.

Diagnosis is made on the basis of a palpable mass, with or without tenderness, and other related symptoms. Radiography or ultrasonography may be used to assist or confirm the diagnosis.

The woman is frequently kept under observation for a month or two because most cysts will resolve on their own and are harmless. Oral contraceptives may be prescribed for 1 to 2 months to suppress ovarian function. If this regimen is effective, a repeat pelvic examination should yield normal findings. If the mass is still present after 60 days of observation and oral contraceptive therapy, a diagnostic laparoscopy or laparotomy may be considered. Tubal or ovarian lesions, ectopic pregnancy, cancer, infection, or appendicitis also must be ruled out before a diagnosis can be confirmed.

Surgery is not always necessary but will be considered if the mass is larger than 6 to 7 cm in circumference; if the woman is over 40 years of age with an adnexal mass, a persistent mass, or continuous pain; or if the woman is taking oral contraceptives. Surgical exploration is also indicated when a palpable mass is found in an infant, a young girl, or a postmenopausal woman. Women may need clear explanations about why the initial therapy is observation. A discussion of the origin and resolution of ovarian cysts may clarify this treatment plan. If a surgical treatment removes or impairs the function of one ovary, the woman needs to be assured that the remaining ovary can be expected to take over ovarian functioning and that pregnancy is still possible.

Women who are taking oral contraceptives should be informed of their preventive effect against ovarian masses.

Uterine Masses

Endometrial polyps are pedunculated (growing on a stalk) overgrowths of the endometrium. They may develop as soft tumors, composed of hyperplastic endometrium, and they can occur as single or multiple growths. Polyps are common, occurring in women between the ages of 12 and 81, and often they are identified incidentally during pelvic ultrasound, curettage, or hysterectomy. Polyps are benign, but they can coexist with carcinoma of the endometrium in about 10% of postmenopausal women. Treatment is curettage, or hysteroscopy and removal, in the postmenopausal woman or if bleeding persists after diagnosis.

Fibroid tumors, or *leiomyomas*, are among the most common benign disease entities in women and are the most common reason for gynecologic surgery. Between 20% and 50% of women develop leiomyomas by 40 years of age. The potential for cancer is minimal. Leiomyomas are more common in women of African heritage.

Fibroid tumors develop when smooth muscle cells are present in whorls and arise from uterine muscles and connective tissue. The size varies from 1 to 2 cm to the size of a 12- to 14-week fetus. Frequently the woman is asymptomatic. Lower abdominal pain, fullness or pressure, menorrhagia, metrorrhagia, or increased dysmenorrhea may occur, particularly with large leiomyomas. As a result, anemia may develop. Ultrasonography revealing masses or nodules can assist and confirm the diagnosis. Leiomyoma is also considered a possible diagnosis when masses or nodules involving the uterus are palpated on a pelvic examination.

The majority of these masses require no treatment and will shrink after menopause. Close observation for symptoms or an increase in size of the uterus or the masses may be the only management most women will require. Routine pelvic examinations every 3 to 6 months are recommended unless new symptoms appear.

If a woman notices symptoms, or pelvic examination reveals that the mass is increasing in size, surgery (myomectomy, dilation and curettage [D & C], or hysterectomy) will be recommended. Otherwise, a hysterectomy is generally performed. The route of surgery is typically via an abdominal incision; however, a laparoscopic procedure may be considered. The mass can be excised or ablated. The choice of surgery depends on the age and reproductive status of the woman and the significance of the noted changes. There are no medications or therapies to prevent fibroids. The use of gonadotropin-releasing hormone (GnRH) agonists results in a 40% to 60% decrease in uterine volume. It may be helpful to shrink the fibroid prior to surgery, especially with a laparoscopic procedure (Spellacy, 1999). If a myomectomy is performed, a woman can preserve her fertility. However, if there is a uterine incision, subsequent children would be born by cesarean.

Endometrial cancer, most commonly a disease of postmenopausal women, has a high rate of cure if detected early. The majority of endometrial cancer occurs in postmenopausal women. Although the overall incidence is lower in African American women than in Caucasian women, the former are often diagnosed in the later stages of the disease process and thus have a poorer survival rate (Brown & Cloutier, 2000). Risk factors include obesity, nulliparity, diabetes, hypertension, and the use of unopposed estrogen; associated factors are a high-fat diet, early menarche or late menopause, and use of tamoxifen.

The hallmark sign is vaginal bleeding in postmenopausal women not treated with HRT. Diagnosis is made occasionally by Pap smear, by endometrial biopsy, by transvaginal ultrasound, or by posthysterectomy pathologic examination of the uterus. Exploratory laparotomy is performed to establish the stage of the cancer. Uterine tissues are biopsied, lymph nodes are sampled, and peritoneal washings are collected for cytology.

Once staging of the cancer is completed, a plan of treatment is proposed. Treatment for all stages of endometrial cancer involves TAH and BSO. This may be adequate treatment for stage I disease without lymph node involvement. Women with stage II may undergo preoperative and postoperative radiation, TAH and BSO, and extensive dissection of the pelvic organs and lymph nodes. Stage III or IV cancer includes all of the previously listed surgical treatment plus external and intracavity radiation. Women with stage IV disease may require surgery to debulk the tumor and hormone therapy with progestins (Brown & Cloutier, 2000).

NURSING CARE MANAGEMENT

Only nurses with special training perform pelvic examinations and Pap smears. In most cases, nursing assessment is directed toward evaluating the woman's understanding of the findings and their implications and her psychosocial response.

The woman needs accurate information on the etiology of the disorder, its symptoms, and treatment options. She should be encouraged to report symptoms and keep appointments for follow-up examination and evaluation. The woman needs realistic reassurance if her condition is benign; she may require counseling and effective emotional support if a malignancy is likely. If the management plan includes surgery, she may need the nurse's support in obtaining a second opinion and making her decision. The nurse can also provide information on available community resources including support groups.

Care of the Woman with Pelvic Relaxation

The muscles of the pelvic floor form a supportive layer that prevents the abdominal and pelvic organs from prolapsing or sagging downward into the genital tract. If these muscles are weakened or damaged, a variety of conditions may develop including cystocele, rectocele, and uterine prolapse. Factors that may contribute to diminished pelvic floor muscle tone include damage to these structures related to childbirth, deterioration with age, metabolic diseases that affect muscle functioning, prolonged lifting, or even chronic coughing due to chronic pulmonary disease (DeLancey, 1999).

Cystocele

A **cystocele** is the downward displacement of the bladder, which appears as a bulge in the anterior vaginal wall. Arbitrary classifications of mild to severe are frequently given. Genetic predisposition, childbearing, obesity, and increased age are factors that may contribute to cystocele.

Women with a cystocele commonly show symptoms of stress incontinence including loss of urine with coughing, sneezing, laughing, or sudden exertion. Vaginal fullness, a bulging out of the vaginal wall, or a dragging sensation may also be noticeable.

If pelvic relaxation is mild, Kegel exercises are helpful in restoring tone (see Chapter 16). The exercises involve contracting and relaxing the pubococcygeal muscle. Women have found these exercises helpful before and after childbirth in maintaining vaginal muscle tone. Estrogen may improve the condition of vaginal mucous membranes—especially in menopausal women. Vaginal pessaries or rings may be used

EVIDENCE-BASED PRACTICE

PELVIC FLOOR MUSCLE TRAINING WITH WEIGHTED VAGINAL CONES

Clinical Question

Are weighted vaginal cones effective in pelvic floor muscle training for women with urinary incontinence?

The Evidence

Pelvic floor muscle training has long been the most common form of conservative treatment for stress urinary incontinence. It is theorized that weighted vaginal cones may help women to train their pelvic floor muscles, thus reducing incontinence. Cones are inserted into the vagina and the pelvic floor is contracted to prevent them slipping out.

Research evidence was summarized from 25 studies involving 1,126 women, 466 of whom received weighted vaginal cones. Cones were better than no active treatment. However, there was little evidence of difference between cones and pelvic floor muscle training (PFMT) or electrostimulation. Because of small sample sizes and wide confidence intervals, certainty is minimized. There was not enough evidence to show that that cones plus PFMT was different from either cones alone or PFMT alone.

Best Practice

Some form of PFMT should be implemented in the care of women with urinary incontinence. This review provides some evidence that weighted vaginal cones are better than no active treatment in women with stress urinary incontinence and may be of similar effectiveness to PFMT and electrostimulation. This conclusion must remain tentative until further larger high quality studies are carried out using comparable and relevant outcome measures.

Reference: Herbison, P., Plevnik, S., Mantle, J. (2002). *Weighted vaginal cones for urinary incontinence.* Cochrane Incontinence Group Cochrane Database of Systematic Reviews.

if surgery is undesirable or impossible, or until surgery can be scheduled. Surgery may be considered for cystoceles considered moderate to severe.

The nurse can instruct the woman in the use of Kegel exercises. Providing information on causes and contributing factors and discussing possible alternative therapies greatly assists the woman.

Rectocele

A rectocele may develop if the posterior vaginal wall is weakened. The anterior wall of the rectum sags forward, ballooning into the vagina, pushing the weakened posterior wall of the vagina in front of it. When the woman strains to have a bowel movement, a pocket of rectum develops that traps stool, and constipation results. The harder a woman with rectocele strains, the larger the pocket becomes. To defecate, women with a rectocele may find it necessary to press the tissue between the vagina and rectum, which elevates the rectocele.

Diagnosis is based on history and physical examination. Decisions about treatment are based on the size of the prolapse, the presence and severity of symptoms, and the woman's individual situation including her overall health status. Surgery is often indicated.

Uterine Prolapse

Because the vagina and the uterus are attached to one another, prolapse of the uterine cervix is associated with prolapse of the upper vagina. The extent of the prolapse is determined by the location of the cervix in the vagina. In severe cases the cervix may prolapse below the vaginal introitus. The woman may report a "dragging" sensation in her groin and a backache over the sacrum, which is caused by pulling on the uterosacral ligaments. Typically these sensations are relieved when the woman lies down. Furthermore, with pronounced prolapse, exposure of the moist vaginal walls may cause a sensation of perineal wetness that the woman might mistake for incontinence. As with cystocele, conservative treatment includes the use of topical or systemic estrogen and vaginal pessaries. Surgery for uterine prolapse often involves hysterectomy and repair of the prolapsed vaginal walls.

Care of the Woman Requiring Gynecologic Surgery

Gynecologic surgeries—particularly hysterectomies—are some of the most common surgical procedures being done in the United States. Many new techniques have been developed for treating a variety of gynecologic and reproductive disorders, and controversy remains as to the high number of procedures being done annually. For these reasons, it is important for the woman considering medical or surgical management of a given gynecologic problem to be well informed.

There are many components to an informed decision to undergo reproductive surgery. Questions that should be addressed include, for example: What are the indications for having the surgery? What are the risks? What is the success rate? Are there other alternative therapies to try before proceeding to surgery? An explanation of the surgical procedure and the reasons it is recommended over other possible therapies should be given to the woman. Effects on childbearing ability and potential impact on sexual performance should be addressed, as well as effects on the general functioning of the body. A discussion of the risks and benefits should be presented, and the risks should include the common risks, the nonserious risks, the rare or unusual complications, and the risk of death.

The question whether a second opinion should be sought regarding recommended treatment is somewhat controversial. In the case of elective surgery, different physicians may have very different opinions. A woman should be encouraged to consult other physicians when there is controversy about a treatment (as in the treatment of early cervical cancer) or when the surgeon is unknown to the woman. A specialist in gynecology is the preferred source for a second opinion. Some third-party payment plans require second opinions. The woman can analyze the information and discuss her concerns with the nurse or physician prior to signing a written consent acknowledging that the information has been given and authorizing the surgery.

Other concerns that may influence the decision to have reproductive surgery may be categorized as general concerns about surgery and specific concerns related to gynecologic surgery. General concerns may include:

- Anesthesia: fear of general anesthesia because of loss of control or fear of "not waking up"; fear of regional anesthesia because of possible postoperative problems and concern about being awake during surgery
- Fear of death or disability
- Concerns about limitation of normal functioning and dependency during recovery
- Financial coverage for hospitalization, and potential financial loss if it is necessary to take extensive time off from work
- Family members: welfare of family members while undergoing surgery (such as child care, loss of wages, help with household work)

Specific concerns related to gynecologic surgery are related to the significance of the reproductive organs for the woman. Surgery to alter or remove reproductive organs may be perceived as a threat to self-concept.

Body image is affected whenever a body part is lost. The degree of mourning for that loss is related to the significance attached to it. Even though there is no outwardly apparent change with a hysterectomy and most other gynecologic procedures, the loss may be felt very strongly. Many women fear postoperative changes such as masculinization, weight gain, loss of sexuality, and permanent loss of the ability to have a child. Reproductive surgery may also be seen as a threat to femininity in any social or cultural group that emphasizes childbearing and motherhood.

Hysterectomy

Hysterectomy is the removal of the uterus. In the United States, approximately 650,000 hysterectomies are performed each year, making it the most common nonpregnancy-related surgical procedure that women in the United States undergo (Kim & Lee, 2001). Removal of the uterus through an abdominal incision is called a *total abdominal hysterectomy (TAH)* and removal of both fallopian tubes and ovaries is called a *bilateral salpingo-oophorectomy (BSO);* when both procedures are done at the same time it is termed a TAH-BSO. When the uterus is removed through the vagina it is termed a *total vaginal hysterectomy (TVH).*

A common technique to perform this surgery is a laparoscopic-assisted vaginal hysterectomy (LAVH). In this technique, the surgeon inserts the laparoscope through an incision near the umbilicus and uses it to assist with visualization and dissection to facilitate vaginal removal of the uterus. The benefit is that the surgeon can achieve results similar to those of a TAH without a large abdominal incision. Theoretically the recovery time should be shorter as compared to a TAH. Some controversy exists because there is often added expense from increased time in the operating room and the risks associated with prolonged anesthesia exposure.

Hysterectomy is the usual treatment for several conditions, although there is no medical consensus about absolute indications. Abdominal hysterectomy is generally recommended for cancer of the cervix, endometrium, or ovary; large fibroids; severe endometriosis; chronic pelvic inflammatory disease (PID); and adenomyosis. TAH is preferred when malignancy is suspected or confirmed because the procedure allows exploration of the abdomen and pelvis to determine the degree and extent of involvement (DiSaia, Walker, & Gold, 1999). This approach is also helpful when large uterine masses are present requiring a larger incision. Disadvantages include more scarring, more postoperative pain, slower recovery, and more problems with bowel function.

Vaginal hysterectomy is generally done for pelvic relaxation, abnormal uterine bleeding, or small fibroids. An anterior and posterior repair of the vaginal walls may also be performed during TVH. Sometimes this repair is done when weakened pelvic supports have displaced one or more of the pelvic organs (such as the urethra, bladder, or rectum), sometimes causing urinary incontinence, constipation, or defecation problems. Advantages include earlier ambulation, less postoperative pain, less anesthesia and operative time, less blood loss, no visible scar, and a shorter hospital stay. This approach is preferred for the elderly, obese, or debilitated woman who is a poor risk for abdominal surgery. The major disadvantage is increased risk of trauma to the bladder.

Removal of the ovaries at time of hysterectomy remains controversial. In premenopausal women, without evidence of ovarian pathology, the ovaries are generally left to avoid forced surgical menopause. Because of the risk of ovarian cancer, some physicians recommend removal of ovaries in all women over 40 years old who undergo hysterectomy. Still others recommend removal of the ovaries in any woman with a family history of ovarian cancer. In any case, removal of the ovaries is not considered routine, and when a BSO is performed in a premenopausal woman, supplemental estrogen replacement therapy is recommended.

Dilation and Curettage

In the United States, dilation and curettage (D&C) is the most frequently performed minor gynecologic procedure. Indications for a D&C may be diagnostic or therapeutic. Diagnostic indications include evaluation for uterine malignancy, infertility evaluation, and investigation of dysfunctional uterine bleeding. Therapeutic indications include elective abortion, treatment of heavy bleeding, incomplete abortion, dysmenorrhea, and removal of polyps. Sometimes D&C is done after hysteroscopy, which is a procedure that allows visualization of the endometrial cavity and minor surgical procedures. Another procedure that can be done at the time of hysteroscopy is an endometrial ablation, which cauterizes endometrial tissue, preventing regeneration and further bleeding. This procedure is not recommended for women who desire pregnancy, and so a simple D&C may be more appropriate. All of these procedures can be done under general anesthesia, intravenous sedation, and/or regional anesthesia, and most are done as an outpatient procedure.

Salpingectomy

The unilateral or bilateral removal of the fallopian tube is called a salpingectomy. Indications include diseases of the tubes, sepsis, malignancy, and ectopic pregnancy of the fallopian tube. Salpingectomy for an ectopic pregnancy is generally an emergency procedure. The developing placental tissue erodes the fallopian tube and can cause rupture and hemorrhage once the tube is completely eroded. This procedure can be done via laparoscopy or via an open abdominal approach.

Oophorectomy

Oophorectomy is the unilateral or bilateral removal of the ovary. Indications include severe PID, malignancy, ectopic pregnancy, and symptomatic ovarian cysts. When both ovaries are removed in a premenopausal woman, abrupt surgical menopause occurs. In this case the woman will experience the same symptoms she might in natural menopause: decreased libido, decreased vaginal lubrication, hot flashes and/or night sweats, and decreased sensation in the lower vaginal tract. These symptoms can be treated with estrogen replacement.

Vulvectomy

A simple vulvectomy is performed for leukoplakia and intractable pruritus, whereas a radical procedure is done for malignant disease. A simple vulvectomy is the removal of the labia majora, labia minora, and clitoris. Radical vulvectomy is the removal of the entire vulva, including the skin and the fat of the femoral triangle, and the pelvic lymph nodes. Skin grafts may be necessary.

This disfiguring procedure is associated with marked psychosexual disturbances. Most women report decreased sexual arousal levels and low self-image. Sexual activity can be resumed within 3 months; however, significant adjustments will be necessary owing to the loss of sensory perception for foreplay. Stimulation of breasts, thighs, buttocks, or anterior abdominal wall can be suggested.

Pelvic Exenteration

A pelvic exenteration is performed for recurrence of cervical cancer. Only about 5% of women with recurrence are candidates for this procedure, which is not performed if there is any evidence of tumor outside of the pelvis, if the cancer has metastasized to the lymph nodes, or if all of the tumor cannot be removed.

Exenteration can be of the anterior or posterior pelvis, or of the total pelvis. Anterior exenteration is the removal of the uterus, ovaries, fallopian tubes, vagina, bladder, urethra, and pelvic lymph nodes. Urine is diverted through an ileal conduit. Posterior exenteration is the removal of the uterus, fallopian tubes, ovaries, descending colon, rectum, and anal canal. A colostomy is created. A total exenteration is a combination of the anterior and posterior procedures. A vagina can be reconstructed from split-thickness skin grafts or a segment of small bowel.

Complications associated with exenteration include intestinal and urinary obstruction, thrombophlebitis, pulmonary embolism, pyelonephritis, hypovolemia, peritonitis, pneumonia, and wound infection.

NURSING CARE MANAGEMENT

Nursing Assessment and Diagnosis

Nursing assessment for all of these surgical procedures includes identifying the woman's physiologic, psychosocial, and sexual needs as she approaches her surgery. Additionally, it is important to understand her learning needs regarding the procedure and its effects. Some factors to consider are the age of the woman, her cultural background and educational level, the attitude of her partner and family, her preoperative status (physically and emotionally), and whether or not this involves a cancer diagnosis. The significance of her reproductive health to her self-image will be reflected in her attitudes about menstruation, childbearing, body image, and sexuality. Many of these procedures have the potential to involve loss, so grieving, anger, sadness, and loss of control are just a few of the feelings the woman may experience.

Nursing diagnoses that may apply to a woman facing gynecologic surgery include the following:

- ***Deficient Knowledge*** related to lack of information about preoperative routines, postoperative activities, and expected postoperative changes

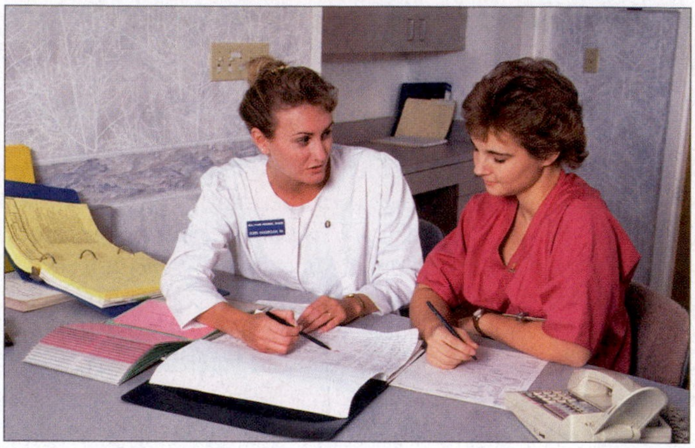

Figure 7–5 ● The nurse provides information for the woman during preoperative teaching.

- ***Fear*** related to the unknown outcome and long-term implications of the surgery

Nursing Plan and Implementation

Preoperative teaching may be brief in the instance of a simple D&C, or quite extensive in the instances of hysterectomy or pelvic exenteration. In any case, preoperative teaching should include information about the procedure, expected preparation, type of anesthesia to be used, possible risks and complications, postoperative care routines, and expected recovery time. See Figure 7–5 ●.

Routine postoperative care includes monitoring of physiologic responses, emotional responses, and nursing interventions to facilitate physical and emotional well-being, specific to the procedure performed. The woman should be aware of potential postoperative complications and when to follow up with her surgeon. Additionally, it is important to discuss those psychosocial issues identified preoperatively, such as support at home, potential for sadness or depression related to the loss she has experienced, and expected sexual and self-image fears. In some instances, it may be necessary to refer the woman to a professional therapist who can help her adjust to these dramatic changes.

Evaluation

Expected outcomes of nursing care include:

- The woman can discuss the reasons for her surgery, the alternatives, and the aspects of self-care after surgery.
- The woman has an uneventful recovery without complications.
- The woman feels she is able to ask questions and obtain support.
- The woman participates in decision making about her care.
- The woman is aware of available resources if she has physical or emotional concerns in the postoperative period.

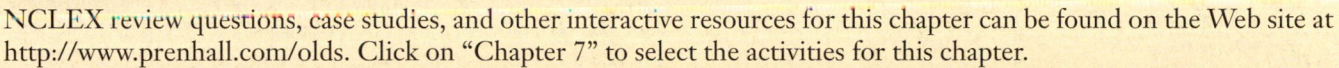

CHAPTER REVIEW

EXPLOREMEDIALINK

NCLEX review questions, case studies, and other interactive resources for this chapter can be found on the Web site at http://www.prenhall.com/olds. Click on "Chapter 7" to select the activities for this chapter.

For tutorials including animations and videos, more NCLEX review questions, and an audio glossary, access the accompanying CD-ROM in this book.

Focus Your Study

- With fibrocystic breast changes, the cysts tend to be round, mobile, and well delineated. The woman generally experiences increased discomfort premenstrually.
- Because of the increased risk of breast cancer, women with fibrocystic changes should understand the importance of monthly breast self-examination (BSE).
- Galactorrhea (nipple discharge not associated with lactation) should be evaluated with cytologic testing.
- Breast cancer affects one in eight women in the United States. Biopsy is essential for a diagnosis, and prompt treatment is critical.
- Endometriosis is a condition in which endometrial tissue occurs outside the endometrial cavity. This tissue bleeds in a cyclic fashion in response to the menstrual cycle. The bleeding leads to inflammation, scarring, and adhesions. The prime symptoms include dysmenorrhea, dyspareunia, and infertility.
- Treatment of endometriosis may be medical, surgical, or a combination. For the woman not desiring pregnancy at present, oral contraceptives are used. Women desiring pregnancy are treated with danazol or the GnRH analogs.
- Toxic shock syndrome, usually caused by a toxin of *Staphylococcus aureus*, is most common in women of childbearing age. There is an increased incidence in women who use tampons or barrier methods of contraception, such as the diaphragm and cervical cap, especially if the woman leaves them in place for extended periods of time.
- Vulvitis is an inflammation of the vulva often caused by external irritants such as tight clothing, feminine hygiene products, and some harsh soaps.
- Vulvar lesions range from slight irritation to vulvar cancer. A common vulvar lesion found in postmenopausal women is atrophic vaginitis. All vulvar lesions should be closely evaluated because cancer of the vulva can have various presentations.
- Pap smear screening is recommended for all women who are sexually active or who have reached the age of 18 years. Several factors put a woman at high risk for an abnormal Pap: intercourse at a young age, multiple partners, history of immunotherapy, long-term COC use, smoking, and previous history of dysplasia. HPV is highly associated with abnormal Pap smears.
- Abnormal uterine bleeding can occur with or without organic pathology. Treatment is geared toward controlling bleeding, preventing anemia, and detecting pathology.
- There are three common forms of pelvic relaxation: A cystocele is a downward displacement of the bladder into the vagina. Often it is accompanied by stress incontinence. Kegel exercises may help restore tone in mild cases. A rectocele is displacement of the rectum into the vagina. Prolapse of the uterus is displacement of the uterine cervix into the vagina.
- Gynecologic surgeries are some of the most common surgical procedures performed in the United States. It is important for the nurse to understand the purpose of the procedure, to know the alternatives to surgery, and to assess the woman's emotional response.

References

American Cancer Society (ACS). (2002). *Breast cancer: Facts and figures 2001–2002.* Atlanta, GA: Author.

Bethesda 2001 Workshop. (2001). NCI Bethesda system 2001: 2001 terminology. *Bethesda system 2001.* Retrieved December 15, 2001, from http://bethesda2001.cancer.gov/terminology.html

Braly, P. S. (1999). Diseases of the uterus. In J. R. Scott, P. J. DiSaia, C. B. Hammond, & W. N. Spellacy (Eds.), *Danforth's obstetrics and gynecology* (8th ed., pp. 837–856). Philadelphia: Lippincott Williams & Wilkins.

Bristow, R. E., & Karlan, B. Y. (1999). Disorders of the uterine cervix. In J. R. Scott, P. J. DiSaia, C. B. Hammond, & W. N. Spellacy (Eds.), *Danforth's obstetrics and gynecology* (8th ed., pp. 805–835). Philadelphia: Lippincott Williams & Wilkins.

Brown, J. S., & Cloutier, A. O. (2000, April). Gynecologic cancers: These cancers challenge screening tools. *American Journal of Nursing*, (*Suppl.*), 32–35.

Centers for Disease Control and Prevention (CDC). (2002). Sexually transmitted diseases treatment guidelines 2002. *Morbidity and Mortality Weekly Report, 51* (RR-6), 1–84.

Corwin, E. J. (1997). Endometriosis: Pathophysiology, diagnosis, and treatment. *Nurse Practitioner, 22*(10), 35–51.

DeLancey, J. O. L. (1999). Pelvic organ prolapse. In J. R. Scott, P. J. DiSaia, C. B. Hammond, & W. N. Spellacy (Eds.), *Danforth's obstetrics and gynecology* (8th ed., pp. 713–736). Philadelphia: Lippincott Williams & Wilkins.

DiSaia, P. J. (1999). Vulvar and vaginal disease. In J. R. Scott, P. J. DiSaia, C. B. Hammond, & W. N. Spellacy (Eds.), *Danforth's obstetrics and gynecology* (8th ed., pp. 779–804). Philadelphia: Lippincott Williams & Wilkins.

DiSaia, P. J., Walker, J. L., & Gold, M. A. (1999). Perioperative care. In J. R. Scott, P. J. DiSaia, C. B. Hammond, & W. N. Spellacy (Eds.), *Danforth's obstetrics and gynecology* (8th ed., pp. 699–712). Philadelphia: Lippincott Williams & Wilkins.

Eschenbach, D. A. (1999). Pelvic infections and sexually transmitted diseases. In J. R. Scott, P. J. DiSaia, C. B. Hammond, & W. N. Spellacy (Eds.), *Danforth's obstetrics and gynecology* (8th ed., pp. 579–600). Philadelphia: Lippincott Williams & Wilkins.

Eskenazi, B., et al. (2002). Serum dioxin concentrations and endometriosis: A cohort study. *Environmental Health Perspectives, 110*(7), 629–634.

Eskin, B. A., & Sepilian, V. (2001). Common benign conditions of the breast. *The Female Patient, 26*(10), 44–49.

Fiorica, J. V. (1999). The breast. In J. R. Scott, P. J. DiSaia, C. B. Hammond, & W. N. Spellacy (Eds.), *Danforth's obstetrics and gynecology* (8th ed., pp. 631–648). Philadelphia: Lippincott Williams & Wilkins.

Howes, D. S. (2001, September 10). Urinary tract infection, female. *eMedicine Journal, 2*(9). Retrieved November 14, 2001, from http://www.imedicine.com/wc.dll?emedclass~ displayTopic~ &BookId=3&Topic= 626&id=2

Hsu, K. (2001, March 5). Endometriosis. *eMedicine Journal, 2*(3). Retrieved November 14, 2001, from http://www.imedicine.com/ wc.dll?emedclass~ displayTopic~ &BookId=3&Topic= 626&id=2

Isacson, C., & Kurman, R. J. (1995). The Bethesda System: A new classification for managing Pap smears. *Contemporary OB/GYN, 40*(6), 67–74.

Kim, K. H., & Lee, K. A. (2001). Symptom experience in women after hysterectomy. *Journal of Obstetric, Gynecologic, and Neonatal Nursing, 30*(5), 472–480.

Love, S. M. (2000). *Dr. Susan Love's breast book.* (3rd ed.). Boulder, CO: Perseus Publishing.

Morrow, M. (2000). The evaluation of common breast problems. *American Family Physician, 61*(8), 2371–2378.

National Cancer Institute (NCI). (2002). *NCI statement on mammography screening.* Bethesda, MD: Author.

Oriel, K. A., & Schrager, S. (1999). Abnormal uterine bleeding. *American Family Physician, 60*(5), 1371–1380.

Richart, R. M. (2002). A sea change in diagnosing and managing HPV and cervical disease—Part I. *Contemporary OB/GYN, 47*(5), 42–56.

Richwald, G. A., & Skaer, T. L. (2001). External genital warts. *The Female Patient, 26*(11), 50–56.

Schenken, R. S. (1999). Endometriosis. In J. R. Scott, P. J. DiSaia, C. B. Hammond, & W. N. Spellacy (Eds.), *Danforth's obstetrics and gynecology* (8th ed., pp. 669–675). Philadelphia: Lippincott Williams & Wilkins.

Scott, L. D., & Hasik, K. J. (2001). The similarities and differences of endometritis and pelvic inflammatory disease. *Journal of Obstetric, Gynecologic, and Neonatal Nursing, 30*(3), 332–341.

Sinaii, N., Cleary, S. D., Ballweg, M. L., Nieman, L. K., & Stratton, P. (2002). High rates of autoimmune and endocrine disorders, fibromyalgia, chronic fatigue syndrome and atopic diseases among women with endometriosis: A survey analysis. *Human Reproduction, 17*(10), 2715–2724.

Solomon, D., Davey, D., Kurman, R., Moriarity, A, O'Connor, D., Prey, M., et al. (2002). Consensus statement:The 2001 Bethesda System—Terminology for reporting results of cervical cytology. *Journal of the American Medical Association, 287*(16), 2114–2119.

Spellacy, W. N. (1999). Utterine leiomyoma. In J. R. Scott, P. J. DiSalia, C.B. Hammond, & W.N. Spellacy (Eds.). *Danforth's obstetrics and gynecology* (8th ed., pp. 857–864), Philadelphia: Lippincott Williams & Wilkins.

Taubes, G. (1997, April). NCI reverses one expert panel, sides will another. *Science, 276* (5309), 27–28.

Uphold, C. R., & Graham, M. V. (1998). *Clinical guidelines in family practice* (3rd ed.). Gainesville, FL: Barmarrae Books.

Williams, J. K., & Parsons, A. (2002). Abnormal uterine bleeding. *The Female Patient, 27*(2), 15–21.

Wright, T. C., Cox, J. T., Massad, L. S., Twiggs, M. D., & Wilkinson, E. J. (2002). Consensus statement: 2001 Consensus guidelines for the management of women with cervical cytological abnormalities. *Journal of the American Medical Association, 287*(16), 2120–2129.

Writing Group for the Women's Health Initiative Investigators. (2002). Risks and benefits of estrogen plus progestin in healthy postmenopausal women: Principal results from the Women's Health Initiative randomized controlled trial. *Journal of the American Medical Association*, 288, 321–333.

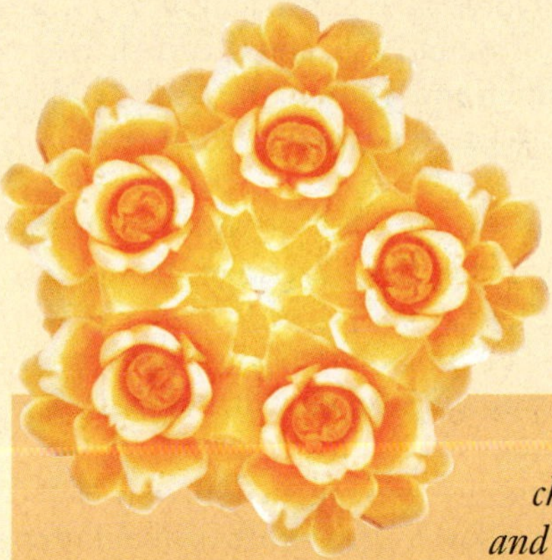

8 Women's Care: Social Issues

I don't think there has ever been a more exciting time for women. There are many challenges that face us: work, wage, and role issues; safety in pregnancy and childbearing; and conflict over women's rights. On the other hand, women have never been more active and involved in issues that affect them. Moreover, the men who care about us and who recognize the importance of fairness for all are beginning to speak out. I am convinced that together, as people of integrity and vision, we are making a difference.

Objectives

- Describe the concept of feminization of poverty.
- Explain the effects of poverty on women's healthcare.
- Identify several factors that affect women's wages.
- Discuss the impact of the Family and Medical Leave Act (FMLA) of 1993 on maternity and paternity leave.
- Describe environmental hazards present in a childbearing woman's workplace.
- Provide several rationales for the economic vulnerability of older women.
- Identify at least four different types of elder abuse.
- Explain the effects of aging on women's healthcare.
- Explain the effects of discrimination on women's access to healthcare.
- Delineate four main types of disabilities.
- Explain the effects of disability on women's healthcare.
- Identify types of discrimination that are commonly faced by lesbian and bisexual women.

Key Terms

Comparable worth 158
Disability 165
Elder abuse 163
Feminization of later life 163
Feminization of poverty 154
Polypharmacy 164

MEDIALINK

Additional resources for this content can be found on the Student CD-ROM and on the Companion Website at www.prenhall.com/olds. Click on "Chapter 8" to select the activities for this chapter.

CD-ROM
- Audio Glossary
- NCLEX Review

Companion Website
- Additional NCLEX Review
- Case Study: Social Issues Affecting Women
- Care Plan Activity: Pregnancy in a Disabled Client

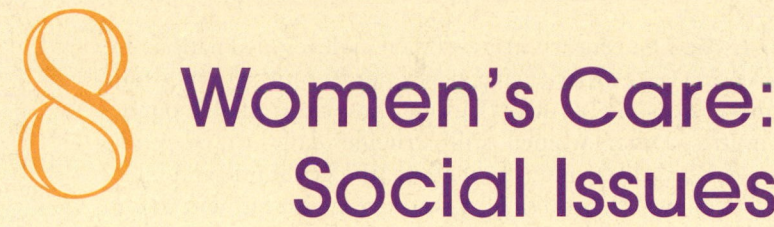

In the 21st century, many women in developed nations are creating and experiencing new opportunities for personal and professional growth. Despite these unparalleled opportunities, other women still struggle daily to overcome poverty, age discrimination, abuse, the economic and interpersonal effects of disability, and unequal treatment due to sexual orientation. Even the most successful and satisfied working women face wage discrimination, lack of safe and nurturing day care for their children, and failure of their governments to support paid maternity and paternity leave.

Every day in their clinical practice, nurses working with women are confronted with these issues and their impact on women's health and well-being. To help nurses better understand their clients' concerns and problems, this chapter addresses some of the serious social issues facing women today.

Social Issues Affecting Women in Poverty

For women living in poverty, life is a day-by-day struggle fraught with anxiety and hardship.

"I never thought this would happen to me. Two months after I became pregnant with our second child, it was over. My husband left us. Suddenly, I am the sole support of myself and my children. Since he left I haven't been able to get a job, so I don't have medical insurance or any benefits to help with this pregnancy. Applying for Medicaid has to be one of the most humiliating experiences I have ever had. I'm an intelligent woman with a college degree, and I couldn't figure out the forms. I felt so dumb. The lines and the impersonal treatment that you hear about are real. I felt like a number, shuttled from one place to the next. I know they don't do it on purpose; they've heard so many awful stories. Still, it hurt. It will take 6 weeks to qualify, and that means I will be more than halfway through my pregnancy. What's more, only two doctors here accept Medicaid, and they are clear across town—three bus transfers with a 2-year-old in tow. I'm thankful that I can get some help, but it is so hard. I never dreamed I'd be in this position. I just never dreamed."

Feminization of Poverty

The harsh economic plight of many women is dramatically reflected in the growing phenomenon referred to as the **feminization of poverty,** a term suggested by Diana Pearce (1993). Simply stated, a growing number of US women live on incomes that fall below the poverty level, which in 2002 was $18,100 for a family of four (Department of Health and Human Services [DHHS], 2002).

Although the number of families living in poverty has declined steadily since 1993, poverty is still a major issue in the United States for female-headed households. Specifically, in 2000, the number of impoverished families reached a 26-year low at 8.6% (US Census Bureau, 2001). However, only 4.8% of families headed by a married couple lived in poverty, compared to a staggering 26.3% of households headed by single mothers. With a divorce rate approaching 50%, an out-of-wedlock birth rate of about 25%, and the median age at first marriage rising for men and women, the reality is that many children will spend at least a portion of their lives in a single-parent family.

Even more disturbing is the number of children in the United States living in poverty. No other age group, not even the elderly, has a higher rate of poverty. Two risk factors are especially significant in documenting poverty in children: female-headed family and race. Although 16.9% of children in the United States live below the poverty level, over half (50.3%) of all children living in female-headed homes fall below the poverty level. The number of children from minority groups who live in female-headed households falling below the poverty level is even more disturbing: 41% of all African American children and 51.1% of all Hispanic children live in poverty (Dalaker & Proctor, 2002). Currently, two thirds of all poor people in the United States are women and children; in other words, women and children account for most of the people living in poverty (Figure 8–1 •).

The feminization of poverty is also evident in the rising trend for women to declare bankruptcy. In 2001 the percentage of women filing for bankruptcy in the United States grew to 30% of applicants. At the same time, new bankruptcy laws were passed that reduce consumer protection and give lenders more leverage to push for repayment. These new laws will inevitably hurt women who are divorced, separated, and widowed since these are the women who disproportionately file for bankruptcy (Warren, 2002).

The feminization of poverty extends beyond the United States. While there are many scales used to measure global poverty, the Purchasing Power Parity (PPP) scale uses calculations based on money available for purchasing. It is estimated that 1.2 billion people live on less than $1 per day, and

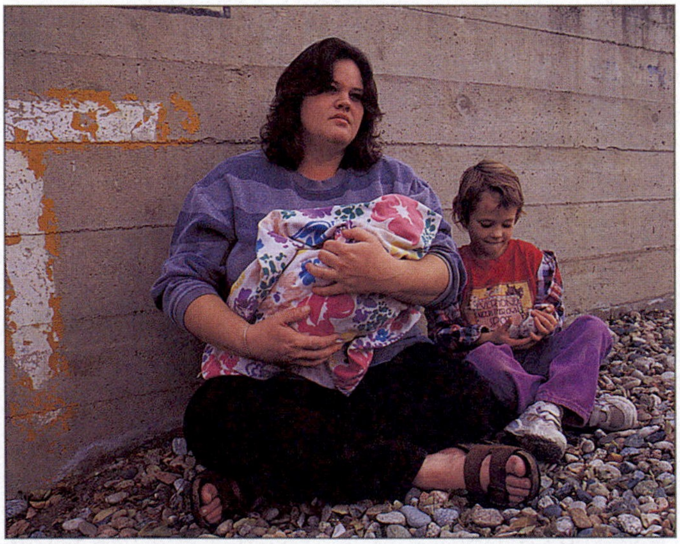

Figure 8–1 • Two thirds of Americans living in poverty are women and children.

MediaLink CASE STUDY: SOCIAL ISSUES AFFECTING WOMEN

an additional 2.8 billion live on less than $2 per day (United Nations Population Fund, 2000). Globally, women must cope with some unique challenges. They typically work more hours than men but are paid less for the same work; they are often expected to bear and raise many children, sometimes in addition to performing a job outside the home; they are frequently abused and beaten in their own homes; and often they have few legal rights.

Both globally and in the United States, poverty has been directly linked to literacy and educational attainment. The literacy rate for females is lower than that for males, and education—when available—is more frequently provided for men even though economic returns on investment in women's education are found to exceed those for men. Also, women who use their skills to increase their income invest more in their children's health and education (United Nations Population Fund, 2000).

Economic Effects of Divorce

The increase in the number of female-headed families is closely associated with divorce. Almost one out of every two marriages ends in divorce. As a result of divorce, a woman's standard of living generally decreases significantly, while a man's increases. This dramatic change in the standard of living is usually associated with the lower earning capacity of women and the fact that women receive custody of the children in 85.1% of cases (US Census Bureau, 2000a). Only about one half of divorced women receive full child support payments; about one fourth receive partial payment, while the remaining one fourth receive nothing at all (DHHS, 1998b). Moreover, these legally awarded payments are frequently inadequate.

Until recently, society has not held men accountable for these payments. This appears to be changing, however. At the national level, the United States Department of Justice is actively investigating and prosecuting individuals who cross state lines to avoid paying child support. In addition, the federal government now intercepts income tax refunds of delinquent parents. To improve access to information on the subject, the DHHS Office of Child Support Enforcement has an Internet home page (http://www.acf.dhhs.gov/programs/cse/) that provides information on the enforcement program. Additionally, under the Personal Responsibility and Work Opportunity Act of 1996, a federal case registry and national directory of new hires was established to help address the problem of nonpayment of child support. Employers are required to report all newly hired employees to state agencies, which then transmit the information to the national directory. This makes it easier to track delinquent parents across state lines. Furthermore, states are required to establish central registries of child support orders and centralized collection and disbursement units. The law also permits states to implement tough collection techniques, including garnishing wages, seizing assets, revoking driver's and professional licenses, and, in some cases, requiring mandatory community service of individuals who are delinquent in making child support payments (DHHS, 1998b).

Factors Contributing to Poverty in Working Women

Women have steadily increased their participation in the labor force. In 1970, 43.3% of women were employed (Fullerton, 1999). In 2002, 60% of females over age 16 were employed (Business Women's Network, 2002).

Along with their participation in the labor market, women have steadily increased their earnings; however, a significant wage discrepancy still exists. In 2002, women employed full-time earned 76.5% of men's medium weekly wages (Business Women's Network, 2002). This disparity is attributed to several factors:

- About one third of women work in a cluster of "pink collar" occupations, which tend to be poorly paid when compared to male-dominated positions requiring comparable levels of responsibility, skill, and education (Fullerton, 1999) (Table 8–1 •).
- Even when women work in upper management positions and in professions dominated by men, such as law, business, or finance, they frequently make less. The wage gap widened between 1995 and 2000 (Business Women's Network, 2002).
- Seventy percent of part-time workers are women. As a result, their wages typically are lower, and they often have no benefits, such as sick leave and health insurance (Business Women's Network, 2002).

For working divorced or single women with children, the issue of child care is especially difficult. Child care is expensive and places a tremendous burden on the single parent's household budget. Moreover, with no partner to bear

Table 8–1 • FIFTEEN LEADING "PINK COLLAR" OCCUPATIONS FOR WOMEN, 2001 (IN THOUSANDS)

Occupation	Number of Women Employed	Percentage
Secretaries	2,366	98.4%
Registered nurses	2,013	93.1%
Bookkeepers/accounting	1,506	92.9%
Nursing aides	1,874	90%
Elementary school teachers	1,828	82.1%
Cashiers	2,288	76.9%
Food servers	1,029	76.4%
Investigators, adjusters	878	75%
Sales workers	925	64.9%
Auditors, accountants	975	58.8%
Secondary school teachers	763	58.5%
Sales supervisors	1,990	44.1%
Cooks	881	42.5%
Janitors	779	36%
Managers/administrators	2,486	31%

Source: Adapted from US Department of Labor. (2001). *2001 report.*

the burden, divorced or single mothers without social support must miss work when their children become ill, causing employers to view them as unreliable or uncommitted. Currently, more enlightened employers are beginning to recognize and accommodate the needs of mothers in the workforce. Like other areas of reform, however, this trend tends to benefit women in better paying, more secure positions far more than it benefits women who are poor and in low-paying positions.

Public Assistance

The US welfare system was originally designed to provide assistance to those in need—in many cases, single female heads of households and their children. Unfortunately, the system often failed to provide adequate assistance to raise families above poverty levels and, in many cases, actually provided disincentives for women to work.

In 1996 growing national concern over the failure of the system led to welfare reform via the passage of the Personal Responsibility and Work Opportunity Reconciliation Act. This comprehensive plan no longer offers unlimited support but requires that an individual work in exchange for time-limited assistance. As one of the provisions of the act, the Aid to Families with Dependent Children (AFDC) program was replaced by the Temporary Assistance for Needy Families (TANF) program. Highlights of the new welfare law include the following (DHHS, 1998a):

- States are granted unprecedented flexibility in designing welfare programs to meet the needs of their recipients, but they must demonstrate measurable results in moving families toward self-sufficiency and work.
- With few exceptions, recipients must work after 2 years on assistance. By fiscal year 2002, 50% of all families in each state must have left the welfare rolls or be engaged in work activities.
- After 5 cumulative years, families become ineligible for cash aid, although states can exempt up to 20% of their cases from the time limit provision. States can also choose to provide noncash assistance and vouchers for families that have reached the time limit using state funds or social security block grant dollars.
- The law provides $14 billion (an increase of $4 billion) in child care funding to enable mothers to have adequate child care as they move into jobs.
- Women on welfare are guaranteed continued healthcare coverage for their families, including at least 1 year of transitional Medicaid as they leave the welfare rolls for work.
- Welfare recipients must meet state work requirements, which include participation in subsidized or unsubsidized employment, community service, on-the-job training, or 12 months of vocational education. Recipients can also meet the requirement by providing child care services to others who are involved in community service.
- As discussed previously, the act also contains several provisions designed to crack down on noncustodial parents who fail to pay child support.
- For unmarried teenage parents, the law has provisions mandating that they live at home (or in an adult-supervised setting) and stay in school in order to receive assistance.

Several trends have emerged as a result of the welfare reform efforts. A report that compared welfare enrollees before and after the TANF changes indicated that more single women on welfare are living with partners. There was an increase in adults on welfare working for pay. Although many of these enrollees faced multiple barriers to employment (poor health, limited education, minimal work experience, and family responsibilities), the number of individuals who gained employment increased from 5% to 20%. Early results of welfare changes are promising in that more recipients are working. There is some concern that individuals who are working may not have engaged in long-term training that could enable them to maintain long-term employment (Zedlewski & Alderson, 2001). Although results appear favorable, it is too early to judge more long-term effects of the welfare reform policy.

Homelessness

For many people the thought of a homeless person conjures up a vision of an older man curled in a doorway or making a home under a bridge. However, this vision is less accurate today than in the past; today's homeless people have very different characteristics. It is estimated that by 2010, 1.7 billion people in the United States will have been homeless at one time in their lives. Homeless families represent the fastest growing group of homeless, having increased to 40%. Many of these families are composed of single mothers and their children. In addition, single childless women make up 14% of the homeless population (US Conference of Mayors, 2001).

FACTORS CONTRIBUTING TO HOMELESSNESS

A major factor contributing to the incidence of homelessness is domestic violence. Research suggests that many homeless women and their children are fleeing from an abusive situation (US Conference of Mayors, 2001).

A second factor contributing to homelessness is the lack of affordable housing. During the past 20 years, housing costs have increased far more than wages or other income sources, especially for women. In many communities, low-income housing has waiting lists of several hundred families. Domestic violence and lack of affordable housing are interrelated factors contributing to women's homelessness. It is estimated that as many as 85% of women return to abusive living situations following unsuccessful attempts to find adequate affordable housing. Many women who have been victims of domestic violence lack rental and employment histories or have poor credit; all are barriers to finding adequate housing and can lead to homelessness (Reif & Krisher, 2000).

Other factors that contribute to homelessness (in order of frequency) include low-paying jobs, substance abuse, untreated mental illnesses, domestic violence, unemployment, poverty, prison release, and changes and cuts in public assistance programs. African Americans make up 50% of the homeless population; 35% are Caucasian, 12% Hispanic, 2% Native American, and 1% Asian (US Conference of Mayors, 2001). The incidence of homelessness is also related to the extent of a woman's social support system. Because middle-class women typically have relatives and friends with more space and resources, they are able to avoid becoming homeless to a greater extent than poorer women. A rising concern exists that the nation's weak economy and the job losses associated with the terrorist attacks of September 11, 2001 are also having a negative impact on the incidence of homelessness (US Conference of Mayors, 2001).

HEALTH RISKS OF HOMELESS WOMEN AND CHILDREN

Homeless women and children experience greater health risks and problems than do people in the general population. Malnutrition predisposes homeless people to a variety of respiratory and nutritional disorders. Moreover, a disproportionately high number of homeless women and children have not received preventive healthcare services, such as screening tests and immunizations.

Homeless women who are pregnant are a special challenge for healthcare providers. Inadequate prenatal care, limited access to general healthcare, poor nutrition, and inadequate housing lead to poor birth outcomes, including an increased incidence of low-birth-weight newborns and a higher rate of infant mortality. In addition, as a group they are at risk for many illnesses that could negatively affect their pregnancies, including substance abuse, sexually transmitted infections, and hepatitis A, B, and C (National Coalition for the Homeless, 1998).

Effects of Poverty on Women's Healthcare

The effects of poverty on women's healthcare are extensive. Since 1981, many funding cuts have reduced or eliminated programs that used to help families in poverty access healthcare. These cuts have come at a time when the benefits of adequate nutrition and prenatal care have been documented to yield significant healthcare benefits for every dollar spent.

Medicaid is the major US program providing healthcare to low-income people in four categories: children, adults in families, the elderly, and blind and disabled people. Traditionally Medicaid has played an important role in financing maternity care, covering the costs of about 40% of births in the United States. It seems likely that the number of women on Medicaid will decrease in the next few years because welfare reform measures eliminate the automatic connection between TANF and Medicaid and significantly decrease the number of women eligible for Medicaid assistance. In addition, newly established policies requiring that women apply separately for Medicaid may cause a drop in the number of enrollees (Gonen, 1998).

Lack of health insurance is also a major problem for the poor. Thirty-seven million Americans have no health insurance, and another 7 to 10 million have inadequate coverage (Gonen, 1998). Decreases in health insurance have led to declines in preventive healthcare that are costing dollars and even lives. Women who do not receive prenatal care are three times more likely to have low-birth-weight babies, and the incidence of low-birth-weight babies is increasing. Women who receive adequate prenatal care are less likely to develop severe complications, such as preterm labor. Moreover, lack of prenatal care is a risk factor for infant morbidity and mortality.

The issue of women and poverty is critical, and the implications for childbearing care are very real. A pregnant woman who is suffering economically may also suffer physically and psychologically. In the end, it is often the children who suffer the most, bearing the physical and psychologic scars of their mothers' struggles.

As healthcare professionals, nurses should be concerned about the issue of women and poverty. The limited resources of these women often frustrates nurses' efforts to provide quality care. Nurses need to explore their own beliefs about poverty and public assistance programs and inform others about the barriers impoverished women face.

When assessing a woman's financial resources, the nurse asks questions in a sensitive manner to identify women at risk for inadequate resources or housing. Counseling can be provided along with an assessment of financial resources. Some women may not have the economic resources to buy infant supplies or other medical supplies that may be needed in the home setting. A nurse who is knowledgeable about community resources and who can provide the woman with follow-up contacts and phone numbers provides an immeasurable service to impoverished clients.

Nurses can also assist impoverished women by working with community groups and organizations and becoming actively involved in the political process. Many nurses use their work experience to present their views to legislators, support various childbearing programs, and alert legislators to legislation that would benefit mothers and families. Finally, nurse researchers can explore medical and social issues related to the impact of poverty on families.

Social Issues Affecting Women in the Workplace

As a result of political and social changes that began in the early 1970s, women's career options have expanded dramatically. Although many women still choose the traditional "women's" careers or choose to stay home full-time to raise children, others are entering occupations that until recently were reserved for men. More women than ever have joined the ranks of lawyers and judges, authors and artists, managers and corporate heads, scientists, engineers, legislators, construction workers, plumbers, and electricians, and thus are sharing in the benefits that come with these positions.

Progress has its costs, however. For example, the woman with both a career and a family may experience tremendous day-to-day stress in attempting to fulfill both her professional and mothering roles. The woman who would like nothing more than to be a stay-at-home mother may be forced by financial pressures to work outside the home and entrust the care of her children to others. Women who do stay at home to raise their children sacrifice earnings, retirement savings, and social security benefits, and have decreased opportunities for social contact and intellectual stimulation. In contrast, the woman who has devoted her prime childbearing years to establishing a career rather than a family may feel a deep sense of loss as she ages.

Several social issues affect women in the workplace. Key among these are wage discrepancy, maternity/paternity leave issues, child care, and environmental hazards.

Wage Discrepancy

The discrepancy between men's and women's wages springs from many factors. In the past, women's wages were purposely set lower than men's simply because it was a woman doing the job. The work of men and women was not valued equally. Unfortunately this belief still lingers, negatively affecting women's wages.

Women's socialization may also contribute to wage discrepancy. Boys are encouraged to develop a competitive spirit first in sports and then in other areas of their lives. They learn that "being a winner" and "knowing how to play the game" are valued qualities. Girls may not be encouraged to develop a competitive spirit; many cultures do not view competitiveness as an important or desirable trait for a girl to have. Some girls learn from parents, the media, their peers, and others that physical attractiveness, not intelligence or hard work, is the key to popularity and success. For a complete discussion on the choices women make regarding employment issues, see S. R. Reis, *Work Left Undone: Choices and Compromises of Talented Females* (Mansfield Center, CT: Creative Learning Press).

Until recently, women's lower level of education was also a significant factor in wage discrepancy. Fortunately, parents, educators, and other concerned citizens have lobbied successfully for programs to encourage girls to explore a wide range of academic pursuits and career options, especially in fields not traditionally seen as welcoming to women. As a result, the Department of Labor has developed a mentoring program that encourages girls to seek nontraditional careers. When girls have more positive experiences in academic settings, they are more likely to pursue higher education and higher paying jobs, which leads to a decrease in wage discrepancy.

Currently, several factors are exerting a positive influence on the issue of wage discrimination.

- The number of women obtaining a college degree continues to increase, and these women influence the work environment as they enter the workforce. Since 1982 more American women have earned bachelor's degrees than American men. Current estimates suggest that 26% of American adults over age 25 have earned a bachelor's degree or higher (US Census Bureau, 2002).
- As noted earlier, more women are entering professions previously dominated by men. For example, the percentage of women lawyers has increased from 15% in 1983 to 29.7% in 2001; during the same period, the percentage of women engineers increased from 13.3% to 17.9%, and the percentage of women physicians increased from 7.6% in 1970 to 24% in 2001 (Society of Women Engineers, 2001; American Medical Association [AMA], 2002).
- Many working women are holding jobs for extended periods and are not as likely to work for short periods. They are gaining more experience in performing their jobs, which has a positive effect on their productivity and chances for promotion. As productivity and job level rise, wages generally rise as well.
- Women have begun to create their own employment opportunities. In 2002, 25% of privately owned businesses were owned by women (Department of Labor, 2002).
- Women have become more involved in the political arena and are raising the issue of wage discrepancy.

Clinical Tip *Speaking out about issues that affect women, children, and families is an integral part of maternal-child nursing. It is difficult for many nurses to do this, so you should practice with friends and family frequently. Be prepared with accurate information, and try various techniques for presenting the information. A friendly, supportive audience helps you get started.*

It may seem difficult to argue against the idea that the same wages should be paid for different types of work that require comparable skills, responsibility, education, and experience. However, this basic premise, which is known as **comparable worth,** is in reality quite controversial. Opponents suggest that, to the extent that job reevaluation results in major increases in women's salaries, comparable worth will increase unemployment and inefficiency, encourage women to remain in female-dominated jobs, decrease US manufacturers' ability to compete with foreign manufacturers, and reallocate limited salary resources away from lower-class, minority men to European American middle-class women. Research suggests, however, that the costs of pay equity adjustments have been overestimated and could be accommodated if phased in gradually and logically (American Federation of Labor-Congress of Industrial Organization, 1998). Moreover, in many companies, comparable worth is a proven success. Major companies such as IBM, AT&T, and Bank of America have instituted some forms of comparable worth. At least 20 states have comparable worth legislation pending or have commissions studying the issue.

Women can combat wage discrimination in several ways. First, women should explore average wages in the community in which they are seeking employment. More wage discrepancies exist when women try to keep their salary information confidential. A high self-esteem and a feeling of self-worth can encourage women to push for wage equity. Women can work collaboratively with community leaders and legislators by informing them of lack of adequate jobs and wage discrepancies. Women can urge legislators to support legislation that enhances equal employment and wages for women. Researchers can investigate variations in salaries across the country by gender and position.

Maternity Leave Issues

Combining a career with childbearing can be a challenging task. Moreover, leaving a job to have a child may result at the very least in lost experience, most commonly in lost benefits, perhaps a lost opportunity for promotion, and sometimes loss of the job completely.

Family options improved somewhat in 1993 when the Family and Medical Leave Act (FMLA) was signed into law by President Bill Clinton. This law permits employees to take up to 12 weeks of unpaid leave from work following the birth or adoption of a child or the placement of a foster child. Employees may also take leave if faced with a personal serious illness or the illness of a spouse, child, or parent. During the leave, health insurance benefits must be continued, and employees are entitled to return to their former position or one considered comparable. Coverage is not mandated for employees who work fewer than 25 hours per week or who have been employed less than 1 year.

Because the FMLA applies only to companies with 50 or more employees, the vast majority of companies and about 25 million employees are not covered by the law. Those employees still must rely on the policies, if any, that their employers have established.

Despite the advances made in this country by the FMLA, the United States fares poorly when compared to maternity leave benefits in other countries. It is one of the few countries that has no legislation requiring a nationally *paid* maternity leave program. In other parts of the world, paid maternity leave is the rule, rather than the exception, and the funding source is often public rather than the private employer. Table 8–2 • compares maternity leave benefits in several countries.

Paternity Leave Issues

The FMLA protects new fathers as well as new mothers; however, studies show that 99% of paternity leave in the United States is unpaid and that fathers who take paternity leave feel stigmatized for taking this benefit. In other studies, men have reported that they would not take paternity leave because they feared it would hinder their careers. Companies often send out subtle messages to men that paternity leave exists only on paper. Those men who do take paternity leave are often seen as pioneers even though the law has been in effect since 1993.

Table 8-2 • MATERNITY LEAVE BENEFITS BY COUNTRY

Country	Length of Leave	Percentage of Pay Covered	Provider of Coverage
Algeria	14 weeks	100	Social Security
Australia	1 year	0	—
Belgium	15 weeks	82% for 30 days, then 75%	Social Security
Brazil	120 days	100	Social Security
Canada	17–18 weeks	55% for 15 weeks	Unemployment insurance
Chile	18 weeks	100	Social Security
China	90 days	100	Employer
Denmark	18 weeks	100	Social Security
Egypt	90 days	100	Social Security/Employer
Ethiopia	90 days	100	Employer
France	16–28 weeks	100	Social Security
Greece	16 weeks	75	Social Security
Italy	5 months	80	Social Security
Jordan	10 weeks	100	Employer
Morocco	12 weeks	100	Social Security
New Zealand	14 weeks	0	—
Pakistan	12 weeks	100	Employer
South Africa	12 weeks	45	Unemployment insurance
United Kingdom	14–18 weeks	90% for 6 weeks, flat rate after	Social Security
United States	12 weeks	0	—
Vietnam	4–6 months	100	Social Security

Source: Adapted from United Nations Statistics Division. (2000). *The World's Women 2000: Trends and statistics.*

One would assume that healthcare workers would have the most flexible maternity and paternity programs, but studies demonstrate that this is not necessarily the case. Of hospitals surveyed, 86% had a defined maternity leave policy, but only 49% had a defined paternity leave policy (AMA, 1999).

Although the global trend supports paid maternity leave, few countries have paid paternity leave. Notable exceptions are Sweden, Norway, and Denmark. Sweden provides paid leave for fathers up to 450 days; Norway allows either parent to take an additional 26 weeks of paid leave after 18 weeks have been given to the mother; and Denmark allows up to 18 weeks of paid leave for either parent (United Nations Statistics Division, 2000).

Obviously, the issue of paternity leave directly affects women. In societies where paternity leave is supported and even paid, the childrearing responsibilities can be more readily divided. Paternity leave benefits enable mothers to return to their careers while fathers care for their infants. While the majority of fathers return to work, it is estimated that 2 million American fathers care for 1.5% of children under the age of 5 on a full-time basis (Baby Center Medical Advisory Board, 2002) (Figure 8–2 •).

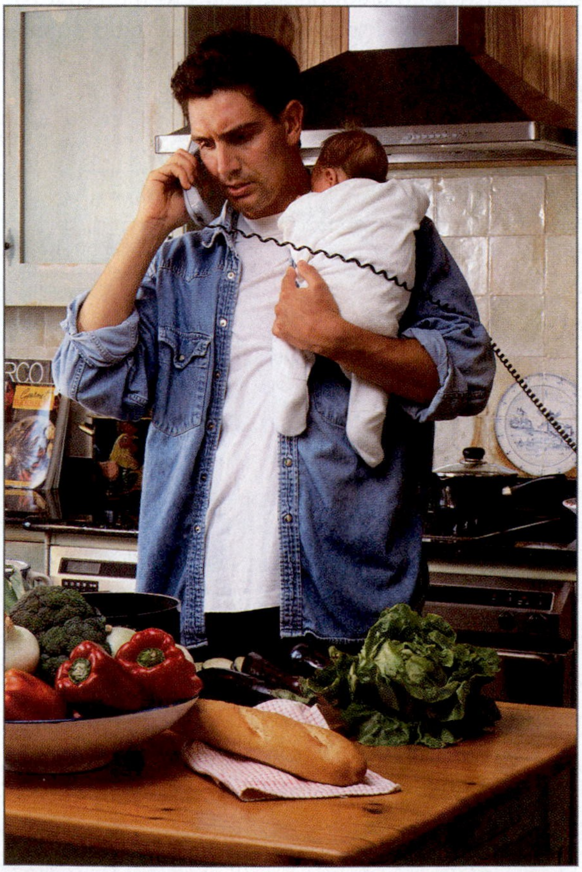

Figure 8–2 • Some women rely on the father to provide full-time child care at home while they pursue their career. Stay-at-home fathers provide only 1.5% of care to children under the age of 5 in the United States.
SOURCE: Corbis RF.

Discrimination Against Pregnant Women

Discrimination against pregnant women remains an issue in some areas, so women need to be aware of their rights, which were established by the Pregnancy Discrimination Act of 1978. This act guarantees the following:

- A pregnant woman cannot be denied a job if she is able to perform major job functions.
- The same procedure for using sick-leave pay or disability benefits must be used for the pregnant woman as for other employees.
- Employee medical coverage must include pregnancy benefits.
- The mother can use all her maternity benefits without penalty.

When a woman is planning a pregnancy, she should acquire information about pregnancy benefits in her work setting. The state in which she lives also has guidelines or regulations about pregnancy.

Child Care

Although some fathers are actively involved in meshing work and family responsibilities, child care remains predominantly a woman's issue, both because of the traditional belief that child care is "women's work," and because of the high percentage of single-parent households headed by a woman.

Access to safe, reliable child care varies. In some areas there is a surplus of child care slots, but in major metropolitan areas availability is an issue. Quality is also a major problem in most areas.

> *In contemplating starting a family, I never dreamed that child care would top my list of primary stressors. The decision to work is hard enough, but then you are faced with the inability to find safe, nurturing child care. The turnover is constant, the settings never ideal. I used to think the trick was to pay more. I was wrong there. It doesn't seem to matter how much you pay or how much you investigate, it is an unending struggle. It leaves you wishing away your children's preschool years, just so you can get past the point in their lives when you are constantly dealing with child care!*

Affordability is also a major problem. In the United States, working women commonly spend 25% of their take-home pay for child care. The average household income before taxes in 2000 was $42,148, yet full-day child care costs from $4,000 to $10,000 per year per child (US Census, Bureau 2001). In addition, the percentage that can be deducted from income taxes is quite small.

Studies have shown the benefits of high-quality child care. For example, a 7-year study by the National Institute of Child Health and Human Development (1998) found that high-quality child care was related to better mother-child relationships, lower levels of insecurity in children, fewer reports of child behavioral problems, higher cognitive and language functioning, and a higher level of school readiness. Low-quality child care was associated with strained maternal-child relationships, higher incidence of insecurity, more problem behaviors, and lower scores on cognitive, language, and school readiness scales. Clearly, the quality of child care affects both children and families.

New trends are emerging to enhance children's development with early childhood education programs. These programs are aimed at providing preschoolers with educational stimulation during the course of the day when they are in a child care setting (Figure 8–3 •). Mothers who have a college education and who work outside of the home are more likely to enroll their children in these types of programs. According to the National Institute of Child Health and Human Development (2002), children enrolled in early educational programs had higher IQ and achievement scores and were more likely to complete school than low-income minority children who were not enrolled in early childhood education programs as preschoolers.

Currently some employers provide some form of support for employees' child care needs through referral programs, on-site or near-site centers, or financial assistance. Other creative approaches to handling child care are also gaining in popularity. These include flex-time scheduling, part-time work, job sharing, and telecommuting (working at home via e-mail, phone, and fax) (Figure 8–4 •).

Another form of child care coverage, which is common among families who have the flexibility to work varying

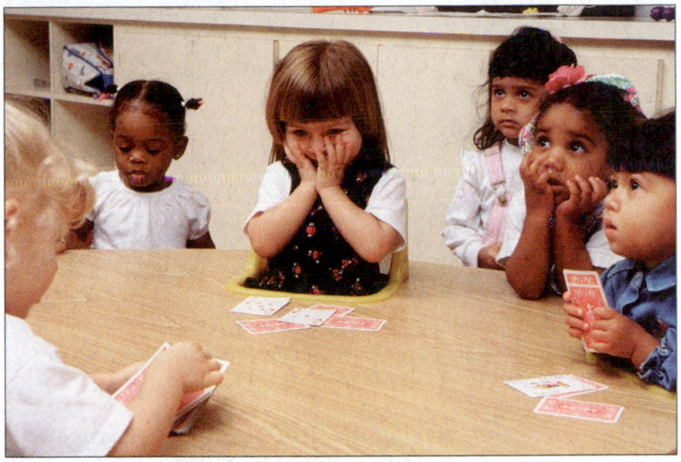

Figure 8–3 • Childhood education centers provide preschoolers with advanced skills for early education and provide care while parents work outside of the home.
SOURCE: Tom and Dee Ann McCarthy/CORBIS.

RESEARCH IN PRACTICE
Evaluating the Health Status of Grandparents Providing Child Care

What is this study about? There is a growing population of older Americans who are either primary custodians of or provide extensive childcare to their grandchildren. These families tend to be low-income, and the grandparents suffer from a variety of health problems related to the stress of caring for a second generation. These problems are exacerbated when a single grandparent–usually the grandmother–is responsible for the well-being of the grandchildren. The purpose of this study is to compare the physical, mental, and functional health status of grandparents providing extensive care to grandchildren with that of custodial grandparents and non-caregivers.

How was this study done? The subjects included 3,260 grandparents that were interviewed in the second wave of the National Survey of Families and Households, a nationally representative panel study. The subjects were categorized into groups based on the extent of the care giving role. The final categories included extensive caregivers, intermediate caregivers, occasional caregivers, non-caregivers, and custodial caregivers. Extensive care was defined as providing 30 or more hours of care per week. Intermediate was defined as 19 to 30 hours per week, occasional was defined as one to nine hours per week, and non-caregiving was defined as no babysitting during an average week. Custodial caregivers reported primary responsibility for grandchildren for six months or more. Measures included a scale describing limitations in activities of daily living, a depression scale, and two variables reflecting change in depressive symptoms or change in self-reported health status. In the last measure, respondents were asked to compare their health status to that of others their age, and whether their health status had changed.

What were the results of the study? Custodial and extensive caregivers had more depressive symptoms than intermediate caregivers. 20% of the extensive caregivers had clinically significant depression, and 40% reported at least one limitation in activities of daily living. The group also rated their own health as "declining." Custodial caregivers had even more limitations in activities of daily living. Married respondents were more likely to have stable health status than single-grandparent caregivers.

What additional questions might I have? What kinds of support do grandparents need in order to maintain their own health while raising their grandchildren? Did the circumstances under which grandparents were required to care for grandchildren affect their health status?

How can I use this study? It appears that even non-custodial grandparents with extensive caregiving responsibilities have a higher risk for depression and limitations in daily activities. This phenomenon involves a growing number of the elderly population. The effects of extensive caregiving should be assessed during health status assessment. The nurse is in a position to determine the impact of these stressors during either adult or child health visits, and to provide support to the grandparents in maintaining their own health.

Source: Minkler, M. & Fuller-Thomson, E. (2001) Physical and mental health status of American grandparents providing extensive child care to their grandchildren. *Journal of the American Medical Womens Association, 56*(4): 199–205.

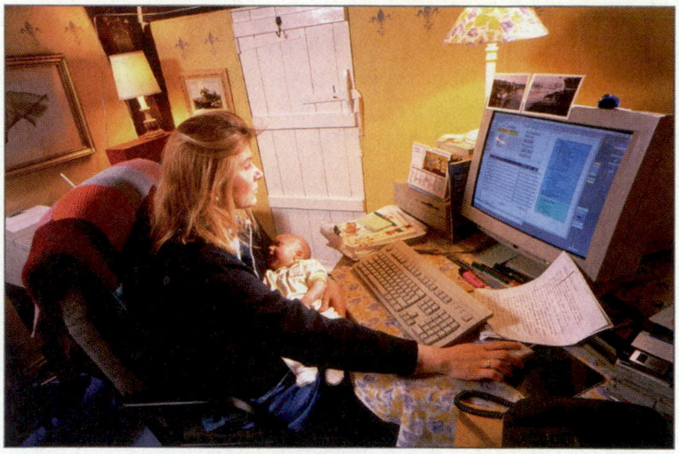

Figure 8–4 • Some mothers are able to combine professional careers with motherhood by telecommuting from a home office.
SOURCE: Getty Images, Inc.

shifts (such as nurses), involves the parents working alternating shifts to eliminate the need for outside child care assistance. While this option has advantages, such as financial benefits, it can be stressful for the parents since caring for the children may interfere with sleeping and other responsibilities.

Environmental Hazards in the Workplace

As more women enter the workforce, they may be exposed to chemicals and environmental pollutants affecting both childbearing and general health. Of the approximately 50,000 chemicals used today in industry, about 500 have been implicated as having potentially hazardous effects on reproduction. For example, exposure to volatile organic compounds, dusts, or pesticides increases the risk of female infertility (Fidler & Bernstein, 1999). Other agents, such as arsenic, formaldehyde, ethylene oxide, and benzene are associated with an increased incidence of spontaneous abortion (Turkington, 2001). Exposure to halogenated hydrocarbons such as polychlorinated biphenyls (PCBs) or anesthetic gases has been linked to both spontaneous abortion and increased incidence of infants born with congenital anomalies.

Other agents have an impact on general health. The incidence of black lung disease in the mining industry and the hazards of exposure to asbestos products are well documented and frightening. Milder chronic respiratory symptoms such as dyspnea, sinusitis, and cough are associated with other industries, including the manufacture of synthetic textiles (Zuskin, Mustajbegovic, Schachter, et al, 1998). Latex allergy is rapidly becoming a significant problem among healthcare workers, with 2% to 15% demonstrating hypersensitivity symptoms ranging from mild contact dermatitis to severe systemic reactions and anaphylactic shock (McGrath, 2000).

Lead exposure is perhaps the oldest known occupational hazard and has been linked to both reproductive and general health hazards. Increased rates of spontaneous abortion, stillbirths, and prematurity have been documented as well as decreased sperm counts and increased abnormal sperm in men who have been exposed to lead. In addition, lead exposure can cause irreversible health effects, such as central nervous system problems and decreased hearing ability (Staudinger & Roth, 1998).

Questions regarding the safety of exposure to video display terminals (VDTs) have arisen in recent years, and various studies have produced contradictory results. However, at present there is no documented evidence of increased risk of spontaneous abortion or overall fetal loss in women whose work exposed them regularly to VDTs (Pealer & Dorman, 1999). Until more is known about the possibility of other biologic effects of chronic exposure to the low-frequency electromagnetic fields found with VDTs, women should avoid chronic exposure. Because the strength of the field decreases significantly with distance, women can decrease their exposure by sitting at least 50 cm (20 inches) from the screen and at least 1 m (3.25 feet) from the sides or back of adjacent machines (electromagnetic field strength is typically higher from the back and sides). Exposure is also decreased by turning off VDTs, printers, and other electrical devices when they are not in use (Pealer & Dorman, 1998).

Nurses have an occupational hazard in the exposure inherent in providing care for sick people. Exposure to toxoplasmosis, rubella, cytomegalovirus, herpes simplex, and hepatitis B may affect pregnancy and fetal outcome (Fidler & Bernstein, 1999). Exposure to HIV infection has also been a concern to healthcare professionals.

Two governmental agencies have primary responsibility for addressing workplace safety. The Occupational Safety and Health Administration (OSHA), part of the Department of Labor, is responsible for creating and enforcing workplace health and safety regulations. The National Institute for Occupational Safety and Health (NIOSH), which is part of the Department of Health and Human Services, is primarily a research agency. However, it also disseminates information on preventing workplace injury and illness, provides training to occupational safety and health professionals, and investigates potentially hazardous working situations when requested by employers or employees (NIOSH, 2001).

Advocacy for Working Women

Before beginning employment, women should inquire about maternity, paternity, and child care benefits in the work setting. Benefit packages that include maternity leave, flexible hours, and on-site discounted child care centers are attractive to many working mothers. Women can support community groups that advocate for fair maternity leave benefits and that support pregnant women in the workplace. Women can also be actively involved in the policy-making process by lobbying their legislators for family leave, maternity and paternity benefits, child care benefits, and job protection. Nurses can play an active role by providing positive reinforcement and support to working women, serving as role models, and participating in establishing policies that support women in the workplace.

Environmental hazards are an area of particular interest and importance to maternal-newborn nurses, both personally and professionally. Nurses need to be aware of the risks that they face in their own environment and the risks that childbearing women face in theirs. Nurses can encourage administrators to investigate potential hazards in their clinical environment, and can encourage clients to take similar action to protect themselves from environmental hazards in their workplaces. The Internet can provide information and resources on specific hazards and preventive strategies to decrease risk of exposure. Nurses can also lobby community leaders and legislators to support positions that protect childbearing women from environmental toxins. Nurse researchers can investigate workforce and environmental hazards, recording, analyzing, and publishing findings.

Social Issues Affecting Older Women

In practically all countries worldwide, women comprise the majority of the older population (over age 60). That proportion increases with age so that, globally, 65% of the oldest old (80 years and older) are women. This phenomenon is called the **feminization of later life** (Ginn, Street, Arber, 2001). It occurs because women have a longer life expectancy than men, especially in developed countries, where the average difference in life expectancy between the sexes is 7 years. In developing countries, the gender gap is narrower (approximately 3 years), most likely because of higher levels of maternal mortality (United Nations Population Fund, 2000). In some developing countries, as Table 8–3 • indicates, the life span for both men and women is still less than 60 years.

Table 8-3 • YEARS OF LIFE EXPECTANCY AT BIRTH FOR SELECTED COUNTRIES, 2001

Country	Male Life Expectancy	Female Life Expectancy
Afghanistan	47	46
Argentina	72	79
Australia	77	83
Canada	76	83
China	70	74
Egypt	62	66
Ethiopia	44	46
France	75	83
India	62	63
Japan	78	84
Mexico	69	75
Russia	62	73
Tanzania	51	53
United Kingdom	75	81
United States	74	80

Source: US Census Bureau. (2001). International Programs Center, International Data Base.

Economic Vulnerability of Older Women

The feminization of later life means that older women are more likely than their male counterparts to be widowed, to live alone, to be disabled, and to be poor. However, of all the elderly in the United States, women of color have the highest poverty rates (US Census Bureau, 2000b). Factors that contribute to the increased economic vulnerability of women include the following (United Nations Population Fund, 2000):

- Women must stretch their financial resources further than men because of their longer life expectancy.
- Older women tend to have less educational preparation than older men.
- Historically women have been economically dependent on men and may have intermittent or nonexistent employment histories.
- Women typically earn less than men and often work in jobs without pension benefits or only limited benefits.
- Intermittent employment decreases women's social security and retirement benefits.
- Women generally have more family caregiving responsibilities than men.
- Women, more often than men, feel the impact of public policies and programs that place undue financial pressures on them.
- Historically, public pension systems have been designed with an expectation that men would be the primary economic providers.

Following widowhood, a middle-class woman faces the risk of "cycling into poverty," especially if her husband had a long, costly illness or if his pension shrinks or ceases following his death. To help keep elderly women from spending their final years in poverty, it is necessary for governments to develop solutions to the economic concerns caused by a fixed income, to deal with problems of pension inequity, and to address the potentially disastrous effects of staggering healthcare costs for the uninsured or underinsured.

Elder Abuse

Elder abuse is any deliberate action or lack of action that causes harm to an elderly person. Elder abuse was first recognized publicly in the mid-1980s. Currently in the United States, the incidence is estimated at 550,000 annually (Young, 2000). Experts anticipate that the problem will continue to grow as the population ages and as illness and financial burdens strain family relationships.

Five different types of elder abuse have been recognized, including psychologic abuse, physical abuse, neglect (by self or caregiver), financial abuse, and abandonment (Table 8–4 •). Multiple forms of abuse may occur simultaneously and tend to intensify with time unless intervention occurs (Young, 2000).

Typically the abuser is a family member or primary caregiver, although the problem of elder abuse by staff in

MEDIALINK NATIONAL CENTER FOR PREVENTION OF ELDER ABUSE

Table 8–4 • DEFINITIONS OF ELDER ABUSE

Physical abuse: Any physical pain or injury that is willfully inflicted upon an elderly person by an individual who cares for, has custody of, or stands in a position of trust with that elder. Includes sexual assault, physical attacks, unreasonable physical restraint, and prolonged deprivation of food and water.

Financial abuse: Any theft or misuse of an elder's money or property by a person in a position of trust.

Neglect: The failure of any person having custody or caring for an elder to provide reasonable care. Reasonable care is defined as the degree of care that a reasonable person in a like position would provide. This includes but is not limited to assistance with personal hygiene; provisions of shelter, food, and clothing; and protection from health and safety hazards. This also includes providing for medical and health needs, except in cases when the elder refuses treatment.

Self-Neglect: Failure to provide for self through inattention or dissipation. The identification of this type of case involves assessing the elder's ability to care for oneself.

Psychologic abuse: The willful infliction of mental suffering, by a person in a position of trust with an elder. This includes but is not limited to verbal assaults, threats, humilitation, intimidation, or isolation of the elder.

Abandonment: The desertion of an elder by any person responsible for the care and custody of that elder, under circumstances in which a reasonable person would continue to provide care.

Source: Adapted from the Elder Abuse Prevention: A Consortium Serving Alameda and Contra Costa Counties, Richmond, CA. (2000). *Definitions of elder abuse.*

nursing homes and long-term care facilities has been well documented. Most elder abuse happens to older (over 80) white women in domestic settings, but on the average, elderly black Americans are abandoned more than older white Americans. Abandonment statistics are much lower for Asians and Hispanics (Young, 2000).

Factors that increase the risk of elder abuse include shared living arrangements, family history of violence, lack of financial resources, dependence, isolation, poor health, and cognitive impairment. Substance abuse and stressful events in the life of the abuser may also contribute to the risk (Young, 2000).

A full discussion of this growing problem, its identification, and treatment is beyond the scope of this textbook. It is imperative, however, that nurses who care for the elderly be alert for signs of abuse and take steps to address the problem when it is identified.

Effects of Aging on Women's Healthcare

Older women face multiple barriers in obtaining adequate healthcare services. Some women have difficulty accessing needed services because of transportation issues. Although public transportation may be available in larger cities, many rural areas do not have any type of public transportation system. Other women may have public transportation available in their communities, but may not be able to use it because of the costs involved.

Lack of health coverage or non-Medicare-covered costs may also be a barrier for some women. Many of these women may opt not to fill prescriptions or receive needed services that their insurance does not cover. For women on limited incomes, paying rent and purchasing food may take priority over obtaining healthcare. Thus nurses must remain aware

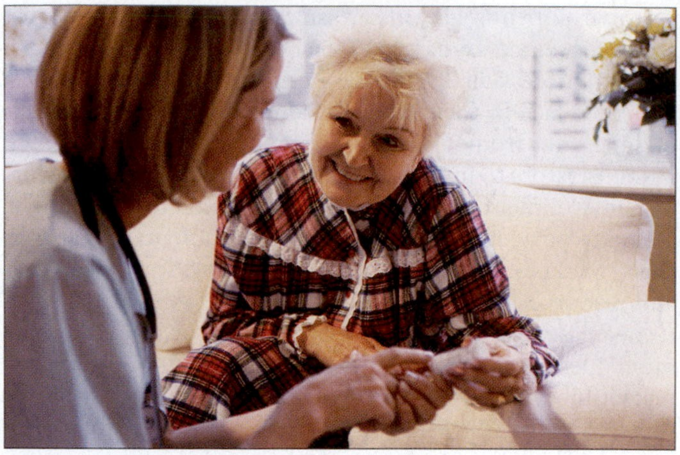

Figure 8–5 • Older women are more likely to have multiple medical conditions that require medication. Careful instructions should be given to prevent medication interactions.
SOURCE: Dann Tardif/CORBIS.

of the possibility that a client's noncompliance may actually be economically driven.

Another barrier for older women is the lack of research and attention paid to chronic diseases in women. Prior to the 1980s, most large-scale studies were based on men. Much of the data and treatment recommendations have been based on studies that excluded female subjects. Research focusing on chronic disease in women, including cardiovascular disease, is a relatively recent development.

Even when research has been conducted on women, practitioners may neglect the complex needs of older women. Many physicians treat older women using a symptom-specific approach instead of a holistic one. This may lead to misdiagnosis. For example, an older woman who complains of hot flashes at her healthcare appointment may be treated for menopausal symptoms without consideration for the possibility that her hot flashes could be attributable to a thyroid disorder. In addition, older women may develop comorbidities. By age 65, half of all women have two or more chronic diseases. These illnesses occur most often in minority and low-income women (Agency for Healthcare Research and Quality, 2002). These clients have an even greater need for a holistic approach to their care because they may be taking multiple drugs. These drugs can interact with each other and themselves become the etiology for the client's symptoms. This phenomenon is known as **polypharmacy.** Thus additional diagnoses warrant more time and attention to the older woman's needs (Figure 8–5 •). Nurses can play a key role in identifying an older woman's concerns and current and past problems, and in alerting the practitioner to specific needs. Coordinating care with all healthcare providers is essential to ensure proper care.

Social Issues Affecting Women with Disabilities

A total of 28.6 million women and girls or 21.3% of all females in the United States have some type of disability (Disability Statistics Center, 2002). Of those women with disabilities, 15.4%

are unable to perform basic care activities for themselves. Women are more likely than men to be disabled because of longer life expectancy rates, and disabilities are most prevalent in women over the age of 85. The majority of women with disabilities (56.6%) are in this age group while another 38.8% are over the age of 65 (Disability Statistics Center, 2002).

Definitions of Disability

Defining disability is often a complex task because of many varying components. In general, a **disability** is a chronic physical or mental health problem or an impairment that restricts an individual's ability to perform one or more activities. For example, *activity limitation* is the inability to perform any major activity. Major activities are age dependent. In middle-aged women, for example, it may be the inability to care for one's home and children. In elderly women, it may be the inability to care for oneself independently. *Work disability* restricts an individual from being able to work. A nurse who sustains a back injury and is unable to return to her position as a staff nurse on labor and delivery is an example of an individual with a work disability. A *severe disability* prohibits an individual from performing basic activities of daily living and requires assistance from another individual to meet basic needs. Approximately 4.7% of the population require personal assistance with one or more self-care or home management activities (McNeil, 2001).

Types of Disabilities

Various types of disability are recognized. *Developmental disabilities* are ongoing and present before the age of 22. They create severe limitations in three or more of the following areas: self-care, receptive and expressive language, learning, mobility, self-direction, ability to live alone, and financial independence. Over 4 million individuals are affected with some type of developmental disability (National Women's Health Information Center, 2002). Mental retardation is the most common (Figure 8–6 •). Other common developmental disabilities include autism, cerebral palsy, epilepsy, and spina bifida.

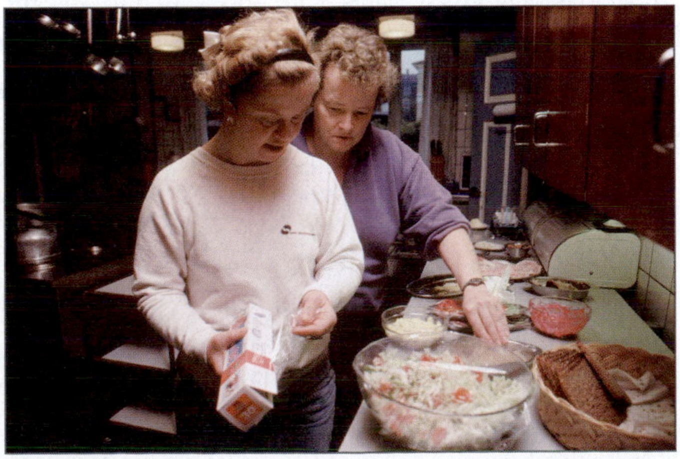

Figure 8–6 • Mental retardation is the most common developmental disability.
SOURCE: Stephanie Maze/CORBIS.

Learning disabilities, such as dyslexia and attention-deficit/hyperactivity disorder, can inhibit educational attainment and employment. *Neurologic disabilities*, including spina bifida and autoimmune diseases, affect 50 million Americans annually (National Women's Health Information Center, 2002). Multiple sclerosis (MS) is a neurologic condition that can cause severe disability through degeneration of nerve fibers in the brain and spinal cord. MS affects a disproportionately high number of women compared to men. Alzheimer dementia is another neurologic disability. *Psychiatric disabilities* can cause significant impairment and significantly alter an individual's quality of life. Women have 50% higher rates of depression, anxiety, panic disorders, and phobias than men (National Women's Health Information Center, 2002). *Sensory disabilities* such as hearing loss and visual impairments can dramatically impair a woman's ability to interact socially and to live independently.

Economic Vulnerability of Women with Disabilities

Since maintaining employment is essential for an individuals' economic well-being, disabilities that prohibit women from working leave them economically vulnerable. In the United States, many people assume that social security benefits keep individuals with disabilities out of poverty, but this is simply not the case. For example, in the year 2000, a woman earning $27,000 a year who suddenly became disabled would be eligible for only about $1250 a month. This may explain why it is estimated that 39.7% of disabled Americans who cannot work currently live in poverty (National Women's Health Information Center, 2002).

Of Americans with disabilities who do work, many can manage no more than part-time employment, which obviously limits their income potential. Even women with disabilities who work full-time may encounter wage disparities. For example, women with disabilities working full-time earn 13% less than full-time workers without disabilities (Disability Statistics Center, 2002).

The Americans with Disabilities Act (ADA) of 1990 was a legislative measure aimed at removing barriers for individuals with disabilities. Although the ADA has brought about some improvements, many barriers to employment still exist, including transportation barriers, architectural obstacles, and discrimination in general.

Violence Against People with Disabilities

Both men and women with developmental disabilities are four to ten times more likely to be victims of crime in general than people without disabilities (Disability Statistics Center, 2002). Women with developmental disabilities are 50% more likely to be sexually assaulted in their lifetime. In general, women with disabilities are more likely to have repeated acts of violence committed against them. Women with disabilities may have difficulties escaping from or fighting off an attacker, may be unable to communicate well enough to report crimes, and/or may be unable to positively identify an attacker because of sensory or cognitive limitations.

Effects of Disability on Women's Healthcare

MediaLink CARE PLAN: PREGNANCY IN DISABLED CLIENT

Women with disabilities need routine gynecologic care and preventive health education like all women, but healthcare services for these women are often suboptimal. Many women with disabilities report they do not obtain routine healthcare services because of barriers they encounter in the healthcare setting. A survey that explored why these women did not get preventive care revealed that 37% had difficulty getting onto the examination table and 29% felt their physician was not empathetic to issues related to their disability (National Women's Health Information Center, 2002).

In addition, many healthcare providers inappropriately assume women with severe disabilities are not sexually active. Based on these false assumptions, many of these women do not get appropriate education in sexually transmitted infection (STI) prevention, STI screening, contraceptive counseling, or preconception counseling.

Social Issues Affecting Lesbian and Bisexual Women

Various social issues affect lesbian and bisexual women, including employment and housing discrimination, parenting issues, and social stigmas, all of which can alter their quality of life. In addition, lesbian and bisexual women's access to and experience of healthcare services is below that of heterosexual women.

Employment Discrimination

Employment discrimination is the most frequent complaint received by the American Civil Liberties Union (ACLU) from gays and lesbians. In 1997 the Employment Non-Discrimination Act was proposed and defeated by one vote. This legislation would have made termination of employment based on sexual orientation illegal. Currently, the House and the Senate are debating a new version of the act. At present, only 11 states and the District of Columbia have laws that protect workers against discrimination based on sexual orientation (Table 8–5 •). Although some local municipalities have followed suit, 80% of states have no legislation in place to prevent employers from firing a woman solely because of her sexual orientation (Robinson, 2002).

Discrimination exists not only in the private sector, but also in the military. The battle over homosexuals in the military has raged on since President Clinton enacted the "don't ask, don't tell" policy in 1994. While this legislation removed sexual orientation as a contraindication to military service, it has been far from successful in protecting gay and lesbian service members from expulsion, and homosexual conduct is

Table 8–5 • US STATES WITH LEGISLATION TO PROTECT HOMOSEXUAL WORKERS AGAINST EMPLOYMENT DISCRIMINATION

California
Connecticut
District of Columbia
Hawaii
Massachusetts
Minnesota
Nevada
New Hampshire
New Jersey
Rhode Island
Vermont
Wisconsin

still grounds for terminating their service. Homosexual conduct includes not only homosexual acts, but also statements that demonstrate a propensity or intent to engage in homosexual acts (Dorn, 1994). In short, lesbian women can serve in the military, but if their sexual orientation becomes known, they can be asked to resign. Indeed, a record number of discharges occurred in 2001. Gay or lesbian discharges totaled 1250, the highest number since 1987, and 30% of discharges for homosexual orientation were women (Servicemembers Legal Defense Network, 2002).

Lesbians face additional discrimination in terms of availability of benefits for their partners who are not legally their spouses. Marriage is not only a personal partnership, but also a legal contract conveying certain rights and responsibilities. While married heterosexuals can receive health insurance coverage, life insurance benefits, retirement pensions, and disability coverage for their partners, lesbian partners—because they are not legally married—cannot. Many lesbians in long-term relationships wish to formalize their union; however, Hawaii and Vermont are currently the only states that recognize same-sex marriage. Only seven states (Washington, Oregon, California, New York, Massachusetts, Connecticut, and Vermont) and the District of Columbia have "domestic partnership" statutes, providing that benefits be paid for same-sex partners. An additional 50 cities and counties, and over 2000 private employers, also offer domestic partnership benefits (ACLU, 2002). Nevertheless, the vast majority of lesbian couples in the United States have no such benefits.

Housing Discrimination

Lesbians also face housing discrimination. The Fair Housing laws apply to broad groups, including pregnant women and families with children; however, same-sex partners do not receive protection under this legislation. Although some cities and counties have enacted this type of legislation, lesbians remain largely unprotected. Additionally, lesbian couples may not be able to report a combined income when purchasing real estate or securing a rental property, rendering them ineligible for property they truly can afford. On the other hand, lesbians may be unfairly disqualified from low-income housing. If one of the partners is working and the other is raising their children, the working partner may not be able to claim her partner or children as dependents—again, because the partners are not legally married.

Parenting Issues

Another inconsistency between heterosexuals and homosexuals involves parenting issues. Many lesbian couples find themselves in the role of coparent, stepparent, or adoptive parent. Legislation in many states makes it difficult for lesbian families to have custody or adopt their partner's children from a previous relationship; however, there have been cases where a lesbian parent's partner has successfully adopted the child. *Second-parent adoption* enables the other parent to adopt the child, legally permitting the child to have the benefit of two legal parents (ACLU, 1999). These types of adoptions ensure stability for the child in case the biologic parent becomes incapacitated or dies. In addition, some agencies that facilitate foreign adoptions routinely disqualify lesbian couples, in some cases because the country involved refuses to permit adoption of its children into homosexual families.

Homosexual couples who may wish to adopt a child together may also face discrimination from both public or private agencies. Currently, 22 states allow for homosexual couples to adopt children legally. These states base adoption decisions on "the best interest of the child." Several states have legislation in place that prohibits homosexual couples from adopting children, including Florida and New Hampshire (ACLU, 1999). Homosexual couples may also have difficulty in serving as foster parents, even though there is an abundance of children who need foster homes and the stability of a family. For example, Arkansas prohibits homosexual couples from serving as foster parents (ACLU, 1999). Although legislation may be in place to protect the rights of homosexual couples who wish to adopt or serve as foster parents, discrimination, legal or not, continues to exist. While many people raise concerns about the effects on children of being raised by same-sex parents, research has not shown any negative effect. In 2002 the American Academy of Pediatrics (AAP) issued a policy statement after reviewing decades of research data that examined children raised by a lesbian or gay parent. No differences were observed between children raised by heterosexual or homosexual parents (AAP, 2002) (Figure 8–7 •).

Social Barriers

Same-sex couples face daily discrimination—and even danger—by mainstream society. At the very least, they may be treated differently or ostracized from business networks, family gatherings, or church or neighborhood functions. At the worst, they may become victims of hate crimes. In 2000, 1300 hate crimes were perpetrated that were based solely on the individuals' sexual orientation (US Department of Justice, 2001). Many lesbians live in fear for their own safety and security, making it more difficult to declare their sexual orientation to outsiders.

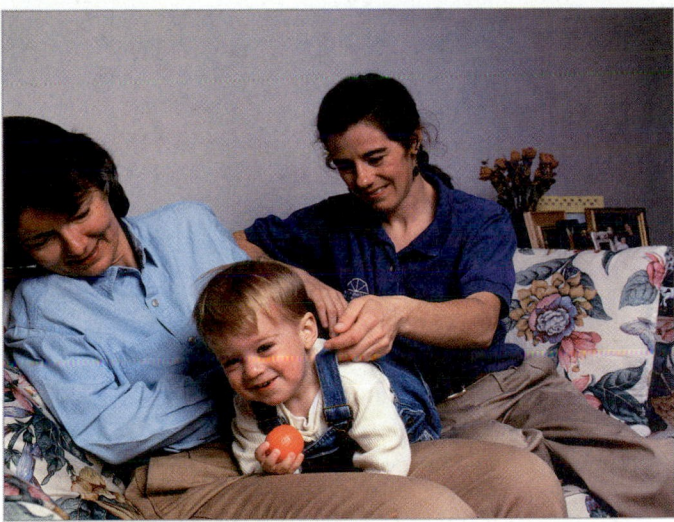

Figure 8–7 • Lesbian families face discrimination that more traditional families do not commonly encounter.
SOURCE: Vanessa Vick/Photo Researchers, Inc.

The road to equality for all women is still largely untraveled, and for lesbians, the burden of discrimination is even greater than for heterosexuals. The last decade introduced multiple legislative efforts to combat discrimination; however, many barriers and inadequacies still exist for this group of women.

Effects of Discrimination on Women's Healthcare

Lesbian and bisexual women may have less access to healthcare services than heterosexual women, and those with access may not use preventive healthcare services as readily because of fear of discrimination. Lesbian and bisexual women are less likely than heterosexual women to have health insurance. In addition, these women face risks from healthcare providers who assume all clients are heterosexual or who are homophobic. Many of these women do not tell their healthcare providers their sexual orientation because of the stigma that still exists. Even worse, fear keeps many in this population from seeking healthcare altogether.

This lack of adequate healthcare is evident when one views the increased risk for cervical and breast cancer within the lesbian population. A national survey found that only 54% of lesbian and bisexual women have had a Pap smear in the last 12 months. Many lesbians believe they are not at risk for cervical cancer even though in one study of women who had no history of sex with men, 14% of them had cervical lesions (Lee, 2000). Further, lesbian and bisexual women are at increased risk for breast cancer because they smoke cigarettes in higher numbers and they are less likely to use oral contraceptives.

CHAPTER REVIEW

EXPLOREMEDIALINK

NCLEX review questions, case studies, and other interactive resources for this chapter can be found on the Web site at http://www.prenhall.com/olds. Click on "Chapter 8" to select the activities for this chapter.

For tutorials including animations and videos, more NCLEX review questions, and an audio glossary, access the accompanying CD-ROM in this book.

Focus Your Study

- The number of women living in poverty is increasing at a rapid rate. Childbearing women seem to be at particular risk because of current trends in the divorce rate, the frequency with which the mother gains custody of children, and factors in the work environment that make it difficult for women to earn a good wage.
- Homeless families represent the fastest growing group.
- Nurses need to be aware of issues affecting the childbearing woman so that they can better understand the client as she comes to the maternal-newborn healthcare setting.
- Women's wages have always been lower than men's because of demand, education, skills, discrimination, and underlying philosophies that deem women's work less valuable. Many people are working to change the wage system by pushing for comparable worth legislation.
- Work benefits that affect women include maternity leave, paternity leave, and child care. The Family and Medical Leave Act ensures leave for childbirth or adoption but applies only to companies with 50 or more employees. Insurance coverage for childbirth varies by company.
- Elder abuse includes physical abuse, financial abuse, neglect, self-neglect, psychologic abuse, and abandonment.
- Older women may face multiple barriers when obtaining healthcare, including transportation difficulties, lack of health coverage, lack of research regarding chronic conditions affecting women, and symptom-specific, rather than holistic care.
- There are multiple types of disabilities. All have the potential for limiting a woman's quality of life and her ability to care for herself.
- Lesbian and bisexual women face various forms of discrimination in their daily lives.

References

Agency for Healthcare Research and Quality (AHRQ). (2002). *AHRQ focus on research: Healthcare for women.* Washington, DC: Author. Retrieved on August 4, 2002 from http://www.ahrq.gov/news/focus/focwomen.htm

American Academy of Pediatrics (AAP). (2002). Technical report: Coparent or second-parent adoption by same-sex parents. *AAP Policy Statement, 109*(2), 341–344.

American Civil Liberties Union (ACLU). (1999). *ACLU fact sheet: Overview of lesbian and gay parenting, adoption and foster care.* New York: Author.

American Civil Liberties Union (ACLU). (2002). *The ACLU's lesbian and gay rights project: What we are and what we do.* New York: Author.

American Federal, State, County & Municipal Employees (AFSCME). (2002). *Protecting the rights of women and working families during an economic crisis.* Washington, DC: Author. Retrieved on September 19, 2002 from http://www.afscme.org

American Federation of Labor-Congress of Industrial Organization (AFL-CIO). (1998). Its time for working women to earn equal pay. Retrieved on December 18, 2002 from www.aflcio.org

American Medical Association (AMA). (1999, April). Parental leave and pediatric residents. *Archives of Pediatrics & Adolescent Medicine, 153*(4), 429–430.

American Medical Association (AMA). (2002). *Women physician statistics.* Washington, DC: Author.

Baby Center Medical Advisory Board. (2002). *Stay-at-home parents.* Retrieved on September 20, 2002 from www.babycenter.com

Business Women's Network. (2002). Women and Diversity, Facts 2002. Washington, DC: Author.

Crenshaw, K. (2000). Mapping the margins: Intersectionality, identity politics, and violence against women of color. 43, Stan L Rev.1241, 1245–1246 as cited in E. Schneider, *Battered women and feminist lawmaking* p. 63, New Haven, CT: Yale University Press.

Dalaker, J., & Proctor, B. D. (2002). *US Census Bureau, current population reports, series P60-210, poverty in the US: 1999.* Washington, DC: US Government Printing Office.

Department of Health and Human Services (DHHS). (1998a, February 24). Annual update of the HHS poverty guidelines. *Federal Register, 63*(36), 9235–9238. Retrieved on December 20, 2002 from wais.access.gpo.gov

Department of Health and Human Services (DHHS). (1998b, March 17). *Child support enforcement: A Clinton administration policy* (Fact Sheet). Retrieved on September 16, 2002 from http://www.hhs.gov/news/press/1998pres/980317b.html

Department of Health and Human Services (DHHS). (1998c, May 27). *The Personal Responsibility and Work Opportunity Reconciliation Act of 1996* (Fact Sheet). Retrieved on September 16, 2002 from http://www.hhs.gov/news/press/1998pres/980509.html

Department of Health and Human Services (DHHS). (1998d). *Searching for the right fit: Homelessness and Medicaid managed care.* Washington, DC: Author.

Department of Health and Human Services (DHHS). (2000, December 6). *New statistics show only small percentage of eligible families receive child care help* (HHS News Release). Washington, DC: Author.

Department of Health and Human Services (DHHS). (2002). Annual update of the HHS poverty guidelines. *Federal Register, 67*, 31. Washington, DC: Author.

Department of Labor. (2002). Women's Bureau Publication on Women-owned businesses, Washington, DC: Author.

Disability Statistics Center. (2002). *How does the Disability Statistics Center define disability?* San Francisco: Author.

Dorn, E. (1994, July 3). *Memorandum for the Assistant Secretary of the Army: Training guidance for DOD policy on homosexual conduct in the armed forces.* Washington, DC: Department of the Army.

Fidler, A. T., & Bernstein, J. (1999). Infertility: From a personal to a public health problem. *Public Health Reports, 114*(6), 494.

Fields, J., & Casper, M. L. (2001). *US Census Bureau, current population reports, series P20-537, America's families and living arrangements: 2000.* Washington, DC: US Census Bureau.

Fullerton, H. N. (1999, November). The labor force: Steady growth, changing composition. *Monthly Labor Review, 122*(11), 19–32.

Ginn, J., Street, D., and Arber, S. (2001). Women, work, and pensions: International issues and prospects. Buckingham, UK: Open University Press.

Gonen, J. S. (1998, January). *Medicaid managed care: The challenge of providing care to low-income women* (Briefing Paper). Washington, DC: Jacob's Institute of Women's Health.

Lee, R. (2000). Healthcare problems of lesbian, gay, bisexual and transgender patients. *Western Journal of Medicine, 172*(6), 403.

McGrath, D. (2000, September 18). The ADA and latex allergy: Nothing to sneeze at. *Healthcare Review, 13*(8), 16.

McNeil, J. M. (2001). Americans with disabilities: Household economic studies. *US Bureau of the Census, Current Populations Reports* (pp. 70–73). Washington, DC: US Government Printing Office.

National Center for Education Statistics (NCES). (2000). *Education attainment* (Table 38–3). Washington, DC: NCES, Office of Education Research and Improvement, US Department of Education. Retrieved on September 16, 2002 from http://nces.ed.gov/pubs2000/coe2000/section3/s_table38_3.html

National Coalition for the Homeless (NCH). (1998, May). *Domestic violence and homelessness* (NCH Fact Sheet No. 8). Retrieved on September 16, 2002 from http://nch.ari.net/domestic.html

National Institute of Child Health and Human Development (NICHD). (1998). *NICHD study of early child care.* Bethesda, MD: Author.

National Institute of Child Health and Human Development (NICHD). (2002). *America's children: Indicators of well-being 2002.* Bethesda, MD: Author.

National Institute for Occupational Safety and Health (NIOSH). (2001, April). *NIOSH facts.* Retrieved on November 22, 2002 from http://www.cdc.gov/niosh/nioshfs.html

National Women's Health Information Center. (2002). *Women with disabilities.* Washington, DC: The Office of Women's Health, US Department of Health and Human Services.

Pealer, L. N., & Dorman, S. M. (1999, September). Video display terminals: Safe use guidelines. *Journal of School Health, 68*(7), 307–327.

Pearce, D. M. (1993). Something old, something new: Women's poverty in the 1990's. In S. Matteo (Ed.), *American women in the nineties.* Boston: Northeastern University Press.

Reif, S. A., & Krisher, L. J. (2000, May-June). Subsidized housing and the unique needs of domestic violence victims. Clearinghouse Rev. 20. Washington, DC: National Network to End Domestic Violence (NNEDV).

Robinson, B. A. (2002). *Employment discrimination against gays and lesbians.* Kingston, Ontario: Ontario Consultants on Religious Tolerance.

Servicemembers Legal Defense Network. (2002, March 14). *Conduct unbecoming: The 8th annual report on "don't ask, don't tell."* Washington, DC: Author Retrieved on September 16, 2002 from http://www.sldn.org/templates/law/record.html?record=473

Shalala, D. (1998, February 6). *Welfare reform.* Remarks presented to the American Enterprise Institute. Washington, DC.

Society of Women Engineers. (2001). *Statistics about women in engineering in the USA.* Chicago: Author.

Staudinger, K. C., & Roth, V. S. (1998, February 15). Occupational lead poisoning. *American Family Physician, 57*(4), 719–726, 731–732.

Turkington, C. A. (2001). Miscarriage. In *Gale encyclopedia of medicine* (2nd ed.). Stanford, CT: Gale Group.

United Nations Population Fund. (2000). *1999 annual report.* New York: Author.

United Nations Statistics Division. (2000). *The world's women 2000: Trends and statistics. Maternity leave benefits, as of 1998.* New York: United Nations.

US Census Bureau. (1997). Labor force, employment, and earnings. In *Statistical abstract of the United States* (117th ed.). Washington, DC: US Department of Commerce, Bureau of the Census.

US Census Bureau. (1998, February 24). *Women's history month: March 1–31. Census Bureau facts for features.* Washington, DC: US Census Bureau Public Information Office.

US Census Bureau. (2000a). *International data base summary of demographic data.* Washington, DC: Author.

US Census Bureau. (2000b, March). *Current population survey.* Washington, DC: Author.

US Census Bureau. (2001, March). *Current population survey.* Washington, DC: Author.

US Census Bureau. (2002). Census Bureau report shows "big payoff" from educational degrees. Retrieved on December 18, 2002 from www.census.gov/press-release/www/2000/cb02-95.html

US Conference of Mayors. (1999). *A status report on hunger and homelessness in America's cities 1999: A 26-city survey December 1999.* New York: Author.

US Conference of Mayors. (2001). *Hanger and homelessness up sharply in major US cities.* New York: Author.

US Department of Commerce. (2001, September 25). *Nation's household income stable in 2000: Poverty level virtually equals record low, Census report* (Press Release). Washington, DC: US Department of Commerce, Bureau of the Census.

US Department of Justice. (2001). *Uniform crime reporting program: 2000 report.* Washington, DC: Author.

US Department of Labor. (2001). Bureau of Labor Statistics, Report on the American Work Force, 2001. Retrieved on October 18, 2002 from www.bls.gov/opub/rtaw/pdf/rtaw2001.pdf

Warren, E. (2002, February 28). *Perspectives on the effects of bankruptcy for women.* Alliance of Independent Feminists Lecture, Harvard Law School.

Young, M. G. (2000, October 30). Recognizing the signs of elder abuse. *Patient Care, 34*(20), 56.

Zedlewski, S. R., & Alderson, D. W. (2001). *Before and after reform: How have families on welfare changed?* Washington, DC: Urban Institute.

Zuskin, E., Mustajbegovic, J., Schachter, E. N., Kern, J., Budak, A., & Godnic-Cvar, J. (1998). Respiratory findings in synthetic textile workers. *American Journal of Industrial Medicine, 33*(3), 263–273.

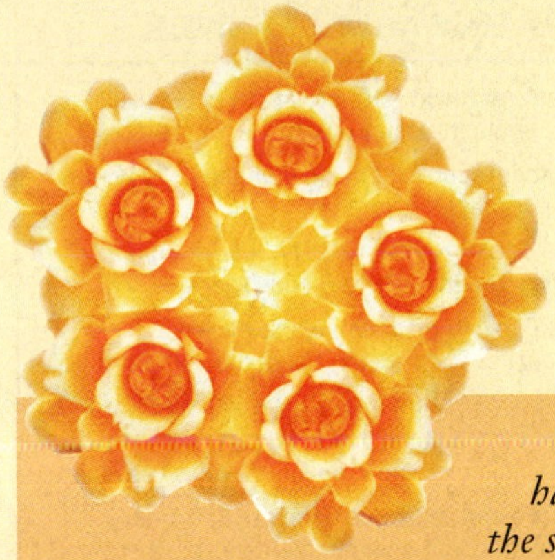

9 Violence Against Women

To my friends I'm living the American dream. My husband is a successful broker; we have a lovely house; we take exotic vacations. Even if I told them about the occasional slap, the shove, the sex when I really didn't want it, they would think it was probably worth putting up with it. Sometimes I do think about leaving, but it would mean admitting I failed. Even as I tell you this, I know it doesn't make sense—he does the hitting, but I feel ashamed. I'm not a battered wife; I can't be. My husband just has a quick temper.

Objectives

- List the social, psychologic, political, and cultural factors that contribute to the occurrence of domestic violence and rape.
- Describe ways in which psychologic, physical, and sexual abuse are used by batterers to maintain power and control in abusive relationships.
- Contrast the myths and the facts about domestic violence and rape.
- Identify the phases of the cycle of violence.
- Compare the characteristics of batterers to the characteristics of rapists.
- Delineate the role of the nurse in caring for women who have experienced battering.
- Articulate proper procedures for the screening, assessment, and documentation of abuse.
- Describe the needs that abused women and children may have, beyond the healthcare setting.
- Compare the types of rape.
- Identify the phases of the rape trauma syndrome.
- Identify drugs commonly used in drug-facilitated sexual assault.
- Explain the reasons why nurses who care for rape survivors should first explore their personal values and beliefs about rape.
- Discuss the nurse's role as client advocate and counselor with domestic violence and rape survivors.
- Summarize the procedures for collecting and preserving physical evidence of sexual assault.
- Discuss the legal responsibilities of the community to prevent and address violence against women.

Key Terms

Cycle of violence 175
Date rape 184
Domestic violence 172
Rape 182
Rape trauma syndrome 184
Vicarious trauma 189

MediaLink

Additional resources for this content can be found on the Student CD-ROM and on the Companion Website at www.prenhall.com/olds. Click on "Chapter 9" to select the activities for this chapter.

CD-ROM
- Audio Glossary
- NCLEX Review
- Video: Spousal Abuse
- Video: Parental Sexual Abuse
- Video: Going Back?

Companion Website
- Additional NCLEX Review
- Case Study: Teenage Rape Victim
- Care Plan Activity: Suspicious Injury and Bruises

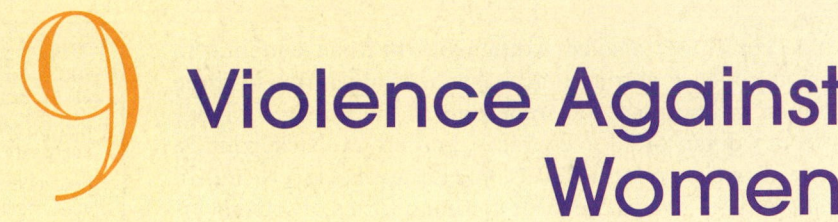

MEDIALINK SPOUSAL ABUSE VIDEO

Violence against women has become endemic in society today. Experts suggest that as many as one in three women will be abused at some time in their lives. Violence affects women of all ages, races, and ethnic backgrounds, from all socioeconomic levels, all educational levels, and all walks of life. Two of the most common forms of societal violence are domestic violence and rape, the topics of this chapter. Perhaps surprisingly, these two types of violence are primarily perpetrated by intimate partners. In one study, nearly two thirds of the women who reported being raped, physically assaulted, and/or stalked since age 18 were victimized by a current or former husband, cohabiting partner, boyfriend, or date (Tjaden & Thoennes, 2000). Further, evidence indicates that a significant proportion of all female homicide victims are killed by their intimate partners.

Violence against women is a major health concern. In addition to injuries sustained during violent episodes, physical, sexual, and psychologic violence are linked to a number of adverse physical and mental health outcomes. Moreover, violence against women costs the healthcare system millions of dollars and thousands of lives each year.

Since the early 1980s healthcare providers and organizations have worked to address this issue. Over the past two decades there have been a number of notable changes in healthcare policy and practices aimed at responding to this issue. In 1990 the Joint Commission on the Accreditation of Hospitals and Healthcare Organizations (JCAHO) mandated the development of protocols for the identification and treatment of women who have been abused by their intimate partners. Healthy People 2010, a national health promotion and disease prevention project, cites intervention and prevention for violent behavior as a national priority, and specifically includes a reduction in violence against women in its summary report objectives. In 1991 the American Nurses Association (ANA) authored a position statement advocating education for all nurses in identifying and preventing violence against women (Table 9–1 •). Significantly, nursing has played and continues to play a key role in developing and evaluating innovative healthcare practices aimed at identifying and reducing violence against women.

Table 9–1 • ACTIONS SUPPORTED BY THE ANA TO COMBAT VIOLENCE AGAINST WOMEN

- Routine education of all nurses and healthcare providers in the skills necessary to prevent violence against women.
- Routine assessment and documentation for physical abuse of all women in any healthcare institution or community setting.
- Targeted assessment of women at increased risk of abuse, including pregnant women and women presenting in emergency rooms.
- Education of all women as to the cycle of violence, the potential for homicide, and community resources for primary, secondary, and tertiary prevention and care.
- Inclusion of the topic of violence against women in every undergraduate nursing curriculum.
- Education of school-age children and adolescents in public schools about relationships without violence and community resources for help.
- Research on violence against women, including the development and evaluation of nursing models for preventive assessment, intervention, and treatment for abused women, their children, and perpetrators of violence.

Source: *American Nurses Association Position Statement Physical Violence Against Women* issued September 6, 1991. http://nursingworld.org/readroom/position/social/scuiol.htm

Historical Factors Contributing to Violence Against Women

Violence against women is not new. Throughout history, for thousands of years in patriarchal societies, women have been victims of violence. Within the institution of marriage, wives were considered the property of husbands, subject to their wishes and demands. A husband had the right—even the duty—to "keep her in line," even to kill her. The phrase "rule of thumb" comes from the judicial restriction that when a man beat his wife, the stick he used could be no larger around than the width of his thumb. Outsiders were expected to "keep out of it"; battering was a family matter.

The legal status of women has improved over the years in many cultures. However, many people still hold to the traditional views of male dominance in marriage or any intimate relationship, which can contribute to the occurrence of domestic violence and rape. Traditionally, rape outside of marriage was not viewed as an act of a man against a woman, but as an act of aggression, the ultimate insult against another man—the woman's husband, father, or brother, whoever was considered her "owner." On conclusion of a battle, rape of the wives and daughters of the losers symbolized the triumph of the conquerors and the humiliation of the vanquished. Unfortunately, women's bodies are still being used to establish dominance, assert authority, and punish the enemy during armed conflicts today.

Domestic Violence

Domestic violence is defined as the collective methods used to exert power and control by one individual over another in an adult intimate relationship. This chapter focuses on domestic violence experienced by women in heterosexual relationships, although gay and lesbian individuals do experience domestic violence in their relationships as well. Among heterosexual couples, estimates indicate that in at least 95% of all domestic violence cases the perpetrators are men. Domestic violence occurs in relationships in which the partners are dating, living together, married, separated, or divorced.

Domestic violence is staggeringly common in the United States. The 2000 National Violence Against Women Survey found that 22% of US women reported physical assault by an intimate male partner. Moreover, the survey found that approximately 1.3 million women are physically assaulted by an intimate partner annually in the United States. Other surveys have found even higher rates of violence. According to the Commonwealth Fund survey (1999), nearly one third of women in the United States report being physically or sexually abused by a husband or boyfriend at some point in their lives. Other figures estimate that a woman is beaten every 9 seconds by her husband, boyfriend, or live-in partner in the United States.

Forms of abuse vary, but are typically described as falling into three categories: psychologic abuse, physical abuse, and sexual abuse. The batterer may use just one or all of these strategies to maintain power and control over his partner's behavior and the relationship.

Psychologic abuse includes a range of behaviors used by the batterer against his female partner, such as:

- **Emotional abuse:** putting her down, making her feel badly about herself, calling her names, negatively comparing her to other women, making unreasonable demands, using things that matter to her against her
- **Isolation:** controlling who she sees and where she goes, using jealousy to justify restricting her actions, interfering with her job, forbidding her to see family and friends, limiting her outside involvement
- **Obfuscation:** denying responsibility for his actions, blaming her, minimizing her concerns, distorting the truth, lying to her
- **Using others:** using the children against her, using visitation to harass her, threatening to take the children away from her, using religion to control her
- **Male privilege:** treating her like a servant, defining rigid men's and women's roles, making all of the decisions or rules in the household
- **Economic abuse:** preventing her from getting or keeping a job, making her ask for money, controlling her money, destroying her property, making all the financial decisions
- **Coercion threats:** making and/or carrying out threats to harm her or her family and friends, threatening to commit suicide, pressuring her to drop charges, threatening negative consequences if she does not cooperate with his wishes, pressuring her with gifts/promises/apologies
- **Intimidation:** making her afraid through looks and gestures, smashing things, harming pets, displaying weapons, yelling, stalking her, driving recklessly

Often, in addition to psychologic abuse, the batterer will use physical and sexual abuse to maintain power and control within the relationship. Physical abuse can include acts such as pushing, shoving, slapping, hitting her with a fist or object, kicking, choking, threatening with a gun or knife, or using a gun or knife against her. Sexual abuse occurs any time the batterer forces or tries to force sex (including vaginal, oral, or anal intercourse). It also includes the forced use of objects, or forcing a woman to have sex with someone else against her will. Figure 9–1 •, the power and control wheel, illustrates how assailants use these tactics in domestic relationships.

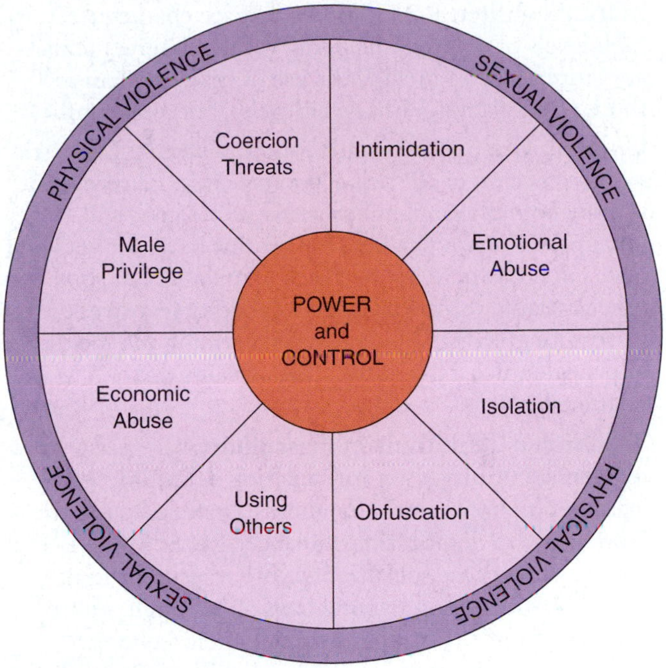

Figure 9–1 • The power and control wheel.
SOURCE: Adapted from the Domestic Abuse Intervention Project, Duluth, Minnesota.

Typically these forms of abuse begin slowly and subtly after some form of commitment, such as engagement, onset of a sexual relationship, marriage, first childbirth, or first statement of commitment. The abuse results in a power imbalance, fear, damage to self-esteem, loss of freedom, and, possibly, injury or death.

Contributing Factors

Domestic violence is a result of the complex and dynamic interaction of social, cultural, political, and psychologic factors. Although none of these factors alone is sufficient to explain why domestic violence occurs, there is substantial research to suggest that the following factors are significantly related to experiences of domestic violence.

- **Childhood experiences.** Children who witness or experience abuse and battering are more likely to become batterers (men) or to be abused (women) in their own relationships. Exposure to domestic violence, however, is not a prerequisite for future abuse. Perhaps more important, not all children who witness violence in the home as children find themselves in abusive relationships as adults.
- **Male dominance in the family.** Worldwide, male economic and decision-making authority in the family is one of the strongest predictors of societies that demonstrate high violence against women, including domestic violence. This notion is also supported by research that demonstrates that men raised in patriarchal families (those that encourage traditional gender roles) are more likely to engage in domestic violence.

- **Marital conflict.** Relationships that are characterized by high levels of conflict, including verbal disagreements, are more likely to include the use of violence than are those relationships with lower levels of marital conflict.
- **Unemployment/low socioeconomic status.** Domestic violence occurs in all socioeconomic classes; however, it is more common in families with low incomes and unemployed men. The reasons for this have not yet been determined. It may not be a lack of income, but some other variable related to living in poverty (eg, stress, frustration, feelings of inadequacy in filling the male role of provider, marital conflict) that explains this relationship.
- **Traditional definitions of masculinity/ hypermasculinity.** Cultures that link definitions of manhood to dominance, toughness, or male honor are more likely to demonstrate violence against women. This may result because socialization into traditional male norms includes telling young boys to be tough, not to shy away from violence, and to hide their feelings, particularly those that are associated with traditional notions of femininity.

Common Myths about Battering and Battered Women

Both professionals and the public believe numerous myths about battering and battered women. These myths often reinforce misunderstanding of battering. Professionals who provide services for battered women need to recognize and counteract these myths. Some commonly accepted myths are discussed here.

- **Battering occurs in a small percentage of the population.** The statistics on reported cases under-represent the true incidence. As many as one in three women may be the victim of assault by her partner in her lifetime; however, it is estimated that only one in ten women will report battering assaults.
- **Battered women provoke men to beat them; women push men beyond the breaking point and incite physical violence.** It is important to recognize that people are individually responsible for their own behavior. Batterers become violent because of their own internal inadequacies, not because of what the women did or did not do.
- **Alcohol and drug abuse cause battering.** Studies do show a relationship between battering incidents and alcohol or drug use by batterers, and many batterers have a history of alcoholism or drug addiction. However, claims that substance abuse *causes* domestic violence are false and only serve to shift the responsibility away from the batterer. Some researchers suggest that batterers use alcohol as an excuse to carry out a violent act and shift the blame from themselves to the alcohol. Others suggest that alcohol or drugs reduce the batterer's inhibitions, increasing the likelihood of violent acts. Battered women sometimes think the abuse will stop if their partners stop drinking or using drugs. Unfortunately, this usually does not happen.
- **Battered women were battered children.** This myth holds true only in a few cases; the majority did not grow up in violent homes. Most women report that their partners were the first person to beat them.
- **Battered women can easily leave the situation.** Leaving is easier said than done. Society encourages women to take greater responsibility for their marriages and children. In addition, battered women may still love their partners or husbands and believe the promises of change, rely on them for financial support, and feel their children need a father. Women with physically abusive partners nearly always experience psychologic abuse as well, and have been told repeatedly by their batterers that the family's problems are their fault. They often are isolated by their abuser from family, friends, and agencies that could assist them. Women may also experience a lack of support from family members, friends, and their religious community. Some family members or friends may send the message that they warned the woman about the batterer and now it is her problem. Others may think that the batterer is a wonderful person, either not believing the woman's accounts or blaming her for the violence she experiences. Many women with children have no place to go, and shelters sometimes have long waiting lists. Moreover, battered women are at greatest risk for injury or domestic homicide when they leave the abuser. A woman may fear for her safety, her children's safety, and the safety of those who help her.
- **Domestic violence is a low-income or minority issue.** Domestic violence occurs among all sectors of society. It happens to women of all socioeconomic statuses, races, ethnicities, and religious faiths. It is true that lower income women are more likely to seek assistance from public agencies, such as hospitals and emergency rooms, because they have fewer private resources than women with greater incomes do. Therefore, they are more likely to be counted in various reporting statistics.
- **Battered women will be safer when they are pregnant.** Battering may occur for the first time during pregnancy or may escalate in intensity if the woman is already being abused (American College of Obstetricians and Gynecologists [ACOG], 1998). The injury is frequently aimed at the breasts, abdomen, or vagina. Many researchers and advocates believe that batterers are threatened by a pregnancy because the fetus interferes with the abuser's ability to maintain power and control within the relationship. Pregnancy is often a time during which a woman receives extra attention from family, friends, and healthcare providers. The intensified violence that some women experience merits serious

attention. Alarmingly, pregnant and recently pregnant women are more likely to be victims of homicide than to die of any other cause (Horon & Cheng, 2001).

> *"Miles hit me for the first time when I was 5 months pregnant. I was stunned. My father never laid a hand on my mother or any of us. I had always been appalled by women who stayed in abusive situations but suddenly I found myself making excuses for him and rationalizing that he hadn't meant it, that he would never do it again. Three months later he shoved me so hard I fell against an end table. I was pretty bruised but I didn't go into labor. Somehow I found the courage to call my dad. He came and got me that night. My baby is 3 months old now and Miles keeps calling, telling me how sorry he is and that he loves me. Oh how I want to believe him when he says he is changed but I just can't take the chance."*

Cycle of Violence

Walker (1984), in an effort to better explain the experience of battered women, developed the theory of the **cycle of violence,** which postulates that battering takes place in a cyclic fashion through three phases.

1. In the *tension-building phase*, the batterer demonstrates power and control. This phase is characterized by anger, arguing, blaming the woman for external problems, and possibly minor battering incidents. As the stress builds and communications break down, the woman often senses growing danger. She may also blame herself for the battering and believe she can prevent the escalation of the batterer's anger by her own actions, hoping that the relationship will somehow change for the better. The length of this phase varies considerably across individual cases, ranging from weeks to years.
2. The *acute battering incident* is typically triggered by some external event or internal state of the batterer. It is an episode of acute violence distinguished by lack of predictability and major destructiveness. The batterer blames the woman for the abuse, and the woman may accommodate him in order to survive, believe that escape is futile, or escape and return when the crisis is over. This is generally the briefest of the three phases, lasting from a few hours to a few days.
3. The *tranquil phase* is also sometimes called the *honeymoon period*. This phase may be characterized by extremely loving, kind, and contrite behaviors by the batterer as he tries to make up with the woman, or it may simply be manifested by an absence of tension and violence. The couple or family is often relieved that the crisis is past, and the woman may accept the batterer's promises and gifts because she is worn down and wants to believe that the violence will not happen again. Without intervention this phase will end at some point, and the cycle of violence will repeat. Over time, the cycle of violence often increases in severity and frequency.

Characteristics of Batterers

Batterers come from all racial, ethnic, and religious groups and all professions, occupations, and socioeconomic strata. They may have only a sixth-grade education, or hold a doctorate. What they have in common are feelings of insecurity, inferiority, powerlessness, and helplessness that conflict with their assumptions of male supremacy. Because they are emotionally immature and aggressive, they have a tendency to express their overwhelming feelings of inadequacy through violence.

Many batterers feel undeserving of their partners, yet they blame and punish the very person they value. Extreme jealousy and possessiveness are the hallmarks of abusers. They characteristically express their ambivalence by alternating episodes of unmerciful beatings with periods of remorse and loving attention. Extremes in behavior and overreacting are typical patterns.

Batterers may be very calculating and select a partner they feel may be vulnerable. Over a period of time they slowly and purposefully isolate the woman, creating a situation of increased dependence.

Battered women often describe their husbands or partners as lacking respect toward women in general, having come from homes where they have witnessed abuse of their mothers or were themselves abused as children, and having a hidden rage that erupts occasionally. Batterers accept conventional "macho" values, yet when they are not angry or aggressive, they appear childlike, dependent, seductive, manipulative, and in need of nurturing. They may be well respected in the community. This is important because it is one of the reasons why women are sometimes not believed or taken seriously when they seek support and assistance from friends, family members, and other resources. This dual personality of batterers reflects the conflict between their belief that they must live up to their macho image and their feelings of inadequacy and insecurity in the role of husband or provider. Combined with low tolerance for frustration and poor impulse control, their pervasive sense of powerlessness leads them to strike out at life's inequities by abusing women.

NURSING CARE MANAGEMENT

Increased publicity, public sensitivity, and heightened awareness of domestic violence are encouraging women with abusive partners to seek resources and community assistance. In the past decade, many communities have

Abuse Assessment Screen

1. **WITHIN THE LAST YEAR**, have you been hit, slapped, kicked, or otherwise physically hurt by someone? YES NO

   If YES, by whom? __________

   Total number of times ______

2. **SINCE YOU'VE BEEN PREGNANT**, have you been hit, slapped, kicked, or otherwise physically hurt by someone? YES NO

   If YES, by whom? __________

   Total number of times ______

MARK THE AREA OF INJURY ON THE BODY MAP
SCORE EACH INCIDENT ACCORDING TO THE FOLLOWING SCALE

	SCORE
1 = Threats of abuse including use of a weapon	______
2 = Slapping, pushing; no injuries and/or lasting pain	______
3 = Punching, kicking, bruises, cuts, and/or continuing pain	______
4 = Beating up, severe contusions, burns, broken bones	______
5 = Head injury, internal injury, permanent injury	______
6 = Use of weapon; wound from weapon	______

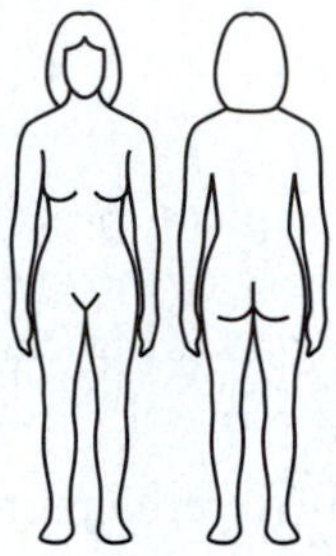

If any of the descriptions for the higher number apply, use the higher number.

3. **WITHIN THE LAST YEAR**, has anyone forced you to have sexual activities? YES NO

   If YES, by whom? __________

   Total number of times ______

Developed by the Nursing Research Consortium on Violence and Abuse.
Readers are encouraged to reproduce and use this assessment tool.

Figure 9–2 • Abuse assessment screen.
SOURCE: Developed by the Nursing Research Consortium on Violence and Abuse. Reprinted from the Web site of the Nursing Network on Violence Against Women International (www.nnvawi.org).

developed domestic violence programs, shelters, and resources for battered women. However, the needs of battered women and their children are still insufficiently met.

Battered women enter the healthcare system in many different settings. Nurses may see them in the physician's office with minor trauma or in the emergency department with multiple severe injuries. Battered women are frequently seen in obstetric services because battering often begins or escalates during pregnancy (ACOG, 1998). Nurses in psychiatric-mental health services frequently counsel women who have been battered, and community health nurses may find battered women during home visits. Unfortunately, emergency departments, hospitals, and social service agencies do not routinely recognize and report battering cases to the legal authorities for action and follow-up, although some states are initiating this policy.

Nurses in many different healthcare settings often come in contact with battered and abused women but fail to recognize them, especially if they have no visible injuries. Nurses who wish to help battered women need advanced knowledge of the dynamics of battered women, assessment skills for recognizing subtle cues of battering, and appropriate intervention skills in counseling and referral.

Working with battered women is sometimes frustrating, and many healthcare providers feel puzzled when women return to their abusive situations. Nurses must realize that they cannot rescue women with abusive partners; women must decide on their own how to handle the situation, which is often incredibly complex and dangerous. The effective nurse provides battered women with information that empowers them in decision making.

Nursing Assessment and Diagnosis

Because domestic violence is so prevalent and yet frequently remains unidentified by healthcare providers, experts and caregivers now advocate *universal screening of all female clients at every healthcare encounter*. Unfortunately, impediments to universal screening exist that range from a lack of institutional or organizational support to the attitudes of individual nurses. Nurses offer a variety of reasons for failing to ask about abuse (Ryan & King, 1998):

- They don't have enough time.
- They believe the question is inappropriate in their health setting (postpartum, general medical unit, etc).
- Their work setting lacks sufficient privacy.
- They believe the myth that only a certain kind of woman is abused.
- They don't want to hear painful stories of abuse.
- There is a difference in ethnicity or age between the nurse and the client, which makes communication difficult.
- They feel inadequate about intervening if the woman discloses abuse.

A majority of the reasons cited by nurses indicate a lack of education about domestic violence in general and a lack of confidence in their own skills specific to domestic violence intervention. This fact underscores the importance of and need for comprehensive domestic violence education and training for healthcare providers, a policy recommendation that was affirmed by the 2000 National Violence Against Women (NVAW) Survey. In addition to factual information about domestic violence and its impact on women's physical and psychologic health, comprehensive education and training should include opportunities to practice skill development (eg, in screening, assessment, empathic listening, diagnosis, planning, and communication across diverse age and ethnic/cultural groups) as well as opportunities to explore one's personal responses, attitudes, and values related to abuse.

Nurses may also be hesitant to ask because they presume the woman may be offended by the questions. However, women are rarely offended by questions about abuse, particularly if prefaced by a statement such as, "Abuse is a major public health problem for women, so we ask all women about it." Showing knowledge about and familiarity with the issue of domestic violence not only increases a nurse's effectiveness in identifying women who have experienced abuse, but also fulfills an important health education function for women who have not experienced abuse.

Three basic screening questions, identified in Figure 9–2 ●, are useful in identifying women who are experiencing abuse. If a woman responds affirmatively to the questions, she is asked to mark the area(s) of injury on the body map. Screening for women experiencing domestic violence must be done privately, with only the nurse and client present, in a safe and quiet place (Figure 9–3 ●). The nurse needs to reassure the woman her responses will be kept confidential. The nurse should also strive for a calm and reassuring tone. While tone, body language, and other nonverbal signs are important in establishing trusting relationships with all women, nurses should be especially aware of these issues in interventions with women from minority groups. Women from minority groups are often sensitized to these cues because they have used them as a survival strategy against discrimination and prejudice in the past.

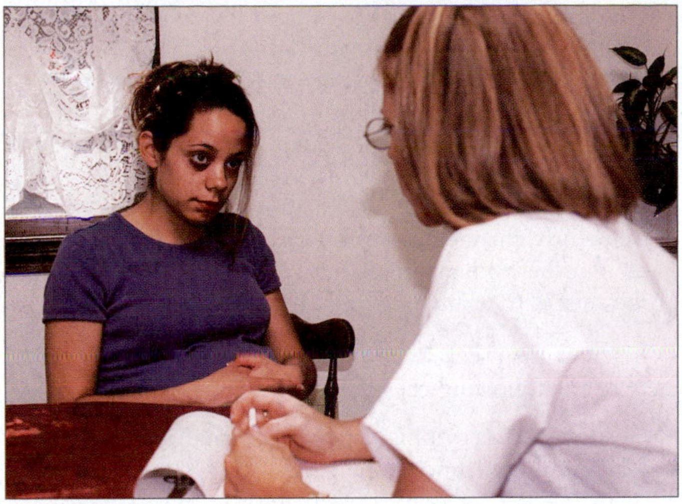

Figure 9–3 ● Screening for domestic violence should be done privately.

A number of signs that may not be related to a woman's presenting injuries can indicate the possibility that a woman is in a violent relationship. While no single one of these signs necessarily indicates abuse, the occurrence of several of these signs certainly merits an at-risk diagnosis. Nurses must exercise their professional judgment and communicate their conclusions to their clients. Signs that may indicate a woman is in an abusive relationship include the following:

- *Neurologic signs*—headaches, including headache following trauma or concussion, tension headache, and migraines; dizziness; paresthesias; unexplained stroke from strangulation; hearing loss; detached retina
- *Gynecologic signs*—dyspareunia (painful intercourse), sexually transmitted infections, frequent vaginal infections, sexual dysfunction, menstrual disorders, pelvic pain
- *Obstetric signs*—late onset of prenatal care, premature labor, low-birth-weight infant, excessive concern over fetal well-being, recurrent therapeutic abortion, recurrent spontaneous abortion
- *Gastrointestinal signs*—dyspepsia, irritable bowel syndrome, globus (sensation of a lump in the throat)
- *Musculoskeletal signs*—arthralgias (painful joints), chronic pain, osteoarthritis, fibromyalgia
- *Psychiatric signs*—anxiety, panic, post-traumatic stress disorder, mood disorders, depression, suicide attempts, somatization, eating disorders, substance abuse, child abuse and neglect

MediaLink CARE PLAN: SUSPICIOUS INJURY AND BRUISES

- *Constitutional signs*—fatigue, weight loss, weight gain, multiple somatic complaints, contusions, abrasions, sleep and appetite disturbances, decreased concentration, frequent use of pain medication or tranquilizers
- *Trauma*—any injury to the female organs, extensive accident history, old fractures, sexual trauma
- *Other signs*—history of missed appointments or frequently changed appointments; low self-esteem, as seen in the woman's dress, her appearance, and the way she relates to healthcare providers

When a woman seeks care for an injury, the nurse should be alert to the following cues of abuse:

- Hesitation in providing detailed information about the injury and how it occurred
- Inappropriate affect for the situation
- Delayed reporting of symptoms
- Pattern of injury consistent with abuse, including multiple injury sites involving bruises, abrasions, or contusions to the head (eyes and back of neck), throat, chest, breast, abdomen, or genitals (Nonbattered women's injuries are usually located at one or two sites and on the extremities, such as sprains and strains. Battered women may have scars and evidence of old injuries that have healed.)
- Inappropriate explanation for the injuries, such as being "accident prone"
- Lack of eye contact
- Signs of increased anxiety in the presence of the possible batterer, who frequently does most of the talking

As with the universal screening, the nurse should conduct the assessment interview in a quiet, private place in which the woman can feel safe. If a man is with the woman, the nurse should tell him to remain in the waiting room while the woman is examined. It is good practice to ask the same of family members or friends because it can be difficult for women in abusive relationships to talk candidly about their situation with others present. When culturally appropriate, it is important to maintain eye contact and avoid excessive note taking. The nurse should assure the woman that her privacy will be respected. It is essential that the nurse remains nonjudgmental, creates a warm, caring climate conducive to sharing, and demonstrates a willingness to talk about violence. A battered woman will often interpret the nurse's willingness to discuss violence as permission for her to discuss it as well.

Assessment is a complex process. It is important for the nurse to gather information about the woman's history of abuse. Getting a sense of the pattern of abuse is key to determining the degree of danger she might face. The nurse can help the woman assess whether or not the cycle of violence is becoming more frequent or severe. Determining whether or not there are weapons in the home, and whether or not her batterer has used or threatened to use weapons might also be warranted. In cases of severe abuse, it is important for the nurse to address the connection between homicide and domestic violence. Finally, the nurse should ask about the presence of sexual abuse within the relationship, another factor that indicates severe abuse.

Equally important, however, the assessment of the woman who may be experiencing abuse should include information about her strengths and her support system. Strengths may include education, employment history, activities in the home, community involvement, and her ability to cope or handle past problems. The woman's support system may include her family, friends, neighbors, and community agencies or organizations. It is helpful to consider assessing a woman's strengths in a cultural context. If the nurse is aware of strong values that a particular cultural group holds, then he or she should look for opportunities to recognize and affirm those strengths as valuable.

Developing Cultural Competence

To provide nursing care to Latina women who are victims of abuse, consider the following:

- Culturally it is often difficult for Latina women to seek help outside their families.
- Some Latina women who experience abuse may perceive it as their lot in life because of the concept of *marianismo* or the myth of martyrdom, which says that it is a woman's duty to sacrifice all for her family, even her own health and well-being (Mattson & Rodriguez, 1999).
- Language can be a powerful barrier to effective communication. Thus it is important to have Spanish-speaking nurses and personnel available.
- Similarly, assessment tools such as that found in Figure 9–2 should be translated into Spanish.
- Latina clients are often receptive to questions about how to screen other women for abuse. When asked, the woman's desire to help another may lead her to relate her own experiences of abuse (Barcelona de Mendoza, 2001).
- Have information available about appropriate community resources including individual and family counseling services in Spanish, shelters with bilingual staff, low-cost services, and the like.
- Community-run interventions designed to raise awareness and provide education can be especially effective if they are culturally sensitive and respectful of differences and individuality.

Clinical Tip *Actually recording a woman's strengths in her medical record and showing her that they are an official part of the record lets her know that the nurse believes that her strengths are as significant as any problems that were noted.*

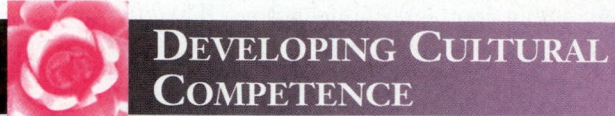

GLOBAL PERSPECTIVES

"In my country [Pakistan], it is OK, yes, to hit your wife or daughter. It is sometimes needed when they are no [sic] doing something right or need to listen better, things like that, you see. It is not like here where it is breaking the law, it is acceptable and sometimes needed."

Examples of circumstances warranting hitting include "like maybe they do not have meal ready or right, or going outside alone, for that is very big punishment, you may hit them with a stick or something. If the woman would look at another man, then they could be hit so much death could occur . . . but it is OK since they brought a great deal of dishonor to the man. If you did not beat her in that case, you would dishonor yourself, you see."

(Excerpt from interview on domestic violence)

During the assessment phase, the nurse begins building a relationship with the woman based on trust, understanding, and advocacy. A woman may feel ashamed and embarrassed about her injuries and her situation. It is important to tell her the purpose of the assessment and to communicate what level of confidentiality she can expect. Clearly, nurses need to be informed about the confidentiality policies of the organization where they work and aware of any mandatory reporting policies that exist. Trust begins as the nurse conveys an attitude of unconditional acceptance, empathy, and positive regard for the woman's worth and dignity. Nurses should show that they recognize the woman's feelings and that they accept her right to feel as she does.

In cases where the woman states she has been beaten, kicked, punched, or attacked but does not identify the assailant, the nurse should record the extent of injuries (eg, size, shape, color, where they are located on her body and so forth), note the woman's exact words, and describe the incident with a diagnosis of probable battering. Full documentation of specific information is critical, as the nurse might be called to testify in court or the medical records might be subpoenaed as evidence in legal proceedings such as custody disputes, stay-away/restraining orders, or other civil or criminal proceedings. Moreover, documenting the abuse works to ensure a woman's continuity of care. Those cases in which the woman states she was beaten by a husband or partner may be diagnosed as battering with all evidence recorded, including the woman's statements. In both cases, taking photographs of the injuries can be of great value. However, to further protect the woman's confidentiality and safety, it is critical that the nurse or other medical personnel do not refer to domestic violence or abuse on any discharge papers.

When abuse or battering is suspected or determined, the nurse should formulate nursing diagnoses based on the assessment findings. Nursing diagnoses related to nonphysical components of abuse or battering may include the following:

- ***Self-Esteem Disturbance*** related to feelings of worthlessness and powerlessness
- ***Health-Seeking Behavior:*** Information about community resources to assist battered women related to an expressed desire to learn about alternatives

Nursing Plan and Implementation

A battered woman needs to reestablish a feeling of control over her world. She needs to regain a sense of predictability by knowing what to expect and how she can interact. The nurse should provide sufficient information about what to expect in terms the woman can understand. Simple explanations about how long she will stay, whom she will see, and what will be done are important. Giving the woman control can be accomplished by asking her permission before any activities or procedures and by providing her with choices whenever possible.

The nurse can encourage the woman to talk about her injuries and home situation by asking, "How did this happen to you?" or saying, "We often see injuries like yours when a woman has been beaten. Has this happened to you?" Directly confronting the injuries and possible battering may provide an opening for the woman who is trying to cope in private. A woman may continue to deny her battering. The nurse should encourage her to talk but should avoid badgering her.

> *No one had ever asked me about my "injuries" until I was in the ER one night and the nurse asked me right out if I had been beaten. It gave me real hope to think that people might see what was happening to me.*

Supportive counseling and reassurance are professional skills nurses use throughout each phase of the nursing process with a battered woman. The nurse should do the following:

- Acknowledge and support the woman for talking about her situation. Reporting abuse is a risk.
- Let the woman work through her story, problems, and situation at her own pace.
- Let the woman know that she is believed and that her feelings are reasonable and normal.
- Anticipate her ambivalence in the love-hate relationship with the batterer. She knows he may be loving and contrite after the incident if she has been through the cycle of violence before.
- Respect the woman's capacity to change and grow when she is ready.
- Assist her in identifying specific problems, and support realistic ideas for reducing or eliminating those problems.

- Help clarify the woman's beliefs and myths, and provide information to change her false beliefs.
- Stress that no one should be abused and that the abuse is not her fault.

The appropriate intervention is not to tell an abused woman what to do, but to help her recognize her options and resources and make her own decisions. Even advising or encouraging a woman to leave an abusive situation is not always in the woman's best interest; leaving the home is a major decision with long-lasting consequences. The woman may be economically unable to leave the situation, especially if she has young children. If the woman leaves and then later returns home, both husband and wife may become more frustrated, increasing the possibility of further beatings and even homicide. The most acceptable course of action is one that the woman freely chooses.

MEDIALINK GOING BACK VIDEO

Teaching for Self-Care

If the woman returns to an abusive situation, the nurse should encourage her to develop an exit, or safety, plan for herself and her children, if she has any. As part of the plan, she should pack a change of clothes for herself and the children, including toilet articles and an extra set of car and house keys. She should store these away from the house with a friend or neighbor. If possible, she should have money, identification papers (driver's license, social security card), checkbook, savings account information, other financial records (such as mortgage papers, automobile title), and information about the children to help her enroll them in school. She should also plan where she will go, regardless of the day or time. The nurse should ensure that the woman has a planned escape route and emergency telephone numbers she can call, including the local police, a phone hotline, and a women's shelter if one is available in the community.

MEDIALINK NATIONAL COALITION AGAINST DOMESTIC VIOLENCE

Community-Based Nursing Care

Besides offering emotional support, medical treatment, and counseling, the nurse should inform any woman who may be in an abusive situation of the services available in the hospital, through agencies, and in the community. The nurse can also provide the woman with the phone number of any local resources, as well as the number for the National Domestic Violence Hotline. In addition to this number, Table 9–2 • provides a range of Internet resources for the nurse to explore and potentially share with the woman who has experienced domestic violence.

Specifically, a woman who has been abused may need

- Medical treatment for injuries
- Temporary shelter to provide a safe environment for herself and her children
- Counseling to raise her self-esteem and help her understand the dynamics of domestic violence
- Legal assistance for protection or prosecution of the batterer
- Financial assistance to provide shelter, food, and clothing
- Job training or employment counseling
- An ongoing support group for herself and her children

Table 9-2 • HOTLINE INFORMATION AND INTERNET-BASED RESOURCES FOR DOMESTIC VIOLENCE

National Domestic Violence Hotline	1-800-799-SAFE 1-800-787-3224 (TDD)
Family Violence Prevention Fund	www.fvpf.org
National Coalition Against Domestic Violence	www.ncadv.org
Nursing Network on Violence Against Women	www.nnvawi.org
Teen Abuse	www.safenetwork.net/teens/teens.html
Lesbian Domestic Violence	www.aabl.org

A network of community agencies can meet the numerous, varied needs of women, children, and batterers. It is important that employees in these agencies understand the complex dynamics of domestic violence as well as how their services and those of other agencies can assist women and their children. An overview of resources available to women with abusive partners and their children is presented in the following sections.

Emergency Department Services

Many battered women are first seen and diagnosed in the emergency departments of their neighborhood hospitals. Emergency department nurses and personnel need to be alert to symptoms of battering, recognize these cues, and encourage women to seek assistance from community agencies. The most innovative and effective domestic violence programs in hospitals and urgent care facilities work collaboratively with domestic violence service agencies, develop a comprehensive community referral network, and work with multidisciplinary intervention teams. Some states require that suspected cases of abuse and battering be reported to the legal authorities or social service agencies.

Shelter

Since domestic violence has been recognized as a major social problem, many community agencies have sought federal and state funds to provide shelters. These shelters differ in the services they provide, depending on the governing body, financial resources and funding agencies, organizational structure, staff qualifications, and range of available community services. Typical shelters provide battered women and their children with a room, beds, food, clothing, and other basic necessities. If professional staff is available, the shelter may offer crisis counseling, individual and group counseling, and information about community agencies such as legal aid, welfare, job training, financial and employment agencies, and women's counseling or support groups.

For safety reasons, the location of most shelters is undisclosed, but they can be contacted through a community crisis line. Admission requirements vary from shelter to shelter, so it is wise for nurses to become familiar with local shelters

RESEARCH IN PRACTICE
Effectiveness of Interventions Targeting Domestic Violence During Pregnancy

What is this study about? The prevalence of abuse during pregnancy is high, and there are serious health consequences for both mother and baby. Pregnancy may be the only time in a healthy woman's life when she regularly sees a healthcare provider, so it is an important window of opportunity for intervention. Most research focuses on recognition of abuse, and not on the effectiveness of interventions. This study evaluated the effectiveness of three levels of intervention for eliminating domestic violence during pregnancy.

How was this study done? Study participants were 329 pregnant, abused Hispanic women who accessed one of two public health prenatal clinics. Potential subjects were identified through a nursing assessment protocol during intake into the clinic. Subjects were randomly assigned to one of three intervention groups. The *brief* intervention consisted of providing a wallet-sized resource card that included phone numbers of local agencies. The women were also provided with a guide for planning for personal safety. The *counseling* intervention consisted of unlimited access to personal counseling services, physically located in the clinic. The counselor provided supportive counseling and education, referral to local services, and assistance in accessing services. The *outreach* intervention consisted of the same unlimited access to a counselor plus the services of a "mentor mother." The mentor mother provided counseling services through personal visits and telephone contacts with the abused women. The frequency and severity of violent episodes was measured with the Severity of Violence Against Women Scale (SVAWS). The women completed the questionnaire on admission to the clinic, at follow-up visits, and at 2, 6, 12, and 18 months after childbirth.

What were the results? Analysis showed that the severity of abuse decreased significantly across time for all three of the intervention groups. The outreach group had significantly fewer violent episodes than the counseling-only group, but was not lower than the brief group. The severity of violent experiences was positively correlated with the use of community resources.

What additional questions might I have? Were specific cultural implications taken into account when designing the interventions? Might culturally sensitive services have increased the effectiveness and/or use of community resources? Did the abuse that was reported start during the pregnancy or was it long-standing?

How can I use this study? It appears that even relatively simple interventions, such as an informational card, can reduce the frequency and severity of abuse during pregnancy. A continued focus on identification of victims of abuse is warranted. Counseling and support for women in accessing community resources may help these women decrease the severity and frequency of abuse during pregnancy.

Source: McFarlane, J., Soeken, K., & Wiist, W. (2000). An evaluation of interventions to decrease intimate partner violence to pregnant women. *Public Health Nursing, 17,* 443–451.

and the resources available if the shelter is full and the woman and her children are in need of a safe place to stay.

Legal Services and Options

During incidents of domestic violence, the woman or her neighbors may summon the police. Family violence typically occurs on the weekend or in late evening, when most social service agencies are closed; therefore, the police department is often one of the first major agencies involved, in addition to those that provide medical services.

Legal options for women with abusive partners vary according to state laws and services. In some states a woman may seek a restraining order from the family court or a domestic relations court to protect herself from the batterer. This restraining order specifies that the man must stay a specified distance away from the woman and may not physically abuse any family members but it does not give him a criminal record. Unfortunately, many abusive men violate the restraining order and continue to stalk, harass, intimidate, and abuse their female partner. If the woman decides to prosecute, and if her case meets the legal requirements for an indictment, the case is usually heard in criminal court, which handles crimes of assault, harassment, and battery. Criminal court hearings may result in a fine, probation, or a jail sentence if the batterer is convicted, giving the man a criminal record. The prosecution process is often lengthy and may last more than a year. Some state judicial systems are introducing other options, such as mandatory counseling for batterers, in lieu of prosecution. Unfortunately, this counseling does not show great promise for permanent change. Divorce is another legal recourse a woman may choose, but divorce often takes several months to a year.

Many women who are abused are unaware of their legal options. They fear further beatings if they prosecute the batterer. Limited financial resources may also keep them from seeking legal assistance. Currently, some communities provide legal advocacy services to help women understand the judicial process, their options within that system, and the possible consequences for the woman, her children, and the batterer.

Financial Services

Once women who have been in a battering relationship leave their homes or seek legal assistance, they usually receive no financial support from the batterer. Without funds, women and their children are at the mercy of community social service agencies, and it usually takes weeks for papers to be processed before any money is forthcoming. Agencies that may provide financial assistance include their county welfare department, federal programs (eg, Temporary Assistance for Needy Families), the United Way, women's support groups, religious organizations, and possibly the Salvation Army. There may be other local groups who assist abused women in other ways, such as by providing food or clothing.

Employment Training or Placement

Some women who experience abuse are full-time mothers who may lack advanced education, training, and job experience. Minimal or out-of-date skills and inadequate transportation often make it difficult for these women to obtain employment with an adequate salary. Women who have children must consider where to place them during working hours as well as the added cost of child care. Often, the woman's choice is restricted to accepting welfare or taking a low-paying job. Either choice usually means lowering the standard of living to mere subsistence.

Some women do seek job training if the opportunities are available, but training provides no guarantee of future job placement. A woman may still have to arrange for financial support and child care while obtaining advanced employment skills or an education.

Counseling

Women who have experienced domestic violence may be offered a variety of counseling services, such as crisis intervention, short-term individual therapy, group therapy, or peer support groups, over an extended period. Specially trained nurses, social workers, psychologists, mental health specialists, or clergy may provide counseling and therapy.

Evaluation

Expected outcomes of nursing care include the following:

- The woman recovers from the effects of physical abuse.
- The woman has the information she needs to make a decision about her future based on thoughtful consideration of alternatives.
- The woman is able to identify community resources available to her and agrees to develop an exit strategy.

Critical Thinking in Practice

Marsha Salvatorri, age 23, has come to the emergency department for an injury to her upper left shoulder. She is accompanied by her boyfriend with whom she lives, Fred Schultz. The nurse asks Marsha to describe the details surrounding the injury to her shoulder. Marsha relates that she is very clumsy and was walking through the house in a hurry when she ran into the door jamb. She says the incident happened 2 hours ago. She complains of discomfort in the shoulder. While relating her story, she often looks at Fred. Fred nods his head in agreement with Marsha's statements. Upon assessment the nurse discovers that Marsha's shoulder is very edematous and bruised. The amount of edema and bruising is not consistent with an injury that happened 2 hours ago. What would you as the nurse do next?

Answers can be found in Appendix I.

Rape

In its broadest sense, rape is involuntary sexual contact with another person. The National Crime Victimization Survey defines it as follows: "**Rape** is forced sexual intercourse and includes both psychological coercion as well as physical force. Forced sexual intercourse means vaginal, anal, or oral penetration by the offender(s)." The rapist may be a stranger, acquaintance, spouse or other relative, or an employer. Rape is an act of violence expressed sexually—most commonly, a man's aggression and rage acted out against a woman.

Rape has been reported against females from age 6 months to 93 years, but it remains one of the most underreported violent crimes in the United States. The National Sexual Violence Resource Center (2000) reports that approximately 70% of rapes and sexual assaults are not reported to the police. Crimes of rape and sexual assault are not uncommon, although estimates do vary. For example, the National Violence Against Women (NVAW) Survey found that one in six surveyed women had been a victim of a completed or attempted rape (Tjaden & Thoennes, 2000). Other estimates are higher, suggesting that one in four women will experience a sexual assault (Rennison, 2000). Even more disturbing, very few rapists are arrested and convicted.

No woman of any age or ethnic background is immune, but findings from the 1999 National Crime Victimization Survey (NCVS) indicate that young women and women who have a low family income are at greater risk of rape or attempted rape (Rennison, 2000). In fact, just over half of female rape victims (54%) were under the age of 18 when they experienced their first attempted or completed rape (Tjaden & Thoennes, 2000). Of those young rape victims, approximately 40% were younger than age 12 when they were first raped, and 60% were between the ages of 12 and 17. Adolescent rape survivors are often reluctant to report a rape for several reasons: embarrassment, feelings of guilt, fear of retribution, lack of knowledge of their legal rights, concerns about confidentiality, lack of funds, and limited access to healthcare. The young adolescent may also avoid disclosing an assault to the authorities because she may be worried about revealing the circumstances, especially if they involved risk-taking behaviors such as underage drinking, drug use, accepting a ride from a stranger, or socializing with older males (Holmes, 1998).

Common Myths about Rape

As with domestic violence, many myths about rape exist. These myths can have a negative impact on women who are assaulted and can hinder their ability to receive optimum healthcare following their attack. Some of the most commonly cited myths include the following:

- **Only certain types of women are raped.** No woman is safe from a rape attempt. Any woman of any age, race, class, religion, occupation, physical disability, sexual identity, or appearance can be raped; rape is a very "democratic" form of violence.

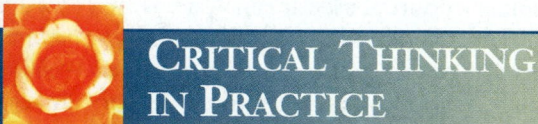

- **Women who party hard, drink, and do drugs are setting themselves up to be raped.** Nobody deliberately "sets herself up" to be raped. This myth is due to a misunderstanding that rape is about sex. Rape is sexual violence and a crime of power. Blaming the victim for the crime is inappropriate and only serves to excuse the behavior of the rapist. Because alcohol and drugs may affect judgment, feelings, and perceptions, as well as lower inhibitions, women may be in a more vulnerable position when they drink. However, it is not a crime to wear particular clothes, show naivete, use poor judgment, or even engage in reckless behavior. The victim's behavior prior to the crime is irrelevant.
- **If a woman just relaxes, it will all be over with soon. She might even find it isn't so bad after all.** Rape is violence using sex as a weapon. Survivors of sexual violence feel very clearly that rape and consensual sex are worlds apart. Rape involves persistent pressure, taking advantage of a person's inability to say "no," calculated drugging with alcohol or other substances, and/or threats, sometimes against the woman's life, her livelihood, her academic career, even her family members and friends. Many survivors recall being in fear for their lives, even if a weapon was not present.
- **Most rapes are interracial.** The overwhelming majority of rapes and other sexual assaults, between 80% and 90%, involve people of the same race, ethnicity, and social class. Unfortunately, media reports tend to play up the race of accused criminals, further encouraging racist misconceptions in our society. When men rape women of other races and ethnicities, it is more often a white assailant raping a woman of color than a man of color raping a white woman (Greensite, 1999).
- **A rapist is easy to spot in a crowd.** There is nothing about men who rape that distinguishes them externally from other men. Rapists come from all races, ethnicities, and socioeconomic groups. They can be large or small, able-bodied or disabled, married or single.
- **Women lie about rape as an act of revenge or guilt.** False rape charges are infrequent. According to the Federal Bureau of Investigation (FBI), false charges are reported at the same rate for rape as for other felonies; that is, about 2% of all rape charges. It is also important to remember that simply because there is not enough evidence to prosecute does not mean the woman was lying.
- **Fighting back incites a rapist to violence.** Most rapists pick out potential victims they believe may be good targets without a fight. They may even test women nonverbally or verbally before determining whether or not to assault. Both verbal and physical resistance may actually lessen the severity of injury in some instances. Recent studies of rape avoidance behavior have shown that women who recognize that they have options for responding to their assailant are less likely to be paralyzed by fear and more likely to resist. However, no one should tell another person what to do in a dangerous situation. Only the woman knows her abilities and can assess the assailant's behavior. Evaluating her options realistically may help the survivor understand that submission is also a viable form of self-protection.

Characteristics of Rapists

Like their victims, rapists come from all ethnic backgrounds, socioeconomic groups, and professions. Clinicians and researchers who work with rapists, both convicted and not convicted, report that a majority of rapists are married and engaged in regular sexual relationships, both inside and outside of marriage. Further, rapists indicate that their sexual needs and interests are being filled. These facts raise an important question. If sexual desire and sexual frustration are not the dominant motive in rape, then why do these men rape?

Unfortunately, so few rapists are actually caught and convicted that a clear characterization of the assailant has not been developed. Far from being lusty, overly amorous, or perverted, the rapist tends to be emotionally weak and insecure and may have difficulty maintaining interpersonal relationships. Many rapists also have trouble dealing with the stresses of daily life. Such men may become angry and overcome by feelings of powerlessness. They then commit the act of rape as an expression of power or anger (Dupre, Hampton, Morrison, et al, 1993).

Types of Rape

Rape has been categorized in different ways, which are not mutually exclusive. Specifically, rape may be categorized according to the rapist's possible motives or purposes for the assault, according to the relationship between the victim and perpetrator, or according to the number of assailants.

- In *power rape*, the purpose of the assault is control or mastery. The male uses sexual intercourse to place a woman in a powerless position so that he can feel dominant, potent, and strong. He often believes his victim enjoys the assault, and he exerts only the amount of force necessary to subdue his victim. Often power rape is a planned stranger attack, but most acquaintance rapes are also power rapes.
- In *anger rape*, the sexual assault is used to express feelings of rage and to retaliate for what he perceives as wrongs against him. These perceived wrongs most often have nothing to do with the rape victim. Considerable brutality and degradation can characterize this type of rape. Attacks on older women often are a form of anger rape.
- In *sadistic rape*, the assailant has an antisocial personality and delights in torture and mutilation. In this type of rape, the victim and assailant are generally strangers, and the assault is planned. Most rape homicides are sadistic rapes.
- In *stranger rape*, also called *blitz rape*, the assailant and victim are strangers, and the rape is sudden and

unexpected. The rapist is more likely to use a weapon and threaten violence or murder.

- In *acquaintance rape*, also called *confidence rape*, the assailant is someone with whom the victim has had previous nonviolent interaction. The attacker uses deception and trust to gain access to the victim and then betrays that trust. Marital rape is included in this category, as is **date rape,** which occurs between a dating couple. In date rape, the male has usually planned to have sex and will do what he feels is necessary if denied. Acquaintance rape is more frequent than stranger rape. Almost 70% of rape and sexual assault victims know the rapist as an acquaintance, friend, relative, or intimate (Rennison, 2000). On college campuses, as many as 80% of rapes are acquaintance rapes. Unfortunately, only about one out of ten victims of acquaintance rape discloses the assault to police, family, healthcare providers, or friends (Rickert & Wiemann, 1998).
- In *gang rape*, the assailants are more commonly younger men responding to peer pressure. Typically, only one or two of the men has a rapist mentality, but they are able to incite the others to commit acts they would not do individually. Often gang rape can escalate to severe violence as the young men seek to outdo each other.

MEDIALINK PARENTAL SEXUAL ABUSE VIDEO

"*I always knew that rape was a terrifying experience physically but I never really thought about the horror that comes from being helpless and in someone else's control.*"

Role of Drugs in Sexual Assault

In some cases, a rapist uses alcohol or other drugs to sedate his intended victim. Flunitrazepam (Rohypnol), a potent sedative-hypnotic that is legal in 80 countries worldwide but illegal in the United States, received considerable attention as the "date rape drug of choice" in the late 1990s. Typically Rohypnol, which dissolves easily and is odorless, is slipped into the drink of an unsuspecting woman. More recently, gamma hydroxybutyrate (GHB), ketamine, and MDMA (Ecstasy) have become popular date rape drugs that are used to incapacitate a woman. Because these drugs frequently produce amnesia, the woman may be unable to remember details of her assault, thereby making prosecution more difficult. She may be left uncertain about the perpetrator's identity, the events of the assault, the presence of birth control, and possible injury or risk for contracting sexually transmitted infections. See Table 9–3 • for indicators of possible date rape drug use.

Table 9–3 • INDICATORS OF POSSIBLE RAPE DRUG USE

- Becoming intoxicated very rapidly, especially after accepting a drink from someone else or drinking a drink she left unattended
- Having just one or two drinks, and then suddenly feeling "very drunk"
- Waking up 8 or more hours later, uncertain but believing she may have been raped because of vaginal soreness, finding herself in an unfamiliar place, or other indicators
- Being told that she suddenly appeared drunk, drowsy, dizzy, or confused, with impaired motor skills, judgment, and amnesia or partial amnesia

Rape Trauma Syndrome

Rape is viewed as a situational crisis, that is, an unanticipated traumatic event that the victim generally is unprepared to handle because it is unforeseen. Following rape, the survivor may experience a cluster of symptoms originally described by Burgess and Holmstrom (1979) as the **rape trauma syndrome.** Burgess and Holmstrom described this syndrome as having two phases: the acute phase and the adjustment, or reorganization, phase. Other authors added a third phase: an intermediate, outward adjustment phase. Recently a fourth phase—integration and recovery—has been suggested (Holmes, 1998). Although the phases of response are discussed individually in the following sections, they often overlap, as do individual responses and their duration.

ACUTE PHASE (DISORGANIZATION)

The acute phase of rape trauma syndrome begins during the rape and may last for a few days or up to 3 weeks. The woman may experience fear, shock, disbelief, and sometimes denial. The woman may feel humiliated, guilty, and unclean; her wish to cleanse herself by bathing or douching may be overpowering, even if she knows that by doing so she is destroying evidence. She may feel angry or anxious, powerless or helpless.

The rape survivor may suppress her emotions or may reveal them by crying, sobbing, or acting tense and restless. Survivors who control or mask their emotions may appear calm, composed, or subdued. Many rape survivors also experience alterations in sleep patterns, such as insomnia, nightmares, or crying out at night.

OUTWARD ADJUSTMENT PHASE (DENIAL)

Once the acute stage has passed, the survivor may appear adjusted. She returns to work or school and resumes her usual roles. But although she appears composed, she is actually coping by denial and suppression. The survivor needs the outward adjustment phase to cope with the experience of rape; it is a means of regaining control of her life. During this time, she may move to a different residence or may institute security measures, such as installing extra locks or requesting an unlisted telephone number. She may buy a weapon or take a course in self-defense. These activities do not resolve her emotional trauma; they simply push it further into her subconscious. In addition she may get less support from others who perceive her as being "over it."

REORGANIZATION

Denial and suppression cannot sustain the survivor for long. As these coping mechanisms deteriorate, she becomes depressed and anxious and feels a strong urge to talk about the rape. At this point, the woman enters the reorganizational phase of the rape trauma syndrome. She must alter her self-concept and resolve her feelings about the rape.

During this phase, the rape survivor may develop phobias. Fears of being indoors or outdoors or of being attacked from behind—depending on how the attack took place—are common. Because of these fears, the woman may alter her lifestyle. If she is afraid of crowds, of being out after dark, or of returning to an empty house, she may become a virtual recluse.

Rape survivors frequently report menstrual or other gynecologic disorders, as well as sexual dysfunction. Some women become totally averse to sexual activity. Those who do try to engage in sex often report a decrease in vaginal lubrication, an inability to be aroused, unusual sensations in the genital area, and an inability to achieve orgasm.

Sleep disorders persist. Survivors report repeated nightmares in which they either relive the rape or thwart the rapist's attempt. In either case the dream contains disturbing violence. The woman repeatedly replays the role of victim until she comes to terms with the experience.

INTEGRATION AND RECOVERY

This final phase brings resolution for the woman. She is able to recognize that the blame for her assault lies with her assailant. She begins to trust others again and begins to feel safe in her life and day-to-day activities. She may be filled with a sense of righteous anger and become an advocate for other women (Holmes, 1998).

SILENT REACTION

Women who do not report the rape go through the phases of the rape trauma syndrome without using available support systems. Their reasons for keeping silent vary. A woman may be embarrassed, she may accept society's "temptress view" and blame herself, or she may fear retaliation. Her experience may be discovered much later, perhaps when she seeks professional help in resolving a different crisis.

Some women seek medical help for their physical injuries without disclosing that a rape was the cause. The nurse who suspects that a woman has been raped should seek validation through sympathetic questioning.

Rape as a Cause of Post-traumatic Stress Disorder

Recent research has demonstrated that rape survivors exhibit high levels of post-traumatic stress disorder (PTSD), the same disorder that developed in many of the veterans of the Vietnam War. To be diagnosed as having PTSD, a person must

- Have been exposed to a traumatic event that triggered feelings of intense fear, horror, or helplessness.
- Reexperience the event in recurrent, intrusive thoughts, images, and perceptions.
- Persistently avoid stimuli associated with the trauma and demonstrate a generalized "numbing" of responsiveness.
- Demonstrate persistent signs of increased arousal, such as exaggerated startle response, difficulty falling asleep, hypervigilance or outbursts of anger, which were not present before the trauma occurred.

PTSD is marked by varying degrees of intensity. One mitigating factor is individual resiliency. Not surprisingly, the intensity of the PTSD is often greatest for women who had psychiatric disorders prior to their assault.

PTSD is difficult to treat. Because the symptoms keep an individual from addressing the problem, she cannot integrate the event into her life, and healing is blocked. Recovery depends on empowering the woman to seek to regain control of her life within the context of healing relationships and professional counseling.

Physical Care of the Rape Survivor

Following rape, repairing tissue damage and preventing complications are primary concerns. As many as 40% of those who are sexually assaulted sustain injuries; of those injured, over one third receive some type of medical care (Tjaden & Thoennes, 2000). About 1% require hospitalization and major surgical repair, while 0.1% are fatal (ACOG, 1997).

Because rape is a crime as well as a traumatic emergency, however, some aspects of healthcare are governed by the need to collect and preserve legal evidence for use in prosecuting the assailant. In so doing, healthcare providers must respect the rights of the rape survivor. Sexual assault survivors have the right to immediate, compassionate, and comprehensive medical-legal examination and treatment by a trained professional who has the experience to anticipate their needs during this time of crisis. Unfortunately, in many communities the treatment of a woman immediately following a rape has been almost as traumatic as the rape itself. To address this concern, many emergency departments use multidisciplinary teams to provide effective care to rape survivors and their families. Sexual assault nurse examiner (SANE) programs and sexual assault response teams (SART) are two examples of successful community programs that coordinate teams of medical, legal, and social service professionals with effective advocacy on behalf of rape survivors.

MEDIALINK HOPE FOR HEALING

DETAILED HISTORY

Obtaining a detailed history is an essential first step in acquiring necessary medical and forensic data, but it can also be a therapeutic tool if done in a sensitive, caring way. Because a rape survivor may appear relaxed and normal when first seen, caregivers may underestimate her needs, but it is essential that she receive immediate attention. Immediately after the woman has received any necessary emergency care, the nurse takes an explicit history of the event in the woman's own words. Many agencies use a standardized forensic chart containing a history flow sheet to record information obtained. The caregiver should use a nonjudgmental approach and must avoid leading or coaching the woman.

COLLECTION OF EVIDENCE

The collection of evidence may, in itself, be traumatic for the woman. It is valuable to have someone available to provide support and act as an advocate. This person may be a family member or close friend, but often it is a nurse. An interpreter should also be provided as necessary.

The woman should receive a thorough explanation of the procedures to be carried out and should sign a consent form. An important legal concept when dealing with rape survivors is the need to preserve the *chain of evidence*, meaning that all physical evidence and specimens must remain in the hands of a professional until they are turned over to a police officer. The evidence that the nurse collects has four primary uses (Ledray, 1999):

1. To confirm recent sexual contact
2. To show that force or coercion was used
3. To identify the assailant
4. To corroborate the survivor's story

Most agencies have special sexual assault kits that contain all necessary supplies for collecting and labeling evidence.

A careful examination of the entire body is necessary. Vaginal and rectal examinations are performed, along with a complete physical examination for trauma. Any lacerations of the vaginal wall are repaired and noted. A colposcope with photographic capability can be used to document injuries to the genitalia.

Clothing

Each piece of clothing is marked, placed in an individual paper bag, sealed, and labeled.

Swabs of Stains and Secretions

Swabs of body stains and secretions are analyzed for semen or sperm. The absence of sperm, however, does not signify that no rape has occurred. Many rapists do not ejaculate because of sexual dysfunction, or they may use a condom. Because victims are often forced to commit fellatio, oral swabs are also examined for semen. Gonorrhea and chlamydia cultures also are taken from vaginal, rectal, and oral cavities.

Hair and Scrapings

Clippings or scrapings of the woman's fingernails are examined for blood or tissue from the assailant. Approximately 20 to 25 hairs are pulled from her head and pubic area to analyze the root structure and identify foreign hairs. Her pubic hair is also combed to check for loose hairs that may have been transferred from the rapist.

Blood Samples

Blood is drawn to test for syphilis and to determine the woman's blood type. Additional blood may be drawn for a pregnancy test if the woman indicates that she wants to take emergency contraception (see discussion in Chapter 5) to prevent pregnancy. She has to have a negative pregnancy test to receive the medication.

Urine Samples

Urine should be collected in cases in which a drug-facilitated sexual assault is suspected and the drug was ingested within 96 hours of the evidentiary exam. It is important to document in the record the time the survivor believes that the drug was ingested and the number of urinations between the ingestion and the exam.

Photographs

Photographs should be taken of injured areas if possible. Prior to taking any photos, the healthcare provider should ask the woman to sign an informed consent form.

PREVENTION OF SEXUALLY TRANSMITTED INFECTIONS

Among women who have been sexually assaulted, trichomoniasis, bacterial vaginosis, gonorrhea, and chlamydia are the most frequently diagnosed infections. Thus, during the initial examination, cultures for *Neisseria gonorrhoeae* and *Chlamydia trachomatis* should be obtained from any body sites of penetration or attempted penetration. However, because these infections are fairly prevalent among sexually active woman, the diagnosis of one or more of these infections following an assault does not necessarily indicate that it was acquired during the assault. If any sexually transmitted infection (STI) is diagnosed, it is treated (Centers for Disease Control and Prevention [CDC], 2002). Most clinicians recommend routine preventive therapy after a sexual assault with follow-up referral to a clinic specializing in the treatment of STIs to evaluate the effectiveness of the therapy. The CDC (2002) recommends a prophylaxis regimen that includes a single dose of ceftriaxone intramuscularly plus a single oral dose of metronidazole and a single oral dose of azithromycin. If the survivor chooses not to receive prophylactic antibiotic treatment, the nurse should instruct her to be seen by her caregiver in 2 weeks for assessment for any STIs. In addition, because hepatitis B is a risk, the woman who has never been immunized should be given hepatitis B immune globulin; she should also begin the hepatitis B three-dose immunization series immediately (ACOG, 1997; CDC, 2002).

If the assailant's HIV status is not known, consideration should be given to offering postexposure prophylaxis with HIV antiviral medications. If postexposure HIV prophylaxis is considered, consultation with an HIV specialist is advised (CDC, 2002).

PREVENTION OF PREGNANCY

The woman is questioned about her menstrual cycle and contraceptive practices. If she is at risk for pregnancy and a pregnancy test is negative, emergency postcoital contraception is offered. (See Chapter 5 for further discussion.)

NURSING CARE MANAGEMENT

Because rape survivors frequently enter the healthcare system by way of the emergency department, nurses are often the first to counsel them. Because the caregiver's values, attitudes, and beliefs will necessarily affect the competence and focus of the care, nurses who work with rape survivors must understand their own attitudes and beliefs about rape and rape survivors and resolve any conflicts that may exist.

In addition to examining their own attitudes and beliefs, nurses must be mindful of the potential for increased complexity of treatment with rape survivors who are members of different ethnic or cultural backgrounds. For example, a woman's membership in a particular ethnic or cultural group could affect her willingness to disclose all the details of a rape, her willingness to follow up with community resources or to seek counseling, and her willingness to prosecute. Being aware of potential cultural differences is important when discussing future courses of action available to rape survivors.

Nursing Assessment and Diagnosis

Policies for admitting and examining rape survivors vary among institutions. A woman who has been raped is under great stress and needs the sensitive care of professionals who are aware of her special needs. The first priority is creating a safe, secure milieu. Professionals should gather admission information in a quiet, private room and reassure the woman that she is not alone, will not be abandoned, and is safe from a second attack.

A full mental status examination should be performed, both for the purpose of planning care and as possible courtroom evidence. Scrupulous documentation is essential because the survivor's medical record is often used in the courtroom to verify her testimony if the rapist is prosecuted.

Examples of nursing diagnoses that may apply to the rape survivor include the following:

- ***Fear*** related to invasion of personal space secondary to rape
- ***Powerlessness*** related to inability to regain sense of control secondary to rape

Nursing Plan and Implementation

Table 9–4 • outlines the general nursing actions that are appropriate during each of the phases of recovery. It is imperative that control be returned to the woman as quickly as possible. The nurse can return control by encouraging the woman to make contact. When feasible, the woman should decide on the sequence of forensic events, such as pulling her own hair (head and pubic), having blood drawn after clothes are collected rather than before, and so forth. In this way the nurse helps her deal with her crisis in small, manageable increments. The nurse should encourage the woman to express her feelings and reassure her that anger and fear are normal, appropriate responses. The nurse can also address expressed or unexpressed guilt by assuring the woman that the rape was not her fault.

Table 9–4 • NURSING ACTIONS APPROPRIATE TO PHASES OF RECOVERY FOLLOWING RAPE

Acute phase	Create a safe milieu. Explain the sequence of events in the healthcare facility. Allow the woman to grieve and express her feelings. Provide care for significant others.
Outward adjustment phase	Provide advocacy and support at the level requested by the woman. Provide assistance to significant others.
Reorganizational phase	Establish a trusting relationship. Assist the woman to understand her role in the assault. Clarify and enhance the woman's feelings. Assist the woman in planning for her future.
Integration and recovery	Acknowledge survivor's success in overcoming trauma; support advocacy efforts.

By explaining the forensic examination and the general sequence of events in the emergency department, the nurse alleviates the client's anxiety related to fear of the unknown. The woman should know what is going to happen and why and how she can assist in each phase of the examination.

MEDIALINK CASE STUDY: TEENAGE RAPE VICTIM

Throughout the experience, the nurse acts as the survivor's advocate, providing support without usurping decision making. The nurse need not agree with all the survivor's decisions but should respect and defend her right to make them.

The family members or friends on whom the survivor calls also need nursing care. Like those of the survivor, the reactions of the family will depend on the values to which they ascribe. Some family members or partners may blame the survivor for the rape and feel angry with her for not having been more careful. They may also incorrectly view the rape as a sexual act rather than as an act of violence. They may feel personally wronged or attacked and see the survivor as being devalued or unclean. Their reactions may compound the survivor's crisis. By spending some time with family members before their first interaction with the survivor, the nurse can reduce their anxiety and help them examine and reconcile their feelings, sparing the woman further trauma. In some cases, the nurse may want to refer them to a sexual assault advocate who can help them address their needs.

Clinical Tip *Strive to listen nonjudgmentally. Impartial listening can often make the difference in a victim's readiness to disclose the full details of the assault and assist her in the recovery process.*

Community-Based Nursing Care

As the woman enters the reorganizational phase, she usually feels a strong urge to discuss and resolve her feelings about herself and her assailant. During this phase, the survivor may benefit from talking with a specially trained rape advocate or counselor. If she is not certain that she wants counseling, or denies any need for counseling, it is appropriate to respect her current wishes and to provide her with referral information for possible future use.

Rape counseling, provided by qualified nurses or other counselors, is a valuable tool in helping the rape survivor come to terms with her assault and its impact on her life. In counseling, the woman is encouraged to explore and identify her feelings and determine appropriate actions to resolve her problems and concerns. It is important for the counselor to assist the woman to realize that the rape was not her fault. The fault lies with the rapist. With the counselor, the woman explores her thoughts and feelings about self-care and celebrates her victories. It is important to emphasize that the loss of control that occurred during the rape was temporary and that the woman does have control over other aspects of her life.

Pregnancy Following Rape

A woman who becomes pregnant as the result of rape needs support and information. In particular, counseling should include information about community resources and all legally available options for dealing with the pregnancy, including keeping the baby, relinquishing it for adoption, or terminating the pregnancy (ACOG, 1997). If the woman carries the pregnancy to term, the nurse should assess the woman carefully for signs of maternal attachment behaviors during the pregnancy and in the postpartal period (Lathrop, 1998). If signs of malattachment develop, counseling may be indicated.

Preventive Education

Local high schools, colleges, or rape awareness groups may offer courses in preventive strategies. Some classes focus on increasing women's awareness of situations in which they are at risk. Others are concerned with changing societal attitudes about rape and rape survivors. Because rape is a considerable risk for any woman, courses in what to do during and after a rape may also be helpful. Nurses who have completed additional education and are thoroughly prepared are well qualified to initiate or participate in preventive instruction.

Rape Crisis Counseling

Most rape crisis counseling centers operate 24 hours a day, 7 days a week. Their services are invaluable. Properly trained telephone counselors can help the woman regain control early in the crisis. Early crisis intervention often encourages the woman to seek professional treatment and assistance. Many rape crisis centers offer free counseling to rape survivors or can refer them to qualified counselors. Information on STIs and pregnancy alternatives may also be obtained from these centers. Table 9–5 • provides a brief list of informational resources for survivors of rape.

Table 9–5 • INFORMATION AND INTERNET-BASED RESOURCES FOR RAPE

Rape, Abuse, and Incest National Network (RAINN)	1-800-656-HOPE www.rainn.org
Sexual Assault Resource Service (SARS)	www.sane-sart.com
Rape Treatment Center: Santa Monica / UCLA Medical Center	www.911rape.org

Evaluation

Expected outcomes of nursing care include the following:

- The woman recovers from the physical effects of the rape.
- The woman is able to verbalize her recognition that rape is a crime of violence expressed sexually.
- The woman is able to identify community resources available to her as she works to adjust psychologically to the assault.
- The woman makes a decision about whether to prosecute her assailant.

Prosecution of the Rapist

Legally, rape, like any criminal action, is considered a crime against the state rather than against the victim. Therefore, prosecution of the assailant is a community responsibility in which the district attorney will act on the victim's behalf. The victim, however, must initiate the process by reporting the crime and pressing charges against her assailant. Once authorities have apprehended the alleged rapist, the judicial system is set into motion.

Procedures vary from state to state. A judge or magistrate generally conducts a hearing to determine whether there is sufficient evidence to hold the defendant over for a grand jury. If so, the grand jury will determine whether the evidence is sufficient to indict the defendant. If not, he is acquitted. If indicted, a defendant must stand trial unless he waives this right. Either a judge or a jury will find the defendant guilty or not guilty, and he will be retained or set free accordingly.

Many rape survivors who have gone through the judicial process refer to it as a second rape—and sometimes a more damaging one. The survivor will be repeatedly asked to identify the assailant and describe the rape in intimate detail. Throughout the pretrial period, the defense attorney may use delaying tactics, further frustrating the survivor and her support system. Publicity may intensify her feelings of humiliation, and if the assailant is released on bail, she may fear retaliation.

During the trial itself, cross-examination by the defense attorney can be a severely degrading experience in which the "victim as temptress" myth may be continually evoked. The defense attorney may try to discredit her testimony, causing her to feel victimized a second time. Fortunately, rape shield laws have become quite common, and nearly every state has passed legislation that prohibits the publicizing of a victim's sexual history. Moreover, despite the difficulties of prosecution, many victims feel a sense of justice in taking their case to court.

The nurse acting as a counselor needs to be aware of the judicial sequence to anticipate rising tension and frustration in the survivor and her support system. They will need consistent, effective support at this crucial time.

Responding to Violence Against Women: Vicarious Trauma

Vicarious trauma, or secondary trauma effect, can occur as a result of working with people who are trauma victims. It refers to a gradual internal transformation that can negatively affect commitment to one's work, reduce any sense of accomplishment, and lead to a questioning of personal belief systems. Nurses who treat and assist domestic violence and rape survivors should be aware of this phenomenon so that they are able to periodically assess the effect of their work on their lives. When the lives of nurses—and indeed of all healthcare professionals—are balanced and there is equal time for self, family, friends, work, play, and rest, then they are better able to provide compassionate and sensitive healthcare.

CHAPTER REVIEW

EXPLOREMEDIALINK

NCLEX review questions, case studies, and other interactive resources for this chapter can be found on the Web site at http://www.prenhall.com/olds. Click on "Chapter 9" to select the activities for this chapter.

For tutorials including animations and videos, more NCLEX review questions, and an audio glossary, access the accompanying CD-ROM in this book.

Focus Your Study

- Domestic violence is common. One in three to one in four women will experience violence at the hands of an intimate partner during their lifetime.
- Batterers use psychologic, physical, and sexual abuse to maintain power and control in abusive relationships.
- Battering occurs in a cyclic pattern called the cycle of violence, which increases in frequency and severity over time.
- Nurses are in an excellent position to intervene and assist battered women by recognizing their cues, diagnosing their problems appropriately, and understanding the complex dynamics of the battering family. The nurse provides information about available community resources, medical attention, and emotional support.
- Estimates suggest that approximately 70% of rapes are not reported to the police. Moreover, just over half (54%) of female rape victims were under the age of 18 when they experienced their first attempted or completed rape.
- Rape is an act of violence acted out sexually. Most rapes are expressions of anger or power.
- Following rape, the survivor will usually experience an assortment of symptoms known as the rape trauma syndrome. Recent research also links the effects of rape to the post-traumatic stress disorder. Nursing actions to assist rape survivors are encompassed in the roles of advocate, educator, and counselor.
- Nurses inform the woman of the sequence of events involved in providing her care and developing the chain of evidence, and support the survivor's decisions.
- Widespread education is needed to abolish societal myths surrounding domestic violence and rape.

References

American College of Obstetricians and Gynecologists (ACOG). (1997). *Sexual assault* (ACOG Educational Bulletin No. 242). Washington, DC: Author.

American College of Obstetricians and Gynecologists (ACOG). (1998). *Mandatory reporting of domestic violence* (ACOG Committee Opinion No. 200). Washington, DC: Author.

American Nurses Association (ANA). (1998). *Culturally competent assessment for family violence*. Washington, DC: American Nurses Publishing.

American Nurses Association (ANA). (1991). *Position statement on physical violence against women*. Washington, DC: Author.

Bachman, R., & Saltzman, L. E. (1995). *Violence against women: Estimates from the redesigned survey*. Bureau of Statistics special report. Washington, DC: US Department of Justice. (NCJ-154348).

Barcelona de Mendoza, V. (2001). Culturally appropriate care for pregnant Latina women who are victims of domestic violence. *Journal of Obstetric, Gynecologic, and Neonatal Nursing, 30*(6), 579–588.

Beckmann, C. R. B., & Groetzinger, L. L. (1989). Treating sexual assault victims: A protocol for health professionals. *The Female Patient, 14*, 78.

Best practices: Innovative domestic violence programs in healthcare settings. (1997, April). The Family Violence Prevention Fund. San Francisco, CA: author.

Bullock, L. F., Sandella, J. A., & McFarlane, J. (1989). Breaking the cycle of abuse: How nurses can intervene. *Journal of Psychosocial Nursing & Mental Health Services, 27*(8), 11–13.

Burge, S. K. (1989). Violence against women as a healthcare issue. *Family Medicine, 21*(5), 368–373.

Burgess, A. W., & Holmstrom, L. L. (1979). *Rape: Crisis and recovery*. Englewood Cliffs, NJ: Prentice Hall.

Campbell, J. (1984). Nursing care of abused women. In J. Campbell & J. Humphreys (Eds.), *Nursing care of victims of family violence*. Reston, VA: Reston Publishing.

Campbell, J. C. (1993). Woman abuse and public policy: Potential for nursing action. *AWHONN's Clinical Issues in Perinatal & Women's Health Nursing, 4*(3), 503–512.

Centers for Disease Control and Prevention (CDC). (2002, May 10). Sexually transmitted diseases treatment guidelines 2002. *Morbidity and Mortality Weekly Report, 51* (RR-6).

Coker, A. L., Smith, P. H., Bethea, L., King, M. R., McKeown, R. E. (2000). Physical health consequences of physical and psychological intimate partner violence. *Archives of Family Medicine, 9*(5), 451–457.

The Commonwealth Fund. (1999, May). *Health concerns across a women's lifespan: The Commonwealth Fund 1998 survey of women's health*. Retrieved December 30, 2002 from www.cmwf.org/program/women/ksc_whsurvey 99_332.osp

DeKeseredy, W. S., Schwartz, M. D., & Tait, K. (1993). Sexual assault and stranger aggression on a Canadian university campus. *Sex Roles, 28*(5–6), 263–277.

Dennis, L. I. (1998). Adolescent rape: The role of nursing. *Issues in Comprehensive Pediatric Nursing, 11*(1), 59–70.

Department of Health & Human Services, Public Health Services. (1990). *Healthy people 2000* (Publication No. PHS 91-50213). Washington, DC: Author.

Dupre, A. R., Hampton, H. L., Morrison, H., & Meeks, G. R. (1993). Sexual assault. *Obstetrical & Gynecological Survey, 48*(9), 640–648.

Fishwick, N. (1993). Nursing care of rural battered women. *AWHONN's Clinical Issues in Perinatal & Women's Health Nursing, 4*(3), 441–448.

Frye, V. (2001, March 21). Examining homicide's contribution to pregnancy-associated deaths. *Journal of the American Medical Association, 285*(11), 1510–1511.

Golan, N. (1978). *Treatment in crisis situations*. New York: Free Press.

Gordon, M. T., & Riger, S. (1989). *The female fear*. New York: Free Press.

Greensite, G. (1999). Rape myths. In *Support for survivors: Training for sexual assault counselors* (pp. 3–9). California Coalition Against Sexual Assault. Sacramento, CA: Author.

Groth, A. N. (1986). The rapist's view. In A. W. Burgess (2000). *Violence through a forensic lens*. King of Prussia, PA: Nursing Spectrum. (Reprinted from Burgess, A. W., & Holmstrom, L. L. [1986]. *Rape: Crisis and recovery*. West Newton, MA: Awab.)

Heise, L. L. (1998). Violence against women: An integrated, ecological framework. *Violence Against Women, 4*(3), 262–291.

Holmes, M. M. (1998). The clinical management of rape in adolescents. *Contemporary OB/GYN, 43*(5), 62–78.

Horon, I. L., & Cheng, D. (2001, March 21). Enhanced surveillance for pregnancy-associated mortality—Maryland, 1993–1998. *Journal of the American Medical Association, 285*(11), 1455–1459.

Kauffold, M. P. (1996, September). The SANE solution: Easing the trauma of rape. *Trustee, 49*(8), 6–9.

Kennedy, P. H. (1993). Sexual abuse within adult intimate relationships. *AWHONN's Clinical Issues in Perinatal & Women's Health Nursing, 4*(3), 391–401.

Koski, S. (1999). Vicarious trauma. In *Support for survivors: Training for sexual assault counselors* (pp. 201–206). California Coalition Against Sexual Assault. Sacramento, CA: Author.

Lathrop, A. (1998). Pregnancy resulting from rape. *Journal of Obstetric, Gynecologic, and Neonatal Nursing, 27*(1), 25–31.

Ledray, L. E. US Department of Justice, Office of Justice Programs, *Office for Victims of Crime. (1999). Sexual Assault Nurse Examiner (SANE) development and operation guide*. Minneapolis, MN: Sexual Assault Resource Service. (NCJ-170609).

Mattson, S., & Rodriguez, E. (1999). Battering in pregnant Latinas. *Issues in Mental Health Nursing, 20*, 405–422.

National Sexual Violence Resource Center (2000). *Overall crime victimization rate decreases 10% but rape increases 20%*. Retrieved May, 2002 from www.nsvr.org/newpress.html

Rennison, C. M. (2000). *Criminal victimization 1999: Changes 1998–1999 with trends 1993–1999*. Washington, DC: Bureau of Justice Statistics, US Department of Justice. (NCJ-182734).

Renshaw, D. C. (1989). Treatment of sexual exploitation. Rape and incest. *Psychiatric Clinics of North America, 12*(2), 257–277.

Responding to drug-facilitated sexual assault: A reference guide for police and medical professionals. (2000). Fairfax, VA: George Mason University Sexual Assault Services.

Rickert, V. I., & Wiemann, C. M. (1998). Date rape: Office-based solutions. *Contemporary OB/GYN, 43*(3), 133–153.

Ryan, J., & King, M. C. (1998). Scanning for violence: Educational strategies for helping abused women. *AWHONN Lifelines, 2*(3), 36–41.

Stenchever, M. A., & Stenchever, D. H. (1991). Abuse of women: An overview. *Women's Health Issues*, 1(4), 187–192.

Tjaden, P., & Thoennes, N. (2000). *Full report of the prevalence, incidence, and consequences of violence against women: Findings from the National Violence Against Women Survey*. Washington, DC: Bureau of Justice Statistics, US Department of Justice.

Voelker, R. (1996, April). Experts hope team approach will improve the quality of rape exams. *Journal of the American Medical Association, 275*(13), 973–974.

Walker, L. (1984). *The battered woman syndrome*. New York: Springer.

THREE

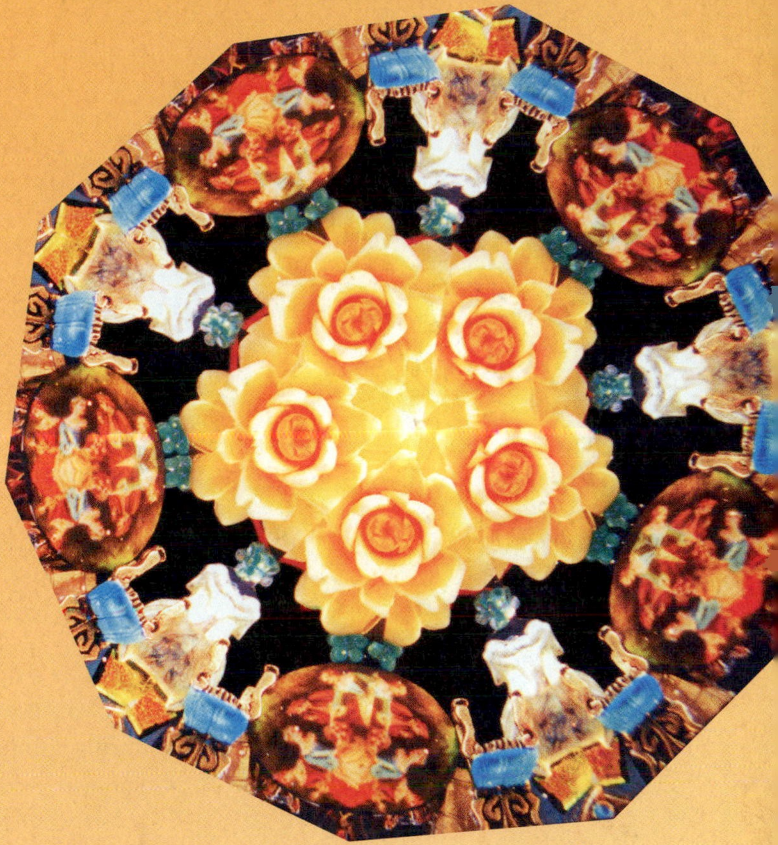

Human Reproduction

The Reproductive System 10

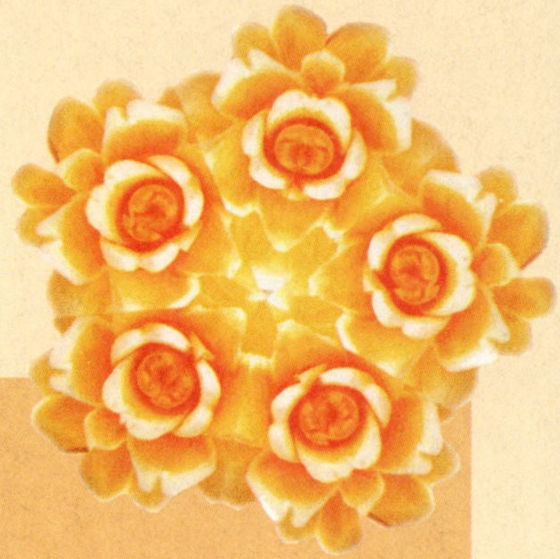

I always thought it was so boring to study anatomy and physiology. Who cares how many bones there are in the pelvis or the muscles involved. But now I'm with mothers having babies, and now it all makes sense.
~ A Nursing Student ~

Objectives

- Describe the differentiation of the male and female reproductive organs during embryonic development.
- Summarize the major changes in the reproductive system that occur during puberty.
- Identify key aspects of the female and male reproductive systems that are important to conception.
- Discuss the significance of specific female reproductive structures during pregnancy and childbirth.
- Summarize the actions of the hormones that affect reproductive functioning.
- Identify the two phases of the ovarian cycle and the changes that occur in each phase.
- Describe the phases of the menstrual cycle, their dominant hormones, and the changes that occur in each phase.

Key Terms

Ampulla 202
Areola 209
Breasts 209
Cervix 201
Conjugate vera 207
Cornua 199
Corpus 199
Corpus luteum 212
Diagonal conjugate 207
Endometrium 200
Estrogens 210
Fallopian tubes 202
Female reproductive cycle (FRC) 210
Fimbria 202
Follicle-stimulating hormone (FSH) 195
Fundus 199
Gonadotropin-releasing hormone (GnRH) 195
Graafian follicle 212
Human chorionic gonadotropin (hCG) 213
Ischial spines 205
Isthmus 202
Luteinizing hormone (LH) 195
Myometrium 200
Nidation 200
Nipple 209
Obstetric conjugate 207
Oocytes 193
Oogenesis 193
Ovulation 212
Ovum 193
Pelvic diaphragm 205

MEDIALINK

Additional resources for this content can be found on the Student CD-ROM and on the Companion Website at www.prenhall.com/olds. Click on "Chapter 10" to select the activities for this chapter.

CD-ROM
- Audio Glossary
- NCLEX Review
- Animation: Female Pelvis
- Activity: Female Reproductive System
- Activity: Ovulation
- Animation: Male Pelvis
- Activity: Male Reproductive System

Companion Website
- Additional NCLEX Review
- Case Study: Sex Education for Teens
- Care Plan Activity: Irregular Menses in a Client With Anxiety

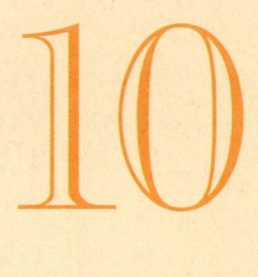

Key Terms

Understanding childbearing requires more than understanding sexual intercourse or the process by which the female and male sex cells unite. The nurse must also become familiar with the structures and functions that make childbearing possible and the phenomena that initiate it. This chapter considers the anatomic, physiologic, and sexual aspects of the female and male reproductive systems. It also provides information regarding basic embryonic development of the reproductive structures. The psychosocial aspects of human sexuality are discussed in Chapter 4.

The female and male reproductive organs are *homologous;* that is, they are fundamentally similar in function and structure. The primary functions of both the female and male reproductive systems are to produce sex cells and transport them to locations where their union can occur. The sex cells, called *gametes,* are produced by specialized organs called *gonads.* A series of ducts and glands within both the male and female reproductive systems contributes to the production and transport of the gametes.

Embryonic Development of Reproductive Structures and Processes

Although the genetic sex of an embryo is determined at fertilization, the male and female reproductive systems are undifferentiated for about the first 8 weeks of gestation. This undifferentiated period is followed by a period of rapid, dramatic changes as the reproductive organs differentiate into recognizable structures.

Ovaries and Testes

During the 5th week of gestation, a primitive gonad arises from the intermediate mesoderm tissue known as gonadal ridges (Figure 10–1 •, top). The gonad develops a medulla (inner part of the organ) and cortex (outer part of the organ), which appear in the underlying mesenchyme (embryonic tissue from which connective and muscle tissue arises; see Table 11–1). In genetic males during the 7th and 8th weeks, the medulla develops into a testis, and the cortex regresses. In genetic females by about the 10th week, the cortex develops into an ovary, and the medulla regresses.

Every egg available for maturation in a woman's reproductive life is present at her birth. During fetal life the ovary produces oogonia, cells that become primitive eggs called **oocytes,** by the process of **oogenesis** (see Chapter 11). No oocytes are formed after fetal development. About 150,000 oocytes are contained in the ovaries at birth. Each oocyte is contained in a small ovarian cavity called a *primitive follicle.*

Every month during a female's reproductive years, one of the oocytes undergoes a process of cellular division and maturation that transforms it into a fertilizable egg, or **ovum.** At ovulation, the ovum is released from its follicle. The remaining follicles and oocytes degenerate over time.

Each testis produces the male gametes, called **spermatozoa** or *sperm,* by a process called **spermatogenesis.** This process is described in Chapter 11. Spermatogenesis of mature sperm does not occur until the onset of puberty.

Figure 10–1 illustrates the embryologic development of the gonads and other internal reproductive organs.

Other Internal Structures

During the undifferentiated period—the first 7 weeks—two pairs of genital ducts develop: the mesonephric and paramesonephric ducts (Cunningham, Gant, Leveno, et al, 2001).

In genetic females the fallopian tubes are formed from the unfused portions of the paramesonephric ducts, and the fused portions give rise to the epithelium and uterine glands. The endometrial stroma and the myometrium (thick layer of smooth muscle in the wall of the uterus) develop from the adjacent mesenchyme.

The vagina is derived from more than one embryologic structure. The vaginal epithelium develops from the endoderm of the urogenital sinus, and the musculature develops from the uterovaginal primordium.

The urethral and paraurethral glands develop from outgrowths of the urethra into the surrounding mesenchyme. Bartholin's glands arise from similar structures.

In genetic males the fetal testes secrete two hormones. The first hormone, testosterone, stimulates the mesonephric ducts to develop into the male genital tract. The other hormone, Müllerian regression factor, suppresses the development of the paramesonephric ducts, which would otherwise develop into the female genital tract.

From the mesonephric ducts comes development of the efferent ductule, vas deferens, epididymis, seminal vesicle, and ejaculatory duct. Both the prostate and the bulbourethral glands develop from endodermal outgrowths of the urethra.

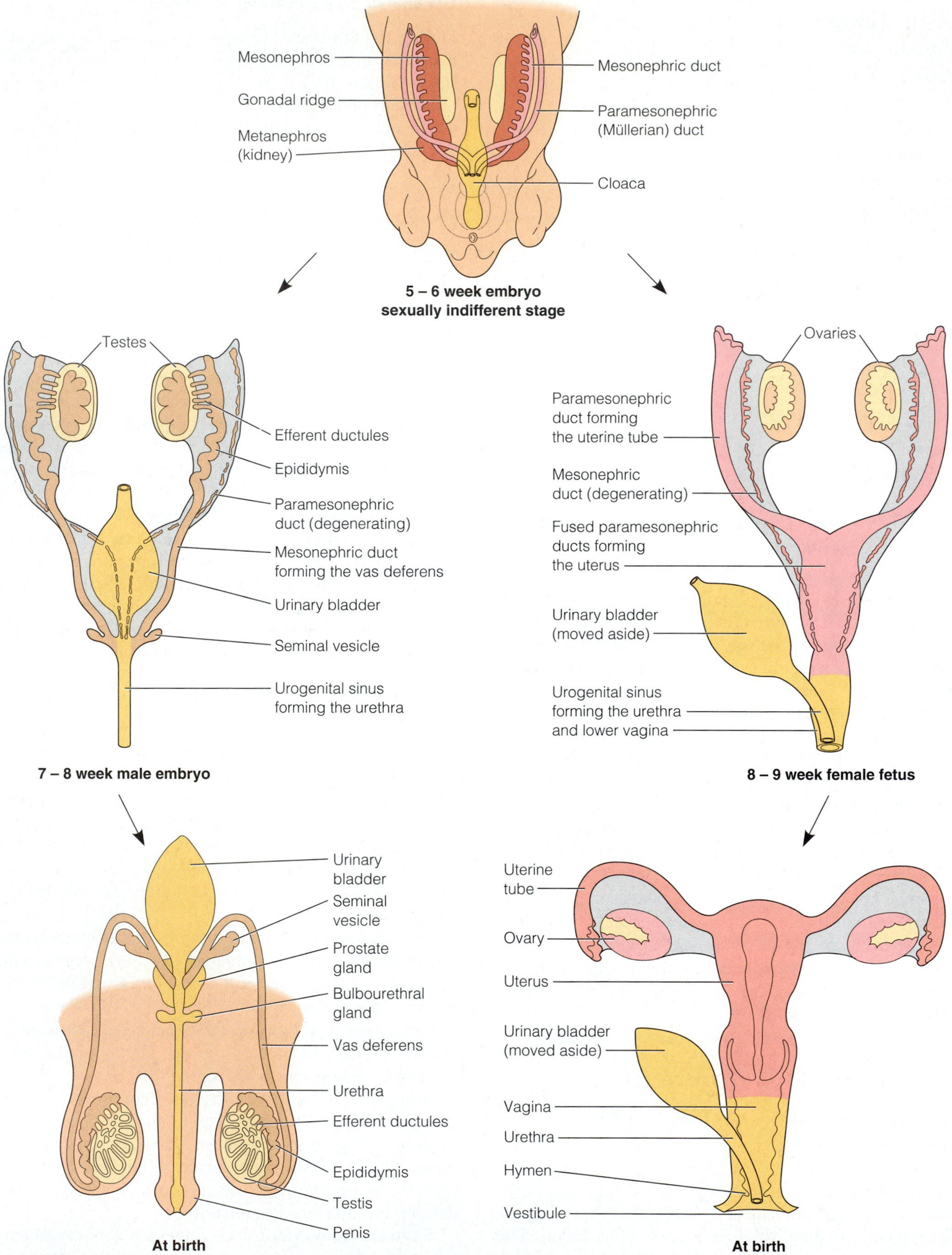

Figure 10-1 • Embryonic differentiation of male and female internal reproductive organs.

External Structures

Genetic males and females possess the same external genitals until the end of the 9th week. By the 12th week, differentiation of the external genitals is complete.

If fetal testosterone is not present, the undifferentiated external genitals are feminized. The phallus becomes the clitoris, and the urogenital folds remain open, forming the labia minora. The labioscrotal folds form the labia majora.

If fetal testosterone is present, the undifferentiated external genitals become masculine. The phallus elongates, forming the penis. The fusion of the urogenital folds on the ventral surface of the penis forms the penile urethra, with the urethral meatus moving forward toward the glans penis.

Puberty

The term **puberty** refers to the developmental period between childhood and attainment of adult sexual characteristics and functioning. Generally, boys mature physically about 2 years later than girls. Puberty lasts from 1.5 to 5 years and involves profound physical, psychologic, and emotional changes. These changes include an altered body image, changing roles, and changing societal expectations and responses as the child matures to an adult.

Major Physical Changes

In both girls and boys, puberty is preceded by an accelerated growth rate called adolescent spurt. Widespread body system changes occur, including maturation of the reproductive organs.

Girls experience a broadening of the hips, then budding of the breasts, the appearance of pubic and axillary hair, and the onset of menstruation, called menarche. The average time between breast development and menarche is 2.3 years.

Boys experience linear growth spurts; an increase in the size of the external genitals; the appearance of pubic, axillary, and facial hair; deepening of the voice; and nocturnal seminal emissions (called wet dreams) without sexual stimulation. These early seminal emissions do not usually contain mature sperm.

The physical changes of puberty present themselves differently in each person. The age at onset and progress of puberty vary widely, physical changes overlap, and the sequence of events can vary from person to person. This diversity results from each individual's response to hormonal stimulation.

Physiology of Onset

Puberty is initiated by the maturation of the hypothalamic-pituitary-gonad complex (the *gonadostat*) and input from the central nervous system. The process, which begins during fetal life, is sequential and complex.

The central nervous system releases a neurotransmitter that stimulates the hypothalamus to synthesize and release **gonadotropin-releasing hormone (GnRH)** (Blackburn, 2003). GnRH is transmitted to the anterior pituitary, where it causes the synthesis and secretion of the gonadotropins **follicle-stimulating hormone (FSH)** and **luteinizing hormone (LH)** (Figure 10–2 ●).

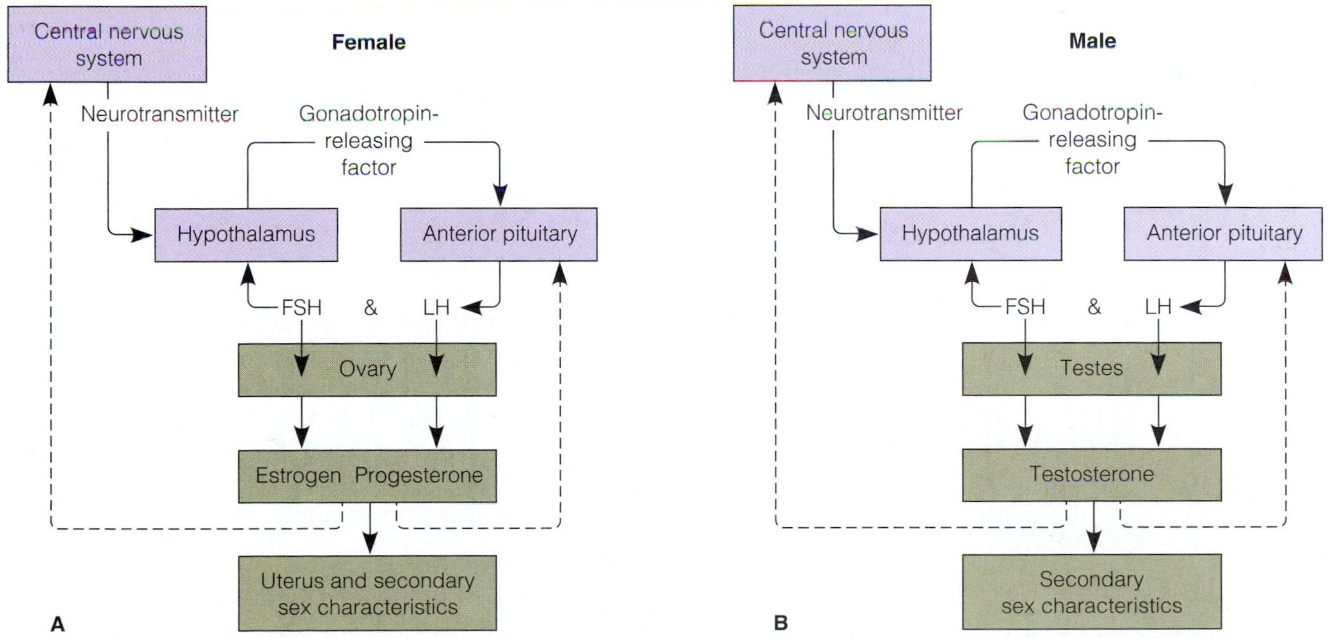

Figure 10–2 ● Physiologic changes leading to onset of puberty. *A,* In females; and *B,* in males. Solid lines illustrate stimulation of hormone production, and broken lines illustrate inhibition. Through a neurotransmitter the central nervous system (CNS) stimulates the hypothalamus, which in turn produces a gonadotropin-releasing factor that causes the anterior pituitary to produce gonadotropins (FSH or LH). These hormones stimulate specific structures in the gonads to secrete steroid hormones (estrogen, progesterone, or testosterone). The rise in pituitary hormone production increases hypothalamus activity. Elevated steroid hormone levels stimulate the CNS and pituitary gland to inhibit hormone production.

Although the gonads do produce small amounts of *androgens* (male sex hormones) and *estrogens* (female sex hormones) before the onset of puberty, FSH and LH stimulate increased secretion of these hormones. Androgens and estrogens influence the development of secondary sex characteristics. FSH and LH stimulate the processes of spermatogenesis and maturation of ova.

Other hormones are involved in the onset of puberty. Although less direct, their action is essential. Abnormally high or low levels of adrenocorticotropic hormone (ACTH), thyroid hormone, or growth hormone (GH) can disrupt the onset of normal puberty (Blackburn, 2003).

Female Reproductive System

The female reproductive system consists of the external and internal genitals and accessory organs of the breasts. The structure of the bony pelvis is also discussed in this section because of its importance in childbearing.

External Genitals

All the external reproductive organs, except the glandular structures, can be directly inspected. The size, color, and shape of these structures vary extensively among races and individuals.

MediaLink WebMD Anatomy

The female external genitals, called the **vulva** or pudendum, include the following structures (Figure 10–3 •):

- Mons pubis
- Labia majora
- Labia minora
- Clitoris
- Urethral meatus and opening of the paraurethral (Skene's) glands
- Vaginal vestibule (vaginal orifice, vulvovaginal glands, hymen, and fossa navicularis)
- Perineal body

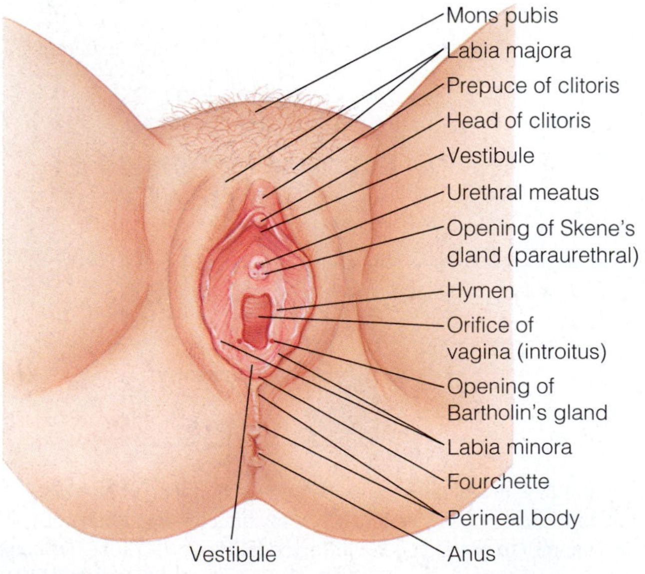

Figure 10–3 • Female external genitals, longitudinal view.

Although they are not actually parts of the female reproductive system, this chapter discusses the urethral meatus and perineal body because of their proximity and relationship to the vulva.

The vulva has a generous supply of blood and nerves. As a woman ages, estrogen secretions decrease, causing gradual atrophy of tissues.

MONS PUBIS

The mons pubis is a softly rounded mound of subcutaneous fatty tissue beginning at the lowest portion of the anterior abdominal wall. Also known as the mons veneris, this structure covers the anterior portion of the symphysis pubis. The mons pubis is covered with pubic hair, typically with the hairline forming a transverse line across the lower abdomen (see Figure 10–3). The hair is short and varies from sparse and fine in the Asian woman to heavy, coarse, and curly in the black woman. The mons pubis protects the pelvic bones, especially during coitus.

LABIA MAJORA

The *labia majora* are longitudinal, raised folds of pigmented skin, one on either side of the vulvar cleft (Figure 10–3). As the pair descend, they narrow, enclosing the vulvar cleft, and merge to form the posterior junction of the perineal skin. Their chief function is to protect the structures lying between them. The labia majora are covered by stratified squamous epithelium containing hair follicles and sebaceous glands with underlying adipose and muscle tissue. Immediately under the skin is a sheet of dartos muscle, which is responsible for the wrinkled appearance of the labia majora.

The inner surface of the labia majora in women who have not had children is moist and looks like a mucous membrane, but after many births it is more skinlike, though not covered with hair (Cunningham et al, 2001). With each pregnancy the labia majora become less prominent.

Because of the extensive venous network in the labia majora, varicosities may occur during pregnancy, and birth trauma or sexual trauma may cause hematomas. The labia majora share an extensive lymphatic supply with the other structures of the vulva, which can facilitate the spread of cancer in the female reproductive organs. Because nerves from the first lumbar and third sacral segment of the spinal cord supply the labia majora, certain regional anesthesia blocks will affect them and cause numbness.

LABIA MINORA

The *labia minora* are soft folds of skin within the labia majora that converge near the anus, forming the *fourchette* (Figure 10–3). Each labium minus has the appearance of a shiny mucous membrane, moist and devoid of hair follicles. The labia minora are rich in sebaceous glands, which lubricate and waterproof the vulvar skin and provide bactericidal secretions. Because sebaceous glands do not open into hair follicles but directly onto the surface of the skin, sebaceous cysts commonly occur in this area. The labia minora are composed of erectile tissue and involuntary muscle tissue. Vulvovaginitis in this area is very irritating because of the many tactile nerve endings. The labia minora increase in size at puberty and decrease after menopause due to changes in estrogen levels.

CLITORIS

The *clitoris*, located between the labia minora, is about 5 to 6 mm long and 6 to 8 mm across. Its tissue is essentially erectile (Figure 10–3). The glans is partially covered by a fold of skin called the *prepuce*, or clitoral hood. This area often looks like an opening to an orifice and may be confused with the urethral meatus. Accidental attempts to insert a catheter in this area produce extreme discomfort. The clitoris has very rich blood and nerve supplies and is the primary erogenous organ of women (Cunningham et al, 2001). In addition, it secretes *smegma*, which along with other vulval secretions has a unique odor that may be sexually stimulating to a man. In some cultures, the clitoris is removed.

URETHRAL MEATUS AND PARAURETHRAL GLANDS

The *urethral meatus* is located 1 to 2.5 cm beneath the clitoris in the midline of the vestibule; it often appears as a puckered, slitlike opening. At times the meatus is difficult to visualize because of the presence of blind dimples, small mucosal folds, or wide variations in location.

The paraurethral glands, or *Skene's glands*, open into the posterior wall of the urethra close to its opening (Figure 10–3). Their secretions help lubricate the vaginal vestibule, facilitating sexual intercourse.

VAGINAL VESTIBULE

The vaginal vestibule is a boat-shaped depression enclosed by the labia majora and visible when they are separated (Figure 10–3). The vestibule contains the vaginal opening, or *introitus*, which is the border between the external and internal genitals.

The *hymen* is a collar or semicollar of tissue that surrounds the vaginal opening. The appearance of the hymen changes during the woman's lifetime. From birth to about 3 years of age, the hymen is fluffy and full, and the tissue appears to fold back on itself and to cover the vaginal opening. These characteristics are due to exposure to estrogen in utero. With the loss of exposure to estrogen after birth, the hymen's appearance begins to change to a thin membranous tissue that is still in a collar or semicollar shape. At approximately 3 years of age, the hymen is thin and membranous, with an absence of tissue beneath the urethra (Cunningham et al, 2001). The hymen is without estrogen stimulation and is hypersensitive to touch. At puberty, under the stimulation of the girl's own increasing estrogen levels, the hymen once again becomes more full. For thousands of years, some societies have perpetuated the belief that the hymen covers the vaginal opening and thus that an intact hymen is a sign of virginity. However, modern studies of female genital anatomy have revealed that the hymen surrounds rather than entirely covers the vaginal opening, and can be broken not only through sexual intercourse, but also through strenuous physical activity, masturbation, menstruation, or the use of tampons, thus dispelling old beliefs.

External to the hymenal tissue at the base of the vestibule are two small papular elevations containing the openings of the ducts of the *vulvovaginal (Bartholin's) glands*. They lie under the constrictor muscle of the vagina. These glands secrete a clear and thick mucus with an alkaline pH that enhances the viability and motility of sperm deposited in the vaginal vestibule. These ducts of the vulvovaginal glands can harbor *Neisseria gonorrhoeae* and other bacteria, which can cause suppuration and abscesses in the Bartholin's glands.

The vestibular area is innervated mainly by the perineal nerve from the sacral plexus. The area is not sensitive to touch generally; however, the hymen contains numerous free nerve endings as receptors to pain.

PERINEAL BODY

The **perineal body** is a wedge-shaped mass of fibromuscular tissue measuring about 4 × 4 × 4 cm, found between the lower part of the vagina and the anal canal (Figure 10–3). The superficial area between the anus and the vagina is referred to as the *perineum*.

The muscles that meet at the perineal body are the external sphincter ani, both levator ani (the superficial and deep transverse perineal), and the bulbocavernosus. These muscles mingle with elastic fibers and connective tissue in an arrangement that allows a remarkable amount of stretching. During the last part of labor, the perineal body thins out until it is just a few centimeters thick. This tissue is often the site of an episiotomy or lacerations during childbirth (see Chapter 27).

Female Internal Reproductive Organs

The female internal reproductive organs—the vagina, uterus, fallopian tubes, and ovaries—are target organs for estrogenic hormones. These organs play a unique part in the reproductive cycle (Figure 10–4 •). The internal reproductive organs can be palpated during vaginal examination and assessed through use of various instruments.

VAGINA

The **vagina** is a muscular and membranous tube that connects the external genitals with the uterus (Figure 10–4). It extends from the vulva to the uterus in a position nearly parallel to the plane of the pelvic brim. The vagina is often referred to as the *birth canal* because it forms the lower part of the axis through which the fetus must pass during birth.

Because the cervix of the uterus projects into the upper part of the anterior wall of the vagina, the anterior wall is approximately 2.5 cm shorter than the posterior wall. Measurements range from 6 to 8 cm for the anterior wall and 7 to 10 cm for the posterior wall.

In the upper part of the vagina, which is called the vaginal vault, there is a recess or hollow around the cervix called the vaginal *fornix*. Because the walls of the vaginal vault are very thin, various structures can be palpated through the walls and fornix of the vaginal vault, including the uterus, a distended bladder, the ovaries, appendix, cecum, colon, and the ureters.

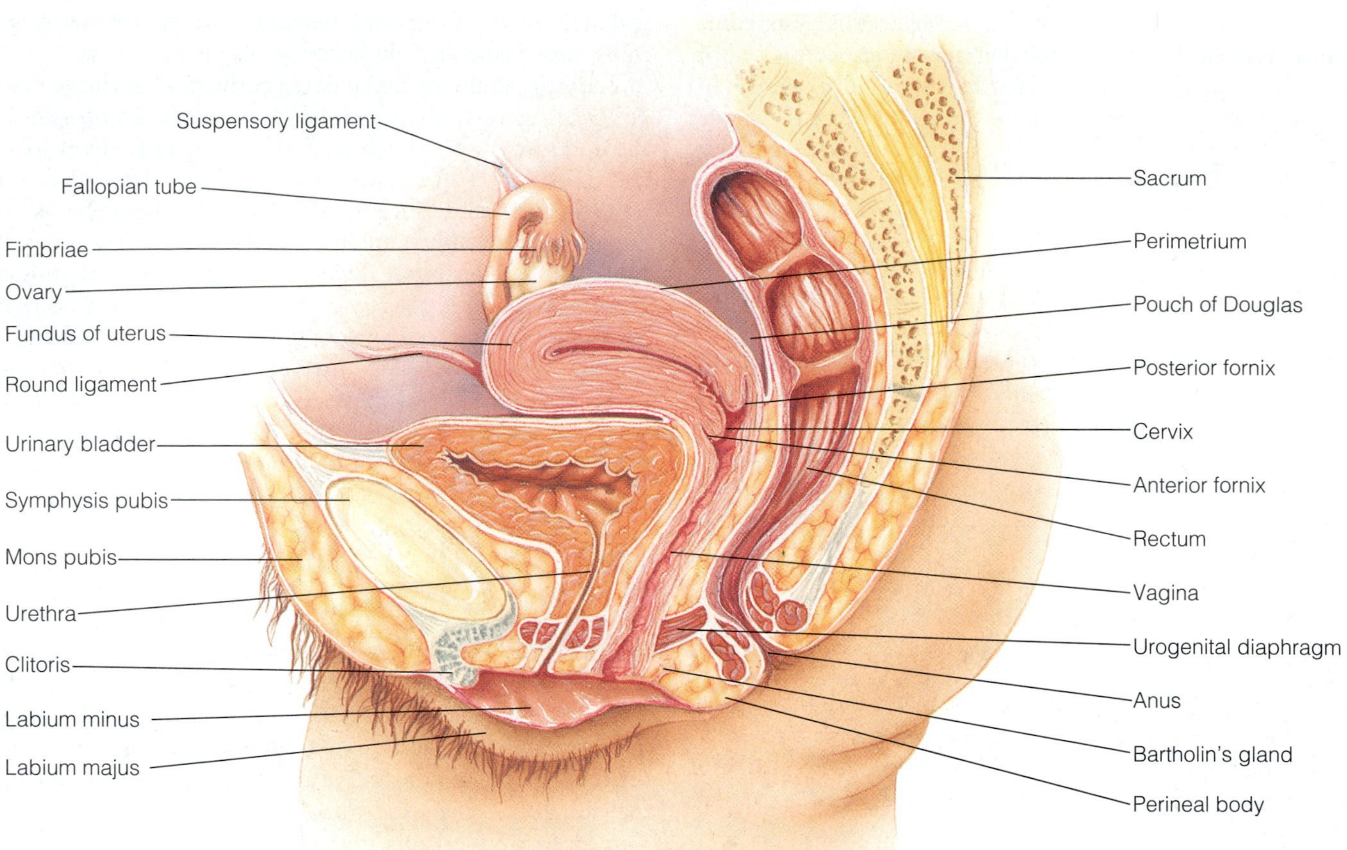

Figure 10–4 • Female internal reproductive organs.

When a woman lies on her back after intercourse, the space in the fornix permits the pooling of semen. The collection of a large number of sperm near the cervix at or near the time of ovulation in the woman increases the chances of pregnancy.

The walls of the vagina are covered with ridges, or rugae, crisscrossing each other. These rugae allow the vaginal tissues to stretch enough for the fetus to pass through during childbirth.

A rich blood supply is needed to maintain a high glycogen content in the epithelial cells as well as to nourish the underlying musculofascial layer, through which the vaginal vault has strong attachments to the cervix. These muscle layers are continuous with the superficial muscle fibers of the uterus. A thin band of striated muscle, the sphincter vaginae, is found at the lowest extremity of the vagina. However, the levator ani is the principal muscle that closes the vagina.

During a woman's reproductive life, the vaginal environment is normally acidic (pH 4.0 to 5.0). Secretion from the vaginal epithelium provides a moist environment. The acidic environment is maintained by a symbiotic relationship between lactic acid-producing bacilli (Döderlein's bacillus or lactobacillus) and the vaginal epithelial cells. These cells contain glycogen, which is broken down by the bacilli into lactic acid. The amount of glycogen is regulated by the ovarian hormones. Any interruption of this process can destroy the normal self-cleansing action of the vagina. Such interruption may be caused by antibiotic therapy, douching, or use of vaginal sprays or deodorants. For further discussion, see Chapter 5.

The acidic vaginal environment is normal only during the mature reproductive years and in the first days of life, when maternal hormones are operating in the infant. A relatively neutral pH of 7.5 is normal from infancy until puberty and after menopause.

Each third of the vagina is supplied by a distinct vascular and lymphatic pattern. Although one would expect venous drainage to go directly to the heart and then the lungs, anastomoses of veins are present and make it possible for a pelvic embolism or carcinoma to bypass the heart and lungs and lodge in the brain, spine, or other remote part of the body.

Vaginal lymphatics drain into the external and internal iliac nodes, the hypogastric nodes, and the inguinal glands. The posterior wall drains into nodes lying in the rectovaginal septum. Any vaginal infection follows these routes.

The pudendal nerve supplies what relatively little somatic innervation there is to the lower third of the vagina.

Thus vaginal sensation during sexual excitement and coitus is minimal, as is vaginal pain during the second stage of labor.

The vagina has the following functions:

- To serve as the passageway for sperm and for the fetus during birth
- To provide passage for the menstrual blood flow from the uterine endometrium to the outside of the body
- To protect against infection from pathogenic organisms

UTERUS

As the core of reproduction and hence continuation of the human race, the uterus, or womb, has been endowed with a mystical aura. Numerous customs, taboos, mores, and values have evolved about women and their reproductive function. Although scientific knowledge has replaced much of this folklore, remnants of old ideas and superstitions persist. To provide effective care, nurses must be cognizant of their own attitudes and beliefs, as well as those of their clients.

The **uterus** is a hollow, muscular, thick-walled organ shaped like an upside-down pear. It lies in the center of the pelvic cavity between the base of the bladder and the rectum and above the vagina (Figure 10–5 •). It is level with or slightly below the brim of the pelvis, with the external opening of the cervix (the external os) about the level of the ischial spines. The mature organ in adult women weighs about 50 to 70 g and is 6 to 8 cm long (Cunningham et al, 2001).

Many uterine anomalies are thought to be congenital. A normal uterus requires two symmetric, parallel, equal-sized paramesonephric ducts to meet in the midline. Their ultimate midline fusion give rise to the fallopian tubes, uterine fundus, cervix, and upper vagina. Anomalies represent the absence of either one or both of the ducts, degrees of failure to fuse, or canalization defects. Uterine malformations such as the uterus bicornuate ("two-horned") and uterus didelphys ("double uterus") are associated with habitual abortion. Because both the urinary and reproductive systems develop from the common urogenital fold in the embryo, anomalies in one system are frequently accompanied by anomalies in the other. Problems of infertility and premature labor and birth are common.

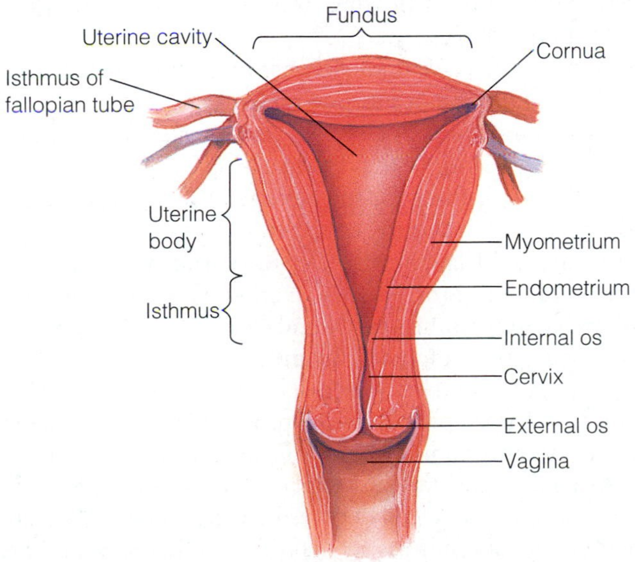

Figure 10–5 • Structures of the uterus.

The body of the uterus can move freely forward or backward. Only the cervix is anchored laterally. Thus the position of the uterus can vary, depending on a woman's posture, number of children borne, bladder and rectal fullness, and even normal respiratory patterns. The axis also varies. Generally, the uterus bends forward, forming a sharp angle with the vagina. There is a bend in the area of the isthmus of the uterus, and from there the cervix points downward. The uterus is said to be anteverted when it is in this position. The anteverted position is considered normal.

The uterus is kept in place by three sets of supports. The upper supports are the broad and round ligaments. The middle supports are the cardinal, pubocervical, and uterosacral ligaments. The lower supports are those structures considered to be the pelvic muscular floor.

The isthmus is a slight constriction in the uterus that divides it into two unequal parts. The upper two thirds of the uterus is the **corpus,** or body, composed mainly of a smooth muscle layer (myometrium). The lower third is the cervix, or neck. The rounded uppermost portion of the corpus that extends above the points of attachment of the fallopian tubes is called the **fundus.** The elongated portion of the uterus where the fallopian tubes enter is called the **cornua.**

The isthmus joins the corpus and the cervix. It is located about 6 mm above the uterine opening of the cervix (the internal os), and it is in this area that the uterine lining changes into the mucous membrane of the cervix; it joins the corpus to the cervix. The isthmus takes on importance in pregnancy because it becomes the lower uterine segment. With the cervix it is a passive segment and not part of the contractile uterus. At birth this thin lower segment, situated behind the bladder, is the site for lower-segment cesarean births (see Chapter 27).

The blood and lymphatic supplies to the uterus are extensive (Figure 10–6 •). The uterus is innervated entirely by the autonomic nervous system. Efferent sympathetic motor nerves arise from the ganglia of the 5th to 10th thoracic vertebrae, come together over the sacrum, and reach the uterus through ganglia that lie near the base of the uterosacral ligaments. These sympathetic motor nerves are believed to cause vasoconstriction and muscular contraction. Even without an intact nerve supply, the uterus can contract adequately for birth. Thus, for example, hemiplegic women have adequate uterine contractions.

Pain of uterine contractions is carried to the central nervous system by the 11th and 12th thoracic nerve roots. Pain from the cervix and upper vagina passes through the ilioinguinal and pudendal nerves. The motor fibers to the uterus arise from the 7th and 8th thoracic vertebrae. Because the sensory and motor levels are separate, epidural anesthesia can be used during labor and birth.

The function of the uterus is to provide a safe environment for fetal development. The uterine lining is cyclically

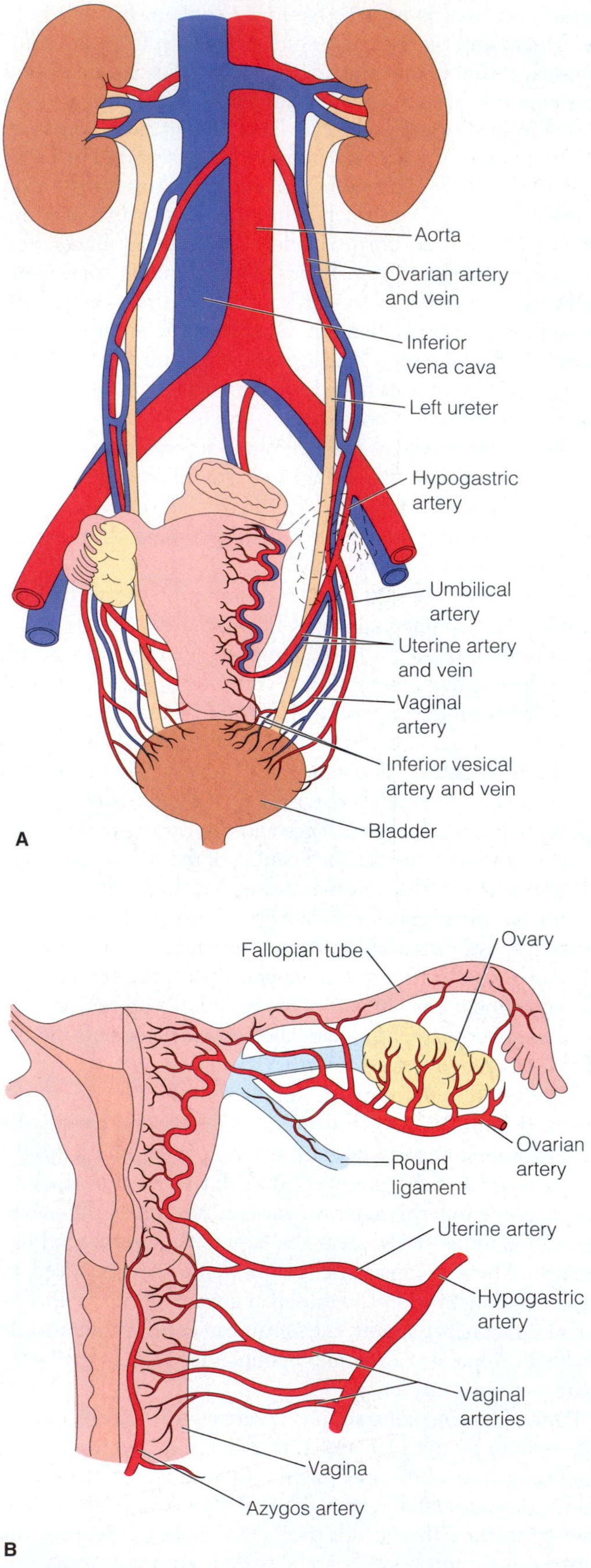

Figure 10–6 • Blood supply to internal reproductive organs: *A,* Pelvic blood supply. *B,* Blood supply to vagina, ovary, uterus, and fallopian tube.

prepared by steroid hormones for implantation of the embryo, a process known as **nidation.** Once the embryo is implanted, the developing fetus is protected until it is expelled.

Both the body of the uterus and the cervix are changed permanently by pregnancy. The body never returns to its prepregnant size, and the external os changes from a circular opening of about 3 mm to a transverse slit with irregular edges.

The Corpus

The uterine corpus is made up of three layers. The outermost layer is the *serosal layer,* or **perimetrium,** which is composed of peritoneum. The middle layer is the *muscular uterine layer,* or **myometrium.** This *muscular uterine layer* is continuous with the muscle layer of the fallopian tubes and with that of the vagina. This characteristic helps the organs present a unified reaction to various stimuli—ovulation, orgasm, or the deposit of sperm in the vagina. These muscle fibers also extend into the ovarian, round, and cardinal ligaments and minimally into the uterosacral ligaments, which helps explain the vague but disturbing pelvic "aches and pains" reported by many pregnant women.

The myometrium has three distinct layers of uterine (smooth) involuntary muscles (Figure 10–7 •). The outer layer, found mainly over the fundus, is made up of longitudinal muscles especially suited to expel the fetus during birth. The middle layer is thick and made up of interlacing muscle fibers in figure-eight patterns. These muscle fibers surround large blood vessels, and their contraction produces a hemostatic action (a tourniquet-like action on blood vessels to stop bleeding after birth). The inner muscle layer is made up of circular fibers, which form sphincters at the fallopian tube attachment sites and at the internal os. The internal os sphincter inhibits the expulsion of the uterine contents during pregnancy but stretches in labor as cervical dilatation occurs. An incompetent cervical os can be caused by a torn, weak, or absent sphincter at the internal os. The sphincters at the fallopian tubes prevent menstrual blood from flowing backward into the fallopian tubes from the uterus.

Although each layer of muscle has been discussed as having a unique function, it must be remembered that the uterine musculature works as a whole. The uterine contractions of labor are responsible for the dilatation of the cervix and provide the major force for the passage of the fetus through the pelvic and vaginal canal at birth.

The innermost layer of the uterine corpus is the *mucosal layer,* or **endometrium,** which is composed of a single layer of columnar epithelium, glands, and stroma. From menarche to menopause, the endometrium undergoes monthly renewal and degeneration in the absence of pregnancy. As it responds to a governing hormonal cycle and prostaglandin influence as well, the endometrium varies in thickness from 0.5 to 5 mm.

The glands of the endometrium produce a thin, watery, alkaline secretion that keeps the uterine cavity moist. This endometrial milk not only assists the sperm as they travel to the fallopian tubes, but also nourishes the developing embryo before it implants in the endometrium (see Chapter 11).

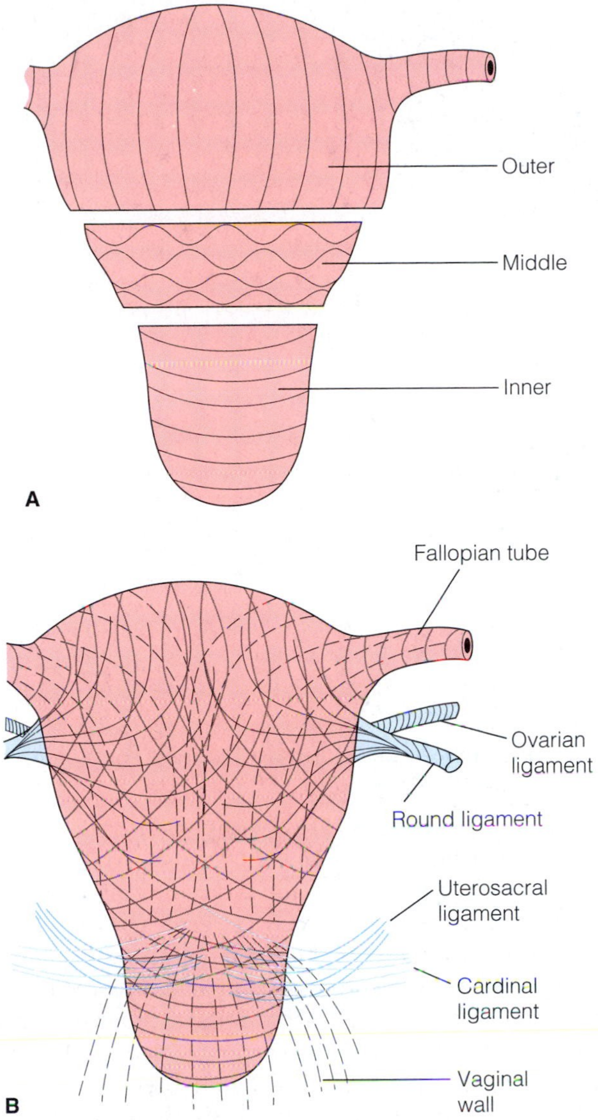

Figure 10–7 • Uterine muscle layers: *A*, Muscle fiber placement. *B*, Interlacing of uterine muscle layers.

The blood supply to the endometrium is unique. In the myometrium, the radial arteries branch off from the arcuate arteries at right angles. Once inside the endometrium, they become the basal arteries supplying the zona basalis (a layer of the endometrium) and ultimately become the coiled arteries supplying the zona functionalis (also part of the endometrium). The straighter basal arteries are smaller than the coiled arteries and are not sensitive to cyclic hormonal control. Hence the zona basalis portion remains intact and is the site of new endometrial tissue generation. The coiled arteries are extremely sensitive to cyclic hormonal control. Their response is alternate relaxation and constriction during the ischemic, or terminal, phase of the menstrual cycle. This response allows for part of the endometrial tissue to remain intact while other endometrial tissue is shed during menstruation.

When pregnancy occurs and the endometrium is not shed, the reticular stromal cells surrounding the endometrial glands become the decidual cells of pregnancy. The stromal cells are highly vascular, channeling a rich blood supply to the endometrial surface.

The Cervix

The narrow neck of the uterus is the **cervix.** Canal-like, it meets the body of the uterus at the internal os and descends about 2.5 cm to connect with the vagina at the external os (Figure 10–5). Thus it provides a protective portal for the body of the uterus. The cervix is divided by its line of attachment into the vaginal and supravaginal areas. The vaginal cervix projects into the vagina at an angle from 45 to 90 degrees. The *supravaginal* cervix is surrounded by the attachments that give the uterus its main support: the uterosacral ligaments, the transverse ligaments of the cervix (Mackenrodt's ligaments), and the pubocervical ligaments.

The vaginal cervix appears pink and ends at the external os. The cervical canal appears rosy red and is lined with columnar ciliated epithelium, which contains mucus-secreting glands. Most cervical cancer begins at this *squamocolumnar junction.* The specific location of the junction varies with age and number of pregnancies. Figure 10–8 • shows this junction at various stages of a woman's life.

Elasticity is the chief characteristic of the cervix. Its ability to stretch is due to the high fibrous and collagenous content of the supportive tissues and also to the vast number of folds in the cervical lining.

The cervical mucosa has three functions:

- To provide lubrication for the vaginal canal
- To act as a bacteriostatic agent
- To provide an alkaline environment to shelter deposited sperm from the acidic vagina

At ovulation, cervical mucus is clearer, thinner, and more alkaline than at other times.

UTERINE LIGAMENTS

The uterine ligaments support and stabilize the various reproductive organs. The ligaments shown in Figure 10–9 • are described in this section.

- The *broad ligament* keeps the uterus centrally placed and provides stability within the pelvic cavity. It is a double layer that is continuous with the abdominal peritoneum.

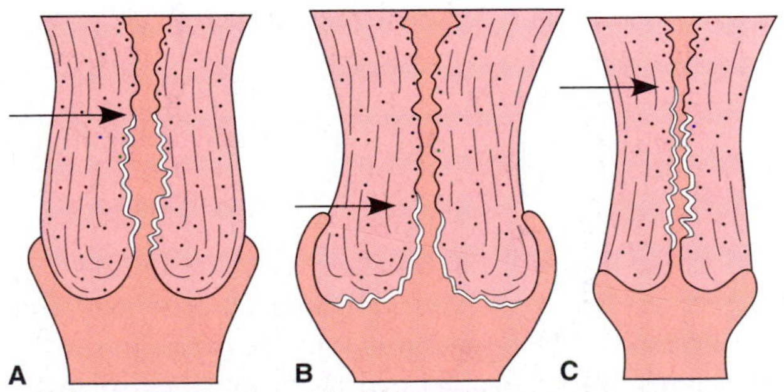

Figure 10–8 • Changes in squamocolumnar junction (arrows) at various stages of life: *A*, Childhood. *B*, Reproductive years. *C*, Postmenopausal years.

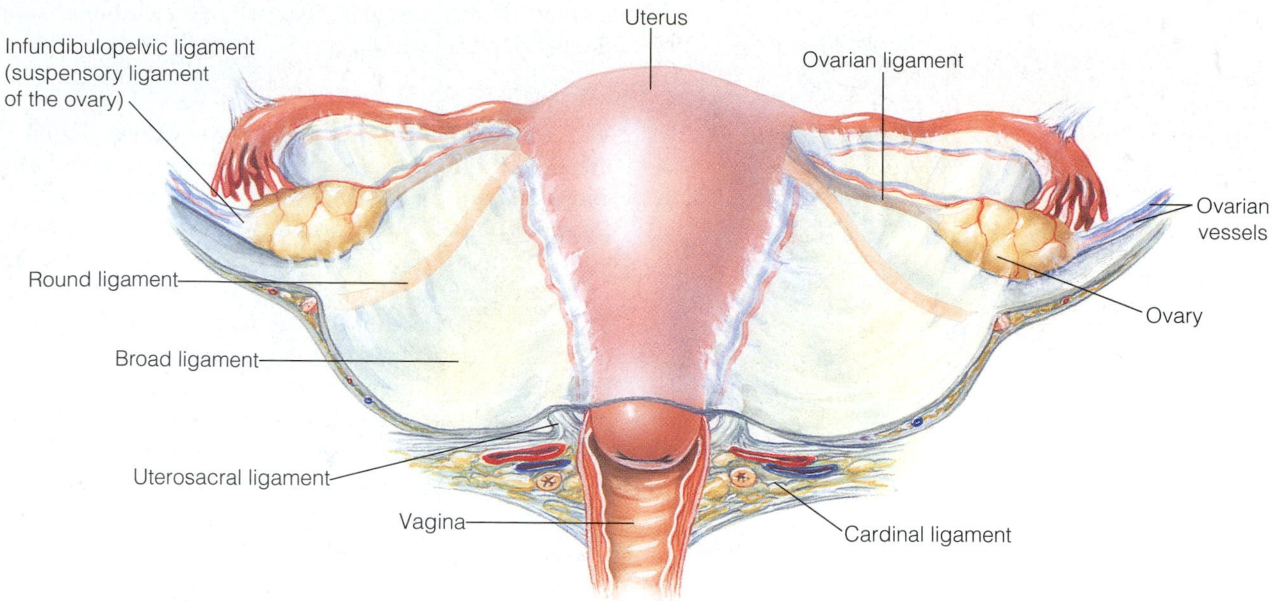

Figure 10–9 • Uterine ligaments.

The broad ligament covers the uterus anteriorly and posteriorly and extends outward from the uterus to enfold and stabilize the fallopian tubes. The round and ovarian ligaments are at the upper border of the broad ligament. At its lower border, the broad ligament forms the cardinal ligaments. Between the folds of the broad ligament are connective tissue, involuntary muscle, blood and lymph vessels, and nerves.

- The *round ligaments* keep the uterus in place. Each of the round ligaments arises from the sides of the uterus near the fallopian tube insertion. They extend outward between the folds of the broad ligament, passing through the inguinal ring and canals and eventually fusing with the connective tissue of the labia majora. The round ligaments are made up of longitudinal muscle and enlarge during pregnancy. During labor the round ligaments steady the uterus, pulling downward and forward, so that the presenting part of the fetus is forced into the cervix.
- The *ovarian ligaments* anchor the lower pole of the ovary to the cornua of the uterus. They are composed of muscle fibers, which allow the ligaments to contract. This contractile ability influences the position of the ovary to some extent, thus helping the fimbriae of the fallopian tubes to "catch" the ovum as it is released each month.
- The *cardinal ligaments* are the chief uterine supports, suspending the uterus from the side walls of the true pelvis. These ligaments, also known as Mackenrodt's ligaments or transverse cervical ligaments, arise from the sides of the pelvic walls and attach to the cervix in the upper vagina. These ligaments prevent uterine prolapse and also support the upper vagina.
- The *infundibulopelvic ligament* suspends and supports the ovaries. Arising from the outer third of the broad ligament, the infundibulopelvic ligament contains the ovarian vessels and nerves.
- The *uterosacral ligaments* provide support for the uterus and cervix at the level of the ischial spines. Arising on each side of the pelvis from the posterior wall of the uterus, the uterosacral ligaments sweep back around the rectum and insert on the sides of the first and second sacral vertebrae. The uterosacral ligaments contain smooth muscle fibers, connective tissue, blood and lymph vessels, and nerves. Providing support for the uterus and cervix at the level of the ischial spines, they also contain sensory nerve fibers that contribute to dysmenorrhea (painful menstruation; see Chapter 4).

FALLOPIAN TUBES

The two **fallopian tubes,** also known as *oviducts* or *uterine tubes,* arise from each side of the uterus and reach almost to the side of the pelvis, where they turn toward the ovaries (Figure 10–10 •). Each tube is approximately 8 to 13.5 cm long. A short section of each fallopian tube is inside the uterus; its opening into the uterus is 1 mm in diameter. The fallopian tubes link the peritoneal cavity with the uterus and vagina. This linkage increases a woman's vulnerability to disease processes.

Each fallopian tube may be divided into three parts: the **isthmus,** the ampulla, and the infundibulum or fimbria. The isthmus is straight and narrow, with a thick muscular wall and an opening (lumen) 2 to 3 mm in diameter. It is the site of tubal ligation (a surgical procedure to prevent pregnancy; see Chapter 5).

Next to the isthmus is the curved **ampulla,** which comprises the outer two thirds of the tube. Fertilization of the secondary oocyte by a spermatozoon usually occurs here. The ampulla ends at the **fimbria,** which is a funnel-like enlargement with many moving fingerlike projections (fim-

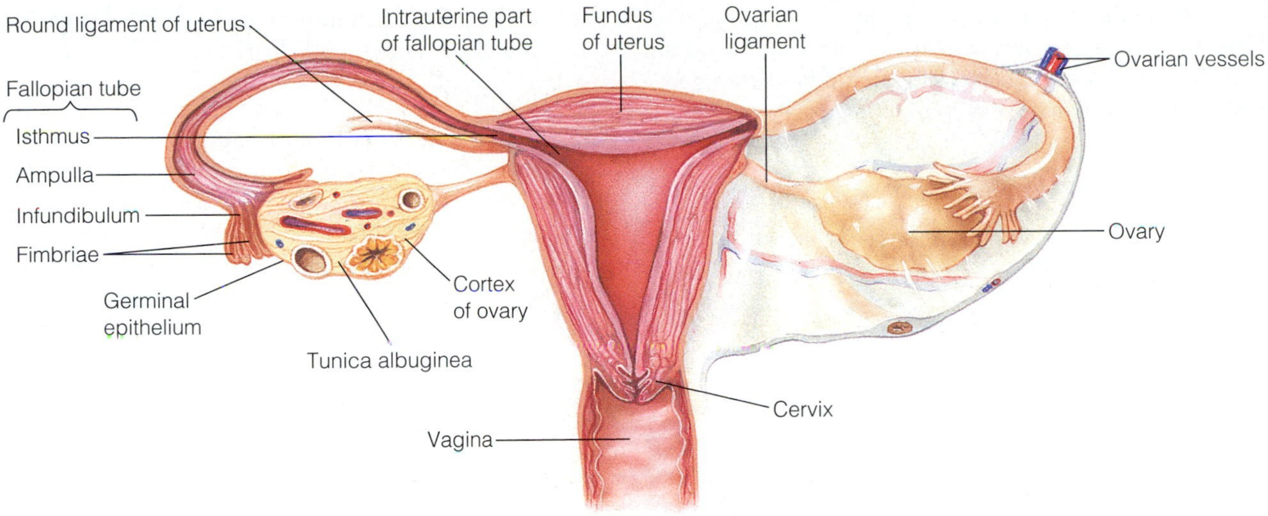

Figure 10–10 • Fallopian tube and ovaries.

briae) reaching out to the ovary. The longest of these, the *fimbria ovarica*, is attached to the ovary to increase the chances of intercepting the ovum as it is released.

The wall of the fallopian tube is made up of four layers: peritoneal (serous), subserous (adventitial), muscular, and mucous tissues. The peritoneum covers the tubes. The subserous layer contains the blood and nerve supply, and the muscular layer is responsible for the peristaltic movement of the tube. The mucosal layer, immediately next to the muscular layer, is composed of ciliated and nonciliated cells, with the number of ciliated cells more abundant at the fimbria. Nonciliated cells are goblet cells that secrete a protein-rich, serous fluid that nourishes the ovum. The constantly moving tubal cilia propel the ovum toward the uterus. Because the ovum is a large cell, this ciliary action is needed to assist the tube's muscular layer peristalsis. Any malformation or malfunction of the tubes could result in infertility, ectopic pregnancy, or even sterility.

A well-functioning tubal transport system involves active fimbriae close to the ovary, peristalsis of the tube created by the muscular layer, ciliated currents beating toward the uterus, and the proximal contraction and distal relaxation of the tube caused by different types of prostaglandins.

A rich blood and lymph supply serves each fallopian tube. Thus the fallopian tubes have an unusual ability to recover from any inflammatory process. The functions of the fallopian tubes are as follows:

- To provide transport for the ovum from the ovary to the uterus (transport through the fallopian tubes varies from 3 to 4 days)
- To provide a site for fertilization
- To serve as a warm, moist, nourishing environment for the ovum or zygote (a fertilized egg; see also Chapter 11)

OVARIES

The *ovaries* are two almond-shaped glandular structures just below the pelvic brim. One ovary is located on each side of the pelvic cavity. Their size varies among women and according to the stage of the menstrual cycle. Each ovary weighs 6 to 10 g and is 1.5 to 3 cm wide, 2 to 5 cm long, and 1 to 1.5 cm thick. The ovaries of girls are small but become larger after puberty. They also change in appearance from smooth-surfaced, dull white organs to pitted gray organs. This pitting is caused by scarring due to ovulation. It is rare for both ovaries to be at the same level in the pelvic cavity. The ovary is held in place by the ovarian, broad, and infundibulopelvic ligaments (Figure 10–9), discussed earlier in the chapter.

There is no peritoneal covering for the ovaries. Although this lack of covering assists the mature ovum to erupt, it also allows easier spread of malignant cells from cancer of the ovaries. A single layer of cuboidal epithelial cells, called the germinal epithelium, covers the ovaries. The ovaries are composed of three layers: the tunica albuginea, the cortex, and the medulla. The *tunica albuginea* is dense and dull white and serves as a protective layer. The *cortex* is the main functional part, containing ova, graafian follicles, corpora lutea, degenerated corpora lutea (corpora albicantia), and degenerated follicles. The *medulla* is completely surrounded by the cortex and contains the nerves and the blood and lymphatic vessels.

The ovaries are the primary source of two important hormones: the estrogens and progesterone. *Estrogens* are associated with characteristics contributing to femaleness, including breast alveolar lobule growth and duct development. The ovaries secrete large amounts of estrogens; the adrenal cortex (extraglandular sites) produces minute amounts of estrogens in nonpregnant women.

Progesterone is often called the *hormone of pregnancy* because its effects on the uterus allow pregnancy to be maintained. The placenta is the primary source of progesterone during pregnancy. This hormone also inhibits the action of prolactin in α-lactalbumin synthesis, thereby preventing lactation during pregnancy (Cunningham et al, 2001).

The interplay between the ovarian hormones and other hormones such as follicle-stimulating hormone (FSH) and luteinizing hormone (LH) is responsible for the cyclic changes that allow pregnancy to occur. The hormonal and physical

MediaLink Activities: Female Reproductive System

changes that occur during the female reproductive cycle are discussed later in this chapter. Between the ages of 45 and 55 years, the woman's ovaries secrete decreasing amounts of estrogen. Eventually, ovulatory activity ceases, and menopause occurs.

Bony Pelvis

The female bony pelvis has two unique functions:

- To support and protect the pelvic contents.
- To form the relatively fixed axis of the birth passage

Because the pelvis is so important to childbearing, its structures should be understood clearly.

BONY STRUCTURE

The pelvis is made up of four bones: two innominate bones, the sacrum, and the coccyx (or tailbone) (Figure 10–11 •). The pelvis resembles a bowl or basin; its sides are the innominate bones, and its back is composed of the sacrum and coccyx. Lined with fibrocartilage and held tightly together by ligaments, the four bones join at the symphysis pubis, the two sacroiliac joints, and the sacrococcygeal joints.

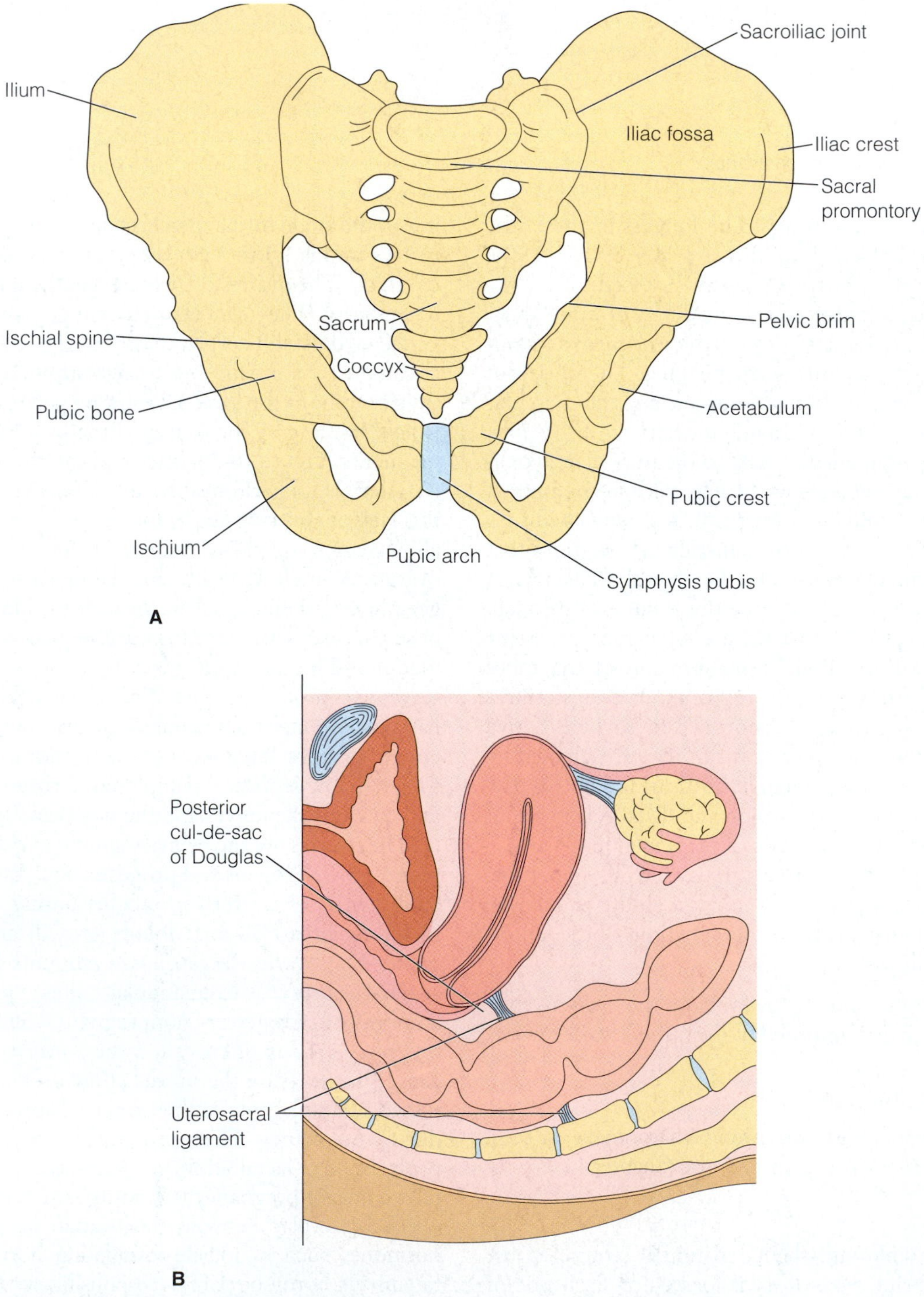

Figure 10–11 • Pelvis: *A,* Pelvic bones. *B,* Midsagittal view in supine position with some ligaments.

The *innominate* bones, also known as the hip bones or os coxae, are made up of three separate bones: the ilium, the ischium, and the pubis. These bones fuse to form a circular cavity, the *acetabulum*, which articulates with the femur.

The *ilium* is the broad, upper prominence of the hip. The *iliac crest* is the margin of the ilium. The ischial spines, the foremost projections nearest the groin, are the site of attachment for ligaments and muscles.

The *ischium*, the strongest bone, lies under the ilium and below the acetabulum. The L-shaped ischium ends in a marked protuberance, the *ischial tuberosity*, on which the weight of a seated body rests. The **ischial spines** arise near the junction of the ilium and ischium and jut into the pelvic cavity. The shortest diameter of the pelvic cavity is located between the ischial spines. The ischial spines can serve as a reference point during labor to evaluate the descent of the fetal head into the birth canal. (See Chapter 22 and Figure 22–7.)

The **pubis** forms the slightly bowed front portion of the innominate bone. Extending medially from the acetabulum to the midpoint of the bony pelvis, the two pubic bones meet to form a joint, the *symphysis pubis*. The triangular space below this junction is known as the pubic arch. The fetal head passes under this arch during birth. The symphysis pubis is formed by heavy fibrocartilage and the superior and inferior pubic ligaments. The mobility of the inferior ligament increases during pregnancy and to a greater extent in subsequent pregnancies than in first pregnancies.

The sacroiliac joints also have a degree of mobility that increases near the end of pregnancy and results in an upward gliding movement. The pelvic outlet may be increased by 1.5 to 2 cm in the squatting, sitting, and dorsal lithotomy positions. These relaxations of the joints are induced by the hormones of pregnancy.

The *sacrum* is a wedge-shaped bone formed by the fusion of five vertebrae. On the anterior upper portion of the sacrum is a projection into the pelvic cavity known as the **sacral promontory.** This projection is another obstetric guide in determining pelvic measurements. (For discussion of pelvic measurements, see Chapter 15.)

The small triangular bone last on the vertebral column is the coccyx. It articulates with the sacrum at the sacrococcygeal joint. The coccyx usually moves backward during labor to provide more room for the fetus.

PELVIC FLOOR

The muscular *pelvic floor* of the bony pelvis is designed to overcome the force of gravity exerted on the pelvic organs. It acts as a supporting structure to the irregularly shaped pelvic outlet, thereby providing stability and support for surrounding structures.

Deep fascia and the levator ani and coccygeal muscles form the part of the pelvic floor known as the **pelvic diaphragm.** Above it is the pelvic cavity; below and behind it is the perineum. The sacrum is located posteriorly.

The levator ani muscle makes up the major portion of the pelvic diaphragm. It consists of four muscles: the iliococcygeus, pubococcygeus, puborectalis, and pubovaginalis muscles. These muscles form a sling for the pelvic structures. The iliococcygeal muscle, a thin muscular sheet underlying the sacrospinous ligament, helps the levator ani support the pelvic organs. Muscles of the pelvic floor are shown in Figure 10–12 • and discussed in Table 10–1 •.

MediaLink ANIMATION: FEMALE PELVIS

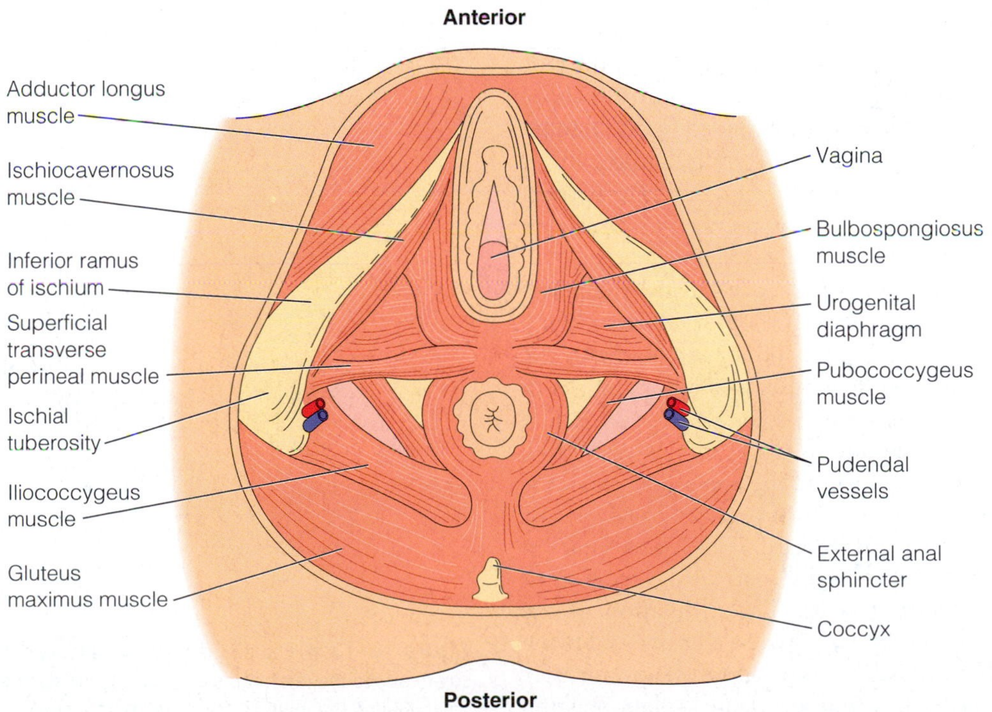

Figure 10–12 • Muscles of the pelvic floor. (The puborectalis, pubovaginalis, and coccygeal muscles cannot be seen from this view.)

Table 10–1 • MUSCLES OF THE PELVIC FLOOR

Muscle	Origin	Insertion	Innervation	Action
Levator ani	Pubis, lateral pelvic wall, and ischial spine	Blends with organs in pelvic cavity	Inferior rectal, 2nd and 3rd sacral nerves, plus anterior rami of 3rd and 4th sacral nerves	Supports pelvic viscera; helps form pelvic diaphragm
Iliococcygeus	Pelvic surface of ischial spine and pelvic fascia	Central point of perineum, coccygeal raphe, and coccyx		Assists in supporting abdominal and pelvic viscera
Pubococcygeus	Pubis and pelvic fascia	Coccyx		
Puborectalis	Pubis	Blends with rectum; meets similar fibers from opposite side		Forms sling for rectum, just posterior to it; raises anus
Pubovaginalis	Pubis	Blends into vagina		Supports vagina
Coccygeus	Ischial spine and sacrospinous ligament	Lateral border of lower sacrum and upper coccyx	3rd and 4th sacral nerves	Supports pelvic viscera; helps form pelvic diaphragm; flexes and abducts coccyx

Endopelvic fascia covers the pelvic diaphragm. The components function as a whole, yet they are able to move over one another. This feature provides an exceptional capacity for dilatation during birth and return to prepregnant condition following birth.

The urogenital triangle (diaphragm) is external to the pelvic diaphragm, in the triangular area between the ischial tuberosities and the hollow of the pubic arch. The most important muscles in this region are the deep transverse perineal muscles, which are flat bands of muscle arising from the ischiopubic rami and intertwining in the midline to form a seam, or raphe. These muscles are modified to encircle both the urinary meatus and the vaginal orifice, forming the urethral and vaginal sphincters.

PELVIC DIVISION

The pelvic cavity is divided into the false pelvis and the true pelvis (Figure 10–13 •). The *false pelvis* is the portion above the pelvic brim, or linea terminalis, bounded by the lumbar vertebrae posteriorly, the iliac fossae laterally, and the lower abdominal wall anteriorly. Its primary function is to support the weight of the enlarged pregnant uterus and direct the presenting fetal part into the true pelvis below.

The **true pelvis** is the portion that lies below the pelvic brim. It is bounded above by the promontory of the sacrum and the upper margins of the pubic bones and below by the pelvic outlet. The true pelvis represents the bony limits of the birth canal. It measures about 5 cm at its anterior wall at the symphysis pubis and about 10 cm at its posterior wall. When a woman is standing upright, the upper portion of the pelvic cavity or canal is directed downward and backward; its lower portion, downward and forward. This forms a curved canal through which the presenting part of the baby must pass during birth (Figure 10–13). The inclination of the pelvis is the angle formed by two planes: a horizontal plane passing through the tip of the coccyx and the superior border of the symphysis pubis, and an inclined plane passing through the sacral promontory and the superior border of the symphysis pubis. This pelvic angle of inclination usually measures 50 to 60 degrees (Figure 10–14 •).

The true pelvis is extremely important in childbearing because its size and shape must be adequate for normal fetal passage during labor and at birth. The relationship of the fetal head to the true pelvic cavity is of critical importance.

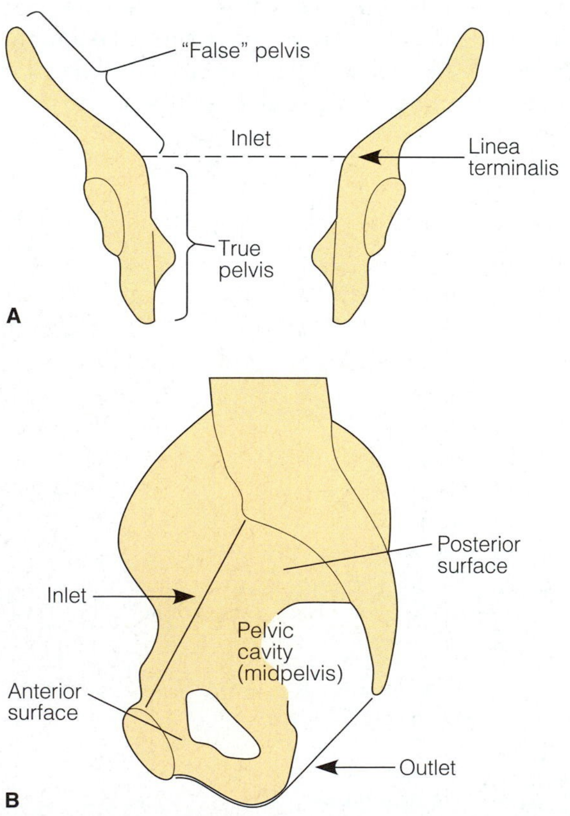

Figure 10–13 • Female pelvis: *A,* The false pelvis is the shallow cavity above the inlet; the true pelvis is the deeper portion of the cavity below the inlet. *B,* The true pelvis consists of the inlet, cavity (midpelvis), and outlet.

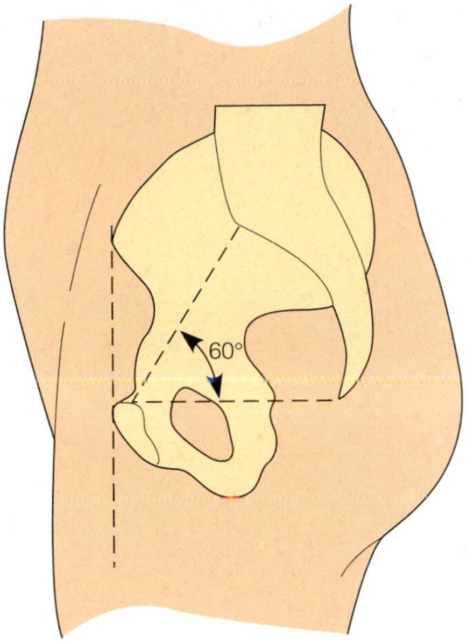

Figure 10–14 • Pelvic angle of inclination while woman is standing.

The true pelvis consists of three parts: the inlet, the pelvic cavity, and the outlet. Associated with each part are distinct measurements that aid in evaluating the adequacy of the pelvis for childbirth. The dimensions of the true pelvis and their obstetric implications are described here. Measurement techniques are discussed in Chapter 15. The effects of inadequate or abnormal pelvic diameters on labor and birth are considered in Chapter 23.

The **pelvic inlet** is the upper border of the true pelvis and typically is round in the female. The size and shape of the pelvic inlet are determined by assessing three anteroposterior diameters: the diagonal conjugate, obstetric conjugate, and conjugate vera. (For an in-depth discussion, see Chapter 15.) The **diagonal conjugate** extends from the subpubic angle to the middle of the sacral promontory and is typically 12.5 cm. The diagonal conjugate can be measured manually during a pelvic examination. The **obstetric conjugate** extends from the middle of the sacral promontory to an area approximately 1 cm below the pubic crest. Its length is estimated by subtracting 1.5 cm from the diagonal conjugate. The fetus passes through the obstetric conjugate, and the size of this diameter determines whether the fetus can move down into the birth canal in order for engagement to occur. The true (anatomic) conjugate, or **conjugate vera,** extends from the middle of the sacral promontory to the middle of the pubic crest (superior surface of the symphysis). One additional measurement, the transverse diameter, helps determine the shape of the inlet. The **transverse diameter** is the largest diameter of the inlet.

The *pelvic cavity* (canal) is a curved canal with a longer posterior than anterior wall. A change in the lumbar curve can increase or decrease the pelvic inclination and can influence the progress of labor because the fetus has to adjust itself to this curved path as well as to the different diameters of the true pelvis.

The **pelvic outlet** is at the lower border of the true pelvis. The size of the pelvic outlet can be determined by assessing the *transverse diameter.* The anteroposterior diameter of the pelvic outlet increases during birth as the presenting part pushes the coccyx posteriorly at the mobile sacrococcygeal joint. Decreased mobility, a large fetal head, and/or a forceful birth can cause the coccyx to break. As the infant's head emerges, the long diameter of the head (occipital frontal) parallels the long diameter of the outlet (anteroposterior).

The transverse diameter (*bi-ischial or intertuberous*) extends from the inner surface of one ischial tuberosity to the other. It is the shortest diameter of the pelvic outlet and becomes even shorter if the woman has a narrowed pubic arch. The pubic arch has great importance because the baby must pass under it during birth. If it is narrow, the baby's head may be pushed backward toward the coccyx, making the extension of the head difficult. This situation, known as *outlet dystocia*, may require the use of forceps or a cesarean birth. The shoulders of a large baby may also get stuck under the pubic arch, making birth more difficult. The clinical assessment of each of these obstetric diameters is discussed further in Chapter 15.

PELVIC TYPES

The Caldwell-Moloy classification of pelves (Figure 10–15 •) is widely used to differentiate types of bony pelves (Caldwell & Moloy, 1933). *Gynecoid, android, anthropoid,* and *platypelloid* are the four basic types. However, variations in the female pelvis are so great that classic types are not usual.

Each type of pelvis has a characteristic shape, and each shape has implications for labor and birth. The types are described briefly here, and their implications for labor and birth are discussed in detail in Chapter 22.

Gynecoid Pelvis

The most common female pelvis is the gynecoid type. The inlet is rounded, with the anteroposterior diameter a little shorter than the transverse diameter. All of the inlet diameters are at least adequate. The posterior segment is broad, deep, and roomy, and the anterior segment is well rounded. The gynecoid midpelvis has nonprominent ischial spines, straight and parallel side walls, and a wide, deep sacral curve. The sacrum is short and slopes backward. All of the midpelvic diameters are at least adequate. The gynecoid pelvic outlet has a wide and round pubic arch; the inferior pubic rami are short and concave. The anteroposterior diameter is long; the transverse diameter, adequate. The capacity of the outlet is adequate. The bones are of medium structure and weight. Approximately 50% of female pelves are classified as gynecoid.

Android Pelvis

The normal male pelvis is the android type; however, it occasionally is seen in females. The inlet is heart shaped. The anteroposterior and transverse diameters are adequate for birth, but the posterior sagittal diameter is too short, and the anterior sagittal diameter is long. The posterior

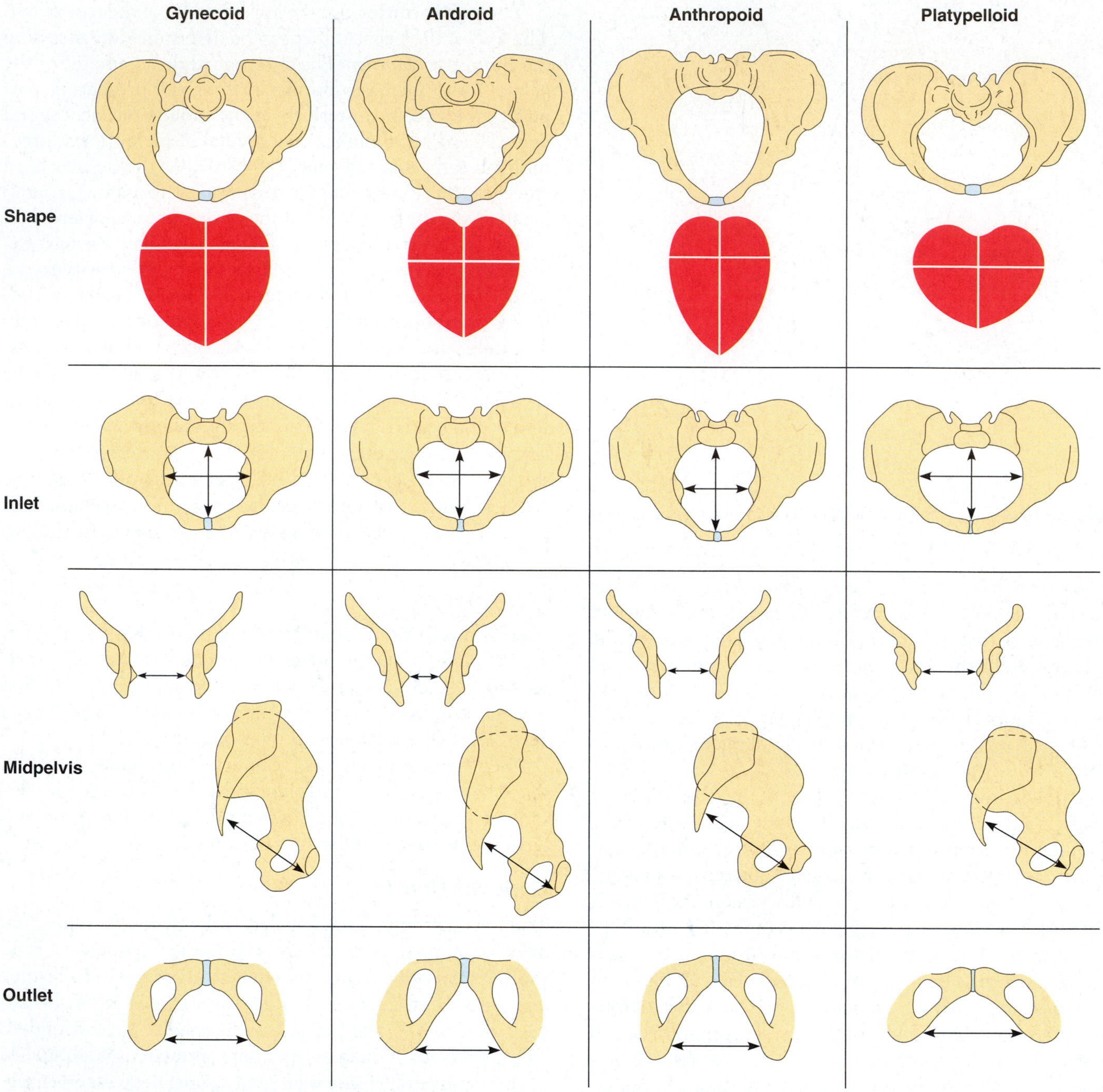

Figure 10–15 • Comparison of Caldwell-Moloy pelvic types.

segment is shallow because the sacral promontory is indented, resulting in a reduced capacity. The anterior segment is narrow, and the forepelvis is sharply angled. The android midpelvis has prominent ischial spines, convergent side walls, and a long, heavy sacrum inclining forward. All of the midpelvic diameters are reduced. The distance from the linea terminalis to the ischial tuberosities is long, yet the overall capacity of the midpelvis is reduced. The android outlet has a narrow, sharp, and deep pubic arch; the inferior pubic rami are straight and long. The anteroposterior diameter is short, and the transverse diameter is narrow. The capacity of the outlet is reduced. The bones are of medium to heavy structure and weight.

Approximately 20% of female pelves are classified as android. The influence of an android pelvis on labor is not favorable. Descent into the pelvis is slow. The fetal head usually engages in the transverse or occipital posterior diameter in asynclitism (oblique presentation) with extreme molding. Arrest of labor is frequent, requiring difficult forceps manipulation (rotation and extraction), and the deep, narrow pubic arch may lead to extensive perineal lacerations. Cesarean birth may be required.

Anthropoid Pelvis

The inlet of an anthropoid pelvis is oval, with a long anteroposterior diameter and an adequate but rather short transverse diameter. Both the posterior and anterior segments are deep; the posterior sagittal diameter is extremely long, as is the anterior sagittal diameter. The anthropoid midpelvis has variable ischial spines, straight side walls, and a narrow and long sacrum that inclines backward. The midpelvic diameters are at least adequate, making its capacity adequate. The anthropoid outlet has a normal or moderately narrow pubic arch; the interior pubic rami are long and narrow. The outlet capacity is adequate, and the bones are of medium weight and structure. Approximately 25% of female pelves are classified as anthropoid.

Platypelloid Pelvis

The platypelloid type refers to the flat female pelvis. The inlet is a distinctly transverse oval, with a short anteroposterior and extremely short transverse diameter. The posterior sagittal and anterior sagittal diameters are short. Both the anterior and posterior segments are shallow. The platypelloid midpelvis has variable ischial spines, parallel side walls, and a wide sacrum with a deep curve inward. Only the transverse diameter is adequate; thus the midpelvic capacity is reduced. The platypelloid outlet has an extremely wide pubic arch; the inferior pubic rami are straight and short. The transverse diameter is wide, but the anteroposterior diameter is short. The outlet capacity may be inadequate. The platypelloid bones are similar to the gynecoid type. Only 5% of female pelves are classified as platypelloid.

Breasts

The **breasts,** or *mammary glands,* considered accessories of the reproductive system, are specialized sebaceous glands. They are conical and symmetrically placed on the sides of the chest. The greater pectoral and anterior serratus muscles underlie each breast. Suspending the breasts are fibrous tissues, called *Cooper's ligaments,* that extend from the deep fascia in the chest outward to just under the skin covering the breast. The left breast is frequently larger than the right. In different racial groups breasts develop at slightly different levels in the pectoral region of the chest (Rebar, 1999).

In the center of each mature breast is the **nipple,** a protrusion about 0.5 to 1.3 cm in diameter. The nipple is composed mainly of erectile tissue, which becomes more rigid and prominent during the menstrual cycle, sexual excitement, pregnancy, and lactation. The nipple is surrounded by the heavily pigmented **areola,** 2.5 to 10 cm in diameter. Both the nipple and areola are roughened by small papillae called *tubercles of Montgomery.* As an infant suckles, these tubercles secrete a fatty substance that helps lubricate and protect the breasts.

The breasts are composed of glandular, fibrous, and adipose tissue. The glandular tissue consists of acini, or

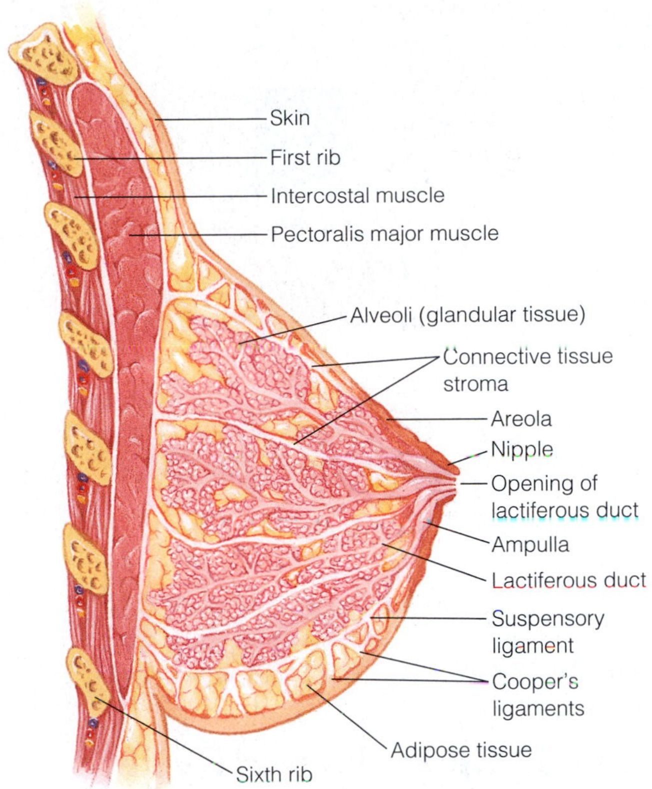

Figure 10–16 • Anatomy of the breast.

alveoli (Figure 10–16 •), which are arranged in a series of 15 to 24 lobes separated from each other by adipose and fibrous tissue.

Each lobe is made up of several lobules, which are made up of many grapelike clusters of alveoli around tiny ducts. They are lined with a single layer of cuboidal epithelium, which secretes the various components of milk. The ducts from several lobules combine to form larger *lactiferous ducts,* or *sinuses,* which open on the surface of the nipple. The smooth muscle of the nipple causes erection of the nipple on contraction.

Cyclic hormonal control of the mature breast is complex. Essentially, estrogenic hormones stimulate the growth and development of the ductal epithelium. Progesterone, in association with estrogen, is responsible for the acinar and lobular development during the luteal phase of menstruation. Adrenal corticosteroids, prolactin, somatotropin (growth hormone), and thyroxine are also necessary for estrogen and progesterone to act.

The arterial, venous, and lymphatic systems communicate medially with the internal mammary vessels and laterally with the axillary vessels. Therefore, in cancer of the breast, metastasis follows the vascular supply both medially and laterally (Figure 10–17 •).

The biologic function of the breasts is to provide nourishment and protective maternal antibodies to infants through the lactation process. They are also a source of pleasurable sexual sensation.

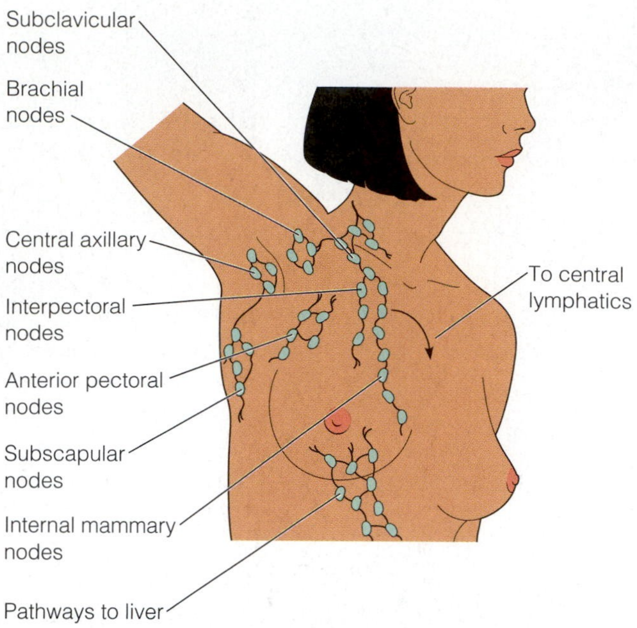

Figure 10–17 • Lymphatic vessels draining the breast.

Female Reproductive Cycle

The **female reproductive cycle (FRC)** is composed of the ovarian cycle, during which ovulation occurs, and the menstrual cycle, during which menstruation occurs. These two cycles take place simultaneously (see Figure 10–18 •).

Effects of Female Hormones

After menarche, a woman undergoes a cyclic pattern of ovulation and menstruation (if pregnancy does not occur) for a period of 30 to 40 years. This cycle is an orderly process under neurohormonal control. Each month, one oocyte matures, ruptures from the ovary, and enters the fallopian tube. The ovary, vagina, uterus, and fallopian tubes are major target organs for female hormones.

The ovaries not only produce mature gametes, but also secrete hormones. Ovarian hormones include the estrogens, progesterone, and testosterone. The ovary is sensitive to follicle-stimulating hormone (FSH) and luteinizing hormone (LH). The uterus is sensitive to estrogen and progesterone. The relative proportions of these hormones control the events of both ovarian and menstrual cycles.

ESTROGENS

Estrogens are hormones that are associated with those characteristics contributing to "femaleness." The major estrogenic effects are due primarily to three estrogens: estrone, β-estradiol, and estriol. β-estradiol is the major estrogen.

Estrogens control the development of the female secondary sex characteristics: breast development, widening of the hips, and deposits of tissue (fat) in the buttocks and mons pubis. Estrogen also influences the growth of body hair in women. In addition, estrogens assist in the maturation of the ovarian follicles and cause the endometrial mucosa to proliferate following menstruation. The amount of estrogens is greatest during the proliferative (follicular or estrogenic) phase of the menstrual cycle. Estrogens also cause the uterus to increase in size and weight because of increased glycogen, amino acids, electrolytes, and water. Blood supply is expanded as well. Under the influence of estrogens, myometrial contractility increases in both the uterus and the fallopian tubes, and uterine sensitivity to oxytocin increases. Estrogens inhibit FSH production and stimulate LH production.

Estrogens have effects on many hormones and other carrier proteins. This explains the increased amount of protein-bound iodine in pregnant women and in women who use oral contraceptives containing estrogen.

Estrogens may increase libido. They decrease the excitability of the hypothalamus, which may cause an increase in sexual desire.

PROGESTERONE

Progesterone is secreted by the corpus luteum and is found in greatest amounts during the secretory (luteal or progestational) phase of the menstrual cycle. It decreases uterine motility and contractility caused by estrogens, thereby preparing the uterus for implantation after the ovum is fertilized. The endometrial mucosa is in a ready state as a result of estrogenic influence. Progesterone causes the uterine endometrium to increase further its supply of glycogen, arterial blood, secretory glands, amino acids, and water. This hormone is often called the *hormone of pregnancy* because its effects on the uterus allow pregnancy to be maintained.

Under the influence of progesterone, the vaginal epithelium proliferates, and the cervix secretes thick, viscous mucus. Breast glandular tissue increases in size and complexity. Progesterone also prepares the breasts for lactation.

The temperature rise of about 0.3C to 0.6C (0.5F to 1.0F) that accompanies ovulation and persists throughout the secretory phase of the menstrual cycle is due to progesterone.

PROSTAGLANDINS

Prostaglandins (PGs) are oxygenated fatty acids that are produced by the cells of the endometrium and are also classified as hormones. Prostaglandins have varied actions in the body. The two primary types of prostaglandins are group E and F. Generally, PGE relaxes smooth muscles and is a potent vasodilator; PGF is a potent vasoconstrictor and increases the contractility of muscles and arteries. Although their primary actions seem antagonistic, their basic regulatory functions in cells are achieved through an intricate pattern of reciprocal events. The discussion here sums up their role in ovulation and menstruation.

Prostaglandin production increases during follicular maturation, is dependent on gonadotropins, and is essential to ovulation. Extrusion of the ovum, resulting from the increased contractility of the smooth muscle in the theca layer of the mature follicle, is thought to be caused by $PGF_{2\alpha}$. Significant amounts of PGs are found in and around the follicle at the time of ovulation.

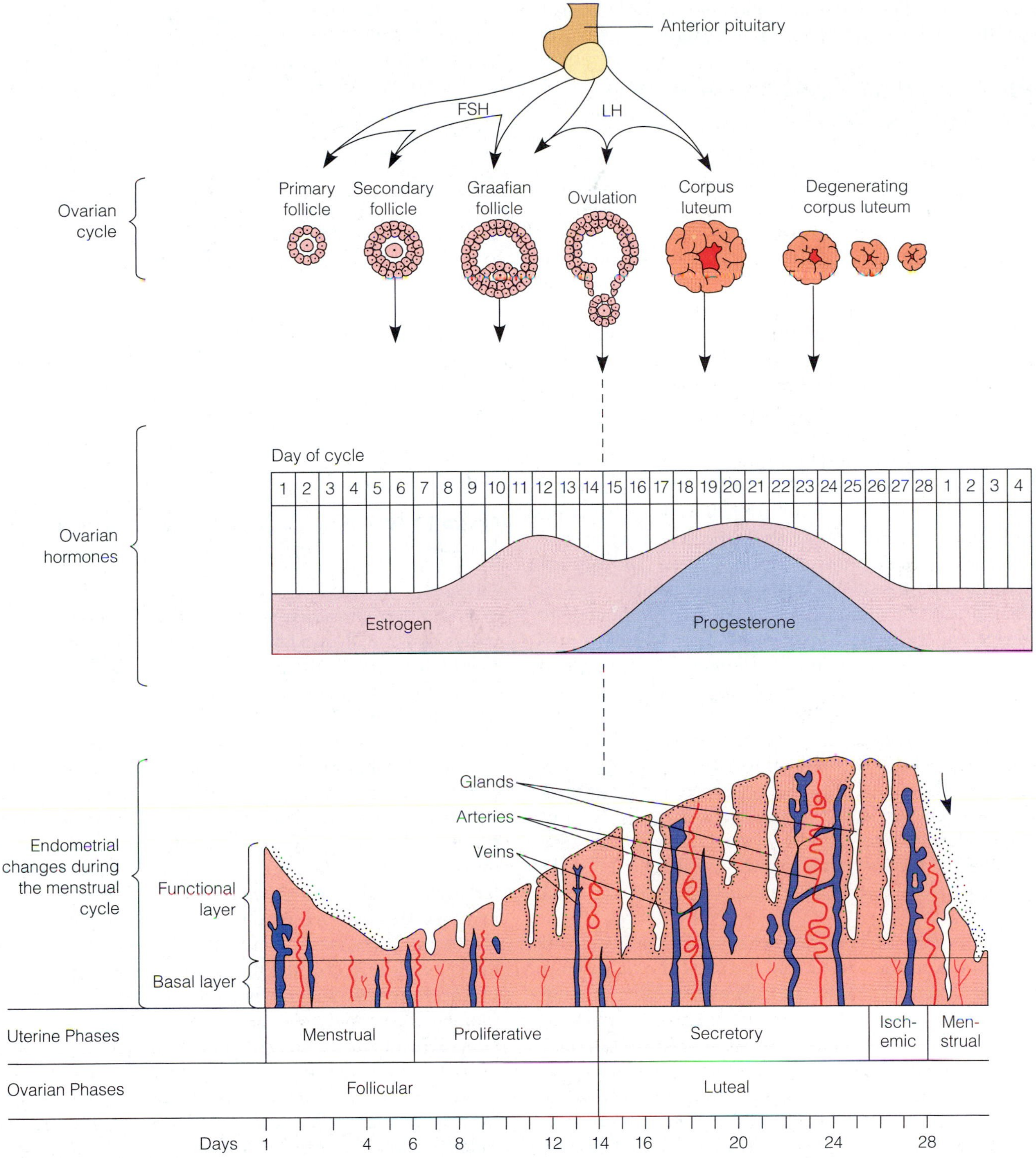

Figure 10–18 • Female reproductive cycle: Interrelationships of hormones, the four phases of the uterine cycle, and the two phases of the ovarian cycle.

Although the exact mechanism by which the corpus luteum degenerates in the absence of pregnancy remains obscure, $PGF_{2\alpha}$ is thought to induce progesterone withdrawal, the lowest point of which coincides with the onset of early menses.

During the late secretory phase, the level of $PGF_{2\alpha}$ is higher than that of PGE (Blackburn, 2003). This event increases vasoconstriction and contractility of the myometrium, which contributes to the ischemia preceding menstruation. A high concentration of PGs may also account for the vasoconstriction of the endometrium venous lacunae allowing for platelet aggregation at vascular rupture points, thereby preventing a rapid blood loss during menstruation. The menstrual flow's high concentration of PGs may also facilitate the process of tissue digestion, which allows for an orderly shedding of the endometrium during menstruation.

Neurohormonal Basis of the Female Reproductive Cycle

The female reproductive cycle is controlled by complex interactions between the nervous and endocrine systems and their target tissues. These interactions involve the hypothalamus, anterior pituitary, and ovaries.

The hypothalamus secretes gonadotropin-releasing hormone (GnRH) to the pituitary gland in response to signals received from the central nervous system. This releasing hormone is often called follicle-stimulating hormone-releasing hormone (FSHRH) or luteinizing hormone-releasing hormone (LHRH) (Blackburn, 2003). This is because, in response to GnRH, the anterior pituitary secretes the gonadotropic hormones *FSH* and *LH.* Each has distinct roles.

MediaLink ACTIVITY: OVULATION

As its name suggests, FSH is primarily responsible for the maturation of the ovarian follicle. As the follicle matures, it secretes increasing amounts of estrogen, which enhance the development of the follicle. (This estrogen also is responsible for the rebuilding/proliferation phase of the endometrium after it is shed during menstruation.)

Final maturation of the follicle will not come about without the action of LH. The anterior pituitary's production of LH increases sixfold to tenfold as the follicle matures. The peak production of LH can precede ovulation by as much as 12 hours (Blackburn, 2003). LH is also responsible for "luteinizing" the increase in production of progesterone by the granulosa cells of the follicle. As a result, estrogen production declines and progesterone secretion continues. Thus, estrogen levels fall a day before ovulation; tiny amounts of progesterone are in evidence. **Ovulation** takes place following the very rapid growth of the follicle—as the sustained high level of estrogen diminishes and progesterone secretion begins.

The ruptured follicle undergoes rapid change, complete luteinization is accomplished, and the mass of cells becomes the **corpus luteum.** The lutein cells secrete large amounts of progesterone with smaller amounts of estrogen. (Concurrently, the excessive amounts of progesterone are responsible for the secretory phase of the uterine cycle.) Seven or 8 days following ovulation the corpus luteum begins to involute, losing its secretory function. The production of both progesterone and estrogen is severely diminished. The anterior pituitary responds with increasingly large amounts of FSH; a few days later, LH production begins. As a result, new follicles become responsive to another ovarian cycle and begin maturing.

Ovarian Cycle

The ovarian cycle has two phases: the *follicular phase* (days 1 to 14) and the *luteal phase* (days 15 to 28 in a 28-day cycle). Figure 10–19 • depicts the changes that the follicle undergoes during the ovarian cycle. In women whose menstrual cycles vary, usually it is only the length of the follicular phase that varies, because the luteal phase is of fixed length. During the follicular phase, the immature follicle matures as a result of FSH. Within the follicle, the oocyte grows. A mature **graafian follicle** appears about the 14th day under dual control of FSH and LH. It is a large structure, measuring about 5 to 10 mm, and produces increasing amounts of estrogen.

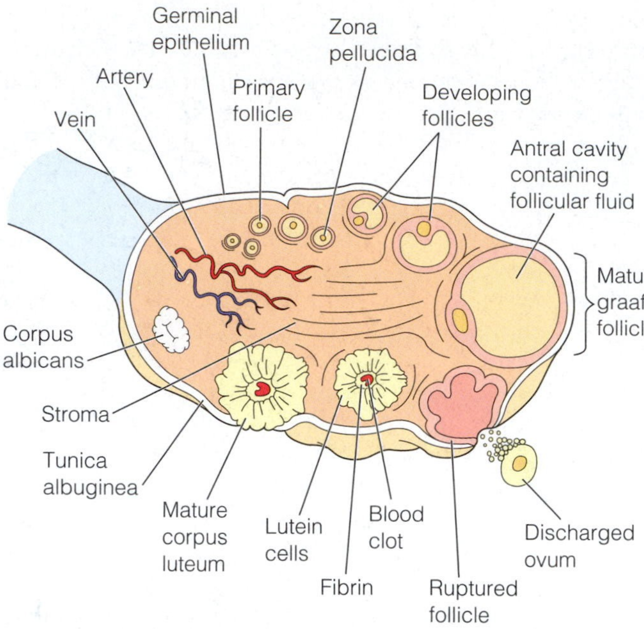

Figure 10–19 • Various stages of development of the ovarian follicles.

In the mature graafian follicle, the cells surrounding the fluid-filled antral cavity are called granulosa cells. The mass of granulosa cells surrounding the oocyte and follicular fluid is called the *cumulus oophorus.* The stromal elements of the ovary are condensed around the follicle in two layers: the theca interna and the theca externa. The theca interna cells resemble the luteal cells of the corpus luteum. In the fully mature graafian follicle, the zona pellucida (oolemma), a thick, elastic capsule, develops around the oocyte. Just before ovulation, the mature oocyte completes its first meiotic division (see Chapter 11 for a description of meiosis). As a result of this division, two cells are formed: a small cell called a *polar body,* and a larger cell called the *secondary oocyte.*

As the graafian follicle matures and enlarges, its walls thin and it travels outward to the surface of the ovary. This surface has a blisterlike protrusion 10 to 15 mm in diameter, where the secondary oocyte, polar body, and follicular fluid are pushed out. The secondary oocyte, which is now considered a mature ovum, is discharged near the fimbria of the fallopian tube and is pulled into the tube to begin its journey toward the uterus. (See Figure 11–6.)

Occasionally ovulation is accompanied by midcycle pain, known as *mittelschmerz.* This pain may be caused by a thick tunica albuginea or by a local peritoneal reaction to the expelling of the follicular contents. Vaginal discharge may increase during ovulation, and a small amount of blood (midcycle spotting) may be discharged as well.

The body temperature increases about 0.3C to 0.6C (0.5F to 1.0F) 24 to 48 hours after the time of ovulation. It remains elevated until the day before menstruation begins. There may be an accompanying sharp basal body temperature drop just before the increase. These temperature changes are useful clinically to determine the approximate time ovulation occurs.

Generally the ovum takes several minutes to travel through the ruptured follicle to the fallopian tube opening. The contractions of the tube's smooth muscle and its ciliary action propel the ovum through the tube. The ovum remains in the ampulla, where it may be fertilized and cleavage can begin. The ovum is thought to be fertile for only 6 to 24 hours. It reaches the uterus 72 to 96 hours after its release from the ovary.

The luteal phase begins when the ovum leaves its follicle. Under the influence of LH the corpus luteum develops from the ruptured follicle. Within 2 or 3 days the corpus luteum becomes yellowish and spherical and increases in vascularity. If the ovum is fertilized and implants in the endometrium, the fertilized egg begins to secrete **human chorionic gonadotropin (hCG),** which is needed to maintain the corpus luteum. The corpus luteum of pregnancy provides progesterone to maintain the pregnancy until the fourth month of pregnancy. If fertilization does not occur, within about a week after ovulation the corpus luteum begins to degenerate, eventually becoming a connective tissue scar called the *corpus albicans.* With degeneration comes a decrease in estrogen and progesterone. This allows for an increase in LH and FSH, which triggers the hypothalamus. Approximately 14 days after ovulation (in an ideal 28-day cycle), in the absence of pregnancy, menstruation begins.

Menstrual Cycle

Menstruation is cyclic uterine bleeding in response to cyclic hormonal changes. Menstruation occurs when the ovum is not fertilized and begins about 14 days after ovulation in a 28-day cycle. The menstrual discharge, also referred to as the *menses* or *menstrual flow,* is composed of blood mixed with cervical and vaginal secretions, bacteria, mucus, leukocytes, and other cellular debris. The menstrual discharge is dark red and has a distinctive odor.

A review of the endometrium and its arterial blood supply will provide further understanding of the menstrual process (Figure 10–20 •). Blood flow from the spiral arterioles in the superficial endometrium is reduced, leading to a lack of blood and oxygen, which in turn produces tissue death (necrosis) and discharge of the superficial endometrium (menses). At the same time, the straight arterioles provide the basal endometrium with sufficient blood flow to maintain this layer of the endometrium and the endometrial glands (or seeds) that are responsible for the generation of the endometrium in the next female reproductive or menstrual cycle (see Figure 10–18). Bleeding is controlled by vasospasm of the straight basal arterioles, resulting in coagulative necrosis at the vessel tips.

Frequently, ovulation does not occur in early menstrual cycles; these are called anovulatory cycles. Early cycles also are often irregular in frequency, amount of flow, and duration. Within several months to 2 to 3 years, a regular cycle becomes established.

Menstrual parameters vary greatly among individuals. Generally, menstruation occurs every 28 days, plus or minus 5 days. Some women normally have cycles as long as 34 to 38 days, which can skew standard calculations of the estimated date of birth (EDB). Emotional and physical factors such as illness, excessive fatigue, stress or anxiety, and rigorous exercise programs can alter the cycle interval. Certain environmental factors such as temperature and altitude may also affect the cycle.

MEDIALINK MENSTRUAL CYCLE CENTRAL

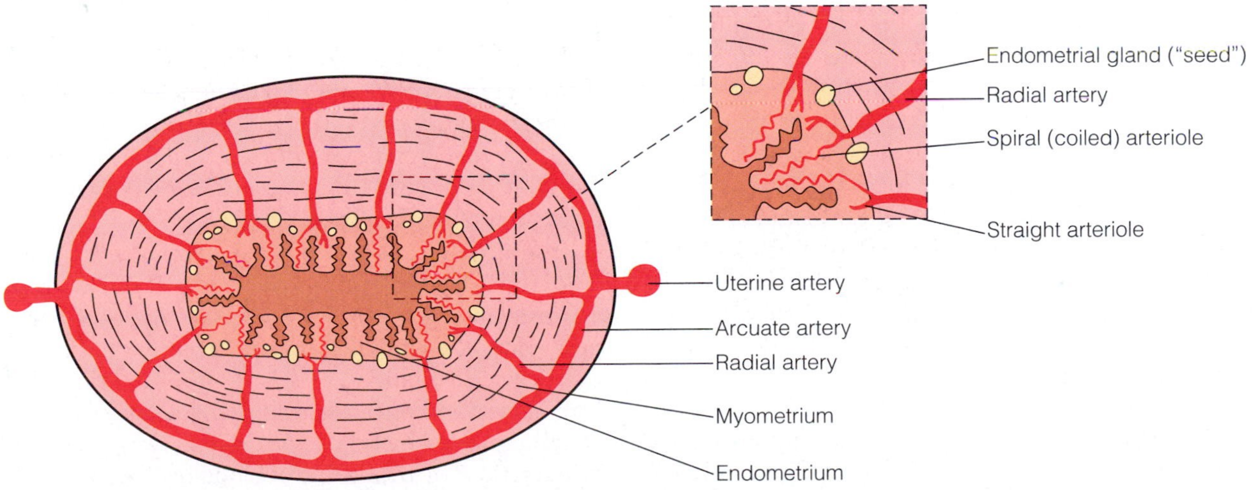

Figure 10–20 • Blood supply to the endometrium (cross-sectional view of the uterus).

Table 10–2 • CHARACTERISTICS OF MENSTRUAL CYCLE AND OVULATION

Menstrual phase (days 1–6)	Estrogen levels are low.
	Cervical mucus is scanty, viscous, and opaque.
	Endometrium is shed.
Proliferative phase (days 7–14)	Endometrium and myometrium thickness increases.
	Estrogen peaks just before ovulation.
	Cervical mucosa at ovulation:
	Is clear, thin, watery, and alkaline.
	Is more favorable to sperm.
	Has elasticity (spinnbarkheit) greater than 5 cm.
	Shows ferning pattern on microscopic exam.
	Just prior to ovulation body temperature drops; then at ovulation basal body temperature increases 0.3C to 0.6C, and mittelschmerz and/or midcycle spotting may occur.
Secretory phase (days 15–26)	Estrogen drops sharply, and progesterone dominates.
	Vascularity of entire uterus increases.
	Tissue glycogen increases, and the uterus is made ready for implantation.
Ischemic phase (days 27–28)	Both estrogen and progesterone levels fall.
	Spiral arteries undergo vasoconstriction.
	Endometrium becomes pale.
	Blood vessels rupture.
	Blood escapes into uterine stromal cells.

The duration of menses is from 2 to 8 days, with the blood loss averaging 30 mL, and the loss of iron averaging 0.5 to 1 mg daily.

The uterine (menstrual) cycle has four phases: the menstrual phase, proliferative phase, secretory phase, and ischemic phase (Table 10–2 •). Menstruation occurs during the *menstrual phase.* Some endometrial areas are shed, while others remain. Some of the remaining tips of the endometrial glands begin to regenerate. The endometrium is in a resting state following menstruation. Estrogen levels are low, and the endometrium is 1 to 2 mm deep. During this part of the cycle the cervical mucosa is scanty, viscous, and opaque.

The *proliferative phase* begins when the endometrial glands enlarge, becoming twisted and longer, in response to increasing amounts of estrogen. The blood vessels become prominent and dilated, and the endometrium increases in thickness sixfold to eightfold. This gradual process reaches its peak just before ovulation. The cervical mucosa becomes thin, clear, watery, and more alkaline, making the mucosa more favorable to spermatozoa. As ovulation nears, the cervical mucous shows increased elasticity, called *spinnbarkheit.* At ovulation, the mucus will stretch more than 5 cm. The cervical mucosa pH increases from below 7.0 to 7.5 at the time of ovulation. On microscopic examination, the mucosa shows a characteristic ferning pattern (Figure 12–4, B). This ferning pattern is a useful aid in assessment of ovulation time (Table 10–3 •). For an in-depth discussion, see Chapter 12 .

The *secretory phase* follows ovulation. The endometrium, under estrogenic influence, undergoes slight cellular growth. Progesterone, however, causes such marked swelling and growth that the epithelium is warped into folds (Figure 10–21 •). The amount of tissue glycogen increases. The glandular epithelial cells begin to fill with cellular debris, and the glands become tortuous and dilate. The glands secrete small quantities of endometrial fluid in preparation for a fertilized ovum. The vascularity of the entire uterus increases greatly, providing a nourishing bed for implantation. If implantation occurs, the endometrium, under the influence of progesterone, continues to develop and becomes even thicker (Figure 10–22 •; see Chapter 11 for an in-depth discussion of implantation).

Table 10–3 • SIGNS OF OVULATION

The cervical mucosa changes in the following ways:

- The amount of mucus increases.
- It appears thin, watery, and clear.
- Spinnbarkheit greater than 5 cm is present.
- A ferning pattern appears on microscopic examination.

Basal body temperature increases 0.3C to 0.6C 24 to 48 hours after ovulation.

Mittelschmerz may be present.

Midcycle spotting may occur.

If fertilization does not occur, the *ischemic phase* begins. The corpus luteum begins to degenerate, and as a result both estrogen and progesterone levels fall. Areas of necrosis appear under the epithelial lining. Extensive vascular changes also occur. Small blood vessels rupture, and the spiral arteries constrict and retract, causing a deficiency of blood in the endometrium, which becomes pale. This ischemic phase is characterized by the escape of blood into the stromal cells of the uterus. The menstrual flow begins, thus beginning the menstrual cycle again. After menstruation, the basal layer re-

MediaLink CARE PLAN: IRREGULAR MENSES

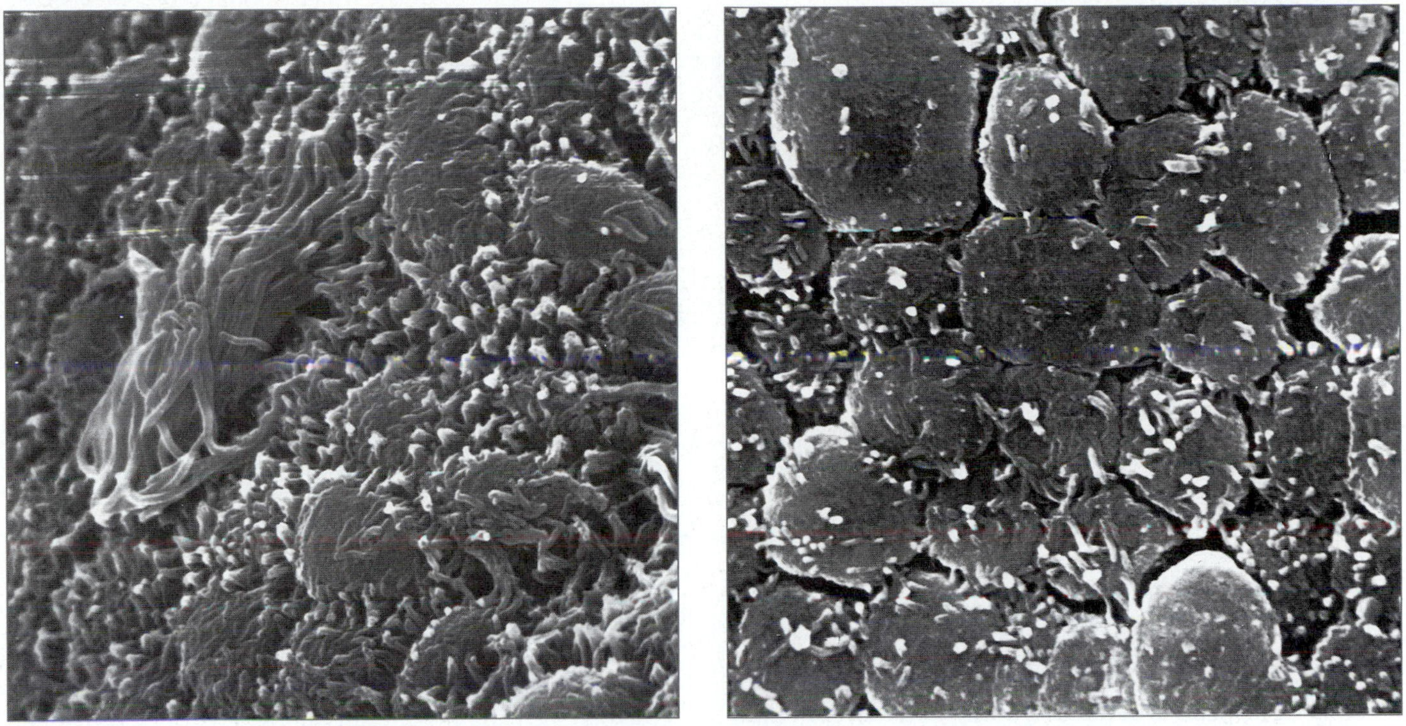

A

B

Figure 10–21 • Scanning electron micrographs of the uterine lining during different phases of the uterine cycle. *A,* During the luteal phase, some of the cells have cilia, and some are secreting droplets. The secreting cells are covered with microvilli. *B,* In the secretory phase, microvilli are still present on the surface of the secreting cells, but the general surface of the lining has a lumpier appearance than during the proliferative phase, and the cilia appear shorter and less numerous. The named phases refer to the uterine condition at the time the photographs were taken.

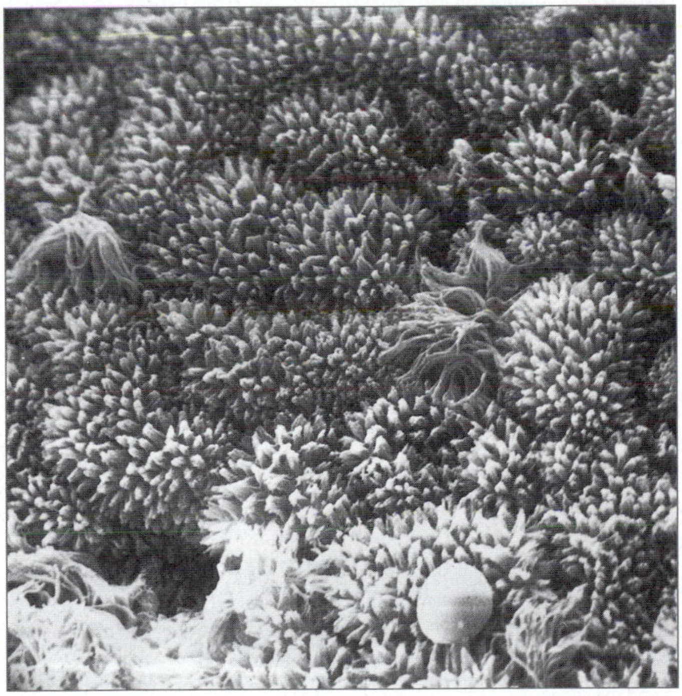

Figure 10–22 • Scanning electron micrograph of the inner lining of the uterus at the time of blastocyst implantation. The blastocyst is an embryo at an early stage of development.

mains so that the tips of the glands can regenerate the new functional endometrial layer. See Table 10–4 • for a summary of the female reproductive cycle.

Male Reproductive System

The primary reproductive functions of the male genitals are to produce and transport the male sex cells (sperm) through and eventually out of the genital tract into the female genital tract. The male reproductive system consists of the external and internal genitals (Figure 10–23 •).

External Genitals

The two external reproductive organs are the penis and the scrotum.

PENIS

The *penis* is an elongated, cylindrical structure consisting of a body, termed the *shaft,* and a cone-shaped end called the *glans.* The penis lies in front of the scrotum.

The shaft of the penis is made up of three longitudinal columns of erectile tissue: the paired *corpora cavernosa* and a third, the *corpus spongiosum.* These columns are covered by a

MEDIALINK ANIMATION: MALE PELVIS

Table 10–4 • SUMMARY OF FEMALE REPRODUCTIVE CYCLE

Ovarian Cycle

Follicular phase (days 1–14): Primordial follicle matures under influence of FSH and LH up to the time of ovulation.

Luteal phase (days 15–28): Ovum leaves follicle; corpus luteum develops under LH influence and produces high levels of progesterone and low levels of estrogen.

Menstrual Cycle

Menstrual phase (days 1–6): Estrogen levels are low, cervical mucus is scant, viscous, and opaque.

Proliferative phase (days 7–14): Estrogen peaks just prior to ovulation. Cervical mucus at ovulation is clear, thin, watery, alkaline, and more favorable to sperm; shows ferning pattern; and has spinnbarkheit greater than 5 cm. At ovulation body temperature drops, then rises sharply and remains elevated under influence of progesterone.

Secretory phase (days 15–26): Estrogen drops sharply, and progesterone dominates.

Ischemic phase (days 27–28): Both estrogen and progesterone levels drop.

MediaLink WebMD Anatomy

dense, fibrous connective tissue and then enclosed by an elastic tissue. The penis is covered by a thin outer layer of skin.

The corpus spongiosum contains the urethra and becomes the glans at the distal end of the penis. The urethra widens within the glans and ends in a slitlike orifice, located in the tip of the glans, called the *urethral meatus.* A circular fold of skin arises just behind the glans and covers it. Known as the *prepuce*, or *foreskin*, it is frequently removed by the surgical procedure of circumcision (Chapter 30). If the corpus spongiosum does not surround the urethra completely, the urethral meatus may occur on the ventral aspect of the penile shaft (hypospadias) or on the dorsal aspect (epispadias).

The penis is innervated by the pudendal nerve. Sexual stimulation causes the penis to elongate, thicken, and stiffen, a process called *erection.* The penis becomes erect when its blood vessels become engorged, a consequence of parasympathetic nerve stimulation. If sexual stimulation is intense enough, the forceful and sudden expulsion of semen occurs through the rhythmic contractions of the penile muscles. This phenomenon is called *ejaculation.*

The penis serves both the urinary and reproductive systems. Urine is expelled through the urethral meatus. The primary reproductive function of the penis is to deposit sperm in the female vagina during sexual intercourse so that fertilization of the ovum can occur.

SCROTUM

The *scrotum* is a pouchlike structure that hangs in front of the anus and behind the penis. Composed of skin and the *dartos muscle*, the scrotum shows increased pigmentation and scattered hairs. The sebaceous glands open directly onto the scrotal surface; their secretion has a distinctive odor. Contraction of the dartos and cremasteric muscles shortens the scrotum and draws it closer to the body, thus wrinkling its outer surface. The degree of wrinkling is greatest in young men and at cold temperatures and is least in older men and at warm temperatures.

Inside the scrotum are two lateral compartments. Each compartment contains a testis with its related structures. Because the left spermatic cord grows longer, the left testis and its scrotal sac hang lower than the right. A ridge (raphe) on the external scrotal surface marks the position of the medial septum and continues anteriorly on the urethral surface of the penis but disappears in the perineal area.

The function of the scrotum is to protect the testes and the sperm by maintaining a temperature lower than that of the body. Spermatogenesis will not occur if the testes fail to descend and thus remain at body temperature. Because it is sensitive to touch, pressure, temperature, and pain, the scrotum defends against potential harm to the testes.

Internal Reproductive Organs

The male internal reproductive organs include the gonads (testes or testicles), a system of ducts (epididymis, vas deferens, ejaculatory duct, and urethra), and accessory glands (seminal vesicles, prostate gland, bulbourethral glands, and

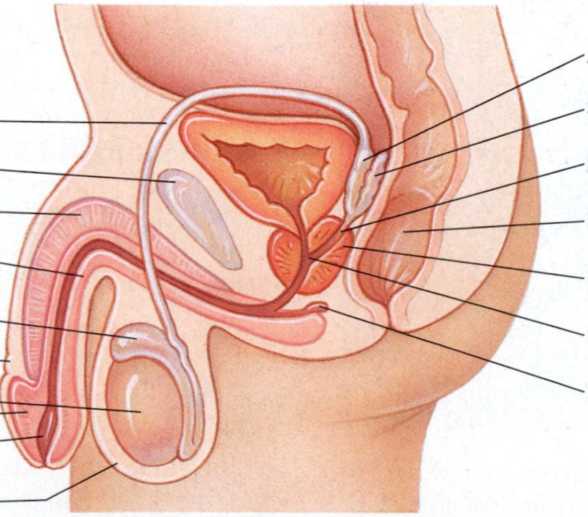

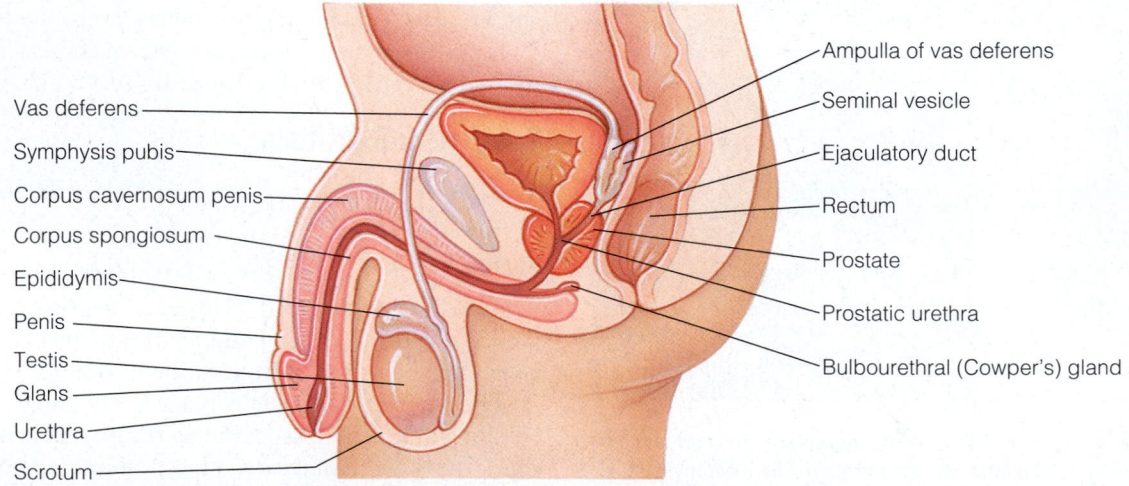

Figure 10–23 • Male reproductive system, sagittal view.

Table 10-5 • SUMMARY OF MALE REPRODUCTIVE ORGAN FUNCTIONS

The testes house seminiferous tubules and gonads.

- Seminiferous tubules contain sperm cells in various stages of development and undergoing meiosis.
- Sertoli's cells nourish and protect spermatocytes (phase between spermatids and spermatozoa).
- Leydig's cells are the main source of testosterone.
- Epididymides provide an area for maturation of sperm and a reservoir for mature spermatozoa.
- The vas deferens connects the epididymis with the prostate gland, then connects with ducts from the seminal vesicle to become an ejaculatory duct.
- Ejaculatory ducts provide a passageway for semen and seminal fluid into the urethra.
- Seminal vesicles secrete yellowish fluid rich in fructose, prostaglandins, and fibrinogen. This provides nutrition that increases motility and fertilizing ability of sperm. Prostaglandins also aid fertilization by making the cervical mucus more receptive to sperm.
- The prostate gland secretes thin, alkaline fluid containing calcium, citric acid, and other substances. Alkalinity counteracts acidity of ductus and seminal vesicle secretions.
- Bulbourethral (Cowper's) glands secrete alkaline, viscous fluid into semen, aiding in neutralization of acidic vaginal secretions.

urethral glands). See Table 10–5 • for a summary of male reproductive organ functions.

TESTES

The *testes* are a pair of oval, compound glandular organs contained in the scrotum (Figure 10–24 •). In the sexually mature male, they are the site of spermatozoa production and the secretion of several male sex hormones.

Each testis is 4 to 6 cm long, 2 to 3 cm wide, and 3 to 4 cm deep and weighs 10 to 15 g. Each is covered by a serous membrane and an inner capsule that is tough, white, and fibrous. The connective tissue sends projections inward to form septa, dividing the testis into 250 to 400 lobules. Each lobule contains one to three tightly packed, convoluted *seminiferous tubules* containing sperm cells in all stages of development.

The seminiferous tubules are surrounded by loose connective tissue, which houses abundant blood and lymph vessels and the *interstitial (Leydig's) cells.* The interstitial cells produce testosterone, the primary male sex hormone. The seminiferous tubules come together to form the 20 or 30 straight tubules, which in turn form an anastomosing network of thin-walled spaces, the rete testis. The rete testis forms 10 to 15 efferent ducts that empty into the duct of the epididymis.

Most of the cells lining the seminiferous tubules undergo *spermatogenesis,* a process of maturation in which spermatocytes become spermatozoa. (See Chapter 11 for further discussion of spermatogenesis .) Sperm production varies among and within the tubules, with cells in different areas of the same tubule undergoing different stages of spermatogenesis. The seminiferous tubules also contain *Sertoli's cells,* which nourish and protect the spermatocytes. The sperm are eventually released from the tubules into the epididymis, where they mature further.

Like the female reproductive cycle, the process of spermatogenesis and other functions of the testes are the result of complex neural and hormonal controls. The hypothalamus secretes releasing factors, which stimulate the anterior pituitary to release the gonadotropins—follicle-stimulating hormone (FSH) and luteinizing hormone (LH). These hormones cause the testes to produce testosterone, which maintains spermatogenesis, increases sperm production by the seminiferous tubules, and stimulates production of seminal fluid.

Testosterone is also responsible for the development of secondary male characteristics and certain behavioral patterns. The effects of testosterone include structural and functional development of the male genital tract, emission and ejaculation of seminal fluid, distribution of body hair, promotion of growth and strength of long bones, increased muscle mass, and enlargement of the vocal cords. The action of testosterone on the central nervous system is thought to produce aggressiveness and sexual drive. The action of testosterone is constant, not cyclic like that of the female hormones. Its production is not limited to a certain number of years, but is thought to decrease with age.

In summary, the primary functions of the testes are to serve as the site of spermatogenesis and to produce testosterone.

EPIDIDYMIS

The *epididymis* (plural, *epididymides*) is a duct about 5.6 m long, although it is convoluted into a compact structure about 3.75 cm long. An epididymis lies behind each testis. It arises from the top of the testis, extends downward, and then passes upward, where it becomes the vas deferens.

The epididymis provides a reservoir where spermatozoa can survive for a long period. When discharged from the seminiferous tubules into the epididymis, the sperm are immobile and incapable of fertilizing an ovum. The spermatozoa remain in the epididymis for 2 to 10 days. As the sperm are transported along the tortuous course of the epididymis, they become both motile and fertile.

VAS DEFERENS AND EJACULATORY DUCTS

The *vas deferens,* also known as the *ductus deferens,* is about 40 cm long and connects the epididymis with the prostate (see Figure 10–23). One vas deferens arises from the posterior border of each testis. It joins the spermatic cord and weaves over and between several pelvic structures until it meets the vas deferens from the opposite side. Each vas deferens terminus expands to form the *terminal ampulla.* It then unites with the seminal vesicle duct (a gland) to form the ejaculatory duct, which enters the prostate gland and ends in the prostatic urethra. The ejaculatory ducts serve as a passageway for semen and fluid secreted by the seminal vesicles. The main function of the vas deferens is to rapidly squeeze the sperm from their storage sites (the epididymis and distal part of the vas deferens) into the urethra.

Men who choose to take total responsibility for birth control may elect to have a vasectomy. In this procedure, the scrotal portion of the vas deferens is surgically incised or cauterized. Although sperm continue to be produced for the

MEDIALINK ACTIVITIES: MALE REPRODUCTIVE SYSTEM

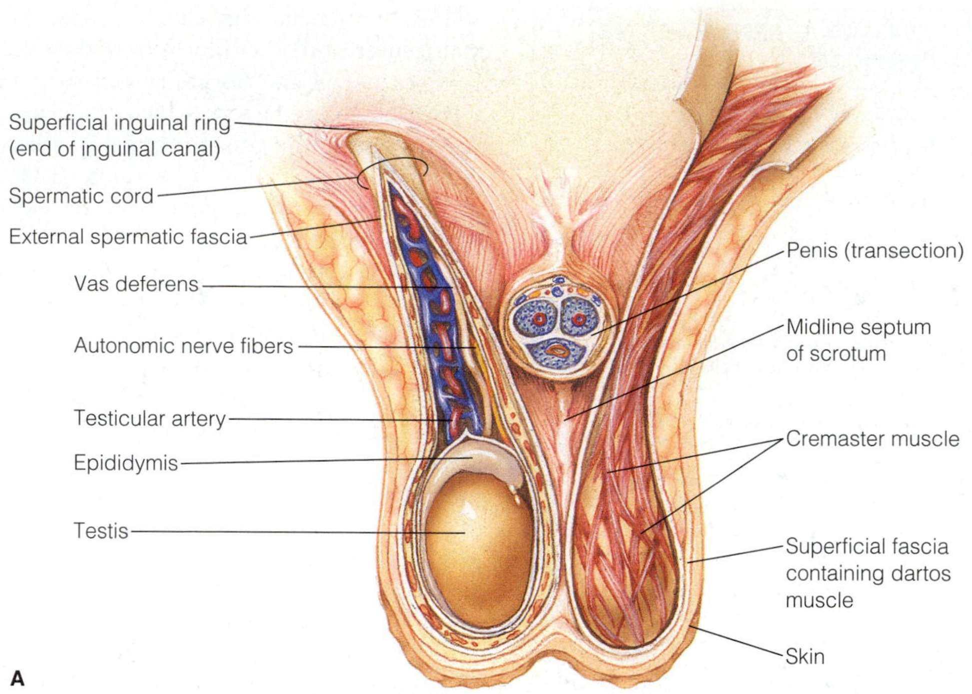

next several years, they can no longer reach the outside of the body. Eventually, the sperm deteriorate and are reabsorbed.

URETHRA

The *male urethra* is a passageway for urine and semen. The urethra begins in the bladder and passes through the prostate gland, where it is called the *prostatic urethra*.

The urethra emerges from the prostate gland to become the *membranous urethra*. It terminates in the penis, where it is called the *penile urethra*. In the penile urethra, goblet secretory cells are present, and smooth muscle is replaced by erectile tissue.

ACCESSORY GLANDS

The male accessory glands are specialized structures under endocrine and neural control. Each secretes a unique and essential component of the total seminal fluid in an ordered sequence.

The *seminal vesicles* are two glands composed of many lobes. Each vesicle is about 7.5 cm long. They are situated between the bladder and rectum and immediately above the base of the prostate. The epithelium lining the seminal vesicles secretes an alkaline, viscous, clear fluid rich in high-energy fructose, prostaglandins, fibrinogen, and amino acids. During ejaculation this fluid mixes with sperm in the ejaculatory ducts. This fluid helps provide an environment favorable to sperm motility and metabolism.

The prostate gland encircles the upper part of the urethra and lies below the neck of the bladder. Made up of several lobes, it measures about 4 cm in diameter and weighs 20 to 30 g. The prostate is made up of both glandular and muscular tissue. It secretes a thin, milky, alkaline fluid containing high levels of zinc, calcium, citric acid, and acid phosphatase. This fluid protects the sperm from the acidic environment of the vagina and the male urethra, which could be spermicidal.

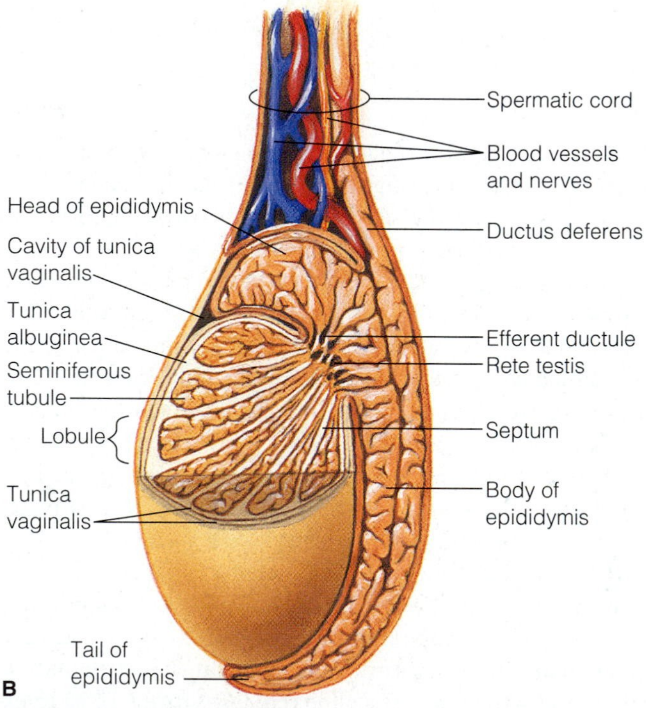

Figure 10–24 • The testes: *A,* External view. *B,* Sagittal view showing interior anatomy.

The *bulbourethral glands (Cowper's glands)* are a pair of small round structures on either side of the membranous urethra. The glands secrete a clear, thick, alkaline fluid rich in mucoproteins that becomes part of the semen. This secretion also lubricates the penile urethra during sexual excitement and neutralizes the acid in the male urethra and the vagina, thereby enhancing sperm motility.

The *urethral glands (Littre's glands)* are tiny mucus-secreting glands found throughout the membranous lining of the penile urethra. Their secretions add to those of the bulbourethral glands.

SEMEN

The male ejaculate, *semen* or *seminal fluid*, is made up of spermatozoa and the secretions of all the accessory glands. The seminal fluid transports viable and motile sperm to the female reproductive tract. Effective transportation of sperm requires adequate nutrients, an adequate pH (about 7.5), a specific concentration of sperm to fluid, and an optimal osmolarity.

A spermatozoon is made up of a head and a tail (Figure 10–25 •). The head's main components are the acrosome and the nucleus. The head carries the male's haploid number of chromosomes (23), and it is the part that enters the ovum at fertilization (Chapter 11). The tail, or *flagellum*, is specialized for motility. The tail is divided into the middle and end piece.

Sperm may be stored in the male genital system up to 42 days, depending primarily on the frequency of ejaculations. The average volume of ejaculate following abstinence for several days is 2 to 5 mL but may vary from 1 to 10 mL. Repeated ejaculation results in decreased volume. Once ejaculated, sperm can live only 2 or 3 days in the female genital tract.

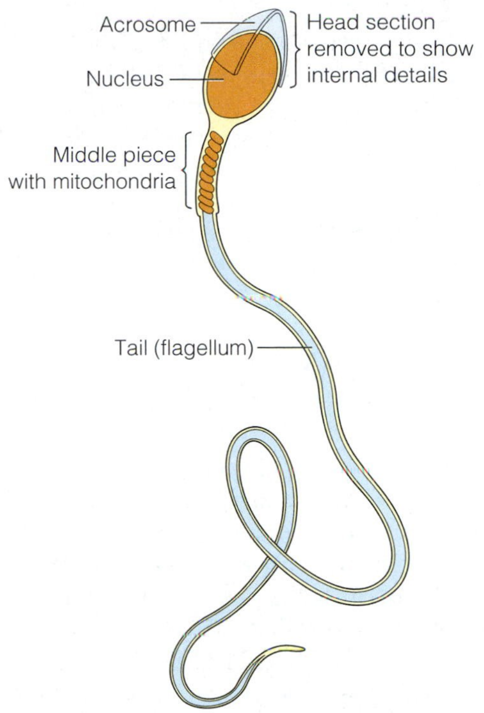

Figure 10–25 • Schematic illustration of a mature spermatozoon.

MEDIALINK CASE STUDY: SEX EDUCATION

CHAPTER REVIEW

EXPLOREMEDIALINK

NCLEX review questions, case studies, and other interactive resources for this chapter can be found on the Web site at http://www.prenhall.com/olds. Click on "Chapter 10" to select the activities for this chapter.

For tutorials including animations and videos, more NCLEX review questions, and an audio glossary, access the accompanying CD-ROM in this book.

Focus Your Study

- The genetic sex of an embryo is determined at fertilization. The male and female reproductive systems are undifferentiated initially. By the 12th week the external genitals are fully differentiated.
- Reproductive activities require complex interactions between the reproductive structures, the central nervous system, and such endocrine glands as the pituitary, hypothalamus, testes, and ovaries.
- At puberty, an alteration in brain sensitivity leads to an increased release of GnRH, which stimulates LH and FSH, leading in the male to an increase in testosterone and in the female to an increase in estrogen and progesterone.
- Estrogen is the principal cause of the events of puberty in females (maturation of ova, enlargement of the uterus and fallopian tubes, deposition of fat in the breasts and hips, and characteristic hair growth).
- Puberty changes for the male (onset of spermatogenesis; enlargement of the penis, scrotum, and testes; voice changes; and characteristic hair

growth) occur as a result of increased testosterone production by the testes.

- The female reproductive system consists of the ovaries, where female germ cells and female sex hormones are formed; the fallopian tubes, which capture the ovum and allow transport to the uterus; the uterus, which is the implantation site for the fertilized ovum (blastocyst); the cervix, which is a protective portal for the body of the uterus and the connection between the vagina and the uterus; and the vagina, which is the passageway from the external genitals to the uterus and provides for discharge of menstrual products to the outside of the body.
- The female reproductive cycle may be described in terms of the ovarian cycle, during which ovulation occurs, and the menstrual cycle, during which menstruation occurs. These two cycles take place simultaneously and are under neurohormonal control. The ovarian cycle has two phases: the follicular phase and the luteal phase. During the follicular phase, the primordial follicle matures under the influence of FSH and LH until ovulation occurs. The luteal phase begins when the ovum leaves the follicle and the corpus luteum develops under the influence of LH. The corpus luteum produces high levels of progesterone and low levels of estrogen.
- The menstrual cycle has four phases: menstrual, proliferative, secretory, and ischemic. Menstruation is the actual shedding of the endometrial lining, when estrogen levels are low. The proliferative phase begins when the endometrial glands begin to enlarge under the influence of estrogen and cervical mucosal changes occur; the changes peak at ovulation. The secretory phase follows ovulation, and, influenced primarily by progesterone, the uterus increases its vascularity to make ready for possible implantation. The ischemic phase is characterized by degeneration of the corpus luteum, decreases in both estrogen and progesterone levels, constriction of the spiral arteries, and escape of blood into the stromal cells of the endometrium.
- The male reproductive system consists of the testes, where male germ cells and male sex hormones are formed; a series of continuous ducts through which spermatozoa are transported outside the body; accessory glands that produce secretions important to sperm nutrition, survival, and transport; and the penis, which serves as the reproductive organ of intercourse.

References

Blackburn, S. T. (2003). *Maternal, fetal, & neonatal physiology: A clinical perspective.* (2nd ed.). St. Louis: Saunders.

Caldwell, W. E., & Moloy, H. C. (1933). Anatomical variations in the female pelvis and their effect on labor with a suggested classification [Historical article]. *American Journal of Obstetrics and Gynecology, 26,* 479–505.

Cunningham, F. G., Gant, N. F., Leveno, K. J., Gilstrap, L. C., Hauth, J. C., & Wenstrom, K. D. (2001). *Williams obstetrics* (21st ed.). New York: McGraw-Hill.

Rebar, R. W. (1999). The breast and the physiology of lactation. In R. K. Creasy & R. Resnik (Eds.), *Maternal-fetal medicine: Principles and practice* (4th ed., pp, 106–121). Philadelphia: Saunders.

11 Conception and Fetal Development

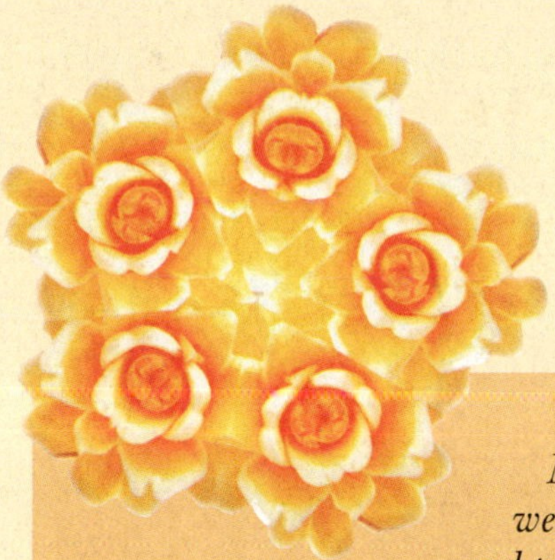

My friends tease me when I say this, but I know the moment my daughter was conceived. My husband and I had both been so busy at work, but we finally went away for a long weekend together. It was wonderful—we got back some of the magic as we took long walks and talked and talked. Until that weekend, whenever we discussed having children it was always "maybe someday." On the second night we decided to skip the diaphragm for the first time ever. Our lovemaking seemed so special that evening, a true reflection of the emotional closeness we had recaptured. I never went back to using the diaphragm after that weekend, but I am convinced that Jennifer is the result of that night together!

Objectives

- Explain the differences between mitotic cellular division and meiotic cellular division.
- Compare the processes by which ova and sperm are produced.
- Describe the process of fertilization.
- Identify the differing processes by which fraternal (dizygotic) and identical (monozygotic) twins are formed.
- Describe in order of increasing complexity the structures that form during the cellular multiplication and differentiation stages of intrauterine development.
- Describe the development, structure, and functions of the placenta during intrauterine life.
- Summarize the significant changes in growth and development of the fetus in utero at 4, 6, 12, 16, 20, 24, 28, 32, 36, and 38 weeks postconception.
- Identify the vulnerable periods during which malformations of the various organ systems may occur, and describe the resulting congenital malformations.

Key Terms

Acrosomal reaction 226
Amnion 231
Amniotic fluid 231
Bag of waters (BOW) 231
Blastocyst 229
Capacitation 226
Chorion 230
Chromosomes 222
Cleavage 229
Cotyledon 233
Decidua basalis 229
Decidua capsularis 229
Decidua vera (parietalis) 229
Diploid number of chromosomes 222
Ductus arteriosus 237
Ductus venosus 237
Ectoderm 230
Embryo 240
Embryonic membranes 230
Endoderm 230
Fertilization 225
Fetus 243
Foramen ovale 237
Gametes 224
Gametogenesis 224
Haploid number of chromosomes 224
Lanugo 231
Meiosis 223
Mesoderm 230
Mitosis 222

MediaLink

Additional resources for this content can be found on the Student CD-ROM and on the Companion Website at www.prenhall.com/olds. Click on "Chapter 11" to select the activities for this chapter.

CD-ROM

- Audio Glossary
- NCLEX Review
- Animation: Cell Division
- Animation: Oogenesis
- Animation: Spermatogenesis
- Animation: Oogenesis and Spermatogenesis Compared
- Activity: Labeling Oogenesis and Spermatogenesis
- Activity: Matching Oogenesis and Spermatogenesis
- Animation: Conception
- Animation: Embryonic Heart Formation and Circulation
- Animation: Formation of Placenta

Companion Website

- Additional NCLEX Review
- Case Study: Teaching About Pregnancy
- Care Plan Activity: Client Fearful of Multiple Gestation

Key Terms

Morula 229
Placenta 233
Postconception age periods 238
Teratogen 245
Trophoblast 229
Umbilical cord 232
Vernix caseosa 244
Wharton's jelly 233
Zygote 224

Each person is unique. Nonetheless, everyone has many if not all of the same "parts," which usually function similarly. The human genome consists of large amounts of chemical deoxyribonucleic acid (DNA) that contains within its structure the genetic information needed to specify all aspects of embryogenesis, development, growth, metabolism, and reproduction. The genome contains, by current estimates, about 50,000 *genes*, which at this point are defined as units of genetic information (Nussbaum, McInnes, & Willard, 2001). Genes are encoded in the DNA that makes up the chromosomes in the nucleus of each cell. Even chromosomes, those determinants of the structure and function of organ systems and traits, are made of the same biochemical substances. How does each person become unique, then? The answer lies in the physiologic mechanisms of heredity, the processes of cellular division, and the environmental factors that influence development from the moment a person is conceived. This chapter explores the processes involved in conception and fetal development—the basis of human uniqueness.

Chromosomes

Human (body) cells contain within their nuclei threadlike bodies known as **chromosomes,** which are composed of strands of *deoxyribonucleic acid (DNA)* and protein. Each chromosome contains two longitudinal halves called *chromatids*, which are joined together at a point called the *centromere* (Figure 11–1, *A* •). Chromosomes are classified according to their length and to the position of their centromere. When the centromere is centrally located, the longitudinal halves are divided into one short arm region and one long arm region, and the chromosome resembles an X. This is the shape of most human chromosomes.

Every body (somatic) cell in the human body contains 46 chromosomes, referred to as the **diploid number of chromosomes.** These are divided into 23 pairs. There are 22 pairs of similar cells in both males and females called *autosomes* and one pair of sex chromosomes (XX in females, XY in males) (Nussbaum et al, 2001). One chromosome of each pair is contributed by the individual's mother, and the other is contributed by the father. The two chromosomes carrying matching genetic information that make up each pair are called *homologous chromosomes* or *homologs.*

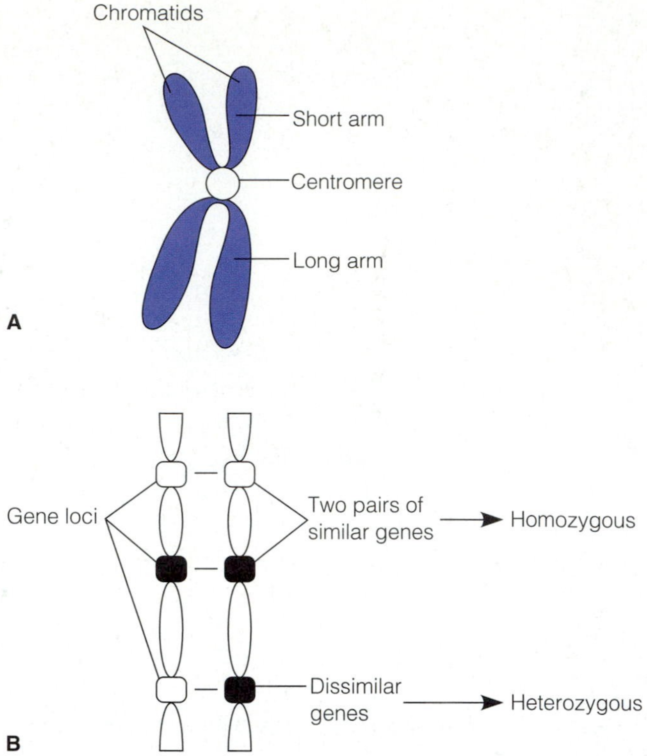

Figure 11–1 • *A,* Chromosomes contain two longitudinal halves called *chromatids,* which are joined together at a point called the *centromere. B,* One pair of homologous chromosomes with similar (homozygous) genes and dissimilar (heterozygous) genes.

Genes are regions in the DNA strands that contain coded information used to determine the unique characteristics—or *traits*—of an individual. Genes in the autosomes determine such traits as hair color or blood type, whereas genes in the sex chromosomes determine the individual's gender. Genes are arranged in linear order on the chromosomes, and can be numbered and studied accordingly.

Each homologous chromosome pair carries genes coding for similar traits in identical locations on the chromosomes. Genes that are similar are called *homozygous* genes, whereas dissimilar genes are referred to as *heterozygous* genes (Figure 11–1, *B*). When an individual is homozygous for a particular trait, he or she has inherited similar genes for that trait from each parent. Genetics is discussed in greater detail in the next chapter.

Cellular Division

Every human begins life as a single cell (fertilized ovum or zygote). This single cell reproduces itself, and in turn each new cell also reproduces itself in a continuing process. The new cells are similar to the cells from which they came.

Cells are reproduced by either mitosis or meiosis, two different but related processes. **Mitosis** results in the production of diploid body (somatic) cells, which are exact copies of the original cell. Mitosis makes growth and development possible, and in mature individuals it is the process by which the body cells continue to divide and replace themselves. **Meiosis** is the cell division process leading to the development of eggs and sperm needed to produce a new organism.

Mitosis

During mitosis, the cell undergoes several changes, ending in cell division. Although mitosis is a continuous process, it is generally divided into five stages: interphase, prophase, metaphase, anaphase, and telophase (see Figure 11–2 •).

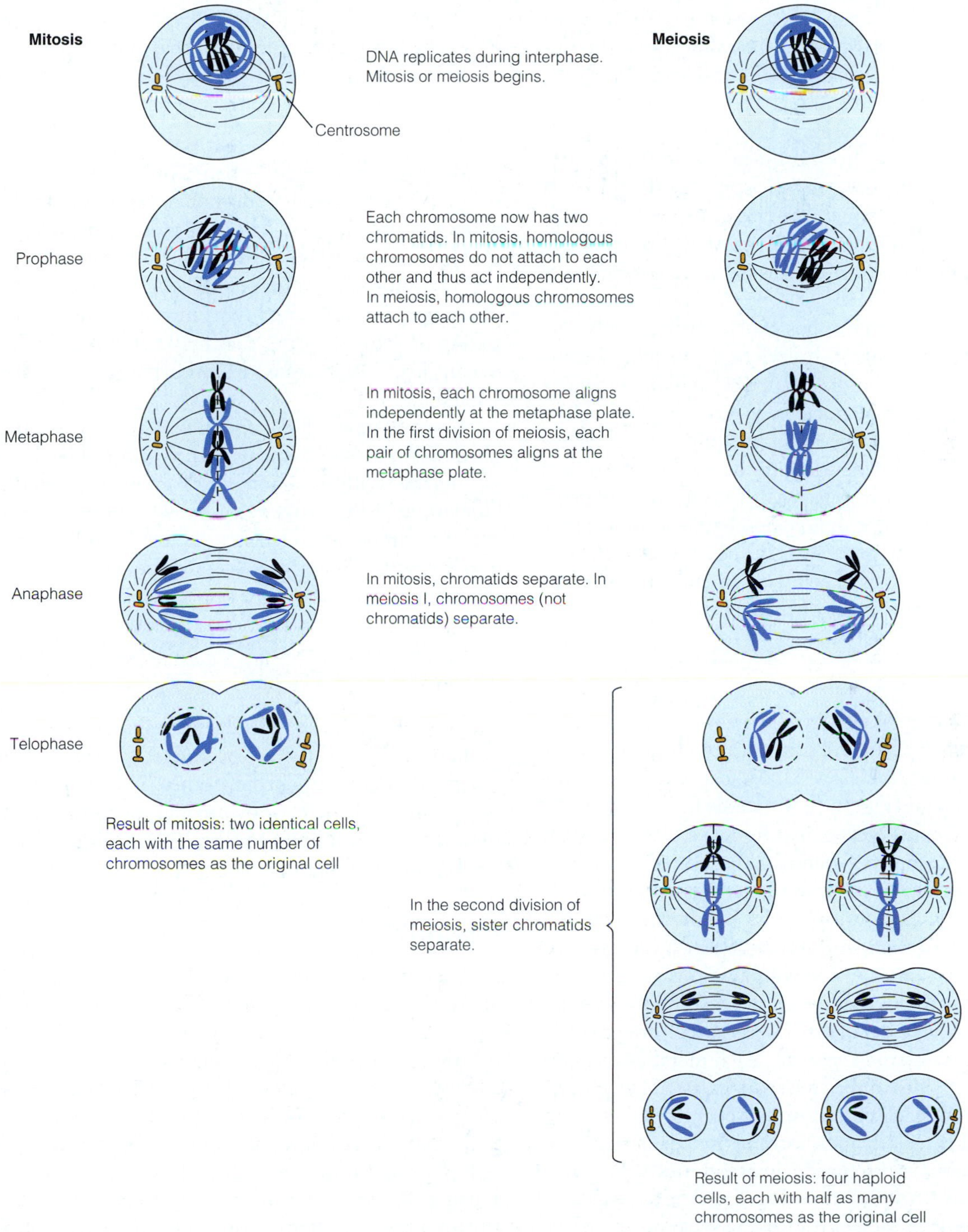

Mitosis
Meiosis
DNA replicates during interphase. Mitosis or meiosis begins.
Centrosome
Prophase
Each chromosome now has two chromatids. In mitosis, homologous chromosomes do not attach to each other and thus act independently. In meiosis, homologous chromosomes attach to each other.
Metaphase
In mitosis, each chromosome aligns independently at the metaphase plate. In the first division of meiosis, each pair of chromosomes aligns at the metaphase plate.
Anaphase
In mitosis, chromatids separate. In meiosis I, chromosomes (not chromatids) separate.
Telophase
Result of mitosis: two identical cells, each with the same number of chromosomes as the original cell
In the second division of meiosis, sister chromatids separate.
Result of meiosis: four haploid cells, each with half as many chromosomes as the original cell

Figure 11–2 • Comparison of mitosis and meiosis.

Before cell division takes place during interphase, the DNA within the chromosomes replicates so that the genes will be doubled. Mitosis begins when the cell enters prophase. During prophase, the chromosomes condense and form the shape we usually recognize as a chromosome. Next comes the appearance of a mitotic apparatus known as a spindle, in which fine threads extend from the top and bottom poles of the nucleus. At each pole of the spindle, a body known as the *centrosome* is formed, so the threads of the spindle extend from one centrosome to the other. Next the nuclear membrane, which separates the nucleus from the cytoplasm, disappears, the nucleus as a separate entity disappears, and the cell enters metaphase (Nussbaum et al, 2001).

During metaphase, the chromosomes line up at the equator (midway between the poles) of the spindle. Metaphase is followed by anaphase, in which the two chromatids of each chromosome separate and move to opposite ends of the spindle, where they cluster in masses near the two poles of the cell.

MediaLink ANIMATION: CELL DIVISION

Telophase is essentially the opposite of prophase. A new nuclear membrane forms, separating each newly formed nucleus from the cytoplasm. The spindle disappears, and the centrioles relocate outside of each new nucleus. Within the nucleus the chromosomes lengthen and become threadlike. As telophase nears completion, a furrow develops in the cell cytoplasm and divides it into two daughter cells, each with its own nucleus. Daughter cells have the same diploid number of chromosomes (46) and the same genetic makeup as the cell from which they came. At the end of mitosis, a cell with 46 chromosomes results in two identical cells, each with 46 chromosomes.

Meiosis

Meiosis is a special type of cell division by which diploid cells give rise to gametes (sperm and ova) with the **haploid number of chromosomes,** which is 23. Meiosis consists of two successive cell divisions (Figure 11–2). In the first division, the chromosomes replicate. Next a pairing takes place between homologous chromosomes (Sadler, 2000). Instead of separating immediately as in mitosis, the similar chromosomes become closely intertwined. At each point of contact, there is a physical exchange of genetic material between the chromatids (arms of the chromosomes). New combinations are provided by the newly formed chromosomes; these combinations account for the wide variation of traits, such as hair or eye color. The chromosome pairs then separate, each member of a pair moving to opposite sides of the cell. (In contrast, during mitosis the chromatids of each chromosome separate and move to opposite poles.) The cell divides, forming two daughter cells, each with 23 double-structured chromosomes—the same amount of DNA as a normal somatic cell. In the second division, the chromatids of each chromosome separate and move to opposite poles of each of the daughter cells. Cell division occurs, resulting in the formation of four cells, each containing 23 single chromosomes, the haploid number of chromosomes. These daughter cells contain only half the DNA of a normal somatic cell (Moore, Persaud, & Shiota, 2000).

MediaLink ANIMATION OOGENESIS

The process of meiosis is important for the following reasons:

- It maintains the *constancy of the chromosome number* from one generation to the next by reducing the chromosome number from diploid to haploid, thereby producing haploid gametes.
- It allows random assortment of *maternal and paternal chromosomes* between the gametes.
- It relocates segments of maternal and paternal chromosomes by *crossing over of chromosome segments*, which "shuffles" the genes and produces a recombination of genetic material.

Mutations may occur during the second meiotic division if two of the chromatids do not move apart rapidly enough when the cell divides. The still-paired chromatids are carried into one of the daughter cells and eventually form an extra chromosome. This condition is referred to as an *autosomal nondisjunction* (chromosomal mutation) and is harmful to the offspring that may result should fertilization occur. The implications of nondisjunction are discussed in Chapter 12.

Another type of chromosomal mutation can occur if chromosomes break during meiosis. If the broken segment is lost, the result is a shorter chromosome; this is known as a deletion. If the broken segment becomes attached to another chromosome, a harmful mutation called a *translocation* is the result. The effects of translocation are described in Chapter 12.

Gametogenesis

Meiosis occurs during **gametogenesis,** the process by which germ cells, or **gametes,** are produced. The gametes must have a haploid number of chromosomes (23) so that when the female gamete (the egg, or ovum) and the male gamete (sperm, or spermatozoon) unite to form the **zygote,** the normal human diploid number of chromosomes (46) is reestablished.

Oogenesis

Oogenesis is the process by which female gametes or ova are produced. As discussed in Chapter 10, the ovaries begin to develop early in the fetal life of the female. All the ova that the female will produce in her lifetime are present at birth. The ovary gives rise to oogonial cells, which develop into oocytes. Meiosis begins in all oocytes before the female infant is born but stops before the first division is complete and remains in this arrested phase until puberty. During puberty the mature primary oocyte continues through the first meiotic division in the graafian follicle of the ovary.

The first meiotic division produces two cells of unequal size with unequal amounts of cytoplasm, but the same number of chromosomes. These two cells are the *secondary oocyte* and a minute first *polar body*. Both the secondary oocyte and

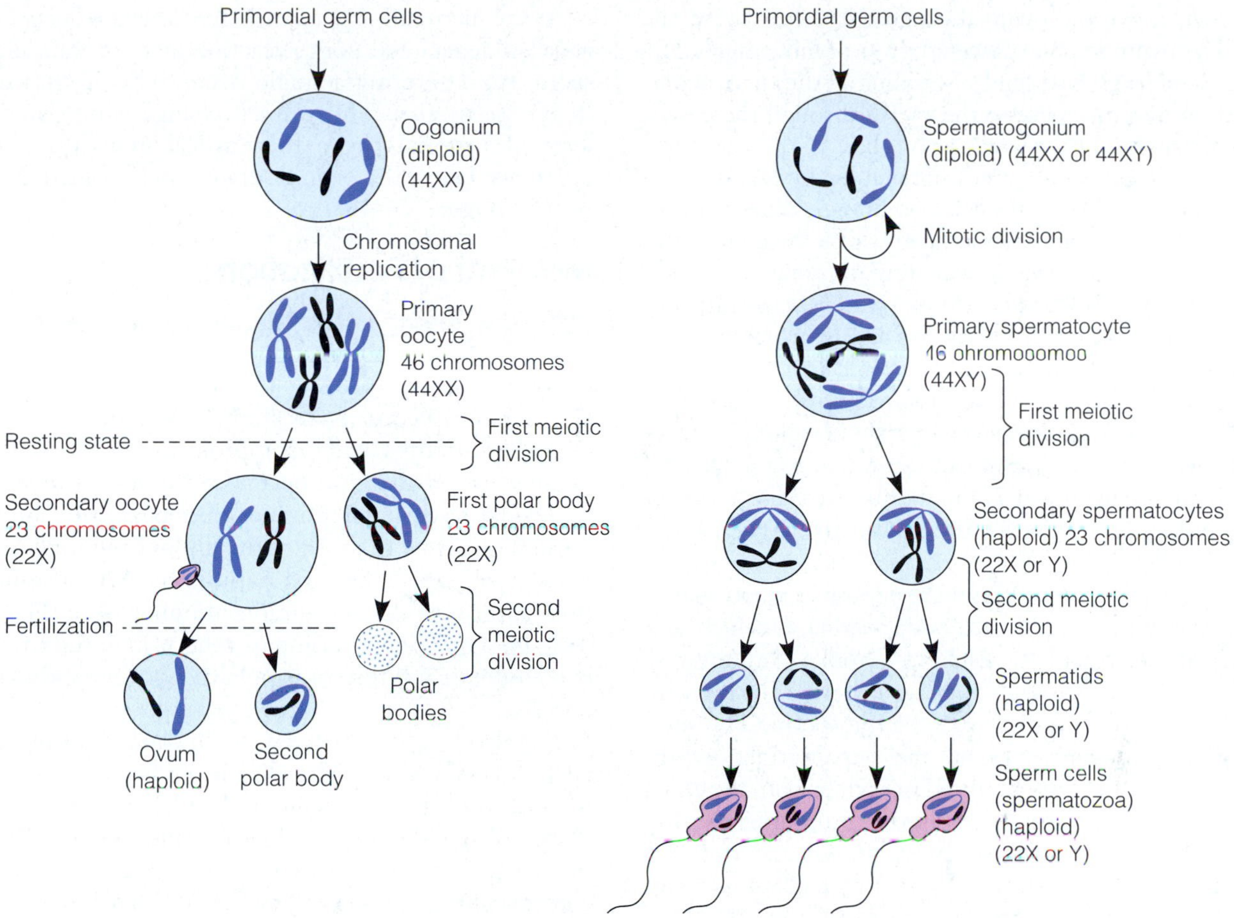

Figure 11–3 • Gametogenesis involves meiosis within the ovary and testis. *A*, During meiosis, each oogonium produces a single haploid ovum once some cytoplasm moves into the polar bodies. *B*, Each spermatogonium, in contrast, produces four haploid spermatozoa.

the first polar body contain 22 double-structured autosomal chromosomes and one double-structured sex chromosome (X). At the time of ovulation, the second meiotic division begins immediately and proceeds as the oocyte moves down the fallopian tube. Again, division is not equal. The secondary oocyte proceeds to metaphase, where its meiotic division is arrested.

When the secondary oocyte completes the second meiotic division after fertilization, the result is a mature ovum with the haploid number of chromosomes and virtually all the cytoplasm. In addition, the second polar body (also haploid) forms at this time (Figure 11–3 •). The first polar body has now also divided, producing two additional polar bodies. Thus when meiosis is completed, four haploid cells have been produced: three small polar bodies, which eventually disintegrate, and one ovum (Sadler, 2000).

Spermatogenesis

During puberty, the germinal epithelium in the seminiferous tubules of the testes begins the process of spermatogenesis, which produces the male gametes (sperm). As the (diploid number) spermatogonium enters the first meiotic division, it is called the *primary spermatocyte.* During this first meiotic division, the spermatogonium replicates and forms two haploid cells termed *secondary spermatocytes,* each of which contains 22 double-structured autosomal chromosomes and either a double-structured X sex chromosome or a double-structured Y sex chromosome. During the second meiotic division they divide to form four spermatids, each with the haploid number of chromosomes (Figure 11–3). The spermatids undergo a series of changes during which they lose most of their cytoplasm and become sperm (spermatozoa). The nucleus becomes compacted into the head of the sperm, which is covered by a cap called an acrosome which is, in turn, covered by a plasma membrane. A long tail is produced from one of the centrioles.

Process of Fertilization

Fertilization is the process by which a sperm fuses with an ovum to form a new diploid cell, or zygote. Following are the events that lead to fertilization.

Preparation for Fertilization

The process of fertilization usually takes place in the ampulla (outer third) of the fallopian tube. During ovulation, high estrogen levels increase peristalsis within the fallopian tubes,

MediaLink ANIMATION: SPERMATOGENESIS

MediaLink Animation: Conception

which helps move the ovum through the tube toward the uterus. The ovum has no inherent power of movement. The high estrogen levels also cause a thinning of the cervical mucus, facilitating movement of the sperm through the cervix, into the uterus, and up the fallopian tube.

The ovum's cell membrane is surrounded by two layers of tissue. The layer closest to the cell membrane is called the *zona pellucida*. It is a clear, noncellular layer whose thickness influences the fertilization rate. Surrounding the zona pellucida is a ring of elongated cells, called the *corona radiata* because they radiate from the ovum like the gaseous corona around the sun. These cells are held together by hyaluronic acid.

The mature ovum and spermatozoa have only a brief time to unite. Ova are considered fertile for about 12 to 24 hours after ovulation. Sperm can survive in the female reproductive tract for 48 to 72 hours but are believed to be healthy and highly fertile for only about the first 24 hours (De Jonge, 2000).

In a single ejaculation, the male deposits approximately 200 to 500 million spermatozoa in the vagina, of which only hundreds of sperm actually reach the ampulla (Brannigan & Lipshultz, 2000). Fructose in the semen, secreted by the seminal vesicles, is the energy source for the sperm. The spermatozoa propel themselves up the female tract by the flagellar movement of their tails. Transit time from the cervix into the fallopian tube can be as short as 5 minutes but usually takes an average of 4 to 6 hours after ejaculation (Cunningham, Gant, Leveno, et al, 2001). Prostaglandins in the semen may increase uterine smooth muscle contractions, which help transport the sperm. The fallopian tubes have a dual ciliary action that facilitates movement of the ovum toward the uterus and movement of the sperm from the uterus toward the ovary.

The sperm must undergo two processes before fertilization can occur: capacitation and the acrosomal reaction. **Capacitation** is the removal of the plasma membrane and glycoprotein coat overlying the spermatozoa's acrosomal area and the loss of seminal plasma proteins. If the glycoprotein coat is not removed, the sperm will not be able to fertilize the ovum (Brannigan & Lipshultz, 2000). Capacitation occurs in the female reproductive tract (aided by uterine enzymes) and is thought to take about 7 hours. Sperm that undergo capacitation take on three characteristics: (1) the ability to undergo the acrosomal reaction, (2) the ability to bind to the zona pellucida, and (3) the acquisition of hypermotility.

MediaLink Case Study: Teaching About Pregnancy

The acrosomal reaction follows capacitation. The acrosomes of the millions of sperm surrounding the ovum release their enzymes (hyaluronidase, a protease called acrosin, and corona-dispersing enzymes) and thus break down the hyaluronic acid in the ovum's corona radiata, the outer layer of the ovum (Brannigan & Lipshultz, 2000). This activity is the **acrosomal reaction.** Hundreds of acrosomes must rupture before enough hyaluronic acid in the corona radiata is cleared for a single sperm to penetrate the zona pellucida of the ovum successfully.

At the moment of penetration by a fertilizing sperm, the zona pellucida undergoes a reaction that prevents additional sperm from entering a single ovum. This is known as the *block to polyspermy*. This cellular change is mediated by release of materials from the cortical granules, organelles found just below the ovum's surface, and is called the *cortical reaction* (Figure 11–4 •).

Moment of Fertilization

After the sperm enters the ovum, a chemical signal prompts the secondary oocyte to complete the second meiotic division, forming the nucleus of the ovum and ejecting the second polar body. Then the nuclei of the ovum and sperm swell and approach each other. The true moment of fertilization occurs as the nuclei unite. Their individual nuclear membranes disappear, and their chromosomes pair up to produce the diploid zygote. Since each nucleus contains a haploid number of chromosomes (23), this union restores the diploid number (46). The zygote contains a new combination of genetic material that results in an individual different from either parent and from anyone else.

It is also at the moment of fertilization that the sex of the zygote is determined. The two chromosomes (the sex chromosomes) of the 23rd pair—either XX or XY—determine the sex of an individual. X chromosomes are larger and bear more genes than Y chromosomes. Females have two X chromosomes, and males have an X and a Y chromosome. Whereas the mature ovum produced by oogenesis can have only one type of sex chromosome—an X—spermatogenesis produces two sperm with an X chromosome and two sperm with a Y chromosome. When each gamete contributes an X chromosome, the resulting zygote is female. When the ovum contributes an X chromosome and the sperm contributes a Y, the resulting zygote is male. As discussed in Chapter 12, certain traits are termed sex-linked because they are controlled by the genes on the X sex chromosome. Two examples of sex-linked traits are color blindness and hemophilia.

Global Perspectives

"My sister, she did not have baby for very, very long time, you see. This is very sad where I am from [Iraq]. Her husband's family wanted him to leave her and we so feared he would. Then my sister became pregnant and it was very nice, we all so happy you see. Then I learned my sister birthed a baby girl and I cried and cried for a week. My mother cried too, so sad all this time no baby come and then finally to have a girl. I still feel sad for her."

(Excerpt from author's interview with Iraqi on childbirth customs in Iraq)

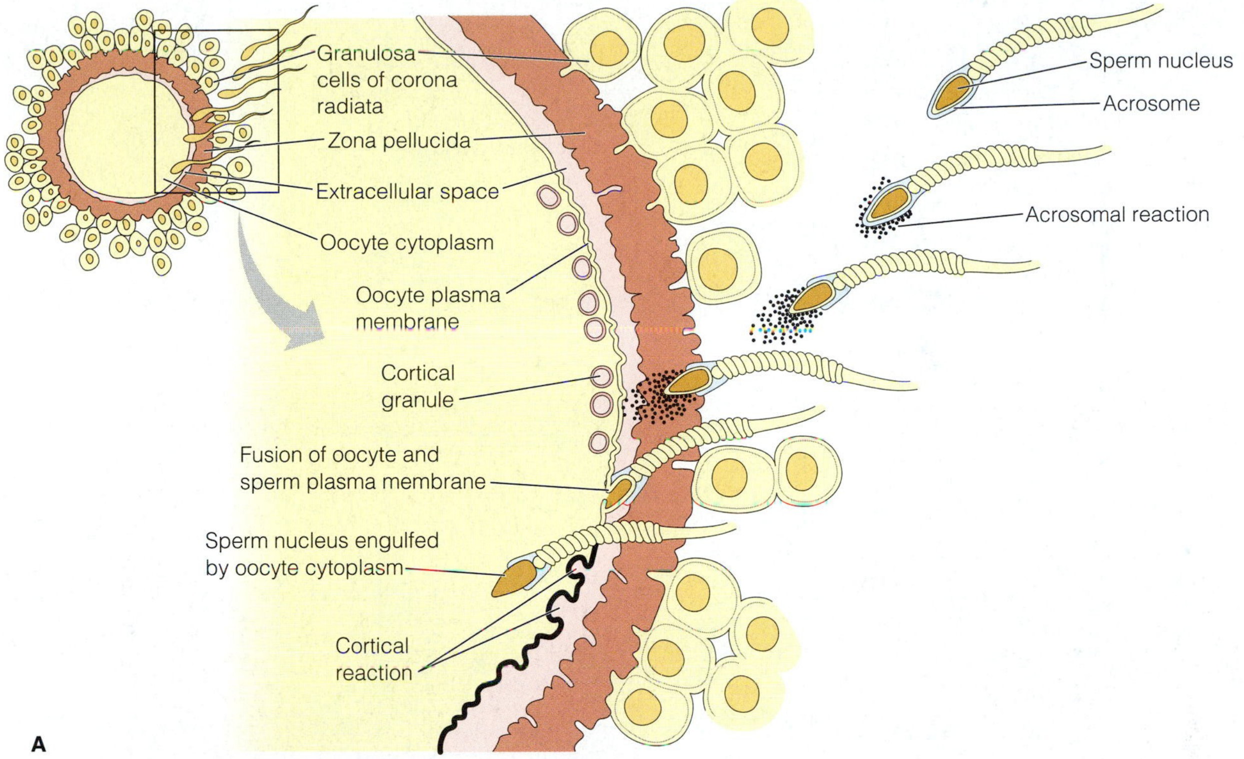

A

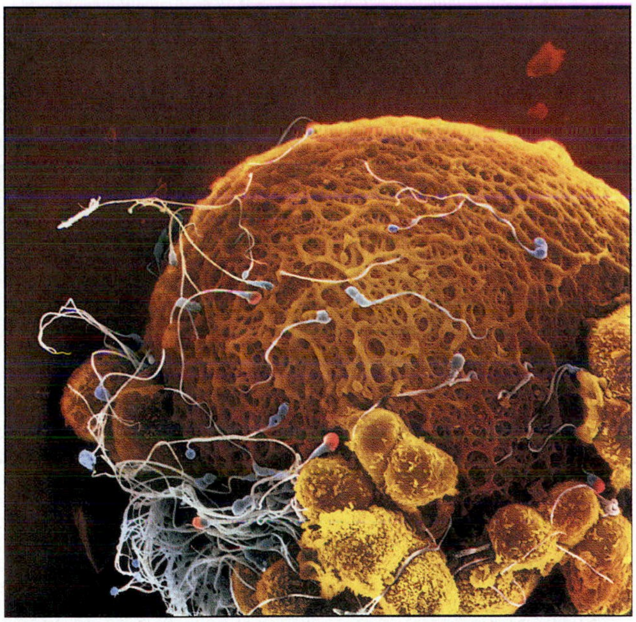

B

Figure 11–4 • Sperm penetration of an ovum. *A,* The sequential steps of oocyte penetration by a sperm are depicted moving from top to bottom. *B,* Scanning electron micrograph of human sperm surrounding a human oocyte (750×). The smaller spherical cells are granulosa cells of the corona radiata.
SOURCE: Scanning electron micrograph from Nilsson, L. (1990). *A child is born.* New York: Dell Publishing.

Twins

Twinning normally occurs in approximately 1 in 80 pregnancies, and triplets in 1 in 8000 pregnancies. Dizygotic twins have been reported to occur more often among black than among white women and more often among white individuals than among women of Asian origin (Chitkara & Berkowitz, 2002). Among all groups, as parity (having given birth to a viable infant) increases so does the chance for multiple births.

Twins may be either fraternal or identical (Figure 11–5 •). If they are fraternal, they are dizygotic, which means they arise from two separate ova fertilized by two separate spermatozoa. There are two placentas, two chorions, and two amnions; however, the placentas sometimes fuse and look as if they are one. Despite their birth relationship, fraternal twins are no more similar to each other than they would be to siblings born singly. They may be the same or different sex.

Dizygotic twinning increases with maternal age up to about 35 years and then decreases abruptly. The chance of dizygotic twins increases with parity, in conceptions that occur in the first 3 months of a relationship, and with increased coital frequency. The chance of dizygotic twinning decreases during periods of malnutrition and during winter and spring for women living in the northern hemisphere. Studies indicate that dizygotic twins tend to occur in certain families, perhaps because of genetic factors that result in elevated serum gonadotropin levels leading to double ovulation (Chitkara & Berkowitz, 2002).

Identical, or monozygotic, twins develop from a single fertilized ovum. They are of the same sex and have the same genotype (appearance). Identical twins usually have a

MediaLink
CARE PLAN: CLIENT FEARFUL OF MULTIPLE GESTATION

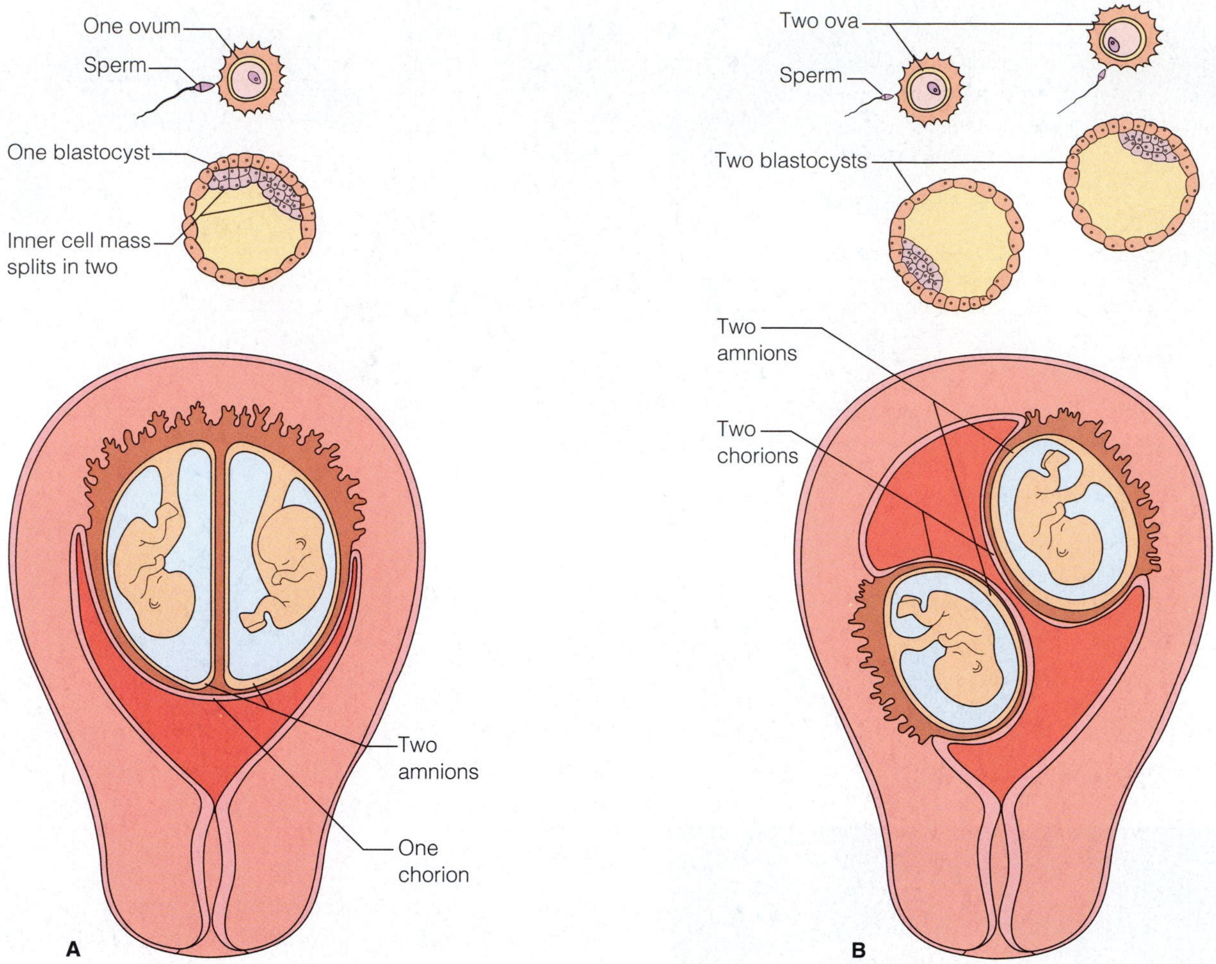

Figure 11–5 • *A,* Formation of identical twins. *B,* Formation of fraternal twins. (Note separate placentas).

common placenta (Figure 11–5). Monozygosity is not affected by environment, race, physical characteristics, or fertility. Monozygotic twins originate from division of the fertilized ovum at different stages of early development, after the zygote consists of thousands of cells.

Complete separation of the cellular mass into two parts is necessary for twin formation. The number of amnions and chorions present depends on the timing of the division.

- If division occurs within 3 days of fertilization (before the inner cell mass and chorion are formed), two embryos, two amnions, and two chorions will develop. This dichorionic-diamniotic situation occurs about 20% to 30% of the time, and there may be two distinct placentas or a single fused placenta.
- If division occurs about 5 days after fertilization (when the inner cell mass is formed and the chorion cells have differentiated but those of the amnion have not), two embryos develop with separate amnionic sacs. These sacs will eventually be covered by a common chorion; thus there will be a monochorionic-diamniotic placenta.
- If the amnion has already developed approximately 7 to 13 days after fertilization, division results in two embryos with a common amnionic sac and a common chorion. This type occurs about 1% of the time (Chitkara & Berkowitz, 2002).

Monozygotic twinning is considered a random event and occurs in approximately 4 per 1000 live births (Chitkara & Berkowitz, 2002). The survival rate of monozygotic twins as a group is 10% lower than that of dizygotic twins, and congenital anomalies are more prevalent. Both twins may have the same malformation.

Preembryonic Stage

The first 14 days of human development, starting on the day the ovum is fertilized (conception), are referred to as the preembryonic stage, or the stage of the ovum. Development after fertilization can be divided into two phases: cellular multiplication and cellular (embryonic membrane) differentiation. This stage is characterized by rapid cellular multiplication and differentiation and the establishment of the embryonic membranes and primary germ layers, discussed earlier. These phases and the process of implantation (nidation), which occurs between them, are discussed next.

Cellular Multiplication

Cellular multiplication begins as the zygote moves through the fallopian tube toward the cavity of the uterus. This transportation takes 3 days or more (Cunningham et al, 2001) and is accomplished mainly by a very weak fluid current in the fallopian tube resulting from the beating action of the ciliated epithelium that lines the tube.

The zygote now enters a period of rapid mitotic divisions called **cleavage,** during which it divides into two cells, four cells, eight cells, and so on. These cells, called *blastomeres,* are so small that the developing cell mass is only slightly larger than the original zygote. The blastomeres are held together by the zona pellucida, which is under the corona radiata. The blastomeres will eventually form a solid ball of 12 to 16 cells called the **morula.** As it enters the uterus, the intracellular fluid in the morula increases, and a central cavity forms within the cell mass.

The inner solid mass of cells is called the **blastocyst.** The outer layer of cells that surround the cavity and have replaced the zona pellucida is the **trophoblast.** Eventually, the trophoblast develops into one of the embryonic membranes, called the chorion. The blastocyst develops into a double layer of cells called the *embryonic disc,* from which the embryo will develop, and the other embryonic membrane, called the amnion. The journey of the fertilized ovum to its destination in the uterus is illustrated in Figure 11–6 •.

Implantation (Nidation)

While floating in the uterine cavity, the blastocyst is nourished by the uterine glands, which secrete a mixture of lipids, mucopolysaccharides, and glycogen. The trophoblast attaches itself to the surface of the endometrium for further nourishment. The most frequent site of attachment is the upper part of the posterior uterine wall (Figure 11–6). Between days 7 and 10 after fertilization, the zona pellucida disappears, and the blastocyst implants itself by burrowing into the uterine lining and penetrating down toward the maternal capillaries until it is completely covered (Ahokas & McKinney, 2000). The lining of the uterus thickens below the implanted blastocyst, and the cells of the trophoblast grow down into the thickened lining, forming processes called *villi.*

Under the influence of progesterone, the endometrium increases in thickness and vascularity in preparation for implantation and nourishment of the ovum. After implantation, the endometrium is called the decidua. The portion of the decidua that covers the blastocyst is called the **decidua capsularis;** the portion directly under the implanted blastocyst is the **decidua basalis;** and the portion that lines the rest of the uterine cavity is the **decidua vera (parietalis)** (Figure 11–6, inset) (Ahokas & McKinney, 2000). The maternal part of the placenta develops from the decidua basalis, which contains large numbers of blood vessels. The chorionic villi (described later) in contact with the decidua basalis will form the fetal portion of the placenta.

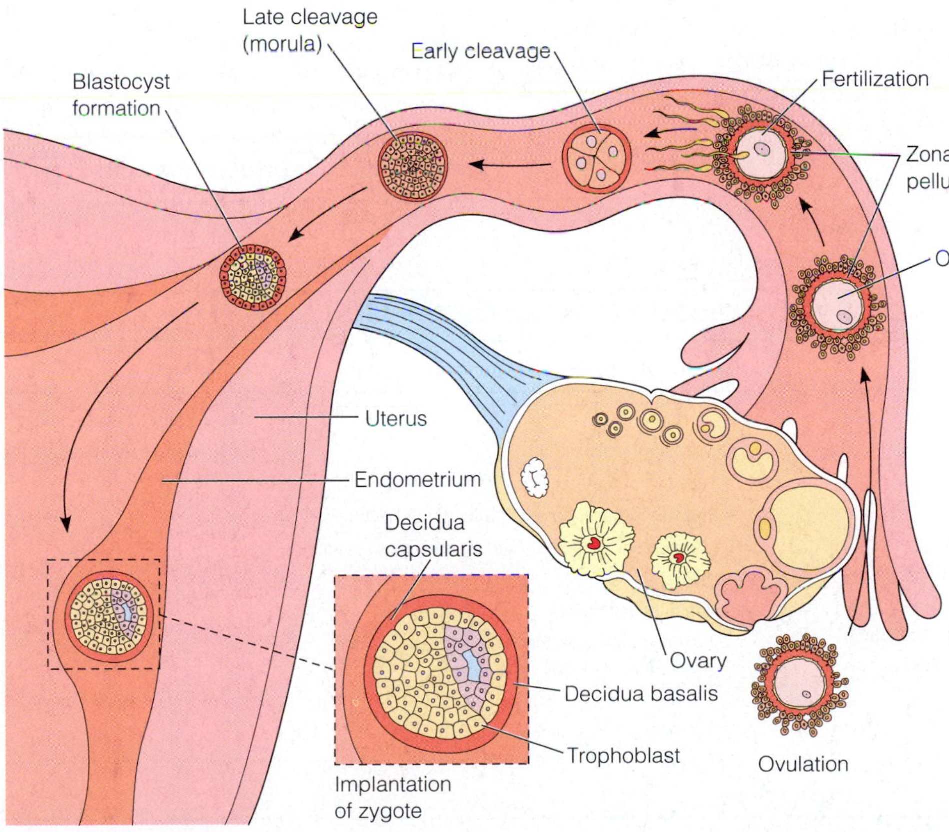

Figure 11–6 • During ovulation, the ovum leaves the ovary and enters the fallopian tube. Fertilization generally occurs in the outer third of the fallopian tube. Subsequent changes in the fertilized ovum from conception to implantation are depicted.

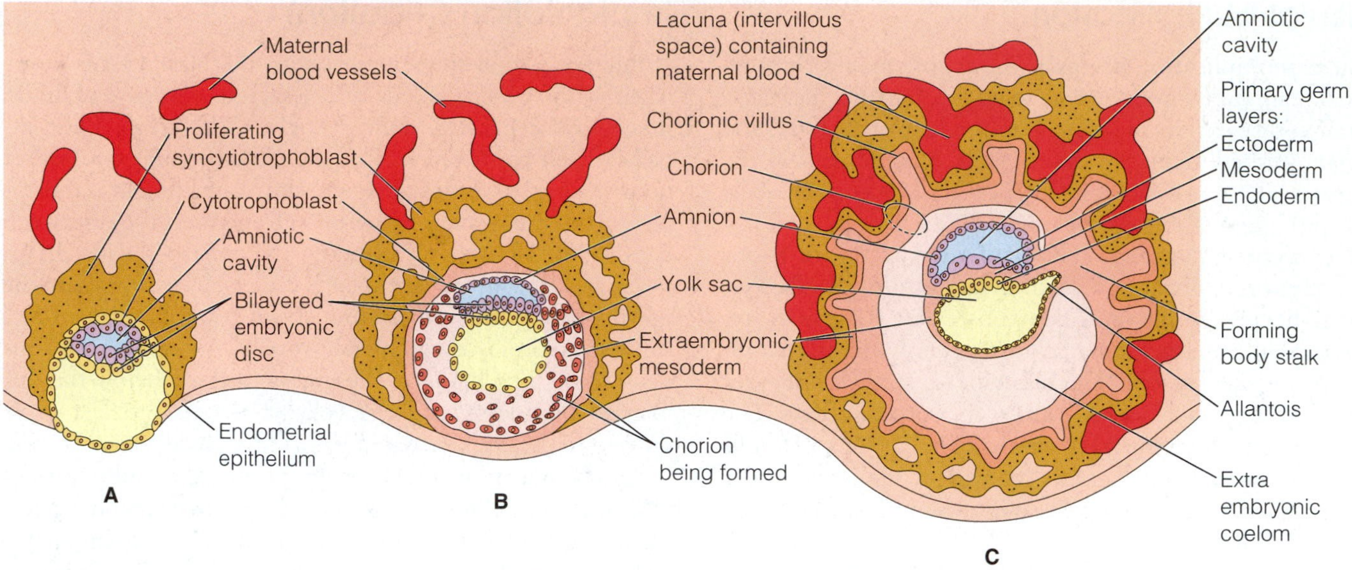

Figure 11–7 • Formation of primary germ layers. *A,* Implantation of a 71/2-day blastocyst in which the cells of the embryonic disc are separated from the amnion by a fluid-filled space. The erosion of the endometrium by the syncytiotrophoblast is ongoing. *B,* Implantation is completed by day 9, and extraembryonic mesoderm is beginning to form a discrete layer beneath the cytotrophoblast. *C,* By day 16, the embryo shows all three germ layers, a yolk sac, and an allantois (an outpouching of the yolk sac that forms the structural basis of the body stalk, or umbilical cord). The cytotrophoblast and associated mesoderm has become the chorion, and chorionic villi are developing.

Cellular Differentiation

PRIMARY GERM LAYERS

About 10 to 14 days after conception, the homogenous mass of blastocyst cells differentiates into the primary germ layers. These layers, the **ectoderm, mesoderm,** and **endoderm** (Figure 11–7 •), are formed at the same time as the embryonic membranes. All tissues, organs, and organ systems will develop from these primary germ cell layers (Table 11–1 • and Figure 11–8 •).

EMBRYONIC MEMBRANES

The **embryonic membranes** begin to form at the time of implantation (Figure 11–9 •). These membranes protect and support the embryo as it grows and develops inside the uterus. The first membrane to form is the **chorion,** the outermost embryonic membrane that encircles the amnion, embryo, and yolk sac. The chorion is a thick membrane that develops from the trophoblast and has many fingerlike projections, called *chorionic villi,* on its surface. These chorionic villi can be used for early genetic

Table 11–1 • DERIVATION OF BODY STRUCTURES FROM PRIMARY CELL LAYERS

Ectoderm	Mesoderm	Endoderm
Epidermis	Dermis	Respiratory tract epithelium
Sweat glands	Wall of digestive tract	Epithelium (except nasal), including pharynx, tongue, tonsils, thyroid, parathyroid, thymus, tympanic cavity
Sebaceous glands	Kidneys and ureter (suprarenal cortex)	Lining of digestive tract
Nails	Reproductive organs (gonads, genital ducts)	Primary tissue of liver and pancreas
Hair follicles	Connective tissue (cartilage, bone, joint cavities)	Urethra and associated glands
Lens of eye	Skeleton	Urinary bladder (except trigone)
Sensory epithelium of internal and external ear, nasal cavity, sinuses, mouth, anal canal	Muscles (all types)	Vagina (parts)
Central and peripheral nervous systems	Cardiovascular system (heart, arteries, veins, blood, bone marrow)	
Nasal cavity	Pleura	
Oral glands and tooth enamel	Lymphatic tissue and cells	
Pituitary gland	Spleen	
Mammary glands		

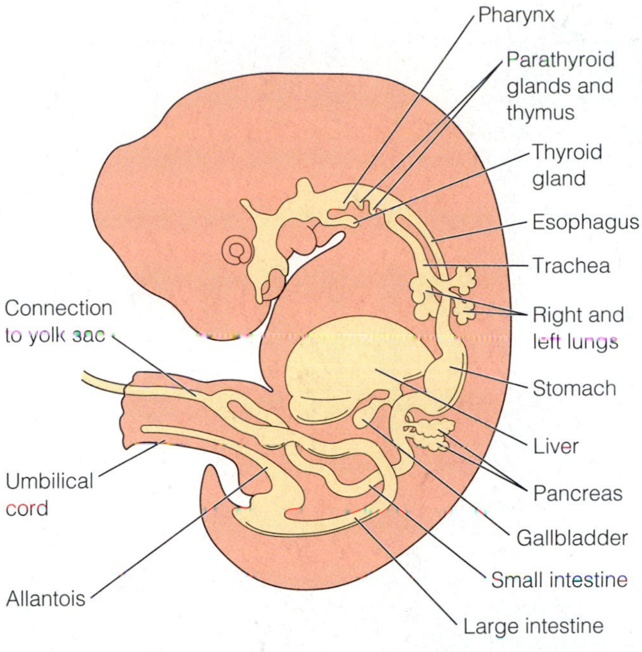

Figure 11–8 • Endoderm differentiates to form the epithelial lining of the digestive and respiratory tracts and associated glands.

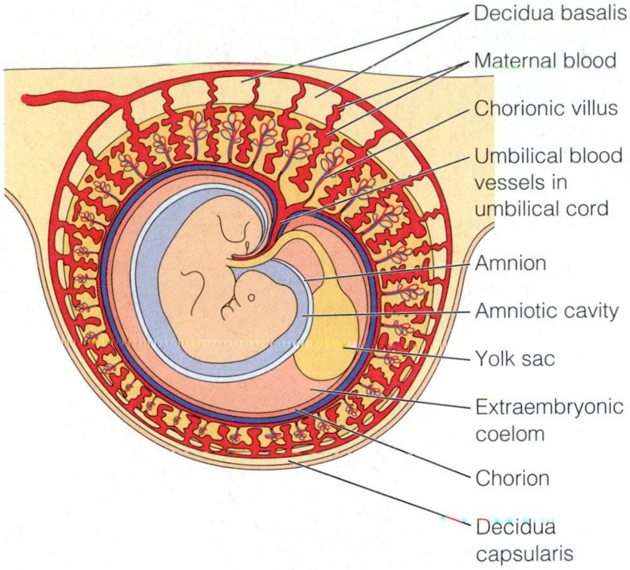

Figure 11–9 • Early development of primary embryonic membranes. At 4 1/2 weeks, the decidua capsularis (placental portion enclosing the embryo on the uterine surface) and decidua basalis (placental portion encompassing the elaborate chorionic villi and maternal endometrium) are well formed. The chorionic villi lie in blood-filled intervillous spaces within the endometrium. The amnion and yolk sac are well developed.

testing of the embryo at 8 to 10 weeks' gestation by chorionic villi sampling (see Chapter 21). As the pregnancy progresses, the villi begin to degenerate, except for those just under the embryo, which grow and branch into depressions in the uterine wall, forming the fetal portion of the placenta. By the fourth month of pregnancy, the surface of the chorion is smooth except at the place of attachment to the uterine wall.

The second membrane, the **amnion,** originates from the ectoderm, a primary germ layer, during the early stages of embryonic development. The amnion is a thin protective membrane that contains amniotic fluid. The space between the amniotic membrane and the embryo is the *amniotic cavity.* This cavity surrounds the embryo and yolk sac, except where the developing embryo (germ layer disc) attaches to the trophoblast via the umbilical cord. As the embryo grows, the amnion expands until it comes in contact with the chorion. These two slightly adherent membranes form the fluid-filled amniotic sac, also called **bag of waters (BOW),** which protects the floating embryo.

AMNIOTIC FLUID

Amniotic fluid functions as a cushion to protect against injury. It also helps control the embryo's temperature, permits symmetric external growth of the embryo, prevents adherence to the amnion, and allows freedom of movement so that the embryo-fetus can change position freely, thus aiding in musculoskeletal development.

The amount of amniotic fluid is about 30 mL at 10 weeks and increases to 350 mL at 20 weeks. After 20 weeks the volume ranges from 700 to 1000 mL . The amniotic fluid volume is constantly changing as the fluid moves back and forth across the placental membrane. As the pregnancy continues, the fetus contributes to the volume of amniotic fluid by excreting urine. The fetus also swallows up to 600 mL of the fluid every 24 hours. Approximately 400 mL of amniotic fluid flows out of the fetal lungs each day (Gilbert & Brace, 1993). Amniotic fluid is slightly alkaline and contains albumin, urea, uric acid, creatinine, lecithin, sphingomyelin, bilirubin, fat, fructose, leukocytes, proteins, epithelial cells, enzymes, and fine hair called **lanugo.** Abnormal variations in amniotic fluid volume are *oligohydramnios* (less than 400 mL of amniotic fluid) and *hydramnios* (more than 2000 mL or amniotic fluid index greater than 97.5 percentile for the corresponding gestational age). Hydramnios is also called *polyhydramnios.* Chapter 27 discusses alterations in amniotic fluid volume . Water and solutes must pass between the amniotic fluid and fetus. Figure 11–10 • summarizes the major pathways of exchange.

Early in the first trimester of pregnancy, amniotic fluid is iso-osmolar with fetal and maternal plasma and is secreted from the developing trophoblast or embryo. Water and solutes move freely across the fetal skin before the time of skin keratinization. After 23 to 25 weeks, thickening of the fetal skin inhibits this diffusion. During the rest of the pregnancy, the fetal kidneys are the major source of fluid

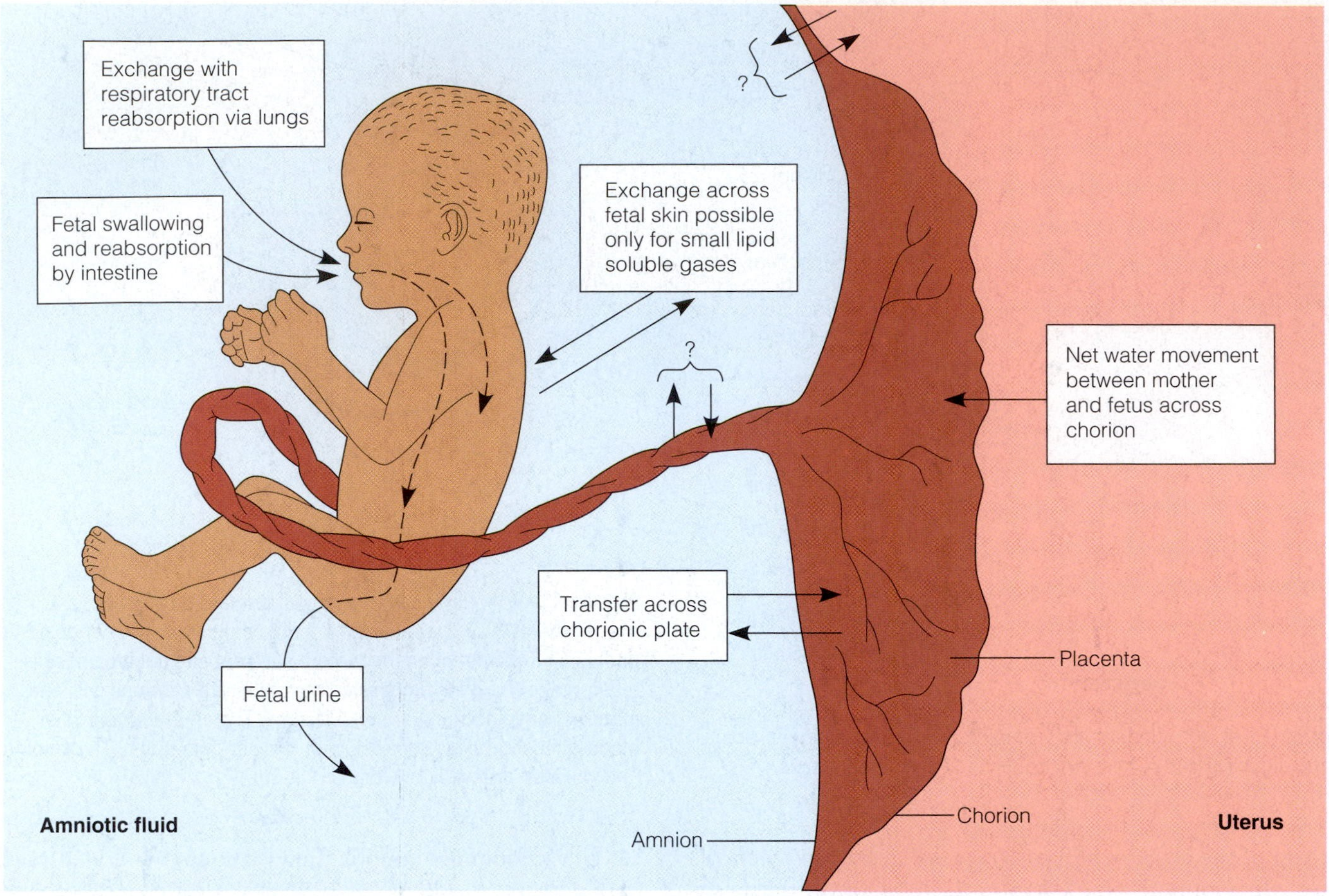

Figure 11–10 • Summary of the significant pathways of water and solute exchange between the amniotic fluid and fetus.
SOURCE: Seeds, A. E. (1980, November). Current concepts of amniotic fluid dynamics. *American Journal of Obstetrics and Gynecology, 138,* 575.

that enters the amniotic sac. Abnormalities of fetal urine production can result in changes in amniotic fluid volume. For example, with obstruction of urine outflow, as in Potter's syndrome, oligohydramnios develops. Conversely, Bartter's syndrome results in a fetal diuresis and hydramnios. The fetal lungs are also significant contributors to amniotic fluid. Fetal breathing movements are associated with the bidirectional flow of fluid through the trachea. Net outflow from the fetal lungs averages 4.3 mL/kg/hr or 10% of body weight per day (Gilbert & Brace, 1993). This outflow of lung and tracheal fluid is used as the basis for amniotic fluid tests of fetal lung maturity.

The major mechanism by which amniotic fluid is removed in the last half of the pregnancy is fetal swallowing, which occurs mostly during periods of fetal breathing movements. In pregnancy when the fetus does not swallow normal amounts of amniotic fluid (as in esophageal atresia and anencephalus), hydramnios will result. A potential route of amniotic fluid removal is by the transmembranous pathway, that is, the movement of fluid across the amniochorion and into the maternal circulation within the uterine wall. Another major regulator of amniotic fluid volume and composition is the intramembranous pathway. This pathway causes amniotic water and/or solutes to be absorbed by the fetal blood that perfuses the fetal surface of the placenta (Gilbert & Brace, 1993).

YOLK SAC

In humans the yolk sac is small and functions only in early embryonic life. It develops as a second cavity in the blastocyst, about day 8 or 9 after conception, and forms primitive red blood cells during the first 6 weeks of development until the embryo's liver takes over the process. As the embryo develops, the yolk sac is incorporated in the umbilical cord, where it can be identified as a degenerate structure after birth.

UMBILICAL CORD

As the placenta is developing, the **umbilical cord** is also being formed from the amnion. The *body stalk,* which attaches the embryo to the yolk sac, contains blood vessels that extend into the chorionic villi. The body stalk fuses with the embryonic portion of the placenta to provide a circulatory pathway from the chorionic villi to the embryo (Figure 11–10). As the body stalk elongates to become the umbilical cord, the vessels in the cord decrease to one large vein and two smaller arteries. About 1% of umbilical cords have only two vessels, an artery and a vein; this condition may be associated with congenital malformations, primarily of the cardiac and gastrointestinal systems. A specialized connective tissue known as **Wharton's jelly** surrounds the blood vessels in the umbilical cord. This tissue, plus the high blood volume pulsating through the vessels, prevents compression of the umbilical cord in utero. The umbilical cord does not have any sensory or motor innervation, so the cutting of the cord after birth is not painful. At term, the average cord is 2 cm (0.8 in) across and about 55 cm (22 in) long. The cord can attach itself to the placenta at various sites. Central insertion into the placenta is considered normal. (Chapter 26 discusses the various attachment sites.)

Umbilical cords appear twisted or spiraled. This is most likely caused by fetal movement (Benirschke, 1999). A true knot in the umbilical cord rarely occurs; if it does, the cord is usually long. More common are so-called false knots caused by the folding of cord vessels. A nuchal cord exists when the umbilical cord encircles the fetal neck.

Development and Functions of the Placenta

The **placenta** is the means of metabolic and nutrient exchange between the embryonic and maternal circulations. Placental development and circulation does not begin until the third week of embryonic development. The placenta develops at the site where the developing embryo attaches to the uterine wall. Expansion of the placenta continues until about 20 weeks, when it covers about half the inside of the uterus. After 20 weeks' gestation, the placenta becomes thicker but not wider. At 40 weeks' gestation, the placenta is about 15 to 20 cm (5.9 to 7.9 in) in diameter and 2.5 to 3.0 cm (1.0 to 1.2 in) in thickness. At that time, it weighs approximately 400 to 600 g (14 to 21 oz).

The placenta has two parts: the maternal portion and the fetal portion. The maternal portion consists of the decidua basalis and its circulation. Its surface is red and fleshlike. The fetal portion consists of the chorionic villi and their circulation. The fetal surface of the placenta is covered by the amnion, which gives it a shiny, gray appearance (Figures 11–11 • and 11–12 •).

MediaLink Animation: Formation of Placenta

Development of the placenta begins with the chorionic villi. The trophoblast cells of the chorionic villi form spaces in the tissue of the decidua basalis. These spaces fill with maternal blood, and the chorionic villi grow into these spaces. As the chorionic villi differentiate, two trophoblastic layers appear: an outer layer called the syncytium (consisting of syncytiotrophoblasts), and an inner layer known as the *cytotrophoblast* (Figure 11–13 •). The cytotrophoblast thins out and disappears about the fifth month, leaving only a single layer of syncytium covering the chorionic villi. The syncytium is in direct contact with the maternal blood in the intervillous spaces. It is the functional layer of the placenta and secretes the placental hormones of pregnancy.

A third, inner layer of connective mesoderm develops in the chorionic villi, forming *anchoring villi.* These anchoring villi eventually form the *septa* (partitions) of the placenta. These septa divide the mature placenta into 15 to 20 segments called **cotyledons** (subdivisions of the placenta made up of anchoring villi and decidual tissue). In each cotyledon, the *branching villi* form a highly complex vascular system that allows compartmentalization of the uteroplacental circulation. The exchange of gases and nutrients takes place across these vascular systems.

Exchange of substances across the placenta is minimal during the first 3 to 5 months of development because of limited permeability. The villous membrane is initially too thick. As the villous membrane thins, the placental permeability increases until about the last month of pregnancy, when permeability begins to decrease as the placenta ages. In

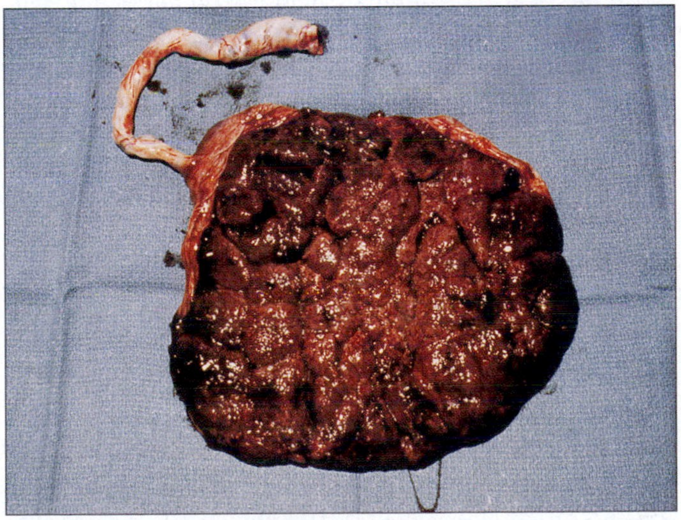

Figure 11–11 • Maternal side of placenta.

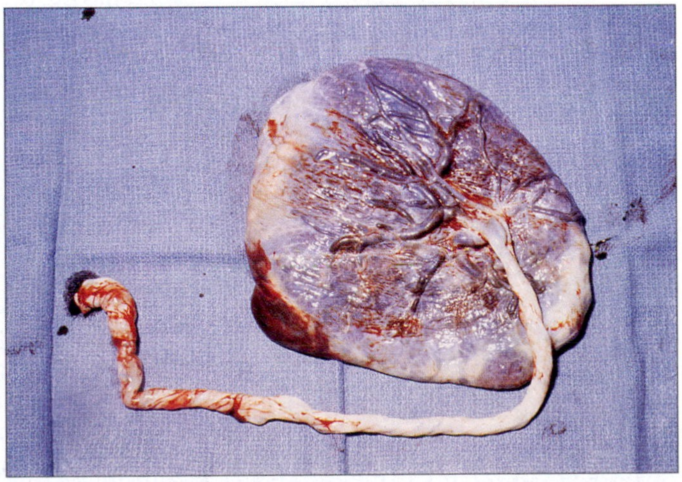

Figure 11–12 • Fetal side of placenta.

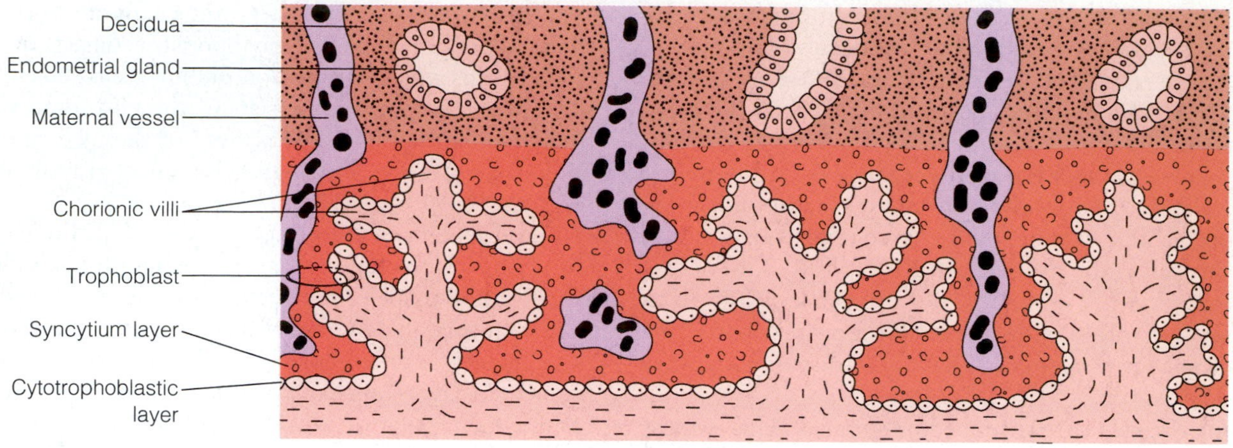

Figure 11–13 • Longitudinal section of placental villus. Spaces formed in the maternal decidua are filled with maternal blood; chorionic villi proliferate into these maternal blood-filled spaces and differentiate into a syncytium layer and a cytotrophoblast layer.

the fully developed placenta, fetal blood in the villi and maternal blood in the intervillous spaces are separated by three to four thin layers of tissue.

Placental Circulation

After implantation of the blastocyst, the cells differentiate into fetal cells and trophoblastic cells. The proliferating trophoblast successfully invades the decidua basalis of the endometrium, first opening the uterine capillaries and later opening the larger uterine vessels. The chorionic villi are an outgrowth of the blastocystic tissue. As these villi continue to grow and divide, the fetal vessels begin to form. The intervillous spaces in the decidua basalis develop as the endometrial spiral arteries are opened.

By the fourth week the placenta has begun to function as a means of metabolic exchange between embryo and mother. The completion of the maternal-placental-fetal circulation occurs about 17 days after conception, when the embryonic heart begins functioning (Benirschke, 1999).

By 14 weeks the placenta is a discrete organ. It has grown in thickness as a result of growth in the length and size of the chorionic villi and accompanying expansion of the intervillous space.

The *cotyledons* of the maternal surface contain branches of a single placental mainstream villus, allowing for some compartmentalization of the uteroplacental circulation. Each cotyledon is a vascular unit containing branching vessels that are distributed throughout a particular lobule and partially separated from other lobules by the cotyledon's thin septal partitions.

The capillaries of the villi are lined with an extremely thin endothelium and are surrounded by a layer of mesenchymal (connective) tissue. This connective tissue is covered by chorionic epithelium consisting of cytotrophoblast and syncytiotrophoblast (Figure 11–13). As previously discussed, the cytotrophoblast thins out and disappears after the fifth month.

In the fully developed placenta's umbilical cord, fetal blood flows through the two umbilical arteries to the capillaries of the villi, and oxygen-enriched blood flows back through the umbilical vein to the fetus (Figure 11–14 •). Late in pregnancy, a soft blowing sound (*funic souffle*) can be heard over the area of the umbilical cord of the fetus. The sound is synchronous with the fetal heartbeat and the flow of fetal blood through the umbilical arteries.

Maternal blood, rich in oxygen and nutrients, spurts from the spiral uterine arteries into the intervillous spaces. These spurts are produced by the maternal blood pressure. The spurt of blood is directed toward the chorionic plate, and as the blood flow loses pressure, it becomes lateral (spreads out). Fresh blood continually enters and exerts pressure on the contents of the intervillous spaces, pushing blood toward the exits in the basal plate. Blood is then drained through the uterine and other pelvic veins. A *uterine souffle* is also heard in the later months of pregnancy. This uterine souffle, which is timed precisely with the mother's pulse and heard just above the mother's symphysis pubis, is caused by the augmented blood flow entering the dilated uterine arteries.

Circulation within the intervillous spaces depends on maternal blood pressure producing a gradient between arterial and venous channels. The lumen of the spiral uterine artery is narrow when it pierces the chorionic plate and enters the intervillous space, resulting in an increased blood pressure. The pressure in the arteries forces the blood into the intervillous spaces and bathes the numerous small villi in oxygenated blood. As the pressure decreases, the blood flows back from the chorionic plate toward the decidua, where it enters the endometrial veins.

Braxton Hicks contractions (Chapter 14) are believed to facilitate placental circulation by enhancing the movement of blood from the center of the cotyledon through the intervillous space. Placental blood flow is thought to be enhanced when the woman is lying on her left side because the vena cava is not compromised. Some evidence exists that lying on either side can enhance blood flow.

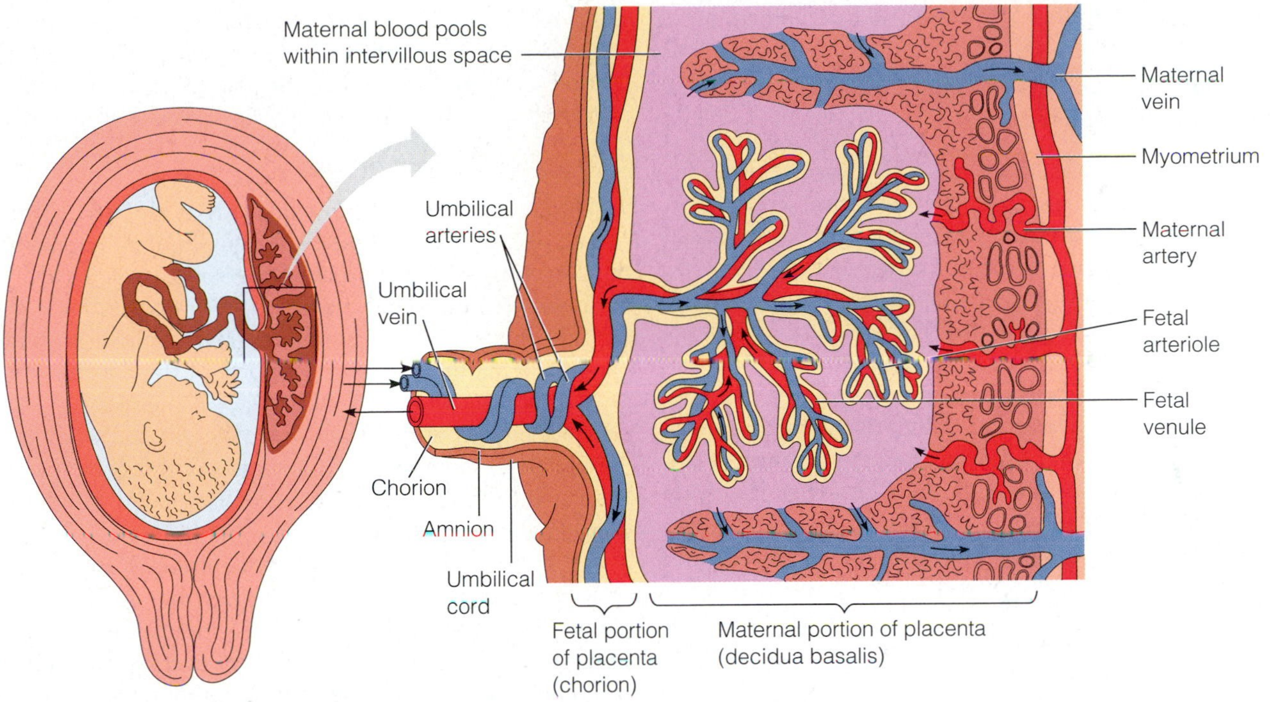

Figure 11–14 • Vascular arrangement of the placenta. Arrows indicate the direction of blood flow. Maternal blood flows through the uterine arteries to the intervillous spaces of the placenta and returns through the uterine veins to maternal circulation. Fetal blood flows through the umbilical arteries into the villous capillaries of the placenta and returns through the umbilical vein to the fetal circulation.

Placental Functions

Placental exchange functions occur only in those fetal vessels that are in intimate contact with the covering syncytial membrane. The syncytium villi have brush borders containing many microvilli, which greatly increase the exchange rate between maternal and fetal circulation (Sadler, 2000).

The placental functions, many of which begin soon after implantation, include fetal respiration, nutrition, and excretion. To carry out these functions, the placenta is involved in metabolic and transfer activities. It also has endocrine functions and special immunologic properties.

METABOLIC ACTIVITIES

The placenta produces glycogen, cholesterol, and fatty acids continuously for fetal use and hormone production. The placenta also produces numerous enzymes required for fetoplacental transfer, and it breaks down certain substances, such as epinephrine and histamine. In addition it stores glycogen and iron.

TRANSPORT FUNCTIONS

The placental membranes actively control the transfer of a wide range of substances by five major mechanisms:

1. *Simple diffusion* moves substances from an area of higher concentration to an area of lower concentration. Substances that move across the placenta by simple diffusion include water, oxygen, carbon dioxide, electrolytes (sodium and chloride), anesthetic gases, and drugs. Insulin and steroid hormones originating from the adrenal glands and thyroid hormones also cross the placenta, but at a very slow rate. The rate of oxygen transfer across the placental membrane is greater than that allowed by simple diffusion, indicating that oxygen is also transferred by facilitated diffusion of some type. Unfortunately many substances of abuse, such as cocaine, cross the placenta via diffusion.
2. *Facilitated transport* involves a carrier system to move molecules from an area of greater concentration to an area of lower concentration. Molecules such as glucose, galactose, and some oxygen are transported by this method. The glucose level in the fetal blood ordinarily is approximately 20% to 30% lower than the glucose level in the maternal blood because glucose is being metabolized rapidly by the fetus. This in turn causes rapid transport of additional glucose from the maternal blood into the fetal blood.
3. *Active transport* can work against a concentration gradient, allowing molecules to move from areas of lower concentration to areas of higher concentration. Amino acids, calcium, iron, iodine, water-soluble vitamins, and glucose are transferred across the placenta this way. The measured amino acid content of fetal blood is greater than that of maternal blood, and calcium and inorganic phosphate occur in greater concentration in fetal blood than in maternal blood (Blackburn, 2003).
4. *Pinocytosis* is important for transferring large molecules, such as albumin and gamma globulin.

Materials are engulfed by amoeba-like cells forming plasma droplets.

5. *Hydrostatic and osmotic pressures* allow the bulk flow of water and some solutes.

Other modes of transfer exist as well. For example, fetal red blood cells pass into the maternal circulation through breaks in the placental membrane, particularly during labor and birth. Certain cells, such as maternal leukocytes, and microorganisms, such as viruses (eg, the human immunodeficiency virus [HIV], which causes acquired immunodeficiency syndrome [AIDS]) and the bacterium *Treponema pallidum* which causes syphilis, can also cross the placental membrane under their own power (Moore et al, 2000). Some bacteria and protozoa infect the placenta by causing lesions and then entering the fetal blood system.

Several factors, including the following, affect transfer rate:

- Molecular size
- Electrical charge
- Lipid solubility
- Placental area
- Diffusion distance
- Maternal-placental-fetal blood flow
- Blood saturation with gases and nutrients
- pK_a of the substance
- Maternal-placental-fetal metabolism of the substance

Substances that have a molecular weight of 1000 daltons or more have difficulty crossing the placenta by simple diffusion. Therefore, heparin, with a molecular weight above 6000, does not cross the placenta, but warfarin sodium (Coumadin), which has a molecular weight in the 300 to 400 range, crosses easily. Electrically charged molecules cross the placenta more slowly. An example is the muscle relaxant succinylcholine. A lipid-soluble substance moves quickly across the placenta into the fetal circulation.

Reduction of the placental surface area, as with abruptio placentae (partial or complete premature separation of a normally implanted placenta), will lessen the area that is functional for exchange. Placental diffusion distance also affects exchange. In conditions such as diabetes and placental infection, edema of the villi increases the diffusion distance, thus increasing the distance the substance has to be transferred.

Changes in blood flow between the fetus and the maternal intervillous space can be influenced by the transfer rate of substances, the ratio of blood on each side of the placenta, and the binding and dissociation abilities of carrier molecules in the blood. Decreased intervillous space blood flow is seen during labor and with certain maternal disease conditions such as hypertension. Mild fetal hypoxia increases the umbilical blood flow, but severe hypoxia results in decreased blood flow.

As the maternal blood picks up fetal waste products and carbon dioxide, it drains back into the maternal circulation through the veins in the basal plate. Fetal blood is hypoxic by comparison; it therefore attracts oxygen from the mother's blood. Affinity for oxygen also increases as the fetal blood gives up its carbon dioxide, which decreases its acidity.

ENDOCRINE FUNCTIONS

The placenta produces hormones that are vital to the survival of the fetus. These include human chorionic gonadotropin (hCG); human placental lactogen (hPL); and two steroid hormones, estrogen and progesterone.

The hormone hCG is similar to luteinizing hormone (LH) and prevents the normal involution of the corpus luteum at the end of the menstrual cycle (see Chapter 10). If the corpus luteum stops functioning before the 11th week of pregnancy, spontaneous abortion occurs. The hCG also causes the corpus luteum to secrete increased amounts of estrogen and progesterone.

After the 11th week, the placenta produces enough progesterone and estrogen to maintain pregnancy. In the male fetus, hCG also exerts an interstitial cell–stimulating effect on the testes, resulting in the production of testosterone. This small secretion of testosterone during embryonic development causes male sex organs to grow. Human chorionic gonadotropin may play a role in the trophoblast's immunologic capabilities (ability to exempt the placenta and embryo from rejection by the mother's system). This hormone is used as a basis for pregnancy tests (for discussion of pregnancy tests, see Chapter 14).

Human chorionic gonadotropin is present in maternal blood serum 8 to 10 days after fertilization, just as soon as implantation has occurred, and is detectable in maternal urine at the time of the missed menses. Chorionic gonadotropin reaches its maximum level at 50 to 70 days' gestation and then begins to decrease as placental hormone production increases.

Progesterone is a hormone essential for pregnancy. It increases the secretions of the fallopian tubes and uterus to provide appropriate nutritive matter for the developing morula and blastocyst. It also appears to aid in ovum transport through the fallopian tube (Ahokas & McKinney, 2000). Progesterone causes decidual cells to develop in the uterine endometrium, and it must be present in high levels for implantation to occur. Progesterone also decreases the contractility of the uterus, thus preventing uterine contractions from causing spontaneous abortion.

Prior to hCG stimulation, the production of progesterone by the corpus luteum reaches a peak about 7 to 10 days after ovulation. Implantation occurs at about the same time as this peak. At 16 days after ovulation, the production of progesterone reaches a level between 25 and 50 mg per day and continues to rise slowly in subsequent weeks (Cunningham et al, 2001). After 10 weeks, the placenta (specifically, the syncytiotrophoblast) takes over the production of progesterone and secretes it in tremendous quantities, reaching levels of more than 250 mg per day late in pregnancy.

By 7 weeks, the placenta produces more than 50% of the estrogens in the maternal circulation. Estrogens serve mainly a proliferative function, causing enlargement of the uterus, breasts, and breast glandular tissue. Estrogens also have a significant role in increasing vascularity and vasodilation, particularly in the villous capillaries, near the end of pregnancy. Placental estrogens increase markedly toward the end of pregnancy, to as much as 30 times the daily production in the middle of a normal monthly menstrual cycle. The primary estrogen secreted by the placenta is different from that secreted by the ovaries. The placenta secretes mainly estriol, whereas the ovaries secrete primarily estradiol. The placenta by itself cannot synthesize estriol. Essential precursors are provided by the adrenal glands of the fetus and are transported to the placenta for the final conversion to estriol.

The hormone hPL (human placental lactogen; sometimes referred to as human chorionic somatomammotropin, or hCS) is similar to human pituitary growth hormone; hPL stimulates certain changes in the mother's metabolic processes. These changes ensure that more protein, glucose, and minerals are available for the fetus. Secretion of hPL can be detected by about 4 weeks. New placental proteins have been identified that may have clinical uses. These include SP 1 (Schwangerschaft's protein), PP 5 (placental protein 5), and others.

IMMUNOLOGIC PROPERTIES

The placenta and embryo are transplants of living tissue within the same species and are therefore considered homografts. Unlike other homografts, the placenta and embryo appear exempt from immunologic reaction by the host. One theory used to explain this phenomenon suggests that trophoblastic tissue is immunologically inert. It may contain a cell coating that masks transplantation antigens, repels sensitized lymphocytes, and protects against antibody formation. The most recent data suggest that there is a suppression of cellular immunity by the placental hormones (progesterone and hCG) during pregnancy.

Development of the Fetal Circulatory System

The circulatory system of the fetus has several unique features that, by maintaining the blood flow to the placenta, provide the fetus with oxygen and nutrients while removing carbon dioxide and other waste products.

Most of the blood supply bypasses the fetal lungs because they do not carry out respiratory gas exchange. The placenta assumes the function of the fetal lungs by supplying oxygen and allowing the fetus to excrete carbon dioxide into the maternal bloodstream. Figure 11–15 • shows the fetal circulatory system. The blood from the placenta flows through the umbilical vein, which enters the abdominal wall of the fetus at the site that, after birth, is the umbilicus (belly button). It divides into two branches, one of which circulates a small amount of blood through the fetal liver and empties into the inferior vena cava through the hepatic vein. The second and larger branch, called the **ductus venosus,** empties directly into the fetal vena cava. This blood then enters the right atrium, passes through the **foramen ovale** into the left atrium, and pours into the left ventricle, which pumps it into the aorta. Some blood returning from the head and upper extremities by way of the superior vena cava is emptied into the right atrium and passes through the tricuspid valve into the right ventricle. This blood is pumped into the pulmonary artery, and a small amount passes to the lungs and provides nourishment only. The larger portion of blood passes from the pulmonary artery through the **ductus arteriosus** into the descending aorta, bypassing the lungs. Finally, blood returns to the placenta through the two umbilical arteries, and the process is repeated.

The fetus receives oxygen via diffusion from the maternal circulation because of the gradient difference of PO_2 of 50 mm Hg in maternal blood in the placenta to a 30 mm Hg PO_2 in the fetus. At term the fetus receives oxygen from the mother's circulation at a rate of 20 to 30 mL/min (Sadler, 2000). Fetal hemoglobin facilitates obtaining oxygen from the maternal circulation because it carries as much as 20% to 30% more oxygen than adult hemoglobin. For further discussion, see Chapter 28.

Fetal circulation delivers the highest available oxygen concentration to the head, neck, brain, and heart (coronary circulation) and a lesser amount of oxygenated blood to the abdominal organs and the lower body. This circulatory pattern leads to cephalocaudal (head-to-tail) development in the fetus.

MEDIALINK
ANIMATION: EMBRYONIC HEART FORMATION AND CIRCULATION

Fetal Heart

The heart of the fetus, as in the adult, is under the control of its own pacemaker. The sinoatrial (SA) node sets the rate and is supplied by the vagus nerve. Bridging the atrium and the ventricle is the atrioventricular (AV) node, also supplied by the vagus nerve. Baseline changes in the fetal heartbeat have been shown to be under the influence of this nerve. Atropine will block this effect.

When the fetus is stressed, the sympathetic nervous system causes the release of norepinephrine, which increases the fetal heart rate. To counteract the increase in blood pressure, baroreceptors, which respond to stretch, are present in the vessel walls at the junction of the internal and external carotid arteries. When stimulated, these receptors, under the influence of the vagus and glossopharyngeal nerves, cause the heart rate to slow.

Chemoreceptors in the fetal peripheral and central nervous systems respond to decreased oxygen tensions and to increased carbon dioxide tensions, leading to fetal tachycardia and an increase in blood pressure. The central nervous system (CNS) also has control over heart rate. Increased activity of the fetus in a wakeful period is exhibited in an *increase in the beat-to-beat variability* of the fetal heart baseline. Sleep patterns demonstrate a *decrease in the beat-to-beat baseline variability.* In cases of severe hypoxia, increased levels of epinephrine and norepinephrine act on the fetal heart to produce a faster and stronger rate.

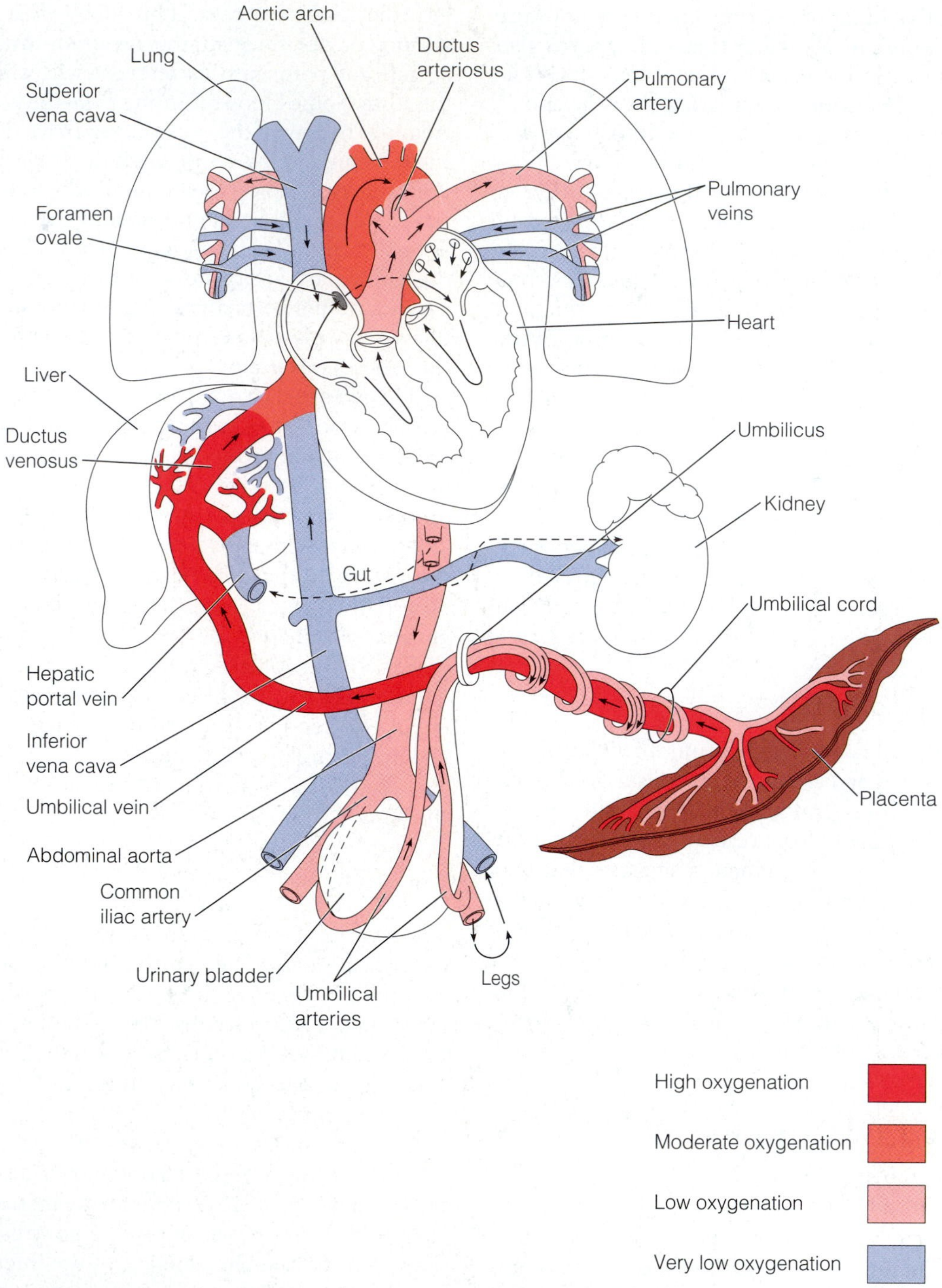

Figure 11–15 • Fetal circulation. Blood leaves the placenta and enters the fetus through the umbilical vein. After circulating through the fetus, the blood returns to the placenta through the umbilical arteries. The ductus venosus, the foramen ovale, and the ductus arteriosus allow the blood to bypass the fetal liver and lungs.

Embryonic and Fetal Development

Pregnancy is calculated to last an average of 10 lunar months: 40 weeks, or 280 days. This period of 280 days is calculated from the beginning of the last normal menstrual period to the time of birth. Estimated date of birth (EDB) is usually calculated by this method. Most fetuses are born within 10 to 14 days of the calculated date of birth. The fertilization age (or postconception age) of the fetus is calculated to be *about* 2 weeks less, or 266 days (38 weeks) or 9½ calendar months. The latter measurement is more accurate because it measures time from the fertilization of the ovum, or conception. The basic events of organ development in the embryo and fetus are outlined in Table 11–2 • . The time periods used in Table 11–2 are **postconception age**

Table 11-2 • SUMMARY OF ORGAN SYSTEM DEVELOPMENT

Age: 2–3 weeks

Length: 2 mm C–R (Crown-to-Rump)

Nervous system: Groove forms along middle back as cells thicken; neural tube forms from closure of neural groove.

Cardiovascular system: Beginning of blood circulation; tubular heart begins to form during third week.

Gastrointestinal system: Liver begins to function.

Genitourinary system: Formation of kidneys beginning.

Respiratory system: Nasal pits forming.

Endocrine system: Thyroid tissue appears.

Eyes: Optic cup and lens pit have formed; pigment in eyes.

Ear: Auditory pit is now enclosed structure.

Age: 4 weeks

Length: 4–6 mm C–R

Weight: 0.4 g

Nervous system: Anterior portion of neural tube closes to form brain; closure of posterior end forms spinal cord.

Musculoskeletal system: Noticeable limb buds.

Cardiovascular system: Tubular heart beats at 28 days and primitive red blood cells circulate through fetus and chorionic villi.

Gastrointestinal system: Mouth: formation of oral cavity; primitive jaws present; esophagotracheal septum begins division of esophagus and trachea. Digestive tract: stomach forms; esophagus and intestine become tubular; ducts of pancreas and liver forming.

Age: 5 weeks

Length: 8 mm C–R

Weight: Only 0.5% of total body weight is fat (to 20 weeks).

Nervous system: Brain has differentiated and cranial nerves are present.

Musculoskeletal system: Developing muscles have innervation.

Cardiovascular system: Atrial division has occurred.

Age: 6 weeks

Length: 12 mm C–R

Musculoskeletal system: Bone rudiments present; primitive skeletal shape forming; muscle mass begins to develop; ossification of skull and jaws begins.

Cardiovascular system: Chambers present in heart; groups of blood cells can be identified.

Gastrointestinal system: Oral and nasal cavities and upper lip formed; liver begins to form red blood cells.

Respiratory system: Trachea, bronchi, and lung buds present.

Ear: Formation of external, middle, and inner ear continues.

Sexual development: Embryonic sex glands appear.

Age: 7 weeks

Length: 18 mm C–R

Cardiovascular system: Fetal heartbeats can be detected.

Gastrointestinal system: Mouth: tongue separates; palate folds. Digestive tract: stomach attains final form.

Genitourinary system: Separation of bladder and urethra from rectum.

Respiratory system: Diaphragm separates abdominal and thoracic cavities.

Eyes: Optic nerve formed; eyelids appear, thickening of lens.

Sexual development: Differentiation of sex glands into ovaries and testes begins.

Age: 8 weeks

Length: 2.5–3 cm C–R

Weight: 2 g

Musculoskeletal system: Digits formed; further differentiation of cells in primitive skeleton; cartilaginous bones show first signs of ossification; development of muscles in trunk, limbs, and head; some movement of fetus now possible.

Cardiovascular system: Development of heart essentially complete; fetal circulation follows two circuits—four extraembryonic and two intraembryonic.

Gastrointestinal system: Mouth: completion of lip fusion. Digestive tract: rotation in midgut; anal membrane has perforated.

Ear: External, middle, and inner ear assuming final forms.

Sexual development: Male and female external genitals appear similar until end of ninth week.

Age: 10 weeks

Length: 5–6 cm C–H (Crown-to-Heel)

Weight: 14 g

Nervous system: Neurons appear at caudal end of spinal cord; basic divisions of brain present.

Musculoskeletal system: Fingers and toes begin nail growth.

Gastrointestinal system: Mouth: separation of lips from jaw; fusion of palate folds. Digestive tract: developing intestines enclosed in abdomen.

Genitourinary system: Bladder sac formed.

Endocrine system: Islets of Langerhans differentiated.

Eyes: Eyelids fused closed; development of lacrimal duct.

Sexual development: Males: production of testosterone and physical characteristics between 8 and 12 weeks.

Age: 12 weeks

Length: 8 cm C–R; 11.5 cm C–H

Weight: 45 g

Musculoskeletal system: Clear outlining of miniature bones (12–20 weeks); process of ossification is established throughout fetal body; appearance of involuntary muscles in viscera.

Gastrointestinal system: Mouth: completion of palate. Digestive tract: appearance of muscles in gut; bile secretion begins; liver is major producer of red blood cells.

Respiratory system: Lungs acquire definitive shape.

Skin: Pink and delicate.

Endocrine system: Hormonal secretion from thyroid; insulin present in pancreas.

Immunologic system: Appearance of lymphoid tissue in fetal thymus gland.

Age: 16 weeks

Length: 13.5 cm C–R; 15 cm C–H

Weight: 200 g

Musculoskeletal system: Teeth beginning to form hard tissue that will become central incisors.

Gastrointestinal system: Mouth: differentiation of hard and soft palate. Digestive tract: development of gastric and intestinal glands; intestines begin to collect meconium.

Genitourinary system: Kidneys assume typical shape and organization.

Skin: Appearance of scalp hair; lanugo present on body; transparent skin with visible blood vessels; sweat glands developing.

Eye, ear, and nose: Formed.

Sexual development: Sex determination possible.

Note: Age refers to postconception age of fetus/conceptus; fertilization age.

(continued on next page)

Table 11-2 • SUMMARY OF ORGAN SYSTEM DEVELOPMENT (CONTINUED)

Age: 18 weeks

Musculoskeletal system: Teeth beginning to form hard tissue (enamel and dentin) that will become lateral incisors.

Cardiovascular system: Fetal heart tones audible with fetoscope at 16–20 weeks.

Age: 20 weeks

Length: 19 cm C–R; 25 cm C–H

Weight: 435 g (6% of total body weight is fat)

Nervous system: Myelination of spinal cord begins.

Musculoskeletal system: Teeth beginning to form hard tissue that will become canine and first molar. Lower limbs are of final relative proportions.

Gastrointestinal system: Fetus actively sucks and swallows amniotic fluid; peristaltic movements begin.

Skin: Lanugo covers entire body; brown fat begins to form; vernix caseosa begins to form.

Immunologic system: Detectable levels of fetal antibodies (IgG type).

Blood formation: Iron is stored and bone marrow is increasingly important.

Age: 24 weeks

Length: 23 cm C–R; 28 cm C–H

Weight: 780 g

Nervous system: Brain looks like mature brain.

Musculoskeletal system: Teeth are beginning to form hard tissue that will become the second molar.

Respiratory system: Respiratory movements may occur (24–40 weeks). Nostrils reopen. Alveoli appear in lungs and begin production of surfactant; gas exchange possible.

Skin: Reddish and wrinkled, vernix caseosa present.

Immunologic system: IgG levels reach maternal levels.

Eyes: Structurally complete.

Age: 28 weeks

Length: 27 cm C–R; 35 cm C–H

Weight: 1200–1250 g

Nervous system: Begins regulation of some body functions.

Skin: Adipose tissue accumulates rapidly; nails appear; eyebrows and eyelashes present.

Eyes: Eyelids open (28–32 weeks).

Sexual development: Males: testes descend into inguinal canal and upper scrotum.

Age: 32 weeks

Length: 31 cm C–R; 38–43 cm C–H

Weight: 2000 g

Nervous system: More reflexes present.

Age: 36 weeks

Length: 35 cm C–R; 42–48 cm C–H

Weight: 2500–2750 g

Musculoskeletal system: Distal femoral ossification centers present.

Skin: Pale; body rounded, lanugo disappearing, hair fuzzy or woolly; few sole creases; sebaceous glands active and helping to produce vernix caseosa (36–40 weeks).

Ears: Ear lobes soft with little cartilage.

Sexual development: Males: scrotum small and few rugae present; descent of testes into upper scrotum to stay (36–40 weeks). Females: labia majora and minora equally prominent.

Age: 38 weeks

Length: 40 cm C–R; 48–52 cm C–H

Weight: 3200+ g (16% of total body weight is fat)

Respiratory system: At 38 weeks, lecithin-sphingomyelin (L/S) ratio approaches 2:1 (indicates decreased risk of respiratory distress from inadequate surfactant production if born now).

Skin: Smooth and pink; vernix present in skinfolds; moderate to profuse silky hair; lanugo hair on shoulders and upper back; nails extend over tips or digits; creases cover sole.

Ears: Ear lobes firmer due to increased cartilage.

Sexual development: Males: rugous scrotum. Females: labia majora well developed and minora small or completely covered.

Sources: Sadler, T. W. (2000). *Langman's Medical Embryology,* (8th ed.) Baltimore: Lippincott Williams & Wilkins, and Moore, K. L., Persaud, T. V. N., & Shiota, K.: *Color Atlas of Clinically Oriented Embryology,* (2nd ed.) Copyright © 2000, Elsevier Science (USA).

periods. During the period from fertilization to the end of the embryonic period (8 weeks), age is often expressed in days but can be given in weeks. During the fetal period (9th week until birth), age is given in weeks (Moore et al, 2000). For a detailed discussion of each body system's development, see Chapter 28.

Human development follows three stages. The preembryonic stage just discussed consists of the first 14 days of development after the ovum is fertilized; the embryonic stage covers the period from day 15 until approximately the eighth week; and the fetal stage extends from the end of the eighth week until birth.

Embryonic Stage

The stage of the **embryo** starts on day 15 (beginning of the third week after conception) and continues until approximately 8 weeks or until the embryo reaches a crown-to-rump (C–R) length of 3 cm (1.2 in). This length is usually reached about 56 days after fertilization (the end of the eighth gestational week). During the embryonic stage, tissue differentiates into essential organs, and the main external features develop (Figure 11–16 •). The embryo is most vulnerable to teratogens during this period.

THREE WEEKS

In the third week, the embryonic disc becomes elongated and pear-shaped, with a broad cephalic end and a narrow caudal end. The ectoderm has formed a long cylindrical tube called the notochord for brain and spinal cord development. The gastrointestinal tract, created from the endoderm, appears as another tubelike structure communicating with the yolk sac. The most advanced organ is the heart. At 3 weeks, a single tubular heart forms just outside the body cavity of the embryo.

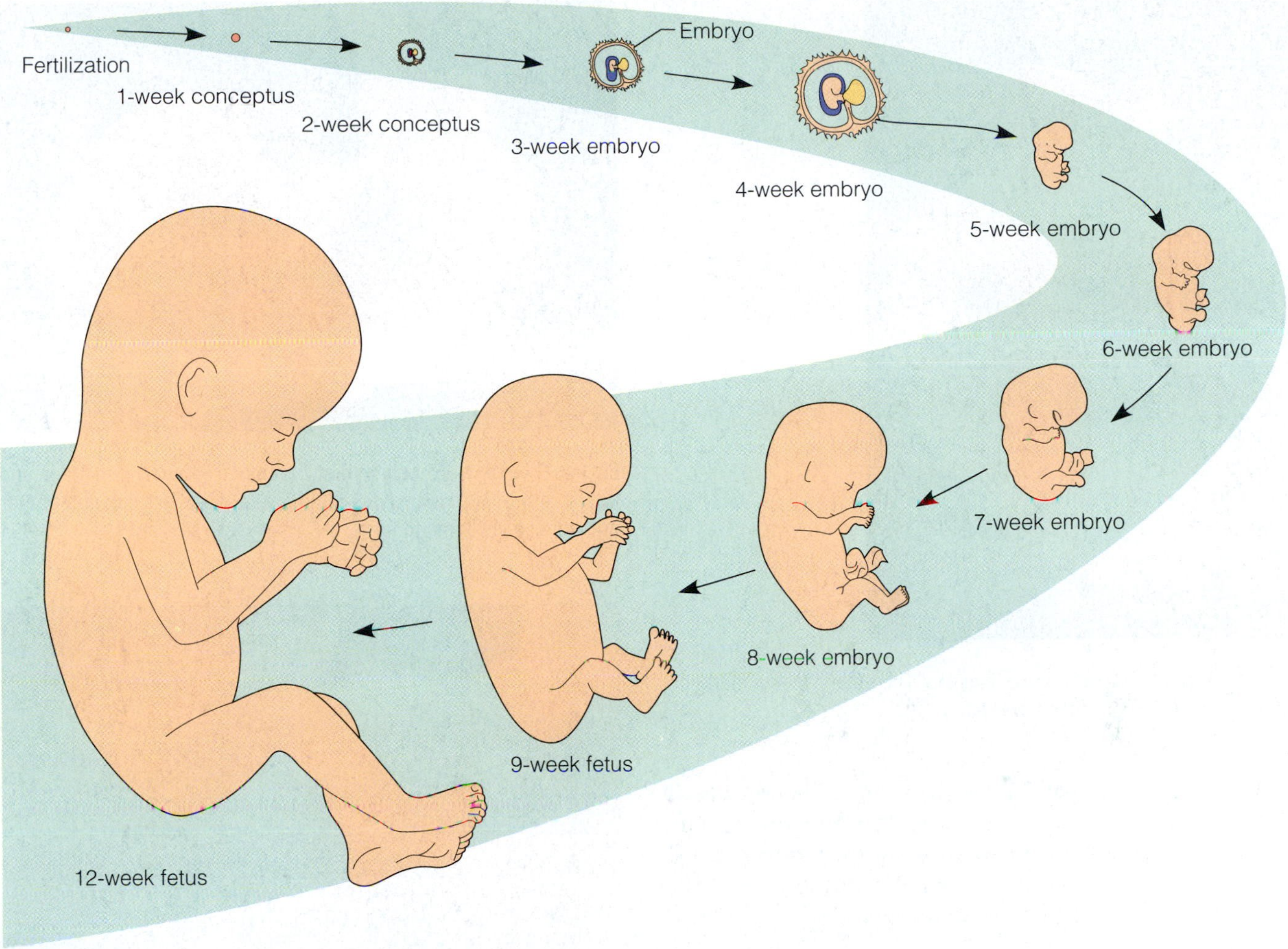

Figure 11–16 • The actual size of a human conceptus from fertilization to the early fetal stage. The embryonic stage begins in the 3rd week after fertilization; the fetal stage begins in the 9th week.

FOUR TO FIVE WEEKS

During days 21 to 32, somites, a series of mesodermal blocks, form on either side of the embryo's midline. The vertebrae that form the spinal column will develop from these somites. Prior to 28 days, arm and leg buds are not visible, but the tail bud is present. The pharyngeal arches—which will form the lower jaw (mandibular arch), hyoid bone, and cartilage of the larynx—develop at this time. The pharyngeal pouches appear now; these pouches will form the eustachian tube and cavity of the middle ear, the tonsils, and the parathyroid and thymus glands. The primordia of the ear and eye are also present (Figure 11–17 •). By the end of 28 days, the tubular heart is beating at a regular rhythm and pushing its own primitive blood cells through the main blood vessels.

During the fifth week, the optic cups and lens vesicles of the eye form and the nasal pits develop. Partitioning in the heart occurs with the dividing of the atrium. The embryo has a marked C-shaped body, accentuated by the rudimentary tail and the large head folded over a protuberant trunk

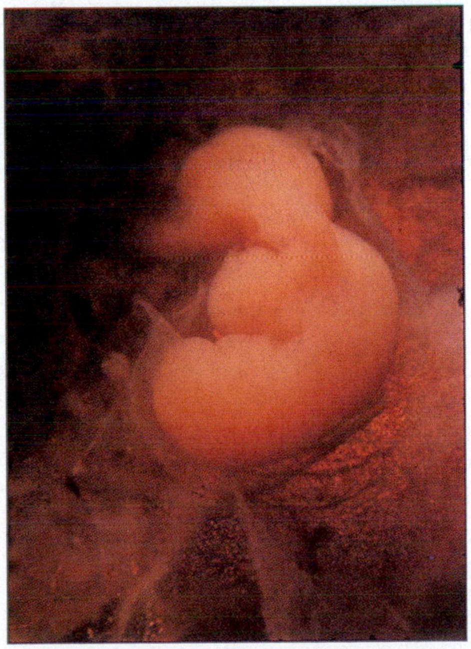

Figure 11–17 • The embryo at 4 weeks. Pharyngeal arches, pharyngeal pouches, and primordia of the ear and eye are present.

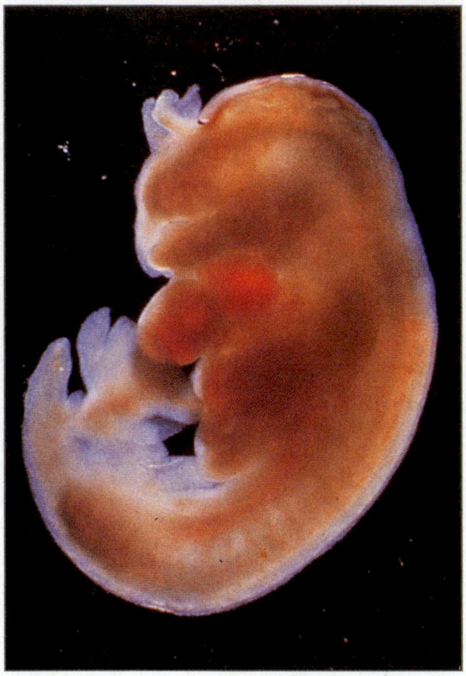

Figure 11–18 • The embryo at 5 weeks. The embryo has a marked C-shaped body and a rudimentary tail.

(Figure 11–18 •). By day 35, the arm and leg buds are well developed, with paddle-shaped hand and foot plates. The heart, circulatory system, and brain show the most advanced development. The brain has differentiated into five areas, and ten pairs of cranial nerves are recognizable.

SIX WEEKS

At 6 weeks, the head structures are more highly developed, and the trunk is straighter than in earlier stages. The upper and lower jaws are recognizable, and the external nares are well formed. The trachea has developed, and its caudal end is bifurcated for beginning lung formation. The upper lip has formed, and the palate is developing. The ears are developing rapidly. The arms have begun to extend ventrally across the chest, and both arms and legs have digits, although they may still be webbed. There is a slight elbow bend in the arm, which is more advanced in development than the leg. Beginning at this stage the prominent tail will recede. The heart now has most of its definitive characteristics, and fetal circulation begins to be established. The liver begins to produce blood cells.

SEVEN WEEKS

At 7 weeks, the head of the embryo is rounded and nearly erect (Figure 11–19 •). The eyes have shifted from their original lateral position to a forward location, where they are closer together, and the eyelids are beginning to form. The palate is nearing completion, and the tongue is developing in the formed mouth. The gastrointestinal and genitourinary tracts undergo significant changes during the seventh week. Prior to this time the rectal and urogenital passages formed one tube that ended in a blind pouch; they now separate into two tubular structures. The intestines enter the extraembryonic coelom in the area of the umbilical cord, called umbilical herniation (Moore et al, 2000). At this point the beginnings of all essential external and internal structures are present.

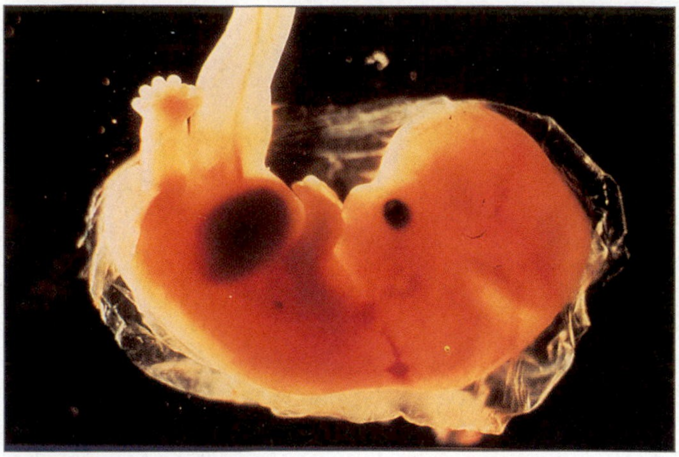

Figure 11–19 • The embryo at 7 weeks. The head is rounded and nearly erect. The eyes have shifted forward and are closer together, and the eyelids begin to form.

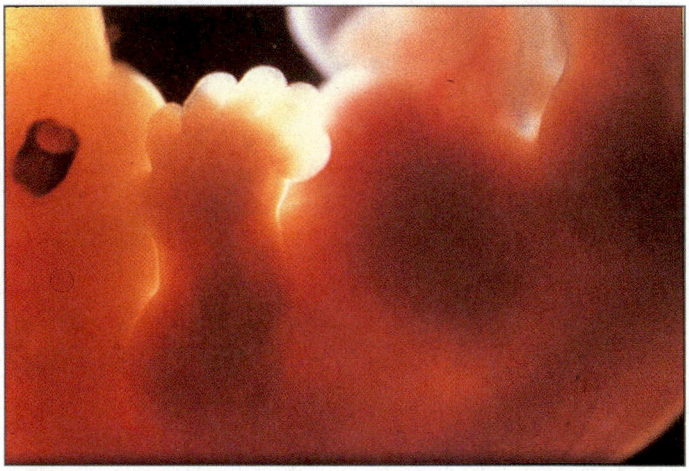

Figure 11–20 • The embryo at 8 weeks. Although only 3 cm in C–R length, the embryo clearly resembles a human being. Facial features continue to develop.

EIGHT WEEKS

At 8 weeks, the embryo is approximately 3 cm (1.2 in) C–R and clearly resembles a human being (Figure 11–20 •). Facial features continue to develop. The eyelids begin to fuse. Auricles of the external ears begin to assume their final shape, but they are still set low (Moore et al, 2000). External genitals appear, but the embryo's sex is not clearly identifiable. The rectal passage opens with the perforation of the anal membrane. The circulatory system through the umbilical cord is well established. Long bones are beginning to form, and the large muscles are now capable of contracting.

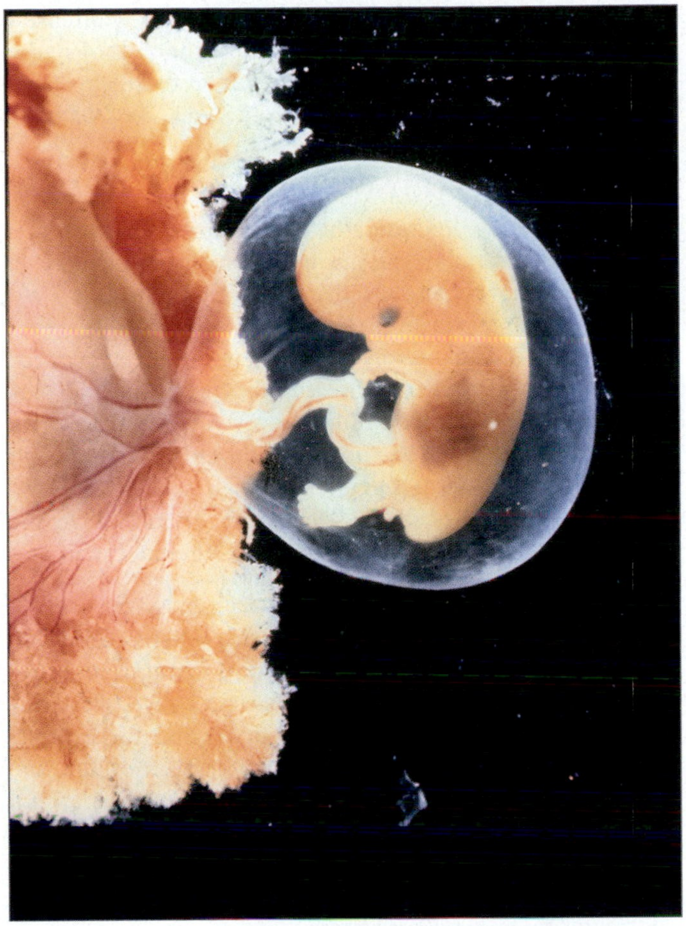

Figure 11–21 • The fetus at 9 weeks. Every organ system and external structure is present.
SOURCE: Nilsson, L. (1990). *A child is born.* New York: Dell Publishing.

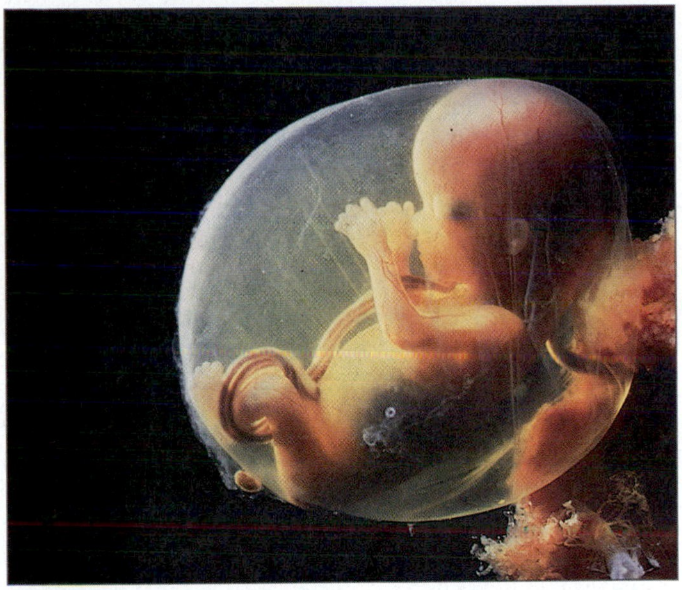

Figure 11–22 • The fetus at 14 weeks. During this period of rapid growth, the skin is so transparent that blood vessels are visible beneath it. More muscle tissue and body skeleton have developed, which holds the fetus more erect.
SOURCE: Nilsson, L. (1990). *A child is born.* New York: Dell Publishing.

Fetal Stage

By the end of the eighth week, the embryo is sufficiently developed to be called a **fetus.** Every organ system and external structure that will be found in the full-term newborn is present. The remainder of gestation is devoted to refining structures and perfecting function.

NINE TO TWELVE WEEKS

By the end of the ninth week, the fetus reaches a C–R length of 5 cm (2 in) and weighs about 14 g. The head is large and comprises almost half of the fetus's entire size (Figure 11–21 •). The neck is distinct from the head and body, and both the head and neck are straighter than in previous stages of development.

By 12 weeks, the fetus reaches an 8 cm (3.2 in) C–R length and weighs about 45 g (1.6 oz). The face is well formed, with the nose protruding, the chin small and receding, and the ears acquiring a more adult shape. The eyelids close at about the tenth week and will not reopen until about 28 weeks. Some reflex movements of the lips suggestive of the sucking reflex have been observed at 3 months. Tooth buds now appear for all 20 of the child's first teeth (baby teeth). The limbs are long and slender, with well-formed digits. The fetus can curl the fingers toward the palm and make a tiny fist. The legs are still shorter and less developed than the arms. The urogenital tract completes its development, well-differentiated genitals appear, and the kidneys begin to produce urine. Red blood cells are produced primarily by the liver. Spontaneous movements of the fetus now occur. Fetal heart tones (the sound of the heart beat) can be ascertained by electronic devices between 8 and 12 weeks. The heart rate is 120 to 160 beats per minute.

THIRTEEN TO SIXTEEN WEEKS

This is a period of rapid growth. At 13 weeks, the fetus weighs 55 to 60 g and is about 9 cm (3.6 in) in C–R length. Lanugo, or fine hair, begins to develop, especially on the head. The skin is so transparent that blood vessels are clearly visible beneath it. More muscle tissue and body skeleton have developed, which hold the fetus more erect (Figure 11–22 •). Active movements are present—the fetus stretches and exercises its arms and legs. It makes sucking motions, swallows amniotic fluid, and produces meconium in the intestinal tract. Bronchial tubes are branching out in the primitive lungs, and sweat glands are developing. The liver and pancreas now begin production of their appropriate secretions. By the beginning of week 16, skeletal ossification is clearly identifiable.

TWENTY WEEKS

The fetus doubles its C–R length and now measures about 19 cm (8 in). Fetal weight is between 435 and 465 g (15.2 to 16.3 oz). Lanugo covers the entire body and is especially prominent on the shoulders. Subcutaneous deposits of brown fat, which has a rich blood supply, make the skin a

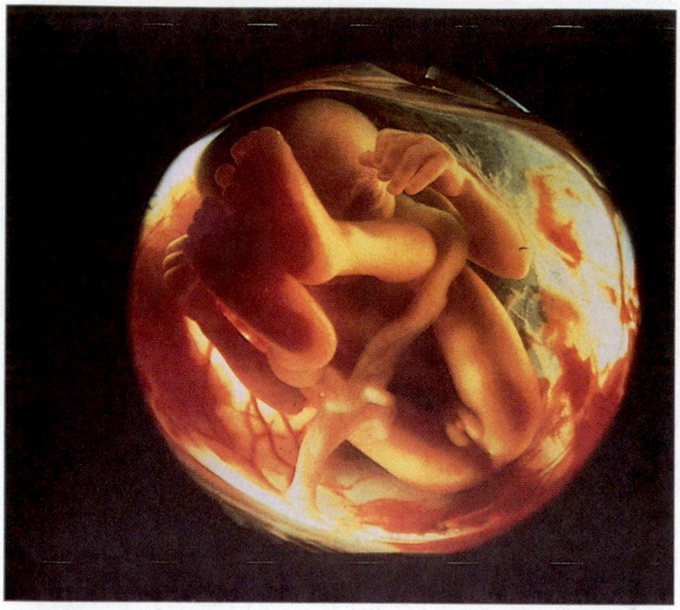

Figure 11–23 • The fetus at 20 weeks. The fetus weighs approximately 435 to 465 g and measures about 19 cm. Subcutaneous deposits of brown fat make the skin less transparent. "Woolly" hair covers the head, and nails have developed on the fingers and toes.
SOURCE: Nilsson, L. (1990). *A child is born.* New York: Dell Publishing.

little less transparent. Nipples now appear over the mammary glands. The head is covered with fine, "woolly" hair, and the eyebrows and eyelashes are beginning to form. The fetus has nails on both fingers and toes (Figure 11–23 •). Muscles are well developed, and the fetus is active. Fetal movement, known as quickening, is felt by the mother. The heartbeat is audible through the fetoscope. Quickening and fetal heartbeat can help in validating the EDB.

TWENTY-FOUR WEEKS

The fetus at 24 weeks reaches a crown-to-heel (C–H) length of 28 cm (11.2 in). It weighs about 780 g (1 lb, 10 oz). The hair on the head is growing long, and eyebrows and eyelashes have formed. The eyes are structurally complete and will soon open. The fetus has a reflex hand grip (grasp reflex) and, by the end of 6 months, a startle reflex. Skin covering the body is reddish and wrinkled, with little subcutaneous fat. Skin on the hands and feet has thickened, with skin ridges on palms and soles forming distinct footprints and fingerprints. The skin over the entire body is covered with a protective cheeselike fatty substance secreted by the sebaceous glands called **vernix caseosa.** The alveoli in the lungs are just beginning to form.

TWENTY-FIVE TO TWENTY-EIGHT WEEKS

At 6 calendar months, the fetal skin is still red, wrinkled, and covered with vernix caseosa. During this time the brain is developing rapidly, and the nervous system is complete enough to provide some degree of regulation of body functions. The eyelids open and close under neural control. If the fetus is a male, the testes begin to descend into the scrotal sac. Even though the lungs are still physiologically immature, they are sufficiently developed to provide gas exchange. A fetus born at this time will require immediate and prolonged intensive care in order to survive and to decrease the risk of major handicap. The fetus at 28 weeks is about 35 to 38 cm (14 to 15 in) long C–H and weighs 1200 to 1250 g (2 lb, 10.5 oz to 2 lb, 12 oz).

TWENTY-NINE TO THIRTY-TWO WEEKS

At 30 weeks, the pupillary light reflex is present (Moore et al, 2000). The fetus is gaining weight from an increase in body muscle and fat and weighs about 2000 g (4 lb, 6.5 oz) with a length of about 38 to 43 cm (15 to 17 in) by 32 weeks of age. The central nervous system (CNS) has matured enough to direct rhythmic breathing movements and partially control body temperature. However, the lungs are not yet fully mature. Bones are now fully developed but are soft and flexible. The fetus begins storing iron, calcium, and phosphorus. In males, the testicles may be located in the scrotal sac but are often still high in the inguinal canal.

THIRTY-FIVE TO THIRTY-SIX WEEKS

The fetus is beginning to get plump with less-wrinkled skin covering the deposits of subcutaneous fat. Lanugo hair is beginning to disappear, and the nails reach the edge of the fingertips. By 35 weeks, the fetus has a firm grasp and exhibits spontaneous orientation to light. By 36 weeks of age, the weight is usually 2500 to 2750 g (5 lb, 12 oz to 6 lb, 11.5 oz), and the C–H length of the fetus is about 42 to 48 cm (16 to 19 in). An infant born at this time has a good chance of surviving but may require some special care, especially if there is intrauterine growth restriction.

THIRTY-EIGHT TO FORTY WEEKS

The fetus is considered full term at 38 weeks and up to 40 weeks after conception. The C–H length varies from 48 to 52 cm (18 to 21 in), with males usually longer than females. Males also usually weigh more than females. The weight at term is about 3000 to 3600 g (6 lb, 10 oz to 7 lb, 15 oz) and varies in different ethnic groups. The skin has a smooth polished look. The only lanugo left is on the upper arms and shoulders. The hair on the head is no longer woolly but coarse and about an inch long. Vernix caseosa is present, with heavier deposits remaining in creases and folds of the skin. The body and extremities are plump, with good skin turgor, and the fingernails extend beyond the fingertips. The chest is prominent but still a little smaller than the head, and mammary glands protrude in both sexes. The testes are in the scrotum or are palpable in the inguinal canals. As the fetus enlarges, amniotic fluid diminishes to about 500 mL or less, and the fetal body mass fills the uterine cavity. The fetus assumes what is referred to as its *position of comfort*, or lie. The head is generally pointed downward, following the shape of the uterus (and also possibly because the head is heavier than the feet). The extremities and often the head are well flexed. After 5 months, feeding patterns, sleeping patterns, and activity patterns become established, so the fetus at term has its own body rhythms and individual style of response. See Table 11–3 • Fetal Development: What parents want to know.

MediaLink FETAL DEVELOPMENT OVERVIEW

Table 11–3 • EMBRYONIC AND FETAL DEVELOPMENT: WHAT PARENTS WANT TO KNOW

4 weeks:	The fetal heart begins to beat.
8 weeks:	All body organs are formed.
8–12 weeks:	Fetal heart tones can be heard by Doppler device.
16 weeks:	Baby's sex can be seen. Although thin, the fetus looks like a baby.
20 weeks:	Heartbeat can be heard with fetoscope. Mother feels movement (quickening). Baby develops a regular schedule of sleeping, sucking, and kicking. Hands can grasp. Baby assumes a favorite position in utero. Vernix (lanolin-like covering) protects the body, and lanugo (fine hair) keeps oil on skin. Head hair, eyebrows, and eyelashes present.
24 weeks:	Weighs 1 lb, 10 oz. Activity is increasing. Fetal respiratory movements begin.
28 weeks:	Eyes begin to open and close. Baby can breathe at this time. Surfactant needed for breathing at birth is formed. Baby is two thirds its final size.
32 weeks:	Baby has fingernails and toenails. Subcutaneous fat is being laid down. Baby appears less red and wrinkled.
38+ weeks:	Baby fills total uterus. Baby gets antibodies from mother.

Table 11–4 • DEVELOPMENTAL VULNERABILITY TIMETABLE

Weeks Since Conception	Potential Teratogen-Induced Malformation
3	Ectromelia (congenital absence of one or more limbs) Ectopia cordis (heart lies outside thoracic cavity)
4	Omphalocele (herniation of abdominal viscera into the umbilical cord) Tracheoesophageal fistula (abnormal connection between trachea and esophagus) (4–5 weeks) Hemivertebra (4–5* weeks)
5	Nuclear cataract Microphthalmia (abnormally small eyeballs) (5–6* weeks) Facial clefts Carpal or pedal ablation (5–6* weeks)
6	Gross septal or aortic abnormalities Cleft lip, agnathia (absence of the lower jaw)
7	Interventricular septal defects Pulmonary stenosis Cleft palate, micrognathia (smallness of the jaw) Epicanthus Brachycephalism (shortness of the head) (7–8* weeks) Mixed sexual characteristics
8	Persistent ostium primum (persistent opening in atrial septum) Digital stunting (shortening of fingers and toes)

*May occur in several time periods after conception.
Source: Modified from Danforth, D. N., & Scott, J. R., (1986). *Obstetrics and Gynecology,* (5th ed., p. 319). Philadelphia: Lippincott.

Factors Influencing Embryonic and Fetal Development

Among factors that may affect embryonic development are the quality of the sperm or ovum from which the zygote was formed, the genetic code established at fertilization, and the adequacy of the intrauterine environment. If the environment is unsuitable before cellular differentiation occurs, all the cells of the zygote are affected. The cells may die, which causes spontaneous abortion, or growth may be slowed, depending on the severity of the situation. When differentiation is complete and the fetal membranes have formed, an injurious agent has the greatest effect on those cells undergoing the most rapid growth. Thus the time of injury is critical in the development of anomalies.

Because organs are formed primarily during embryonic development, the growing organism is considered most vulnerable to hazardous agents during the first months of pregnancy. Table 11–4 • lists potential malformations related to the time of insult. Any agent, such as a drug, virus, or chemicals, that can cause development of abnormal structures in an embryo is referred to as a **teratogen.** It is important to remember that the effects of teratogens depend on the (1) maternal and fetal genotype, (2) stage of development when exposure occurs, and (3) dose and duration of exposure of the agent. Chapter 14 discusses the effects of specific teratogenic agents on the developing fetus.

Adequacy of the maternal environment is also important during the periods of rapid embryonic and fetal development. Maternal nutrition can affect brain development. The period of maximum brain growth and myelination begins with the fifth lunar month before birth and continues during the first 6 months after birth, when there is a twofold increase in myelination (Volpe, 2000). Amino acids, glucose, and fatty acids are considered to be the primary dietary factors in brain growth. A subtle type of damage that affects the associative capacity of the brain, possibly leading to learning disabilities, may be caused by nutritional deficiency at this stage. Maternal nutrition may

CRITICAL THINKING IN PRACTICE

Melodie Chong, in her third week of pregnancy, develops a fever of 104F but refuses to take any medication because she is afraid that drugs will harm her baby. Is she correct?

See Appendix I for possible responses.

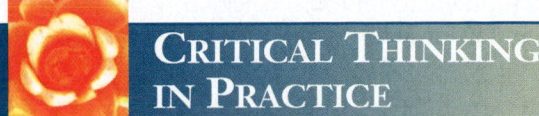

also predispose to the development of adult coronary heart disease, hypertension, and diabetes in babies who were small or disproportionate at birth. Maternal nutrition is discussed in depth in Chapter 18.

Another prenatal influence on the intrauterine environment is maternal hyperthermia associated with sauna baths or hot tub use. Studies of the effects of maternal hyperthermia during the first trimester have raised concern about possible central nervous system defects and failure of neural tube closure. The effects of maternal substance abuse on fetal development are discussed in Chapters 19 and 32.

Research in Practice
Effect of Vegetarian Diet on Mother and Baby

What is this study about? The impact of diet during pregnancy is well known, and nurses are in a unique position to help mothers understand the effects of their dietary choices. Less well known, though, are the effects of special diets, including those without meat. This study undertook the investigation of the effects of a vegetarian diet on both the mother and her baby. A vegetarian diet was defined as one without meat or fish.

How was this study done? Data were collected from charts for all mothers who presented for delivery at a hospital in Great Britain. Conducted over a one-year period, this resulted in 5942 subjects. Guidelines for classifying the mothers as vegetarians were developed, and the attending midwife entered the classification into the records. Outcomes of interest were defined as gestation at delivery, pre- and postdelivery hemoglobin, live births, birth weight, Apgar score, gender, admission to neonatal unit, smoking, breastfeeding at discharge, and stillbirth rate. Results were reported as percentages, and tested for statistical differences between the vegetarian mothers and the nonvegetarian mothers.

What were the results of the study? Only a small proportion—4.9%—of the studied mothers were vegetarian. This small sample makes it difficult both to achieve statistical significance and to draw meaningful conclusions. However, some differences were found in the two groups of mothers. Vegetarian mothers were much less likely to smoke—10.3% of the vegetarian mothers as opposed to 24.4% of the nonvegetarians. Babies clearly benefit from lower smoking rates, so this finding is encouraging. Vegetarian mothers were also more likely to be breastfeeding successfully at discharge than nonvegetarian mothers.

What additional questions might I have? Would a larger sample detect more significant differences? Were these mothers well educated in their diet? What challenges were presented to these mothers as they managed their pregnancy on a vegetarian diet? How can the nurse support mothers in their dietary choices?

How can I use this study? The nurse is in a key position to counsel mothers about the effects of their diet. Vegetarian mothers can have healthy outcomes despite their dietary restrictions.

Source: Hudson, P., & Buckley, R. (2000). Vegetarian diets: Are they good for pregnant women and their babies? *Practicing Midwife, 3*(7), 22–23.

Chapter Review

ExploreMediaLink

NCLEX review questions, case studies, and other interactive resources for this chapter can be found on the Web site at http://www.prenhall.com/olds. Click on "Chapter 11" to select the activities for this chapter.

For tutorials including animations and videos, more NCLEX review questions, and an audio glossary, access the accompanying CD-ROM in this book.

Focus Your Study

- Humans have 46 chromosomes, which are divided into 23 pairs—22 pairs of autosomes and one pair of sex chromosomes.
- Mitosis is the process by which additional somatic (body) cells are formed. It provides growth and development of the organs and replacement of body cells.

- Meiosis is the process by which gametes (ova and sperm) are formed. It occurs during gametogenesis (oogenesis and spermatogenesis) and consists of two successive cell divisions (reduction division), which produce a gamete with 23 chromosomes (22 chromosomes and 1 sex chromosome)—the haploid number of chromosomes.
- Gametes must have a haploid number (23) of chromosomes so that when the female gamete (ovum) and the male gamete (spermatozoon) unite to form the zygote, the normal human diploid number of chromosomes (46) is reestablished.
- An ovum is considered fertile for about 12 to 24 hours after ovulation, and the sperm is believed to be capable of fertilizing the ovum for about 24 hours after it is deposited in the female reproductive tract.
- Fertilization usually takes place in the ampulla (outer third) of the fallopian tube. Both capacitation and the acrosomal reaction must occur for the sperm to fertilize the ovum. Capacitation is the removal of the plasma membrane, which exposes the acrosomal covering of the sperm head. The acrosomal reaction is the deposit of hyaluronidase in the corona radiata, which allows the sperm head to penetrate the ovum.
- Sex chromosomes are referred to as X and Y. Females have two X chromosomes, and males have an X and a Y chromosome. Y chromosomes are carried only by the sperm. To produce a female child, both the mother and the father contribute an X chromosome. To produce a male child, the mother contributes an X chromosome and the father contributes a Y chromosome.
- Twins are either dizygotic (fraternal) or monozygotic (identical). Dizygotic twins arise from two separate ova fertilized by two separate spermatozoa. Monozygotic twins develop from a single ovum fertilized by a single spermatozoon.
- Intrauterine development first proceeds via cellular multiplication in which the zygote undergoes rapid mitotic division called cleavage. As a result of cleavage, the zygote divides and multiplies into cell groupings called blastomeres, which are held together by the zona pellucida. The blastomeres will eventually become a solid ball of cells called the morula. When a cavity forms in the morula cell mass, the inner solid cell mass is called the blastocyst.
- Implantation usually occurs in the upper part of the posterior uterine wall when the blastocyst burrows into the uterine lining.
- After implantation, the endometrium is called the decidua. Decidua capsularis is the portion that covers the blastocyst. Decidua basalis is the portion that is directly under the blastocyst. Decidua vera is the portion that lines the rest of the uterine cavity.
- Embryonic membranes are called the amnion and the chorion. The amnion is formed from the ectoderm and is a thin protective membrane that contains the amniotic fluid and the embryo. The chorion is a thick membrane that develops from the trophoblast and encloses the amnion, embryo, and yolk sac.
- Amniotic fluid cushions the fetus against mechanical injury, controls the embryo's temperature, allows symmetric external growth, prevents adherence to the amnion, and permits freedom of movement.
- Primary germ layers will give rise to all tissues, organs, and organ systems. The three primary germ cell layers are ectoderm, endoderm, and mesoderm.
- The placenta, which develops from the chorionic villi and the decidua basalis, has two parts. The maternal portion, consisting of the decidua basalis, is red and flesh-looking; the fetal portion, consisting of chorionic villi, is covered by the amnion and appears shiny and gray. The placenta is made up of 15 to 20 segments called cotyledons.
- The placenta serves metabolic functions, endocrine functions (production of hPL, hCG, estrogen, and progesterone), and immunologic functions. It acts as the fetus's respiratory organ, is an organ of excretion, and aids in the exchange of nutrients.
- The umbilical cord contains two umbilical arteries, which carry deoxygenated blood from the fetus to the placenta, and one umbilical vein, which carries oxygenated blood from the placenta to the fetus. The umbilical cord has a central insertion into the placenta.
- Wharton's jelly, a specialized connective tissue, prevents compression of the umbilical cord in utero.
- The fetal circulatory system provides for oxygenation of the fetus while bypassing the fetal lungs.
- Stages of fetal development include the preembryonic stage (the first 14 days of human development starting at fertilization), the embryonic stage (from day 15 after fertilization, or the beginning of the third week, until approximately 8 weeks after conception), and the fetal stage (from 8 weeks until birth at approximately 38 weeks postconception).
- Significant events that occur during the embryonic stage are that at 4 weeks the fetal heart begins to beat and at 6 weeks fetal circulation is established.
- The fetal stage is devoted to refining structures and perfecting function. The following are some significant developments during the fetal stage:

  At 8 to 12 weeks, all organ systems are formed and now require maturation.

At 16 weeks, the sex of the fetus can be determined visually.

At 20 weeks, fetal heartbeat can be auscultated by a fetoscope, and the mother can feel movement (quickening).

At 24 weeks, vernix caseosa covers the entire body.

At 26 to 28 weeks, the eyes reopen.

At 32 weeks, skin appears less wrinkled and red because subcutaneous fat has been laid down.

At 35 weeks, fingernails reach the ends of fingers.

At 38 weeks, vernix caseosa is apparent only in creases and folds of skin, and lanugo remains on upper arms and shoulders only.

- The embryo is particularly vulnerable to teratogenesis during the first 8 weeks of cell differentiation and organ system development.

References

Ahokas, R. A., & McKinney, E. T. (2000). Development and physiology of the placenta and membranes. In J. J. Sciarra & T. J. Watkins (Eds.), *Gynecology and obstetrics* (Vol. 2, chap. 11, pp. 1–21). Philadelphia: Lippincott Williams & Wilkins.

Benirschke, K. (1999). Normal development. In R. K. Creasy & R. Resnik (Eds.), *Maternal-fetal medicine* (4th ed., pp. 63–71). Philadelphia: Saunders.

Blackburn, S. T. (2003). *Maternal, fetal, & neonatal physiology: A clinical perspective.* (2nd ed.). St. Louis: Saunders.

Brannigan, R. E., & Lipshultz, L. I. (2000). Sperm transport and capacitation. In J. J. Sciarra & T. J. Watkins (Eds.), *Gynecology and obstetrics* (Vol. 5, chap. 45, pp. 1-9). Philadelphia: Lippincott Williams & Wilkins.

Chitkara, U., & Berkowitz, R. L. (2002) Multiple gestations. In S. G. Grabbe, G. R. Niebyl, & J. L. Simpson (Eds.), *Obstetrics: Normal and problem pregnancies.* (4th ed.). New York: Churchill Livingstone.

Cunningham, F. G., Gant, N. G., Leveno, K. J., Gilstrap, L. C., III, Hauth, J. C., & Wenstrom, K. D. (2001). *Williams obstetrics* (21st ed.). New York: McGraw-Hill.

De Jonge, C. J. (2000). Egg transport and fertilization. In J. J. Sciarra & T. J. Watkins (Eds.), *Gynecology and obstetrics* (Vol. 5, chap. 46, pp. 1–7). Philadelphia: Lippincott Williams & Wilkins.

Gilbert, W. M., & Brace, R. A. (1993). Amniotic fluid volume and normal flows to and from the amniotic cavity. *Seminars in Perinatology, 17*(3), 150–157.

Moore, K. L., Persaud, T. V. N., & Shiota, K. (2000). *Color atlas of clinical embryology* (2nd ed.). Philadelphia: Saunders.

Nussbaum, R. L., McInnes, R. R., & Willard, H. F. (2001). *Thompson & Thompson genetics in medicine* (6th ed.). Philadelphia: Saunders.

Sadler, T. W. (2000). *Langman's medical embryology* (8th ed.). Philadelphia: Lippincott Williams & Wilkins.

Volpe, J. J. (2000). *Neurology of the newborn* (4th ed.). Philadelphia: Saunders.

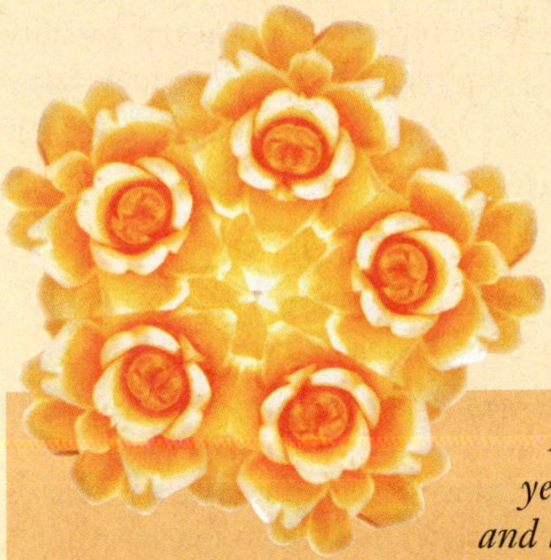

12 Special Reproductive Concerns

As we sat in the waiting room at the in vitro clinic, I felt great apprehension. For 4 years we had been unable to conceive. I'd been through two surgeries, dozens of blood tests, and hormone drugs that made me irrational and emotional. It was difficult at times—I blamed myself, felt out of control, and had surprisingly painful reactions to seeing mothers with babies. After many long talks we decided that if in vitro didn't work for us, we would adopt. Still, we felt that we wanted to experience childbirth together.

We were on the brink of the most expensive infertility treatment—the last resort for most infertile couples. Every month's treatment would involve huge and potentially uninsured costs; numerous injections, many of which I would have to administer to myself; egg retrieval; four or five ultrasounds; a dozen blood tests; and only a 30% to 50% chance of conceiving a child. Is this the right thing? Is this the right clinic for us? After so many disappointments did I dare get my hopes up again?

A young nurse burst into the office, excited and out of breath. She'd just come from the lab, having done a blood test, and had discovered that a client was pregnant. Watching the thrill and caring of the nurse's face helped me to decide. Yes, I was in the right place. Yes, it was worth hoping again. Even if in vitro didn't work for us, we had to try.

Objectives

- Identify the components of fertility.
- Describe the elements of the preliminary investigation of infertility.
- Summarize the indications for the tests and associated treatments, including assisted reproductive technologies, that are done in an infertility work-up.
- Summarize the physiologic and psychologic effects of infertility.
- Describe the nurse's roles as counselor, educator, and advocate during infertility evaluation and treatment.
- Discuss the indications for preconceptual chromosomal analysis and prenatal testing.
- Identify the characteristics of autosomal dominant, autosomal recessive, and X-linked recessive disorders.
- Compare prenatal and postnatal diagnostic procedures used to determine the presence of genetic disorders.
- Explore the emotional impact on a couple undergoing genetic testing or coping with the birth of a baby with a genetic disorder, and explain the nurse's role in supporting the family undergoing genetic counseling.

Key Terms

Autosomes 268
Basal body temperature (BBT) 252
Chromosomes 268
Endometrial biopsy 254
Ferning capacity 257
Gamete intrafallopian transfer (GIFT) 263
Genotype 271
Huhner test 258
Hysterosalpingography (HSG) 258
Infertility 250
In vitro fertilization (IVF) 263
Karyotype 268
Laparoscopy 258
Mendelian (single-gene) inheritance 271
Monosomies 270
Mosaicism 270

MediaLink

Additional resources for this content can be found on the Student CD-ROM and on the Companion Website at www.prenhall.com/olds. Click on "Chapter 12" to select the activities for this chapter.

CD-ROM
- Audio Glossary
- NCLEX Review
- Activity: Ovulation

Companion Website
- Additional NCLEX Review
- Case Study: Infertility
- Care Plan Activity: Infertile Couple

Key Terms

Nonmendelian (multifactorial) inheritance 271
Pedigree 272
Phenotype 271
Spinnbarkheit 255
Subfertility 250
Therapeutic insemination 262
Transvaginal ultrasound 255
Trisomies 269
Tubal embryo transfer (TET) 263
Zygote intrafallopian transfer (ZIFT) 263

Most couples who want children conceive with little difficulty. Pregnancy and childbirth usually take their normal course, and a healthy baby is born. But some less fortunate couples are unable to fulfill their dream of having a healthy baby because of infertility or genetic problems.

This chapter explores two particularly troubling reproductive problems facing some couples: the inability to conceive, and the risk of bearing babies with genetic problems.

Infertility

Infertility is defined as lack of conception despite unprotected sexual intercourse for at least 12 months (Bopp & Seifer, 2000). Infertility has a profound emotional, psychologic, and economic impact on both the affected couple and society. Approximately 10% to 15% of couples in their reproductive years are infertile (Gordon & Speroff, 2002). *Sterility* is a term applied when there is an absolute factor preventing reproduction. **Subfertility** is used to describe a couple having difficulty conceiving because both partners have reduced fertility.

Public perception is that the incidence of infertility is increasing, but in fact there has been no significant change in the proportion of infertile couples in the United States. What has changed is the composition of the infertile population; the infertility diagnosis has increased in the age group 25 to 44 because of delayed childbearing and the entry of the baby-boom cohort into this age range in Western society (Bopp & Seifer, 2000).

The perception that infertility is on the rise may be related to the following factors:

- The deferring of pregnancy and then the desire to have a family shortly after marriage
- The increase in assisted reproduction techniques
- The increase in availability and use of infertility services
- The increase in insurance coverage of some ethnic groups for diagnosis of and treatment for infertility
- The increased number of childless women over 35 seeking medical attention for infertility

MediaLink INFERTILITY

Essential Components of Fertility

Understanding the elements essential for normal fertility can help the nurse identify the many factors that may cause infertility. The following components must be present for normal fertility.

Female partner:

1. The cervical mucus must be favorable to the survival of spermatozoa and allow passage to the upper genital tract.
2. The fallopian tubes must be patent and have normal fimbria with peristaltic movements toward the uterus to facilitate normal transport and interaction of ovum and sperm.
3. The ovaries must produce and release normal ova in a regular cyclic fashion.
4. There must be no obstruction between the ovaries and the uterus.
5. The endometrium must be in a physiologic state to allow implantation of the blastocyst and to sustain normal growth and development.
6. Adequate reproductive hormones must be present.

Male partner:

1. The testes must produce spermatozoa of normal quality, quantity, and motility.
2. The male genital tract must not be obstructed.
3. The male genital tract secretions must be normal.
4. Ejaculated spermatozoa must be deposited in the female vagina in such a manner that they reach the cervix.

These normal components are correlated with possible causes of deviation in Table 12–1 •. With the intricacies of the normal male and female reproductive cycle, it is an impressive phenomenon that the majority of couples in the United States are able to conceive. The remaining couples suffer infertility due to a male factor (35%), a female factor (45%), or either an unknown cause (unexplained infertility) or a problem with both partners (20%) (Gordon & Speroff, 2002). Professional intervention can help approximately 65% of infertile couples achieve pregnancy.

Couples should be referred for infertility evaluation if they have been unable to conceive after at least 1 year of attempting to achieve pregnancy. In women over 35 years of age, it may be appropriate to refer the couple after only 6 to 9 months of unprotected intercourse without conception. At 25 years of age, when couples are the most fertile, the average length of time needed to achieve conception is 5.3 months. The average 20- to 30-year-old American couple has intercourse one to three times a week, a frequency that should be sufficient to achieve pregnancy if all other factors are satisfactory. In about 20% of cases, conception occurs within the first month of unprotected intercourse (Cowan, 2002).

Table 12–1 • POSSIBLE CAUSES OF INFERTILITY

Necessary Norms	Deviations from Normal
Female	
Favorable cervical mucus	Cervicitis, cervical stenosis, use of coital lubricants, antisperm antibodies (immunologic response)
Clear passage between cervix and tubes	Myomas, adhesions, adenomyosis, polyps, endometritis, cervical stenosis, endometriosis, congenital anomalies (eg, septate uterus, DES exposure)
Patent tubes with normal motility	Pelvic inflammatory disease, peritubal adhesions, endometriosis, IUD, salpingitis (eg, chlamydia, recurrent STIs), neoplasm, ectopic pregnancy, tubal ligation
Ovulation and release of ova	Primary ovarian failure, polycystic ovarian disease, hypothyroidism, pituitary tumor, lactation, periovarian adhesions, endometriosis, premature ovarian failure, hyperprolactinemia, Turner syndrome
No obstruction between ovary and tubes	Adhesions, endometriosis, pelvic inflammatory disease
Endometrial preparation	Anovulation, luteal phase defect, malformation, uterine infection, Asherman syndrome
Male	
Normal semen analysis	Abnormalities of sperm or semen, polyspermia, congenital defect in testicular development, mumps after adolescence, cryptorchidism, infections, gonadal exposure to x-rays, chemotherapy, smoking, alcohol abuse, malnutrition, chronic or acute metabolic disease, medications (eg, morphine, ASA, ibuprofen), cocaine, marijuana use, constrictive underclothing, heat
Unobstructed genital tract	Infections, tumors, congenital anomalies, vasectomy, strictures, trauma, varicocele
Normal genital tract secretions	Infections, autoimmunity to semen, tumors
Ejaculate deposited at the cervix	Premature ejaculation, impotence, hypospadias, retrograde ejaculation (eg, diabetic), neurologic cord lesions, obesity (inhibiting adequate penetration)

Nurse's Role During Initial Investigation

The easiest and least intrusive infertility testing approach is used first. Extensive testing is avoided until data confirm that the timing of intercourse and the length of coital exposure have been adequate. The nurse informs the couple of the most fertile times to have intercourse during the menstrual cycle. Teaching the couple factors that influence fertility, the signs and timing of ovulation, and the most effective times for intercourse within the cycle may solve the problem before extensive testing needs to be initiated (Table 12–2 •). Primary assessment, including a comprehensive history (with a discussion of genetic conditions) and physical examination for any obvious causes of infertility, is done before a costly, time-consuming, and emotionally trying investigation is initiated. During the first visit for the preliminary investigation, the nurse explains the basic infertility work-up. The basic investigation for the couple depends on the individuals' history and usually includes assessment of ovarian function, cervical mucus adequacy and receptivity to sperm, sperm adequacy, tubal patency, and the general condition of the pelvic organs. Because approximately 35% of infertility is related to a male factor, a semen analysis should be one of the first diagnostic tests prior to moving on to the more invasive diagnostic procedures involving the woman (Cowan, 2002).

The mutual desire to have children is a cornerstone of many marriages. A fertility problem is a deeply personal, emotion-laden area in a couple's life. The self-esteem of one or both partners may be threatened if the inability to conceive is seen as a lack of virility or femininity (Leon, 2000). It is never easy to discuss one's sexual activity, especially when potentially irreversible problems with fertility may exist. The nurse can provide comfort to couples by offering a sympathetic ear, a nonjudgmental approach, and appropriate information and instructions throughout the diagnostic and therapeutic process. Because counseling includes discussion of very personal matters, nurses who are comfortable with their own sexuality are more capable of establishing rapport and eliciting relevant information from couples with fertility problems.

The first interview should involve both partners and include a comprehensive history and a physical examination. Table 12–3 • lists the items in a complete infertility physical work-up and laboratory evaluation for both partners. Figure 12–1 • outlines the historical database, diagnostic tests usually performed, and healthcare interventions in cases of infertility.

Table 12–2 • FERTILITY AWARENESS

Avoid douching and artificial lubricants. Prevent alteration of pH of vagina and introduction of spermicidal agents.

Promote retention of sperm. The male superior position with female remaining recumbent for at least 1 hour after intercourse maximizes the number of sperm reaching the cervix.

Avoid leakage of sperm. Elevate the woman's hips with a pillow after intercourse. Avoid getting up to urinate for 1 hour after intercourse.

Maximize the potential for fertilization. Have intercourse one to three times per week at intervals no less than 48 hours.

Avoid emphasizing conception during sexual encounters to decrease anxiety and potential sexual dysfunction.

Maintain adequate nutrition and reduce stress. Using stress-reduction techniques and good nutritional habits increases sperm production.

Explore other methods to increase fertility awareness, such as home assessment of cervical mucus and basal body temperature (BBT) recordings.

Seek counsel and advice from valued friend or family member.

Consider incorporating culturally appropriate methods to enhance fertility.

Table 12–3 • INITIAL INFERTILITY PHYSICAL WORK-UP AND LABORATORY EVALUATIONS

Female	Male
Physical Examination	**Physical Examination**
Assessment of height, weight, blood pressure, temperature, and general health status	General health (assessment of height, weight, blood pressure)
Endocrine evaluation of thyroid for exophthalmos, lid lag, tremor, or palpable gland	Endocrine evaluation (eg, presence of gynecomastia)
Optic fundi evaluation for presence of increased intracranial pressure, especially in oligomenorrheal or amenorrheal women (possible pituitary tumor)	Visual fields evaluation for bitemporal hemianopia
Reproductive features (including breast and external genital area)	Abnormal hair patterns
Physical ability to tolerate pregnancy	**Urologic Examination**
Pelvic Examination	Presence or absence of phimosis
Papanicolaou smear	Location of urethral meatus
Culture for gonorrhea if indicated and possibly chlamydia or mycoplasma culture (opinions vary)	Size and consistency of each testis, vas deferens, and epididymis
Signs of vaginal infections (Chapter 6)	Presence of varicocele
Shape of escutcheon (eg, does pubic hair distribution resemble that of a male?)	**Rectal Examination**
Size of clitoris (enlargement caused by endocrine disorders)	Size and consistency of the prostate with microscopic evaluation of prostate fluid for signs of infection
Evaluation of cervix: old lacerations, tears, erosion, polyps, condition and shape of os, signs of infections, cervical mucus (evaluate for estrogen effect of spinnbarkheit and cervical ferning)	Size and consistency of seminal vesicles
Bimanual Examination	**Laboratory Examination**
Size, shape, position, and motility of uterus	Complete blood count
Presence of congenital anomalies	Sedimentation rate if indicated
Presence of endometriosis	Serology
Evaluation of adnexa: ovarian size, cysts, fixations, or tumors	Urinalysis
Rectovaginal Examination	Rh factor and blood grouping
Presence of retroflexed or retroverted uterus	Semen analysis
Presence of rectouterine pouch masses	If indicated, testicular biopsy, buccal smear
Presence of possible endometriosis	Hormonal assays, FSH, LH, prolactin
Laboratory Examination	
Complete blood count	
Sedimentation rate if indicated	
Serology	
Urinalysis	
Rh factor and blood grouping	
If indicated, thyroid function tests, prolactin levels, glucose tolerance test, hormonal assays including estradiol, LH, progesterone, FSH, DHEA, androstenedione, testosterone, 17-OHP.	

Tests of the Woman's Fertility

After a thorough history and physical examination, both partners may undergo tests to identify causes of infertility. A thorough evaluation of the woman's fertility includes assessment of the hypothalamic-pituitary axis in terms of ovulatory function, as well as structure and function of the cervix, uterus, fallopian tubes, and ovaries.

EVALUATION OF OVULATORY FACTORS

Ovulation problems account for approximately 15% of couples' infertility (Gordon & Speroff, 2002). For review of the characteristics of the female reproductive cycle, see Table 12–4 • and Figure 12–2 •. For an in-depth discussion, see Chapter 10.

Basal Body Temperature Recording

One basic test of ovulatory function is the **basal body temperature (BBT)** recording, which aids in identifying

Table 12–4 • FEMALE REPRODUCTIVE CYCLE

Ovarian Cycle	Menstrual Cycle
Follicular phase (days 1–14): Primordial follicle matures under influence of FSH and LH up to the time of ovulation.	*Menstrual phase* (days 1–6): Estrogen levels are low; cervical mucus is scant, viscous, and opaque.
Luteal phase (days 15–28): Ovum leaves follicle, corpus luteum develops under LH influence and produces high levels of progesterone and low levels of estrogen.	*Proliferative phase* (days 7–14): Estrogen peaks just prior to ovulation. Cervical mucus at ovulation is clear, thin, watery, alkaline, and more favorable to sperm; shows ferning pattern; and has spinnbarkheit greater than 8 cm. At ovulation body temperature drops, then rises sharply and remains elevated under influence of progesterone.
	Secretory phase (days 15–26): Estrogen drops sharply and progesterone dominates.
	Ischemic phase (days 27–28): Both estrogen and progesterone levels drop.

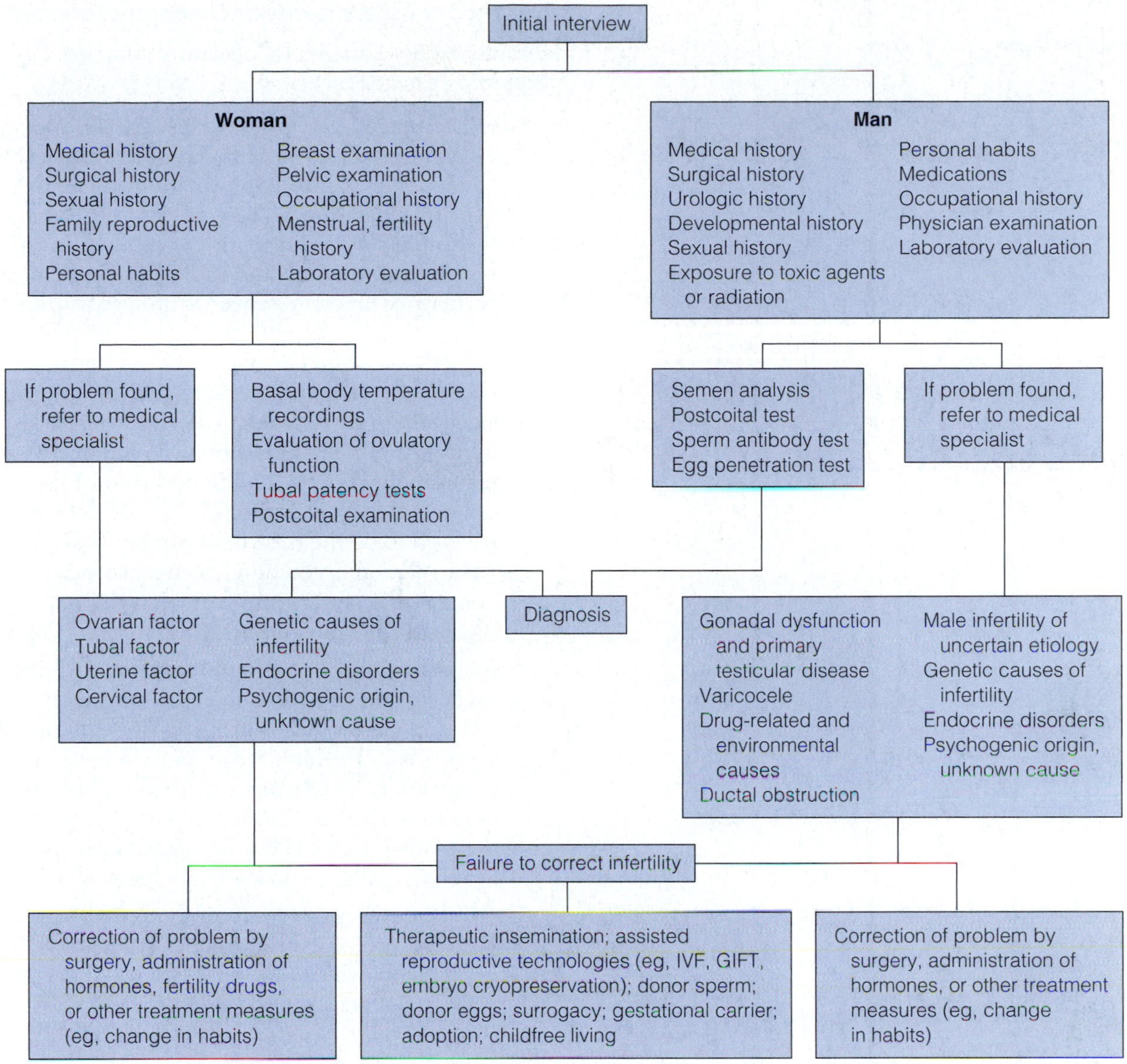

Figure 12–1 • Flow chart for management of the infertile couple.

follicular and luteal phase abnormalities. At the initial visit, the nurse instructs the woman in the technique of recording BBT on a special form. The woman is instructed to begin a new chart on the first day of every monthly cycle. The temperature can be taken with a standard oral or rectal thermometer calibrated by tenths of a degree, making slight temperature changes readily apparent. A special kind of thermometer (BBT) may be used to measure temperature only between 35.6C (96F) and 37.8C (100F). In addition to the traditional glass/mercury thermometer, tympanic thermometry, which provides a reading in only a few seconds, may also be a valid method. Computerized or digitalized BBT devices ("the Rabbit," Fertil-A-Chron) have been developed to identify the fertile period more accurately at home.

The woman records daily variations on a temperature graph. The temperature graph typically shows a biphasic pattern during ovulatory cycles, whereas in anovulatory cycles it remains monophasic. The woman uses the readings on the temperature graph to detect ovulation and direct the timing of intercourse (Figure 12–3 •, *A*).

Basal temperature for females in the preovulatory (follicular) phase is usually below 36.7C (98F). As ovulation approaches, production of estrogen increases and at its peak may cause a slight drop, then rise, in the basal temperature. The slight drop in temperature before ovulation is often difficult to capture on the BBT chart. After ovulation, there is a surge of luteinizing hormone (LH), which stimulates production of progesterone by the corpus luteum, causing a 0.3C to 0.6C (0.5F to 1.0F) sustained rise in basal temperature. Immediately before or coincident with the onset of menses, the temperature falls below 98F. These changes in the basal temperature create the typical biphasic pattern.

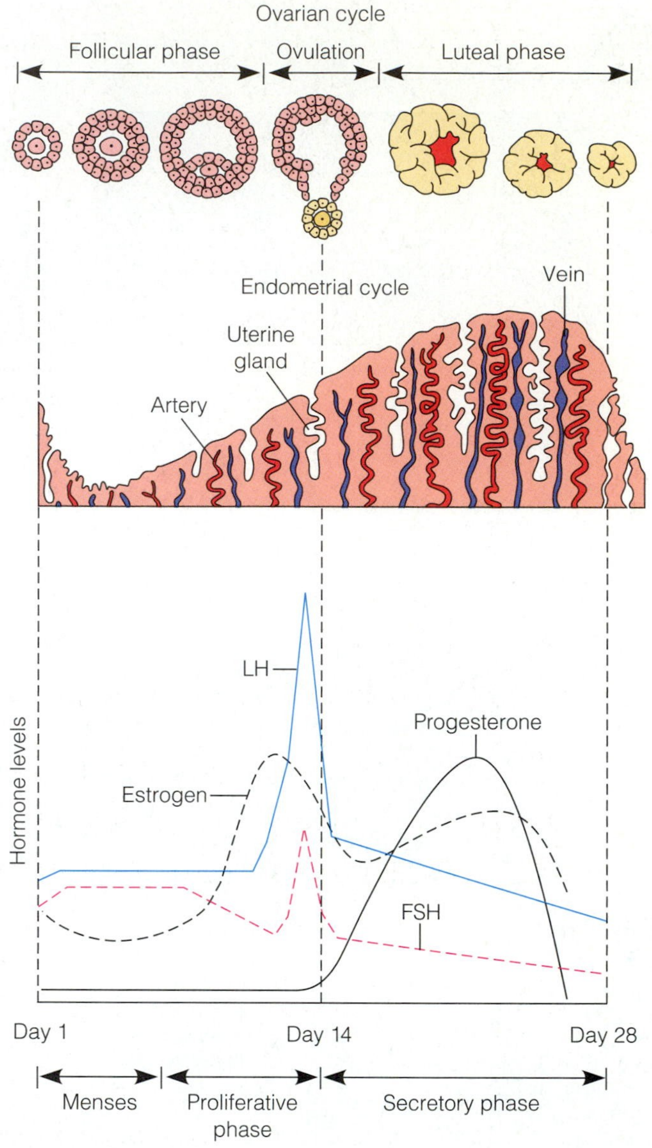

Figure 12–2 • Sequence of events in a normal reproductive cycle showing the relationship of hormone levels to events in the ovarian and endometrial cycles.

Figure 12–3, *B* shows a biphasic ovulatory BBT chart. Progesterone is thermogenic (produces heat), thereby maintaining the temperature increase during the second half of the menstrual cycle (luteal phase). Temperature elevation does not predict the day of ovulation but provides supportive evidence of ovulation about a day after it has occurred. Actual release of the ovum probably occurs 24 to 36 hours prior to the first temperature elevation (estrogen peak) (Gordon & Speroff, 2002).

Based on serial BBT charts, the clinician might recommend sexual intercourse *every other day* beginning 3 to 4 days prior to and continuing for 2 to 3 days after the expected time of ovulation. See Client Teaching: Methods of Determining Ovulation on page 256.

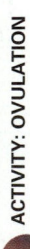

MediaLink Activity: Ovulation

Hormonal Assessments of Ovulatory Function

Hormonal assessments of ovulatory function fall into the following categories:

1. *Gonadotropin levels (FSH, LH).* Baseline hormonal assessment of follicle-stimulating hormone (FSH) and LH provides valuable information concerning normal ovulatory function. Measured on cycle day 3, FSH is the single most valuable test in assessing ovarian reserve and function and should always be measured, particularly in women over 35, to predict the potential for successful treatment with ovulation induction treatment cycles. LH levels may be measured early in the cycle to rule out disorders associated with androgen excess, causing a disruption in normal follicular development and oocyte maturation. Daily sampling of serum LH at midcycle can detect the LH surge. The day of the LH surge is believed to be the time of maximum fertility. Urine LH ovulation prediction kits are also available for home use to better time postcoital testing, insemination, and coitus.
2. *Progesterone assays.* Progesterone levels furnish the best evidence of ovulation and corpus luteum function. Serum levels begin to rise with the LH surge and peak about 8 days later. A level of 5 ng/mL 3 days after the LH surge generally confirms ovulation (Cowan, 2002). On day 21 (7 days postovulation) a level of 10 ng/mL or higher generally indicates an adequate luteal phase.
3. *Prolactin.* Elevated levels of the anterior pituitary hormone prolactin are a frequent cause of ovulatory dysfunction, which may range from a luteal phase defect to anovulation to amenorrhea.
4. *Thyroid-stimulating hormone (TSH).* Thyroid hormone is necessary for most body functions, not only metabolism but also specific tissue activities. TSH stimulates prolactin secretion by the pituitary gland. Hypothyroidism may have a dramatic effect on ovulatory function and cause menstrual irregularities and bleeding problems.
5. *Androgen levels (testosterone, DHEAS, androstenedione).* Androgen excess can originate from the adrenal glands, ovaries, or peripheral tissue. Despite the origin, it usually results in specific clinical symptoms such as acne, hirsutism, virilization, and ovulatory dysfunction—which can range from oligomenorrhea to anovulation to amenorrhea.

Endometrial Biopsy

Endometrial biopsy provides information about the effects of progesterone produced by the corpus luteum after ovulation and endometrial receptivity. The biopsy is performed not earlier than 10 to 12 days after ovulation and

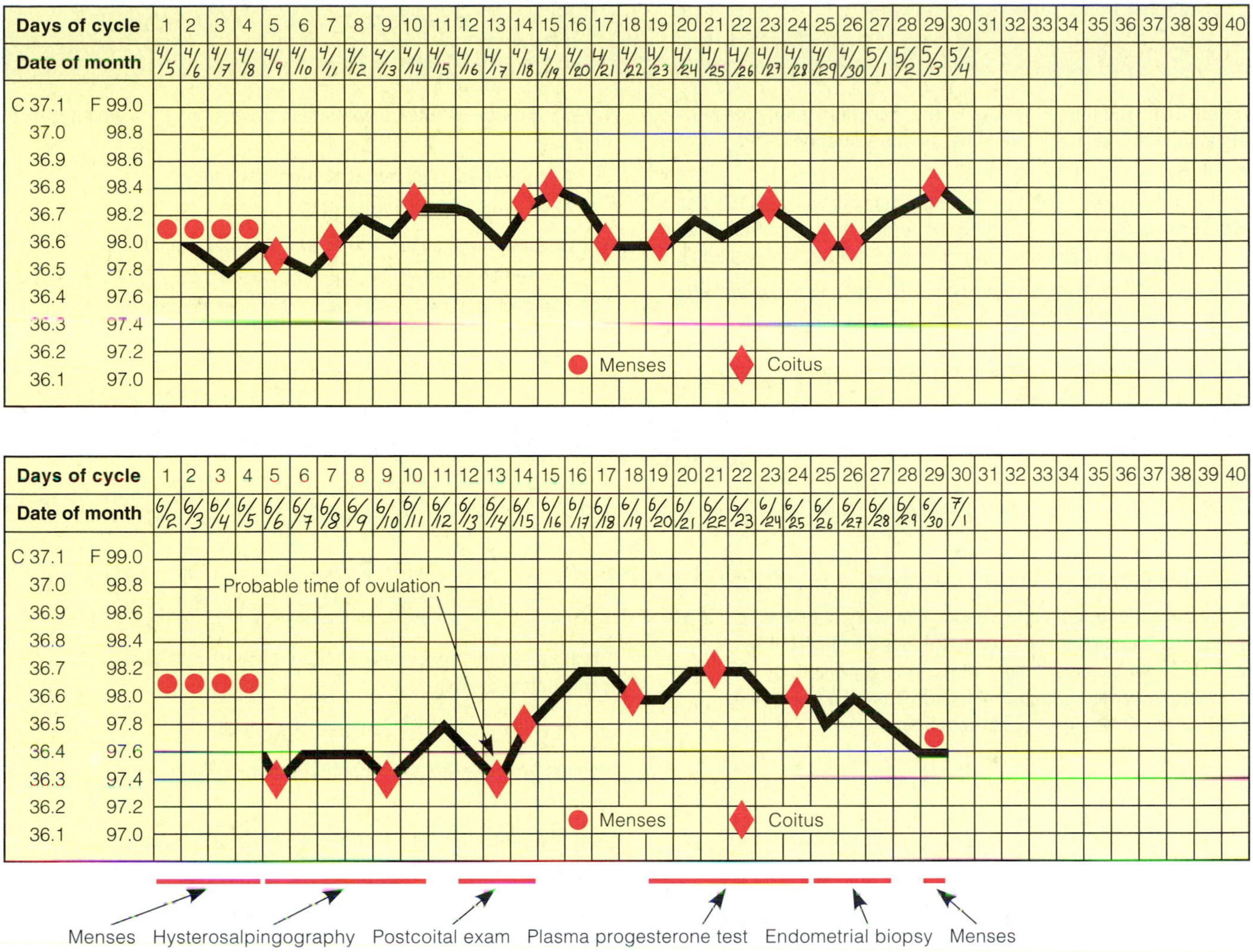

Figure 12–3 • *A,* A monophasic, anovulatory basal body temperature (BBT) chart. *B,* A biphasic BBT chart illustrating probable time of ovulation, the different types of testing, and the time in the cycle that each would be performed.

involves removing a sample of endometrium with a small pipette attached to suction (Cowan, 2002). The woman should be informed that some pelvic discomfort, cramping, and vaginal spotting is normal during and following the procedure. The onset of menses following biopsy should be reported for accurate interpretation of the biopsy report.

A dysfunction may exist if the endometrial lining does not show the expected amount of secretory tissue for that day of the woman's menstrual cycle. A repeat biopsy is indicated to confirm luteal phase dysfunction. Serum progesterone levels may also be used in conjunction with endometrial biopsy to confirm adequate luteal phase function.

Transvaginal Ultrasound

Transvaginal ultrasound is an invaluable adjunct in diagnosis and treatment of infertility. It is the method of choice for follicular monitoring of women undergoing ovulation induction cycles, for timing ovulation for insemination and intercourse, for retrieving oocytes for in vitro fertilization (IVF), and for monitoring early pregnancy.

The use of transvaginal color flow Doppler to investigate uterine blood flow may in the future help the endocrinologist evaluate the adequacy of the developing follicle, further assessing oocyte maturity and endometrial development and patterns, and improve the diagnosis of luteal phase defect (Widrich, 2002).

EVALUATION OF CERVICAL FACTORS

The mucus cells of the endocervix consist predominantly of water. As ovulation approaches, the ovary increases its secretion of estrogen and produces changes in the cervical mucus. The amount of mucus increases tenfold, and the water content rises significantly. At ovulation, mucus elasticity, or **spinnbarkheit,** increases, and the viscosity decreases. Excellent spinnbarkheit exists when the mucus can be stretched 8 to 10 cm or longer. Mucus elasticity is determined by using two

Client Teaching — Methods of Determining Ovulation

Assessment The nurse focuses on the woman's knowledge and beliefs about her own body functions, mucus secretions, and menstrual cycle.

Nursing Diagnosis The key nursing diagnosis will probably be ***Health-Seeking Behaviors:*** Methods of determining ovulation related to a desire to plan a pregnancy (or to practice natural family planning)

Nursing Plan and Implementation The teaching plan includes information on expected changes in cervical mucus and body temperature related to menstrual cycle, how to recognize that ovulation has occurred, and self-care methods for determining fertility days.

Client Goals At the completion of the teaching the woman will be able to

1. Accurately identify cervical mucus changes.
2. Accurately take and record BBT.
3. Discuss the changes in BBT and cervical mucus that indicate ovulation has occurred.
4. Summarize physical symptoms that may indicate ovulation has occurred.

Teaching Plan

CONTENT	TEACHING METHOD
Basal Body Temperature (BBT) Method	
Describe the expected findings with an ovulatory (biphasic) cycle and stress the need to monitor BBT for 3 to 4 months to establish a pattern. BBT can be used to time intercourse if pregnancy is desired or as a method of natural family planning. Describe the timing of intercourse to achieve or avoid pregnancy.	Choose a private location, free of distractions for the discussion. Create a supportive, comfortable atmosphere by attitude and communication style. *Briefly* explain why BBT can predict ovulation. Use pictures or graphs to demonstrate the BBT changes that indicate ovulatory and ovulatory cycles. Learning is best accomplished when content is broken down into smaller steps.
Describe the procedure for measuring BBT: • Using a BBT thermometer, the woman chooses one site (oral, vaginal, or rectal), which she uses consistently. • The woman takes her temperature for 5 minutes every day before arising and before starting any activity, including smoking. • The result is then recorded immediately on a BBT chart, and the temperature dots for each day are connected to form a graph. • She then shakes the thermometer down in preparation for use the next day.	Show the woman the BBT thermometer and demonstrate its use. *Note:* A tympanic (ear) electric thermometer may also be used. Provide a blank chart. Ask the woman to chart 3 days' findings using temperature results you identify.
Explain that certain situations can disturb body temperature such as large alcohol intake, sleeplessness, fever, warm climate, jet lag, shift work, or the use of an electric blanket.	Provide a handout summarizing the procedure. Provide frequent opportunities for questions and discussion.
Cervical Mucus Method	
Explain that cervical mucus changes throughout a woman's menstrual cycle and that the quality of the mucus can be used to predict ovulation. Describe the various characteristics of the cervical mucus throughout the menstrual cycle. Stress that it may take several cycles for the woman to become familiar with the pattern.	Discuss the characteristics of the mucus and the rationale for the changes. Explore the woman's feelings about using the procedure.
Describe the procedure for assessing cervical mucus changes: • Every day when she uses the bathroom the woman checks her vagina, either by dabbing the vaginal opening with toilet paper or by putting a finger in the opening.	Show pictures of the mucus changes including spinnbarkheit of different degrees of elasticity. Encourage the woman to ask questions.

Client Teaching METHODS OF DETERMINING OVULATION *(continued)*

- She notes the wetness (presence of mucus), collects some mucus, determines its color and consistency, and records her findings on a chart.
- She washes her hands before and after the procedure.

Stress that the presence and consistency of the mucus are altered by vaginal infection, vaginal medications, spermicides, lubricants, douching, sexual arousal, and semen.

Provide a written handout describing the process and findings so that the woman has information readily available.

EVALUATION

Evaluate the learning by providing time for discussion, questions, and practice using the charts and thermometer. Ask the woman to describe the selected procedure in her own words.

glass slides (Figure 12–4 •, *A*) or by grasping some mucus at the external os and stretching it in the vagina toward the introitus. (See Client Teaching: Methods of Determining Ovulation.)

The **ferning capacity** (crystallization) (Figure 12–4, *B*) of the cervical mucus also increases as ovulation approaches. Ferning is caused by decreased levels of salt and water interacting with the glycoproteins in the mucus during the ovulatory period and is thus an indirect indication of estrogen production. To test for ferning, mucus from the cervical os is spread on a glass slide, allowed to air dry, and then examined under the microscope. Within 24 to 48 hours postovulation, rising levels of progesterone cause a marked decrease in the quantity of cervical mucus and an increase in viscosity and cellularity, resulting in absence of spinnbarkheit and ferning capacity and consequently sperm survival.

To be receptive to sperm, cervical mucus must be thin, clear, watery, profuse, alkaline, and acellular. As shown in

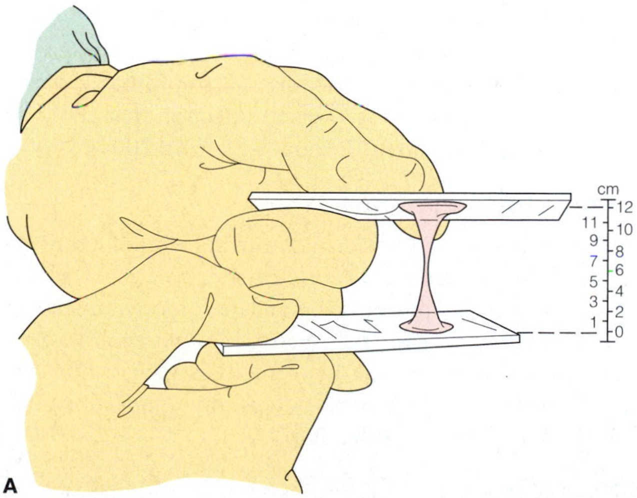

A

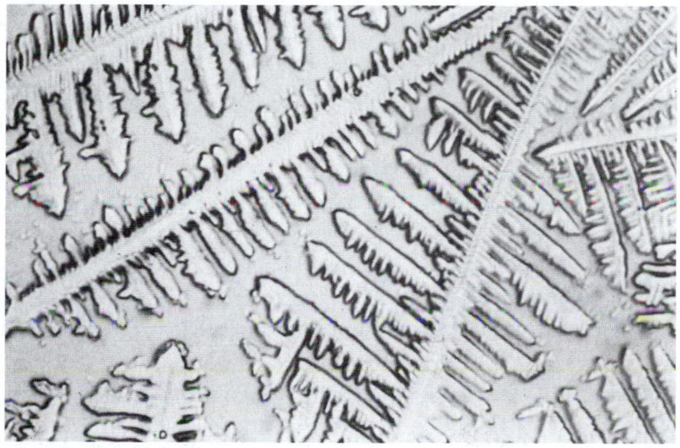

B

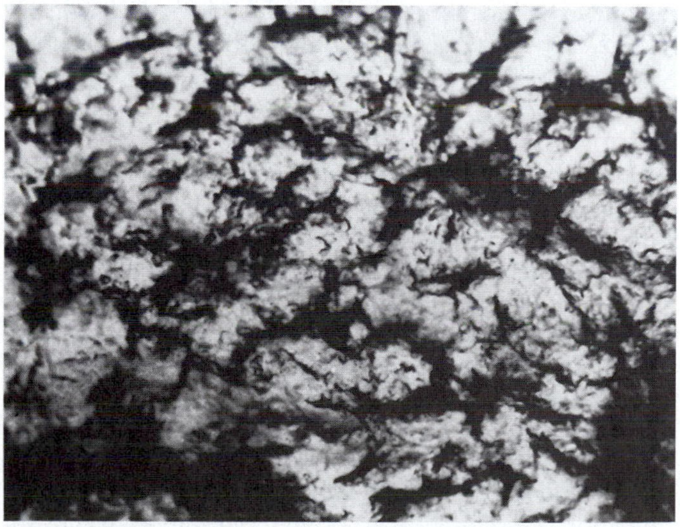

C

Figure 12–4 • *A,* Spinnbarkheit (elasticity). *B,* Ferning pattern. *C,* Lack of ferning pattern.
SOURCE: Speroff, L. et al. (1994). *Clinical gynecologic endocrinology and infertility* (5th ed., p. 818). Baltimore, MD: Williams & Wilkins.

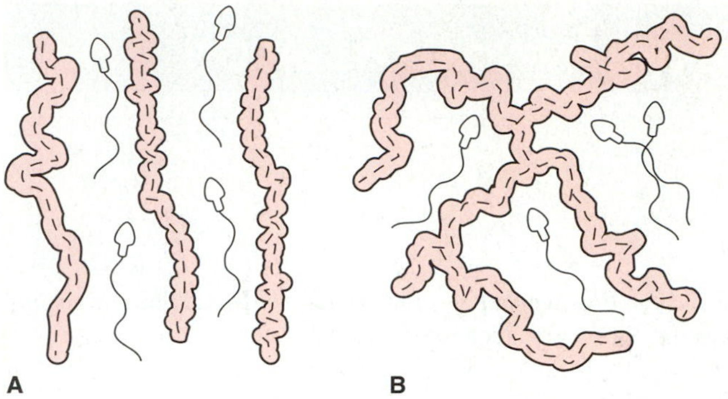

Figure 12–5 • Sperm passage through cervical mucus. *A*, Appearance at the time of ovulation with channels favoring efficient sperm penetration and migration upward. *B*, Unfavorable mazelike configuration found at other times of the menstrual cycle.
SOURCE: Corson, S. (1990). *Conquering infertility* (p. 16). A guide for couples (4th ed.). Vancouver, BC: EMIS-Canada.

Figure 12–5 •, the mazelike microscopic mucoid strands align in a parallel manner to allow for easy sperm passage. The mucus is termed *inhospitable* if these changes do not occur.

Cervical mucus inhospitable to sperm survival can have several causes, some of which are treatable. For example, estrogen secretion may be inadequate for the development of receptive mucus. Cervical infection, another cause of mucosal hostility to sperm, can be treated, depending on the type of infection. Cone biopsy, electrocautery, or cryosurgery of the cervix may remove large numbers of mucus-producing glands, creating a "dry cervix" that decreases sperm survival. Finally, treatment with clomiphene citrate may have deleterious effects on cervical mucus due to its antiestrogenic properties. Therapy with supplemental estrogen for approximately 6 days before expected ovulation is sometimes employed to encourage formation of suitable spinnbarkheit. However, intrauterine insemination (IUI) is more often the most appropriate therapy to overcome these obstacles. Profuse mucus is necessary for a hospitable sperm environment.

The cervix can also be the site of secretory immunologic reactions in which antisperm antibodies are produced, causing agglutination or immobilization of sperm. The most widely used serum sperm bioassay to detect specific classes of antibodies in serum and seminal fluid is direct immunobead testing (IBT) (Spear, 2002). The treatment for antisperm antibodies may include IUI of the male's washed sperm to bypass the cervical factor.

The *postcoital test (PCT)*, also called the **Huhner test,** is performed 1 or 2 days before the expected date of ovulation as determined by previous BBT charts, the length of prior cycles, or urinary LH kit. This examination evaluates the cervical mucus, sperm motility, sperm-mucus interaction, and the sperm's ability to negotiate the cervical mucus barrier.

The couple can have intercourse 2 to 8 hours before examination (Gordon & Speroff, 2002). If the results are abnormal, the test should be repeated at the optimal time of 2 to 3 hours after intercourse. A small plastic catheter attached to a 10-mL syringe is placed in the cervix. Mucus is aspirated from the endocervical canal, measured, and examined microscopically for signs of infection, spinnbarkheit, ferning, number of active spermatozoa per high-power field (HPF), and number of sperm with poor or no motility. The focus of the postcoital exam is on the timing of intercourse and may promote sexual difficulties for some infertile couples.

EVALUATION OF UTERINE STRUCTURES AND TUBAL PATENCY

Tubal patency tests are usually done after BBT evaluation, semen analysis, and the other less invasive tests. Tubal patency and uterine structure are usually evaluated by hysterosalpingography. Other invasive tests of the tubes' function are laparoscopy and hysteroscopy. Hysteroscopy may be performed earlier in the evaluation if the woman's history suggests the potential for tubal or adhesive disease or uterine abnormalities.

Hysterosalpingography

Hysterosalpingography (HSG), or hysterogram, involves an instillation of a radiopaque substance into the uterine cavity. As the substance fills the uterus and fallopian tubes and spills into the peritoneal cavity, it is viewed with x-ray techniques. This procedure can reveal tubal patency and any distortions of the uterine cavity. In addition, the water-based dye used in HSG may have a therapeutic effect. This effect may be caused by the flushing of debris, breaking of adhesions, or induction of peristalsis by the instillation.

The hysterosalpingogram should be performed in the follicular phase of the cycle to avoid interrupting an early pregnancy. This timing also avoids the lush secretory changes in the endometrium that occur after ovulation, which may prevent the passage of the dye through the tubes and present a false picture of cornual obstruction. HSG causes moderate discomfort. The pain is referred from the peritoneum (which is irritated by the subdiaphragmatic collection of gas) to the shoulder. The cramping may be decreased if the radiopaque dye is warmed to body temperature before instillation. Women can take an over-the-counter prostaglandin synthesis inhibitor (such as ibuprofen) 30 minutes prior to the procedure to decrease the pain, cramping, and discomfort. HSG can also cause serious recurrence of pelvic inflammatory disease, so prophylactic antibiotics are recommended to prevent infection that could be triggered by the procedure (Gordon & Speroff, 2002).

Hysteroscopy

Hysteroscopy allows the physician to further evaluate any areas of suspicion within the uterine cavity revealed by HSG. It is often done in conjunction with a laparoscopy but can be done independently in the office and does not require general anesthesia. A fiberoptic instrument is placed into the uterus for further evaluation of polyps, myomata (fibroids), or structural variations (Valle, 2002).

Laparoscopy

Laparoscopy enables direct visualization of the pelvic organs and is usually done 6 to 8 months after HSG unless symptoms or findings suggest the need for earlier evaluation. Diagnostic laparoscopy is an outpatient procedure requiring the use of general anesthesia. Generally, a three-puncture approach is used; entry is made through the umbilical area, and supporting instruments are inserted in two suprapubic incisions. The peritoneal cavity is distended with carbon dioxide gas, and the pelvic organs can be directly visualized with a fiberoptic instrument. Tube patency can be assessed by instilling dye into the uterine cavity through the cervix. The pelvis is evaluated for endometriosis, adhesions, organ fixations, pelvic inflammatory disease, tumors, and cysts. The intraperitoneal gas is usually manually expressed at the end of the procedure. In routine preanesthesia instructions, the woman is told that she may have some discomfort from organ displacement and shoulder to chest pain caused by gas in the abdomen. She should be informed that she can resume normal activities as tolerated after 24 hours. Using postoperative pain medication and assuming a supine position may help relieve residual shoulder and chest discomfort caused by any remaining gas.

Tests of the Man's Fertility

The semen analysis is the single most important diagnostic study of the man. It should be done early in the couple's evaluation and prior to invasive testing of the woman. Although a postcoital test can provide information about sperm viability, it does not provide sufficient information concerning normal seminal parameters.

To obtain accurate results, the specimen is collected after 2 to 3 days of abstinence and usually by masturbation to avoid contamination or loss of any ejaculate. If the man has difficulty producing sperm by masturbation, special medical grade condoms are available to collect the sperm during intercourse. Regular or nonlatex condoms should not be used because they contain spermicidal agents, and sperm can be lost in the condom. Most lubricants also are spermicidal and should not be used unless approved by the andrology laboratory. There may be seasonal as well as incidental variability in count and motility seen in successive semen samples from the same individual. Thus, a repeat semen analysis may be required to assess the man's fertility potential adequately; a minimum of two separate analyses is recommended for confirmation. In the case where a known testicular insult has occurred, such as infection, high fevers, or surgery, a repeat analysis may not be done for at least 2.5 months to allow for new sperm maturation.

Semen analysis provides information about sperm motility and morphology as well as a determination of the absolute number of spermatozoa present (Table 12–5 •). Although it is known that low numbers and motility may indicate compromised fertility, other parameters such as morphology, motion patterns, and progression are important prognostic indicators. Values previously thought to indicate subfertility may in fact be compatible with normal fertility when these factors are considered. An infertile specimen is one that reveals fewer than 20 million sperm per mL, less than 50% motility at 6 hours, or less than 30% normal sperm forms.

Table 12–5 • NORMAL SEMEN ANALYSIS

Factor	Value
Volume	$>$ 2 mL
pH	7 to 8
Total sperm count	$>$ 20 million m/L
Liquefaction	Complete in 1 hour
Motility	50% or greater forward progression
Normal forms	30% or greater
Round cells	$<$ 5 million/mL
White cells	$<$ 1 million/mL

Source: Carson, S. L. (1998). *Conquering infertility: A guide for couples* (4th ed.). Vancouver, BC: EMIS-Canada.

Some studies have indicated that the quality of sperm decreases with increased age. Infants born to 50- to 60-year-old fathers are at risk for trisomy 21 (Gordon & Speroff, 2002).

A variety of environmental factors can affect male fertility. Causes of increased scrotal heat, such as jockey shorts, hot tubs, or occupations requiring long hours of sitting, are thought to decrease fertility potential, but there are no clinical studies to substantiate this belief. Heavy use of marijuana, alcohol, or cocaine within 2 years of testing can depress sperm count and testosterone levels; cigarette smoking may depress sperm motility. Neurologic ejaculatory dysfunction can be caused by alpha blockers, phentolamine, methyldopa, guanethidine, and reserpine. Lead and pesticide exposure can also reduce sperm count (Gordon & Speroff, 2002).

Spermatozoa have been shown to possess intrinsic antigens that can provoke male immunologic infertility. This is especially apparent following vasectomy reversals or genital trauma, such as testicular torsion, in which autoimmunity to sperm develops (the man produces antibodies to his own sperm). Research now indicates that it is the actual presence of antibodies on the spermatozoal surface, not just the presence of antibodies in the serum, that affects sperm function and thus leads to subfertility. Treatment for antisperm antibodies is directed toward preventing the formation of antibodies or arresting the underlying mechanism that compromises sperm function. Therapies such as immunosuppression with corticosteroids and IUI have not proved effective. The treatment of choice for clinically significant antisperm antibodies is IVF and IUI (Spear, 2002).

Tests such as the hamster sperm penetration assay (SPA), hemizona (HZA), acrosome reaction assay, and sperm density evaluation may be performed, but their usefulness is controversial. If the man's history indicates, he may be referred to a urologist for further testing.

Methods of Managing Infertility

Methods of managing infertility include pharmacologic agents, therapeutic insemination, in vitro fertilization, and other assisted reproductive techniques. In addition, many couples choose adoption as their preferred response to infertility.

Table 12–6 • DRUGS COMMONLY USED TO TREAT INFERTILITY

Drugs	Indications: Women	Indications: Men
Clomiphene citrate (Clomid, Serophene)	Polycystic ovarian disease (3 days, beginning day 5 of bleeding) Hyperandrogenemia (with no neoplasia) Premature follicular rupture	Low levels of gonadotropins Hypothalamic hypogonadism
Bromocriptine mesylate (Parlodel)	Hyperprolactinemia (functional or pituitary adenoma)	Hyperprolactinemia (functional or pituitary adenoma)
Progesterone	Luteal phase dysfunction	
hMG, menotropins (FSH and LH) (Pergonal) with hCG	Hypothalamic ovulatory dysfunction (after failure of clomiphene) Hypopituitarism Polycystic ovarian disease (rarely) Luteinized unruptured follicle syndrome (after failure of hCG alone) Inadequate cervical mucus In vitro fertilization, GIFT, ZIFT Controlled superovulation	Hypothalamic-pituitary failure due to Kallmann syndrome or delayed puberty Hypogonadotropic hypogonadism (deficiency of FSH and LH)
hCG	Luteinized unruptured follicle syndrome Induction of ovulation	
FSH, urofollitropin (Metrodin) with hCG	Polycystic ovarian disease	
C,FSH, follitropin (Gonal-F, Follistim) with hCG	In vitro fertilization, GIFT, ZIFT	
GnRH (Factrel)	Hypothalamic ovulatory dysfunction (pulsed infusion)	Hypothalamic-pituitary failure due to Kallmann syndrome or delayed puberty (pulsed infusion)
GnRH agonist Leuprolide acetate (Lupron) Nafarelin acetate (Synarel)	Endometriosis Premature follicular rupture In vitro fertilization, GIFT, ZIFT	Hypogonadotropic gonadism

Source: Adapted from Shane, J. (1993). Evaluation and treatment of infertility. *Clinical Symposia, 45*, 2.

PHARMACOLOGIC AGENTS

The pharmacologic treatment chosen depends on the specific cause of the infertility. Table 12–6 • lists some of the drugs commonly used and indications for use.

Clomiphene Citrate

In the presence of normal ovaries, a normal prolactin level, and an intact pituitary gland, *clomiphene citrate* (Clomid, Serophene) is often used. See Drug Guide: Clomiphene Citrate. Clomiphene citrate acts by competing with estrogen receptor sites at the level of the hypothalamus, the pituitary, and the ovary, thus increasing secretion of FSH and LH, which stimulates follicular growth. This medication induces ovulation in 80% of women by actions at both the hypothalamic and ovarian levels; 40% of these women will become pregnant. Approximately 8% of women develop multiple gestation pregnancies, almost exclusively twins (Usadi & Fritz, 2002).

The woman is informed that if ovulation occurs, it is expected to occur 5 to 9 days after the last dose. The presence of ovulation and evaluation of the response to therapy is assessed by BBT or urinary LH kit monitoring for in-home use, ultrasound evaluation, and possibly progesterone assays in conjunction with an endometrial biopsy.

After the first treatment cycle, a pelvic exam should be done to rule out ovarian enlargement or hyperstimulation. The risk of ovarian hyperstimulation is reported to be 10% but is rarely as severe as that reported with menotropins (gonadotropin therapy, discussed shortly). Ovarian enlargement and abdominal discomfort (bloating) may result from follicular growth and the formation of multiple corpus lutea. Persistence of ovarian cysts is a contraindication for subsequent treatment cycles. Other side effects include hot flashes, abdominal distention, bloating, breast discomfort, nausea and vomiting, vision problems, headache, and dryness or loss of hair (Usadi & Fritz, 2002). Some women experience severe mood swings (Bambi-Hitler syndrome). Supplemental low-dose estrogen may be given to ensure appropriate quality and quantity of cervical mucus, or IUI may be employed to overcome this obstacle.

The nurse determines if the couple has been advised to have sexual intercourse every other day for 1 week beginning 5 days after the last day of medications. The nurse also reminds couples that if the woman doesn't have a period she must be checked for pregnancy before another trial of clomiphene is started.

Women can assess the presence of ovulation and possible response to clomiphene therapy by doing BBT and urinary LH tests. The woman should be knowledgeable about side effects and call her healthcare provider if they occur. When visual disturbances (flashes, blurring, spots) occur, the woman should avoid bright lighting. This side effect disappears within a few days or weeks after discontinuation of therapy (Gordon & Speroff, 2002). The occurrence of hot

DRUG GUIDE Clomiphene Citrate (Clomid, Serophene)

• Overview of Action

Clomiphene citrate stimulates follicular growth by stimulating the release of FSH and LH. Ovulation is expected to occur 5 to 9 days after last dose. Used when anovulation is caused by hypothalamic dysfunction, luteal phase dysfunction, or oligo-ovulation, and for in vitro fertilization protocols.

• Route, Dosage, Frequency

Administered orally. Fifty mg/day from cycle day 3 to day 7 or day 5 to day 9 then for 5 consecutive days of the menstrual cycle. Usually start with 50 mg/day and increase dose 50 mg if no response, to a maximum of 250 mg (Usadi & Fritz, 2002). May need to give estrogen simultaneously if decrease in cervical mucus occurs.

• Contraindications

Presence of ovarian enlargement, ovarian cysts, hyperstimulation syndrome, liver disease, visual problems, pregnancy.

• Side Effects

Antiestrogenic effects may cause decrease in cervical mucus production and endometrial lining development. Other side effects include vasomotor flushes; abdominal distention and ovarian enlargement secondary to follicular growth and development and multiple corpus luteum formation; bloating, pain, soreness, breast discomfort; nausea and vomiting; visual symptoms (spots, flashes); headaches, dryness or loss of hair; multiple pregnancies.

• Nursing Considerations

Determine if couple has been advised to have sexual intercourse every other day for 1 week beginning 5 days after the last day of medications.

Instruct couple on use of BBT chart to assess whether ovulation has occurred, or instruct on the use of urinary LH kits to predict the onset of LH surge. Also inform couple that plasma progesterone, cervical mucus, and postcoital test may be done. Remind couples that if the woman doesn't have a period, she must be checked for the possibility of pregnancy before another trial of clomiphene citrate is started.

flashes may be due to the antiestrogenic properties of clomiphene. The woman can obtain some relief through increasing intake of fluids and using fans.

Human Menopausal Gonadotropins

Therapy using *human menopausal gonadotropins (hMG)*, which include menotropins (Pergonal, Humegon, Repronex) and urofollitropin (Fertinex), is indicated as a first line of therapy for the anovulatory infertile woman with low to normal levels of gonadotropins (FSH and LH) and as a second line of therapy in women who fail to ovulate or conceive with clomiphene citrate therapy and in women undergoing assisted reproduction to induce superovulation. Menotropin is a mixture of FSH and LH, and urofollitropin is a further purified form and contains only FSH. Because hMG is inactive, it must be given by intramuscular injection. Immediately prior to injection, the powder is reconstituted with diluent. More recently, however, recombinant FSH has been produced through genetic engineering, giving rise to more consistent preparation. It has been approved by the Food and Drug Administration (FDA) for use where ovulation induction therapy is indicated. Recombinant FSH is homogenous and free of contaminants by proteins (unlike urinary menotropins) and thus allows for subcutaneous administration. It is marketed under the names Gonal-F (follitropin alpha) and Follistim (follitropin beta). Current investigations using recombinant LH are being tested and are expected to be FDA approved for clinical use in the near future. It is thought that the use of recombinant gonadotropins will eventually become the preferred preparation and that the use of urinary preparations will be phased out.

Normal functioning of the pituitary is not necessary with menotropins or urofollitropin because their mechanisms of action are direct stimulation of follicular development in the ovary, thus totally bypassing the hypothalamic-pituitary axis. However, normal ovarian reserve and functioning are necessary to ensure that follicles can be stimulated by FSH and LH. As previously described, the single most valuable test to assess ovarian reserve and function is the FSH level, with elevated levels being a poor prognostic sign for conception and pregnancy.

Menotropins (FSH, LH) are the primary preparations used for therapy. Urofollitropin (FSH only) is indicated for women who have excessive androgen production, such as those with polycystic ovary disease (PCO). Clients with PCO have high endogenous LH levels. Urofollitropin, which is predominantly FSH, is used to equalize the hormonal ratio and induce ovulation.

Gonadotropin therapy requires close observation with serum estradiol levels and ultrasound. Follicle development must be monitored to minimize the risk of multiple pregnancy and to avoid ovarian hyperstimulation syndrome. The daily dose of medication given is titrated based on serum estradiol and ultrasound findings. Then once follicle maturation has occurred, human chorionic gonadotropin (hCG) may be administered by intramuscular injection to stimulate ovulation. The couple is advised to have intercourse 24 to 36 hours after hCG administration and for the next 2 days. Women who elect to have hMG medication usually have passed through all other forms of management without conceiving. Strong emotional support and thorough education are needed because of the numerous office visits and injections. Often the male partner is instructed, with return demonstration, to administer the daily injections (Leibowitz & Hoffman, 2000).

Bromocriptine

High prolactin levels may impair production of FSH and LH or block their action on the ovaries. When hyperprolactinemia accompanies anovulation, the infertility may be treated with bromocriptine. This medication acts directly on the prolactin-secreting cells in the anterior pituitary. It inhibits the pituitary's secretion of prolactin—thus preventing suppression of the pulsatile secretion of FSH and LH. This restores normal menstrual cycles and induces ovulation by allowing FSH and LH production. If treatment is successful, the tests of ovulatory function will indicate that ovulation is occurring with a normal luteal phase. Bromocriptine should be discontinued if pregnancy is suspected or at the anticipated time of ovulation because of its possible teratogenic effects. Other side effects, which include nausea, diarrhea, dizziness, headache, and fatigue, can be attributed to the dopaminergic action of bromocriptine. To mimimize side effects for women who are extremely sensitive, treatment may be initiated with a dose of 1.25 mg, slowly building tolerance toward the usual dose of 2.5 mg bid. Intravaginal administration also has been shown to decrease the occurrence of side effects.

Danazol

When endometriosis is determined to be the cause of the infertility, *danazol* (Danocrine) may be given to suppress ovulation and menstruation and to effect atrophy of the ectopic endometrial tissue. Temporary suppression has been shown to result in healing of the endometriosis. The treatment regimen may last for 6 to 12 months or longer, depending on the severity of the disease. Other pharmacologic treatments involve use of the oral contraceptives or oral medroxyprogesterone acetate, and gonadotropin-releasing hormone (GnRH) agonists (Leibowitz & Hoffman, 2000). For in-depth discussion of the management and care needed for endometriosis, see Chapter 7.

Other Pharmacologic Agents

Gonadotropin-releasing hormone (GnRH) is a therapeutic tool for inducing ovulation, but its use is limited to women who have insufficient endogenous release of GnRH. Administration is usually by continuous intravenous infusion accomplished by a portable infusion pump with a pulsatile mechanism worn on a belt around the waist. The length of treatment varies from 2 to 4 weeks, and hCG is also given to stimulate ovulation. The risk of multiple gestation and hyperstimulation of the ovaries is less than with hMG therapy, and the treatment is also less expensive (Gordon & Speroff, 2002). Significant client education and support are necessary for effective use of the pump. Some women find the pump cumbersome.

Treatment of luteal phase defects may include the use of progesterone to augment luteal phase progesterone levels or the use of ovulation induction agents, such as clomiphene citrate or menotropins (discussed previously), which will augment proliferative phase FSH production of the developing follicle. Women with luteal phase defects have been found to have decreased FSH production in the proliferative phase. This is associated with a decline in luteal phase progesterone and estrogen production and is manifested by an out-of-phase endometrial biopsy. It is also common to use progesterone supplementation in conjunction with these ovulation induction agents if the drug alone does not correct the luteal phase. Occasionally, hCG therapy may be used in the luteal phase to stimulate corpus luteum production of progesterone.

THERAPEUTIC INSEMINATION

The term **therapeutic insemination** has replaced the previously used term *artificial insemination.* The procedure involves depositing sperm at the cervical os or in the uterus by mechanical means. *Therapeutic donor insemination (TDI)* is the current term for use of donor semen, and *therapeutic husband insemination (THI)* is the current term for use of the husband's semen.

THI is generally indicated for such seminal deficiencies as oligospermia (low sperm count), asthenospermia (decreased motility), and teratospermia (low percentage, abnormal morphology); for anatomic defects that are accompanied by inadequate deposition of sperm, such as hypospadias (a congenital abnormal male urethral opening on the underside of the penis); and for ejaculatory dysfunction, such as retrograde ejaculation.

THI is also indicated in unexplained infertility and some cases of female factor infertility, specifically infertility due to cervical factors, such as scant or inhospitable mucus, persistent cervicitis, or cervical stenosis. In such cases, *intrauterine insemination (IUI)* would be indicated in order to bypass the cervical factor. Because the seminal fluid contains high levels of prostaglandins, IUI prevents the violent reaction of nausea, severe cramps, abdominal pain, and diarrhea that can result from the absorption of prostaglandins by the cervical lining. Sperm preparation for IUI involves washing sperm from the seminal plasma. IUI, with or without ovulation induction therapy, is an option for many couples before more aggressive treatments such as in vitro fertilization are employed.

TDI is considered in cases of azoospermia (absence of sperm), severe oligospermia or asthenospermia, inherited male sex-linked disorders, and autosomal dominant disorders (Gordon & Speroff, 2002). In the past several years, indications for donor insemination have expanded to include single women or lesbians desirous of pregnancy. Some states have specified the parental rights of the single woman and the donor, but most are silent on this issue.

Intracytoplasmic sperm injection (ICSI), microsurgical epididymal sperm aspiration (MESA), and testicular sperm aspiration (TESA) are procedures that address severe male factor infertility. ICSI is a microscopic procedure to inject a single sperm into the outer layer of an ovum so that fertilization will occur. MESA and TESA involve the retrieval of sperm from the gonadal tissue of men who have azoospermia or an ejaculatory disorder.

TDI has become more complicated and expensive in the last decade because of the need for strict screening and processing procedures to prevent transmission of a genetic defect or sexually transmitted infection to the offspring or recipient. Guidelines established by the American Fertility Society (1994) include mandatory medical and infectious disease screening of both the donor and recipient, the need for informed consent from all parties, the need to limit the number of pregnancies per donor, and the need to establish an accurate means of record keeping. Finally, because of the risk of transmitting infectious disease, donated sperm must be frozen and quarantined for 6 months from the time of acquisition and the donor must be retested before sperm can be released for use.

Numerous factors must be evaluated before TDI is performed. Has every possible effort been made to diagnose and treat the cause of the male infertility? Do tests indicate normal ovulation and sperm/ovum transport in the woman? Has the couple had an opportunity to discuss this option with an infertility counselor to explore the issues of secrecy, disclosure, and potential feelings of loss that the couple (particularly the male partner) may feel because of their inability to have a genetic child? After making the decision, the couple should allow themselves time to assess their concerns further and explore their feelings individually and together to ensure that this option is acceptable to both.

IN VITRO FERTILIZATION

In vitro fertilization (IVF) is selectively used in cases in which infertility has resulted from tubal factors, mucus abnormalities, male infertility, unexplained infertility, male and female immunologic infertility, and cervical factors. In IVF, a woman's eggs are collected from her ovaries, fertilized in the laboratory, and placed into her uterus after normal embryo development has begun. If the procedure is successful, the embryo continues to develop in the uterus, and pregnancy proceeds naturally.

The potential for a successful pregnancy with IVF is maximized by replacing three to four embryos (rather than one). For this reason, fertility drugs are used to induce ovulation. Follicular development and oocyte maturity are monitored frequently with ultrasound and hormonal assays. Monitoring usually begins around cycle day 5, and medications are titrated according to individual response. When the follicles appear mature, hCG is given to stimulate final egg maturation and control the induction of ovulation. Egg retrieval is performed approximately 35 hours later.

In the majority of cases, egg retrieval is performed by a transvaginal approach under ultrasound guidance. It is an outpatient procedure performed with intravenous sedation and a cervical block for anesthesia. A needle guide that helps direct the aspirating needle through the posterior vaginal wall into the follicle is attached to the vaginal ultrasound probe. Many follicles can be aspirated with only one puncture, and the procedure generally lasts no more than 30 minutes. The woman usually tolerates the procedure well and is discharged to home within 2 hours with instructions for limited activity for 24 hours.

Once the eggs are fertilized and progress to the embryo stage, the embryos are placed in the uterus. After the procedure, the woman is advised to engage in only minimal activity for 12 to 24 hours, and progesterone supplementation is prescribed.

Success with IVF depends on many factors, the two most important of which are the woman's age and the indication. Women with an average of three cycles of IVF have a good chance of achieving pregnancy. Many couples find the emotional, physical, and financial costs of going beyond three cycles too great. Clinical delivery rates reported by the Society of Assisted Reproductive Technology (SART) in 1999 were 31.1% per embryo transfer for women regardless of age or indication (American Society for Reproductive Medicine, 2002). The increase in maternal and neonatal morbidity associated with IVF because of the multiple gestation rates remains an issue. Differences in successful IVF may exist between various ethnic groups (Sharara & McClamrock, 2000).

OTHER ASSISTED REPRODUCTIVE TECHNIQUES

Other assisted reproductive techniques include procedures for transferring gametes, zygotes, or embryos; cryopreservation of embryos; IVF using donor oocytes; micromanipulation techniques; and use of a gestational carrier (Kingsberg, Applegarth, & Janata, 2000).

Gamete Intrafallopian Transfer

Gamete intrafallopian transfer (GIFT) involves the retrieval of oocytes by laparoscopy; immediate placement of the oocytes in a catheter with washed, motile sperm; and placement of the gametes into the fimbriated end of the fallopian tube. Fertilization occurs in the fallopian tube as with normal conception (in vivo), rather than in the laboratory (in vitro). The fertilized egg then travels through the fallopian tube to the uterus for implantation as in normal reproduction. This practice is acceptable to the Roman Catholic Church.

GIFT has proven to be a very effective therapy for couples whose infertility results from various seminal deficiencies, unexplained factors, cervical factors, immunologic factors, and endometriosis when less aggressive means of therapy have failed. In cases of male factor infertility, GIFT offers an opportunity for the egg and an adequate concentration of sperm to meet in the fallopian tube; with coitus, in contrast, sperm with low count or motility may never reach the tube.

The major prerequisite for GIFT is the presence of at least one normal fallopian tube. It is not an appropriate therapy for any woman with a history of pelvic inflammatory disease, tubal disease, or ectopic gestation because the passage of the fertilized ova to the uterus is slowed, thereby increasing the chance of sustaining an ectopic tubal pregnancy.

From the GIFT technology evolved several other transfer procedures such as **zygote intrafallopian transfer (ZIFT)** and **tubal embryo transfer (TET).** In these procedures eggs are retrieved and incubated with the man's sperm. However, the eggs are transferred back to the woman's body at a much earlier stage of cell division than in IVF and, as in GIFT, are placed in the fallopian tube or tubes and not in the uterus. In TET, the placement is done at the embryo stage. These procedures allow fertilization to be documented, which is not possible with GIFT, and the pregnancy rate is theoretically increased when the fertilized ovum is placed in the fallopian tube. When considering IVF and the transfer procedures, several factors must be weighed. IVF success rates approximate those that have been achieved with the transfer procedures, and IVF is a much less invasive and costly procedure. For these reasons, the transfer procedures have lost some acceptance and IVF techniques are more often used. However, GIFT may be more acceptable to adherents of some religions, since fertilization does not occur outside the woman's body.

Embryo Cryopreservation

Research has shown that replacing three to four embryos in a treatment cycle offers the best chances for pregnancy. Replacing more than four only increases the chance for a multiple pregnancy. To minimize this risk, excess embryos may be stored using freezing, or cryopreservation. Should a pregnancy not ensue, frozen embryos can be thawed. After they are maintained in culture for a short time to confirm resumption of growth, they are replaced in the woman's uterus at the appropriate time in her menstrual cycle. Thus freezing affords the couple another attempt at pregnancy without having to undergo stimulation and egg retrieval again.

Ethical issues to consider in this situation include the following: Who has legal custody of the embryos? How long can they be frozen? What options do the couple have in the event of divorce, if one or both partners die, or if they do not wish to use the embryos at a later date? These issues must be addressed with all couples so that they may make informed decisions when executing their consent forms and legal statements. Perinatal nurses need to be involved in establishing standards and guidelines for assisted reproduction technologies. Clinically, the perinatal nurse is instrumental in providing support, education, and counseling to couples considering assisted reproductive methods. The nurse assesses the couple for personal, marital, and parenting difficulties and initiates interventions that help establish family roles and bonds. Follow-up care mechanisms can be set, thereby aiding in individual growth, marital stability, and family development.

In Vitro Fertilization Using Donor Oocytes

The use of donor eggs, a natural extension of IVF, is reserved for women who do not produce viable eggs because of premature ovarian failure, surgical removal of the ovaries, advanced maternal age, or inherent oocyte defects but who do have a functional uterus. Women with normal ovarian function may also benefit from egg donation if they have an autosomal dominant or sex-linked genetic disorder such as hemophilia or Duchenne muscular dystrophy.

Oocyte donors may be either known or anonymous. In either case, both donors and recipients undergo extensive psychologic evaluation and counseling to ensure that all parties have explored and discussed potential issues and are comfortable with the process. The nurse functions as a case manager by coordinating the many tests, procedures, and educational and counseling sessions that are involved for the donor and recipient couple.

Once donor eggs are available, they are inseminated with the sperm of the recipient's partner. After fertilization has occurred and embryo development has begun, the embryos are placed in the recipient's uterus. Pregnancies can be achieved and maintained in these women with an estrogen/progesterone replacement protocol. When pregnancy occurs, hormonal support is continued until the placenta is capable of supporting the pregnancy, usually at 10 to 12 weeks.

Micromanipulation and Blastomere Analysis

Micromanipulation allows individual eggs and sperm to be handled through the use of very fine, specialized instruments. Using the micromanipulators allows the clinician to handle cells under the microscope with magnification of 200 to 400 times and to inject a sperm cell directly into an egg. This procedure, known as intracytoplasmic sperm injection (ICSI), has revolutionized the treatment of severe male factor infertility. The procedure has achieved fertilization in cases of extremely low sperm concentrations, in cases of absence of motility, and in cases where previous IVF therapy failed.

Assisted embryo hatching is another micromanipulation procedure that has proved to be an effective adjunct therapy in IVF. It is indicated for women in whom the normal "hatching" process may be impeded because of a hardening or thickening of the zona pellucida. Assisted hatching involves creating a small opening in the zona pellucida of the embryo using micromanipulators. The small opening may facilitate the natural hatching process, allowing the embryo to escape from the zona pellucida and interact with the endometrium for implantation.

Other recent advances in micromanipulation allow a single cell to be removed from the embryo for genetic study. Couples at risk for having a detectable single gene or chromosomal anomaly may wish to undergo such preimplantation genetic testing, called *blastomere analysis*. The single cell is obtained from a six- to eight-cell embryo by a process known as blastomere biopsy (Gordon & Speroff, 2002). The genetic content of the cell is examined using the polymerase chain reaction (PCR) technique. The cell's DNA is amplified 1,000,000 times and examined so that embryos affected with genetic disease are not placed in the mother. Results of genetic testing on the preimplantation embryos are available in 4 to 24 hours, so unaffected embryos may still be placed during the required biologic window of time without the need for cryopreservation.

The diagnosis of genetic disorders before implantation provides couples with the option of forgoing the attempt to establish a pregnancy and thereby avoiding a difficult decision about terminating an affected pregnancy (Simpson, 2002a). This technology also raises several issues, including the following:

- Identification of couples at risk. There is a need for criteria that identify couples at risk for diseases that

RESEARCH IN PRACTICE
Disclosure Decisions of Parents Who Conceive Using Donor Eggs

What is this study about? The application of donor egg technology has allowed thousands of parents to conceive. The growth in this technology has often outpaced a critical examination of its impact on families and society. There is no generally accepted boundary for whether children conceived using donor egg technology should be informed about their origins. There is little to guide the practitioner in helping parents make decisions about disclosure. The purpose of this study was to identify the variables that influence the disclosure decision. The authors also compared the variables influencing those who make the decision to disclose with the variables influencing those who make a nondisclosure decision.

How was this study done? A mixed method was used for this descriptive study. A convenience sample included 48 couples who had conceived as a result of donor egg technology. A Disclosure Decision Interview Guide, developed by the authors, was used to interview the parents. The Family Environment Scale was used to assess parental perceptions of the current family environment; the Social Support Appraisals Scale was used to explore social support. Both family environment and social support were hypothesized to be variables in the disclosure decision. Additional data were collected on demographics that might influence the disclosure decision. Surveys were mailed to participants, and interviews were conducted with those who returned surveys. At least one parent participated from each of 31 families that completed the study.

What were the results of the study? All of the parents identified the disclosure decision as a difficult one. The majority of these parents reported that they intended disclosure. Themes that emerged from these parents included beliefs that a child has a right to know and concerns that secrets in families lead to dysfunction. Parents that did not intend to disclose generated themes of knowing no compelling reason to disclose and perceived potential harm to the family. Some parents were undecided, focusing on concerns about timing of the disclosure and concerns about the child's possible reaction.

What additional questions might I have? Can we determine the impact on children of the disclose/nondisclose decision? How do parents feel about their decision after they have actually acted upon it? Do these parents have similar responses as families in other situations (eg, adoptions) that require a disclosure decision?

How can I use this study? Parents who use donor egg technology often look to healthcare professionals to guide the many decisions that accompany this experience. The nurse can help parents consider the implications of the disclosure decision and suggest strategies for living with their choices.

Source: Hahn, S., & Craft-Rosenberg, J. (2002). The disclosure decisions of parents who conceive children using donor eggs. *Journal of Obstetric, Gynecologic, and Neonatal Nursing, 31*(3), 283–293.

constitute significant hardship and suffering so that "wrongful birth" cases can be avoided.

- Availability of and access to centers providing blastomere analysis. Should society provide access for those at risk for genetic transfer of disease but without the financial resources to pay for the services?
- Analysis of blastomeres for sex gene testing when a genetic disorder carried on the sex chromosomes is suspected. In X-linked diseases, the only way to prevent the disorder is to select against the blastomere with the Y chromosome.
- Identification of late-onset diseases. The Human Genome Project has aided in the identification of genetic markers for late-onset disease. Couples may wish to choose to implant blastomeres that do not carry these markers.

In Vitro Fertilization Using a Gestational Carrier

A *gestational carrier* is a woman who has contracted with the infertile woman or couple to carry an embryo/fetus that is not genetically her own offspring. This must be distinguished from surrogate motherhood, wherein the gestational mother makes a genetic contribution to the child.

IVF using a gestational carrier is appropriate for the infertile woman who is genetically sound but unable to carry a pregnancy due to (1) congenital absence or surgical removal of her uterus; (2) a reproductively impaired uterus, myomas, uterine synechiae (adhesion of uterus), or any other congenital abnormalities; or (3) a medical condition that might be life threatening during pregnancy, such as diabetes, immunologic problems, or a severe heart, kidney, or liver disease (Pergament & Fiddler, 2000).Use of a gestational carrier allows a couple with any of these conditions to have their own biologic pregnancy (Pergament & Fiddler, 2000). All participants are required to have medical and psychologic screening as well as legal counsel prior to acceptance into the program.

Adoption

As infertile couples consider various alternatives for resolving their infertility, adoption may emerge as their preferred response. They may seek adoption after aggressive infertility treatments have failed, or because of ethical or spiritual values that prompt them to parent a child in need. As couples begin to consider adoption, an important aspect of this exploration is the reading of books, magazines, and informational Web sites on adoption, attending adoption support groups and conferences, and meeting with adoptive parents to discuss their experiences with adoption.

The adoption of an infant can be difficult and frustrating, often involving long waiting periods, continual setbacks, and high costs. Thus, many couples seek international adoptions

Complementary and Alternative Therapies

Common Treatments for Infertility

Couples experiencing infertility may seek out alternative treatments. Some common treatments include acupuncture and herbs.

Acupuncture: Acupuncture is a therapy used in traditional Chinese medicine (TCM), and has become a very popular complementary treatment. Acupuncture involves inserting sterile needles into specific points on the body to control the flow of chi, or life energy (Gottlieb, 2000). Acupuncture treatment would focus on balancing the flow of chi in the kidneys and adrenal glands. Several clinical studies have shown acupuncture to be effective in treating infertility in both men and women (Sinclair, 2000; Siterman, Eltes, Wolfson, et al, 2000; Beal, 1999; Paulus, Zhang, Strehler, et al, 2002; Tiran & Mack, 2000).

Herbal Treatments: Herbs frequently recommended to treat infertility include ginseng and astragalus. Herbalists cite the healing and hormone-balancing effects of these herbs (Gladstar, 1993). Ginseng has historically been used in TCM to enhance male virility and fertility (Sinclair, 2000). Several studies also cite ginseng, as well as astragalus, in enhancing in vitro sperm motility (Chen, Xu, Chen, et al, 1999; Hong, Ku, & Wu, 1992).

The nurse should be alert for signs that the couple is pursuing complementary therapies out of desperation, and may not be using their best judgment.

or consider adopting older children, children with handicaps, or children of mixed parentage because the adoption process in such cases is quicker, more children are available, and the available children are perceived to have a critical need for timely intervention. The nurse can assist couples considering adoption by providing information on community resources for adoption as well as by providing support throughout the adoption process. Couples also need support if they choose to remain childless.

Pregnancy After Infertility

The feeling of being infertile does not necessarily disappear with pregnancy. Although there may be initial ecstasy, the couple may also face a whole new arena of fear and anxieties, and the parents-to-be often do not know where they "fit in." They may feel a great sense of loss and isolation because those who have had no trouble conceiving cannot relate to the physical and emotional pain they endured to achieve the pregnancy. Contact with their past "infertile" support system may vanish when peers learn the couple has resolved their infertility (Braverman & English, 1992).

Although the desperation to become pregnant may have superseded the couple's ability to acknowledge their concerns about undergoing various treatments or procedures, questions about the repeated cycle of fertility drugs or the achievement of pregnancy through IVF technology or cryopreservation may now arise. The expectant couple may be very concerned about the potential of these treatments for adverse effects on the fetus (Greenfeld, 2002). Couples may need much reassurance throughout the pregnancy to allay these anxieties.

The nurse can assist couples who experience pregnancy after infertility by acknowledging their past experience of infertility treatment; validating their fears and anxieties as they face childbirth classes, birth, and parenting issues; and providing education and support regarding what to anticipate physically and emotionally throughout the pregnancy. These interventions will go a long way toward normalizing the experience for the couple.

NURSING CARE MANAGEMENT

Infertility therapy taxes a couple's financial, physical, and emotional resources. Treatment can be costly and often insurance coverage is limited. Years of effort and numerous evaluations and examinations may take place before a conception occurs, if one occurs at all. In a society that values children and considers them to be the natural result of marriage, infertile couples may face a myriad of tensions and discrimination.

The clinic nurse needs to be constantly aware of the emotional needs of the couple confronting infertility evaluation and treatment. Often an intact marriage will become stressed with the intrusive but necessary infertility procedures and treatments. Constant attention to temperature charts and instructions about their sex life from a person outside the relationship naturally affect the spontaneity of a couple's interactions. Tests and treatments may heighten feelings of frustration or anger between the couple. The need to share this intimate area of a relationship, especially when one or the other is identified as "the cause" of infertility, may precipitate feelings of guilt or shame. Infertility often becomes a central focus for role identity, especially for women (Greenfeld, 2002). The couple may experience feelings of loss of control, feelings of reduced competency and defectiveness, loss of status and ambiguity as a couple, a sense of social stigma, stress on the marital and sexual relationship, and a strained relationship with healthcare providers.

The nurse's roles can be summarized as those of counselor, educator, and advocate. Tasks of the infertile couple and appropriate nursing interventions are summarized in Table 12–7 •. Throughout the evaluation process, nurses can play a key role in lessening the stress these couples must endure by providing them with appropriate resources and accurate information about what treatment entails and what physical, emotional, and financial demands they can

MediaLink CARE PLAN: INFERTILE COUPLE

Table 12–7 • TASKS OF THE INFERTILE COUPLE

Tasks	Nursing Interventions
Recognize how infertility affects their lives and express feelings (may be negative toward self or mate)	Supportive: help to understand and facilitate free expression of feelings
Grieve the loss of potential offspring	Help to recognize feelings
Evaluate reasons for wanting a child	Help to understand motives
Decide about management	Identify alternatives; facilitate partner communication

Source: Sawatzky, M. (1981). Tasks of the infertile couple. *Journal of Obstetric, Gynecologic, and Neonatal Nursing, 10,* 132.

anticipate throughout the process (Greenfeld, 2002). The nurse's ability to assess and respond to emotional and educational needs is essential to give infertile couples control and help them negotiate the treatment process (Hammond, 2001). An assessment tool such as an infertility questionnaire (Table 12–8 •) may be helpful. Extensive and repeated explanations and written instruction may be necessary because the couple's anxiety often overwhelms their ability to retain all the information given. It is important to use a nursing framework that recognizes the multidimensional needs of the infertile individual or couple within physical, social, psychologic, spiritual, and environmental contexts.

Infertility may be perceived as a loss by one or both partners. Affected individuals have described this as loss of their relationship with spouse, family, or friends; their health; their status or prestige; their self-esteem and self-confidence; their security; and the potential child. Only one such loss may lead to depression and, in many cases, the crisis of infertility evokes feelings of all these losses (Greenfeld, 2002). Each couple passes through several stages, not unlike those identified by Kübler-Ross: surprise, denial, anger, isolation, guilt, grief, and resolution. The impact of these feelings on the couple and how fast they move into resolution, if ever, may depend on the cause and duration of treatment. Each partner may progress through the stages at different rates (Sandelowski, 1994). Nonjudgmental acceptance and a professional, caring attitude on the nurse's part can go far to dissipate the negative emotions the couple may experience while going through these stages.

This is also a time when the nurse may assess the quality of the couple's relationship: Are they able and willing to communicate verbally and share feelings? Are they mutually supportive? The answers to these questions may help the nurse identify areas of strength and weakness and construct an appropriate plan of care. Availability of mental health professionals for referral is helpful when the emotional issues become too disruptive in the couple's relationship or life. Couples should be made aware of infertility support and education organizations such as RESOLVE, which may help meet some of these needs and validate their feelings. Finally, individual or group counseling with other infertile couples may help the couple resolve feelings brought about by their own difficult situation.

Table 12–8 • INFERTILITY QUESTIONNAIRE

Self-Image

1. I feel bad about my body because of our inability to have a child.
2. Since our infertility, I feel I can do anything as well as I used to.
3. I feel as attractive as before our infertility.
4. I feel less masculine/feminine because of our inability to have a child.
5. Compared with others, I feel I am a worthwhile person.
6. Lately, I feel I am sexually attractive to my wife/husband.
7. I feel I will be incomplete as a man/woman if we cannot have a child.
8. Having an infertility problem makes me feel physically incompetent.

Guilt/Blame

1. I feel guilty about somehow causing our infertility.
2. I wonder if our infertility problem is due to something I did in the past.
3. My spouse makes me feel guilty about our problem.
4. There are times when I blame my spouse for our infertility.
5. I feel I am being punished because of our infertility.

Sexuality

1. Lately I feel I am able to respond to my spouse sexually.
2. I feel sex is a duty, not a pleasure.
3. Since our infertility problem, I enjoy sexual relations with my spouse.
4. We have sexual relations for the purpose of trying to conceive.
5. Sometimes I feel like a "sex machine," programmed to have sex during the fertile period.
6. Impaired fertility has helped our sexual relationship.
7. Our inability to have a child has increased my desire for sexual relations.
8. Our inability to have a child has decreased my desire for sexual relations.

Note: The questionnaire is scored on a Likert scale, with responses ranging from "strongly agree" to "strongly disagree." Each question is scored separately, and the mean score is determined for each section (Self-Image, Guilt/Blame, and Sexuality). The total mean score is then divided by 3. A final mean score of greater than 3 indicates distress.

Source: From AWHONN. (1985). Bernstein, J., Potts, N., and Mattox, J. H., Assessment of psychological dysfunction association with infertility. *Journal of Obstetric, Gynecologic, and Neonatal Nursing.* 14 (Suppl.), 64S, Table 1. Washington, DC: Author.

MEDIALINK CASE STUDY: INFERTILITY

Genetic Disorders

Even when conception has been achieved, families can have special reproductive concerns. The desired and expected outcome of any pregnancy is the birth of a healthy, "perfect" baby. Parents experience grief, fear, and anger when they discover that their baby has been born with a defect or a genetic disease. They may also experience feelings of guilt and blame when the baby is perceived to have inherited a disorder from one parent. These feelings, if not expressed and dealt with openly, can create strife within the family.

Regardless of the type or scope of the problem, parents will have many questions: "What did I do?" "What caused it?" "How do I cope with it?" "Will it happen again?" The nurse must anticipate the parents' questions and concerns, direct the family to the appropriate resources, and support the family. To do so, the nurse must have a basic knowledge of genetics and genetic counseling.

MEDIALINK GENETICS

Chromosomes and Chromosomal Analysis

All hereditary material is carried on tightly coiled strands of DNA known as **chromosomes.** The chromosomes carry the genes, the smallest unit of inheritance, as discussed in greater detail in Chapter 11 .The Human Genome Project, which began in 1988, has made remarkable advances toward determining the exact DNA sequence of human genes.

All *somatic (body) cells* contain 46 chromosomes, which is the *diploid* number; the sperm and egg contain half as many (23) chromosomes, or the *haploid* number (see Chapter 11). There are 23 pairs of homologous chromosomes (a matched pair of chromosomes, one inherited from each parent). Twenty-two of the pairs are known as **autosomes** (nonsex chromosomes), and one pair is the sex chromosome, X or Y. A normal female has a 46, XX chromosome constitution, the normal male, 46, XY (Figures 12–6 • and 12–7 •).

The **karyotype,** or pictorial analysis of an individual's chromosomes, is usually obtained from specially treated and stained peripheral blood lymphocytes. Although the use of peripheral blood is an easy, convenient method of obtaining chromosomes, almost any tissue can be examined to get this information. After birth, for example, a piece of the placenta taken from a site near the insertion of the cord and deep enough to include chorion can be sent for karyotyping of the fetus.

Chromosome abnormalities can occur in either the autosomes or the sex chromosomes and can be divided into two categories: abnormalities of number and abnormalities of structure. Even small alterations in chromosomes can cause problems, especially those associated with delayed growth and development. The child does not need to have obvious major malformations to be affected. Some of these abnormalities can also be passed on to other offspring. Thus in some cases chromosomal analysis is appropriate even if clinical manifestations are mild. Whatever the case, too much or too little genetic material usually produces adverse effects on a child's growth and development. The Human Genome Project has already led to the identification of the gene associated with certain abnormalities such as fragile X and cystic fibrosis (Williams, 2000).

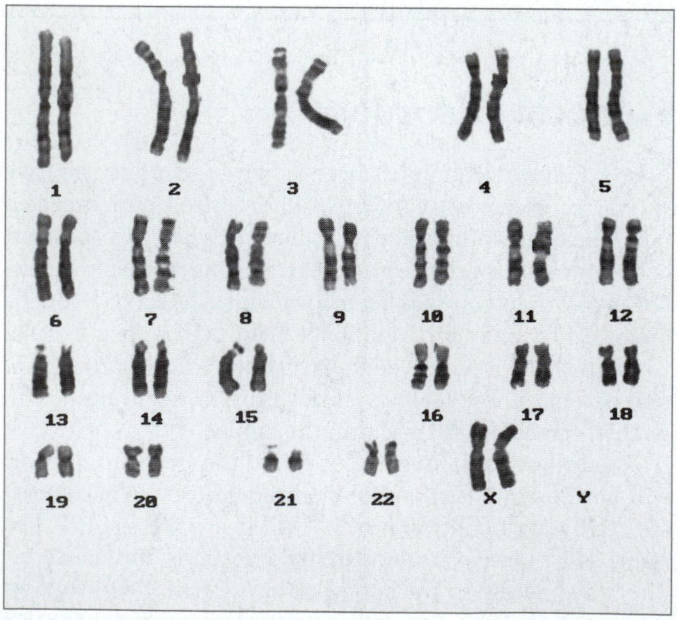

Figure 12–6 • Normal female karyotype.
SOURCE: Courtesy of David Peakman, Reproductive Genetics Center, Denver, CO.

Autosomal Abnormalities

As noted, abnormalities of autosomes may involve variations in either number or structure.

ABNORMALITIES OF CHROMOSOME NUMBER

Abnormalities of chromosome number are most commonly seen as trisomies, monosomies, and as mosaicism. In all three cases, the abnormality is most often caused by nondisjunction, which occurs when paired chromosomes fail to separate

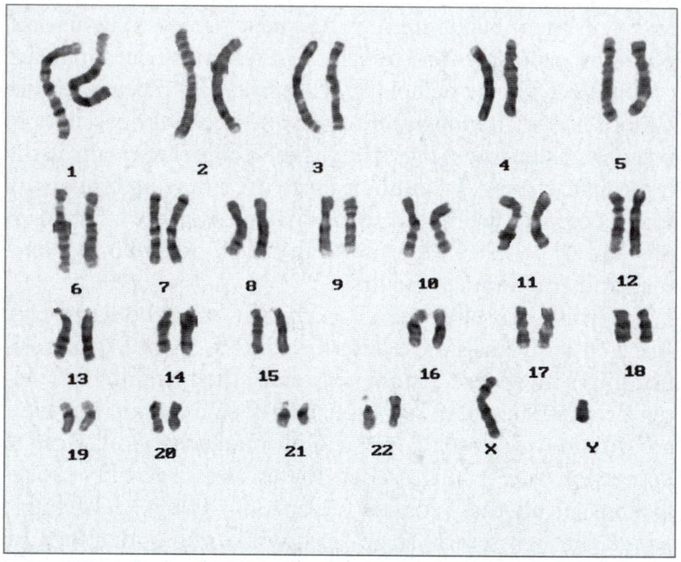

Figure 12–7 • Normal male karyotype.
SOURCE: Courtesy of David Peakman, Reproductive Genetics Center, Denver, CO.

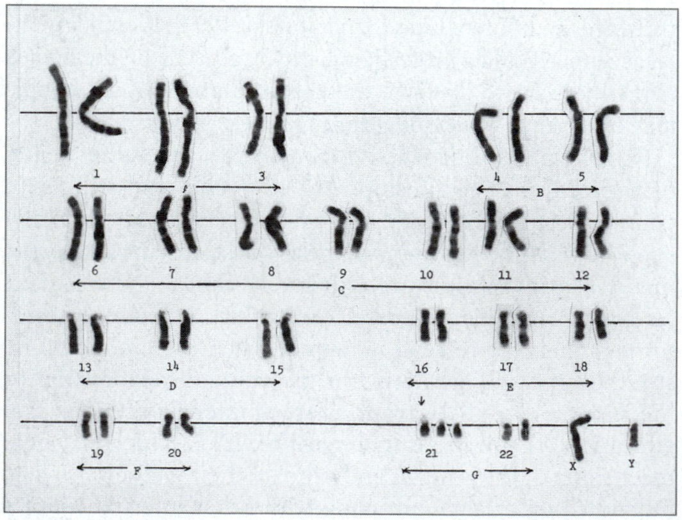

Figure 12–8 • Karyotype of a male who has trisomy 21, Down syndrome. Note the extra chromosome 21.
SOURCE: Courtesy of Dr. Arthur Robinson, National Jewish Hospital and Research Center, Denver, CO.

Table 12-9 • CHROMOSOMAL SYNDROMES

Altered chromosome: 21 Genetic defect: trisomy 21 (Down syndrome) (secondary nondisjunction or 14/21 unbalanced translocation) Incidence: average 1 in 700 live births, incidence variable with age of woman	**Characteristics:** CNS: mental retardation; hypotonia at birth Head: flattened occiput; depressed nasal bridge; mongoloid slant of eyes; epicanthal folds; white specking of the iris (Brushfield spots); protrusion of the tongue; high, arched palate; low-set ears Hands: broad, short fingers; abnormalities of finger and foot; dermal ridge patterns (dermatoglyphics); transverse palmar crease (simian line) Other: congenital heart disease
Altered chromosome: 18 Genetic defect: trisomy 18 Incidence: 1 in 3000 live births	**Characteristics:** CNS: mental retardation; severe hypotonia Head: prominent occiput; low-set ears; corneal opacities; ptosis (drooping of eyelids) Hands: third and fourth fingers overlapped by second and fifth fingers; abnormal dermatoglyphics; syndactyly (webbing of fingers) Other: congenital heart defects; renal abnormalities; single umbilical artery; gastrointestinal tract abnormalities; rocker-bottom feet; cryptorchidism; various malformations of other organs
Altered chromosome: 13 Genetic defect: trisomy 13 Incidence: 1 in 5000 live births	**Characteristics:** CNS: mental retardation; severe hypotonia; seizures Head: microcephaly; microphthalmia and/or coloboma (keyhole-shaped pupil); malformed ears; aplasia of external auditory canal; micrognathia (abnormally small lower jaw); cleft lip and palate Hands: polydactyly (extra digits); abnormal posturing of fingers; abnormal dermatoglyphics Other: congenital heart defects; hemangiomas; gastrointestinal tract defects; various malformations of other organs
Altered chromosome: 5p Genetic defect: deletion of short arm of chromosome 5 (cri du chat, or cat cry, syndrome) Incidence: 1 in 20,000 live births (Figure 12–10)	**Characteristics:** CNS: severe mental retardation; a catlike cry in infancy Head: microcephaly; hypertelorism (widely spaced eyes); epicanthal folds; low-set ears Other: failure to thrive; various organ malformations
Altered chromosome: XO (sex chromosome) Genetic defect: only one X chromosome in female (Turner syndrome) Incidence: 1 in 300–7000 live female births (Figure 12–11)	**Characteristics:** CNS: no intellectual impairment; some perceptual difficulties Head: low hairline; webbed neck Trunk: short stature; cubitus valgus (increased carrying angle of arm); excessive nevi (congenital discoloration of skin due to pigmentation); broad shieldlike chest with widely spaced nipples; puffy feet; no toenails Other: fibrous streaks in ovaries; underdeveloped secondary sex characteristics; primary amenorrhea; usually infertile; renal anomalies; coarctation of the aorta
Altered chromosome: XXY (sex chromosome) Genetic defect: extra X chromosome in male (Klinefelter syndrome) Incidence: 1 in 1000 live male births, approximately 1%–2% of institutionalized males	**Characteristics:** CNS: mild mental retardation Trunk: occasional gynecomastia (abnormally large male breasts); eunuchoid body proportions (lack of male muscular and sexual development) Other: small, soft testes; underdeveloped secondary sex characteristics; usually sterile

during cell division. If nondisjunction occurs in either the sperm or the egg before fertilization, the resulting zygote (fertilized egg) will have an abnormal chromosome makeup in all of the cells (trisomy or monosomy). If nondisjunction occurs after fertilization, the developing zygote will have cells with two or more different chromosome makeups, evolving into two or more different cell lines (mosaicism).

Trisomies are the product of the union of a normal gamete (egg or sperm) with a gamete that contains an extra chromosome. The individual will have 47 chromosomes and be trisomic (have three copies of the same chromosome) for whichever chromosome is extra. Down syndrome (formerly called mongolism) is the most common trisomy abnormality seen in children (Figure 12–8 •). The presence of the extra chromosome 21 produces distinctive clinical features (Table 12–9 •). With the advent of modern surgical techniques and antibiotics, children with Down syndrome are now living into their fifth or sixth decade of life.

The other two common trisomies are trisomy 18 and trisomy 13 (Table 12–9). The prognosis for both trisomy 13 or 18 is extremely poor. Most children (70%) die within the first 3 months of life as a result of complications related to respiratory and cardiac abnormalities. However, 10% survive the first year of life; therefore, the family needs to plan for the possibility of long-term care of a severely affected infant and for family support.

Monosomies occur when a normal gamete unites with a gamete that is missing a chromosome. In this case, the individual will have only 45 chromosomes and is said to be monosomic. Monosomy of an entire autosomal chromosome is incompatible with life.

Mosaicism occurs after fertilization and results in an individual with two different cell lines, each having a different chromosomal number. Mosaicism tends to be more common in the sex chromosomes, but when it does occur in the autosomes, it is most common in Down syndrome. An individual with many of the classic signs of Down syndrome but with normal or near-normal intelligence should be investigated for the possibility of mosaicism.

ABNORMALITIES OF CHROMOSOME STRUCTURE

Abnormalities of chromosome structure involve only parts of the chromosome and generally occur in two forms: translocation, and deletions or additions.

Some children born with Down syndrome have trisomy 21, whereas others have an abnormal rearrangement of chromosomal material known as *translocation*. Clinically, the two types of Down syndrome are indistinguishable. What is of major importance to the family is that the two different types have significantly different risks of occurrence. In families with one child with trisomy 21, the risk of a second child also having the disorder is 1 in 700 live births. In contrast, the risk of a second child with a balanced translocation type of Down syndrome is 1 in 500 live births. The only way to distinguish between the two is to do a chromosome analysis.

The translocation occurs when the carrier parent has 45 chromosomes, usually with one chromosome fused to another. A common translocation is one in which a particle of chromosome 14 breaks and fuses to chromosome 21. The parent has one normal 14, one normal 21, and one 14/21 chromosome. Since all the chromosomal material is present and functioning normally, the parent is clinically normal. This individual is known as a *balanced translocation carrier*. When a person who is a balanced translocation carrier has a child with a person who has a structurally normal chromosome constitution, the child can have a normal number of chromosomes, be a carrier, or have an extra chromosome 21 (Figure 12–9 •). Such a child has an *unbalanced translocation* and has Down syndrome.

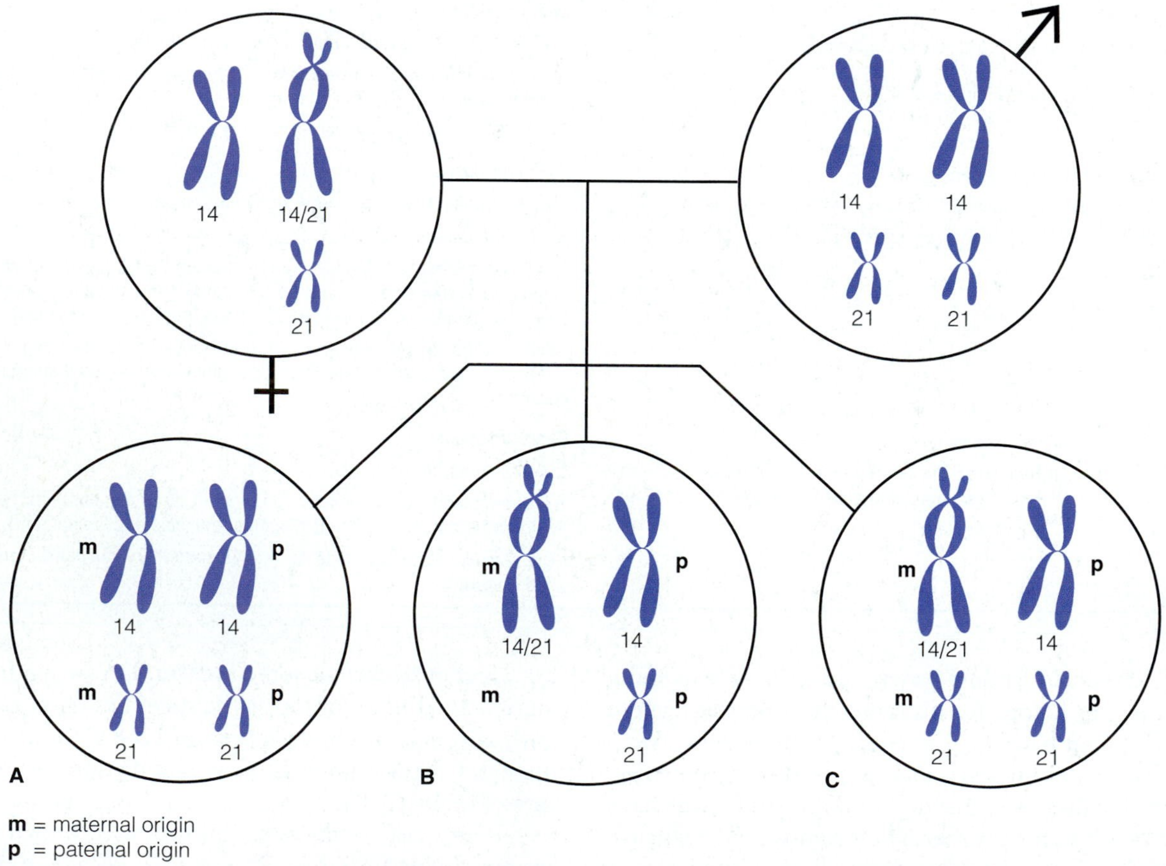

Figure 12–9 • Diagram of various types of offspring when mother has a balanced translocation between chromosomes 14 and 21 and father has a normal arrangement of chromosomal material. *A*, Normal offspring. *B*, Balanced translocation carrier. *C*, Unbalanced translocation. Child has Down syndrome.

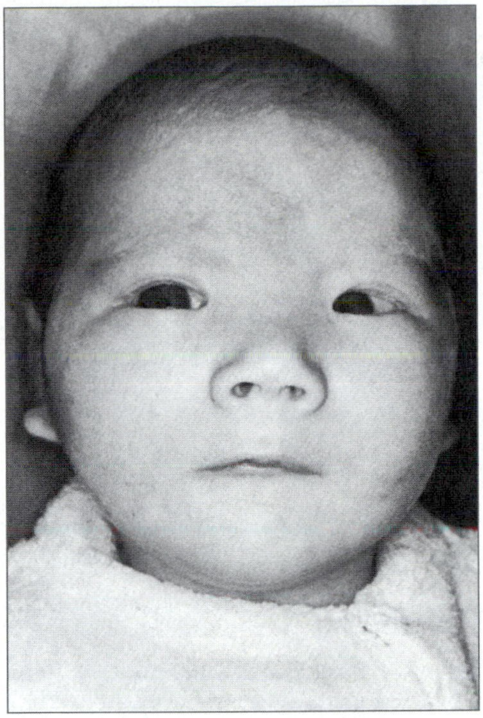

Figure 12–10 • Infant with cri du chat syndrome resulting from deletion of part of the short arm of chromosome 5. Note characteristic faces with hypertelorism, epicanthus, and retrognathia.
SOURCE: Reprinted from Thompson, J. S., & Thompson, M. W.: Genetics in Medicine, 5th ed., ©1991, with permission from Elsevier Science.

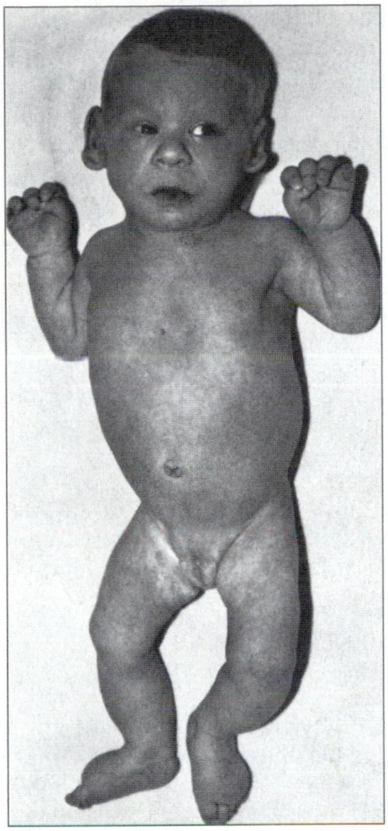

Figure 12–11 • Infant with Turner syndrome at 1 month of age. Note the prominent ears.
SOURCE: Reprinted from Lemli, L. Smith, D. W. (1963). The XO syndrome: A study of the differential phenotype in 25 patients. *Journal of Pediatrics,* 63, 577, with permission from Elsevier Science.

The other type of structural abnormality seen is caused by *additions* or *deletions* of chromosomal material. Any portion of a chromosome may be lost or added, generally leading to some adverse effect. Depending on how much chromosomal material is involved, the clinical effects may be mild or severe. Many types of additions and deletions have been described, such as a deletion of the short arm of chromosome 5 (cri du chat, or cat cry, syndrome; Figure 12–10 •) or the deletion of the long arm of chromosome 18 (Edwards syndrome). Table 12–9 lists other chromosomal syndromes.

Sex Chromosome Abnormalities

To better understand abnormalities of the sex chromosomes, the nurse should know that in females, at an early embryonic stage, one of the two normal X chromosomes becomes inactive. The inactive X chromosome forms a dark-staining area known as the *Barr body*, or sex chromatin body. The normal female has one Barr body because one of her two X chromosomes has been inactivated. The normal male has no Barr bodies because he has only one X chromosome.

The most common sex chromosome abnormalities are Turner syndrome in females (45,XO with no Barr bodies present) and Klinefelter syndrome in males (47,XXY with one Barr body present). See Figure 12–11 • and Table 12–9 for clinical descriptions of these abnormalities.

The mosaic form of the XO chromosome is associated with daughters of women who took the drug diethylstilbestrol (DES) during pregnancy. The fertility of women with the mosaic form of the XO chromosome may not be impaired; however, there is a higher percentage of uterine malformation and hormonal difficulty associated with it, and hence a high degree of miscarriage.

Modes of Inheritance

Many inherited diseases are produced by an abnormality in a single gene or pair of genes. In such instances the chromosomes are grossly normal. The defect is at the gene level. Some of these gene defects can be detected by new technologies, including DNA and other biochemical assays.

There are two major categories of inheritance: **mendelian (single-gene) inheritance** and **nonmendelian (multifactorial) inheritance.** Each single-gene trait is determined by a pair of genes working together. These genes are responsible for the observable expression of the traits (eg, brown eyes, dark skin), referred to as the **phenotype.** The total genetic makeup of an individual is referred to as the **genotype** (pattern of the genes on the chromosomes).

One of the genes for a trait is inherited from the mother; the other, from the father. Individuals who have two identical genes at a given locus are considered to be *homozygous* for that trait. Individuals are considered to be *heterozygous* for a particular trait when they have two different alleles (alternate forms of the same gene) at a given locus on a pair of homologous chromosomes.

The best known modes of single-gene inheritance are autosomal dominant, autosomal recessive, and X-linked (sex-linked) recessive. There is also a less common, X-linked dominant mode of inheritance, and a new identified mode of inheritance, the fragile X syndrome.

AUTOSOMAL DOMINANT INHERITANCE

An individual is said to have an autosomal dominantly inherited disorder if the disease trait is heterozygous. That is, the abnormal gene overshadows the normal gene of the pair to produce the trait. The following occurs in autosomal dominant inheritance:

- An affected individual generally has an affected parent. The family **pedigree** (graphic representation of a family tree) usually shows multiple generations having the disorder.
- Affected individuals have a 50% chance of passing on the abnormal gene to each of their children (Figure 12–12 •).
- Males and females are equally affected, and a father can pass the abnormal gene on to his son. This is an important principle when distinguishing autosomal dominant disorders from X-linked disorders.
- Autosomal dominant inherited disorders have varying degrees of presentation. This is an important factor when counseling families concerning autosomal dominant disorders. Although a parent may have a mild form of the disease, the child may have a more severe form.

Autosomal dominant conditions such as phocomelia (a developmental anomaly characterized by the absence of the upper portion of the limbs) can have very minimal expression in a parent but severe effects in a child. Other common autosomal dominantly inherited disorders are Huntington disease, polycystic kidney disease, neurofibromatosis (von Recklinghausen disease), and achondroplastic dwarfism.

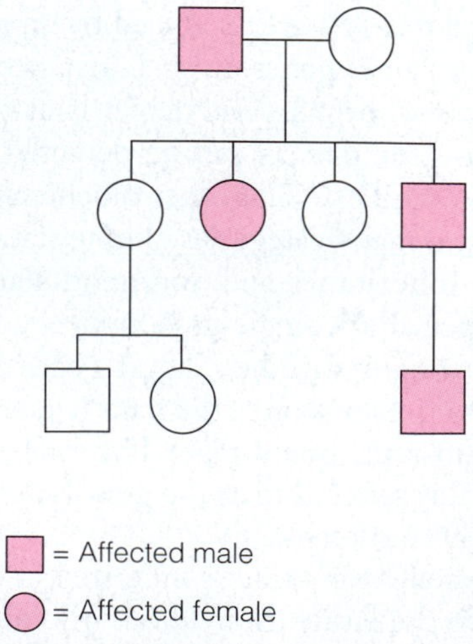

Figure 12–12 • Autosomal dominant pedigree. One parent is affected. Statistically, 50% of offspring will be affected, regardless of sex.

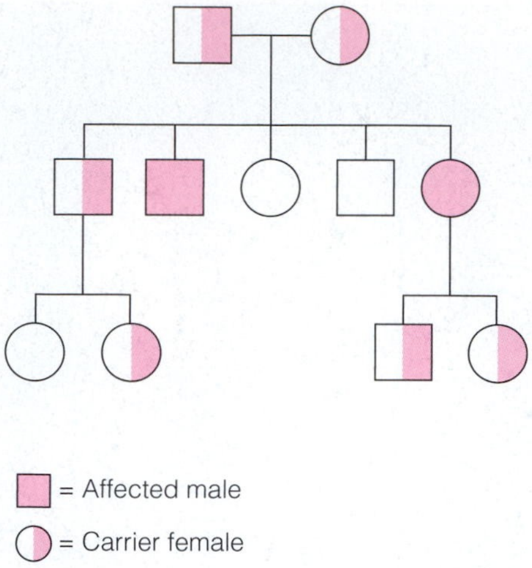

Figure 12–13 • Autosomal recessive pedigree. Both parents are carriers. Statistically, 25% of offspring will be affected, regardless of sex.

AUTOSOMAL RECESSIVE INHERITANCE

In an autosomal recessively inherited disorder, the individual must have two abnormal genes to be affected. The notion of a *carrier state* is appropriate here. A carrier is an individual who is heterozygous for the abnormal gene and clinically normal. It is not until two carriers mate and pass on the same abnormal gene that affected children may appear. It is essential to remember the following facts about autosomal recessive inheritance:

- An affected individual has clinically normal parents, but both parents are carriers of the abnormal gene (Figure 12–13 •).
- There is a 25% chance of carrier parents passing the abnormal gene on to any of their offspring. Each pregnancy has a 25% chance of resulting in an affected child.
- If the child of two carrier parents is clinically normal, there is a 50% chance that the child is a carrier of the gene.
- Both males and females are equally affected.
- There is an increased history of consanguineous matings (as between cousins).

Some common autosomal recessive inherited disorders are cystic fibrosis, phenylketonuria (PKU), galactosemia, sickle cell anemia, Tay-Sachs disease, and most metabolic disorders.

X-LINKED RECESSIVE INHERITANCE

X-linked, or sex-linked, disorders are those for which the abnormal gene is carried on the X chromosome. Thus an X-linked disorder is manifested in a male who carries the abnormal gene on his X chromosome. His mother is considered to be a carrier when the normal gene on one X chromosome overshadows the abnormal gene on the other X chromosome. The following occurs in X-linked recessive inheritance:

- There is no male-to-male transmission. Affected males are related through the female line (Figure 12–14 •).

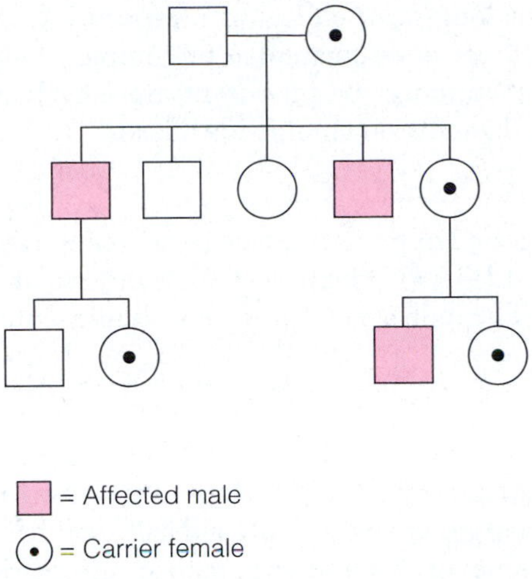

Figure 12–14 • X-linked recessive pedigree. The mother is the carrier. Statistically, 50% of male offspring will be affected, and 50% of female offspring will be carriers.

- There is a 50% chance that a carrier mother will pass the abnormal gene to each of her sons, who will thus be affected. There is a 50% chance that a carrier mother will pass the normal gene to each of her sons, who will thus be unaffected. There is a 50% chance that a carrier mother will pass the abnormal gene to each of her daughters, who become carriers.
- Fathers affected with an X-linked disorder cannot pass the disorder to their sons, but all their daughters become carriers of the disorder.

Common X-linked recessive disorders are hemophilia, Duchenne muscular dystrophy, and some forms of color blindness.

X-LINKED DOMINANT INHERITANCE

X-linked dominant disorders are extremely rare, the most common being vitamin D-resistant rickets. When X-linked dominance does occur, the pattern is similar to X-linked recessive inheritance except that heterozygous females may also be affected. It is essential to remember that in X-linked dominant inheritance there is no male-to-male transmission. Affected fathers will have affected daughters, but since they pass only the Y chromosome to male offspring, any sons will not be affected.

FRAGILE X SYNDROME

The fragile X syndrome is a common inherited form of mental retardation second only to Down syndrome among all cases of moderate mental retardation in males. Fragile X syndrome is a CNS disorder linked to a "fragile site" on the X chromosome. Fragile X syndrome is characterized by moderate mental retardation, large protuberant ears, and large testes after puberty. The carrier females are not dysmorphic (having abnormal features), but about one third are mildly retarded.

MULTIFACTORIAL INHERITANCE

Many common congenital malformations, such as cleft palate, heart defects, spina bifida, dislocated hips, clubfoot, and pyloric stenosis, are caused by an interaction of many genes and environmental factors. They are therefore multifactorial in origin. It is essential to remember that in multifactorial inheritance:

- The malformations may vary from mild to severe. For example, spina bifida may range in severity from mild, as spina bifida occulta, to more severe, as a myelomeningocele. It is believed that the more severe the defect, the greater the number of genes present for that defect.
- There is often a sex bias. Pyloric stenosis is more common in males, whereas cleft palate is more common among females. When a member of the less commonly affected sex shows the condition, a greater number of genes must usually be present to cause the defect.
- In the presence of environmental factors (such as seasonal changes, altitude, radiation exposure, chemicals in the environment, or exposure to toxic substances) that affect the parents, fewer genes may be needed to manifest the disease in the offspring.
- In contrast to single-gene disorders, there is an additive effect in multifactorial inheritance. The more family members who have the defect, the greater the risk that the next pregnancy will also be affected (Simpson, 2002b).

Although most congenital malformations are multifactorial, a careful family history should always be taken because occasionally cleft lip and palate, certain congenital heart defects, and other malformations can also be inherited as autosomal dominant or recessive traits. Other disorders thought to be within the multifactorial inheritance group are diabetes, hypertension, some heart diseases, and mental illness.

Nongenetic Conditions

Although most malformations present at birth may be attributed to genetic defects or environmental insult during pregnancy, such as exposure to a drug or an infectious agent, some cannot be adequately explained by these mechanisms. However, the nurse must avoid false reassurances following the birth of a baby with a malformation. Telling parents that "it won't happen again" can put any healthcare professional in jeopardy. Instead, a referral to a genetic center is warranted with any birth defect.

Prenatal Diagnostic Tests

Parent-child and family-planning counseling have become a major responsibility of professional nurses. To be effective counselors, nurses need to have the most current knowledge available concerning prenatal diagnosis. Appropriate counseling should occur before prenatal screening is done. It is essential that the couple be completely informed as to the known and potential risks of each of the genetic diagnostic procedures. The prescreening counseling should include the conditions detectable by the screen, diagnostic test available if screen is positive, risk to mother and child of the test performed, accuracy of the test, and limitations of the test

(Graves, Miller, & Sellers, 2002). The nurse needs to recognize the emotional impact on the family of a decision to undergo or not to undergo a genetic diagnostic procedure.

The ability to diagnose certain genetic diseases by various diagnostic tools has enormous implications for the practice of preventive healthcare. Several methods are available for prenatal diagnosis, although some are still experimental.

GENETIC ULTRASOUND

Ultrasound may be used to assess the fetus for genetic or congenital problems. With ultrasound, one can visualize the fetal head for abnormalities in size, shape, and structure. (For a detailed discussion of ultrasound technology, see Chapter 21.) Craniospinal defects (anencephaly, microcephaly, hydrocephalus), gastrointestinal malformations (omphalocele, gastroschisis), renal malformations (dysplasia or obstruction), and skeletal malformations (caudal regression, conjoined twins) are only some of the disorders that have been diagnosed in utero by ultrasound.

Screening by ultrasound for congenital anomalies is best done at 18 to 20 weeks, when fetal structures have completed development. There is no information documenting harm to the fetus or long-term effects with exposure to ultrasound. However, there is no guarantee of complete safety; therefore, the practitioner and the parents must evaluate the risks against the benefits on an individual basis.

GENETIC AMNIOCENTESIS

A major method of prenatal diagnosis is genetic amniocentesis (Figure 12–15 •). The procedure is described in Chapter 21. The indications for genetic amniocentesis include the following:

- **Maternal age 35 or older.** Women 35 or older are at greater risk for having children with chromosome abnormalities. Half of the chromosomal abnormalities due to maternal age are trisomy 21, and half are other abnormalities of chromosome number, such as trisomy 13, 18, XXX, or XXY. The risk of having a live-born infant with a chromosome problem is 1 in 200 for a 35-year-old woman; the risk for trisomy 21 is 1 in 365. At age 45 the risks are 1 in 20 and 1 in 40, respectively (Newberger, 2000).
- **Previous child born with a chromosomal abnormality.** Young couples who have had a child with

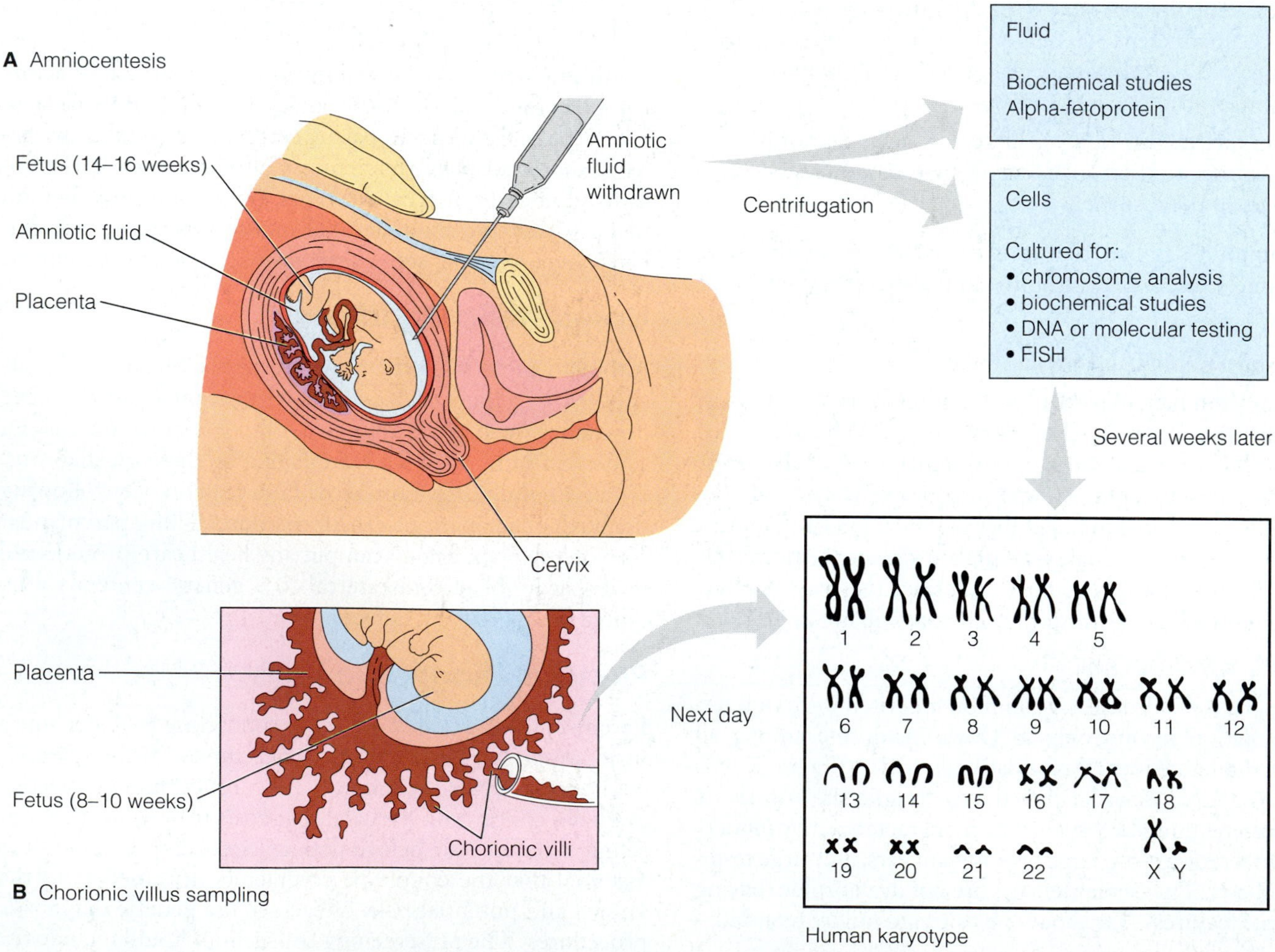

Figure 12–15 • *A,* Genetic amniocentesis for prenatal diagnosis is done at 14 to 16 weeks' gestation. *B,* Chorionic villus sampling is done at 8 to 10 weeks, and the cells are karyotyped within 48 to 72 hours.

trisomy 21, 18, or 13 have approximately a 1% to 2% risk of a future child having a chromosome abnormality.

- **Parent carrying a chromosomal abnormality (balanced translocation).** For example, a woman who carries a balanced 14/21 translocation has a risk of approximately 10% to 15% that her children will be affected with the unbalanced translocation of Down syndrome; if the father is a carrier, there is a 2% to 5% risk.
- **Mother carrying an X-linked disease.** In families in which the woman is a known or possible carrier of an X-linked disorder, such as Duchenne muscular dystrophy or hemophilia, genetic amniocentesis, chorionic villus sampling, or percutaneous umbilical cord sampling may be appropriate options. For a known female carrier, the risk of having an affected male fetus is 50%. Now DNA testing may make it possible to distinguish affected males from nonaffected males in some disorders. In disorders where female carriers can be distinguished from noncarriers, only the carrier females would be offered prenatal diagnosis.
- **Parents carrying an inborn error of metabolism that can be diagnosed in utero.** Metabolic disorders detectable in utero include Fabry disease, galactosemia, Gaucher disease, homocystinuria, Hunter syndrome, Hurler disease, Krabbe disease, Lesch-Nyhan syndrome, maple syrup urine disease, Niemann-Pick disease, Pompe disease, and Tay-Sachs disease.
- **Both parents carrying an autosomal recessive disease.** When both parents are carriers of an autosomal recessive disease, there is a 25% risk for each pregnancy that the fetus will be affected. Diagnosis is made by testing the cultured amniotic fluid cells (enzyme level, substrate level, product level, or DNA) or the fluid itself. Autosomal recessive diseases identified by amniocentesis are hemoglobinopathies such as sickle cell anemia, thalassemia, and cystic fibrosis.
- **Family history of neural tube defects.** Genetic amniocentesis is available to those couples who have had a child with neural tube defects or who have a family history of these conditions, which include anencephaly, spina bifida, and myelomeningocele. Neural tube defects are usually multifactorial traits; for example, folic acid deficiency in the first few weeks of pregnancy is a risk factor.

CHORIONIC VILLUS SAMPLING

Chorionic villus sampling (CVS) is a technique used in selected regional centers. Its diagnostic capability is similar to that of amniocentesis. Its advantages are that diagnostic information is available at 8 to 10 weeks' gestation and that products of conception are tested directly. (For further discussion, see Chapter 21.)

PERCUTANEOUS UMBILICAL BLOOD SAMPLING

Percutaneous umbilical blood sampling (PUBS) is a technique used for obtaining blood that allows for more rapid chromosome diagnosis, for genetic studies, or for transfusion for Rh isoimmunization or hydrops fetalis. (For more in-depth discussion, see Chapter 21.)

ALPHA-FETOPROTEIN (AFP AND AFP3)

The maternal circulation or amniotic fluid is tested for Alpha-fetoprotein (AFP). Maternal serum AFP (MSAFP) is elevated in infants with open neural tube defect, anencephaly, omphalocele, or gastroschisis, and in multiple gestation (Graves et al, 2002). Low MSAFP has been associated with Down syndrome. MSAFP is tested at 15 to 22 weeks' gestation (Graves et al, 2002). Ultrasound and amniocentesis are offered with low or high MSAFP. Inaccurate dating is the most common cause for abnormal AFP; therefore, ultrasound dating is very important. With high MSAFP, normal amniotic fluid AFP, and normal ultrasound, there is an increased risk for preterm labor, perinatal death, and intrauterine growth restriction.

IMPLICATIONS OF PRENATAL DIAGNOSTIC TESTING

It is imperative that counseling precede any procedure for prenatal diagnosis. Many questions and points must be considered if the family is to reach a satisfactory decision. See Table 12–10 • and Developing Cultural Competence.

With the advent of diagnostic techniques such as amniocentesis, at-risk couples who would not otherwise have a first child or additional children can decide to conceive. Following prenatal diagnosis, a couple can decide not to have a child with a genetic disease. For many couples, prenatal diagnosis is not a solution because they choose not to prevent the genetic disease by aborting the fetus. The decision whether or not to use prenatal diagnosis can be made only by the family. Even when termination is not an option, prenatal diagnosis can give parents an opportunity to prepare for the birth of a child with special needs, contact other families with a child with similar problems, or contact support services before the birth.

Table 12–10 • COUPLES WHO MAY BENEFIT FROM PRENATAL DIAGNOSIS
Women age 35 or over at time of birth
Couples with a balanced translocation (chromosomal abnormality)
Family history of known or suspected mendelian genetic disorder (eg, cystic fibrosis, hemophilia A & B, Duchenne muscular dystrophy)
Couples with a previous child with chromosomal abnormality
Couples in which either partner or a previous child is affected with, or in which both partners are carriers for, a diagnosable metabolic disorder
Family history of birth defects and/or mental retardation (eg, neural tube defects, congenital heart disease, cleft lip and/or palate)
Ethnic groups at increased risk for specific disorders (see Developing Cultural Competence)
Couples with history of two or more first trimester spontaneous abortions
Women with an abnormal maternal serum alpha-fetoprotein (MSAFP or AFP3) test
Women with a teratogenic risk secondary to an exposure or maternal health condition (eg, diabetes)

Developing Cultural Competence

Genetic Screening Recommendations for Various Ethnic and Age Groups

Background of Population at Risk	Disorder	Screening Test	Definitive Test
Ashkenazic Jewish, French-Canadians, Cajuns	Tay-Sachs Disease	Decreased serum hexosaminidase-A	CVS* or amniocentesis for hexosaminidase-A assay
African; Hispanic from Caribbean, Central America, or South America; Arabs; Egyptians; Asian Indians	Sickle cell anemia	Presence of sickle cell hemoglobin; confirmatory hemoglobin electrophoresis	CVS or amniocentesis for genotype determination; direct molecular studies
Greek, Italian	Beta-thalassemia	Mean corpuscular volume < 80%; confirmatory hemoglobin electrophoresis	CVS or amniocentesis for genotype determination (direct molecular studies or indirect RFLP† analysis)
Southeast Asian (Vietnamese, Loatian, Cambodian), Filipino	Alpha-thalassemia	Mean corpuscular volume < 80%; confirmatory hemoglobin electrophoresis	CVS or amniocentesis for genotype determination (direct molecular studies)
Women over age 35 (all ethnic groups)	Chromosomal trisomies	None	CVS or amniocentesis for cytogenetic analysis
Women of any age (all ethnic groups; particularly suggested for women from British Isles, Ireland)	Neural tube defects and selected other anomalies	Maternal serum alpha-fetoprotein (MSAFP)	Amniocentesis for amniotic fluid, alpha-fetoprotein, and acetylcholinesterase assays
Ashkenazic Jewish	Gaucher disease	Decrease glucocerebrosidase	CVS
Caucasians (Northern Europeans, Celtic population), Ashkenazic Jewish	Cystic fibrosis	Delta F508 amino acid mutation	CVS or amniocentesis for genotype determination; definitive diagnosis for all fetuses not possible

*Chorionic villus sampling.

†Restriction fragment length polymorphism.

Every pregnancy has a 3% to 4% risk for resulting in an infant with a birth defect. When an abnormality is detected or suspected, an attempt is made to determine the diagnosis by assessing the family health history (via the pedigree) and the pregnancy history, and by evaluating the fetal anomaly or anomalies via ultrasound. Experts on a specific disorder are consulted, and healthcare professionals can then present the parents with information and options. Families with a baby having a lethal anomaly, such as trisomy 13 or 18, may wish to consider nonaggressive intervention.

Treatment of prenatally diagnosed disorders may begin during the pregnancy, thus possibly preventing irreversible damage. For example, a galactose-free diet may be given to a mother carrying a fetus with galactosemia. In light of the philosophy of preventive healthcare, information on what data can be obtained prenatally should be made available to all couples who are expecting a baby or who are contemplating pregnancy.

Postnatal Diagnosis

Questions concerning genetic disorders (cause, treatment, and prognosis) are most often first discussed in the newborn nursery or during the infant's first few months of life. When a child is born with anomalies, has a stormy neonatal period, or does not progress as expected, a genetic evaluation may well be warranted. Accurate diagnosis and an optimal treatment plan incorporate:

- Complete and detailed histories to determine whether the problem is prenatal (congenital), postnatal, or familial in origin.
- Thorough physical examination, including dermatoglyphic analysis (Figure 12–16 ●).
- Laboratory analysis, which includes chromosome analysis; enzyme assay for inborn errors of metabolism (see Chapter 32 for further discussion on these specific tests); DNA studies (both direct and by linkage); and antibody titers for infectious teratogens, such as toxoplasmosis, rubella, cytomegalovirus, and herpes virus (see Chapter 19) (Mahowald, McKusick, Scheuerle, et al, 2001).

To make an accurate diagnosis, the geneticist consults with other specialists and reviews the current literature. This lets the geneticist evaluate all the available information before arriving at a diagnosis and plan of action.

The Human Genome Project will have significant implications for the identification and management of inherited disorders. Once genes have been identified, it will be possible to detect their presence in carriers and lead

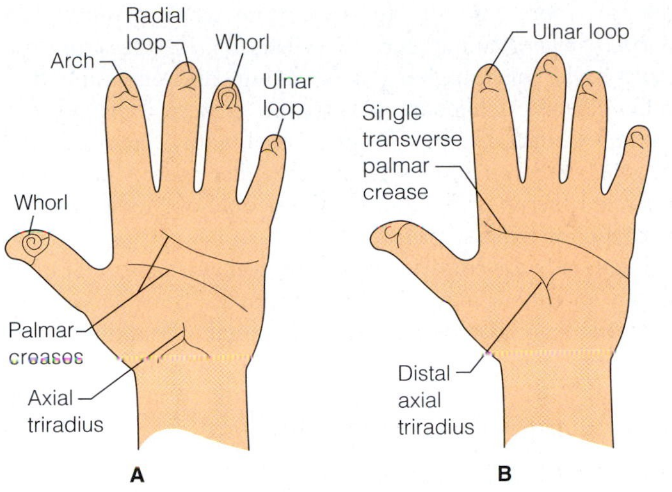

Figure 12–16 • Dermatoglyphic patterns of the hands in *A*, a normal individual and *B*, a child with Down syndrome. Note the single transverse palmar crease, distally placed axial triradius, and increased number of ulnar loops.

to better genetic counseling. New genetic material might be inserted into cells to provide important missing information (gene transfer) as may be possible in cystic fibrosis, or medications can be specifically designed to target the disease on a molecular level (Stribley, Rehman, Niu, et al, 2002).

However, concerns have been voiced about ethical considerations with genetic research. What guidelines are needed to protect children and families so that genetic testing does not lead to discrimination in future employment or health insurance? Who should be tested for genetic diseases, and who should have access to the results? Since children cannot yet give informed consent for genetic testing (see Chapter 1 for discussion of informed consent), it is recommended that children and adolescents should have genetic testing *only* when medical treatment could help if the disease is identified, or when another family member might benefit from the knowledge for their own health and the child will not be harmed by the testing (American Academy of Pediatrics, Committee on Genetics, 2000; Drenkard & Ferguson, 2002). Whenever genetic testing is performed, counseling about the results must be available. Some nurses are choosing special educational programs to enable them to work in the growing field of genetics and healthcare (Tinkle & Cheek, 2002).

Genetic Counseling

Genetic counseling is a communication process in which the genetic counselor, physician, or specially trained and certified nurse tries to provide a family with the most complete and accurate information on the occurrence or the risk of recurrence of a genetic disease in that family (Pagon, Hanson, Neufeld-Kaiser, et al, 2001). Genetic counseling is thus an appropriate course of action for any family wondering, "Will it happen to us?" or "Will it happen again?"

REFERRAL

Genetic counseling referral is advised for any of the following categories:

- **Congenital abnormalities, including mental retardation.** Any couple who has a child or a relative with a congenital malformation may be at an increased risk and should be so informed. If mental retardation of unidentified cause has occurred in a family, there may be an increased risk of recurrence. In some cases, the genetic counselor will identify the cause of a malformation as a teratogen (see Chapter 16). The family should be aware of teratogenic substances so they can avoid exposure during any subsequent pregnancy.
- **Familial disorders.** Families should be told that certain diseases may have a genetic component and that the risk of their occurrence in a particular family may be higher than that for the general population. Such disorders as diabetes, heart disease, cancer, and mental illness fall into this category.
- **Known inherited diseases.** Families may know that a disease is inherited but not know the mechanism or the specific risk for them. An important point to remember is that family members who are not at risk for passing on a disorder should be as well informed as family members who are at risk.
- **Metabolic disorders.** Any families at risk for having a child with a metabolic disorder or biochemical defect should be referred for genetic counseling. Because most inborn errors of metabolism are autosomal recessively inherited ones, a family may not be identified as at risk until the birth of an affected child. Carriers of the sickle cell trait can be identified before pregnancy is begun, and the risk of having an affected child can be determined. Prenatal diagnosis of an affected fetus is available on an experimental basis only.

Global Perspectives

In the United States, marriage between related individuals is generally taboo. In Western medicine, there is a concern that a child conceived by people who are related by blood may have an increased risk for birth defects. This has not, however, been supported by recent research unless the relationship is closer than first cousins. In many other cultures, marriage of first cousins and others who are related by blood is acceptable and even common. Egypt has a high rate of consanguineous (blood relationship) marriages. Reasons for consanguineous marriage include: "increase family links," "they knew each other and everything would be clear before marriage," "customs and traditions," and "less cost." The most common type of consanguineous marriage in Egypt is between first cousins.

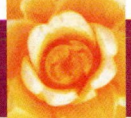

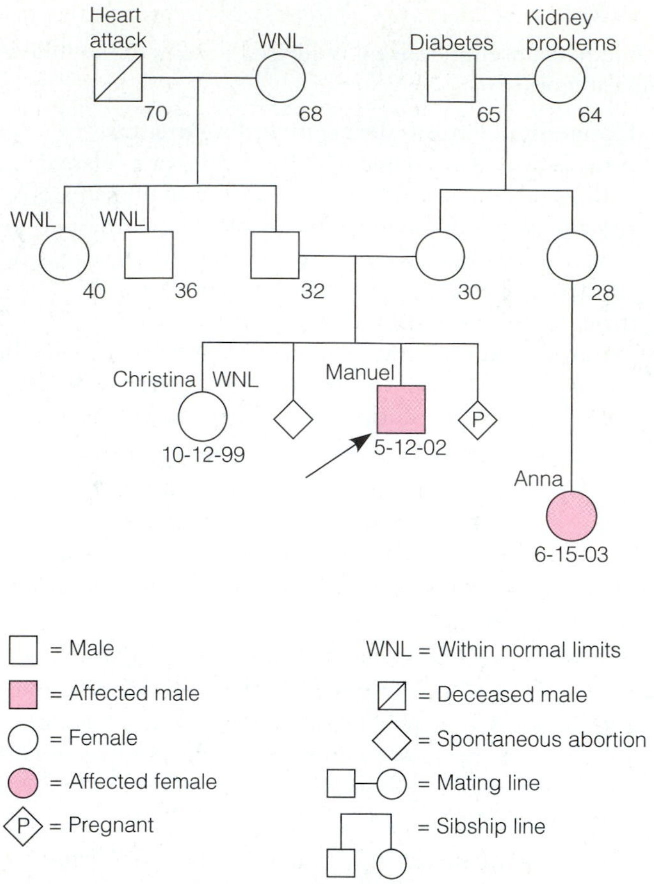

Figure 12–17 • Screening pedigree. Arrow indicates the nearest family member affected with the disorder being investigated. Numbers refer to the ages of family members.

- **Chromosomal abnormalities.** As discussed previously, any couple who has had a child with a chromosomal abnormality may be at an increased risk of having another child similarly affected. This group includes families in which there is concern for a possible translocation.

After the couple has been referred to the genetic clinic, they are sent a form requesting information on the health status of various family members. This information assists the genetic counselor in creating the family's pedigree. Together, the pedigree and health history facilitate identification of other family members who might also be at risk for the same disorder (Figure 12–17 •). The family being counseled may wish to notify those relatives at risk so that they, too, can be given genetic counseling. When done correctly, the family history and pedigree are two of the most powerful and useful tools for determining a family risk.

INITIAL SESSION

During the initial session, the counselor gathers additional information about the pregnancy, the affected child's growth and development, and the family's understanding of the problem. The counselor also elicits information concerning ethnic background and family origin. Many genetic disorders are more common among certain ethnic groups or in particular geographic areas. For example, families from the British Isles are at higher risk of having children with neural tube defects; Ashkenazi Jews (from eastern Europe) and French Canadians are at higher risk for Tay-Sachs disease; people of African descent for sickle cell anemia; Mennonites for maple syrup urine disease; and people of Mediterranean heritage for thalassemias.

Generally the child is given a physical examination. Other family members may also be examined. If any laboratory tests, such as chromosomal analysis, metabolic studies, or vital titers, are indicated, they are performed at this time. The genetic counselor may then give the family some preliminary information based on the data at hand.

FOLLOW-UP COUNSELING

When all the data have been carefully examined and analyzed, the family returns for a follow-up visit. At this time, the parents are given all the information available, including the medical facts, diagnosis, probable course of the disorder, and any available management; the inheritance pattern for this particular family and their risk of recurrence; and the options or alternatives for dealing with the risk of recurrence. The remainder of the counseling session is spent discussing the course of action that seems appropriate to the family in view of their risk and family goals (Pagon et al, 2001).

Among those options or alternatives are prenatal diagnosis and early detection and treatment and, in some cases, adoption, therapeutic insemination, or delayed childbearing.

The family may consider therapeutic donor insemination (TDI), discussed earlier in this chapter. This alternative is appropriate in several instances; for example, if the man has an autosomal dominant disease, TDI would decrease to zero the risk of having an affected child (if the sperm donor is not at risk) because the child would not inherit any genes from the affected parent. If the man is affected with an X-linked disorder and does not wish to continue the gene in the family (all his daughters will be carriers), TDI would be an alternative to terminating all pregnancies with a female fetus. If the man is a carrier for a balanced translocation and if termination of pregnancy is against family ethics, TDI is an appropriate alternative. TDI is also appropriate if both parents are carriers of an autosomal recessive disease. TDI lowers the risk to a very low level or to zero if a carrier test is available. Finally, TDI may be appropriate if the family is at high risk for a multifactorial disorder.

Couples who are young and at risk may decide to delay childbearing for a few years. Medical science and medical genetics are continually making breakthroughs in early detection and treatment. These couples may find in a few years that prenatal diagnosis will be available or that a disease can be detected and treated early to prevent irreversible damage.

When the parents have completed the counseling sessions, the counselor sends them and their physician a letter detailing the contents of the sessions. The family keeps this document for reference. See Table 12–11 •.

Table 12–11 • NURSING RESPONSIBILITIES IN GENETIC COUNSELING

Identify families at risk for genetic problems.
Determine how the genetic problem is perceived and what information is desired before proceeding.
Assist families in acquiring accurate information about the specific problem.
Act as liaison between family and genetic counselor.
Assist the family in understanding and dealing with information received.
Provide information on support groups.
Aid families in coping with this crisis.
Provide information about known genetic factors.
Assure continuity of nursing care to the family.

NURSING CARE MANAGEMENT

In both prospective and retrospective genetic counseling, timely nursing intervention is a crucial factor. During annual exams and other clinical appointments, the nurse should interview all women of childbearing age to determine any family history or other risk factors for genetic disorders. If the woman is planning to conceive, genetic counseling should be encouraged prior to discontinuation of contraception.

In retrospective counseling, the nurse has a key role in preventing recurrence. Although one cannot expect a family who has just learned that their child has a birth defect or a genetic abnormality to assimilate any information concerning future risks, the couple should never be "put off" from counseling for too long a period. Otherwise, they risk conceiving another affected child. The perinatal nurse frequently has the first contact with the family that has a newborn with a congenital abnormality. At the birth of an affected child, the nurse can inform the parents that before they attempt having another child, genetic counseling is available. The family nurse practitioner and family-planning nurse are also in an excellent position to reach at-risk families before the birth of another baby with a congenital problem.

After genetic counseling, the nurse with the appropriate knowledge of genetics is in an ideal position to help families review what has been discussed during the sessions and to answer any additional questions they might have. As the family returns to the daily aspects of living, the nurse can provide helpful information on the day-to-day aspects of caring for the child, answer questions as they arise, support parents in their decisions, and refer the family to other health and community agencies (Lewis, 2001).

The family may return to the genetic counselor a number of times to air their questions and concerns. It is desirable for the nurse working with the family to attend many or all of these counseling sessions. Because the nurse has already established a rapport with the family, the nurse can act as a liaison between the family and the genetic counselor. Hearing directly what the genetic counselor says helps the nurse clarify issues for the family, which in turn helps them formulate questions.

Additionally, if the couple is considering having more children or if siblings want information concerning their affected brother or sister, the nurse should recommend that the family return for another follow-up visit with the genetic counselor. Appropriate options can again be defined and discussed, and any new information available can be given to the family. Many genetic centers employ public health nurses to provide such follow-up care.

Nurses must be careful not to assume a diagnosis, determine carrier status or recurrence risks, or provide genetic counseling without adequate information and training. Inadequate, inappropriate, or inaccurate information may be misleading or harmful. Healthcare professionals need to learn the appropriate referral systems and options for care in their region.

CHAPTER REVIEW

EXPLOREMEDIALINK

NCLEX review questions, case studies, and other interactive resources for this chapter can be found on the Web site at http://www.prenhall.com/olds. Click on "Chapter 12" to select the activities for this chapter.

For tutorials including animations and videos, more NCLEX review questions, and an audio glossary, access the accompanying CD-ROM in this book.

Focus Your Study

- A couple is considered infertile when they do not conceive after 1 year of unprotected coitus.
- At least 8% of couples in the United States are infertile.
- A thorough history and physical of both partners is essential as a basis for infertility investigation.
- General fertility investigations include evaluation of ovarian function, cervical mucus adequacy and receptivity to sperm, sperm number and function, tubal patency, general condition of the pelvic organs, and certain laboratory tests.
- Among cases of infertility, 35% involve male factors, 45% involve female factors, or 20% have no identifiable cause or have multifactorial causes.
- Medications may be prescribed to induce ovulation, facilitate cervical mucus formation, reduce antibody concentration, increase sperm count and motility, and suppress endometriosis.
- The emotional aspect of infertility may be more difficult for the couple than the testing and therapy.
- The nurse needs to be prepared to provide accurate information about infertility and dispel myths.
- The nurse assesses coping responses and initiates counseling referrals as indicated.
- In autosomal dominant disorders, an affected parent has a 50% chance of having an affected child. Such disorders equally affect both males and females. The characteristic presentation will vary in each individual with the gene. Some of the common autosomal dominant inherited disorders are Huntington disease, polycystic kidney disease, and neurofibromatosis (von Recklinghausen disease).
- Autosomal recessive disorders are characterized by both parents being carriers; each offspring has a 25% chance of having the disease, a 25% chance of not being affected, and a 50% chance of being a carrier. Males and females are equally affected. Some common autosomal recessive inheritance disorders are cystic fibrosis, phenylketonuria (PKU), galactosemia, sickle cell anemia, Tay-Sachs disease, and most metabolic disorders.
- X-linked recessive disorders are characterized by no male-to-male transmission; effects limited to males; a 50% chance that a carrier mother will pass the abnormal gene to her sons; a 50% chance that her daughters will be carriers; and a 100% chance that daughters of affected fathers will be carriers. Common X-linked recessive disorders are hemophilia, some forms of color blindness, and Duchenne muscular dystrophy.
- Multifactorial inheritance disorders include cleft lip and palate, spina bifida, dislocated hips, clubfoot, and pyloric stenosis.
- Some genetic conditions that can currently be diagnosed prenatally are neural tube and cranial defects, renal malformations, hemophilia, fragile X syndrome, thalassemia, cystic fibrosis, and many inborn errors of metabolism such as Tay-Sachs disease. This list expands daily as new technology allows more conditions to be detected.
- The chief tools of prenatal diagnosis are ultrasound, maternal serum alpha-fetoprotein testing, amniocentesis, chorionic villus sampling, and percutaneous umbilical blood sampling.
- Based on sound knowledge about common genetic problems, the nurse should prepare the family for counseling and act as a resource person during and after the counseling sessions. Many nurses with advanced training are entering the field of genetic counseling.

References

American Academy of Pediatrics, Committee on Genetics. (2000). Molecular genetic testing in pediatric practice: A subject review. *Pediatrics, 106,* 1494–1497.

American Fertility Society. (1994). *Infertility: Questions and answers.* Washington, DC: American Fertility Society, Office of Government Relations.

American Society for Reproductive Medicine. (2002). Assisted reproductive technology in the United States: 1999 results generated from the American Society for Reproductive Medicine/Society for Assisted Reproductive Technology Registry. *Fertility and Sterility, 78*(5), 918–931.

Beal, M. W. (1999). Acupuncture and acupressure. Applications to women's reproductive healthcare. *Journal of Nurse Midwifery, 44*(3), 217–230.

Bopp, B. L., & Seifer, D. B. (2000). Age and reproduction. In J. J. Sciarri & T. J. Watkins (Eds.), *Gynecology and obstetrics* (Vol. 5, chap. 72, pp. 1–26). Philadelphia: Lippincott Williams & Wilkins.

Braverman, A., & English, M. (1992). Creating brave new families with advanced reproductive technologies. *Clinical Issues in Perinatal Women's Health Nursing, 3*(2), 353–363.

Chen, J. C., Xu, M. X., Chen, L. D., Chen, Y. N., & Chiu, T. H. (1999). Effect of Panax notoginseng extracts on inferior sperm motility in vitro. *American Journal of Chinese Medicine, 27,* 123–128.

Cowan, B. D. (2002). Evaluation of the female for infertility. In D. B. Seifer & R. L. Collins (Eds.), *Office-based infertility practice.* New York: Springer.

Drenkard, K., & Ferguson, S. (2002). Genetic testing and discrimination: Case example-Virginia. *Pediatric Nursing, 28*(1), 71–73.

Giarelli, E., & Jacobs, L. A. (2000). Issues related to the use of genetic material and information. *Oncology Nursing Forum, 27*, 459–467.

Gladstar, R. (1993). *Herbal healing for women.* New York: Simon & Schuster.

Gordon, J. D., & Speroff, L. (2002). *Handbook for clinical gynecologic, endocrinology and infertility.* Philadelphia: Lippincott Williams & Wilkins.

Gottlieb, B. (2000). *Alternative cures: The most effective natural home remedies for 160 health problems.* Emmaus, PA: Rodale Press.

Graves, J. C., Miller, K. E., & Sellers, A. (2002). Maternal serum triple analyte screening in pregnancy. *American Family Physician, 65*(5), 915–920.

Greenfeld, D. A. (2002). Coping with infertility: Practical psychosocial issues. In D. B. Seifer & R. L. Collins (Eds.), *Office-based infertility practice.* New York: Springer.

Hammond, K. (2001). How to help an infertile couple. *The Nurse Practitioner, 26*(Supp. 1), 1–15.

Hong, C. Y., Ku, J., & Wu, P. (1992). Astragalus membranaceus stimulates human sperm motility in vitro. *American Journal of Chinese Medicine, 20*, 289–294.

Johnson, C. L. (1996). Regaining self-esteem: Strategies and interventions for the infertile woman. *Journal of Obstetric, Gynecologic, and Neonatal Nursing, 25*(4), 291–295.

Kingsberg, S. A., Applegarth, L. D., & Janata, J. W. (2000). Embryo donation programs and policies in North America: Survey results and implications for health and mental health professionals. *Fertility and Sterility, 73*(2), 215–220.

Leibowitz, D., & Hoffman, D. (2000). Fertility drug therapies: Past, present, and future. *Journal of Obstetric, Gynecologic, and Neonatal Nursing, 29*(2), 201–210.

Leon, I. G. (2000). Psychology of reproduction: Pregnancy, parenthood, and parental ties. In J. J. Sciarri & T. J. Watkins (Eds.), *Gynecology and obstetrics* (Vol. 6, chap. 62, pp. 1–29). Philadelphia: Lippincott Williams & Wilkins.

Lewis, J. A. (2001). The human genome and public policy: A nursing perspective. *Journal of Obstetric, Gynecologic, and Neonatal Nursing, 30*(5), 541–545.

Mahowald, M. B., McKusick, V. A., Scheuerle, A. S., & Aspinwall, T. J. (2001). *Genetics in the clinic: Clinical, ethical, and social implications for primary care.* St. Louis, MO: Mosby.

Newberger, D. S. (2000). Down syndrome: Prenatal risk assessment and diagnosis. *American Family Physician, 62*(4), 825–832, 837–838.

Pagon, R. A., Hanson, N. B., Neufeld-Kaiser, W., & Covington, M. L. (2001). Genetic consultation. *Western Journal of Medicine, 174*(6), 397–399.

Paulus, W. E., Zhang, M., Strehler, E., El-Danasouri, I., & Sterzik, K. (2002). Influence of acupuncture on the pregnancy rate in patients who undergo assisted reproduction therapy. *Fertility and Sterility, 77*(4), 721–724.

Pergament, E., & Fiddler, M. (2000). Indications and patient selection for preimplantation-related chromosome abnormalities. In J. J. Sciarri & T. J. Watkins (Eds.), *Gynecology and obstetrics* (Vol.5, chap. 107, pp. 1–7). Philadelphia: Lippincott Williams & Wilkins.

Sandelowski, M. (1994). On infertility. *Journal of Obstetric, Gynecologic, and Neonatal Nursing, 23*(9), 749–752.

Sawatzky, M. (1981). Tasks of the infertile couple. *Journal of Obstetric, Gynecologic, and Neonatal Nursing, 10*, 132–133.

Shane, J. M. (1993). Evaluation and treatment of infertility. *Clinical Symposia, 45*, 2–32.

Sharara, F. I., & McClamrock, H. D. (2000). Differences in in-vitro fertilization (IVF) outcome between white and black women in an inner-city university-based IVF program. *Fertility and Sterility, 73* (6), 1170–1173.

Simpson, J. L. (2002a). Genetic counseling and prenatal diagnosis. In S. G. Gabbe, J. R. Niebyl, & J. L. Simpson (Eds.), *Obstetrics: Normal and problem pregnancies* (4th ed., pp. 187–219). Philadelphia, PA: Churchill Livingstone.

Simpson, J. L. (2002b). Polygenic/multifactorial inheritance. In J. J. Sciarri (Ed.), *Gynecology and obstetrics* (Vol. 5, chap. 75, pp. 1–9). Hagerstown, MD: Harper & Row.

Sinclair, S. (2000). Male infertility: Nutritional and environmental considerations. *Alternative Medicine Review, 5*(1), 28–38.

Siterman, S., Eltes, F., Wolfson, V., Lederman, H., & Bartoov, B. (2000). Does acupuncture treatment affect sperm density in males with very low sperm count? A pilot study. *Andrologia, 32*(1), 31–39.

Spear, K. A. (2002). Evaluation of the male for infertility. In D. B. Seifer & R. L. Collins (Eds.), *Office-based infertility practice.* New York: Springer.

Stribley, J. M., Rehman, K. S., Niu, H., & Christman, G. M. (2002). Gene therapy and reproductive medicine. *Fertility and Sterility, 77*(4), 645–657.

Tinkle, M. B., & Cheek, D. J. (2002). Human genomics: Challenges and opportunities. *Journal of Obstetric, Gynecologic, and Neonatal Nursing, 31*(2), 178–187.

Tiran, D., & Mack, S. (2000). *Complementary therapies for pregnancy and childbirth* (2nd ed.). Philadelphia: Harcourt Publishers Limited.

Usadi, R. S., & Fritz, M. A. (2002). Induction of ovulation with clomiphene citrate. In J. J. Sciarri (Ed.), *Gynecology and obstetrics* (Vol. 5, chap. 68, pp. 1–12). Hagerstown, MD: Harper & Row.

Valle, R. F. (2002). Hysteroscopy and infertility. In J. J. Sciarri (Ed.), *Gynecology and obstetrics* (Vol. 1, chap. 121, pp. 1–18). Hagerstown, MD: Harper & Row.

Widrich, T. (2002). Role of ultrasonography in infertility. In D. B. Seifer & R. L. Collins (Eds.), *Office-based infertility practice.* New York: Springer.

Williams, J. K. (2000). Impact of genome research on children and their families. *Journal of Pediatric Nursing, 15*(4), 207–211.

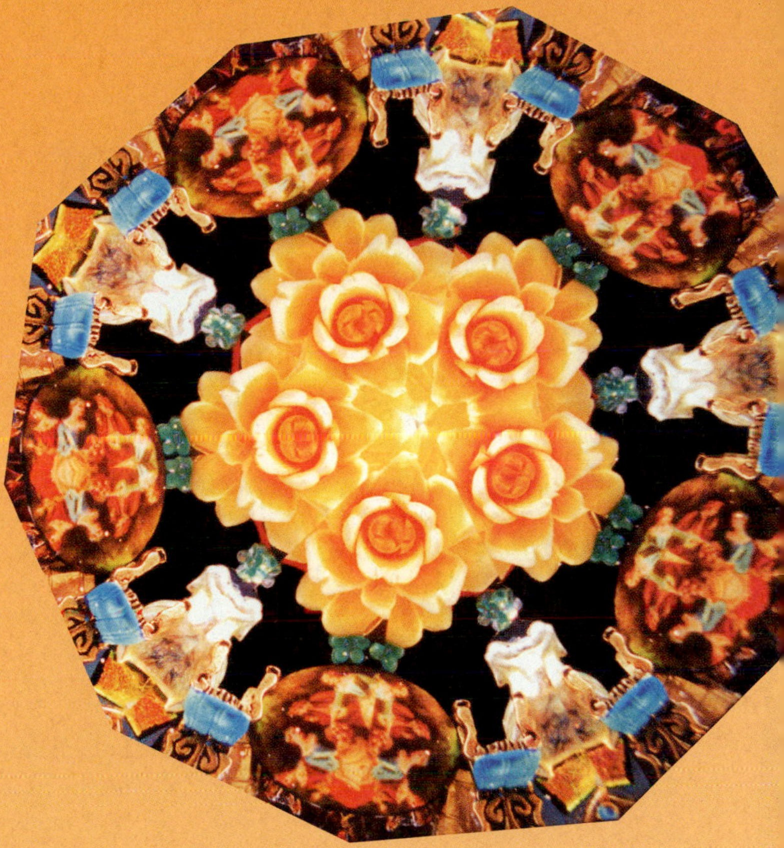

FOUR

Pregnancy

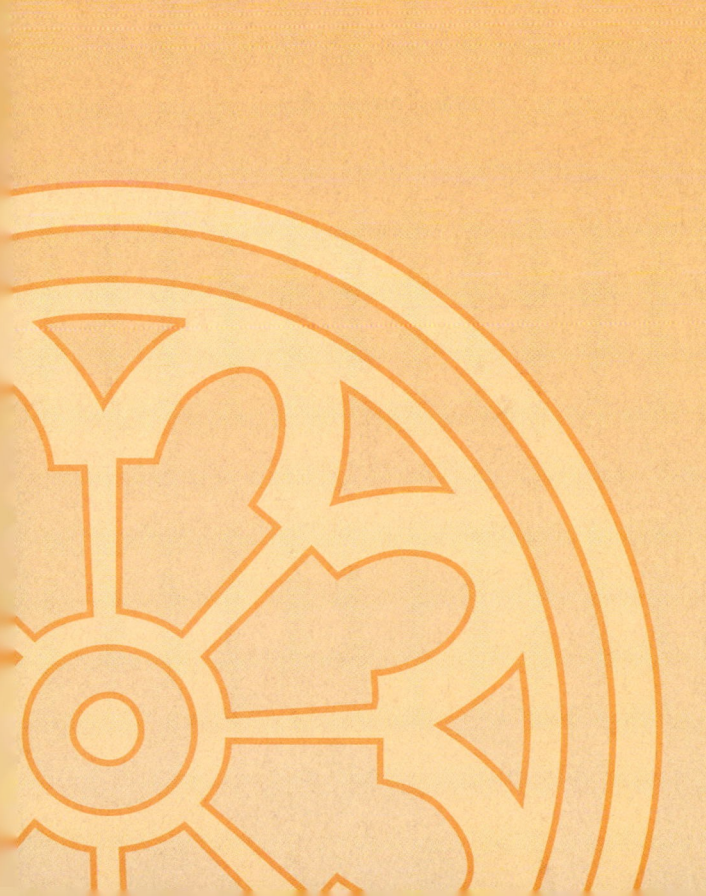

Preparation for Parenthood

13

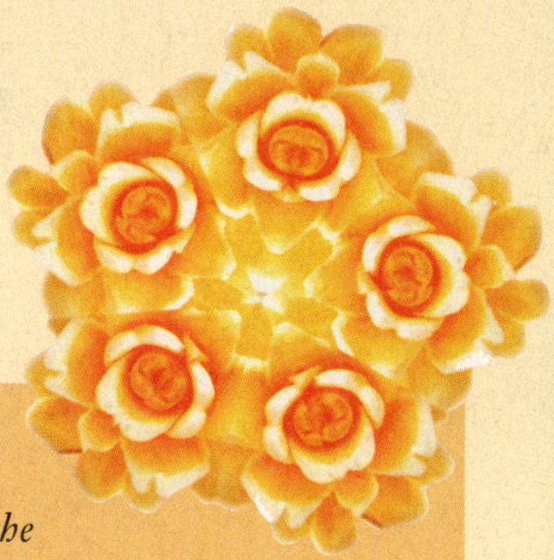

I couldn't wait to begin our childbirth classes. Attending the classes with the other expectant parents made the pregnancy and upcoming labor seem so much more real. Our childbirth educator helped ease our anxiety and gave us guidance on how to make the most of the birth. I still keep in contact with a few of my classmates and send an annual holiday greeting card with my son's photograph to our instructor.

Objectives

- Apply the nursing process to help couples prepare for childbirth.
- Identify the various issues related to preconception counseling, pregnancy, labor, and birth that require decision making by parents.
- Discuss the basic goals of childbirth education.
- Summarize the role of the doula/labor companion during labor and birth.
- Describe the types of prenatal education programs available to expectant couples and their families.
- Delineate the childbirth educator's role in promoting relaxation for pregnant women.
- Compare methods of childbirth preparation.

MediaLink

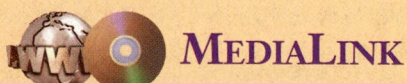

Additional resources for this content can be found on the Student CD-ROM and on the Companion Website at www.prenhall.com/olds. Click on "Chapter 13" to select the activities for this chapter.

CD-ROM
- Audio Glossary
- NCLEX Review

Companion Website
- Additional NCLEX Review
- Case Study: Preparing for Pregnancy
- Care Plan Activity: Preconception Counseling

Key Terms

Birth plan 287
Disassociation relaxation 295
Doula 290
Effleurage 296
Prenatal education 290
Progressive relaxation 295
Touch relaxation 295

Preparation for parenthood begins with one's own birth into a family. Attitudes, feelings, and fears about pregnancy, birth, and parenthood are molded by numerous factors, including relationships within and outside one's own family, cultural conditioning, personal history, and discussions with healthcare providers, friends, and other women.

A person's experiences with parenting or children may have been pleasant or uncomfortable. A person's information about parenthood and related areas may or may not be accurate. Because people bring their beliefs and fears with them to the childbearing period, the nurse can do much to correct misconceptions and calm fears about pregnancy, childbirth, and early parenting. While some women may approach labor and birth with great excitement and anticipation, others may view it as a fearful, unpleasant experience. One way that a couple can cope with feelings about impending parenthood is to assume an active, participatory role during the preconception, prenatal, intrapartal, and postpartal periods. This involvement offers them a degree of control over what could otherwise be an overwhelming experience.

Some of the decisions that the childbearing family must consider are presented in this chapter. These include the decision to have a baby, choice of care provider, type of childbirth preparation, place of birth, activities during the birth, method of infant feeding, and choices surrounding the care of the newborn. The chapter also considers the role of the nurse, who provides information that enables the family to make informed decisions.

Throughout this chapter the term "childbearing family" is used to include all family types. In today's society, the childbearing family may be composed of a man and a woman joined by marriage or simply by mutual personal commitment, a single woman living alone or with a friend or family member, or a lesbian couple. No matter what the family structure and configuration, the expectant woman and her support person have similar concerns and educational needs during this time.

Today's professional nurse has many opportunities to help the childbearing family make the decisions that are part of pregnancy and birth. The nurse can help families seek preconceptual counseling, select a healthcare provider, find prenatal classes that meet their needs, and make informed choices. Even more important, as the family works through these decisions, the nurse is able to affirm their decision-making abilities and their ability to take on parenting roles. For first-time parents in particular, the decisions may seem numerous, complicated, and sometimes overwhelming. The nurse has a unique opportunity to help these families establish a pattern of decision making that will serve them well in their years as parents (Figure 13–1 •).

MEDIALINK CARE PLAN: PRECONCEPTION COUNSELING

Preconception Counseling

One of the first questions a couple should ask before conception is whether they wish to have children. This involves consideration of each person's goals, expectations of their relationship, and desire to be a parent. At times one individual wishes to have a child while the other does not. In such situations, an open discussion is essential to reach a mutually acceptable decision. In some cases, professional counseling for the couple may be necessary.

Couples who wish to have a child face a decision about the timing of pregnancy. At what point in their lives do they believe it would be best to become parents? Pregnancy comes as a surprise even when the decision about timing is made, but at least the couple has some control over it.

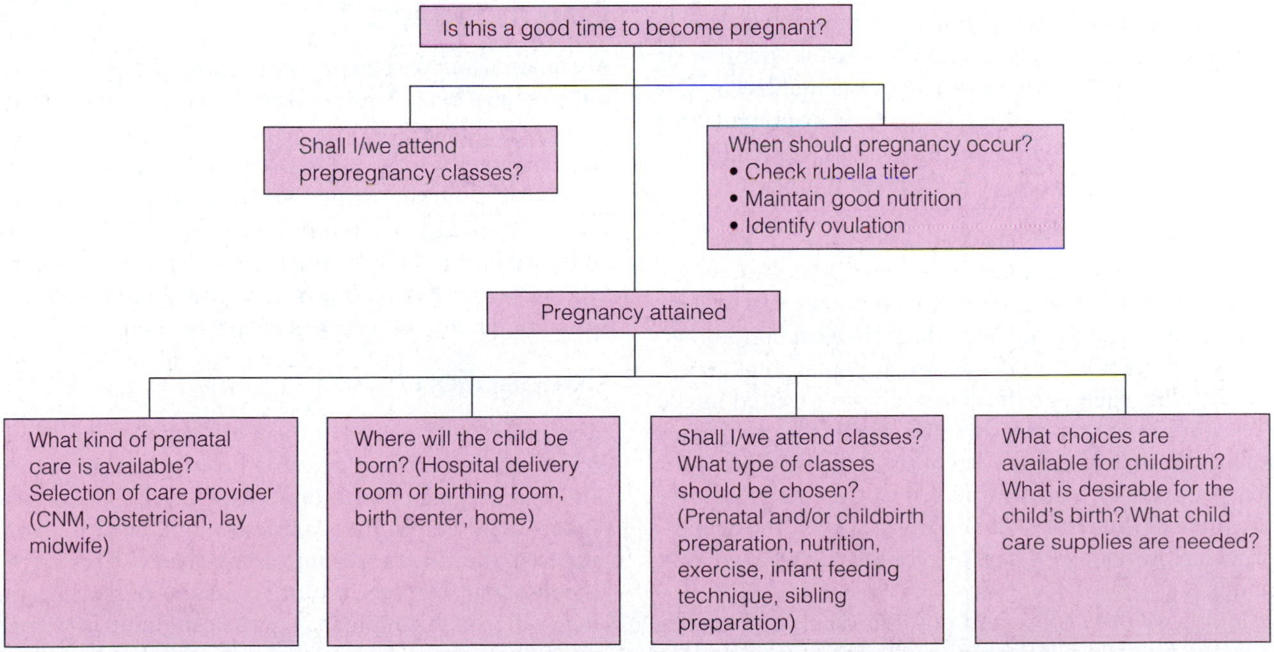

Figure 13–1 • Pregnancy decision tree.

MediaLink CASE STUDY: PREPARING FOR PREGNANCY

For couples who have religious beliefs that do not support contraception or who feel that family planning is unnatural and wrong, planning the timing of pregnancy is unacceptable and irrelevant. These couples can still take steps to ensure that they are in the best possible physical and mental health when pregnancy occurs.

Ideally, the decision to become pregnant and have a child should be a conscious one; however, this is not always the case. Of all pregnancies in the United States, 9.2% are unplanned (Ventura, Mosher, Curtin, et al, 2000). Couples with unplanned pregnancies may need additional support from the nurse such as information about community resources available for the couple and their infant. Encouragement and reassurance are especially needed for these families.

Preconception Health Measures

The nurse working with a woman or couple during the preconception period explains about known or suspected health risks. The nurse advises the woman to cease smoking if possible, or to limit her cigarette intake. Cigarette smoking has been associated with low birth weight, spontaneous abortion, abruptio placentae, placenta previa, sudden infant death syndrome, and reduced infant lung functioning (Chin, 2001; Gawley & Cupples, 2002). Cigarette smokers also have a higher incidence of ectopic pregnancy than nonsmokers (Chin, 2001). Secondhand smoke has been found to increase the risk of small-for-gestational-age infants; therefore, partners of pregnant women should refrain from smoking in the woman's presence (Dejin-Karlsson, Hanson, Ostergren, et al, 1998).

The effects of caffeine are less clearly understood; however, as a precaution the woman is advised to avoid caffeine or limit her intake. Alcohol, social drugs, and street drugs pose a real threat to the fetus. A woman who uses any prescription or over-the-counter medications needs to discuss the implications of their use with her healthcare provider. It is best to avoid using any medication if possible. Because of the possible teratogenic effects of environmental hazards in the workplace, the nurse urges the couple contemplating pregnancy to determine whether they are exposed to any environmental hazards at work or in their community.

PHYSICAL EXAMINATION

It is advisable for both partners to have a physical examination to identify any health problems so that they can be corrected if possible. These might include medical conditions, such as high blood pressure or obesity; problems that pose a threat to fertility, such as certain sexually transmitted infections; or conditions that keep the individual from achieving optimal health, such as anemia or colitis. If the family history indicates previous genetic disorders, or if the couple is planning pregnancy when the woman is over age 35, the healthcare provider may suggest that the couple consider genetic counseling.

In addition to the history and physical exam, the woman may have the following laboratory tests: urinalysis, complete blood count, Rh factor, venereal disease research laboratory (VDRL) test, Pap smear, gonorrhea culture, chlamydia screen, and rubella and hepatitis screens (Andolsek & Ketton, 2000). Women who are nonimmune to rubella should be counseled about the possible effects on the fetus should infection occur during the first trimester of pregnancy. Women may choose to receive the vaccine and then wait 3 months before conceiving to eliminate the risk of prenatal infection. Women should be counseled to use contraception during the 3-month time period to prevent pregnancy. Prior to conception, the woman is also advised to have a dental examination and any necessary dental work to avoid exposure to x-rays and the risk of infection.

NUTRITION

Prior to conception it is advisable for the woman to be at an average weight for her body build and height. The nurse can discuss nutrition and recommend that the woman follow a nutritious diet that contains ample quantities of all the essential nutrients. Some nutritionists advocate emphasizing the following nutrients: calcium, protein, iron, B complex vitamins, vitamin C, magnesium, and folic acid. Folic acid supplementation should be initiated prior to conception since it decreases the incidence of neural tube defects in infants. (See discussion in Chapter 18.) Excessive intake of certain vitamins can cause severe fetal problems and should be avoided.

EXERCISE

A woman is advised to establish a regular exercise plan beginning at least 3 months before she plans to attempt to become pregnant. The exercise should be one she enjoys and will continue. It needs to provide some aerobic conditioning and some general toning. Exercise improves the woman's circulation and general health and tones her muscles. Once an exercise program is well established, the woman is generally encouraged to continue it during pregnancy.

Contraception

A woman who takes birth control pills is advised to stop the pill and have two or three normal menses before attempting to conceive. This allows the natural hormonal cycle to return and facilitates dating the subsequent pregnancy. A woman using an intrauterine device is advised to have it removed and wait 1 month before attempting to conceive. This allows the endometrium to be resterilized. During the waiting period, she can use barrier methods of contraception (condoms, diaphragm, or cervical cap with a spermicide).

Conception

Most preconception recommendations focus on helping the couple attain their best possible health state so that they do not enter pregnancy with unnecessary risks. Conception is a personal and emotional experience and, even if a couple is prepared, they may feel some ambivalence. This is a normal response, but they may require reassurance that the ambivalence will pass. A couple may get so caught up in preparation and in their efforts to "do things right" that they lose sight of the pleasure they derive from each other and their lives together and cease to value the joy of spontaneity in their relationship. It is often helpful for the healthcare provider to remind an overly zealous couple that moderation is always appropriate and that there is value in "taking time to smell the roses."

Childbearing Decisions

Parents face several decisions about their childbirth experience. A method that has assisted many couples in making these choices is called a birth plan. In the **birth plan,** prospective parents identify aspects of the childbearing experience that are most important to them. (A sample birth plan is presented in Figure 13–2 •.) The birth plan helps identify available options and becomes a tool for communication among the expectant parents, the healthcare providers, and the healthcare professionals at the birth setting. The plan can also specify options the couple might wish to avoid (England & Horowitz, 1998).

The birth plan also helps pregnant women and couples set priorities. Using the plan, they identify areas that they want to incorporate in their own birth experience. Then they can take the birth plan to a visit with their certified nurse-midwife or other care provider and use it in discussing and comparing their wishes with the philosophy and beliefs of the provider. It is imperative that the couple discusses their preferences at a prenatal visit prior to labor. Sometimes couples may include requests that need clarification. For example, if the couple states they do not want any external monitoring, the provider needs to explain that intermittent monitoring could be provided but that eliminating all monitoring during labor could jeopardize both the mother and the fetus. They can also take the birth plan to the birth setting and use it as a basis for communicating their wishes during the childbirth experience.

There are many more choices that pregnant women and couples make. Some of these are explored in Table 13–1 •. Although most birth experiences are close to the desired experience, at times expectations cannot be met. This may be due to unavailability of some choices in the community or to unexpected problems during pregnancy or birth. It is important for nurses to help expectant parents keep sight of what is realistic for their situation.

Sample Birth Plan

Choice	*Choice*
Care provider:	Position during birth:
Certified nurse-midwife	On side
Obstetrician	Hands and knees
Family physician	Kneeling
Lay midwife	Squatting
Birth setting	Birthing chair
Hospital:	Birthing bed
Birthing room	Other:
Delivery room	Family present (sibs)
Birth center	Filming of birth (videotaping)
Home	Photography of birth
Support during labor and birth:	Leboyer
Partner present	Episiotomy
Doula present	No sterile drapes
During labor:	Partner to cut umbilical cord
Ambulate as desired	Hold baby immediately after birth
Shower if desired	Breastfeed immediately after birth
Wear own clothes	No separation after birth
Use hot tub	Save the placenta
Use own rocking chair	Collect cord blood for banking
Have perineal prep	Newborn care:
Have enema	Eye treatment for the baby
Water birth	Vitamin K injection
Electronic fetal monitor	Heptovac injection
Membranes:	Breastfeeding
Rupture naturally	Formula feeding
Amniotomy if needed	Pacifier use
Labor stimulation if needed	Glucose water
Medication:	Circumcision
Identify type desired	Postpartum care:
Fluids or ice as desired	Short stay
Music during labor and birth	48-hour stay after vaginal birth
Massage	Home visits after discharge
Therapeutic touch	Home doula
Healing touch	Other:

Figure 13–2 • Birth plan for childbirth choices. The columns list various choices that the couple may consider during their childbirth experience. Once the couple has considered each of the choices, they may circle the items they desire.

Care Provider

MEDIALINK CHILDBIRTH SOLUTIONS

One of the first decisions facing expectant parents is the selection of a healthcare provider. The nurse assists them by explaining the various options and outlining what can be expected from each. A thorough understanding of the differences of education preparation, skill level, practice style, and general philosophy and characteristics of practice of certified nurse-midwives, obstetricians, family practice physicians, and lay midwives is essential. The nurse can encourage expectant parents to investigate the care provider's credentials, basic and special education and training, fee schedule, and availability to new clients; this is often accomplished by telephoning the provider's office.

The nurse can also help the woman/couple develop a list of interview questions for their first visit to a care provider. These could include the following:

- Who is in practice with you, or who covers for you when you are unavailable?
- At what point after admission do you come to the hospital or birth setting to provide support?
- How do your partners' philosophies compare to yours?
- How do you feel about my partner, other support person, or other children coming to the prenatal visits?
- What weight gain do you recommend and why?
- What are your feelings about (fill in special desires for the birth event, such as different positions assumed during labor, avoidance of an episiotomy, induction of labor, other people present during the birth, pain control measures, breastfeeding immediately after the birth, no separation of infant and parents following birth, and so on)?

Table 13–1 • BENEFITS AND RISKS OF SOME CONSUMER DECISIONS DURING PREGNANCY, LABOR, AND BIRTH

Issue	Benefits	Risks
Breastfeeding	• No additional expense • Contains maternal antibodies • Decreases incidence of infant otitis media, vomiting, and diarrhea, hospitalizations during the first year of life, and allergies • Easier to digest than formula • Immediately after birth, promotes uterine contractions and decreases incidence of postpartum hemorrhage • Promotes maternal-infant bonding	• Transmission of maternal infections to newborn, such as HIV • Irregular ovulation and menses can cause false sense of security and nonuse of hormonal contraceptives • Increased nutritional requirement in mother
Perineal prep	• May decrease risk of infection • Facilitates episiotomy repair	• Nicks can be portal for bacteria • Discomfort as hair grows back
Enema	• May facilitate labor • Increases space for infant in pelvis • May increase strength of contractions • May prevent contamination of sterile field	• Increases discomfort and anxiety

Ambulation during labor	• Comfort for laboring woman
	• May assist in labor progression by
	  • Stimulating contractions
	  • Allowing gravity to help descent of fetus
	  • Giving sense of independence and control
		• Cord prolapse will rupture membranes unless engagement has occurred
		• Birth of infant in undesirable locations (hallways, outdoors, waiting area)
		• Inability to monitor fetal heart rate

Electronic fetal monitoring	• Helps evaluate fetal well-being • Helps identify fetal stress • Useful in diagnostic testing • Helps evaluate labor progress	• Supine postural hypotension • Intrauterine perforation (with internal uterine pressure device) • Infection (with internal monitoring) • Decreases personal interaction with mother because of attention paid to the machine • Mother is unable to ambulate or change her position freely
Whirlpool (jet hydrotherapy)	• Increased relaxation • Decreased anxiety • Stimulation of labor • Provides pain relief • Slight decrease in BP • Increased diuresis • Decreased incidence of vacuum and forceps deliveries • Increased pain threshold • Higher satisfaction with birth • Decreased use of pain medication	• May slow contractions if used before active labor is established • Possible risk of infection if membranes are ruptured • Slight increase in maternal temperature and pulse in tub • Hypothermia • Increases FHR by 10–20 BPM (Teschendorf & Evans, 2000)
Analgesia	• Maternal relaxation facilitates labor	• All drugs reach the fetus in varying degrees and with varying effects
Episiotomy	• Decreases irregular tearing of perineum • Easier to repair for practitioner	• Increased pain after birth and for 1–3 months following birth • Dyspareunia • Infection • Increased frequency of 3rd- and 4th-degree lacerations (Low, Seng, Murtland, et al, 2000)

Note: For additional information regarding these issues, refer to Chapter 26.

- If a cesarean is necessary, can my partner be present?
- What are your feelings regarding complementary treatments during labor (herbs to augment labor, use of acupressure/massage/hypnosis, use of oils for perineal massage, and so on)?

Expectant parents also need to discuss the qualities they want in a care provider for the newborn. They may want to visit several before the birth to select someone who will meet their needs and those of their child.

Birth Setting

The nurse can help expectant parents choose a birth setting by suggesting they tour facilities and talk with nurses there, as well as talk with friends or acquaintances who are recent parents. Questions that may be asked of new parents include the following:

- What kind of support did you receive during labor? Was it what you wanted?
- If the setting has both labor and delivery rooms and birthing rooms, was a birthing room available when you wanted it?
- Were you encouraged to be mobile during labor or to do what you wanted to do (walking, sitting in a rocking chair, remaining in bed, sitting in a hot tub, standing in a shower, and so on)?
- Was your labor partner or coach treated well?
- Were you allowed to take an active role in decision making throughout the birth process?

- If you had a doula, was her role respected? Was she welcome in the birth setting?
- Was your birth plan respected? Did you share it with the facility before the birth? If something did not work, why do you think there were problems?
- Did the nurse offer suggestions regarding comfort measures?
- Did the healthcare team provide emotional support?
- How were medications handled during labor? Were you comfortable with this?
- Were siblings welcomed in the birth setting? At the birth? After the birth?
- Did you feel you were given ample time to spend with your baby immediately after childbirth?
- Was the nursing staff helpful after the baby was born? Did you receive self-care and infant care information? Was it in a usable form? Did you have a choice about what information you got? Did they let you decide what information you needed?
- Did you feel your choice of feeding method was supported?

The nurse helps expectant parents understand the array of choices available to them. The nurse can encourage them to consider options early in the pregnancy to allow time for talking with other parents and touring facilities.

> *What I've seen time and again is that the technology of the hospital overwhelms patients' natural instincts; they are intimidated, afraid of appearing stupid or clumsy or sentimental in a surrounding that seems too efficient and immaculate and intelligent.*
>
> ~ A MIDWIFE'S STORY ~

Nurses involved in childbirth education need to include the concept of individuality when providing information to expectant parents about the process of childbirth and their own pattern of coping. The wave of the future in childbirth education is to encourage women to incorporate their natural responses into coping with the pain of labor and birth. Alternative self-care activities should be explored with the expectant couple to identify preferences.

Nurses should encourage expectant women and couples to personalize the birth setting. The woman might plan, for example, to bring items from home to enhance relaxation and comfort, such as warm socks, slippers, bath powder, lotion, or a favorite blanket. She may wish to bring photographs of children, parents, or friends who cannot be there to share the birth experience. Many expectant parents enjoy listening to tapes of favorite music or watching home videotapes or favorite films. Such personalization of the birth setting may give expectant parents feelings of increased serenity and empowerment.

> ***Clinical Tip*** *Call the birthing facilities in your community and inquire about what choices are available in each facility so that you can answer expectant parents' questions.*

Labor Support Person

Some of the first formal childbirth preparation classes were patterned after a book entitled *Husband Coached Childbirth* by Dr. Robert Bradley, published in 1965. Since that time, husbands and other partners of expectant women have been very involved in acting as "coaches" or support persons during childbirth classes, labor, and birth. While some men or support persons welcome the role and look forward to providing emotional and physical support, others do not. Some men may become anxious and fearful. They may express feelings of helplessness during the birthing process or

EVIDENCE-BASED PRACTICE

EFFECTS OF HOME-LIKE SETTING FOR BIRTH

Clinical Question

What effects do home-like birth settings have on labor and birth outcomes compared to conventional hospital care?

The Evidence

A review of six trials involving almost 9000 women was conducted. In home-like birth settings, there were lower rates of intrapartum analgesia/anesthesia, lower rates of augmented labor, lower rates of episiotimies, lower rates of operative delivery, and greater satisfaction with care, when compared to hospital-like birth settings. A non-statistically significant trend towards higher perinatal mortality was evident in the home-like setting. However, women in home-like settings were more likely to have vaginal/perineal tears. There was no difference in the likelihood of having a non-intact perineum.

One trial found a greater incidence of sore nipples and mastitis in the home-like setting, but no difference was evident in the number who had discontinued breastfeeding at 6-8 weeks.

Best Practice

Home-like birth settings offer important benefits for mother. Of utmost importance is the need for monitoring for complications.

Reference: Hodnett, E. D.. Home-like versus conventional institutional settings for birth (Cochrane Review). In: The Cochrane Library, Issue 3, 2002. Oxford: Update Software.

become frustrated that techniques learned in prenatal education classes do not appear to be working (Chapman, 2000). These feelings can be related to past experiences and/or cultural factors. In these situations, the nurse provides encouragement and support to both the woman and her support person. A recent study identified women's satisfaction with childbirth as being directly affected by four key factors: the relationship with the caregiver, the support she received from caregivers, personal expectations, and her involvement with decision making (Hodnett, 2002). Clearly, the role of the nurse cannot be overestimated.

When the partner is not actively involved in supportive, attentive care, most women look to another woman for empathy and help (Robotti & Inman, 1998). Out of this need for companionship and special support in the birthing journey, the role of the **doula** has evolved. *Doula* is a Greek word that means "woman's servant." In the birthing environment, a doula is a companion who provides support but does not perform any clinical tasks. The doula provides emotional, physical, and informational support and acts as an advocate for the woman and her family by verbalizing their wishes to the nurses and physicians or certified nurse-midwives. A doula may also be trained to provide support and care during the postpartum period and in this role is called a *home doula* (Robotti & Inman, 1998). The doula may accompany the childbearing couple on a volunteer basis or may be paid a fee by the family. Another support person who has been involved in labor and birthing is a monitrice. *Monitrice* is a French word that refers to a specially trained nurse who provides assessment, nursing care, and support. The role of monitrice is not common in the United States.

MEDIALINK DOULAS OF NORTH AMERICA

Siblings at Birth

Some couples decide to have their other children present at the birth. Children who will attend a birth can be prepared through books, audiovisual materials, models, discussion, and sibling classes. Nurses can assist parents with sibling preparation by helping them understand the stresses a child may experience. For example, the child may feel left out when there is a new child to love or disappointed if a brother is born when a sister is expected.

It is imperative that the child has his or her own support person or coach whose sole responsibility is tending to the needs of that child. The support person should be familiar to the child, warm, sensitive, flexible, knowledgeable about the birth process, and comfortable with sexuality and birth. This person must be prepared to interpret what is happening to the child and to intervene when necessary. The support person should not be one who would hesitate to leave the birthing room (such as a maternal grandmother) but should be amenable to the child's desire to leave. The support person for the child should assume responsibility for providing distractions when needed. Trips to the cafeteria, visits to the nursery window, outdoor walks, and other age-appropriate activities should be available for the child.

Children should be given the option of relating to the birth in whatever manner they choose as long as it is not disruptive. Children should understand that it is their own choice to be there and that they may stay or leave the room as they choose. To help children recognize their needs and desires, the nurse may wish to elicit exactly what they expect from the experience. Children need to feel free to ask questions and express feelings.

In general, the presence of siblings at birth engenders feelings of interest and the desire to nurture "our" baby, as opposed to jealousy and rivalry directed at "Mom's" baby. The mother does not disappear mysteriously into the hospital and return with a demanding outsider. Instead, the family attending the birth together finds a new opportunity for closeness and growth by sharing in the birth of a new member.

GLOBAL PERSPECTIVES

In most Middle Eastern countries, childbirth is exclusively attended to by women. A woman in labor is most commonly surrounded by female relatives and friends. It is customary for the husband to be excluded from the delivery room. In Iran, full segregation is mandated by law. Women can only be cared for by female healthcare providers.

Classes for Family Members During Pregnancy

Childbirth classes are routinely taught by certified childbirth educators (CBEs or CCEs). These are individuals who have received specific educational preparation related to pregnancy, labor, birth, and postpartum/newborn care and issues. Many CBEs are also registered nurses; however, nursing training is not required. The majority of the certification programs do, however, require witnessing a minimum number of births.

Prenatal education programs provide important opportunities to share information about pregnancy, childbirth, coping mechanisms, and choices available for the woman and her support person. The content of each class is generally directed by the overall goals of the program. For example, in classes that aim to provide preconception information, preparations for becoming pregnant would be the major topics. Other classes may be directed toward childbirth choices available today, preparation of the mother for pregnancy and birth, preparation for cesarean birth, preparation for vaginal birth after cesarean, preparation for couples who desire an unmedicated birth, and preparation of specific people such as grandparents or siblings for the birth. The nurse who knows the types of prenatal programs available in the community can direct expectant parents to programs that meet their special needs and learning goals. Childbirth preparation classes usually contain information about changes in the woman and the developing baby. See Table 13–2 ●.

Table 13–2 • POSSIBLE CONTENT OF CLASSES FOR CHILDBIRTH PREPARATION

Early Classes (First Trimester)

- Early gestational changes
- Self-care during pregnancy
- Fetal development, environmental dangers for the fetus
- Sexuality in pregnancy
- Birth settings and types of care providers
- Nutrition, rest, and exercise suggestions
- Relief measures for common discomforts of pregnancy
- Psychologic changes in pregnancy
- Information for getting pregnancy off to a good start
- Danger signs that warrant immediate medical attention
- Feeding choices/benefits of breastfeeding

Later Classes (Second and Third Trimesters)

- Preparation for birth process
- Postpartum self-care
- Birth choices (episiotomy, medications, fetal monitoring, perineal prep, enema, etc.)
- Relaxation techniques
- Breathing techniques
- Infant stimulation
- Newborn safety issues, such as car seats and sleeping positions
- Alternative therapies in pregnancy and labor

Adolescent Preparation Classes

- Stresses specific to adolescents
- Newborn care
- Health dangers for the baby
- Weight gain issues and nutrition
- How to recognize when baby is ill
- Baby care: Physical and emotional
- Sexuality
- Peer relationships

Breastfeeding Programs

- Advantages and disadvantages
- Medical benefits of breastfeeding
- Maternal nutrition
- Techniques of breastfeeding
- Methods of breast preparation
- Involvement of fathers in feeding process
- Cultural considerations

From the expectant parents' point of view, class content is best presented in chronology with the pregnancy (Figure 13–3 •). It is important that the classes begin by identifying the parents' needs, goals, and learning styles. Although both parents expect to learn breathing and relaxation techniques and infant care, fathers usually expect facts and mothers expect coping strategies. Stamler (1998) examined other maternal expectations from childbirth classes. Women's goals included obtaining a sense of being prepared, knowing what to expect from the experience, and learning about the hospital procedures. They expected an environment supportive of practicing newly learned techniques and the freedom to ask questions and receive explanations. Classes may be divided into early and late classes so specific needs can be addressed.

Early Classes: First Trimester

Early prenatal classes may include prepregnant women and couples as well as those in early pregnancy. In addition to the topics listed in Table 13–2, the classes cover early gestational

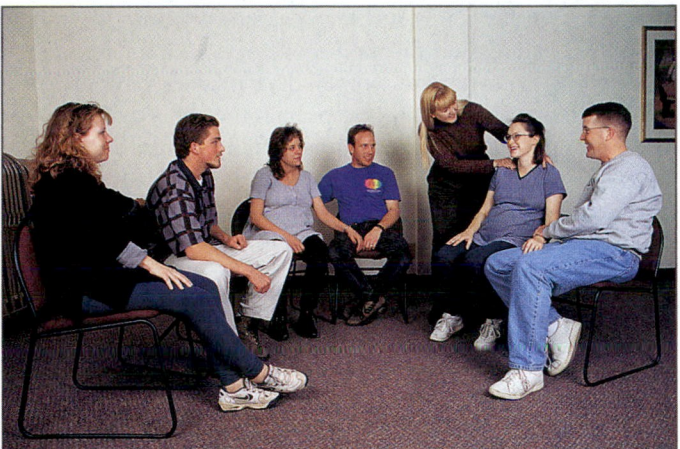

Figure 13–3 • In a group setting with a nurse-instructor, expectant parents share information about pregnancy and childbirth.

changes; self-care during pregnancy; fetal development and environmental dangers for the fetus; sexuality in pregnancy; birth settings and types of care providers; nutrition, rest, and exercise suggestions; common discomforts of pregnancy and relief measures; psychologic changes in pregnancy for the woman and man; and getting the pregnancy off to a good start by following a healthful lifestyle, learning methods of coping with stress, and avoiding alcohol and smoking. Early classes should provide information about factors that place the woman at risk for preterm labor and about how to recognize symptoms of preterm labor. Early classes should also present the advantages and disadvantages of formula feeding or breastfeeding. The majority of women (50% to 80%) have made their infant feeding decision before the sixth month of pregnancy.

Later Classes: Second and Third Trimesters

The later classes focus on preparation for the birth, infant care and feeding, postpartum self-care, birth choices (episiotomy, medications, fetal monitoring, perineal prep, enema, and so forth), and newborn safety issues. Because many parents purchase a car seat before birth, later classes should also include information about the importance of car seats, how they work, and how to select an approved car seat (Bull & Sheese, 2000).

Infant stimulation concepts can easily be incorporated into childbirth preparation classes. This will aid in the development of parenting skills and enhance prenatal and neonatal bonding. Johnson, Molby, Scallan, et al (2000) conducted a follow-up study 7 years after parents had completed an infant stimulation program and found that participants had better parenting skills and higher self-esteem. Stimulation methods that can be used include tactile, vestibular, auditory, and visual stimulation.

Tactile stimulation can be discussed when maternal physiology is being presented. As the uterine wall thins during the pregnancy, the mother and father are better able to feel the baby, and the fetus can sense the parents' stroking and patting through the abdominal wall. *Effleurage* (a light, stroking movement made with the fingertips) can also be used over the abdominal wall to provide tactile stimulation to the fetus. Vestibular stimulation through movement of the fetus is provided while the expectant woman does the pelvic-tilt exercise. Rocking in a rocking chair is also a comfortable way to provide relaxation for the expectant woman and vestibular stimulation for the fetus. Auditory stimulation can be provided by playing music. Classical music (such as Vivaldi, Mozart, Beethoven, and Bach) is found to be pleasing to the fetus. In the prenatal period, actual visual stimulation for the fetus is not possible.

Adolescent Parenting Classes

Adolescents have special learning needs during pregnancy. Areas of special concern for teens include altered body image, relationships with peers, caring for the new baby, normal infant behavior, and weight gain issues (Lesser & Escoto-Lloyd, 1999). Pregnant teens face a myriad of both psychologic and physical risks throughout pregnancy. Prenatal education and mentoring are essential. Often teenage mothers face pregnancy and childbirth without adequate support from a partner or parents. Prenatal education classes specifically designed for teens can provide a forum for verbalization of fears and concerns. The nurse can also identify community resources for young mothers and their infants. Teenagers also have concerns about labor and birth issues, specifically pain in labor, sexuality issues, and life changes that occur after pregnancy (Flynn, 1999).

Breastfeeding Programs

Programs offering information on breastfeeding are increasing. For decades, a primary source of information has been La Leche League. Information can also be obtained from lactation consultants, peer counselors, labor and postpartum nurses, birthing centers, hospitals, and health clinics. Rates of breastfeeding in the United States are well below the *Healthy People 2010* objective of 75%. Breastfeeding education and support is positively correlated to successful breastfeeding. In one study, women who attended childbirth education classes and those who received postpartum breastfeeding instructions were more likely to continue breastfeeding beyond 6 weeks postpartum (Deshpande & Gazmararian, 2000). Breastfeeding programs that are taught by other women from the same cultural background appear to be the most effective (Riordan & Gill-Hopple, 2001).

The father's support and encouragement of the mother is vital, so it is important to include him in the educational program and involve him in the decision making. Some fathers may feel negative and resentful about breastfeeding and need opportunities in the prenatal period for discussion and sharing of information. The decision to breastfeed is strongly related to the father's feeding preference.

Sibling Preparation: Adjustment to a Newborn

The birth of a new sibling is a significant event in a child's life. Positive adjustment can be enhanced by attendance at formal sibling preparation classes (Figure 13–4 •). Typically, the classes are attended by children ages 3 to 12 years. Children younger than 3 tend to have shorter attention spans and may have difficulty participating in the class; however, many facilities will allow younger children to attend, especially if an older sibling is enrolled in the class. These classes can assist with decreasing sibling rivalry and reducing children's anxiety. They help children feel that they are part of the birthing process. The classes also enable parents to identify children's concerns related to the new baby. They provide a means to facilitate communication and explore children's feelings. They also provide an educational foundation for children to learn about pregnancy, birth, infant behavior, and baby care (Storr & Robinson, 1998).

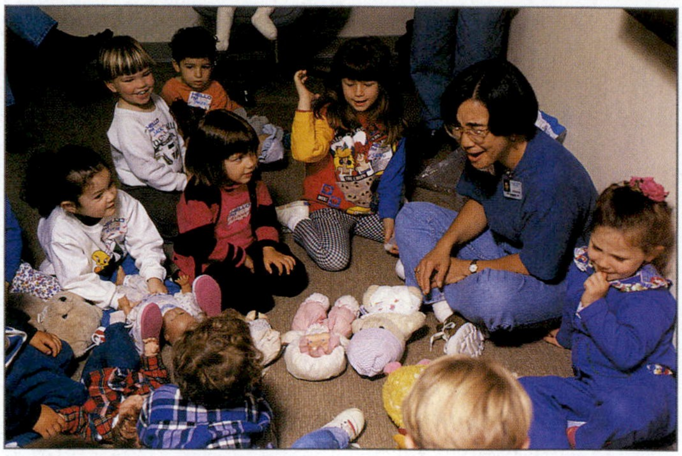

Figure 13–4 • It is especially important that siblings be well prepared when they are going to be present at the birth. However, even siblings who will not be present at the birth can benefit from information about birth and the new baby ahead of time.

Typically, parents and their children attend the class together. Many activities are devised to help each child feel special. Time is usually allotted at the end of the class for talking with parents about coping skills and providing hints about dealing with sibling jealousy. Class content typically includes care and behavior of new babies, a practice session holding anatomically correct dolls, changing diapers, and a tour of the "bedroom" and the nursery where Mom and baby will stay. Many times, a newborn is held up at the nursery window so the children can see a "real baby." Some facilities give the children a special gift for attendance or a trip to the cafeteria for a special treat.

Sibling preparation can be addressed through a formal class like the one just described, or in a less formal way by preparing a booklet for parents that addresses issues affecting both parents and children. Also, several excellent books and videos are available to help children prepare for a new sibling.

Classes for Grandparents

Grandparents are an important source of support and information for prospective and new parents. They are now being included in the birthing process more frequently. Prenatal programs for grandparents can address current roles, transitioning to a new role, beliefs regarding childbirth, and ways to support the new family unit. Grandparents can also benefit from educational information such as the benefits of breastfeeding, and updates on infant care, such as proper infant sleep positions and when to introduce foods. Grandparents who will be integral members of the labor and birth team need information about being coaches.

Education of the Family Having Cesarean Birth

Cesarean birth is an alternative method of birth via an abdominal and uterine incision.

Preparation for Cesarean Birth

Because one out of every four or five births is a cesarean, preparation for this possibility should be an integral part of every childbirth education curriculum. The instructor should treat cesarean birth as a normal event and present factual information that allows expectant parents to make choices and be full participants in their birth experience. The instructor can emphasize the similarities between cesarean and vaginal births to minimize undertones of "normal" versus "abnormal" birth. This helps diminish the feelings of anger, loss, and grief that often accompany cesarean births.

Cesarean birth classes should cover what the parents can expect to happen during a cesarean birth, what they will feel, and what they can do. All pregnant women and couples should be encouraged to discuss with their certified nurse-midwife/physician what the approach would be in the event of a cesarean. They can also discuss their needs and preferences regarding the following:

- Participating in the choice of anesthetic
- Father (or significant other) being present during the birth
- Planning initial contact with their newborn

> *As a nurse midwife, I felt extremely disappointed when I learned I would have to have a cesarean birth with my second child. I had great expectations about how much easier my second birth would be, and how I would "do everything different this time." I was amazed at how satisfied and happy I was immediately after the cesarean birth. During the birth, I asked the physician if the baby was almost out and how things were progressing. In the end, I had a beautiful, healthy baby and it turned out to be even a better experience than my first birth. I always try to comfort women who have medically indicated cesarean births by telling them it is still an amazing experience and a wonderful* birthday!

Preparation for Repeat Cesarean Birth

When expectant parents are anticipating a repeat cesarean birth, they have time to plan and prepare. Many hospitals or local groups (such as C-Sec, Inc.) provide preparation classes for cesarean birth. Parents who have had previous negative experiences need an opportunity to describe what contributed to their feelings. They should be encouraged to identify what they would like to change and to list interventions that would make the experience more positive. Those who have had positive experiences need reassurance that their needs and desires will be met in the same manner. In addition, all parents are encouraged to air any fears or anxieties.

A specific concern of the woman facing a repeat cesarean is anticipation of pain. She needs reassurance that subsequent cesareans are often less painful than the first. If her first cesarean was preceded by a long or strenuous labor, she will not experience the same fatigue. Giving this information will help her cope more effectively with all stressful stimuli, including pain. The nurse can remind the woman that she has already had experience with how to prevent, cope with, and alleviate painful stimuli.

Preparation for Parents Desiring Vaginal Birth after Cesarean Birth

Parents who are anticipating a vaginal birth after cesarean birth (VBAC) have unique needs. Because they may have unresolved questions and concerns about the last birth, it is helpful to begin the series of classes with an informational session. During this session, they can ask questions, share experiences, and begin to form bonds with one another. The nurse can supply information regarding the criteria necessary to attempt a trial of labor and identify decisions regarding the birth experience. Some childbirth educators find it helpful to have the parents prepare two birth plans: one for vaginal birth and one for cesarean birth. The preparation of the two plans seems to help parents take more control of the birth experience and tends to increase the positive aspects of the experience.

After an informational session, the classes may be divided according to the needs of the expectant parents. Those with recent coached childbirth experiences may need only refresher classes, whereas others may need complete training. Some parents may choose to attend regular classes after participating in the informational session.

Methods of Childbirth Preparation

Various methods of childbirth preparation are taught in North America. The most common methods of this type are Lamaze (psychoprophylactic), Kitzinger (sensory memory), Bradley (partner-coached childbirth), and HypnoBirthing. See Table 13–3 • for differentiating characteristics of each method.

The programs in prepared childbirth share some similarities. All have an educational component to help eliminate fear and teach coping mechanisms. The classes vary in coverage of subjects related to the maternity cycle, but all teach relaxation techniques and all prepare the participants for what to expect during labor and birth. Most methods also feature exercises to condition muscles and use breathing

Table 13-3 • SUMMARY OF SELECTED CHILDBIRTH PREPARATION METHODS

Method	Purpose or Philosophy	Goals	Techniques	Class Content
Bradley	To have the best, safest, and most rewarding birth experience as possible.	• Natural childbirth. • Active participation of the husband as coach. • Excellent nutrition. • Breastfeeding, beginning at birth.	• Working in harmony with your body using breath control and deep abdominopelvic breathing (Bradley, 1974) • Promoting general body relaxation (Bradley, 1974)	• Nutrition • Coach's role • Introduction to stages of labor • Birth planning • Variations and complications of labor • Postpartum preparation • Advanced first- and second-stage techniques • Preparation for your new family
Lamaze	Childbirth education empowers women to make informed choices in healthcare, to assume responsibility for their health, and to trust their inner wisdom.	• Birth is normal, natural, and healthy. • The experience of birth profoundly affects women and their families. • Women's inner wisdom guides them through birth. • Women have the right to give birth free from routine medical interventions.	• Disassociation relaxation • Controlled muscular relaxation • Breathing patterns	• Nutrition • Gestational changes • Labor and birth techniques for easing pain • Breathing techniques • Positioning during labor
Kitzinger	• Sheila Kitzinger campaigns for women to have the information they need to make choices about childbirth. • She is a strong believer in the benefits of home birth for women who are not at high risk.	• Uses sensory memory to help the woman understand and work with her body in preparation for birth.	• Uses chest breathing in conjunction with abdominal relaxation • Incorporates elements of the Stanislavsky method of acting in a way to teach relaxation	• Antenatal care • Birth plans • Therapeutic touch during labor • Post-traumatic stress following childbirth • Breastfeeding
HypnoBirthing	HypnoBirthing is about eliminating fear and experiencing birth in a stress-free, calm, and gentle environment that most resembles nature's own design.	• With both mind and body relaxed, the muscles of the uterus work in complete neuromuscular harmony. • When in a relaxed state, the body releases endorphins, the body's natural anesthesia.	• Relaxation techniques • Deep breathing • Slow breathing • Breathing your baby down • Maintaining comfort and eliminating pain	• HynoBirthing philosophy • Rapid, progressive relaxation/deepening techniques for transition • Visualizations for labor • Composing a birth plan • Early signs of labor • Birthing companion's integral role in labor • Pushing techniques • Postnatal bonding of parents with baby

patterns needed in labor. The greatest differences among the methods lie in the theories of why they work and in the relaxation techniques and breathing patterns they teach.

There are several advantages to these methods of childbirth preparation. The most important is that the baby may be healthier because of the reduced need for analgesics and anesthetics. Another is the satisfaction of the parents, for whom childbirth becomes a shared and profound emotional experience over which they feel a sense of control. In addition, each method has been shown to shorten labor. All nurses must know how these methods differ, so that they can support each birth experience effectively.

The International Childbirth Education Association (ICEA) is a well-known organization that provides antepartum education. Although this is not a method of preparation, it offers education and resources to the childbirth educator with a philosophy grounded in providing support to the individual couple's choices and decisions (ICEA, 2000). Many couples find ICEA classes appealing because they discuss all alternatives and choices that are available. Many hospital-based childbirth education programs now use this approach.

MEDIALINK INTERNATIONAL CHILDBIRTH EDUCATION ASSOCIATION

Body-Conditioning Exercises

Some body-conditioning exercises, such as the pelvic tilt, pelvic rock, and Kegel exercises, are taught in childbirth preparation classes. Other exercises strengthen the abdominal muscles for the expulsive phase of labor. (See Chapter 16 for a description of recommended exercises.)

Relaxation Exercises

Relaxation during labor allows the woman to conserve energy and allows the uterine muscles to work more efficiently. Without practice it is very difficult to relax the whole body in the midst of intense uterine contractions. However, many people can quickly master one or more of the following exercises.

Table 13–4 • TOUCH RELAXATION

Practice is vital to the following exercises, which require that the pregnant woman and her partner work very closely together. Tell the woman, "With practice you will train yourself to release not only in response to your partner's touch but also to the touch of doctors or nurses as they examine you. This technique will also help you to be more comfortable with your own body."

Goals

(For her) To recognize and release tension in response to partner's touch; to be able to do this automatically and spontaneously.
(For partner) To recognize her tension in its very early stages; to learn how to touch in a firm yet sensitive way; to concentrate on her problem areas.

Tools

(For her) Conscious relaxation, comfortable positioning, and trust.
(For partner) Sensitivity, patience, and warm hands!

Procedure

She tenses.
Partner touches.
She immediately releases toward touch.
Partner strokes, "drawing" tension from her.
She releases all residual tension.

Sequence

- Contract muscles of the scalp and raise eyebrows. Partner cups hands on either side of the scalp. Immediately release tension in response to the pressure of your partner's touch. Then release any residual tension as your partner strokes your head.
- Frown, wrinkle nose, and squeeze eyes shut. Partner rests hands on brow and then strokes down over temples. Release.
- Grit teeth and clench jaw. Partner rests hands on either side of jaw. Release.
- Press shoulder blades back. Partner rests hands on front of shoulders. Release.
- Pull abdominal wall toward spine. Partner rests hands on sides of abdomen and then strokes down over her hips. Partner might also stroke the lower curve of abdomen across pubic symphysis. Release.
- Press thighs together. Partner touches outside of each leg. Relax and let legs move apart. Partner strokes firmly down outside of leg with light strokes up on inner thigh.
- Press legs outward, still flexed but forcing thighs apart. Partner rests hands with fingers pointing downward, on inner thighs. Firmly strokes down to knees, then lightly strokes upward on outside of leg. Release.
- Tense arm muscles. Partner places hands on the upper arm and shoulder area, one on the inside and one on the outside of the arm. Strokes down to the elbow and then down forearm to wrist, and over fingertips. Release. Repeat with other arm.
- Tighten leg muscles, being careful not to cramp them. Partner touches foot around the instep, firmly without tickling. Release whole leg. Partner moves hands up, placing one on either side of the thigh, stroking down to the knee then down the calf to the foot and over the toes. Release. Repeat with other leg.
- Change to the Sims, lateral or side-lying position. Raise chin, contracting the muscles at the back of the neck. Partner rests hand on nape of neck and massages. Release.
- Curl into fetal position, drawing shoulders forward. Partner applies pressure to back of shoulders. Strokes upper back. Release.
- Hollow the small of back by arching back. Partner rests hands against either side of spine and follows with stroking down over buttocks. Release.
- Press buttocks together. Partner rests one hand on each buttock. After initial release, strokes down toward thighs.

Source: O'Halloran, S. (1984). *Pregnant and prepared: A guide to preparing for childbirth* (p.45), Wayne, NJ: Avery Publishing Group.

PROGRESSIVE RELAXATION

In **progressive relaxation** exercises, the woman learns how to tense and then relax one muscle group at a time. An example follows:

- Lie down on your back or side. (The left side position is best for pregnant women.)
- Tighten your muscles in both feet. Hold the tightness for a few seconds, and then relax the muscles completely, letting all the tension drain out.
- Tighten your lower legs, hold for a few seconds, then relax the muscles, letting all the tension drain out.
- Continue tensing and relaxing parts of your body, moving up the body as you do so.

TOUCH RELAXATION

Another type of relaxation exercise, called **touch relaxation,** requires cooperation between the woman and her coach. It is particularly useful in working together during labor. An example is provided in Table 13–4 •.

DISASSOCIATION RELAXATION

An additional exercise, **disassociation relaxation,** is used in both Lamaze and Bradley methods. The woman is taught to become familiar with the sensation of contracting and relaxing the voluntary muscle groups throughout her body. She then learns to contract a specific muscle group and relax the rest of her body. This process of isolating the action of one group of voluntary muscles from the rest of the body is called *neuromuscular disassociation.* The exercise conditions the woman to relax uninvolved muscles while the uterus contracts, creating an active relaxation pattern (Table 13–5 •).

Although it is not possible to simulate the pain of uterine contractions, the coach may use one of two methods to induce some discomfort so the woman can practice the relaxation exercises:

1. The coach places both hands in a grasping position firmly on the upper arm and turns them in opposite directions to create a burning sensation. This is begun slowly and gently and increased at the direction of the woman as she continues to practice relaxation breathing techniques (Figure 13–5 •).
2. The coach places a hand on the woman's inner thigh just above the knee and pinches the area.

While practicing, the coach checks the woman's neck, shoulders, arms, and legs for relaxation. As tense areas are found, the coach encourages the woman to relax those particular body parts. The woman learns to respond to her own perceptions of tense muscles and also to the suggestion from others. The suggestion can come verbally or from touch. The exercises are usually practiced each day so that they become comfortable and easy to do.

Table 13–5 • DISASSOCIATION RELAXATION

The uterus, an involuntary muscle over which you have no control, will work most efficiently and effectively when the rest of your body is free from tension. The following exercises will give you further practice in conscious release. They will also give you and your partner a way to evaluate your progress.

Goals

During pregnancy, disassociation relaxation will teach you consciously to release certain sets of muscles, while contracting others, and to disassociate yourself from voluntary tension. During labor, this technique will release all voluntary muscles of your body at will, while the uterus contracts. This conserves energy and fights fatigue.

Tools

Body awareness, touch release, and concentration.

Procedure

Partner gives consistent suggestions.
Partner checks relaxation using touching.

Example

Partner: "Contraction begins."
Mother: Relaxation breath (following with a comfortable rate of breathing).
Partner: [See suggested patterns.]
Mother: Relaxation breath.

Sequence

"Contract right arm. Hold. Release."
"Contract left arm. Hold. Release."
"Contract right leg. Hold. Release."
"Contract left leg. Hold. Release."
"Contract both arms. Hold. Release."
"Contract both legs. Hold. Release."
"Contract right side (arm and leg). Hold. Release."
"Contract left side (arm and leg). Hold. Release."
"Contract right arm and left leg. Hold. Release."
"Contract left arm and right leg. Hold. Release."

For Variety

"Contract right arm and left leg."
"Release left leg. Contract right leg. Release right arm. Contract left arm."
"Release."

Source: O'Halloran, S. (1984). *Pregnant and prepared: A guide to preparing for childbirth.* (pp.45–46) Wayne, NJ: Avery Publishing Group.

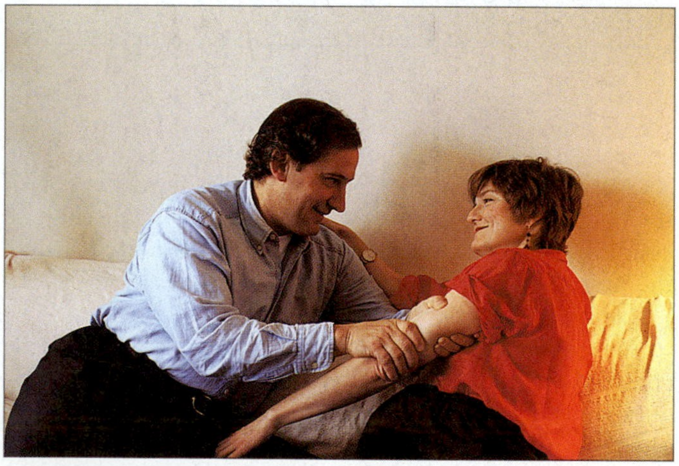

Figure 13–5 • To help the woman practice relaxing in the presence of discomfort, the coach can induce discomfort by "twisting" the skin of her upper arm or by pinching her inner thigh.

OTHER RELAXATION TECHNIQUES

A specific type of cutaneous stimulation called abdominal **effleurage** is used prior to the transitional phase of labor (Figure 13–6 •). This light abdominal stroking effectively relaxes the woman experiencing mild to moderate pain. Deep pressure over the sacrum is more effective for relieving back pain.

Additional modalities that may be used to promote relaxation in labor include guided imagery, hypnosis, meditation, music, massage, aromatherapy, therapeutic touch, biofeedback, transcutaneous electrical nerve stimulation unit (TENS unit), acupressure, and acupuncture. In addition to these measures, the nurse can promote relaxation by encouraging and supporting the client's controlled breathing.

Individualization is essential when choosing appropriate relaxation techniques. The nurse should encourage techniques that are comfortable for the woman. Some techniques that may be beneficial are as follows:

- Vocalization or "sounding" to relieve tension in pregnancy and labor.
- Massage (light touch) to facilitate relaxation.
- Breathing in any manner that seems to bring relief. No specific pattern is followed.
- Use of warm water for showers or bathing during labor.
- Visualization (imagery).
- Relaxing music and subdued lighting.

Breathing Techniques

Breathing techniques are a key element of most childbirth preparation programs. They help keep the mother and her unborn baby adequately oxygenated and help the mother relax and focus her attention appropriately (Table 13–6 •). Breathing techniques are best taught during the final trimester of pregnancy when the expectant mother's attention is focused on the birth experience. The nurse then supports the mother's use of breathing techniques during labor. Breathing techniques are described in detail in Chapter 24.

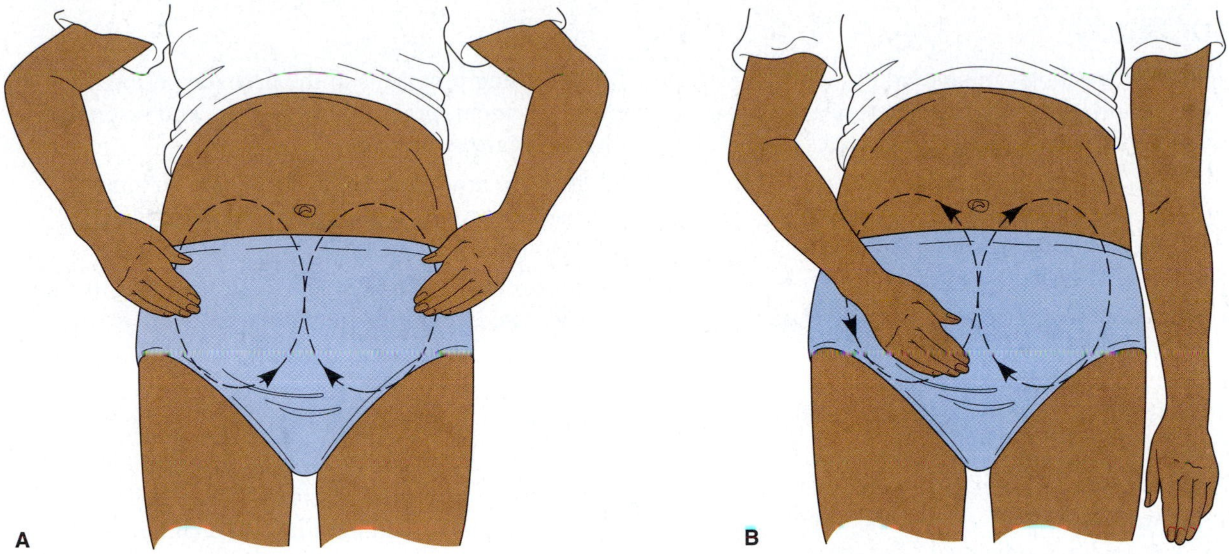

Figure 13-6 • Effleurage is light stroking of the abdomen with the fingertips. *A,* Starting at the symphysis, the woman lightly moves her fingertips up and around in a circular pattern. *B,* An alternative approach involves using one hand in a figure-eight pattern. This light stroking can also be done by the support person.

Table 13-6 • GOALS OF BREATHING TECHNIQUES
• Provide adequate oxygenation of mother and baby, open maternal airways, and avoid inefficient use of muscles.
• Increase physical and mental relaxation.
• Decrease pain and anxiety.
• Provide a means of focusing attention.
• Control inadequate ventilation patterns that are related to pain and stress.
• Provide a sense of control for the mother.

Clinical Tip *Practice the techniques for relaxation yourself. This practice will prepare you to help expectant parents and laboring women.*

Vocalization Techniques

With the increased use of analgesics and epidural anesthesia, many nurses have become unfamiliar with and may be uncomfortable about natural sounds made by laboring women. Vocalization or *sounding* during uterine contractions can be encouraged to promote relaxation and relieve tension. The nurse should encourage the woman to relax, drop her jaw to her chest, and make low-pitched sounds. Suggesting that the woman try to sound like a man or a mother bear can help her to produce the appropriate pitch. These low, moaning sounds open the glottis helping the woman to relax, breathe freely, and feel confident and strong. In contrast, high-pitched sounds can promote tension, closure, and a feeling of fear.

CHAPTER REVIEW

EXPLOREMEDIALINK

NCLEX review questions, case studies, and other interactive resources for this chapter can be found on the Web site at http://www.prenhall.com/olds. Click on "Chapter 13" to select the activities for this chapter.

For tutorials including animations and videos, more NCLEX review questions, and an audio glossary, access the accompanying CD-ROM in this book.

Focus Your Study

- Preconception counseling can be used to identify risk factors and unhealthy behaviors before a pregnancy occurs. Healthful lifestyle changes can be employed.
- Childbearing decisions include the care provider, the birth setting, support persons, and whether to include siblings in the birth experience.
- Prenatal education programs vary in their goals, content, leadership techniques, and method of teaching. The major childbirth preparation methods are Lamaze, Kitzinger, Bradley, and HypnoBirthing.
- Prenatal classes may be offered early or late in the pregnancy. The class content varies depending on the type of class and the individual offering it. Expectant parents tend to want information in chronologic sequence with the pregnancy.
- Breastfeeding programs in the prenatal period offer encouragement, practical instruction, and resources for the breastfeeding family.
- Siblings are now included in the whole birthing process, and classes for them are available from many sources.
- Grandparents have unique information needs that are addressed in grandparents' classes.
- Information regarding cesarean birth is included in antepartal classes to help prepare all parents for this alternative method of birth.
- Most childbirth classes include information on body-toning exercises, relaxation techniques, breathing method, and vocalization techniques.

References

Andolsek, K. M., & Ketton, G. M. (2000). Risk assessment. *Primary Care: Clinicals in Office Practice, 27*(1), 71–103.

Bradley, R. A. (1974). *Husband-coached childbirth.* New York: Harper Row.

Bull, M. J., & Sheese, J. (2000). Update for the pediatrician on child passenger safety: Five principles for safer travel. *Pediatrics, 106*(5, part 1), 1113–1116.

Chapman, L. L. (2000). Expectant fathers and labor epidurals. *American Journal of Maternal-Child Nursing,* 25(3), 133–138.

Chin, H. G. (2001). *On call obstetrics and gynecology* (2nd ed.). Philadelphia: W. B. Saunders.

Dejin-Karlsson, E., Hanson, B. S., Ostergren, P. O., Sjoberg, N. O., & Marshal, K. (1998). Does passive smoking in early pregnancy increase the risk of small for gestational age infants? *American Journal of Public Health, 88,* 1523–1527.

Deshpande, A. D., & Gazmararian, J. A. (2000). Breast-feeding education and support: Association with the decision to breastfeed. *Effective Clinical Practice, 3*(3), 116–122.

England, P., & Horowitz, R. (1998). *Birthing from within.* Albuquerque, NM: Pantera Press.

Flynn, L. (1999). The adolescent parenting program: Improving outcomes through mentorship. *Public Health Nursing, 16*(3), 182–189.

Gawley, S., & Cupples, M. E. (2002). Smoking in pregnancy: The size of our challenge. *Ulster Medical Journal, 71*(1), 17–21.

Hodnett, E. D. (2002). Pain and women's satisfaction with the experience of childbirth: A systematic review. *American Journal of Obstetrics and Gynecology, 186* (Suppl. 5 Nature), S160–172.

International Childbirth Education Association (ICEA). (2000). ICEA philosophy statement. *International Journal of Childbirth Education, 15,* 1.

Johnson, Z., Molby, B., Scallan, E., Fitzpatrick, P., Keegan, T., & Byrne, P. (2000). Community mothers programme: Seven year follow-up of a randomized controlled trial of non-professional intervention in parenting. *Journal of Public Health Medicine, 22*(3), 337–342.

Klerman, L. V., & Rooks, J. P. (1999). A simple, effective method that midwives can use to help pregnant women stop smoking. *Journal of Nurse Midwifery, 44*(2), 118–123.

Lesser, J., & Escoto-Lloyd, S. (1999). Health-related problems in a vulnerable population: Pregnant teens and adolescent mothers. *Nursing Clinics of North America, 34*(2), 289–299.

Low, L. K., Seng, J. S., Murtland, T. L., & Oakley, D. (2000). Clinician-specific episiotomy rates: Impact on perineal outcomes. *Journal of Nurse Midwifery and Women's Health, 45*(2), 87–93.

Olds, S. B. (1997). Care of the childbearing family. In J. Luckman (Ed.), *Saunders manual of nursing care.* Philadelphia: Saunders.

Polomeno, V. (1999). Perinatal education and grandparents: Creating an interdependent family environment; Part II; The pilot study. *Journal of Perinatal Education, 8*(3), 1–11.

Riordan, J., & Gill-Hopple, K. (2001). Breastfeeding care in multicultural populations. *Journal of Obstetric, Gynecologic, and Neonatal Nursing, 30*(2), 216–223.

Robotti, S. B., & Inman, M. A. (1998). *Childbirth instructor magazine's guide to careers in birth.* Hoboken, NJ: Wiley, John & Sons, Inc.

Scott, J. A., & Binns, C. W. (1999). Factors associated with the initiation and duration of breastfeeding: A review of the literature. *Breastfeeding Review,* 7(1), 5–16.

Stamler, L. L. (1998). The participants' view of childbirth education: Is there congruency with an enablement framework for patient education? *Journal of Advanced Nursing, 28*(5), 939–947.

Storr, G. B., & Robinson, P. (1998). Preparing kids for the new baby. *Canadian Nurse, 94*(3), 33–35.

Teschendorf, M., & Evans, C. P. (2000). Hydrotherapy during labor: An example of developing a practice policy. *American Journal of Maternal Child Nursing, 25*(4), 198–203.

Ventura, S. J., Mosher, W. D., Curtin, S. A., Abma, J. C., & Henshaw, S. (2000). Trends in pregnancy rates for the United States: 1976–1997: An update. *National Vital Statistics Reports, 49*(4), 1–10.

14 Physical and Psychologic Changes of Pregnancy

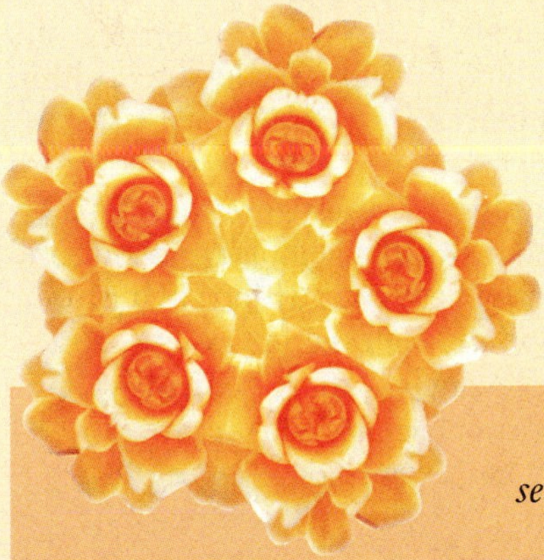

The atmosphere of approval in which I was bathed—even by strangers on the street, it seemed—was like an aura I carried with me. . . . This is what women have always done.

Adrienne Rich, Of Woman Born

Objectives

- Identify the anatomic and physiologic changes that occur during pregnancy.
- Relate the physiologic and anatomic changes that occur in the body systems during pregnancy to the signs and symptoms that develop in the woman.
- Compare subjective (presumptive), objective (probable), and diagnostic (positive) changes of pregnancy.
- Contrast the various types of pregnancy tests.
- Discuss the emotional and psychologic changes that commonly occur in a woman, her partner, and her family during pregnancy.
- Summarize cultural factors that may influence a family's response to pregnancy.

Key Terms

Ballottement 309
Braxton Hicks contractions 300
Chadwick's sign 300
Chloasma (melasma gravidarum) 303
Colostrum 301
Couvade 317
Goodell's sign 300
Hegar's sign 308
Linea nigra 303
McDonald's sign 308
Morning sickness 307
Mucous plug 300
Physiologic anemia of pregnancy 302
Quickening 308
Striae 301
Supine hypotensive syndrome (vena caval syndrome, aortocaval compression) 302

MediaLink

Additional resources for this content can be found on the Student CD-ROM and on the Companion Website at www.prenhall.com/olds. Click on "Chapter 14" to select the activities for this chapter.

CD-ROM
- Audio Glossary
- NCLEX Review

Companion Website
- Additional NCLEX Review
- Case Study: Prenatal Education
- Care Plan Activity: Preparing Siblings for New Baby

Through modern technology and highly evolved research methods, we know a great deal about how pregnancy occurs and what happens to the fetus and the woman's body during gestation. Yet no matter how much we learn about this event, it never ceases to amaze us. First, it is nothing short of a miracle that the union of two microscopic entities—an ovum and a sperm—can produce a living being. Second, the woman's body must undergo extraordinary physical changes to sustain a pregnancy. A pregnant woman's body changes in size and shape, and all her organ systems modify their functions to create an environment that protects and nurtures the growing fetus.

Pregnancy is divided into three trimesters, each a 3-month period. Each trimester has its own predictable developments in both the fetus and the mother. This chapter describes both obvious and subtle physical and psychologic changes caused by pregnancy. It also discusses the various cultural factors that can affect a woman's well-being during pregnancy.

Anatomy and Physiology of Pregnancy

The changes that occur in the pregnant woman's body are caused by several factors. Many changes are the result of hormonal influences, some are caused by the growth of the fetus inside the uterus, and some are a result of the mother's physical adaptation to the changes that are occurring.

Reproductive System

UTERUS

The changes in the uterus during pregnancy are phenomenal. Before pregnancy the uterus is a small, almost solid, pear-shaped organ measuring approximately 7.5 × 5 × 2.5 cm and weighing about 60 g (2 oz). At the end of pregnancy the dimensions are approximately 28 × 24 × 21 cm, with an organ weight of approximately 1100 g (2.5 lb). Its capacity increases from 10 mL to 5000 mL (5 L) or more (Cunningham, Gant, Leveno, et al, 2001).

The enlargement of the uterus is primarily a result of an increase in size (hypertrophy) of the preexisting myometrial cells. Only a limited increase in cell number (hyperplasia) occurs. The amount of fibrous tissue between the muscle bands increases markedly, which adds to the strength and elasticity of the muscle wall.

The uterine walls become considerably thicker during the first few months of pregnancy than during the nonpregnant state. The initial changes are stimulated by increased estrogen and progesterone levels and not by mechanical distention (enlargement) by the fetus, placenta, and amniotic fluid. In general, the uterus enlarges more around the placental insertion site and in the upper portion of the uterus, the *fundus* (Cunningham et al, 2001). After approximately the third month, the uterine contents begin to exert intrauterine pressure. The myometrial hypertrophy continues during the first few months of pregnancy. Then the musculature begins to distend, resulting in a thinning of the muscle wall to a thickness of about 1.5 cm or less at term (38 through 41 weeks of gestation). The ease of palpating the fetus through the abdominal wall attests to this thinning.

The circulatory requirements of the uterus increase as the uterus enlarges and the fetus and placenta develop. The size and number of the blood and lymphatic vessels within the uterine layers increase greatly. By the end of pregnancy, one sixth of the total maternal blood volume is contained within the vascular system of the uterus.

Braxton Hicks contractions—irregular contractions of the uterus—occur intermittently throughout pregnancy. They may be palpated bimanually beginning about the fourth month of pregnancy. These contractions help stimulate the movement of blood through the intervillous spaces of the placenta. In late pregnancy as these contractions increase in frequency, they can become uncomfortable and may be confused with true labor contractions.

> **Clinical Tip** *Beginning early in pregnancy, have the woman feel her uterus periodically so that she becomes familiar with the size and the way it feels. As her pregnancy progresses she then will be more likely to identify Braxton Hicks contractions and preterm labor, should it occur.*

CERVIX

The major component of cervical tissue is connective tissue, which is rearranged as pregnancy progresses. At term its strength is one twelfth of its prepregnant strength, facilitating cervical changes during labor (Cunningham et al, 2001).

Estrogen stimulates the glandular tissue of the cervix, which increases in cell number and becomes hyperactive. The endocervical glands occupy about half the mass of the cervix at term, as compared to a small fraction in the nonpregnant state. They secrete a thick, tenacious mucus, which accumulates and thickens to form the **mucous plug** that seals the endocervical canal and prevents the ascent of bacteria or other substances into the uterus. This plug is expelled when cervical dilatation begins. The hyperactive glandular tissue also causes an increase in the normal physiologic mucorrhea, at times resulting in a profuse discharge. Increased vascularization causes both the softening of the cervix (**Goodell's sign**) and a blue-purple discoloration of the cervix (**Chadwick's sign**). Increased vascularization is a result of hypertrophy and engorgement of the vessels below the growing uterus.

OVARIES

The ovaries cease ovum production during pregnancy. Many follicles develop temporarily but never to the point of maturity. The cells lining these follicles, the thecal cells, become active in hormone production and have been called the interstitial glands of pregnancy.

During early pregnancy human chorionic gonadotropin (hCG) maintains the corpus luteum, which persists and produces hormones until about weeks 6 to 8 of pregnancy. The corpus luteum engulfs approximately a third of the ovary at its peak of hypertrophy. By the middle of pregnancy it has regressed to almost complete obliteration. The corpus luteum secretes progesterone to maintain the endometrium until the placenta produces enough progesterone to maintain the pregnancy; then the corpus luteum disintegrates slowly.

VAGINA

The vaginal epithelium undergoes hypertrophy, increased vascularization, and hyperplasia during pregnancy. As with the cervical changes, these changes are estrogen induced and result in a thickening of mucosa, a loosening of connective tissue, and an increase in vaginal secretions. The secretions are thick, white, and acidic (pH 3.5 to 6.0). The acid pH plays a significant role in preventing infections. However, it also favors the growth of yeast organisms, resulting in moniliasis, a common vaginal infection during pregnancy.

As in the uterus, the smooth muscle cells of the vagina hypertrophy, with an accompanying loosening of the supportive connective tissue. By the end of pregnancy, the vaginal wall and perineal body have become sufficiently relaxed to permit distention of the tissues and passage of the infant.

Because the blood flow to the vagina increases, it may show the same blue-purple color (Chadwick's sign) seen in the cervix.

Breasts

Soon after the woman first misses her menstrual period, estrogen- and progesterone-induced changes occur in the mammary glands. Increases in breast size and nodularity are the result of glandular hyperplasia and hypertrophy in preparation for lactation. By the end of the second month, superficial veins are prominent, nipples are more erectile, and pigmentation of the areola is obvious. Pigmentation tends to be more pronounced in women with dark complexions. Hypertrophy of Montgomery's follicles is noted within the primary areola. **Striae** (purplish stretch marks that slowly turn silver after childbirth) may develop as the pregnancy progresses. Breast changes are often most noticeable in the woman who is pregnant for the first time.

Colostrum, an antibody-rich, yellow secretion, may be expressed manually by the 12th week and may leak from the breasts during the last trimester of pregnancy. Colostrum gradually converts to mature milk during the first few days following childbirth.

Respiratory System

Pulmonary function is modified throughout pregnancy. Pregnancy induces a small degree of hyperventilation as the tidal volume (amount of air breathed with ordinary respiration) increases steadily throughout pregnancy. There is a 30% to 40% rise from nonpregnant values in the volume of air breathed each minute. Between weeks 16 and 40, oxygen consumption increases approximately 15% to 20% to meet the increased needs of the mother as well as those of the fetus and placenta. The vital capacity (maximum amount of air that can be moved in and out of the lungs with forced respiration) increases slightly, while lung compliance (elasticity) and pulmonary diffusion remain constant. Measurements of airway resistance show a marked decrease in pregnancy in response to elevated progesterone levels. The diaphragm is elevated and the subcostal angle is increased as a result of pressure from the enlarging uterus. This change causes the rib cage to flare, with a decrease in the vertical diameter and increases in the anteroposterior and transverse diameters. The circumference of the chest may increase by as much as 6 cm. The increase compensates for the elevated diaphragm, and there is no significant loss of intrathoracic volume. Breathing changes from abdominal to thoracic as pregnancy progresses. Overall, pulmonary function is not impaired by pregnancy. Many women experience an increased awareness of the need to breathe, however, starting early in pregnancy. This may be perceived as dyspnea and is thought to be due to the increased tidal volume, which causes a slight decrease in blood P_{CO_2}. Actual lung disease may be aggravated by pregnancy due to the increased need for oxygen by the woman and her fetus (Cunningham et al, 2001).

Nasal stuffiness and congestion, referred to as rhinitis of pregnancy, are not uncommon. Epistaxis (nosebleeds) may also occur. They are primarily the result of estrogen-induced edema and vascular congestion of the nasal mucosa.

Cardiovascular System

The growing uterus exerts pressure on the diaphragm, pushing the heart upward and to the left and rotating it forward. This lateral displacement makes the heart appear somewhat enlarged on x-ray examination. A systolic murmur can be heard in 90% of pregnant women, and the first and third heart sounds are louder.

Blood volume progressively increases throughout pregnancy, beginning in the first trimester and peaking near term at about 40% to 45% above nonpregnant levels. This increase is due to increases in both plasma and erythrocytes. No increase occurs in pulmonary capillary wedge pressure or in central venous pressure despite the increase in blood volume. This is due to decreases in both systemic vascular resistance and pulmonary vascular resistance, which enable the circulation to adapt to higher blood volume while maintaining normal vessel pressures. Cardiac output begins to increase early in pregnancy and peaks at 20 to 24 weeks' gestation at 30% to 50% above prepregnant levels. It then remains elevated for the duration of the pregnancy (Cruikshank, Wigton, & Hays, 1996).

During pregnancy, organ systems receive additional blood flow according to their increased workload. Thus blood flow to the uterus and kidneys increases, whereas hepatic and cerebral flow remains unchanged.

The pulse rate frequently increases during pregnancy, although the amount varies from almost no increase to an increase of 10 to 15 beats per minute. The blood pressure decreases slightly during pregnancy, reaching its lowest point during the second trimester. The blood pressure then gradually increases during the third trimester and is near prepregnant levels at term (when the baby is due).

The femoral venous pressure slowly rises as the uterus exerts increasing pressure on return blood flow. There is an increased tendency toward stagnation of blood in the lower extremities, with a resulting dependent edema and tendency toward varicose vein formation in the legs, vulva, and rectum late in pregnancy. In addition to the effects of increased femoral venous pressure, a reduction of plasma colloid osmotic pressure resulting from a reduction in plasma albumin further maintains the presence of fluid in the extravascular space. The pregnant woman becomes more prone to develop postural hypotension because of the increased blood volume in the lower extremities.

During pregnancy the enlarging uterus may put pressure on the vena cava when the woman is supine, resulting in **supine hypotensive syndrome,** also called **vena caval syndrome** or **aortocaval compression.** This pressure interferes with returning blood flow and produces a marked decrease in blood pressure with accompanying dizziness, pallor, and clamminess, which can be corrected by having the woman lie on her left side. Research indicates that the enlarging uterus may press on the aorta and its collateral circulation as well (Cunningham et al, 2001) (Figure 14–1 •).

The total erythrocyte volume increases by about 30% in women who receive iron supplementation but increases only about 18% without iron supplements (Cruikshank et al, 1996). This increase is necessary to transport the additional oxygen required during pregnancy. The increase in plasma volume averages about 50%. Because the plasma volume increase is greater than the erythrocyte increase, however, the hematocrit, which measures the portion of whole blood that is composed of erythrocytes, decreases slightly. This decrease is sometimes referred to as the **physiologic anemia of pregnancy** (pseudoanemia).

Iron is necessary for hemoglobin formation, and hemoglobin is the oxygen-carrying component of erythrocytes. Thus the increase in erythrocyte levels results in an increased need for iron by the pregnant woman. Even though the gastrointestinal absorption of iron is moderately increased during pregnancy, it is usually necessary to add supplemental iron to the diet to meet the expanded red blood cell and fetal needs.

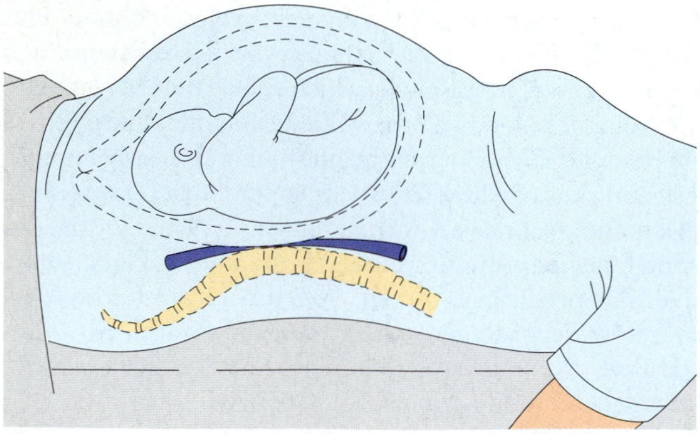

Figure 14–1 • Vena caval syndrome. The gravid uterus compresses the vena cava when the woman is supine. This reduces the blood flow returning to the heart and may cause maternal hypotension.

Leukocyte production equals or is slightly greater than the increase in blood volume. The average cell count is 5000 to 12,000/mm^3, with an occasional woman developing a physiologic leukocytosis of 15,000/mm^3. During labor and the early postpartum period, these levels may reach 25,000/mm^3. The reason for this dramatic increase remains unknown, but similar leukocyte changes occur with physiologic stress such as vigorous exercise. It probably represents the return to the circulation of mature leukocytes that had been shunted out of the circulatory system (Cunningham et al, 2001).

The platelet count does not change much in pregnancy, but the plasma fibrinogen has been known to increase by as much as 50%. The increased fibrinogen accounts for the nonpathologic rise of the sedimentation rate. Although the clotting time of the pregnant woman does not differ significantly from that of the nonpregnant woman, blood factors VII, VIII, IX, and X are increased so that pregnancy becomes a somewhat hypercoagulable state. These changes, coupled with venous stasis in late pregnancy, place the pregnant woman at increased risk of developing venous thrombosis.

Gastrointestinal System

Many of the discomforts of pregnancy are attributed to changes in the gastrointestinal system. Nausea and vomiting during the first trimester are associated with the hCG secreted by the implanted blastocyst and with a change in carbohydrate metabolism that occurs in early pregnancy. Peculiarities of taste and smell are common and can further aggravate gastrointestinal discomfort. Gum tissue may become hyperemic and softened and may bleed when only mildly traumatized. The secretion of saliva may increase or become excessive (ptyalism).

During the second half of pregnancy, numerous gastrointestinal symptoms are attributable to the pressure of the growing uterus and smooth muscle relaxation due to elevated progesterone levels. The intestines are displaced laterally and posteriorly and the stomach superiorly. Heartburn (pyrosis) is caused by the reflux of acidic secretions from the stomach into the lower esophagus as a result of relaxation of the cardiac sphincter. Gastric emptying time and intestinal motility are delayed, leading to frequent complaints of bloating and constipation, which can be aggravated by the smooth muscle relaxation and increased electrolyte and water reabsorption in the large intestine. Hemorrhoids frequently develop if constipation is a problem or, in the second half of pregnancy, from pressure on vessels below the level of the uterus.

Only minor liver changes occur with pregnancy. Plasma albumin concentrations and serum cholinesterase activity decrease with normal pregnancy as with certain liver diseases.

The emptying time of the gallbladder is prolonged during pregnancy as a result of smooth muscle relaxation from progesterone. Hypercholesterolemia may follow, and it can predispose the woman to gallstone formation. Pruritus (itching) caused by retained bile salts may also occur (Cunningham et al, 2001).

Urinary Tract

During the first trimester, the growing uterus puts pressure on the bladder, producing urinary frequency until the second trimester when the uterus becomes an abdominal organ. Near term, when the presenting part engages in the pelvis, pressure is again exerted on the bladder. This pressure can impair the drainage of blood and lymph from the hyperemic bladder, rendering it more susceptible to infection and trauma. The bladder, normally a convex organ, becomes concave from the external pressure, and its capacity is greatly reduced.

Dilation of the kidneys and ureter may occur, most frequently on the right side above the pelvic brim, due to the lie of the uterus. This dilation is accompanied by elongation and curvature of the ureter. There appears to be no single factor accounting for this anatomic variation; instead a combination of ureteral atonia and hypoperistalsis, probably caused by pressure from the enlarging fetus with some progesterone effects, seems to be involved. The presence of amino acids and glucose in the urine in conjunction with the tendency toward ureteral atonia and stasis of urine in the ureters may increase the risk of urinary tract infection.

The glomerular filtration rate (GFR) and renal plasma flow (RPF) increase early in pregnancy. The GFR rises by as much as 50% by the beginning of the second trimester and remains elevated until birth. The increase in RPF is slightly less and decreases somewhat during the third trimester (Cunningham et al, 2001). The mechanism for these rises remains unclear.

An increased renal tubular reabsorption rate compensates for the increased glomerular activity. Amino acids and water-soluble vitamins are excreted in greater amounts than in the nonpregnant woman. Glycosuria is not uncommon or necessarily pathogenic during pregnancy but is merely a reflection of the kidneys' inability to reabsorb all of the glucose filtered by the glomeruli. However, pregnancy can be diabetogenic, so the possibility of diabetes mellitus cannot be disregarded.

The increased renal function during pregnancy results in an increased clearance of urea and creatinine and in a lowering of the blood urea and nonprotein nitrogen values. Because of this, measurement of creatinine clearance provides an accurate test of renal functioning during pregnancy.

Skin and Hair

Changes in skin pigmentation commonly occur during pregnancy. These changes are thought to be stimulated by increased estrogen, progesterone, and α-melanocyte-stimulating hormone levels.

Pigmentation of the skin increases primarily in areas that are already hyperpigmented: the areolae, the nipples, the vulva, the perianal area, and the linea alba. The linea alba refers to the midline of the abdomen from the pubic area to the umbilicus and above. During pregnancy increased pigmentation may cause this area to darken. It is then referred to as the **linea nigra** (Figure 14–2 •). Some women also develop facial **chloasma** (or **melasma gravidarum**), the "mask of pregnancy." This is an irregular pigmentation of the cheeks, forehead, and nose that occurs in many women during pregnancy and is accentuated by sun exposure. Similar changes may occur in women who are taking oral contraceptives. Facial melasma is more prominent in dark-haired women and is occasionally disfiguring. Fortunately, it fades or at least regresses soon after birth when the hormonal influence of pregnancy has stopped.

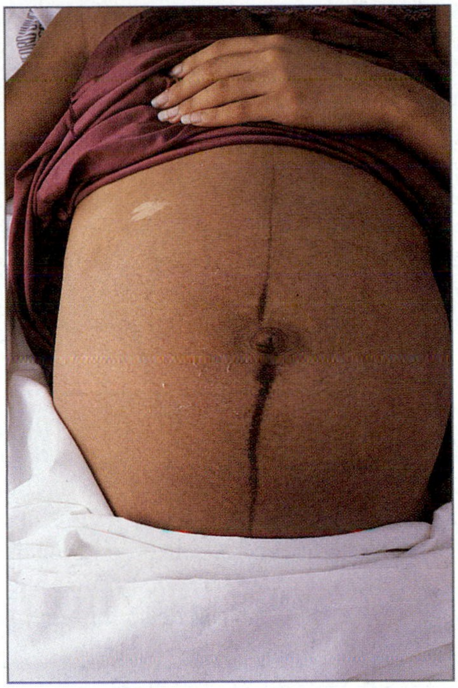

Figure 14–2 • Linea nigra.

Striae, or stretch marks, are reddish, wavy, depressed streaks that may occur over the abdomen, breasts, and thighs as pregnancy progresses. They are caused by reduced connective tissue strength due to elevated adrenal steroid levels.

Vascular spider nevi may develop on the chest, neck, face, arms, and legs. They are small, bright-red elevations of the skin radiating from a central body. They may be caused by increased subcutaneous blood flow in response to increased estrogen levels. This condition is of no clinical significance and disappears after pregnancy ends.

The rate of hair growth may decrease during pregnancy, and the number of hair follicles in the resting or dormant phase also decreases. After birth the number of hair follicles in the resting phase increases sharply, and the woman may notice increased shedding of hair for 1 to 4 months. Practically all hair is replaced within 6 to 12 months, however (Cunningham et al, 2001).

Finally, the sweat and sebaceous glands are frequently hyperactive during pregnancy. Some women may notice heavy perspiration, night sweats, and/or the development of acne even if they have never experienced these symptoms before.

Musculoskeletal System

No demonstrable changes occur in the teeth of the pregnant woman. No demineralization takes place. The fairly common occurrence of dental caries during pregnancy has led to the myth "a tooth for every pregnancy." The dental caries that may accompany pregnancy are likely to be caused by inadequate oral hygiene and dental care.

The sacroiliac, sacrococcygeal, and pubic joints of the pelvis relax in the later part of the pregnancy, presumably as a result of hormonal changes. This often causes a waddling gait. A slight separation of the symphysis pubis can often be demonstrated on radiologic examination.

As the pregnant woman's center of gravity gradually changes, the lumbodorsal spinal curve is accentuated, and the woman's posture changes (Figure 14–3 •). This posture change compensates for the increased weight of the uterus anteriorly and frequently results in low backache. Late in pregnancy, aches in the neck, shoulders, and upper extremities may occur because of shoulder slumping and anterior flexion of the neck accompanying the lumbodorsal lordosis. Paresthesias of the extremities may occur late in pregnancy as a result of pressure on peripheral nerves.

Often pressure of the enlarging uterus on the abdominal muscles causes the rectus abdominis muscle to separate, producing *diastasis recti*. If the separation is severe and muscle tone is not regained postpartally, subsequent pregnancies will not have adequate support, and the woman's abdomen may appear pendulous.

Eyes

Two changes generally occur in the eyes during pregnancy. First, intraocular pressure decreases, probably as a result of increased vitreous outflow. Second, a slight thickening of the cornea occurs, which is generally attributed to fluid retention. Although these changes are not readily perceived, some pregnant women experience difficulty wearing previously comfortable contact lenses (Cunningham et al, 2001). The change in the corneas generally disappears by 6 weeks postpartum.

Central Nervous System

Pregnant women frequently describe decreased attention, concentration, and memory during and shortly after pregnancy, but few studies have explored this phenomenon. One study did compare a group of pregnant women against a control group, finding a decline in memory that could not be attributed to depression, anxiety, sleep deprivation, or other physical changes of pregnancy. This memory loss disappeared soon after childbirth. Another study found that sleep problems are common in pregnancy. These include difficulty going to sleep, frequent awakenings, fewer hours of night sleep, and reduced sleep efficiency (Cunningham et al, 2001).

Metabolism

Most metabolic functions accelerate during pregnancy to support the additional demands of the growing fetus and its support system. The expectant mother must meet her own tissue replacement needs, those of the fetus, and those preparatory for labor and lactation. No other event in life induces such profound metabolic changes.

WEIGHT GAIN

Growth of the uterus and its contents, and of the breasts, and increases in intravascular fluids account for most of the

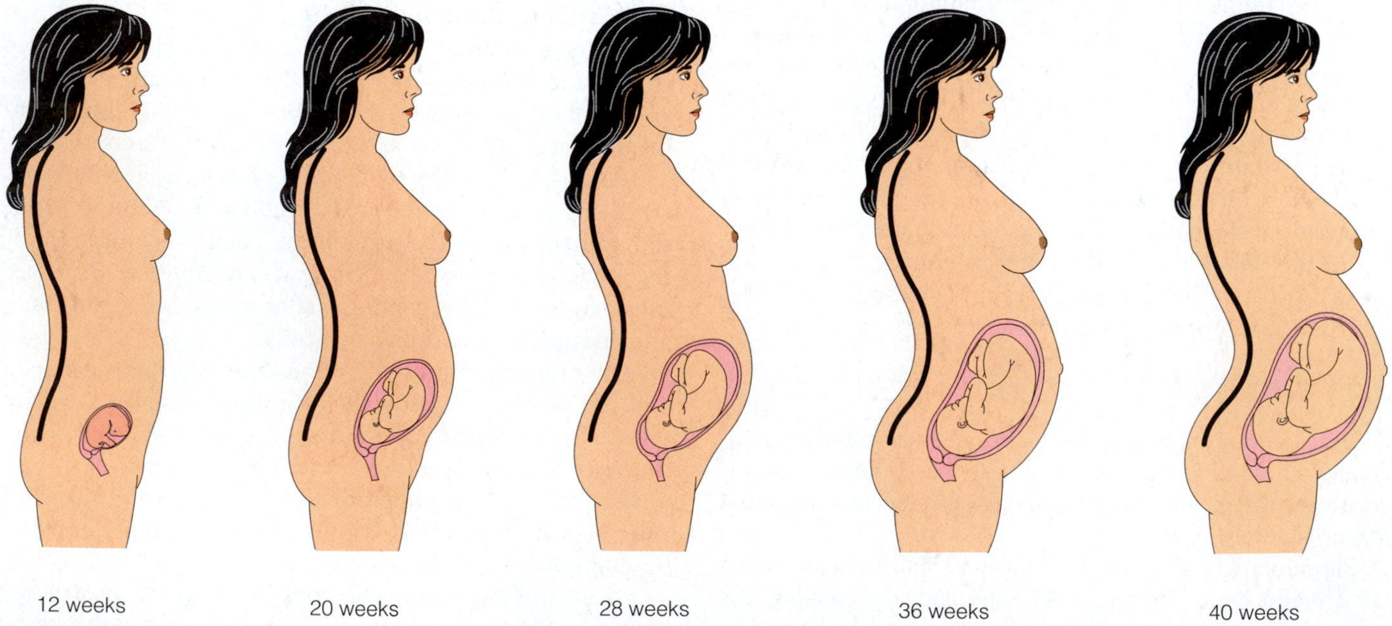

Figure 14–3 • Postural changes during pregnancy. Note the increasing lordosis of the lumbosacral spine and the increasing curvature of the thoracic area.

weight gain in pregnancy. In addition, extra water, fat, and protein are stored; these are usually called *maternal reserves.*

The recommended total weight gain during pregnancy for a woman of normal weight prior to pregnancy is 11.5 to 16 kg (25 to 35 lb); for women who were overweight before becoming pregnant, the recommended gain is 6.8 to 11.5 kg (15 to 25 lb). Underweight women are advised to gain the weight needed to reach their ideal weight plus 11.5 to 16 kg (25 to 35 lb) (Mattson & Smith, 2000). Weight may decrease slightly during the first trimester due to nausea, vomiting, and food intolerances of early pregnancy. The lost weight is soon regained, and an average increase of 1.6 to 2.3 kg (3.5 to 5 lb), 5.5 to 6.8 kg (12 to 15 lb), and 5.5 to 6.8 kg (12 to 15 lb) occurs in the first, second, and third trimesters, respectively.

Adequate nutrition and weight gain are important during pregnancy. Maternal nutrition is discussed in detail in Chapter 18.

WATER METABOLISM

Increased water retention is a basic chemical alteration of pregnancy. Several interrelated factors cause this phenomenon. The increased level of steroid sex hormones affects sodium and fluid retention. The lowered serum protein also influences the fluid balance, as do the increased intracapillary pressure and permeability. The extra water is needed for the products of conception—the fetus, placenta, and amniotic fluid—and the mother's increased blood volume, interstitial fluids, and enlarged organs.

NUTRIENT METABOLISM

The fetus makes its greatest protein and fat demands during the second half of gestation, doubling in weight in the last 6 to 8 weeks. The increased protein retention that begins in early pregnancy is initially used for hyperplasia and hypertrophy of maternal tissues, such as the uterus and breasts. Protein must also be stored during pregnancy to maintain a constant level within the breast milk and to avoid depletion of maternal tissues.

Fats are more completely absorbed during pregnancy, resulting in a marked increase in the serum lipids, lipoproteins, and cholesterol and decreased elimination through the bowel. Fat deposits in the fetus increase from about 2% at midpregnancy to almost 12% at term. The excess nitrogen and lipidemia are considered to be a preparation for lactation. In addition, the woman's body switches from glucose metabolism to lipid metabolism once glucose from food intake has been used up. This leads to an increased tendency to develop ketosis between meals and overnight. The demand for carbohydrate increases, especially during the last two trimesters. Intermittent glycosuria is not uncommon during pregnancy. When it is not accompanied by a rise in blood sugar levels, glycosuria is a physiologic entity secondary to the increased glomerular filtration rate. Fasting blood sugar levels tend to fall slightly, returning to more normal levels by the sixth postpartal month. The oral glucose tolerance test shows no change with pregnancy.

The possibility of diabetes must not be overlooked during pregnancy. Plasma levels of insulin increase during pregnancy (probably due to hormonal changes that cause increased tissue resistance), and rapid destruction of insulin takes place within the placenta. Insulin production must be increased by the mother during the second trimester, and any marginal pancreatic function quickly becomes apparent. The diabetic woman often experiences increased exogenous insulin demands during pregnancy.

The demand for iron during pregnancy is accelerated, and the pregnant woman needs to guard against anemia. Iron is necessary for the increase in erythrocytes, hemoglobin, and blood volume, as well as for the increased tissue demands of both woman and fetus.

Iron transfer takes place at the placenta in only one direction—toward the fetus. It has been demonstrated that approximately five sixths of the iron stored in the fetal liver is assimilated during the last trimester of pregnancy. This stored iron in the fetal liver compensates in the first 4 months of neonatal life for the normal inadequate amounts of iron available in breast milk and non-iron-fortified formulas.

The progressive absorption and retention of calcium during pregnancy has been noted. The maternal plasma concentration of bound calcium decreases as the levels of bindable plasma proteins fall. Approximately 30 g of calcium is retained in maternal bone for fetal deposition late in pregnancy.

Pregnancy produces little change in the metabolism of most other minerals, other than retention of amounts needed for fetal growth.

Vitamin metabolism does not change appreciably with pregnancy. (See Chapter 18 for the mother's requirements of minerals and vitamins.)

COMPLEMENTARY AND ALTERNATIVE THERAPIES

HERBS DURING PREGNANCY

Pharmaceutical companies continue to refuse to include children and babies in their studies of drug safety, claiming excessive costs and other research problems. As a result, very few over-the-counter or prescription drugs can claim to be safe for pregnant women and nursing mothers. The same can be said for herbal medicines. Although herbs have been researched extensively in Europe and Asia, there has been little clinical research done in the United States on the use of herbs in pregnancy. Every pregnant or nursing woman must be extremely cautious about everything she ingests—foods, liquids, medications, and herbs. If a problem warrants intervention, she and her primary healthcare provider should discuss the benefits and risks of all treatments, synthetic and natural.

More information about the use of herbs in pregnancy can be found in Chapter 3.

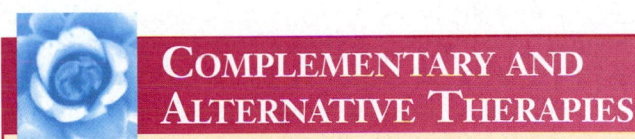

Endocrine System

THYROID

Pregnancy influences the thyroid gland's size and activity. Often a palpable change is noted, which represents an increase in vascularity and hyperplasia of glandular tissue. Total serum thyroxine (T_4) increases in early pregnancy, and thyroid-stimulating hormone (TSH) decreases. The elevated levels of total T_4 continue until several weeks postpartum, although the level of free serum T_4 returns to normal after the first trimester (Cunningham et al, 2001). Increased thyroxine-binding capacity is evidenced by an increase in serum protein-bound iodine (PBI), probably due to the increased levels of circulating estrogens.

The basal metabolic rate (BMR) increases by as much as 20% to 25% during pregnancy. The increased oxygen consumption is due primarily to fetal metabolic activity.

PARATHYROID

The concentration of the parathyroid hormone and the size of the parathyroid glands increase, paralleling the fetal calcium requirements. Parathyroid hormone concentration reaches its highest level of approximately twofold between 15 and 35 weeks of gestation, returning to a normal or even subnormal level before childbirth.

PITUITARY

During pregnancy, the pituitary gland enlarges somewhat, but it returns to normal size after birth. There is no significant change in the posterior lobe of the gland, although the anterior lobe increases in weight with each successive pregnancy.

Pregnancy is made possible by the hypothalamic stimulation of the anterior pituitary hormones: follicle-stimulating hormone (FSH), which stimulates follicle growth within the ovary, and luteinizing hormone (LH), which effects ovulation. Pituitary stimulation prolongs the corpus luteal phase of the ovary, which maintains the secretory endometrium for development of the pregnancy.

Two additional pituitary hormones, thyrotropin and adrenotropin, alter maternal metabolism to support the pregnancy. Prolactin, also an anterior pituitary secretion, is responsible for initial lactation. Its levels increase tenfold during pregnancy and then, somewhat surprisingly, decrease after childbirth, even in breastfeeding women. (Continued lactation depends on the suckling of the infant.)

The posterior pituitary contains the mechanism for the release of oxytocin and vasopressin, which exert oxytocic, vasopressor, and antidiuretic effects. The main effects of oxytocin are the promotion of uterine contractility and the stimulation of milk ejection from the breasts. Vasopressin causes vasoconstriction, which results in increased blood pressure; it also has an antidiuretic effect and plays an important role in the regulation of water balance. Vasopressin secretion is controlled by changes in plasma osmolarity and blood volume.

ADRENALS

Little structural change occurs in the adrenal glands during a normal pregnancy. Estrogen-induced increases in the levels of circulating cortisol result primarily from lowered renal excretion. The circulating cortisol levels regulate carbohydrate and protein metabolism. A normal level resumes 1 to 6 weeks postpartum.

The adrenals secrete increased levels of aldosterone by the early part of the second trimester. The levels of secretion are even more elevated in the woman on a sodium-restricted diet. This increase in aldosterone in a normal pregnancy may be the body's protective response to the increased sodium excretion associated with progesterone (Cunningham et al, 2001).

PANCREAS

The pregnant woman has increased insulin needs. The islets of Langerhans are stressed to meet this increased demand, and a latent deficiency may become apparent during pregnancy, producing symptoms of gestational diabetes (Chapter 19 .)

HORMONES IN PREGNANCY

Several hormones are required to maintain pregnancy. Most of these are produced initially by the corpus luteum; production is then assumed by the placenta. (For an in-depth discussion of placental hormones, see Chapter 11 .)

Human Chorionic Gonadotropin

The trophoblast secretes human chorionic gonadotropin (hCG) in early pregnancy. This hormone stimulates progesterone and estrogen production by the corpus luteum to maintain the pregnancy until the placenta is developed sufficiently to assume that function.

Human Placental Lactogen

Also called human chorionic somatomammotropin (hCS), human placental lactogen (hPL) is produced by the syncytiotrophoblast. This hormone is an antagonist of insulin; it increases the amount of circulating free fatty acids for maternal metabolic needs and decreases maternal metabolism of glucose to favor fetal growth.

Estrogen

Secreted originally by the corpus luteum, estrogen is produced primarily by the placenta as early as the seventh week of pregnancy. Estrogen stimulates uterine development to provide a suitable environment for the fetus. It also helps to develop the ductal system of the breasts in preparation for lactation.

Progesterone

Progesterone, also produced initially by the corpus luteum and then by the placenta, plays the greatest role in maintaining pregnancy. It maintains the endometrium and also inhibits spontaneous uterine contractility, thus preventing early spontaneous abortion due to uterine activity. In addition, progesterone helps develop the acini and lobules of the breasts in preparation for lactation.

Relaxin

Relaxin is detectable in the serum of a pregnant woman by the time of the first missed menstrual period. Relaxin inhibits uterine activity, diminishes the strength of uterine contractions, aids in the softening of the cervix, and has the long-term effect of remodeling collagen. Its primary source is the corpus luteum, but small amounts are believed to be produced by the placenta and uterine decidua throughout pregnancy.

PROSTAGLANDINS IN PREGNANCY

Prostaglandins (PGs) are lipid substances that can arise from most body tissues but occur in high concentrations in the female reproductive tract and are present in the decidua during pregnancy. The exact functions of PGs during pregnancy are still unknown, although it has been proposed that they are responsible for maintaining reduced placental vascular resistance. Decreased PG levels may contribute to hypertension and preeclampsia. Prostaglandins are also believed to play a role in the complex biochemistry that initiates labor, although their specific functions are still being defined.

Signs of Pregnancy

Many of the changes women experience during pregnancy are used to diagnose the pregnancy itself. They are called the subjective (or presumptive) changes, the objective (or probable) changes, and the diagnostic (or positive) changes of pregnancy.

Subjective (Presumptive) Changes

The subjective changes of pregnancy are the symptoms the woman experiences and reports. They can be caused by other conditions (Table 14–1 •) and therefore cannot be considered proof of pregnancy. The following can be diagnostic clues when other signs and symptoms of pregnancy are also present.

Amenorrhea is the earliest symptom of pregnancy. In a healthy woman whose menstrual cycles are regular, missing one or more menstrual periods leads to the consideration of pregnancy.

Nausea and vomiting of pregnancy (NVP) are experienced by almost half of all pregnant women during the first 3 months of pregnancy and result from elevated human chorionic gonadotropin (hCG) levels and changed carbohydrate metabolism. The woman may feel merely a distaste for food or may suffer extreme vomiting, which may be accompanied by dehydration and ketosis. Because these symptoms frequently occur in the early part of the day and disappear within a few hours, they are commonly called **morning sickness.** In reality, symptoms may occur at any time. This gastrointestinal disturbance usually appears about 6 weeks after the first day of the last menstrual period (LMP) and usually disappears spontaneously 6 to 12 weeks later, although it may be prolonged in some instances. Research suggests that women who experience NVP often have a more favorable pregnancy outcome than those who do not.

> *I simply was not prepared to deal with the nausea. I was tired all the time and queasy, too. I only vomited a few times but there were many more times when I was sure I would lose everything! I kept telling myself that nausea was a good sign of a healthy pregnancy but it sure made it hard to go to work. Fortunately I was a week or two into my second trimester when it passed and the rest of my pregnancy was a breeze.*

Table 14-1 • DIFFERENTIAL DIAGNOSIS OF PREGNANCY—SUBJECTIVE CHANGES

Subjective Changes	Possible Alternative Causes
Amenorrhea	Endocrine factors: early menopause; lactation; thyroid, pituitary, adrenal, ovarian dysfunction
	Metabolic factors: malnutrition, anemia, climatic changes, diabetes mellitus, degenerative disorders, long-distance running
	Psychologic factors: emotional shock, fear of pregnancy or sexually transmitted infection, intense desire for pregnancy (pseudocyesis), stress
	Obliteration of endometrial cavity by infection or curettage
	Systemic disease (acute or chronic), such as tuberculosis or malignancy
Nausea and vomiting	Gastrointestinal disorders
	Acute infections such as encephalitis
	Emotional disorders such as pseudocyesis or anorexia nervosa
Urinary frequency	Urinary tract infection
	Cystocele
	Pelvic tumors
	Urethral diverticula
	Emotional tension
Breast tenderness	Premenstrual tension
	Chronic cystic mastitis
	Pseudocyesis
	Hyperestrogenism
Quickening	Increased peristalsis
	Flatus ("gas")
	Abdominal muscle contractions
	Shifting of abdominal contents

Excessive fatigue may be noted within a few weeks after the first missed menstrual period and may persist throughout the first trimester.

Urinary frequency is experienced during the first trimester as the enlarging uterus exerts pressure on the bladder. The increased vascularization and pelvic congestion that occur in each pregnancy can also cause frequent voiding. This symptom decreases during the second trimester, when the uterus is an abdominal organ, but reappears during the third trimester, when the presenting part descends into the pelvis.

Changes in the breasts are frequently noted in early pregnancy. Some women report significant breast changes prior to missing their first menses. Engorgement of the breasts due to the hormone-induced growth of the secretory ductal system results in the subjective symptoms of tenderness and tingling, especially of the nipple area. The veins also become more visible and form a bluish pattern beneath the skin in fair-skinned women.

Quickening, or the mother's perception of fetal movement, occurs about 18 to 20 weeks after the LMP in a primigravida (a woman who is pregnant for the first time) but may occur as early as 16 weeks in a multigravida (a woman who has been pregnant more than once). Quickening is a fluttering sensation in the abdomen that gradually increases in intensity and frequency.

> ***Clinical Tip*** *Some women suggest that it is easiest to imagine the fluttering associated with quickening by letting the outer tips of the eyelashes brush a finger and then imagining that same sensation deep inside the abdomen.*

Objective (Probable) Changes

An examiner can perceive the objective changes that occur in pregnancy. They are more diagnostic than the subjective symptoms. However, their presence does not offer a definite diagnosis of pregnancy (Table 14–2 •).

Changes in the pelvic organs caused by increased vascular congestion are the only physical signs detectable within the first 3 months of pregnancy. These changes are noted on pelvic examination. There is a softening of the cervix, called Goodell's sign. Chadwick's sign is the deep red to purple or bluish coloration of the mucous membranes of the cervix, vagina, and vulva due to increased vasocongestion of the pelvic vessels. **Hegar's sign** is a softening of the isthmus of the uterus, the area between the cervix and the body of the uterus, which occurs at 6 to 8 weeks of pregnancy. This area may become so soft that on a bimanual exam there seems to be nothing between the cervix and the body of the uterus (Figure 14–4 •). *Ladin's sign* is a soft spot anteriorly in the middle of the uterus near the junction of the body of the uterus and cervix (Figure 14–5, *A* •). **McDonald's sign** is an ease in flexing the body of the uterus against the cervix.

Table 14–2 • DIFFERENTIAL DIAGNOSIS OF PREGNANCY—OBJECTIVE CHANGES

Objective Changes	Possible Alternative Causes
Changes in pelvic organs	Increased vascular congestion
Goodell's sign	Estrogen-progestin oral contraceptives
Chadwick's sign	Vulvar, vaginal, cervical hyperemia
Hegar's sign	Excessively soft walls of nonpregnant uterus
Uterine enlargement	Uterine tumors
Braun von Fernwald's sign	Uterine tumors
Piskacek's sign	Uterine tumors
Enlargement of abdomen	Obesity, ascites, pelvic tumors
Braxton Hicks contractions	Hematometra, pedunculated, submucous, and soft myomas
Uterine souffle	Large uterine myomas, large ovarian tumors, or any condition with greatly increased uterine blood flow
Pigmentation of skin	Estrogen-progestin oral contraceptives
Chloasma (Melasma)	Melanocyte hormonal stimulation
Linea nigra	
Nipples/areola	
Abdominal striae	Obesity, pelvic tumor
Ballottement	Uterine tumors/polyps, ascites
Pregnancy tests	Increased pituitary gonadotropins at menopause, choriocarcinoma, hydatidiform mole
Palpation for fetal outline	Uterine myomas

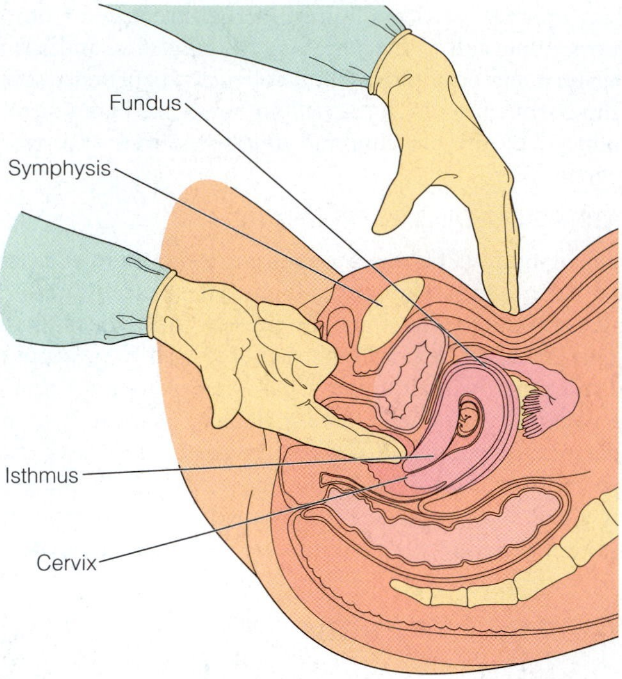

Figure 14–4 • Hegar's sign, a softening of the isthmus of the uterus, can be determined by the examiner during a vaginal examination.

The uterus assumes an irregular globular shape during the early months of pregnancy. Irregular softening and enlargement at the site of implantation, known as *Braun von Fernwald's sign*, occurs about the fifth week (Figure 14–5, *B*). Occasionally an almost tumorlike, asymmetric enlargement occurs, called *Piskacek's sign* (Figure 14–5, *C*). Generalized enlargement and softening of the body of the uterus are present after the eighth week of pregnancy. The fundus of the uterus is palpable just above the symphysis pubis at approximately 10 to 12 weeks' gestation and at the level of the umbilicus at 20 to 22 weeks' gestation (Figure 14–6 •).

Enlargement of the abdomen during the childbearing years is usually regarded as evidence of pregnancy, especially if the enlargement is progressive and is accompanied by a continuing amenorrhea. It is generally more pronounced in a woman whose abdominal musculature has lost some of its tone because of previous childbirth.

As mentioned earlier, *Braxton Hicks* contractions are irregular, ordinarily painless contractions that occur at irregular intervals throughout pregnancy but are felt with abdominal palpation after week 28. As the woman approaches the end of the pregnancy, these contractions often become more uncomfortable and are then called *false labor.*

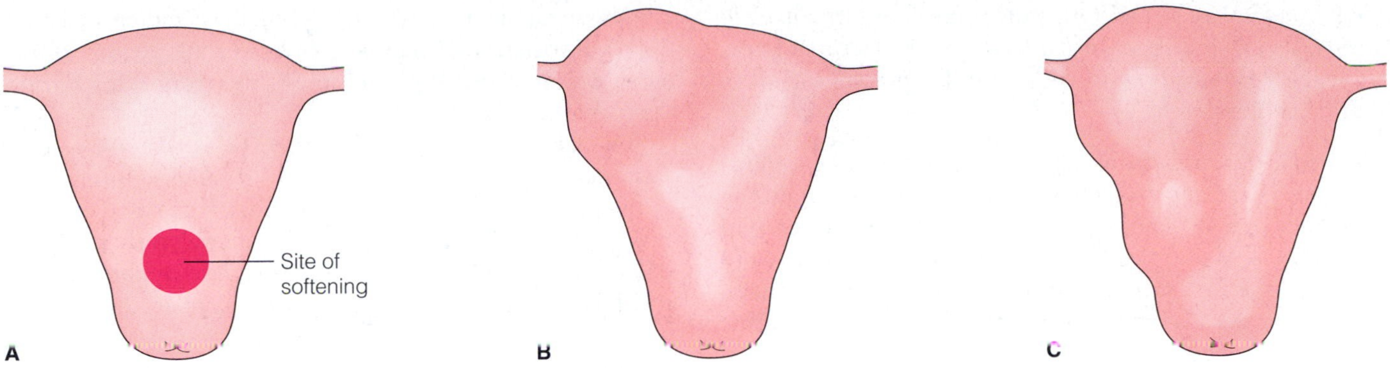

Figure 14–5 • Early uterine changes of pregnancy. ***A,*** Ladin's sign, a soft spot anteriorly in the middle of the uterus near the junction of the body of the uterus and the cervix. ***B,*** Braun von Fernwald's sign, irregular softening and enlargement at the site of implantation. ***C,*** Piskacek's sign, a tumorlike, asymmetric enlargement.

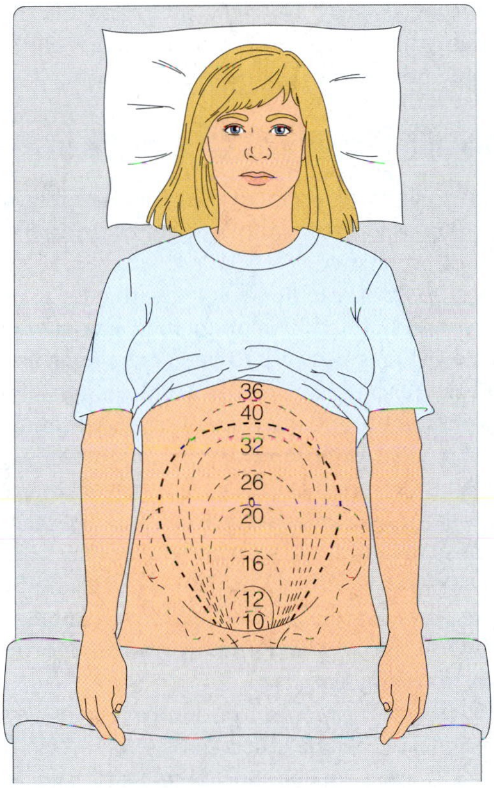

Figure 14–6 • Approximate height of the fundus at various weeks of pregnancy.

Uterine souffle may be heard when auscultating the abdomen over the uterus. It is a soft blowing sound at the same rate as the maternal pulse and is due to the increased uterine vascularization and the blood pulsating through the placenta. It is sometimes confused with the *funic souffle*, which is a soft blowing sound of blood pulsating through the umbilical arteries. The funic souffle is at the same rate as the fetal heart rate.

Changes in pigmentation of the skin and the *appearance of abdominal striae* are common manifestations in pregnancy. Facial melasma (chloasma) occurs in varying degrees after week 16. The pigmentation of the nipple and areola may darken, especially in primigravidas and dark-haired women. The Montgomery glands of the areola may become enlarged. The skin in the midline of the abdomen may develop a pigmented line, the linea nigra. As pregnancy progresses, striae appear on the abdomen and buttocks.

The *fetal outline* may be identified by palpation in many pregnant women after 24 weeks of gestation, becoming easier to distinguish as term approaches. **Ballottement** is the passive fetal movement elicited by pushing up against the cervix with two fingers. This pushes the fetal body up and, as it falls back, the examiner feels a rebound.

Pregnancy tests are based on analysis of maternal blood or urine for the detection of hCG, the hormone secreted by the trophoblast. These tests are not considered positive signs of pregnancy because the similarity of hCG and the pituitary-secreted luteinizing hormone (LH) occasionally results in cross-reactions. In addition, certain conditions other than pregnancy can cause elevated levels of hCG.

CRITICAL THINKING IN PRACTICE

At 33 weeks' gestation, Elena Martinez, G2P1, who is 5 feet 4 inches tall and who weighs 144 lb (prepregnancy weight of 120 lb), is examined by her certified nurse-midwife. At that time her fundal height is measured as 33 cm. Because of a vacation trip, she is not seen again by her midwife until 36 weeks' gestation. At that time her fundus measures 35 cm and she weighs 147 lb. Elena asks you if there is something wrong with her baby's growth. What is your assessment?

Answer may be found in Appendix I.

CLINICAL PREGNANCY TESTS

A variety of assay techniques are available to detect hCG during early pregnancy.

- *Hemagglutination-inhibition test* (Pregnosticon R), an immunoassay, is based on the fact that no clumping of cells occurs when the urine of a pregnant woman is added to the hCG-sensitized red blood cells of sheep.

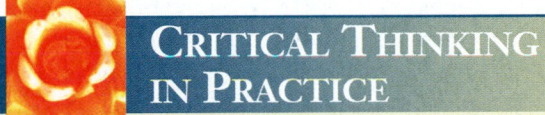

- *Latex agglutination test* (Gravindex and Pregnosticon slide test), also an immunoassay, is based on the fact that latex particle agglutination is inhibited in the presence of urine containing hCG.

The hemagglutination-inhibition test and the latex agglutination tests are approximately 95% accurate in diagnosing pregnancy and 98% accurate in determining the absence of pregnancy. The tests become positive approximately 10 to 14 days after the first missed menstrual period. The specimen used for the tests is the first early morning midstream urine because it is adequately concentrated for accuracy. The presence of protein substances (such as blood) in the specimen should be avoided because false-positive results may occur.

Several pregnancy tests are done on maternal serum, including the following:

- *β-subunit radioimmunoassay* (RIA) uses an antiserum with specificity for the β-subunit of hCG in blood plasma. This is a very accurate pregnancy test that becomes positive a few days after presumed implantation, thereby permitting earlier diagnosis of pregnancy. This test is also used in the diagnosis of ectopic pregnancy or trophoblastic disease. However, because it requires several hours to perform and has only limited sensitivity, it is being replaced by other, simpler tests such as the immunoradiometric assay.
- *Immunoradiometric assay* (IRMA) (Neocept; Pregnosis) uses a radioactive antibody to identify the presence of hCG in the serum. This test can identify very low concentrations of hCG and requires only about 30 minutes to perform.
- *Enzyme-linked immunosorbent assay* (ELISA) (Model Sensichrome, Quest Confidot) does not use radioisotopes but a substance that results in a color change after binding. A blue color develops, the intensity of which is related to the amount of hCG present. The test is sensitive and quick. It can detect hCG levels as early as 7 to 9 days after ovulation and conception, which is 5 days before the first missed period (Buster & Carson, 1996).
- *Fluoroimmunoassay* (FIA) (Opus hCG; Stratus hCG) uses an antibody tagged with a fluorescent label to detect serum hCG. The test, which takes about 2 to 3 hours to perform, is extremely sensitive and is used primarily to identify and follow hCG concentrations.

OVER-THE-COUNTER PREGNANCY TESTS

Home pregnancy tests are available over the counter at a reasonable cost. These enzyme immunoassay tests are quite sensitive and detect even low levels of hCG in urine. Many physicians and nurse-midwives use them in the office to confirm pregnancy for their clients because they are less expensive and faster than time-consuming clinical pregnancy tests.

Home pregnancy test instructions are quite explicit and should be followed carefully. Best results are obtained with the first morning-voided urine if using tests based on polyclonal antibodies, although tests based on monoclonal antibodies can be used on any voided specimen (Curran, 2000). Furthermore, because the newer kits require only a short wait (usually 3 to 5 minutes), the margin for error is very small.

The false-positive rate of these tests is quite low, but the false-negative results are higher and should be followed up in the presence of pregnancy symptoms. Kits based on monoclonal antibodies can detect a pregnancy as early as the day of a missed period while the polyclonal tests are best used 12 to 14 days after the first missed period (Curran, 2000). If the results are negative, the woman should repeat the test in 1 week if she has not started her menstrual period. A false-negative result may lead to delays in beginning prenatal care or in the use of drugs that may be harmful to the fetus. It is important that women using the home kits understand that a positive result merely indicates growing trophoblastic tissue and not necessarily a uterine pregnancy. If the woman delays seeking prenatal care after pregnancy is confirmed, an early ectopic pregnancy may be missed.

Diagnostic (Positive) Changes

The positive signs of pregnancy are completely objective, cannot be confused with pathologic states, and offer conclusive proof of pregnancy.

The *fetal heartbeat* can be detected with a fetoscope by approximately weeks 17 to 20 of pregnancy. With the electronic Doppler device it is possible to detect the fetal heartbeat as early as weeks 10 to 12. The fetal heart rate is between 120 and 160 beats per minute and must be counted and compared with the maternal pulse for differentiation. Auscultation of the abdomen may reveal sounds other than that of the fetal heart. The maternal pulse, emanating from the abdominal aorta, may be unusually loud, or a uterine souffle may be heard.

Fetal movement is actively palpable by a trained examiner after about 20 weeks' gestation. The movements vary from a faint flutter in the early months to more vigorous movements late in pregnancy.

Visualization of the fetus by ultrasound confirms a pregnancy. The gestational sac can be observed by 4 to 5 weeks' gestation (2 to 3 weeks after conception). Fetal parts and fetal heart movement can be seen as early as 8 weeks. Recently, ultrasound using a vaginal probe has been used to detect a gestational sac as early as 10 days after implantation (Cunningham et al, 2001).

Psychologic Response of the Expectant Family to Pregnancy

Pregnancy is a developmental challenge, a turning point, in a family's life and therefore is accompanied by stress and anxiety whether the pregnancy is desired or not. Pregnancy confirms one's biologic capabilities to reproduce. It is evidence of one's participation in sexual activity and as such is an affirmation of one's sexuality. For beginning families, pregnancy is the transition period from childlessness to parenthood. If the pregnancy terminates in the birth of a child, the couple enters a new stage of their life together, one that is irreversible and characterized by awesome responsibilities.

The expectant couple may be unaware of the physical, emotional, and cognitive states peculiar to pregnancy. The couple may anticipate no problem from such a normal event as pregnancy and therefore may be confused and distressed by new feelings and behaviors that are generally considered normal.

If the expectant woman is married or has a stable partner, she no longer is only a mate but also must assume the role of mother. Her partner will also assume a parenting role. Career goals and mobility may be altered or thwarted for one or both partners. Each partner begins to see the other in a different light. Their relationship takes on a different meaning to them and within the larger family and community. Their lifestyle changes. With each pregnancy, routines and family dynamics are altered, requiring readjustment and realignment.

If a pregnant woman is without a stable partner, she will still experience changes in role identity and psychobiologic maturation. She must deal alone with the role changes, fears, and adjustments of pregnancy or seek support from family and friends. She also faces the reality of planning for the future as a single parent. Even if the pregnant woman plans to relinquish her infant, she must still deal with the adjustments of pregnancy. She is no longer a separate individual; she must consider the needs of another being who depends on her totally, at least during the pregnancy. This adjustment can be especially difficult without a good support system.

In most pregnancies, whether of a mother with a supportive partner, a single mother, or a relinquishing mother, finances are an important consideration. Traditional lore relegates to the father the role of primary breadwinner, and indeed finances are often a very real concern for fathers. However, in today's society even pregnant women with stable partners recognize the financial impact of a child and may feel concern about financial issues. For the single mother, finances may be a major source of concern.

Decisions about financial matters need to be made at this time. Will the woman work during the pregnancy and return to work after the baby is born? Who will provide child care if she works? Decisions may also need to be made about the division of tasks within the home. Any differences of opinion must be discussed openly and resolved so that the family can meet its members' needs.

The couple must face the realities of labor and birth. Many nonparents have little idea what labor entails. Their information is frequently based on contacts with visual or print media and on experiences related to them by family members or friends, and these tales are often fraught with myths and exaggerations. Classes in prepared childbirth can help them address this lack of information or misinformation.

Labor is threatening in many respects. Pain, disfigurement, disruption of bodily function, and even death are potential threats for the woman. The partner faces the threat of the woman's disfigurement, impairment of her health, or her death. Both fear that the baby may be ill or disfigured. The expectant couple is subject to anxiety during this period because no one can provide total reassurance about the outcome.

Pregnancy can be viewed as a developmental stage with its own distinct developmental tasks. It can be a time of support or conflict for a couple, depending on the amount of adjustment each is willing to make to maintain the family's equilibrium. Family dynamics are an important factor in adjusting to pregnancy. Family strengths include the ability of the couple to talk about issues that are important to them, to resolve conflicts and make compromises, and to seek and receive assistance and support from loved ones.

During pregnancy, the couple plans together for the first child's arrival, collecting information on how to be parents. At the same time, each continues to participate in some separate activities with friends or family members. The availability of social support is an important factor in psychosocial well-being during pregnancy. Most pregnant women turn to their partners as their primary source of social support. In particular, a woman needs support from her partner that affirms that she is valued and that her baby will be welcomed and accepted (Logsdon, 2000–2001). The broader social network often is a major source of advice for the pregnant woman. However, evidence indicates that both sound and unsound information is given.

Although individual activities are important, some conflict may arise if the couple's activities become too divergent. Thus they may find it necessary to limit their outside associations.

The expectant mother and her partner both face significant changes during pregnancy and must deal with major psychosocial adjustments (Table 14–3 •). Other family members, especially other children of the woman or couple, and the grandparents-to-be, must also adjust to the pregnancy.

In late pregnancy, the concerns of expectant fathers tend to focus most on the health of the unborn child and the safety of the mother. The expectant mothers' concerns center on the health of the baby and their ability to handle labor and birth. Couples typically agree on the primary concern, the health of the unborn child. Nurses can use this focus as a springboard for discussing other concerns. Couples can then come to understand the differences between their second most important concerns. A woman worries about how she will handle labor and birth, but has little concern for her own safety; the father's expression of his fear for her safety can be seen as evidence that he cares enough to worry about her. This response may allow the mother to depend on him more during the vulnerable time of late pregnancy and birthing. Sharing his views gives the father a chance to express his love and concern for mother and child, encouraging the development of stronger marital and paternal relationships (White, 1998a, 1998b).

For some couples, pregnancy is more than a developmental stage; it is a crisis. *Crisis* can be defined as a disturbance or conflict in which the individual cannot maintain a state of equilibrium. Pregnancy can be considered a *maturational crisis* because it is a common event in the normal growth and development of the family. During such a crisis, the individual or family is in disequilibrium. Egos weaken, usual defense mechanisms lose their effectiveness, unresolved material from the past reappears, and relationships shift. The period of disequilibrium and disorganization is marked by abortive attempts to solve the perceived problems. If the

MEDIALINK CASE STUDY: PRENATAL EDUCATION

Table 14-3 • PARENTAL REACTIONS TO PREGNANCY

First Trimester	Second Trimester	Third Trimester
Mother's Reactions	**Mother's Reactions**	**Mother's Reactions**
Informs father secretively or openly. Feels ambivalent toward pregnancy, anxious about labor and responsibility of child. Is aware of physical changes, daydreams of possible miscarriage. Develops special feelings for and renewed interest in her own mother, with formation of a personal identity.	Remains regressive and introspective, projects all problems with authority figures onto partner, may become angry as if lack of interest is sign of weakness in him. Continues to deal with feelings as a mother and looks for furniture as something concrete. May have other extreme of anxiety and wait until 9th month to look for furniture and clothes for baby. Feels movement and is aware of fetus and incorporates it into herself. Dreams that partner will be killed, telephones him often for reassurance. Experiences more distinct physical changes; sexual desires may increase or decrease.	Experiences more anxiety and tension, with physical awkwardness. Feels much discomfort and insomnia from physical condition. Prepares for birth, assembles layette, picks out names. Dreams often about misplacing baby or not being able to give birth, fears birth of deformed baby. Feels ecstasy and excitement, has spurt of energy during last month.
Father's Reactions	**Father's Reactions**	**Father's Reactions**
Differ according to age, parity, desire for child, economic stability. Acceptance of pregnant woman's attitude or complete rejection and lack of communication. Is aware of his own sexual feelings, may develop more or less sexual arousal. Accepts, rejects, or resents mother-in-law. May develop new hobby outside of family as sign of stress.	If he can cope, will give her extra attention she needs; if he cannot cope, will develop a new time-consuming interest outside of home. May develop a creative feeling and a "closeness to nature." May become involved in pregnancy and buy or make furniture. Feels for movement of baby, listens to heartbeat, or remains aloof, with no physical contact. May have fears and fantasies about himself being pregnant, may become uneasy with this feminine aspect in himself. May react negatively if partner is too demanding, may become jealous of physician and of physician's importance to partner and her pregnancy.	Adapts to alternative methods of sexual contact. Becomes concerned over financial responsibility. May show new sense of tenderness and concern, treats partner like doll. Daydreams about child as if older and not newborn, dreams of losing partner. Renewed sexual attraction to partner. Feels he is ultimately responsible for whatever happens.

crisis is unresolved, it will result in maladaptive behaviors in one or more family members and possible disintegration of the family. Families who are able to resolve a maturational crisis successfully will return to normal functioning and can even strengthen the bonds in the family relationship.

Mother

Pregnancy is a condition that alters body image and also necessitates a reordering of social relationships and changes in roles of family members. The way a particular woman meets the stresses of pregnancy is influenced by her emotional makeup, her sociologic and cultural background, and her acceptance or rejection of the pregnancy. However, many women manifest similar psychologic and emotional responses during pregnancy, including ambivalence, acceptance, introversion, mood swings, and changes in body image.

INTENDEDNESS

Large-scale surveys such as the Pregnancy Risk Assessment Monitoring Systems (PRAMS) have included questions about whether women's pregnancies have been intended (Klerman, 2000). Interest in the large number of unintended pregnancies revealed by the studies has resulted in Institute of Medicine reports and objectives listed in *Healthy People 2000* and *Healthy People 2010* to decrease unintended pregnancies. However, researchers have not considered the nuances among such terms as *intended* and *unintended*, *planned* and *unplanned*, and *wanted*, *unwanted*, or *mistimed*. This makes the data hard to interpret. For example, a pregnancy can be mistimed, unintended, and wanted all at the same time, with prospective parents who are happy to find themselves expecting. In addition, contraceptive failure does not always lead to the report of unintended pregnancy. Further research is needed to clarify these concepts and to distinguish between terms that define attitudes and those that define behaviors (Klerman, 2000).

AMBIVALENCE

Initially, even if the pregnancy is planned, the mother may experience a sense of surprise that conception has actually occurred. This may be coupled with a feeling that pregnancy is desirable "some day" but "not now." Such ambivalence may be related to feelings that the timing is somehow "wrong," worries about the need to modify existing relationships or career plans, fears about assuming a new role, unresolved emotional conflicts with the woman's own mother,

RESEARCH IN PRACTICE
Women's Lived Experiences of Pregnancy

What is this study about? The passage from pregnancy to the maternal role has been studied extensively, but the nature of the experience from the mother's point of view is not well described. Most research focuses on childbirth preparation, physiologic changes, and biomedical interventions. The purpose of this study was to develop an understanding of the lived experiences of women during pregnancy.

How was this study done? This qualitative study used a phenomenological approach to develop an understanding of the pregnancy experience. In-depth interviews were conducted with 40 women, including both primiparous and multiparous mothers. The subjects were purposefully selected for the study, and were interviewed in early and late pregnancy, and during and after the birth. Each woman was asked to describe her experience of pregnancy in depth. Interviews were transcribed verbatim and analyzed using accepted qualitative analysis techniques. Meanings were labeled and organized into themes, which were further categorized to develop an exhaustive description of the experience.

What were the results of the study? Themes were classified into three categories: the desire for a perfect child, an altered mode of being, and striving for family communion. The desire for a perfect child focused the mother on health-related behavior, both for self and for the unborn baby. Mothers reported that they no longer took their health for granted, and were more willing to change their own health behaviors. They consciously made even difficult changes in their own lives if they believed it would avoid harm to the baby. In addition, the women believed that labor and birth would be easier if they were in good physical health. Self-concept changed for these women as their bodies changed and the physiologic signs of pregnancy became more obvious. The discomforts associated with pregnancy were seen as an expected part of the experience. Variations in mood also characterized the pregnancy process, as well as the onset of specific worries about their health, the baby's health, and the family's health. Although all of the women reported that the child was welcome in their lives, the importance of the child as a member of the family evolved gradually. The pregnancy brought about changes in relationships, particularly with their partner. These women wanted the whole family to want the child as much as they did, but expressed concern about how the baby would affect siblings, partners, and extended family.

What additional questions might I have? Are these experiences different when the pregnancy is unplanned or unwanted? Were there any significant differences between the experiences of the primiparous women and the multiparous women?

How can I use this study? Understanding the experience of pregnancy from the mother's point of view can help the nurse develop interventions to support the mother as she moves from pregnancy to parenthood. Recognition of both the positive and troublesome aspects of pregnancy allows for empathy and individualized care planning. It also appears that pregnancy is an ideal time for health teaching and for motivating changes in health behaviors.

Source: Bondas, T., & Eriksson, K. (2001). Women's lived experiences of pregnancy: A tapestry of joy and suffering. *Qualitative Health Research, 11*(6), 824–840.

and fears about pregnancy, labor, and birth. Indirect evidence of ambivalence includes complaints about prolonged or frequent depression, considerable physical discomfort, significant dissatisfaction with body shape, excessive mood swings, and difficulty accepting the life changes resulting from the pregnancy (Lederman, 1996).

Such feelings may be even more pronounced if the pregnancy is unintended or unwanted. Women who view their pregnancy as unwanted are more likely to delay prenatal care and to experience complications. The support and opinion of the woman's current partner, even if he is not the father of the child, have a major impact on pregnancy wantedness. Financial and emotional support from the partner are essential to the woman's positive attitude (Kroelinger & Oths, 2000). Involving the partner in the prenatal care may help promote a supportive attitude. During the early months, the pregnant woman may consider the possibility of a therapeutic abortion if the pregnancy is unwanted. In the event of religious conflicts about induced abortion, the woman may experience guilt feelings about her thoughts or may tend to focus on the possibility of spontaneous abortion (miscarriage). Even when the pregnancy is planned, thoughts of abortion and miscarriage arise. Concurrently, the pregnant woman may feel guilty for having such negative thoughts and may worry that in some way these thoughts will harm the baby.

ACCEPTANCE

Acceptance of pregnancy is influenced by many factors. Lower acceptance tends to be related to an unplanned pregnancy and greater evidence of fear and conflict. The woman carrying an unplanned pregnancy tends to experience more physical discomfort and depression. When a pregnancy is well accepted, the woman demonstrates feelings of happiness and pleasure in the pregnancy. She experiences less physical discomfort and shows a high degree of tolerance for the discomforts associated with the third trimester (Lederman, 1996).

Conflicts about adapting to pregnancy are no more pronounced for older pregnant women (age 35 and older) than for younger ones. Moreover, older pregnant women tend to be less concerned about the normal physical changes of pregnancy and are confident about handling issues that arise during pregnancy and parenting. This may be because mature pregnant women have more experience with problem solving. However, mature pregnant women may have fewer pregnant peers and thus may have fewer people with whom to share concerns and expectations (Stark, 1997).

For some women, an unintended pregnancy has more psychologic and social advantages than disadvantages. It provides purpose and direction to life and allows a woman to test the devotion and love of her partner and family (Moos, Petersen, Meadows, et al, 1997).

> *I didn't expect to get pregnant, but my baby seems like a gift from God. Suddenly I feel like I have a purpose in life. I know I have to do the right things so the baby will be okay. Being pregnant made me grow up in a hurry, but I don't regret it—not at all.*

During the *first trimester,* evidence of pregnancy is often limited to amenorrhea and to the word of the caregiver that the pregnancy test was positive. Unless the woman has the opportunity to see the gestational sac during an ultrasound, her baby may not seem real. Consequently, she may tend to focus on herself and her pregnancy. In an effort to verify her condition, a woman may become minutely conscious of changes in her body that could validate the pregnancy.

The *second trimester* is relatively tranquil. Morning sickness generally passes, the threat of spontaneous abortion diminishes, and the woman begins to accept the reality of her pregnancy. It is not unusual for an enthusiastic primigravida to don maternity clothes at the beginning of this trimester even when it is not truly necessary. The clothing serves as a verification of her pregnant state.

The highlight of the second trimester is quickening, which generally occurs about week 20—midway through the pregnancy. Actual perception of fetal movement frequently produces dramatic changes in the woman. She now perceives her baby as a real person and generally becomes excited about the pregnancy even if she hasn't been prior to this time.

As quickening and her altered physical appearance confirm her pregnant state, the woman adjusts to the idea of change and begins to prepare for her new role and her new set of relationships—with her partner and family, the child-to-be and other children, friends, and loved ones. When the pregnancy is well accepted, the woman takes pleasure in the sensations of pregnancy and attempts to picture her baby in order to know him or her better. She may seek out other women who are pregnant or have recently given birth. She feels well, is excited, and may exhibit the "glow" so often attributed to pregnant women.

The *third trimester* combines a sense of pride with anxiety about what is to come in order for the child to be born. During this time, the special prerogatives of pregnancy may be most marked. As her protruding abdomen proclaims her advanced pregnancy, the woman may find that others become more solicitous, that a chair may be offered in a crowded room, that others may carry her parcels. The woman may actually need this help, she may simply enjoy the attention as a privilege of pregnancy, or she may reject it if she fears that such gestures indicate she is helpless.

During the final trimester, physical discomforts again increase, and adequate rest becomes a necessity. The woman makes final preparation for the baby and may spend long periods considering names for the child. During this time she worries more about the health and safety of her unborn child and may have concerns that she will not behave well during childbirth.

The woman may feel vulnerable to rejection, loss, or insult. She may worry about a variety of things and may withdraw into the security and quiet of her home. Toward the end of this period many women report bursts of energy in which they vigorously clean and organize their homes ("nesting").

INTROVERSION

Introversion, or turning in on oneself, is a common occurrence in pregnancy. An active, outgoing woman may become less interested in previous activities and more concerned with needs for rest and time alone. This concentration of attention permits the woman to plan, adjust, adapt, build, and draw strength in preparation for her child's birth. As she becomes more aware of herself, her partner may feel she is being overly sensitive. Her partner may perceive her introversion and passivity as exclusionary and may in turn become unable to interact with her, either verbally or physically, or to provide the affection, support, and consideration she requires. This change may result in disequilibrium and stress for the entire family. It is essential that the couple work together to establish new, mutually acceptable patterns of response to overcome these blocks to communication.

Fantasies about the unborn child are quite common among pregnant women. However, the themes of the fantasies (baby's appearance, gender, traits, impact on parents, and so forth) vary by trimester and also differ between women pregnant for the first time and women who already have children (Sorenson & Schuelke, 1999).

MOOD SWINGS

> *I don't know if this is really considered a problem or not, but at times it seems like a problem. I'm really subject to drastic mood changes. That or I'll be extremely emotional. For no reason at all I'll start crying or just laugh till I can hardly breathe. I don't know why; and if I can't understand it, it's twice as hard for John, especially if I'm bummed out or crying. It don't [sic] seem normal for a person to cry for no reason, and I never did it before.*
>
> QUOTED IN RP LEDERMAN
> *PSYCHOSOCIAL ADAPTATION IN PREGNANCY,* 1996

Throughout pregnancy, the emotions of many women are characterized by mood swings, from great joy to deep despair. Frequently, the woman will become tearful with little apparent cause. When asked why she is crying, she may find it difficult or impossible to give a reason. The situation may be extremely unsettling for the partner, causing him to feel confused and inadequate. Because the man may feel unable to handle the woman's tears, he often reacts by withdrawing and ignoring the problem. Because the pregnant woman needs increased love and affection, she may perceive his reaction as unloving and nonsupportive. Once the couple understands that this behavior is characteristic of pregnancy, it becomes easier for them to deal with it more effectively—although it will be a source of stress to some extent throughout pregnancy.

CHANGES IN BODY IMAGE

Pregnancy produces marked changes in a woman's body within a relatively short period of time. With these changes, women also experience changes in body image. The degree of this change is related to a certain extent to personality factors, social network responses, and attitudes toward pregnancy. Changes in body image are normal but can be very stressful for the pregnant woman. Explanation and discussion of the changes may help both the woman and her partner deal with the stress associated with this aspect of pregnancy.

PSYCHOLOGIC TASKS OF THE MOTHER

Rubin (1984) identified four major tasks that the pregnant woman undertakes to maintain her intactness and that of her family and at the same time incorporate her new child into the family system. These tasks form the basis for a mutually gratifying relationship with her baby:

1. *Ensuring safe passage through pregnancy, labor, and birth.* The pregnant woman feels concern for both her unborn child and herself. She seeks competent maternity care to provide a sense of control. She may also seek knowledge from literature, observation of other pregnant women and new mothers, and discussion with others. The pregnant woman also seeks to ensure safe passage by engaging in self-care activities related to diet, exercise, alcohol consumption, and so forth. In the third trimester, as her movements slow and her body mass increases, she becomes aware of external threats in the environment—a toy on a stair, the awkwardness of an escalator—that pose a threat to her intactness and represent hazards to be overcome. She may worry if her partner is late or if she is home alone. Sleep becomes difficult, and she begins to long for the baby's birth, even though it, too, is frightening.
2. *Seeking of acceptance of this child by others.* The birth of a child alters a woman's primary support group, her family, and her secondary affiliative groups. The family generally makes the transition, and the woman slowly and subtly alters her secondary network to meet the needs of her pregnancy. In this adjustment the woman's partner is the most important figure. The partner's support and acceptance influence her completion of her maternal tasks and the formation of her maternal identity. If there are other children in the home, the mother also works to ensure their acceptance of the coming child. Accepting the coming change in exclusive relationships—woman and partner or mother and first child—can be stressful, and the woman will often work to maintain some special time with her partner or older child. Achieving social acceptance of the child and of herself as mother may be more difficult for the adolescent mother or single woman. The child to come is not always wanted, and the woman often must direct her energies to changing this situation.
3. *Seeking of commitment and acceptance of self as mother to the infant (binding-in).* During the first trimester, the child remains a rather abstract concept. With quickening, however, the child begins to become a real person, and the mother begins to develop bonds of attachment. The mother experiences the movement of the child within her in an intimate, exclusive way, and out of this experience bonds of love form. The mother develops a fantasy image of her ideal child. This binding-in process, characterized by its strong emotional component, motivates the pregnant woman to become competent in her role and provides satisfaction for her in her role of mother (Mercer, 1995). This possessive love increases her maternal commitment to protect her fetus now and her child after she or he is born.
4. *Learning to give of oneself on behalf of one's child.* Childbirth involves many acts of giving. The man "gives" a child to a woman; she in turn "gives" a child to the man. Life is given to an infant; a sibling is given to older children of the family. The woman begins to develop a capacity for self-denial and learns to delay immediate personal gratification to meet the needs of another. Baby showers and baby gifts are acts of giving that help the mother's self-esteem while also helping her acknowledge the separateness and needs of the coming baby.

Accomplishment of these tasks helps the expectant woman develop her self-concept as mother. The expectant mother who was well nurtured by her own mother may view her mother as a role model and emulate her; the woman who views her own mother as a "poor mother" may worry that she will make similar mistakes (Lederman, 1996). A woman's self-concept as mother expands with actual experience and continues to grow through subsequent childbearing and childrearing. Occasionally, a woman never accepts the mother role but plays the role of babysitter or older sister.

Father

Until fairly recently, the expectant father was often viewed as a "bystander" or observer of his partner's pregnancy. He was necessary for conception, for bill paying, and for providing male guidance as his child matured. This view has changed, and the father of today is expected to fulfill the role of nurturing, caring, involved parent as well as provider. In response to societal pressures, the influence of the feminist movement, and the economic pressures that result in more women employed outside the home, shared parenting and breadwinning have become more commonplace. Many men have actively sought to be more involved in the experience of childbirth and parenting.

Expectant fathers experience many of the same feelings and conflicts experienced by expectant mothers when the pregnancy has been confirmed. Initially, expectant fathers may feel pride in their virility, which pregnancy confirms, but also have ambivalent feelings. The extent of ambivalence depends on many factors, including the father's relationship with his partner, his previous experience with pregnancy, his age, his economic stability, and whether the pregnancy was planned. Research suggests that expectant fathers who have more self-actualizing behaviors, exercise regularly, use more stress management techniques, and have good interpersonal support tend to find pregnancy less stressful and feel more confident about parenting (Walker, Fleschler, & Heaman, 1998).

The expectant father must first deal with the reality of the pregnancy and then struggle to gain recognition as a parent from his partner, family, friends, coworkers, society—and from his baby as well. The expectant mother can help her partner be a participant and not merely a helpmate to her if she has a definite sense of the experience as their pregnancy and their infant and not her pregnancy and her infant.

Men whose partners are pregnant following a previous pregnancy loss may experience a variety of emotions attributable to the loss. These emotions might include an increased sense of risk, feelings of increased concern about the outcome of the current pregnancy, the recognition that something could go wrong again, and the sense that increased vigilance is essential. These fathers may also feel an increased need to be involved more actively in the current pregnancy (Armstrong, 2001).

In general, the expectant father faces psychologic stress as he makes the transition from nonparent to parent or from parent of one to parent of two or more. Sources of stress include financial issues, unexpected events during pregnancy, concern that the baby will not be healthy and normal, worry about the pain the partner will experience in childbirth, and his role during labor and birth. Other sources of stress for expectant fathers include concern over the changing relationship with their partner, diminished sexual responsiveness in their partner or in themselves, change in relationships with their family or male friends, and their ability to parent.

The expectant father must establish a fatherhood role just as the woman develops a motherhood role. Fathers who are most successful at this generally like children, are excited about the prospect of fatherhood, are eager to nurture a child, have confidence in their ability to be a parent, and share the experiences of pregnancy and childbirth with their partners (Lederman, 1996).

FIRST TRIMESTER

After the initial excitement of the announcement of the pregnancy to friends and relatives and their congratulations, an expectant father may begin to feel left out of the pregnancy. He is also often confused by his partner's mood changes and perhaps bewildered by his responses to her changing body. He may resent the attention given to the woman and the need to change their relationship as she experiences fatigue and a decreased interest in sex.

During this time, his child is a "potential baby." Fathers often picture interacting with a child of 5 or 6 rather than a newborn. Even the pregnancy itself may seem unreal until the woman shows more physical signs.

SECOND TRIMESTER

The father's role in the pregnancy is still vague in the second trimester, but his involvement can be increased by his watching and feeling fetal movement. It is helpful if the father, as well as the mother, has the opportunity to hear the fetal heartbeat. That requires a visit to the nurse-midwife's or physician's office. Involvement of fathers in antepartal care is increasing as fathers become more comfortable with this new role. For many men, seeing the infant on ultrasound is an important experience in accepting the reality of the pregnancy.

Like expectant mothers, expectant fathers need to confront and resolve some of their own conflicts about the fathering they received. A father needs to sort out those behaviors in his own fathering that he wants to imitate and those he wishes to avoid. This process usually occurs gradually as the pregnancy progresses.

> *Don't get me wrong. I love my dad and I know he did his best to provide for us but he worked long hours and was gone a lot. I don't think I ever had any kind of meaningful conversation with him until recently when Anita got pregnant. Once he found out he was going to be a grandfather he started talking about what he had missed out on when my sister and I were growing up. He is determined to be a wonderful grandpa. I think a part of him sees it as a second chance.*

Evidence suggests that the father-to-be's anxiety is lessened if both parents agree on the support role the man is to assume during pregnancy and on his projected paternal role. For example, if both see his role as that of breadwinner, the man's stress is low. However, if the man views his role as that of breadwinner and the woman expects him to be actively involved in preparations and child care, his stress increases. Thus the ability of the couple to negotiate a mutually agreeable role for the man may provide a significant coping mechanism for expectant fathers (Diemer, 1997).

The woman's appearance begins to alter at this time too, and men react differently to the physical change. For some it decreases sexual interest; for others it may have the opposite effect. Both partners experience a multitude of emotions, and it continues to be important for them to communicate and accept each other's feelings and concerns. In situations in which the expectant mother's demands dominate the relationship, the expectant father's resentment may increase to the point that he is spending more time at work, involved in a hobby, or with his friends. The behavior is even more likely if the expectant father did not want the pregnancy and/or if the relationship was not a good one prior to the pregnancy.

THIRD TRIMESTER

If the couple have communicated their concerns and feelings to one another and grown in their relationship, the third trimester is a special and rewarding time. A more clearly defined role evolves at this time for the expectant father, and it becomes more obvious how the couple can prepare together for the coming event. They may become involved in childbirth education classes and make concrete preparations for the arrival of the baby, such as shopping for a crib, car seat, and other equipment. If the expectant father has developed a detached attitude about the pregnancy prior to this time, however, it is unlikely that he will become a willing participant even though his role becomes more obvious.

Concerns and fears may recur. Many men are afraid of hurting the unborn baby during intercourse. The father may also begin to have anxiety and fantasies about what could happen to his partner and the unborn baby during labor and birth and feels a great sense of responsibility. The questions asked earlier in pregnancy emerge again. What kind of parents will he and his partner be? Will he really be able to help his partner in labor? Can they afford to have a baby?

COUVADE

The term **couvade** traditionally referred to the observance of certain rituals and taboos by the male to signify the transition to fatherhood. This observance affirms his psychosocial and biophysical relationship to the woman and child. These taboos may have taken specific form—for example, the man may have been forbidden to eat certain foods or carry certain weapons before and immediately after the birth. More recently, the term has been used to describe the unintentional development of physical symptoms, such as fatigue, increased appetite, difficulty sleeping, depression, headache, or backache by the partner of the pregnant woman. Men who demonstrate couvade syndrome tend to have a higher degree of paternal role preparation and be involved in more activities related to this preparation.

Siblings

The introduction of a new baby into the family is often the beginning of sibling rivalry. Sibling rivalry results from children's fear of change in the security of their relationships with their parents. Some of the behaviors demonstrating feelings of sibling rivalry may even be directed toward the mother during the pregnancy as she experiences more fatigue and less patience with her toddler, for example. Parents who recognize the situation early in pregnancy and begin constructive actions can help minimize the problems of sibling rivalry.

Preparation of the young child begins several weeks prior to the anticipated birth and is designed according to the age and experience of the child. Because they do not have a clear concept of time, young children should not be told too early about the pregnancy. From the toddler's point of view "several weeks" is an extremely long time. The mother may let the child feel the baby moving in her uterus, explaining that this is "a special place where babies grow." The child can help the parents put the baby clothes in drawers or prepare the baby's room.

The concept of consistency is important in dealing with young children. They need reassurance that certain people, special things, and familiar places will continue to exist after the new baby arrives. The crib is an important though transient object in a child's life. If it is to be given to the new baby, the parents should thoughtfully help the child adjust to this change. Any move from crib to bed or from one room to another should precede the baby's birth by at least several weeks. If the new baby must share a room with siblings, the parents must discuss this with the siblings.

Some parents advocate cosleeping or bed sharing (one or both parents sleeping with their baby or young child), and so the crib is less of an issue. Cosleeping, which is common in many non-Western cultures, is on the increase in the United States. In fact a recent study reports that approximately 12.8% of infants regularly share an adult bed at night while almost 50% of the infants in the study had spent at least some time sleeping in an adult bed at night in the preceding two weeks. Among the group studied, African American infants were four times more likely to cosleep than white infants and Asian/other infants were three times more likely to do so than white infants (National Institute of Child Health and Human Development, 2003). However, the practice has sparked controversy in the United States. Opinion varies sharply about the advantages and risks of the practice, especially in light of an American Academy of Pediatrics policy statement (2000) recommending against cosleeping because of the increased risk of sudden infant death syndrome (SIDS). (See discussion in Chapter 36.) Parents who choose to cosleep must make decisions about the sleeping arrangements of other siblings following the birth of the baby.

If the child is ready for toilet training, it is most effectively done several months before or after the baby's arrival. Parents should know that the older, toilet-trained child may regress to wetting or soiling because he or she sees the new baby getting attention for such behavior. The older, weaned child may want to drink from the breast or bottle again after the new baby comes. If the new mother anticipates these behaviors, they will be less frustrating during her early postpartum days.

During the pregnancy, older children should be introduced to a new baby for short periods to get an idea of what a new baby is like. This introduction dispels fantasies that the new arrival will be big enough to be a playmate. Pregnant women may also find it helpful to bring their children to a prenatal visit after they have been told about the expected baby. The children are encouraged to become involved in prenatal care and to ask any questions they may have. They are also given the opportunity to hear the baby's heartbeat, either with a stethoscope or with the Doppler. This helps make the baby more real to them.

If siblings are school-age children, the pregnancy should be viewed as a family affair. Teaching about the pregnancy should be based on the child's level of understanding and interest. Overeager parents may go into lengthier and more indepth responses than the child is able to understand. Some children are more curious than others. Books at their level of

MEDIALINK CARE PLAN: PREPARING SIBLINGS FOR NEW BABY

understanding can be made available in the home. Involvement in family discussions, attendance at sibling preparation classes, encouragement to feel fetal movement, and an opportunity to listen to the fetal heart supplement the learning process and help make the school-age child feel part of the pregnancy. Sibling preparation classes assist in the transition process for both parents and children. After attending the classes, children often exhibit less anxiety and increased ability to express their feelings.

Older children or adolescents may appear to have a sophisticated knowledge base, but it may be intermingled with many misconceptions. Thus the parents should make opportunities to discuss their concerns and should involve the children in preparation for the new baby.

Even after the birth, siblings need to feel that they are part of a family affair. Changes in hospital regulations allowing siblings to be present at the birth or to visit their mother and the new baby facilitate this process. On arrival at home, siblings can share in "showing off" the new baby.

Sibling preparation for the arrival of a new baby is essential, but other factors are equally important. These include the amount of parental attention focused on the new arrival, the amount of parental attention given the older child after the birth of the new arrival, and parental skill in dealing effectively with regressive and/or aggressive behavior.

Grandparents

The first relatives told about a pregnancy are usually the grandparents. Although relationships with parents can be very complex, this period in a family's life most often promotes a closer relationship between the expectant couple and their parents. Usually the expectant grandparents become increasingly supportive of the expectant couple, even if conflicts previously existed.

Grandparents may be unsure about the amount of involvement they are "allowed" during the pregnancy and childbearing process. Most want to be helpful; some may bestow advice and/or gifts unsparingly. Because grandparenting can occur over a wide span of years, people's response to this role can vary considerably. For some, this new role may occur at a relatively young age, and the connotation of aging that accompanies the role may affect their response to the pregnancy. The younger grandparent may also be involved in work and other activities and may not demonstrate as much interest as the young couple would like.

It can be difficult for even sensitive grandparents to know how much involvement the couple wants. Expectant couples want to feel in control of their new situation, which may be initially difficult in their changing roles. Grandparents find that this factor, as well as changing roles in their own lives (eg, retirement, financial concerns, menopause of the expectant grandmother, death of a friend), may contribute to conflicts in the changing family structure. Some parents of expectant couples may already be grandparents and have already developed their own style of grandparenting, which will be an important factor in how they respond to the pregnancy.

Childbearing and childrearing practices are very different for today's childbearing couple. It helps family cohesiveness for young couples to share with interested grandparents what today's practices are and why they feel they are effective. At the same time, it is important for young couples to listen to any differences expectant grandparents want to explain. When grandparents give advice, it helps to remember that they care. When their recommendations seem effective, it is significant to grandparents that young couples do listen and follow their advice.

Occasionally young couples feel they are receiving more advice than they can tolerate. Too often they perceive parents' suggestions as criticizing their ability to prepare adequately for the childbearing process—and later as criticizing their care of the newborn. It is useful for the young couple to discuss the problem and agree on a plan of action. The role of the helping grandparents when the new baby is brought home needs to be clarified before the event to ensure a comfortable situation for all.

In some areas, classes for grandparents provide information about changes in birthing and parenting practices. These classes help familiarize grandparents with new parents' needs and may offer suggestions for ways in which the grandparents can support the childbearing woman or couple.

Cultural Values and Pregnancy

A universal tendency exists to create ceremonial rituals and rites around important life events. Thus pregnancy, childbirth, marriage, and death are often tied to ritual (Spector, 2000). The rituals, customs, and practices of a group are a reflection of the group's values. Consequently the identification of cultural values is useful in planning and providing culturally sensitive care.

Generalizations about cultural characteristics or cultural values are difficult because not every individual in a culture may display these characteristics. Just as variations are seen among cultures, variations are also seen within cultures. These variations are often related to social and economic factors such as class, income, and education. For example, because of their exposure to the American culture, a third-generation Cambodian American family might have very different values and beliefs from those of a traditional Cambodian family who has recently immigrated to America. For this reason, the nurse needs to supplement a general knowledge of cultural values and practices with a complete assessment of the individual's values and practices. Developing Cultural Competence summarizes the key actions a nurse can take to become more culturally aware.

Cultural assessment is an important aspect of prenatal care (see Figure 2–8 •). Healthcare professionals are becoming increasingly aware of the importance of addressing cultural, physiologic, and psychologic needs in the prenatal assessment in order to provide culture-specific healthcare during pregnancy. The nurse needs to identify the main beliefs, val-

DEVELOPING CULTURAL COMPETENCE

Nurses who are interacting with expectant families from a different culture or ethnic group can provide more effective, culturally sensitive nursing care by

- Critically examining their own cultural beliefs
- Identifying personal biases, attitudes, stereotypes, and prejudices
- Making a conscious commitment to respect the values and beliefs of others
- Using sensitive, current language when describing others' cultures
- Learning the rituals, customs, and practices of the major cultural and ethnic groups with whom they have contact
- Including cultural assessment and assessment of the family's expectations of the healthcare system as a routine part of prenatal nursing care
- Incorporating the family's cultural practices into prenatal care as much as possible
- Fostering an attitude of respect for and cooperation with alternative healers and caregivers whenever possible
- Providing for the services of an interpreter if language barriers exist
- Learning the language (or at least several key phrases) of at least one of the cultural groups with whom they interact
- Recognizing that ultimately it is the woman's right to make her own healthcare choices
- Evaluating whether the client's healthcare beliefs have any potential negative consequences for her health

ues, and behaviors that relate to pregnancy and childbearing. This includes information about ethnic background, amount of affiliation with the ethnic group, patterns of decision making, religious preferences, language, communication style, and common etiquette practices. The nurse can also explore the woman's (or family's) expectations of the healthcare system. Once this information is gathered, the nurse can then plan and provide care that is appropriate and responsive to the family's needs. These topics are discussed in detail in Chapter 2 .

CHAPTER REVIEW

EXPLOREMEDIALINK

NCLEX review questions, case studies, and other interactive resources for this chapter can be found on the Web site at http://www.prenhall.com/olds. Click on "Chapter 14" and select the activities for this chapter.

For tutorials including animations and videos, more NCLEX review questions, and an audio glossary, access the accompanying CD-ROM in this book.

Focus Your Study

- Virtually all systems of a woman's body are altered in some way during pregnancy. Blood pressure decreases slightly during pregnancy. It reaches its lowest point in the second trimester and gradually increases to near normal levels in the third trimester. The enlarging uterus may exert pressure on the vena cava when the woman lies supine, causing a drop in blood pressure. This is called the vena caval syndrome or supine hypotension.
- A physiologic anemia may occur during pregnancy because the total plasma volume increases more than the total number of erythrocytes. This produces a drop in the hematocrit.
- The glomerular filtration rate increases during pregnancy. Glycosuria may be caused by the body's inability to reabsorb all the glucose filtered by the glomeruli.

- Changes in the skin include the development of chloasma; linea nigra; darkened nipples, areolae, and vulva; striae; and spider nevi.
- Insulin needs increase during pregnancy. A woman with a latent deficiency state may respond to the increased stress on the islets of Langerhans by developing gestational diabetes mellitus.
- The subjective (presumptive) signs of pregnancy are those symptoms experienced and reported by the woman, such as amenorrhea, nausea and vomiting, fatigue, urinary frequency, breast changes, and quickening.
- The objective (probable) signs of pregnancy can be perceived by the examiner but may be caused by conditions other than pregnancy.
- The diagnostic (positive) signs of pregnancy can be perceived by the examiner and can be caused only by pregnancy.
- During pregnancy the expectant woman may experience ambivalence, acceptance, introversion, emotional lability, and changes in body image.
- Rubin (1984) identified four developmental tasks for the pregnant woman: (1) ensuring safe passage through pregnancy, labor, and birth; (2) seeking acceptance of this child by others; (3) seeking commitment and acceptance of self as mother to the infant; and (4) learning to give of oneself on behalf of one's child.
- Fathers also face a series of adjustments as they accept their new role.
- Siblings of all ages require assistance in dealing with the birth of a new baby.
- Cultural values, beliefs, and behaviors influence a couple's response to childbearing and the healthcare system.
- A cultural assessment should focus on factors that will influence the practices of the childbearing family with regard to their health needs.

References

American Academy of Pediatrics (AAP). (2000). Policy statement: Changing concepts of sudden infant death syndrome: Implications for infant sleep environment and sleep position. *Pediatrics, 105*(3), 650–656.

American College of Obstetricians and Gynecologists (ACOG). (1998). Cultural competency in health care (ACOG Committee Opinion No. 201). Washington, DC: Author.

Armstrong, D. (2001). Exploring fathers' experiences of pregnancy after a prior perinatal loss. *American Journal of Maternal Child Nursing, 26*(1), 147–153.

Beckman, C. R. B., & Dysart, D. (2000). The challenge of multicultural medical care. *Contemporary OB/GYN, 45*(12), 12–33.

Blackburn, S. T., & Loper, D. L. (1992). *Maternal, fetal, and neonatal physiology: A clinical perspective.* Philadelphia: Saunders.

Bodo, K., & Gibson, N. (1999a). Childbirth customs in Orthodox Jewish traditions. *Canadian Family Physician, 45,* 682–686.

Bodo, K., & Gibson, N. (1999b). Childbirth customs in Vietnamese traditions. *Canadian Family Physician, 45,* 690–697.

Buster, J. E., & Carson, S. A. (1996). Endocrinology and diagnosis of pregnancy. In S. G. Gabbe, J. R. Niebyl, & J. L. Simpson (Eds.), *Obstetrics: Normal and problem pregnancies* (3rd ed.). New York: Churchill Livingstone.

Choudhry, U. K. (1997). Traditional practices of women from India: Pregnancy, childbirth, and newborn care. *Journal of Obstetric, Gynecologic, and Neonatal Nursing, 26*(5), 533–539.

Conley, L. J. (1990). Childbearing and childrearing practices in Mormonism. *Neonatal Network, 9*(3), 41–48.

Cruikshank, D. P., Wigton, T. R., & Hays, P. M. (1996). Maternal physiology in pregnancy. In S. G. Gabbe, J. R. Niebyl, & J. L. Simpson (Eds.), *Obstetrics: Normal & problem pregnancies* (3rd ed.). New York: Churchill Livingstone.

Cunningham, F. G., Gant, N. F., Leveno, K. J., Gilstrap, L. C., III, Hauth, J. C., & Wenstrom, K. D. (2001). *Williams obstetrics* (21st ed.). New York: McGraw-Hill.

Curran, C. (2000). Hormonal pregnancy testing: Am I or aren't I? An update on pregnancy tests. *Professional Care of Mother & Child, 10*(5), 121–122.

D'Avanzo, C. E. (1992). Bridging the cultural gap with Southeast Asians. *American Journal of Maternal Child Nursing, 17*(4), 204–208.

Diemer, G. A. (1997). Expectant fathers: Influence of perinatal education on stress, coping, and spousal relations. *Research in Nursing & Health, 20*(4), 281–293.

Gennaro, S., Kamwendo, L. A., Mbweza, E., & Kershbaumer, R. (1998). Childbearing in Malawi, Africa. *Journal of Obstetric, Gynecologic, and Neonatal Nursing, 27*(2), 191–196.

Hyde, A.(1998, September). From mutual pretense awareness to open awareness: Single pregnant women's public encounters in an Irish context. *Qualitative Health Research, 8*(5), 634–643.

Institute of Medicine. (1990). *Nutrition during pregnancy: I. Weight gain.* Washington, DC: National Academy Press.

Klerman, L. V. (2000, September). The intendedness of pregnancy: A concept in transition. *Maternal & Child Health Journal, 4*(3), 155–162.

Kroelinger, C. D., & Oths, K. S. (2000). Partner support and pregnancy wantedness. *Birth, 27*(2), 112–119.

Lederman, R. P. (1996). *Psychosocial adaptation in pregnancy* (2nd ed.). New York: Springer.

Logsdon, M. C. (2000–2001). Helping hands: Exploring the cultural implications of social support during pregnancy. *AWHONN Lifelines, 4*(6), 29–32.

Long, C. R., & Curry, M. A. (1998, May-June). Living in two worlds: Native American women and prenatal care. *Health Care for Women International, 19*(3), 205–215.

Mattson, S. (1995). Culturally sensitive perinatal care for Southeast Asians. *Journal of Obstetric, Gynecologic, and Neonatal Nursing, 24*(4), 335–341.

Mattson, S., & Smith, J. E. (2000). *Core curriculum for maternal-newborn nursing* (2nd ed.). Philadelphia: Saunders.

Mercer, R. T. (1995). *Becoming a mother.* New York: Springer.

Moos, M. K., Petersen, R., Meadows, K., Melvin, C. L., & Spitz, A. M. (1997). Pregnant women's perspectives on intendedness of pregnancy. *Women's Health Issues,* 7(6), 385–392.

National Institute of Child Health and Human Development. (2003, January 13). NIH News Release. Retrieved on January 19, 2003 from http://www.nih.gov/new/releases/bed_shaving.cfm

Pearce, C. W. (1998, November). Seeking a healthy baby: Hispanic women's views of pregnancy and prenatal care. *Clinical Excellence for Nurse Practitioners,* 2(6), 352–361.

Rubin, R. (1984). *Maternal identity and the maternal experience.* New York: Springer.

Sorenson, D. S., & Schuelke, P. (1999). Fantasies of the unborn among pregnant women. *American Journal of Maternal Child Nursing,* 24(2), 92–97.

Spector, R. E. (2000). *Cultural diversity in health and illness* (5th ed.). Norwalk, CT: Appleton & Lange.

Stark, M. A. (1997). Psychosocial adjustment during pregnancy: The experience of mature gravidas. *Journal of Obstetric, Gynecologic, and Neonatal Nursing,* 26(2), 206–211.

Walker, L. O., Fleschler, R. G., & Heaman, M. (1998). Is a healthy lifestyle related to stress, parenting confidence, and health symptoms among new fathers? *Canadian Journal of Nursing Research,* 30(3), 21–36.

White, M. B. (1998a, June). Men's concerns during pregnancy, part 1: Evaluating the role of the expectant father. *International Journal of Childbirth Education,* 13(2), 14–17.

White, M. B. (1998b, September). Men's concerns during pregnancy, part 2: Implications for the expectant couple. *International Journal of Childbirth Education,* 13(3), 21–25.

Antepartal Nursing Assessment 15

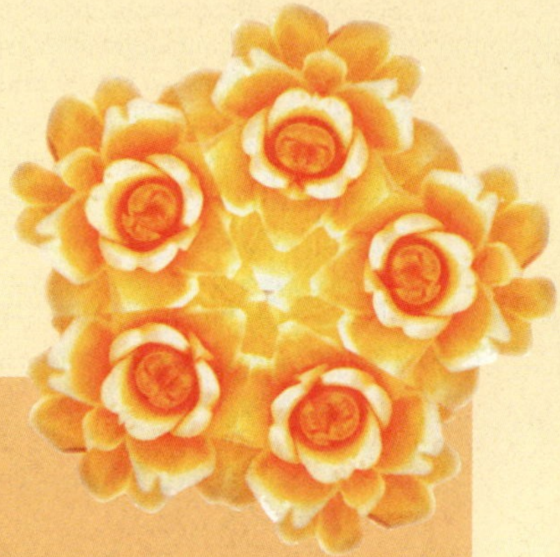

My daughter, one of the authors of this book, invited me to write a few paragraphs. What would I write about? How about comparing the father's role at childbirth when she was born to the role of today's father? The father of the 1940s. . . . Main objective: Get your wife to the hospital on time. No delays. You're not schooled in delivering babies. Next, check her in and find the father's waiting lounge. You won't be needed until the baby is born. Fathers are really useless at this time. Try not to be nervous. Coffee is available. Lots and lots of coffee. This hospital is very considerate.

It seems babies are never born in the daytime. It's always at night. You're tired. Maybe you can pace. It's hard to pace in a room 10 feet square. Delivery may take anywhere from 20 minutes to 20 hours. Hope it's not 20 hours.

More coffee, more pacing, no sleep. What a drain on the father. . . . The baby finally comes. Two hours later the doctor remembers the father is waiting. "It's a beautiful, healthy baby girl. Mother and baby are doing fine. You can see them now, but only for 5 minutes." What a relief. The pressure is finally off. Isn't nature wonderful? . . .

Today's father, my son. Schooled in Lamaze. Drives his wife to the hospital. Coaches her through her labor. Helps her find a comfortable position to birth their baby. His camera is ready. The baby is born. He cuts the cord. What a relief. The pressure is finally off. Isn't nature wonderful?

MediaLink

Additional resources for this content can be found on the Student CD-ROM and on the Companion Website at www.prenhall.com/olds. Click on "Chapter 15" to select the activities for this chapter.

CD-ROM
- Audio Glossary
- NCLEX Review

Companion Website
- Additional NCLEX Review
- Case Study: Initial Prenatal Assessment
- Care Plan Activity: Initial Assessment of Primigravida

Objectives

- Summarize the essential components of a prenatal history.
- Define common obstetric terminology found in the history of maternity clients.
- Identify factors related to the father's health that should be recorded on the prenatal record.
- Describe the normal physiologic changes one would expect to find when performing a physical assessment on a pregnant woman.
- Explain the use of Nägele's rule to determine the estimated date of birth.
- Develop an outline of the essential measurements that can be determined by clinical pelvimetry.
- Describe areas that should be evaluated as part of the initial assessment of psychosocial factors related to a woman's pregnancy.
- Relate the danger signs of pregnancy to their possible causes.

Key Terms

Abortion 323
Antepartum 323
Diagonal conjugate 342
Estimated date of birth (EDB) 339
Gestation 323
Gravida 323
Intrapartum 323
Multigravida 323
Multipara 323
Nägele's rule 339
Nulligravida 323
Nullipara 323
Obstetric conjugate 342
Para 323

Key Terms

Postpartum 323
Postterm labor 323
Preterm or premature labor 323
Primigravida 323
Primipara 323
Risk factors 326
Stillbirth 323
Term 323

Today nurses are assuming a more important role in prenatal care, particularly in the area of assessment. The certified nurse-midwife has the education and skill to perform in-depth prenatal assessments. The nurse practitioner may share the assessment responsibilities with a physician. An office nurse, whose primary role may be to counsel and meet the psychologic needs of the expectant family, performs assessments in those areas.

The nurse should establish an environment of comfort and open communication with each prenatal visit, conveying concern for the woman as an individual and being available to listen and discuss the woman's concerns and desires. A supportive atmosphere coupled with the information found in the prenatal assessment guides in this chapter will enable the nurse to identify needed areas of education and counseling.

Initial Client History

The course of a pregnancy depends on a number of factors, including the past pregnancy history (if this is not a first pregnancy), prepregnancy health of the woman, presence of disease states, emotional status, and past healthcare. Ideally, healthcare before the advent of pregnancy has been adequate, and antenatal care will be a continuation of that established care. One important method of determining the adequacy of a woman's prepregnancy care is a thorough history.

Definition of Terms

The following terms are used in recording the obstetric history of maternity clients:

- **Antepartum:** Time between conception and onset of labor, usually used to describe the period during which a woman is pregnant; used interchangeably with *prenatal.*
- **Intrapartum:** Time from onset of labor until the birth of the infant and placenta.
- **Postpartum:** Time from birth until the woman's body returns to an essentially prepregnant condition.
- **Gestation:** The number of weeks since the first day of the last menstrual period (LMP).
- **Abortion:** Birth that occurs before 20 weeks' gestation or the birth of a fetus-neonate who weighs less than 500 g (Cunningham, Gant, Leveno, et al, 2001).
- **Term:** The normal duration of pregnancy (38 to 42 weeks' gestation).
- **Preterm or premature labor:** Labor that occurs after 20 weeks but before the completion of 37 weeks of gestation.
- **Postterm labor:** Labor that occurs after 42 weeks of gestation.
- **Gravida:** Any pregnancy, regardless of duration, including present pregnancy.
- **Nulligravida:** A woman who has never been pregnant.
- **Primigravida:** A woman who is pregnant for the first time.
- **Multigravida:** A woman who is in her second or any subsequent pregnancy.
- **Para:** Birth after 20 weeks' gestation, regardless of whether the infant is born alive or dead.
- **Nullipara:** A woman who has not given birth at more than 20 weeks' gestation.
- **Primipara:** A woman who has had one birth at more than 20 weeks' gestation, regardless of whether the infant is born alive or dead.
- **Multipara:** A woman who has had two or more births at more than 20 weeks' gestation.
- **Stillbirth:** A fetus born dead after 20 weeks' gestation.

The terms *gravida* and *para* refer to pregnancies, not to the fetus. Thus twins, triplets, and other multiple fetuses count as one pregnancy and one birth.

The following examples illustrate how these terms are applied in clinical situations:

1. Jean Sanchez has one child born at 38 weeks and is pregnant for the second time. At Jean's initial prenatal visit, the nurse indicates her obstetric history as "gravida 2 para 1 ab 0." Jean Sanchez's present pregnancy terminates at 16 weeks' gestation. She is now "gravida 2 para 1 ab 1."
2. Liz Buehl is pregnant for the fourth time. She has a toddler born at 35 weeks. She lost one pregnancy at 10 weeks' gestation and gave birth to another infant stillborn at term. At her prenatal assessment the nurse records Liz Buehl's obstetric history as "gravida 4 para 2 ab 1."

To provide more comprehensive data, a more detailed approach is used in some settings. Using the detailed system, *gravida* keeps the same meaning, but the meaning of *para* changes because the detailed system counts *each infant born* rather than the number of pregnancies carried to viability (Cunningham et al, 2001; Varney, 1997). Thus, for example, twins count as *one* pregnancy but *two* babies. A useful acronym for remembering the system is TPAL.

MEDIALINK AWHONN

Name	Gravida	Term	Preterm	Abort	Living Child
Jean Sanchez	2	1	0	0	1
Liz Buehl	4	1	1	1	1

Figure 15–1 • The TPAL approach provides more detailed information about the woman's pregnancy history.

T: number of *term* infants born; that is, the number of infants born at the completion of 37 weeks' gestation or beyond, whether living or stillborn.

P: number of *preterm* infants born; that is, the number of infants born after 20 weeks' but before the completion of 37 weeks' gestation, whether living or stillborn.

A: number of pregnancies ending in either spontaneous or therapeutic *abortion*.

L: number of currently *living* children to whom the woman has given birth.

Using this approach, the nurse would have initially classified Jean Sanchez (described in the first example) as "gravida 2 para 1001." Following her spontaneous abortion, she would be "gravida 2 para 1011." Liz Buehl would be described as "gravida 4 para 1111" (Figure 15–1 •).

Client Profile

The history is essentially a screening tool that identifies the factors that may detrimentally affect the course of a pregnancy. For optimal prenatal care, the nurse should obtain the following information for each maternity client at the first prenatal assessment:

1. Current pregnancy
   - First day of last normal menstrual period (LMP). Is she sure of date or uncertain?
   - Presence of cramping, bleeding, or spotting since LMP
   - Woman's opinion about time when conception occurred and when infant is due
   - Woman's attitude toward pregnancy (Is pregnancy planned? Wanted?)
   - Results of pregnancy test, if completed
   - Any discomforts since LMP, such as nausea, vomiting, urinary frequency, fatigue, breast tenderness
2. Past pregnancies
   - Number of pregnancies
   - Number of abortions, spontaneous or induced
   - Number of living children
   - History of previous pregnancies: length of pregnancy, length of labor and birth, type of birth (vaginal, forceps or vacuum-assisted birth, cesarean), type of anesthesia used (if any), woman's perception of the experience, complications (antepartal, intrapartal, postpartal)
   - Neonatal status of previous children: Apgar scores, birth weights, general development, complications, feeding patterns (breast or formula)
   - Loss of a child (miscarriage, elective or medically indicated abortion, stillbirth, neonatal death, relinquishment, death after the neonatal period). What was the experience like for her? What coping skills helped? How did her partner, if involved, respond?
   - Blood type and Rh factor (If Rh negative, was medication received after birth to prevent sensitization?)
   - Prenatal education classes, resources (books)
3. Gynecologic history
   - Date of last Pap smear; any history of abnormal Pap results?
   - Previous infections: vaginal, cervical, tubal, sexually transmitted
   - Previous surgery
   - Age of menarche
   - Regularity, frequency, and duration of menstrual flow
   - History of dysmenorrhea
   - Sexual history
   - Contraceptive history (If birth control pills were used, did pregnancy immediately follow cessation of pills? If not, how long after?)
   - Date of last Pap smear, any history of abnormal Pap smear
4. Current medical history
   - Weight (prepregnant and current)
   - Blood type and Rh factor, if known
   - General health, including nutrition (dietary practices such as vegetarianism; if so, which kind of vegetarian? Vegan?), regular exercise program (type, frequency, duration)
   - Any medications being taken currently (including nonprescription, homeopathic, or herbal medications) or taken since the onset of pregnancy
   - Previous or present use of alcohol, tobacco, or caffeine (Ask specifically about the amounts of alcohol, cigarettes, and caffeine [specify coffee, tea, colas, chocolate] consumed each day.)
   - Illicit drug use or abuse (Ask about specific drugs such as cocaine, crack, marijuana.)

- Drug allergies and other allergies
- Potential teratogenic insults to this pregnancy, such as viral infections, medications, x-ray examinations, surgery, or cats in home (possible source of toxoplasmosis)
- Presence of disease conditions, such as diabetes, hypertension, asthma, cardiovascular disease, renal problems, or thyroid disorders
- Record of immunizations (especially rubella)
- Presence of any abnormal symptoms

5. Past medical history
   - Childhood diseases
   - Past treatment for any disease condition: Any hospitalizations? History of hepatitis? Rheumatic fever? Pyelonephritis?
   - Surgical procedures
   - Presence of bleeding disorders or tendencies (Has she received blood transfusions?)
6. Family medical history
   - Presence of diabetes, cardiovascular disease, hypertension, hematologic disorders, tuberculosis, preeclampsia-eclampsia
   - Occurrence of multiple births
   - History of congenital diseases or deformities
   - History of mental illness
   - Occurrence of cesarean births and cause, if known
   - Cause of death of deceased parents or siblings
7. Religious/cultural history
   - Does the woman wish to specify a religious preference on her chart? Does she have any religious beliefs or practices that might influence her healthcare or that of her child, such as prohibition against receiving blood products, dietary considerations, circumcision rites, or other practices?
   - What practices are important to maintain her spiritual well-being?
   - Are there practices in her culture or that of her partner that might influence her care or that of her child?
8. Occupational history
   - Occupation
   - Physical demands (Does she stand all day, or are there opportunities to sit and elevate her legs? Does she do any heavy lifting?)
   - Exposure to lead, chemicals, or other harmful substances
   - Opportunity for regular meals and breaks for nutritious snacks
   - Provision for maternity or family leave
9. Partner's history
   - Presence of genetic conditions or diseases
   - Age
   - Significant health problems
   - Previous or present alcohol intake, drug use, or tobacco use
   - Blood type and Rh factor
   - Occupation
   - Educational level; methods by which he learns best
   - Attitude toward the pregnancy
10. Personal information
    - Age
    - Educational level; methods by which she learns best
    - Race or ethnic group (to identify need for prenatal genetic screening or counseling)
    - Housing; stability of living conditions
    - Economic level
    - Any history of emotional or physical deprivation or abuse of herself or children (Does she experience any abuse in her current relationship? Ask specifically whether she has been hit, slapped, kicked, or hurt within the past year or since she has been pregnant. Ask whether she is afraid of her partner or anyone else. If yes, of whom is she afraid?)
    - History of emotional problems. Ask specifically about depression in general, postpartum depression, anxiety, and so forth.
    - Support systems
    - Overuse or underuse of healthcare system
    - Acceptance of pregnancy
    - Personal preferences about the birth (expectations of both the woman and her partner, presence of others, and so on) (See Chapter 13 .)
    - Plans for care of child following birth
    - Feeding preference for the baby (breast or formula)

Obtaining Data

In many instances, nurses use a questionnaire like the one shown in Figure 15–2 • to obtain information. The woman should complete the questionnaire in a quiet place with a minimum of distractions.

The nurse can obtain further information in a direct interview, which allows the pregnant woman to expand or clarify her responses to questions and gives the nurse and client the opportunity to begin developing a good relationship. The expectant father should be encouraged to attend the initial and subsequent prenatal assessments. He is often able to contribute information to the history and may use the opportunity to ask questions and express concerns that may be of particular importance to him.

RESEARCH IN PRACTICE
Measuring Prenatal Drug Exposure

What is this study about? Prenatal drug exposure is an increasing obstetric and pediatric problem. Accurate measurement of prenatal drug exposure is complicated and relies heavily on maternal report. The reliable and valid measurement of prenatal drug exposure is critical if the effects of this exposure are to be accurately determined. This study had as its goal the identification of issues related to accurately measuring prenatal drug exposure and the development of reliable measurement methods.

How was this study done? Subjects in this study were 248 volunteers from an inner-city obstetric or pediatric clinic. Data were collected for a 2-year period. Seventy-seven percent of the subjects were low income, and 81% were unmarried. The clinic routinely performs toxicology screens for its obstetric clients at the first prenatal visit and again at birth. If the screen was positive or if the mother reported drug use, they were recruited to the study. A chemical dependency counselor made a hospital or home visit after discharge to interview participants for an in-depth drug use history. The clinical interview was a standardized, structured interview. Actual drug use was determined via toxicology screen at the initial prenatal visit, during each prenatal care visit, at birth, and during the postpartum interview.

What were the results of the study? While only 57% of the subjects reported alcohol or drug use during the prenatal period, urine toxicology screens yielded a 72% positive rate. At birth, urine toxicology screens were positive for 71% of the mothers and 59% of the newborns. Postpartum clinical interviews provided valuable data, particularly for multiple drug use, which is not detected by urine toxicology. Issues relative to determining prenatal drug exposure were identified during the measurement process. Substantial variations in the amount and frequency of drug exposure existed in this sample, so categorizing newborns as "exposed" or "not exposed" may underestimate fetal exposure. Likewise, drug exposure is not constant throughout gestations, and the ultimate effects may depend on the stage of fetal development at the time of exposure. Polydrug exposure was also an issue in this sample, and this problem has been inadequately addressed in previous measurements. No single source of information provided a complete picture of maternal drug use. Without multiple sources of drug exposure data, the incidence of fetal exposure to drugs is most likely underestimated. Toxicology screens have serious limitations, but these can be mediated somewhat by maternal self-report and structured interviewing by a professional.

What additional questions might I have? Was there a relationship between drug exposure and neonatal outcomes in this sample? Are these issues prevalent in all populations, or just those that are low income? Were there identifiable risk factors that might indicate the potential for prenatal drug exposure?

How can I use this study? In populations at high risk for prenatal drug exposure, nurses should consider using multiple sources of data to identify both the frequency and amount of fetal drug exposure. More sensitive measurement methods are needed to accurately determine if drug exposure may be occurring during pregnancy, so that preventive interventions can be used to reduce fetal risk.

Source: Bergin, C., Cameron, C., Fleitz, R., & Patel, A. (2001). Measuring prenatal drug exposure. *Journal of Pediatric Nursing, 16*(4), 245–255.

> *I didn't know what to expect when I went for my first prenatal visit. I'm clean now and wanted to be honest, but I was afraid they would yell if I told them about some of the really dumb things I did in high school—the drinking, the marijuana, the sex and stuff. I really liked the nurse-midwife who was taking care of me, so I decided to be straight with her—for the baby's sake, you know. She was great about everything and really made me feel okay.*

Prenatal High-Risk Screening

A highly significant part of the prenatal assessment is the screening for high-risk factors. **Risk factors** are any findings that have been shown to have a negative effect on pregnancy outcome, either for the woman or her unborn child. Many risk factors can be identified during the initial prenatal assessment; others may be detected during subsequent prenatal visits. It is important that high-risk pregnancies be identified early so that appropriate interventions can be instituted immediately.

All risk factors do not threaten the pregnancy to the same degree. Thus many agencies use a risk-scoring sheet to determine the degree of risk. The sheet is initiated at the first visit and becomes a permanent part of the woman's record. Information may be updated throughout the pregnancy as necessary. It is always possible that a pregnancy may begin as low risk and change to high risk because of complications. Risk is also assessed intrapartally and postpartally.

Table 15–1 • is an example of one risk-scoring protocol that evaluates the woman for factors that increase her risk of spontaneous preterm birth. Table 15–2 • identifies the major prenatal risk factors currently recognized. The table describes maternal and fetal/neonatal implications should the risk be present in the pregnancy. In addition to the factors listed, the perinatal health team also needs to evaluate such psychosocial factors as ethnic background; occupation and education; financial status; environment, including living arrangements and location; and the woman's and her family's or significant other's concept of health, which might influence her attitude toward seeking healthcare.

Name ____________________ Age ________

Address ____________________ Home Phone ________

What was the last year of schooling completed? ________

How old were you when your menstrual periods started? ________

How many days does a normal period last? ________

How many days are there between periods? ________

Do you have cramping with your periods? yes ____ no ____

Is the pain: minimal ________
moderate ________
severe ________

What was the date of your last normal menstrual period? ________

Have you had bleeding or spotting since your last menstrual period? yes ____ no ____

Have you been on birth control pills? yes ____ no ____

If yes, when did you stop taking them? ________

How many previous pregnancies have you had? ________

How many living children do you have? ________

Have you had any abortions or stillbirths? yes ____ no ____

If yes, how many? ________

Were any of your previous babies born prematurely?

yes ____ no ____

List the birth weight of all previous children.

1. ________ 3. ________

2. ________ 4. ________

Did any of your children have problems immediately after birth?

yes ____ no ____

If yes, check the problems that occurred:

____ Respiratory ____ Feeding

____ Jaundice ____ Heart

____ Bleeding

Did you have any problems with:

previous pregnancies? yes ____ no ____

If yes, what was the problem? ________

previous labors? yes ____ no ____

If yes, what was the problem? ________

previous postpartal periods: yes ____ no ____

If yes, what was the problem? ________

Are you Rh negative: yes ____ no ____

Did you receive Rh immune globulin after each pregnancy? yes ____ no ____

What is your present weight? ________

Are you presently taking any prescription or nonprescription drugs?

yes ____ no ____

If yes, please list the medications:

1. ________ 3. ________

2. ________ 4. ________

Do you smoke? yes ____ no ____

If yes, how many cigarettes per day? ________

How much alcohol do you consume each day? ________

each week? ________

How much caffeine do you consume each day? ________

If you have had any of the following diseases, place a check beside it.

____ Chickenpox
____ Mumps
____ Measles (3 day)
____ Measles (2 week)
____ Asthma
____ Hepatitis
____ High blood pressure
____ Heart disease
____ Respiratory disease
____ Kidney disease
____ Frequent bladder infections

If any of the following are present in your family, place a check beside the item.

____ Diabetes
____ Cardiovascular disease
____ High blood pressure
____ Breast cancer
____ Preeclampsia-eclampsia
____ Multiple pregnancies
____ Congenital disorder

The following questions pertain to the father of this child.

What is the father's age? ________

Does he take prescription or nonprescription drugs?

yes ____ no ____

If yes, please list the medications:

1. ________ 3. ________

2. ________ 4. ________

What is his alcohol intake each day? ________

each week? ________

Figure 15–2 • Sample prenatal questionnaire.

Table 15-1 • SYSTEM FOR DETERMINING RISK OF SPONTANEOUS PRETERM BIRTH

Points Assigned	Socioeconomic Factors	Previous Medical History	Daily Habits	Aspects of Current Pregnancy
1	Two children at home Low socioeconomic status	Abortion × 1 Less than 1 year since last birth	Works outside home	Unusual fatigue
2	Maternal age 18–20 years or > 40 years Single parent	Abortion × 2	Smokes more than 10 cigarettes per day	Gain of less than 5 kg by 32 weeks
3	Very low socioeconomic status Height < 150 cm Weight < 45 kg	Abortion × 3	Heavy or stressful work Long, tiring trip	Breech at 32 weeks Weight loss of 2 kg Head engaged at 32 weeks Febrile illness
4	Maternal age < 18 years	Pyelonephritis		Bleeding after 12 weeks Effacement Dilatation Uterine irritability
5		Uterine anomaly Second trimester abortion DES exposure Cone biopsy		Placenta previa Hydramnios
10		Preterm birth Repeated second trimester abortion		Twins Abdominal surgery

Note: The score is computed by adding the number of points given any item. The score is computed at the first visit and again at 22 to 26 weeks' gestation. A total score of 10 or more places the woman at high risk of spontaneous preterm birth.

Source: Adapted from Creasy, R.K., Gummer, B.A., & Liggins, G.C. (1980). A system for predicting spontaneous preterm birth. *Obstetrics & Gynecology, 55,* 692.

Initial Prenatal Assessment

The assessment focuses on the woman holistically by considering physical, cultural, and psychosocial factors that influence her health. At the initial visit the woman may be concerned with the diagnosis of pregnancy. However, during this visit she and her primary support person are also evaluating the health team that she has chosen. The establishment of the nurse-client relationship will help the woman evaluate the health team and also provide the nurse with a basis for developing an atmosphere that is conducive to interviewing, support, and education. Because many women are excited and anxious at the first antepartal visit, the initial psychosocial-cultural assessment is general.

As part of the initial psychosocial-cultural assessment the nurse discusses with the woman any religious, cultural, or socioeconomic factors that influence the woman's expectations of the childbearing experience. It is especially helpful if the nurse is familiar with common practices of various religious and cultural groups who reside in the community. Gathering these data in a tactful, caring way can help make the childbearing woman's experience a positive one.

After the history is obtained, the nurse prepares the woman for the physical examination. The physical examination begins with assessment of vital signs; then the woman's body is examined. The pelvic examination is performed last.

Before the examination, the woman should provide a clean urine specimen. When her bladder is empty, the woman is more comfortable during the pelvic examination, and the examiner can palpate the pelvic organs more easily. After the woman has emptied her bladder, the nurse asks her to disrobe and gives her a gown and sheet or some other protective covering.

Increasing numbers of nurses, such as certified nurse-midwives and other nurses in advanced practice, are pre-

Clinical Tip *In a clinic or office setting, gowns and goggles for the healthcare provider are not usually necessary because splashing of body fluids is unlikely. Gloves are worn for procedures that involve contact with body fluids such as drawing blood for lab work, handling urine specimens, and conducting pelvic examinations.*

CRITICAL THINKING IN PRACTICE

Karen Blade, a 23-year-old, G1P0, is 10 weeks pregnant when she sees the certified nurse-midwife (CNM) for her first prenatal exam. She has been experiencing some mild nausea and fatigue but otherwise is feeling well. She asks the CNM about continuing with her routine exercises (walking 3 miles a day and lifting light weights). She also asks about using the heated pool and a hot tub. What should she be told?

Answers can be found in Appendix I.

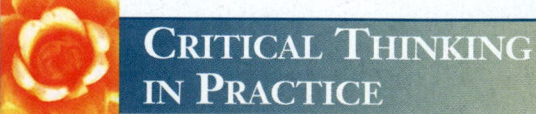

Table 15–2 • PRENATAL HIGH-RISK FACTORS

Factor	Maternal Implications	Fetal/Neonatal Implications
Social-Personal		
Low income level and/or low educational level	Poor antenatal care or late antenatal care Poor nutrition ↑ risk of preeclampsia	Low birth weight Intrauterine growth restriction (IUGR)
Poor diet	Inadequate nutrition/inadequate weight gain ↑ risk anemia ↑ risk preeclampsia	Fetal malnutrition Prematurity Small for gestational age
Living at high altitude	↑ hemoglobin	Prematurity IUGR ↑ hemoglobin (polycythemia)
Multiparity > 3	↑ risk antepartum or postpartum hemorrhage	Anemia Fetal death
Weight < 45.5 kg (100 lb)	Poor nutrition Cephalopelvic disproportion Prolonged labor	IUGR Hypoxia associated with difficult labor and birth
Weight > 91 kg (200 lb)	↑ risk hypertension ↑ risk cephalopelvic disproportion ↑ risk diabetes	↓ fetal nutrition ↑ risk macrosomia
Age < 16	Poor nutrition Poor antenatal care ↑ risk preeclampsia ↑ risk cephalopelvic disproportion	Low birth weight ↑ fetal demise
Age > 35	↑ risk preeclampsia ↑ risk cesarean birth Psychosocial issues	↑ risk congenital anomalies ↑ chromosomal aberrations
Smoking one pack/day or more	↑ risk hypertension ↑ risk cancer	↓ placental perfusion → ↓ O_2 and nutrients available Low birth weight IUGR Preterm birth
Use of addicting drugs	↑ risk poor nutrition ↑ risk of infection with IV drugs ↑ risk HIV, hepatitis C ↑ risk abruptio placentae	↑ risk congenital anomalies ↑ risk low birth weight Neonatal withdrawal Lower serum bilirubin
Excessive alcohol consumption	↑ risk poor nutrition Possible hepatic effects with long-term consumption	↑ risk fetal alcohol syndrome
Preexisting Medical Disorders		
Diabetes mellitus	↑ risk preeclampsia, hypertension Episodes of hypoglycemia and hyperglycemia ↑ risk cesarean birth	Low birth weight Macrosomia Neonatal hypoglycemia ↑ risk congenital anomalies ↑ risk respiratory distress syndrome
Cardiac disease	Cardiac decompensation Further strain on mother's body ↑ maternal death rate	↑ risk fetal demise ↑ perinatal mortality
Anemia: hemoglobin < 11 g/dL < 32% hematocrit	Iron deficiency anemia Low energy level Decreased oxygen-carrying capacity	Fetal death Prematurity Low birth weight
Hypertension	↑ vasospasm ↑ risk CNS irritability → convulsions ↑ risk CVA ↑ risk renal damage	↓ placental perfusion → low birth weight Preterm birth
Thyroid disorder Hypothyroidism Hyperthyroidism	↑ infertility ↓ BMR, goiter, myxedema ↑ risk postpartum hemorrhage ↑ risk preeclampsia Danger of thyroid storm	↑ spontaneous abortion ↑ risk congenital goiter Mental retardation → cretinism ↑ incidence congenital anomalies ↑ incidence preterm birth ↑ tendency to thyrotoxicosis
Renal disease (moderate to severe)	↑ risk renal failure	↑ risk IUGR ↑ risk preterm birth

(continued on next page)

Table 15-2 • PRENATAL HIGH-RISK FACTORS (CONTINUED)

Factor	Maternal Implications	Fetal/Neonatal Implications
DES exposure	↑ infertility, spontaneous abortion ↑ cervical incompetence ↑ risk breech presentation	↑ spontaneous abortion ↑ risk preterm birth
Obstetric Considerations		
Previous Pregnancy		
Stillborn	↑ emotional/psychologic distress	↑ risk IUGR ↑ risk preterm birth
Habitual abortion	↑ emotional/psychologic distress ↑ possibility diagnostic work-up	↑ risk abortion
Cesarean birth	↑ possibility repeat cesarean birth Risk of uterine rupture	↑ risk preterm birth ↑ risk respiratory distress
Rh or blood group sensitization	↑ financial expenditure for testing	Hydrops fetalis Icterus gravis Neonatal anemia Kernicterus Hypoglycemia
Large baby	↑ risk cesarean birth ↑ risk gestational diabetes ↑ risk instrument-assisted birth	Birth injury Hypoglycemia
Current Pregnancy		
Rubella (first trimester)		Congenital heart disease Cataracts Nerve deafness Bone lesions Prolonged virus shedding
Rubella (second trimester)		Hepatitis Thrombocytopenia
Cytomegalovirus		IUGR Encephalopathy
Herpesvirus type 2	Severe discomfort Concern about possibility of cesarean birth, fetal infection	Neonatal herpesvirus type 2 Hepatitis with jaundice Neurologic abnormalities
Syphilis	↑ incidence abortion	↑ fetal demise Congenital syphilis
Urinary tract infection	↑ risk preterm labor Uterine irritability	↑ risk preterm birth
Abruptio placentae and placenta previa	↑ risk hemorrhage Bed rest Extended hospitalization	Fetal/neonatal anemia Intrauterine hemorrhage ↑ fetal demise
Preeclampsia/eclampsia	See hypertension	↓ placental perfusion → low birth weight
Multiple gestation	↑ risk postpartum hemorrhage	↑ risk preterm birth ↑ risk fetal demise
Elevated hematocrit (> 41%)	Increased viscosity of blood	Fetal death rate 5 times normal rate
Spontaneous premature rupture of membranes	↑ uterine infection	↑ risk preterm birth ↑ fetal demise

pared to perform physical examinations. The nurse who has not yet fully developed these specific assessment skills assesses the woman's vital signs, explains the procedures to allay apprehension, positions her for examination, and assists the examiner as necessary. Each nurse is responsible for operating at the expected standard for a professional with that individual nurse's skill and knowledge base.

Thoroughness and a systematic procedure are the most important considerations when performing the physical portion of an antepartal examination (see the Initial Prenatal Assessment Guide on the next page). To promote completeness, the Initial Prenatal Assessment Guide is organized into three columns that address the areas to be assessed, the variations or alterations that may be observed, and nursing responses to the data. The nurse should be aware that certain organs and systems are assessed concurrently with other systems during the physical portion of the examination.

Nursing interventions based on assessment of the normal physical and psychosocial changes, as well as the cultural influences associated with pregnancy and client teaching and counseling needs that have been mutually defined, are discussed further in Chapter 16.

Assessment Guide — Initial Prenatal Assessment

PHYSICAL ASSESSMENT/ NORMAL FINDINGS	ALTERATIONS AND POSSIBLE CAUSES*	NURSING RESPONSES TO DATA†
➤ VITAL SIGNS		
Blood pressure (BP): 90–140/60–90 mm Hg	High BP (essential hypertension; renal disease; pregestational hypertension, apprehension or anxiety associated with pregnancy diagnosis, exam, or other crises; preeclampsia if initial assessment not done until after 20 weeks' gestation)	BP > 140/90 requires immediate consideration; establish woman's BP; refer to physician if necessary. Assess woman's knowledge about high BP; counsel on self-care and medical management.
Pulse: 60–90 beats/min; rate may increase 10 beats/min during pregnancy	Increased pulse rate (excitement or anxiety, cardiac disorders)	Count for 1 full minute; note irregularities.
Respirations: 16–24 breaths/min (or pulse rate divided by four); pregnancy may induce a degree of hyperventilation; thoracic breathing predominant	Marked tachypnea or abnormal patterns	Assess for respiratory disease.
Temperature: 36.2–37.6C (98–99.6F)	Elevated temperature (infection)	Assess for infection process or disease state if temperature is elevated; refer to physician or CNM.
➤ WEIGHT		
Depends on body build	Weight < 45 kg (100 lb) or > 91 kg (200 lb); rapid, sudden weight gain (preeclampsia)	Evaluate need for nutritional counseling; obtain information on eating habits, cooking practices, foods regularly eaten, income limitations, need for food supplements, pica and other abnormal food habits. Note initial weight to establish baseline for weight gain throughout pregnancy.
➤ SKIN		
Color: Consistent with racial background; pink nail beds	Pallor (anemia); bronze, yellow (hepatic disease; other causes of jaundice)	The following tests should be performed: complete blood count (CBC), bilirubin level, urinalysis, and blood urea nitrogen (BUN).
	Bluish, reddish, mottled; dusky appearance or pallor of palms and nail beds in dark skinned women (anemia)	If abnormal, refer to physician.
Condition: Absence of edema (slight edema of lower extremities is normal during pregnancy)	Edema (preeclampsia); rashes, dermatitis (allergic response)	Counsel on relief measures for slight edema. Initiate preeclampsia assessment; refer to physician.
Lesions: Absence of lesions	Ulceration (varicose veins, decreased circulation)	Further assess circulatory status; refer to physician if lesion is severe.
Spider nevi common in pregnancy	Petechiae, multiple bruises, ecchymosis (hemorrhagic disorders; abuse)	Evaluate for bleeding or clotting disorder. Provide opportunities to discuss abuse if suspected.
Moles	Change in size or color (carcinoma)	Refer to physician.
Pigmentation: Pigmentation changes of pregnancy include linea nigra, striae gravidarum, melasma		Assure woman that these are normal manifestations of pregnancy and explain the physiologic basis for the changes.
Café-au-lait spots	Six or more (Albright syndrome or neurofibromatosis)	Consult with physician.

*Possible causes of alterations were placed in parentheses.

†This column provides guidelines for further assessment and initial nursing intervention.

(Continued on next page)

ASSESSMENT GUIDE: INITIAL PRENATAL ASSESSMENT *continued*

PHYSICAL ASSESSMENT/ NORMAL FINDINGS	ALTERATIONS AND POSSIBLE CAUSES*	NURSING RESPONSES TO DATA†
➤ NOSE		
Character of mucosa: Redder than oral mucosa; in pregnancy nasal mucosa is edematous in response to increased estrogen, resulting in nasal stuffiness (rhinitis of pregnancy) and nosebleeds	Olfactory loss (first cranial nerve deficit)	Counsel woman about possible relief measures for nasal stuffiness and nosebleeds (epistaxis); refer to physician for olfactory loss.
➤ MOUTH		
May note hypertrophy of gingival tissue because of estrogen	Edema, inflammation (infection); pale in color (anemia)	Assess hematocrit for anemia; counsel regarding dental hygiene habits. Refer to physician or dentist if necessary. Routine dental care appropriate during pregnancy (no x-ray studies, no nitrous anesthesia).
➤ NECK		
Nodes: Small, mobile, nontender nodes	Tender, hard, fixed, or prominent nodes (infection, carcinoma)	Examine for local infection; refer to physician.
Thyroid: Small, smooth, lateral lobes palpable on either side of trachea; slight hyperplasia by third month of pregnancy	Enlargement or nodule tenderness (hyperthyroidism)	Listen over thyroid for bruits, which may indicate hyperthyroidism. Question woman about dietary habits (iodine intake). Ascertain history of thyroid problems; refer to physician.
➤ CHEST AND LUNGS		
Chest: Symmetric, elliptic, smaller anteroposterior (AP) than transverse diameter	Increased AP diameter, funnel chest, pigeon chest (emphysema, asthma, chronic obstructive pulmonary disease [COPD])	Evaluate for emphysema, asthma, pulmonary disease (COPD).
Ribs: Slope downward from nipple line	More horizontal (COPD) Angular bumps Rachitic rosary (vitamin C deficiency)	Evaluate for COPD. Evaluate for fractures. Consult physician. Consult nutritionist.
Inspection and palpation: No retraction or bulging of intercostal spaces (ICS) during inspiration or expiration; symmetric expansion.	ICS retractions with inspiration, bulging with expiration; unequal expansion (respiratory disease)	Do thorough initial assessment. Refer to physician.
Tactile fremitus	Tachypnea, hyperpnea, Cheyne-Stokes respirations (respiratory disease)	Refer to physician.
Percussion: Bilateral symmetry in tone	Flatness of percussion, which may be affected by chest wall thickness	Evaluate for pleural effusions, consolidations, or tumor.
Low-pitched resonance of moderate intensity	High diaphragm (atelectasis or paralysis), pleural effusion	Refer to physician.
Auscultation: Upper lobes—bronchovesicular sounds above sternum and scapulas; equal expiratory and inspiratory phases	Abnormal if heard over any other area of chest	Refer to physician.
Remainder of chest: Vesicular breath sounds heard; inspiratory phase longer (3:1)	Rales, rhonchi, wheezes; pleural friction rub; absence of breath sounds; bronchophony, egophony, whispered pectoriloquy	Refer to physician.

*Possible causes of alterations were placed in parentheses.

†This column provides guidelines for further assessment and initial nursing intervention.

➤

ASSESSMENT GUIDE: INITIAL PRENATAL ASSESSMENT *continued*

PHYSICAL ASSESSMENT/ NORMAL FINDINGS	ALTERATIONS AND POSSIBLE CAUSES*	NURSING RESPONSES TO DATA†
➤ BREASTS		
Supple; symmetric in size and contour; darker pigmentation of nipple and areola; may have supernumerary nipples, usually 5–6 cm below normal nipple line	"Pigskin" or orange-peel appearance, nipple retractions, swelling, hardness (carcinoma); redness, heat, tenderness, cracked or fissured nipple (infection)	Encourage monthly self-examination; instruct woman how to examine her own breasts.
Axillary nodes unpalpable or pellet sized	Tenderness, enlargement, hard node (carcinoma); may be visible bump (infection)	Refer to physician if evidence of inflammation.
Pregnancy changes: 1. Size increase noted primarily in first 20 weeks. 2. Become nodular. 3. Tingling sensation may be felt during first and third trimester; woman may report feeling of heaviness. 4. Pigmentation of nipples and areolae darkens. 5. Superficial veins dilate and become more prominent. 6. Striae seen in multiparas. 7. Tubercles of Montgomery enlarge. 8. Colostrum may be present after 12th week. 9. Secondary areola appears at 20 weeks, characterized by series of washed-out spots surrounding primary areola. 10. Breasts less firm, old striae may be present in multiparas.		Discuss normalcy of changes and their meaning with the woman. Teach and/or institute appropriate relief measures. Encourage use of supportive, well-fitting brassiere.
➤ HEART		
Normal rate, rhythm, and heart sounds ***Pregnancy changes:*** 1. Palpitations may occur due to sympathetic nervous system disturbance. 2. Short systolic murmurs that increase in held expiration are normal due to increased volume.	Enlargement, thrills, thrusts, gross irregularity or skipped beats, gallop rhythm or extra sounds (cardiac disease)	Complete an initial assessment. Explain normalcy of pregnancy-induced changes. Refer to physician if indicated.
➤ ABDOMEN		
Normal appearance, skin texture, and hair distribution; liver nonpalpable; abdomen nontender ***Pregnancy changes:*** 1. Purple striae may be present (or silver striae on a multipara) as well as linea nigra.	Muscle guarding (anxiety, acute tenderness); tenderness, mass (ectopic pregnancy, inflammation, carcinoma)	Assure woman of normalcy of diastasis. Provide initial information about appropriate prenatal and postpartum exercises. Evaluate woman's anxiety level. Refer to physician if indicated.
	*Possible causes of alterations were placed in parentheses.	†This column provides guidelines for further assessment and initial nursing intervention.

(Continued on next page)

Assessment Guide: INITIAL PRENATAL ASSESSMENT *continued*

PHYSICAL ASSESSMENT/ NORMAL FINDINGS	ALTERATIONS AND POSSIBLE CAUSES*	NURSING RESPONSES TO DATA†
➤ ABDOMEN *(continued)*		
2. Diastasis of the rectus muscles late in pregnancy.		
3. Size: Flat or rotund abdomen; progressive enlargement of uterus due to pregnancy. 10–12 weeks: Fundus slightly above symphysis pubis. 16 weeks: Fundus halfway between symphysis and umbilicus. 20–22 weeks: Fundus at umbilicus. 28 weeks: Fundus three finger breadths above umbilicus. 36 weeks: Fundus just below ensiform cartilage.	Size of uterus inconsistent with length of gestation (intrauterine growth restriction [IUGR], multiple pregnancy, fetal demise, hydatidiform mole)	Reassess menstrual history regarding pregnancy dating. Evaluate increase in size using McDonald's method. Use ultrasound to establish diagnosis.
4. Fetal heart rate: 110–160 beats/min may be heard with Doppler at 10–12 weeks gestation; may be heard with fetoscope at 17–20 weeks.	Failure to hear fetal heartbeat with Doppler (fetal demise, hydatidiform mole)	Refer to physician. Administer pregnancy tests. Use ultrasound to establish diagnosis.
5. Fetal movement palpable by a trained examiner after the 18th week.	Failure to feel fetal movements after 20 weeks' gestation (fetal demise, hydatidiform mole)	Refer to physician for evaluation of fetal status.
6. Ballottement: During fourth to fifth month fetus rises and then rebounds to original position when uterus is tapped sharply.	No ballottement (oligohydramnios)	Refer to physician for evaluation of fetal status.
➤ EXTREMITIES		
Skin warm, pulses palpable, full range of motion; may be some edema of hands and ankles in late pregnancy; varicose veins may become more pronounced; palmar erythema may be present	Unpalpable or diminished pulses (arterial insufficiency); marked edema (preeclampsia)	Evaluate for other symptoms of heart disease; initiate follow-up if woman mentions that her rings feel tight. Discuss prevention and self-treatment measures for varicose veins; refer to physician if indicated.
➤ SPINE		
Normal spinal curves: Concave cervical, convex thoracic, concave lumbar	Abnormal spinal curves; flatness, kyphosis, lordosis	Refer to physician for assessment of cephalopelvic disproportion (CPD).
In pregnancy, lumbar spinal curve may be accentuated	Backache	May have implications for administration of spinal anesthetics; see Chapter 16 for relief measures.
Shoulders and iliac crests should be even	Uneven shoulders and iliac crests (scoliosis)	Refer very young women to a physician; discuss back-stretching exercise with older women.
➤ REFLEXES		
Normal and symmetric	Hyperactivity, clonus (preeclampsia)	Evaluate for other symptoms of preeclampsia.
	*Possible causes of alterations were placed in parentheses.	†This column provides guidelines for further assessment and initial nursing intervention.

➤

Assessment Guide: INITIAL PRENATAL ASSESSMENT *continued*

PHYSICAL ASSESSMENT/ NORMAL FINDINGS	ALTERATIONS AND POSSIBLE CAUSES*	NURSING RESPONSES TO DATA†
➤ PELVIC AREA		
External female genitals: Normally formed with female hair distribution; in multiparas, labia majora loose and pigmented; urinary and vaginal orifices visible and appropriately located	Lesions, hematomas, varicosities, inflammation of Bartholin's glands; clitoral hypertrophy (masculinization)	Explain pelvic examination procedure (see Procedure 7–1). Encourage woman to minimize her discomfort by relaxing her hips. Provide privacy.
Vagina: Pink or dark pink, vaginal discharge odorless, nonirritating; in multiparas, vaginal folds smooth and flattened; may have episiotomy scar	Abnormal discharge associated with vaginal infections	Obtain vaginal smear. Provide understandable verbal and written instructions about treatment for woman and partner, if indicated.
Cervix: Pink color; os closed except in multiparas, in whom os admits fingertip	Eversion, reddish erosion, nabothian or retention cysts, cervical polyp; granular area that bleeds (carcinoma of cervix); lesions (herpes, human papilloma virus [HPV]) Presence of string or plastic tip from cervix (intrauterine device [IUD] in uterus)	Provide woman with a hand mirror and identify genital structures for her; encourage her to view her cervix if she wishes. Refer to physician if indicated. Advise woman of potential serious risks of leaving an IUD in place during pregnancy; refer to physician for removal.
Pregnancy changes: 1–4 weeks' gestation: Enlargement in anteroposterior diameter		
4–6 weeks' gestation: Softening of cervix (Goodell's sign), softening of isthmus of uterus (Hegar's sign); cervix takes on bluish coloring (Chadwick's sign)	Absence of Goodell's sign (inflammatory conditions, carcinoma)	Refer to physician.
8–12 weeks' gestation: Vagina and cervix appear bluish violet in color (Chadwick's sign)		
Uterus: Pear shaped, mobile; smooth surface	Fixed (pelvic inflammatory disease [PID]); nodular surface (fibromas)	Refer to physician.
Ovaries: Small, walnut shaped, nontender (ovaries and Fallopian tubes are located in the adnexal areas)	Pain or movement of cervix (PID); enlarged or nodular ovaries (cyst, tumor, tubal pregnancy, corpus luteum of pregnancy)	Evaluate adnexal areas; refer to physician.
➤ PELVIC MEASUREMENTS		
Internal measurements: 1. Diagonal conjugate at least 11.5 cm (Figure 15–7)	Measurement below normal	Vaginal birth may not be possible if deviations are present.
2. Obstetric conjugate estimated by subtracting 1.5–2 cm from diagonal conjugate	Disproportion of pubic arch	
3. Inclination of sacrum	Abnormal curvature of sacrum	
4. Motility of coccyx; external intertuberosity diameter > 8 cm	Fixed or malposition of coccyx	

*Possible causes of alterations were placed in parentheses.

†This column provides guidelines for further assessment and initial nursing intervention.

(Continued on next page)

ASSESSMENT GUIDE: INITIAL PRENATAL ASSESSMENT *continued*

PHYSICAL ASSESSMENT/ NORMAL FINDINGS	ALTERATIONS AND POSSIBLE CAUSES*	NURSING RESPONSES TO DATA†
➤ ANUS AND RECTUM		
No lumps, rashes, excoriation, tenderness; cervix may be felt through rectal wall	Hemorrhoids, rectal prolapse; nodular lesion (carcinoma)	Counsel about appropriate prevention and relief measures; refer to physician for further evaluation.
➤ LABORATORY EVALUATION		
Hemoglobin: 12–16 g/dL; women residing in areas of high altitude may have higher levels of hemoglobin	<11 g/dL (anemia)	Note: Wear gloves when drawing blood. Hemoglobin < 12 g/dL requires nutritional counseling; < 11 g/dL requires iron supplementation.
ABO and Rh typing: Normal distribution of blood types	Rh negative	If Rh negative, check for presence of anti-Rh antibodies. Check partner's blood type; if partner is Rh positive, discuss with woman the need for antibody titers during pregnancy, management during the intrapartal period, and possible need for Rh immune globulin. (See Chapter 20).
Complete blood count (CBC)		
Hematocrit: 38%–47% physiologic anemia (pseudoanemia) may occur	Marked anemia or blood dyscrasias	Perform CBC and Schilling differential cell count.
Red blood cells (RBC): 4.2–5.4 million/μL		
White blood cells (WBC): 5,000–12,000/μL	Presence of infection; may be elevated in pregnancy and with labor	Evaluate for other signs of infection.
Differential		
Neutrophils: 40%–60%		
Bands: up to 5%		
Eosinophils: 1%–3%		
Basophils: up to 1%		
Lymphocytes: 20%–40%		
Monocytes: 4%–8%		
Syphilis tests: Serologic tests for syphilis (STS), complement fixation test, veneral disease research laboratory (VDRL) test—nonreactive	Positive reaction STS—tests may have 25%–45% incidence of biologic false-positive results; false results may occur in individuals who have acute viral or bacterial infections, hypersensitivity reactions, recent vaccinations, collagen disease, malaria, or tuberculosis	Positive results may be confirmed with the fluorescent treponemal antibody-absorption (FTA-ABS) tests; all tests for syphilis give positive results in the secondary stage of the disease; antibiotic tests may cause negative test results.
Gonorrhea culture: Negative	Positive	Refer for treatment.
Urinalysis (u/a): Normal color, specific gravity; pH 4.6–8.0	Abnormal color (porphyria, hemoglobinuria, bilirubinemia); alkaline urine (metabolic alkalemia, *Proteus* infection, old specimen)	Repeat u/a; refer to physician.

*Possible causes of alterations were placed in parentheses.

†This column provides guidelines for further assessment and initial nursing intervention.

Assessment Guide: INITIAL PRENATAL ASSESSMENT *continued*

PHYSICAL ASSESSMENT/ NORMAL FINDINGS	ALTERATIONS AND POSSIBLE CAUSES*	NURSING RESPONSES TO DATA†
➤ LABORATORY EVALUATION (*continued*)		
Negative for protein, red blood cells, white blood cells, casts	Positive findings (contaminated specimen, kidney disease)	Repeat u/a; refer to physician.
Glucose: Negative (small degree of glycosuria may occur in pregnancy)	Glycosuria (low renal threshold for glucose, diabetes mellitus)	Assess blood glucose level; test urine for ketones.
Rubella titer: Hemagglutination-inhibition (HAI) test—1:10 indicates woman is immune	HAI titer < 1:10	Immunization will be given on postpartum or within 6 weeks after childbirth. Instruct woman whose titers are > 1:10 to avoid children who have rubella.
Hepatitis B screen for hepatitis B surface antigen (HbsAg); negative	Positive	If negative, consider referral for hepatitis B vaccine. If positive, refer to physician. Infants born to women who test positive are given hepatitis B immune globulin soon after birth followed by first dose of hepatitis B vaccine.
HIV screen: Offered to all women; encouraged for those at risk; negative	Positive	Refer to physician.
Illicit drug screen: Offered to all women; negative	Positive	Refer to physician.
Sickle cell screen for clients of African descent: Negative	Positive; test results would include a description of cells	Refer to physician.
Pap smear: Negative	Test results that show atypical cells	Refer to physician. Discuss with the woman the meaning of the findings and the importance of follow-up.

CULTURAL ASSESSMENT	VARIATIONS TO CONSIDER*	NURSING RESPONSES TO DATA†
Determine the woman's fluency in English.	Woman may be fluent in a language other than English.	Work with a knowledgeable translator to provide information and answer questions.
Ask the woman how she prefers to be addressed.	Some women prefer informality; others prefer to use titles.	Address the woman according to her preference. Maintain formality in introducing oneself if that seems preferred.
Determine customs and practices regarding prenatal care:	Practices are influenced by individual preference, cultural expectations, or religious beliefs.	Honor a woman's practices and provide for specific preferences unless they are contraindicated because of safety.
• Ask the woman if there are certain practices she expects to follow when she is pregnant.	Some women believe that they should perform certain acts related to sleep, activity, or clothing.	Have information printed in the language of different cultural groups that live in the area.
• Ask the woman if there are any activities she cannot do while she is pregnant.	Some women have restrictions or taboos they follow related to work, activity, sexual, environmental, or emotional factors.	

*Possible causes of alterations were placed in parentheses.

†This column provides guidelines for further assessment and initial nursing intervention.

(Continued on next page)

Assessment Guide: Initial Prenatal Assessment *continued*

CULTURAL ASSESSMENT	VARIATIONS TO CONSIDER*	NURSING RESPONSES TO DATA†
• Ask the woman whether there are certain foods she is expected to eat or avoid while she is pregnant. Determine whether she has lactose intolerance.	Foods are an important cultural factor. Some women may have certain foods they must eat or avoid; many women have lactose intolerance and have difficulty consuming sufficient calcium.	Respect the woman's food preferences, help her plan an adequate prenatal diet within the framework of her preferences, and refer to a dietitian if necessary.
• Ask the woman whether the gender of her caregiver is of concern.	Some women are comfortable only with a female caregiver.	Arrange for a female caregiver if it is the woman's preference.
• Ask the woman about the degree of involvement in her pregnancy that she expects or wants from her support person, mother, and other significant people.	A woman may not want her partner involved in the pregnancy. For some the role falls to the woman's mother or a female relative or friend.	Respect the woman's preferences about her partner or husband's involvement; avoid imposing personal values or expectations.
• Ask the woman about her sources of support and counseling during pregnancy.	Some women seek advice from a family member, *curandera,* tribal healer, and so forth.	Respect and honor the woman's sources of support.
➤ PSYCHOLOGIC STATUS		
Excitement and/or apprehension, ambivalence	Marked anxiety (fear of pregnancy diagnosis, fear of medical facility)	Establish lines of communication. Active listening is useful. Establish trusting relationship. Encourage woman to take active part in her care.
	Apathy; display of anger with pregnancy diagnosis	Establish communication and begin counseling. Use active listening techniques.
➤ EDUCATIONAL NEEDS		
May have questions about pregnancy or may need time to adjust to reality of pregnancy		Establish educational, supporting environment that can be expanded throughout pregnancy.
➤ SUPPORT SYSTEMS		
Can identify at least two or three individuals with whom woman is emotionally intimate (partner, parent, sibling, friend)	Isolated (no telephone, unlisted number); cannot name a neighbor or friend whom she can call upon in an emergency; does not perceive parents as part of her support system	Institute support system through community groups. Help woman to develop trusting relationship with healthcare professionals.
➤ FAMILY FUNCTIONING		
Emotionally supportive Communications adequate Mutually satisfying Cohesiveness in times of trouble	Long-term problems or specific problems related to this pregnancy, potential stressors within the family, pessimistic attitudes, unilateral decision making, unrealistic expectations of this pregnancy or child	Help identify the problems and stressors, encourage communication, and discuss role changes and adaptations.
	*Possible causes of alterations were placed in parentheses.	*Possible causes of alterations were placed in parentheses.

(Continued on next page)

ASSESSMENT GUIDE: INITIAL PRENATAL ASSESSMENT *continued*

CULTURAL ASSESSMENT	VARIATIONS TO CONSIDER*	NURSING RESPONSES TO DATA†
➤ ECONOMIC STATUS		
Source of income is stable and sufficient to meet basic needs of daily living and medical needs	Limited prenatal care; poor physical health; limited use of healthcare system; unstable economic status	Discuss available resources for health maintenance and the birth. Institute appropriate referral for meeting expanding family's needs—food stamps and so forth.
➤ STABILITY OF LIVING CONDITIONS		
Adequate, stable housing for expanding family's needs	Crowded living conditions; questionable supportive environment for newborn	Refer to appropriate community agency. Work with family on self-help ways to improve situation.
	* Possible causes of alterations were placed in parentheses.	† This column provides guidelines for further assessment and initial nursing intervention.

Determination of Due Date

Childbearing families generally want to know the "due date," or the date around which childbirth will occur. Historically, the due date has been called the *estimated date of confinement (EDC)*. The concept of confinement is, however, rather negative, and there is a trend in the literature to avoid it by referring to the birth date as the *estimated date of delivery (EDD)*. However, childbirth educators often stress that babies are not "delivered" like a package; they are *born*. In keeping with a view that emphasizes the normality of the process, we have chosen to refer to the due date as the **estimated date of birth (EDB)** throughout this text.

To calculate the EDB, it is helpful to know the first day of the woman's last menstrual period (LMP). However, some women have episodes of irregular bleeding or fail to keep track of menstrual cycles. Thus other techniques also help determine how far along a woman is in her pregnancy, that is, at how many weeks' gestation she is. Other techniques that can be used include evaluating uterine size, determining when quickening occurs, using ultrasound, and auscultating the fetal heart rate.

NÄGELE'S RULE

The most common method of determining the EDB is **Nägele's rule.** To use this method, begin with the first day of the LMP, subtract 3 months, and add 7 days. For example,

First day of LMP	November 21
Subtract 3 months	– 3 months
	August 21
Add 7 days	+ 7 days
EDB	August 28 (of the next year)

It is simpler to change the months to numeric terms:

November 21 becomes	11–21
Subtract 3 months	– 3
	8–21
Add 7 days	+ 7
EDB	8–28 (of next year)

A gestation calculator or "wheel" permits the caregiver to calculate the EDB even more quickly (Figure 15–3 ●).

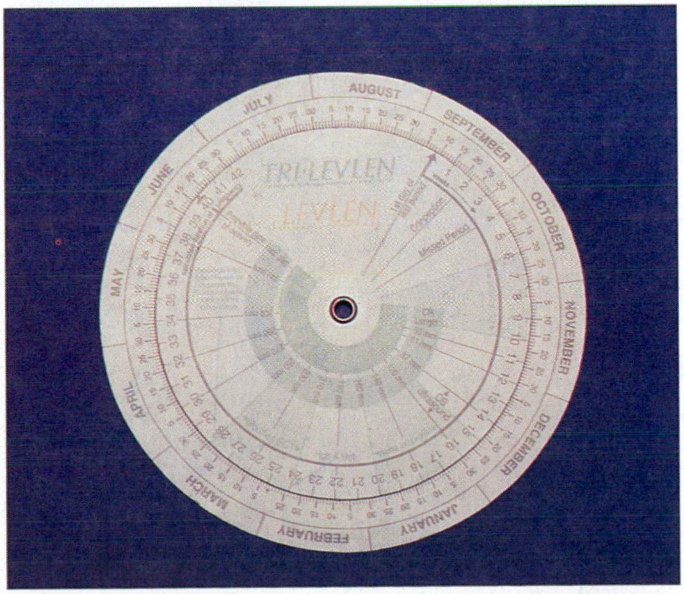

Figure 15–3 ● The EDB wheel can be used to calculate the due date. To use it, place the arrow labeled "1st day of last period" on the date of the woman's LMP. Then read the EDB at the arrow labeled 40. In this case the LMP is September 8th and the EDB is June 17th.

If a woman with a history of menses every 28 days remembers her LMP and was not taking oral contraceptives prior to becoming pregnant, Nägele's rule may be a fairly accurate determiner of her predicted birth date. However, if her cycle is irregular or 35 to 40 days in length, the time of ovulation may be delayed by several days. Ovulation usually occurs 14 days before the onset of the next menses, not 14 days after the previous menses. In such cases a sonogram is done to visualize the gestational sac and obtain measurements of the embryo/fetus. (See discussion of ultrasound on the next page.)

Thus Nägele's rule, while helpful, is not foolproof. It is of no use in calculating EDB for (1) women with markedly irregular periods that include one or more months of amenorrhea, (2) women who are amenorrheic but ovulating and conceive while breastfeeding, or (3) women who conceive before regular menstruation is established following discontinuation of oral contraceptives or termination of a pregnancy (Varney, 1997).

Uterine Assessment

PHYSICAL EXAMINATION

When a woman is examined in the first 10 to 12 weeks of her pregnancy and the nurse practitioner, certified nurse-midwife, or physician thinks that her uterine size is compatible with her menstrual history, uterine size may be the single most important clinical method for dating her pregnancy. In many cases, however, women do not seek obstetric care until well into their second trimester, when it becomes much more difficult to evaluate specific uterine size. In the case of the obese woman, it is most difficult to determine uterine size early in pregnancy because the uterus is more difficult to palpate.

FUNDAL HEIGHT

Fundal height may be used as an indicator of uterine size, although this method cannot be used late in pregnancy. A centimeter tape measure is used to measure the distance from the top of the symphysis pubis over the curve of the abdomen to the top of the uterine fundus (McDonald's method) (Figure 15–4 •). Fundal height in centimeters correlates well with weeks of gestation between 22 to 24 weeks and 34 weeks. At 26 weeks' gestation, for example, fundal height is probably about 26 cm. Typically ±2 cm is considered normal. To be most accurate, fundal height should be measured by the same examiner each time. The woman should empty her bladder before the examiner takes the measurement (Cunningham et al, 2001). Maternal position (trunk elevation, knee flexion) also influences fundal height measurement. If the woman is very tall or very short, fundal height will differ. In the third trimester, variations in fetal weight decrease the accuracy of fundal height measurements. Unfortunately, this method of dating a pregnancy can be quite inaccurate in the following situations:

- Obese women (because of difficulty palpating the fundus accurately)

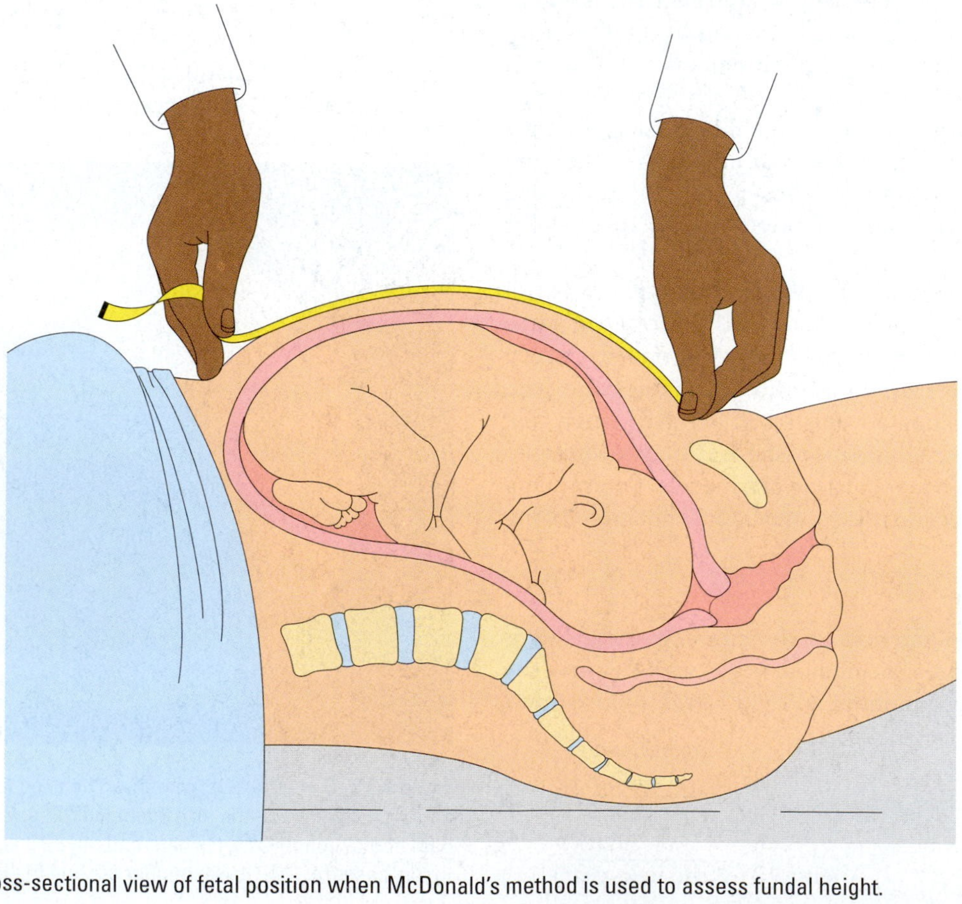

Figure 15–4 • A cross-sectional view of fetal position when McDonald's method is used to assess fundal height.

- Women with uterine fibroids (because uterine size may be distorted)
- Women who develop hydramnios (because the excess fluid increases uterine size, leading the examiner to conclude the fetus is larger than it is)

Measurements of fundal height from month to month and week to week may yield other information, as well. For example, a lag in the progression of fundal height may indicate intrauterine growth restriction (IUGR); a sudden increase in height may indicate the presence of twins or hydramnios.

Fetal Development

QUICKENING

Fetal movements felt by the mother—*quickening*—may give some indications that the fetus is nearing 20 weeks' gestation. However, quickening may be experienced between 16 and 22 weeks' gestation, so this is not a completely accurate method. Because multiparous women have experienced quickening before, they often report it earlier than a primigravida does.

FETAL HEARTBEAT

The ultrasonic Doppler device (Figure 15–5 •) is the primary tool for assessing fetal heartbeat. It may detect fetal heartbeat at about 10 to 12 weeks' gestation. If an ultrasonic Doppler is not available, a special type of stethoscope called a *fetoscope* may be used. The fetal heartbeat can be detected by fetoscope as early as week 16 and almost always by 19 or 20 weeks of gestation. In the case of twins or the obese woman, it may be later before the fetal heartbeat can be detected.

> *I went with my son and daughter-in-law to one of her prenatal appointments and I got to hear my first grandbaby's heartbeat. It made me cry. How wonderful of her to include me.*

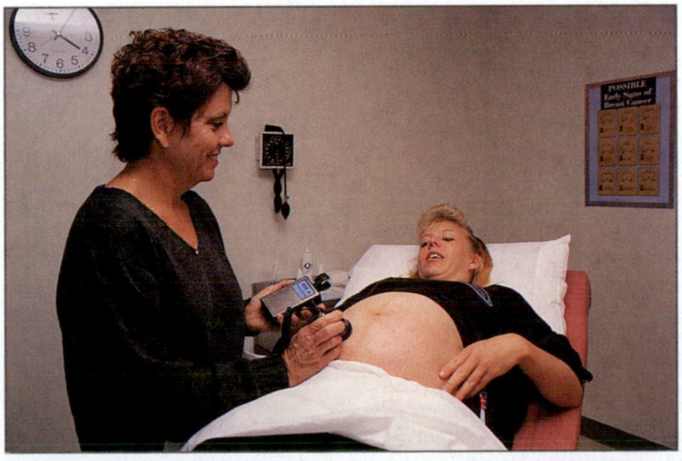

Figure 15–5 • Listening to the fetal heartbeat with a Doppler device.

ULTRASOUND

In the first trimester, ultrasound scanning can detect a gestational sac as early as 5 to 6 weeks after the LMP, fetal heart activity by 6 to 7 weeks, and fetal breathing movement by 10 to 11 weeks of pregnancy. Crown-to-rump measurements can be made for assessment of fetal age until the fetal head can be defined. Biparietal diameter measurements can be made by approximately 12 to 13 weeks and are most accurate between 20 and 30 weeks, when rapid growth in biparietal diameter occurs. (See Chapter 21 for an in-depth discussion of ultrasound scanning of the fetus.)

Assessment of Pelvic Adequacy

By performing a series of assessments and measurements, the examiner assesses the pelvis vaginally to determine whether the size and shape are adequate for a vaginal birth. This procedure, *clinical pelvimetry*, is performed by physicians and by advanced practice nurses such as certified nurse-midwives or nurse practitioners. For a detailed description of clinical pelvimetry, refer to a nurse-midwifery text. This section provides general information about the assessment of the inlet, midpelvis, and outlet. These terms are defined in Chapter 10.

PELVIC INLET

The important anteroposterior diameters of the inlet for childbearing are the diagonal conjugate, the obstetric conjugate, and the conjugata vera, or true conjugate (Figure 15–6 •).

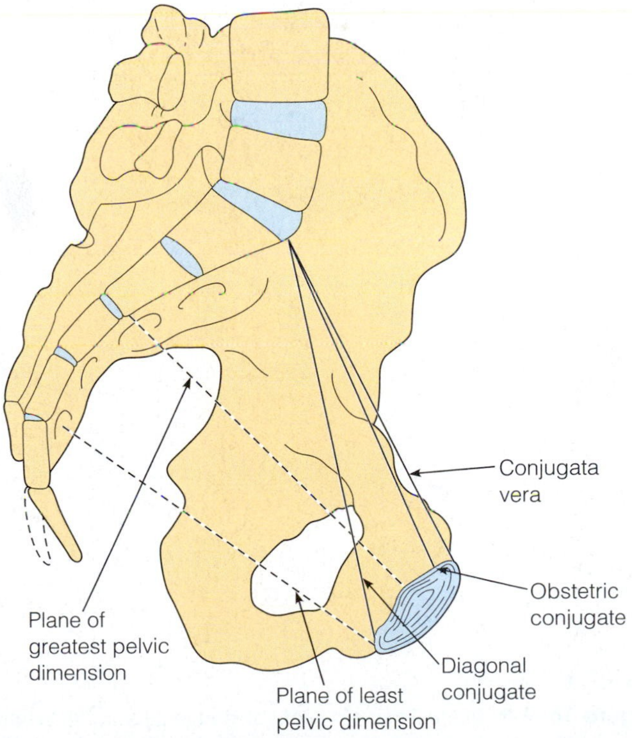

Figure 15–6 • Anteroposterior diameters of the pelvic inlet and their relationship to the pelvic planes.

Other diameters are the transverse (approximately 13.5 cm) and the oblique (averages 12.75 cm).

The anteroposterior diameters of the pelvic inlet may be assessed. To measure the **diagonal conjugate,** the distance from the lower border of the symphysis pubis to the sacral promontory, the examiner inserts a gloved hand into the vagina with index and middle finger extended. The thumb remains extended outside the vagina. The examiner then attempts to reach from the lower border of the symphysis pubis to the sacral promontory with the middle finger. The clinician should determine the length of the finger before attempting this. The diagonal conjugate can then be measured by marking the place where the proximal part of the hand makes contact with the pubis (Figure 15–7, *A* •). Then the examiner measures the distance (which normally measures at least 11.5 cm). The **obstetric conjugate** is the smallest and thus the most important anteroposterior diameter through which the fetus must pass. It extends from the middle of the sacral promontory to the upper inner point on the symphysis. Because it cannot be measured manually (but only by x-ray examination), it is estimated by subtracting 1.5 to 2 cm from the length of the diagonal conjugate. It should measure 10 cm or more in order for an average size baby (7.5 to 8 lb) to pass through without difficulty. The true conjugate extends from the upper border of the symphysis pubis to the middle of the sacral promontory. It can be determined by subtracting 1 cm from the diagonal conjugate.

PELVIC CAVITY (MIDPELVIS)

Important midpelvic measurements include the plane of least dimension, or midplane (anteroposterior diameter, normally

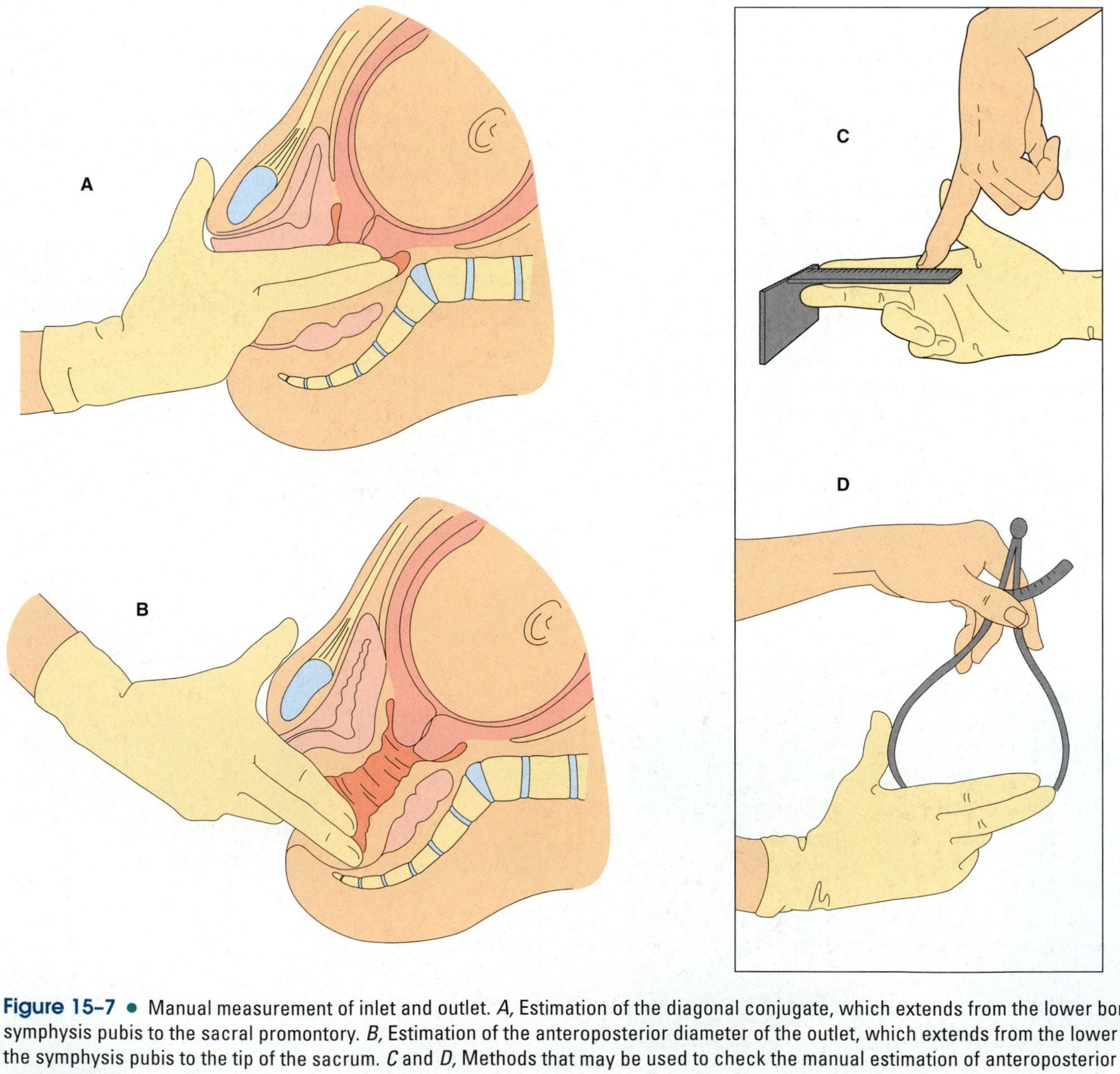

Figure 15–7 • Manual measurement of inlet and outlet. *A,* Estimation of the diagonal conjugate, which extends from the lower border of the symphysis pubis to the sacral promontory. *B,* Estimation of the anteroposterior diameter of the outlet, which extends from the lower border of the symphysis pubis to the tip of the sacrum. *C* and *D,* Methods that may be used to check the manual estimation of anteroposterior measurements.

11.5 to 12 cm; posterior sagittal diameter, 4.5 to 5 cm; and transverse diameter [interspinous], 10 cm). It is shown in Figure 15–6. The planes of the midpelvis cannot be accurately measured by clinical examination. An evaluation of adequacy is made based on the prominence of the ischial spines and degree of convergence of the side walls.

Location of the sacrospinous ligament, a firm ridge of tissue, makes location of the ischial spines easier. When this ligament is located, the examiner should run the fingers along it laterally toward the anterior portion of the pelvis. The spines may range from a small, firm bump like the knuckle of a finger (termed *not encroaching*) to a very prominent bone (called *encroaching*).

The sacrosciatic notch should admit two fingers. A wide notch means that the sacrum curves posteriorly, giving the anteroposterior diameter of the midpelvis a greater length. A narrow notch indicates a decreased diameter. The width of the sacrosciatic notch is more accurately evaluated through x-ray examination but can be estimated through vaginal examination.

The length of the sacrospinous ligament is measured by tracing the ligament from its origin on the ischial spines to its insertion on the sacrum. It is usually 4 cm, or two to three finger breadths long.

The capacity of the cavity can be assessed by sweeping the fingers down the side walls bilaterally to evaluate the shape of the pelvic side walls. They may be termed *convergent* (closer together at the outlet than the inlet, like a funnel), *divergent* (side walls farther apart at the outlet, which typically means the pubic arch will have a wide angle), or *straight* (normal finding). The curvature, inclination, and hollowness of the sacrum help indicate the capacity of the posterior pelvis. It is estimated digitally by palpating the sacrococcygeal junction and by inching up toward the promontory. The examiner then estimates the hollowness of the sacrum. A flat or shallow sacrum has less room; a hollow sacrum is considered normal.

The plane of greatest pelvic dimensions represents the largest portion of the pelvic cavity and has no obstetric significance.

PELVIC OUTLET

The anteroposterior diameter of the pelvic outlet (9.5 to 11.5 cm), which extends from the lower border of the symphysis pubis to the tip of the sacrum, can be measured digitally (Figure 15–7, *B*). The transverse diameter of the outlet is measured by placing the fist between the ischial tuberosities. It usually measures 8 to 10 cm (Figure 15–8 •). The posterior sagittal diameter, the third important outlet diameter, normally measures at least 7.5 cm.

The mobility of the coccyx is determined by pressing down on it with the forefinger and middle finger during the initial vaginal examination. An immobile coccyx can decrease the diameter of the outlet.

The subpubic angle is estimated by palpating the bony structure externally with two fingers placed side by side at the border of the symphysis (Figure 15–9 •). It should be 85 to 90 degrees. The angle is probably less if the examiner cannot separate his or her fingers.

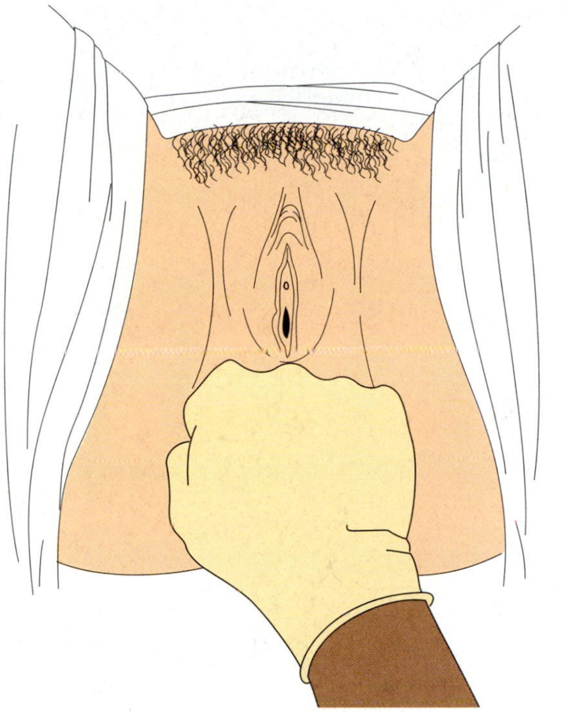

Figure 15–8 • Use of a closed fist to measure the outlet. Most examiners know the distance between their first and last proximal knuckles. If they don't, they can use a measuring device.

The length and shape of the pubic rami affect the transverse diameter of the outlet. The pubic ramus is expected to be short and concave inward, as opposed to straight and long.

The height and inclination of the symphysis pubis are measured, and the contour of the pubic arch is estimated. Excessively long or angulated bone structure shortens the diameter of the obstetric conjugate. Height can be determined by placing the index finger of the gloved hand up to the superior border of the symphysis. The examiner should measure the length of the first phalanx of the index finger (normally about 2.5 cm). Inclination can be determined by externally placing one finger on the top of the symphysis while the internal finger palpates the internal margin. An imaginary line is drawn between the fingers, and the angle is estimated.

A posterior inclination with the lower border of the pubis slanting inward decreases the anteroposterior diameter. The anteroposterior sagittal diameter is the most significant diameter of the outlet because it is the shortest diameter through which the infant must pass. Estimating the contour of the pubic arch provides information on the width of the angle at which these bones come together. The pubic arch has obstetric importance; if it is narrow, the infant's head may be pushed backward toward the coccyx, making extension of the fetal head difficult, which may lengthen the second stage of labor.

MediaLink CARE PLAN: INITIAL ASSESSMENT OF PRIMIGRAVIDA

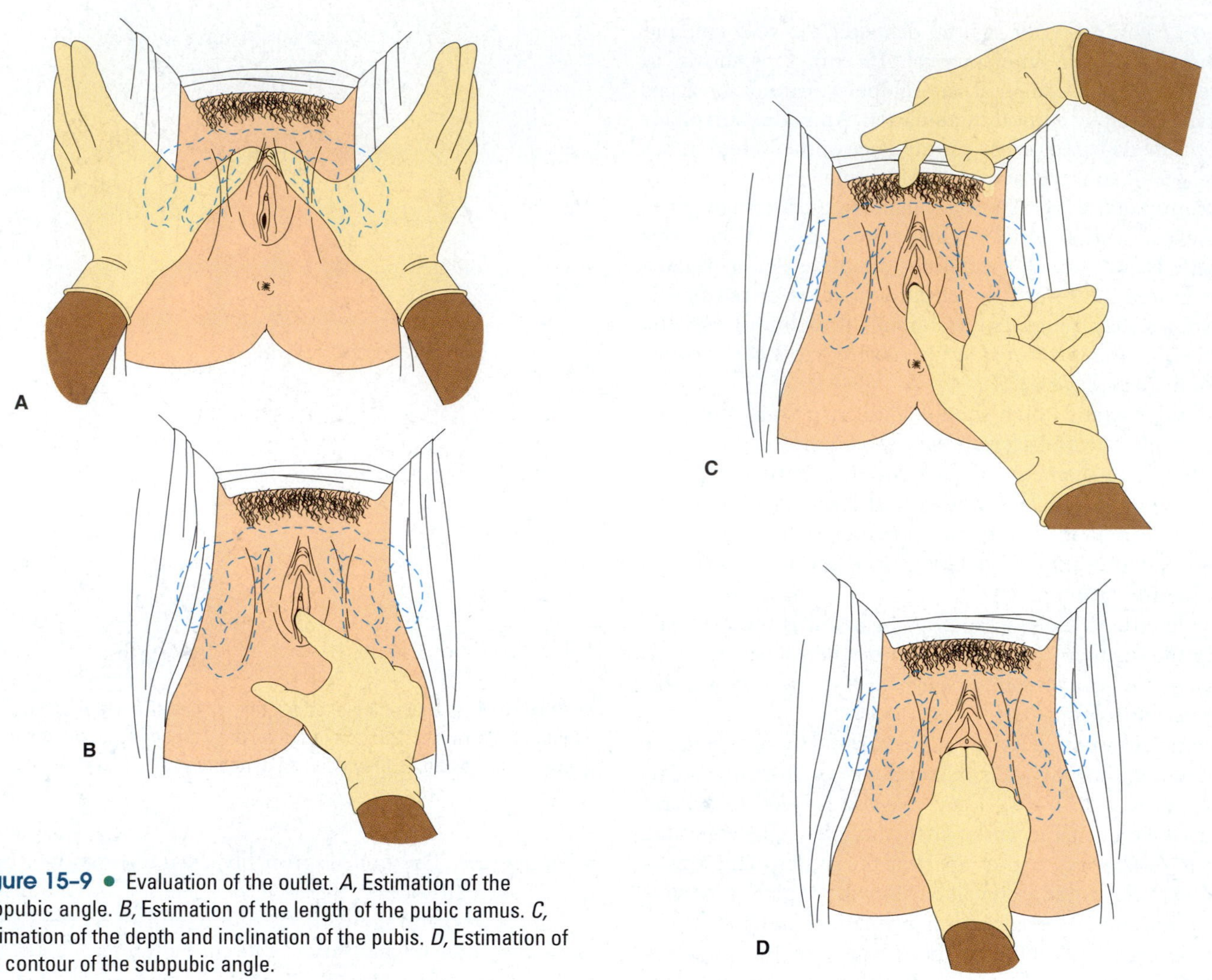

Figure 15–9 • Evaluation of the outlet. *A,* Estimation of the subpubic angle. *B,* Estimation of the length of the pubic ramus. *C,* Estimation of the depth and inclination of the pubis. *D,* Estimation of the contour of the subpubic angle.

Subsequent Client History

At subsequent prenatal visits, the nurse continues to gather data about the family's adjustment to the pregnancy and the course of the pregnancy to date. The nurse asks the pregnant woman how she thinks the pregnancy is progressing. In what ways is it the same as her expectations, and how is it different? The nurse also asks about the adjustment of the support person and expectations of the support person and other children, if any, in the family. As the pregnancy progresses, the nurse asks about preparations the family has made for the new baby. Taking time to address psychosocial issues is necessary in helping the nurse assess the family's success in meeting their developmental tasks.

The nurse also asks specifically whether the woman has experienced any discomfort, especially the kinds of discomfort that are often seen at specific times during a pregnancy. The nurse inquires about physical changes that relate directly to the pregnancy, such as the woman's perception of fetal movement. Other pertinent information includes any exposure to contagious illnesses, medical treatment and therapy prescribed for nonpregnancy problems since the last visit, and any prescription or over-the-counter medications that were not prescribed as part of the woman's prenatal care.

The danger signs that a woman should report immediately are generally discussed during the initial prenatal visit and reviewed when she comes for her second prenatal visit. Many caregivers also provide printed information on the subject written in lay terms. Table 15–3 • identifies the danger signs of pregnancy and possible causes for each.

Periodic prenatal examinations offer the nurse an opportunity to assess the childbearing woman's psychologic needs and emotional status. If the woman's partner attends the prenatal visits, his needs and concerns can also be identified.

The interchange between the nurse and woman will be facilitated if it takes place in a friendly, trusting environment. The nurse should give the woman sufficient time to ask questions and to air concerns. If the nurse provides the time and demonstrates genuine interest, the woman will feel more at ease bringing up questions that she may believe are silly or concerns that she has been afraid to verbalize. The nurse who has an accurate understanding of all the changes of preg-

COMPLEMENTARY AND ALTERNATIVE THERAPIES

YOGA DURING PREGNANCY

The following advice is important for women who practice yoga during pregnancy (Fontaine, 2000):

- During pregnancy, some yoga poses or positions are contraindicated. In particular pregnant women should avoid those poses that put pressure on the uterus as well as any extreme stretching positions.
- Because of the changed center of gravity that occurs as pregnancy progresses, women need to be especially careful to maintain balance when doing stretching.
- Pregnant women should avoid stomach-lying for any poses. After 20 weeks' gestation, women should lie on their left side rather than their back for floor positions.
- Pregnant women should immediately stop any pose that is uncomfortable.
- Warning signs that indicate the need to contact the physician or certified nurse-midwife immediately include the following: dizziness, extreme shortness of breath, sudden swelling, vaginal bleeding.

Table 15-3 • DANGER SIGNS IN PREGNANCY

The woman should report the following danger signs in pregnancy immediately.

Danger Sign	Possible Cause
Sudden gush of fluid from vagina	Premature rupture of membranes
Vaginal bleeding	Abruptio placentae, placenta previa
	Lesions of cervix or vagina "Bloody show"
Abdominal pain	Premature labor, abruptio placentae
Temperature above 38.3C (101F) and chills	Infection
Dizziness, blurring of vision, double vision, spots before eyes	Hypertension, preeclampsia
Persistent vomiting	Hyperemesis gravidarum
Severe headache	Hypertension, preeclampsia
Edema of hands, face, legs, and feet	Preeclampsia
Muscular irritability, convulsions	Preeclampsia, eclampsia
Epigastric pain	Preeclampsia, ischemia in major abdominal vessel
Oliguria	Renal impairment, decreased fluid intake
Dysuria	Urinary tract infection
Absence of fetal movement	Maternal medication, obesity, fetal death

nancy is most able to answer questions and provide information. See the foldout color chart, "Maternal-Fetal Development," for vivid illustrations of some of this information.

The nurse should also be sensitive to religious, spiritual, cultural, and socioeconomic factors that may influence a family's response to pregnancy, as well as to the woman's expectations of the healthcare system. The nurse can avoid stereotyping clients simply by asking each woman about her expectations for the antepartal period. Although many women's responses may reflect what are thought to be traditional norms, other women will have decidedly different views or may have expectations that represent a blending of beliefs or cultures.

During the prenatal period, it is essential that the nurse begin assessing the developing readiness of the woman (and her partner, if possible) to take on the responsibilities of parenthood successfully. Table 15–4 • identifies areas for assessment and provides some sample questions the nurse might use to obtain necessary information. If the woman's responses are primarily negative, the nurse can plan interventions for the prenatal and postpartal periods.

Subsequent Prenatal Assessment

The Subsequent Prenatal Assessment Guide, which begins on page 348, provides a systematic approach to the regular physical examinations the pregnant woman should undergo for optimal prenatal care and a model for evaluating both the pregnant woman and the expectant father, if he is involved in the pregnancy.

Clinical Tip *When assessing blood pressure, have the pregnant woman sit up with her arm resting on a table so that her arm is at the level of her heart. Expect a decrease in her blood pressure from baseline during the second trimester because of normal physiologic changes. If this decrease doesn't occur, evaluate further for signs of preeclampsia.*

The woman's individual needs and the assessment of her risks should determine the frequency of subsequent visits. Generally, the recommended frequency of prenatal visits is as follows:

- Every 4 weeks for the first 28 weeks of gestation
- Every 2 weeks until 36 weeks' gestation
- After week 36, every week until childbirth

During the subsequent antepartal assessments, most women demonstrate ongoing psychologic adjustment to pregnancy and ever-improving coping skills. However, some

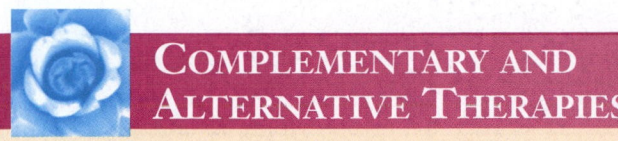

Table 15-4 • GUIDE TO PRENATAL ASSESSMENT OF PARENTING

Areas Assessed	Sample Questions
I. Perception of complexities of mothering	
A. Desires baby for itself Positive: 1. Feels positive about pregnancy Negative: 1. Wants baby to meet own needs such as someone to love her, someone to get her out of unhappy home	1. Did you plan on getting pregnant? 2. How do you feel about being pregnant? 3. Why do you want this baby?
B. Expresses concern about impact of mothering role on other roles (wife, career, school) Positive: 1. Realistic expectations of how baby will affect job, career, school, and personal goals 2. Interested in learning about child care Negative: 1. Feels pregnancy and baby will make no emotional, physical, or social demands on self 2. Has no insight that mothering role will affect other roles or lifestyle	1. What do you think it will be like to take care of a baby? 2. How do you think your life will be different after you have your baby? 3. How do you feel this baby will affect your job, career, school, and personal goals? 4. How will the baby affect your relationship with your boyfriend or husband? 5. Have you done any reading, baby-sitting, or made any things for a baby?
C. Gives up routine habits because "not good for baby" (eg, quits smoking, adjusts time schedule) Positive: 1. Gives up routines not good for baby (quits smoking, adjusts eating habits)	
II. Attachment	
A. Strong feelings regarding sex of baby. Why? Positive: 1. Verbalizes positive thoughts about the baby Negative: 1. Baby will be like negative aspects of self and partner	1. Why do you prefer a certain sex? (Is reason inappropriate for a baby?) 2. Note comments client makes about baby not being normal and why client feels this way.
B. Interested in data regarding fetus (eg, growth and development, heart tones) Positive: 1. As above Negative: 1. Shows no interest in fetal growth and development, quickening, and fetal heart tones 2. Expresses negative feelings about fetus by rejecting counseling regarding nutrition, rest, hygiene	
C. Fantasies about baby Positive: 1. Follows cultural norms regarding preparation 2. Time of attachment behaviors appropriate to her history of pregnancy loss Negative: 1. Bonding conditional depending on sex, age of baby, and/or labor and birth experience 2. Woman considers only own needs when making plans for baby 3. Exhibits no attachment behaviors after critical period of previous pregnancy 4. Failure to follow cultural norms regarding preparation	1. What did you think or feel when you first felt the baby move? 2. Have you started preparing for the baby? 3. What do you think your baby will look like—what age do you see your baby at? 4. How would you like your new baby to look?
III. Acceptance of child by significant others	
A. Acknowledges acceptance by significant other of the new responsibility inherent in child Positive: 1. Acknowledges unconditional acceptance of pregnancy and baby by significant others 2. Partner accepts new responsibility inherent with child 3. Timely sharing of experience of pregnancy with significant others	1. How does your partner feel about this pregnancy? 2. How do your parents feel? 3. What do your friends think? 4. Does your partner have a preference regarding the baby's sex? Why? 5. How does your partner feel about being a father? 6. What do you think he'll be like as a father? 7. What do you think he'll do to help you with child care?

Table 15-4 • GUIDE TO PRENATAL ASSESSMENT OF PARENTING (CONTINUED)

Areas Assessed	Sample Questions
Negative: 1. Significant others not supportively involved with pregnancy 2. Conditional acceptance of pregnancy depending on sex, race, age of baby 3. Decision making does not take in needs of fetus (eg, spends food money on new car) 4. Takes no/little responsibility for needs of pregnancy, woman/fetus	8. Have you and your partner talked about how the baby might change your lives? 9. Who have you told about your pregnancy?
B. Concrete demonstration of acceptance of pregnancy/baby by significant others (eg, baby shower, significant other involved in prenatal education)	
Positive: 1. Baby shower 2. Significant other attends prenatal class with client	1. Note if partner attends clinic with client (degree of interest; eg, listens to heart tones). Significant other plans to be with client during labor and birth. 2. Is your partner contributing financially?
IV. Ensures physical well-being	
A. Concerns about having normal pregnancy, labor and birth, and baby	
1. Preparing for labor and birth, attends prenatal classes, interested in labor and birth	1. What have you heard about labor and birth?
2. Aware of danger signs of pregnancy	2. Note data about client's reaction to prenatal class.
3. Seeks and uses appropriate healthcare (eg, time of initial visit, keeps appointments, follows through on recommendations)	
Negative: 1. Denies signs and symptoms that might suggest complications of pregnancy 2. Verbalizes extreme fear of labor and birth—refuses to talk about labor and birth 3. Misses appointments, fails to follow instructions, refuses to attend prenatal classes	
B. Family/client decisions reflect concern for health of mother and baby (eg, use of finances, time)	
Positive: 1. As above	

Note: When "Negative" is not listed in a section, the reader may assume that negative is the absence of positive responses.

Source: Modified and used with permission of the Minneapolis Health Dept, Minneapolis, MN.

women may exhibit signs of psychologic problems. These signs may include one or more of the following:

- Increasing anxiety
- Depression or feelings of sadness
- Inability to establish communication
- Inappropriate responses or actions
- Denial of pregnancy
- Inability to cope with stress
- Intense preoccupation with the sex of the baby
- Failure to acknowledge quickening
- Failure to plan and prepare for the baby (for example, living arrangements, clothing, feeding methods)
- Indications of substance abuse

If the woman's behavior indicates possible psychologic problems, the nurse should provide ongoing support and counseling and also refer the woman to appropriate professionals.

Assessment Guide — Subsequent Prenatal Assessment

PHYSICAL ASSESSMENT/ NORMAL FINDINGS	ALTERATIONS AND POSSIBLE CAUSES*	NURSING RESPONSES TO DATA†
➤ VITAL SIGNS		
Temperature: 36.2–37.6C (98–99.6F)	Elevated temperature (infection)	Evaluate for signs of infection. Refer to physician.
Pulse: 60–90/min Rate may increase 10 beats/min during pregnancy	Increased pulse rate (anxiety, cardiac disorders)	Note irregularities. Assess for anxiety and stress.
Respiration: 16–24/min.	Marked tachypnea or abnormal patterns (respiratory disease)	Refer to physician.
Blood pressure: 90–140/60–90 (falls in second trimester)	>140/90 or increase of 30 mm systolic and 15 mm diastolic (preeclampsia)	Assess for edema, proteinuria, and hyperreflexia. Refer to physician. Schedule appointments more frequently.
➤ WEIGHT GAIN		
First trimester: 1.6–2.3 kg (3.5–5 lb)	Inadequate weight gain (poor nutrition, nausea, IUGR)	Discuss appropriate weight gain.
Second trimester: 5.5–6.8 kg (12–15 lb)	Excessive weight gain (excessive caloric intake, edema, preeclampsia)	Provide nutritional counseling. Assess for presence of edema or anemia.
Third trimester: 5.5–6.8 kg (12–15 lb)		
➤ EDEMA		
Small amount of dependent edema, especially in last weeks of pregnancy	Edema in hands, face, legs, and feet (preeclampsia)	Identify any correlation between edema and activities, blood pressure, or proteinuria. Refer to physician if indicated.
➤ UTERINE SIZE		
See Assessment Guide: Initial Prenatal Assessment for normal changes during pregnancy	Unusually rapid growth (multiple gestation, hydatidiform mole, hydramnios, miscalculation of EDB)	Evaluate fetal status. Determine height of fundus (page 340). Use diagnostic ultrasound.
➤ FETAL HEARTBEAT		
120–160/min	Absence of fetal heartbeat after 20 weeks' gestation (maternal obesity, fetal demise)	Evaluate fetal status.
Funic souffle		
➤ LABORATORY EVALUATION		
Hemoglobin: 12–16 g/dL Pseudoanemia of pregnancy	< 11 g/dL (anemia)	Provide nutritional counseling. Hemoglobin is repeated at 7 months' gestation. Women of Mediterranean heritage need a close check on hemoglobin because of possibility of thalassemia.

*Possible causes of alterations are placed in parentheses.

†This column provides guidelines for further assessment and initial nursing intervention.

➤

ASSESSMENT GUIDE: SUBSEQUENT PRENATAL ASSESSMENT *continued*

PHYSICAL ASSESSMENT/ NORMAL FINDINGS	ALTERATIONS AND POSSIBLE CAUSES*	NURSING RESPONSES TO DATA†
➤ **LABORATORY EVALUATION (*continued*)**		
Triple screen (also called multiple marker screening [MMS]) serum test done at 16–18 weeks' gestation. Evaluates three factors—maternal serum alpha-fetoprotein (MSAFP), estriol, and hCG: normal levels	Evaluated MSAFP (neural lube defect, underestimated gestational age, multiple gestation, Rh disease). Low level (trisomy 21 [Down syndrome], trisomy 18). Elevated hCG combined with lower than normal estriol and MSAFP (Down syndrome) (ACOG, 2000)	Refer to physician.
Indirect Coombs test done on Rh− women: Negative (done at 28 weeks' gestation)	Rh antibodies present (maternal sensitization has occurred)	If Rh− and unsensitized, Rh immune globulin given (see Chapter 20). If Rh antibodies present, Rh immune globulin not given; fetus monitored closely for isoimmune hemolytic disease.
50-g 1-hour glucose screen (done between 24 and 28 weeks gestation)	Plasma glucose level > 140 mg/dL (gestational diabetes mellitus [GDM])	Discuss implications of GDM. Refer for a diagnostic 100-g oral glucose tolerance test.
	Note: Some facilities use level > 130 mg/dL, which identifies 90% of women with GDM (American Diabetes Association, 2000)	
Urinalysis: See Assessment Guide: Initial Prenatal Assessment for normal findings	See Assessment Guide: Initial Prenatal Assessment for deviations	Repeat urinalysis at 7 months' gestation. Repeat dipstick test at each visit.
Protein: Negative	Proteinuria, albuminuria (contamination by vaginal discharge, urinary tract infection, preeclampsia)	Obtain dipstick urine sample. Refer to physician if deviations are present.
Glucose: Negative	Persistent glycosuria (diabetes mellitus)	Refer to physician.
Note: Glycosuria may be present due to physiologic alterations in glomerular filtration rate and renal threshold		
Screening for Group B streptococcus (GBS): Rectal and vaginal swabs obtained at 35–37 weeks' gestation for all pregnant women (Centers for Disease Control and Prevention [CDC], 2002).	Positive culture (maternal infection)	Explain maternal and fetal/neonatal risks (see Chapter 20). Refer to physician or CNM for therapy.

CULTURAL ASSESSMENT	VARIATIONS TO CONSIDER*	NURSING RESPONSES TO DATA†
Determine the mother's (and family's) attitudes about the sex of the unborn child.	Some women have no preference about the sex of the child; others do. In many cultures, boys are especially valued as firstborn children.	Provide opportunities to discuss preferences and expectations; avoid a judgmental attitude to the response.
Ask about the woman's expectations of childbirth. Will she want someone with her for the birth? Whom does she choose? What is the role of her partner?	Some women want their partner present for labor and birth; others prefer a female relative or friend.	Provide information on birth options but accept the woman's decision about who will attend.

*Possible causes of alterations are placed in parentheses.

†This column provides guidelines for further assessment and initial nursing intervention.

(Continued on next page)

ASSESSMENT GUIDE: SUBSEQUENT PRENATAL ASSESSMENT *continued*

CULTURAL ASSESSMENT	VARIATIONS TO CONSIDER*	NURSING RESPONSES TO DATA†
	Some women expect to be separated from their partner once cervical dilation has occurred (Andrews & Boyle, 1998).	Explore reasons for not preparing for the baby. Support the mother's preferences and provide information about possible sources of assistance if the decision is related to a lack of resources.
Ask about preparations for the baby. Determine what is customary for the woman.	Some women may have a fully prepared nursery; others may not have a separate room for the baby.	

PSYCHOSOCIAL ASSESSMENT	VARIATIONS TO CONSIDER*	NURSING RESPONSES TO DATA†
➤ EXPECTANT MOTHER		
Psychologic status	Increased stress and anxiety	Encourage woman to take an active part in her care.
First trimester: Incorporates idea of pregnancy; may feel ambivalent, especially if she must give up desired role; usually looks for signs of verification of pregnancy, such as increase in abdominal size or fetal movement	Inability to establish communication; inability to accept pregnancy; inappropriate response or actions; denial of pregnancy; inability to cope	Establish lines of communication. Establish a trusting relationship. Counsel as necessary. Refer to appropriate professional as needed.
Second trimester: Baby becomes more real to woman as abdominal size increases and she feels movement; she begins to turn inward, becoming more introspective		
Third trimester: Begins to think of baby as separate being; may feel restless and may feel that time of labor will never come; remains self-centered and concentrates on preparing place for baby		
Educational needs Self-care measures and knowledge about the following:	Inadequate information	Provide information and counseling.
Health promotion		
Breast care		
Hygiene		
Rest		
Exercise		
Nutrition		
Relief measures for common discomforts of pregnancy		
Danger signs in pregnancy (Table 15–3)		

*Possible causes of alterations are placed in parentheses.

†This column provides guidelines for further assessment and initial nursing intervention.

ASSESSMENT GUIDE: SUBSEQUENT PRENATAL ASSESSMENT *continued*

PSYCHOSOCIAL ASSESSMENT	VARIATIONS TO CONSIDER*	NURSING RESPONSES TO DATA†
➤ EXPECTANT MOTHER ***(continued)***		
Sexual activity: Woman knows how pregnancy affects sexual activity	Lack of information about effects of pregnancy and/or alternative positions during sexual intercourse	Provide counseling.
Preparation for parenting: Appropriate preparation	Lack of preparation (denial, failure to adjust to baby, unwanted child)	Counsel. If lack of preparation is due to inadequacy of information, provide information (Chapter 16).
Preparation for childbirth ***Client aware of the following:*** 1. Prepared childbirth techniques		If couple chooses particular technique, refer to classes (see Chapter 13 for description of childbirth preparation techniques).
2. Normal processes and changes during childbirth		Encourage prenatal class attendance. Educate woman during visits based on current physical status. Provide reading list for more specific information.
3. Problems that may occur as a result of drug and alcohol use and of smoking	Continued abuse of drugs and alcohol; denial of possible effect on self and baby	Review danger signs that were presented on initial visit.
Woman has met other physician or nurse-midwife who may be attending her birth in the absence of primary caregiver	Introduction of new individual at birth may increase stress and anxiety for woman and partner	Introduce woman to all members of group practice.
➤ EXPECTANT FATHER		
Impending labor	Lack of information	Provide appropriate teaching, stressing importance of seeking appropriate medical assistance.
Client knows signs of impending labor: 1. Uterine contractions that increase in frequency, duration, and intensity 2. Bloody show 3. Expulsion of mucous plug 4. Rupture of membranes		
➤ EXPECTANT FATHER		
Psychologic status		
First trimester: May express excitement over confirmation of pregnancy and of his virility; concerns move toward providing for financial needs; energetic, may identify with some discomforts of pregnancy and may even exhibit symptoms	Increasing stress and anxiety; inability to establish communication; inability to accept pregnancy diagnosis; withdrawal of support; abondonment of the mother	Encourage expectant father to come to prenatal visits. Establish lines of communication. Establish trusting relationship.

*Possible causes of alterations are placed in parentheses.

†This column provides guidelines for further assessment and initial nursing intervention.

(Continued on next page)

Assessment Guide: SUBSEQUENT PRENATAL ASSESSMENT *continued*

PSYCHOSOCIAL ASSESSMENT	VARIATIONS TO CONSIDER*	NURSING RESPONSES TO DATA†
➤ **EXPECTANT FATHER** (*continued*)		
Second trimester: May feel more confident and be less concerned with financial matters; may have concerns about wife's changing size and shape, her increasing introspection		Counsel. Let expectant father know that it is normal for him to experience these feelings.
Third trimester: May have feelings of rivalry with fetus, especially during sexual activity; may make changes in his physical appearance and exhibit more interest in himself; may become more energetic; fantasizes about child but usually imagines older child; fears mutilation and death of woman and child		Include expectant father in pregnancy activities as he desires. Provide education, information, and support. Increasing numbers of expectant fathers are demonstrating desire to be involved in many or all aspects of prenatal care, education, and . preparation.

*Possible causes of alterations are placed in parentheses.

†This column provides guidelines for further assessment and initial nursing intervention.

Chapter Review

EXPLOREMediaLink

NCLEX review questions, case studies, and other interactive resources for this chapter can be found on the Web site at http://www.prenhall.com/olds. Click on "Chapter 15" to select the activities for this chapter.

For tutorials including animations and videos, more NCLEX review questions, and an audio glossary, access the accompanying CD-ROM in this book.

Focus Your Study

- A complete history forms the basis of prenatal care and is reevaluated and updated as necessary throughout the pregnancy.
- The initial prenatal assessment is a careful and thorough physical examination and cultural and psychosocial assessment designed to identify variations and potential risk factors.
- Laboratory tests completed at the initial visit, such as a complete blood count, ABO and Rh typing, urinalysis, Pap smear, chlamydia culture, gonorrhea culture, rubella titer, and various blood screens (such as rapid plasma reagin [RPR], HIV, and hepatitis B), provide information about the woman's health during early pregnancy and also help detect potential problems.
- The estimated date of birth can be calculated using Nägele's rule. Using this approach, one begins with the first day of the last menstrual period, subtracts 3 months, and adds 7 days. A "wheel" may also be used to calculate the EDB.
- Accuracy of the EDB may be evaluated by physical examination to assess uterine size, measurement of fundal height, and ultrasound. Perception of quickening and auscultation of fetal heartbeat are

also useful tools in confirming the gestation of a pregnancy.

- The diagonal conjugate is the distance from the lower posterior border of the symphysis pubis to the sacral promontory. The obstetric conjugate is estimated by subtracting 1.5 to 2.0 cm from the length of the diagonal conjugate.
- As part of the assessment of the pelvic cavity (midpelvis), the prominence of the ischial spines is assessed, the sacrosciatic notch and the length of the sacrospinous ligament are measured, and the shape of the pelvic side walls is evaluated. Finally, the hollowness of the sacrum is determined.
- The anteroposterior diameter of the pelvic outlet is determined, the mobility of the coccyx is assessed, the suprapubic angle is estimated, and the contour of the pubic arch is evaluated to assess the adequacy of the pelvic outlet.
- The nurse begins evaluating the woman psychosocially during the initial prenatal assessment. This assessment continues and is modified throughout the pregnancy.
- Cultural and ethnic beliefs may strongly influence the woman's attitudes and apparent cooperation with care during pregnancy.

References

American College of Obstetricians and Gynecologists (ACOG). (2000). *Planning your pregnancy and birth* (3rd ed.). Washington, D.C.: Author.

American Diabetes Association. (2000). Position statement: Gestational diabetes mellitus. *Diabetes Care, 23* (Suppl. 1), 1–6.

Andrews, M. M., & Boyle, J. S. (1998). *Transcultural concepts in nursing care* (2nd ed.). Glenview, IL: Scott, Foresman/ Little, Brown.

Centers for Disease Control and Prevention. (2002). Prevention of perinatal group B streptococcal disease: Revised guidelines from the CDC. *Morbidity and Mortality Weekly Reports, 51*(RR-11), 1–22.

Cunningham, F. G., Gant, N. F., Leveno, K. J., Gilstrap, L. C., III, Hauth, J. C., & Wenstrom, K. D. (2001). *Williams obstetrics* (21st ed.). New York: McGraw-Hill.

Fontaine, K. L. (2000). *Healing practices: Alternative therapies for nursing.* Upper Saddle River, NJ: Prentice Hall Health.

Milunsky, A., Ulcickas, M., Rothman, K. J., Willett, W., Jick, S. S., & Jick, H. (1992, August 19). Maternal heat exposure and neural tube defects. *Journal of the American Medical Association, 268*(7), 882–885.

Varney, H. (1997). *Varney's midwifery* (3rd ed.). Sudbury, MA: Jones & Bartlett.

The Expectant Family: Needs and Care 16

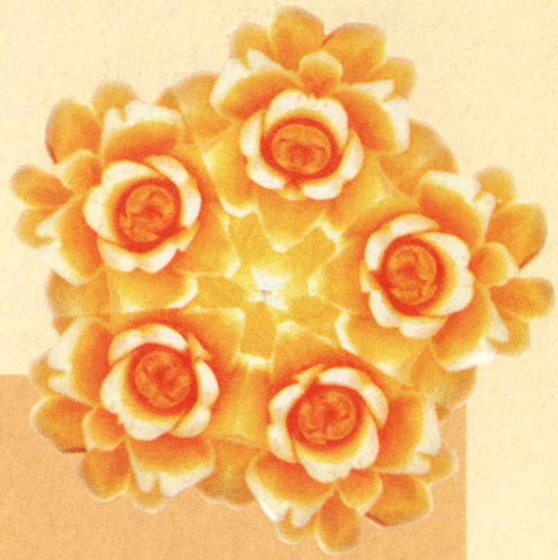

I don't know how I timed it, but my nursing program OB rotation finishes up right about my due date. Watching all the births during my rotation has been really exciting. The labor and delivery nurses laugh and say my hormones should be hopping now, but I think this baby is subliminally telling me that we won't "hatch" until I take my last final exam!

Objectives

- Describe the significance of using the nursing process to promote health in the woman and her family during pregnancy.
- Describe actions the nurse can take to help maintain the well-being of the expectant father and siblings during a family's pregnancy.
- Discuss the significance of cultural considerations in managing nursing care during pregnancy.
- Explain the causes of the common discomforts of pregnancy.
- Summarize appropriate measures to alleviate the common discomforts of pregnancy.
- Delineate self-care actions a pregnant woman and her family can take to maintain and promote well-being during each trimester of pregnancy.
- Describe factors that have contributed to the increased incidence of pregnancy in women over age 35.
- Compare similarities and differences in the needs of expectant women in various age groups.

MediaLink

Additional resources for this content can be found on the Student CD-ROM and on the Companion Website at www.prenhall.com/olds. Click on "Chapter 16" to select the activities for this chapter.

CD-ROM

- Audio Glossary
- NCLEX Review

Companion Website

- Additional NCLEX Review
- Case Study: First Trimester Client
- Care Plan Activity: Common Discomforts of Pregnancy

Key Terms

Fetal alcohol syndrome (FAS) 384
Fetal movement record (FMR) 369
Kegel exercises 377
Leukorrhea 363
Lightening 368
Nipple preparation 369
Pelvic tilt 375
Ptyalism 364
Teratogens 381

From the moment a woman finds out that she is pregnant, she faces a future marked by dramatic changes. Her appearance will be altered. Her relationships will change. She will experience a variety of unique physical changes throughout the pregnancy. Even her psychologic state will be affected. In coping with these changes she needs to make adjustments in her daily life.

Her family must also adjust to the pregnancy. Roles and responsibilities of family members will change as the woman's ability to perform certain activities changes. They too must adapt psychologically to the situation.

The expectant woman and her family will probably have many questions about the pregnancy and its impact on her and the other members of the family. In addition, the daily activities and healthcare practices of the woman become of concern when she and her family realize that what she does can affect the well-being of the unborn child.

Nurses caring for pregnant women need a clear understanding of pregnancy and the changes it brings if they are to be effective in managing nursing care. With this in mind, Chapter 14 provided a database for the nurse by presenting material related to the normal physical, psychologic, social, and cultural changes of pregnancy. Chapter 15 then used that database to begin a discussion of nursing care management by focusing on client assessment. This chapter further addresses nursing care management as it relates to the needs of the expectant woman and her loved ones.

Nursing Care During the Prenatal Period

Nursing Diagnosis

The nurse may see a pregnant woman only once every 4 to 6 weeks during the first several months of her pregnancy. To ensure continuity of care, therefore, a written care plan that incorporates assessment data, nursing diagnoses, and client goals is essential.

The nurse can anticipate that, for many women with a low-risk pregnancy, certain nursing diagnoses will be made more frequently than others will. Nursing diagnoses will, of course, vary from woman to woman and according to the time in the pregnancy. Examples of common nursing diagnoses include the following:

- ***Constipation*** related to the physiologic effects of pregnancy
- ***Altered Sexuality Patterns*** related to discomfort during late pregnancy

After formulating an appropriate diagnosis, the nurse establishes related goals to guide the nursing plan and interventions.

Nursing Plan and Implementation

Once nursing diagnoses have been identified, the next step is to establish priorities of nursing care. Sometimes priorities of care are based on the most immediate needs or concerns perceived by the woman. For example, during the first trimester, a woman is probably not ready to hear about labor and birth because she is likely to have more immediate concerns, such as nausea or concerns about sexual intimacy with her partner.

At other times priorities may develop as a result of findings during a prenatal visit. For example, the nurse may stress the need for frequent rest periods for a woman who is showing signs of preeclampsia (a pregnancy complication discussed in Chapter 20). However, the woman may feel well physically and find it difficult to accept the nurse's emphasis on rest. It is the responsibility of medical and nursing professionals to help the woman and her family understand the significance of a problem and to plan appropriate interventions to deal with it.

The intervention methods most used by nurses in caring for the expectant woman and her family are communication techniques and teaching-learning strategies. These intervention methods are often used in groups, such as early pregnancy classes and childbirth education classes, but the nurse in the prenatal setting also applies these techniques with individuals.

COMMUNITY-BASED NURSING CARE

Prenatal care, especially for women with low-risk pregnancies, is community based, typically in a clinic or private office. The healthcare community recognizes the value of providing a primary care nurse in these settings to coordinate care for each childbearing family. The nurse in a clinic or health maintenance organization (HMO) may be the only source of continuity for the woman, who may see a different physician or certified nurse-midwife at each visit. The nurse can be extremely effective in working with the expectant family by answering their questions; providing them with complete information about pregnancy, appropriate prenatal self-care measures, and community resources or referral agencies; and supporting the healthcare activities of the woman and her family. Communities often have a wealth of services and educational opportunities available for pregnant women and their families, and the knowledgeable nurse can help the woman access these services. This allows the family to assume equal responsibility with healthcare providers in working toward their common goal of a positive childbearing experience.

Home Care

Home care can be of benefit to any pregnant woman, but it is especially effective in removing barriers for women who have difficulty accessing healthcare. These barriers may include lack of locally available healthcare facilities, problems with transportation to the facility, or schedule conflicts with available appointment times because of employment hours or family responsibilities.

In-home nursing assessments vary according to the scope of practice of the nurse and include current history and those screening procedures typically completed in an office or clinic: vital signs, weight, urine screen, physical activity, and dietary intake. Advanced practice nurses can also assess reflexes, perform tests of fetal well-being, and even do cervical examinations.

Once the assessments are completed, the nurse can determine the level of follow-up home care or telephone contact needed.

A prenatal home care visit or phone contact can also be useful for women who anticipate a short inpatient stay after childbirth. At the prenatal contact, the nurse explains the postpartum program and answers any questions the woman or her family has.

Although the use of home care for women with uncomplicated pregnancies is growing, it is most often used for women with prenatal complications that can be managed without hospitalization if effective nursing assessment and care are provided in the home (see Chapters 19 and 20).

TEACHING FOR SELF-CARE

Throughout the prenatal period the nurse provides informal and formal teaching to the childbearing family designed to help the family carry out self-care when appropriate and to report changes that may indicate a possible health problem. The teaching is most effective if timed to coincide with the woman's (couple's) readiness and needs (Table 16–1 •). The nurse also provides anticipatory guidance to help the family plan for changes that will occur following childbirth. The expectant couple should discuss issues that could be possible sources of postpartal stress. Issues to be resolved beforehand may include the sharing of infant and household chores, help in the first few days, reapportionment of family finances, options for baby-sitting to allow the mother (and couple) some free time, the mother's return to work after the baby's birth, and sibling rivalry.

Table 16–1 • TOPICS FOR CLIENT TEACHING DURING PREGNANCY

All Three Trimesters
Discomforts of pregnancy (see Table 16–4)
Nutrition and weight gain
Sexual activity
Sibling preparation
First Trimester
Attitude toward pregnancy
Exercise and rest
Smoking; use of alcohol and other drugs
Traveling
Fetal growth and development
Danger signals associated with spontaneous abortion
Employment
Early pregnancy classes
Second Trimester
Concerns related to changes in body
Fetal growth and development
Fetal movement
Clothing
Care of skin and breasts
Beginning preparation for care of the infant (equipment and room)
Decisions about infant feeding
Third Trimester
Exercise and rest
Traveling
Danger signals
Preparation for labor and birth
Completion of preparation in home for new baby
Decisions about the infant (circumcision, method of feeding, and so forth)
Decision making for the early postpartum period
Education about psychologic and physical expectations in the early postpartum period

Care of the Pregnant Woman's Family

Relieving the expectant woman's discomforts, maintaining her physical health, and providing anticipatory guidance are important parts of nursing care management. In addition, the nurse helps meet the needs of the woman's family to better maintain the harmony and integrity of the family unit. The nurse does this by providing support and prenatal education. If the nurse is effective, family members may gain greater problem-solving ability, self-esteem, self-confidence, and ability to participate in healthcare.

Although the father of the baby is generally present, his presence cannot be assumed. If he is not a part of the family structure, it is important to assess the woman's support system to determine what significant persons in her life will play a major role during this childbearing experience.

When the father is part of the family or support system, providing anticipatory guidance to him is a necessary part of any plan of care. He may need information about the anatomic, physiologic, and emotional changes that occur during pregnancy and postpartum, the couple's sexuality and sexual response, and the reactions that he may experience. He may wish to express his feelings about breastfeeding versus formula-feeding, the sex of the child, and other topics. If it is culturally acceptable to the couple and personally acceptable to him, the nurse refers the couple to expectant parents' classes. These classes provide valuable information about pregnancy and childbirth using a variety of teaching strategies such as discussion, films, demonstrations with educational models, and written handouts. Some classes even give fathers the opportunity to get a "feel" for pregnancy by wearing a pregnancy simulator (Figure 16–1 •).

The nurse assesses the father's intended degree of participation during labor and birth and his knowledge of what to expect. If the couple prefers that his participation be minimal or restricted, the nurse supports their decision and does not try to impose personal values. Research suggests that, despite the current trend for fathers to attend prenatal childbirth classes, positive childbirth experiences are not always the outcome (Greenhalgh, Slade, & Spiby, 2000). Thus it is important for caregivers to be respectful of personal preferences. With this type of consideration and collaboration, the father is less apt to develop feelings of alienation, helplessness, and guilt during the pregnancy. The relationship between the couple may be strengthened

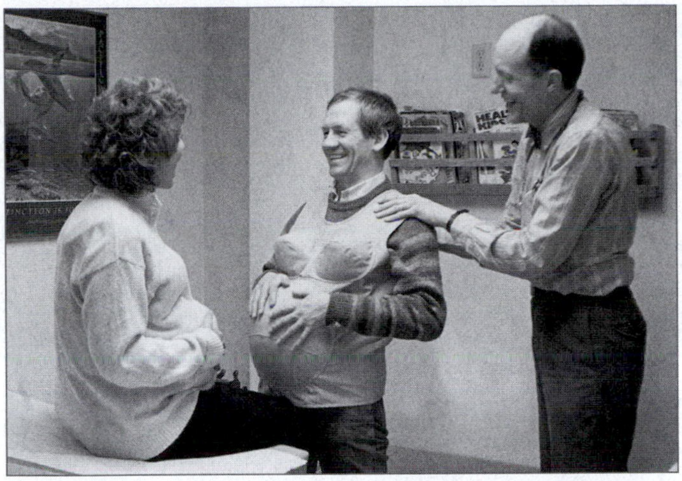

Figure 16–1 • The Empathy Belly is a pregnancy simulator that allows males and females to experience some of the symptoms of pregnancy. The "belly," which weighs 33 lb, produces symptoms such as shortness of breath, bladder pressure, shift in the center of gravity with resulting waddling gait, increased lordosis and backache, and fatigue. It can also simulate fetal kicking movements.
SOURCE: Photograph courtesy of Birthways, Inc. at empathybelly.org

and his self-esteem raised. He is then better able to provide physical and emotional support to his partner during labor and birth.

In the plan for prenatal care, the nurse also considers the effect of the pregnancy on any other children the couple may have. For example, the nurse may initiate a discussion about the ambivalence that older children may feel about the pregnancy. Parents who are unprepared for the older child's feelings of anger, jealousy, and rejection may respond inappropriately in their confusion and surprise. The nurse emphasizes that open communication between parents and children (or acting out feelings with a doll if the child is too young to verbalize) helps children master their feelings and may prevent them from hurting the baby when they are unsupervised. Children may feel less neglected and more secure if they know that their parents are willing to listen to their expressions of sadness or to help with their anger and aggressiveness.

Parents may be encouraged to bring their children to antepartal visits. Seeing what is involved and listening to the fetal heartbeat may make the pregnancy more real to siblings. Many agencies also provide sibling classes geared to different ages and levels of understanding.

Relationship changes with in-laws should be addressed as well as the woman's or couple's expectations of the grandparents. Although some grandparents are eager to assist with child care by baby-sitting, others are not. The parents should also give some thought to the best ways of dealing with possible conflicts with the grandparents over childraising approaches. Couples resolve these issues in different ways; however, postpartal adjustment is easier for a couple who agrees on the issues beforehand than for a couple who does not confront and resolve these issues.

Cultural Considerations in Pregnancy

As discussed in Chapter 2, culturally competent nursing care is critical to the provision of quality healthcare. In the United States the Caucasian population is decreasing while the population of other ethnic or minority groups, such as the Latino population, is increasing. Moreover, in many countries throughout the world diversity is increasing as more stable or prosperous areas experience an influx of immigrants seeking a more secure life. Consequently, prenatal care should always include a cultural assessment. This assessment helps the nurse better understand the client's health beliefs and practices.

DEVELOPING CULTURAL COMPETENCE

In caring for pregnant women of Native American descent, it is helpful to consider the following general points (Cesario, 2001):

- Because there are more than 500 federally recognized tribes in the United States, it is difficult to summarize common cultural characteristics of Native Americans.
- Many Native American tribes are matrilineal. Women are respected and heeded in decision making and the children belong to the clan of their mother.
- Three-generation extended families are common and the grandparents and aunts and uncles often assume primary responsibility for discipline and education of the children. Thus it is important to learn whether a new mother will be the primary caregiver for her infant.
- Many tribes are "present-oriented," viewing events such as childbearing as part of the rhythms of life. Thus, during pregnancy a Native American woman is often focused on the pregnancy itself and not on issues that will follow such as contraception or childrearing practices. This has implications for the focus of the teaching a nurse offers.

CRITICAL THINKING IN PRACTICE

Rosario Gonzalez is a 33-year-old G1P0 of Mexican American descent. She is 9 weeks pregnant when she sees the nurse at her first prenatal visit. Ms. Gonzalez is a stockbroker who works 50 to 55 hours per week. Her pregnancy history reveals that this is her first pregnancy. She states that she smokes about half a pack of cigarettes each day and has wine occasionally with meals. What are some questions the nurse should ask to increase her awareness of Ms. Gonzalez's cultural beliefs and practices? What teaching must the nurse include about Ms. Gonzalez's lifestyle?

Answer can be found in Appendix I.

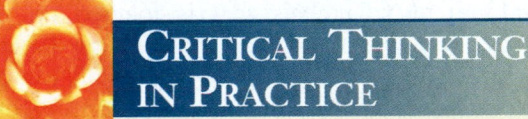

Table 16–2 • CULTURAL BELIEFS AND PRACTICES DURING PREGNANCY

Here are a few examples of cultural beliefs and practices related to pregnancy. It is important not to make assumptions about a client's beliefs, because cultural norms vary greatly within a culture and from generation to generation. The nurse should observe the client carefully and take the time to ask questions. Clients will benefit greatly from the nurse's increased awareness of their cultural beliefs and practices.

Belief or Practice	Nursing Consideration
Home Remedies	
Pregnant women of Native American background may use herbal remedies. An example is the dandelion, which contains a milky juice in its stem believed to increase breast milk flow in mothers who choose to breastfeed (Spector, 2000). Clients of Chinese descent may drink ginseng tea for faintness after childbirth or as a sedative when mixed with bamboo leaves. Some people of African heritage may use self-medication for pregnancy discomforts—for example, laxatives to prevent or treat constipation (Spector, 2000).	Find out what medications and home remedies your client is using, and counsel your client regarding overall effects. It is common for individuals to avoid telling healthcare workers about home remedies; the client may feel this will be judged unfavorably. Phrase your questions in a sensitive, accepting way.
Nutrition	
Some women of Italian background may believe that it is necessary to satisfy desires for certain foods in order to prevent congenital anomalies. Also, they may believe that they must eat food that they smell, or else the fetus will move "inside," which will result in a miscarriage. Pregnant women of African descent may continue the tradition of eating clay, dirt, or starch, which they believe will benefit the mother and fetus (Spector, 2000).	Discuss the client's beliefs and practices in regard to nutrition during pregnancy. Obtain a diet history from the client. Discuss the importance of a well-balanced diet during pregnancy, with consideration of the client's cultural beliefs and practices. In some cases, you might want to suggest remedies that may be more effective—for example, eating high-fiber foods to reduce constipation. If the home remedy is not harmful, there is no reason to ask a client to discontinue this practice.
Alternative Healthcare Providers	
Pregnant women of Mexican background may choose to seek out the care of a *partera* (midwife) for prenatal and intrapartal care. A partera speaks their language, shares a similar culture, and can care for pregnant women at home or in a birthing center instead of a hospital. Some people in Hispanic-American communities may use the *curandero*, the folk healer. The *curandero* frequently uses herbs, massage, and religious artifacts for treatment (Spector, 2000).	Discuss the variety of choices of healthcare providers available to the pregnant woman. Contrast the benefits and risks of different settings for prenatal care and birth. Provide reassurance that the goal of healthcare during pregnancy and birth is a healthy outcome for mother and baby, with respect for the specific cultural beliefs and practices of the client.
Exercise	
Pregnant women of Italian descent may fear changing their body position in certain ways because they believe this may cause the fetus to develop abnormally (Spector, 2000). Some people of European, African, and Mexican descent believe that reaching over the head during pregnancy can harm the baby.	Ask your client whether there are any activities she is afraid to do because of the pregnancy. Assure her that reaching over her head will not harm the baby, and evaluate other activities related to their effect on the pregnancy.
Spirituality	
Native Americans may want to include the medicine man (traditional healer) in their healthcare during pregnancy. The traditional healer may use feathers, corn meal, grasses, rocks, or medicine bags in healing rituals (Cesario, 2001). Some people of European background may tend to pay more attention to spirituality in their life to alleviate fears and ensure a safe birth.	Encourage the use of support systems and spiritual aids that provide comfort for the mother.

Based on the cultural assessment, the nurse can adapt to the specific healthcare needs of each perinatal client. Using the nursing process, the nurse can then formulate a transcultural nursing diagnosis that is focused on the cultural needs of the specific woman. The nursing diagnosis should reflect cultural sensitivity and build on the strengths of the client, such as "anxiety related to culturally unusual expectations for behavior and treatment" (Mattson, 2000a, p. 76).

A major goal of transcultural nursing is to understand and assist people of diverse cultural groups with their healthcare needs. Culturally competent nurses recognize that each childbearing family, shaped by culture and life experience, has expectations of both its members and the healthcare system during pregnancy and birth. Callister (2001) states that providing culturally competent care includes:

- Understanding the dimensions of culture
- Moving to a holistic approach
- Seeking to increase knowledge, change attitudes, and hone clinical skills
- Building on women's strengths (p. 210)

Pregnancy and childbirth are recognized as special or transitional events in virtually all cultures (Mattson, 2000d). Additionally, specific actions during pregnancy are often determined by cultural beliefs. According to Mattson (2000d), these beliefs can be divided into two types:

- Prescriptive beliefs or requirements that describe expected behaviors
- Restrictive beliefs, which are stated negatively and limit behaviors

Thus, these activities are viewed as having the potential to impact the outcome of the pregnancy either positively or negatively. Table 16–2 • describes activities that are encouraged (prescriptive) or forbidden (restrictive) by specific cultures. The table is not meant to be all-inclusive

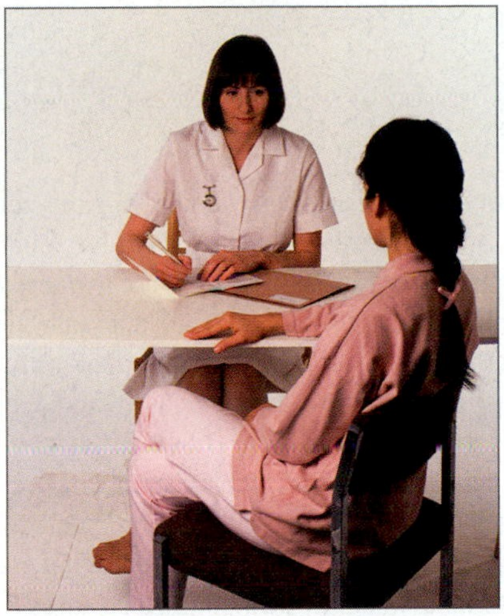

Figure 16–2 • The culturally competent nurse respects the culture and values of the pregnant women.
SOURCE: Antonia Deutsch/Dorling Kindersley Media Library.

but rather to offer a few examples of cultural activities that may be important to some clients during the prenatal period.

In working with clients of another culture, the healthcare professional should be as open as possible to other beliefs. If certain activities are not harmful, there is no need to impose one's beliefs and practices upon a person of another culture. If the activities are proving to be harmful, the nurse can consult or work with someone within the culture or someone aware of the cultural beliefs and values to see whether the client's behavior can be modified. (See Figure 16–2 •.)

In providing effective, culturally sensitive care, nurses can use the following strategies (Mattson, 2000b):

- Take actions that help break down language barriers.
- Explain the reasons for suggestions made to the woman or couple.
- Integrate folk treatments and Western medicine as much as possible.
- Enlist the family caretaker and others as needed.
- Get permission or consent to act from the right person.
- Provide printed materials in the client's language.

To provide culturally competent healthcare, nurses may need to seek outside resources. A number of helpful Web sites exist that healthcare professionals can use to promote culturally competent care. See Table 16–3 •.

In order for the nurse to evaluate if the care provided is culturally competent, it is important to have measurable outcomes of care. Willis (1999) has identified measurable outcomes of culturally competent care as the following:

- Clients demonstrate increased self-esteem and self-reliance.

Table 16–3 • WEB SITES THAT ARE HELPFUL IN PROVIDING CULTURALLY COMPETENT CARE

- Office of Minority Health of the US Department of Health and Human Services (www.omhrc.gov)
- National Center for Cultural Competence (www.dml.georgetown.edu/depts/pediatrics/gucdc/cultural.html)
- Diversity Rx Web Site (www.diversityrx.org)
- Bureau of Primary Health Care (www.bphc.hrsa.gov)

- Clients adopt behaviors that promote health and wellness.
- Clients view healthcare providers as culturally competent, collaborative professionals.
- Clients use healthcare services appropriately.
- Clients and families demonstrate positive and effective coping strategies.

Relief of the Common Discomforts of Pregnancy

Healthcare professionals often refer to the common discomforts of pregnancy as minor. These discomforts, however, are not minor to the pregnant woman.

Most of the discomforts of pregnancy are a result of physiologic and anatomic changes and are fairly specific to either the first trimester or to the second and third trimesters. Table 16–4 • identifies the common discomforts of pregnancy, their possible causes, and the self-care measures that might relieve the discomfort.

Clinical Tip *At each prenatal visit, focus your teaching on changes or possible discomforts the woman might encounter during the coming month and the next trimester. If the pregnancy is progressing normally, spend a few minutes describing her baby at this stage of development.*

First Trimester

The dramatic hormonal changes of the first trimester account for many of the discomforts experienced in this period. These discomforts tend to abate by the beginning of the fourth month of pregnancy.

NAUSEA AND VOMITING

Nausea and vomiting of pregnancy (NVP) are early, very common symptoms. These symptoms appear sometime after the first missed menstrual period and usually cease by the fourth missed menstrual period. Research indicates that approximately 70% to 85% of pregnant women experience NVP (Jewell & Young, 2001). These symptoms last, on average, 35 days. Of those women experiencing NVP,

RESEARCH IN PRACTICE
Chinese Women's Perceptions of the Effectiveness of Antenatal Education

What is this study about? Preparation for childbearing occurs both formally and informally. Western countries initiated formal antenatal education in response to a need to improve maternal-infant outcomes. Other cultures rely more exclusively on informal preparation provided from extended family members. Most research has focused on maternal preparation for labor and birth, but little has focused on preparation for motherhood. Even less attention has been given to this preparation in non-Western cultures. This study examined the attitudes of Chinese women toward antenatal motherhood preparation and the perceived effectiveness of formalized parenting education programs for this group.

How was this study done? This exploratory, qualitative study involved both participant observation and structured interview. The structure and process of five antenatal classes that focused on motherhood were observed. Eleven women who attended the classes were interviewed in two focus groups, using a semistructured interview guide. Mothers were included if they were married and primiparous, and had given birth to a healthy baby at 38 to 42 weeks' gestation. Transcripts of the focus groups were analyzed for themes through content analysis.

What were the results of the study? Findings from the focus groups and observational data fell into two common themes. The theme of structure included several subcategories. There was a perception of an unfavorable environment for the classes, both in terms of size and physical comfort of the room. The mothers noted that audiovisual aids helped stimulate interest and enhanced learning, but were often based on Western values and were not applicable to their situation. The subjects also criticized the length of the classes, and suggested shorter class sessions that reduced information overload. A second theme was class process. The mothers noted that lecture with minimal interaction was the norm, and did not feel it was an effective way to learn the information. Although the mothers felt that content was appropriate in general, the topic of common neonatal problems seemed less relevant to these women, and presentation of uncommon neonatal problems provoked anxiety. The subjects were more positive about the midwives who presented the classes, and described them as warm in their teaching. Learning about the complex emotional responses to motherhood helped these mothers prepare for mood changes they could expect, and helped their husbands understand their mood alterations more empathetically. The mothers also agreed that the antenatal period was the best time for personal preparation for becoming a mother. These mothers also reported feeling guilty if they were not successful at breastfeeding, and felt they had been given unrealistic preparation for breastfeeding problems.

What additional questions might I have? Are there similar concerns for women of Western cultures? Did these women find alternative sources of parenting education? If so, what were they? Additional research linking antenatal education to actual parenting skill would be helpful.

How can I use this study? Participants in antenatal classes have a variety of needs for information and support. Cultural sensitivity is needed to ensure prospective parents are getting the help they need prior to parenthood. Nurses are in a position to determine the needs of potential parents and provide information and support to them in a way that is structured effectively and includes appropriate processes.

Source: Ho, I., & Holroyd, E. (2002). Chinese women's perceptions of the effectiveness of antenatal education in the preparation for motherhood. *Journal of Advanced Nursing, 38*(1), 74–85.

about 80% report that the nausea lasts all day (Lacroix, Eason, & Melzak, 2000). Some women develop an aversion only to specific foods. Many experience nausea on arising in the morning, and others experience nausea only in the evening.

The exact cause of NVP is unknown but is believed to be multifactorial. Research has identified possible hormonal, metabolic, neurologic, and psychosomatic factors contributing to its development. Human chorionic gonadotropin (hCG) is often cited as a major factor because it begins to be present in the body at about the time symptoms of morning sickness usually begin, and hCG levels are subsiding when the discomfort of nausea and vomiting usually ends. Evidence also suggests that nausea is linked to rising estrogen levels, which are similar to rising hCG levels (Cunningham, Gant, Leveno, et al, 2001). Changes in carbohydrate metabolism, fatigue, and emotional factors may also play a role in the development of NVP.

Teaching for Self-Care

Treatment of nausea and vomiting is not always successful, but the symptoms can be reduced. The nurse must assess the onset, frequency, and duration of symptoms and actual nutritional intake to be helpful in suggesting methods of relief. Physical assessment of the woman should include particular attention to skin color, texture, and turgor as well as vital signs and bowel sounds. For some women, simply avoiding the odor of certain foods or other conditions that precipitate the problem may relieve nausea. If nausea occurs most frequently during early morning, the woman may find it helpful to eat dry crackers or toast before arising and to rise from bed slowly. Rising slowly and avoiding sudden position changes throughout the day may also help prevent nausea due to hypotensive episodes. In addition, the nurse can suggest that the woman avoid brushing her teeth right after eating, because this, too, may trigger vomiting. Occasionally the woman is advised to stop taking prenatal vitamins with

Table 16-4 • SELF-CARE MEASURES FOR COMMON DISCOMFORTS OF PREGNANCY

Discomfort	Influencing Factors	Self-Care Measures
First Trimester		
Nausea and vomiting	Increased levels of human chorionic gonadotropin Changes in carbohydrate metabolism Emotional factors Fatigue	Avoid odors or causative factors. Eat dry crackers or toast before arising in morning. Have small but frequent meals. Avoid greasy or highly seasoned foods. Take dry meals with fluids between meals. Drink carbonated beverages.
Urinary frequency	Pressure of uterus on bladder in both first and third trimesters	Void when urge is felt. Increase fluid intake during the day. Decrease fluid intake *only* in the evening to decrease nocturia.
Fatigue	Specific causative factors unknown May be aggravated by nocturia due to urinary frequency	Plan time for a nap or rest period daily. Go to bed earlier. Seek family support and assistance with responsibilities so that more time is available to rest.
Breast tenderness	Increased levels of estrogen and progesterone	Wear well-fitting, supportive bra.
Increased vaginal discharge	Hyperplasia of vaginal mucosa and increased production of mucus by the endocervical glands due to the increase in estrogen levels	Promote cleanliness by daily bathing. Avoid douching, nylon underpants, and pantyhose; cotton underpants are more absorbent; powder can be used to maintain dryness if not allowed to cake.
Nasal stuffiness and nosebleed (epistaxis)	Elevated estrogen levels	May be unresponsive, but cool-air vaporizer may help; avoid use of nasal sprays and decongestants.
Ptyalism (excessive, often bitter salivation)	Specific causative factors unknown	Use astringent mouthwashes, chew gum, or suck hard candy.
Second and Third Trimesters		
Heartburn (pyrosis)	Increased production of progesterone, decreasing gastrointestinal motility and increasing relaxation of cardiac sphincter, displacement of stomach by enlarging uterus, thus regurgitation of acidic gastric contents into the esophagus	Eat small and more frequent meals. Use low-sodium antacids. Avoid overeating, fatty and fried foods, lying down after eating, and sodium bicarbonate.
Ankle edema	Prolonged standing or sitting Increased levels of sodium due to hormonal influences Circulatory congestion of lower extremities Increased capillary permeability Varicose veins	Practice frequent dorsiflexion of feet when prolonged sitting or standing is necessary. Elevate legs when sitting or resting. Avoid tight garters or restrictive bands around legs.
Varicose veins	Venous congestion in the lower veins that increases with pregnancy Hereditary factors (weakening of walls of veins, faulty valves) Increased age and weight gain	Elevate legs frequently. Wear supportive hose. Avoid crossing legs at the knees, standing for long periods, garters, and hosiery with constrictive bands.
Hemorrhoids	Constipation (see following discussion) Increased pressure from gravid uterus on hemorrhoidal veins	Avoid constipation. Apply ice packs, topical ointments, anesthetic agents, warm soaks, or sitz baths; gently reinsert into rectum as necessary.
Constipation	Increased levels of progesterone, which cause general bowel sluggishness Pressure of enlarging uterus on intestine Iron supplements Diet, lack of exercise, and decreased fluids	Increase fluid intake, fiber in the diet, and exercise. Develop regular bowel habits. Use stool softeners as recommended by physician.
Backache	Increased curvature of the lumbosacral vertebrae as the uterus enlarges Increased levels of hormones, which cause softening of cartilage in body joints Fatigue Poor body mechanics	Use proper body mechanics. Practice the pelvic-tilt exercise. Avoid uncomfortable working heights, high-heeled shoes, lifting heavy loads, and fatigue.
Leg cramps	Imbalance of calcium/phosphorus ratio Increased pressure of uterus on nerves Fatigue Poor circulation to lower extremities Pointing the toes	Practice dorsiflexion of feet to stretch affected muscle. Evaluate diet. Apply heat to affected muscles. Arise slowly from resting position.

(continued on next page)

Table 16-4 • SELF-CARE MEASURES FOR COMMON DISCOMFORTS OF PREGNANCY–continued

Discomfort	Influencing Factors	Self-Care Measures
Second and Third Trimesters		
Faintness	Postural hypotension Sudden change of position causing venous pooling in dependent veins Standing for long periods in warm area Anemia	Avoid prolonged standing in warm or stuffy environments. Evaluate hematocrit and hemoglobin.
Dyspnea	Decreased vital capacity from pressure of enlarging uterus on the diaphragm	Use proper posture when sitting and standing. Sleep propped up with pillows for relief if problem occurs at night.
Flatulence	Decreased gastrointestinal motility leading to delayed emptying time Pressure of growing uterus on large intestine Air swallowing	Avoid gas-forming foods. Chew food thoroughly. Get regular daily exercise. Maintain normal bowel habits.
Carpal tunnel syndrome	Compression of median nerve in carpal tunnel of wrist Aggravated by repetitive hand movements	Avoid aggravating hand movements. Use splint as prescribed. Elevate affected arm.

iron until the nausea and vomiting decreases because iron can aggravate the symptoms. In such cases, the woman should take a folic acid supplement until she can restart the vitamins (Chez & Niebyl, 2000).

Generally, it is helpful to eat small meals every 2 to 3 hours during the day and to avoid greasy or highly seasoned foods. Food may be salted to taste. The salt increases the palatability of the food and replaces any chloride lost when the woman vomits hydrochloric acid from the stomach. Eating dry meals and taking all liquids, including soups, between meals may help some women by avoiding overdistention of the stomach. Sudden changes in blood sugar levels can be avoided if the small meals are high in low-fat protein or complex carbohydrates. Some women find that slowly sipping herbal tea (peppermint, chamomile, raspberry leaf, or spearmint) or a carbonated beverage helps reduce nausea.

More recently, some women have obtained relief from NVP by using acupressure wristbands. Research suggests that Sea-Bands with acupressure buttons are a safe, effective treatment (Steele, French, Gatherer-Boyles, et al, 2001). (See Figure 16–3 •.) As an alternative to the wristbands, women can be taught to use acupressure to a pressure point located in the wrist.

In addition to common self-care measures (see Complementary and Alternative Therapies: Ginger and Acupressure for Morning Sickness), some women find 25 mg pyridoxine (vitamin B_6) taken three times a day helpful in reducing symptoms; if vitamin B_6 is not effective, caregivers often recommend doxylamine (Unisom), an over-the-counter antihistamine (Chez & Niebyl, 2000). Although some nausea is common, the woman who suffers from extreme nausea coupled with vomiting requires further assessment. She should be advised to contact her care provider if she vomits more than once per day or shows signs of dehydration, such as dry mouth, decreased amounts of highly concentrated urine, and the like. In such cases, the physician or certified nurse-midwife (CNM) may order antiemetics. However, antiemetics should be avoided if at all possible during the first trimester because of the danger of teratogenic effects on embryo development.

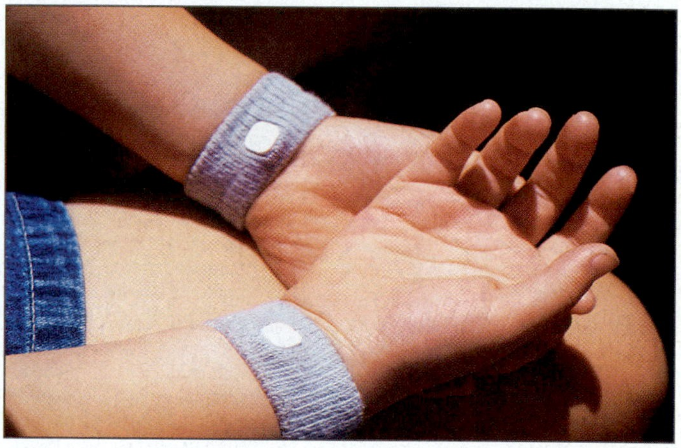

Figure 16–3 • Acupressure wristbands are sometimes used to help relieve nausea during early pregnancy.
SOURCE: © 2000–2003 Custom Medical Stock Photo—All Rights Reserved.

Nausea and vomiting generally cease by the fourth month of pregnancy. If they do not, hyperemesis gravidarum (a complication of pregnancy discussed in Chapter 20) must be considered.

URINARY FREQUENCY

Urinary frequency is a common discomfort of pregnancy. It occurs early in pregnancy and again during the third trimester because of the pressure of the enlarging uterus on the bladder. Coughing or sneezing in the last month may even cause leakage of urine. Although the glomerular filtration rate increases in pregnancy, it does not cause a significant increase in urine output. Urinary frequency is considered normal during the first and third trimesters; however, the nurse should advise the woman to contact her healthcare provider if she experiences any signs of bladder in-

Complementary and Alternative Therapies

Ginger and Acupressure for Morning Sickness

Ginger and acupressure are among the most frequently used alternative therapies for the nausea and vomiting of morning sickness.

Ginger: Ginger is widely used in traditional Chinese medicine but without contraindications in pregnancy (Blumenthal, Goldberg, & Brinckmann, 2000). Many clinical trials have confirmed the effectiveness and safety of ginger (Aikins Murphy, 1998; Fulder & Tenne, 1996; Jewell & Young, 2000; Vutyavanich, Kraisarin, & Ruangsri, 2001; Weidner & Sigwart, 2001); yet Skidmore-Roth (2001) cites that it is an abortifacient (abortion-inducing), when used in large doses. Although no specific clinical studies are cited in this latter source, ginger should be used with caution during pregnancy, and the dosage should not exceed 1 g of dried root daily (Hardy, 2000). Ginger is available in many forms, including capsules, candied, or as a tea. See Complementary and Alternative Therapies later in this chapter for more information on the use of herbs during pregnancy.

Acupressure: Acupressure, like acupuncture, is a therapy based on the ancient philosophy of traditional Chinese medicine. Acupressure involves the application of pressure using fingers or thumbs to stimulate and balance the body's healing energy known by the Chinese as chi. A specific acupressure point that relieves nausea is located on the forearm, three finger widths above the wrist closest to the palm, toward the elbow. The point is pressed firmly for 30 seconds every couple of minutes (Gottlieb, 2000). A motion sickness wristband (brand names include Sea-Band and Acuband) can be purchased that puts gentle pressure on this acupressure point (Steele, French, Gatherer-Boyles, et al, 2001).

fection such as painful urination (dysuria), burning with voiding, or blood in the urine (hematuria).

Teaching for Self-Care

There are no methods of decreasing the frequency of urination in pregnancy. Fluid intake should never be decreased to prevent frequency. The woman should be encouraged to maintain an adequate fluid intake: at least 2000 mL per day. She should also be encouraged to empty her bladder frequently (approximately every 2 hours while awake).

Frequent bladder emptying helps decrease the incidence of leakage of urine. Because frequency often results in several trips to the bathroom each night, it is important to remind the woman to consider safety factors in the home, such as a clear path to the bathroom, the use of a night-light, and the like. The woman who leaks urine may choose to wear pantyliners during the day. If she does, she should change them as soon as they become damp to avoid perineal excoriation and to avoid contamination of the perineum from the rectal area if the pads move back and forth as she walks. Tightening of the pubococcygeus muscle, which supports internal organs and controls voiding, can help maintain good perineal tone. This procedure, known as Kegel exercise, is discussed later in this chapter.

FATIGUE

Marked fatigue, often out of proportion to the woman's normal pattern, is so common in early pregnancy that it is considered a presumptive sign of pregnancy. The sleep-inducing effects of progesterone may play a role in the development of this sign (Cunningham et al, 2001). It is aggravated if the woman has to arise several times each night because of urinary frequency. Typically, it resolves soon after the end of the first trimester.

Teaching for Self-Care

Scheduling activities to allow for napping is helpful. Women should be encouraged to use every opportunity available to rest, including going to bed earlier in the evening. The woman's partner, if he is involved in the pregnancy, needs to understand that the fatigue is normal and will subside. He can be encouraged to assume more home responsibilities to support the woman and enable her to rest.

BREAST TENDERNESS

Sensitivity of the breasts occurs early and continues throughout the pregnancy. Increased levels of estrogen and progesterone contribute to the soreness and tingling felt in the breasts and to the increased sensitivity of the nipples.

Teaching for Self-Care

A well-fitting, supportive brassiere gives the most relief for this discomfort. The qualities of a properly supportive brassiere are discussed in Breast Care, later in this chapter.

INCREASED VAGINAL DISCHARGE

Increased whitish vaginal discharge, called **leukorrhea**, is common in pregnancy. It occurs as the result of hyperplasia of vaginal mucosa and increased production of mucus by the endocervical glands. In addition, the increased acidity of the secretions encourages the growth of *Candida albicans*, and the woman is thus more susceptible to monilial vaginitis.

Teaching for Self-Care

Cleanliness is important in preventing excoriation and vaginal infections. Daily bathing is adequate; douching is generally avoided during pregnancy. However, if the pregnant woman is seriously bothered by the discharge, she may find it helpful to use an occasional gentle douche of warm water that is made mildly acidic with vinegar (Cunningham et al, 2001). The woman should avoid nylon underpants and pantyhose because they retain heat and moisture in the genital area; absorbent cotton underpants should be worn to help prevent problems. The nurse can advise the pregnant woman to report any change in vaginal discharge, any irritation in the perineal area, and intense vaginal itching. These changes frequently indicate vaginal infections.

NASAL STUFFINESS AND EPISTAXIS

Once pregnancy is well established, elevated estrogen levels may produce edema of the nasal mucosa, resulting in nasal stuffiness, nasal discharge, and obstruction (rhinitis of pregnancy). *Epistaxis* (nosebleed) may also result.

Teaching for Self-Care

Cool air vaporizers and normal saline nose drops may be helpful. However, the problem is often unresponsive to treatment. Women experiencing these problems find it difficult to sleep and may resort to medicated nasal sprays and decongestants to relieve the problem. Such interventions may provide relief initially but can actually increase the nasal stuffiness over time. The use of any medication in pregnancy should be avoided if possible.

PTYALISM

Ptyalism is a rare discomfort of pregnancy in which excessive, often bitter, saliva is produced. Its cause has not been established, although stimulation of the salivary glands by the ingestion of starch has been suggested as a possible cause (Cunningham et al, 2001). Effective treatments are limited.

Teaching for Self-Care

Using astringent mouthwashes, chewing gum, or sucking on hard candy may minimize the problem of ptyalism. It may also be helpful to reduce or limit starch intake.

Second and Third Trimesters

It is difficult to classify discomforts as specifically occurring in the second or third trimester since their timing varies because of individual variations in women. The symptoms discussed in this section usually do not appear until the third trimester in primigravidas but may occur earlier with each succeeding pregnancy.

HEARTBURN (PYROSIS)

Heartburn is the regurgitation of acidic gastric contents into the esophagus. It creates a burning or irritating sensation in the esophagus and radiates upward, sometimes leaving a bad taste in the mouth. Heartburn appears to be primarily a result of the displacement of the stomach by the enlarging uterus. The increased production of progesterone in pregnancy, decreases in gastrointestinal motility, and relaxation of the cardiac (esophageal) sphincter also contribute to heartburn.

Teaching for Self-Care

Heartburn is aggravated by overeating, ingesting fatty and fried foods, and lying down soon after eating. The woman should therefore avoid these situations. The woman should be encouraged to drink an adequate amount of fluid (eight to ten 8-oz glasses) each day and to eat smaller, more frequent meals to accommodate the decreased size of her stomach. Good posture is important because it allows more room for the stomach to function. Some women choose complementary approaches to relieving their heartburn. See Complementary and Alternative Therapies: Meadowsweet for Heartburn.

> **COMPLEMENTARY AND ALTERNATIVE THERAPIES**
>
> **MEADOWSWEET FOR HEARTBURN**
>
> Meadowsweet has traditionally been used as a pain reliever (the analgesic substance *salicin* was first isolated from meadowsweet leaves in 1827); it also provides relief for heartburn (Blumenthal, 2000). However, because it contains salicylates, a woman with a sensitivity to aspirin should not take meadowsweet. See Complementary and Alternative Therapies later in this chapter for more information on the use of herbs during pregnancy.

The caregiver may recommend a low-sodium antacid, such as aluminum hydroxide (Amphojel) or a combination of aluminum hydroxide and magnesium hydroxide (Maalox). Because aluminum alone tends to cause constipation, and magnesium alone is associated with diarrhea, the combined approach is more desirable. Sodium bicarbonate (baking soda) and Alka-Seltzer should be avoided because of the potential for electrolyte imbalance.

If maternal heartburn is severe, not relieved by antacids, and accompanied by gastrointestinal reflux, an antisecretory agent (H_2-blocker) such as ranitidine (Zantac), cimetidine (Tagamet), or omeprazole (Losec) may be necessary. Research to date has not linked these medications with an excessive risk of birth defects, preterm birth, or intrauterine growth restriction. Moreover, up to 85% of pregnant women who experience acid reflux use at least one of these medications to control it ("Good News for Pregnant Women with Heartburn," 1999).

ANKLE EDEMA

Most women experience ankle edema in the last part of pregnancy because of the increasing difficulty of venous return from the lower extremities. Prolonged standing or sitting and warm weather increase the edema. It is also associated with varicose veins. Ankle edema becomes a concern only when accompanied by hypertension or proteinuria or when the edema is not postural in origin.

Teaching for Self-Care

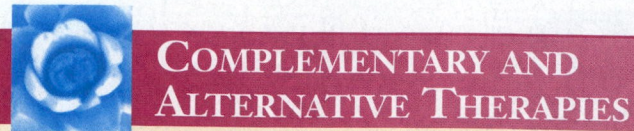

The aggravating conditions just mentioned should be avoided. If the woman has to sit or stand for long periods, frequent dorsiflexion of her feet will help contract muscles, thereby squeezing the fluid back into circulation. The pregnant woman should not wear tight garters or other restrictive bands around her legs. During rest periods, the woman should elevate her legs and hips as described in the following section on varicose veins.

VARICOSE VEINS

Varicose veins are a result of weakening of the walls of veins or faulty functioning of the valves. Poor circulation in the lower extremities predisposes the woman to varicose veins in the legs and thighs, as does prolonged standing or sitting. The weight of the gravid uterus on the pelvic veins aggravates the development of varicosities in the legs and pelvic area by preventing good venous return. Increased maternal age, excessive weight gain, a large fetus, heredity, and multiple pregnancy can all contribute to the problem.

Vulvar varicosities may also be a problem in pregnancy, although they are less common. Varicosities in the vulva and perineum cause aching and a sense of heaviness.

Treatment of varicose veins by surgery or by the injection method is not recommended during pregnancy (Cunningham et al, 2001). The woman should be aware that treatment might be needed after pregnancy because the problem will be aggravated by a succeeding pregnancy.

Teaching for Self-Care

Regular exercise, such as swimming, cycling, or walking, promotes venous return, which helps prevent varicosities. Avoiding factors that contribute to venous stasis is also helpful. The pregnant woman should avoid standing or sitting for prolonged periods. She should also avoid crossing her legs at the knees because of the pressure on her veins. She should not wear garters or hosiery with constricting bands, such as knee-high hose. However, supportive hose or elastic stockings may be extremely helpful. Supportive hose should be put on in the morning and should be washed daily with soap and warm water to help retain elasticity. In addition, some women advocate the use of complementary care in relieving varicose veins. See Complementary and Alternative Therapies: Horse Chestnut for Varicose Veins.

The pregnant woman should be encouraged to elevate her legs level with her hips when she sits. She can enhance comfort by supporting the entire leg rather than simply propping her feet up on a stool, which may lead to hyperextension of the knees. The woman who sits or stands for long periods should walk around frequently to promote venous return to the heart. She can also be encouraged to dorsiflex her feet, hold the position for 3 seconds, then release, with 8 to 10 repetitions several times each day. Venous return is most effectively promoted if the woman lies down with her feet elevated several times a day. To avoid difficulty related to pressure of the uterus on the vena cava, the woman can lie with her legs elevated on pillows and a pillow placed under one hip to displace the uterus to one side (Figure 16–4 •).

Wearing two sanitary pads inside the underpants can provide support for vulvar varicosities. Elevation of only the legs aggravates vulvar varicosities by creating stasis of blood in the pelvic area. Therefore, it is important that the pelvic area also be elevated to promote venous drainage into the trunk of the body. More than one firm pillow under the hips may be needed to accomplish this elevation. Near the end of pregnancy, this position may be extremely awkward; the woman may best relieve uterine pressure on the pelvic veins by resting on her side. Blocks may also be placed under the foot of her bed to elevate it slightly.

FLATULENCE

Flatulence results from decreased gastrointestinal motility, leading to delayed emptying, and from pressure upon the large intestine by the growing uterus. Air swallowing may also contribute to the problem.

Teaching for Self-Care

The woman should be advised to avoid gas-forming foods and to chew her food thoroughly. Regular bowel habits and exercise can also decrease flatulence.

Complementary and Alternative Therapies

Horse Chestnut for Varicose Veins

Horse chestnut seed extract may be helpful in preventing or reducing varicose veins (Blumenthal, 2000; Gottlieb, 2000). It is available in oral form (capsules, tincture, etc), as well as topical (gel) form. It is reported to combine well with other herbs that improve peripheral circulation, such as ginkgo leaf and bilberry fruit (Morgan & Bone, 1998). See Complementary and Alternative Therapies later in this chapter for more information on the use of herbs during pregnancy.

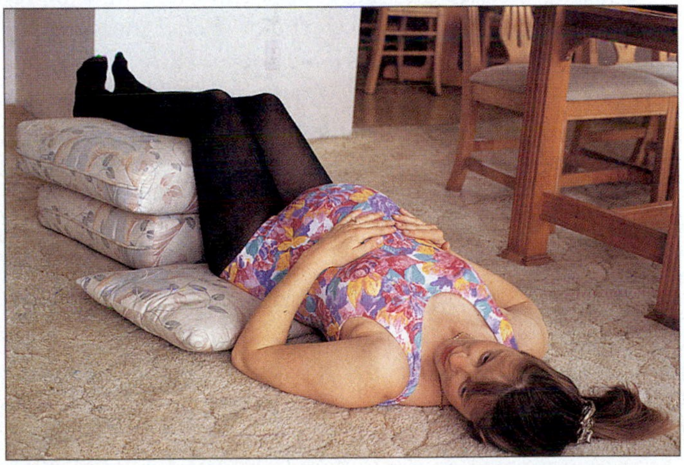

Figure 16–4 • Swelling and discomfort from varicosities can be decreased by lying down with the legs and one hip elevated (to avoid compression of the vena cava).

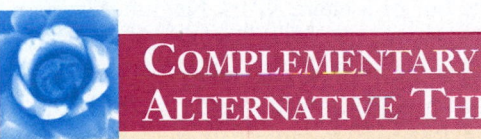

HEMORRHOIDS

Hemorrhoids are varicosities of the veins in the lower end of the rectum and anus. In the nonpregnant state, the straining that occurs with constipation usually causes hemorrhoids. During pregnancy, the gravid uterus presses on the veins and interferes with venous circulation. As the pregnancy progresses, the straining that accompanies constipation can contribute to the development of hemorrhoids.

Hemorrhoids may not bother some women until the second stage of labor, when the hemorrhoids appear as they push just before birth. Hemorrhoids that occur in pregnancy or at birth usually become asymptomatic after the early postpartal period.

Symptoms of hemorrhoids include itching, swelling, pain, and bleeding. Internal hemorrhoids are located above the anal sphincter and are responsible for bleeding, usually with defecation. They are not usually painful unless they protrude from the anus. External hemorrhoids are located outside the anal sphincter. They are not usually the source of bleeding or pain; however, thrombosis of the hemorrhoids can occur, and in that case they become extremely painful. The thrombosis may resolve itself in 24 hours, or the physician can treat it by incising and evacuating the blood clot. Women who have hemorrhoids prior to pregnancy frequently experience more difficulties with them during pregnancy.

Teaching for Self-Care

Relief can be achieved by gently and carefully reinserting the hemorrhoids. The woman lies on her side or in the knee to chest position. She places some lubricant on her finger and presses against the hemorrhoids, pushing them inside. She holds them in place for 1 to 2 minutes and then gently withdraws her finger. The anal sphincter should then hold them inside the rectum. The woman will find it especially helpful if she can then maintain a side-lying (Sims') position for a time, so this procedure is best done before bed or prior to a daily rest period.

Avoiding constipation is important in preventing or relieving the discomfort of hemorrhoids. Relief measures for existing hemorrhoid symptoms include ice packs, use of topical ointments and anesthetic agents, and warm soaks.

The woman should contact her healthcare provider if the hemorrhoids become hardened and noticeably tender to touch. Rectal bleeding that is more than spotting following defecation should also be reported.

CONSTIPATION

Conditions in pregnancy that predispose the woman to constipation include general bowel sluggishness caused by increased progesterone and steroid metabolism; displacement of the intestines, which increases with the growth of the fetus; and oral iron supplements, which most pregnant women need.

Teaching for Self-Care

Increased fluid intake (at least 2000 mL/day), adequate roughage or bulk in the diet, regular bowel habits, and adequate daily exercise can often maintain good bowel function in women who have not had previous problems. Some women find it helpful to drink a warm beverage or glass of prune juice in the morning. Women should leave sufficient time following breakfast so that the natural action of the body will produce defecation.

In severe or preexisting cases of constipation, the woman may need a mild laxative, stool softeners, or suppositories as recommended by her caregiver.

BACKACHE

Many pregnant women experience backache due primarily to the increased curvature of the lumbosacral vertebrae that occurs as the uterus enlarges and becomes heavier. Circulating steroid hormones cause a softening and relaxation of pelvic joints, contributing to the problem. If the woman does not learn how to correct this curvature, the strain on the muscles and ligaments will cause backache.

Teaching for Self-Care

An exercise called the pelvic tilt (discussed later in this chapter) can help restore proper body alignment. As the anterior pelvis is tilted upward, the curvature of the back is automatically decreased, relieving much of the discomfort. If proper body alignment is maintained throughout pregnancy, backaches can be relieved or even prevented. See Exercises to Prepare for Childbirth, later in this chapter.

The use of proper posture and good body mechanics throughout pregnancy is important. The pregnant woman should avoid bending over to lift or pick up items from the floor. The strain is felt in the muscles of the back. Leg muscles should be used to do the work instead. The woman can keep her back straight by bending her knees to lower her body into the squatting position (Figure 16–5 •). She should place her feet 12 to 18 inches apart to maintain body balance. When lifting a heavy object, such as a child, she should place one foot flat on the floor, slightly in front of the other foot, and lower herself to the other knee. The object is held close to her body for lifting. This same principle of keeping the back straight and bending the knees applies when the woman sits down or gets out of a chair. Work heights that require constant bending can contribute to backache and should be adjusted as necessary. See Complementary and Alternative Therapies: Physical Modalities for Relief of Backache and Other Pregnancy-Related Muscular Pain for information on other relief measures.

A pendulous abdomen contributes to backache by increasing the curvature of the spine. The use of a supportive maternity girdle is discussed later in this chapter, as is the role of high-heeled shoes in increasing the lumbosacral curvature.

LEG CRAMPS

Leg cramps are painful muscle spasms in the gastrocnemius muscles. They occur most frequently at night after the woman has gone to bed but may occur at other times. Ex-

COMPLEMENTARY AND ALTERNATIVE THERAPIES

PHYSICAL MODALITIES FOR RELIEF OF BACKACHE AND OTHER PREGNANCY-RELATED MUSCULAR PAIN

Massage Therapy for Low Back Pain: Massage often helps relieve the low back pain associated with pregnancy. During the first 4 months of pregnancy, the body should be massaged with a gentle, soft touch. The best position for lumbar massage is with the woman sitting on a stool, resting her arms on a table, and leaning her forehead against her arms. The person doing the massage kneels on the floor behind her, which enhances the ability to apply an effective amount of pressure to the back muscles.

Yoga: Many women find that the regular practice of yoga builds and tones muscles, increases flexibility, improves endurance, and promotes a state of relaxation. One of the many applications of yoga is in pregnancy and childbirth. In fact, many of the techniques taught in childbirth classes, such as focus, relaxation, and systematic breathing, have their roots in yoga. The gentle stretching of the poses helps ease the muscle aches of pregnancy and strengthens the muscles that will be used during childbirth. The breathing techniques may lessen the shortness of breath that often accompanies advanced pregnancy.

Yoga practiced while pregnant is slightly different from regular yoga in that some poses are contraindicated. These poses are the extreme stretching positions and any position that puts pressure on the uterus. Full forward bends will probably be uncomfortable for both woman and baby. A woman's center of balance has shifted completely, and thus she must be careful with balance poses. Pregnant women should never lie on the stomach for any pose. If any pose feels uncomfortable, the woman should stop at once. If she experiences dizziness, sudden swelling, extreme shortness of breath, or vaginal bleeding, she should see her midwife or doctor immediately.

Reflexology for Sciatica: Reflexology is a field of therapy that uses specific touch techniques to stimulate "reflex points and areas" on the feet, hands, and ears. Reflexologists believe that each of these points corresponds to a specific part of the body. The growing baby can put pressure on the large sciatic nerve. The pressure inflames the nerve, causing severe lower back pain that radiates into the legs. Reflexology may help this condition. The reflex points for the sciatic nerve are on the heel. A woman in her second or third trimester can press gently and release with her thumbs to stimulate first one whole heel, then the other. Each heel can be worked for a minute or two twice a day until the pain is gone.

Women who are in the first trimester of pregnancy should not have reflexology that stimulates the uterine points on the hands, feet, or ears. In general, it's best for pregnant women to receive reflexology that uses light, gentle pressure (Gottlieb, 2000).

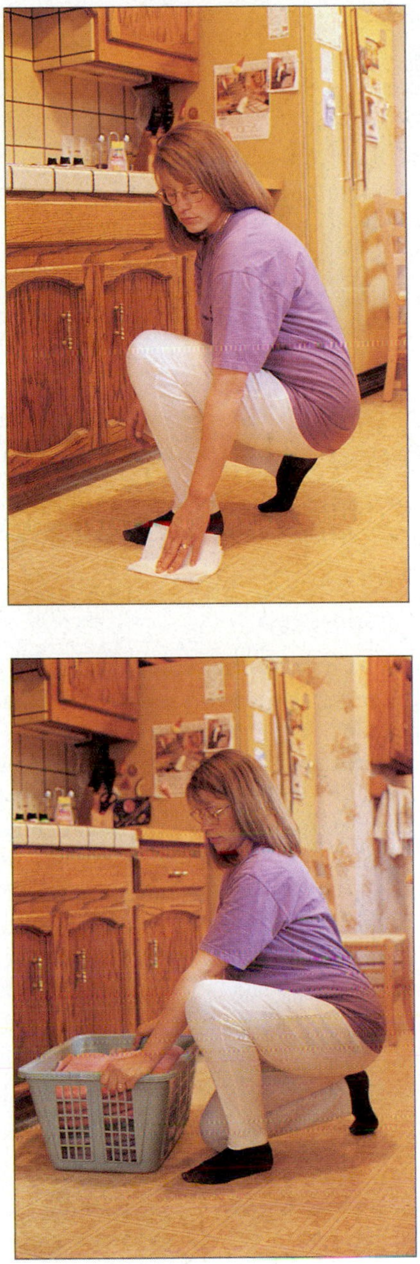

Figure 16–5 • When picking up objects from floor level or lifting objects, the pregnant woman must use proper body mechanics.

tension of the foot can often cause leg cramps. The nurse should warn the pregnant woman not to extend the foot during childbirth preparation exercises or during rest periods.

The exact cause of leg cramps is not known. Proposed contributing factors include an inadequate calcium intake, an imbalance in the calcium/phosphorus ratio, pressure of the enlarged uterus on the pelvic nerves leading to the legs, or pressure on the pelvic vessels causing impaired circulation.

Leg cramps are more common in the third trimester because of increased weight of the uterus on the nerves supplying the lower extremities. Fatigue and poor circulation in the lower extremities contribute to this problem.

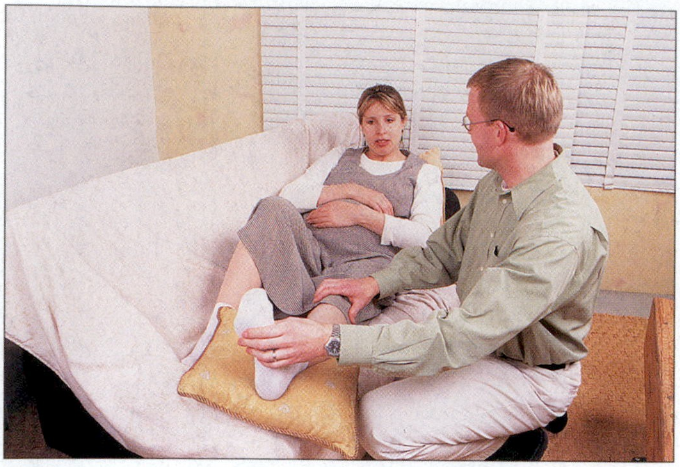

Figure 16–6 ● The expectent father can help relieve the woman's painful leg cramps by flexing her foot and straightening her leg.

Teaching for Self-Care

The woman can achieve immediate relief of the muscle spasm by stretching the muscle. With the woman lying on her back, another person can press the woman's knee down to straighten her leg while pushing her foot toward her leg (Figure 16–6 ●). The woman may also stand and put her foot flat on the floor. Massage and warm packs can be used to alleviate discomfort from leg cramps. Stretching exercises before bedtime may help prevent leg cramps. The caregiver may recommend that the woman drink no more than a pint of milk daily and take calcium carbonate or that she drink a quart of milk daily and take aluminum hydroxide gel. The gel absorbs phosphorus and eliminates it directly through the intestinal tract. The treatment recommendations depend on the frequency of the leg cramps.

CARE PLAN: COMMON DISCOMFORTS OF PREGNANCY
MEDIALINK

FAINTNESS

Many pregnant women occasionally feel faint, especially in warm, crowded areas. Faintness is caused by a combination of changes in the blood volume and postural hypotension due to venous pooling of blood in the dependent veins. Sudden change of position or standing for prolonged periods can cause this sensation, and fainting can occur.

Teaching for Self-Care

The nurse should first be certain that the pregnant woman understands the symptoms of faintness. These include slight dizziness, a "swirling" or "floating" sensation, and a decreased ability to hear or focus attention. If a woman feels faint from prolonged standing or from being in a warm, crowded room, she should sit down and lower her head between her knees. If this procedure does not help, the woman should be assisted to an area where she can lie down and get fresh air. When arising from a resting position, she should move slowly. Women whose jobs require standing in one place for long periods should march in place regularly to increase venous return from the legs.

SHORTNESS OF BREATH

Shortness of breath occurs as the uterus rises into the abdomen and causes pressure on the diaphragm. This problem worsens in the last trimester as the enlarged uterus presses directly on the diaphragm, decreasing vital capacity. The primigravida experiences considerable relief from shortness of breath in the last few weeks of pregnancy, when **lightening** occurs, and the fetus and uterus move down in the pelvis. Because the multigravida does not usually experience lightening until labor, shortness of breath will continue throughout her pregnancy.

Teaching for Self-Care

During the day, sitting straight in a chair and using proper posture when standing help provide relief. If distress is great at night, the woman can sleep propped up in bed with several pillows behind her head and shoulders.

DIFFICULTY SLEEPING

Sleep disturbances are common during pregnancy, especially in the late third trimester (Mindell & Jacobson, 2000). Although the pregnant woman may experience difficulty sleeping for many of the same psychologic reasons as the nonpregnant woman, many physical factors also contribute to this problem. The enlarged uterus may make it difficult to find a comfortable position for sleep, and an active fetus may aggravate the problem. The other discomforts of pregnancy such as urinary frequency, shortness of breath, and leg cramps may also be contributing factors.

Teaching for Self-Care

The nurse should conduct a thorough assessment of the sleep habits of the pregnant woman and offer information about habits and activities that help promote restful sleep (Mindell & Jacobsen, 2000). The pregnant woman may find it helpful to drink a warm (caffeine-free) beverage before bed and may benefit from a soothing backrub given by her partner or a family member. Pillows may be used to provide support for her back, between her legs, or for her upper arm when she lies on her side. Relaxation techniques may also help. The woman should avoid caffeine products, stimulating activity, and sleeping medication.

ROUND LIGAMENT PAIN

As the uterus enlarges during pregnancy, the round ligaments stretch, hypertrophy, and lengthen as the uterus rises up in the abdomen. Round ligament pain is attributed to this stretching.

Teaching for Self-Care

The woman may feel concern when she first experiences round ligament pain because it is often intense and causes a "grabbing" sensation in the lower abdomen and inguinal area. The nurse should warn women of this possible discomfort. Few treatment measures really alleviate this discomfort, but understanding the cause will help decrease anxiety. Once the caregiver has ascertained that the cause of the discomfort is not related to a medical complication such as appendicitis or gallbladder disease, the woman may find that a heating pad applied to the abdomen brings some relief. She may also benefit from bringing her knees up on her abdomen.

CARPAL TUNNEL SYNDROME

Carpal tunnel syndrome (CTS) results from compression of the median nerve in the carpal tunnel of the wrist. The syndrome is commonly bilateral but may be more pronounced in the dominant hand and is characterized by numbness, tingling, or burning in the fleshy part of the palm near the thumb. During pregnancy, approximately one fourth of women experience symptoms of CTS (Cunningham et al, 2001). The syndrome is aggravated by repetitive hand movements, such as typing, and may disappear following birth. Treatment involves splinting, avoiding aggravating movements, and in some cases injecting steroids into the carpal tunnel. Surgery is indicated in severe cases.

Teaching for Self-Care

Although the condition is not preventable, the woman should be advised to avoid aggravating activities and use her splint as directed.

Promotion of Self-Care During Pregnancy

The pregnant woman is faced with the important responsibility of maintaining her health not only for her sake but also for the sake of her fetus. Nurses can help promote maternal and fetal well-being by providing expectant couples with accurate and complete information about health behaviors that can affect pregnancy and childbirth. Some women prefer to gather their own information. The nurse can refer these women to a variety of sources, including the National Women's Health Information Center, which is sponsored by the US Public Health Service's Office on Women's Health.

Fetal Activity Monitoring

Many caregivers encourage pregnant women to monitor their unborn child's well-being by regularly assessing fetal activity beginning at 28 weeks' gestation. Research has documented a good positive correlation between maternal perception of fetal movement and fetal movement confirmed by ultrasound monitoring (Christensen & Rayburn, 1999; Cunningham et al, 2001). Vigorous fetal activity generally provides reassurance of fetal well-being, whereas a marked decrease in activity or cessation of movement may indicate possible fetal compromise requiring immediate evaluation. Sound, drugs, cigarette smoking, fetal sleep state, and time of day affect fetal activity. At times, a healthy fetus may be minimally active or inactive.

A variety of methods for assessing fetal activity have been developed. They focus on having the woman keep a **fetal movement record (FMR),** such as the Cardiff Count-to-Ten Method (Figure 16–7 •). A FMR is a noninvasive technique that enables the pregnant woman to monitor and record fetal well-being easily and without expense. The woman's perceptions of fetal movements and her commitment to completing a movement record may vary. Ideally, when the woman understands the purpose of the assessment, how to complete the form, whom to call with questions, and what to report, and has the opportunity for follow-up during each visit, she will see this as an important activity. See client Teaching: What to Tell the Pregnant Woman about Assessing Fetal Activity.

> *I like doing the fetal movement counts each day. It gives me a "time out," when I can focus on my baby and really enjoy this very special time in my life.*

Breast Care

Whether the pregnant woman plans to formula-feed or breastfeed her infant, proper support of the breasts is important to promote comfort, retain breast shape, and prevent back strain, particularly if the breasts become large and pendulous. The sensitivity of the breasts in pregnancy is also relieved by good support.

A well-fitting, supportive brassiere has the following qualities:

- The straps are wide and do not stretch (elastic straps soon lose their tautness due to the weight of the breasts and frequent washing).
- The cup holds all breast tissue comfortably.
- The brassiere has tucks or other devices that allow it to expand, thus accommodating the enlarging chest circumference.
- The brassiere supports the nipple line approximately midway between the elbow and shoulder. At the same time, the brassiere is not pulled up in the back by the weight of the breasts.

Cleanliness of the breasts is important, especially as the woman begins producing colostrum. Colostrum that crusts on the nipples should be removed with warm water. The woman planning to breastfeed should not use soap on her nipples because of its drying effect.

Nipple preparation, begun during the third trimester, helps prevent soreness during the early days of breastfeeding. Nipple preparation promotes the distribution of the natural lubricants produced by Montgomery's tubercles and helps develop the protective layer of skin over the nipple. Women who are planning to breastfeed can begin by going braless when possible and by exposing their nipples to sunlight and air. Rubbing the nipples removes

Sample Cardiff–Count–to–Ten scoring card

Month: ________ Week of gestation at beginning of month: ________

	9:00 AM	9:30	10:00	10:30	11:00	11:30	12:00 PM	12:30	1:00	1:30	2:00	2:30	3:00	3:30	4:00	4:30	5:00	5:30	6:00	6:30	7:00	7:30	8:00	8:30	9:00
1																									
2																									
3																									
4																									
5																									
6																									
7																									
8																									
9																									
10																									
11																									
12																									
13																									
14																									
15																									
16																									
17																									
18																									
19																									
20																									
21																									
22																									
23																									
24																									
25																									
26																									
27																									
28																									
29																									
30																									
31																									

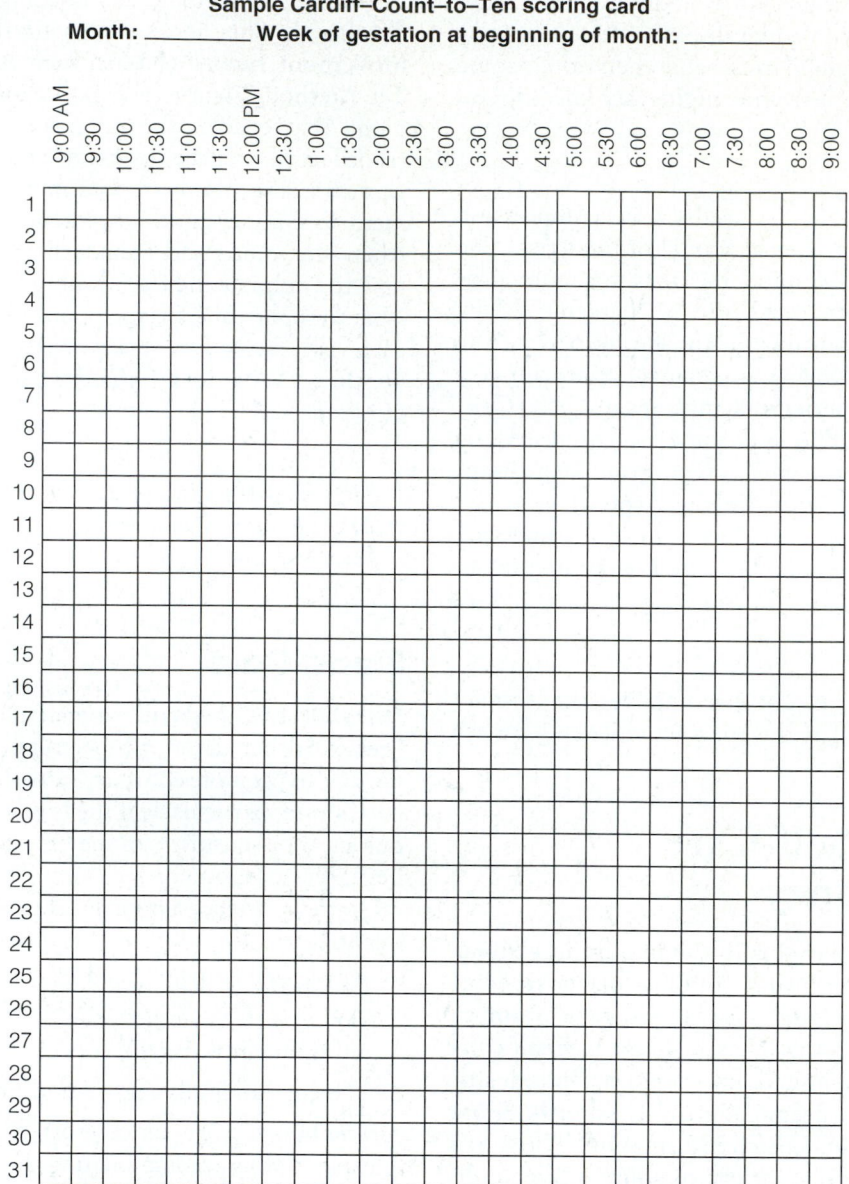

Figure 16–7 • An adaptation of the Cardiff Count-to-Ten scoring card for fetal movement assessment.

protective lubrication and should be avoided, but rolling the nipple may be beneficial. This is done by grasping the nipple between thumb and forefinger and gently rolling and pulling on it. A woman with a history of preterm labor is advised not to do this because nipple stimulation triggers the release of oxytocin. (See Chapter 20 for further discussion .)

Nipple rolling is more difficult for women with flat or inverted nipples, but it is still a useful preparation for breastfeeding. True nipple inversion, which is rare, is usually diagnosed during the initial antepartal assessment. Occasionally, a nipple appears inverted at all times. In other cases, the nipple appears normal initially, but pressure on the areola with the examiner's thumb and finger causes the nipple to retract. The normal or flat nipple protrudes when this is done (Figure 16–8 •).

Some women with truly inverted nipples may benefit from wearing special breast shields for the last 3 months of pregnancy (Figure 16–9 •). Others gain no benefit from them (Chez & Friedmann, 2000). These shields tend to absorb moisture and can cause a rash, so they should not be worn more than a few hours at a time. Alternatively, women with flat or inverted nipples who wish to breastfeed may find it helpful to stimulate the nipple or nipples postpartally by using an electric breast pump before having the baby latch on (Chez & Friedmann, 2000).

Oral stimulation of the nipple by the woman's partner during sex play is also an excellent technique for toughening the nipple in preparation for breastfeeding. The couple who enjoys this stimulation should be encouraged to continue it throughout the pregnancy, except when the woman has a history of preterm labor, as discussed earlier.

CLIENT TEACHING — WHAT TO TELL THE PREGNANT WOMAN ABOUT ASSESSING FETAL ACTIVITY

Assessment The nurse focuses on the woman's prior knowledge and former use of fetal movement assessment methods, the week of gestation, and her communication and ability to understand and process information.

Nursing Diagnosis The key nursing diagnosis will probably be

Health-Seeking Behaviors: Information on assessing fetal activity related to an expressed desire to monitor her baby's well-being.

Nursing Plan and Implementation The teaching plan provides general information about fetal movement and assessment methods the pregnant woman can use at home.

Client Goals At the completion of the teaching session the woman will

- Discuss the types of fetal assessment methods, reasons for assessment, how to accomplish the assessment, and methods of record keeping.
- Demonstrate the use of a fetal movement record.
- Identify resources to call if questions arise.
- Agree to bring the fetal movement record to each prenatal visit.

Teaching Plan

CONTENT	TEACHING METHOD
Explain that fetal movements are first felt around 18 weeks' gestation. From that time the fetal movements get stronger and easier to detect. A slowing or stopping of fetal movement may be an indication that the fetus needs some attention and evaluation.	Describe procedures and demonstrate how to assess fetal movement. Sit beside woman and show her how to place her hand on the fundus to feel fetal movement.
Explain procedure for Cardiff Count-to-Ten method or for the Daily Fetal Movement Record (DFMR). For both methods, advise the woman to	Provide a written teaching sheet for the woman's use at home.
• Beginning at about 27 weeks gestation, keep a daily record of fetal movement.	Demonstrate how to record fetal movements on Cardiff Count-to-Ten scoring card or on DFMR.
• Try to begin counting at about the same time each day, about 1 hour after a meal if possible.	Watch woman fill out record as examples are provided. Encourage her to complete the record each day and bring it with her to each prenatal visit. Assure her that the record will be discussed at each prenatal visit, and questions may be addressed at that time if desired.
• Lie quietly in a side-lying position.	
Using the Cardiff card, have the woman place an X for each fetal movement until she has recorded 10. Movement varies considerably, but most women feel fetal movement at least 10 times in 3 hours (see Figure 16–7).	
Using the DFMR have the woman count three times a day for 20 to 30 minutes each session. If there are fewer than three movements in a session, have the woman count for 1 hour or more.	
Explain when to contact the care provider:	Provide the woman with a name and phone number in case she has further questions.
If there are fewer than 10 movements in 3 hours	
If overall the fetus's movements are slowing, and it takes much longer each day to note 10 movements	
If there are no movements in the morning	
If there are fewer than 3 movements in 8 hours	

EVALUATION

Evaluate learning by having the woman explain the method and by asking the woman to fill the card in using a fictitious situation. At each prenatal visit review the expectant woman's record. Review of the record provides opportunities for questions and clarification.

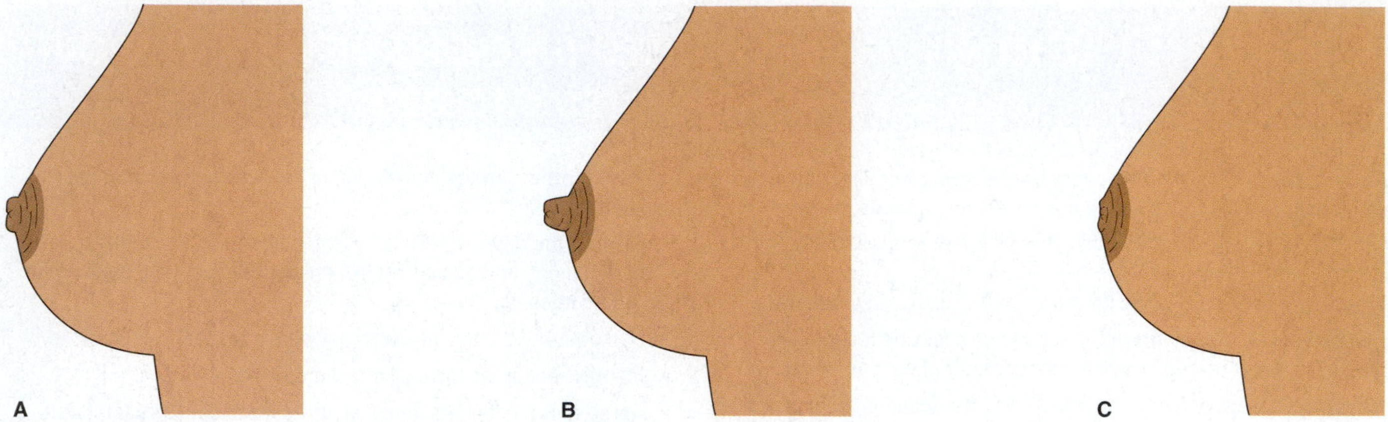

Figure 16–8 • *A,* When not stimulated, normal and inverted nipples often look alike. *B,* When stimulated, the normal nipple protrudes. *C,* When stimulated, the inverted nipple retracts. However, great variation exists; in some women, for example, one or both nipples always appear inverted, even when not stimulated.

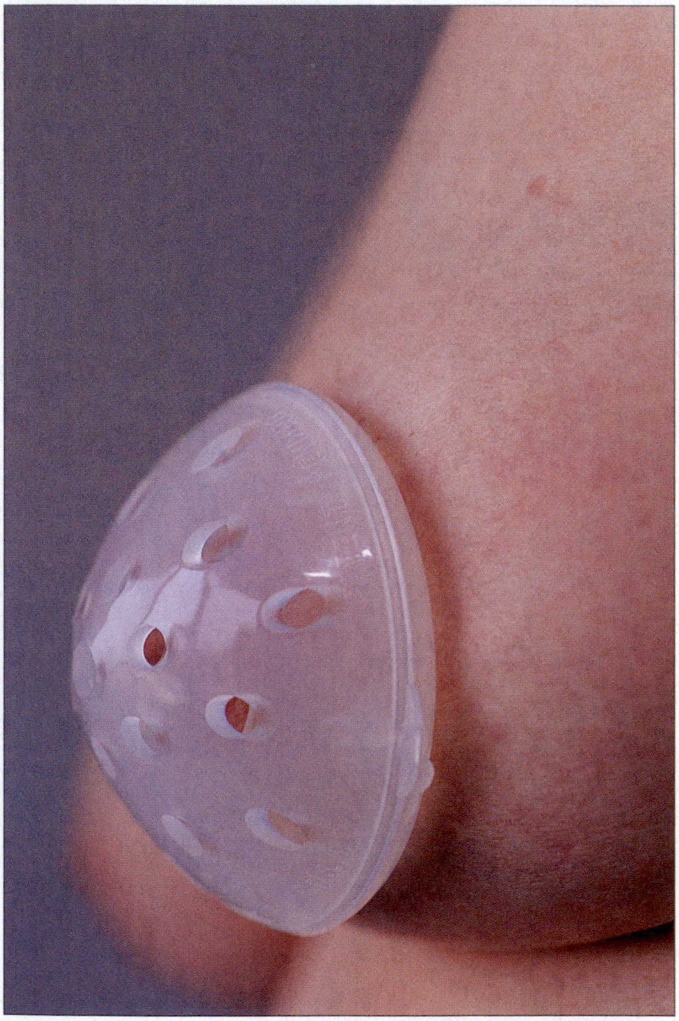

Figure 16–9 • This breast shield is designed to increase the protractility of inverted nipples. Worn the last 3 to 4 months of pregnancy, they exert gentle pulling pressure at the edge of the areola, gradually forcing the nipple through the center of the shield. They may be used after birth if necessary.

Table 16–5 • provides a list of Web sites available for women who want more information on breastfeeding.

Clothing

Traditionally, maternity clothes have been constructed with fuller lines to allow for the increase in abdominal size during pregnancy. Skirts and slacks have soft elastic waistbands and a stretchable panel over the abdominal area. However, maternity wear has changed in recent years and now also includes clothes that are more fitted, with less attempt to hide the pregnant abdomen (Cunningham et al, 2001). Maternity clothing is expensive, however, and is worn for a relatively short time. Women can economize by sharing clothes with friends, sewing their own garments, or buying used maternity clothing.

Clothing should be loose and nonconstricting. Maternity girdles are seldom worn today and are not necessary for most women. They are sometimes used by women athletes, such as runners, dancers, or gymnasts, who maintain a light workout schedule during pregnancy. Women with large, pendulous abdomens may also benefit from a well-fitting, supportive girdle. Without this support, the pendulous abdomen increases the curvature of the spine and is a source of backache and general discomfort. Tight leg bands on girdles should be avoided.

High-heeled shoes aggravate back discomfort by increasing the curvature of the spine. They should not be worn if the woman experiences backache or problems with her balance. Shoes should fit properly and feel comfortable.

Bathing

Daily bathing is important because of the increased perspiration and mucoid vaginal discharge that occurs during pregnancy. The woman may take either a shower or a tub bath, according to her preference. Caution is needed during tub baths because balance becomes a problem as

Table 16–5 • WEB SITES FOR INFORMATION ABOUT BREASTFEEDING

Web Site	Usefulness
www.lalecheleague.org	Home page of the LaLeche League. Offers useful information on all aspects of breastfeeding.
www.aap.org	Home page of the American Academy of Pediatrics. Offers information on a variety of issues related to infant care. Also provides information about medications that will pass into breast milk.
www.nomotc.org	Home page of the National Organization of Mothers of Twins Club. Provides useful information about caring for multiple births, including successful breastfeeding.
www.breastfeeding.com	Contains a wide range of information such as choosing nursing bras and breast pumps, getting started breastfeeding, and frequently asked questions. Also contains a link to video clips about breastfeeding.
www.babyfriendly.org	Home page for UNICEF UK Baby Friendly Initiative. Contains information for practitioners and for parents with a British focus.

pregnancy advances. Rubber tub mats and handgrips are valuable safety devices. Moreover, vasodilation due to the warm water may cause the woman to experience some faintness when she attempts to get out of the tub. Thus she may require assistance, especially in the third trimester. To avoid introducing infection, tub baths are contraindicated in the presence of vaginal bleeding or when the membranes are ruptured.

Employment

Because increasing numbers of women of childbearing age are part of the workforce, it is important to be aware of the effects of occupation on pregnancy. Pregnant women who are employed in jobs that require prolonged standing do have a higher incidence of preterm birth (Cunningham et al, 2001). Research also suggests that pregnant women who engage in physically demanding work have an increased incidence of preterm birth, fetal growth restriction, and hypertension (Mozurkewich, Luke, Avni, et al, 2000).

Major deterrents to employment during pregnancy include fetotoxic hazards in the environment, excessive physical strain, overfatigue, and medical or pregnancy-related complications. In the last half of pregnancy, occupations involving balance should be adjusted to protect the mother.

Fetotoxic hazards in the environment are always a concern to the expectant couple. If the pregnant woman or the woman contemplating pregnancy is working in industry, she should contact her company physician or nurse about possible hazards in her work environment and should do her own reading and research on environmental hazards as well.

Travel

If medical or pregnancy complications are not present, there are no restrictions on travel. Pregnant women should avoid travel if there is a history of bleeding or preeclampsia or if multiple births are anticipated.

Travel by automobile can be especially fatiguing, aggravating many of the discomforts of pregnancy. The pregnant woman needs frequent opportunities to get out of the car and walk. (A good pattern to follow is to stop every 2 hours and walk around for approximately 10 minutes.) The American College of Obstetricians and Gynecologists (ACOG, 1998) has formulated guidelines for the use of seat belts during pregnancy. These guidelines state that the pregnant woman should use a properly positioned three-point restraint. She should wear both lap and shoulder belts. The lap belt should fit snugly and be positioned under the abdomen and across the upper thighs. The shoulder belt should be positioned snugly between the breasts. Seat belts play an important role in preventing maternal mortality with subsequent fetal loss (Cunningham et al, 2001). Fetal loss in car accidents is also caused by placental separation as a result of uterine distortion. Use of the shoulder belt decreases the risk of traumatic flexion of the woman's body, thus decreasing the risk of placental separation. Studies suggest that most pregnant women use car seat belts but are not well informed about their correct use during pregnancy (Johnson & Pring, 2000; Tyroch, Kaups, Rohan, et al, 1999). Thus, it clearly is important for nurses to provide information about car safety early in the prenatal period.

As pregnancy progresses, travel by airplane or train is generally recommended for long distances. However, those women who have medical or obstetric complications such as poorly controlled diabetes, sickle cell disease, or preeclampsia, and those women with placental abnormalities or who are at risk for preterm birth are advised to avoid flying during pregnancy (ACOG, 2002). Prior to flying, the pregnant woman should check with her particular airline to see if it has any travel restrictions. Currently, flying is considered safe up to 36 weeks' gestation in the absence of any obstetric or medical complications. To avoid the development of phlebitis or blood clots, pregnant women should wear support hose while flying. They should also be advised to request an aisle seat and walk about the plane at regular intervals. The availability of medical care at her destination is an important consideration for the near-term woman who travels.

Activity and Rest

Exercise during pregnancy helps maintain maternal fitness and muscle tone, leads to improved self-image, increases energy, improves sleep, relieves tension, helps control weight gain, promotes regular bowel function, and is associated with improved postpartum recovery. Normal participation in regular exercise can continue and in fact is encouraged throughout an uncomplicated pregnancy. Physically fit women who run or do aerobic exercise regularly during pregnancy have been found to have less fetal distress during labor, shorter active labors, fewer cesarean births, and less meconium-stained amniotic fluid (Cunningham et al, 2001). In particular, nulliparous women who participate in regular exercise during the first and second trimesters have a lower risk of cesarean birth (Bungum, Peaslee, Jackson, et al, 2000).

Before beginning an exercise program, a pregnant woman should be examined by her certified nurse-midwife or physician. A pregnant woman who is already in an exercise program can discuss her degree of participation with her caregiver. Women should also seek the opinion of their healthcare provider about taking part in strenuous sports, such as skiing and horseback riding. In general, the skilled sportswoman is no longer discouraged from participating in these activities if her pregnancy is uncomplicated. Pregnancy is not the time, however, to learn a new or strenuous sport.

High-risk activities requiring balance and coordination, such as skydiving, mountain climbing, ice skating, surfing, and racquetball, should be avoided. In addition, women who are or may become pregnant should be advised not to scuba dive. Research suggests that diving below 30 feet increases the risk of spontaneous abortion (miscarriage), fetal malformation, fetal growth restriction, and preterm labor (Clapp, 2001). Certain conditions do contraindicate exercise. Absolute contraindications to exercise include the following (ACOG, 2002):

- Rupture of the membranes
- Preeclampsia-eclampsia
- Incompetent cervix (cerclage)
- Persistent vaginal bleeding in the second or third trimesters
- Multiple gestation at risk for preterm labor
- History of preterm labor in the prior or current pregnancy
- Placenta previa after 26 weeks' gestation
- Chronic medical conditions that might be negatively impacted by vigorous exercise such as significant heart disease or restrictive lung disease

Research related to the effects of maternal exercise on the fetus is varied and contradictory. Exercise can lead to increased maternal core temperature and hyperthermia. However, research suggests that the incidence of neural tube defects or other birth defects is not increased in the pregnancies of women who continue to exercise, even vigorously, during early pregnancy (ACOG, 1994).

Uterine blood flow is reduced during exercise as blood is shunted from visceral organs to muscles. The fetus does seem able to withstand this stress, however, without developing hypoxia. For most healthy pregnant women with no additional risk factors for preterm labor, exercise does not increase the incidence of preterm labor and birth or baseline uterine activity (ACOG, 1994). Benefits to the fetus of a sustained maternal program of moderate weight-bearing exercise include improved fetoplacental growth and a decreased incidence of fetal distress during labor. Research indicates that the children of mothers who exercised regularly during pregnancy have a decrease in fat mass and improved neurologic development through the fifth year of life (Clapp, 2001).

The following guidelines are helpful in counseling pregnant women about exercise:

- Even mild to moderate exercise is beneficial during pregnancy. Regular exercise—at least 30 minutes of moderate exercise daily or at least most days of the week—is preferred (ACOG, 2002).
- Research suggests that women who exercised regularly before pregnancy can safely maintain moderate intensity, weight-bearing exercise for 60 minutes per day, 5 days per week without risk to the fetus (Clapp, 2001).
- After the first trimester, women should avoid exercising in the supine position. In most pregnant women, the supine position is associated with decreased cardiac output. Because uterine blood flow is reduced during exercise as blood is shunted from the visceral organs to the muscles, the remaining cardiac output is further decreased. Similarly, women should avoid standing motionless for prolonged periods (ACOG, 2002).
- Because decreased oxygen is available for aerobic exercise during pregnancy, women should modify the intensity of their exercise based on their symptoms, should stop when they become fatigued, and should avoid exercising to the point of exhaustion. Non-weight-bearing exercises, such as swimming or cycling, are recommended because they decrease the risk of injury and provide fitness with comfort (ACOG, 1994).
- As pregnancy progresses and the center of gravity changes, especially in the third trimester, exercises in which the loss of balance or falling could pose a risk to mother or fetus (eg, gymnastics, downhill skiing, horseback riding) are best avoided. Similarly, the woman should avoid any type of exercise that has a high potential for physical contact such as basketball, soccer, and ice hockey because it could result in trauma to the woman or her fetus (ACOG, 2002).
- A normal pregnancy requires an additional 300 kcal per day. Women who exercise regularly during pregnancy should be careful to ensure that they consume an adequate diet.
- To augment heat dissipation, especially during the first trimester, pregnant women who exercise should wear appropriate clothing, ensure adequate hydration, and avoid the prolonged overheating associated with vigorous exercise in hot, humid weather because of the possible teratogenic effects of hyperthermia on the fetus (Hefferman, 2000). For the same reason, they should avoid hot tubs and saunas.
- Women should avoid reaching their maximum physical effort during pregnancy. Thus, as a general rule, their pulse rates should not exceed 140 beats per minute (Shrock, 2000).

CRITICAL THINKING IN PRACTICE

Constance Petrowski, a 24-year-old G1P0, is 11 weeks pregnant when she sees the nurse-midwife for her first prenatal exam. She is a world-class marathon runner. Because of her low body fat, her menses have always been irregular, and it had not occurred to Constance that she might be pregnant. Constance tells the certified nurse-midwife that she has just begun serious training for a marathon that is to take place when Constance is about 22 weeks pregnant. Constance says she has been told that it is fine to continue any physical activity at which one is proficient and says that she would like to compete in the marathon because she believes she has a chance to come in as one of the top three women runners. What should the nurse tell Constance about competing in the marathon?

Answers can be found in Appendix I.

In addition to the previously discussed recommendations, the nurse may suggest that the woman wear a supportive bra and appropriate shoes when exercising. She should be advised to warm up and stretch to help prepare the joints for activity and cool down with a period of mild activity to help restore circulation and avoid pooling of blood. A moderate, rhythmic exercise routine involving large muscle groups such as swimming, cycling, walking, or cross-country skiing is best. Jogging or running is acceptable for women already conditioned to these activities as long as they avoid exercising at maximum effort and overheating.

Warning signs include the following: pain of any kind, vaginal bleeding, uterine contractions, decreased or absent fetal movement, fluid loss from the vagina, dizziness, headache, dyspnea before exertion, and muscle weakness (ACOG, 2002; Clapp, 2001). The woman should stop exercising if any of these symptoms occur and contact her caregiver.

Adequate rest in pregnancy is important for both physical and emotional health. Women need more sleep throughout pregnancy, particularly in the first and last trimesters, when they tire easily. Without adequate rest, pregnant women have less resilience.

Finding time to rest during the day may be difficult for women who work outside the home or have small children. The nurse can help the expectant mother examine her daily schedule to develop a realistic plan for short periods of rest and relaxation.

Sleeping becomes more difficult during the last trimester because of the enlarged abdomen, increased frequency of urination, and greater activity of the fetus. Finding a comfortable position becomes difficult for the pregnant woman. Figure 16–10 • shows a position most pregnant women find comfortable. Progressive relaxation techniques similar to those taught in prepared childbirth classes can help prepare the woman for sleep.

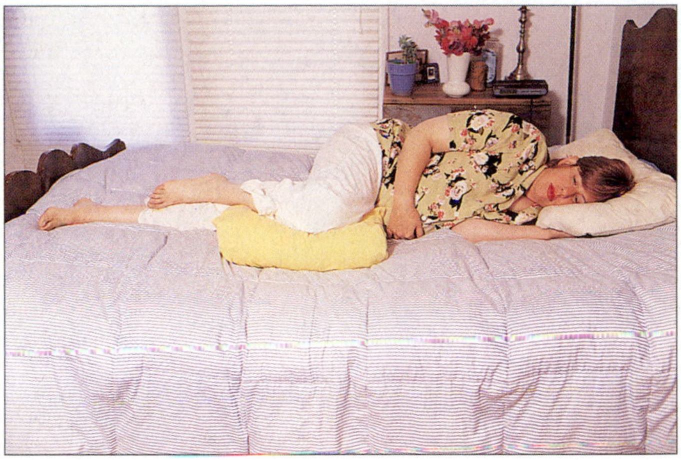

Figure 16–10 • Position for relaxation and rest as pregnancy progresses.

Exercises to Prepare for Childbirth

Certain exercises help strengthen muscle tone in preparation for birth and promote more rapid restoration of muscle tone after birth. The woman can reduce some physical changes of pregnancy considerably by faithfully practicing prescribed body-conditioning exercises. Many body-conditioning exercises for pregnancy are taught; a few of the more common ones are discussed here.

The **pelvic tilt,** or pelvic rocking, helps prevent or reduce back strain and strengthens abdominal muscle tone. To do the pelvic tilt, the pregnant woman lies on her back and puts her feet flat on the floor. This bent position of the knees helps prevent strain and discomfort. She decreases the curvature in her back by pressing her spine toward the floor. With her back pressed to the floor, the woman tightens her buttocks and abdominal muscles as she tucks in her buttocks. The pelvic tilt can also be performed on hands and knees (Figure 16–11 •), while sitting in a chair, or while standing with the back against a wall. The body alignment achieved when the pelvic tilt is correctly done should be maintained as much as possible throughout the day.

Clinical Tip *Doing the pelvic tilt on hands and knees may aggravate back strain. Teach women with a history of minor back problems to do the pelvic tilt only in the standing position.*

ABDOMINAL EXERCISES

A basic exercise to increase abdominal muscle tone is tightening abdominal muscles with each breath. It can be done in any position, but it is best learned while the woman lies supine. With knees flexed and feet flat on the floor, the woman expands her abdomen and slowly takes a deep breath. As she slowly exhales, she gradually pulls in her abdominal muscles until they are fully contracted. She relaxes for a few seconds and then repeats the exercise.

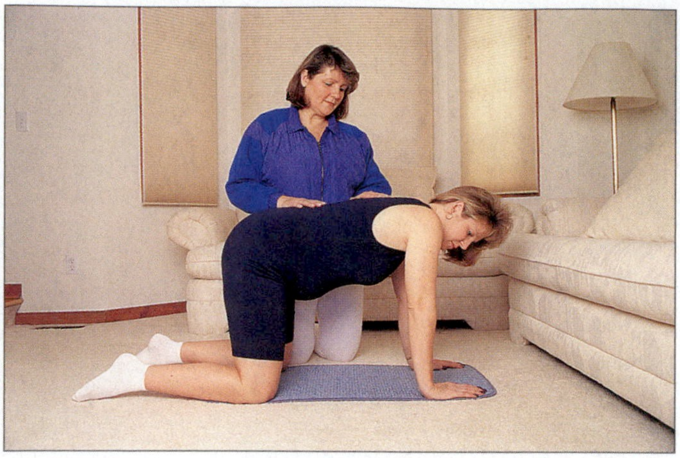

A

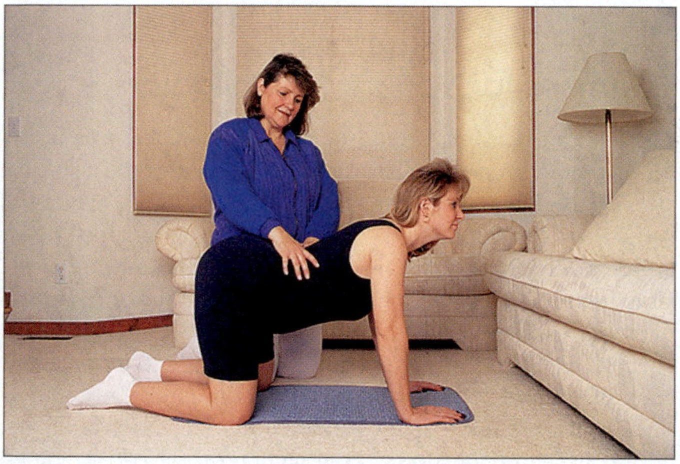

B

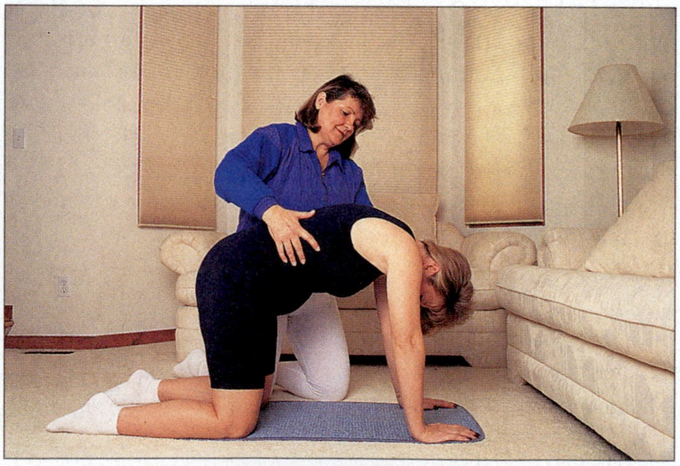

C

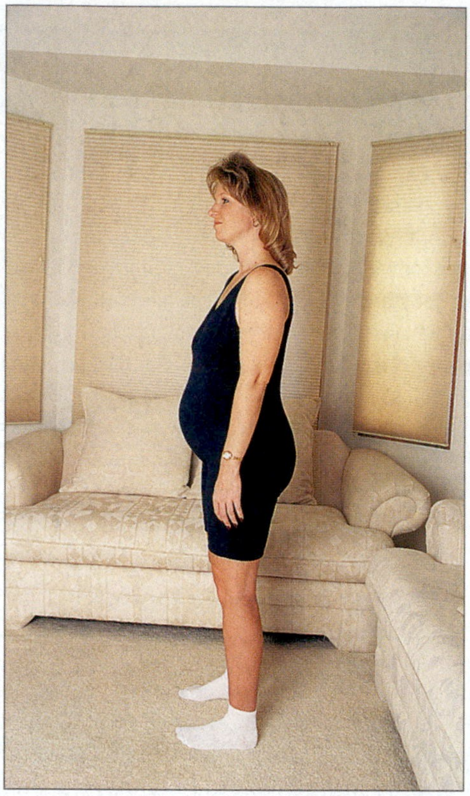

D

Figure 16–11 • *A,* Starting position when the pelvic tilt is done on hands and knees. The back is flat and parallel to the floor, the hands are under the head, and the knees are directly under the buttocks. *B,* A prenatal yoga instructor offers pointers for proper positioning for the first part of the tilt: head up, neck long and separated from the shoulders, buttocks up, and pelvis thrust back, allowing the back to drop and release on an inhaled breath. *C,* The instructor helps the woman assume the correct position for the next part of the tilt. It is done on a long exhalation, allowing the pregnant woman to arch her back, drop her head loosely, push away from her hands, and draw in the muscles of her abdomen to strengthen them. Note that in this position the pelvis and buttocks are tucked under, and the buttock muscles are tightened. *D,* Proper posture. The knees are slightly bent but not locked, the pelvis and buttocks are tucked under, thereby lengthening the spine and helping support the weighty abdomen. With her chin tucked in, this woman's neck, shoulders, hips, knees, and feet are all in a straight line perpendicular to the floor. Her feet are parallel. This is also the starting position for doing the pelvic tilt while standing.

Partial sit-ups strengthen abdominal muscle tone and are done according to individual comfort levels. When doing a partial sit-up, the woman lies on the floor as just described (Figure 16–12 •). This exercise is done with the knees bent and the feet flat on the floor to avoid undue strain on the lower back. She stretches her arms toward her knees as she slowly pulls her head and shoulders off the floor to a comfortable level. (If she has poor abdominal muscle tone, she may not be able to pull up very far.) She then slowly returns to the starting position, takes a deep breath, and repeats the exercise. To strengthen the oblique abdominal muscles, she repeats the process, but stretches the left arm to the side of her right knee, returns to the floor, takes a deep breath, and then reaches with the right arm to the left knee.

These exercises can be done approximately five times in a sequence, and the sequence can be repeated several times

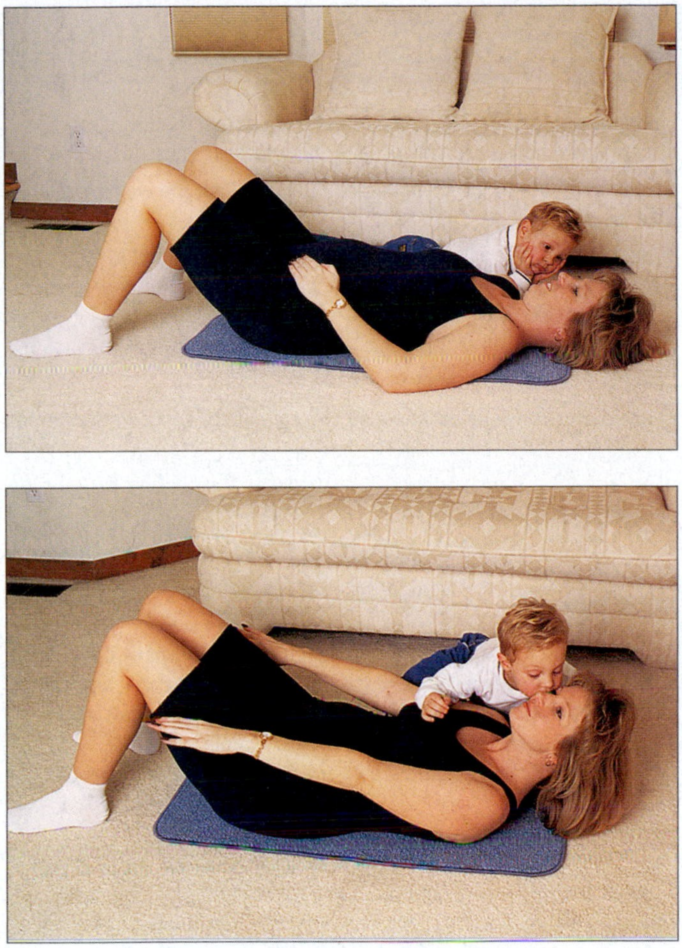

Figure 16–12 • The pregnant woman can strengthen her abdominal muscles by doing partial sit-ups.

during the day as desired. It is important that the woman do the exercises slowly to prevent muscle strain and overtiring.

PERINEAL EXERCISES

Perineal muscle tightening, also referred to as **Kegel exercises,** strengthens the pubococcygeus muscle and increases its elasticity (Figure 16–13 •). This muscle helps support the pelvic organs, including the uterus and bladder. A strong pubococcygeus muscle helps prevent stress incontinence, cystocele, rectocele, and uterine prolapse in women following childbirth.

The woman can feel the specific muscle group to be exercised by stopping urination midstream. However, doing Kegel exercises while urinating is discouraged because this practice has been associated with urinary stasis and urinary tract infection.

Childbirth educators sometimes use the following technique to teach Kegel exercises. They tell the woman to think of her perineal muscles as an elevator. When she relaxes, the elevator is on the first floor. To do the exercises, she contracts, bringing the elevator to the second, third, and fourth floors. She keeps the elevator on the fourth floor for a few seconds, and then gradually relaxes the area. If the exercise is

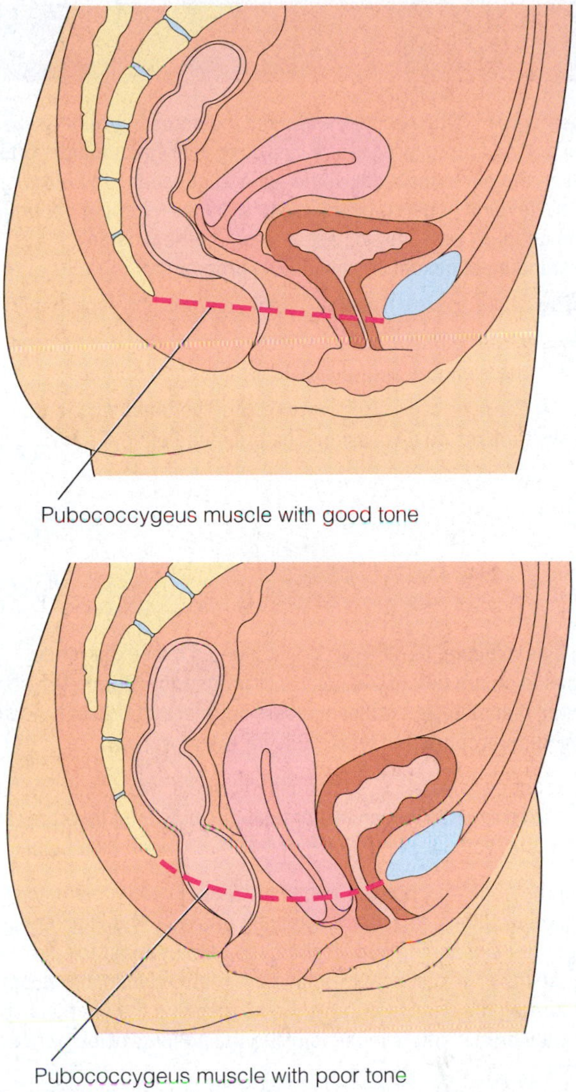

Figure 16–13 • Kegel exercises. The woman tightens the pubococcygeus muscle to improve support to the pelvic organs.

properly done, the woman does not contract the muscles of the buttocks and thighs.

Kegel exercises can be done at almost any time. Some women use ordinary events—for instance, stopping at a red light—as a cue to remember to do the exercise. Others do Kegel exercises while waiting in a checkout line, talking on the telephone, or watching television.

INNER THIGH EXERCISES

The pregnant woman should assume a cross-legged sitting position whenever possible. This "tailor sit" stretches the muscles of the inner thighs in preparation for labor and birth.

Sexual Activity

As a result of the physiologic, anatomic, and emotional changes of pregnancy, the couple usually have many questions and concerns about sexual activity during pregnancy. Often these questions are about possible injury to the baby

CLIENT TEACHING SEXUAL ACTIVITY DURING PREGNANCY

Assessment Occasionally a woman indicates her beliefs about sexual activity during pregnancy by asking a direct question. Often, however, the nurse must ask some general questions to determine the woman's level of understanding. In many cases teaching about this topic is coupled with ongoing assessment of the woman's understanding of sexual activity during pregnancy.

Nursing Diagnosis The key nursing diagnosis will probably be

Health-Seeking Behaviors: Information on sexuality during pregnancy related to the woman's expressed desire for clarification.

Nursing Plan and Implementation The teaching plan generally focuses on discussion. The presence of both partners may be beneficial in fostering communication between them and is acceptable unless personal or cultural factors indicate otherwise.

Client Goals At the completion of the teaching the woman will be able to

- Relate the changes in sexuality and sexual response that may occur during pregnancy to changes in technique, frequency, and response that may be indicated.
- Explore personal attitudes, beliefs, and expectations about sexual activity during pregnancy.
- Cite maternal factors that would contraindicate sexual intercourse.

Teaching Plan

CONTENT	TEACHING METHOD
Begin by explaining that the pregnant woman may experience changes in desire during the course of pregnancy. During the first trimester, discomforts such as nausea, fatigue, and breast tenderness may make intercourse less desirable for many women. In the second trimester, as symptoms decrease, desire may increase. In the third trimester, discomfort and fatigue may lead to decreased desire in the woman.	Universal statements that give permission, such as "Many couples experience changes in sexual desire during pregnancy. What kind of changes have you experienced?" are often effective in starting discussion. Depending on the woman's (or couple's) level of knowledge and sophistication, part or all of this discussion may be necessary.
Explain that men may notice changes in their level of desire, too. Among other things, this change may be related to feelings about their partner's changing appearance, their belief about the acceptability of sexual activity with a pregnant woman, or concern about hurting the woman or fetus. Some men find the changes of pregnancy erotic; others must adjust to the notion of their partners as mothers.	If the partner is present, approach him in the same nonjudgmental way used above. If not, ask the woman if she has noticed any changes in her partner or if he has expressed any concerns.
Explain that the woman may notice that orgasms are much more intense during the last weeks of pregnancy and may be followed by cramping. Because of the pressure of the enlarging uterus on the vena cava, the woman should not lie flat on her back for intercourse after about the fourth month. If the couple prefer that position, a pillow should be placed under her right hip to displace the uterus. Alternate positions such as side-by-side, female superior, or vaginal rear entry may become necessary as her uterus enlarges.	Deal with any specific questions about the physical and psychologic changes that the couple may have.
Stress that sexual activities that both partners enjoy are generally acceptable. It is not advisable for couples who favor anal sex to go from anal penetration to vaginal penetration because of the risk of introducing *Escherichia coli* into the vagina.	Discussion about various sexual activities requires that you be comfortable with your sexuality and that you be tactful.
Suggest that alternative methods of expressing intimacy and affection such as cuddling, holding and stroking each other, and kissing may help maintain the couple's feelings of warmth and closeness. If the man feels desire for further sexual release, his partner may help him masturbate to ejaculation, or he may prefer to masturbate in private. Advise the woman who is interested in masturbation as a form of gratification that the orgasmic contractions may be especially intense in later pregnancy.	The couple may be content with these approaches to meeting their sexual needs, or they may require assurance that such approaches are indeed "normal."

(continued)

CLIENT TEACHING SEXUAL ACTIVITY DURING PREGNANCY *(continued)*

Stress that sexual intercourse is contraindicated once the membranes are ruptured or if bleeding is present. Women with a history of preterm labor may be advised to avoid intercourse because the oxytocin that is released with orgasm stimulates uterine contractions and may trigger preterm labor. Because oxytocin is also released with nipple stimulation, fondling the breasts may also be contraindicated in those cases.	An explanation of the contraindications accompanied by their rationale provides specific guidelines that most couples find helpful.
A discussion of sexuality and sexual activity should stress the importance of open communication so that the couple feel comfortable expressing their feelings, preferences, and concerns.	Some couples are skilled at expressing their feelings about sexual activity. Others find it difficult and can benefit from specific suggestions. The nurse should provide opportunities for discussion throughout the talk. Specific handouts on sexual activity are also helpful for couples and may address topics that were not discussed.

EVALUATION

Evaluate the learning by assessing the woman's (or couple's) response to information throughout the discussion. Ask the woman to express information such as the contraindications to intercourse in her own words. Follow-up sessions and questions from the woman also provide information about teaching effectiveness.

or the woman during intercourse and about changes in the desire each partner feels for the other.

In the past, couples were frequently warned to avoid sexual intercourse during the last 6 to 8 weeks of pregnancy to prevent complications such as infection or premature rupture of the membranes. However, these fears seem to be unfounded. In a healthy pregnancy, there is no medical reason to limit sexual activity. Intercourse is contraindicated for medical reasons such as multiple pregnancy, threatened spontaneous abortion, incompetent cervix, partner with a sexually transmitted infection, or a maternal history of miscarriage following orgasm (Shrock, 2000). Most caregivers also advise against intercourse when the membranes are ruptured and in women with a history of preterm labor.

The expectant mother may experience changes in sexual desire and response. Often these are related to the various discomforts that occur throughout pregnancy. For instance, during the first trimester, fatigue or nausea and vomiting may decrease desire, and breast tenderness may make the woman less responsive to fondling of her breasts. During the second trimester, many of the discomforts have lessened, and with the vascular congestion of the pelvis the woman may experience even greater sexual satisfaction than she experienced prior to pregnancy.

During the third trimester, interest in coitus may again decrease as the woman becomes more uncomfortable and fatigued. In addition, shortness of breath, painful pelvic ligaments, urinary frequency, and decreased mobility may lessen sexual desire and activity. If they are not already using them, the couple should consider coital positions other than male superior, such as side-by-side, female superior, and vaginal rear entry.

Sexual activity does not have to include intercourse. Cuddling, kissing, and being held can satisfy many of the nurturing and sexual needs of the pregnant woman. The warm, sensual feelings that accompany these activities can be an end in themselves. Her partner, however, may need to masturbate more frequently than before.

The sexual desires of men are also affected by many factors in pregnancy. These include the previous relationship with the partner, acceptance of the pregnancy, attitudes toward the partner's change of appearance, and concern about hurting the expectant mother or baby. Some men may withdraw from sexual contact because of a belief that sex with a pregnant woman is immoral. This may be especially true for the couple whose religious beliefs teach that sexual intercourse is only for procreation. Some men find it difficult to view their partners as sexually appealing while they are adjusting to the concept of her as a mother. Other men feel their partner's pregnancy is arousing and experience feelings of increased happiness, intimacy, and closeness.

The expectant couple should be aware of their changing sexual desires, the normality of these changes, and the importance of communicating these changes to each other so that they can make nurturing adaptations. The nurse has an important role in addressing the sexuality concerns of the expectant couple. The couple must feel free to express concerns about sexual activity, and the nurse must be able to respond and give anticipatory guidance in a comfortable manner. See Client Teaching: Sexual Activity During Pregnancy.

Dental Care

Proper dental hygiene is important in pregnancy. In fact, research suggests a link between periodontal disease in pregnant women and preterm birth and low-birth-weight infants (Carl, Roux, & Matacale, 2000). In spite of such discomforts as nausea and vomiting, gum hypertrophy and tenderness, possible ptyalism, and heartburn, it is important for pregnant women to maintain regular oral hygiene.

Ensuring a healthy oral environment is essential to overall health. Women should be advised to do the following (Mills & Moses, 2002):

- Have extensive dental work done before becoming pregnant if possible.
- Eat a healthy diet including foods high in protein, calcium, phosphorus, and vitamins C, A, and D.
- Take prenatal vitamins daily.
- Maintain good oral hygiene by brushing at least twice a day and flossing daily.
- Use an antibacterial fluoride mouth rinse.
- If morning sickness occurs, brush teeth following vomiting to prevent tooth erosion caused by stomach acids.
- Have teeth cleaned every 6 months.

The pregnant woman is encouraged to have a dental checkup early in her pregnancy. The woman should inform her dentist of her pregnancy so that she is not exposed to teratogenic substances. The second trimester is considered the most appropriate time for minor dental treatments such as general repairs and extractions, preferably under local anesthetic (Carl et al, 2000). Dental x-ray examinations and extensive dental work should be delayed when possible until after birth. Extensive dental care during pregnancy requires consultation between the dentist and the woman's healthcare professional.

Immunizations

All women of childbearing age need to be fully aware of the risks of receiving specific immunizations if pregnancy is possible. Expectant women, especially those who intend to travel internationally, should be aware of the immunizations that are contraindicated during pregnancy. Immunizations with attenuated live viruses, such as rubella vaccine, should not be given in pregnancy because of the possible teratogenic effect of the live viruses on the developing embryo. Vaccinations using killed viruses can be used (Stevenson, 1999). Recommendations for immunizations during pregnancy are summarized in Table 16–6 •.

Complementary and Alternative Therapy

As discussed in Chapter 3, many women are electing to use complementary and alternative medicine (CAM), such as homeopathy, herbal medicine, acupressure, acupuncture, biofeedback, therapeutic touch, massage, and chiropractic, as part of a holistic approach to their healthcare regimens. However, they often choose not to report use of alternative approaches to their healthcare provider (Eisenberg, Davis, Ettner, et al, 1998). Therefore, the nurse must inquire about the use of CAM as part of a routine antepartal assessment. It is important that nurses working with pregnant women and their families develop a general understanding of the more commonly used therapies to be able to answer questions and provide resources as needed.

Nurses caring for pregnant women can develop printed materials describing the use of homeopathic remedies and herbs during pregnancy and identifying those that may present a risk. It is especially important that women choosing these complementary approaches consult someone who is knowledgeable, well trained, and experienced in the specific therapy, and that they buy their herbs or homeopathic remedies from reputable manufacturers (Belew, 1999). See Complementary and Alternative Therapies: Homeopathy and

Table 16–6 • RECOMMENDATIONS FOR IMMUNIZATION DURING PREGNANCY

Live virus vaccines	**Inactivated bacterial vaccines**	**Hyperimmune globulins**
Measles—contraindicated	Pneumococcal—same as nonpregnant	Hepatitis B—postexposure prophylaxis: give along with hepatitis B vaccine initially, then vaccine alone at 1 and 6 mo
Mumps—contraindicated	Meningococcal—same as nonpregnant	Rabies—postexposure prophylaxis
Varicella-zoster—contraindicated	Hemophilus—same as nonpregnant	Tetanus—postexposure prophylaxis
Live bacterial vaccine	Cholera—risks vs benefits	Varicella—consider for postexposure within 96 h
Typhoid (Ty21a)—risks vs benefits		
Poliomyelitis—no longer recommended		
Yellow fever—high-risk areas only		
Inactivated virus vaccines	**Toxoids**	**Pooled immune serum globulins**
Influenza—after first trimester request	Tetanus-diphtheria—same as nonpregnant	Hepatitis A—postexposure prophylaxis
Rabies—same as nonpregnant		Measles—postexposure prophylaxis
Hepatitis A and B—same as nonpregnant		
Enhanced poliomyelitis (IPV-e)—risk of exposure		
Japanese encephalitis—weigh risks vs benefits		

Source: Cunningham, T. G., Gant, N. F., & Leveno, K. J. (2001). *Williams Obstetrics,* 21st ed. New York: McGraw-Hill. Reproduced with permission of The McGraw-Hill Companies.

Table 16-7 • COMMON HERBS TO AVOID IN PREGNANCY*

Aloe spp.	Kava kava
Black cohosh	Licorice
Buckthorn	Ma huang
Cascara sagrada	Pennyroyal
Chamomile, Roman	Rue
Chaste tree berry	Sage
Dong quai	Senna
Feverfew	St. John's Wort
Goldenseal	Stinging nettle
Gotu kola	Tansy
Guggul	Wormwood
Horehound	Yarrow
Horseradish (fresh)	
Use with caution:	
Garlic	
Ginger	
Turmeric	

*Avoid excessive consumption relative to usual and customary food use.

Source: Hardy, M. (2000). Herbs of special interest to women. *Journal of the American Pharmaceutical Association, 40* (2), 234–242.

COMPLEMENTARY AND ALTERNATIVE THERAPIES

HOMEOPATHY AND HERBAL MEDICINE

Homeopathy: Homeopathy means "like suffering." Homeopathic medicine is based on the theory that a miniscule amount of a substance can cure symptoms in a sick person that are similar to the symptoms the substance causes in healthy people. Thus, for example, ipecac, which induces vomiting, may be used to treat a person who is vomiting, such as a pregnant woman with severe nausea and vomiting (Brennan, 1999). Currently, homeopathic practitioners use about 2000 plant, animal, and mineral substances.

Homeopathic therapies are available for pregnancy-related symptoms such as musculoskeletal disorders, anemia, nausea, ptyalism, pica, threatened miscarriage, and preterm labor. According to homeopathic theory, homeopathic remedies either help an individual or have no effect. However, a healing crisis or aggravation of symptoms can occur if the remedy is given in too high a potency or repeated too frequently (Brennan, 1999). More information about homeopathy can be found on our companion Web site.

Herbal Medicine: Herbal medicine uses therapies derived from plants. Many have been used for centuries in different parts of the world and are well recognized. In fact, countries such as Germany, Canada, England, and France recognize the benefits of scores of herbs and include information about their use as part of formal educational programs for physicians and pharmacists.

In the United States, herbs are categorized as dietary supplements rather than drugs and are often used by pregnant women. It is best to advise pregnant women interested in using herbs to follow three basic principles: (1) if at all possible, avoid the use of herbs, even tonic herbs, during the first trimester (with the exception of ginger in amounts less than 1 g daily); (2) avoid standardized or highly concentrated extracts because the risk of side effects tends to be higher than with whole plant extracts; and (3) do not take essential oils internally (Belew, 1999). In addition, pregnant women need to avoid certain categories of herbs such as abortifacient (abortion-inducing) herbs, herbs that induce menstruation, nervous system stimulants, stimulant laxatives, and so forth. Lists identifying common herbs that women are advised to avoid or use with caution during pregnancy and location are available; an example is shown in Table 16–7.

Herbal Medicine. Table 16–7 • identifies common herbs that pregnant women should avoid or use with caution.

For a reliable source of information about herbs, homeopathic therapies, and other alternative options, consumers or healthcare providers can contact the National Center for Complementary and Alternative Medicine Web site (http://nccam.nih.gov) and the Office of Dietary Supplements Web site (http://odp.od.nih.gov/ods/).

Teratogenic Substances

Substances that adversely affect the normal growth and development of the fetus are called **teratogens.** Many of these effects are readily apparent at birth, but others may not be identified for years. A well-known example is the development of cervical cancer in adolescent females whose mothers took diethylstilbestrol (DES) during pregnancy.

Known teratogens include chemicals, viruses, environmental factors, physical factors, and drugs (Cunningham et al, 2001). Medications are perhaps the most likely documented teratogens, but other factors can also harm the fetus, including certain infections such as rubella, syphilis, herpesvirus type 2, toxoplasmosis, and cytomegalovirus (CMV). During pregnancy, women need to have adequate information available and a realistic perspective on potential environmental hazards. Factors that are suspected to be hazardous to the general population should obviously be avoided if possible.

MEDICATIONS

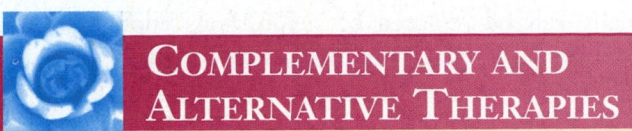

The use of medications in pregnancy, including prescription, over-the-counter (OTC), and herbal and homeopathic remedies, is of great concern. Studies have demonstrated that the average pregnant woman takes many more medications than commonly believed, including OTC drugs as well as prescription drugs (Cunningham et al, 2001). Many pregnant women need medication for therapeutic purposes, such as the treatment of infections, allergies, or other pathologic processes. In these situations, the problem can be extremely complex. Known teratogenic agents are not prescribed and usually can be replaced by medications considered safe. Even when a woman is highly motivated to avoid taking any medications, she may have taken potentially teratogenic medications before her pregnancy was diagnosed, especially if she had an irregular menstrual cycle.

The greatest potential for gross abnormalities in the fetus occurs during the first trimester of pregnancy, when fetal organs are first developing. The classic period of teratogenesis in a woman with a 28-day cycle extends from day 31 after the last menstrual period (17 days after fertilization) to day 71 (54 days after fertilization) (Niebyl, 1999). Many factors influence teratogenic effects, including the specific identity and dose of the teratogen, the state of embryo development, and the genetic sensitivity of the mother and fetus (ACOG, 1997c). For example, the commonly prescribed acne medication isotretinoin (Accutane) is associated with a high incidence of spontaneous abortion and congenital malformations if taken early in pregnancy. Valproic acid, an anticonvulsant, is associated with an increased risk of spina bifida (Cunningham et al, 2001).

To provide information for caregivers and clients, the Food and Drug Administration (FDA) has developed the following classification system for medications administered during pregnancy:

Category A. Controlled studies in women have demonstrated no associated fetal risk. Few drugs fall into this category. Vitamin C is cited as a category A drug as long as its use does not exceed the recommended dietary allowance.

Category B. Either animal studies show no risk, but there are no controlled studies in women; or animal studies indicate a risk, but controlled human studies fail to demonstrate a risk. The penicillins fall into this category.

Category C. Either (1) no adequate studies, either in animals or women, are available; or (2) animal studies show teratogenic effects, but no controlled studies in women are available. Many drugs fall into this category, and the lack of information poses a problem for caregivers. Zidovudine, a drug used to decrease perinatal transmission of human immunodeficiency virus (HIV), falls into this category.

Category D. Evidence of human fetal risk does exist, but the benefits of the drug in certain situations are thought to outweigh the risks. Examples in this category include tetracycline, vincristine, lithium, and hydrochlorothiazide.

Category X. The demonstrated fetal risks clearly outweigh any possible benefit. An example of a drug in this category is isotretinoin (Accutane), the acne medication, which can cause multiple central nervous system (CNS), facial, and cardiovascular anomalies.

If a woman has taken a drug in category D or X, she should be informed of the risks associated with that drug and of her alternatives. Similarly, a woman who has taken a drug in the safer categories can be reassured (Cunningham et al, 2001). For up-to-date information on the risks associated with specific drugs, women can contact drug information centers, either by telephone or by using online databases such as reprotox.org, which charges a fee for the service.

The FDA system, while useful, has been criticized because the letter system suggests a risk grading that is not necessarily accurate. More important, not all drugs in a category have the same risk level. Currently the FDA is working to develop a new labeling system (Whitney, 1999).

Although the first trimester is the critical period for teratogenesis, some medications are known to have teratogenic effect when taken in the second and third trimesters. For example, tetracycline taken in late pregnancy is commonly associated with staining of teeth in children and has been shown to depress skeletal growth, especially in preterm infants. Sulfonamides taken in the last weeks of pregnancy are known to compete with bilirubin attachment of protein-binding sites, increasing the risk of jaundice in the newborn (Niebyl, 1999). Warfarin (Coumadin), a commonly prescribed anticoagulant, is associated with CNS defects following fetal exposure during the second and third trimesters (Cunningham et al, 2001). Because heparin does not cross the placenta, it is safer for the fetus than warfarin and other anticoagulants.

Pregnant women should avoid all medication if possible. If a medication is necessary during pregnancy, the benefits must clearly outweigh the risks. If no alternative exists, it is wisest to select a well-known medication rather than a newer drug whose potential teratogenic effects may not be known. When possible, the oral form of the drug should be used, and it should be prescribed in the lowest possible therapeutic dose for the shortest time possible. Finally, the caregiver should carefully consider the multiple components of the medication.

A woman clearly has a right to the most comprehensive information available concerning medications. The nurse can assist her by suggesting appropriate references and helping her research information. Some excellent reference books on drugs and pregnancy are currently available and should be part of the library of every office and clinic that provides prenatal care. In addition, several online databases that provide information on teratogens are available for convenient reference.

The nurse should remind the woman of the need to check with her caregiver about medications she was taking when pregnancy occurred and about any nonprescription drugs she is contemplating using. Any medication with possible teratogenic effects must be avoided.

TOBACCO

Smoking has been linked to higher infertility rates in both men and women. In women, smoking has been identified as a factor in ovulatory, tubal function, and implantation disorders, as well as oocyte depletion and early pregnancy loss. In men, smoking has been linked to impaired sperm concentration and changes in sperm motility and morphology (ACOG, 1997b).

Smoking during pregnancy is one of the most important, modifiable causes of poor pregnancy outcomes in the United States. Smoking accounts for 20% of the births of infants with low birth weights, 8% of all preterm births, and 5% of perinatal deaths (Orleans, Barker, Kaufman, et al, 2001). For women with a twin pregnancy, this effect is even more pronounced (Pollack, Lantz, & Frohna, 2000). In addition, mothers who smoke have an increased risk of spontaneous abortion, preterm birth, placentae previa, abruptio placentae, and premature rupture of membranes. This risk is related to the number of cigarettes smoked (ACOG, 1997b). Smoking has also been linked to an increased risk of cleft lip and palate in the newborn (Chung, Kowalski, Kim, et al, 2000). Research also links maternal smoking, both during pregnancy and afterward, with an increased risk of sudden infant death syndrome (SIDS). Maternal smoking exposes young children to other risks of secondhand smoke including middle ear infections, acute and chronic respiratory tract illnesses, and decreased lung function (Orleans et al, 2001).

The specific mechanism by which smoking affects the fetus is not known. However, the main ingredients in cigarette smoke that account for the adverse effects in the fetus are carbon monoxide and nicotine which decrease the availability of oxygen to maternal and fetal tissue (ACOG, 1997b).

Currently, there are 14 million women of childbearing age (15 to 45 years) in the United States who smoke cigarettes. In one year, up to one million of these women will become pregnant (Goldenberg & Dolan-Mullen, 2000; Todd, Bradshaw-LaSala, & Neil-Urban, 2001). Approximately 15% to 29% of women smoke during pregnancy (ACOG, 2000). Women who smoke tend to stop smoking or at least reduce their intake once pregnancy is confirmed. Unfortunately, a majority of women who quit smoking during their pregnancy resume after birth; this percentage is lower for women who quit earlier in pregnancy. This finding suggests that although women are aware of the potential impact of smoking on the fetus, they may be less knowledgeable about the effects of passive smoke on the baby.

Studies demonstrate that any decrease in smoking during pregnancy improves fetal outcome, and researchers continue to explore approaches designed to help women quit smoking. The three critical components of an effective smoking cessation program have been found to be assessment, education, and support (Maloni, 2001). ACOG (2000) suggests a 5- to 15-minute intervention, with women who smoke fewer than 20 cigarettes a day, to be most effective. This program and other programs encourage healthcare providers to use the five A's:

- Ask about tobacco use.
- Advise to quit smoking.
- Assess willingness to quit.
- Assist with modifying smoking behavior.
- Arrange for follow-up care (ACOG, 2000; Maloni, 2001).

The nurse can play an important role in counseling women about the importance of smoking cessation during pregnancy, and can be actively involved in offering smoking cessation programs.

If smoking cessation efforts are not successful, the healthcare provider might consider the pharmacologic approaches of nicotine gum (FDA category C) or a transdermal system (FDA category D). However, these approaches are somewhat controversial. They should be offered only if the pregnant woman has failed at prior attempts to quit smoking and continues to smoke 10 to 15 cigarettes per day. In this case, the potential benefit of stopping smoking outweighs the unknown risk of nicotine replacement (ACOG, 2000; Cunningham et al, 2001).

Many educational resources are available for healthcare providers and consumers on smoking cessation programs. Organizations and Web sites that might be helpful include the following:

- American Lung Association: www.lungusa.org
- March of Dimes: www.modimes.org
- American Cancer Society: www.cancer.org
- Healthy Mothers, Healthy Babies: www.hmhb.org

EVIDENCE-BASED PRACTICE

SMOKING INTERVENTIONS DURING PREGNANCY

Clinical Question

What are the effects of smoking cessation programs implemented during pregnancy on the health of the fetus and infant, on the mother, and on the family?

The Evidence

Smoking remains one of the few potentially preventable prenatal factors associated with low birth weight, very preterm birth, and perinatal death.

A review of 37 randomized and quasi-randomized trials that included 16,916 women revealed a significant reduction in smoking in the intervention groups (odds ratio 0.53, 95% confidence interval 0.47 to 0.60). Smoking cessation produced a reduction in low birth weight, a reduction in preterm birth, and an increase in mean birth weight. Smoking cessation programs in pregnancy appear to reduce smoking, low birth weight, and preterm birth, but no effect was detected for very low birth weight or perinatal mortality.

Best Practice

Because smoking cessation programs have been shown to increase smoking cessation, increase mean birth weight, and reduce low birth weight, they need to be implemented in all maternity care settings. Assessment of smoking behavior and support for smoking cessation and relapse prevention should be routine in antenatal care.

Interventions involving additional group sessions during pregnancy have been reported as being extremely poorly attended in virtually all trials where they were planned, and it is recommended that they be abandoned.

Source: Lumley, J., Oliver, S., & Waters, E. (2002). *Interventions for promoting smoking cessation during pregnancy.* Cochrane Pregnancy and Childbirth Group, Cochrane Database of Systematic Reviews.

ALCOHOL

Alcohol is now considered one of the primary teratogens in the Western world. Fetuses of women who are heavy drinkers are at increased risk for developing **fetal alcohol syndrome (FAS),** which is characterized by growth restriction, behavioral disturbances, craniofacial abnormalities, and brain, cardiac, and spinal defects. FAS is also the major cause of mental retardation in the United States (Cunningham et al, 2001).

The effects of moderate consumption of alcohol during pregnancy are not clearly known, but research suggests there is an increased incidence of lower birth weight and of some neurologic effects, such as attention deficit disorder. Evidence suggests that the risk of teratogenic effects increases proportionately with increased average daily intake of alcohol. Although an occasional drink during pregnancy does not carry any known risk, no safe level of drinking during pregnancy has been identified, and caregivers should recommend that pregnant women abstain from all alcohol during pregnancy (Niebyl, 1999).

Alcohol passes the placental barrier within minutes after consumption, with fetal blood alcohol levels becoming equivalent to maternal blood alcohol levels. The effects of alcohol consumption vary according to the stage of fetal development. During the first trimester, alcohol probably alters embryonic development; throughout pregnancy, alcohol may interfere with cell division and growth; in the third trimester, the time of most rapid brain growth, alcohol may alter CNS development and contribute to growth retardation (Cunningham et al, 2001). The risk of neurologic damage is lessened if heavy drinking ceases in the third trimester. Decreased consumption of alcohol in mid-pregnancy is associated with a lower incidence of growth retardation.

Assessment of alcohol intake should be a chief part of each woman's medical history, with questions asked in a direct, nonjudgmental manner. All women should be counseled about the role of alcohol in pregnancy. When pregnant women become aware of the risk of alcohol to the fetus, most usually attempt to modify their alcohol consumption. If heavy consumption is involved, these women should be referred early to an alcoholic treatment program. Because the drug disulfiram (Antabuse), which is often used in the treatment of alcoholism, is a suspected teratogen, a woman in such a program should inform her counselor if she becomes pregnant.

Counseling pregnant women about the effects of alcohol during pregnancy has been effective in reducing drinking among pregnant women and it should, of course, continue. Because the most profound impact of alcohol occurs in the first weeks after conception, however, nurses and other healthcare providers will see the most dramatic decrease in the effects of alcohol during pregnancy by increasing their teaching efforts in the period prior to conception.

CAFFEINE

Current research reveals no evidence that moderate levels of caffeine are linked to birth defects. However, caffeine ingestion at high levels may increase the risk of spontaneous abortion (Cunningham et al, 2001; Cnattingius, Signorello, Anneren, et al, 2000). Maternal coffee consumption also decreases iron absorption and may increase the risk of anemia (Niebyl, 1999). In the United Kingdom, the Food Standards Agency has recommended that women limit their caffeine intake to 300 mg per day. The average cup of brewed coffee has 100 mg, a cup of tea has 50 mg, a regular cola drink has up to 40 mg, and a normal-sized chocolate bar has up to 50 mg (Reuters Medical News, 2001). Until more definitive data are available, nurses should advise women of common sources of caffeine, including coffee, tea, colas, and chocolate, and suggest they use good judgment in moderating their caffeine intake.

MARIJUANA

Research reveals that approximately 15% of pregnant women use marijuana. The prevalence of marijuana use in our society raises concerns about its effect on the fetus, but to date no teratogenic effects of marijuana use during pregnancy have been documented (Cunningham et al, 2001). Research on marijuana use in pregnancy is difficult, however, because it is an illegal drug. Unreliability of reporting, lack of a representative population, inability to determine strength or composition of the marijuana used, presence of herbicides, and use of other drugs at the same time are major factors complicating the research being done.

COCAINE

During pregnancy, cocaine and marijuana are the most commonly used illicit substances (Askin & Diehl-Jones, 2001; Blatt, Meguid, & Church, 2000). Estimates suggest that there are 45,000 cocaine-exposed babies born per year in the United States (Askin & Diehl-Jones, 2001). A woman who uses cocaine is at increased risk for acute myocardial infarction, cardiac arrhythmias, ruptured ascending aorta, seizures, cerebrovascular accidents, hypertension, bowel ischemia, and sudden death (Cunningham et al, 2001). During pregnancy, cocaine use has been related to abruptio placentae, preterm birth, fetal distress, meconium-stained amniotic fluid, low birth weight, neonatal irritability, SIDS, and developmental delays as a toddler (Blatt et al, 2000). Several congenital anomalies in the newborn have been linked to maternal cocaine use, including genitourinary anomalies, congenital heart defects, limb reduction defects, CNS anomalies, prune belly syndrome (congenital absence of abdominal muscles), and segmental intestinal atresia (Cunningham et al, 2001).

As cocaine becomes more widely used by women of childbearing age, healthcare providers need to be alert to early signs of cocaine use. Six factors are associated with cocaine use during pregnancy (Askin & Diehl-Jones, 2001):

1. Poor prenatal care
2. Use of other illicit substances
3. Signs of maternal malnourishment
4. Use of alcohol or cigarettes
5. Lower socioeconomic status
6. Testing positive for a sexually transmitted infection

It is often difficult for a healthcare provider to face the fact that a client may be using cocaine, but ongoing alertness and an open, nonjudgmental approach are important in early detection. Maternal urine screening for cocaine is valuable, but because cocaine is metabolized rapidly, the drug screen is negative within 24 to 48 hours after cocaine use. Thus it is probable that many abusers are missed. However, the newborn may also be screened to document maternal cocaine use. Newborn urine will stay positive for cocaine for 3 to 5 days after maternal use. Newborn meconium or hair will test positive for maternal cocaine use starting at the 16th week of pregnancy (Askin & Diehl-Jones, 2001; Blatt et al, 2000). It is important for the nurse to promote early detection of fetal exposure to cocaine in order to provide appropriate newborn care.

Evaluation

Throughout the antepartal period, evaluation is an essential part of effective nursing care. As nurses ask questions of the pregnant woman and her family or make observations of physical changes, they are evaluating the results of previous interventions. In evaluating the effectiveness of the interventions, the nurse should not be afraid to try creative solutions if they are logical and carefully thought out. This is especially important in dealing with families from other cultures. If a practice is important to a woman and not harmful, the culturally competent nurse will not discourage it.

In completing an evaluation, the nurse must also recognize situations that require referral for further evaluation. For example, a woman who has gained 4 lb in 1 week probably does not require counseling about nutrition; she needs further assessment for preeclampsia. The nurse who has a sound knowledge of theory will recognize this and act immediately.

The ongoing and cyclic nature of the nursing process is especially evident in the prenatal setting. However, throughout the course of pregnancy nurses can use certain criteria to determine the quality of care provided. In essence, nursing care has been effective if the following have been met:

- The common discomforts of pregnancy are quickly identified and are relieved or lessened effectively.
- The woman is able to discuss the physiologic and psychologic changes of pregnancy.
- The woman implements appropriate self-care measures, if they are indicated, during pregnancy.
- The woman avoids substances and situations that pose a risk to her well-being or that of her child.
- The woman seeks regular prenatal care.

Care of the Expectant Couple Over 35

Today an increasing number of women are choosing to have their first baby after age 35 (see Table 16–8 •). In fact, approximately 10% of first pregnancies occur in women who are age 35 or older (Cunningham et al, 2001). Many factors contribute to this trend, including the following:

Table 16–8 • PREGNANCY IN WOMEN OVER AGE 35

- Couples who choose pregnancy at a later age are usually financially secure and have made a thoughtful, planned choice.
- If the woman has no existing health problems, her risk during pregnancy is not appreciably higher than that of the general population.
- The decreased fertility of women over age 35 may make conception more difficult.
- The incidence of Down syndrome increases somewhat in women over age 35 and significantly in those over age 40.
- The couple may choose to have amniocentesis or chorionic villus sampling to gain information about the health of their fetus.

- The availability of effective birth control methods
- The expanded roles and career options available for women
- The increased number of women obtaining advanced education, pursuing careers, and delaying parenthood until they are established professionally
- The increased incidence of later marriage and second marriage
- The high cost of living, which causes some young couples to delay childbearing until they are more secure financially
- The increased number of women in this older reproductive age group due to the baby boom between 1946 and 1964
- The increased availability of specialized fertilization procedures, which offers opportunities for women who had previously been considered infertile

There are advantages to having a first baby after the age of 35. Single women or couples who delay childbearing until they are older tend to be well educated and financially secure. Usually their decision to have a baby was deliberately and thoughtfully made (Figure 16–14 •). Because of their greater

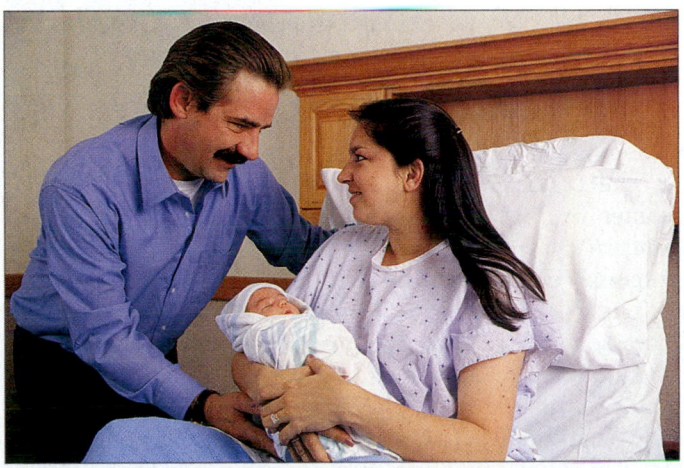

Figure 16–14 • For many older couples, the decision to have a child may be a very rewarding one.

life experiences, they are also more aware of the realities of having a child than younger women and they recognize what it means to have a baby at their age (Windridge & Berryman, 1999). Many of the women have experienced fulfillment in their careers and feel secure enough to take on the added responsibility of a child. Some women are ready to make a change in their lives, desiring to stay home with a new baby. Those who plan to continue working tend to be more able to afford good child care.

Medical Risks

Historically, medical professionals considered women who were over 30 at the time of their first pregnancy, and especially those who were 35 or older, at higher risk for maternal or fetal complications. This age-related concern began to change during the 1980s, when studies comparing healthy pregnant women over 35 years of age with healthy younger women did not confirm these beliefs. In addition, adverse pregnancy outcomes in this age group have been linked to socioeconomic status, which can, in turn, influence a woman's health status and her access to care (Cunningham et al, 2001). However, the current medical literature does report *some* adverse pregnancy outcomes associated with advanced maternal age.

In the United States and Canada over the past 30 years, the risk of fetal death has declined dramatically for women of all ages as a result of advances in maternal health and obstetric practice. However, the risk for fetal death remains highest among teenagers and among women age 40 or older (National Center for Health Statistics, 1999). Moreover, in both the United States and Canada, the risk of maternal mortality increases with maternal age. For women age 40 or older, the risk of dying from a pregnancy-related or pregnancy-aggravated cause is five times higher than the risk for women ages 20 to 24 years (Hoyert, Danel, & Tully, 2000). Women over 35 are more likely to have chronic medical conditions. Preexisting medical conditions, such as hypertension or diabetes, probably play a more significant role than age in maternal well-being and the outcome of pregnancy. The incidence of low-birth-weight infants and preterm births is higher among women age 35 or older (Tough, Newburn-Cook, Johnston, et al, 2002). In addition, placenta previa, abruptio placentae, spontaneous abortion, macrosomia, and congenital malformations occur more frequently in pregnant women over 35 (Cunningham et al, 2001).

The cesarean birth rate is also increased in pregnant women over 35. This practice may be related to increased concern by the woman and physician about the pregnancy outcome (Cunningham et al, 2001).

The risk of conceiving a child with Down syndrome does increase with age, especially over 35. Amniocentesis is routinely offered to all women over age 35 to permit the early detection of several chromosomal abnormalities, including Down syndrome. Routine genetic testing has not been offered to couples in which the only risk is advanced paternal age, because there is not sufficient evidence to determine a specific paternal age at which to start genetic testing. However, advanced paternal age does affect autosomal dominant diseases, such as neurofibromatosis, achondroplasia, and Marfan syndrome (ACOG, 1997a). Research has also focused on the use of multiple marker screening to detect Down syndrome and trisomy 18. Also called a triple screening test, this involves a blood test to detect levels of specific serum markers, namely alpha-fetoprotein (AFP), human chorionic gonadotropin (hCG), and unconjugated estriol. When these tests in combination show certain patterns of increase or decrease, they are considered positive, and the woman is advised to consider amniocentesis. Although these tests are not as definite as amniocentesis in detecting abnormalities, they are safer and less expensive (Cunningham et al, 2001).

Special Concerns of the Expectant Couple Over 35

No matter what their age, most expectant couples have concerns regarding the well-being of the fetus and their ability to parent. The older couple has additional concerns related to their age, especially the closer they are to 40 or more. Some couples are concerned about whether they will have enough energy to care for a new baby. Of greater concern is their ability to deal with the needs of the older child when they too are older.

> “*I didn't really think I would get married but then I met Antonio and fell hard. I was 35 and he was 43, a widower with no children. We both really wanted a baby, so here I am 36 and pregnant. How I pray that this baby will be healthy.*”

The financial concerns of an older couple are usually different from those of a younger couple. The older couple is generally more financially secure than the younger couple. However, when their "baby" is ready for college, the older couple may be near retirement and might not have the means to provide for their child.

While considering their financial future and future retirement, the older couple may be forced to face their own mortality. Certainly this is not uncommon in midlife, but instead of confronting this issue at 40 to 45 years of age or later, the older expectant couple may confront the issue several years earlier as they consider what will happen as their child grows.

The older couple facing pregnancy following a late or second marriage or after therapy for infertility may find themselves somewhat isolated socially. They may feel "different" because they are often the only couple in their peer group expecting their first baby. In fact, many of their peers are likely to be parents of adolescents or young adults and may be grandparents as well.

The response of older couples who already have children to learning that the woman is pregnant may vary greatly depending on whether the pregnancy was planned or unexpected. Other factors influencing their response include the attitudes of their children, family, and friends to the pregnancy; the impact on their lifestyle; and the financial implications of having another child. Sometimes couples who had previously been married to other mates will choose to have a child together. The concept of blended family applies to situations in which "her" children, "his" children, and "their" children come together as a new family group.

Healthcare professionals may treat the older expectant couple differently from the way they would a younger couple. Older women may be asked to submit to more medical procedures, such as amniocentesis and ultrasound, than younger women. An older woman may be prevented from using a birthing room or birthing center even if she is healthy because her age is considered to put her at risk.

The woman who has delayed pregnancy may be concerned about the limited amount of time that she has to bear children. When pregnancy does not occur as quickly as she hoped, the older woman may become increasingly anxious as time slips away on her "biological clock." When an older woman becomes pregnant but experiences a spontaneous abortion, her grief for the loss of her unborn child is exacerbated by her anxiety about her ability to conceive again in the time remaining to her.

NURSING CARE MANAGEMENT

Nursing Assessment and Diagnosis

In working with a woman in her 30s or 40s who is pregnant, the nurse makes the same assessments as are appropriate in caring for any woman who is pregnant. These include assessing physical status, the woman's understanding of pregnancy and the changes that accompany it, any health teaching needs that exist, the degree of support the woman has available to her, and her knowledge of infant care. In addition, the nurse explores the woman's and her partner's attitudes about the pregnancy and their expectations of the impact a baby will have on their lives.

The nursing diagnoses that are applicable to any pregnant woman apply to the pregnant woman who is over the age of 35. Examples of other nursing diagnoses that may apply include the following:

- ***Decisional Conflict*** related to unexpected pregnancy
- ***Impaired Social Interaction*** related to changes associated with pregnancy

Nursing Plan and Implementation

Once an older couple has decided to have a child, it is the nurse's responsibility to respect and support them in this decision. As with any client, the nurse needs to discuss risks, identify concerns, and promote strengths. The woman's age should not be made an issue. To promote a sense of well-being, the nurse should treat the pregnancy as "normal" unless specific health risks are identified.

As the pregnancy continues, the nurse should identify and discuss concerns the woman may have related to her age or to specific health problems. The older woman who has made a conscious decision to become pregnant often has carefully thought through potential problems and may actually have fewer concerns than a younger woman or one with an unplanned pregnancy.

Childbirth education classes are important in promoting adaptation to the event of childbirth for expectant couples of any age. However, older expectant couples, who are still in the minority, often feel uncomfortable in classes where the majority of participants are much younger. Because of the differences in age and life experiences, many of the needs of the older couple may not be met in the class. The nurse teaching a childbirth education class should try to anticipate the informational needs of the older couple. At the same time, the nurse should not make the couple feel uncomfortable by drawing attention to their age. Fortunately, classes for expectant parents over age 35 are now available in many communities. Women who are over 35 years of age and having their first baby tend to be better educated than other healthcare consumers. These clients frequently know the kind of care and services they want and are assertive in their interactions with the healthcare system. The nurse should neither be intimidated by these clients nor assume that they do not need anticipatory guidance and support. Instead, the nurse should support the couple's strengths and be sensitive to their individual needs.

MEDIALINK CHILDBIRTH.ORG

A particularly difficult issue older expectant couples face is the possibility of bearing an unhealthy child. Because of the risk of Down syndrome in these families, amniocentesis is encouraged. Chorionic villus sampling may also be suggested if available in the area. The decision to have amniocentesis can be difficult to make merely on the basis of its possible risks to the fetus. But that becomes almost a minor concern when the couple thinks of the implications of the possible findings of Down syndrome or other chromosomal abnormalities. The finding of abnormalities means that the couple may be faced with an even more difficult decision about continuing the pregnancy.

A couple's decision to have amniocentesis is usually related to their beliefs and attitudes about abortion. Generally, amniocentesis is not even considered by couples who are strongly opposed to abortion for any reason. Health professionals must respect the couple's decision, take a nonjudgmental approach, and provide them with emotional support throughout the pregnancy.

The decision to have an abortion is a painful one even when couples are not opposed to abortion on political or philosophic grounds. Even though the couple may believe that terminating a high-risk pregnancy is right for their family, they may feel a great deal of ambivalence about amniocentesis. If the results are such that the couple elects to have an abortion, they will usually feel much grief for their loss.

Many health professionals assume that the couple who agrees to amniocentesis will also elect to have an abortion if Down syndrome or another condition is diagnosed. This is not necessarily the case. Some couples choose not to have an abortion after being informed that their unborn child has genetic abnormalities.

For the couple who agrees to amniocentesis, the first few months of pregnancy are a difficult time. Amniocentesis cannot be done until 14 weeks of pregnancy, and the chromosomal studies take roughly 2 weeks to complete. Their fear that the fetus is at risk may delay the successful completion of the psychologic tasks of early pregnancy.

The nurse can support couples who decide to have amniocentesis in several ways:

- The nurse should make sure that the couple is aware of the risks of amniocentesis and why it is being performed.
- The nurse who is present during the amniocentesis procedure can offer comfort and emotional support to the expectant woman. The nurse can also provide information about the procedure as it is being performed.
- The nurse can facilitate a support group for women during the difficult waiting period between the procedure and the results.
- If the results indicate that the fetus has Down syndrome or another genetic abnormality, the nurse can ensure that the couple has complete information about the condition, its range of possible manifestations, and its developmental implications.
- The nurse can support the couple in their decision about continuing or terminating the pregnancy. It is essential that the nurse and other health professionals involved with the couple not impose their philosophic or political beliefs about abortion on the couple. The decision is the couple's, and it should be based on their belief system and a nonbiased presentation of risks and choices from caregivers.

Amniocentesis is discussed further in Chapter 21.

Evaluation

Expected outcomes of nursing care include the following:

- The woman and her partner are knowledgeable about the pregnancy and make appropriate healthcare choices.
- The expectant couple is able to cope successfully with the pregnancy and its implications for the future.
- The woman receives effective healthcare throughout her pregnancy and during birth and the postpartum period.
- The woman and her partner develop skills in child care and parenting as necessary.

CHAPTER REVIEW

EXPLOREMEDIALINK

NCLEX review questions, case studies, and other interactive resources for this chapter can be found on the Web site at http://www.prenhall.com/olds. Click on "Chapter 16" to select the activities for this chapter.

For tutorials including animations and videos, more NCLEX review questions, and an audio glossary, access the accompanying CD-ROM in this book.

Focus Your Study

- Providing anticipatory guidance about childbirth, the postpartum period, and childrearing is a primary responsibility of the nurse caring for women in an antepartal setting.
- The nurse assesses the expectant father's knowledge level and intended degree of participation and then works with the couple to help ensure a satisfying experience.
- Culturally based practices and forbidden activities may have a major impact on the childbearing family.
- The common discomforts of pregnancy occur as a result of physiologic and anatomic changes. The nurse provides the woman with information about self-care activities aimed at reducing or relieving discomfort.
- To make appropriate self-care choices and ensure healthful habits, a pregnant woman requires accurate information about a range of subjects from exercise to sexual activity, from bathing to immunization.

- Maternal assessment of fetal activity keeps the woman "in touch" with her fetus and provides ongoing assessment of fetal status.
- Teratogenic substances are substances that adversely affect the normal growth and development of the fetus.
- A pregnant woman should avoid taking nonessential medications or using over-the-counter preparations during pregnancy.
- Evidence confirms that smoking, consuming alcohol, or using social drugs during pregnancy may be harmful to the fetus.
- Childbirth among women over 35 is becoming increasingly common. It poses fewer health risks than previously believed and offers advantages for the woman or couple who makes the choice.
- A major risk for the older expectant couple relates to the increased incidence of Down syndrome in children born to women over age 35. Amniocentesis can provide information as to whether the fetus has Down syndrome. The couple can then decide whether they wish to continue the pregnancy.

References

Aikins Murphy, P. (1998). Alternative therapies for nausea and vomiting of pregnancy. *Obstetrics and Gynecology, 91*(1), 149–155.

American College of Obstetricians and Gynecologists (ACOG). (1994). *Exercise during pregnancy and the postpartum period* (ACOG Technical Bulletin No. 189). Washington, DC: Author.

American College of Obstetricians and Gynecologists (ACOG). (1997a). *Advanced paternal age* (ACOG Committee Opinion No. 189). Washington, DC: Author.

American College of Obstetricians and Gynecologists (ACOG). (1997b). *Smoking and women's health* (ACOG Educational Bulletin No. 240). Washington, DC: Author.

American College of Obstetricians and Gynecologists (ACOG). (1997c). *Teratology* (ACOG Educational Bulletin No. 236). Washington, DC: Author.

American College of Obstetricians and Gynecologists (ACOG). (1998). *Obstetrical aspects of trauma management* (ACOG Educational Bulletin No. 251). Washington, DC: Author.

American College of Obstetricians and Gynecologists (ACOG). (2000). *Smoking cessation during pregnancy* (ACOG Educational Bulletin No. 260). Washington, DC: Author.

American College of Obstetricians and Gynecologists (ACOG). (2001). *Air travel during pregnancy* (ACOG Committee Opinion No. 264). Washington, DC: Author.

American College of Obstetricians and Gynecologists (ACOG). (2002). *Exercise during pregnancy and the postpartum period* (ACOG Technical Bulletin No. 267). Washington, DC: Author.

Andrews, M., & Boyle, J. (Eds.). (1999). *Transcultural concepts in nursing care* (3rd ed.). Philadelphia: Lippincott.

Askin, D. F., & Diehl-Jones, B. (2001). Cocaine: Effects of in utero exposure on the fetus and neonate. *Journal of Perinatal and Neonatal Nursing, 14*(4), 83–102.

Beckman, C. R., & Dysart, D. (2000). The challenge of multicultural medical care. *Contemporary OB/GYN, 45*(12), 12–33.

Belew, C. (1999). Herbs and the childbearing woman: Guidelines for midwives. *Journal of Nurse Midwifery, 44*(3), 231–253.

Blatt, S. D., Meguid, V., & Church, C. C. (2000). Prenatal cocaine: What's known about outcomes? *Contemporary OB/GYN, 45*(9), 67–81.

Blumenthal, M; Goldberg, A; Brinckmann, J. (Eds.). (2000). *Herbal Medicine: Expanded Commission E monographs*, Newton, MA: Integrative Medicine Communications.

Brennan, P. (1999). Homeopathic remedies in prenatal care. *Journal of Nurse Midwifery, 44*(3), 291–299.

Bungum, T. J., Peaslee, D., Jackson, A. W., & Perez, M. A. (2000). Exercise during pregnancy and type of delivery in nulliparae. *Journal of Obstetric, Gynecologic, and Neonatal Nursing, 29*(3), 258–264.

Callister, L. C. (2001). Culturally competent care of women and newborns: Knowledge, attitude, and skills. *Journal of Obstetric, Gynecologic, and Neonatal Nursing, 30*(2), 209–215.

Carl, D. L., Roux, G., & Matacale, R. (2000). Exploring dental hygiene and perinatal outcomes: Oral health implications for pregnancy and early childhood. *AWHONN Lifelines, 4*(1), 22–27.

Cesario, S. K. (2001). Care of the Native American woman: Strategies for practice, education, and research. *Journal of Obstetric, Gynecologic, and Neonatal Nursing, 30*(1), 13–19.

Chez, R. A., & Friedmann, A. K. (2000). Offering effective breastfeeding advice. *Contemporary OB/GYN, 45*(8), 32–50.

Chez, R. A., & Murphy, P. (2000). Management of nausea and vomiting in pregnancy: Alternative therapies. *Contemporary OB/GYN, 45*(4), 55–64.

Chez, R. A., & Niebyl, J. (2000). Management of nausea and vomiting in pregnancy: Traditional therapies. *Contemporary OB/GYN, 45*(3), 130–136.

Christensen, F. C., & Rayburn, W. F. (1999). Fetal movement counts. *Obstetrics and Gynecology Clinics of North America, 26*(4), 607–621.

Chung, K. C., Kowalski, C. P., Kim, H. M., & Buchman, S. R. (2000). Maternal cigarette smoking during pregnancy and the risk of having a child with cleft lip/palate. *Plastic and Reconstructive Surgery, 105*(2), 485–491.

Clapp, J. F., III. (2001). Recommending exercise during pregnancy. *Contemporary OB/GYN, 46*(1), 30–50.

Clapp, J. F., III, Kim, H., Burciu, B., & Lopez, B. (2000). Beginning regular exercise in pregnancy: Effect on fetoplacental growth. *American Journal of Obstetrics and Gynecology, 183*(6), 1484–1488.

Cnattingius, S., Signorello, L.B., Anneren, G., Clausson, B., Ekbom, A., Ljunger, E., et al. (2000). Caffeine intake and the risk of first-trimester spontaneous abortion. *New England Journal of Medicine, 343*(25), 1839–1845.

Cunningham, F. G., Gant, N. F., Leveno, K. J., Gilstrap, L. C., III, Hauth, J. C., & Wenstrom, K. D. (2001). *Williams obstetrics* (21st ed.). New York: McGraw-Hill.

Eisenberg, D. M., Davis, R. B., Ettner, S. L., Appel, S., Wilkey, S., Van Rompey, M., et al. (1998). Trends in alternative medicine use in the United States, 1990-1997. *Journal of the American Medical Association, 280*(18), 1569–1575.

Fulder, S., & Tenne, M. (1996). Ginger as an anti-nausea remedy in pregancy: The issue of safety. *HerbalGram, 38*, 47–50.

Gallo, M., Sarkar, M., Au, W., Pietrzak, K., Comas, B., Smith, M., et al. (2000). Pregnancy outcome following gestational exposure to echinacea. *Archives of Internal Medicine, 160*, 3141–3143.

Goldenberg, R. L., & Dolan-Mullen, P. (2000). Convincing pregnant patients to stop smoking. *Contemporary OB/GYN, 45*(11), 35–44.

Good news for pregnant women with heartburn. (1999). *Contemporary OB/Gyn, 44*(12), 50.

Gottlieb, B. (2000). *Alternative cures.* Emmaus, PA: Rodale Press.

Greenhalgh, R., Slade, P., Spiby, H. (2000). Fathers' coping styles, antenatal preparation, and experiences of labor and the postpartum. *Birth, 27*(3), 177–84.

Hardy, M. (2000). Herbs of special interest to women. *Journal of the American Pharmaceutical Association, 40*(2), 234–242.

Hefferman, A. E. (2000). Herbs of special interest to women. *Journal of the American Pharmaceutical Association, 40*(2), 234–242.

Hoyert, D. L., Danel, I., & Tully, P. (2000). Maternal mortality, United States and Canada, 1982–97. *Birth, 27*(1), 4–11.

Jewell, D., & Young, G. (2001). Interventions for nausea and vomiting in early pregnancy (Cochrane Review). In: *The Cochrane Library, 4,* Oxford: Update Software.

Johnson, H. C., & Pring, D. W. (2001). Car seatbelts in pregnancy: The practice and knowledge of pregnant women remain causes for concern. *British Journal of Obstetrics and Gynaecology, 107,* 644–647.

Lacroix, R., Eason, E., & Melzak, R. (2000). Nausea and vomiting during pregnancy: A prospective study of its frequency, intensity, and patterns of change. *American Journal of Obstetrics and Gynecology, 182*(4), 931–937.

Maloni, J. A. (2001). Preventing low birthweight: How smoking cessation counseling can help. *AWHONN Lifelines, 5*(1), 3235.

Mattson, S. (2000a). Ethnocultural considerations in the childbearing period. In S. Mattson, & J. E. Smith (Eds.), *Core curriculum for maternal-newborn nursing* (2nd ed.). Philadelphia: W. B. Saunders.

Mattson, S. (2000b). Providing culturally competent care: Strategies and approaches for perinatal clients. *AWHONN Lifelines, 4*(5), 37–39.

Mattson, S. (2000c). Striving for cultural competence: Providing care for the changing face of the U.S. *AWHONN Lifelines, 4*(3), 48–52.

Mattson, S. (2000d). Working toward cultural competence: Making the first steps through cultural assessment. *AWHONN Lifelines, 4*(4), 41–43.

Mills, L. W., & Moses, D. T. (2002). Oral health during pregnancy. *American Journal of Maternal Child Nursing, 27*(5), 275–280.

Mindell, J. A., & Jacobson, B. J. (2000). Sleep disturbances during pregnancy. *Journal of Obstetric, Gynecologic, and Neonatal Nursing, 29*(6), 590–597.

Morgan, M., & Bone, K. (1998). *Professional review: Horsechestnut Medicinal Herb, 65,* 1–4.

Mozurkewich, E. M., Luke, B., Avni, M., & Wolf, F. M. (2000). Working conditions and adverse pregnancy outcome: A meta-analysis. *Obstetrics & Gynecology, 95*(4), 623–635.

National Center for Health Statistics. (1999, December 15). *Infant mortality rates vary by race and ethnicity* (News release). Hyattsville, MD: Author.

Niebyl, J. R. (1999). Teratology and drugs in pregnancy. In J. R. Scott, P. J. DiSaia, C. B. Hammond, & W. N. Spellacy, (Eds.), *Danforth's obstetrics and gynecology* (8th ed., pp. 197–212.). Philadelphia: Lippincott Williams & Wilkins.

Orleans, C. T., Barker, D. C., Kaufman, N. J., & Marx, J. F. (2001). Helping pregnant smokers quit: Meeting the challenge in the next decade. *Western Journal of Medicine, 174*(4), 276–281.

Pollack, H., Lantz, P. M., & Frohna, J. G. (2000). Maternal smoking and adverse birth outcomes among singletons and twins. *American Journal of Public Health, 90*(3), 395–400.

Shrock, P. (2000). Exercise and physical activity during pregnancy. In J. J. Sciarra, (Ed.), *Gynecology and Obstetrics* (Vol. 2, chap. 8, pp. 1–17). Philadelphia: Lippincott Williams & Wilkins.

Reuters Medical News. (2001). UK advises pregnant women on caffeine intake. *Medscape.* Retrieved October 16, 2001, from http://womenshealth.medscape.com/reuters/prof/2001/10/10.11/20011010plcy002.html

Skidmore-Roth, L. (2001). *Mosby's handbook of herbs & natural supplements.* St. Louis, MO: Mosby.

Spector, R. E. (2000). *Cultural diversity in health and illness* (5th ed.). Upper Saddle River, NJ: Prentice Hall Health.

Steele, N. M., French, J., Gatherer-Boyles, J., Newman, S., & Leclaire, S. (2001). Effect of acupressure by Sea-Bands on nausea and vomiting of pregnancy. *Journal of Obstetric, Gynecologic, and Neonatal Nursing, 30*(1), 6170.

Stevenson, A. M. (1999). Immunizations for women and infants. *Journal of Obstetric, Gynecologic, and Neonatal Nursing, 28*(5), 534–544.

Tedesco, P., & Cicchetti, J. (2001). Like cures like: Homeopathy. *American Journal of Nursing, 101*(9), 43–49.

Todd, S. T., Bradshaw-LaSala, K., & Neil-Urban, S. (2001). An integrated approach to prenatal smoking cessation interventions. *American Journal of Maternal Child Nursing, 26*(4), 185–190.

Tough, S. C., Newburn-Cook, C., Johnston, D. W., Svenson, L. W., Rose, S., & Belitok, J. (2002). Delayed childbearing and its impact on population rate changes in lower birth weight, multiple birth, and preterm delivery. *Pediatrics, 109*(3), 399–403.

Tyroch, A. H., Kaups, K. L., Rohan, J., Song, S., & Beingesser, K. (1999). Pregnant women and car restraints: Beliefs and practices. *Journal of Trauma: Injury, Infection, and Critical Care, 46*(2), 241–244.

Underwood-Gichia, J. E. (2000). Mothers and others: African-American women's preparation for motherhood. *American Journal of Maternal Child Nursing, 25*(2), 86–91.

US Census Bureau. (1998). *Resident population of the U.S.: Estimates by sex, race, and Hispanic origin.* Washington, DC: Government Printing Office.

Vutyavanich, T., Kraisarin, T., & Ruangsri, R. (2001). Ginger for nausea and vomiting in pregnancy: Randomized, double-mashed, placebo-controlled trial. *Obsetrics and Gynecology, 97*(4), 577–582.

Weidner, M. S., & Sigwart, K. (2001). Investigation of the teratogenic potential of a *Zingiber officinale* extract in the rat. *Reproductive Toxicology, 15*(1), 75–80.

Whitney, J. L. (1999). Drug labeling and pregnancy update: What has the FDA done lately? *Contemporary OB/GYN, 44*(1), 85–95.

Willis, W. O. (1999). Culturally competent nursing care during the perinatal period. *Journal of Perinatal and Neonatal Nursing, 13*(3), 45–59.

Windridge, K. C., & Berryman, J. C. (1999). Women's experiences of giving birth after 35. *Birth, 26*(1), 16–23.

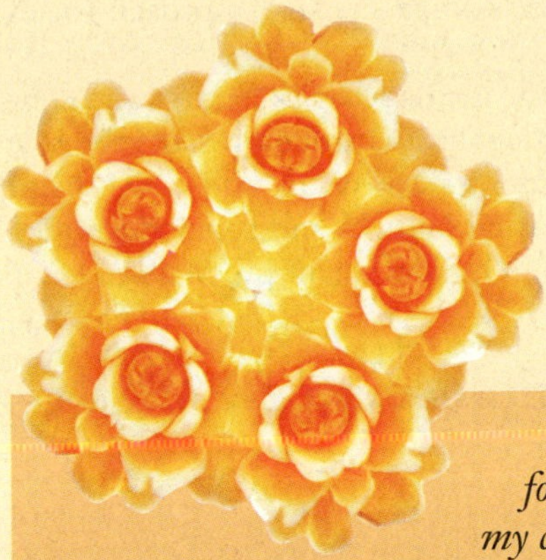

17 Adolescent Pregnancy

I am a freshman in college, and so is my daughter. I had her when I was 15, and that forced me to grow up in a hurry. For years I've thought about being a nurse, and now is my chance. Please understand, my daughter is very precious to me, but a part of me knows that if I had it to do over, I would change so much of my life—if only I had known!

Objectives

- Briefly discuss the physical and psychosocial changes of adolescence.
- Compare the three stages of adolescence: early adolescence, middle adolescence, and late adolescence.
- Summarize the developmental tasks of adolescence and the impact that pregnancy superimposes on these tasks.
- Describe the major factors that contribute to teenage pregnancy.
- Identify the impact of cultural factors on the desirability of early pregnancy.
- Identify the physical, psychologic, and sociologic risks faced by an adolescent who is pregnant.
- Describe successful community approaches to adolescent pregnancy prevention.
- Delineate characteristics of the fathers of children of adolescent mothers.
- Discuss the reactions of the adolescent's family and social support groups to her pregnancy.
- Formulate a plan of care to meet the needs of a pregnant adolescent.

Key Terms

Early adolescence 393
Emancipated minors 400
Late adolescence 393
Middle adolescence 393

MediaLink

Additional resources for this content can be found on the Student CD-ROM and on the Companion Website at www.prenhall.com/olds. Click on "Chapter 17" to select the activities for this chapter.

CD-ROM
- Audio Glossary
- NCLEX Review

Companion Website
- Additional NCLEX Review
- Case Study: Adolescent Pregnancy
- Care Plan Activity: Adolescent Pregnancy

Adolescent pregnancy is a multifaceted issue with no single cause or cure. For a teen, pregnancy comes at a time when her physical development and the developmental tasks of adolescence are incomplete. She is not prepared physically, psychologically, or economically for parenthood. Thus both she and her child are at high risk. The negative socioeconomic impact on society is also significant.

Approximately 900,000 teenage girls (ages 15 to 19) in the United States become pregnant each year, and most of these pregnancies are unplanned (Preventing Teenage Pregnancy, 2002). Of these pregnancies, about one third are terminated by therapeutic abortion, and about 14% end in miscarriage. More than half the teens who become pregnant give birth and keep their babies. Very few adolescents give up their babies for adoption (Singh & Darroch, 2000).

The US birth rate (number of births per 1000 women) for adolescents ages 15 to 19 has dropped steadily over the past decade, from 62.1 per 1000 females in 1991 to 45.9 in 2001, a 26% decline (National Center for Health Statistics, 2002) (Figure 17–1 •). This continuing decline is extremely encouraging. However, the US teenage birth rate remains the highest of any industrialized nation (National Campaign to Prevent Teen Pregnancy, 2000). The incidence of sexual activity among teens in other countries is as high as in the United States. Research suggests that these countries may have lower adolescent pregnancy rates because of family influences, a greater openness about sexuality, better access to contraceptives, and a more comprehensive approach to sex education.

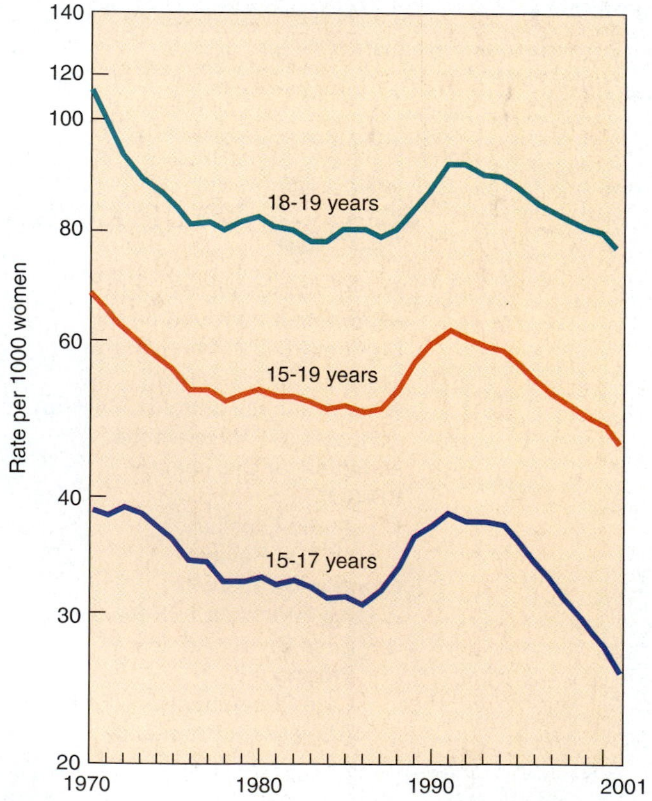

Figure 17–1 • Birth rates for teenagers by age: United States, 1970–2001.
SOURCE: Martin, J. A., Park, M. M., & Sutton, P. D. (2002). Births: Preliminary data for 2001. *National Vital Statistics Report, 50*(10), 1–20.

This chapter explores the incidence, risk factors, and consequences of adolescent pregnancy. It then presents the role of the nurse in meeting the special needs and concerns of pregnant adolescents and their families and concludes with a discussion of efforts to prevent adolescent pregnancy.

Overview of Adolescence

Physical Changes

Puberty, that period during which an individual becomes capable of reproduction, is a maturational process that can last from 1.5 to 6 years and generally coincides with adolescence. The major physical changes of puberty include a growth spurt, weight change, and the appearance of secondary sexual characteristics. *Menarche*, or the time of the first menstrual period, usually occurs in the last half of this maturational process, with the average age between 12 and 13.

The initial menstrual cycles are usually irregular and often anovulatory for the first 12 to 18 months; however, this is not true for all females. Some adolescents do not use contraception during this time because they falsely assume that they cannot get pregnant. Even if their initial menstrual cycles are anovulatory, there is no certainty about when the first ovulatory cycle will occur; thus, contraception is important during this time for all adolescents who are sexually active.

Psychosocial Development

Although it is well documented that the onset of puberty now occurs at a younger age than it did 50 years ago, there are no data to indicate that psychosocial development, particularly cognitive development, occurs at an earlier age. Developmental tasks of adolescence have been described by many writers and are based on a variety of classic theories. These tasks are issues that individuals may struggle with at other times in their lives, but they are especially significant during adolescence to help ensure a successful transition from childhood to adulthood. The following are major developmental tasks of this period (Steinberg, 2002):

- Developing an identity
- Gaining autonomy and independence
- Developing intimacy in a relationship
- Developing comfort with one's own sexuality
- Developing a sense of achievement

Resolving these tasks is a developmental process that occurs over time. This developmental process is reflected in the behaviors of youths during early, middle, and late adolescence. Although average ages for the completion of tasks have been identified, these ages are somewhat arbitrary and are affected by many factors such as culture, religion, and socioeconomic status.

In **early adolescence** (age 14 and under), the teen still sees authority as resting with the parents. She perceives her locus of control as external; that is, her destiny is controlled by others, such as parents and school authorities. However, she begins the process of "leaving the family" by spending more time with friends, especially friends of the same sex. Conformity to peer group standards is reflected in her behavior and in the clothes she wears. During this phase, the adolescent has a rich fantasy life. In addition, she is struggling to become comfortable with her changing body and body image and to fit this image with her fantasy life. Much time is spent in front of the mirror. The adolescent in this phase is very egocentric and is a concrete thinker. She has only minimal ability to see herself in the future or foresee the consequences of her behavior.

Middle adolescence (15 to 17 years) is the time for challenging authority. Experimentation with drugs, alcohol, and sex is a common method of rebellion. As the middle adolescent seeks independence, she turns increasingly to her peer group, identifying with and conforming to them in her choice of dress, makeup, hairstyle, and music. These years are often a time of great turmoil for the family as the adolescent struggles for independence and challenges the family's values and expectations.

The middle adolescent wants to be treated as an adult. However, fear of adult responsibility may cause fluctuation in behavior. At times she seems like a child; at other times she is surprisingly mature. She is beginning to move from concrete thinking to formal operational thought but is not yet able to anticipate the long-term implications of all her actions. She may even believe that she is invincible and will not suffer negative consequences from risk-taking behaviors.

In **late adolescence** (18 to 19 years), the young woman is more at ease with her individuality and decision-making ability. She can think abstractly and anticipate consequences. During this time, she becomes more confident of her personal identity. The late adolescent is capable of formal operational thought. She is learning to solve problems, to conceptualize, and to make decisions. These abilities help her see herself as having control, which leads to the ability to understand and accept the consequences of her behavior.

Table 17–1 • describes successful resolution of each of the developmental tasks of adolescence and identifies high risk factors for adolescent pregnancy.

Table 17–1 • DEVELOPMENTAL TASKS OF ADOLESCENCE

Tasks	Description of Successful Resolution	High-Risk Factors for Teen Pregnancy
Developing an identity	As individuals enter puberty, their physical appearance begins to change, and others begin to respond differently to them. The media present idealized images of the teenage female. Self-esteem may fluctuate, and hormonal changes create awareness of sexual desire. Adolescents experience confusion about their self-image. This is a time of experimentation until they become comfortable with who they are.	If the young adolescent feels she cannot live up to parents' expectations or is in a dysfunctional family situation, she may adopt a negative identity. She may become rebellious and actively involved in risk-taking behaviors, such as substance abuse and early sexual activity.
Gaining independence	Adolescents gradually move away from parental control and are influenced by peers. Eventually, they develop values that help govern their behavior responsibly without extrinsic control of peers or parents.	Peer pressure is highest during early and middle adolescence. If peers are involved in antisocial behavior, this influences their behavior and all other developmental tasks. Substance abuse and sexual activity are common in these groups.
Developing emotional intimacy in relationships	Adolescents begin to develop a close emotional attachment with another individual. They can share innermost feelings and have empathy for the other. This usually begins with a friend of the same sex and eventually develops into a trusting and loving relationship with someone of the opposite sex.	Sexual activity may be an attempt to meet needs for intimacy. This is a problem for victims of neglect or abuse. Although sexual intercourse has become a common adolescent experience, emotional intimacy is not associated with the majority of dating relationships, and most teenage marriages end in divorce.
Developing comfort with their sexuality	Puberty causes a new awareness of sexual desire and new meaning about physical contact with others. Adolescents learn to express sexual feelings appropriately and comfortably in a relationship.	Many young adolescent females who become sexually involved at an early age do so for a variety of reasons that do not lead to comfort with their own sexuality: peer pressure, pressure from an older male partner, rebellion against parents, sexual abuse and its consequences.
Gaining a sense of achievement	Adolescents begin to look toward the future and compare talents, work skills, and/or academic achievement with reality in preparing for adult working roles.	Those who drop out of school prematurely tend to be from economically disadvantaged backgrounds. Data show that early sexual experimentation by adolescents correlates with poor school performance whatever their background (Stevens-Simon, Kelly, Singer, et al, 1996). Use of contraception is more likely among adolescent females who are high academic achievers and have a future orientation (Alan Guttmacher Institute, 2002).

Source: Adapted from Steinberg, L. (2002). *Adolescence*, (6th ed.). New York: McGraw-Hill.

Factors Contributing to Adolescent Pregnancy

Teenagers rarely plan pregnancy. Those who are sexually active become pregnant because they lack a firm commitment not to do so. *Pregnancy risk taking* (sexual activity without use of pregnancy prevention measures) is believed to stem from a complex variety of factors, the most important of which are discussed next.

Peer Pressure to Engage in Sexual Activity

Among American adolescents, there is tremendous peer pressure to become sexually active. In a 1996 survey, 61% of adolescent girls reported that their partner was pressuring them to have sex, while 41% reported that they had engaged in sex because they wanted to be popular (Figure 17–2 •). In addition to this direct pressure from their peers, adolescents encounter sexual images and innuendo almost everywhere they turn—in magazines, pop music, music videos, television, and movies. These images feed the adolescent's rich fantasy life, and may glamorize unprotected intercourse as proof of "true love." At the same time, media aimed at teens largely ignores issues of sexual responsibility, and fails to convey the physical, emotional, financial, and social costs of pregnancy risk-taking behavior.

Lack of Knowledge about Sexuality and Contraception

Accurate sex education is not part of many adolescents' learning experiences, and pregnancy risk taking has been linked to lack of knowledge about contraception. Because of teens' lack of knowledge about sexuality, many healthcare providers advocate sex education in schools, and at a younger age than previously provided. Others feel that sex education is the responsibility of the parents and are concerned that sex education in the schools will promote sexual activity. Review of research on sex education, however, demonstrates that it does not increase initiation of sexual activity at an earlier age (Doniger, Adams, Utter, et al, 2001).

About three fourths of adolescents do use some form of contraception (often a condom) the first time they have sexual intercourse (Graydanus, Patel, & Rimsza, 2001). More encouragingly, statistics have demonstrated an increased use of condoms among the adolescent population, probably because of the tremendous educational efforts related to the human immunodeficiency virus (HIV) (Santelli, Linburg, Abma, et al, 2000). Once adolescents have their first sexual experience, however, subsequent sexual experiences may occur infrequently. As a result, they do not consistently use contraceptives (Graydanus et al, 2001). When asked why they didn't use birth control, the most common response by teens is that they did not plan or expect to have sex (National Campaign to Prevent Teen Pregnancy, 2000). Other factors reducing contraceptive use include lack of access or availability, cost of supplies, and concerns about confidentiality.

Emotional Factors

For some adolescents, a pregnancy meets relationship needs or age-related goals (Montgomery, 2001). Thus, the girl may deliberately or subconsciously plan to get preg-

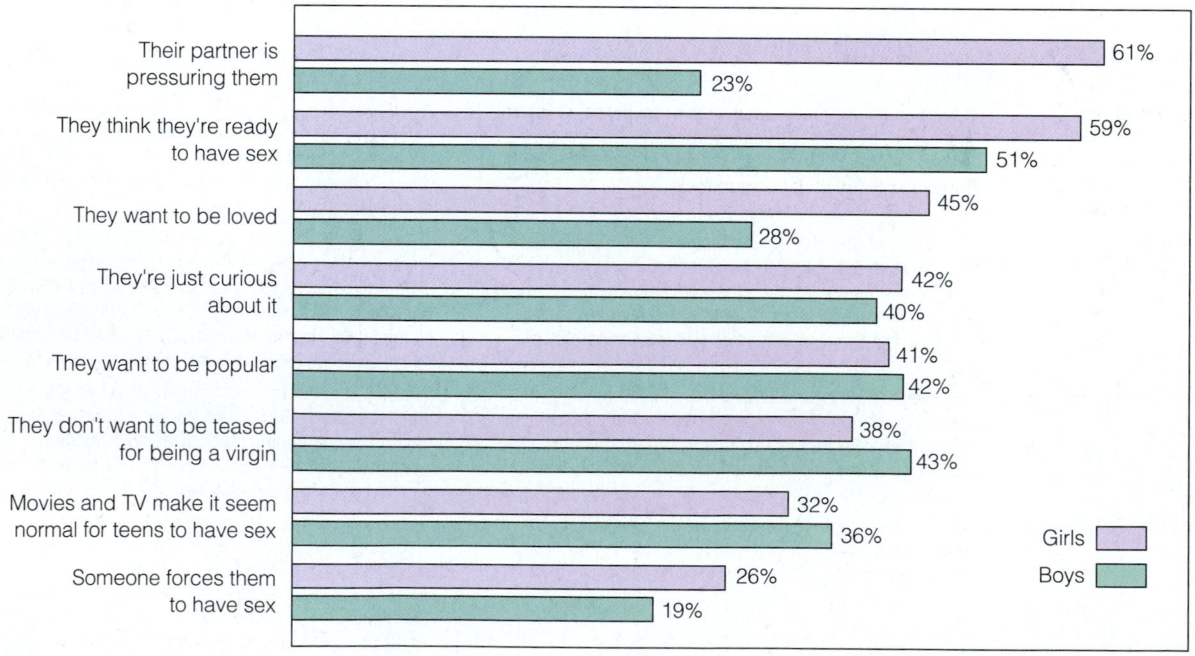

Figure 17–2 • Why teens have sex.
SOURCE: *The 1996 Kaiser Family Foundation Survey on Teens and Sex: What They Say. Teens Today Need to Know, and Who They Listen To,* Chart 3, *Girls' and Boys' Views Differ on Why Teens Have Sex.* Kaiser Family Foundation/Princeton Survey Research Associates, June 24, 1996. This information was reprinted with permission of the Henry J. Kaiser Family Foundation of Menlo Park, California. The Kaiser Family Foundation is an independent health care philanthropy and is not associated with Kaiser Permanente or Kaiser Industries.

nant for a variety of reasons: to punish her father or mother, to escape from an undesirable home situation, to gain attention, or to feel that she has someone to love and to love her. In these cases, pregnancy may in a sense be the young woman's form of delinquency. Like delinquent males, pregnant adolescents often have a history of troubled family relationships, poor school achievement, and exposure to drug abuse.

Whereas most teens have their first experience of sexual intercourse during middle or late adolescence, those who become sexually active at an earlier age tend to have been physically, emotionally, or sexually abused at a young age (Adams & East, 1999). In fact, maltreatment of any kind is a high-risk contributor to early-teen pregnancy (Stock, Bell, Boyer, et al, 1997).

Teenage pregnancy can result from an incestuous relationship. In the very young adolescent, incest or sexual abuse should always be suspected as a possible cause of pregnancy. In middle adolescence, the psychologic turmoil experienced by the incest victim may obliterate thought of the risk of pregnancy. Late adolescents may fear the possibility of pregnancy, but for a variety of psychologic reasons may deny the reality. Teenage pregnancy could also be caused by other nonvoluntary sexual experiences, such as acquaintance rape.

Socioeconomic Factors

Compared with poor teens, middle-class teens with future goals (ie, college or job) tend to use birth control more consistently. If they do become pregnant, they are more likely to have an abortion. Adolescents who do not have such goals or who lack access to middle-class opportunities, in contrast, tend to maintain their pregnancies. Eighty-five percent of births to unmarried teens occur to those from families who are poor or near poor (Alan Guttmacher Institute, 2002). Recent revisions of welfare policies (see Chapter 8) are expected to reduce teen pregnancy rates in this group, although the true reduction may be in the welfare of children of adolescent mothers.

The adolescent birth rate is higher among African American and Hispanic teens than white teens. However, pregnancy rates in all of these groups are decreasing steadily (Mims, 1998; Santelli et al, 2000). To some degree, the higher teen pregnancy rate in these groups reflects the impact of poverty, as a disproportionately higher number of African American and Hispanic youths live in poverty.

Other Factors

In addition to the high-risk factors already discussed, the younger the teen when she first gets pregnant, the more likely she will have another pregnancy in her teens (Key, Barbosa, & Owens, 2001). Moreover, the likelihood of repeat pregnancies increases when the teen is living with her sexual partner and has dropped out of school. Similarly, siblings of adolescent parents have been found to be at higher risk for earlier sexual activity and adolescent pregnancy.

International Perspective

Currently more than 15 million births—slightly more than 10% of all births worldwide—are to women under age 20. In many parts of North Africa, Asia, and the Middle East, early childbearing is, fortunately, declining; however, little has changed in sub-Saharan Africa and Latin America (Alan Guttmacher Institute, 1998). Cultural factors often play a significant role in the desirability of early pregnancy. Specifically, adolescent women are more likely to welcome a pregnancy in a country where Islam is the predominant religion, where large families are desired, where social change is slow in coming, and where most childbearing occurs within marriage. Early pregnancy is less desired in countries where the reverse is true.

Among industrialized countries, adolescent pregnancy rates for girls ages 15 to 19 years vary from a low of 12 pregnancies per 1000 adolescents in the Netherlands to a high of 102 pregnancies per 1000 in the Russian Federation. Most western European countries and Japan have low rates (fewer than 40 per 1000), whereas the United States joins four other countries—Belarus, Bulgaria, Romania, and the Russian Federation—that have pregnancy rates of greater than 70 per 1000 adolescents (Alan Guttmacher Institute, 2002). Despite these seemingly high rates, the trend toward lower adolescent birth rates and pregnancy rates over the past 25 years is widespread and occurs in most industrialized countries. The reasons for this decrease may be related to the increased recognition of the importance of education along with an ever-increasing desire in many young people to attain education. In addition, in many parts of the world, young women now have goals in their life beyond marriage and motherhood (Singh & Darroch, 2000).

The Adolescent Mother

Physiologic Risks

Adolescents over age 15 who receive early, thorough prenatal care are at no greater risk during pregnancy than women over 20 years. Unfortunately, many adolescents fail to seek early prenatal care. Those who do seek care may fail to cooperate with recommendations. In addition, teenage mothers are more likely to smoke than older pregnant women and less likely to gain sufficient weight during their pregnancy. Thus risks for pregnant adolescents include preterm births, low-birth-weight (LBW) infants, preeclampsia-eclampsia and its sequelae, iron deficiency anemia, and cephalopelvic disproportion (CPD). In the adolescent age group, prenatal care is the critical factor that most influences pregnancy outcome.

DEVELOPING CULTURAL COMPETENCE

Throughout the world, the higher a woman's educational level, the more likely she is to delay marriage and childbirth.

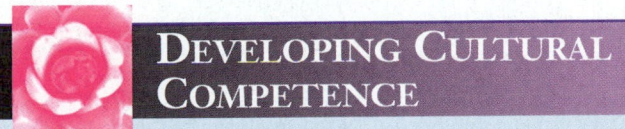

Iron deficiency anemia is a problem in all pregnant women. The adolescent who begins her pregnancy already anemic, however, is at increased risk and must be followed closely and counseled carefully regarding nutrition during pregnancy. The increased risk of CPD is a concern in adolescent pregnancy, especially with the early adolescent, because of a lack of pelvic maturity.

Teenagers 15 to 19 years old have a high incidence of sexually transmitted infections, including herpesvirus, syphilis, and gonorrhea. The incidence of chlamydial infection is also increased in this age group. The presence of such infections during a pregnancy greatly increases the risk to the fetus (refer to Chapter 20). Other problems seen in adolescents are alcohol and drug use. By the time pregnancy is confirmed in young women, the fetus may already be harmed by these substances.

Psychologic Risks

The most profound psychologic risk to the adolescent who maintains her pregnancy is the interruption of progress in her developmental tasks. Although adolescents have become sexually active at an earlier age and the incidence of adolescent pregnancy has increased, the developmental tasks of this age group remain the same. Add to this the tasks of pregnancy, and the young woman has an overwhelming amount of psychologic work to do, the success of which will affect her own and her newborn's future.

Table 17–2 • identifies typical behaviors of the early, middle, and late adolescent when she becomes aware of her pregnancy. In reviewing these behaviors, the nurse should realize that other factors may influence the age at which the behaviors are seen.

Table 17–3 • identifies the early adolescent's response to the developmental tasks of pregnancy. The early adolescent's response reflects her level of development, with pregnancy as an interruption of the normal process of development. The middle and late adolescents respond differently, reflecting their maturational progress through the developmental tasks. In addition to her maturational level, the amount of nurturing the pregnant adolescent receives is also a critical factor in the way she handles pregnancy and motherhood.

Sociologic Risks

A substantial body of research indicates that the adolescent mother is at higher risk for social and economic disadvantages than her teenage counterpart who is not pregnant and lives in the same social environment. Being forced into adult roles before completing adolescent developmental tasks causes a series of events that affects the adolescent's entire life. These events may result in a prolonged dependence on parents, lack of stable relationships with the opposite sex, and lack of economic and social stability.

Many teen mothers drop out of school during their pregnancy. This tendency may have as much to do with low academic achievement and low academic commitment as it does with the pregnancy. Many never complete their education. Lack of education reduces the quality of jobs available to

Table 17–2 • INITIAL REACTION TO AWARENESS OF PREGNANCY

Age	Adolescent Behavior	Nursing Implications
Early adolescent (14 and under)	Fears rejection by family and peers. Enters healthcare system with an adult, most likely mother (parents still seen as locus of control). Value system still closely reflects that of parents, so still turns to parents for decision or approval of decision. Pregnancy probably not result of intimate relationship. Is self-conscious about normal adolescent changes in body. Self-consciousness and low self-esteem likely to increase with rapid breast enlargement and abdominal enlargement of pregnancy.	Be nonjudgmental in approach to care. Focus on needs and concerns of adolescent, but if parent accompanies daughter, include parent in plan of care. Encourage both to express concerns and feelings regarding pregnancy and options: abortion, maintaining pregnancy, adoption. Be realistic and concrete in discussing implications of each option. During physical exam of adolescent, respect increased sense of modesty. Explain in simple and concrete terms physical changes that are produced by pregnancy versus puberty. Explain each step of physical exam in simple and concrete terms.
Middle adolescent (15–17 years)	Fears rejection by peers and parents. Unsure in whom to confide. May seek confirmation of pregnancy on own with increased awareness of options and services, such as over-the-counter pregnancy kits and Planned Parenthood. If in an ongoing, caring relationship with partner (peer), may choose him as confidant. Economic dependence on parents may determine if and when parents are told. Future educational plans and perception of parental support or lack of support are significant factors in decision regarding termination or maintenance of the pregnancy. Possible conflict in parental and own developing value system.	Be nonjudgmental in approach to care. Reassure the adolescent that confidentiality will be maintained. Help adolescent identify significant individuals in whom she can confide to help make a decision about the pregnancy. Be aware of state laws regarding requirement of parental notification if abortion intended. Also be aware of state laws regarding requirements for marriage: usually, minimum age for both parties is 18; 16- and 17-year-olds are, in most states, allowed to marry only with consent of parents. Encourage adolescent to be realistic about parental response to pregnancy.
Late adolescent (18–19 years)	Most likely to confirm pregnancy on own and at an earlier date due to increased acceptance and awareness of consequences of behavior. Likely to use pregnancy kit for confirmation. Relationship with father of baby, future educational plans, and own value system are among significant determinants of decision about pregnancy.	Be nonjudgmental in approach to care. Reassure the adolescent that confidentiality will be maintained. Encourage adolescent to identify significant individuals in whom she can confide. Refer to counseling as appropriate. Encourage adolescent to be realistic about parental response to pregnancy.

Table 17-3 • THE EARLY ADOLESCENT'S RESPONSE TO THE DEVELOPMENTAL TASKS OF PREGNANCY

Stage	Developmental Tasks of Pregnancy	Early Adolescent's Response to Pregnancy	Nursing Implications
First trimester	Pregnancy confirmation. Seeking early prenatal care as a confirmation tool. Begins to evaluate her diet and general health habits. Initial ambivalence common. Usually supportive partner.	May delay confirmation of pregnancy until late part of first trimester or later. Reasons for delay may include lack of awareness that she is pregnant, fear of confiding in anyone, or denial. Rapid enlargement and sensitivity of breasts are embarrassing and frightening to early adolescent—may be perceived as changes of puberty. If confiding in mother, may be experiencing family turmoil in response to pregnancy.	Explain physiologic changes of pregnancy versus those associated with puberty. Explain that ambivalence is normal with any pregnancy, but recognize it as a much greater concern with adolescent pregnancy. Emphasize need for good nutrition as important for her well-being as much as infant's (prevention of preeclampsia and anemia). Use simple explanations and lots of audiovisuals. Have adolescent listen to fetal heart rate (FHR) with Doppler.
Second trimester	Changes in physical appearance begin, and fetal movement is experienced, causing pregnancy to be experienced as a reality. Begins wearing maternity clothes to accommodate the physical changes. As a result of quickening she perceives her fetus as a real baby and begins preparing for the maternal role and new relationships with her partner and members of her family.	Some teenagers may delay validation of pregnancy until now, with family turmoil occurring at this time. Abdominal enlargement and quickening may be perceived as loss of control over body image. May try to maintain prepregnant weight and wear restrictive clothing to control and conceal changing body. Becomes dependent on her own mother for support. Egocentric; unable to develop a maternal role at this time.	Continue to discuss importance of good nutrition and adequate weight gain as noted above. Discuss ways of utilizing common teenage clothing (large sweatshirts, blouses) to promote comfort but preserve adolescent image to some degree. Discuss plans being made for baby, continued educational plans, and role of teen's parents.
Third trimester	At end of second trimester begins to view fetus as separate from self. Buys baby clothes and supplies. Prepares a place for the baby. Realistic about what baby is like. Prepares to give birth to infant. Anxiety increases as labor and birth approach and has concerns about well-being of fetus.	May focus on "wanting it to be over." May have trouble individuating fetus. May have fantasies, dreams, or nightmares about childbirth. Natural fears of labor and birth greater than with older primigravida. Probably has not been in a hospital, and may associate this with negative experiences.	Assess whether adolescent is preparing for baby by buying supplies and preparing a place in the home. Childbirth education important. Provide hospital tour. Assess for discomforts of pregnancy, such as heartburn and constipation. Adolescent may be uncomfortable mentioning these and other problems.

these women. Childbearing at an early age is a strong predictor of need for public assistance, especially in lower socioeconomic groups and when the pregnant adolescent's family will not support her (National Campaign to Prevent Teen Pregnancy, [NCPTP] 2000).

Adolescent mothers frequently fail to establish a stable family, especially if they have a second child while still an adolescent. Their family structure tends to be a single-parent, matriarchal family structure, often the same type in which the adolescent herself was raised.

Some pregnant adolescents choose to marry the father of the baby, who may also be a teen. Unfortunately, the majority of adolescent marriages end in divorce. This fact is not surprising because pregnancy and marriage interrupt the partners' "childhood" and basic education. Failure to be self-supporting logically follows lack of education and lost career goals. Lack of maturity in dealing with an intimate relationship also contributes to marital breakdown in this age group.

In the United States, the results of teenage childbearing cost taxpayers $7 billion each year (NCPTP, 2002). Simply delaying these births could result in significant savings because of the improvement in both education and occupational status of these young women.

In general, children of teenage mothers are at a developmental disadvantage compared to children whose mothers were older at the time of their birth. Many factors contribute to these differences, but the strongest evidence indicates that the adverse social and economic conditions facing teenage mothers are significant factors. These factors result in high rates of family instability. Consequently, their children tend to have behavioral problems, do not do as well in school, and are less likely to complete high school. There are also higher rates of abuse and neglect than among those who delay childbearing (Koniak-Griffin, Anderson, Verzemnieks, et al, 2000).

The increased incidence of maternal complications, premature birth, and LBW babies among adolescent mothers also has an impact on society because many of these mothers are on welfare. The need for increased financial support for good prenatal care and nutritional programs remains critical.

Partners of Adolescent Mothers

Almost half of the fathers of infants of adolescent mothers are not teens themselves, but are 20 years of age or older. Of these men, approximately one fifth are 6 years or more older than the adolescent mother (Taylor, Chavez, Adams, et al, 1999). The poorer the adult father's education, the greater the risk of his paternity, possibly because these men are seeking intellectual and emotional equals. Often the older partners of pregnant adolescents are similar to adolescent fathers socioeconomically. They have experienced early school failure, are unemployed, and are no more likely to support the mother than adolescent fathers (Roye & Balk, 1996). Psychosocial development of these adult fathers is also more similar to that of an adolescent father than to that of adult men who have not fathered a child. Adult paternity also tends to be higher when the teenage mother is born outside the United States, which may reflect cultural norms (Taylor, Chavez, Chabra, et al, 1997).

When the father is an adolescent, he, too, generally has not yet completed the developmental tasks of his age group and is no better prepared psychologically to deal with the consequences of pregnancy than the adolescent mother. Consequently, the adolescent who attempts to assume his responsibility as a father faces many of the same psychologic and sociologic risks as the adolescent mother. The mother and father are generally from similar socioeconomic backgrounds and have similar educational levels.

Although not married, many adolescent couples are involved in meaningful relationships. Adolescent fathers may be very involved in the pregnancy and may be present for the birth. Unfortunately, research indicates that there is decreasing contact with the mother and infant over time, even when fathers are involved in the birth (Taylor et al, 1999).

Some adolescent fathers face negative reactions from people, including their own family and the family of the young woman. Feelings of anger, shame, and disappointment may be aimed at them. Even at the time of childbirth, the mother of the pregnant adolescent may discourage the presence of the adolescent father.

The lack of responsibility shown by some unwed fathers has caused a shift in cultural and community attitudes. Fathers are being included on birth certificates far more frequently today than in the past. This helps ensure the father's rights and encourages him to meet his responsibilities to his child. In addition, legal paternity gives children access to military and social security benefits and to medical information about their fathers.

In some situations, the pregnant adolescent may not want to identify or contact the father of the baby, and the father

Research in Practice

Gender Differences in Teen Parents' Perceptions of Their Responsibilities

What is this study about? Increasing paternal involvement in parenting requires an understanding of male perceptions about parental responsibilities. This qualitative study investigated the differences in teen mothers and their partners relative to knowledge of child development and expectations regarding parental roles. Paternal responses to governmental efforts to promote involvement of unmarried fathers through child support payments and establishing legal paternity were also explored.

How was this study done? Seven pairs of unmarried teen mothers and their male partners agreed to participate in focus group interviews. Five of the couples were Mexican American and two were African American. The mothers were, on average, 16.7 years old and the fathers averaged 19.3 years of age. The mothers' focus group was separate from the fathers' focus group. A structured interview guide was used to collect data, and tape-based analysis was used to evoke and code themes. The coded responses of both groups were compared to identify gender-based similarities and differences.

What were the results of the study? In general, adolescent mothers were better able to identify established norms for developmental progress of children than were the fathers. Mothers seemed to be more willing to tolerate a delay in developmental progress than fathers, who appeared to view developmental delays as a parental weakness rather than a potentially normal variation in child development. The fathers, however, expressed greater willingness to learn about child development. The greatest differences were in attitudes toward discipline of young children. Mothers preferred nonphysical methods of discipline, whereas the fathers preferred physical methods of discipline for children younger than 3 and nonphysical methods as the child matured.

The groups differed with respect to expectations of parental role behaviors as well. While both groups agreed that father-child interactions were important, mothers tended to emphasize emotional commitment whereas fathers emphasized specific behaviors. Surprisingly, neither teen mothers nor fathers were enthusiastic about establishing legal paternity of the child, although the fathers expressed interest in establishing biologic paternity. The mothers implied that establishing legal paternity might trade greater economic security for less control over the child. The adolescent mothers saw child support payments as compensation for assuming child care responsibilities and as a way to ensure the father's continuing involvement with the child. Conversely, the fathers wanted to ensure biologic paternity before committing either emotional or financial resources to their children.

What additional questions might I have? What might have been the results if the girls and boys had been interviewed together? Would a more ethnically diverse sample have yielded the same results?

How can I use this study? Nurses can use parenting classes, support groups, and individual counseling to ensure that both adolescent mothers and fathers have the information they need to nurture a child effectively. Understanding the different needs of mothers and fathers, as well as their differences in understanding and perceptions of the parental role, can help nurses design programs that will be effective in preparing these teens for parental responsibilities.

Source: Dallas, C., Wilson, T., & Salgado, V. (2000). Gender differences in teen parents' perceptions of parental responsibilities. *Public Health Nursing, 17,* 423–433.

may not readily acknowledge paternity. Those situations include rape, exploitative sexual relations, incest, and casual sexual relations. If healthcare providers suspect any of the first three causes, further investigation into the situation is important for the well-being of the pregnant adolescent, and referral to other resources should be made as appropriate.

In situations in which the adolescent father wants to assume some responsibility, healthcare providers should support him in his decision. It is important, however, that the pregnant adolescent have the opportunity to decide whether she wants the father to participate in her healthcare.

If the adolescents perceive that they have a caring relationship, the adolescent father may want to be supportive and protective but probably does not understand the physical and psychologic changes that his partner is experiencing. The young man will need education regarding pregnancy, childbirth, child care, and parenting.

Although the adolescent father may have been included in the healthcare of the young woman throughout the pregnancy, it is not unusual for her to want her mother as her primary support person during labor and birth. This is especially true with younger adolescents. It is important both to support her wishes and also to acknowledge and support the adolescent father's wishes as appropriate.

As a part of counseling, the nurse should assess the young man's stressors, his support systems, his plans for involvement in the pregnancy and childbearing, and his future plans. He should be referred to social services for an opportunity to be counseled regarding his educational and vocational future. When the father is involved in the pregnancy, the young mother feels less deserted, more confident in her decision making, and better able to discuss her future.

Reactions of Family and Social Supports to Adolescent Pregnancy

The reactions of family members and social supports to adolescent pregnancy are as varied as the motivation and cause of the pregnancy. In families who foster educational and career goals for their children, adolescent pregnancy is often a shock. Anger, shame, and sorrow are common reactions. The majority of pregnant adolescents from these families are most likely to use contraception or choose abortion, with the exception of those teens whose cultural and religious beliefs prevent them from seeking an abortion.

In populations in which adolescent pregnancy is more prevalent and more socially acceptable, family and friends may be more supportive of the adolescent parents. In many cases, friends as well as the teen's mother are present at the birth. The expectant couple may also have friends who are already teen parents. For some male partners of these adolescent mothers, pregnancy and the birth of a baby are seen as a sign of adult status and increased sexual prowess—a sense of pride.

The mother of the pregnant adolescent is usually among the first to be told about the pregnancy. She typically becomes involved with decision making, especially with the younger adolescent, about issues such as maintaining the pregnancy, abortion, and dealing with the father-to-be and his family. As discussed previously, the pregnant adolescent may not want to identify or contact the father of the baby, especially in situations where rape or other exploitative sex was involved, or with casual sexual relationships. Family input in these matters is important in the adolescent's decision making.

Once the decision about the pregnancy has been made, it is usually the mother who helps the teen access healthcare and accompanies her to her first visit. If the pregnancy is maintained, the mother may participate in prenatal care classes and can be an excellent support system for her daughter. She should be encouraged to participate if the mother-daughter relationship is positive. If the baby's father is involved in the pregnancy, he and the pregnant teen's mother may be able to work together to support the teenage mother. The pregnant teen's mother should be updated on obstetric practice to clarify any misconceptions she might have. During labor and birth, the mother may be a key figure for her daughter. Drawing on her own experience, she can offer reassurance and instill confidence in the adolescent.

Research suggests that a supportive relationship between a teenage mother and her own parents leads to an increased sense of mastery and life satisfaction, decreased depression, and decreased anxiety in the young woman. In addition, a continuing, good relationship with a significant other leads to increased self-esteem in the young mother (Stevenson, Maton, & Teti, 1999).

The relationship between an adolescent and her parents can be turbulent without the superimposed stress of adolescent parenting. One of the developmental tasks of this time is the need to gain autonomy and independence; therefore, conflicts between mother and daughter are no surprise, especially with the struggle between the teen's need for independence and the increased dependence that results from her need for financial and psychologic support in giving birth and caring for the new infant. The younger the adolescent when she gives birth, however, the more she needs support from her mother (Stevenson et al, 1999). Children of adolescent parents experience more negative outcomes, including more aggressive behavior at a young age, when the adolescent is in constant conflict with her mother and becomes less involved in parenting.

> *Miranda left for college back East in September. She was just 18 and I thought she had the world in front of her. At Thanksgiving she came home to tell us she was 4 months pregnant and planned to keep the baby even though she and Tony had broken up and he wanted no part of fatherhood. She finished the semester, then moved back home and transferred to a state college near us. Tina was born two days after her mom finished the spring semester. Now Miranda's life is a juggling act—part-time job, part-time school, full-time mom. We help all we can. I am so sorry that my child has lost out on so much but I am so proud of the woman she has become.*

NURSING CARE MANAGEMENT

In working with adolescents, the nurse should remember that they often think differently than adults. Adolescents, especially younger adolescents, tend to be more concrete thinkers and may not plan ahead for more than a few days. As a result, nurses need to recognize that missed appointments are not unusual. Missed appointments may also be caused by other factors such as a lack of transportation, especially for those teens who are not old enough to drive. Many adolescents have never before accessed healthcare without a parent. If they are unable to share their concerns with a parent, they must be highly motivated to seek healthcare independently for purposes of contraception, treatment of sexually transmitted infections, diagnosis of pregnancy, or prenatal care.

Nursing Assessment and Diagnosis

The nurse needs to establish a database to plan interventions for the adolescent mother and family. Areas of assessment include history of family health and personal physical health, developmental level and impact of pregnancy, and emotional and financial support. The nurse also assesses the family and social support network and the father's degree of involvement in the pregnancy.

As with all pregnant women, it is important that the caregiver have information on the teen's general physical health. This may be the first time many adolescents have ever provided a health history. The nurse may find it helpful to ask very specific questions and give examples if the young woman appears confused about a question. The nurse may find that the teen's mother is best able to answer questions about family history because the adolescent is often unaware of this information.

The following areas should be assessed:

- Family and personal health history
- Medical history
- Menstrual history
- Obstetric and gynecologic history
- Substance abuse history

It is important to assess the maturational level of each individual. The adolescent's development level and the impact of pregnancy are reflected in the degree to which the teen recognizes the realities and responsibilities involved in pregnancy and parenting. The mother's self-concept (including body image), her relationship with the significant adults in her life, her attitude toward her pregnancy, and her coping methods in the situation are just a few of the significant factors that need to be assessed.

The socioeconomic status of the pregnant teen often places the baby at risk throughout life, beginning with conception. It is essential that the nurse assess family and social support as well as the extent of financial support.

Adolescent lifestyles and support systems vary greatly. It is imperative that the interdisciplinary health team have information about the expectant adolescents' feelings and perceptions about themselves, their sexuality, and the coming baby; their knowledge of, attitude toward, and anticipated ability to care for and support the infant; and their maturational level and needs.

The nursing diagnoses that are applicable to any pregnant woman apply to the pregnant adolescent. Other nursing diagnoses are influenced by the adolescent's age, support systems, socioeconomic situation, health, and maturity. Examples of nursing diagnoses more specific to the pregnant adolescent may include the following:

- ***Altered Nutrition:*** Less than Body Requirements related to poor eating habits
- ***Self-Esteem Disturbance*** related to unanticipated pregnancy

Nursing Plan and Implementation

Early, thorough prenatal care is the strongest and most critical determinant for reducing risk for the adolescent mother and her newborn. Nurses working with pregnant adolescents may need to act as advocates to help adolescent mothers meet this challenge successfully.

Community-Based Nursing Care

Many new and innovative community-based agencies have evolved to provide care for high-risk clients throughout the childbearing experience and beyond. For example, an Early Intervention Program in California provides a planned program that includes preparation for motherhood classes and a series of focused prenatal and postpartum home visits made by specially educated public health nurses as well as monthly home visits for the infant's first year of life. Early results demonstrate a reduced rate of preterm births and fewer days of infant hospitalization (Koniak-Griffin, Mathenge, Anderson, et al, 1999). Nurses in all community-based agencies can help adolescents access the healthcare system as well as social services and other support services (ie, food banks and The Special Supplemental Food Program for Women, Infants, and Children [WIC]).

Nurses working with pregnant adolescents are also involved extensively in counseling and client teaching. During their interactions, several challenges typically arise, including safeguarding the client's confidentiality, winning her trust, and helping to build her sense of self-esteem. These and other challenges of adolescent prenatal care are discussed here.

Issues of Confidentiality and Consent to Care

Most states in the United States have passed legislation that confirms the right of some minors to assume the rights of adults. These adolescents are referred to as **emancipated**

minors. An adolescent may be considered emancipated if he or she is self-supporting and living away from home, married, pregnant, a parent, or in the military. The pregnant adolescent, even if very young, is considered emancipated and has the right and responsibility to consent to healthcare for herself and later for her child. She is entitled to respect and confidentiality in her dealings with healthcare providers. Only with her consent can other adults, including her parents, be included in communication.

Development of a Trusting Relationship with the Pregnant Adolescent

The first visit to the clinic or office may be fraught with anxiety on the part of the young woman. She may be nervous not only because of her situation, but also because this may well be her first exposure to the healthcare system since early childhood. Making this experience as positive as possible for the young woman will encourage a favorable attitude toward healthcare and increase the likelihood that she will return for follow-up visits, whether she chooses to terminate or maintain the pregnancy.

Depending on how young the adolescent is, this may be her first pelvic examination, an anxiety-provoking experience for any woman. The nurse can help provide a thorough explanation of the procedure. A gentle and thoughtful examination technique will help the young woman to relax.

> ***Clinical Tip*** *During the initial pelvic examination, with the consent of the examiner, offer the teen the opportunity to visualize her external genitalia and cervix with a handheld mirror. A mirror is helpful in enabling the young woman to see her cervix, thus educating her about her anatomy. It also gives her an active role in the exam if she so desires.*

Developing a trusting relationship with the pregnant adolescent is essential. Honesty and respect for the individual and a caring attitude promote self-esteem. As the nurse develops a trusting relationship with the young woman, the nurse's attitudes about self-care and responsibility affect the adolescent's maturation process.

Promotion of Self-Esteem and Problem-Solving Skills

The nurse assists the adolescent in her decision-making and problem-solving skills so that she can proceed with her developmental tasks and begin to assume responsibility for her own as well as her newborn's life. An overview of what the young woman will experience over the prenatal course, along with thorough explanations and rationale for each procedure as it occurs, will foster the adolescent's understanding and give her some measure of control. Actively involving the young woman in her care gives her a sense of participation and responsibility (Figure 17–3 ●).

Adolescents tend to be egocentric, and even if they realize that their health-related behaviors affect their fetus, they might not feel that this is important. In light of this fact, it is often more helpful to emphasize the effects of these practices on the client *herself*. Because of their immature cognitive development, they also need help in problem solving, in visualizing themselves in the future, and in imagining what the consequences of their actions might be.

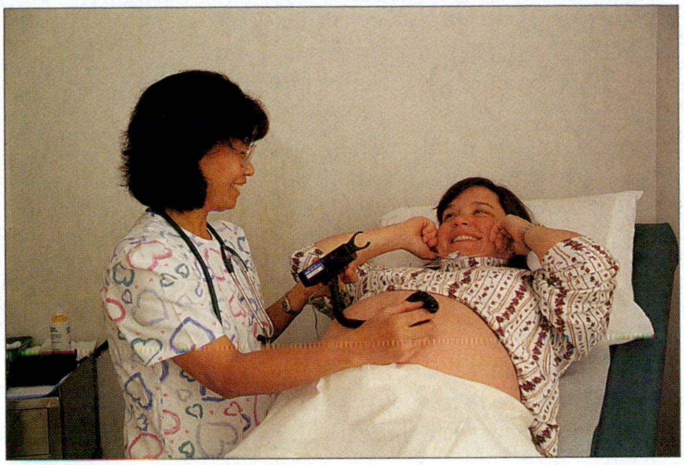

Figure 17–3 ● The nurse gives a young mother an opportunity to listen to her baby's heartbeat.

Promotion of Physical Well-Being

Baseline weight and blood pressure measurements will be valuable in assessing weight gain and predisposition to preeclampsia-eclampsia. The adolescent may be encouraged to take part in her care by measuring and recording her weight. The nurse may use this time as an opportunity for assisting the young woman in problem solving: "Have I gained too much or too little weight?" "What influence does my diet have on my weight?" "How can I change my eating habits?"

The nurse can also introduce the subject of nutrition during measurement of baseline and subsequent hemoglobin and hematocrit values. Because the adolescent is at risk for anemia, she will need education regarding the importance of iron in her diet. Indeed, basic education about nutrition is a critical component of care for pregnant teens.

Preeclampsia-eclampsia is one of the most common, serious complications of pregnancy in general. It also represents the most prevalent medical complication of pregnant

> **CRITICAL THINKING IN PRACTICE**
>
> Rachel Kalaras is an 18-year-old G1P0 who is 16 weeks pregnant when she arrives for her prenatal visit. When discussing her plans for the pregnancy, Rachel indicates that she is considering adoption. She has not discussed this plan with anyone but is seeking information about the process of relinquishment. What should you consider in discussing this issue with Rachel?
>
> **Answers can be found in Appendix I.**

adolescents. Preeclampsia-eclampsia is typically characterized by high blood pressure, proteinuria, and edema. In adult women, a blood pressure reading of 140/90 is often used as evidence of hypertension. However, it is sometimes difficult to recognize hypertension in adolescent females. Women ages 14 to 20 years without evidence of high blood pressure usually have diastolic readings between 50 and 66 mm Hg. Gradual increases from the prepregnant diastolic readings, along with excessive weight gain, proteinuria, and sudden edema, must be evaluated as precursors to preeclampsia. Blood pressure readings of 140/90 mm Hg are not acceptable as the determinant of preeclampsia in teens. This is one reason why early prenatal care is vital to the effective management of the adolescent.

Adolescents have an increased incidence of sexually transmitted infections (STIs). The initial prenatal examination should include gonococcal and chlamydial cultures and wet prep for *Candida*, *Trichomonas*, and *Gardnerella*. Tests for syphilis should also be done. Education about STIs is important, as is careful observation for herpetic lesions or other symptoms throughout the young woman's pregnancy. Although today's teens are knowledgeable about AIDS, they know much less about other STIs, especially with regard to symptoms and risk reduction. If the adolescent's history indicates that she is at increased risk for HIV, she should be given information about it and offered HIV screening.

The nurse should also discuss substance abuse with adolescents. It is important to review the risks associated with the use of tobacco, caffeine, drugs, and alcohol. The young woman should be aware of the effects of these substances on her development as well as on the development of the fetus.

Ongoing care should include the same assessments that the older woman receives. Special attention should be paid to evaluating fetal growth by determining when quickening occurs and by measuring fundal height, fetal heart tones, and fetal movement. Comparing the dates of auscultating fetal heart tones with the date of the last menstrual period and quickening can be helpful in determining correct estimates of time of birth. If, when measuring fundal height, there is a question of size-date discrepancy by 2 cm either way, an ultrasound is warranted to establish fetal age so that instances of intrauterine growth restriction (IUGR) may be diagnosed and treated early. To ensure the most accurate dating possible, an ultrasound is also warranted early in pregnancy if the date of the last menstrual period is not known.

Promotion of Family Adaptation

The nurse assesses the family situation during the first prenatal visit and ascertains the level of involvement the adolescent desires from each of her family members and the father of the child, as well as her perception of their present support. A sensitive approach to daughter-mother relationships helps motivate their communication. If the mother and daughter agree, the mother should be included in the client's care.

The nurse should also help the mother assess her daughter's needs and assist her in meeting them. Some adolescents become more dependent during pregnancy, and some become more independent. The mother can ease and encourage her daughter's self-growth by understanding how best to respond and support the adolescent.

Finally, the father of the adolescent's infant should not be forgotten in promoting the family's successful adaptation to the pregnancy. He should be included in prenatal visits, classes, health teaching, and in the birth itself to the extent that he wishes and that is acceptable to the teenage mother. He should also have the opportunity to express his feelings and concerns and to have his questions answered.

Facilitation of Prenatal Education

Some school systems are currently attempting to meet prenatal education needs in a variety of ways. The most effective method appears to be mainstreaming the pregnant adolescent in academic classes with her peers and adding classes appropriate to her needs during pregnancy and initial parenting experiences. Classes about growth and development, beginning with the newborn and early infancy, can help teenage parents have more realistic expectations of their infants and may help decrease child abuse. Mainstreaming pregnant adolescents in school is also an ideal way to help them complete their education while learning the skills they need to cope with childbearing and parenting. Vocational guidance in this setting is also most beneficial to their future.

As stated previously, early adolescents especially tend to be oriented to the present and to be concrete thinkers. As a result, teaching needs to be simple, direct, and responsive to their more immediate needs. For example, teaching about preparation for birth is most effective in the last weeks of pregnancy when this topic is of greater concern and teens are more motivated to practice breathing and relaxation techniques for labor.

Although some childbirth educators believe that older couples can be role models for pregnant adolescents, most believe that prenatal classes with other teens are generally preferable even though these classes can be challenging to teach (Figure 17–4 •). Attendance may be sporadic. The pregnant teen may be accompanied by her mother, her boyfriend, or her girlfriends. Those who bring girlfriends may bring a different one each time. In such cases, giggling and side con-

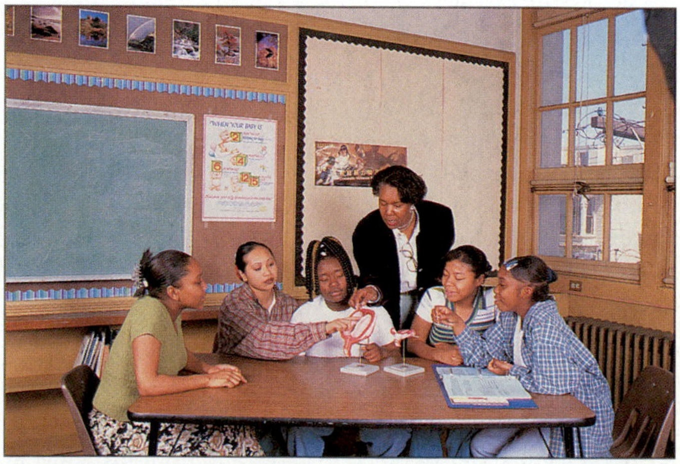

Figure 17–4 • Young adolescents may benefit from prenatal classes designed specifically for them.

versations may occur. Such activity reflects the short attention span of the teen and is fairly typical. Thus, to keep the attention of the participants, it is important to use a variety of teaching strategies, including age-appropriate audiovisual aids, demonstrations, and games.

Goals for prenatal classes may include some or all of the following:

- Providing anticipatory guidance about pregnancy
- Preparing the participants for labor and birth
- Helping participants identify the problems and conflicts of teenage pregnancy and parenting
- Increasing self-esteem
- Providing information about available community resources
- Helping participants develop more adaptive coping skills

During prenatal classes, nurses can also share information on the benefits of breastfeeding. Adolescents who learn about the advantages of breastfeeding during the prenatal period are almost three times as likely to initiate breastfeeding as those who do not (Volpe & Bear, 2000).

Topics on parenting, although sometimes included in prenatal classes for adolescents, tend to be less effective, again because adolescents tend to be oriented to the present. Parenting skills are crucial, but adolescents generally are not ready to learn about these skills until birth makes the newborn a reality.

Hospital-Based Nursing Care

The adolescent in labor has the same care needs as any pregnant woman. However, the importance of a sustained presence for her cannot be overemphasized. The nurse must be readily available and should answer questions simply and honestly, using lay terminology. The nurse can also help the adolescent's support people understand their roles in assisting the teen. If the father is involved, the nurse can encourage him to work within his own level of comfort to play an active role in all phases of the birth process, perhaps by feeding ice chips to the mother, timing her contractions, and coaching her with her breathing. The nurse can also let the couple know that holding hands, back rubs, and supportive touching are acceptable and therapeutic. Chapter 24 provides further information on care of the adolescent during labor and birth.

During the postpartum period, most teens do not foresee that they will become sexually active in the near future and are often adamant about the fact that they will not become pregnant again for an extended period. However, the statistics demonstrate a different reality. Thus, contraception remains a critical part of the national effort to decrease adolescent pregnancy. Prior to discharge, it is important for the nurse to provide information about the resumption of ovulation and the importance of contraception. It is especially helpful to do this teaching with the sexual partner present. Several safe and effective contraceptive options are available for adolescents. The barrier method of condoms and spermicidal foam is an attractive option from the perspective that it is good at preventing pregnancy and addresses issues of sexually transmitted infection. Regardless of the method chosen, the use of a condom should be encouraged. Additional options are combined oral contraceptives, the contraceptive patch, a vaginal ring, Lunelle, Depo-Provera, and Norplant. The last two have limited long-term effectiveness in adolescents, as they tend to miss appointments for Depo-Provera and dislike the side effects of Norplant. Intrauterine devices (IUDs) are not recommended for adolescents (Graydanus, Patel, & Rimsza, 2001; Lim, Rieder, Coupey, et al, 1999) and many teens are not comfortable with a diaphragm.

As part of discharge planning, the nurse should ensure that the teen is aware of community resources available to assist her and her family. Postpartum classes and new-mother support groups, especially with peers, can be extremely beneficial. Such classes address a variety of topics, including postpartum adaptation, infant and child development, and parenting skills.

MediaLink CARE PLAN: ADOLESCENT PREGNANCY

Prevention of Adolescent Pregnancy

Beginning in the 1980s, the federal government allocated millions of dollars for abstinence-only sex education programs because of the belief of some legislators that abstinence was the only method of prevention that would work or would be accepted by the general public. These programs have had limited success because adolescent pregnancy is a complex issue with many contributing factors.

National Campaign to Prevent Teen Pregnancy

A new national effort to prevent teen pregnancy was initiated in 1996 with the establishment of the National Campaign to Prevent Teen Pregnancy. Its purpose is to reduce teenage pregnancy by one third by the year 2005 (National Campaign to Prevent Teen Pregnancy, 2000). The National Campaign is a private, nonprofit organization made up of a broad spectrum of religious, political, social, human services, health, and academic organizations. The Association of Women's Health, Obstetric, and Neonatal Nurses (AWHONN) is one of the professional organizations that joined this group and made a commitment to focus on adolescent pregnancy prevention.

Accomplishments of the National Campaign to date include legislative proposals from bipartisan groups in Congress to allocate money to fund better evaluation of adolescent pregnancy prevention programs and for one-time incentive grants for communities. The National Campaign has also developed partnerships with powerful entertainment leaders such as *People* magazine, ABC Television, and Warner Brothers to help the message of pregnancy prevention reach adolescents (National Campaign to Prevent Teen Pregnancy, 2000).

One of the first actions of the National Campaign was to commission a task force to do a comprehensive review of the incidence of adolescent pregnancy and its impact on the nation. At the same time, another task force was commissioned to review the research on the effectiveness of pregnancy prevention programs. The purpose of these task forces was to provide accurate information based on fact and research. In the first year, the National Campaign summarized the results in several publications. Not surprisingly, they have found that adolescent pregnancy is a multifaceted problem with no easy answers. The best approach in local areas needs to be based on strong, community-wide involvement with a variety of programs directed at multiple causes of the problem. The National Campaign to Prevent Teen Pregnancy publishes a regular newsletter and maintains an active Web site (www.teenpregnancy.org) to communicate their work and disseminate information.

Current Community Challenges

One of the major problems in local communities continues to be intense conflict among different groups about how to approach adolescent pregnancy prevention. Some groups feel that abstinence is the only answer, whereas others feel that abstinence programs will not work with the many teens who are already sexually active. The latter groups feel that sex education and easy availability of contraception are the answers. Ironically, a comprehensive review of research suggests that neither of the proposed solutions, individually or together, is as effective in reducing the teen pregnancy rate as many believe. The risk factors most closely associated with teen birth rates appear to be poverty, low educational achievement, poor self-esteem, family dysfunction, and high-risk behaviors in general. Thus, communities and groups continue to sponsor pregnancy prevention programs that focus on a variety of risk factors such as early sexual activity, parental communication, and substance abuse (Aquiline & Bragadottir, 2000; McBride & Gienapp, 2000). As a result of site visits to communities that have launched programs for adolescent pregnancy prevention, members of the National Campaign concluded that adults must "agree to disagree" and individual groups must be encouraged to move ahead with their different programs because a variety of approaches are needed.

The cause or motivation for pregnancy varies somewhat from one community to another. In inner-city areas where there are higher rates of poverty, low self-esteem, school failure, early behavioral problems, and delinquent behaviors, emphasis on programs that promote self-esteem, deal with these social ills, and provide hope for these youth will be critical. However, similar characteristics have been identified by the National Campaign's task forces in successful programs, no matter what type of offering or community. Some of the critical characteristics include the following:

- Involvement of adolescents in planning programs
- The need for good role models from the same cultural and racial backgrounds
- The need for long-term and intensive programs
- The need to focus on the adolescent males

CHAPTER REVIEW

EXPLOREMEDIALINK

NCLEX review questions, case studies, and other interactive resources for this chapter can be found on the Web site at http://www.prenhall.com/olds. Click on "Chapter 17" to select the activities for this chapter.

For tutorials including animations and videos, more NCLEX review questions, and an audio glossary, access the accompanying CD-ROM in this book.

Focus Your Study

- Pregnancy rates for teens ages 15 to 19 have decreased from 62.1 per 1000 females in 1991 to 45.9 in 2001, a 26% decline. Although this is a significant improvement, the US teenage pregnancy rate is the highest of any industrialized nation.
- Many factors contribute to the high teenage pregnancy rate, including earlier age of first sexual intercourse, lack of knowledge about conception, lack of easy access to contraception, lessened stigma associated with adolescent pregnancy in some

populations, poverty, early school failure, and early childhood sexual abuse.

- The major psychologic risk the pregnant adolescent faces is the interruption of her own developmental tasks.
- Physical risks of adolescent pregnancies include preterm births, low-birth-weight infants, cephalopelvic disproportion, iron deficiency anemia, and preeclampsia and its sequelae.
- Almost half of the fathers of infants of adolescent mothers are age 20 or older, but they are often similar to adolescent fathers psychosocially and are no more likely to be able to support the mother.
- Factors affecting an adolescent's response to pregnancy include her degree of achievement of the developmental tasks of adolescence (which can be closely associated with age), as well as cultural, religious, and socioeconomic factors.
- Nurses working with pregnant adolescents face many challenges including safeguarding the client's confidentiality, winning her trust, and helping to build her sense of self-esteem.
- Often the adolescent has little understanding of pregnancy, childbirth, or parenting. Consequently, education is a primary responsibility of the nurse.
- Adolescent pregnancy prevention programs should be multifaceted, target males as well as females, and involve community-wide approaches.

References

Acgs, G. (1996). The impact of welfare on young mothers' subsequent childbearing decisions. *Journal of Human Resources, 31*(4), 898–907.

Adams, J., & East, P. (1999). Past physical abuse is significantly correlated with pregnancy as an adolescent. *Journal of Pediatric & Adolescent Gynecology, 12*(3), 133–138.

Alan Guttmacher Institute. (1998). *Facts in brief: Teen sex and pregnancy.* Retrieved December 2, 1999 from http://www.guttmacher.org/pubs/fb_teen_sex.html

Alan Guttmacher Institute. (2002). *Facts in brief: Teenagers' sexual and reproductive health.* Retrieved September 21, 2002 from http://www.agi-usa.org/pubs/fb_teens.html

Aquiline, M., & Bragadottir, H. (2000). Adolescent pregnancy. Teen perspectives on prevention. *American Journal of Maternal Child Nursing, 25*(4), 192–197.

Clark, L. R., Cohall, A. T., & Joffe, A. (1998). Beyond the birds and the bees: Talking to teens about sex. *Contemporary OB/GYN, 43*(4), 35–61.

Cockey, C. D. (1997). Preventing teen pregnancy: It's time to stop kidding around. *AWHONN Lifelines, 1*(3), 32–40.

Doniger, A., Adams, E., Utter, C., & Riley, J. (2001). Impact evaluation of the "not me, not now" abstinence-oriented, adolescent pregnancy prevention communications program, Monroe County, New York. *Journal of Health Communication, 6*(1), 45–60.

East, P. L. (1996). Do adolescent pregnancy and childbearing affect younger siblings? *Family Planning Perspectives, 28*(4), 148–153.

Graydanus, D., Patel, D., & Rimsza, M. (2001). Contraception in the adolescent: An update. *Pediatrics, 107*(3), 526–573.

Jacoby, M., Gorenflo, D., Black, E., Wunderlick, C., & Eyler, A. (1999). Rapid repeat pregnancy and experiences of interpersonal violence among low-income adolescents. *American Journal of Preventive Medicine, 16*(4): 318–321.

Key, J. D., Barbosa, G. A. & Owens, V. J. (2001). The second chance club: Repeat adolescent pregnancy prevention with a school-based intervention. *Journal of Adolescent Health, 28*(3), 167–169.

Koniak-Griffin, D., Anderson, N., Verzemnieks, I., & Brecht, M. (2000). A public health nursing early intervention program for adolescent mothers: Outcomes from pregnancy through 6 weeks postpartum. *Nursing Research, 49*(3), 130–138.

Koniak-Griffin, D., Mathenge, C., Anderson, N. L. R., & Verzemnieks, I. (1999). An early intervention program for adolescent mothers: A nursing demonstration project. *Journal of Obstetric, Gynecologic, and Neonatal Nursing, 28*(1), 51–59.

Landry, D. J., & Forrest, J. D. (1995). How old are US fathers? *Family Planning Perspectives, 27*(4), 159–161, 165.

Lim, S., Rieder, J., Coupey, S., & Bijur, P. (1999). Depot medroxyprogesterone acetate use in inner-city, minority adolescents: Continuation rates and characteristics of long term users. *Archives of Pediatric and Adolescent Medicine, 153*(10), 1068–1072.

Long, S. H., Marquis, M. S., & Harrison, E. R. (1994). The costs and financing of perinatal care in the United States. *American Journal of Public Health, 84*(9), 1473–1478.

Maynard, R. A. (Ed.). (1996). *Kids having kids: A Robin Hood Foundation special report on costs of adolescent childbearing.* New York: Robin Hood Foundation.

Maynard, R. A. (Ed.). (1997). *Kids having kids: Economic costs and social consequences of teen pregnancy.* Washington, DC: Urban Institute Press.

McBride, D., & Gienapp, A. (2000). Using randomized designs to evaluate client-centered programs to prevent adolescent pregnancy. *Family Planning Perspectives, 32*(5), 227–235.

Mills, C. B. (1997). Taking time to care: Making ways to help teen parents. *AWHONN Lifelines, 1*(5), 70–72.

Mims, B. (1998). Afrocentric perspective of adolescent pregnancy in African American families: A literature review. *ABNF Journal, 9*(4), 80–88.

Montgomery, K. (2001). Planned adolescent pregnancy: What they needed. *Issues in Comprehensive Pediatric Nursing, 24*(1), 19–29.

Moore, K., Miller, B., Glei, D., & Morrison, D. R. (1995). *Adolescent sex, contraception and childbearing: A review of recent research.* Washington, DC: Child Trends.

Moore, K., & Sugland, B. (1996). *Next steps and best bets: Approaches to preventing adolescent childbearing.* Washington, DC: Child Trends.

National Campaign to Prevent Teen Pregnancy. (NCPTP): (2000). *Fact sheet report.* Washington, DC: Author.

National Campaign to Prevent Teen Pregnancy. (2002). United States birth rates for teens 15–19. Retrieved September 22, 2002 from www.teenpregnancy.org

National Center for Health Statistics. (2002). Births: Preliminary data for 2001. *National Vital Statistics Report, 50*(10), 1–20.

Philliber, S., & Namerow, P. (1995, December). *Trying to maximize the odds: Using what we know to prevent teen pregnancy.* Paper presented at technical assistance workshop to support the Teen Pregnancy Prevention Program, Division of Reproductive Health, Centers for Disease Control and Prevention, Atlanta, GA.

Preventing Teenage Pregnancy. (2002, June10). U. S. Department of Health and Human Services Press Release. Retrieved October 20, 2002 from www.hhs.gov/news/press/2002pres/teenpreg.html

Roye, C. F., & Balk, S. J. (1996). The relationship of partner support to outcomes for teenage mothers and their children: A review. *Journal of Adolescent Health, 19*(2), 86–93.

Santelli, J., Linburg, L., Abma, J., & McNeely, C. (2000). Adolescent sexual behaviors: Estimates and trends from four nationally representative surveys. *Family Planning Perspectives, 32*(4), 156–165, 194.

Sells, C. W., & Blum, R. W. (1996). Morbidity and mortality among US adolescents: An overview of data and trends. *American Journal of Public Health, 86*(4), 513–519.

Singh, S., & Darroch, E. (2000). Adolescent pregnancy and childbearing: Levels and trends in developed countries. *Family Planning Perspectives, 32*(1), 14–23.

Smith, C. (1996). The link between childhood maltreatment and teenage pregnancy. *Social Work Research, 20*(3), 131–141.

Smith, P. B., & Weinman, M. L. (1995). Cultural implications for public health policy for pregnant Hispanic adolescents. *Health Values: The Journal of Health Behavior, Education, & Promotion, 19*(1), 3–9.

Spieker, S. J., & Bensley, L. (1994). Roles of living arrangements and grandmother social support in adolescent mothering and infant attachment. *Developmental Psychology, 30*(1), 102–111.

Steinberg, L. (2002). *Adolescence* (6th ed.). New York: McGraw-Hill.

Stevenson, W., Maton, K., & Teti, D. M. (1999). Social support, relationship quality, and well being among pregnant adolescents. *Journal of Adolescence, 22*(1), 109–121.

Stevens-Simon, C., Kelly, L., & Singer, D. (1999). Preventing repeat adolescent pregnancies with early adoption of the contraceptive implant. *Family Planning Perspectives, 31*(2), 88–93.

Stevens-Simon, C., Kelly, L., Singer, D., & Cox, A. (1996). Why pregnant adolescents say they did not use contraceptives prior to conception. *Journal of Adolescent Health, 19*(1), 48–53.

Stock, J. L., Bell, M. A., Boyer, D. K., & Connell, F. A. (1997). Adolescent pregnancy and sexual risk-taking among sexually abused girls. *Family Planning Perspectives, 29*(5), 200–203, 227.

Taylor, D., Chavez, G., Adams, E., Chabra, A., & Shah, R. (1999). Demographic characteristics in adult paternity for first births to adolescents under 15 years of age. *Journal of Adolescent Health, 24*(4), 251–258.

Taylor, D., Chavez, G., Chabra, A., & Boggess, J. (1997). Risk factors for adult paternity in births to adolescents. *Obstetrics & Gynecology, 89*(2), 199–205.

US Department of Health and Human Services. (1995, September). *Report to Congress on out-of-wedlock childbearing.* Washington, DC: Author.

Volpe, E., & Bear, M. (2000). Enhancing breastfeeding initiation in adolescent mothers through the Breastfeeding Educated and Supported Teen (BEST) Club. *Journal of Human Lactation, 16*(3), 196–200.

Wilcox, B. L., Limber, S. P., O'Bierne, H., & Bartels, C. L. (1996, November 18). *Adolescent abstinence promotion programs: An evaluation of evaluations.* Paper presented at the biennial meeting of the American Public Health Association, New York, NY.

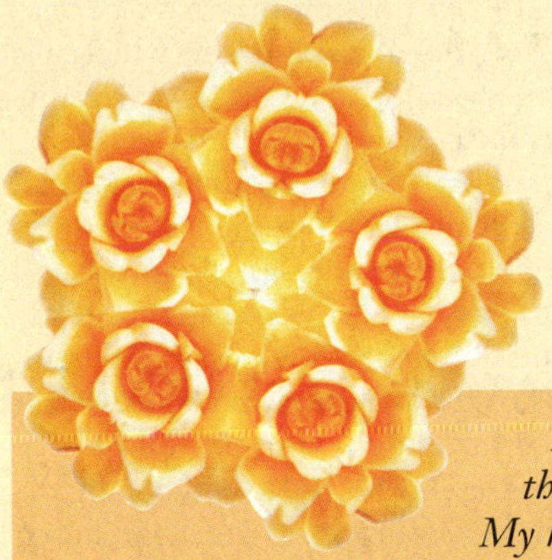

18 Maternal Nutrition

I'm trying to be very careful about what I eat. I've had more salads and fresh fruit than I can remember. Sometimes, though, I get a "cookie attack" and indulge myself. My husband says I should eat oatmeal cookies so I could feel that my cravings were nutritionally sound!

Objectives

- Identify the role of specific nutrients in the diet of the pregnant woman.
- Compare nutritional needs during pregnancy, postpartum, and lactation with nonpregnant requirements.
- Discuss effects of maternal nutrition on fetal outcomes.
- Evaluate adequacy and pattern of weight gain during different stages of pregnancy.
- Plan adequate prenatal vegetarian diets based on nutritional requirements of pregnancy.
- Describe ways in which various physical, psychosocial, and cultural factors can affect nutritional intake and status.
- Compare recommendations for weight gain and nutrient intakes in the pregnant adolescent with those for the mature pregnant adult.
- Describe basic factors a nurse should consider when offering nutritional counseling to a pregnant adolescent.
- Compare nutritional counseling issues for breastfeeding and formula-feeding mothers.
- Formulate a nutritional care plan for pregnant women based on a diagnosis of nutritional problems.

Key Terms

Adequate intake (AI) 408
Calorie 411
Folic acid 417
Kilocalorie 411
Lactase deficiency (lactose intolerance) 421
Lacto-ovovegetarians 418
Lactovegetarians 418
Pica 421
Recommended dietary allowance (RDA) 408
Vegans 418

MediaLink

Additional resources for this content can be found on the Student CD-ROM and on the Companion Website at www.prenhall.com/olds. Click on "Chapter 18" to select the activities for this chapter.

CD-ROM
- Audio Glossary
- NCLEX Review

Companion Website
- Additional NCLEX Review
- Case Study: Maternal Weight Gain
- Care Plan Activity: Maternal Nutrition

MEDIALINK CASE STUDY: MATERNAL WEIGHT GAIN

A woman's nutritional status prior to and during pregnancy can significantly influence her own health and that of her unborn child. In most prenatal clinics and offices, nurses provide nutritional counseling directly or work closely with dietitians in providing any necessary nutritional assessment and teaching.

This chapter focuses on the nutritional needs of a normal pregnant woman. Special sections consider the nutritional needs of the pregnant adolescent and the woman after birth.

Many factors influence a woman's ability to achieve good prenatal nutrition, including the following:

- **General nutritional status prior to pregnancy.** Good prenatal nutrition is the result of proper eating throughout life, not just during pregnancy, although pregnancy may motivate a woman to improve poor eating habits. Nutritional deficits at conception and during the early prenatal period may influence the outcome of the pregnancy.
- **Maternal age.** An expectant adolescent must meet the nutritional needs for her own growth in addition to the nutritional needs of pregnancy.
- **Maternal parity.** A mother's nutritional needs and the outcome of her pregnancy are influenced by the number of pregnancies she has had and by the intervals between them.

A mother's nutritional status does affect her fetus. Factors influencing fetal well-being are interrelated, but nutrient deficiencies alone can produce measurable effects on cell and organ growth of the developing fetus. Fetal growth occurs in three overlapping stages: (1) growth by increase in cell number, (2) growth by increase in cell number and cell size, and (3) growth by increase in cell size alone. The nutritional problems that interfere with cell division may have permanent consequences. If the nutritional insult occurs when cells are mainly enlarging, the changes are usually reversible when normal nutrition resumes.

Growth of fetal and maternal tissues requires increased quantities of nutrients. These are listed in the *dietary reference intakes (DRIs)* as specific allowances for pregnant and lactating women (Table 18–1 •). The DRIs distinguish between pregnant women and pregnant adolescents because of the greater nutrient needs of the adolescent. The DRIs are subdivided into the **recommended dietary allowance (RDA)** and **adequate intake (AI)**. A RDA is the daily dietary intake that is considered sufficient to meet the nutritional requirements of nearly all individuals in a specific life stage and gender group. An AI is a value cited for a nutrient when there is not sufficient data to calculate an estimated average requirement.

The pregnant woman can obtain most of the recommended nutrients by eating a well-balanced diet each day. The basic food groups and recommended amounts during pregnancy and lactation are presented in Table 18–3 •.

Maternal Weight

Prepregnancy Weight

Prepregnancy weight is an important factor for both mothers and their babies. Women who are underweight before pregnancy, especially younger adolescents, have a higher risk of giving birth to a low-birth-weight infant than women who begin pregnancy at normal weight for height. On the other hand, women who are obese before pregnancy have an increased risk of pregnancy-related complications such as gestational diabetes mellitus, high blood pressure, and

Table 18–1 • DIETARY REFERENCE INTAKES (DRI's) FOR NONPREGNANT FEMALES AND FOR PREGNANT AND

	Age	Vitamin A (μg/d)	Vitamin D (μg/d)	Vitamin E (mg/d α-tocopherol)	Vitamin K (μg/d)	Vitamin C (mg/d)	Thiamine (mg/d)	Riboflavin (mg/d)
Females	9–13 y	600	5*	11	60*	45	0.9	0.9
	14–18 y	700	5*	15	75*	65	1.0	1.0
	19–30 y	700	5*	15	90*	75	1.1	1.1
	31–50 y	700	5*	15	90*	75	1.1	1.1
	50–70 y	700	10*	15	90*	75	1.1	1.1
	> 70 y	700	15*	15	90*	75	1.1	1.1
Pregnancy	≤ 18 y	750	5*	15	75*	80	1.4	1.4
	19–30 y	770	5*	15	90*	85	1.4	1.4
	31–50 y	770	5*	15	90*	85	1.4	1.4
Lactation	≤ 18 y	1,200	5*	19	75*	115	1.4	1.6
	19–30 y	1,300	5*	19	90*	120	1.4	1.6
	31–50 y	1,300	5*	19	90*	120	1.4	1.6

*Values are adequate intakes (AIs) rather than recommended dietary allowances (RDAs). All other values on chart are RDAs.

Source: All data is from the Institute of Medicine (1997–2001). Dietary reference intakes, Washington, D.C. National Academy Press. Also available as http://www.nap.edu.

hospitalization. Their babies are at increased risk for prematurity and congenital malformations. Moreover, as these babies grow up they are more likely to be obese and have obesity-related health problems such as cardiovascular disease, hypertension, and diabetes (March of Dimes, 2002).

Maternal Weight Gain

Maternal weight gain is another important factor in fetal growth and in infant birth weight. An adequate weight gain over time indicates an adequate caloric intake. It does not, however, ensure that the woman has a sufficient nutrient intake. The diet may not be of high enough nutritional quality even though its caloric content supports the recommended weight gain. The pregnant woman must maintain the nutritional quality of her diet as her weight gain progresses.

Weight gain, even in women with a healthy pregnancy outcome, tends to be quite variable. Optimal weight gain depends on the woman's weight for height (body mass index [BMI]) and her prepregnant nutritional state. The Institute of Medicine (IOM, 1992) recommends weight gain in terms of optimum ranges based on prepregnant BMI (Table 18–2 •). Studies examining these recommendations have demonstrated that women who fail to reach the lower end of the IOM recommended weight gain ranges have a higher risk of having a low-birth-weight infant while women who gained above the IOM recommended upper limit are more likely to retain the weight 10 to 18 months postpartum (Salzberg, 2002).

The pattern of weight gain during pregnancy is also important. For example, inadequate prenatal weight gain during the second trimester is closely associated with reduced birth weight in the newborn. For women of normal weight, the recommended pattern consists of a gain of 1.6 to 2.3 kg (3.5 to 5 lb) during the first trimester, followed by an average gain of 0.5 kg (1 lb) per week during the last two trimesters. The rate of weight gain in the second and third trimesters needs to be slightly higher for underweight women and slightly lower (0.7 lb per week) for overweight women (IOM, 1990). A maternal weight gain of 1.5 lb per week has been suggested for normal-weight women during the second half of a twin pregnancy. Underweight women should strive for a gain of 1.75 lb per week after 20 weeks' gestation.

The average maternal weight gain is distributed as follows:

5.0 kg (11 lb)	Fetus, placenta, amniotic fluid
0.9 kg (2 lb)	Uterus
1.8 kg (4 lb)	Increased blood volume
1.4 kg (3 lb)	Breast tissue
2.3 to 4.5 kg (5 to 10 lb)	Maternal stores

Table 18–2 • RECOMMENDED TOTAL WEIGHT GAIN RANGES FOR PREGNANT WOMEN

	Recommended Total Gain	
Pregnancy Weight-for-Height Category	lb	kg
Low (BMI <19.8)	28–40	12.5–18
Normal (BMI 19.8–26)	25–35	11.5–16
High (BMI >26.0–29.0)	15–25	7.0–11.5
Obese (BMI >29.0)	>15	≥7.0

Note: For singleton pregnancies. The range for women carrying twins is 16–20 kg (35–45 lb). Young adolescents (<2 years after menarche) and African American women should strive for gains at the upper end of the range. Short women (<157 cm or <62 in) should strive for gains at the lower end of the range.

Source: Institute of Medicine Subcommittee for a Clinical Application Guide (1992). *Nutrition during pregnancy and lactation: An implementation guide* (p. 44). Washington, DC: National Academy Press.

LACTATING FEMALES

Niacin (mg/d)	Vitamin B_6 (mg/d)	Folate (μg/d)	Vitamin B_{12} (μg/d)	Calcium (mg/d)	Phosphorus (mg/d)	Magnesium (mg/d)	Iron (mg/d)	Zinc (mg/d)	Iodine (μg/d)	Selenium (μg/d)
12	1.0	300	1.8	1,300*	1,250	240	8	8	120	40
14	1.2	400	2.4	1,300*	1,250	360	15	9	150	55
14	1.3	400	2.4	1,000*	700	310	18	8	150	55
14	1.3	400	2.4	1,000*	700	320	18	8	150	55
14	1.5	400	2.4	1,200*	700	320	8	8	150	55
14	1.5	400	2.4	1,200*	700	320	8	8	150	55
18	1.9	600	2.6	1,300*	1,250	400	27	12	220	60
18	1.9	600	2.6	1,000*	700	350	27	11	220	60
18	1.9	600	2.6	1,000*	700	360	27	11	220	60
17	2.0	500	2.8	1,300*	1,250	360	10	13	290	70
17	2.0	500	2.8	1,000*	700	310	9	12	290	70
17	2.0	500	2.8	1,000*	700	320	9	12	290	70

Table 18-3 • DAILY FOOD PLAN FOR PREGNANCY AND LACTATION

Food Group	Nutrients Provided	Food Source	Recommended Daily Amount During Pregnancy	Recommended Daily Amount During Lactation
Dairy products	Protein; riboflavin; vitamins A, D, and others; calcium; phosphorus; zinc; magnesium	Milk—whole, 2%, skim, dry, buttermilk Cheeses—hard, semisoft, cottage Yogurt—plain, low-fat Soybean milk—canned, dry	Four (8 oz) cups (five for teenagers) used plain or with flavoring, in shakes, soups, puddings, custards, cocoa Calcium in 1 cup milk equivalent to 1½ cups cottage cheese, 1½ oz hard or semisoft cheese, 1 cup yogurt, 1½ cups ice cream (high in fat and sugar)	Four (8 oz) cups (five for teenagers); equivalent amount of cheese, yogurt, and so forth
Meat and meat alternatives	Protein; iron; thiamine, niacin, and other vitamins; minerals	Beef, pork, veal, lamb, poultry, animal organ meats, fish, eggs; legumes; nuts, seeds, peanut butter, grains in proper vegetarian combination (vitamin B_{12} supplement needed)	Three servings (one serving = 2 oz), combination in amounts necessary for same nutrient equivalent (varies greatly)	Two servings
Grain products, whole grain or enriched	B vitamins; iron; whole grain also has zinc, magnesium, and other trace elements; provides fiber	Breads and bread products such as cornbread, muffins, waffles, hotcakes, biscuits, dumplings, cereals, pastas, rice	Six to 11 servings daily: one serving = one slice bread, ¾ cup or 1 oz dry cereal, ½ cup rice or pasta	Same as for pregnancy
Fruits and fruit juices	Vitamins A and C; minerals; raw fruits for roughage	Citrus fruits and juices, melons, berries, all other fruits and juices	Two to four servings (one serving for vitamin C): one serving = one medium fruit, ½–1 cup fruit, 4 oz orange or grapefruit juice	Same as for pregnancy
Vegetables and vegetable juices	Vitamins A and C; minerals; provides roughage	Leafy green vegetables; deep yellow or orange vegetables such as carrots, sweet potatoes, squash, tomatoes; green vegetables such as peas, green beans, broccoli; other vegetables such as beets, cabbage, potatoes, corn, lima beans	Three to five servings (one serving of dark green or deep yellow vegetable for vitamin A): one serving = ½–1 cup vegetable, two tomatoes, one medium potato	Same as for pregnancy
Fats	Vitamins A and D; linoleic acid	Butter, cream cheese, fortified table spreads; cream, whipped cream, whipped toppings; avocado, mayonnaise, oil, nuts	As desired in moderation (high in calories): one serving = 1 tbsp butter or enriched margarine	Same as for pregnancy
Sugar and sweets		Sugar, brown sugar, honey, molasses	Occasionally, if desired	Same as for pregnancy
Desserts		Nutritious desserts such as puddings, custards, fruit whips, and crisps; other rich, sweet desserts and pastries	Occasionally, if desired	Same as for pregnancy
Beverages		Coffee, decaffeinated beverages, tea, bouillon, carbonated drinks	As desired, in moderation	Same as for pregnancy
Miscellaneous		Iodized salt, herbs, spices, condiments	As desired	Same as for pregnancy

Note: The pregnant woman should eat regularly, three meals a day, with nutritious snacks of fruit, cheese, milk, or other foods between meals if desired. (More frequent but smaller meals are also recommended.) Four to 6 (8 oz) glasses of water and a total of 8 to 10 (8 oz) cups total fluid intake should be consumed daily. Water is an essential nutrient.

Adequate maternal weight gain contributes to the tissue expansion and growth of both the mother and the developing fetus. Inadequate weight gain has been associated with preterm birth and its related problems for the newborn (Salzberg, 2002). Moreover, research suggests that women who gain an insufficient amount of weight are less likely to have spoken to a physician at the beginning of pregnancy about weight gain and tend to be less knowledgeable about the importance of adequate weight gain (Strychar, Chabot, Champagne, et al, 2000).

Because of the association between maternal weight gain and pregnancy outcome, most caregivers pay close attention

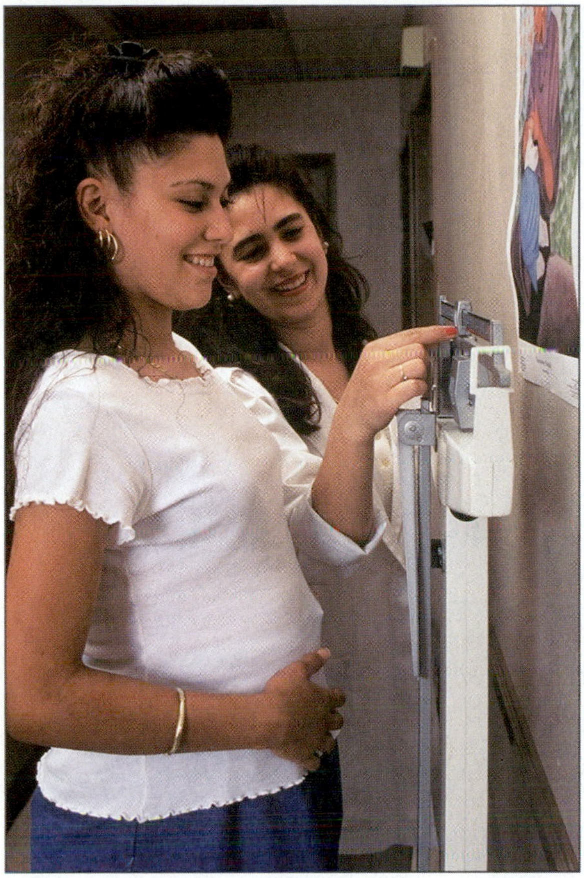

Figure 18–1 • It is important to monitor a pregnant woman's weight over time.
SOURCE: Michael Newman/Photo Edit

to weight gain during pregnancy (Figure 18–1 •). Weight gain charts can be useful in monitoring the rate of weight gain over time. If a significant deviation from the anticipated pattern occurs, the cause should be determined and appropriate interventions planned with the woman.

As mentioned earlier, weight gain alone does not guarantee adequate nutrition. A diet may be high in energy (calories) but low in vitamins, minerals, or complex carbohydrates and protein. Pregnancy is not a time to diet, and severe caloric restriction during pregnancy can result in maternal ketosis. Counseling the pregnant woman to eat according to the Food Guide Pyramid (Figure 18–2 •) places less emphasis on the amount of her weight gain and more on the quality of her intake.

> ***Clinical Tip*** *Weight varies with time of day, amount of clothing, inaccurate scale adjustment, or weighing error. Do not overemphasize a single weight but pay attention to the pattern of weight gain.*

Nutritional Requirements

The requirements for calories and almost all nutrients increase during pregnancy, although the amount of increase varies with each nutrient. These increases reflect the additional requirements of both the mother and the developing fetus (see Table 18–1).

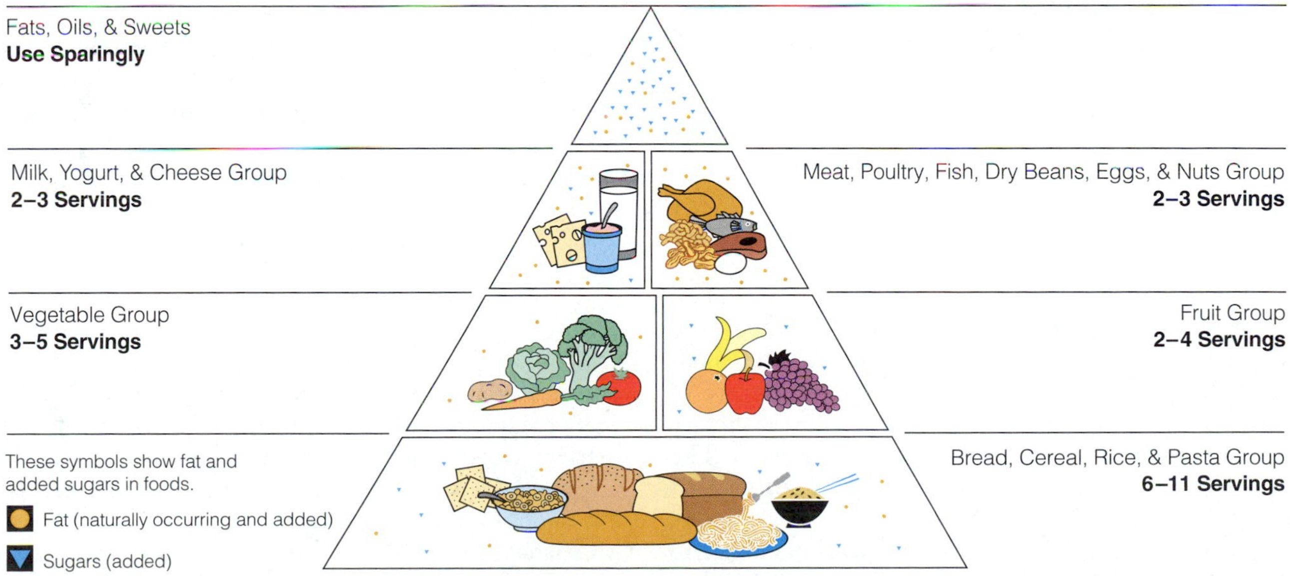

Figure 18–2 • The Food Guide Pyramid provides a quick reference for people interested in healthy eating. The largest portion of the pyramid is devoted to grains, rice, bread, and pasta, whereas the smallest portion is devoted to fats, oils, and sweets, which should be used sparingly.
SOURCE: US Department of Agriculture; US Department of Health and Human Services.

Calories

The term **calorie** (cal) stands for the amount of heat required to raise the temperature of 1 gram of water 1 degree centigrade. The **kilocalorie** (kcal) is equivalent to 1000 cal and is the unit used to express the energy value of food.

Energy requirements remain the same during the first trimester but increase by 300 kcal per day during the second and third trimesters. Women with a twin pregnancy should add an additional 300 kcal, for a total of 600 kcal above nonpregnant levels (American College of Obstetricians and Gynecologists [ACOG], 1998a). Weight gains should be monitored regularly, and dietary recommendations should be individualized to help the pregnant woman meet her caloric needs. Prepregnant weight, height, maternal age, activity, and health status all affect caloric requirements.

See Client Teaching: Helping the Pregnant Woman Add 300 kcal to Her Diet for basic nutritional information and suggestions for increasing caloric intake.

Carbohydrates

Carbohydrates provide the body's primary source of energy as well as fiber necessary for proper bowel functioning. If the carbohydrate intake is not adequate, the body uses protein for energy. Protein then becomes unavailable for growth needs. In addition, protein breakdown leads to ketosis. Ketosis can be a problem, especially in diabetic women, because of glycosuria, reduced alkaline reserves, and lipidemia.

The carbohydrate and caloric needs of the pregnant woman increase, especially during the last two trimesters. Carbohydrate intake promotes weight gain and growth of the fetus, placenta, and other maternal tissues. Dairy products, fruits, vegetables, and whole grain cereals and breads all contain carbohydrates.

Protein

During pregnancy, the woman needs increased amounts of protein to provide amino acids for fetal development, blood volume expansion, and growth of other maternal tissues, such as the breasts and uterus. Protein also contributes to the body's overall energy metabolism. The recommendation for protein during pregnancy is 60 g, an increase of about 14 g over nonpregnant levels. The quality of dietary protein is as important as the total amount consumed. The quality is determined by the complex of amino acids that makes up the protein. Proteins are said to be complete when they are made up of all the amino acids necessary to sustain growth and are considered incomplete when they lack some of the necessary amino acids. Proteins of animal origin are generally complete, and proteins of plant origin are incomplete.

Table 18–4 • AMOUNT OF PROTEIN IN COMMON FOODS

Food	Protein (g)
Dairy Products	
Milk, 8 oz	8
Cheese: cheddar, Swiss, and so forth, 1 oz	7
Cottage cheese ¼ cup	7
Meat and Meat Alternatives	
Meat, fish, poultry, 1 oz	7
Egg, 1	7
Cooked dry beans and peas, ½ cup	7
Cooked soybeans, ½ cup	11
Peanut butter, 2 tbsp	7
Peanuts (3 tbsp), cashews/almonds (5 tbsp)	7
Breads and Cereals	
Bread, 1 slice	2
Buns, biscuits, muffins, 1	2
Cooked cereals and grains, ½ cup	2
Breakfast cereal, 1 oz	2
Vegetables and Fruits	
Vegetables, ½ cup	0.5–1
Fruits and juices, ½ cup	0.5

To obtain high-quality protein in the diet, it is best to eat a variety of foods. Animal products, such as lean meats, fish, poultry, and eggs, are sources of high-quality, complete protein. Dairy products are also important protein sources. A quart of milk supplies 32 g of protein, more than half the average daily protein requirement. Milk can be incorporated into the diet in a variety of dishes, including soups, puddings, custards, sauces, yogurt, and beverages such as hot chocolate and fruited milk drinks. Various kinds of hard and soft cheeses and cottage cheese are also excellent protein sources, although cream cheese is categorized as a fat source only. Table 18–4 • provides information on the protein content of common foods.

Women who have allergies to milk, who have lactose intolerance, or who practice vegetarianism may find soy milk acceptable. It can be used in cooked dishes or as a beverage. Soy cheeses are also available.

Fat

Fats are valuable sources of energy for the body. Fats are more completely absorbed during pregnancy, resulting in a marked increase in serum lipids, lipoproteins, and cholesterol and decreased elimination of fat through the bowel. Fat deposits in the fetus increase from about 2% at midpregnancy to almost 12% at term. However, fat requirements are unchanged during pregnancy and should account for about 30% of the total daily caloric intake (Salzberg, 2002). US dietary guidelines recommend that less than 10% of fat calories should be saturated fat (US Department

CLIENT TEACHING — HELPING THE PREGNANT WOMAN ADD 300 KCAL TO HER DIET

Assessment The nurse recognizes that the notion of "eating for two" may cause a woman to overestimate the amount of food she should consume during pregnancy. The nurse assesses the pregnant woman's knowledge of basic nutrition, including the use of the Food Guide Pyramid (Figure 18–2), and assesses her awareness of the best way to increase the nutrients in her diet.

Nursing Diagnosis The key nursing diagnosis will probably be ***Health-Seeking Behaviors:*** Information on recommended dietary changes in pregnancy related to an expressed desire to maintain good nutrition.

Nursing Plan and Implementation The teaching plan focuses on providing information about the Food Guide Pyramid and about the most effective way to use the additional 300 kcal that a woman needs daily during pregnancy.

Client Goals At the completion of the teaching the woman will be able to

1. Identify the Food Guide Pyramid categories and the foods included in each
2. Cite the increase in kilocalories indicated during pregnancy.
3. Discuss the most nutritionally sound way to use the additional calories.
4. Use the information she has gained to plan a nutritionally sound sample menu.

Teaching Plan

CONTENT	TEACHING METHOD
Describe the basic food groups, which include the following: Grains: 6 to 11 servings (one serving = 1 slice bread, ½ hamburger roll, 1 oz dry cereal, 1 tortilla, ½ cup pasta, rice, grits) Fruits: Two to four servings; one should be a good source of vitamin C (one serving = 1 medium-sized piece of fruit, ½ cup juice). Vegetables: Three to five servings (one serving = 1 cup raw vegetable, 1 cup green leafy vegetable, ½ cup cooked vegetable) Dairy: Two to three servings (one serving = 1 cup milk or yogurt, 1.5 oz hard cheese, 2 cups cottage cheese, 1 cup pudding made with milk) Meats and alternatives: Two to three servings (one serving = 2 oz cooked lean meat, poultry, or fish; 2 eggs; ½ cup cottage cheese; 1 cup cooked legumes [kidney, lima, garbanzo, or soybeans, split peas]; 6 oz tofu; 2 oz nuts or seeds; 4 tbsp peanut butter)	Ask woman if she has received nutritional information using this approach before. Discuss her understanding of it. Use that information to plan the amount of detail you will use. Use a chart or colorful handout to explain the basic food groups and to give examples of equivalent foods.
Point out that not all foods that are nutritionally equivalent have the same number of calories; it is important to consider that when making food choices. Explain the Food Guide Pyramid.	Use a calorie-counting guide to compare the calories in a variety of foods that are equivalent, such as 2 oz beef and 2 oz fish or 1 cup low-fat milk and 1 cup whole milk.
The Food Guide Pyramid is designed to represent the food groups needed to make a balanced diet. The grain, fruit, and vegetable groups are at the base of the pyramid and should account for the majority of the food selections. Fewer servings of dairy and meat or meat alternative are required in the diet, and these groups fall in the middle portion of the pyramid. The very top of the pyramid represents fats, oils, and sweets. These items do not have a high nutritional value and should be used sparingly.	Use a similar approach to evaluate the calories in fats, oils, and sweets, but also evaluate their nutrient content, especially levels of nutrients such as vitamin C, iron, and calcium.
Emphasize that a woman only has to add 300 kcal/day during pregnancy. This can be achieved by adding two milk servings and one serving of meat or alternative. Because of the varying caloric value, a woman needs to consider the advisability of using low-fat milk, lean cuts of meat, or fish broiled or baked instead of fried.	In planning the woman's diet to get optimum nutrition without too many additional calories, it is often helpful to ask her to plan and evaluate a sample menu.
Foods can be combined. For example, 1 cup spaghetti with a 2 oz meatball would count as 1 serving meat, ¾ cup spaghetti = 1 grain, and ¼ cup tomato sauce = ½ serving vegetable.	Provide handouts on which the woman can list the foods she has eaten and check off the corresponding nutrient categories. Have her bring her completed handouts to a subsequent visit.

(continued on next page)

CLIENT TEACHING — HELPING THE PREGNANT WOMAN ADD 300 KCAL TO HER DIET (continued)

EVALUATION

Evaluate the learning by providing time for discussion, questions, and practice using the calorie-counting guide.

Teaching has been effective if all the identified goals are achieved and if the woman seems comfortable planning her diet to provide for the best nutrition possible.

of Agriculture & US Department of Health and Human Services, 1990).

When dairy products are used as a regular part of the diet, it may be helpful to select items that have a reduced fat content. Selecting lean cuts of meats, fish, and poultry will also help decrease dietary fat.

Minerals

The woman can increase minerals needed for the growth of new tissue during pregnancy by improving mineral absorption and increasing mineral intake.

CALCIUM AND PHOSPHORUS

Calcium and phosphorus are involved in the mineralization of fetal bones and teeth, energy and cell production, and acid-base buffering. Calcium is absorbed and used more efficiently during pregnancy. Some additional calcium and phosphorus are required early in pregnancy, but most of the fetus's bone calcification occurs during the last 2 or 3 months. Teeth begin to form at about 8 weeks' gestation and are formed by birth. The 6-year molars begin to calcify just before birth. Additional calcium is stored in the maternal skeleton as a reserve for lactation.

The identified adequate intake for calcium for the pregnant or lactating woman 19 years of age or older is 1000 mg per day. For those 18 years of age and younger, the requirement increases to 1300 mg per day to compensate for the additional needs of the mother. If calcium intake is not adequate, fetal needs will be met at the mother's expense by demineralization of maternal bone. Maternal calcium supplementation during the second and third trimesters has been shown to increase fetal bone mineralization in women whose dietary calcium intake is inadequate (Koo, Walters, Esterlitz, et al, 1999).

Food is the preferred source of calcium because food provides other nutrients as well. A diet that includes 4 cups of milk or an equivalent dairy alternative (see Table 18–2) and a variety of other foods will provide sufficient calcium. Smaller amounts of calcium are supplied by legumes, nuts, dried fruits, and dark green leafy vegetables (such as kale, broccoli, collard greens, and beet greens). It is important to remember that some of the calcium in beet greens, spinach, and Swiss chard is bound with oxalic acid, which makes it less available to the body. Larger amounts of these foods need to be consumed if they are substituted for dairy sources of calcium (Table 18–5 ●).

The recommended dietary allowance (RDA) for phosphorus does not change from that of a nonpregnant woman

Table 18-5 ● FOODS THAT PROVIDE COMPARABLE AMOUNTS OF CALCIUM

Food	Amount
Dairy Products	
Milk	8 oz
Cheese, cheddar	1½ oz
Pudding, vanilla	1 cup
Fruits	
Figs	10
Raisins	2 cups
Vegetables	
Broccoli	2½ cups
Collards	1 cup
Kale	3 cups
Mustard greens	3½ cups
Turnip greens	1½ cups
Fish	
Salmon, canned, with bones	2⁄3 cup
Sardines	6
Nuts	
Almonds	4 oz
Brazil nuts	½ cup
Miscellaneous	
Molasses, blackstrap	2 tbsp

Source: Data from Pennington, J. A. T. (1989). *Bowes and Church's food values of portions commonly used,* (15th ed.). Philadelphia: Lippincott.

age 19 or older: 700 mg per day. Similarly, for females age 18 and younger it remains stable at 1250 mg per day. Phosphorus is readily supplied through calcium- and protein-rich foods, especially milk, eggs, and meat.

IODINE

Iodine is an essential part of the thyroid hormone thyroxine. Inorganic iodine is excreted in the urine during pregnancy. Enlargement of the thyroid gland may occur if iodine is not replaced by adequate dietary intake or additional supplement. Iodine deficiency is the most widespread nutritional cause of impaired brain development. This can result in cretinism and lesser degrees of retardation.

A woman can meet the iodine requirement of 220 mg per day by using iodized salt. Seafood is also a good source of iodine. Plant sources vary because they reflect the iodine content of the soil in which they grow. When sodium is restricted, the physician may prescribe an iodine supplement.

SODIUM

The sodium ion is essential for proper metabolism and the regulation of fluid balance. Sodium intake in the form of salt is never entirely curtailed during pregnancy, even when hypertension or preeclampsia is present. The woman can obtain moderate sodium intake (2 to 3 g) by using fresh food lightly seasoned to taste during cooking. The use of extra salt at the table should be avoided. Salty foods, such as potato chips, ham, sausages, and sodium-based seasonings, can be eliminated to avoid excessive intake.

ZINC

Zinc is a part of numerous enzymes and is involved in protein metabolism and the synthesis of DNA and RNA. It is essential for normal fetal growth and development as well as milk production during lactation. Zinc absorption increases during pregnancy (Fung, Ritchie, Woodhouse, et al, 1997). The RDA during pregnancy for women age 19 and older is 11 mg per day. This increases to 12 mg during lactation. Best sources of zinc are meats, shellfish, and poultry. Good sources include whole grains and legumes.

MAGNESIUM

Magnesium is essential for cellular metabolism and structural growth. The RDA for pregnancy is 320 mg. Good sources include milk, whole grains, dark green vegetables, nuts, and legumes.

IRON

Iron requirements increase during pregnancy because of the growth of the fetus and placenta and the expansion of maternal blood volume. Anemia in pregnancy is mainly caused by low iron stores, although it may also result from inadequate intake of other nutrients, such as vitamins B_6 and B_{12}, folic acid, ascorbic acid, copper, and zinc. Women with poor diet histories, frequent conceptions, or records of prior iron depletion are particularly at risk.

Iron deficiency anemia is associated with a higher incidence of low-birth-weight infants and preterm birth (Salzberg, 2002). Iron deficiency anemia is generally defined as a decrease in the oxygen-carrying capacity of the blood. This significantly reduces the hemoglobin per deciliter of blood, the volume of packed red cells per deciliter of blood (hematocrit), or the number of erythrocytes.

The normal hematocrit in the nonpregnant woman is 38% to 47%. In the pregnant woman, the level may drop to as low as 34%, even when nutrition is adequate. This condition is called the physiologic anemia of pregnancy (see Chapter 14). Fetal demands for iron further contribute to symptoms of anemia in the pregnant woman. The fetal liver stores iron, especially during the third trimester. The infant will need this stored iron during the first 4 months of life to compensate for the normally inadequate levels of iron in breast milk and non-iron-fortified formulas. To prevent anemia, the woman must balance iron requirements and intake. Doing so is a problem for nonpregnant women and a greater one for pregnant women. Although the rate of absorption increases during pregnancy, it is still important to select foods high in iron to increase the daily intake (Bothwell, 2000). Lean meats, dark green leafy vegetables, eggs, and whole grain and enriched breads and cereals are the foods usually depended on for their iron content. Other iron sources include dried fruits, legumes, shellfish, and molasses.

Iron absorption is generally higher for animal products than for vegetable products. However, the woman may enhance absorption of iron from nonmeat sources by combining them with meat or a food rich in vitamin C. In addition, the use of iron-fortified foods is a cost-effective and efficient way to increase iron intake (Bothwell, 2000).

The most iron that can reasonably be obtained from the average diet is about 15 to 18 mg per day. However, the recommended intake for iron during pregnancy is 27 mg per day. Thus during pregnancy a supplement of simple iron salt, such as ferrous gluconate, ferrous fumarate, or ferrous sulfate, is needed. The Centers for Disease Control and Prevention (CDC) recommends a daily supplement of 30 mg elemental iron beginning at the first prenatal visit. Iron deficiency anemia is treated with a daily ferrous iron supplement of 60 to 120 mg. When the hematocrit becomes normal for the stage of pregnancy, the dose of iron should be decreased to 30 mg per day (CDC, 1998).

A prenatal iron supplement helps women with depleted iron reserves meet their iron requirement during pregnancy. However, it is helpful to remember that iron supplementation may interfere with zinc status (O'Brien, Zavaleta, Caulfield, et al, 1999). Also, iron supplements often cause gastrointestinal discomfort, especially if taken on an empty stomach. Once the woman begins taking an iron supplement, taking it after a meal may help reduce gastrointestinal discomfort. In addition, iron is often constipating, so it is important for the woman to consume sufficient fluids and roughage in her diet to combat this effect.

Vitamins

Vitamins are organic substances necessary for life and growth. They are found in small amounts in specific foods and generally cannot be synthesized by the body in adequate amounts.

Vitamins are grouped according to their solubility. Those that dissolve in fat are A, D, E, and K; those soluble in water include vitamin C and the B complex vitamins. An adequate intake of all vitamins is essential during pregnancy; however, several are required in larger than normal amounts to fulfill specific needs.

A balanced diet generally provides necessary vitamins without the need for supplementation. Despite this, many people who are concerned about nutrition have become involved in the practice of taking exceptionally large doses—megadoses—of vitamins. However, in vitamin therapy, more is not necessarily better. Megadoses of vitamins, especially vitamins A, D, C, and B_6, have been documented to have a negative effect on the fetus. Furthermore, excessive intake of one vitamin may interfere with the body's use of another vitamin. For example, excessive intake of vitamin C may block the body's use of vitamin B_{12}. Consequently, although it is important to meet the recommended dietary allowances of vitamins during pregnancy, megadoses are best avoided.

FAT-SOLUBLE VITAMINS

The fat-soluble vitamins A, D, E, and K are stored in the liver and thus are available should the dietary intake become inadequate. They are not excreted in the urine, so excessive consumption of these vitamins, particularly vitamins A and D, can lead to toxicity. Symptoms of fat-soluble vitamin toxicity include nausea, gastrointestinal upset, dryness and cracking of the skin, and loss of hair.

Vitamin A

Vitamin A is involved in the growth of epithelial cells, which line the entire gastrointestinal tract and compose the skin. Vitamin A plays a role in the metabolism of carbohydrates and fats. The body cannot synthesize glycogen in the absence of vitamin A, and the body's ability to handle cholesterol is also affected. In addition, the protective layer of tissue surrounding nerve fibers does not form properly if vitamin A is lacking. Probably the best known function of vitamin A is its effect on vision in dim light. A person's ability to see in the dark depends on the eye's supply of retinol, a form of vitamin A. In this manner, vitamin A prevents night blindness. Vitamin A is associated with the formation and development of healthy eyes in the fetus.

If maternal stores of vitamin A are adequate, the overall effects of pregnancy on the woman's vitamin A requirements are not remarkable. The blood serum level of vitamin A decreases slightly in early pregnancy, rises in late pregnancy, and falls before the onset of labor. Thus the RDA for vitamin A is 770 μg per day for pregnant women age 19 and older.

Deficiencies of vitamin A are not common. However, an inadequate maternal intake has been associated with preterm birth, intrauterine growth restriction, and decreased birth weight (IOM, 1990). Although routine supplementation with vitamin A is not recommended, supplementation with 5000 IU is indicated for women whose dietary intake may be inadequate, specifically strict vegetarians and recent emigrants from countries where deficiency of vitamin A is endemic (ACOG, 1998b).

Rich plant sources of vitamin A include deep green and yellow or deep orange vegetables and some fruits; animal sources include liver, egg yolk, cream, butter, fortified margarine, and milk.

Vitamin D

Vitamin D is best known for its role in the absorption and utilization of calcium and phosphorus in skeletal development. To supply the needs of the developing fetus, the pregnant woman should have a vitamin D intake of 5 μg per day.

Main food sources of vitamin D include fortified milk, margarine, butter, liver, and egg yolks. Drinking a quart of vitamin D–fortified milk daily provides the vitamin D needed during pregnancy.

Excessive intake of vitamin D is not usually a result of eating but of taking high-potency vitamin preparations. Overdoses during pregnancy can cause hypercalcemia or high blood calcium levels due to withdrawal of calcium from the skeletal tissue. Symptoms of toxicity include excessive thirst, loss of appetite, vomiting, weight loss, irritability, and high blood calcium levels.

Vitamin E

The major function of vitamin E, or tocopherol, is as an antioxidant. Vitamin E takes on oxygen, thus preventing other nutrients from undergoing chemical changes. For example, vitamin E helps spare vitamin A by preventing its oxidation in the intestinal tract and the tissues. It decreases the oxidation of polyunsaturated fats, thus helping to retain the flexibility and health of the cell membrane. In protecting the cell membrane, vitamin E affects the health of all cells in the body.

Vitamin E is also involved in certain enzymatic and metabolic reactions. It is an essential nutrient for the synthesis of nucleic acids required in the formation of red blood cells in the bone marrow. Vitamin E is beneficial in treating certain types of muscular pain and intermittent claudication, in surface healing of wounds and burns, and in protecting lung tissue from the damaging effects of smog. These functions may help explain the abundant claims and cures attributed to vitamin E, many of which have not been scientifically proved.

The newborn's need for vitamin E has been widely recognized. Human milk provides adequate vitamin E, whereas cow's milk is lower in vitamin E content. Deficiency symptoms of vitamin E are related to long-term inability to absorb fats. In humans, malabsorption problems exist in cases of cystic fibrosis, liver cirrhosis, postgastrectomy, obstructive jaundice, pancreatic problems, and sprue.

The recommended intake of vitamin E is 15 mg per day for pregnant women. Vitamin E is widely distributed in foodstuffs, especially vegetable fats and oils, whole grains, greens, and eggs.

Some pregnant women massage vitamin E oil on the abdominal skin to make it supple and possibly prevent permanent stretch marks. It is questionable whether taking high doses orally will accomplish this goal or satisfy any other claims related to vitamin E's role in reproduction or virility. In addition, excessive intake of vitamin E has been associated with abnormal coagulation in the newborn.

Vitamin K

Vitamin K, or menadione as used synthetically in medicine, is an essential factor for the synthesis of prothrombin; its function is thus related to normal blood clotting. Synthesis occurs in the intestinal tract by the *Escherichia coli* normally inhabiting the large intestine. However, the body's need for vitamin K is not totally met through synthesis. Green leafy vegetables and liver are excellent sources. The requirement for vitamin K does not increase during pregnancy. It is 90 μg per day.

Intake of vitamin K is usually adequate in a well-balanced prenatal diet. Secondary problems may arise if an illness results in malabsorption of fats or if antibiotics are used for an extended period. Antibiotics inhibit vitamin K synthesis by destroying intestinal *E coli.*

WATER-SOLUBLE VITAMINS

Water-soluble vitamins are excreted in the urine. Only small amounts are stored, so there is little protection from dietary inadequacies. Thus adequate amounts must be ingested daily. During pregnancy, the concentration of water-soluble vitamins in the maternal serum falls, whereas high concentrations are found in the fetus.

Vitamin C

The requirement for vitamin C (ascorbic acid) is increased in pregnancy from 75 to 85 mg per day. The major function of vitamin C is to aid the formation and development of connective tissue and the vascular system. Ascorbic acid is essential to the formation of collagen. Collagen is like a cement that binds cells together, just as mortar holds bricks together. If the collagen begins to disintegrate due to lack of ascorbic acid, cell functioning is disturbed, and cell structure breaks down, causing muscular weakness, capillary hemorrhage, and eventual death. These are symptoms of scurvy, the disease caused by vitamin C deficiency. Newborns of women who have taken megadoses of vitamin C may experience a rebound form of scurvy.

Maternal plasma levels of vitamin C progressively decline throughout pregnancy, with values at term being about half those at midpregnancy. It appears that ascorbic acid concentrates in the placenta; levels in the fetus are 50% or more above maternal levels.

A nutritious diet should meet the pregnant woman's needs for vitamin C without additional supplementation. Common food sources of vitamin C include citrus fruit, tomatoes, cantaloupe, strawberries, potatoes, broccoli, and other leafy green vegetables. Ascorbic acid is readily destroyed by water and oxidation. Therefore, foods containing vitamin C should have limited exposure to air, heat, and water during storage and cooking.

The B Vitamins

The B vitamins include thiamine (B_1), riboflavin (B_2), niacin, folic acid, pantothenic acid, vitamin B_6, and vitamin B_{12}. These vitamins serve as vital coenzyme factors in many reactions, such as cell respiration, glucose oxidation, and energy metabolism. Consequently, the quantities needed invariably increase as caloric intake increases to meet the metabolic and growth needs of the pregnant woman.

The *thiamine* requirement increases from the prepregnant level of 1.1 mg per day to 1.4 mg per day. Sources include pork, liver, milk, potatoes, enriched breads, and cereals.

Riboflavin deficiency is manifested by *cheilosis* (fissures and cracks of the lips and the corners of the mouth) and other skin lesions. It may also be a risk factor for preeclampsia independent of other factors (Wacker, Fruhauf, Schultz, et al, 2000). During pregnancy, women may excrete less riboflavin and still require more because of increased energy and protein needs. Thus the recommended intake of riboflavin increases by 0.3 mg per day, to 1.4 mg per day for pregnant women age 19 and older. Sources include milk, liver, eggs, enriched breads, and cereals.

Niacin requirements increase by 4 mg per day during pregnancy to 18 mg. Sources of niacin include meat, fish, poultry, liver, whole grains, enriched breads, cereals, and peanuts.

Folic acid, or folate, is required for normal growth, reproduction, and lactation and prevents the macrocytic, megaloblastic anemia of pregnancy. Megaloblastic anemia due to folic acid deficiency is seldom found in the United States, but those caring for pregnant women must be aware that it does occur. An inadequate intake of folic acid has also been associated with neural tube defects (NTDs) (spina bifida, anencephaly). Research indicates that up to 70% of spina bifida and anencephaly could be prevented by adequate intake of folic acid (Ahluwalia & Daniel, 2001; CDC, 2000). Consequently, all women of childbearing age should consume 400 μg of folic acid daily to reduce the risk of a pregnancy affected by NTDs.

It is important for nurses working with pregnant women to be aware that folic acid deficiency can be present in the absence of overt anemia. Folic acid cannot be synthesized by the human body but must be acquired from dietary sources. The best food sources are fresh green leafy vegetables, orange juice, liver, peanuts, yeast preparations, and whole grain breads and cereals. However, folic acid can be made inactive by oxidation, ultraviolet light, and heating. Thus, it can be easily lost during improper storage and cooking. To prevent unnecessary loss, foods should be stored covered to protect them from light, cooked with only a small amount of water, and not overcooked.

No allowance has been set for *pantothenic acid* in pregnancy but 5 mg per day is considered an adequate intake. Sources include meats, egg yolk, legumes, and whole grain cereals and breads.

Vitamin B_6 (pyridoxine) is associated with amino acid metabolism; thus a higher-than-average protein intake requires increased pyridoxine intake. The RDA for vitamin B_6 during pregnancy is 1.9 mg per day, an increase of 0.6 mg over the allowance for nonpregnant women. Generally the slightly increased need can be supplied by dietary sources, which include wheat germ, yeast, fish, liver, pork, potatoes, and lentils.

Vitamin B_{12}, or *cobalamin*, is the cobalt-containing vitamin found only in animal sources. Rarely is B_{12} deficiency found in women of reproductive age. Vegans (see later discussion of vegetarian diets) can develop a deficiency, however, so it is essential that their dietary intake be supplemented with this vitamin. A deficiency may also be due to a congenital inability to absorb vitamin B_{12} resulting in pernicious anemia; however, infertility is a complication of this type of anemia.

Occasionally, vitamin B_{12} levels decrease during pregnancy but increase again after birth. The RDA during pregnancy is 2.6 µg per day, an increase of 0.2 µg.

Folic acid and iron are the only nutritional supplements generally recommended during pregnancy. The increased need for other vitamins and minerals can usually be met with an adequate diet. To avoid possible deficiencies, however, many healthcare professionals still recommend a daily vitamin supplement.

MediaLink PRACTICAL GUIDE TO VEGANISM

Clinical Tip *More women are consuming over-the-counter vitamin, mineral, and food supplements today than in the past. Ask about the use of any over-the-counter supplements to help avoid potentially harmful excess intakes.*

Fluid

The nutrient water is essential for life and is found in all body tissues. It is necessary for many biochemical reactions. It also serves as a lubricant, acts as a medium of transport for carrying substances in and out of the body, and aids in the regulation of body temperature. A pregnant woman should consume at least 8 to 10 (8 oz) glasses of fluid each day, of which 4 to 6 glasses should be water. Other beverages such as juices and milk can contribute water as well as other nutrients to the diet. Sodas and diet sodas should be used in moderation because they do not contribute to the nutritional value of the diet.

Caffeine is found in beverages, foods, and medications. Its use during pregnancy remains controversial (Cnattingius, Signorello, Anneren, et al, 2000; Eskenazi, 1999). It is a central nervous system stimulant and passes readily to the fetus, who is unable to metabolize it effectively (IOM, 1990). Caffeinated beverages also have a diuretic effect, which may be counterproductive to increasing fluid intake. However, no conclusive evidence has been found linking caffeine consumption to birth defects or spontaneous abortion. At this time, most healthcare providers advise pregnant women to limit their daily intake of caffeine to moderate amounts (see Chapter 16).

Critical Thinking in Practice

Jaya Singh, a 28-year-old G1P0, is 14 weeks pregnant. The rate and total amount of her weight gain during the first trimester have been consistent with recommendations. She has gained an average of 0.5 kg (1 lb) per week during both of the past 2 weeks. Her appetite is good, and she consumes three meals per day and snacks between meals on occasion.

Jaya has altered her diet because she is concerned about excessive weight gain. She told the nurse that she has decreased her intake from the bread and dairy groups in order to limit her calorie intake. Because she has omitted most dairy products, she has increased her consumption of salads and broccoli to provide calcium sources.

A diet history revealed the following:

Grain	3–4 servings, mainly cereal and rice
Fruit	2–4 servings, fresh fruit
Vegetables	3–5 servings, salads, peas, corn, broccoli
Meat	4–5 servings, beef, pork, chicken
Dairy	occasionally cheese, ice cream, pudding
Fats, oils, sweets	occasionally salad dressings, margarine, desserts
Beverages	8–10 servings, soda, juices, water

After assessing her diet history, what is your evaluation of Jaya's diet? How could you counsel her?

Answers can be found in Appendix I.

Vegetarianism

Vegetarianism is the dietary choice of many people for religious, health, ethical, and economic reasons. There are several types of vegetarians. **Lacto-ovovegetarians** include milk, dairy products, and eggs in their diet. **Lactovegetarians** include dairy products but no eggs. **Vegans** are strict vegetarians who will not eat any food from animal sources.

In their position statement on vegetarian diets, the American Dietetic Association stated that "appropriately planned vegetarian diets are healthful, are nutritionally adequate, and provide health benefits in the prevention and treatment of certain diseases" (ADA, 1997). People following vegetarian diets tend to have lower blood pressure; a lower incidence of coronary artery disease, lung cancer, and colorectal cancer; and lower morbidity and mortality rates from chronic degenerative diseases than do nonvegetarians (ADA, 1997).

The expectant woman who is lacto-ovovegetarian can obtain ample and complete proteins from dairy products and

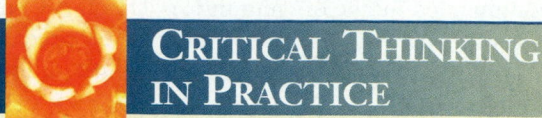

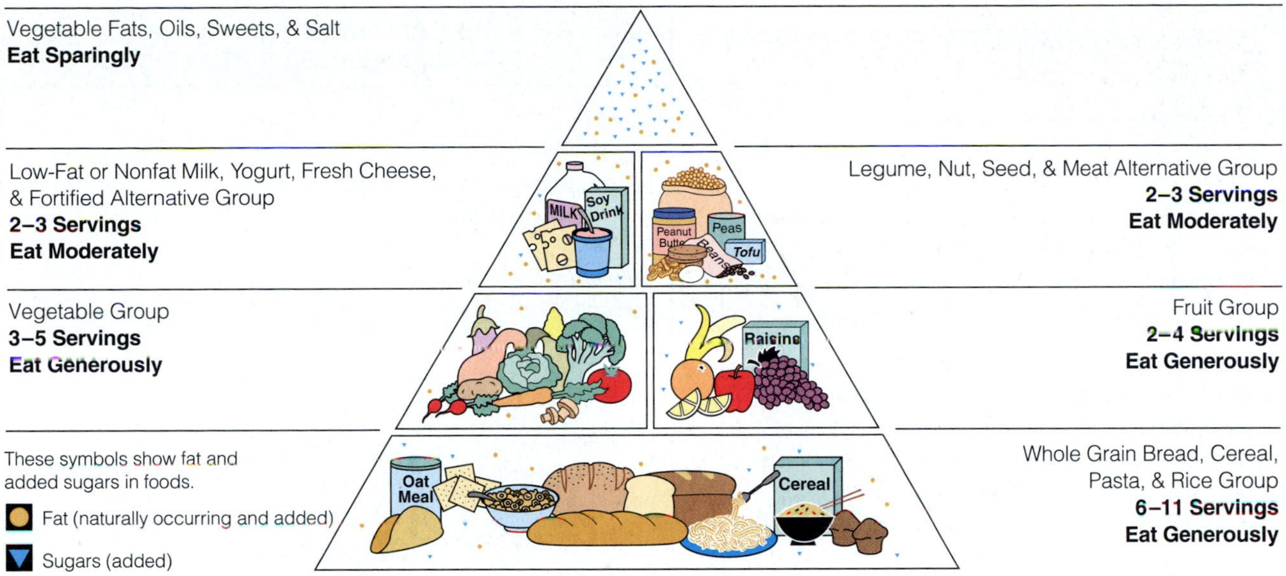

Figure 18–3 • The vegetarian food pyramid.
SOURCE: Adapted from The Health Connection, 55 West Oak Ridge Drive, Hagerstown, MD 21740-7390.

eggs. Plant protein quality may be improved if consumed with these animal proteins. If the diet contains fewer than four servings of milk and dairy products, calcium supplementation may be necessary.

If the woman follows a vegan diet, careful planning is necessary to obtain complete proteins and sufficient calories. Adequate dietary protein can be obtained by consuming a varied diet with adequate caloric intake and complementary amino acids. Complete proteins may be obtained by eating different types of plant-based proteins such as beans and rice, peanut butter on whole grain bread, and whole grain cereal with soy milk, either in the same meal or over the course of a day. Protein and amino acid supplements are not recommended (IOM, 1990). Obtaining sufficient calories to achieve adequate weight gains can be difficult because vegan diets tend to be higher in fiber and therefore filling. Low prepregnancy weight and optimum pregnancy weight gains are often a problem. Supplementation with energy-dense foods helps provide increased energy intake to prevent the body from using protein for caloric needs.

Because vegans use no animal products, a daily supplement of 4 mg of vitamin B_{12} is necessary. If soy milk is used, only partial supplementation may be needed. If no soy milk is taken, daily supplements of 1200 mg of calcium and 10 mg of vitamin D are needed.

A vegan diet may be low in iron and zinc because the best sources of these minerals are found in animal products. In addition, a high-fiber intake may reduce mineral (calcium, iron, and zinc) bioavailability. The nurse should emphasize the use of foods containing these nutrients.

Figure 18–3 • depicts the vegetarian food pyramid. A guide to vegetarian food groups is provided in Table 18–6 •.

Factors Influencing Nutrition

Besides having knowledge of nutritional needs and food sources, the nurse needs to be aware of other factors that affect a client's nutrition. What are the age, lifestyle, dietary practices, and culture of the pregnant woman? What food beliefs and habits does she have? What a person eats is also determined by availability, economics, and symbolism. These and other factors influence the expectant mother's acceptance of the nurse's intervention.

Table 18–6 • VEGETARIAN FOOD GROUPS

Food Group	Mixed Diet	Lacto-ovovegetarian	Lacto-vegetarian	Vegan
Grain	Bread, cereal, rice, pasta	Bread, cereal, rice, pasta	Bread, cereal, rice, pasta	Bread, cereal, rice, pasta
Fruit	Fruit, fruit juices	Fruit, fruit juices	Fruit, fruit juices	Fruit, fruit juices
Vegetable	Vegetables, vegetable juices	Vegetables, vegetable juices	Vegetables, vegetable juices	Vegetables, vegetable juices
Dairy and dairy alternatives	Milk, yogurt, cheese	Milk, yogurt, cheese	Milk, yogurt, cheese	Fortified soy milk, rice milk
Meat and meat alternatives	Meat, fish, poultry, eggs, legumes, tofu, nuts, nut butters	Eggs, legumes, tofu, nuts, nut butters	Legumes, tofu, nuts, nut butters	Legumes, tofu, nuts, nut butters

Complementary and Alternative Therapies

Nutritional Content of Herbs

Several herbs are good sources of various vitamins and minerals. Like other "whole" foods, herbs contain all the necessary nutrients and enzymes to increase bioavailability versus isolated substances (such as in vitamin and mineral supplements).

Dandelion root and herb: Contains high concentrations of vitamins A and C, beta carotene, and potassium (Blumenthal, 2000; Kemper, 1999).

Oat straw: Rich in calcium and magnesium, plus iron, manganese, and zinc (Blumenthal, 2000; Skidmore-Roth, 2001). Note that this is the same plant from which we derive oatmeal.

Raspberry leaf: Contains vitamin C and naturally chelated iron (Skidmore-Roth, 2001).

It is best to advise pregnant women interested in using herbs to follow three basic principles: (1) if at all possible, avoid the use of herbs, even tonic herbs, during the first trimester (with the exception of ginger in amounts less than 1 g daily); (2) avoid standardized or highly concentrated extracts because the risk of side effects tends to be higher than with whole plant extracts; and (3) do not take essential oils internally (Belew, 1999).

Table 18-7 • ABNORMALITIES THAT MAY INDICATE AN UNDISCLOSED EATING DISORDER

Somatic
Arrested growth
Marked change or frequent fluctuation in weight
Inability to gain weight
Fatigue
Constipation or diarrhea
Susceptibility to fractures
Delayed menarche
Hypokalemia, hyperphosphatemia, metabolic acidosis or alkalosis, or high serum amylase levels
Behavioral
Change in eating habits
Difficulty eating in social settings
Reluctance to be weighed
Depression
Social withdrawal
Absence from school or work
Deceptive or secretive behavior
Stealing (eg, to obtain food)
Substance abuse
Excessive exercise

Source: Becker, A. E., Grinspoon, S. K., Klibanski, A., & Herzog, D. B. (1999). Eating disorders. *New England Journal of Medicine, 340,* 1092–1098.

Eating Disorders

Millions of men and women are affected by eating disorders each year, but eating disorders are most common in adolescent girls and young women. These psychologic disorders can have a major impact on a pregnant client's physiologic and emotional well-being.

Anorexia nervosa is an eating disorder that is characterized by an extreme fear of weight gain and fat. People with this problem have distorted body images and perceive themselves as fat even when they are extremely underweight. Their dietary intake is very restrictive in both variety and quantity. They may also engage in excessive exercise to prevent weight gain.

Bulimia nervosa, another eating disorder, is characterized by bingeing (secretly consuming large quantities of food in a short period of time) and purging. Self-induced vomiting is the most common method of purging; laxatives and/or diuretics may also be used. Individuals with bulimia often maintain normal or near-normal weight for their height, so it is often difficult to know whether bingeing and purging occur.

Although pregnancies occur most often in women of normal weight, the underweight woman can conceive (Hofeldt, 1999). The presence of an eating disorder can be difficult to detect because of the secretive nature of the behaviors. Many women will decrease or discontinue their eating disorder behaviors during pregnancy, only to resume them postpartum (Morrill & Nickols-Richardson, 2001). Table 18-7 • identifies abnormalities that may indicate an eating disorder.

Women with eating disorders who become pregnant are at risk for a variety of complications. The consequences of the restricting, bingeing, and purging behaviors characteristic of eating disorders can result in a lack of nutrients available for the fetus. This, in turn, can lead to an increased risk of low-birth-weight infants, miscarriage, premature birth, and prenatal death which have been observed in women with anorexia nervosa or bulimia (Becker, Grinspoon, Klibanski, et al, 1999).

Pregnancy can be an especially difficult time for the woman with an eating disorder even if she has long desired a child. For someone who already struggles with eating and body image, the consumption of additional food and the expectations that she will gain additional weight can result in feelings of fear and guilt (Reiff & Reiff, 2000). When working with a pregnant woman with an eating disorder, education and individualized meal plans can help the woman increase her dietary intake while maintaining a sense of control. It is important to address (1) the baby's health, (2) the mother's emotional well-being, and (3) the mother's physical health (Reiff & Reiff, 2000).

The treatment needs of a woman with an eating disorder can best be met by a team approach that includes medical, nutritional, and psychiatric practitioners who are familiar with eating disorders. The pregnant woman with an eating disorder needs to be closely monitored and supported throughout her pregnancy to help ensure the best possible outcome.

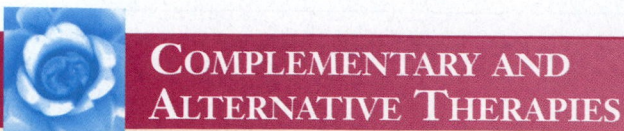

"I developed anorexia during my sophomore year in college. My parents were shocked when they saw me at Thanksgiving and, fortunately, they got me some help. For the past several years I have maintained my weight in the low normal range and feel OK about it. Now I am expecting my first child. It is so hard to think of gaining 25 to 30 pounds but I am working very hard to eat properly for my baby. I have reconnected with my therapist so that I can be sure I keep my head on straight about the importance of good nutrition. I don't think people realize how tough eating disorders are to overcome but I will NOT jeopardize my child, I just won't!"

Lactase Deficiency (Lactose Intolerance)

Some individuals have difficulty digesting milk and dairy products. This condition, known as **lactase deficiency,** or **lactose intolerance,** results from an inadequate amount of the enzyme lactase, which breaks down the milk sugar lactose into smaller digestible substances.

Lactase deficiency is found primarily in many people of African, Mexican, Native American, Ashkenazic Jewish, and Asian descent although it is found in other cultural groups as well. In the United States, 30 to 50 million people have lactose intolerance. Furthermore up to 75% of African Americans and Native Americans are lactose intolerant as are 90% of Asian Americans (National Digestive Diseases Information Clearinghouse, 2002). People who are not affected are mainly of Northern European heritage. Symptoms may include abdominal distention, discomfort, nausea, vomiting, loose stools, and cramps. When counseling pregnant women who might be intolerant of milk and milk products, the nurse should be aware that tolerances vary between individuals and even a partial serving of milk or dairy products can produce symptoms. Lactase deficiency need not be a problem for pregnant women, as the enzyme is available over the counter in tablets or drops. In addition, specially treated cow's milk is now available in most large grocery stores.

Pica

Pica is the persistent craving and eating of substances such as ice, freezer frost, cornstarch, laundry starch, baby powder, clay, dirt, and other nonnutritive substances. Most women who eat such substances do so only during pregnancy.

Iron deficiency anemia is the most common concern with pica. The ingestion of laundry starch or certain types of clay may contribute to iron deficiency by replacing iron-containing foods from the diet or by interfering with iron absorption. In fact, research indicates that women with pica, regardless of substance, tend to have lower hemoglobin levels at birth than women who do not have pica (Rainville, 1998). Women with pica that involves eating ice or freezer frost often have poor weight gain because of lack of appetite, whereas the ingestion of starch may be associated with excessive weight gain. Other adverse effects of pica include constipation, fecal impaction (often related to the consumption of clay), decreased absorption of nutrients, and a contraction of tooth fillings leading to increased dental caries (Salzberg, 2002).

Nurses should be aware of pica and its implications for the woman and her fetus. Assessment for pica is an important part of the nutritional history. However, women may be embarrassed about their cravings or reluctant to discuss them for fear of criticism. It is helpful if the nurse uses a nonjudgmental approach and explains the possible harmful effects. Reeducation of the expectant woman is important in helping her to decrease or eliminate this practice. Some women are able to switch to eating nonfat powdered milk instead of laundry starch and frozen fruit pops instead of ice. Others find that sucking on hard lemon or mint candies helps decrease the craving (Salzberg, 2002).

Common Discomforts of Pregnancy

Gastrointestinal functioning can be altered at various times throughout pregnancy, resulting in nausea, vomiting, heartburn, and constipation. Although these changes can be uncomfortable for the woman, they are seldom a major problem. Minor dietary modifications may provide relief for some individuals (see Chapter 16, Table 16–4).

Cultural, Ethnic, and Religious Influences

Cultural, ethnic, and, occasionally, religious backgrounds determine one's experiences with food and influence food preferences and habits (Figure 18–4 •). People of different nationalities are accustomed to eating foodstuffs available in their country of origin and prepared in a manner consistent with the customs and traditions of their ethnic and cultural group. In addition, the laws of certain religions allow particular foods, prohibit others, and direct the preparation and serving of meals. (See Developing Cultural Competence.)

In each culture, certain foods have symbolic significance. Generally, these symbolic foods are related to major life experiences such as birth, death, or developmental milestones. Although generalizations have been made about the food

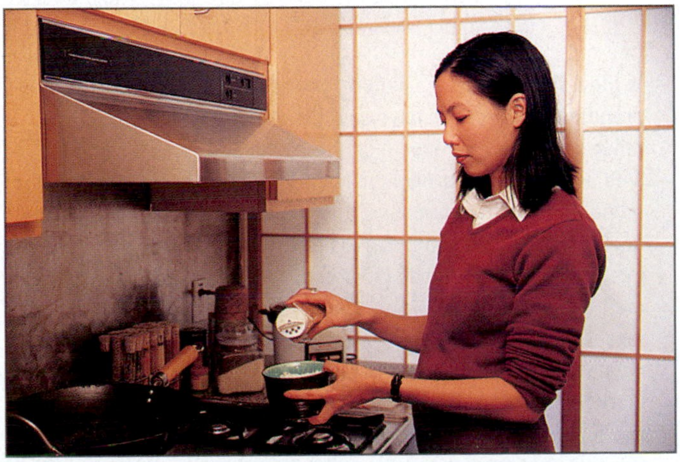

Figure 18–4 • Cultural factors affect food preferences and habits.

MEDIALINK CARE PLAN: MATERNAL NUTRITION

Developing Cultural Competence

The kosher diet followed by many Jewish people forbids the eating of pig products and shellfish. Certain cuts of meat from sheep and cattle are allowed as are fish with fins and scales. In addition, many Jews believe that meat and milk should not be mixed and eaten at the same meal.

practices of ethnic and religious groups, there are many variations. Food customs will differ among groups in various regions of the same country, among families within local regions, and among individuals within the same family. The extent to which the use of traditional ethnic foods and customs are continued is affected by the recency of immigration, the extent of exposure to other cultures, and the availability, quality, and cost of the traditional foods.

When working with a pregnant woman from any ethnic background, the nurse needs to understand the cultural influences on the woman's eating habits and to identify beliefs she may have about foods and pregnancy. Talking with the client can enable the nurse to determine the level of influence that traditional food customs exert. Only then can the nurse provide dietary advice in a manner that is meaningful to the client.

Psychosocial Factors

The sharing of food has long been a symbol of friendliness, warmth, and social acceptance in many cultures. Food is also symbolic of motherliness; that is, taking care of the family and feeding them well is a part of the traditional mothering role. Some foods and food-related practices are associated with status. Certain items may be prepared "just for company." Other foods are served only on special occasions—holidays such as Thanksgiving, for example.

MEDIALINK UNICEF

Global Perspectives

In the traditional Navajo culture, consuming certain foods when pregnant is believed to have specific effects on the baby. On the other hand, certain foods must be avoided. Although some beliefs are no longer strongly followed, others live on as cultural taboos for pregnant women. It is believed that eating a great deal of fat while pregnant can result in a difficult labor, while eating Navajo onions causes women to have many children. Pregnant women are advised to avoid excessive sweets because sweets result in the baby "not being strong." If a pregnant woman swallows chewing gum, it is believed to result in birthmarks on the baby. Pregnant women are also cautioned to avoid peeling apples or potatoes when pregnant since it is believed this results in the baby having a flat face.

SOCIOECONOMIC FACTORS

Socioeconomic level may be a determinant of nutritional status. Poverty-level families are unable to afford the same foods that higher income families can. Thus, pregnant women with low incomes are frequently at risk for inadequate intake of nutrients.

EDUCATION

Knowledge about the basic components of a balanced diet is essential. The nurse must present written and oral communication in a manner consistent with a client's level of comprehension. Often educational level is related to economic status, but even people on very limited incomes can prepare well-balanced meals if their knowledge of nutrition is adequate.

PSYCHOLOGIC FACTORS

Emotions directly affect nutritional well-being. For example, food may be used as a substitute for the expression of emotions such as anger or frustration, or as a way of expressing feelings of joy. The expectant woman's attitudes and feelings about her pregnancy may influence her food consumption. The woman who is depressed or who does not wish to be pregnant may manifest these feelings by loss of appetite or by an overindulgence of certain foods.

The Pregnant Adolescent

Nutritional care of the pregnant adolescent is of particular concern to healthcare professionals. Many adolescents are nutritionally at risk due to a variety of complex and interrelated emotional, social, and economic factors that may adversely affect dietary intake. The increased energy and nutrient demands of pregnancy place the pregnant adolescent at even greater risk.

Nutritional Concerns

GENERAL CONCERNS

Pregnant adolescents as a group are considered at risk nutritionally. Nutritional status is an important, modifiable variable in any pregnancy, but especially in adolescent pregnancy because teens are more likely than older women to be underweight at the onset of pregnancy and to gain less weight during pregnancy. Good maternal weight gain during adolescent pregnancy significantly improves fetal growth and reduces mortality.

Important nutrition-related factors to assess in pregnant adolescents include low prepregnant weight, low weight gain during pregnancy, younger age with regard to menarche, smoking, excessive prepregnant weight, anemia, unhealthy lifestyle (drugs, alcohol use), chronic disease, and history of an eating disorder. Each of these factors can independently affect the adolescent's nutrient intake and, consequently, the status of the pregnancy.

The psychosocial development of adolescents often results in a compromised nutritional intake. As adolescents become more independent, they make more of their own food choices; these may be influenced, either positively or negatively, by peer acceptance. For example, adequate weight gain may be difficult in the face of social pressures to be thin. The pregnant adolescent without a strong sense of self-esteem may therefore have trouble consuming a diet that will support adequate weight increase.

Physiologic maturation plays a role in the development of a body image and self-concept. Weight gain and changes in body appearance occur as growth and development progress. This may be difficult for some adolescent girls to accept and can lead to a negative self-concept and possible restrictive food choices. In some cases, a negative body image can be a contributing factor in the development of eating disorders. In determining nutrient needs for pregnant adolescents, the nurse needs to consider the number of years that have passed since menstruation began. Adolescent women generally are considered physiologically mature about 4 years after menarche because linear growth is usually completed by this time. Their nutritional needs would be similar to those of other "adult" women.

Adolescents who become pregnant fewer than 4 years after menarche, however, are at a high biologic risk because of their physiologic and anatomic immaturity. They are most likely to be growing, which can impact the fetus's development. Nutritional needs for these young women will be higher than for those whose growth has been completed.

Little information is currently available on the nutritional needs of pregnant adolescents. Estimates are usually obtained by using the DRI for nonpregnant teenagers (ages 11 to 14 or 15 to 18) and adding nutrient amounts recommended for all pregnant women (see Table 18–1). Although the DRIs are based on chronologic age, they are probably the best available figures to use if the pregnant female is still growing. If mature, the pregnant adolescent has nutritional needs approaching those reported for pregnant adults. However, young adolescents (13 to 15 years) need to gain more weight than older adolescents (16 years or older) to produce babies of equal size. Thus in determining the optimum weight gain for a pregnant adolescent, the nurse needs to consider the following:

- Recommended weight gain for a normal pregnancy
- Amount of weight gain expected during the postmenarcheal year during which the pregnancy occurs

These values would be added together to obtain a recommended weight gain for the pregnant adolescent. Young adolescents (2 years after menarche) should strive for a weight gain at the upper end of the range of weight gain for adults (see Table 18–3).

SPECIFIC NUTRIENT CONCERNS

Caloric needs of pregnant adolescents vary widely. Major factors in determining caloric needs include whether growth has been completed and the physical activity level of the individual. Figures as high as 50 kcal/kg have been suggested for young, growing teens who are very active physically. However, many pregnant adolescents have difficulty consuming enough calories (Giddens, Krug, Tsang, et al, 2000). A satisfactory weight gain will confirm adequacy of caloric intake in most cases.

An inadequate iron intake is a major concern with the adolescent diet. Iron needs are high for the pregnant teen due to the requirement for iron by the enlarging maternal muscle mass and blood volume. Iron supplements—providing 30 to 60 mg of elemental iron—are indicated.

Calcium is another nutrient that demands special attention from pregnant adolescents. Inadequate intake of calcium is frequently a problem in this age group. Adequate calcium intake is needed to support normal growth and development of the fetus as well as growth and maintenance of calcium stores in the adolescent. Calcium supplementation is indicated for teens with an aversion to or intolerance of milk unless other dairy products or significant calcium sources are consumed in sufficient amounts.

Because folic acid plays a role in cell reproduction, it is also an important nutrient for pregnant teens. As previously indicated, a supplement is often suggested for pregnant females, whether adult or teenager.

Other nutrients and vitamins must be considered when evaluating the overall nutritional quality of the teenager's diet. Nutrients that have frequently been found to be deficient in this age group include zinc, magnesium, folate, and vitamins A, D, E, and B_6. Inclusion of a wide variety of foods—especially fresh foods—is helpful in obtaining adequate amounts of trace minerals, fiber, and other vitamins. A low-dose vitamin and mineral supplement may be necessary when the diet is not adequate (IOM, 1990).

DIETARY PATTERNS

Healthy adolescents often have irregular eating patterns. Many skip breakfast, and most tend to be frequent snackers. Teens rarely follow the traditional three-meals-a-day pattern; their day-to-day intake often varies drastically; and they eat food combinations that may seem bizarre to adults. Despite this, adolescents usually achieve a better nutritional balance than most adults would expect.

> "*My mom is so cool. She has hung in with me throughout this pregnancy even though I know she feels bad about it—she thinks my life will be harder and I guess she is right. She is really working to make sure that I eat right so that I have a healthy baby but instead of nagging, she has turned this into something we are doing together. We have taken a couple of cooking classes and experimented with different recipes. Last week we made some great but healthy snacks and I brought them to my friend Cari's birthday party. Those snacks just disappeared!*"

In assessing the diet of the pregnant adolescent, the nurse should consider the eating pattern over time, not simply a single day's intake. This pattern is critical because of the irregularity of most adolescent eating patterns. Once the pattern is identified, counseling can be directed toward correcting deficiencies.

Counseling Issues

A positive approach to nutritional counseling for the pregnant adolescent is more effective than a negative one. The nurse must be ready to suggest nutrient-dense foods that pregnant teens can choose in many places and at any time. If an adolescent's family member does most of the meal preparation, it may be useful to include that person in the discussion if the adolescent agrees. Involving the expectant father in counseling may be beneficial. The pregnant teenager will soon become a parent, and her understanding of nutrition will influence not only her well-being but also that of her child. However, teens tend to live in the present, and counseling that stresses long-term changes may be less effective than more concrete approaches. Messages should emphasize that the pregnant teen is eating for her own health and that of the baby and should focus on foods themselves rather than on nutrients. In many cases, classes with other teens are effective. In a group atmosphere, adolescents often work together to plan adequate meals including foods that are their special favorites.

Postpartum Nutrition

Nutritional needs will change following the birth. Nutrient requirements will vary depending on whether the mother decides to breastfeed. An assessment of postpartal nutritional status is necessary before the nurse provides nutritional guidance.

Postpartal Nutritional Status

Postpartal nutritional status is determined primarily by assessing the new mother's weight, hemoglobin and hematocrit levels, clinical signs, and dietary history.

As previously discussed, an ideal weight gain for the normal-weight woman during pregnancy is between 11.5 and 16 kg (25 and 35 lb). After birth, there is a weight loss of approximately 10 to 12 lb. Additional weight loss will be most rapid during the first few weeks after birth as the uterus returns to normal size, tissue fluids are released, and maternal blood volume returns to normal. The mother's weight will then begin to stabilize. Weight loss may also be affected by lactation. Individual weight loss of women who breastfeed will vary but tends to be greater than that of women who do not if breastfeeding continues for at least 6 months.

The rate of postpartum weight loss is influenced by many factors. Some women approach their prepregnancy weight several weeks after birth; most approach this weight about 6 months later. The amount of weight gained during pregnancy is a major determinant of weight loss after childbirth. Generally, the more weight gained during pregnancy, the more is lost postpartum.

It is important to evaluate the mother's current weight, ideal weight for her height, weight before pregnancy, and weight before the birth. Women who are interested in weight reduction should be referred to a dietitian. Different guidelines for weight loss are used for breastfeeding mothers and nonbreastfeeding mothers.

Hemoglobin and erythrocyte values vary after birth, but they should return to normal levels within 2 to 6 weeks. Hematocrit levels should rise gradually due to hemoconcentration as extracellular fluid is excreted. The hematocrit is usually checked at the postpartum visit to detect any anemia. Mothers can be encouraged to eat a diet high in iron. Iron supplements are generally prescribed for 2 to 3 months following birth to replenish supplies depleted by pregnancy.

The nurse assesses any clinical symptoms the new mother may be experiencing. Food cravings and aversions typically drop significantly during the postpartal period and do not usually pose a problem. However, constipation is a common problem following birth. The nurse can encourage the woman to maintain a high fluid intake to keep the stool soft. Dietary sources of fiber and physical exercise are also helpful in preventing constipation.

The nurse obtains specific information on diet and eating habits directly from the woman. Visiting the mother during mealtimes provides an opportunity for unobtrusive nutritional assessment. Which foods has a woman selected? Has she avoided fruits and vegetables? Is her diet nutritionally sound? A comment focusing on a positive aspect of her meal selection may initiate a discussion of nutrition.

The dietitian should be informed about any woman whose cultural or religious beliefs require specific foods. Appropriate meals can then be prepared for her. The nurse may also refer women with unusual eating habits or numerous questions about food or nutrition to a dietitian. In all cases, the nurse should provide literature on nutrition so that the woman will have a source of appropriate information at home.

Nutritional Care of Formula-Feeding Mothers

After birth, the formula-feeding mother's dietary requirements return to prepregnancy levels (see Table 18–1). If the mother has a good understanding of nutritional principles, it is sufficient to advise her to reduce her daily caloric intake by about 300 kcal and to return to prepregnancy levels for other nutrients.

If the mother has a poor understanding of nutrition, this is an opportunity to teach her the basic principles and the importance of a well-balanced diet. Her eating habits and dietary practices will eventually be reflected in the diet of her child.

If the mother has gained excessive weight during pregnancy (or perhaps was overweight before pregnancy), referral to a dietitian is appropriate. The dietitian can design weight reduction diets to meet nutritional needs and food preferences. Weight loss goals of 1 to 2 lb per week are usually suggested.

In addition to learning how to meet her own nutritional needs, the new mother will usually be interested in learning how to provide for her infant's nutritional needs. A discussion of infant feeding, which includes topics such as selecting infant formulas, formula preparation, and vitamin and mineral supplementation, is appropriate and generally well received.

Nutritional Care of Breastfeeding Mothers

Nutrient needs increase during breastfeeding. Table 18–1 lists the DRIs during breastfeeding for specific nutrients. Table 18–2 includes a sample daily food guide for lactating women. A few key nutrients need further discussion.

CALORIES

One of the most important factors in the breastfeeding woman's diet is calories. An inadequate caloric intake can reduce milk volume. However, milk quality generally remains unaffected. The breastfeeding mother should increase her caloric intake by 200 kcal over the pregnancy requirements (that is, a 500-kcal increase from her prepregnancy requirement). This results in a total of about 2500 to 2700 kcal per day for most women.

Depending on her own dietary preferences, the breastfeeding mother can use the general Food Guide Pyramid or the vegetarian food pyramid to assess her dietary intake. She should strive to include a variety of foods from each food group. Her caloric intake needs to provide enough energy to sustain lactation. After her weight stabilizes several weeks following childbirth, weight loss should not exceed more than 1 lb per week.

PROTEIN

An adequate protein intake is essential while breastfeeding because protein is an important component of breast milk. An intake of 65 g per day during the first 6 months of breastfeeding and 62 g per day thereafter is recommended. As in pregnancy, it is important that the woman consume adequate nonprotein calories to prevent the use of protein as an energy source.

CALCIUM

Calcium is also an important nutrient in milk production, and increases over nonpregnancy needs are expected. Requirements during breastfeeding remain the same as requirements during pregnancy: 1000 mg per day. An inadequate intake of calcium from food sources necessitates the use of calcium supplements.

IRON

Iron needs during lactation are not substantially different from those of nonpregnant women because iron is not a principal component of breast milk. However, as previously mentioned, continued supplementation of the mother for 2 to 3 months after parturition is advisable to replenish maternal stores depleted by pregnancy.

FLUIDS

Liquids are especially important during lactation because inadequate fluid intake may decrease milk volume. The recommended fluid intake of 8 to 10 (8 oz) glasses daily can be met by the consumption of water, juices, milk, and soups.

“*For me, the hardest part of breastfeeding was drinking enough fluid. I am not a big water person and they told me to go easy on caffeine beverages. Once I started adding a slice of lemon to my water, I found it a lot easier. My baby is 13 months old now and I have stopped breastfeeding, but I still drink the water with lemon. I think I have developed a good new habit!*”

Counseling Issues

In addition to counseling mothers on how to meet their increased nutrient needs during breastfeeding, nurses should discuss a few issues related to infant feeding. For example, many mothers are concerned about how specific foods they eat will affect their babies during breastfeeding. Generally, there are no foods the nursing mother must avoid except those to which she might be allergic. Occasionally, however, some breastfeeding mothers find that their babies are affected by certain foods. Onions, turnips, cabbage, chocolate, spices, and seasonings are commonly listed as offenders. The best advice to give the breastfeeding mother is to avoid those foods she suspects cause distress in her infant. For the most part, however, she should be able to eat any nourishing food she wants without fear that her baby will be affected. For further discussion of successful infant feeding, see Chapter 31.

NURSING CARE MANAGEMENT

Nursing Assessment and Diagnosis

The nurse needs to assess nutritional status in order to plan an optimal diet with each woman. The nurse may gather data by consulting the woman's chart and by interviewing her. Information is obtained about the following:

- The woman's height and weight and her weight gain during pregnancy
- Pertinent laboratory values, especially hemoglobin and hematocrit
- Clinical signs that have possible nutritional implications, such as constipation, anorexia, or heartburn
- Diet history to determine the woman's views on nutrition as well as her specific nutrient intake

The nurse can obtain a diet history by asking the woman to complete a 24-hour diet recall, in which she lists everything consumed in the previous 24 hours, including foods, fluids, and any supplements. At least 3 days of diet recalls should be done to compensate for daily variations. Diet may also be evaluated using a food frequency questionnaire. The questionnaire lists common categories of foods and asks the woman how frequently in a day (or week) she consumes foods from the list. Common categories include vegetables, fruits, milk or cheese, meat or poultry, fish, desserts or sweets, coffee or tea, and alcoholic beverages. This method may be less reliable because it requires the individual to be accurate about her intake.

Clinical Tip *When completing a diet history it is as important to identify the foods a woman avoids as it is to determine which foods she eats.*

In some instances, the nurse will ask the woman to keep a food record or diary of everything she eats for a specified period of time (such as a week). This provides a clearer picture of nutritional patterns and may prompt the woman to make changes if the diary reveals areas of deficiency or excess.

During the data-gathering process, the nurse has an opportunity to discuss important aspects of nutrition in the context of the family's needs and lifestyle. The nurse also seeks information about psychologic, cultural, and socioeconomic factors that may influence food intake.

The nurse can use a nutritional questionnaire to gather and record important facts. This information provides a database the nurse can use to develop an intervention plan to fit the woman's individual needs. The sample questionnaire shown in Figure 18–5 • has been filled in to demonstrate this process.

Once the data are obtained, the nurse begins to analyze the information, formulate appropriate nursing diagnoses, and develop client goals. For a woman during the first trimester, for example, the diagnosis may be ***Altered Nutrition: Less than Body Requirements*** related to nausea and vomiting. In many cases the diagnosis may be related to excessive weight gain. In such cases the diagnosis might be ***Altered Nutrition: More than Body Requirements*** related to excessive calorie intake. Although these diagnoses are broad, the nurse must be specific in addressing issues such as inadequate intake of nutrients such as iron, calcium, or folic acid; problems with nutrition due to a limited food budget; problems related to physiologic alterations, such as anorexia, heartburn, or nausea; and behavioral problems related to excessive dieting, anorexia nervosa, or bulimia. In some instances, the diagnosis ***Health-Seeking Behavior*** may seem most appropriate, especially if the woman asks for information about nutrition.

Nursing Plan and Implementation

After the nursing diagnosis is made, the nurse can plan an approach to correct any nutritional deficiencies or improve the overall quality of the diet.

Teaching for Self-Care

In counseling the pregnant woman, the nurse needs to avoid "talking down" to her or "preaching" to her. The nurse should present information in a clear, logical way, using appropriate language but avoiding jargon. Examples are often helpful in clarifying material. The nurse should also answer all questions appropriately and clearly.

When a person requires nutritional counseling, a dietary change usually is necessary. Change is often difficult,

RESEARCH IN PRACTICE
Comparing Pregnant Women's Nutritional Knowledge to Actual Dietary Intake

What is this study about? Nutritional intake during pregnancy directly affects maternal weight gain, and indirectly affects the weight of the baby. Inadequate nutritional intake has been linked to low birth weight, premature birth, and congenital defects. This researcher investigated the linkage between the nutritional knowledge of low- and middle-income mothers and their actual nutritional intake and weight gain.

How was this study done? This descriptive study evaluated the nutritional knowledge of 82 low- and middle-income women using a self-completed questionnaire. The women in the study were all attending either childbirth education classes or a free prenatal clinic. The questionnaire included demographic information and an assessment of knowledge of the Food Guide Pyramid. The mothers were also asked to complete a 2-day dietary recall. The questionnaire was scored and each subject's knowledge was classified as accurate or, if inaccurate, whether estimates of daily intake were low or high. Dietary records were categorized according to the Food Guide Pyramid food groups and analyzed by computer software to determine nutritional content.

What were the results of the study? The average age of subjects was 25 years, and most (77%) were primiparous. Most women had inadequate general nutritional knowledge. While 85% reported familiarity with the Food Guide Pyramid, few correctly identified the number of servings for each food group. These women's dietary intake did not meet all of the nutritional requirements of pregnancy. In particular, vitamin D, folate, calcium, iron, and phosphorus were less than the RDA recommendations. Fat, vitamin A, and sodium were all greater than the recommended allowances. Women in this study had a high intake of fried and processed foods, and drank an average of only two glasses of water per day. Significant differences were found between women's nutritional knowledge and actual dietary intake for breads, fruits, and vegetables, but not for meat or milk. The subjects tended to eat more than the recommended amount of breads and less than the recommended amount of fruits and vegetables.

What additional questions might I have? How accurate is the self-report dietary recall? What relationships were found between nutritional knowledge, nutritional intake, and actual outcomes?

How can I use this study? Pregnant women, particularly in low- and middle-income groups, may not have adequate knowledge of good nutrition and the recommended intake for various food groups. Women need to be encouraged to learn and practice recommended nutritional intake during pregnancy. Nurses are in a key position to both educate and encourage women to use good nutritional practices during pregnancy.

Source: Fowles, R. (2002). Comparing pregnant women's nutritional knowledge to their actual dietary intake. *American Journal of Maternal Child Nursing, 27*(3), 171–177.

NUTRITIONAL QUESTIONNAIRE

Name Susan Longmont　　Date 8-15-03

Age 20

Ethnic group Caucasian

Religion Protestant

Gravida i　　Para 0　　EDB 3-21-04

Age of youngest child? NA

Birth weights of previous children? NA

Usual nonpregnant weight 115　　Present weight 125

Weight gain during last pregnancy? NA

Vitamin supplements? none

Current medications? aspirin for headache

Do you smoke? yes　　How much per day? 1-1½ packs

Eating patterns:

1. How many meals per day? 2　　when 12:30 pm 6:30 pm
2. How many snacks per day? 3　　when 10:30 am 4:00 pm 10:00 pm
3. What other foods are important to your usual diet? chocolate and candy bars
4. Amount per day 4 bars/week
5. Do you have any different food preferences now? no
6. Do you eat nonfoods such as:

		Amount
laundry starch	no	NA
ice	yes	10 cubes/day
other (name)	no	NA

7. What foods do you dislike or do not eat? spinach and dried beans
8. For added information complete a typical daily intake (24 hour recall is suggested).

Do you have special problems in food preparation such as:

1. Physical disability　　yes ____　　no ✓　　Explain ____
2. Cooking appliances　　yes ____　　no ✓　　Explain ____
3. Refrigeration of food　　yes ____　　no ✓　　Explain ____

Who does the meal planning? I do.　　shopping? We both do.

cooking? I do most of the time but my husband likes to help.

Are there transportation problems? We have only one car but we go in the evening.

Financial situation: My husband is working and going to school. I am not working.　　Food stamps yes　　WIC no

Do you have any previous nutritional problems? No. I have never paid much attention to food before, but now I have lots of questions.

Are there any problems with this pregnancy? Nausea Yes, in the morning.

Constipation No　　Other NA

Assessment by the nurse following the completion of the questionnaire.

Basic estimated nutrient and caloric value of typical daily intake.

Please circle one of the following:

Protein intake was	low	**adequate**	high
Caloric intake was	low	adequate	**high**
Calcium intake was	**low**	adequate	high
Iron intake was	**low**	adequate	high
Vitamin C intake was	low	**adequate**	high

Figure 18–5 ● Sample nutritional questionnaire used in nursing management of a pregnant woman.

however. Counseling will be more effective if the nurse understands the client's values and explains the needed change in a way that is meaningful to the client. Because the pregnant woman must follow the plan, it should be developed in cooperation with her, be suitable for her financial level and background, and be based on reasonable, achievable goals.

The following example demonstrates one way a nurse can implement a plan with a client based on the nursing diagnosis.

Diagnosis: ***Altered Nutrition: Less than Body Requirements*** related to low intake of calcium

Client goal: The woman will increase her intake of calcium to the DRI level.

Implementation:

1. Plan with the woman additional milk or dairy products that she can reasonably add to the diet (specify amounts).
2. Encourage the use of other calcium sources, such as leafy green vegetables and legumes.
3. Plan for the addition of powdered milk in cooking and baking.
4. If none of the above are realistic or acceptable, consider the use of calcium supplements.

Most families can benefit from guidance about food purchasing and preparation. The nurse should advise women to plan food purchases thoughtfully by preparing menus and a grocery list before shopping. It is also helpful to advise clients to monitor sales, compare brands, and be selective when purchasing "convenience" foods, which tend to be expensive. Other techniques for keeping food costs down without jeopardizing quality include buying food in season, using bulk foods when appropriate, using whole grain or enriched products, buying lower grade eggs (grading has no relation to the egg's nutritional value but indicates color of the shell and delicacy of flavor), and avoiding fancy grades of food and foods in elaborate packaging.

Community-Based Nursing Care

Food is a significant portion of a family's budget, and meeting nutritional needs may be a challenge for families on limited incomes. Community-based services offered through clinics, local agencies, schools, and volunteer organizations are effective in addressing these needs. Increasingly, nurses play an important role in managing such community-based services, especially those services focusing on client education. In addition, most communities offer special assistance to qualifying families to meet their nutritional needs. The Food Stamp Program provides stamps or coupons for participating households whose net monthly income is below a specified level. These stamps can be used to purchase food for the household each month.

The Special Supplemental Food Program for Women, Infants, and Children (WIC) is designed to assist low-income pregnant or breastfeeding women and their children under 5 years of age. The program provides food assistance, nutrition education, and referrals to healthcare providers. The food distributed, including dried beans and peas, peanut butter, eggs, cheese, milk, fortified adult and infant cereals, juice, and iron-fortified infant formula, is designed to provide good sources of iron, protein, and certain vitamins for individuals with an inadequate diet. Research indicates that participation in the WIC program during pregnancy and infancy is associated with a reduced risk of infant death (Moss & Carver, 1998). In addition, the WIC program is credited with helping reduce the incidence of low birth weight in infants and in decreasing the incidence of anemia in the infants and young children of low-income families.

Evaluation

Once a plan has been developed and implemented, the nurse and client may wish to identify ways of evaluating its effectiveness. Evaluation may involve keeping a food journal, writing out weekly menus, returning weekly for weighing, and the like. If anemia is a special problem, periodic hematocrit assessments are also indicated.

Women with serious nutritional deficiencies are referred to a dietitian. The nurse can then work closely with the dietitian and the client to improve the pregnant woman's health by modifying her diet.

Chapter Review

ExploreMediaLink

NCLEX review questions, case studies, and other interactive resources for this chapter can be found on the Web site at http://www.prenhall.com/olds. Click on "Chapter 18" to select the activities for this chapter.

For tutorials including animations and videos, more NCLEX review questions, and an audio glossary, access the accompanying CD-ROM in this book.

Focus Your Study

- Maternal weight gains averaging 11.5 to 16 kg (25 to 35 lb) for a normal-weight woman are associated with the best reproductive outcomes.
- If the diet is adequate, folic acid and iron are the only supplements generally recommended during pregnancy.
- Women should not restrict caloric intake to reduce weight during pregnancy.
- Pregnant women should be encouraged to eat regularly and to eat a wide variety of foods, especially fresh and lightly processed foods.
- Taking megadoses of vitamins during pregnancy is unnecessary and potentially dangerous.
- Pregnant women who eat vegetarian diets should place special emphasis on obtaining ample complete proteins, calories, calcium, iron, vitamin D, vitamin B_{12}, and zinc through food sources or supplementation if necessary.
- Evaluation of physical, psychosocial, and cultural factors that affect food intake is essential before the nurse can determine nutritional status and plan nutritional counseling.
- Adolescents who become pregnant less than 4 years after menarche have higher nutritional needs and are considered to be at high biologic risk.
- Weight gains during adolescent pregnancy must accommodate recommended gains for a normal pregnancy plus necessary gains due to growth.
- After childbirth, the nonbreastfeeding mother's dietary requirements return to prepregnancy levels.
- Breastfeeding mothers require an additional 200 calories above pregnancy intake and increased fluid intake to maintain ample milk volume.

References

Ahluwalia, I. B., & Daniel, K. L. (2001). Are women with recent live births aware of the benefits of folic acid? *Morbidity and Mortality Weekly Report, 50* (RR-6), 3–14.

American College of Obstetricians and Gynecologists (ACOG). (1998). *Vitamin A supplementation during pregnancy* (ACOG Committee Opinion No. 196). Washington, DC: Author.

American Dietetic Association (ADA). (1997). Position of ADA: Vegetarian diets. *Journal of the American Dietetic Association, 97,* 1317–1321.

Becker, A. E., Grinspoon, S. K., Klibanski, A., & Herzog, D. B. (1999). Eating disorders. *New England Journal of Medicine, 340,* 1092–1098.

Belew, C. (1999). Herbs and the childbearing woman: Guidelines for midwives. *Journal of Nurse-Midwifery, 44*(3), 231–246.

Blumenthal, M. (2000). *Herbal medicine: Expanded Commission E Monographs.* Austin, TX: American Botanical Council.

Bothwell, T. H. (2000). Iron requirements in pregnancy and strategies to meet them. *American Journal of Clinical Nutrition,* 72 (Suppl.), 257–264.

Centers for Disease Control and Prevention (CDC). (1998, April 3). Recommendations to prevent and control iron deficiency in the United States. *Morbidity and Mortality Weekly Report, 47* (RR-3), 1–36.

Centers for Disease Control and Prevention (CDC). 2000. *Folic acid now.* Birth Defects and Pediatric Genetics Branch, National Center for Environmental Health, Atlanta, GA: Author.

Cnattingius, S., Signorello, L. B., Anneren, G., Clausson, B., Ekbom, A., Ljuner, E., et al. (2000). Caffeine intake and the risk of first-trimester spontaneous abortion. *New England Journal of Medicine, 343,* 1839–1845.

Eskenazi, B. (1999). Caffeine—filtering the facts. *New England Journal of Medicine, 341,* 688–689.

Food and Nutrition Board—Institute of Medicine. (1997). *Dietary reference intakes for calcium, phosphorus, magnesium, vitamin D, and fluoride.* Washington, DC: National Academy Press.

Food and Nutrition Board—Institute of Medicine. (1998). *Dietary reference intakes for thiamin, riboflavin, niacin, vitamin B6, folate, vitamin B12, pantothenic acid, biotin, and choline.* Washington, DC: National Academy Press.

Food and Nutrition Board—Institute of Medicine. (2000). *Dietary reference intakes for vitamin C, vitamin E, selenium, and carotenoids.* Washington, DC: National Academy Press.

Fung, E. B., Ritchie, L. D., Woodhouse, L. R., Roehl, R., & King, J. C. (1997). Zinc absorption in women during pregnancy and lactation: A longitudinal study. *American Journal of Clinical Nutrition, 66*(1), 80–88.

General Accounting Office. (1992, May). *Early intervention: Federal investments like WIC can produce savings* (Document HRD 92–19). Washington, DC: Author.

Giddens, J. B., Krug, S. K., Tsang, R. C., Guo, S., Miodovnik, M., & Prada, J. A. (2000). Pregnant adolescent and adult women have similarly low intakes of selected nutrients. *Journal of the American Dietetic Association, 100,* 1334–1340.

Hofeldt, F. D. (1999). Gynecology, endocrinology, and osteoporosis. In P. S. Mehler & A. E. Anderson (Eds.), *Eating disorders: A guide to medical care and complications* (pp. 118–131). Baltimore, MD: John Hopkins University Press.

Institute of Medicine (IOM), Subcommittee for a Clinical Application Guide. (1992). *Nutrition during pregnancy and lactation: An implementation guide.* Washington, DC: National Academy Press.

Institute of Medicine (IOM), Subcommittee on Dietary Intake and Nutrient Supplements During Pregnancy, Committee on Nutrition Status During Pregnancy and Lactation, Food and Nutrition Board. (1990). *Nutrition during pregnancy: Weight gain and nutrient supplements.* Washington, DC: National Academy Press.

Kemper, K. J. (1999, November). Longwood Herbal Task Force and the Center for Holistic Pediatric Education and Research; Monograph on Dandelion (*Taraxacum offinalis*).

Klebanoff, M. A., Levine, R. J., DerSimonian, R., Clemns, J. D., & Wilkins, D. G. (1999). Maternal serum paraxanthine, a caffeine metabolite, and the risk of spontaneous abortion. *New England Journal of Medicine, 341,* 1639–1644.

Koo, W. W. K., Walters, J. C., Esterlitz, J., Levine, R. J., Bush, A. J., & Sibai, B. (1999). Maternal calcium supplementation and fetal bone mineralization. *Obstetrics & Gynecology, 94*, 577–582.

Lemone P. (1999). Vitamins and minerals. *Journal of Obstetric, Gynecologic, and Neonatal Nursing, 28*, 520–533.

March of Dimes. (2002). *Nutrition today matters tomorrow: A report from the March of Dimes task force on nutrition and optimal human development.* Washington, DC: Author.

Morrill, E. S., & Nickols-Richardson, H. M. (2001). Bulimia nervosa during pregnancy: A review. *Journal of the American Dietetic Association, 101*, 448–454.

Moss, N., & Carver, K. (1998). The effect of WIC and medicaid on infant mortality in the United States. *American Journal of Public Health, 88* (9), 1354–1361.

National Digestive Diseases Information Clearinghouse (NIDDK). (2002). *Lactose intolerance.* Retrieved October 1, 2002, from http://www.niddk.nih.gov/health/digest/pubs/lactose/lactose.html

O'Brien, K. O., Zavaleta, N., Caulfield, L., Yang, D. X., & Abrams, S. A. (1999). Influence of prenatal iron and zinc supplements on supplemental iron absorption, red blood cell iron incorporation, and iron status in pregnant Peruvian women. *American Journal of Clinical Nutrition, 69*, 509–515.

Rainville, A. J. (1998). Pica practices of pregnant women are associated with lower maternal hemoglobin level at delivery. *Journal of the American Dietetic Association, 98*(3), 293–296.

Reiff, D. W., & Reiff, K. K. L. (2000). *Eating disorders: Nutrition in the recovery process.* Gaithersburg, MD: Aspen Publishers.

Reifsnider, E., & Gill, S. L. (2000). Nutrition for the childbearing years. *Journal of Obstetric, Gynecologic, and Neonatal Nursing, 29*, 43–55.

Salzberg, H. S. (2002). Nutrition in pregnancy. In J. J. Sciarra (Ed.), *Gynecology and obstetrics* (vol. 2, chap. 7). Philadelphia: Lippincott Williams & Wilkins.

Skidmore-Roth, L. (2001). *Mosby's handbook of herbs & natural supplements*. St. Louis, MO: Mosby.

Strychar, I. M., Chabot, C., Champagne, F., Ghadirian, P., Leduc, L., Lemonnier, M. C., et al. (2000). Psychosocial and lifestyle factors associated with insufficient and excessive maternal weight gain during pregnancy. *Journal of the American Dietetic Association, 100*, 353–356.

US Department of Agriculture & US Department of Health and Human Services. (1990). *Nutrition and your health: Dietary guidelines for Americans* (3rd ed.). (Home and Garden Bulletin No. 232). Washington, DC: Authors.

Wacker, J., Fruhauf, J., Schultz, M., Chiwora, F. M., Volz, C. J., & Becker, K. (2000). Riboflavin deficiency and preeclampsia. *Obstetrics & Gynecology, 96*, 38–44.

19 Pregnancy at Risk: Pregestational Problems

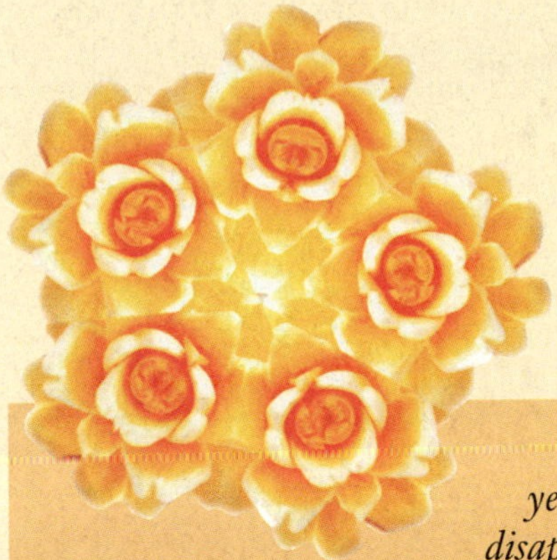

Today is the anniversary of my Julie's death. She died of a heroin overdose. During the years before her death, we tried everything to help her, but nothing worked. She would disappear, sometimes for weeks, and then reappear filled with good intentions to kick her habit—but she never could. She was 29 when I lost her, and 3 months pregnant with our grandchild. I miss her so. I don't know if my heart will ever mend.

Objectives

- Summarize the effects of alcohol and illicit drugs on the childbearing woman and her fetus/newborn.
- Discuss the pathology, treatment, and nursing care of pregnant women with diabetes.
- Discriminate among the four major types of anemia associated with pregnancy with regard to signs, treatment, and implications for pregnancy.
- Discuss acquired immunodeficiency syndrome (AIDS), including care of the pregnant woman with HIV/AIDS, neonatal implications, and ramifications for the childbearing family.
- Describe the effects of various heart disorders on pregnancy, including their implications for nursing care.
- Compare the effects of selected gestational medical conditions on pregnancy.

Key Terms

Acquired immunodeficiency syndrome (AIDS) 451

Crack 434

Gestational diabetes mellitus (GDM) 438

Human immunodeficiency virus (HIV) 451

Macrosomia 440

MEDIALINK

Additional resources for this content can be found on the Student CD-ROM and on the Companion Website at www.prenhall.com/olds. Click on "Chapter 19" to select the activities for this chapter.

CD-ROM
- Audio Glossary
- NCLEX Review

Companion Website
- Additional NCLEX Review
- Case Study: Client With Gestational Diabetes
- Care Plan Activity: Antepartal Client at Risk

Pregnancy is biologically, physiologically, and psychologically stressful, even for healthy women. For women with preexisting (pregestational) conditions such as substance abuse, diabetes, HIV infection, and cardiac disease it may be life threatening. For these women, pregestational counseling is especially important to identify early interventions designed to diminish the adverse effects of pregnancy on both the mother and fetus. In some cases, interventions prior to conception may be critical (deWeerd, Thomas, Cikot, et al, 2002).

Prenatal care is aimed toward identification, assessment, and care management of women whose pregnancies are at risk because of potential or existing complications. This chapter focuses on women with pregestational medical disorders and their possible effects on the outcome of pregnancy. Chapter 20, in turn, focuses on medical disorders that develop during pregnancy.

Care of the Woman Practicing Substance Abuse

Substance abuse occurs when an individual experiences difficulties with work, family, social relations, and/or health as a result of alcohol or drug use. Research indicates that approximately 6.9% of people in the United States use illicit drugs (March of Dimes, 2002). In general, the rate of illicit drug use among pregnant women is less than half the rate as among nonpregnant women. Specifically, approximately 3% of pregnant women use an illicit drug during pregnancy. However, illicit drug usage varies greatly by age. In 1999 and 2000, about 12.9% of pregnant females ages 15 to 17 used illicit drugs compared to 5.5% of females ages 18 to 25, and 1.3% of women ages 26 to 44 (Substance Abuse and Mental Health Services Administration [SAMHSA], 2002). See Figure 19–1 •.

Because women of childbearing age (15 to 44 years) make up a substantial proportion of the drug-using population, the problem has major significance for women and children. In testimony to these statistics is the increasing number of drug-exposed infants being born throughout the United States. Indiscriminate use of drugs during pregnancy, particularly in the first trimester, may adversely affect the health of the woman and the growth and development of her fetus. Drugs that are commonly misused include tobacco, alcohol, cocaine, marijuana, amphetamines, barbiturates, hallucinogens, club drugs, heroin, and other narcotics. Tobacco is discussed in Chapter 16 as a teratogenic substance. Table 19–1 • identifies common addictive drugs and their effects on the fetus and newborn.

Drug use during pregnancy may be the most frequently missed diagnosis in all of maternity care. Substance-abusing women typically do not seek prenatal care until late in their pregnancy. They may be noncompliant or they may present in labor with no history of prenatal care. Even when they do seek care early, physicians and nurses may fail to ask the woman about drug and alcohol use because of their own lack of knowledge, discomfort, or biases. When asked, women may deny use of illegal substances out of fear or shame. Although some clinics perform routine or random drug screens, consent from the client is required.

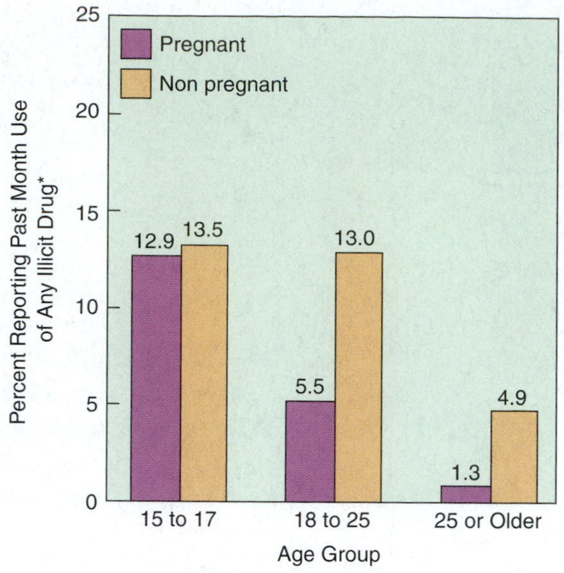

*Refers to marijuana/hashish, cocaine (including crack), inhalants, hallucinogens, heroin, or perscription-type drugs used nonmedically.

Figure 19–1 • Percentages of females ages 15 to 44 reporting past month use of any illicit drugs by pregnancy status and age , 1999 and 2000.

SOURCE: Substance Abuse and Mental Health Services Administration (SAMHSA). (2002). *The NHSDA Report: Substance use among pregnant women during 1999 and 2000.* Washington, DC: Author.

Clinical Tip *Keep in mind that approximately 1 of 10 women in the United States, regardless of socioeconomic status or ethnic background, is currently abusing a substance. If you consider that possibility with every woman, you will ask the important questions about drug use and be alert for signs of substance abuse.*

Providing prenatal care to chemically dependent women presents multiple dilemmas and challenges to clinicians. However, pregnancy represents a period in most women's lives when they recognize the need for and are receptive to caring and responsive interventions. By optimizing the prenatal experience of chemically dependent women, maternal-fetal outcomes will be improved and the groundwork laid for the ongoing therapeutic services that are needed to maintain the health and well-being of the mother and child (McComish, Greenberg, Ager, et al, 2000).

The substance-abusing woman who seeks prenatal care may not voluntarily reveal her addiction, so caregivers should be alert for a history or physical signs that suggest

Table 19–1 • POSSIBLE EFFECTS OF SELECTED DRUGS OF ABUSE/ADDICTION ON FETUS AND NEWBORN

Maternal Drug	Effect on Fetus/Newborn
Depressants	
Alcohol	Mental retardation, microcephaly, midfacial hypoplasia, cardiac anomalies, intrauterine growth restriction (IUGR), potential teratogenic effects, fetal alcohol syndrome (FAS), fetal alcohol effects (FAE)
Narcotics	
Heroin	Withdrawal symptoms, convulsions, IUGR, tremors, irritability, sneezing, vomiting, fever, diarrhea, and abnormal respiratory function
Methadone	Fetal distress, meconium aspiration; with abrupt termination of the drug, severe withdrawal symptoms, preterm labor, rapid labor, abruption
Barbiturates	Withdrawal symptoms
Phenobarbital	Withdrawal symptoms Fetal growth restriction
"T's and Blues" (combination of the following)	
Talwin (narcotic)	Safe for use in pregnancy; depresses respiration if taken close to time of birth
Amytal (barbiturate)	See barbiturates
Tranquilizers	
Phenothiazine derivatives	Withdrawal, extrapyramidal dysfunction, delayed respiratory onset, hyperbilirubinemia, hypotonia or hyperactivity, decreased platelet count
Diazepam (Valium)	Hypotonia, hypothermia, low Apgar score, respiratory depression, poor sucking reflex, possible cleft lip
Antianxiety drugs	
Lithium	Congenital anomalies
Stimulants	
Amphetamines	
Amphetamine sulfate (Benzedrine)	Generalized arthritis, learning disabilities, poor motor coordination, transposition of the great vessels, cleft palate
Dextroamphetamine sulfate (Dexedrine)	Congenital heart defects, biliary atresia, limb reduction defects
Cocaine	Cerebral infarctions, microcephaly, learning disabilities, poor state organization, decreased interactive behavior, CNS anomalies, cardiac anomalies, genitourinary anomalies, sudden infant death syndrome (SIDS)
Nicotine (half to one pack cigarettes/day)	Increased rate of spontaneous abortion, increased incidence of placental abruption, SGA, small head circumference, decreased length, SIDS, attention-deficit/hyperactivity disorder, (ADHD) in school-age children
Psychotropics	
PCP ("angel dust")	Withdrawal symptoms Newborn behavioral and developmental abnormalities
LSD	Chromosomal breakage?
Marijuana	IUGR ?

substance abuse (Table 19–2 •). Because substance abuse has increased rapidly in the past decade, it is helpful to discuss the specific substances that are abused to increase understanding of this serious problem.

Substances Commonly Abused During Pregnancy

The substances most commonly abused during pregnancy are alcohol, cocaine/crack, marijuana, phencyclidine, MDMA (Ecstasy), and heroin. In this section, we also discuss the prescription drug methadone, which can have negative effects on pregnancy outcome.

ALCOHOL

Alcohol abuse has increased dramatically among women in the United States. The incidence is highest among women 20 to 40 years old; alcoholism is also seen in teenagers. An estimated 12% of pregnant women use alcohol in a given month. However, that number decreases significantly by trimester (see Figure 19–2 •). This figure is of concern because birth defects that are related to prenatal fetal exposure to alcohol can occur in the first 3 to 8 weeks' gestation, often before the woman even knows that she is pregnant (SAMHSA, 2002).

Chronic abuse of alcohol can undermine maternal health by causing malnutrition (especially folic acid and thiamine deficiencies), bone marrow suppression, increased incidence of infections, and liver disease. As a result of alcohol dependence, the woman may have withdrawal seizures in the intrapartal period as early as 12 to 48 hours after she stops drinking. Delirium tremens may occur in the postpartal period, and the newborn may suffer withdrawal syndrome.

The effects of alcohol on the fetus may result in a group of signs referred to as fetal alcohol syndrome (FAS). The syndrome has characteristic physical and mental abnormalities that vary in severity and combination. (See discussion in Chapter 32.) There is no definitive answer as to how much alcohol a woman can safely consume during pregnancy. Consequently, the expectant woman should "play it safe" by avoiding alcohol completely. Even low levels of alcohol cannot be recommended (Cunningham, MacDonald, Gant, et al, 2001).

The nursing staff in the maternal-newborn unit must be aware of the manifestations of alcohol abuse so that they can

Table 19-2 • POSSIBLE SIGNS OF SUBSTANCE ABUSE

History
- History of vague or unusual medical complaints
- Family history of alcoholism or other addiction
- History of childhood physical, sexual, or emotional abuse
- History of cirrhosis, pancreatitis, hepatitis, gastritis, sexually transmitted infections, or unusual infections such as cellulitis or endocarditis
- History of high-risk sexual behavior
- Psychiatric history of treatment and/or hospitalization

Physical Signs
- Dilated or constricted pupils
- Inflamed nasal mucosa
- Evidence of needle "track marks" or abscesses
- Poor nutritional status
- Slurred speech or staggering gait
- Odor of alcohol on breath

Behavioral Signs
- Memory lapses, mood swings, hallucinations
- Pattern of frequently missed appointments
- Frequent accidents, falls
- Signs of depression, agitation, euphoria
- Suicidal gestures

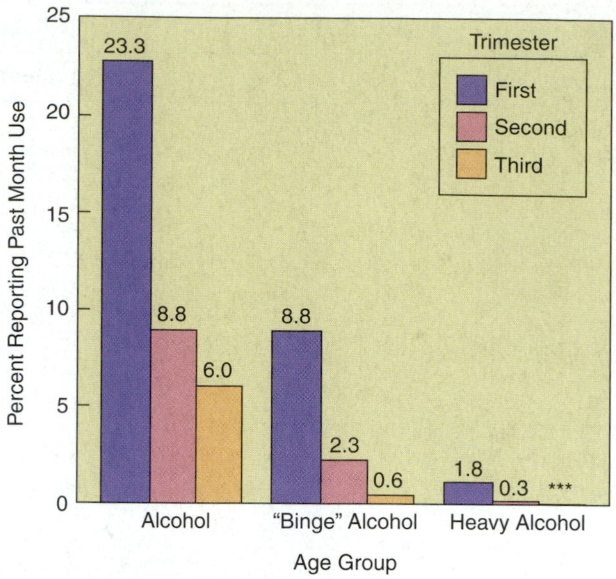

Figure 19-2 • Percentages of pregnant females ages 15 to 44 reporting past month alcohol use, by trimester, 1999 and 2000.
SOURCE: Substance Abuse and Mental Health Services Administration (SAMHSA). (2002). *The NHSDA Report: Substance use among pregnant women during 1999 and 2000.* Washington, DC: Author.

prepare for the client's special needs. The care regimen includes sedation to decrease irritability and tremors, seizure precautions, intravenous fluid therapy for hydration, and preparation for an addicted newborn. Although high doses of sedatives and analgesics may be necessary for the woman, caution is advised because these can cause fetal depression.

Breastfeeding generally is not contraindicated, although alcohol is excreted in breast milk. Excessive alcohol consumption may intoxicate the infant and inhibit maternal letdown reflex. Discharge planning for the alcohol-addicted mother and newborn should be correlated with the social service department of the hospital.

COCAINE/CRACK

Cocaine use appears to have reached its peak during the 1990s, but it continues to be of concern for the childbearing family (Bergin, Cameron, Fleitz, et al, 2001). Cocaine acts at the nerve terminals to prevent the reuptake of dopamine and norepinephrine, which in turn results in vasoconstriction, tachycardia, and hypertension. Placental vasoconstriction decreases blood flow to the fetus.

Cocaine is usually taken in three ways: snorting, smoking, and intravenous injection. **Crack** is a form of freebase cocaine that is made up of baking soda, water, and cocaine mixed into a paste and microwaved to form a rock. The rock can then be smoked. Many women, especially those in low-income areas, favor this form of the drug over other forms because it is cheaper and readily available. In addition, smoking crack leads to a quicker, more intense high because the drug is absorbed through the large surface area of the lungs.

The onset of effects of cocaine occurs rapidly, but the euphoria lasts only about 30 minutes. Irritability, depression, pessimism, fatigue, and a strong desire for more cocaine usually follow this profound euphoria and excitement. This pattern often leads the user to take repeated doses to sustain the effect. Cocaine metabolites may be present in the urine of a pregnant woman for up to 4 to 7 days following use.

The cocaine user is difficult to identify prenatally. Because cocaine is an illegal substance, many women are reluctant to volunteer information about their drug use. The nurse who is familiar with the woman may recognize subtle signs of cocaine use, including mood swings and appetite changes, and withdrawal symptoms such as depression, irritability, nausea, lack of motivation, and psychomotor changes.

Major adverse maternal effects of cocaine use include seizures and hallucinations, pulmonary edema, respiratory failure, and cardiac problems. Women who use cocaine have an increased incidence of spontaneous first trimester abortion, abruptio placentae, intrauterine growth restriction (IUGR), preterm birth, and stillbirth (March of Dimes, 2002).

Exposure of the fetus to cocaine in utero increases the risk of IUGR, small head circumference, cerebral infarctions, shorter body length, altered brain development, malformations of the genitourinary tract, and lower Apgar scores at birth. Newborns who were exposed to cocaine in utero may have neurobehavioral disturbances, marked irritability, an exaggerated startle reflex, labile emotions, and an increased risk of sudden infant death syndrome (SIDS). These newborns have poor interactive behaviors, have difficulty responding appropriately to voices, and fail to respond well to consoling behaviors. These complications may interfere with maternal-infant attachment and increase the infant's risk of abuse and neglect (Singer, Hawkins, Huang, et al, 2001).

Cocaine does cross into the breast milk and may cause such symptoms in the breastfeeding infant as extreme irritability, vomiting, diarrhea, dilated pupils, and apnea. Thus women who continue to use cocaine following childbirth should avoid breastfeeding.

MARIJUANA

Typically, pregnant women use marijuana in conjunction with alcohol and tobacco. Men who smoke marijuana may have decreased sperm counts and may develop gynecomastia (enlarged breasts); women may experience menstrual cycle irregularities. To date, however, there is no evidence that marijuana has any teratogenic effects on the fetus. The impact of heavy marijuana use on pregnancy is difficult to evaluate because of the variety of social factors that may influence the results.

Infants exposed to marijuana in utero have been reported to have increased fine tremors, prolonged startles, irritability, and poor habituation to visual stimuli, but these symptoms were not present in follow-up at 12 and 24 months of age (Cunningham et al, 2001).

PHENCYCLIDINE (PCP)

Phencyclidine (PCP) is a popular hallucinogen that can be smoked, taken orally, or injected intravenously. The onset of effects occurs in 2 to 4 minutes and lasts about 4 to 6 hours, with no withdrawal state. The drug causes confusion, delirium, and hallucinations and may produce feelings of euphoria. Signs of PCP use include constricted pupils, ataxia, nystagmus, double vision (diplopia), dizziness, and diaphoresis. The greatest risk for the pregnant woman is overdose or a psychotic response. Signs of overdose include hypertension, hyperthermia, diaphoresis, and possible coma, which may jeopardize fetal well-being.

PCP has been associated with neurobehavioral problems in the newborn but there are no good long-term studies that document this fact (Cunningham et al, 2001).

MDMA (ECSTASY)

MDMA (methylenedioxymethamphetamine), better known as Ecstasy, is the most commonly used of a group of drugs referred to as *club drugs*, so called because they have become popular among adolescents and young adults who frequent dance clubs and "raves." Other club drugs include flunitrazepam (Rohypnol), gamma hydroxybutyrate (GHB), and ketamine hydrochloride. PCPs and LSD are sometimes classified as club drugs as well.

MDMA is the third most widely used illicit drug after marijuana and amphetamines. Surveys reveal that 11.7% of high school seniors, 8% of sophomores, and 5.2% of eighth graders state that they have used MDMA at least once in their lives. Similarly 13.1% of individuals ages 18 to 25 report trying MDMA at least once (Office of National Drug Control Policy, 2002). It has been widely perceived as "safe" because of a relatively low incidence of adverse reactions. However, adverse responses are very unpredictable and the incidence is growing (Gowing, Henry-Edwards, Irvine, et al, 2002).

MDMA is taken by mouth usually in tablet form. Its effects last for about 4 to 6 hours. MDMA use is appealing because it produces euphoria and feelings of empathy for others (thus it is also called the "hug drug"). The most common significant side effects include hyperthermia (elevated body temperature) and hyponatremia (low blood sodium). Other side effects include hypertension and heart or kidney failure. Deaths have occurred among users. Repeated use of Ecstasy is associated with mood, sleep, and anxiety disorders, memory deficits, increased impulsiveness, and attention problems, which may last for up to 2 years following cessation of use. In addition, because MDMA may deplete levels of serotonin, users may increase their risk of neurologic and psychiatric problems (Montoya, Sorrentino, Lukas, et al, 2002).

Little is yet known about the effects of MDMA on pregnancy. Preliminary research using rats suggests that prenatal use of MDMA may be associated with long-term impaired memory and learning (Broening, Morford, Inman-Wood, et al, 2001). However, the impact of the timing of Ecstasy exposure during brain development may be a critical issue (Cockey, 2001).

HEROIN

Heroin is an illicit central nervous system (CNS) depressant narcotic that alters perception and produces euphoria. It is an addictive drug that is generally administered intravenously. Pregnancy in women who use heroin is considered high risk because of the associated increased incidence of poor nutrition, iron deficiency anemia, and preeclampsia-eclampsia (see Chapter 20). There is also an increased rate of breech position, abnormal placental implantation, abruptio placentae, preterm labor, premature rupture of the membranes (PROM), and meconium staining. Heroin users also have a higher incidence of sexually transmitted infection because many must rely on prostitution to support their drug habit. They also are at increased risk of HIV infection because they may use nonsterile needles or share needles when administering the drug.

The fetus of a heroin-addicted woman is at increased risk for IUGR and withdrawal symptoms after birth. The newborn frequently shows signs of heroin addiction, such as restlessness; lack of habituation; shrill, high-pitched cry; irritability; fist sucking; vomiting; and seizures. Signs of withdrawal usually appear within 72 hours and may last for several days. The newborn may exhibit poor consolability for 3 months or more. These behaviors may interfere with successful maternal-infant attachment and increase the potential for parenting problems or abuse in an already high-risk mother.

METHADONE

Methadone is the most commonly used drug in the treatment of women who are dependent on opioids such as heroin. Methadone blocks withdrawal symptoms and the craving for street drugs. Dosage should be individualized at the lowest possible therapeutic level. Methadone does cross the placenta and prenatal exposure has been associated with prematurity, rapid labor, abruptio placentae, decreased birth weight, and fetal distress (Wang, 1999). The newborn may experience withdrawal symptoms that are more severe than those associated with heroin.

Clinical Therapy

Antepartal care of the substance-abusing woman involves medical, socioeconomic, and legal considerations. The use of a team approach allows for the comprehensive management necessary to provide safe labor and childbirth for the woman and her fetus.

The management of drug addiction may include hospitalization as necessary to initiate detoxification. "Cold turkey" withdrawal is not advisable during pregnancy because of potential risk to the fetus. Maintenance and support therapy are best individualized to the woman's history and condition.

Urine screening may also be done regularly throughout pregnancy if the woman is known or suspected to be abusing drugs. This testing is helpful in identifying the type and amount of drug being abused and in providing objective feedback to the woman (McComish et al, 2000).

NURSING CARE MANAGEMENT

Nursing Assessment and Diagnosis

Nurses and other healthcare providers should make it a practice to screen all pregnant women for substance abuse. Because illicit drug users seldom use only one drug, it is necessary to complete a thorough drug and alcohol abuse history (American College of Obstetricians and Gynecologists [ACOG], 1999). Several simple screening tools are available. In addition, the nurse should be alert for clues in the history or appearance of the woman that suggest substance abuse (refer to Table 19–2). If abuse is suspected, the nurse needs to ask direct questions, beginning with less threatening questions about the use of tobacco, caffeine, and over-the-counter medications. The nurse can then progress to questions about alcohol consumption and finally to questions focusing on past and current use of illicit drugs. The nurse who is matter-of-fact and nonjudgmental in approach is more likely to elicit honest responses.

Nursing assessment of the woman who is known to abuse substances focuses on her general health status, with specific attention to nutritional status, susceptibility to infections, and evaluation of all body systems. The nurse also assesses the woman's understanding of the impact of substance abuse on herself and her pregnancy. Some women are reluctant to discuss their substance abuse; others are quite open about it. Once the nurse establishes a relationship of trust, the nurse can gain information to use in planning the woman's ongoing care.

Nursing diagnoses that may apply to the woman practicing substance abuse include the following:

- ***Altered Nutrition: Less than Body Requirements*** related to inadequate food intake secondary to substance abuse
- ***Risk for Infection*** related to use of inadequately cleaned syringes and needles secondary to IV drug use
- ***Risk for Altered Health Maintenance*** related to a lack of information about the impact of substance abuse on the fetus

Nursing Plan and Implementation

Preventing substance abuse during pregnancy is the ideal nursing goal and is best accomplished through education. Unfortunately, many women who abuse substances do not receive regular healthcare and may not seek care until far along in their pregnancy or at the onset of labor.

The nurse's role in providing prenatal care for the woman who is practicing substance abuse focuses on ongoing assessment and client teaching. Unfortunately, some maternal-newborn nurses have only limited knowledge about substance abuse and are negative and punitive rather than positive and supportive toward women who abuse substances during pregnancy. It is essential that nurses caring for childbearing families develop the knowledge and skill necessary to identify pregnant women who abuse substances. To provide care that is truly effective, it is equally important that nurses develop and maintain a nonjudgmental, nonpunitive, positive attitude when caring for these women.

When the nurse encounters a pregnant woman who screens positive for substance abuse, the nurse should review for the woman what the screen revealed and express concern for the health of the mother and infant. The nurse can then go on to state the belief that the mother is concerned about the baby's health and stress the need for the woman to stop using drugs or alcohol during pregnancy. The nurse can then discuss possible strategies to help the woman quit (addiction treatment programs, 12-step programs, individual counseling) and suggest a referral for more in-depth assessment by a specialist. If feasible, the nurse can make an appointment while the woman is in the office or clinic. Nurses should also be aware of treatment options available for women who lack financial resources. Finally the nurse should make a follow-up appointment to see the woman again after her drug or alcohol assessment. The knowledgeable nurse can provide information about the relationship between substance abuse and existing health problems and the implications for the woman's unborn child. By establishing a relationship of trust and support, the nurse may foster the woman's cooperation.

Preparation for labor and birth should be part of the prenatal planning. Fear, tension, or discomfort may be relieved through nonnarcotic psychologic support and careful explanation of the labor process. If pain medication is necessary, it should not be withheld, however, because the notion that it will contribute to further addiction is not correct. Preferred methods of pain relief include the use of psychoprophylaxis and regional or local anesthetics, such as pudendal block and local infiltration. These techniques decrease the risk of additional fetal respiratory depression. Immediate intensive care should be available for the newborn, who will probably have respiratory depression, be small for gestational age (SGA), and be premature. For care of the addicted newborn, see Chapter 32.

Evaluation

Expected outcomes of nursing care include the following:

- The woman is able to describe the impact of substance abuse on herself and her unborn child.
- The woman successfully gives birth to a healthy infant.
- The woman agrees to cooperate with referral to social services (or other appropriate community agency) for follow-up care after discharge.

Care of the Woman with Diabetes Mellitus

Diabetes mellitus, an endocrine disorder of carbohydrate metabolism, results from inadequate production or utilization of insulin.

Normal Glucose Homeostasis

After consumption of a meal, the body metabolizes carbohydrates into glucose. Insulin, produced by the beta cells of the islets of Langerhans in the pancreas, lowers blood glucose levels by enabling the glucose to move from the blood into muscle and liver cells, where it is stored as glycogen. When several hours have passed since a meal, falling blood glucose levels stimulate the pancreas to release glucagon, which in turn stimulates breakdown of liver glycogen stores into glucose, which is returned to the bloodstream. Glucagon can also stimulate the synthesis of glucose directly from amino acids in stored body proteins.

CRITICAL THINKING IN PRACTICE

Patti Chang, a 35-year-old G3P2, is a well-educated, active Chinese American woman with no history of glucose intolerance. Her two children were born healthy at 36 weeks' gestation. She receives the usual 50-g glucose tolerance test at 26 weeks' gestation, and her plasma level is 160 mg/dL. She seems irritated and frustrated when her obstetrician tells her that it would be best to perform a 3-hour fasting glucose tolerance test. After the physician leaves the room, Patti asks the nurse the following questions: "Will the glucose hurt my baby? What will the treatment be?" How will the nurse answer the questions? Why does Patti seem so upset?

Answers can be found in Appendix I.

Carbohydrate Metabolism in Normal Pregnancy

Carbohydrate metabolism is affected early in pregnancy by a rise in serum levels of estrogen, progesterone, and other hormones. These hormones stimulate maternal insulin production and increase tissue response to insulin; therefore, anabolism (building up) of glycogen stores in the liver and other tissues occurs.

In the second half of pregnancy, the woman demonstrates prolonged hyperglycemia and hyperinsulinemia (increased secretion of insulin) following a meal. Although the mother is producing more insulin, placental secretion of human placental lactogen (hPL) and prolactin (from the decidua), as well as elevated levels of cortisol (an adrenal hormone) and glycogen, cause increased maternal peripheral resistance to insulin. This resistance helps ensure that there is a sustained supply of glucose available for the fetus. This glucose is transported across the placenta to the fetus, who uses it as a major source of fuel. Maternal amino acids are also actively transported by the placenta from the mother to her fetus. These amino acids are used by the fetus for protein synthesis and as a source of energy. In addition to ensuring that glucose is available to the fetus, the increased maternal resistance to insulin also means that the pregnant woman has a lower peripheral uptake of glucose to meet her own needs. This results in a catabolic (destructive) state during fasting periods (eg, during the night and after meal absorption). Because increasing amounts of circulating maternal glucose are being diverted to the fetus, maternal fat is metabolized (lipolysis) during fasting periods much more readily than in a nonpregnant person. This process is called *accelerated starvation.* Ketones may be present in the urine as a result of lipolysis.

The delicate system of checks and balances that exists between glucose production and glucose use is stressed by the growing fetus, who derives energy from glucose taken from the mother and by maternal resistance to the insulin her body produces. This stress is referred to as the diabetogenic effect of pregnancy. Thus any preexisting disruption in carbohydrate metabolism is augmented by pregnancy, and any diabetic potential may precipitate gestational diabetes mellitus.

Pathophysiology of Diabetes Mellitus

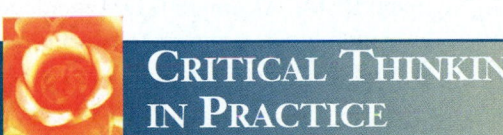

In diabetes mellitus, the pancreas does not produce sufficient amounts of insulin to allow necessary carbohydrate metabolism. With inadequate amounts of insulin, glucose cannot enter the cells but remains circulating in the blood. The body cells become energy depleted while the blood glucose level remains elevated. Fats and proteins in the body tissues are then oxidized by the cells as a source of energy. This results in wasting of fat and muscle tissue of the body, negative nitrogen balance due to protein breakdown, and ketosis due to fat metabolism. The strong osmotic force of the glucose concentration in the blood pulls water from the cells into the blood, which results in cellular dehydration. The high level of glucose in the blood eventually spills over into the urine, producing glycosuria. Osmotic pressure of the glucose in the urine prevents reabsorption of water into the kidney tubules, causing extracellular dehydration.

These pathologic developments cause the four cardinal signs and symptoms of diabetes mellitus: polyuria, polydipsia, weight loss, and polyphagia. *Polyuria* (frequent urination) results because water is not reabsorbed by the renal tubules because of the osmotic activity of glucose. *Polydipsia* (excessive thirst) is caused by dehydration from polyuria. *Weight loss* (seen in insulin-dependent diabetes, also called type 1 diabetes) is due to the use of fat and muscle tissue for energy. *Polyphagia* (excessive hunger) is caused by tissue loss and a state of starvation, which results from the inability of the cells to utilize the blood glucose. Diagnosis of diabetes is based on the presence of clinical symptoms and laboratory tests showing elevated glucose levels in the blood, glycosuria, and ketoacidosis.

Classification of Diabetes Mellitus

States of altered carbohydrate metabolism have been classified several different ways. Table 19–3 • shows the classification of diabetes mellitus based on its cause. This classification contains four main categories: type 1 diabetes, type 2 diabetes, other specific types, and gestational diabetes mellitus. Type 1 diabetes develops because of β-cell destruction and generally results in an absolute insulin deficiency. Type 2 diabetes, which is the most common form, results from a combination of an insulin secretory defect and insulin resistance (Caughron & Smith, 2002).

Table 19-3 • ETIOLOGIC CLASSIFICATION OF DIABETES MELLITUS

I. Type 1 diabetes* (β-cell destruction, usually leading to absolute insulin deficiency)
   A. Immune mediated
   B. Idiopathic
II. Type 2 diabetes* (may range from predominantly insulin resistance with relative insulin deficiency to a predominantly secretory defect with insulin resistance)
III. Other specific types†
IV. Gestational diabetes mellitus

*Patients with any form of diabetes may require insulin treatment at some stage of their disease. Such use of insulin does not classify the patient.

†The more detailed classification, which can be found in medical-surgical texts and the original source, provides eight subcategories of type.

Source: Adapted from the 1999 Report of the Expert Committee on the Diagnosis and Classification of Diabetes Mellitus, *Diabetes Care,* Suppl. 5.

Table 19-4 • WHITE'S CLASSIFICATION OF DIABETES IN PREGNANCY

Class	Criterion
A	Chemical diabetes
B	Maturity onset (age over 20 years), duration under 10 years, no vascular lesions
C_1	Age 10 to 19 years at onset
C_2	10 to 19 years' duration
D_1	Under 10 years at onset
D_2	Over 20 years' duration
D_3	Benign retinopathy
D_4	Calcified vessels of legs
D_5	Hypertension
E	No longer sought
F	Nephropathy
G	Many failures
H	Cardiopathy
R	Proliferating retinopathy
T	Renal transplant (added by Tagatz and colleagues of the University of Minnesota)

Source: White, P. (1978). Classification of obstetric diabetes. *American Journal of Obstetrics and Gynecology, 130,* 228. Used with permission.

Table 19–4 • shows White's classification of diabetes in pregnancy. This classification is useful for describing the extent of the disease.

Gestational diabetes mellitus GDM is defined as carbohydrate intolerance of variable severity with onset or first recognition during pregnancy. It results from (1) an unidentified preexistent disease, (2) the unmasking of a compensated metabolic abnormality by the added stress of pregnancy, or (3) a direct consequence of the altered maternal metabolism stemming from changing hormonal levels. When GDM is diagnosed, the goal of treatment is to decrease the likelihood of fetal macrosomia, shoulder dystocia, birth trauma, and cesarean birth (ACOG, 2001a). (See discussion in Fetal-Neonatal Risks.) Although GDM incidence rates vary, many of these individuals progress to overt type 2 diabetes mellitus with time (ACOG, 2001a).

Influence of Pregnancy on Diabetes

Pregnancy can affect diabetes significantly. First, the physiologic changes of pregnancy can drastically alter insulin requirements. Second, pregnancy may accelerate the progress of vascular disease secondary to diabetes.

The disease may be more difficult to control during pregnancy because insulin requirements are changeable. Insulin need frequently decreases early in the first trimester. Levels of hPL, an insulin antagonist, are low; energy demands of the embryo are minimal; and the woman may be consuming less food because of nausea and vomiting. Nausea and vomiting may also cause dietary fluctuations, which can increase the risk of hypoglycemia or insulin shock. Insulin requirements usually begin to rise late in the first trimester as glucose use and glycogen storage by the woman and fetus increase. As a result of placental maturation and production of hPL and other hormones, insulin requirements may double or quadruple by the end of pregnancy.

Increased energy needs during labor may require more insulin to balance intravenous glucose. After delivery of the placenta, insulin requirements usually decrease abruptly with loss of hPL in the maternal circulation.

Other factors contribute to the difficulty in controlling the disease. As pregnancy progresses, the renal threshold for glucose decreases. There is an increased risk of ketoacidosis, which may occur at lower serum glucose levels in the pregnant woman with diabetes than in the nonpregnant woman with diabetes. The vascular disease that accompanies diabetes may progress during pregnancy. Hypertension may occur. Nephropathy may result from renal blood vessel impairment, and retinopathy may develop (from occlusion of the microscopic blood vessels of the eye).

The primary concern for the pregnant woman who has diabetes is control of circulating blood glucose levels. If control can be achieved and maintained, diabetes generally does not worsen during pregnancy. The woman's health status may even improve because of close medical supervision.

Influence of Diabetes on Pregnancy Outcome

The pregnancy of a woman who has diabetes carries a higher risk of complications, especially perinatal mortality and congenital anomalies. The risk has been reduced by the recent recognition of the importance of tight metabolic control (blood glucose between 70 mg/dL and 120 mg/dL). New techniques for monitoring blood glucose, delivering insulin, and monitoring the fetus have also reduced perinatal mortality.

MATERNAL RISKS

Maternal health problems in diabetic pregnancy have been greatly reduced by the team approach to preconception planning and early prenatal care and by the increased emphasis on maintaining tight control of blood glucose levels. The prognosis for the pregnant woman with gestational, type 1, or type 2 diabetes that has not resulted in significant vascular damage is positive. However, diabetic pregnancy still carries higher risks for complications than normal pregnancy.

Hydramnios, or an increase in the volume of amniotic fluid, occurs in 10% to 20% of pregnant women with diabetes. It is thought to be a result of excessive fetal urination because of fetal hyperglycemia (Dashe, Nathan, McIntire, et al, 2000). *Preeclampsia-eclampsia* occurs more often in diabetic pregnancies, especially when diabetes-related vascular changes already exist.

Hyperglycemia due to insufficient amounts of insulin can lead to *ketoacidosis* as a result of the increase in ketone bodies (which are acidic) in the blood released when fatty acids are metabolized. Ketoacidosis usually develops slowly, but it may develop more rapidly in the pregnant woman because of the hyperketonemia associated with accelerated starvation in the fasting state. The tendency for higher postprandial glucose levels because of decreased gastric motility and the contrainsulin effects of hPL also predispose the woman to ketoacidosis. If the ketoacidosis is not treated, it can lead to coma and death of both mother and fetus.

Another risk to the pregnant woman with diabetes is a difficult labor (*dystocia*), caused by fetopelvic disproportion if fetal macrosomia exists. The pregnant woman with diabetes is also at increased risk for recurrent monilial vaginitis and urinary tract infections because of increased glycosuria, which contributes to a favorable environment for bacterial growth. If untreated, asymptomatic bacteriuria can lead to pyelonephritis, a serious kidney infection.

Several studies have demonstrated that pregnancy worsens *retinopathy* in women with diabetes. Most investigators agree that during diabetic pregnancy, good control of blood glucose levels and the use of laser photocoagulation (a treatment used to prevent retinal hemorrhage when the retina shows changes in the blood vessels) when indicated minimize the risk of the negative effects of pregnancy (Cunningham et al, 2001). Hence, women with preexisting diabetes should be referred to an ophthalmologist for evaluation during pregnancy.

FETAL-NEONATAL RISKS

Many of the problems of the newborn result directly from high maternal plasma glucose levels. In the presence of severe maternal ketoacidosis, the risk of fetal death increases to 50% (Spellacy, 1999). Fetal enzyme systems cease functioning in an acidic environment.

The incidence of *congenital anomalies* in diabetic pregnancies is 5% to 10% and is the major cause of death for infants of diabetic mothers. Research suggests that this increased incidence of congenital anomalies is related to multiple factors including high glucose levels in early pregnancy (Schaefer-Graf, Buchanan, Xiang, et al, 2000). The anomalies often involve the heart, central nervous system, and skeletal system. Septal defects, coarctation of the aorta, and transposition of the great vessels are the most common heart lesions seen. Central nervous system anomalies include hydrocephalus, meningomyelocele, and anencephaly. One anomaly, *sacral agenesis*, appears only in infants of diabetic mothers. In sacral agenesis, the sacrum and lumbar spine fail to develop and the lower extremities develop incompletely. To reduce the incidence of congenital anomalies, preconception counseling and strict diabetes control before conception and in the early weeks of pregnancy are indicated.

Characteristically, infants of diabetic mothers in White's classes A, B, and C (see Table 19–4) are large for gestational age (LGA) as a result of high levels of fetal insulin production stimulated by the high levels of glucose crossing the placenta from the mother. Sustained fetal hyperinsulinism and hyperglycemia ultimately lead to excessive growth, called **macrosomia,** and deposition of fat. If born vaginally, the macrosomic infant is at increased risk for birth trauma such as fractured clavicle or brachial plexus injuries due to shoulder dystocia. To prevent such injuries, cesarean birth may be indicated if birth weight is expected to exceed 4500 g (ACOG, 2001a).

After birth, the umbilical cord is severed, and thus the generous maternal blood glucose supply is eliminated. However, continued islet cell hyperactivity leads to excessive insulin levels and depleted blood glucose (hypoglycemia) in 2 to 4 hours. Macrosomia can be significantly reduced by tight maternal blood glucose control.

Infants of diabetic mothers with vascular involvement may demonstrate *intrauterine growth restriction (IUGR).* This occurs because vascular changes in the mother decrease the efficiency of placental perfusion, and the fetus is not as well sustained in utero.

Respiratory distress syndrome appears to result from inhibition, by high levels of fetal insulin, of some fetal enzymes necessary for surfactant production. Polycythemia in the newborn is due primarily to the diminished ability of glycosylated hemoglobin in the mother's blood to release oxygen. *Hyperbilirubinemia* is a result of the inability of immature liver enzymes to metabolize the increased bilirubin resulting from the polycythemia. Hypocalcemia, characterized by signs of irritability or even tetany, may occur. The cause of these low calcium levels in infants of diabetic mothers is not known.

MEDIALINK CASE STUDY: CLIENT WITH GESTATIONAL DIABETES

Clinical Therapy

DETECTION AND DIAGNOSIS OF GESTATIONAL DIABETES

Gestational diabetes is more common than pregestational diabetes. It is estimated to occur in 3% to 6% of pregnancies. Therefore, screening for its detection is a standard part of prenatal care. If diabetes is suspected, further testing is undertaken for diagnosis.

All pregnant women, regardless of risk factors, should be screened for diabetes toward the end of the second trimester (24 to 28 weeks) using a 1-hour, 50-g oral glucose tolerance test. Women with risk factors (age over 40; family history of diabetes in a first-degree relative; a prior macrosomic, malformed, or stillborn infant; obesity; hypertension; or glucosuria) should be screened earlier in pregnancy (ACOG, 2001a). The oral glucose load is administered without regard to time of day or time of last meal, and venous plasma glucose is measured 1 hour later. A plasma level that is equal to or greater than 130 to 140 mg/dL (depending on the lab used) indicates a need for further diagnostic testing.

During pregnancy, if the 1-hour oral glucose screen indicates that a woman might have gestational diabetes, diagnosis is made using a 3-hour, 100-g oral glucose tolerance test (OGTT). To do this test, the woman eats an unrestricted diet, consuming at least 150 g of carbohydrates per day for at least 3 days before her scheduled test. She then ingests 100-g oral glucose solution in the morning after an overnight fast. Plasma glucose is measured fasting and at 1, 2, and 3 hours. The woman should remain seated and not smoke throughout the test. Gestational diabetes is diagnosed if two or more of the following values are met or exceeded:

Fasting	95 mg/dL
1 hour	180 mg/dL
2 hour	155 mg/dL
3 hour	140 mg/dL

If only one value is elevated, many clinicians recommend exercise and nutrition counseling and then either repeat the 3-hour OGTT in 1 month or perform periodic glucose monitoring (ACOG, 2001a). In cases of borderline values and the presence of risk factors, some clinicians repeat the testing at 32 weeks' gestation.

LABORATORY ASSESSMENT OF LONG-TERM GLUCOSE CONTROL

Glycosylated hemoglobin (HbA_{1c}) is a laboratory test that loosely reflects glucose control over the previous 4 to 8 weeks. It measures the percentage of glycohemoglobin in the blood. Glycohemoglobin, or HbA_{1c}, is the hemoglobin to which a glucose molecule is attached. The test is not reliable for screening for gestational diabetes or for close daily control, but it is useful as an indicator of overall blood glucose control. Women with abnormal HbA_{1c} values greater than 10% are at most significant risk for having a fetus with malformations (Cunningham et al, 2001).

ANTEPARTAL MANAGEMENT OF DIABETES

The major goals of medical care for a pregnant woman with diabetes—whether gestational or pregestational—are (1) to maintain a physiologic equilibrium of insulin availability and glucose utilization during pregnancy and (2) to ensure an optimally healthy mother and newborn. To achieve these goals, good prenatal care using a team approach is a top priority. The team consists of an obstetrician, an endocrinologist, a perinatologist, a diabetes nurse-educator, a perinatal nurse, a nutritionist, a social worker, and, most important, the diabetic woman and her partner if he is involved in the pregnancy. Education of the couple and their active involvement in managing her care are essential for a good outcome.

For the woman with gestational diabetes, the diagnosis may be a shock, leaving her frightened and anxious (Langer & Langer, 2000). She needs clear explanation and teaching to enlist her participation in ensuring a good outcome. The diabetes nurse-educator plays a major role in this counseling.

Diet therapy and regular exercise form the cornerstone of intervention for GDM. Insulin therapy is indicated when dietary management is unable to achieve a 1-hour postprandial blood glucose value less than 130 to 140 mg/dL, a 2-hour postprandial level less than 120 mg/dL, or a fasting glucose less than 95 mg/dL. In most instances, the overt diabetic manifestation disappears postpartum, though subtle manifestations of impaired insulin secretory capacity may remain.

The woman with pregestational diabetes needs to understand changes she can expect during pregnancy; thus she should receive such teaching in preconception counseling. At the initial prenatal visit, height, weight, and vital signs are assessed along with a thorough assessment of thyroid and cardiac function. Thyroid function is assessed because there is a 5% to 10% incidence of hyper- or hypothyroidism in women with type 1 diabetes (Caughron & Smith, 2002). Special attention is given to dating the pregnancy. Laboratory data are obtained, and the diabetes is classified using White's criteria. Women should be screened for diabetic neuropathy, and a funduscopic examination is done to detect any retinopathy. In some cases, the woman may be referred to an ophthalmologist for further evaluation.

Dietary Regulation

The pregnant woman requires about 300 calories per day more than she does when she is not pregnant to meet increased metabolic demands. In general, women need approximately 30 kcal/kg of ideal body weight (IBW) during the first trimester and 35 to 36 kcal/kg IBW during the second and third trimesters. If ketonuria develops or the woman complains of hunger, the number of calories may be increased. Dietary guidelines are similar for women with gestational and pregestational diabetes. Approximately 40% to 50% of the calories should come from complex carbohydrates, 15% to 20% from protein, and 20% to 30% from fats (Curet, 2000).

This caloric intake is divided among three meals and three snacks. The prebedtime snack is the most important and must include both protein and complex carbohydrates to prevent hypoglycemia at night. Because it is so important that the pregnant woman follow these guidelines, a nutritionist works out meal plans based on the woman's lifestyle, culture, and food preferences and teaches her food exchanges so she can vary and plan her own meals. Cookbooks for people with diabetes are available and can be a great help.

Glucose Monitoring

Glucose monitoring is an essential part of diabetes management for determining the need for insulin and assessing glucose control. Many physicians have the woman come in for a weekly assessment of her fasting glucose levels and one or two postprandial levels. In addition, frequent self-monitoring of glucose levels is paramount in maintaining good glucose control. Self-monitoring is discussed on page 446.

Insulin Administration

Whether the woman with gestational diabetes needs additional insulin (over her own body production) depends on how well her blood glucose levels can be maintained by diet alone. Individuals with pregestational diabetes usually have type 1 diabetes, requiring insulin administration. Whether the client has gestational or pregestational diabetes, human insulin should be used because it is the least likely to cause an allergic response. If the woman has previously used bovine or porcine insulin, she may require smaller doses of human insulin to achieve the same pharmacologic effect. Insulin is given either in multiple injections or by continuous subcutaneous infusion. Multiple injections are used more commonly and with excellent results. Most women will need a mixture of intermediate and regular insulin. Some clinicians have moved away from the use of regular insulin, replacing it with a fast-acting human analog called lispro. Lispro is associated with better glucose control (Jovanovic, 2000). Often a four-dose approach is used, with regular insulin or lispro taken before each meal and NPH or Lente insulin added at bedtime (Curet, 2000). Other clinicians vary the NPH and regular insulin patterns slightly but still prefer a four-dose approach. It is important to remember that the amount of insulin needed usually increases during each trimester of pregnancy.

Oral hypoglycemics are never used during pregnancy because they cross the placenta, may be teratogenic, and stimulate fetal insulin production (ACOG, 2001a).

Evaluation of Fetal Status

Information about the well-being, maturation, and size of the fetus is important for planning the course of the pregnancy and the timing of birth. Because pregnancies complicated by diabetes are at increased risk of neural tube defects, maternal serum *α-fetoprotein (AFP)* screening is offered at weeks 16 to 20 of gestation (see Chapter 21).

Daily maternal evaluation of *fetal activity*, begun at about 28 weeks, is effective and simple to do. The woman is taught a particular method for counting fetal movements (see Chapter 16). She records the results on a special card, and brings the card to each subsequent office visit.

Nonstress testing (NST) is usually begun weekly at about 28 weeks. If evidence of IUGR, preeclampsia, oligohydramnios, or poorly controlled blood glucose exists, testing may begin as early as 26 weeks and may be done more often. NSTs are increased to twice weekly at 32 weeks' gestation. If the NST is nonreactive, a fetal biophysical profile or *contraction stress test* is performed (ACOG, 2001a). If the woman requires hospitalization (for example, to control glycemia or for complications), NSTs may be done daily.

Ultrasound at 18 weeks establishes gestational age and diagnoses multiple pregnancy or congenital anomalies. It is repeated at 28 weeks to monitor fetal growth for IUGR or macrosomia. Some physicians order *fetal biophysical profiles* (ultrasound evaluation of fetal well-being in which fetal breathing movements, fetal activity, reactivity, muscle tone, and amniotic fluid volume are assessed) as part of an ongoing evaluation of fetal status.

INTRAPARTAL MANAGEMENT OF DIABETES MELLITUS

During the intrapartal period, medical therapy includes the following:

- *Timing of birth.* Most diabetic pregnancies are allowed to go to term, with spontaneous labor, thereby decreasing the risk of respiratory distress in the newborn. Some clinicians do opt to induce labor in a woman at term to avoid problems related to an aging placenta. Cesarean birth may be indicated if evidence of fetal distress exists. Birth before term may be indicated for diabetic women with vascular changes and worsening hypertension or if evidence of IUGR exists (Landon, 2000). In pregnancies in which there is evidence of fetal macrosomia, fetal compromise, or elevated maternal HbA_{1c}, amniocentesis is done for lecithin/sphingomyelin (L/S) ratio and the presence of phosphatidylglycerol (PG). Whereas levels of 2:1 for the L/S ratio indicate fetal lung maturity in the nondiabetic pregnancy, levels of up to 3.5:1 L/S ratio have been found necessary at some centers before low risk of respiratory distress syndrome (RDS) is achieved. The presence of phosphatidylglycerol seems to enhance lecithin activity, and its presence is considered favorable for lung maturity. Fetal lung maturity must be weighed against other considerations when deciding time of childbirth. If preterm labor occurs, tocolytic therapy (use of medications in an attempt to halt preterm labor) (Chapter 20 ∞) and β-sympathomimetic drugs should not be administered because they may worsen maternal glucose control (Cunningham et al, 2001).
- *Labor management.* The degree of prenatal maintenance of normal maternal glucose levels (euglycemia) and the maintenance of maternal euglycemia during labor are important in preventing neonatal hypoglycemia. Maternal insulin requirements often decrease dramatically during labor. Consequently, maternal glucose levels are measured hourly to determine insulin need. (See Figure 19–3 •.) The primary goal in controlling maternal glucose levels intrapartally is to prevent neonatal hypoglycemia (Curet, 2000). In some cases, no insulin is necessary. Long-acting insulin should be reduced or stopped and regular insulin should be used to meet most or all of the woman's identified needs. Often two intravenous lines are used, one with a 5% dextrose solution and one with a saline solution. The saline solution is then available if a bolus is needed or for piggybacking insulin. Insulin clings to the plastic intravenous bag and tubing. To ensure that the woman receives the desired dose, the intravenous tubing must be flushed with insulin before the prescribed amount is added. During the second stage of labor and the immediate postpartum period, the woman may not need additional insulin. The intravenous insulin is discontinued with the completion of the third stage of labor.

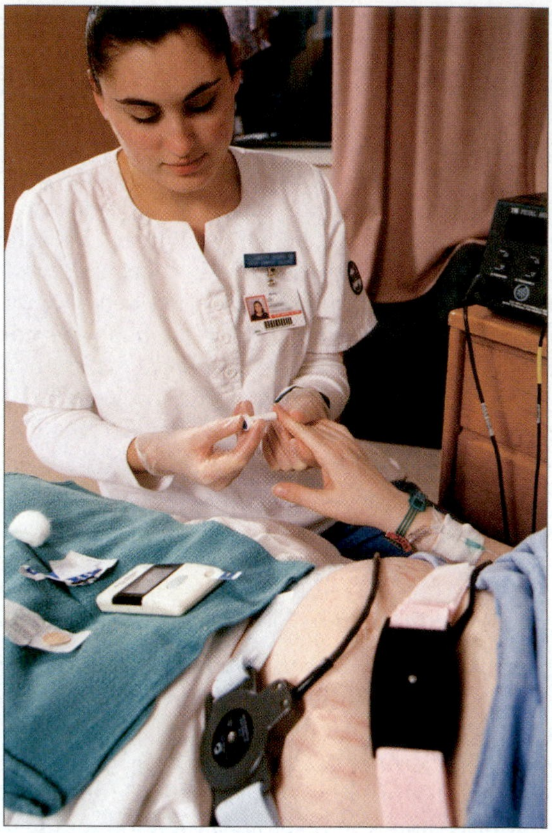

Figure 19–3 • During labor the nurse closely monitors the blood glucose levels of the woman with diabetes mellitus.

POSTPARTAL MANAGEMENT OF DIABETES MELLITUS

Maternal insulin requirements fall significantly postpartally because the levels of hPL, progesterone, and estrogen fall after placental separation, and their anti-insulin effect ceases, resulting in decreased blood glucose levels. The diabetic mother may require no insulin for the first 24 hours or only one fourth to one half her previous dose. Then, reestablishment of insulin needs based on blood glucose testing is necessary. Diet and exercise levels must also be redetermined. Consequently, the woman with diabetes that is not controlled by diet alone may need insulin for a time (Kjos, 2000).

Women with GDM who did not require insulin during pregnancy generally do not need it during the postpartum period. Clinicians routinely discontinue insulin for women with GDM following childbirth and then monitor blood glucose levels. If elevated glucose levels develop, oral antihyperglycemic agents may be tried if the woman is not breastfeeding (Curet, 2000). Antihyperglycemics are contraindicated during breastfeeding. The woman should be reassessed 6 weeks postpartum to determine whether her glucose levels are normal. If her levels are normal, she should be reassessed at a minimum of 3-year intervals (American Diabetes Association, 2000).

Diabetic control and the establishment of parent-child relationships in light of neonatal needs are the priorities of this period. If her newborn must be cared for in a special care nursery, the mother needs support and information about the baby's condition. Every effort must be made to provide as much contact as possible between the parents and their newborn.

Breastfeeding is encouraged as beneficial to both mother and baby. The composition of breast milk is not altered by diabetes, and infants of mothers with diabetes gain weight appropriately. The lactating mother with diabetes often has a sense of well-being and diminished insulin needs even while increasing caloric intake. Blood glucose levels may be lower because glucose is transferred from serum to breast to be converted to lactose, and energy is expended in milk production. Caloric needs increase during lactation to 500 to 800 kcal above prepregnant requirements. Insulin must be adjusted according to individual needs. Home blood glucose monitoring should continue for the insulin-dependent diabetic.

The woman and her partner, if he is involved, should receive information on family planning. Barrier methods of contraception (diaphragm and condom) used with spermicide are safe, effective, and inexpensive and are the method of choice for insulin-dependent diabetic women. The use of combined oral contraceptives (COCs) by women with diabetes is controversial. Some evidence suggests that women with diabetes may be at greater risk for COC complications such as myocardial infarction and thrombophlebitis. Many physicians who prescribe low-dose COCs to women with diabetes restrict them to women who have no vascular disease and who do not smoke. The progesterone-only pill may also be used as may Depo-Provera. Many couples who have completed their families choose elective sterilization.

> *It's hard to realize that I have gestational diabetes and to know that it increases my chances of getting diabetes later. My grandmother had diabetes, so I always thought of it as an old person's disease. All the finger sticks, watching my diet, and keeping track has taken some getting used to. I'll be glad when our baby is born and I can put this behind me, at least for now.*

NURSING CARE MANAGEMENT

The Clinical Pathway on page 444 for a woman with diabetes mellitus summarizes nursing management during the antepartum, intrapartum, and postpartum periods.

Nursing Assessment and Diagnosis

Whether diabetes has been diagnosed before pregnancy occurs or the diagnosis is made during pregnancy (GDM), careful assessment of the disease process and the woman's understanding of diabetes is important. Thorough physical examination, including assessment for vascular complications, any signs of infectious conditions, and urine and blood testing for glucose, is essential at the first prenatal visit. Follow-up visits are usually scheduled twice a month during the first two trimesters and weekly during the last trimester.

Assessment also yields vital information about the woman's ability to cope with the combined stress of pregnancy and diabetes and her ability to follow a recommended regimen of care. It is necessary to determine the woman's knowledge about diabetes and self-care before formulating a teaching plan.

Nursing diagnoses that may apply to the pregnant woman with diabetes mellitus include the following:

- ***Risk for Altered Nutrition: More than Body Requirements*** related to imbalance between intake and available insulin
- ***Risk for Injury*** related to possible complications secondary to hypoglycemia or hyperglycemia
- ***Altered Family Processes*** related to the need for hospitalization secondary to GDM.

Nursing Plan and Implementation

Prepregnancy counseling may be provided by a nurse and a physician, using a team approach. Ideally, the couple is seen prior to pregnancy so that the diabetes can be assessed by ophthalmologic evaluation, electrocardiographic study, and a 24-hour urine collection for creatinine clearance and protein excretion. Prepregnancy counseling about the importance of tight glucose control is cost-effective in preventing congenital anomalies. If the diabetes is of recent onset without vascular complications, the outcome of pregnancy should be good, provided that glucose levels are controlled.

Community-Based Nursing Care

In many cases, women with GDM are stabilized in the hospital, and necessary teaching for self-care is begun. Women with preexisting diabetes may also require hospitalization for stabilization of their diabetes. In either case, the majority of ongoing teaching and supervision of pregnant women with diabetes is then carried out by nurses in clinics, community agencies, and the women's homes.

Effective Insulin Use

The nurse ensures that the couple understands the purpose of the insulin, the types of insulin the woman is to use, the number of doses she is to receive daily, and the correct procedure for its administration. The woman's partner is also instructed about insulin administration in case it should be necessary for him to give it. For some highly motivated women whose glucose levels are not well controlled with multiple injections, the continuous insulin infusion pump may improve glucose control.

CLINICAL PATHWAY FOR A WOMAN WITH DIABETES MELLITUS

Category	Antepartal Management	Intrapartal Management*	Postpartal Management*
Referral	• Perinatologist • Endocrinologist • Neonatologist • Social worker • Psych clinical nurse practitioner • Diabetes nurse educator • Dietary/nutritionist • Physical therapy, occupational therapy	• Obtain prenatal record	• Home nursing referral if indicated • Diabetes nurse educator **➤ Expected Outcomes** Appropriate resources identified and utilized
Assessment	• Electronic fetal monitoring as indicated • Nonstress test as indicated • Ultrasound as indicated • Amniocentesis for lung maturity at 34–36 weeks • α-fetoprotein (done usually at 18–20 weeks)	• Assess for signs and symptoms (s/sx) of hypoglycemia (sweating, periodic tingling, disorientation, shakiness, pallor, clammy skin, irritability, hunger, headache, and blurred vision) during labor • Continuous electronic fetal monitoring • Assess glucose levels with glucometer as ordered or if s/sx of hypoglycemia occur	• Assess glucose levels with glucometer—generally insulin requirements fall significantly in the postpartum phase • Continue normal postpartum assessment q8h • Feeding technique with newborn: should be progressing • Vital signs assessment: q8h; all WNL; report temperature > 38C (100.4F) • Continue assessment of comfort level **➤ Expected Outcomes** Assessment findings indicate control of blood sugar levels with related complications minimized. Fetal growth and development unimpaired
Teaching/ psychosocial	• Room orientation • Notify RN of s/sx of hyper/hypoglycemia, uterine contractions, decreased fetal movement, vaginal leaking and/or bleeding, dysuria • Assess family status and/or additional psychosocial needs • Evaluation of client learning needs • Importance of following diet • Tour of ICN • Prebirth teaching for vaginal and/or cesarean (CS) • Evaluation of teaching effectiveness	• Evaluation of teaching effectiveness • Continuing evaluation of ongoing learning needs	• Complete normal postpartum teaching **➤ Expected Outcomes** Client verbalizes/demonstrates understanding of diabetic and healthcare education
Nursing care management and reports	• CBC • UA/dipstick for protein and ketones • Biochemistry profile • Glycosylated hemoglobin level (Hb_{A1C}) daily • 24-hour urine for protein and creatinine clearance • Finger stick blood sugar (BS), every AM, before meals, and 2 hours after meals • Vital signs q4h • Fundal height weekly • Daily weight	• Glucose levels monitored as directed	• Continue sitz bath prn • May shower if ambulating without difficulty • DC buffalo cap if present **➤ Expected Outcomes** Labs/reports reflect stable, controlled blood sugar Maternal/fetal well-being maintained Active involvement of client in plan of care for diabetic management
Activity	• Bed rest with bathroom privileges • Diversional activity	• Bed rest as tolerated	• Up ad lib **➤ Expected Outcomes** Level of activity has not exacerbated condition
Comfort	• Assess for discomfort • Provide comfort measures as needed	• Assess for discomfort • Provide comfort measures as needed	• Continue with pain management techniques **➤ Expected Outcomes** Optimal comfort maintained

*Interventions for a woman with a normal labor and birth and during the early postpartum period may be found in those appropriate clinical pathways.

CLINICAL PATHWAY FOR A WOMAN WITH DIABETES MELLITUS *CONTINUED*

Category	Antepartal Management	Intrapartal Management*	Postpartal Management*
Nutrition	• American Dietetic Association (ADA) per order • Encourage fluids	• Ice chips Hard candy, prn	• Encourage breastfeeding • Increase calorie needs 500–800 kcal • Continue diet and fluids ➤ **Expected Outcomes** Nutritional needs met, with emphasis on diabetic control
Elimination	• Review measures to prevent UTI	➤ **Expected Outcomes** Monitor and record intake and output	➤ **Expected Outcomes** Intake and output WNL
Medications	• IV ____ @ ____ mL/h/heparin lock • Insulin as ordered →__________ • Prenatal vitamins and iron	• Two IV lines are usually used, one with 5% dextrose solution and one with a saline solution (saline line is used for insulin if needed) • The IV insulin is usually discontinued with completion of 3rd stage of labor	• May take own prenatal vitamins • Rh immune globulin and rubella vaccine administered if indicated ➤ **Expected Outcomes** BS levels within acceptable medical parameters
Discharge planning/ home care	• Explain purpose of scheduled tests and procedures • Include family in diabetic teaching • Assess family support	• Assess family support	• Review discharge instruction sheet and check list • Describe postpartum warning signs and when to call CNM/physician • Provide prescriptions • Gift pack given to woman • Arrangements made for baby pictures if desired • Postpartum visit scheduled • Newborn check scheduled ➤ **Expected Outcomes** Discharge teaching completed with emphasis on follow-up healthcare needs and adequate support network
Family involvement	• Identify available support persons • Assess family perceptions of situation	• Involve support persons in care	• Evidence of parental bonding behaviors apparent • Involve support persons in care: teaching • Plans being made for providing support to mother following discharge ➤ **Expected Outcomes** Family utilizes resources
Date			

*Interventions for a woman with a normal labor and birth and during the early postpartum period may be found in those appropriate clinical pathways.

Note: BS, blood sugar; heparin lock, intravenous catheter that allows intermittent access; CBC=complete blood count, ICN, intensive care nursery; IV, intravenous; PRN, as needed or as desired; q8h - every 8 hours; Q4h every 4 hours; RN registered nurse; s/sx, signs/symptoms; UA, urinalysis UTI, urinary tract infection, WNL, within normal limits.

The nurse teaches the client how and when to monitor her blood sugar, the desired range of blood sugar levels, and the importance of good control (Figure 19–4 •). Most women use a glucose meter because it provides a more accurate reading. The nurse teaches the client to follow the manufacturer's directions exactly, to wash hands thoroughly before puncturing her finger, and to touch the blood droplet, not her finger, to the test pad on the strip.

With a blood glucose meter, an electronic eye measures the blood sugar, and a digital reading is given. The blood droplet should cover the test pad because uncovered portions

Clinical Tip *When teaching a pregnant woman to do her own blood glucose testing, have gloves available and put them on if it becomes necessary to help the woman obtain a blood sample. The woman does not need to wear gloves during the procedure.*

Also be sure to wear gloves when doing finger sticks for blood glucose levels, when testing the urine for ketones, when starting an IV for insulin therapy, or when drawing blood for other laboratory tests.

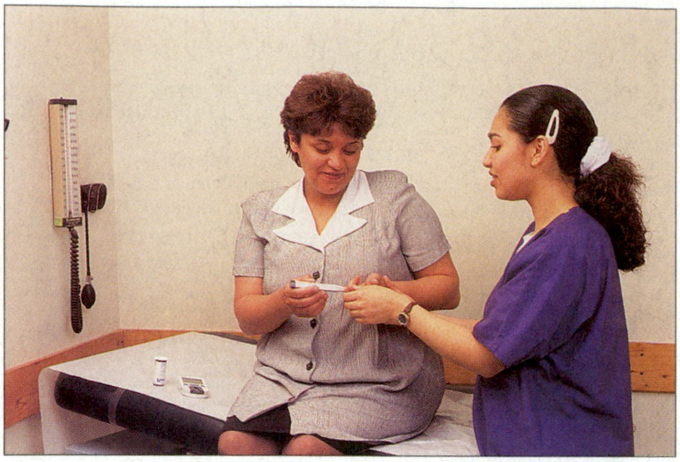

Figure 19–4 • The nurse teaches the pregnant woman with gestational diabetes mellitus how to do home glucose monitoring.

MEDIALINK CARE PLAN: ANTEPARTAL CLIENT AT RISK

are read as low sugar. The glucose meter is a portable pocket-sized device that is more accurate than the visual, color comparison method. Some meters are able to store and recall a specified number of readings, which helps ensure the accuracy of recorded results.

The nurse may offer the client the following tips regarding finger puncture:

- Various spring-loaded devices are available that make puncturing easier.
- Hanging the arm down for 30 seconds increases blood flow to the fingers.
- Warming the hands under running water increases blood flow to them.
- The sides of fingers should be punctured instead of the ends because the ends contain more pain-sensitive nerves.

Clients with diabetes need to keep a record of each blood sugar reading as a guide for management. Specific record sheets are available for this purpose and should be brought to each visit.

Planned Exercise Program

Exercise is encouraged for the woman's overall well-being. If she is used to a regular exercise program, she is encouraged to continue. She is advised to exercise after meals (when blood sugar levels are high), to wear diabetic identification, to carry a simple sugar such as hard candy (because of the possibility of exercise-induced hypoglycemia), to monitor her blood glucose levels regularly, and to avoid injecting insulin into an extremity that will soon be used during exercise.

If she has not been following a regular exercise plan, she is encouraged to begin gradually. Because exercise can alter metabolism, the woman's blood glucose should be well controlled before she begins an exercise program. Women with GDM should not use unusual, strenuous, and excessive exercise in an attempt to reduce glucose levels (ACOG, 2001a).

Teaching for Self-Care

Using the information gained during the nursing assessment of the pregnant woman with diabetes, the nurse provides appropriate teaching to the woman and her family so that the woman can meet her own healthcare needs as much as possible.

- *Glucose monitoring.* Home blood glucose monitoring is the most accurate and convenient way to determine insulin dose and assess control. It should be taught at the first visit after the diagnosis of gestational diabetes has been established. The woman with pregestational diabetes may already be monitoring her own blood sugar. Women are taught to perform the procedure four to six times per day—generally at least a fasting blood sugar before breakfast, then a postprandial test 2 hours after each meal. Women are encouraged to maintain blood sugars in the normal ranges as follows: fasting (before eating or taking insulin), 70 to 100 mg/dL; 2 hours after each meal, less than 120 mg/dL (ADA, 2000b). New technology that is capable of automatically and painlessly monitoring blood glucose levels is currently being investigated and shows great promise.
- *Symptoms of abnormal blood glucose levels.* The pregnant diabetic woman must recognize symptoms of changing glucose levels—whether hypoglycemia or hyperglycemia accompanied by ketoacidosis—and take appropriate action by immediately checking her capillary blood glucose level. Hypoglycemia may develop fairly rapidly. Symptoms include sweating, periodic tingling, disorientation, shakiness, pallor, clammy skin, irritability, hunger, headache, and blurred vision. If the pregnant woman is hypoglycemic with a blood glucose level less than 65-70 mg/dL, she is advised to take 20 g of carbohydrate, wait 20 minutes, and then retest her glucose level. She can obtain the necessary carbohydrate by drinking 1 cup of skim milk, ½ cup orange or apple juice, or ½ cup cola or by eating 1 tbsp honey or brown sugar (Cleveland Clinic, 2003). Many people overtreat their symptoms by continuing to eat. This can cause a rebound hyperglycemia. The woman should carry a snack at all times and should have other fast sources of glucose (simple carbohydrates such as hard candy) at hand so that she can treat an insulin reaction when milk is not available. Family members are also taught how to inject glucagon in the event that food does not work or is not feasible, for instance, in the presence of severe morning sickness.

Hyperglycemia and ketoacidosis typically develop more slowly and tend to occur more commonly during the second half of pregnancy. Because most problems for the fetus are related to maternal hyperglycemia, this is a serious situation. Symptoms include polyuria, polydipsia,

dry mouth, fatigue, nausea, hot flushed skin, rapid deep breathing, abdominal cramps, acetone breath, headache, drowsiness, depressed reflexes, oliguria or anuria, stupor, or coma. Hyperglycemia is treated with insulin.
- *Smoking.* Smoking has harmful effects on the maternal vascular system and the developing fetus and is contraindicated for both pregnancy and diabetes.
- *Travel.* Insulin can be kept at room temperature while traveling. Insulin supplies should be kept with the traveler and not packed in the baggage. Most airlines can supply special meals if notified a few days before departure. The woman should wear a diabetic identification bracelet or necklace. In addition, the woman should check with her physician for any instructions or advice before leaving.
- *Support groups.* Many communities have diabetes support groups or education classes, which can be helpful to women with newly diagnosed diabetes.
- *Cesarean birth.* Chances for a cesarean birth increase if the pregnant woman is diabetic because of the risk of fetal macrosomia and shoulder dystocia. This possibility should be anticipated—enrollment in cesarean birth preparation classes may be suggested. Many hospitals offer classes, and information is available through other organizations. The couple may prefer simply to discuss cesarean birth with the nurse and their obstetrician and read some books on the topic.

Hospital-Based Nursing Care

Hospitalization may become necessary during the pregnancy to evaluate blood glucose levels and adjust insulin dosages. In such cases, nurses monitor the woman's status and continue to provide teaching so that the woman is knowledgeable about her condition and its management. During the intrapartal period, the nurse must have a clear understanding about the impact of labor on the condition. The nurse carefully monitors the woman's status, maintains her intravenous fluids, is alert for signs of hypoglycemia, and provides the care indicated for any woman in labor. If a cesarean birth is indicated, the nurse provides appropriate care as described in Chapter 27.

Evaluation

Expected outcomes of nursing care include the following:

- The woman is able to discuss her condition and its possible impact on her pregnancy, labor and birth, and postpartal period.
- The woman participates in developing a healthcare regimen to meet her needs and follows it throughout her pregnancy.
- The woman avoids developing hypoglycemia or hyperglycemia.
- The woman gives birth to a healthy newborn.
- The woman is able to care for her newborn.

Care of the Woman with Anemia

Anemia indicates inadequate levels of hemoglobin (Hb) in the blood. *Anemia* is defined as hemoglobin less than 12 g/dL in nonpregnant women and less than 10 g/dL in pregnant and postpartum women (Cunningham et al, 2001). Race, altitude, smoking, and medications can affect the normal limits of hemoglobin. The lower limit of normal tends to be higher for women who smoke and those who live at higher altitudes because their bodies require a greater quantity of red blood cells to maintain their tissue oxygen levels. For example, a pregnant woman who lives in Denver, Colorado (elevation 5280 feet), would be considered anemic if her hemoglobin dropped below 10.5 g/dL. Similarly, the lower limit of normal for a pregnant woman who smokes ½ to 1 pack of cigarettes per day would increase by 0.3 g/dL to 10.3 g/dL (Varney, 1997). Reference tables are available that indicate these adjustments in the lower level of normal hemoglobin.

The common anemias of pregnancy are due either to insufficient hemoglobin production related to nutritional deficiency in iron or folic acid during pregnancy, or to hemoglobin destruction in inherited disorders, specifically sickle cell anemia and thalassemia.

Iron Deficiency Anemia

Dietary iron is needed to synthesize hemoglobin. Because hemoglobin is necessary to transport oxygen, a deficiency of iron may affect the body's transport of oxygen.

Iron deficiency anemia is the most common medical complication of pregnancy, primarily as a consequence of expansion of plasma volume without normal expansion of maternal hemoglobin mass (Cunningham et al, 2001). Approximately 200 mg of iron will be conserved due to the functional amenorrhea of pregnancy, but a pregnant woman needs approximately 1000 mg more iron intake during the pregnancy. Between 300 and 400 mg of iron is transferred to the fetus; 500 mg is needed for the increased red blood cell mass in the woman's own increased circulating blood volume; another 100 mg is needed for the placenta; and about 280 mg is needed to replace the 1 mg of iron lost daily through feces, urine, and sweat.

The greatest need for increased iron intake occurs in the second half of pregnancy. When the iron needs of pregnancy are not met, maternal hemoglobin falls below 11 g/dL. Serum ferritin levels, indicating iron stores, are below 12 mg/L.

Many women begin pregnancy in a slightly anemic state. In pregnancy, mild anemia can rapidly become more severe; therefore, it needs immediate treatment.

MATERNAL RISKS

The woman with iron deficiency anemia may be asymptomatic, but she is more susceptible to infection, may tire easily, has an increased chance of preeclampsia and postpartal hemorrhage, and tolerates poorly even minimal blood loss during birth. Healing of an episiotomy or an incision may be delayed. If the anemia is severe (Hb less than 6 g/dL), cardiac failure may ensue.

FETAL-NEONATAL RISKS

There is evidence of increased risk of low birth weight, prematurity, stillbirth, and neonatal death in infants of women with severe iron deficiency (maternal Hb less than 6 g/dL). The infant is not iron deficient at birth due to active transport of iron across the placenta, even when maternal iron stores are low. However, these babies do have lower iron stores and are at increased risk for developing iron deficiency during infancy.

CLINICAL THERAPY

The first goal of healthcare is to prevent iron deficiency anemia. If it occurs, the goal is to return low iron and hemoglobin levels to normal. To prevent anemia, the Centers for Disease Control and Prevention (CDC, 1998) recommends starting low-dose (30 mg/day) supplements of iron at the first prenatal visit. In addition, the woman should be encouraged to eat an iron-rich diet. To prevent constipation, the most common side effect of iron supplementation, a stool softener may be necessary.

If anemia is diagnosed, the dosage should be increased to 60 to 120 mg per day of iron. If the woman remains anemic after one month of therapy, further evaluation is indicated. With a twin pregnancy, a larger dose is needed. If a large dose of oral iron causes vomiting, diarrhea, or constipation, or if the anemia is discovered late in pregnancy, parenteral iron may be needed.

Complementary and Alternative Therapies

Stinging Nettle to Prevent Anemia

Stinging nettle *(Urtica dioica)* is sometimes recommended to pregnant women at risk for iron deficiency anemia who have difficulty consuming adequate amounts of iron. Nettles are a good source of iron and also contain high levels of calcium, magnesium, potassium, phosphorus, vitamin C, beta-carotene, and B-complex vitamins. Because of the high levels of vitamin C found in the plant, its use helps facilitate the absorption of iron in the gastrointestinal tract. Stinging nettle can be consumed fresh as a cooked green leafy vegetable or added to soups. However, it is more commonly prepared as a tea. The tea is prepared by placing 2 teaspoons of dried or fresh stinging nettle in a cup and adding boiling water. The mixture is allowed to steep for several minutes. Cinnamon and honey may be added to improve the taste. The woman is advised to drink 1 to 2 cups per day.

Source: Brill, S. (1994). *Identifying and harvesting edible and medicinal plants in wild (and not so wild) places.* New York: William Morrow.

NURSING CARE MANAGEMENT

Nursing Assessment and Diagnosis

The main presenting symptom of iron deficiency anemia may be fatigue. Nutritional history usually gives evidence of poor dietary intake of iron. Physical examination reveals pallor of skin and conjunctiva. Laboratory studies show hemoglobin values below 10 g/dL, serum ferritin levels below 12 mg/L, and possibly microcytic and hypochromic red blood cells (a late finding).

Nursing diagnoses that may apply to a pregnant woman with iron deficiency anemia include the following:

- ***Altered Nutrition: Less than Body Requirements*** related to inadequate intake of iron-containing foods
- ***Constipation*** related to daily intake of iron supplements

Nursing Plan and Implementation

The nurse stresses the importance of an iron-rich diet and of iron supplements during pregnancy. Supplements are indicated because dietary sources cannot meet the extra requirements. The woman is taught to take iron tablets with vitamin C (eg, orange juice) to increase absorption. Iron absorption is reduced by 40% to 50% if the tablets are taken with meals. However, gastrointestinal upset is more likely if they are taken on an empty stomach. The client may tolerate the iron better if she starts with small doses and gradually increases the dosage over several days. She is informed that her stool will turn black and may be more formed. She is also advised to keep the tablets out of the reach of children because ingestion may be fatal to a young child.

Evaluation

Expected outcomes of nursing care include the following:

- The woman is able to identify the risks associated with iron deficiency anemia during pregnancy.
- The woman takes her iron supplements as recommended.
- The woman's hemoglobin levels remain normal or return to normal during her pregnancy.

Folic Acid Deficiency Anemia

Folate deficiency is the most common cause of megaloblastic anemia during pregnancy, affecting between 1% and 4% of pregnant women in the United States. It is more prevalent with twin pregnancies.

Folic acid is needed for DNA and RNA synthesis and cell duplication. In its absence, immature red blood cells fail to divide, become enlarged (megaloblastic), and are fewer in number. Even more significantly, an inadequate intake of folic acid has been associated with neural tube defects (NTDs) (spina bifida, anencephaly, meningomyelocele) in the fetus or newborn. With the tremendous cell multiplication that occurs in pregnancy, an adequate amount of folic acid is crucial. However, increased urinary excretion of folic acid and fetal uptake can rapidly result in folic acid deficiency.

CLINICAL THERAPY

Diagnosis of folic acid deficiency anemia may be difficult, and it is usually not detected until late in pregnancy or the early puerperium. This is because serum folate levels normally fall as pregnancy progresses. Even though folate levels are lower with deficiency, they will fluctuate with diet. Measurement of erythrocyte folate status is more reliable but indicates folate status of several weeks previously. Women with true folic acid deficiency anemia often present with nausea, vomiting, and anorexia. Hemoglobin levels as low as 3 to 5 g/dL may be found. Typically the blood smear reveals that the newly formed erythrocytes are macrocytic.

Folic acid deficiency during pregnancy is prevented by a daily supplement of 0.4 mg of folate. Treatment of deficiency consists of 1-mg folic acid supplement. Because iron deficiency anemia almost always coexists with folic acid deficiency, the woman also needs iron supplements.

NURSING CARE MANAGEMENT

The nurse can help the pregnant woman avoid folate deficiency by teaching her food sources of folic acid and cooking methods for preserving folic acid. The best sources are fresh leafy green vegetables, orange juice, other citrus fruits and juices, red meats, fish, poultry, and legumes. As much as 50% to 90% of folic acid can be lost by cooking in large volumes of water. Microwave cooking destroys more folic acid than conventional cooking.

The Food and Drug Administration (FDA) requires the addition of folic acid for all foods labeled "enriched." Even with this addition, the US Public Health Service recommends that all women of childbearing age (15 to 45 years) consume 0.4 mg of folic acid daily. This recommendation is important because half of all US pregnancies are unplanned and NTDs occur very early in pregnancy (3 to 4 weeks after conception), before most women realize they are pregnant (Mersereau, 2000). Nurses can play a crucial role in helping young women become aware of this important recommendation.

Sickle Cell Anemia

Sickle cell anemia (HbSS) is a recessive autosomal disorder in which the normal adult hemoglobin, hemoglobin A (HbA), is abnormally formed. It occurs primarily in people of African descent and occasionally in people of Southeast Asian or Mediterranean origin (ie, Greeks, Italians, Arabs, and Turks) (ACOG, 2000b). The anemia is characterized by acute, recurring episodes of tissue, abdominal, and joint pain. Individuals with the disorder are homozygous for the sickle cell gene. They inherit from each parent an allele causing an amino acid substitution in the two beta protein chains in the hemoglobin molecule. This abnormal hemoglobin is called hemoglobin S (HbS). Heterozygous individuals are carriers for sickle cell anemia but are usually asymptomatic. This condition is called sickle cell trait (HbSA). One of the beta protein chains formed in their hemoglobin is normal; the other has the amino acid substitution. Sickle cell trait occurs in 1 out of 12 African Americans; sickle cell anemia is found in 1 out of 576 (Cunningham et al, 2001).

Hemoglobin S causes the red blood cells to be sickle or crescent shaped. In conditions of low oxygenation, normal hemoglobin is soluble, but HbS becomes semisolid and distorts the red blood cell shape. These erythrocytes easily interlock and clog capillaries, particularly in organs characterized by slow flow and high oxygen extraction, such as the spleen, bone marrow, and placenta. This phenomenon, called *sickling*, varies in frequency depending on the amount of the S hemoglobin in the red blood cells (there is seldom a crisis with levels below 40%) and other hemoglobin factors. Diagnosis is confirmed by hemoglobin electrophoresis or a test to induce sickling in a blood sample. Prenatal diagnosis of sickle cell disease is also available now (ACOG, 2000b).

MATERNAL RISKS

Women with sickle cell trait have a good prognosis for pregnancy if they have adequate nutrition and prenatal care. They are, however, at increased risk for nephritis, bacteriuria, and hematuria, and tend to become anemic.

Women with sickle cell anemia have considerably more risk during pregnancy. Low oxygen pressure—caused by high temperature, dehydration, infection, or acidosis, for example—may precipitate a vaso-occlusive crisis. The crisis produces sudden attacks of pain that may be general or localized in bones or joints, lungs, abdominal organs, or the spinal cord. The pain is due to ischemia in the tissues from occluded capillaries. Vaso-occlusive crises occur more often in the second half of pregnancy.

Maternal mortality due to sickle cell anemia is rare. However, 50% to 67% of pregnant women with sickle cell anemia develop infections, often urinary tract infections or pulmonary infections, because of impaired immune functioning (Cunningham et al, 2001). Congestive heart failure or acute renal failure may also occur.

FETAL-NEONATAL RISKS

The incidence of fetal death during and immediately following an attack has decreased greatly in recent years but is still high. Perinatal mortality is estimated to be 18% (Cunningham et al, 2001). Prematurity and intrauterine growth restriction (IUGR) are also associated with sickle cell anemia. Fetal death is believed to be due to sickling attacks in the placenta.

CLINICAL THERAPY

Because the woman with sickle cell anemia maintains her hemoglobin levels by intense erythropoiesis, additional folic acid supplements (1.0 mg/day) are required. Maternal infection should be treated promptly because dehydration and fever can trigger sickling and crisis. Vaso-occlusive crisis is best treated by a perinatal team in a medical center. Proper management requires close observation and evaluation of all symptoms. The term *sickle cell crisis* should be applied only after all other possible causes for the pain are excluded (Cunningham et al, 2001).

Rehydration with intravenous fluids, administration of oxygen, antibiotics and analgesics, and monitoring of fetal heart rate are important aspects of therapy. Antiembolism stockings are used postpartally.

If vaso-occlusive crisis occurs during labor, the previous therapies are instituted and the woman is kept in a left lateral position. Oxytocics may be used if needed to promote labor. Episiotomy and outlet forceps are recommended to shorten the second stage of labor.

Several antisickling agents are being researched, and in the future sickle cell crisis may be prevented.

NURSING CARE MANAGEMENT

Nursing Assessment and Diagnosis

The woman with sickle cell anemia usually relates a history of frequent illnesses and recurrent abdominal and joint pains and is found to be extremely anemic. The woman may appear undernourished and have long, thin extremities. Ulcers are often present on her ankles. Anemia may be severe.

A diagnosis of sickle cell anemia is confirmed by hemoglobin electrophoresis or a test to induce sickling in a blood sample. The woman is assessed for infection, which is associated with one third of sickle cell crises in adults. Infections most often seen during pregnancy or postpartum are pneumonia, urinary tract infections, puerperal endomyometritis, and osteomyelitis.

Fetal status is assessed during a crisis by electronic fetal monitoring. During labor, the woman's vital signs are assessed frequently and continuous fetal heart rate monitoring is initiated. Compatible blood should be available for transfusion. Oxygen is administered if necessary. The woman is assessed for joint pains and other signs of sickle cell crisis.

Nursing diagnoses that might apply to the pregnant woman with sickle cell anemia include the following:

- ***Pain*** related to the effects of sickle cell crisis
- ***Risk for Altered Health Maintenance*** related to lack of understanding of the need to avoid exposure to infection secondary to the risk of a sickle cell crisis

Nursing Plan and Implementation

The nursing goal for a pregnant woman with sickle cell disease is to provide effective health teaching to help prevent a sickle cell crisis, improve the anemia, and prevent infection. The nurse teaches the woman to increase hydration, use good hygiene, avoid people with infections, seek immediate treatment for infection, and take folic acid supplements (see Figure 19–5 •). As stated earlier, folic acid is important because of its role in red blood cell production; therefore, folic acid supplements are essential. Bed rest is sometimes recommended to decrease the chance of preterm labor. Other nursing interventions are aimed at facilitating the medical therapy and alleviating anxiety through support and education.

Partners should be screened to evaluate their sickle cell status. If both partners have either sickle cell trait or sickle cell disease, genetic counseling is warranted.

Evaluation

Expected outcomes of nursing care include the following:

- The woman is able to describe her condition and identify its possible impact on her pregnancy, labor and childbirth, and postpartal period.
- The woman takes appropriate healthcare measures to avoid a sickle cell crisis.

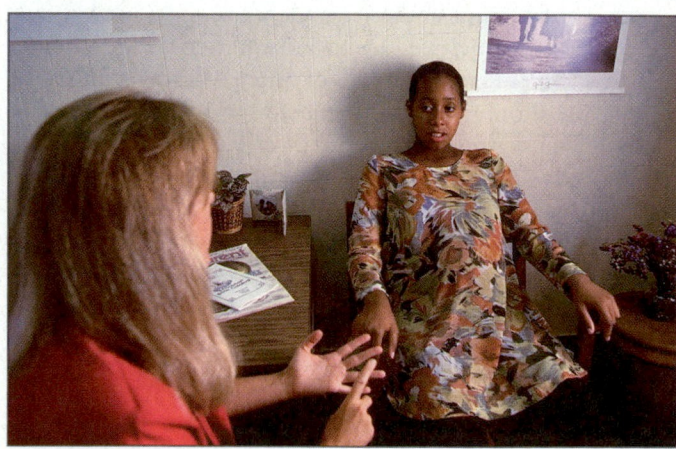

Figure 19–5 • Health teaching is an important part of nursing care for the pregnant woman with sickle cell anemia.
SOURCE: Mark Richards/Photo Edit

- The woman gives birth to a healthy infant.
- The woman and her caregivers quickly identify and successfully manage any complications that arise.

Thalassemia

The thalassemias are a group of autosomal recessive disorders characterized by a defect in the synthesis of the alpha or beta chains in the hemoglobin molecule. The one most frequently encountered in the United States is β-thalassemia. Symptoms are caused by the shortened lifespan of the red blood cells, which result in active erythropoiesis in the liver, spleen, and bones. This produces hepatosplenomegaly and sometimes bony malformations. The thalassemias are seen most often in persons from Greece, Italy, or southern China and are also known as Mediterranean anemia and Cooley anemia. Early identification of thalassemia and preventive management avoids missed diagnosis and unnecessary treatment for iron deficiency anemia (ACOG, 2000b). Prenatal genetic diagnosis is now available for this disorder.

If the woman is heterozygous for β-thalassemia, half of the beta chains are formed normally. This is β-thalassemia minor, or β-thalassemia trait. Mild anemia is usually the only symptom.

Persons born homozygous for the disease have β-thalassemia major. Because newborns have fetal hemoglobin (HbF), which does not have beta chains, no symptoms are present for several months. Once infants with β-thalassemia major start producing adult type hemoglobin (HbA), they develop severe anemia and are dependent on transfusions, from which they eventually develop iron overload. Iron chelation therapy must be instituted soon after chronic transfusions are begun because excess iron damages the liver and heart. Without chelation therapy, these children do not live past the second or third decade, and those who reach puberty are often amenorrheic and infertile.

MATERNAL-FETAL-NEONATAL RISKS

The woman with β-thalassemia minor has mild anemia with small (microcytic) red cells. This mild anemia must be distinguished from iron deficiency anemia because a woman with β-thalassemia minor should not receive iron therapy unless she is also deficient in iron. A woman with iron deficiency anemia typically has low serum iron and serum ferritin levels, whereas the woman with β-thalassemia minor has normal levels. Beta-thalassemia minor varies in degree of severity from extremely mild (minima) anemia, which results in a relatively smooth pregnancy, to a more symptomatic form (intermedia). Pregnancy is rare in women with β-thalassemia major. If it does occur, the woman generally has severe anemia, needs transfusion therapy, and is at risk for congestive heart failure. These women are generally cared for by a perinatologist in a facility that can accommodate high-risk pregnancies.

CLINICAL THERAPY

Folic acid supplements are indicated for women with thalassemia, but iron supplements are not given. Those with thalassemia intermedia and thalassemia major may need transfusion and chelation therapy. They should avoid exposure to infections and seek treatment promptly if an infection develops. Their care is similar to that of women with sickle cell anemia.

NURSING CARE MANAGEMENT

The woman with thalassemia needs to understand her disease and the possibility of transmitting it to her offspring. These clients have lived with thalassemia since childhood but may have questions regarding its effect on pregnancy outcome and their own prognosis.

Care of the Woman with Acquired Immunodeficiency Syndrome (AIDS)

Acquired immunodeficiency syndrome (AIDS), caused by the **human immunodeficiency virus (HIV),** is one of today's major health concerns. As of June 2001, a total of 767,023 cases of AIDS was reported in the United States (CDC, 2002a). Homosexual and bisexual males are still the largest group of infected individuals. Women account for almost 17% of the cases. Rates among black and Latino women are significantly higher than among white women. Although fewer than one fourth of US women are African American or Latino, these groups accounted for 76.5% of all female AIDS cases in 2001. In 2001, the cumulative pediatric total of AIDS cases was 8589, including both males and females under the age of 13 (CDC, 2002a). Of these pediatric cases, the vast majority were infants born to mothers who were infected with HIV during the prenatal or intrapartum period or while breastfeeding. Fortunately the number of new pediatric AIDS cases is declining rapidly. The decline is associated with (1) the implementation of universal counseling about the risks of transmission from mother to fetus, (2) voluntary testing of pregnant women for the presence of HIV, and (3) the use of zidovudine therapy for infected pregnant women and their infants.

Homosexual intercourse is the primary method of transmission in men (45% of cases), whereas intravenous drug use is the means of transmission for 15% of cases. In HIV-infected women, almost equal numbers acquire the disease through heterosexual sex or intravenous drug use (CDC, 2001b).

Pathophysiology of HIV/AIDS

HIV found in blood, semen, vaginal fluid, and breast milk has been implicated in disease transmission, although the virus has been isolated in urine, tears, cerebrospinal fluid, lymph nodes, brain tissue, and bone marrow. HIV shedding has also been detected in the genital tract of women.

Once infected with the virus, the individual develops antibodies that can be detected with enzyme-linked immunosorbent assay (ELISA) and confirmed with the Western blot test. Antibodies can be detected in most individuals within 6 months after exposure, but in rare circumstances the latent period is longer. An asymptomatic period lasting from a few months to as long as 17 years (with a median length of 10 years) follows seroconversion (CDC, 2002b). The majority of infected pregnant women fall into this category.

The diagnosis of AIDS is made when an individual is HIV positive and is identified as having one of several specific opportunistic infections. AIDS can also be diagnosed without laboratory evidence of HIV infection when one of the opportunistic infections is definitively diagnosed and there is no other known cause for the immune deficiency.

Maternal Risks

AIDS-defining diseases that are more common in women than men include wasting syndrome, esophageal candidiasis, and herpes simplex virus disease. Kaposi's sarcoma is rare in women. Non-AIDS-defining gynecologic conditions, such as vaginal *Candida* infections and cervical pathology, are prevalent among women at all stages of HIV infection.

Many women who are HIV positive choose to avoid pregnancy because of the risk of infecting the fetus and the likelihood of dying before the child is raised. Women who are asymptomatic and who do become pregnant should be advised that pregnancy is not believed to accelerate the progression of HIV/AIDS. In contrast, women with low CD4 counts who are symptomatic have been reported to have accelerated progression of the disease during pregnancy (Stratton, Tuomata, Abboud, et al, 1999). The use of zidovudine (ZDV), formerly called azidothymidine (AZT), during pregnancy significantly reduces the risk of transmitting HIV to the fetus, and most medications used to treat HIV can be taken safely during pregnancy.

Fetal-Neonatal Risks

HIV transmission can occur during pregnancy and through breast milk; however, it is believed that at least half of all infection occurs during labor and birth. Beginning in the early 1990s, rates of mother-to-child transmission of HIV began to decrease in Europe and the United States, possibly because of changes in clinical management. For HIV-infected pregnant women who receive no prophylactic medication, the rate of transmission to the newborn is about 15% to 25%. However, for HIV-infected pregnant women who receive prophylactic therapy with ZDV, give birth by elective cesarean at 38 weeks (prior to rupture of membranes), and avoid breastfeeding, the rate of transmission drops to less than 2% (CDC, 2002b). These decreases in transmission are dramatic and impressive.

Following birth, infants will often have a positive antibody titer, which reflects the passive transfer of maternal antibodies and does not indicate HIV infection. Although infected infants are usually asymptomatic at birth, they are likely to be premature, low birth weight, and small for gestational age (SGA). However, these findings are associated with several socioeconomic factors and may not be unique to HIV infection (Stratton et al, 1999). The signs of AIDS in infants may include failure to thrive, hepatosplenomegaly, interstitial lymphocytic pneumonia, recurrent infections, cell-mediated immunodeficiency, evidence of Epstein-Barr virus, and neurologic abnormalities. Recurrent bacterial infections are common in children with AIDS; Kaposi's sarcoma is rare. Encephalopathy, characterized by delayed developmental milestones or the loss of acquired skills, including cognitive abilities, is found in 50% to 90% of children with AIDS. Treatments that prevent the central nervous system effects of HIV have yet to be identified. The prognosis for an infected child remains poor.

Clinical Therapy

Early knowledge of a woman's HIV status is important for her well-being and that of her child. Thus the revised CDC screening guidelines for pregnant women state that HIV screening should be emphasized as a routine part of all prenatal care. To this end, the recommendation that all pregnant women should be tested for HIV has been strengthened while continuing to ensure that testing of pregnant women and their infants is voluntary and informed (CDC, 2001a). Initial testing is done using ELISA, followed by a confirmatory Western blot assay. Women who test positive should be counseled about the implications of the diagnosis for themselves and their fetus in order to ensure an informed reproductive choice. The care of the woman who chooses to continue her pregnancy should focus on stabilizing the disease, preventing opportunistic infections and transmission of the virus from mother to fetus, and providing psychosocial and educational support.

Antiretroviral therapy should be recommended to all infected pregnant women to reduce the rate of perinatal transmission. A triple therapy approach is recommended during the prenatal period. It includes ZDV, a nucleoside analog, plus a second nucleoside analog such as zalcitabine, didanosine, or lamivudine combined with a protease inhibitor such as indinavir, ritonavir, or saquinavir. Alternatively, the ZDV and second nucleoside analog can be combined with a nonnucleoside analog such as nevirapine or delavirdine (Cunningham et al, 2001). Treatment recommendations have also been developed for the mother and infant for the intrapartum and postpartum periods. The decision about which regimen is most appropriate should be determined following discussion with the woman about the risks and benefits based on her individual HIV status.

HIV-infected women should be evaluated and treated for other sexually transmitted infections and for conditions oc-

Complementary and Alternative Therapies

Garlic Supplements Interfere with HIV Medication

Garlic has been well regarded as a natural way of combating elevated cholesterol levels. This has made it attractive to many HIV-positive individuals on combination drug therapy because increased cholesterol is a side effect of treatment. However, research has revealed that garlic supplements may actually interfere with the effectiveness of the HIV medication saquinavir, a protease inhibitor, which is usually prescribed in combination with other HIV medications.

The study was conducted with nine healthy, HIV-negative volunteers. Blood analysis revealed that the blood concentrations of saquinavir decreased by over 50% when the volunteers took garlic caplets twice daily for 3 weeks. Moreover, even after a 10-day period with no garlic, the participants' blood levels were about 35% lower than the expected baseline.

At present, researchers do not know what impact the garlic supplements would have on a combined medication regimen but they do recommend that individuals on saquinavir *avoid* taking garlic supplements.

Sources: National Institutes of Health News Release. (2001, December 5). Retrieved November 17, 2002, from www.nih.gov/news

Piscitelli, S.C., et al. (2001, December 3). The effect of garlic supplements on the pharmacokinetics of saquinavir. *Clinical Infectious Diseases* electronic edition.

curring more commonly in women with HIV, such as tuberculosis, cytomegalovirus, toxoplasmosis, and cervical dysplasia. HIV-infected women with no history of hepatitis B should receive the hepatitis vaccine, which is not contraindicated prenatally, as well as the pneumococcal vaccine and an annual flu shot. In addition to routine prenatal laboratory tests, a platelet count and a complete blood count with differential should be obtained at the first prenatal visit and repeated each trimester to identify anemia, thrombocytopenia, and leukopenia, which are associated both with HIV infection and with antiviral therapy.

The woman with HIV also should be assessed regularly for serologic changes that indicate the disease is progressing. This is determined by the absolute CD4+ T-lymphocyte count, which provides the number of helper T4 cells. When CD4+ counts fall to 200/mm^3 or lower, opportunistic infections such as *Pneumocystis carinii* pneumonia are more likely to develop, and prophylaxis should be instituted (CDC, 1999).

At each prenatal visit, asymptomatic HIV-infected women are monitored for early signs of complications, such as weight loss in the second or third trimester or fever. The woman is asked about signs of vaginal infection. Her mouth is inspected for signs of infections such as thrush (candidiasis) or hairy leukoplakia; her lungs are auscultated for signs of pneumonia; and her lymph nodes, liver, and spleen are palpated for signs of enlargement. Each trimester the woman should have a visual examination and a funduscopic examination to detect such complications as toxoplasmosis retinitis. Further discussion of therapy for the pregnant woman who is HIV positive or who has AIDS may be found in journal articles and specialty texts.

A pregnancy complicated by HIV infection, even if asymptomatic, is considered high risk, and the fetus is monitored closely. Weekly nonstress testing is begun at 32 weeks' gestation, and serial ultrasounds are done to detect intrauterine growth restriction. Biophysical profiles are also indicated (see Chapter 21). Invasive procedures such as amniocentesis are avoided when possible to prevent the contamination of a noninfected infant.

The American College of Obstetricians and Gynecologists (ACOG, 2000b) recommends that scheduled cesarean birth should be discussed with HIV-positive pregnant women. This procedure may be done as early as 38 weeks' gestation to decrease the risk of rupture of the membranes. Other authorities have expressed concern that cesarean birth may increase the HIV-infected woman's risk of complications following surgery. They suggest that the use of combined antiretroviral therapy reduces the risk of vertical transmission of infection significantly (Cunningham et al, 2001).

Intrapartal care is similar to that for all pregnant women, although strict adherence to universal precautions is crucial to avoid nosocomial infection. To prevent exposure of an uninfected infant to HIV during labor and birth, invasive procedures such as vaginal examinations following rupture of the membranes, fetal scalp electrode monitoring, fetal scalp sampling, and vacuum extraction should be done only after carefully evaluating the risks and benefits (ACOG, 2000b).

Women who are HIV positive are at increased risk for complications such as intrapartal or postpartal hemorrhage, postpartal infection, poor wound healing, and infections of the genitourinary tract. Thus they need careful monitoring and appropriate therapy as indicated.

Following childbirth, the HIV-positive woman should be referred to a physician knowledgeable about treating individuals with HIV infection. Because of the profound implications of HIV infection for the woman, her family, the fetus/newborn, and her healthcare providers, screening is recommended for all pregnant women, but especially those at increased risk, including the following: prostitutes; women with multiple sexual partners; women whose current or previous sex partners have been bisexual, have abused IV drugs, had hemophilia, or tested positive for HIV; women who are or have been IV drug users; and women from countries where heterosexual transmission is common. In addition, clinics located in areas with a large HIV-positive population may require routine HIV screening of all prenatal clients.

MediaLink AIDS in Pregnancy

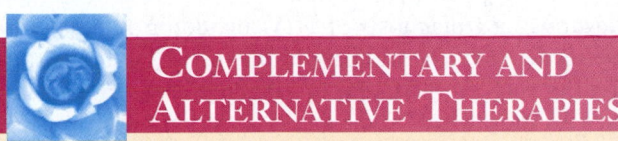

NURSING CARE MANAGEMENT

Nursing Assessment and Diagnosis

A woman who tests positive for HIV may be asymptomatic or may present with any of the following signs or symptoms: fatigue, anemia, malaise, progressive weight loss, lymphadenopathy, night sweats, diarrhea, fever, neurologic dysfunction, cell-mediated immunodeficiency, or evidence of Kaposi's sarcoma (purplish, reddish brown lesions, either externally or internally).

If a woman tests HIV positive or is involved in a relationship or an activity that places her at high risk, the nurse should assess the woman's knowledge level about the disease, its implications for her and her fetus, and self-care measures the woman can take.

Examples of nursing diagnoses that might apply for an HIV-positive pregnant woman include the following:

- ***Risk for Altered Health Maintenance*** related to lack of information about HIV/AIDS and its long-term implications for the woman and her unborn child
- ***Risk for Infection*** related to altered immunity secondary to HIV/AIDS
- ***Ineffective Family Coping*** related to the implications of a positive HIV test in one of the family members

> *"I've been a nurse for 30 years now, and I've never seen anything change nursing practice more than HIV/AIDS has. Nursing students today will take universal precautions for granted because they won't know any other way, but I can remember when we could touch more freely. I remember drying a newly born infant and stroking him—my hands warm against his skin. I remember a time when people didn't think twice before trying to stop bleeding or give other first aid at an accident scene. I know this way is safer, but a part of me mourns what we have lost."*

Nursing Plan and Implementation

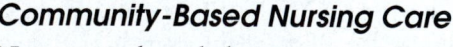

Community-Based Nursing Care

Nurses need to help women understand that HIV/AIDS is a fatal disease. HIV infection can be avoided if women avoid sharing intravenous drug needles and practice safe sex, including insisting that their sex partners wear a latex condom for each act of intercourse.

Women at risk for AIDS should be offered premarital and prepregnancy screening for HIV antibodies (ACOG, 2001b). They should be given clear information about the implications of a diagnosis of HIV, including societal attitudes. Access to information about the disease and about the test results empowers women by enabling them to make informed decisions about their sexual activities and about becoming pregnant.

A detailed drug and sexual history of each prenatal client is the first step in perinatal HIV/AIDS prevention. All women should be offered HIV counseling. The following are counseling guidelines for HIV testing:

- The nurse should discuss HIV testing during the normal prenatal assessment.
- The nurse should assure the woman of confidentiality, explaining the difference between anonymity and confidentiality.
- The nurse should provide an environment that is private, comfortable, and nonjudgmental.
- The nurse should provide the woman with information about AIDS, including pathophysiology, mode of transmission of HIV, high-risk behaviors, and methods of decreasing transmission, such as practicing safe sex and not sharing needles.
- If the woman chooses to have an antibody test for HIV (ELISA, Western blot), written consent should be obtained.
- Posttest counseling should be provided. A negative test means that no HIV antibodies were found; it does not ensure that the woman has not been infected with the virus, because antibodies may not be detected for 6 weeks to 6 months after exposure.
- If test results are positive, supportive follow-up is necessary. This includes an explanation of the implications for the woman and her unborn child as well as the value of ZDV therapy, recommended medical therapy, follow-up of sex partners, transmission prevention, discussion of immediate posttest plans, and referral to appropriate psychologic and educational services. The nurse should tell the woman not to donate blood or blood products and not to share toothbrushes, razors, and other implements that could be contaminated with blood.

This information can be overwhelming to the woman who is HIV positive and should be provided orally and in writing. She will need more than one counseling session to absorb the information. The initial reaction may be one of shock or denial, so it is important for the nurse to allow her a little time to think and to give her empathy and support. The nurse needs to stress that being HIV positive does not mean that the woman has AIDS but that she can transmit the virus to others (by sexual contact, sharing IV drug needles, and donating blood) and to her fetus during pregnancy or childbirth or by breastfeeding. Most people develop AIDS within 10 years of being infected with HIV. It is currently impossible to prevent AIDS from developing in people who are HIV positive or to predict when they will develop the disease.

In monitoring the asymptomatic HIV-positive pregnant woman, the nurse should be alert for nonspecific symptoms such as fever, weight loss, fatigue, persistent candidiasis, diarrhea, cough, skin lesions, and behavior changes. Laboratory findings—such as decreased hemoglobin, hematocrit, and T4 lymphocytes; elevated erythrocyte sedimentation rate (ESR); and abnormal complete blood count, differential, and platelets—may indicate complications or progression of the disease.

Education about optimal nutrition and maintenance of wellness are important and should be reviewed frequently with the woman.

Hospital-Based Nursing Care

The Clinical Pathway for a Woman with HIV/AIDS beginning on page 456 summarizes essential nursing management during the antepartum, intrapartum, and postpartum periods.

In community and hospital settings, the nurse faces the important task of taking the precautions necessary to protect staff, other clients, and families from exposure to HIV while meeting the needs of the childbearing woman with this infection.

In 1987 the CDC stated that the prevalence of AIDS and the risk of exposure faced by healthcare workers is significant enough that *precautions should be taken with all clients* (not only those with known HIV infection), especially in dealing with blood and body fluids. These are now called *universal precautions.*

Nurses who deal with childbearing families are exposed to blood and body fluids and should pay careful attention to the CDC guidelines, which are addressed in introductory nursing courses in preparation for clinical practice. Protocols have been established for postexposure treatment of caregivers who experience a needle stick or exposure to the body fluids of a person with HIV or a person whose HIV status is not known. The effectiveness of such therapy, using a combined drug approach, depends on starting therapy rapidly. Thus such exposure should be reported immediately.

Teaching for Self-Care

The psychologic implications of HIV/AIDS for the childbearing family are staggering. The woman is faced with the knowledge that she and her newborn, if infected, have a decreased life expectancy. If her infant is not infected, she must face the probability that others will raise her child. She may have feelings of fear, helplessness, anger, and isolation. If she shares her diagnosis with others, she may face rejection and condemnation. The couple must deal with the impact of the illness on the partner, who may or may not be infected, and on other children. Dealing with the tasks and responsibilities of a newborn may be especially difficult if the woman is physically depleted or if she is trying to come to grips with the long-term implications of her condition.

The nonjudgmental, supportive nurse plays an essential role in preserving confidentiality and the client's right to privacy. In addition, the nurse can help ensure that the woman receives complete, accurate information about her condition and ways she might cope. This usually involves a referral to social services for follow-up care.

Evaluation

Expected outcomes of nursing care include the following:

- The woman discusses the implications of her positive HIV antibody screen (or diagnosis of AIDS), its implications for herself and her unborn child, the method of transmission, and treatment options.
- The woman uses information regarding referral to social services (or other agency) for follow-up assistance and counseling.
- The woman begins to verbalize her feelings about her condition and its implications in an atmosphere she finds supportive.

Care of the Woman with Heart Disease

A healthy woman with a normal heart has adequate cardiac reserve to adjust easily to the demands of pregnancy. The woman with heart disease, however, has decreased cardiac reserve, making it more difficult for her heart to accommodate the higher workload of pregnancy. Approximately 1% of pregnant women are at risk because of pregestational heart disease. Heart disease ranks fourth after hypertension, hemorrhage, and infection as a cause of maternal mortality.

Types of Maternal Heart Disease

Currently, cardiac disease complicates about 1% of pregnancies (Martin & Foley, 2002). Although rheumatic heart disease used to predominate, at least half of all cases of heart disease currently encountered during pregnancy are caused by congenital heart defects (Cunningham et al, 2001). Other less common causes of heart disease in pregnancy include Marfan syndrome, peripartum cardiomyopathy, and Eisenmenger syndrome. All can cause significant maternal mortality. Mitral valve prolapse is usually asymptomatic but is addressed here because of its frequent occurrence during pregnancy.

CONGENITAL HEART DEFECTS

Congenital heart defects have become a more common finding in pregnant women as improved surgical techniques enable females born with heart defects to live to childbearing age. The exact pathology depends on the specific defect. Congenital defects most often seen in pregnant women include tetralogy of Fallot, atrial septal defect, ventricular septal defect, patent ductus arteriosus, and coarctation of the aorta. When surgical repair can be accomplished with no remaining

CLINICAL PATHWAY FOR A WOMAN WITH HIV/AIDS

Category	Antepartal Management	Intrapartal Management*	Postpartal Management*
Referral	• Perinatologist • Internist • Social worker • Psych clinical nurse practitioner • Dietary/nutritionist • Infectious disease consult	• Obtain prenatal record	• Home nursing referral if indicated **➤ Expected Outcomes** Appropriate resources identified and utilized

Assessment	• Obtain course of present pregnancy
	• Assess estimated gestational age
	• Assess any sensitivity to medications
	• Obtain history of any infections
	• Obtain complete physical examination to include:
	  • Fetal size, fetal status (FHR), and fetal maturity
	  • Signs of fatigue, weakness, recurrent diarrhea, pallor, night sweats
	  • Lymphadenopathy
	  • Present weight and amount of weight gain or weight loss
	  • Presence of nonproductive cough, fever, sore throat, chills, shortness of breath (*Pneumocystis carinii* pneumonia)
	  • Dark purplish marks or lesions, especially on the lower extremities (Kaposi's sarcoma)
	  • Oral, gingival lesions
	• Obtain diagnostic studies:
	  • Ultrasound
	  • Fetal maturity studies (L/S ratio, PG creatinine)
	  • Hemoglobin and hematocrit
	  • WBC
	  • HIV-I
	  • CD4+ T lymphocyte count
	  • ESR
	  • Differential
	  • Platelet count
		• Assess for signs of infection	• Monitor daily Hct
			• Continue normal postpartum assessment q8h
			• Feeding technique with newborn: should be progressing
			• TPR assessment: q8h; all WNL; report temperature > 38C (100.4F)
			• Continue assessment of comfort level
			➤ Expected Outcomes
			Potential/actual health problems and complications identified and minimized

Teaching/ psychosocial	• Room orientation • Explain signs and symptoms (s/sx) of worsening disease and importance of notifying RN • Explain s/sx of labor • Increase awareness of fetal monitoring • Evaluation of client teaching	• Tour of ICN • Discuss with woman: a. Mode of childbirth b. Postpartum expectation	• Implement normal postpartum teaching and psychosocial support **➤ Expected Outcomes** Client verbalizes/demonstrates understanding and incorporation of teaching
Nursing care management and reports	• Assess emotional response so that support and teaching can be planned accordingly • Weigh woman • Obtain food history • Establish rapport • Provide opportunities to talk without interruption • Monitor for signs of infection • Maintain appropriate isolation precautions	• Ongoing monitoring of blood pressure • Electronic fetal monitoring in place • Try to have same nurses caring for woman during her hospitalization • Maintain appropriate isolation precautions • Monitor for signs of infection Provide supportive care	• Continue sitz baths prn • May shower if ambulating without difficulty • DC heparin lock (saline lock) if present • Maintain appropriate isolation precautions • Monitor for signs of infection **➤ Expected Outcomes** Maternal/fetal well-being maximized Active involvement of client in plan of care to include physical, emotional, and spiritual needs
Activity	• Decreased stimulation in room • Limit visitors	Encourage position change and activity as tolerated	• Up ad lib **➤ Expected Outcome** Level of activity has not exacerbated condition

*Interventions for a woman with a normal labor and birth and during the early postpartum period may be found in those appropriate clinical pathways.

CLINICAL PATHWAY FOR A WOMAN WITH HIV/AIDS *CONTINUED*

Category	Antepartal Management*	Intrapartal Management*	Postpartal Management*
Comfort	• Assess for discomfort • Provide comfort measures as needed	• Assess for discomfort • Provide comfort measures as needed	• Continue with pain management techniques ➤ **Expected Outcome** Optimal comfort maintained
Nutrition	• Plan high-protein, high-calorie diet	• Ice chips; popsicles	• Continue diet and fluids ➤ **Expected Outcome** Nutritional needs met with emphasis on appetite enhancement and reduction of deficiencies
Elimination			➤ **Expected Outcome** Intake and output WNL
Medications		• Continuous IV infusion	• May take own prenatal vitamins • Rh immune globulin administered if indicated • Rubella vaccine administered if indicated ➤ **Expected Outcomes** Perfusion and hydration supported Ongoing treatments maintained

Discharge planning/ home care	• Assess home care needs
	• If the client is asymptomatic, the primary nursing activity is client teaching regarding
	  • Disease process
	  • Screening and healthcare for sex partners as appropriate
	  • Impact of disease on pregnancy
	  • Methods of HIV transmission
	  • Precautions to take in preventing the spread of infection
	  • Options in regard to pregnancy
	  • Available community resources
	  • Signs and symptoms to report to healthcare provider including common discomforts of pregnancy such as nausea and fatigue and complications such as premature rupture of membranes, vaginal bleeding, and preterm labor
	  • Importance of regular prenatal visits
	• Provide teaching regarding nutritional needs
	• Refer to community resources
	• Discuss disease process, impact on pregnancy, and pregnancy options
	• Provide support and counseling
			• Review discharge instruction sheet and check list
			• Describe postpartum warning signs and when to call CNM/physician
			• Provide prescriptions and gift pack
			• Arrangements made for baby pictures
			• Postpartum visit scheduled
			• Newborn check scheduled
			• Discuss the implications of breastfeeding (current information suggests that the virus may be spread in breast milk)
			• Provide information on transmission of HIV and measures to prevent infection. Discuss household safety issues (eg, it is acceptable to use same dishes, safe to sleep in same bed, safe to use same bathroom, can hold and hug children, should avoid using razors and toothbrushes and should wear gloves and use 10% bleach solution to clean spills of body fluids or disinfect bathroom). Inform the woman that sexual abstinence is safest; otherwise latex condoms should be used.
			➤ **Expected Outcomes**
			Discharge teaching completed with emphasis on follow-up continuing healthcare needs, adequate support network

Family Involvement	• Assess woman's major concerns re: losing fetus, relationship with other children, relationship with partner • Assess support systems	• Encourage family member to stay with the woman as long as possible throughout labor and childbirth	• Family members urged to visit • Continue to involve support persons in teaching • Shows parental bonding behaviors • Plans made for providing support to mother following discharge. Support persons verbalize understanding of need for woman to rest, eat nutritionally, recover. ➤ **Expected Outcomes** Family demonstrates resource utilization, integration of newborn into family, helpful coping skills
Date			

*Interventions for a woman with a normal labor and birth and during the early postpartum period may be found in those appropriate clinical pathways.

BSI, body substance isolation; ESR erythrocyte sedimentation rate; FHR, fetal heart rate; hct hematocrit ICN, intensive care nursery; IV, intravenous; L/S ratio, Lecithin/sphingomyelin ratio; PG, phosphotidyl glycerol; Q8h every 8 hours; s/sx, signs/symptoms; WBC, white blood count; WNL, within normal limits.

evidence of organic heart disease, pregnancy may be undertaken with confidence. In such cases, antibiotic prophylaxis is recommended to prevent subacute bacterial endocarditis at the time of birth. When congenital heart disease is associated with cyanosis, whether the defect was originally uncorrected or the correction failed to relieve the cyanosis, the woman should be counseled to avoid pregnancy because the risk to both her and the fetus would be high. She also needs to know that there is about a 2% to 4% chance that the baby will inherit the disorder because most congenital heart defects are believed to be polygenetic and multifactorial in origin (Cunningham et al, 2001).

RHEUMATIC HEART DISEASE

Rheumatic heart disease has declined rapidly in the last four decades, because of prompt identification of pharyngeal infections caused by group A β-hemolytic streptococcus and the availability of penicillin for treatment. Rheumatic fever, which may develop in untreated streptococcal infections, is an inflammatory connective tissue disease that can involve the heart, joints, central nervous system, skin, and subcutaneous tissue. When the heart is affected, mitral valve stenosis is the most common and serious lesion. Aortic valve involvement, manifested by aortic insufficiency, is the second most common problem. The tricuspid and pulmonic valves are rarely affected.

The increased blood volume of pregnancy, coupled with the pregnant woman's need for increased cardiac output, stresses the heart of a woman with mitral valve stenosis. She may develop dyspnea, orthopnea, and pulmonary edema and is at increased risk for congestive heart failure (CHF). Even the woman who has no symptoms at the onset of pregnancy is at risk for CHF.

MARFAN SYNDROME

Marfan syndrome is an autosomal dominant disorder of connective tissue in which there may be serious cardiovascular involvement—usually dissection or rupture of the aorta. Because maternal mortality rate may be as high as 25% to 50%, a pregnant woman with Marfan syndrome needs very careful cardiovascular assessment and counseling regarding her prognosis for pregnancy (Cunningham et al, 2001). Because of its inheritance pattern, there is a 50% chance that the disease will be passed on to offspring.

PERIPARTUM CARDIOMYOPATHY

Peripartum cardiomyopathy is a dysfunction of the left ventricle that occurs in the last month of pregnancy or the first 5 months postpartum in a woman with no previous history of heart disease. This is a relatively rare but serious condition, which occurs in 1 in 3000 to 4000 live births. Mortality rates range from 18% to 56% (Martin & Foley, 2002). The symptoms are related to CHF: dyspnea, orthopnea, chest pain, palpitations, weakness, and edema. The cause is unknown, although symptoms are often attributable to chronic hypertension, mitral stenosis, obesity, or viral myocarditis. The condition usually presents with anemia and infection; consequently, treatment focuses on underlying abnormalities. Digitalis, diuretics, vasodilators, anticoagulants, sodium restriction, and strict bed rest are often part of the treatment. Peripartum cardiomyopathy may resolve with bed rest as the heart gradually returns to normal size. Subsequent pregnancy is strongly discouraged because the disease tends to recur during pregnancy.

EISENMENGER SYNDROME

Eisenmenger syndrome is not a congenital defect, but a complication that can develop with cardiac lesions characterized by left-to-right shunting (as with atrial septal defects or ventricular septal defects). This shunting can result in progressive pulmonary hypertension. As pulmonary vascular resistance increases, the shunting becomes bidirectional or reverses to right-to-left shunting. This condition cannot be corrected surgically and is associated with maternal mortality rates of 30% to 50% (Cunningham et al, 2001).

MITRAL VALVE PROLAPSE

Mitral valve prolapse (MVP) is usually an asymptomatic condition that is found in approximately 3% of women of childbearing age (Martin & Foley, 2002). The condition is more common in women than in men and seems to be inherited. In MVP, the mitral valve leaflets tend to prolapse into the left atrium during ventricular systole because the chordae tendineae that support them are long and thin. As a result, some mitral regurgitation may occur. On auscultation a midsystolic click and a late systolic murmur are heard.

Women with MVP usually tolerate pregnancy well, and the prognosis is excellent. Most women require assurance that they can continue with normal activities. A few women experience symptoms such as palpitations, chest pain, and dyspnea, which are usually due to arrhythmias. They are often treated with propranolol hydrochloride (Inderal). Limiting caffeine intake also helps decrease palpitations. Women should be given antibiotic prophylaxis if there is mitral valve regurgitation, valvular damage, or other risk factors (Cunningham et al, 2001).

Clinical Therapy

The primary goal of medical management is early diagnosis and ongoing treatment of the woman with cardiac disease. Echocardiogram, chest x-ray, electrocardiogram, auscultation of heart sounds, and sometimes cardiac catheterization are essential for establishing the type and severity of the heart disease. The severity of heart disease can also be determined by the individual's ability to perform ordinary physical activity. The following classification of functional capacity for those with cardiac disease has been standardized by the Criteria Committee of the New York Heart Association (1994):

- *Class I.* Individuals with cardiac disease but with no resulting limitation of physical activity and no symptoms of cardiac insufficiency. Ordinary physical activity causes no undue fatigue, dyspnea, or palpitations; anginal pain is not present.
- *Class II.* Individuals with cardiac disease that results in slight limitation of physical activity. They are

RESEARCH IN PRACTICE
Studying Pregnancy Outcomes in Women with Heart Disease

What is this study about? The maternal and neonatal risks associated with pregnancy in women with heart disease have not been clearly identified. The circulatory changes of pregnancy may result in compromised health or even death for the mother and/or baby. Available risk estimates are based on retrospective studies, studies with limited populations, or studies that were focused on specific cardiac lesions. The purpose of this study was to prospectively evaluate the frequency of cardiac complications related to pregnancy, and to determine risk predictors for this population. The study also undertook the development of a validated risk index to evaluate the risk of cardiac complications during pregnancy for women who are pregnant or are considering pregnancy in the presence of cardiac disease.

How was this study done? There were 562 women with 617 pregnancies enrolled in this prospective study. The women were all receiving care in one of 13 Canadian cardiac or obstetric teaching hospitals. The women had either congenital or acquired cardiac lesions, or had experienced documented cardiac arrhythmias that required treatment prior to pregnancy. The sample did not include women with isolated mitral valve prolapse classified as mild or moderate. Baseline data, including demographic and behavioral characteristics as well as physiologic indicators, were recorded at the initial prenatal visit. Follow-up data were obtained from clinical visits during the second and third trimesters, the peripartum period, and at 6 weeks and 6 months postpartum. Data were also collected about the physiologic condition of the newborns. A total of 546 women with 599 pregnancies completed the study. Complications were classified as primary cardiac, secondary cardiac, neonatal, or obstetric. Statistical analysis resulted in descriptive statistics as well as identification of predictors of cardiac events.

What were the results of the study? The live birth rate in these pregnancies was 98%, of which 27% were by cesarean. Most of the cesarean births were for obstetric indications; maternal cardiac status was the indication in 4%. A primary cardiac event occurred in 80 completed pregnancies, or 13%. Pulmonary edema and cardiac arrhythmia accounted for most of these. Maternal stroke or cardiac death occurred in 1% of the pregnancies. The four characteristics that were identified as predictors of primary cardiac events were prior cardiac event, cyanosis, left heart obstruction, and reduced systemic ventricular systolic function. There was no association between cardiac events and the administration of cardiac medications, including aspirin and anticoagulants. The method of childbirth was not associated with the cardiac event rate. However, the use of anticoagulants throughout pregnancy was a predictor of neonatal events, which occurred in 20% of these pregnancies. The most common neonatal events were premature labor and/or birth and small-for-gestational-age birth weight. Additionally, maternal smoking was confirmed as a predictor of neonatal events.

What additional questions might I have? Since some of the women had more than one pregnancy, was the cardiac event rate different for first and subsequent pregnancies? Did the type of delivery affect the rate of neonatal events?

How can I use this study? The neonatal mortality rate and rate of preterm labor for these women were higher than that reported for a general obstetric population. When these risk factors are present, prepregnant women should be counseled to consider treatment prior to conception. Women who are already pregnant and who have identified risk factors should be referred to an appropriate center for ongoing care and treatment during the pregnancy. Women with these risk factors should have an increased frequency of prenatal visits and monitoring.

Source: Siu, S., Sermer, M., Colman, J., Alvarez, A., Mercier, L., Morton, B., et al. (2001). Prospective multicenter study of pregnancy outcomes in women with heart disease. *Circulation, 104*(5), 515–521.

comfortable at rest but ordinary physical activity causes fatigue, dyspnea, palpitation, or anginal pain.

- *Class III.* Individuals with cardiac disease that results in marked limitation of physical activity. They are comfortable at rest but less than ordinary physical activity results in fatigue, dyspnea, palpitation, or anginal pain.
- *Class IV.* Individuals with cardiac disease that results in the inability to carry on any physical activity without experiencing discomfort. Even at rest, they may experience symptoms of cardiac insufficiency or anginal pain; discomfort increases with any physical activity.

Women in classes I and II usually experience a normal pregnancy and have few complications, whereas those in classes III and IV are at risk for more severe complications, which may affect both maternal and fetal outcomes. Preconception counseling is important for these women in order to optimize maternal and fetal outcomes.

Because anemia increases the work of the heart, it should be diagnosed early and treated. Infection also increases the cardiac workload, so even minor infections should be treated thoroughly. To reduce the risk of pyelonephritis, monthly screening for asymptomatic bacteriuria is indicated, with antibiotic therapy as needed.

As pregnancy progresses, it is important to minimize cardiac workload and promote tissue perfusion. Consequently, the woman's activity should be limited. Weight gain may also be limited and a daily sodium intake of only 2 to 4 g is recommended (Mason & Bobrowski, 1998).

DRUG THERAPY

Besides the iron and vitamin supplements prescribed during pregnancy, the pregnant woman with heart disease may need additional drug therapy to maintain health. Antibiotics, usually penicillin if not contraindicated by allergy, are used to prevent recurrent bouts of rheumatic fever and subsequent heart valve damage. Antibiotics are also recommended during labor and the early postpartum period for either acquired or congenital disease to prevent bacterial endocarditis. If the woman develops coagulation problems, the anticoagulant heparin may be used. Heparin offers the greatest safety to the fetus because it does not cross the placenta. The thiazide diuretics and furosemide (Lasix) may be used to treat congestive heart failure if it develops. Digitalis glycosides and common antiarrhythmic drugs may be used to treat cardiac failure and arrhythmias. These agents do cross the placenta but have no reported teratogenic effect; however, they have not been adequately studied to establish their safety in pregnancy (Cunningham et al, 2001).

LABOR AND CHILDBIRTH

Spontaneous natural labor with adequate pain relief is usually recommended for clients in classes I and II. Special attention should be given to the prompt recognition and treatment of any signs of heart failure (see Figure 19–6 •). Those in classes III and IV may need to be hospitalized prior to onset of labor for cardiovascular stabilization. They may also require invasive cardiac monitoring during labor.

Use of low forceps or vacuum assistance provides the safest method of birth, with lumbar epidural anesthesia to reduce the stress of pushing. Cesarean is used only if fetal or maternal indications exist, not on the basis of heart disease alone.

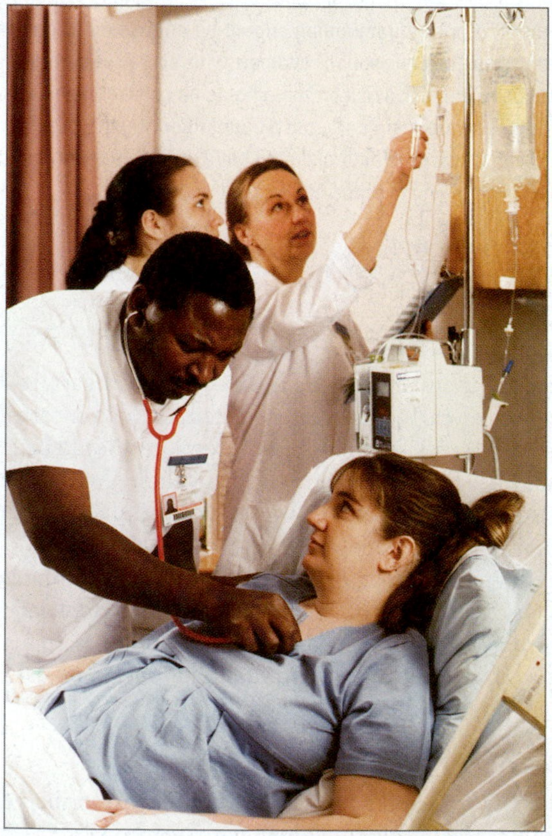

Figure 19–6 • When a woman with heart disease begins labor, the nursing students and instructor caring for her monitor her closely for signs of congestive heart failure.

NURSING CARE MANAGEMENT

Nursing Assessment and Diagnosis

The nurse assesses the stress of pregnancy on the functional capacity of the heart during every antepartal visit. The nurse notes the category of functional capacity assigned to the woman; takes the woman's pulse, respirations, and blood pressure; and compares them to the normal values expected during pregnancy and to the woman's previous values. The nurse then determines the woman's activity level, including rest, and any changes in the pulse and respirations that have occurred since previous visits. The nurse also identifies and evaluates other factors that would increase strain on the heart. These might include anemia, infection, anxiety, lack of support system, and household and career demands.

The following symptoms, if they are progressive, are indicative of CHF, the heart's signal of its decreased ability to meet the demands of pregnancy:

- Cough (frequent, with or without hemoptysis)
- Dyspnea (progressive, upon exertion)
- Edema (progressive, generalized, including extremities, face, eyelids)
- Heart murmurs (heard on auscultation)
- Palpitations
- Rales (auscultated in lung bases)

Progressiveness of the cycle is the critical factor, because some of these same symptoms are seen to a minor degree in a pregnancy without cardiac problems.

Nursing diagnoses that might apply to the pregnant woman with heart disease include the following:

- ***Decreased Cardiac Output:*** Easy fatigability
- ***Impaired Gas Exchange*** related to pulmonary edema secondary to cardiac decompensation
- ***Fear*** related to the effects of the maternal cardiac condition on fetal well-being

Nursing Plan and Implementation

Nursing care is directed toward maintaining a balance between cardiac reserve and cardiac workload.

Antepartum Period

Nursing actions are designed to meet the physiologic and psychosocial needs of the pregnant woman with heart disease. The priority of nursing actions varies according to the severity of the disease process and the individual needs of the woman as determined by nursing assessment.

The woman and her family should thoroughly understand her condition and its management and should recognize signs of potential complications. This will increase their understanding and decrease anxiety. When the nurse provides explanations, uses printed material, and offers frequent opportunities to ask questions and discuss concerns, the woman is better able to meet her own healthcare needs and seek assistance appropriately.

As part of health teaching, the nurse explains the purposes of the dietary and activity changes that are required. A diet is instituted that is high in iron, protein, and essential nutrients but low in sodium, with adequate calories to ensure normal weight gain. Such a diet best meets the nutrition needs of the client with cardiac disease. Excessive weight gain is avoided because it taxes the heart. To help preserve her cardiac reserves, the woman may need to restrict her activities. In addition, 8 to 10 hours of sleep and frequent daily rest periods are essential. The nurse can encourage the woman to rest in the side-lying position to promote optimal placental perfusion. Because upper respiratory infections may tax the heart and lead to decompensation, the woman must avoid contact with sources of infection and report symptoms of infection immediately.

During the first half of pregnancy, the woman is seen approximately every 2 weeks to assess cardiac status. During the second half of pregnancy, the woman is seen weekly. These assessments are especially important between weeks 28 and 30, when the blood volume reaches maximum amounts. If symptoms of cardiac decompensation occur, prompt medical intervention is indicated to correct the cardiac problem.

Intrapartum Period

Labor and birth exert tremendous stress on the woman and her fetus. This stress could be fatal to the fetus of a woman with cardiac disease because the fetus may be receiving an inadequate oxygen and blood supply. Thus the intrapartal care of a woman with cardiac disease is aimed at reducing the amount of physical exertion and accompanying fatigue.

The nurse evaluates maternal vital signs frequently to determine the woman's response to labor. A pulse rate greater than 100 beats per minute or respirations greater than 24 per minute may indicate beginning cardiac decompensation, especially if accompanied by dyspnea, and require further evaluation. The nurse also auscultates the woman's lungs frequently for rales and carefully observes for other signs of developing decompensation.

To ensure cardiac emptying and adequate oxygenation, the nurse encourages the laboring woman to assume either a semi-Fowler's position with lateral tilt or side-lying position with her head and shoulders elevated. Oxygen by mask, diuretics to reduce fluid retention, sedatives and analgesics, prophylactic antibiotics, and digitalis may also be used as indicated by the woman's status.

The nurse remains with the woman to support her. It is essential that the nurse keep the woman and her family informed of labor progress and management plans, collaborating with them to fulfill their wishes for the birth experience as much as possible. The nurse needs to maintain an atmosphere of calm to lessen the anxiety of the woman and her family.

Continuous electronic fetal monitoring is used to provide ongoing assessment of the fetus's response to labor. To prevent overexertion and the accompanying fatigue, the nurse encourages the woman to sleep and relax between contractions and provides her with emotional support and encouragement. During pushing, the nurse encourages the woman to use shorter, more moderate open glottis pushing (see Chapter 24), with complete relaxation between pushes. The nurse monitors vital signs closely during the second stage.

Postpartum Period

The postpartal period is a significant time for the woman with cardiac disease. After birth, the intra-abdominal pressure and the venous pressure are reduced, the splanchnic vessels engorge, and blood flow to the heart increases. As extravascular fluid returns to the bloodstream for excretion, cardiac output and blood volume increase. This physiologic adaptation places great strain on the heart and may lead to decompensation, especially in the first 48 hours postpartum.

So that the healthcare team can detect any possible problems, the woman may remain in the hospital longer than the low-risk woman postpartally. Her vital signs are monitored frequently, and she is assessed for signs of decompensation. She stays in the semi-Fowler's or side-lying position, with her head and shoulders elevated, and begins a gradual, progressive activity program. Appropriate diet and stool softeners facilitate bowel movement without undue strain.

The postpartum nurse gives the woman opportunities to discuss her birth experience and helps her deal with any feelings or concerns that cause her distress. The nurse also encourages maternal-infant attachment by providing frequent opportunities for the mother to interact with her child.

Because there is no evidence that cardiac output is compromised during lactation, the only concern about breastfeeding for women with cardiovascular disease is related to medications that the mother may be taking. These must be evaluated for their ability to pass into the milk and for any effect of the drug on lactation. The nurse can assist the breastfeeding mother to a comfortable side-lying position with her head moderately elevated or to a semi-Fowler's position. To conserve the mother's energy, the nurse should position the newborn at the breast and be available to burp the baby and reposition him or her at the other breast. The nurse can also encourage family members to provide the new mother with support and assistance as needed to help her avoid becoming fatigued.

In addition to providing the normal postpartum discharge teaching, the nurse stresses that follow-up for the new mother is imperative. Moreover, the nurse should ensure that the woman and her family understand the signs of possible problems resulting from her heart disease or from other postpartal complications. For women with heart disease, postpartum complications such as hemorrhage, thromboembolism, anemia, and infection pose a real threat and may even precipitate heart failure.

MEDIALINK HEART DISEASE AND PREGNANCY

Table 19–5 • LESS COMMON MEDICAL CONDITIONS AND PREGNANCY

Condition	Brief Description	Maternal Implications	Fetal/Neonatal Implications
Rheumatoid arthritis	Chronic inflammatory disease believed to be caused by a genetically influenced antigen-antibody reaction. Symptoms include fatigue, low-grade fever, pain and swelling of joints, morning stiffness, pain on movement. Treated with salicylates, physical therapy, and rest. Corticosteroids used cautiously if not responsive to above.	Usually there is remission of rheumatoid arthritis symptoms during pregnancy, often with a relapse postpartum. Anemia may be present due to blood loss from salicylate therapy. Mother needs extra rest, particularly to relieve weight-bearing joints, but needs to continue range-of-motion exercises. If in remission, may stop medication during pregnancy.	Possibility of prolonged gestation and longer labor with heavy salicylate use. Possible teratogenic effects of salicylates.
Epilepsy	Chronic disorder characterized by seizures; may be idiopathic or secondary to other conditions, such as head injury, metabolic and nutritional disorders such as PKU or vitamin B_6 deficiency, encephalitis, neoplasms, or circulatory interferences. Treated with anticonvulsants.	Vast majority of pregnancies in women with seizure disorders are uneventful and have an excellent outcome. Women with more frequent seizures before pregnancy may have exacerbations during pregnancy, but this may be related to nausea and vomiting, lack of cooperation with drug regimen, or sleep deprivation. During pregnancy the woman should continue to be treated with the medication that best controls her seizures. Folic acid therapy should be started prior to conception if possible. Folic acid and vitamin D are indicated throughout pregnancy (Crawford, 2001).	Certain anticonvulsant medications are associated with increased incidence of congenital anomalies, especially cleft lip and heart defects, although the incidence has decreased in recent years. This may be due to the fact that the current ability to determine blood levels of medications has led to more accurate dosages and the resultant use of a single medication; consequently multiple medications are used less often (Crawford, 2001).
Hepatitis B	Hepatitis B, caused by the hepatitis B virus (HBV), is a major, growing health problem. Groups at risk include those from areas with a high incidence (primarily developing countries), illegal IV drug users, prostitutes, homosexuals, those with multiple sex partners, or occupational exposure to blood, although many infected people have no identifiable source of infection. HBV transmission is blood borne, primarily sexually and perinatally transmitted. Because of the dramatic increase and the difficulty of vaccinating high-risk individuals before they become infected, the CDC now recommends (1) testing all pregnant women for the presence of hepatitis B surface antigen (HBsAG); (2) routine vaccination of all newborns; (3) vaccination of older children at high risk for hepatitis B; (4) vaccination of children age 11–12 years who have not previously received the vaccine; (5) vaccination of adolescents and adults at high risk for infection (CDC, 1998).	Hepatitis B does not usually affect the course of pregnancy. However, chronic HBV carriers have a great potential for infecting others when exposure to blood and body fluids occurs. In addition, chronic carriers may develop long-term sequelae, such as chronic liver disease and liver cancer. Approximately 4000 to 5000 deaths are caused annually by liver disease associated with chronic HBV infection. It is now recommended that all pregnant women be tested for the presence of hepatitis B surface antigen (HBsAg). A woman who is negative may be given the hepatitis vaccine.	Perinatal transmission most often occurs at or near the time of childbirth. More important, the risk of becoming a chronic carrier of the HBV is inversely related to the age of the individual at the time of initial infection (Shiraki, 2000). Therefore infants infected perinatally have the highest risk of becoming chronically infected if not treated. Recommendations now include routine vaccination of all neonates born to HBsAg-negative women and immunoprophylaxis to all newborns of HBsAg-positive women.
Hyperthyroidism (thyrotoxicosis)	Enlarged, overactive thyroid gland; increased T_4:TBG ratio and increased BMR. Symptoms include muscle wasting, tachycardia, excessive sweating, and exophthalmos. Treatment by antithyroid drug propylthiouracil (PTU) while monitoring free T_4 levels. Surgery used only if drug intolerance exists.	Mild hyperthyroidism is not dangerous. Increased incidence of preeclampsia and postpartum hemorrhage if not well controlled. Serious risk related to thyroid storm characterized by high fever, tachycardia, sweating, and congestive heart failure. Now occurs rarely. When diagnosed during pregnancy, may be transient or permanent.	Neonatal thyrotoxicosis is rare. Even low doses of antithyroid drug in mother may produce a mild fetal/neonatal hypothyroidism; higher dose may produce a goiter or mental deficiencies. Fetal loss not increased in euthyroid women. If untreated, rates of abortion, intrauterine death, and stillbirth increase. Breastfeeding contraindicated for women on antithyroid medication because it is excreted in the milk (may be tried by woman on low dose if neonatal T_4 levels are monitored).

The nurse plans with the woman an activity schedule that is gradual, progressive, and appropriate to her needs and home environment. The nurse provides appropriate health teaching, including information about resumption of sexual activity and contraception. Visiting nurse or homemaker assistance referrals may be necessary, depending on the woman's status.

Evaluation

Expected outcomes of nursing care include the following:

- The woman is able to discuss her condition and its possible impact on her pregnancy, labor and birth, and the postpartal period.

Table 19–5 • CONTINUED

Condition	Brief Description	Maternal Implications	Fetal/Neonatal Implications
Hypothyroidism	Characterized by inadequate thyroid secretions (decreased T_4:TBG ratio), elevated TSH, lowered BMR, and enlarged thyroid gland (goiter). Symptoms include lack of energy, excessive weight gain, cold intolerance, dry skin, and constipation. Treated by thyroxine replacement therapy.	Long-term replacement therapy usually continues at same dosage during pregnancy as before. Weekly nonstress test (NST) after 35 weeks' gestation.	If mother untreated, fetal loss 50%; high risk of congenital goiter or true cretinism. Therefore newborns are screened for T_4 level. Mild TSH elevations present little risk because TSH does not cross the placenta.
Maternal phenylketonuria (PKU) (hyperphenylalaninemia)	Inherited recessive single gene anomaly causing a deficiency of the liver enzyme needed to convert the amino acid phenylalanine to tyrosine, resulting in high serum levels of phenylalanine. Brain damage and mental retardation occur if not treated early.	Low phenylalanine diet is mandatory before conception and during pregnancy. The woman should be counseled that her children will either inherit the disease or be carriers, depending on the zygosity of the father for the disease. Treatment at a PKU center is recommended.	Risk to fetus if maternal treatment not begun preconception. In untreated women increased incidence of fetal mental retardation, microcephaly, congenital heart defects, and growth retardation. Fetal phenylalanine levels are approximately 50% higher than maternal levels.
Multiple sclerosis	Neurologic disorder characterized by destruction of the myelin sheath of nerve fibers. The condition occurs primarily in young adults, more commonly in females, and is marked by periods of remission; progresses to marked physical disability in 10 to 20 years.	Associated with remission during pregnancy, but with slightly increased relapse rate postpartum (Haas, 2000). Rest is important; help with child care should be planned. Uterine contraction strength is not diminished, but because sensation is frequently lessened, labor may be almost painless.	Increased evidence of a genetic predisposition. Therefore reproductive counseling is recommended.
Systemic lupus erythematosus (SLE)	Chronic autoimmune collagen disease, characterized by exacerbations and remissions; symptoms range from characteristic rash to inflammation and pain in joints, fever, nephritis, depression, cranial nerve disorders, and peripheral neuropathies.	Women are generally advised that SLE should be in remission for at least 5–7 months before conceiving. Pregnancy does not appear to alter the long-term prognosis of women with SLE, but maternal morbidity and mortality increase. They also face an increased risk of renal or CNS deterioration after pregnancy. (Yasmeen, Wilkins, Field, et al, 2001)	Increased incidence of spontaneous abortion, stillbirth, prematurity, and IUGR. Infants born to women with SLE may have characteristic skin rash, which usually disappears by 12 months. Infants are at increased risk for complete congenital heart block, a condition that can be diagnosed prenatally. Fetal echocardiography is then performed to rule out other cardiac defects (Shillingford & Weiner, 2001).
Tuberculosis (TB)	Infection caused by *Mycobacterium tuberculosis;* inflammatory process causes destruction of lung tissue, increased sputum, and coughing. Associated primarily with poverty and malnutrition and may be found among refugees from countries where TB is prevalent. Treated with isoniazid and either ethambutol or rifampin or both.	The incidence of tuberculosis has begun to increase significantly since the late 1980s, and it is increasingly associated with HIV infection (Simpkins et al, 1996). If TB inactive due to prior treatment, relapse rate no greater than for nonpregnant women. When isoniazid is used during pregnancy, the woman should take supplemental pyridoxine (vitamin B6). Extra rest and limited contact with others is required until disease becomes inactive.	If maternal TB is inactive, mother may breastfeed and care for her infant. If TB is active, newborn should not have direct contact with mother until she is noninfectious. Isoniazid crosses the placenta, but most studies show no teratogenic effects. Rifampin crosses the placenta. Possibility of harmful effects still being studied.

- The woman participates in developing an appropriate healthcare regimen and follows it throughout her pregnancy.
- The woman gives birth to a healthy infant.
- The woman does not develop congestive heart failure, thromboembolism, or infection.
- The woman is able to identify signs and symptoms of possible postpartum complications.
- The woman is able to care effectively for her newborn infant.

Other Medical Conditions and Pregnancy

A woman with a preexisting medical condition should be aware of the possible impact of pregnancy on her condition, as well as the impact of her condition on the outcome of her pregnancy. Table 19–5 • discusses some of the less common medical conditions vis-à-vis pregnancy.

Chapter Review

ExploreMediaLink

NCLEX review questions, case studies, and other interactive resources for this chapter can be found on the Web site at http://www.prenhall.com/olds. Click on "Chapter 19" to select the activities for this chapter.

For tutorials including animations and videos, more NCLEX review questions, and an audio glossary, access the accompanying CD-ROM in this book.

Focus Your Study

- Almost any health problem that a person can have when not pregnant can coexist with pregnancy. Some problems, such as anemias, may be exacerbated by pregnancy. Others, such as collagen disease, may go into temporary remission with pregnancy. Regardless of the health problem, careful healthcare is needed throughout pregnancy to improve the outcome for mother and fetus.
- The diagnosis of high-risk pregnancy can shock an expectant couple. Providing emotional support, teaching about the condition and prognosis, and educating for self-care are important nursing measures that help the client cope.
- Substance abuse (either drugs or alcohol) not only is detrimental to the mother's health but also may have profound lasting effects on the fetus.
- The key point in the care of the pregnant woman with diabetes is scrupulous maternal plasma glucose control. This is best achieved by home blood glucose monitoring, multiple daily insulin injections, regular exercise, and a careful diet. To reduce incidence of congenital anomalies and other problems in the newborn, the woman should be euglycemic (have a normal blood glucose) throughout the pregnancy. Women with diabetes, even more than most other clients, need to be educated about their conditions and involved with their own care.
- Anemia indicates inadequate levels of hemoglobin (Hb) in the blood. Anemia is defined as hemoglobin less than 12 g/dL in nonpregnant women and less than 10 g/dL in pregnant and postpartum women. Iron deficiency anemia is the most common form of anemia. Other anemias include folic acid deficiency, sickle cell anemia, and thalassemia.
- HIV infection, which is transmitted via blood and body fluids, may also be transmitted transplacentally to the fetus. Currently, there is no definitive therapy for HIV/AIDS. Nurses should employ blood and body fluid precautions (universal precautions) in caring for all women to avoid potential spread of infection.
- Cardiac disease during pregnancy requires careful assessment, limitation of activity, and knowing and reporting signs of impending cardiac decompensation by both client and nurse.

References

American Academy of Pediatrics (AAP) & American College of Obstetricians and Gynecologists (ACOG). (1997). *Guidelines for perinatal care* (4th ed.). Elk Grove Village, IL: Author.

American College of Obstetricians and Gynecologists (ACOG). (1999). *Psychosocial risk factors: Perinatal screening and intervention* (ACOG Educational Bulletin No. 255). Washington, DC: Author.

American College of Obstetricians and Gynecologists (ACOG). (2000a). *Genetic screening for hemoglobinopathies* (ACOG Committee Opinion No. 238). Washington, DC: Author.

American College of Obstetricians and Gynecologists (ACOG). (2000b). *Scheduled cesarean delivery and the prevention of vertical transmission of HIV infection* (ACOG Committee Opinion No. 234). Washington, DC: Author.

American College of Obstetricians and Gynecologists (ACOG). (2000c). *Smoking cessation during pregnancy* (ACOG Educational Bulletin No. 260). Washington, DC: Author.

American College of Obstetricians and Gynecologists (ACOG). (2001a). *Gestational diabetes* (ACOG Practice Bulletin No. 30). Washington, DC: Author.

American College of Obstetricians and Gynecologists (ACOG). (2001b). *Human immunodeficiency virus: Ethical guidelines for obstetricians and gynecologists* (ACOG Committee Opinion No. 255). Washington, DC: Author.

American Diabetes Association (2000). Position statement: Gestational diabetes mellitus. *Diabetes Care, 23* (Suppl. 1), 577–579.

Bergin, C., Cameron, C. E., Fleitz, R. S., & Patel, A. V. (2001). Measuring prenatal drug exposure. *Journal of Pediatric Nursing: Nursing Care of Children & Families, 16*(4), 245–255.

Botto, L. D., Moore, C. A., Khoury, M. J., & Erickson, J. D. (1999). Neural tube defects. *New England Journal of Medicine, 341*(20), 1509–1510.

Broening, H. W., Morford, L. L., Inman-Wood, S. L., Fukumura, M., & Vorhees, C. V. (2001). 3,4-methylenedioxymethamphetamine (Ecstasy)-inducing learning and memory impairments depend on the age of exposure during early development. *Journal of Neuroscience, 21*(9), 3228–3235.

Carpenter, C. C. J., Fischl, M. A., Hammer, S. M., Hirsch, M. S., Jacobsen, D. M., Katzenstein, D. A., et al. (1998). Antiretroviral therapy for HIV infection in 1998. *Journal of the American Medical Association, 280*(1), 78–85.

Caughron, K. F., & Smith, E. L. Diabetes mellitus. Selected Guidelines. *Medscape* Retrieved March 29, 2002 from www.medscape.com/viewarticle/426920_print

Centers for Disease Control and Prevention (CDC). (2002a). Health, United States, 2002. Hyattsville, MD: Author.

Centers for Disease Control and Prevention (CDC). (2002b). Sexually transmitted diseases treatment guidelines 2002. *Morbidity and Mortality Weekly Report, 47*(RR-6), 1–84.

Centers for Disease Control and Prevention (CDC). (2001b). *U.S. HIV and AIDS cases reported through December 2000* (Year-end edition, Vol.12, No.2). Retrieved November 17, 2002 from http://www.cdc.gov/hiv/stats/hasr1202.htm

Centers for Disease Control and Prevention (CDC). (2001a). Revised recommendations for HIV screening of pregnant women. *Morbidity and Mortality Weekly Report, 50*(RR-19), 59–86.

Centers for Disease Control and Prevention (CDC). (1999). USPHS/IDSA guidelines for the prevention of opportunistic infection in persons infected with human immunodeficiency virus. *Morbidity and Mortality Weekly Report, 48*(RR-10), 1–10.

Centers for Disease Control and Prevention. (1998). Guidelines for the use of antiretroviral agents in pediatric infection. *Morbidity and Mortality Weekly Report, 47*(RR-4), 1–43.

Classen, S. R., Paulson, P. R., & Zacharias, S. R. (1998). Systemic lupus erythematosus: Perinatal and neonatal implications. *Journal of Obstetric, Gynecologic, and Neonatal Nursing, 27*(5), 493–500.

Cleveland Clinic, (2003). Hypoglycemia. Retrieved February 3, 2003 from http://www.clevelandclinic.org/health/health-info/docs/0000/0098.asp

Cockey, C. D. (2001). On the edge. Prenatal ecstasy use and long-term memory loss. *AWHONN Lifelines, 5*(4), 23.

Crawford, P. (2001). Epilepsy and pregnancy. *Seizure, 10*(3), 212–219.

Criteria Committee of the New York Heart Association. (1994). *Nomenclature and criteria for diagnosis of diseases of the heart and great vessels* (9th ed.). Dallas, TX: American Heart Association.

Cunningham, F. G., Gant, N. F., Leveno, K. J., Gilstrap, L. C., III, Hauth, J. C., & Wenstrom, K. D. (2001). *Williams obstetrics* (21st ed.). New York: McGraw-Hill.

Curet, L. B. (2000). Obstetric management of diabetes mellitus in pregnancy. In J. J. Sciar, (Ed.), *Maternal and fetal medicine* (Vol 3, chap. 14, pp. 1–10).

Dashe, J. S., Nathan, L., McIntire, D. D., & Leveno, K. J. (2000). Correlation between amniotic fluid glucose concentration and amniotic fluid volume in pregnancy complicated by diabetes. *American Journal of Obstetrics and Gynecology, 182*(4), 901–904.

de Weerd, S., Thomas, C. M., Cikot, R. J., Steegers-Theunissen, R. P., de Boo, T. M., & Steegers, E. A. (2002). Preconception counseling improves folate status of women planning pregnancy. *Obstetrics & Gynecology, 99*(1), 45–51.

Friedman, J. M., & Polifka, J. E. (1996). *The effects of drugs on the fetus and nursing infant.* Baltimore, MD: John Hopkins University Press.

Gowing, L. R., Henry-Edwards, S. M., Irvine, R. J., & Ali, R. L. (2002). The health effects of ecstasy: A literature review. *Drug and Alcohol Review, 21*(1), 53–62.

Guralnick, M. J. (1997). *The effectiveness of early intervention.* Baltimore, MD: Paul Brookes.

Haas, J. (2000). High dose IVIG in the post partum period for prevention of exacerbations in MS. *Multiple Sclerosis, 6* (Suppl. 2), S18–20.

Hsu, H. W., Moye, J., Jr., Kunches, L., Ng, P., Shea, B., Caldwell, B., et al. (1992). Perinatally acquired human immunodeficiency virus infection: Extent of clinical recognition in a population-based cohort [Massachusetts Pediatric HIV Surveillance Working Group]. *Pediatric Infectious Disease Journal, 11*(11), 941–945.

Idrogo, M. A., & Mazze, R. S. (1998). Gestational diabetes: Implications for women's health. *The Female Patient, 23*(5), 19–34.

Jensen, C. E., Tuck, S. M., & Wonke, B. (1995). Fertility in beta thalassemia major: A report of 16 pregnancies, preconceptual evaluation and a review of the literature. *British Journal of Obstetrics and Gynaecology, 102*(8), 625–629.

Jovanovic, L. (2000). Role of diet and insulin treatment of diabetes in pregnancy. *Clinical Obstetrics and Gynecology, 43*(1), 46–55.

Kjos, S. L. (2000). Postpartum care of the women with diabetes. *Clinical Obstetrics and Gynecology, 43*(1), 65–74.

Landesman, S. H., Kalish, L. A., Burns, D. N., Minkoff, H., Fox, H. E., Zorrilla, C., et al. (1996, June 20). Obstetrical factors and the transmission of human immunodeficiency virus type 1 from mother to child: The Women and Infants Transmission Study. *New England Journal of Medicine, 334*(25), 1617–1623.

Landon, M. B. (2000). Obstetric management of pregnancies complicated by diabetes mellitus. *Clinical Obstetrics and Gynecology, 43*(1), 65–74.

Langer, N., & Langer, O. (2000). Comparison of pregnancy mood profiles in gestational diabetes and preexisting diabetes. *Diabetes Educator, 26*(4), 667–672.

March of Dimes. (2002). *Cocaine use during pregnancy. For professionals and researchers.* Retrieved November 17, 2002, from www.marchofdimes.com

Margono, F., Mroueh, J., Garely, A., White, D., Duerr, A., & Minkoff, H. L. (1994). Resurgence of active tuberculosis among pregnant women. *Obstetrics & Gynecology, 83*(6), 911–914.

Martin, S. R., & Foley, M. R. (2002). Adult-onset heart disease in pregnancy. *Contemporary OB/GYN, 47*(11), 74–92.

Mason, B. A., & Bobrowski, R. A. (1998). Cardiac disease. *Contemporary OB/GYN, 43*(8), 15–26.

McComish, J. F., Greenberg, R., Ager, J., Chruscial, H., & Laken, M. A. (2000). Survival analysis of three treatment modalities in a residential substance abuse program for women and children. *Outcomes Management for Nursing Practice, 4*(2), 71–77.

Mersereau, P. W. (2000). Preventing neural tube defects: A national campaign. *Small Talk, 12*(2), 1–5.

Montoya, A. G., Sorrentino, R., Lukas, S. E., & Price, B. H. (2002). Long-term neuropsychiatric consequences of "ecstasy" (MDMA): A review. *Harvard Review of Psychiatry, 10*(4), 212–220.

Office of National Drug Control Policy. (2002). Club drugs. *Drug Facts.* Retrieved November 17, 2002, from www.whitehousedrugpolicy.gov

Pearson, D. A., McGrath, N. M., Nozyce, M., Nichols, S. L., Raskino, C., Brouwers, P., et al. (2000). Predicting HIV disease progression in children using measures of neuropsychological and neurological functioning. Pediatric AIDS clinical trials 152 study team. *Pediatrics, 106*(6), E76.

Perinatal HIV Guidelines Working Group Members: US Public Health Service Task Force recommendations for the use of antiretroviral drugs in pregnant women infected with HIV-1 for maternal health and for reducing perinatal HIV-1 transmission in the United States. (2000, February 25). Retrieved January 24, 2001, from http://www.hivatis.org?list

Schaefer-Graf, U. M., Buchanan, T. A., Xiang, A., Songster, G., Montoro, M., & Kjos, S. L. (2000). Patterns of congenital anomalies and relationship to initial maternal fasting glucose levels in pregnancies complicated by type 2 and gestational diabetes. *American Journal of Obstetrics and Gynecology, 182*(2), 313–320.

Shields, L. E., Gan, E. A., Murphy, H. F., Sahn, D. J., & Moore, T. R. (1993). The prognostic value of hemoglobin A1c in predicting fetal heart disease in diabetic pregnancies. *Obstetrics & Gynecology, 81*(6), 954–957.

Shillingford, A. J., & Weiner, S. (2001). Maternal issues affecting the fetus. *Clinics in Perinatology, 28*(1), 31–70.

Shiraki, K. (2000). Perinatal transmission of hepatitis B virus and its prevention. *Journal of Gastroenterology & Hepatology, 15* (Suppl.), 11–15.

Simpkins, S. M., Hench, C. P., & Bhatia, G. (1996). Management of the obstetric patient with tuberculosis. *Journal of Obstetric, Gynecologic, and Neonatal Nursing, 25*(5), 305–312.

Singer, L.T., Hawkins, S., Huang, J., Davillier, M., & Baley, J. (2001). Developmental outcomes and environmental correlates of very low birthweight, cocaine-exposed infants. *Early Human Development, 64*(2), 91–103.

Smith, J. A., Espeland, M., Bellevue, R., Bonds, D., Brown, A. K., & Koshy, M. (1996). Pregnancy in sickle cell disease: Experience of the cooperative study of sickle cell disease. *Obstetrics & Gynecology, 87*(2), 199–204.

Spellacy, W. N. (1999). Diabetes mellitus and pregnancy. In J. R. Scott, P. J. Di Saia, C. B. Hammord, & W. N. Spellacy (Eds.). *Danforth's obstetrics and gynecology* (8th ed., pp. 301–308). Philadelphia: Lippincott Williams and Wilkins.

Stratton, P., Tuomata, R. E., Abboud, R., Rodriguez, E., Rick, K., Pitt, J., et al. (1999). Obstetric and newborn outcomes in a cohort of HIV-infected pregnant women: A report of the women and infants transmission study. *Journal of Acquired Immune Deficiency Syndromes, 20*(2), 179–186.

Substance Abuse and Mental Health Services Administration (SAMHSA), Office of Applied Studies. *National household survey on drug abuse, 1999 computer assisted interview.* Retrieved April 17, 2002 from http://www.samhsa.gov/oas/nhsda.htm

Substance Abuse and Mental Health Services Administration (SAMHSA), Office of Applied Studies. (2002). *The NHSDA Report: Substance use among pregnant women during 1999 and 2000.* Washington, DC: Author.

Tamada, J. A., Garg, S., Jovanovic, L., Pitzer, K. R., Fermi, S., & Potts, R. O. (1999). Noninvasive glucose monitoring: Comprehensive clinical results. *Journal of the American Medical Association, 282*(19), 1839–1844.

Varney, H. (1997). *Varney's midwifery.* Boston: Jones & Bartlett.

Wang, E. C. (1999). Methadone treatment during pregnancy. *Journal of Obstetric, Gynecologic, and Neonatal Nursing, 28*(6), 615–622.

Yasmeen, S., Wilkins, E. E., Field, N. T., Sheikh, R. A., & Gilbert, W. M. (2001). Pregnancy outcomes in women with systemic lupus erythematosus. *Journal of Maternal-Fetal Medicine, 10*(2), 91–96.

20 Pregnancy at Risk: Gestational Onset

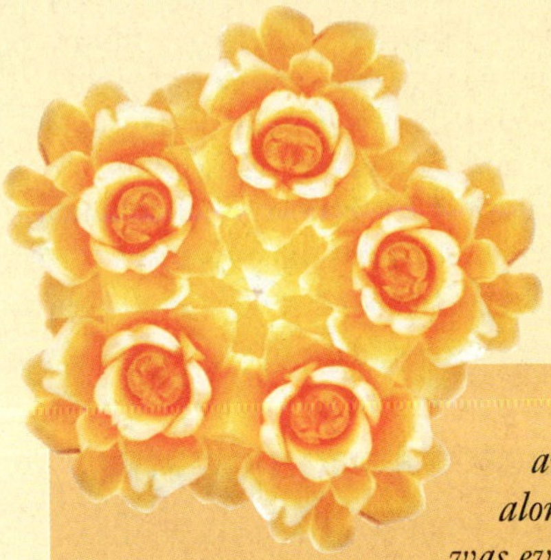

Not long ago, my husband and I happily found out that we were expecting our second child, and although we had experienced it before, we anxiously looked forward to each exciting step along the way. On my second routine prenatal visit, however, we were told that no heartbeat was evident and that I appeared to be nowhere near my then estimated 14 weeks. An ultrasound verified what my doctor had suspected: There was no viable pregnancy—I had miscarried. I was suddenly overwhelmed with a feeling of great loss. But after my D & C, that feeling of loss turned to one of fear and uncertainty as my doctor informed me that no fetal development had existed; I had had a molar pregnancy.

As my doctor told me about the disease and explained the potential risks, it occurred to me that the possibility existed that I might never have another child. Suddenly, my healthy, happy toddler became the most important thing in my life—how blessed I was to have her!

Although some anxiety still exists, I now approach my weekly follow-up visits with a renewed sense of being. It will be at least another year before my husband and I might again rejoice in the anticipation of a second child; but for now we rejoice more fully in the precious one we have.

Objectives

- Contrast the etiology, medical therapy, and nursing interventions for the various bleeding problems associated with pregnancy.
- Identify the medical therapy and nursing interventions indicated in caring for a woman with an incompetent cervix.
- Discuss the medical therapy and nursing care of a woman with hyperemesis gravidarum.
- Discuss the nursing care for a woman experiencing premature rupture of the membranes or preterm labor.
- Describe the development and course of hypertensive disorders associated with pregnancy.
- Explain the cause and prevention of hemolytic disease of the newborn secondary to Rh incompatibility.
- Compare Rh incompatibility to ABO incompatibility with regard to occurrence, treatment, and implications for the fetus/newborn.
- Summarize the effects of surgical procedures on pregnancy, and explain ways in which pregnancy may complicate diagnosis of conditions that require surgery.
- Discuss the implications of trauma due to accidents or battering for the pregnant woman and her fetus.
- Describe the effects of infections on the woman and her unborn child.

MediaLink

Additional resources for this content can be found on the Student CD-ROM and on the Companion Website at www.prenhall.com/olds. Click on "Chapter 20" to select the activities for this chapter.

CD-ROM
- Audio Glossary
- NCLEX Review
- Animation: Early Premature Labor

Companion Website
- Additional NCLEX Review
- Case Study: Client with Preeclampsia
- Care Plan Activity: Client at Risk for Preterm Labor

Key Terms

Abortion 468
Eclampsia 490
Ectopic pregnancy 471
Erythroblastosis fetalis 506
Gestational trophoblastic disease (GTD) 474
HELLP syndrome 492
Hydatidiform mole 474
Hydrops fetalis 506
Hyperemesis gravidarum 478
Incompetent cervix 476
Miscarriage 468
Preeclampsia 490
Premature rupture of membranes (PROM) 479
Preterm labor (PTL) 483
Rh immune globulin (RhoGAM) 508
Tocolysis 485

Pregnancy is usually a normal, uncomplicated experience. In some cases, however, problems arise during the pregnancy that place the woman and her unborn child at risk. Regular prenatal care serves to detect these potential complications quickly so that effective care can be provided. This chapter focuses on problems that primarily occur during pregnancy, those with a gestational onset.

Care of the Woman at Risk Because of Bleeding During Pregnancy

During the first and second trimesters of pregnancy the major cause of bleeding is **abortion.** This is the expulsion of the fetus prior to viability, which is considered 20 weeks' gestation or weight of less than 500 g (Cunningham, Gant, Leveno, et al, 2001). Abortions are either spontaneous, occurring naturally, or induced, occurring as a result of artificial or mechanical interruption. **Miscarriage** is a lay term applied to spontaneous abortion.

Other complications that can cause bleeding in the first half of pregnancy are ectopic pregnancy and gestational trophoblastic disease. In the second half of pregnancy, particularly in the third trimester, the two major causes of bleeding are placenta previa and abruptio placentae.

General Principles of Nursing Intervention

Spotting is relatively common during pregnancy and can occur following sexual intercourse or exercise as a result of trauma to the highly vascular cervix. However, the woman is advised to report any spotting or bleeding that occurs during pregnancy so that it can be evaluated.

It is often the nurse's responsibility to make the initial assessment of bleeding. In general, the following nursing measures should be implemented for pregnant women being evaluated for bleeding during pregnancy:

- Monitor blood pressure and pulse frequently.
- Observe woman for indications of shock, such as pallor, clammy skin, perspiration, dyspnea, or restlessness.
- Count and weigh pads to assess amount of bleeding over a given time period; save any tissue or clots expelled.
- If pregnancy is of 12 weeks' gestation or beyond, assess fetal heart tones with a Doppler.
- Prepare for intravenous (IV) therapy. There may be standing orders to start IV therapy on bleeding clients.
- Prepare equipment for examination.
- Have oxygen therapy available.
- Collect and organize all data, including antepartal history, onset of bleeding episode, laboratory studies (hemoglobin, hematocrit, Rh status, and hormonal assays).
- Obtain an order to type and cross-match for blood if there is evidence of significant blood loss.
- Assess coping mechanisms and support system of woman in crisis. Give emotional support to enhance her coping abilities by continuous, sustained presence, by clear explanation of procedures, and by communicating her status to her family. Most important, prepare the woman for possible fetal loss. Assess her expressions of anger, denial, guilt, depression, or self-blame.
- Assess the family's response to the situation.

Spontaneous Abortion (Miscarriage)

Many pregnancies end in the first trimester as a result of spontaneous abortion. Statistics are inaccurate because some women abort without being aware that they were pregnant during the early weeks of gestation, when the bleeding may be seen as a heavy menstrual period. If these very early abortions are included, the actual incidence of spontaneous abortion may be as high as 60% (Rosevear, 1999). However, when only clinically recognized pregnancies are considered, the incidence falls to approximately 20% (Athey & Spielvogel, 2000). About 1% of childbearing couples have experienced two previous miscarriages (Hill, 1999).

When a spontaneous abortion occurs, the woman and her family may search for a cause so that they can plan knowledgeably for future family expansion. However, even with current technology and medical advances, a direct cause cannot always be determined.

A majority of first trimester spontaneous abortions are related to chromosomal abnormalities. Other causes include teratogenic drugs, faulty implantation due to abnormalities of the female reproductive tract, a weakened cervix, placental abnormalities, chronic maternal diseases, endocrine imbalances, and maternal infections. Some people believe that psychic trauma, alcohol consumption, and accidents are primary causes of abortion, but statistics do not support this belief.

The pathophysiology of spontaneous abortion differs according to the cause. In most cases, embryonic death occurs, which results in loss of human chorionic gonadotropin (hCG) and decreased progesterone and estrogen levels. The uterine decidua is then sloughed off (vaginal bleeding), and the uterus becomes irritable, contracts, and usually expels the embryo/fetus. In late spontaneous abortion, the cause is usually a maternal factor, for example, incompetent cervix or maternal disease, and fetal death may not precede the onset of abortion.

Spontaneous abortion can be extremely distressing to the couple desiring a child. Chances for carrying the next pregnancy to term after one spontaneous abortion are as good as they are for the general population. Thereafter, however, chances of successful pregnancy decrease with each succeeding abortion. Following two to three consecutive losses, a woman and her partner should be evaluated and are candidates for genetic counseling (Hill, 1999).

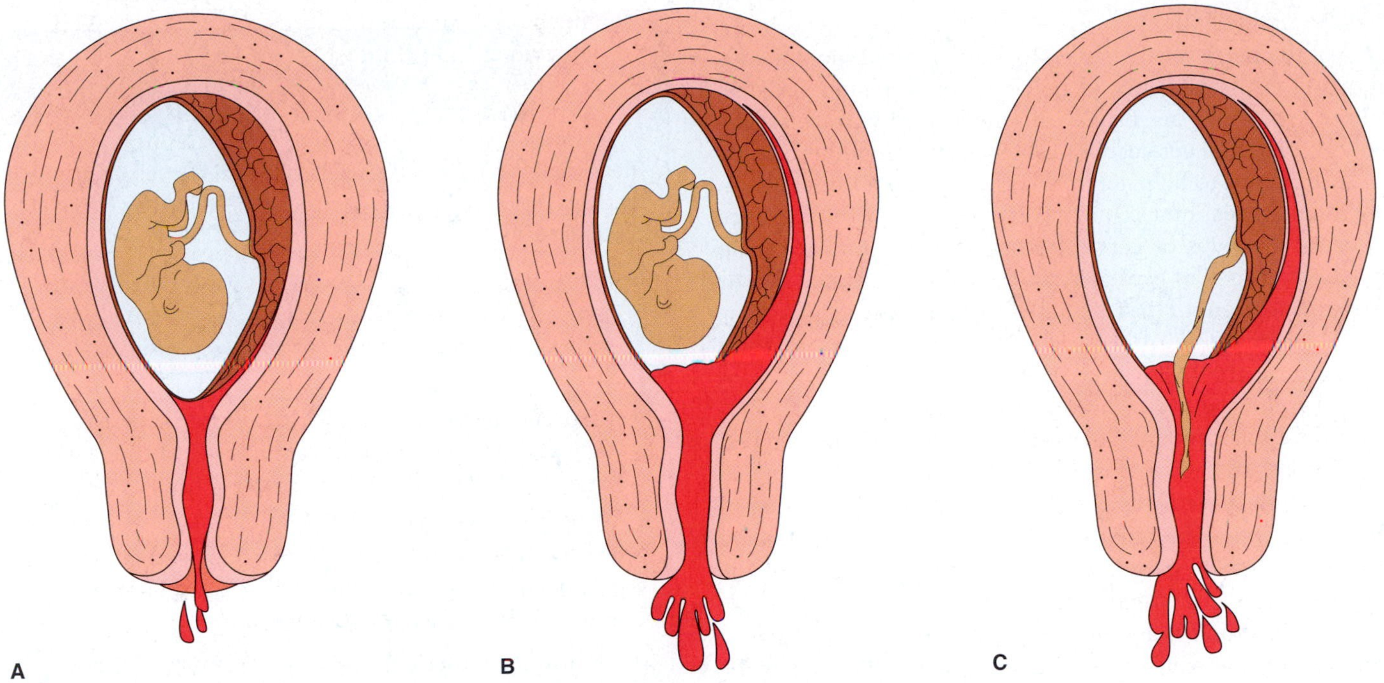

Figure 20–1 • Types of spontaneous abortion. *A,* Threatened. The cervix is not dilated, and the placenta is still attached to the uterine wall, but some bleeding occurs. *B,* Imminent. The placenta has separated from the uterine wall, the cervix has dilated, and the amount of bleeding has increased. *C,* Incomplete. The embryo/fetus has passed out of the uterus; however, the placenta remains.

CLASSIFICATION

Spontaneous abortions are subdivided into the following categories so that they can be differentiated clinically:

- **Threatened abortion** (Figure 20–1, *A* •). Unexplained bleeding, cramping, or backache indicate that the fetus may be in jeopardy. Bleeding may persist for days. The cervix is closed. It may be followed by partial or complete expulsion of pregnancy, or it may resolve without threatening the fetus. Evaluation for hydatidiform mole or ectopic pregnancy (discussed shortly) is advisable.
- **Imminent abortion** (Figure 20–1, *B*). Bleeding and cramping increase. The internal cervical os dilates. Membranes may rupture. The term *inevitable abortion* also applies.
- **Incomplete abortion** (Figure 20–1, *C*). Part of the products of conception are retained, most often the placenta. The internal cervical os is dilated.
- **Complete abortion.** All the products of conception are expelled. The uterus is contracted and the cervical os may be closed.
- **Missed abortion.** The fetus dies in utero but is not expelled. Uterine growth ceases, breast changes regress, and the woman may report a brownish vaginal discharge. The cervix is closed. Diagnosis is made based on history, pelvic examination, and a drop in hCG levels or a negative pregnancy test and may be confirmed by ultrasound if necessary. If the fetus is retained beyond 4 weeks, fetal autolysis (breakdown of cells or tissue) results in the release of thromboplastin, and disseminated intravascular coagulation (DIC) may develop.
- **Recurrent pregnancy loss, formerly called habitual abortion.** Abortion occurs consecutively in three or more pregnancies.
- **Septic abortion.** Presence of infection. Septic abortion is less common since the availability of legal abortion. May occur with prolonged, unrecognized rupture of the membranes, pregnancy with intrauterine device (IUD) in utero, or attempts by inadequately prepared individuals to terminate a pregnancy.

ETIOLOGY

Numerous factors have been implicated as possible causes for recurrent pregnancy loss. They include genetic factors such as a trisomy or a balanced translocation in one of the parents (see Chapter 12), polycystic ovary syndrome, maternal metabolic abnormalities, uterine anatomic abnormalities, and problems with maternal antibody responses (American College of Obstetricians and Gynecologists [ACOG], 2001). Other possible causes include thyroid abnormalities; severe maternal illness such as poorly controlled diabetes mellitus, cyanotic heart disease, inflammatory bowel disease, and phenylketonuria; incompetent cervix (discussed later); maternal infections; environmental chemicals such as benzene, formaldehyde, pesticides, and anesthetic gases; exposure to radiation; chemotherapy; presence of an IUD; and trauma (Simpson & Carson, 2002). In approximately 50% of couples, after a thorough evaluation, the cause of recurrent pregnancy loss remains unexplained.

CLINICAL THERAPY

One of the more reliable indicators of potential spontaneous abortion is the presence of pelvic cramping and backache. These symptoms are usually absent in bleeding caused by polyps, ruptured cervical blood vessels, or cervical erosion.

Evaluations to help determine the cause of vaginal bleeding include speculum examination to determine the presence of cervical polyps or cervical erosion, ultrasound scanning for the presence of cardiac activity and a gestational sac, or crown-rump length that is small for gestational age. Laboratory determination of hCG level can confirm a pregnancy, but because the hCG level falls slowly after fetal death, it cannot confirm a live embryo/fetus. Hemoglobin and hematocrit levels are obtained to assess blood loss. Blood is typed and cross-matched for possible replacement needs.

Although there is no evidence that supports the value of restricting physical activity (Rosevear, 1999), the therapy prescribed for the pregnant woman with bleeding often includes bed rest, abstinence from coitus, and perhaps sedation. If bleeding persists and abortion is imminent or incomplete, the woman may be hospitalized, IV therapy or blood transfusions may be started to replace fluid, and dilation and curettage (D & C) or suction evacuation is performed to remove the remainder of the products of conception. If the woman is Rh negative and not sensitized, Rh immune globulin (RhoGAM) is given within 72 hours. (See discussion on Rh sensitization later in this chapter.)

In missed abortions, the products of conception eventually are expelled spontaneously. If this does not occur within 1 month to 6 weeks after fetal death, hospitalization is necessary. Suction evacuation, or D & C, is done if the pregnancy is in the first trimester. Beyond 12 weeks' gestation, induction of labor by IV oxytocin and intra-amniotic prostaglandin $F_{2\alpha}$, intravaginal prostaglandin E_2, or intravaginal misoprostol (a synthetic prostaglandin E_1 analog) may be used to expel the dead fetus.

Recent studies have indicated that dysfunctional folate metabolism is linked to failed pregnancies. The current recommendation is for periconceptual supplementation with folic acid. (See discussion of folate supplementation in Chapter 18.)

DEVELOPING CULTURAL COMPETENCE

Remember that individual responses to fetal loss following miscarriage may vary greatly and may be influenced by ethnic or cultural norms.

- Miscarriage may be viewed in many ways. For example, it may be seen as a punishment from God, as the result of the evil eye or of a hex or curse by an enemy, or as a natural part of life.
- When grieving over a pregnancy loss, women from some cultures and ethnic groups may show their emotions freely, crying and wailing, whereas other women may hide their feelings behind a mask of stoicism.
- In some cultures the woman's partner is her primary source of support and comfort. In others, the woman turns to her mother or close female relatives for comfort.
- Avoid falling into the trap of stereotyping women according to culture. Individual responses are influenced by many factors including the degree of assimilation into the dominant culture.

NURSING CARE MANAGEMENT

Nursing Assessment and Diagnosis

The nurse assesses the amount and appearance of any vaginal bleeding and monitors the woman's vital signs and degree of discomfort. The woman's blood type and antibody status should be identified to determine the need for Rh immune globulin (see page 508). If the pregnancy is 10 to 12 weeks or more, fetal heart rate should be assessed by Doppler. The nurse also assesses the responses of the woman and her family to this crisis and evaluates their coping mechanisms and ability to comfort each other.

Nursing diagnoses that may apply include the following:

- ***Fear*** related to the risk of pregnancy loss.
- ***Pain*** related to abdominal cramping secondary to threatened abortion.
- ***Anticipatory Grieving*** related to expected loss of unborn child.

Nursing Plan and Implementation

Community-Based Nursing Care

If a woman in her first trimester of pregnancy begins cramping or spotting, she may be evaluated on an outpatient basis if the bleeding is not heavy. Providing emotional support is an important task for nurses caring for women who have spontaneously aborted. Couples who approached the pregnancy with feelings of joy and a sense of expectancy now feel grief, sadness, and possibly anger.

Because many women, even with planned pregnancies, feel some ambivalence initially, guilt is a common emotion. The woman may harbor negative feelings about herself, ranging from lowered self-esteem resulting from a belief that she is lacking or abnormal in some way, to a notion that the abortion may be a punishment for some wrongdoing.

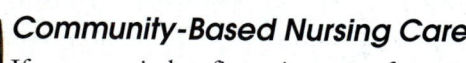

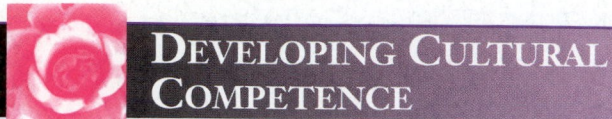

The nurse can offer invaluable psychologic support to the woman and her family by encouraging them to verbalize their feelings, allowing them the privacy to grieve, and listening sympathetically to their concerns about this pregnancy and future ones. The nurse can aid in decreasing any feelings of guilt or blame by supplying the woman and her family with information regarding the causes of spontaneous abortion and possibly referring them to clergy or other healthcare professionals for additional help, such as a genetic counselor if there is a history of habitual abortions.

The grieving period following a spontaneous abortion usually lasts 6 to 24 months. Many couples can be helped during this period by an organization or support group established for parents who have lost a fetus or newborn.

> *We lost our baby together. I know, you could say I never really had a baby, except during those few hours when it was already over and done with, but I guess these things aren't entirely logical. I loved my baby. . . . Absorbed in pain and self-pity, still I was flooded with adoration for this tiny, not yet shaped baby who had lived in me.*
>
> —A MIDWIFE'S STORY

The physical pain of the cramps and the amount of bleeding may be more severe than a couple anticipates, even when they are prepared for the possibility of an abortion. Nurses need to be aware that couples feel unprepared for their first experience of spontaneous abortion. Nurses should offer support in dealing with the physical experience by explaining why the discomfort is occurring and by offering analgesics for pain relief.

Hospital-Based Nursing Care

A suction D & C is performed if the woman experiences an incomplete or missed abortion. This can be performed on an outpatient basis, and, barring any complications, the woman can return home a few hours after the procedure with instructions for self-care. An Rh-negative woman with a negative antibody screen should be given Rh immune globulin prior to discharge.

Throughout the procedure the nurse monitors the woman's physical status and provides emotional support. The nurse also answers any questions the woman or her partner may have and provides referrals to community agencies as needed.

Teaching for Self-Care

If the woman had a D & C, someone should remain with her for the first 12 to 24 hours. The pregnant woman is instructed to report all episodes of heavy bleeding, fever, chills, foul-smelling vaginal discharge, or abdominal tenderness to her healthcare provider. The woman who experiences a pregnancy loss requires information about possible causes of the loss and the chances of recurrence with a future pregnancy. She may also require information about the grief process so she is prepared for it when she goes home. In addition, she should receive information about available resources, including support groups to help her cope with her feelings related to the loss of the pregnancy. The woman's partner or a family member should be included in the educational process when possible to assist him or her in personal grief work as well as to provide tools to help support the woman through the loss.

COMPLEMENTARY AND ALTERNATIVE THERAPIES

HERBS USED FOR PREVENTION OF MISCARRIAGE

Three herbs are frequently used by herbalists for the prevention of miscarriage: black haw, cramp bark, and false unicorn root. (Note that black haw and cramp bark are sometimes considered synonymous, as they are part of the same family. black haw is *Viburnum prunifolium* and cramp bark is *Viburnum opulus.*)

Black Haw: This herb is administered in tincture; tea, or capsule/tablet form, it has a uterine relaxant effect (Skidmore-Roth, 2001).

Cramp Bark: A "cousin" plant to black haw, cramp bark is reported to also have a relaxant effect on the uterine muscles.

False Unicorn Root: Considered a uterine tonic, this root is administered in tincture or dried root form. These three herbs are frequently combined in formulas. They should only be administered by a qualified herbalist. Refer back to "Complementary and Alternative Therapies: Homeopathy and Herbal Medicine" in Chapter 16 (page 381) for reminders about the use of herbs during pregnancy.

Evaluation

Expected outcomes of nursing care include the following:

- The woman is able to explain spontaneous abortion, the treatment measures employed in her care, and long-term implications for future pregnancies.
- The woman suffers no complications.
- The woman and her partner are able to begin verbalizing their grief and to recognize that the grieving process usually lasts several months.

Ectopic Pregnancy

Ectopic pregnancy is an implantation of a fertilized ovum in a site other than the endometrial lining of the uterus. It may result from a number of different causes. Risk factors for ectopic pregnancy include tubal damage caused by pelvic inflammatory disease; previous pelvic or tubal surgery; endometriosis; previous ectopic pregnancy; presence of an IUD; high levels of progesterone, which can alter the motility of the egg in the fallopian tube; congenital anomalies of the tube; use of ovulation-inducing drugs; primary infertility; smoking; advanced maternal age; and douching (Mashburn, 1999).

The incidence of ectopic pregnancy in the United States has risen dramatically from 4.5 per 1000 pregnancies in 1970 to 19.7 per 1000 pregnancies in 2000 (Gracia & Barnhardt, 2001).

In spite of the increasing incidence of ectopic pregnancies, the mortality rate has declined almost 90%. This decrease can be credited to better diagnostic methods, which allow detection prior to tubal rupture (Lipscomb, Stovall, & Ling, 2000).

The actual pathogenesis of ectopic pregnancy occurs when the fertilized ovum is prevented or slowed in its progress down the tube. The fertilized ovum implants in either the fallopian tube or the ovary, peritoneal cavity, cervix, or uterine cornua (Figure 20–2 •). The most common location for implantation of an ectopic pregnancy is the ampulla of the tube.

Initially, the normal symptoms of pregnancy may be present, specifically, amenorrhea, breast tenderness, and nausea. The normal clinical signs of early pregnancy such as the bluish discoloration of the cervix (Chadwick's sign) and the softening of the isthmus (Hegar's sign) may be noted on physical exam. The hormone hCG is present in the blood and urine. With an ectopic implantation, the trophoblastic cells grow into the adjacent tissue, often the tubal wall, and arterial vessels. This results in internal hemorrhage. The faulty implantation of the placenta causes fluctuation of hormone levels. Hormones first stimulate the endometrial lining of the uterus to grow, but fluctuation in levels cannot support the endometrium, and vaginal bleeding ensues. The implanted ovum quickly begins to rupture the fallopian tube if it is implanted there. The woman may experience one-sided lower abdominal pain or diffuse lower abdominal pain and vasomotor disturbances such as fainting or dizziness. In about 50% of cases, referred right shoulder pain occurs from blood irritating the subdiaphragmatic phrenic nerve.

In many instances, the symptoms are not obvious. One fourth of ectopic pregnancies may involve uterine enlargement. Physical examination usually reveals adnexal tenderness; an adnexal mass is palpable in approximately one half of the cases.

If internal hemorrhage is profuse, the woman rapidly develops signs of hypovolemic shock. More commonly, the bleeding is slow (chronic), and the abdomen gradually becomes rigid and very tender. If bleeding into the pelvic cavity has been extensive, vaginal examination causes extreme pain, and a mass of blood may be palpated in the cul-de-sac of Douglas.

Laboratory tests may reveal low hemoglobin and hematocrit levels and rising leukocyte levels. In a normal pregnancy β-hCG titers double every 48 hours from 3 to 6 weeks' gestation. Ectopic pregnancies are associated with β-hCG titers that increase more slowly.

CLINICAL THERAPY

It is important to differentiate an ectopic pregnancy from other disorders with similar clinical presenting pictures. Consideration must be given to possible spontaneous abortion, ruptured corpus luteum cyst, appendicitis, salpingitis, torsion of the ovary, ovarian cysts, and urinary tract infection.

The following measures are used to establish the diagnosis of ectopic pregnancy and assess the woman's status:

- A careful assessment of menstrual history, particularly the last menstrual period (LMP).
- Careful pelvic exam to identify any abnormal pelvic masses and tenderness.
- Laboratory testing as described previously.
- Ultrasonography. In a normal pregnancy, transvaginal ultrasound should detect an intrauterine gestational sac when the β-hCG is greater than 1500 mIU/mL. By transabdominal scan, an intrauterine sac may not be identified until the β-hCG levels reach 6500 mIU/mL. Confirming an intrauterine pregnancy nearly eliminates the diagnosis of ectopic pregnancy.
- Laparoscopy. If the presence or absence of an ectopic pregnancy cannot be confirmed by other measures, laparoscopic intervention may be necessary for both diagnosis and treatment.

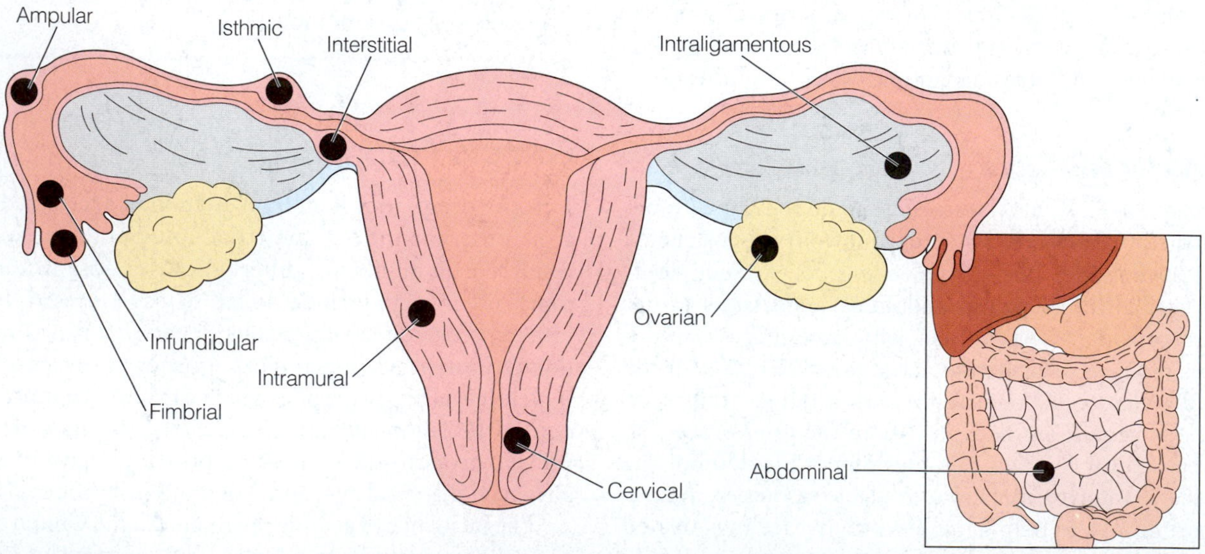

Figure 20–2 • Various implantation sites in ectopic pregnancy. The most common site is within the fallopian tube, hence the name "tubal pregnancy."

Once an ectopic pregnancy is confirmed, therapy options are reviewed with the woman. Recent developments in medical management of ectopic pregnancy include the use of methotrexate, potassium chloride, hyperosmolar glucose, dactinomycin, prostaglandins, and mifepristone. Methotrexate, dactinomycin, prostaglandins, and mifepristone may be given orally, intramuscularly, or intravenously. The others may be injected into the ectopic sac. Only methotrexate has been studied extensively enough to be routinely used as an alternative to surgery (Lipscomb et al, 2000).

Medical management using methotrexate is indicated for the woman who desires future pregnancy if her ectopic pregnancy is unruptured and of 3.5 cm size or less and if her condition is stable. In addition, there must be no fetal cardiac motion and no evidence of maternal thrombocytopenia, leukopenia, kidney disease, or liver disease. The medication is administered intramuscularly. As an outpatient, the woman is monitored for increasing abdominal pain. β-hCG titers are monitored regularly. β-hCG titers increase for 1 to 4 days and then decrease. As many as 25% to 30% of women require a second dose of methotrexate (Cunningham et al, 2001).

If surgery is indicated and the woman desires future pregnancies, a laparoscopic linear salpingostomy will be performed to evacuate the ectopic pregnancy gently and preserve the tube. If the tube is ruptured or if future childbearing is not an issue, laparoscopic salpingectomy (removal of the tube) is performed. If the woman is in shock and unstable, an abdominal incision will be made. During surgery, the most important risk to be considered is potential hemorrhage. Bleeding must be controlled, and replacement therapy should be on hand. The Rh-negative nonsensitized woman is given Rh immune globulin to prevent sensitization.

NURSING CARE MANAGEMENT

Nursing Assessment and Diagnosis

When the woman with a suspected ectopic pregnancy is admitted to the hospital, the nurse assesses the appearance and amount of vaginal bleeding. The nurse monitors vital signs, particularly blood pressure and pulse, for evidence of developing shock.

It is also the nurse's responsibility to assess the woman's emotional status and coping abilities and to evaluate the couple's informational needs. If surgery is necessary, the nurse performs the ongoing assessments appropriate for any client postoperatively.

Nursing diagnoses that may apply for a woman with an ectopic pregnancy include the following:

- ***Anticipatory Grieving*** related to the loss of the pregnancy
- ***Pain*** related to abdominal bleeding secondary to tubal rupture
- ***Health-Seeking Behavior:*** Information about the treatment of ectopic pregnancy related to an expressed desire to gain better understanding of the condition and its long-term implications

Nursing Plan and Implementation

Community-Based Nursing Care

Women with ectopic pregnancy are often seen initially in a clinic or office setting. Nurses need to be alert to the possibility of ectopic pregnancy if a woman presents with complaints of abdominal pain and lack of menses for 1 to 2 months. Once an initial evaluation is complete, if no ultrasound is available, the woman should be referred to another facility where ultrasound is available. The nurse plays an important role in monitoring the woman's condition and in providing her with information.

A woman with a confirmed ectopic pregnancy who meets the criteria for methotrexate administration is followed as an outpatient. The nurse should advise the woman that some abdominal pain is common following the injection but it is generally mild and lasts only 24 to 48 hours. More severe pain might indicate treatment failure and should be evaluated. The woman should also report heavy vaginal bleeding, dizziness, or tachycardia. In addition, the nurse should stress the need to return for follow-up β-hCG testing.

For all women treated for ectopic pregnancy, a follow-up phone call by the nurse may be especially welcome. It gives the woman the opportunity to ask any questions she may have. In addition, the nurse can use the opportunity to assist the woman in dealing with her grief.

Hospital-Based Nursing Care

Once a diagnosis of ectopic pregnancy is made and surgery is scheduled, the nurse starts an IV as ordered and begins preoperative teaching. The nurse should report signs of developing shock to the physician immediately and initiate interventions. If the woman is experiencing severe abdominal pain, the nurse can administer appropriate analgesics and evaluate their effectiveness.

Teaching for Self-Care

Teaching is an important part of nursing care. The woman may want her condition and various procedures explained. She may need instruction about measures to prevent infection, symptoms to report (pain, bleeding, fever, chills), and her follow-up visit.

The woman and her family will need emotional support during this difficult time. Their feelings and responses to this crisis will probably be similar to those that occur in cases of spontaneous abortion. As a result, similar nursing actions are required.

Evaluation

Expected outcomes of nursing care include the following:

- The woman is able to explain ectopic pregnancy, treatment alternatives, and implications for future childbearing.

- The woman and her caregivers detect possible complications early and manage them appropriately.
- The woman and her partner are able to begin verbalizing their loss and recognize that the grieving process usually lasts several months.

Gestational Trophoblastic Disease

As discussed in Chapter 11, the trophoblast is the outermost layer of embryonic cells, and gives rise to the chorion. **Gestational trophoblastic disease (GTD)** is the pathologic proliferation of trophoblastic cells, and includes partial or complete hydatidiform mole, invasive mole (chorioadenoma destruens), and choriocarcinoma.

Hydatidiform mole (molar pregnancy) is a condition in which a proliferation of trophoblastic cells results in the formation of a placenta characterized by *hydropic* (fluid-filled) grapelike clusters. The significance of this disease for the woman who has it is the loss of the pregnancy and the possibility, though remote, of developing choriocarcinoma, a form of cancer, from the trophoblastic tissue.

Molar pregnancies are classified into two types, complete and partial, both of which meet the preceding criteria. Little is known about the cause of either type, but some of the pathophysiology has been clarified. The *complete mole* develops from an anuclear ovum that contains no maternal genetic material, an "empty" egg. In most cases, a haploid sperm, 23X, fertilizes this anuclear egg and duplicates before the first cell division. The conceptus then contains in its cells a 46XX chromosomal set of totally paternal origin (Szulman, 2000). The hydropic vesicles that form from the chorionic villi are avascular in the complete mole. No embryonic or fetal tissue or membranes are found. Choriocarcinoma seems to be associated primarily with the complete mole (Secki, Fisher, Salerno, et al, 2000).

In contrast to the complete mole, the *partial mole* usually has a triploid karyotype, that is, 69 chromosomes. Most often, a normal ovum with 23 chromosomes is fertilized by two sperm (dispermy) or by a sperm that has failed to undergo the first meiosis and therefore contains 46 chromosomes. In about one fifth of the cases, the ovum does not undergo reduction division, so it contains 46 chromosomes and is fertilized by a normal sperm.

In partial molar pregnancy, the villi are often vascularized and may be hydropic only in sections of the placenta rather than universally as with a complete mole. Often partial moles are recognized only after spontaneous abortion, or they may go unnoticed. Unlike the complete mole, the fetus usually survives to 8 or 9 weeks' gestation and occasionally longer. Twin pregnancies in which a normal fetus coexists with a molar pregnancy have been reported (Berman, DiSaia, & Brewster, 1999).

GTD occurs in about 1 in 1000 pregnancies (see Developing Cultural Competence). The incidence of molar pregnancy increases with extremes in maternal age and has a familial tendency. The risk of repeat molar pregnancy has been reported as 1% after one molar pregnancy (Berman et al, 1999; Rosevear, 1999). *Invasive mole* (chorioadenoma destruens) is similar to a complete mole but involves the uterine myometrium. Treatment is the same as for a complete mole.

Choriocarcinoma is invasive, malignant trophoblastic disease that is usually metastatic and can be fatal. It is discussed in more detail shortly.

DEVELOPING CULTURAL COMPETENCE

- The incidence of ectopic pregnancy is higher for nonwhite women than for whites in every age category.
- The incidence of preeclampsia is also related to genetic predisposition. Women of African American descent are at higher risk.
- Until recently, researchers thought that the incidence of GTD was significantly higher in women of Asian ancestry. However, population-based studies show that the incidence of GTD in most of the world is similar to that found in the United States—about 1 in 1000 pregnancies (Cunningham et al, 2001).

CLINICAL THERAPY

Diagnosis of hydatidiform mole is often suspected in the presence of the following signs:

- Vaginal bleeding is almost universal with molar pregnancies and may occur as early as the fourth week or as late as the second trimester. It is often brownish, "like prune juice," due to liquefaction of the uterine clot, but it may be bright red.
- Anemia occurs frequently due to the loss of blood.
- Hydropic vesicles may be passed and, if so, are diagnostic (Figure 20–3 •). With a partial mole, the vesicles are often smaller and may not be noticed by the woman.
- Uterine enlargement greater than expected for gestational age is a classic sign, present in about 50% of cases. In the remainder of cases, the uterus is appropriate or small for the gestational stage. Enlargement is due to the proliferating trophoblastic tissue and to a large amount of clotted blood.
- Absence of fetal heart sounds in the presence of other signs of pregnancy is a classic sign of molar pregnancy. (Only rarely has a viable fetus been born in a partial molar pregnancy.)
- Markedly elevated serum hCG may be present due to continued secretion by the proliferating trophoblastic tissue. (Normally hCG levels increase from the time of implantation, peak at 60 to 70 days, and then decline slowly, reaching a low point at 100 to 130 days [Cunningham et al, 2001]).
- Very low levels of maternal serum α-fetoprotein (MSAFP) are found.

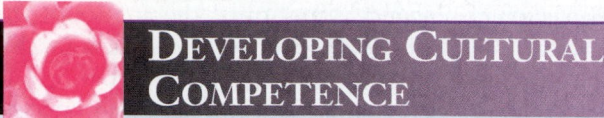

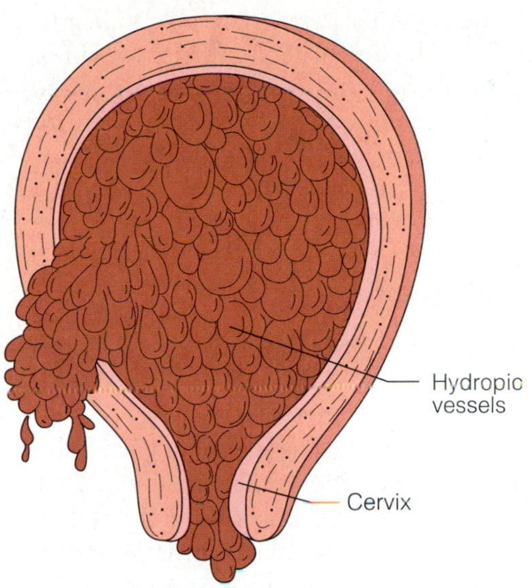

Figure 20–3 • Hydatidiform mole. A common sign is vaginal bleeding, often brownish (the characteristic "prune juice" appearance) but sometimes bright red. In this figure, some of the hydropic vessels are being passed. This occurrence is diagnostic for hydatidiform mole.

- Hyperemesis gravidarum may occur, probably as a result of the high levels of hCG.
- Preeclampsia (discussed shortly) may be seen, especially if the molar pregnancy continues into the second trimester. Because preeclampsia is a disease of late pregnancy, if symptoms occur in the first half of pregnancy, molar pregnancy must be considered as the first diagnosis.
- Rarely, hyperthyroidism results from production of thyrotropin by molar tissue. It produces thyrotoxicosis, which may precipitate a clinical emergency.

Ultrasound is the primary means of diagnosing a molar pregnancy, usually after 6 to 8 weeks, when the vesicular enlargement of the villi can be identified.

Therapy begins with suction evacuation of the mole and curettage of the uterus to remove all fragments of the placenta. Early evacuation decreases the possibility of other complications. If the woman is older and has completed her childbearing, or if there is excessive bleeding, hysterectomy may be the treatment of choice to reduce the incidence of malignant sequelae.

Complications associated with hydatidiform mole that require medical recognition and therapy include the following:

- Anemia
- Hyperthyroidism
- Infection, usually seen with late diagnosis and spontaneous abortion of the mole
- Disseminated intravascular coagulation (DIC)
- Trophoblastic embolization of the lung, usually seen after molar evacuation of a significantly enlarged uterus (this creates a cardiorespiratory emergency)
- Ovarian cysts, which may be small or large enough to displace the uterus

Malignant GTD, usually choriocarcinoma, develops following evacuation of a mole in 20% of women. To detect this serious problem early and initiate treatment, follow-up care is essential. Follow-up for women who have had a mole evacuated consists of baseline chest x-ray examination to detect metastasis and a repeat x-ray if chemotherapy is necessary. Continued high or rising hCG levels in women who have had molar pregnancy but are not currently pregnant suggest secretion of hCG by metastatic trophoblastic cells. Thus, radioimmunoassay hCG values should be determined every week until negative two consecutive times, then should be monitored monthly for 1 year. If hCG plateaus or rises during this time or metastases are detected, chemotherapy is started immediately (Berman et al, 1999). In addition, the woman has physical exams with a pelvic exam every 4 weeks until remission and then every 3 months for 1 year.

Effective contraception is needed during this time to prevent pregnancy and the resulting confusion about the cause of changes in hCG levels. In addition, pregnancy could mask an hCG rise associated with malignant GTD.

Several systems have been proposed for classifying clients with metastatic gestational neoplasms. The World Health Organization (WHO) is used most widely and categorizes clients as low risk, intermediate risk, or high risk. Treatment at a center specializing in GTD is advised. Once pregnancy has been ruled out, full physical examination, chest x-ray, abdominopelvic computed tomography (CT) scan, and brain CT scan are done to rule out metastatic spread. Chemotherapy is then begun using methotrexate alone or in combination with other chemotherapy agents.

After treatment, careful follow-up monitoring of hCG levels is important. Malignant GTD is curable if diagnosed early and treated appropriately. Malignant sequelae appear to be increased with repetitive moles.

NURSING CARE MANAGEMENT

Nursing Assessment and Diagnosis

It is important for nurses involved in antepartal care to be aware of symptoms of hydatidiform mole and observe for them at each antepartal visit. The classic symptoms used to diagnose molar pregnancy are found more frequently with the complete than with the partial mole. The partial mole may be difficult to distinguish from a missed abortion prior to evacuation.

When the woman is hospitalized for evacuation of the mole, the nurse should monitor vital signs and vaginal bleeding for evidence of hemorrhage. In addition, the nurse determines whether abdominal pain is present and assesses the woman's emotional state and coping ability.

Nursing diagnoses that may apply to a woman with a hydatidiform mole include the following:

- ***Fear*** related to the possible development of choriocarcinoma
- ***Health-Seeking Behavior:*** Information about the need for regular monitoring of hCG levels related to an expressed desire to understand the long-term implications of the disease
- ***Anticipatory Grieving*** related to the loss of the pregnancy

Nursing Plan and Implementation

Community-Based Nursing Care

When molar pregnancy is suspected, the woman needs emotional support. The nurse can relieve some of the woman's anxiety by answering questions about the disease process and explaining what ultrasound and other diagnostic procedures will entail. If a molar pregnancy is diagnosed, the nurse supports the childbearing family as they deal with their grief about the lost pregnancy. Healthcare counselors, the hospital chaplain, or their own clergy may be of assistance in helping them deal with this loss.

Hospital-Based Nursing Care

When the woman is hospitalized for evacuation of the mole, explanation of the curettage procedure is necessary. Although the physician is responsible for providing this explanation, the woman and her partner may have many questions and concerns that the nurse can discuss with them. The nurse may also clarify areas of confusion or misunderstanding.

Typed and cross-matched blood must be available for surgery because of previous blood loss and the potential for hemorrhage. Oxytocin is administered to keep the uterus contracted and prevent hemorrhage. In addition, acute renal failure, a syndrome of rapid onset, may occur when significant hemorrhage results in absolute loss of fluid volume. Following surgery, the nurse carefully observes the woman's urinary output, watches for further signs of bleeding, and assesses for any signs of infection.

If the woman is Rh negative and not sensitized, she is given Rh immune globulin to prevent antibody formation. (See discussion on Rh sensitization later in this chapter.)

Teaching for Self-Care

The woman needs to know the importance of the follow-up visits. She is advised to use contraception to delay becoming pregnant again until after the follow-up program is completed.

Evaluation

Expected outcomes of nursing care include the following:

- The woman has a smooth recovery following successful evacuation of the mole.
- The woman is able to explain GTD, its treatment, follow-up, and long-term implications for pregnancy.
- The woman and her partner are able to begin verbalizing their grief at the loss of their anticipated child.
- The woman is able to discuss the importance of follow-up assessment and indicates her willingness to cooperate with the regimen.

Placenta Previa

In *placenta previa,* the placenta is improperly implanted in the lower uterine segment, sometimes over the internal os. As the lower uterine segment contracts and the cervix dilates in the later weeks of pregnancy, the placental villi are torn from the uterine wall, thus exposing the uterine sinuses at the placental site. Bleeding begins, but because its amount depends on the number of sinuses exposed, it may initially be either scanty or profuse. The classic symptom is painless vaginal bleeding usually occurring after 20 weeks' gestation. See Chapter 26 for an in-depth discussion of placenta previa.

Abruptio Placentae

Abruptio placentae is the premature separation of a normally implanted placenta from the uterine wall. It occurs prior to birth, usually during the labor process. It is characterized by maternal pain disproportionate to the strength of uterine contractions and may or may not be accompanied by obvious bleeding. See Chapter 26 for an in-depth description of abruptio placentae.

Care of the Woman with an Incompetent Cervix

Many questions remain unanswered about **incompetent cervix.** The classic definition presents cervical incompetence as painless dilatation of the cervix without contractions because of a structural or functional defect of the cervix. It occurs in 0.1% to 2% of pregnancies (Norwitz, 2002). The woman is usually unaware of contractions and presents with advanced effacement and dilatation and, possibly, bulging membranes. The emerging view is that cervical incompetence and cervical resistance to labor occur as a continuum from complete incompetence through, perhaps, excessive competence demonstrated by those women who have prolonged labors (Iams, 1999).

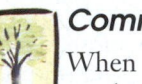

Factors that may contribute to the tendency for the cervix to dilate prematurely can be divided into three categories: congenital factors, acquired factors, and biochemical (hormonal) factors. Congenitally incompetent cervix may be found in women exposed to diethylstilbestrol (DES) or those with a bicornuate uterus. Acquired cervical incompetence may be related to inflammation, infection, subclinical uterine activity, cervical trauma, cone biopsy or late second trimester elective abortions, or increased uterine volume (as with a multiple gestation). The hormone relaxin may be an endocrine cause of cervical incompetence. Researchers suggest that the increased relaxin levels related to ovulation induction may contribute to connective tissue changes in the cervix (Iams, 1999; Landy, 1999).

A woman's obstetric history may give her healthcare provider an indication of increased risk for incompetent cervix. Factors include repetitive second trimester losses, previous preterm birth, progressively earlier births with each subsequent pregnancy, short labors, previous elective abortion or cervical manipulation, DES exposure, or other uterine anomaly. These women will benefit from close surveillance of cervical length with transvaginal ultrasound beginning at about 18 weeks' gestation. Cervical effacement occurs from the internal os out and can be seen on ultrasound as "funneling." Alteration is apparent in transvaginal scan when fundal pressure is applied or the woman assumes a standing position. In addition, women at risk for incompetent cervix need to be informed early in pregnancy of warning signs of impending birth, such as lower back pain, pelvic pressure, and changes in vaginal discharge.

Incompetent cervix has been managed by a variety of methods. Women who are at risk and have cervical lengths of 25 to 30 mm may be managed conservatively with bed rest, avoidance of heavy lifting, and no coitus. Cervical cerclage has become the standard treatment for those who have had previous losses (see Figure 20–4 •). An elective cervical cerclage may be placed late in the first trimester or early in the second trimester. A cervical cerclage involves using a heavy suture to reinforce the cervix at the level of the internal os. The McDonald cerclage utilizes a purse-string technique high up on the cervix to tie it closed. The Shirodkar method uses a submucosal band placed at the level of the internal os. An emergency, urgent "rescue" cerclage may be performed for women who have advanced effacement or dilatation and intact membranes although they may be prolapsing. In this situation, tocolytics (drugs that stop labor), broad-spectrum antibiotics, and anti-inflammatory agents are given perioperatively and for ongoing treatment (Novy, Gupta, Wothe, et al, 2001).

Cerclage should not be placed if intra-amniotic infection, fetal death, fetal anomaly, vaginal bleeding, or premature rupture of the membranes exists. Vaginal cultures should be done to identify bacterial vaginosis, group B streptococcus, or sexually transmitted infections.

An uncomplicated elective cerclage may be done on an outpatient basis or the woman may be hospitalized and discharged after 24 to 48 hours. An emergency cerclage, however, requires hospitalization for 5 to 7 days or longer. After 37 completed weeks' gestation, the suture may be cut and vaginal birth permitted, or the suture may be left in place and a cesarean birth performed to avoid repeating the procedure in subsequent pregnancies.

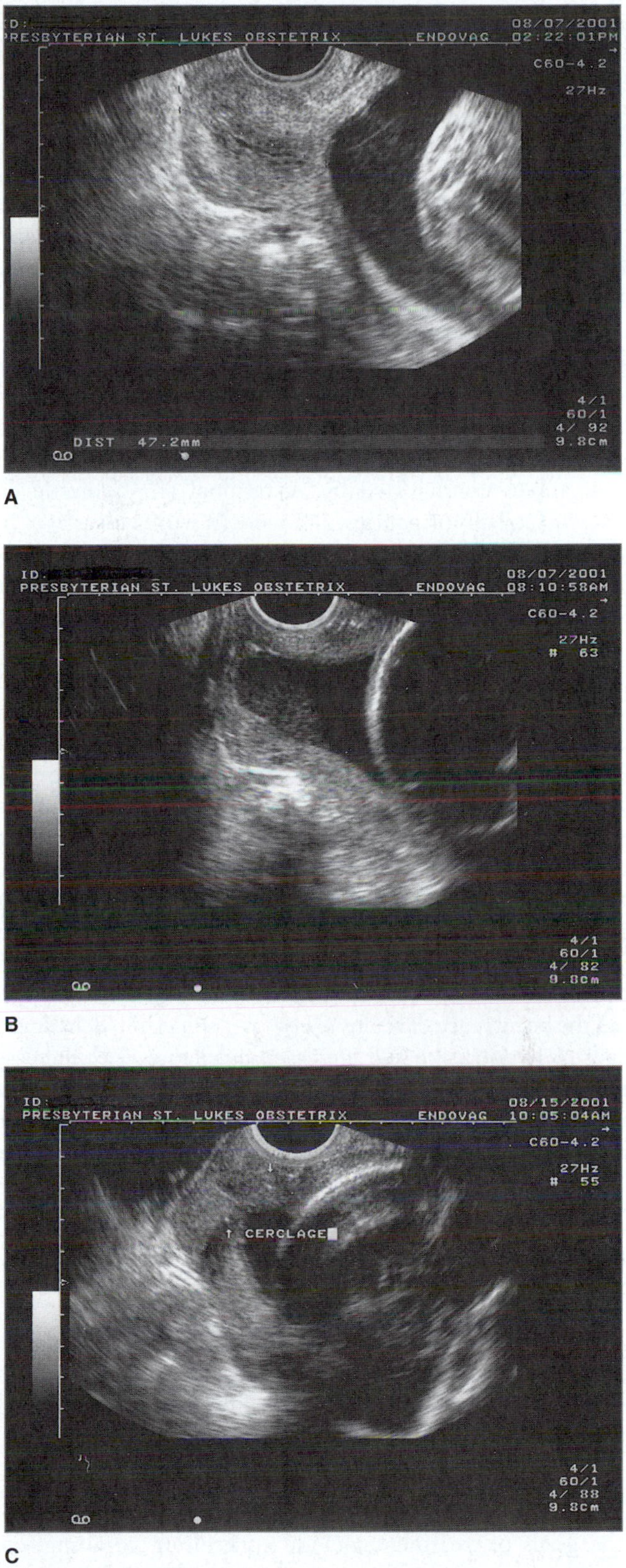

Figure 20–4 • Endovaginal ultrasound of the cervix. *A,* Normal cervix measuring 47.2 mm. *B,* Woman at 24 weeks' gestation with chorioamnionitis and preterm labor. Cervix is fully effaced and dilated 2 cm. *C,* Arrow indicates stitch placement of McDonald cerclage. Cervix is 18.5 cm in length.
SOURCE: Courtesy of Debbie McGee, MSN, PNNP, RDMS.

Care of the Woman with Hyperemesis Gravidarum

Nausea and vomiting of mild to moderate intensity are common during early pregnancy, affecting between 50% and 70% of pregnant women (Eliakim, Abulafia, & Sherer, 2000). It most commonly occurs between 5 and 12 weeks and usually subsides by the end of the first trimester or early second trimester (Steele, French, Gatherer-Boyles, et al, 2001). **Hyperemesis gravidarum** is a relatively rare condition, occurring in about 1% of all pregnancies, in which nausea and vomiting are so severe that they affect hydration and nutritional status. Dehydration, electrolyte imbalances, acidosis, weight loss, ketonuria, and possibly hepatic and renal damage are attributable to hyperemesis (Eliakim et al, 2000).

Hyperemesis can be a temporarily disabling condition in which affected women may need multiple hospitalizations and face disruption of work, family, or social routines. In rare instances, the psychologic impact is so extreme that a woman may request pregnancy termination (Nelson-Piercy, Fayers, & de Swiet, 2001). It occurs more frequently in nulliparous women, adolescents, women with a multiple gestation, women with increased body weight, certain ethnic groups, pregnancies complicated by gestational trophoblastic disease, or fetal abnormalities, and women with a history of hyperemesis in a previous pregnancy (Eliakim et al, 2000).

The cause of hyperemesis during pregnancy is still unclear, but human chorionic gonadotropin (hCG) plays a role. A temporary suppression of thyroid-stimulating hormone occurs in normal pregnancy and is correlated with the rise in hCG. Other mechanisms that may relate to hyperemesis are displacement of the gastrointestinal tract, hypofunction of the anterior pituitary gland and adrenal cortex, abnormalities of the corpus luteum, *Helicobacter pylori* infection, and psychologic factors. Interestingly, hyperemesis is rare in populations of developing countries.

In severe cases, the pathology of hyperemesis begins with dehydration. This leads to fluid-electrolyte imbalance and alkalosis from the loss of hydrochloric acid. More prolonged vomiting can result in loss of predominantly alkaline intestinal juices and the occurrence of acidosis. Hypovolemia from dehydration leads to hypotension and increased pulse rate, with increased hematocrit and blood urea nitrogen levels and decreased urine output. Severe potassium loss (hypokalemia) interferes with the ability of the kidneys to concentrate urine and disrupts cardiac functioning. Starvation causes muscle wasting and severe protein and vitamin deficiencies. Jaundice, hyperpyrexia, and peripheral neuritis may develop. If inadequately or incorrectly treated, complications such as Wernicke encephalopathy, esophageal rupture, or even maternal death may occur.

The diagnostic criteria for hyperemesis include a history of intractable vomiting in the first half of pregnancy, dehydration, ketonuria, and a weight loss of 5% of prepregnancy weight.

Clinical Therapy

The goals of treatment include controlling vomiting, correcting dehydration, restoring electrolyte balance, and maintaining adequate nutrition. If the woman with intractable nausea and vomiting does not respond to frequent small meals of simple carbohydrates and the occasional use of antiemetics, she may require intravenous (IV) fluids on an outpatient basis. If the woman's symptoms do not improve, hospitalization may be necessary.

The initial work-up should include an ultrasound to exclude the possibility of molar pregnancy. Initially the woman is given nothing by mouth; IV fluids are administered to correct dehydration. Potassium chloride is typically added to the IV infusion to prevent hypokalemia. Replacement of thiamine and pyroxidine (vitamin B_6) is important to correct deficiencies of these vitamins and prevent peripheral neuropathy. Administration of dextrose solution prior to the correction of thiamine deficiency could lead to Wernicke encephalopathy (loss of memory, confusion) (Power, Holzman, & Schulkin, 2001). Desired urine output is a minimum of 1000 mL/24 hours.

As long as 50 years ago, corticosteroids were used for the treatment of hyperemesis. Recent studies suggest that steroids can play a beneficial role in the treatment of severe hyperemesis gravidarum. It is thought that corticosteroids exert an antiemetic effect by working on a trigger zone located in the brain stem (Nelson-Piercy et al, 2001).

Complementary therapies have also been tried in treating hyperemesis because they may offer relief for nausea and vomiting of pregnancy. Ginger has been used for its beneficial effects on motion sickness. Although there is little data available on its use for hyperemesis, a small randomized trial demonstrated that ginger significantly reduced the number of vomiting episodes during treatment (Vutyavanich, Kraisarin, & Ruangsri, 2001). The use of acupuncture or Sea-Bands with acupressure may cause a reduction in the severity of symptoms (Knight, Mudge, Openshaw, et al, 2001; Steele et al, 2001).

If the woman does not respond to this management, total parenteral nutrition may be used to meet the caloric and nutritional needs of the woman and her fetus. When the woman's condition has improved, oral feedings are started. Six small dry feedings followed by clear liquids is one suggested treatment. Another method is 1 oz of water offered each hour, followed as tolerated by clear, then nourishing liquids, progressing on succeeding days to low-fat soft and regular diets.

NURSING CARE MANAGEMENT

Nursing Assessment and Diagnosis

When a woman is hospitalized for control of vomiting, the nurse must regularly assess the amount and character of further emesis, intake and output, fetal heart rate, maternal vital signs, initial weight, evidence of jaundice or bleeding, and the woman's emotional state.

Nursing diagnoses that may apply to the woman with hyperemesis gravidarum include the following:

- ***Altered Nutrition: Less than Body Requirements*** related to persistent vomiting secondary to hyperemesis
- ***Fear*** related to the effects of hyperemesis or its treatment on fetal well-being

Nursing Plan and Implementation

Community-Based Nursing Care

The initial evaluation of the woman is designed to distinguish between morning sickness, which is amenable to self-care, and real nutritional risk. The nurse should take this opportunity to evaluate possible family and lifestyle stressors. It is wise to include both the woman and her family in the discussion of strategies to reduce nausea and vomiting she can try at home, including such tactics as small carbohydrate meals, total avoidance of fatty foods, resting with her feet up and head elevated, or slowly sipping carbonated beverages when nauseated. Herbal tea, such as spearmint, peppermint, raspberry, chamomile, or ginger root, may be helpful. Odors, exposure to fresh air, very hot or cold liquids, ice, and straws should be avoided. If the nausea and vomiting progress to a point where oral intake is not tolerated and dehydration is evident, medical intervention is required.

Home Care

Parenteral therapy provided at home in collaboration with a physician and registered dietitian is sometimes used to allow the woman to remain in her home and help decrease healthcare costs. It also gives the nurse an opportunity to observe family interactions and evaluate the home environment. This assessment is often useful in determining the pregnant woman's level of support, any significant stressors in her life, her understanding of nutrition and self-care measures, and so forth.

Hospital-Based Care

Nursing care should be supportive and directed at maintaining a relaxed, quiet environment away from food odors or offensive smells. Once oral feedings are started, food should be attractively served. Oral hygiene is important because the mouth is dry and may be irritated from vomitus. Weight gain or loss should be monitored regularly. Because emotional factors have been found to play a major role in this condition, psychotherapy may be recommended. With proper treatment, the prognosis is favorable.

Teaching for Self-Care

As part of client teaching, the nurse should review actions the woman can take to prevent or decrease nausea. These are discussed in Chapter 16.

Evaluation

Expected outcomes of nursing care include the following:

- The woman is able to explain hyperemesis gravidarum, its therapy, and its possible effects on her pregnancy.
- The woman's condition is corrected, and possible complications are avoided.

Global Perspectives

On Smith Island, a small island in the Chesapeake Bay in Maryland, there are no healthcare providers and no medical facilities. When an islander is in labor, she typically travels 45 minutes by boat and another 45 minutes by car to reach the nearest hospital. Although several women have died en route to the hospital from pregnancy-induced complications, islanders view pregnancy as a normal process and are not afraid even though medical assistance is so remote. Childbirth education is nonexistent on the island and the women rarely share childbirth experiences with younger women because they do not want to scare them. Moreover, pregnant women are protected by the community and are shielded from emotional events, including funerals and sad news.

Care of the Woman with Premature Rupture of Membranes

Spontaneous rupture of the membranes prior to the onset of labor is known as **premature rupture of membranes (PROM).** Some authorities define PROM as the rupture of the bag of waters any time before the onset of labor; others require that a specific period elapse without labor, generally between 1 and 12 hours. *Preterm PROM* has been described as rupture before 37 weeks' gestation. Prolonged rupture of the membranes is rupture more than 24 hours before birth. In the United States, PROM complicates more than 130,000 pregnancies each year and is associated with more than one third of the preterm births (Edwards, Locksmith, & Duff, 2000).

Although the cause of PROM is unknown, it is thought that PROM occurs because of multiple, interrelated factors. An incompetent cervix may be the cause of second trimester PROM (Hassan, Romero, Maymon, et al, 2001). Cervicitis, urinary tract infection (UTI), amniocentesis, placenta previa, abruptio placentae, hydramnios, trauma, multiple pregnancy, and maternal genital tract anomalies may also result in PROM. It has also been suggested that nulliparous women who work outside the home have an increased risk of occupational fatigue and PROM as the hours worked increase (Newman, Goldenberg, Moawad, et al, 2001). Other risk factors include smoking, substance abuse, connective tissue disorders, fetal anomalies, and lower socioeconomic status; however, in most cases the cause is undefined (Garite, 1999).

Once membranes have ruptured, labor may occur within a relatively short time. The latency period, the period of time between rupture of membranes and the onset of labor, decreases with increasing gestational age. When PROM occurs before 26 weeks, approximately 50% of women will begin labor within 1 week. Between 80% and 90% of those women who rupture membranes between 28 and 34 weeks will give birth within 7 days (Garite, 1999).

Maternal Risks

Maternal risk is related to infection, specifically *chorioamnionitis* (intra-amniotic infection resulting from bacterial invasion and inflammation of the membranes before birth) and *endometritis* (infection of the endometrium postpartally that may be related to chorioamnionitis or may occur independently). Chorioamnionitis occurs in about 3% to 15% of all cases of PROM, but in 15% to 25% of cases of preterm PROM (Garite, 1999). Collection of amniotic fluid by amniocentesis permits analysis of the fluid for subclinical chorioamnionitis. Gram stain, white cell count, glucose concentration, interleukin-6 concentration, and culture of the fluid are useful in determining treatment. Also, fluid gathered either by amniocentesis or from fluid that has pooled in the vagina can be analyzed for fetal lung maturity. When the fetal lungs are mature, the risk of serious pulmonary complication in newborns is minimal and labor is allowed to progress naturally (Edwards, Duff, & Ross, 2000).

Abruptio placentae occurs more frequently in women with PROM. It is not clear whether infection causes inflammation of the decidua, which facilitates premature separation, or whether the bleeding episode contributes to a weakening of the membranes, which eventually leads to rupture (McGregor, 1999). Childbirth may be complicated by malpresentation and reduced amniotic fluid volume (Svigos, Robinson, & Vigneswaran, 1999).

Fetal-Neonatal Risks

The most significant cause of neonatal morbidity and mortality is prematurity and its associated complications such as respiratory distress syndrome, necrotizing enterocolitis, and intraventricular hemorrhage (see Chapter 32). Neonatal infection (sepsis) occurs in 2% to 4% of newborns, but the preterm infant is much more likely to develop sepsis and die than a baby born at term. Fetal hypoxia may occur from cord prolapse or cord compression. In cases of early, prolonged PROM, the oligohydramnios that occurs may result in fetal pulmonary hypoplasia, facial anomalies, limb position defects, and fetal growth restriction (Garite, 1999; Svigos et al, 1999).

Clinical Therapy

Any time a woman complains of watery vaginal discharge or a sudden gush of fluid, rupture of the membranes must be considered. The woman should be questioned about the time of initial loss of fluid; if continuous leaking is occurring; the color, consistency, and amount of the fluid; and any odor noted. These questions not only help to determine whether there is blood, meconium, or vernix present, but also may help to differentiate PROM from increased vaginal secretions associated with infection or preterm labor, urinary incontinence, normal leukorrhea of pregnancy, or the passage of the mucous plug.

During the initial physical inspection, any fluid leaking from the vaginal introitus can be checked with nitrazine paper. This test relies on the fact that amniotic fluid is more alkaline (pH 7.0 to 7.5) than normal vaginal secretions (pH 4.5 to 5.5). A color change in the paper to blue-green or blue is highly suggestive of ruptured membranes. Factors that can yield a false-positive result are contamination of the fluid with blood, semen, urine, or antiseptic cleansers. The elevated pH associated with bacterial vaginosis can also lead to misleading results. If there is copious fluid leaking from the vaginal introitus, the diagnosis of PROM is considered confirmed.

If further evaluation is required, a sterile speculum exam is done. Unless the woman is in active labor, direct digital exam of the cervix or vagina is avoided until a management plan has been determined. Speculum exam relies on gross pooling of amniotic fluid in the vaginal vault. The woman can be asked to "bear down," performing a Valsalva maneuver, if fluid is not visualized in the vagina. The woman may also remain in a supine position for several hours to allow collection of fluid to occur; the exam is then repeated. In addition to performing a nitrazine test on the fluid, a fern test can be performed by applying a thin sample of secretions onto a clean slide and looking for microscopic evidence of a fernlike pattern (see Chapter 21). Vaginal cultures for group B streptococcus, chlamydia, and gonorrhea may be obtained at this time. Ultrasound can be used to look for reduced amniotic fluid.

In situations in which the diagnosis of PROM cannot be made with any certainty, an amniocentesis may be performed to instill either indigo carmine or Evan's blue dye. A tampon is inserted in the vagina for several hours and then is inspected for blue tinged fluid. The woman should be warned that as the dye is absorbed, it will temporarily change her urine to a green color.

Concurrently, fetal well-being should be assessed through a fetal heart rate tracing or biophysical profile. In addition, the gestational age of the fetus must be calculated in order to decide on a management plan (see Table 20–1 •). At greater than 36 weeks' gestation, labor will begin in 50% of women within 12 hours. Labor induction may be delayed for 12 to 24 hours unless a situation exists that would preclude expectant management.

Management of PROM in the absence of infection and gestation of less than 37 weeks is usually conservative. Amniocentesis may be done to evaluate for intra-amniotic infection. Fetal lung maturity studies will also be done if the fetus is nearing 34 weeks' gestation (American Academy of Pediatrics [AAP] & American College of Obstetricians and Gynecologists [ACOG], 1997). The woman is hospitalized on bed rest. An admission, complete blood count (CBC), C-reactive protein (CRP), and urinalysis are obtained. Regular nonstress tests (NSTs) or biophysical profiles are used to monitor fetal well-being. Maternal blood pressure, pulse, and temperature are assessed every 4 hours. Regular laboratory evaluations should be performed to detect maternal infection. After initial treatment and observation, if the fetus has not reached viability or if leaking of fluid ceases, some women may be followed at home (Garite, 1999). The woman

Table 20-1 • CURRENTLY USED PLANS FOR WOMEN WITH PREMATURE RUPTURE OF MEMBRANES

Preterm
Expectant management (observation); birth when labor or clinical infection develops
Fetal pulmonary status determined by amniotic fluid testing; birth if fetus is mature
Risk of infection determined by amniotic fluid Gram stain, white cell count, glucose and culture; maternal white cell count and C-reactive protein, assessment for maternal fever or uterine tenderness; assessment for fetal well-being through electronic fetal monitoring or ultrasound for biophysical profile scoring; birth if infection develops
Administration of corticosteroids, with or without birth in 48 hours after first dose; tocolytics as needed
Birth after an arbitrary latent period (eg, 16–72 hours)
Assess for group B streptococci, chlamydia, or *Neisseria gonorrhoeae*; treatment indicated if positive
Combinations of the above
Term
Induction if spontaneous labor does not begin in approximately 12 hours, or if cervix is ripe, or if there are other complications (eg, preeclampsia)
Expectant management for women with uncomplicated pregnancies and cervix unfavorable for induction

is advised to continue bed rest (with bathroom privileges), monitor her temperature four times a day, and avoid intercourse, douches, and tampons ("pelvic rest"). The woman is advised to contact her physician and return to the hospital if she has fever, uterine tenderness or contractions, increased leakage of fluid, decreased fetal movement, or a foul vaginal discharge. Weekly NSTs should be continued.

Authorities disagree regarding the ideal management of preterm PROM. Prophylactic antibiotics are often administered for the first 48 hours while awaiting culture results. The use of prophylactic antibiotics for preterm PROM can prolong the interval from rupture of membranes to childbirth by as much as several weeks. In addition, the neonatal mortality rate is significantly lower in neonates whose mothers received antibiotics (Bar, Maayan-Metsger, Hod, et al, 2000). The use of broad-spectrum antibiotics in women with PROM also seems to decrease the incidence of postpartum endometritis and neonatal sepsis.

If vaginal cultures are positive, antibiotics will be continued for at least 7 days. If amniotic fluid studies indicate a low glucose level, high white blood cell (WBC) count, a positive Gram stain, or organisms in the fluid, immediate birth is indicated. When a cervical cerclage is in place, it should be removed promptly.

Betamethasone, a corticosteroid, decreases the likelihood of neonatal respiratory distress syndrome, necrotizing enterocolitis, intraventricular hemorrhage, and perinatal death in infants who are born prematurely (Canterino, Verma, Visintainer, et al, 2001; Shelton, Boggess, Murtha, et al, 2001). Recently, there has been a great deal of controversy regarding antenatal administration of single course betamethasone (12 mg IM with a second dose in 24 hours) versus multiple courses repeated at 7-day intervals. Corticosteroids have been associated with increased maternal and neonatal infection, decreased neonatal birth weight, reduction of brain size, maternal and fetal adrenal suppression, and psychomotor delay and behavioral problems. Data on these effects are not conclusive, but until there is additional data from clinical trials, the recommendation is that repeat courses of corticosteroids should not be used routinely (National Institutes of Health [NIH] Consensus Development Panel, 2001). See Drug Guide: Betamethasone.

Use of tocolytics is generally not indicated in the woman who has ruptured membranes. Short-term use of tocolytics may be considered, however, to allow a course of steroids to be given.

NURSING CARE MANAGEMENT

Nursing Assessment and Diagnosis

Determining the duration of the rupture of membranes is a significant component of the antepartal assessment. The nurse asks the woman when her membranes ruptured and when contractions began because the risk of infection may be directly related to the time involved. Gestational age is determined to prepare for the possibility of a preterm birth. The nurse observes the mother for signs and symptoms of infection, especially by reviewing her white blood cell count, CRP, temperature, and pulse rate, and the character of her amniotic fluid. If the mother has a fever, the nurse checks hydration status. Fetal heart rate tracings should be watched for tachycardia, loss of variability, or decelerations. When a preterm or cesarean birth is anticipated, the nurse evaluates the childbirth preparation and coping abilities of the woman and her partner.

Nursing diagnoses that may be used for the woman with PROM include the following:

- ***Risk for Infection*** related to premature rupture of membranes
- ***Impaired Gas Exchange*** in the fetus related to compression of the umbilical cord secondary to prolapse of the cord
- ***Risk for Ineffective Individual Coping*** related to unknown outcome of the pregnancy

Nursing Plan and Implementation

Nursing actions should focus on the woman, her partner, and the fetus. Uterine activity and fetal response to the labor are evaluated, but vaginal exams are not done unless absolutely necessary. The woman is encouraged to rest on her right or left side to promote optimal uteroplacental

DRUG GUIDE Betamethasone (Celestone Solupan)

• Overview of Maternal-Fetal Action

Studies have provided ample evidence that glucocorticoids such as betamethasone are capable of inducing pulmonary maturation and decreasing the incidence of respiratory distress syndrome in preterm infants. The mechanism by which corticosteroids accelerate fetal lung maturity is unclear, but it is related to the stimulation of enzyme activity by the drug. The enzyme is required for biosynthesis of surfactant by the type II pneumocytes. Surfactant is of major importance to the proper functioning of the lung in that it decreases the surface tension of the alveoli. Glucocorticoids also increase the rate of glycogen depletion, which leads to thinning of the interalveolar septa and increases the size of the alveoli. The thinning of the epithelium brings the capillaries into closer proximity with the air spaces and improves oxygen exchange.

• Route, Dosage, Frequency

Prenatal maternal intramuscular injections of 12 mg of betamethasone are given once a day for 2 days. Dexamethasone may also be given in doses of 6 mg every 12 hours for four doses (NIH Consensus Development Panel, 2001). To obtain maximum results, birth should be delayed for at least 24 hours after completing the first round of treatment. The effect of corticosteroids may be transient. Currently, it is suggested that repeat courses of corticosteroids should not be used routinely.

• Contraindications

Inability to delay birth

Adequate L/S ratio

Presence of a condition that necessitates immediate birth (eg, maternal bleeding)

Presence of maternal infection, diabetes mellitus (relative contraindication)

Gestational age greater than 34 completed weeks

• Maternal Side Effects

Increased risk for infection has not been supported in large studies. There may, however, be some increase in the incidence of infection in women with premature rupture of the membranes. Maternal hyperglycemia may occur during corticosteroid administration. Insulin-dependent diabetics may require insulin infusions for several days to prevent ketoacidosis. Corticosteroids possibly may increase the risk of pulmonary edema, especially when used concurrently with tocolytics (Iams, 1996a; NIH Consensus Development Panel, 2001).

• Effects on Fetus/Newborn

Lowered cortisol levels at birth, but rebound occurs by 2 hours of age

Hypoglycemia

Increased risk of neonatal sepsis

Animal studies have shown serious fetal side effects such as reduced head circumference, reduced weight of the fetal adrenal and thymus glands, and decreased placental weight. Human studies have not shown these effects, however.

• Nursing Considerations

Assess for presence of contraindications.

Provide education regarding possible side effects.

Administer betamethasone deep into gluteal muscle, avoiding injection into deltoid (high incidence of local atrophy) (Dexamethasone may be administered IM or IV.)

Periodically evaluate BP, pulse, weight, and edema.

Assess lab data for electrolytes and blood glucose.

Although concomitant use of betamethasone and tocolytic agents has been implicated in increased risk of pulmonary edema, the betamethasone has little mineral corticoid activity; therefore, it probably doesn't add significantly to the salt and water retention effects of beta-adrenergic agonists. Other causes of noncardiogenic pulmonary edema should also be investigated if pulmonary edema develops during administration of betamethasone to a woman in preterm labor.

perfusion. Comfort measures may help promote rest and relaxation. The nurse must also ensure that hydration is maintained, particularly if the woman's temperature is elevated.

Teaching for Self-Care

Education is another important aspect of nursing care. The couple needs to understand the implications of PROM and all treatment methods. It is important to address side effects and alternative treatments. The couple needs to know that although the membranes are ruptured, amniotic fluid continues to be produced. Accurate information about neonatal outcomes for the given gestational age will help the woman and those she looks to for support have a more realistic view of the situation. This is often done in conjunction with a tour of the nursery by a care provider experienced in the care of high-risk newborns such as a neonatologist or a neonatal nurse practitioner. Providing psychologic support for the couple is critical. The nurse may reduce anxiety by listening empathetically, relaying accurate information, and providing explanations of procedures. It may be necessary to prepare the couple for a cesarean birth, a preterm newborn, and the possibility of fetal or neonatal demise.

Evaluation

Expected outcomes of nursing care include the following:

- The woman's risk of infection and cord prolapse are decreased.
- The couple is able to discuss the implications of PROM and all treatment options.
- The pregnancy is maintained without trauma to the mother or fetus.

Care of the Woman at Risk Due to Preterm Labor

Labor that occurs between 20 and 37 completed weeks of pregnancy is referred to as **preterm labor (PTL).** Prematurity continues to be the number one perinatal and neonatal problem in the United States today—it is estimated that the incidence of preterm birth is more than 11% of all births in the United States, up more than 20% since 1981 (Heaman, Sprague, & Stewart, 2000; Andrews, Hauth, & Goldenberg, 2000). Moreover, 15% of births from socioeconomically underprivileged populations occur prior to 37 weeks' gestation (AAP & ACOG, 1997). Despite new diagnostic and therapeutic technologies, efforts to prevent preterm birth have been largely ineffective.

Table 20–2 • presents a list of risk factors for spontaneous preterm birth.

Table 20-2 • RISK FACTORS FOR SPONTANEOUS PRETERM LABOR

Multiple gestation	Cervical shortening < 1 cm
DES exposure	Uterine irritability
Known cervical incompetence	Age (< 18 or > 35)
Polyhydramnios	Low socioeconomic status
Uterine anomaly	Cigarettes—more than 10/day
Cervix dilated > 1 cm at 32 weeks	Substance abuse
Second trimester abortion	Low maternal weight
Fetal abnormality	Poor weight gain
Febrile illness	More than 2 first trimester abortions
Bleeding after 12 weeks	Non-white race
History of pyelonephritis or other maternal infection	Cervical cerclage in situ
Maternal medical disease	In vitro fertilization (singleton or multiple gestation)
Previous preterm birth	STD (trichomoniasis, chlamydia,)
Previous preterm labor with term birth	Anemia
Abdominal surgery during 2nd or 3rd trimester	Abdominal trauma
History of cone biopsy	Foreign body (IUD)
Uteroplacental ischemia	Bacterial vaginosis, *E. coli* (ascending intrauterine infection)
Stress	Periodontal disease
Inadequate prenatal care	

Maternal Risks

The initial cause of preterm labor—for example, antepartum hemorrhage, trauma, or maternal infection—may pose a risk to the pregnant woman. In addition, the treatment itself is another area of significant risk. Beta-sympathomimetic drugs cause a myriad of maternal side effects including pulmonary edema, especially in women with multiple gestations or chorioamnionitis. Diabetes, cardiac disease, and thyrotoxicosis may contribute to maternal risk with the administration of this class of drugs. Other widely used drugs such as magnesium sulfate, prostaglandin synthesis inhibitors, and calcium channel blockers also may have severe maternal consequence.

Bed rest is frequently prescribed for women having preterm contractions although no evidence supports its use to prevent PTL (Maloni, Brezinski-Tomasi, & Johnson, 2001). Bed rest in general is associated with adverse physiologic effects including maternal thromboembolism and decreased muscle mass. It is also linked with psychologic effects that extend to the entire family. Financial loss, child care issues, disruption of routines, depression, anxiety, and family/marital stress are among the problems that the woman and her family face.

Fetal-Neonatal Risks

Mortality increases for neonates born before 37 weeks' gestation. Although the preterm infant is faced with many maturational deficiencies (fat storage, heat regulation, immaturity of organ systems), the most critical factor is the lack of development of the respiratory system—to the extent that life cannot be supported. In some instances, such as severe maternal diabetes or serious isoimmunization, continuation of the pregnancy may be more life threatening to the fetus than the hazards of prematurity. See Chapter 32 for in-depth consideration of the preterm newborn.

Clinical Therapy

The prevention and treatment of preterm labor has been widely studied. Preterm birth prevention programs, which were implemented in the 1980s and early 1990s, focused on identifying women who were at high risk for PTL. Once identified, those women were educated about signs and symptoms of PTL and had weekly contact with a nurse or other healthcare provider. However, these educational programs did not significantly prevent preterm birth. One contributing factor is that risk assessment screenings have poor ability to predict those women who will eventually develop PTL and give birth early. Up to 60% of preterm births occur in women who would initially be scored at low risk. Nevertheless, the screening tests currently used, such as fetal fibronectin (fFN), cervical length, and Bishop's score, have not been recommended for use in asymptomatic, low-risk women (Iams, Goldenberg, Mercer, et al, 2001). Another presumption of these programs was that reduction in PTL could be achieved by early identification and treatment with tocolytic agents. It has been found that these agents have limited effectiveness and may only delay birth for up to 48 hours (Heaman et al, 2000).

MediaLink Animation: Early Premature Labor

RESEARCH IN PRACTICE
Preterm Birth Prevention

What is this study about? The cornerstone of preterm birth prevention is early detection. The expectant mother must be able to identify subtle symptoms of preterm labor in order to seek care quickly. Only a small portion of the pregnant population is formally educated about the signs of preterm labor, some of which may be subtle and precede the onset of actual preterm labor by days or weeks. Preterm labor symptoms are similar to many of the expected discomforts of a normal pregnancy, and so may make recognition even more elusive. The purpose of this study was to explore women's experiences with the onset of preterm labor-related symptoms. The goal was to understand events that lead to the recognition of preterm labor and prompt the mother to seek healthcare intervention.

How was this study done? This qualitative design used grounded theory to conceptualize major themes. The sample included 30 women who were admitted to the hospital with diagnosed preterm labor. None of the women had experienced preterm labor before, and all of the mothers' pregnancies were less than 35 weeks' gestation. All of the subjects were in a tertiary hospital setting, where interviews were conducted. The semistructured interview was tape recorded and transcribed. A constant comparative method of analysis was used to identify themes.

What were the results of the study? An overriding theme was identified in the experiences of these women. This theme was related to resolving the uncertainty of preterm labor symptoms, and recognizing and responding to the possibilities. The onset of preterm labor was subtle, and identification involved a process of recognizing and naming the symptoms as other than normal signs of pregnancy. Women described the sensations associated with preterm labor but often failed to associate them with contractions or labor. The women often attributed the symptoms to events or personal situations, creating a reassuring meaning for the symptoms. Although these women initially used self-care measures to deal with their symptoms, many did seek precautionary healthcare advice. The mothers engaged healthcare assistance when their experience was associated with a high level of uncertainty about the meaning of the symptoms. Admission to the hospital occurred when the woman and her provider agreed that the symptom pattern might be preterm labor.

What additional questions might I have? Would there be differences for women who had previously had a preterm labor? What kind of education needs to be added to routine prenatal classes to help mothers recognize the symptoms of preterm labor?

How can I use this study? Every expectant woman needs information about the early signs of preterm labor. Expectant women can benefit from guidance to help them identify the symptoms of preterm labor, make timely contact with their provider, and know when to access the healthcare system.

Source: Weiss, M., Saks, N., & Harris, S. (2002). Resolving the uncertainty of preterm symptoms: Women's experiences with the onset of preterm labor. *Journal of Obstetric, Gynecologic, and Neonatal Nursing 31*(1), 66–76.

Prompt diagnosis of preterm labor is difficult because many of its symptoms are also common in normal pregnancy. These include the following:

- Abdominal pain
- Back pain
- Pelvic pain
- Menstrual-like cramps
- Vaginal bleeding
- Increased vaginal discharge (may be pinkish stained or mucus-like in consistency)
- Pelvic pressure
- Urinary frequency
- Diarrhea

Some women have frequent contractions without changes in the cervix. In these women, a clinical assay for fFN may aid in diagnosis. Fetal fibronectin is an extracellular matrix protein that is normally found in the fetal membranes and the decidua. The presence of fFN after 20 weeks' gestation is abnormal until near term, when it appears again. A negative fFN in a woman with preterm contractions is associated with a very low risk of birth within 7 days. A positive test is associated with recent sexual intercourse, vaginal examination, bacterial vaginosis, and vaginal bleeding, and is not very specific in predicting those women who will give birth imminently (Giles, Bisits, Knox, et al, 2000). Assessing cervical length by transvaginal ultrasonography is another diagnostic tool. A cervical length of at least 30 mm (3 cm) is good evidence that the woman is not in preterm labor (Creasy & Iams, 1999). A woman suspected of being in preterm labor should have a digital cervical examination and be monitored with an electronic fetal monitor for a minimum of 1 to 2 hours to detect uterine contractions. At the end of this time, the cervix should be reexamined, preferably by the same person, to determine whether there has been any change in effacement or dilatation. An endovaginal ultrasound of cervical length is also useful in assessing whether uterine activity is causing cervical change. Figure 20–4 compares a cervix of normal length with one indicative of preterm labor. A cerclage is in place.

Maternal bacterial infection has been implicated as a causative factor of PTL with the strongest evidence pointing to upper genital tract infections. The microbial colonization may even precede conception and ascend from the cervix and vagina into the uterus (Andrews et al, 2000). Bacterial vaginosis (BV) and group B streptococcus (GBS) are two of the lower genital tract infections that have received considerable attention because of their potential relationship to PTL. Research indicates that women colonized with GBS at birth were 3 times more likely to have a preterm birth than those women who were not colonized (Feikin, Thorsen, Zywicki, et al, 2001). BV has been consistently determined to be a risk factor for preterm birth. Although only 30% of women with BV give birth prematurely, they have approximately two times the likelihood of doing so as do uninfected women (Andrews et al, 2000).

Preterm labor is also associated with urinary tract infections, so it is prudent to obtain a clean catch or catheterized urine specimen to identify and treat infection. Women with a positive culture should be retested following therapy to ensure that the infection is resolved. Because asymptomatic bacteriuria is common during pregnancy, women with frequent UTIs can be given low-dose suppression therapy with daily antibiotics.

Table 20–3 • summarizes common criteria for diagnosing preterm labor.

No attempt is made to stop labor if any of the following conditions exist (Creasy & Iams, 1999):

- Fetal demise
- Lethal fetal anomaly
- Severe preeclampsia/eclampsia
- Hemorrhage/abruptio placentae
- Chorioamnionitis
- Severe fetal growth restriction
- Fetal maturity
- Acute fetal distress

The initial management of preterm labor is directed toward maintaining good uterine perfusion, detecting uterine contractions, and assessing fetal well-being. Maternal laboratory studies include complete blood count (CBC), C-reactive protein (CRP), vaginal cultures, and urine cultures. Amniotic fluid cultures are sometimes done to rule out intra-amniotic infection as a cause of PTL.

The goal of clinical therapy is to prevent preterm labor from advancing to a point that no longer responds to medical treatment. Hydration has long been used to decrease the frequency of uterine contractions, but there has been no scientific support for the practice. IV hydration with large quantities of hypertonic fluids increases the risk of pulmonary edema and should be used with caution.

Tocolysis is the use of medications in an attempt to stop labor. If the cervix is dilated more than 4 to 5 cm or if there is subclinical amnionitis, the effect of tocolytics on labor is reduced. If labor cannot be arrested, the priority becomes successful preterm birth and management of its psychologic effect on the woman and her partner.

Drugs currently used for tocolysis include beta-adrenergic agonists (also called β-mimetics or β-agonists),

Table 20-3 • CRITERIA FOR DIAGNOSIS OF PRETERM LABOR

Gestation 20–37 weeks
and
Documented uterine contractions (4/20 minute, 8/60 minute)
and
Documented cervical change
or
Cervical effacement of 80%
or
Cervical dilatation 1 cm

Source: American Academy of Pediatrics and American College of Obstetricians and Gynecologists. *Guidelines for perinatal care,* 5th edition. Elk Grove Village, IL and Washington, DC, © AAP/ACOG, October, 2002.

magnesium sulfate ($MgSO_4$), calcium channel blockers, and prostaglandin synthetase inhibitors. These drugs, along with other tocolytic agents, prolong pregnancy a mean of 48 hours (Tsatsaris, Papatsonis, Goffinet, et al, 2001). Although the delay of childbirth by 48 hours in itself may not improve neonatal outcome, it may permit the administration of betamethasone for fetal surfactant induction or allow for the transport of the mother to a tertiary care facility. Such a facility can generally provide better equipment and services, and more experienced, highly trained staff. Studies have shown that in utero transport of a preterm fetus for birth at a tertiary care center is associated with improved neonatal outcomes (Chien, Whyte, Aziz, et al, 2001).

Beta-mimetics are often chosen as the first-line tocolytic agent. The use of β-mimetics does pose a significant risk to the mother in preterm labor. Beta-mimetics, which may be administered intravenously, intramuscularly, subcutaneously, or orally, can significantly affect maternal cardiovascular and metabolic physiology. The most serious effects include hypotension, cardiac arrhythmia, tachycardia, palpitations, myocardial ischemia, pulmonary edema, and maternal hyperglycemia.

Magnesium sulfate, long used in the treatment of preeclampsia, has gained favor in the treatment of preterm labor because it is effective and has fewer side effects than beta-adrenergic agonists. The usual recommended loading dose is 4 to 6 g intravenously in 100 mL of IV fluid over 15 to 20 minutes (Cunningham et al, 2001). The maintenance dose is then 1 to 4 g/hour titrated to deep tendon reflexes and serum magnesium levels. The therapy is maintained for 12 to 24 hours at the lowest rate to significantly diminish contractions. The maternal serum level that is usually necessary for tocolysis seems to be 5.5 to 7.5 mg/dL.

Side effects with the loading dose may include flushing, a feeling of warmth, headache, nystagmus, nausea, dry mouth, and dizziness. Other side effects include lethargy and sluggishness and a risk of pulmonary edema if the woman has predisposing conditions such as multiple gestation, infection, or hydramnios; has had excessive IV fluid administration; or has concurrent β-sympathomimetic therapy. See

Drug Guide: Magnesium Sulfate for other side effects. Fetal side effects may include hypotonia and lethargy that persist for 1 or 2 days following birth.

Of the calcium channel blockers approved for use in the United States, nifedipine appears to have the most clinical promise as a tocolytic. Nifedipine acts by reducing the flow of extracellular calcium ions into the intracellular space of the myometrial smooth muscle cells, thereby inhibiting contractile activity. Nifedipine is well absorbed either orally or sublingually. The most common side effects are related to arterial vasodilation, that is, hypotension, tachycardia, facial flushing, and headache. Because the mechanism of action of nifedipine is different from the beta-adrenergic drugs, coadministration of nifedipine and terbutaline or ritodrine may prove beneficial in the treatment of preterm labor. Because both $MgSO_4$ and nifedipine block calcium, however, coadministration of them has been implicated in serious maternal side effects related to low calcium levels.

Prostaglandins enhance the formation of myometrial gap junctions and stimulate the influx of intracellular calcium ions needed for muscle contraction. Prostaglandin synthetase inhibitors, therefore, are a logical choice for tocolysis. Indomethacin, sulindac, or celecoxib are the prostaglandin synthetase inhibitors most often used to suppress labor. Maternal side effects are few. Dyspepsia, nausea, vomiting, depression, and dizzy spells may occur. On rare occasions, psychosis or renal failure may result. These drugs are best administered with an antacid or taken with meals to reduce the chance of gastrointestinal (GI) upset. Prostaglandin synthetase inhibitors are generally not used in women with drug-induced asthma, coagulation disorders, hepatic or renal insufficiency, or peptic ulcer disease.

MEDIALINK PRETERM LABOR

Indomethacin crosses the placenta readily, and oligohydramnios and premature closure of the fetal ductus arteriosus may occur with long-term use. Consequently the drug, which is no longer widely used, is not recommended after 32 weeks' gestation for a course of therapy longer than 48 hours. Indomethacin has been associated with necrotizing enterocolitis and grades III and IV intravascular hemorrhage (IVH) in the neonate. Research suggests that the risk of necrotizing enterocolitis is not increased when it is used as a single agent, but that when combined with another tocolytic, the risk is increased (Parilla, Grobman, Holtzman, et al, 2000). At extremely preterm gestations, there is a greater likelihood of receiving combined tocolytic therapy. The risk for IVH increases with decreasing gestational age at birth. In the presence of subclinical chorioamnionitis, a woman is also more likely to receive more than one tocolytic agent for recalcitrant preterm labor. Chorioamnionitis is associated with an increased risk of intraventricular hemorrhage in the neonate and may be the cause of IVH rather than the therapy itself (Suarez, Grobman, & Parilla, 2001).

The National Institutes of Health Consensus Development Panel (2001) recommends that corticosteroids (typically betamethasone or dexamethasone) be administered antenatally to women at risk of preterm birth because of their beneficial effect on fetal lung maturation. Any women who are candidates for tocolysis are candidates for antenatal corticosteroids, regardless of fetal gender, race, or availability of surfactant therapy for the newborn, especially between 24 and 34 weeks' gestation.

NURSING CARE MANAGEMENT

Nursing Assessment and Diagnosis

During the antepartal period, the nurse identifies the woman at risk for preterm labor by noting the presence of predisposing factors. The primary areas for ongoing assessment are change in risk status for preterm labor, educational needs of the woman and her loved ones, and the woman's responses to medical and nursing interventions.

Nursing diagnoses that may apply to the woman with preterm labor include the following:

- ***Health-Seeking Behavior:*** Information about the causes, identification, and treatment of preterm labor related to an expressed desire to understand the condition and its implications
- ***Fear*** related to early labor and birth
- ***Ineffective Individual Coping*** related to need for constant attention to pregnancy

Nursing Plan and Implementation

Community-Based Nursing Care

Once uterine activity stops, the woman is sometimes placed on oral tocolysis. She may then be discharged and followed by home care nurses or as part of a specialized prematurity prevention program. (See Evidence-Based Practice on p. 488.)

Home Care

Home care frequently involves programs that combine home monitoring of uterine activity with daily contact between the woman and a nurse. The monitor consists of a contraction sensor belt the woman wears around her abdomen. A small electronic recorder worn at the waist collects and transmits uterine activity data via the telephone to be interpreted by a nurse at a receiving center. The woman also receives in-depth education about the signs and symptoms of preterm labor and how to palpate for contractions. If uterine activity is excessive or if symptoms are reported, the woman is referred to her certified nurse-midwife or physician for prompt evaluation.

Once at home, the woman usually receives weekly or biweekly visits from the home care nurse. During visits from the home care nurse, physical assessments similar to those done in the hospital are completed. Weekly cervical exams may be performed to enhance detection of preterm labor.

DRUG GUIDE MAGNESIUM SULFATE ($MgSO_4$)

• Pregnancy Risk Category: B

• Overview of Obstetric Action

$MgSO_4$ acts as a CNS depressant by decreasing the quantity of acetylcholine released by motor nerve impulses and thereby blocking neuromuscular transmission. This action reduces the possibility of convulsion, which is why $MgSO_4$ is used in the treatment of preeclampsia. Because magnesium sulfate secondarily relaxes smooth muscle, it may decrease the blood pressure, although it is not considered an antihypertensive. $MgSO_4$ may also decrease the frequency and intensity of uterine contractions; as a result it is also used as a tocolytic in the treatment of preterm labor.

• Route, Dosage, Frequency

$MgSO_4$ is generally given intravenously to control dosage more accurately and prevent overdosage. An occasional physician still prescribes intramuscular administration. However, it is painful and irritating to the tissues and does not permit the close control that IV administration does. The intravenous route allows for immediate onset of action. It must be given by infusion pump for accurate dosage.

• For Treatment of Preterm Labor

Loading dose: 4–6 g $MgSO_4$ in 100 mL solution administered over a 15- to 20-minute period (Cunningham et al, 2001).

Maintenance dose: 1–4 g/hour via infusion pump.

• For Treatment of Preeclampsia

Loading dose: 6 g $MgSO_4$ is administered over a 20-minute period.

Maintenance dose: 2 g/hour via infusion pump (Hallak, 1999).

Note: $MgSO_4$ is excreted via the kidneys. Because women in preterm labor typically have normal renal function, they generally require higher levels of magnesium to achieve a therapeutic range than women who have preeclampsia and may have compromised renal function. Maintenance dose may need to be adjusted based on serum magnesium levels.

• Maternal Contraindications

Diagnosed maternal myasthenia gravis is the only absolute contraindication to the administration of $MgSO_4$. A history of myocardial damage or heart block is a relative contraindication to use of the drug because of the effects on nerve transmission and muscle contractility. Extreme care is necessary in administration to women with impaired renal function because the drug is eliminated by the kidneys, and toxic magnesium levels may develop quickly.

• Maternal Side Effects

Most maternal side effects are dose related. Lethargy and weakness related to neuromuscular blockade are common. Sweating, a feeling of warmth, flushing and nasal congestion may be related to peripheral vasodilation. Other common side effects include nausea and vomiting, constipation, visual blurring, headache, and slurred speech. Signs of developing toxicity include depression or absence of reflexes, oliguria, confusion, respiratory depression, circulatory collapse, and respiratory paralysis. Rapid administration of large doses may cause cardiac arrest.

• Effects on Fetus/Neonate

The drug readily crosses the placenta. Some authorities suggest that transient decrease in FHR variability may occur; others report that no change occurred. In general, $MgSO_4$ therapy does not pose a risk to the fetus. Occasionally, the newborn may demonstrate neurologic depression or respiratory depression, loss of reflexes, and muscle weakness. Ill effects in the newborn may actually be related to fetal growth retardation, prematurity, or perinatal asphyxia.

• Nursing Considerations

1. Monitor the blood pressure closely during administration.
2. Monitor maternal serum magnesium levels as ordered (usually every 6–8 hours). Therapeutic levels are in the range of 4–8 mg/dL. Reflexes often disappear at serum magnesium levels of 9–12 mg/dL; respiratory depression occurs at levels of 15–17 mg/dL; cardiac arrest occurs at levels above 30 mg/dL (Hallak, 1999).
3. Monitor respirations closely. If the rate is less than 12/minute, magnesium toxicity may be developing, and further assessments are indicated. Many protocols require stopping the medication if the respiratory rate falls below 12/minute.
4. Assess knee jerk (patellar tendon reflex) for evidence of diminished or absent reflexes. Loss of reflexes is often the first sign of developing toxicity. Also note marked lethargy or decreased level of consciousness and hypotension.
5. Determine urinary output. Output less than 30 mL/hour may result in the accumulation of toxic levels of magnesium.
6. If the respirations or urinary output fall below specified levels or if the reflexes are diminished or absent, no further magnesium should be administered until these factors return to normal.
7. The antagonist of magnesium sulfate is calcium. Consequently, an ampule of calcium gluconate should be available at the bedside. The usual dose is 1 g given IV over a period of about 3 minutes.
8. Monitor fetal heart tones continuously with IV administration.
9. Continue $MgSO_4$ infusion for approximately 24 hours after birth as prophylaxis against postpartum seizures if given for preeclampsia.
10. If the mother has received $MgSO_4$ close to birth, the newborn should be closely observed for signs of magnesium toxicity for 24–48 hours.

Note: Protocols for magnesium sulfate administration may vary somewhat according to agency policy. Consequently, individuals are referred to their own agency protocols for specific guidelines.

EVIDENCE-BASED PRACTICE

SOCIAL SUPPORT DURING HIGH-RISK PREGNANCY

Clinical Question

Does social support during pregnancy for women at increased risk of low birth weight and premature babies improve medical and/or psychologic outcomes?

The Evidence

Evidence was assembled from 14 trials involving over 11,000 women. Studies were generally of good to excellent quality. This evidence indicated that social support programs for at-risk pregnant women did not improve medical outcomes (low birth weight and prematurity). The programs were, however, associated with increased maternal satisfaction with antenatal care, reduced anxiety about their babies, and reports of feeling less burdened.

Best Practice

Previous studies have suggested a relationship between life stress and the development of pregnancy complications, with social support as a mediating influence. Current research evidence does not support this relationship. Instead, it appears that social support is insufficient to improve poor pregnancy outcomes in high-risk pregnancy groups.

Although pregnant women certainly need the support of caring family members, friends, and health professionals, such support is unlikely to improve medical outcomes (ie, low birth weight or prematurity). Social support programs do appear, however, to improve psychologic outcomes. Such programs need to set realistic target outcomes and acknowledge that, presumably, medical outcomes will not be improved.

Source: Hodnett, E. D. (2002). Support during pregnancy for women at increased risk of low birth weight babies (Cochrane Review). In *The Cochrane Library* (Issue 3). Oxford: Update Software.

MEDIALINK CARE PLAN: CLIENT AT RISK FOR PRETERM LABOR

Consideration of the woman's ability to care for herself, the impact of the changes in relationships that will occur, and care of any young children in the home are among the issues that affect the woman's ability to cope effectively with this situation. The home care nurse needs to be alert to any signs that the woman is failing to achieve the emotional and developmental tasks of pregnancy, such as lack of maternal attachment. An individualized nursing management plan helps focus on each woman's specific needs. Although current evidence does not show that increased social support or home uterine activity monitoring are effective in preventing preterm birth (Svigos et al, 1999), these therapies continue to be widely used.

Teaching for Self-Care

Once the woman at risk for preterm labor has been identified, she needs to be taught about the importance of recognizing the onset of labor. Increasing the woman's awareness of the subtle symptoms of preterm labor is one of the most important teaching objectives of the nurse (see Client Teaching: Preterm Labor). Signs and symptoms of preterm labor include the following:

- Uterine contractions that occur every 10 minutes or less with or without pain
- Mild menstrual-like cramps felt low in the abdomen
- Constant or intermittent feelings of pelvic pressure that may feel like the baby pressing down
- Rupture of membranes
- Low, dull backache, which may be constant or intermittent
- A change in the vaginal discharge (an increase in amount, a change to more clear and watery, or a pinkish tinge)
- Abdominal cramping with or without diarrhea

The woman is also taught to evaluate contraction activity once or twice a day. She does so by lying down tilted to one side with a pillow behind her back for support. The woman places her fingertips on the fundus of the uterus (which is above the umbilicus after 20 weeks' gestation). She checks for contractions (hardening or tightening in the uterus) for about 1 hour. It is important for the pregnant woman to know that uterine contractions occur occasionally throughout the pregnancy. If they occur every 10 minutes for 1 hour, however, the cervix could begin to dilate, and labor could continue.

The nurse ensures that the woman knows when to report signs and symptoms. If contractions occur every 10 minutes (or less) for 1 hour, if any of the other signs and symptoms are present for 1 hour, or if clear fluid begins leaking from the vagina, she should telephone her physician/nurse-midwife, clinic, or hospital birthing unit and make arrangements to be checked for ongoing labor.

If the woman experiences any preterm labor symptoms for more than 15 minutes while physically active, she should be instructed to do the following:

- Empty her bladder.
- Lie down tilted toward her side.
- Drink 3 to 4 (8 oz) cups of fluid.
- Palpate for uterine contractions, and if contractions occur 10 minutes apart or less for 1 hour, notify the healthcare provider.
- Soak in a warm tub bath with the uterus completely submerged.
- Rest for 30 minutes after the symptoms have subsided, and gradually resume activity.
- Call her healthcare provider if symptoms persist, even if uterine contractions are not palpable.

CLIENT TEACHING PRETERM LABOR

Assessment During the antepartal period, the woman is usually screened for factors that place her at risk for preterm labor. You may then assess the woman's understanding of the danger of preterm labor, the signs of preterm labor, and the actions she can take to prevent it. If she is on a home monitoring program, assess the woman's understanding of the purpose and rationale for the program.

Nursing Diagnosis The key nursing diagnosis will probably be ***Knowledge Deficit*** related to lack of information about the risks of preterm labor and the self-care measures to prevent it.

Nursing Plan and Implementation Your teaching will focus on the risks of preterm labor, the functions of and procedures for home monitoring, and self-care activities to decrease the risk of preterm labor.

Client Goals At the completion of teaching the woman will be able to:

Discuss the risks of preterm labor.

Describe the purpose of home monitoring.

Demonstrate the correct procedures for doing home monitoring.

Explain self-care measures that help decrease the risk of preterm labor.

Teaching Plan

CONTENT	TEACHING METHOD
• Describe the dangers of preterm labor, especially the risk of prematurity in the infant, and all the potential problems.	Discuss the risks specifically. Many people understand in a general way that prematurity can be dangerous, but they fail to understand how the baby is affected.
• Stress the value of home monitoring in evaluating uterine activity on a regular basis. Emphasize that many of the early symptoms of labor, such as backache and increased bloody show, may be subtle initially. Home monitoring can often detect increased uterine activity in the early stages before cervical changes progress to the point where it is impossible to stop labor. Studies have demonstrated that home uterine monitoring programs offer little or no significant difference in preterm delivery compared with clients followed by daily contact with the nurse and no home uterine monitoring (Creasy & Iams, 1999).	Use handouts during the discussion. Help the woman clearly understand the value of the program because, to be successful, it requires a real commitment on her part.
If the woman is to be part of a home monitoring program, the monitoring nurse will usually do the initial teaching. Be prepared to reinforce the information provided and answer questions that may arise.	Teach the woman how to palpate for uterine contractions. Do a demonstration and ask for a return demonstration.
• Summarize self-care measures, such as maintaining generous fluid intake (2 to 3 quarts daily), voiding every 2 hours, avoiding lifting and overexertion, avoiding nipple stimulation or orgasm, limiting sexual activity, and cooperating with activity restrictions and bed rest requirements.	Use a handout during the discussion. Provide opportunities for discussion. If the woman has concerns about certain recommendations, try to modify the approach to best meet her needs.

Evaluation

At the end of the teaching session the woman will be able to discuss the risks of preterm labor, demonstrate home monitoring techniques and explain their rationale, and implement self-care activities to decrease the risks of preterm labor.

Caregivers need to be aware that the woman is knowledgeable and attuned to changes in her body and to take her call seriously. When a woman is at risk for preterm labor, she may have many episodes of contractions and other signs or symptoms. If she is treated positively, she will feel freer to report problems as they arise. Other preventive measures the woman might follow are presented in Table 20–4 ●.

Hospital-Based Nursing Care

Providing supportive nursing care to the woman in preterm labor is important during hospitalization. This care consists of promoting bed rest, monitoring vital signs, measuring intake and output, and continuously monitoring fetal heart rate (FHR) and uterine contractions. Placing the woman on her left side facilitates maternal-fetal circulation. Vaginal

Table 20-4 • SELF-CARE MEASURES TO PREVENT PRETERM LABOR

Rest two or three times a day lying on your left side.
Drink 2 to 3 quarts of water or fruit juice each day. Avoid caffeine drinks. Filling a quart container and drinking from it will eliminate the need to keep track of numerous glasses of fluid.
Empty your bladder at least every 2 hours during waking hours.
Avoid lifting heavy objects. If small children are in the home, work out alternatives for picking them up, such as sitting on a chair and having them climb on your lap.
Avoid prenatal breast preparation such as nipple rolling or rubbing nipples with a towel. This is not meant to discourage breastfeeding but to avoid the potential increase in uterine irritability.
Pace necessary activities to avoid overexertion.
Sexual activity may need to be curtailed or eliminated.
Find pleasurable ways to help compensate for limitations of activities and boost the spirits.
Try to focus on 1 day or 1 week at a time rather than on longer periods of time.
If on bed rest, get dressed each day and rest on a couch rather than becoming isolated in the bedroom.

Source: Prepared in consultation with Susan Bennett, RN, ACCE, Coordinator of the Prematurity Prevention Program.

examinations are kept to a minimum. If tocolytic agents are being administered, the mother and fetus are monitored closely for any adverse effects.

Whether preterm labor is arrested or proceeds, the woman and her partner, if he is involved, experience intense psychologic stress. Decreasing the anxiety associated with the unknown and the risk of a preterm newborn is a primary aim of the nurse. The nurse also recognizes the stress of prolonged bed rest and of lack of sexual contact and helps the couple find satisfactory ways of dealing with these stresses. With empathetic communication, the nurse can facilitate the couple's expression of their feelings, which commonly include guilt and anxiety, thereby helping the couple identify and implement coping mechanisms. The nurse also keeps the couple informed about the labor progress, the treatment regimen, and the status of the fetus so that their full cooperation can be elicited. In the event of imminent vaginal or cesarean birth, the couple should be offered brief but ongoing explanations to prepare them for the actual birth process and the events following the birth. The nurse may also offer to arrange consultation for the woman and her support person with the neonatologist, social worker, or hospital chaplain if requested.

Evaluation

Expected outcomes of nursing care include the following:

- The woman can discuss the cause, diagnosis, and treatment of preterm labor.
- The woman affirms that her fears about early labor are decreased.
- The woman states that she feels comfortable in her ability to cope with her situation and has resources to call on if needed.
- The woman can identify signs and symptoms of preterm labor that need to be reported to her caregiver.
- The woman can describe appropriate self-care measures to initiate in the event that she experiences any preterm labor.
- The woman successfully gives birth to a healthy infant.

Care of the Woman with a Hypertensive Disorder

Hypertension is the most common medical disorder in pregnancy, accounting for up to 15% of prenatal hospitalizations. The incidence of hypertension among pregnant women ranges from 3% to 10% (MacKay, Berg, & Atrash, 2001) and it is the third leading cause of all pregnancy-related death. Various attempts have been made to classify hypertensive disorders. The following classification is recommended by the NIH (2000):

- Preeclampsia-eclampsia
- Chronic hypertension
- Chronic hypertension with superimposed preeclampsia
- Gestational (or transient) hypertension

The pathophysiology and collaborative care of women with these disorders are quite different; thus, each is discussed separately.

Preeclampsia and Eclampsia

Preeclampsia is the most common hypertensive disorder in pregnancy. It is estimated that 50,000 women die from preeclampsia each year worldwide (Pipkin, 2001). Blood pressure normally increases in the first trimester, decreases in the second trimester, and returns to nonpregnant values by the end of the third trimester. In contrast, **preeclampsia** is clinically defined as an increase in blood pressure after 20 weeks' gestation accompanied by proteinuria (NIH, 2000). Edema is no longer included in the definition because it is a common feature in normal pregnancy. However, sudden onset of severe edema warrants close evaluation to rule out preeclampsia or other pathologic processes such as renal disease (Higgins & de Swiet, 2001).

Eclampsia is the occurrence of a seizure in a woman with preeclampsia who has no other cause for seizure. Women who are going to develop preeclampsia usually become hypertensive before they develop proteinuria. In any event, the onset of hypertension in pregnancy warrants close observation.

PATHOPHYSIOLOGY OF PREECLAMPSIA

Preeclampsia has been called a "disease of theories" because the true mechanisms behind the pathogenesis are unknown. The only cure for this disease is birth of the fetus and re-

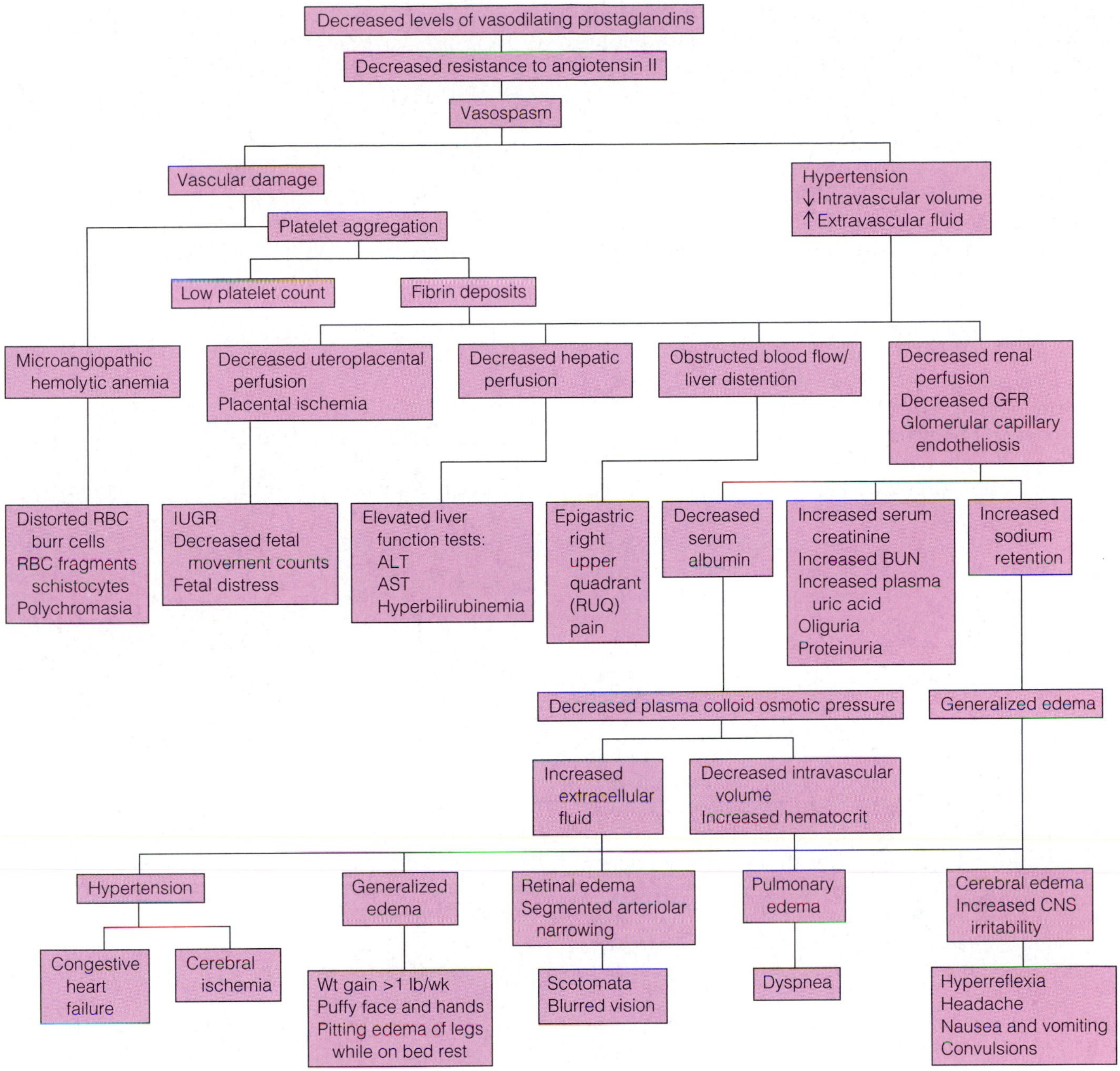

Figure 20–5 • Clinical manifestations and possible pathophysiology of preeclampsia-eclampsia.

moval of the placenta. Key features of preeclampsia involve the failure of the uterine spiral arteries to transform from thick-walled muscular vessels to saclike flaccid vessels, exaggerated inflammatory response, and inappropriate endothelial-cell activation (Dekker & Sibai, 2001; NIH, 2000). Characteristics include maternal vasospasm resulting in decreased perfusion to virtually all organs, including the placenta (see Figure 20–5 •), a decrease in plasma volume, activation of the coagulation cascade, and alterations in glomerular capillary endothelium. The increased platelet activation and markers of endothelial activation can predate clinically evident preeclampsia by weeks or even months (Roberts & Cooper, 2001).

Women who develop preeclampsia become more sensitive to pressor agents (substances that increase blood pressure) rather than less sensitive to them, as in normal pregnancy. This response has been linked to the ratio between the prostaglandins prostacyclin and thromboxane. Prostacyclin, a vasodilator produced by endothelial cells, decreases blood pressure, prevents platelet aggregation, and promotes uterine blood flow. Thromboxane, produced by platelets, causes vessels to constrict and platelets to clump together (NIH, 2000). Prostacyclin is decreased in preeclampsia, allowing the potent vasoconstrictor and platelet-aggregating effects of thromboxane to dominate. These hormones are produced partially by the placenta, which would help explain the reversal of the condition when the placenta is removed and why the incidence is increased when there is a larger than normal placental mass, such as in hydrops, multiple pregnancy, or hydatidiform mole. There also seems to be an increased risk of preeclampsia in women with preexisting vascular disease.

Recently, attention has been directed to another theory, which postulates that uteroplacental ischemia acts as a trigger for preeclampsia, with other factors playing contributory roles. Although the prostacyclin-thromboxane imbalance may provide an explanation for the clinical features of preeclampsia, this theory is now being challenged as the primary cause. In the woman with preeclampsia, in addition to a reduced production of the vasoactive substance prostacyclin, there is also a decreased production of nitric oxide. Nitric oxide is a potent vasodilator and important regulator of maternal blood pressure. Nitric oxide synthesis in the placenta may play a meaningful role in maintaining a low-pressure, high-flow placental system and also may prevent intervillous thrombosis. The loss of normal vasodilatation of uterine arterioles results in decreased placental perfusion (Figure 20–6 •), potentially leading to fetal growth restriction and chronic hypoxia or distress.

Decreased renal perfusion is associated with preeclampsia. With a reduction in glomerular filtration rate (GFR), serum levels of creatinine, blood urea nitrogen (BUN), and uric acid begin to rise from normal pregnant levels, while urine output diminishes. For each 50% decrease in GFR, serum creatinine and BUN plasma levels double, while sodium is retained in increased amounts. Sodium retention results in increased extracellular volume and increased sensitivity to angiotensin II. The typical kidney lesion of preeclampsia involves swollen glomerular capillary endothelial cells containing fibrin deposits. Stretching of the capillary walls allows the large protein molecules, primarily albumin, to escape into the urine, decreasing serum albumin.

Edema is usually more profound in preeclampsia than in normal pregnancy although some of the most severe forms of the disease may occur without edema. The pathologic basis of edema is twofold:

1. The higher salt retention draws out intravascular fluid.
2. Plasma colloid osmotic pressure decreases due to serum albumin loss through edematous renal glomeruli and damaged vascular endothelium. This causes fluid movement to extracellular spaces.

The decreased intravascular volume causes increased viscosity of the blood and a corresponding rise in hematocrit.

MediaLink HELLP Syndrome Society

HELLP SYNDROME

HELLP syndrome (*h*emolysis, *e*levated *l*iver enzymes, and *l*ow *p*latelet count) is sometimes associated with severe preeclampsia, although it may occur before the signs and symptoms of preeclampsia develop. Ninety percent of

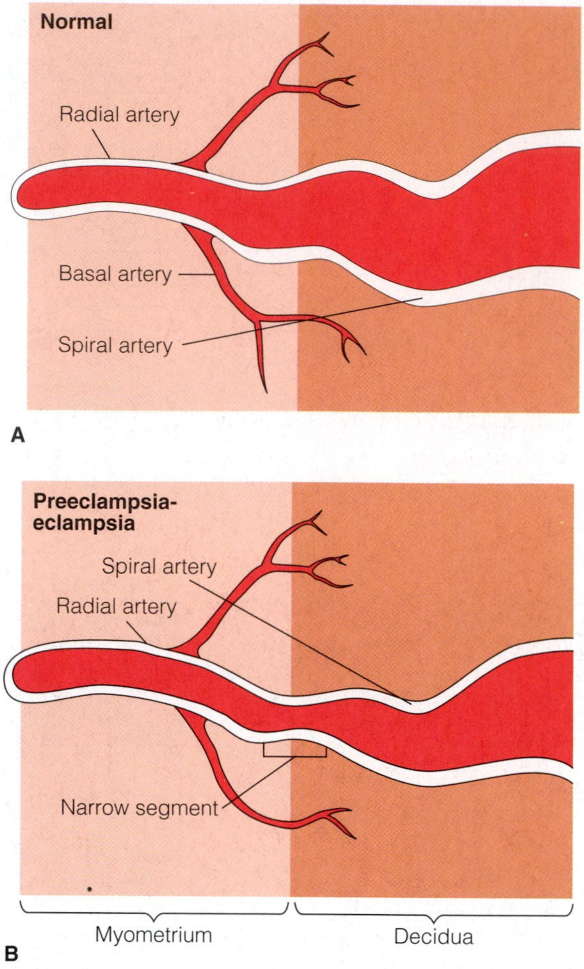

Figure 20–6 • *A,* In a normal pregnancy, the passive quality of the spiral arteries permits increased blood flow to the placenta. *B,* In preeclampsia, vasoconstriction of the myometrial segment of the spiral arteries occurs.

women with HELLP syndrome present with symptoms before 36 weeks' gestation.

The hemolysis that occurs is termed *microangiopathic hemolytic anemia*. It is thought that red blood cells are distorted or fragmented during passage through small, damaged blood vessels. Elevated liver enzymes occur from blood flow that is obstructed due to fibrin deposits. Hyperbilirubinemia and jaundice may also be seen. Liver distention causes epigastric pain. Thrombocytopenia is a frequent finding in preeclampsia. Vascular damage is associated with vasospasm, and platelets aggregate at sites of damage, resulting in low platelet count (less than 100,000/mm^3).

Symptoms may include nausea, vomiting, malaise, flu-like symptoms, or epigastric pain (Magann & Martin, 2000). This may lead to misdiagnoses of gastroenteritis, hepatitis, gallbladder disease, pyelonephritis, renal disease, or thrombocytopenia purpura. Regardless of their blood pressure or the presence of protein in their urine, women presenting with the preceding symptoms should have a CBC with platelet count and liver enzymes drawn. Perinatal morbidity and mortality with HELLP syndrome are high; therefore, the possibility of HELLP should be considered carefully.

Women with HELLP syndrome are best cared for in a tertiary care center. Initially, the mother's condition should be assessed and stabilized, especially if her platelets are very low. The fetus is also assessed using a nonstress test and biophysical profile. All women with true HELLP syndrome should give birth regardless of gestational age.

MATERNAL RISKS

Preeclampsia can impact most organ systems, causing serious complications. Central nervous system changes include hyperreflexia, headache, and eclamptic seizure. Seizures of eclampsia are the result of cerebral edema and occur in 1% of all affected women. The cause of the cerebral edema is most likely related to endothelial permeability changes and loss of protective cerebral autoregulation. Intracerebral hemorrhage is a rare complication, but the most common cause of death in preeclamptic women. Increased intraocular pressure can cause retinal detachment, but spontaneous reattachment usually occurs with reduction in blood pressure and diuresis.

Acute tubular necrosis may result from underperfusion of the kidneys. This is associated with hypovolemia and renal vasoconstriction. Although many women with preeclampsia will have oliguria, most do not develop acute tubular necrosis. One of the more common problems related to preeclampsia is pulmonary edema due to increased capillary permeability.

Thrombocytopenia complicates severe preeclampsia in about 10% of women. The exact mechanism is not fully understood, but platelet consumption is believed to be related to endothelial damage and activation of thrombin. Abruptio placentae is a risk associated with preeclampsia. The release of procoagulants, such as thromboplastin, can result in acute disseminated intravascular coagulation (DIC).

Subcapsular hematoma of the liver is a rare but important occurrence in women with preeclampsia and HELLP syndrome. In addition to the signs of preeclampsia, physical examination may reveal hepatomegaly and peritoneal irritation. Rupture of a subcapsular hematoma is a life-threatening event. The woman may complain of right shoulder pain or severe epigastric pain persisting for several hours before circulatory collapse is evident. This is a surgical emergency requiring a multidisciplinary approach to management. Maternal and fetal mortality is over 50%, and women who survive are at risk for adult pulmonary distress syndrome, pulmonary edema, and acute renal failure in the postoperative period.

Vaginal birth is preferable to cesarean birth in women with preeclampsia or HELLP syndrome. Aggressive induction of labor should take place regardless of the favorability of the cervix. Cesarean birth is considered if vaginal birth does not take place within a reasonable amount of time, usually 24 hours, or for the usual obstetric indications (NIH, 2000).

Women who have preeclampsia complicated by HELLP syndrome do tend to have a somewhat longer clinical and hematologic recovery time than those who do not develop HELLP.

FETAL-NEONATAL RISKS

Infants of women with preeclampsia during pregnancy tend to be small for gestational age (SGA) because of intrauterine growth restriction. The cause is related specifically to maternal vasospasm and hypovolemia, which result in fetal hypoxia and malnutrition. Placental abruption secondary to hypertension may result in fetal hypoxia or even death. In addition, the newborn may be premature because the treatment for the maternal condition may require early childbirth.

Perinatal mortality associated with preeclampsia is approximately 10%, and that associated with eclampsia is 20%. When preeclampsia is superimposed on chronic hypertension, perinatal mortality may be higher.

At birth, the newborn may be oversedated because of medications administered to the woman. The newborn may also have hypermagnesemia due to treatment of the woman with large doses of magnesium sulfate.

CLINICAL MANIFESTATIONS AND DIAGNOSIS

The most commonly occurring clinical manifestations and diagnoses are discussed here.

Mild Preeclampsia

The diagnosis of mild preeclampsia is made based on the presence of hypertension and proteinuria. Previously, it had been recommended that an increase in blood pressure of 30 mm Hg systolic and 15 mm Hg diastolic be used as a diagnostic criterion. However, it has been found that, in the absence of other symptoms, women in this group are not likely to suffer adverse outcome. Therefore, 140/90 mm Hg is commonly used for diagnosis.

With mild preeclampsia, proteinuria is generally between 300 mg/L (1+ dipstick) and 1 g/L (2+ dipstick). This is measured in a midstream clean-catch or catheter-derived urine specimen.

The gold standard for the measurement of proteinuria is the 24-hour urine. Excretion of more than 300 mg of protein in a 24-hour period is considered abnormal. This correlates approximately with a dipstick protein reading of 1+ (30 mg/dL) or greater if specific gravity is less than 1.030 or 2+ if the specific gravity is higher. Protein measurement may vary throughout the 24-hour period, partly related to urine concentration. This can be adjusted for with the use of a protein/creatinine ratio rather than the simple protein concentration alone (Higgens & de Swiet, 2001). Also, protein concentrations may be elevated in women with urinary tract infections.

Although edema is no longer considered a diagnostic criterion, generalized edema, seen as puffy face, hands, and dependent areas such as the ankles and lower legs, may be present. Edema is identified by a weight gain of more than 1.5 kg/month (3.3 lb) in the second trimester or more than 0.5 kg/week (1.1 lb) in the third trimester. Edema is assessed on a 1+ to 4+ scale.

Severe Preeclampsia

Severe preeclampsia may develop suddenly. The following clinical signs are often present (AAP & ACOG, 1997):

- Blood pressure of 180/110 or higher on two occasions at least 6 hours apart while the woman is on bed rest
- Proteinuria ≥ 5 g/L in 24 hours or 3+ or greater on two random urine samples collected at least 4 hours apart
- Oliguria: urine output ≤ 500 mL in 24 hours
- Cerebral or visual disturbances
- Pulmonary edema or cyanosis
- Epigastric or right upper quadrant pain
- Impaired liver function (elevated hepatic enzymes–alanine aminotransferase (ALT) (new name for SGPT) or aspartate aminotransferase (AST) (new name for SGOT))
- Thrombocytopenia
- Fetal growth restriction

Other signs or symptoms that may be present include headache, blurred vision or scotomata (spots before the eyes), narrowed segments on the retinal arterioles when examined with an ophthalmoscope, retinal edema (retinas appear wet and glistening) on funduscopy, dyspnea due to pulmonary edema, moist breath sounds on auscultation, pitting edema of lower extremities while on bed rest, epigastric pain, hyperreflexia, nausea and vomiting, irritability, and emotional tension.

Eclampsia

Eclampsia, characterized by convulsion or coma, may occur before the onset of labor, during labor, or early in the postpartal period. Late postpartal eclampsia (convulsions occurring more than 48 hours following birth) occurs rarely but has been documented. Some women experience only one convulsion, especially if it occurs late in labor or during the postpartal period. Others may have from 2 to 20 or more. Unless they occur extremely frequently, the woman often regains consciousness between convulsions.

CLINICAL THERAPY

The goals of medical management are prevention of cerebral hemorrhage, convulsion, hematologic complications, and renal and hepatic diseases; and birth of an uncompromised newborn as close to term as possible. Reduction of elevated blood pressure is essential in accomplishing these goals.

Antepartal Management

The only known cure for preeclampsia is birth of the infant. Recent research has focused on preventing preeclampsia in at-risk women through the use of low-dose (50 to 150 mg daily) aspirin begun between 12 and 18 weeks' gestation. Aspirin is known to block the action of an enzyme, cyclooxygenase, essential to the production of prostaglandins. This results in lowered levels of thromboxane, the vasoconstrictor. At the same time, levels of the vasodilator prostacyclin are not significantly affected. However, research has failed to show significant reduction in preeclampsia in women treated with low-dose aspirin therapy. The most likely explanation is that the prostacyclin/thromboxane imbalance is not the only pathogenic biochemical pathway. It is unclear whether a different dose used at a different time during pregnancy might have a more beneficial effect (Dekker & Sibai, 2001). Thus, widespread prophylactic use of aspirin is not yet indicated. However, it is reasonable to use low-dose aspirin in women with a history of fetal loss after the first trimester, a previous episode of severe fetal growth restriction in a previous pregnancy, or a history of severe early-onset preeclampsia.

Several dietary approaches have been suggested, including supplementation with calcium, magnesium, fish oil, and vitamins C and E. It has been suggested that the frequency of preeclampsia-eclampsia is higher in women with low nutritional calcium intake. The Cochrane Library on calcium supplementation reviewed nine studies and over 6000 women. The review shows that calcium supplementation does not improve perinatal outcome, but may decrease the frequency of near-term preeclampsia in populations with low baseline calcium intake (Dekker & Sibai, 2001). Neither magnesium nor fish oil supplements has been shown to be beneficial in the reduction of preeclampsia. A recent study has shown some benefit from supplementation with vitamins C and E, but further investigation is needed for confirmation (Dekker & Sibai, 2001; NIH, 2000).

HOME CARE OF MILD PREECLAMPSIA. In general, women with proteinuric preeclampsia should be admitted to the hospital. However, with changes in healthcare, more attention has been given to decreasing inpatient hospital days for women whose symptoms allow.

A woman should be considered for management at home if she meets the following criteria: blood pressure ≤ 150/100, proteinuria less than 1 g/24 hours or < 3+ dipstick, platelet count greater than 120,000 mm^3, and normal fetal growth if not at term or showing signs of complicating factors such as vaginal bleeding. She must have a basic understanding of her condition, be able to recognize the signs and symptoms of worsening preeclampsia (Table 20–5 •), be able to accurately count fetal movements, be cooperative, and know when to call the doctor. She is not restricted to bed rest but is encouraged to rest frequently, especially in the left lateral position.

The woman monitors her blood pressure, weight, and urine protein daily. Weight gains of 1.4 kg (3 lb) in 24 hours or 1.8 kg (4 lb) in a 3-day period are generally cause for concern. Remote NSTs are performed on a daily to biweekly basis. Companies that provide this service have equipment that allows phone transmission of blood pressure readings as well as fetal monitor tracings. This eliminates concerns about in-

Table 20–5 • SIGNS AND SYMPTOMS OF WORSENING PREECLAMPSIA

Increasing edema, especially of hands and face (If on bed rest, observe for sacral edema.)
Worsening headache
Epigastric pain
Visual disturbances
Decreasing urinary output
Nausea/vomiting
Bleeding gums
Disorientation
Generalized complaints of not feeling well

accurate reporting on the part of the woman. Nursing contact varies from daily to weekly, depending on physician request. Laboratory testing regularly evaluates platelet counts, uric acid and BUN, liver enzymes, and 24-hour urine specimens for creatinine clearance and total protein. Estimates of fetal growth and amniotic fluid volume should be made at the time preeclampsia is diagnosed and repeated every 3 weeks if normal. Any woman with worsening symptoms or severe preeclampsia should be hospitalized.

HOSPITAL CARE OF MILD PREECLAMPSIA. The woman is placed on bed rest, primarily in the left lateral recumbent position, to decrease pressure on the vena cava, thereby increasing venous return, circulatory volume, and placental and renal perfusion. Improved renal blood flow helps decrease angiotensin II levels, promotes diuresis, and lowers blood pressure.

Her diet should be well balanced and nutritious. Sodium intake should be moderate, not to exceed 6 g/day. Excessively salty foods should be avoided, but strict sodium restriction and diuretics are no longer used in treating preeclampsia.

Tests to evaluate fetal status are done more frequently as a pregnant woman's preeclampsia progresses. These tests are described in detail in Chapter 21. Monitoring fetal well-being is essential to achieving a safe outcome for the fetus. The following tests are used:

- Fetal movement record
- Nonstress test
- Ultrasonography at least every 3 to 4 weeks for serial determination of growth
- Biophysical profile
- Serum creatinine determinations
- Amniocentesis to determine fetal lung maturity
- Doppler velocimetry beginning at 30 to 32 weeks to screen for fetal compromise

Maternal well-being is monitored by the following:

- Blood pressure four times daily
- Daily weight and daily evaluation for worsening edema, persistent headache, visual changes, or epigastric pain

COMPLEMENTARY AND ALTERNATIVE THERAPIES

HERBS AND SUPPLEMENTS USED TO TREAT HYPERTENSION

There are several herbs and supplements that are used by herbalists to help reduce hypertension: burdock, dandelion, hawthorn, and the supplement coenzyme Q10.

Burdock (Seeds): Burdock seeds (not the root) are used for their hypotensive and diuretic properties. It is administered in extract, tincture, and tea form. Note that the chemical constituents in the root appear to be stronger than in the seeds, and may be a uterine stimulant—so pregnant women should be advised against using this portion of the burdock plant.

Dandelion: Dandelion root is used as an antihypertensive. It is also used as a diuretic, thereby reducing the effects of hypertension. It is administered in extract, tincture, capsule, and tea form.

Hawthorn (Leaf and Flower): The hawthorn leaf and flower are frequently used in cardiac disorders, including hypertension. It is administered in extract, tincture, capsule, and tea form. Note that potential uteroactivity has been found in the use of hawthorn berries, so the pregnant woman should be advised against using this part of the hawthorn plant (Blumenthal, 2000).

These herbs should only be administered by a qualified herbalist. Refer back to "Complementary and Alternative Therapies: Homeopathy and Herbal Medicine" in Chapter 16 for reminders about the use of herbs during pregnancy.

Coenzyme Q10: Coenzyme Q10 is a fat-soluble vitamin-like compound known as ubiquinone (Skidmore-Roth, 2001). It is used to treat a variety of cardiac disorders, including hypertension.

Note: Licorice in any form should be avoided, as it has a hypertensive effect.

- Daily urine dipstick for protein; 24-hour urine for total protein and creatinine
- CBC with platelet count every 2 days
- Serum creatinine, uric acid, and liver function tests (AST, ALT, LDH, bilirubin) one to two times per week

SEVERE PREECLAMPSIA. If the uterine environment is considered detrimental to fetal growth and maturation, birth may be the treatment of choice for both mother and fetus even if the fetus is immature. Other medical therapies for severe preeclampsia include the following:

- **Bed rest.** Bed rest must be complete. Stimuli that may bring on a convulsion should be reduced.
- **Diet.** A high-protein, moderate-sodium diet is given as long as the woman is alert and has no nausea or indication of impending convulsion.
- **Anticonvulsants.** Magnesium sulfate ($MgSO_4$) is the treatment of choice for convulsions because of its CNS-depressant action. In fact, research indicates that the use

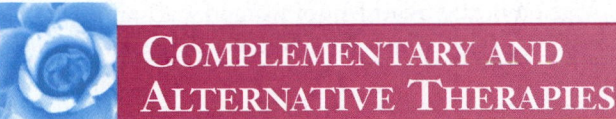

of $MgSO_4$ in the treatment of women with preeclampsia cut the risk of eclampsia and possible maternal death by 50% (Sheth & Chalmers, 2002). It is more effective and has fewer risks than phenytoin and diazepam (Dekker & Sibai, 2001). Blood levels of $MgSO_4$ should be maintained at therapeutic levels (levels vary according to laboratory). Excessive blood levels may produce respiratory paralysis or cardiac arrest. (See Drug Guide: Magnesium Sulfate on page 487.)

- **Corticosteroids.** Betamethasone or dexamethasone is often administered to the woman whose fetus has an immature lung profile. The benefits of corticosteroids in women with HELLP syndrome were first recognized when the drugs were given for fetal lung maturity enhancement to women with preterm gestations. Antepartum platelet counts stabilized or increased, while hepatic enzymes and LDH stabilized or decreased. In addition, neonatal benefits may include fewer grade III and IV intraventricular hemorrhages, less necrotizing enterocolitis, less retinopathy of prematurity, and fewer neonatal deaths (Magann & Martin, 2000). Dexamethasone, which has the potency 1.25 times that of betamethasone, is often chosen for use with HELLP syndrome. Dexamethasone may be administered intravascularly which may also impact its effectiveness (Isler, Barrilleaux, Magann, et al, 2001). Therapy must be administered 24 to 48 hours prior to birth to maximize the beneficial effect.
- **Fluid and electrolyte replacement.** The goal of fluid intake is to achieve a balance between correcting hypovolemia and preventing circulatory overload. Fluid intake may be oral or supplemented with intravenous (IV) therapy. Intravenous fluids may be started "to keep lines open" in case they are needed for drug therapy, even when oral intake is adequate. Criteria vary for determining appropriate fluid intake. Electrolytes are replaced as indicated by daily serum electrolyte levels. Women with preeclampsia are at risk for hyponatremia (low blood sodium), which is indicative of low serum osmolality. A rapid decrease in serum osmolality can cause seizures as a result of cerebral dysfunction. It is imperative that serum sodium levels be evaluated to assess the need for fluid restriction and the switch from IV administration to an isotonic sodium chloride administration (Magriples, Laifer, & Hayslett, 2001).
- **Antihypertensives.** In general, antihypertensive therapy is given for diastolic blood pressures of 105 to 110 or above. The therapeutic goal is to maintain the diastolic blood pressure between 90 and 100 mm Hg. Decreasing the diastolic below 90 mm Hg may decrease uterine blood flow, causing fetal compromise. Methyldopa is often used for long-term control of mild to moderate hypertension in pregnancy because it is effective and has a well-documented fetal and maternal safety record. Hydralazine is the most commonly used drug for the treatment of acute hypertension in pregnancy and is generally administered by IV boluses ("Treating Hypertension in Pregnancy," 2001). Labetalol is used as a second-line IV drug, but should be avoided in women with asthma or congestive heart failure. Oral nifedipine acts rapidly and has favorable hemodynamic effects, but has not been approved for treating hypertensive emergencies. Care should also be taken when using any calcium channel blocker with $MgSO_4$. If these medications are not successful in controlling blood pressure, sodium nitroprusside may be indicated for an acute emergency (NIH, 2000).

ECLAMPSIA. Eclampsia is defined as the occurrence of either seizure or coma associated with pregnancy and not caused by other neurologic disease. The overall incidence is about 1 in 1600 pregnancies, but it becomes much more common as term approaches (Hallak, 1999). Seizures may be focal, multifocal, or generalized. The etiology of the seizure is most likely related to cerebral vasospasm, edema, hemorrhage, ischemia, and hypertensive or metabolic encephalopathy. Many women experience an increase in deep tendon reflexes (DTRs) before seizure, but seizures may also occur without hyperreflexia. The woman with preeclampsia should be monitored for signs and symptoms of impending eclampsia: scotomata, which can appear as dark spots or flashing lights in the field of vision; blurred vision; epigastric pain; vomiting; persistent or severe headache, generally frontal in location; neurologic hyperactivity; pulmonary edema; or cyanosis.

If a seizure occurs, nursing assessment should include time of onset, progress of the seizure, body involvement, duration, presence of incontinence, status of the fetus, and signs of placental abruption. The airway should be maintained and oxygen administered during the seizure. The woman is positioned on her side to avoid aspiration. Suctioning may be necessary to keep the airway clear; a tongue blade should not be inserted into the back of the throat because it may stimulate the gag reflex. To prevent injury, side rails should be up and padded, but the woman should not be restrained.

A bolus of 4 to 6 g $MgSO_4$ is administered intravenously over 5 minutes in an attempt to break the seizure. Magnesium failures require the addition of a second agent, such as 10 mg of diazepam administered intravenously up to a maximum of 30 mg. Phenytoin (Dilantin) may be used for seizure prevention: A bolus of 10 mg/kg of body weight is piggybacked to a main line and infused at a rate no greater than 50 mg/minute. A second bolus of 5 mg/kg of phenytoin is given 2 hours later with maintenance doses beginning 12 hours later and repeated every 8 to 12 hours based on serum levels of the drug. The therapeutic range of phenytoin is 10 to 20 mg/mL.

During a seizure, fetal bradycardia may occur. If possible, the fetus is allowed to recover before birth. The seizure increases uterine irritability and may cause a precipitous birth. Therefore a minimum ratio of one nurse to one client is imperative to assess fetal and maternal status. While she is still unconscious, the woman should be observed for onset of labor. The woman is also observed for signs of placental separation (see Chapter 25). She should be checked every 15 minutes for vaginal bleeding, which may or may not be present with abruptio placentae. The abdomen is palpated for uterine rigidity.

Following a seizure, frequent auscultation of maternal lungs is required to assess for complications from aspiration and to rule out pulmonary edema, which is common in eclamptic clients. The woman is watched for circulatory and renal failure and for signs of cerebral hemorrhage. Furosemide (Lasix) may be given in low doses for pulmonary edema; digitalis may be given for circulatory failure. An indwelling Foley catheter is often inserted and intake and output are monitored hourly.

A woman may have a single convulsion or many convulsions, usually followed by a period of coma. She may be combative and confused as she awakens, but having a family member at her side helps to reduce her agitation. Also, it is important to avoid bright light, noises, and frequent disturbances.

The most serious complication, cerebral hemorrhage, arises from uncontrolled hypertension. Loss of vision, which is usually temporary, is a sign of impending hemorrhage. Blood pressure control with IV hydralazine has been the preferred treatment until after birth because of extensive experience with its use and rare reports of adverse fetal effects. Intravenous options are labetalol, diazoxide, or nitroprusside. Nitroprusside has been restricted to hypertensive crises when childbirth is imminent and other medications have not worked. Fetal cyanide poisoning may occur if the drug is continued and birth is delayed. Use of nitroprusside requires an arterial line because of its quick action and profound effects on blood pressure.

Intrapartum Management

PREECLAMPSIA. Labor may be induced by intravenous oxytocin when there is evidence of fetal maturity and cervical readiness. In very severe cases, cesarean birth may be necessary regardless of fetal maturity.

The woman may receive both intravenous oxytocin and $MgSO_4$ simultaneously. Because $MgSO_4$ has a depressant action on smooth muscle, uterine contractions may diminish, and labor may be augmented with oxytocin. Equipment and IV lines for both fluids must be checked frequently to ensure that they are being administered at the proper rate. Infusion pumps should be used to guarantee accuracy. Bags and tubing must be labeled carefully.

Meperidine (Demerol) or fentanyl may be given intravenously for pain relief in labor. An epidural, spinal, or combined spinal-epidural can be safely administered to the woman with preeclampsia. Hypotension can be avoided by careful attention to technique and careful volume expansion (NIH, 2000).

Childbirth in the Sims' position should be considered. If the lithotomy position is used, a wedge should be placed under the right buttock to displace the uterus. The wedge should also be used if birth is by cesarean. Oxygen is administered to the woman during labor if the need is indicated by fetal response to the contractions.

ECLAMPSIA. Often the woman with eclampsia is cared for in an intensive care unit until labor begins or is induced. Invasive hemodynamic monitoring of either central venous pressure (CVP) or pulmonary artery wedge pressure (PAWP) may be instituted using a Swan-Ganz catheter. Both these procedures carry risk to the woman, and the decision to use them should be made judiciously. Invasive hemodynamic monitoring may be indicated for the woman with the following:

- Urine output less than 30 mL/hr for 3 hours with lack of response to an intravenous fluid bolus
- Pulmonary edema resulting in impaired maternal oxygenation
- Administration of a vasoactive drug, such as nitroprusside or dopamine

When the woman's vital signs have stabilized, urinary output is good, and the maternal and fetal hypoxic and acidotic states are alleviated, birth of the fetus should be considered. Birth is the only known cure for preeclampsia-eclampsia. If the newborn will be preterm, it may be necessary to transfer the woman to a tertiary center for childbirth. The woman and her partner deserve careful explanation about the status of the fetus and woman and the treatment they are receiving. Plans for childbirth and further treatment must be discussed with them.

A pediatrician, neonatologist, or neonatal nurse practitioner must be available to care for the newborn at birth. This caregiver must be aware of all amounts and times of medication the woman has received during labor.

Postpartum Management

The woman with preeclampsia usually improves rapidly after childbirth, although seizures can still occur during the first 48 hours postpartum. A woman who has required $MgSO_4$ antepartally will continue to receive the infusion for about 24 hours postpartum. Antihypertensive medication may also be required for a time.

Postpartum nurses should be acutely aware of the possibility of a worsening of the maternal condition in the immediate postpartum period. The potential for HELLP syndrome, liver rupture, or seizure continues. Twenty-five percent of cases of eclampsia occur postpartum; therefore, caregivers should not be lulled into a false sense of security once birth has occurred (Abramaovici & Sibai, 1999).

When a woman's blood pressure (BP) remains above 150/100 for 2 to 3 days postpartum, antihypertensive therapy should be used. Blood pressure should then be monitored at least weekly during the postpartum period. If blood pressure fails to return to normal by 12 weeks postpartum, further evaluation is indicated to rule out underlying causes for hypertension (NIH, 2000).

The risk of recurrence depends upon several factors. When preeclampsia occurs before 30 weeks' gestation, the recurrence rate may be as high as 40%, but if it occurs after 36 weeks, the risk decreases to about 10%. African American women have a substantially greater risk, as do women who have underlying cardiovascular disease or diabetes, or have had preeclampsia as a multipara. Women who have had one episode of HELLP syndrome carry a 5% risk of recurrence. Women who have had a normotensive previous pregnancy are at increased risk when they conceive with a new partner.

Selective screening should be done for inherited coagulopathies (clotting disorders) in women who have had early-onset preeclampsia or a poor pregnancy history related to repeated miscarriages, intrauterine growth restriction, fetal demise, or prior history of a thrombotic event (NIH, 2000; Ninia, 2000). This information is important in client counseling and management not only related to future pregnancies, but also to assess their risk for thrombotic episodes outside of pregnancy.

NURSING CARE MANAGEMENT

See the Clinical Pathway for a Woman with Preeclampsia-Eclampsia for a detailed summary of nursing care management.

Nursing Assessment and Diagnosis

An essential part of nursing assessment is to obtain a baseline blood pressure early in pregnancy. Arterial blood pressure varies with position and is highest when the woman is sitting, intermediate when she is supine, and lowest when she is in the left lateral recumbent position. Therefore it is important that the woman be in the same position when the blood pressure is measured each visit.

Blood pressure is taken and recorded at each antepartal visit. If the blood pressure rises or if the normal slight decrease in blood pressure expected between 8 and 28 weeks of pregnancy does not occur, the woman should be followed closely.

Blood pressure elevations should be based on at least two determinations not more than one week apart. To minimize errors in blood pressure measurements and improve reproducibility, the following precautions should be taken when measuring blood pressure (Higgins & de Swiet, 2001; Zhang, Klebanoff, & Roberts, 2001):

- Take blood pressure measurements while the woman is seated, with feet supported and her arm at the level of the heart.
- Use Korotkoff phase V (sound disappearance) to measure the diastolic pressure.
- Calibrate the mercury sphygmomanometer and use the nearest 2 mm measurement.
- If using an electronic device, use one that has been validated for pregnancy.

When blood pressure and other signs indicate that the preeclampsia is worsening, hospitalization is necessary to monitor the woman's condition closely. The nurse then assesses the following:

- *Blood pressure.* Blood pressure should be determined every 1 to 4 hours, more frequently if indicated by medication or other changes in the woman's status.
- *Temperature.* Temperature should be determined every 4 hours, every 2 hours if elevated or if PROM has occurred.
- *Pulse and respirations.* Pulse rate and respirations should be determined along with blood pressure.
- *Fetal heart rate.* The fetal heart rate should be determined with the blood pressure or monitored continuously with the electronic fetal monitor if the situation indicates.
- *Urinary output.* Every voiding should be measured. Frequently, the woman will have an indwelling catheter. In this case, hourly urine output can be assessed. Output should be 700 mL or greater in 24 hours or at least 30 mL per hour.
- *Urine protein.* Urinary protein is determined hourly if an indwelling catheter is in place or with each voiding. Readings of 3+ or 4+ indicate loss of 5 g or more protein in 24 hours.
- *Urine specific gravity.* Specific gravity of the urine should be determined hourly or with each voiding. Readings over 1.040 correlate with oliguria and proteinuria.
- *Edema.* The face (especially eyelids and cheekbone area), fingers, hands, arms (ulnar surface and wrist), legs (tibial surface), ankles, feet, and sacral area are inspected and palpated for edema. The degree of pitting is determined by pressing over bony areas.
- *Weight.* The woman is weighed daily at the same time, wearing the same robe or gown and slippers. Weighing may be omitted if the woman is to maintain strict bed rest, or a bed scale may be used.
- *Pulmonary edema.* The woman is observed for coughing. The lungs are auscultated for moist respirations.
- *Deep tendon reflexes.* The woman is assessed for evidence of hyperreflexia in the brachial, wrist, patellar, or Achilles

Clinical Tip *Common errors in measuring blood pressure (BP) include the following:*

- Incorrect cuff size—a cuff that is too small results in a falsely elevated BP, whereas one that is too large falsely lowers BP.
- Elevating the arm above the level of the heart, such as occurs when a woman lies on her left side using her right arm for a BP measurement, will falsely lower the BP 10 to 20 mm Hg.
- Korotkoff's phase—when BP is checked during pregnancy, the disappearance of the sound (phase V) is the preferred indicator rather than the muffling of the sound (phase IV).
- Anxiety, exercise, and smoking can elevate BP. Wait 10 minutes after the woman's arrival to check a resting BP.

CLINICAL PATHWAY FOR A WOMAN WITH PREECLAMPSIA-ECLAMPSIA

Category	Antepartal Management	Intrapartal Management*	Postpartal Management*
Referral	• Perinatologist • Nephrologist • Social worker • Psych clinical nurse practitioner • Dietary/nutritionist	• Obtain prenatal record	• Home nursing referral if indicated ➤ **Expected Outcomes** Appropriate resources identified and utilized
Assessment	• Electronic fetal monitoring (EFM) _ q4h _ q8h _ Continuous • NST: _ qd • Ultrasound as indicated • Assess for headache, visual disturbances, epigastric pain, edema, DTRs, clonus, and protein in urine • Assess for signs of low platelets/DIC: petechiae, bleeding gums, bruising, hematuria	• Assess prenatal BP readings and compare to baseline reading • Assess for headache, visual disturbances, epigastric pain, edema, DTRs, clonus, and protein in urine, output • Assess for low platelets/DIC	• BP q4h for first 48h then q8h until discharge • Platelet counts and liver function tests as indicated • Monitor daily Hct • Continue normal postpartum assessment q8h • Feeding technique with newborn: should be progressing • TPR assessment: q8h; all WNL: report temperature > 38C (100.4F) • Continue assessment of comfort level • Assess for headache, visual disturbances, epigastric pain, edema, DTRs, clonus, and protein in urine ➤ **Expected Outcomes** Findings indicate hypertension reduced or stabilized Unstable/escalating hypertension identified in timely manner
Teaching/ psychosocial	• Room orientation • Explain signs and symptoms (s/sx) of worsening disease and importance of notifying RN • Explain s/sx of labor • Increase pt awareness of fetal monitoring, importance of bed rest and lying on left side • Evaluation of client teaching	• Tour of ICN • Discuss with woman: a. Mode of childbirth b. Progression of disease and possible use of $MgSO_4$ prior to birth c. Postpartum expectation	• Implement normal postpartum teaching and psychosocial support (see Chapter 35) ➤ **Expected Outcomes** Verbalizes/demonstrates understanding of teaching Incorporates teaching of BP management into self-care

Nursing care management and reports	• CBC daily
	• Biochemical profile
	• U/A/Dipstick for protein and ketones with each void as well as specific gravity
	• 24-hour urine for total protein and creatinine clearance
	• VS q4h or more frequently if indicated
	• I&O q8h; fluid restriction __ mL as ordered
	• DTR and clonus q4h; report 3+ or 4+ results
	• Daily weight
	• Seizure precautions
	  • Headache, visual distress, epigastric pain → report abnormal findings
	  • Edema (ongoing)
	  • Auscultate lungs for moist respirations and report
	  • Assess hourly for vaginal bleeding and/or uterine irritability or contractions
	  • Observe for alertness, mood changes, and signs of impending convulsion or coma
	  • Assess emotional response so that support and teaching can be planned accordingly
		• Ongoing monitoring of blood pressure
		• Ongoing monitoring of edema
		• Assess urine for proteinuria every shift
		• Electronic fetal monitoring in place
		• Assess woman for worsening signs of preeclampsia (placental separation, pulmonary edema, renal failure, and fetal distress)
		• Try to have same nurses caring for woman during her hospitalization
		• Lab assessments, $MgSO_4$ levels q 4 to 24 hr depending on woman's status
			• Continue sitz bath prn
			• May shower if ambulating without difficulty
			• DC buffalo cap (heparin lock) if present
			• Continue to monitor VS, breath sounds, edema, epigastric pain, DTRs, clonus, and protein in urine until return to normal limits
			➤ **Expected Outcomes**
			Hypertension reduced or controlled
			Maternal/fetal complications quickly identified and minimized
			Feels safe in environment and remains injury free

CLINICAL PATHWAY FOR A WOMAN WITH PREECLAMPSIA-ECLAMPSIA *CONTINUED*

Category	Antepartal Management	Intrapartal Management*	Postpartal Management*
Comfort	• Assess for discomfort • Provide comfort measures as needed	• Assess for discomfort • Provide comfort measures as needed	• Continue with pain management techniques ➤ **Expected Outcomes** Comfort level is maintained
Activity	• BR with BRP • Decreased stimulation in room • Limit visitors • Encourage left lateral recumbent position	• Positioned on side • Encouraged to push while lying on side • Birth is in a side-lying position if possible	• Up ad lib when VS have stabilized ➤ **Expected Outcomes** Level of activity has not exacerbated condition
Nutrition	• Regular diet	• Ice chips	• Continue diet and fluids ➤ **Expected Outcomes** Nutritional needs met
Elimination	• Report urine output < 30 mL/hr or urine specific gravity > 1.040	• Monitor urine output	• Monitor urine output • I/O recorded for 48h after birth ➤ **Expected Outcomes** Intake and output WNL
Medications	• Heparin lock or IV • If gestational age indicates: • Cetestone Soluspan or dexamethasone • $MgSO_4$ per infusion pump if indicated • Antihypertensive medication if indicated • Assess home care needs	• Continuous IV infusion • $MgSO_4$ per infusion pump if indicated • Antihypertensive medication if indicated	• Continue $MgSO_4$ and antihypertensive meds as indicated • May take own prenatal vitamins • RhoGAM and rubella vaccine administered if indicated ➤ **Expected Outcomes** Hypertensive crisis prevented Pain level controlled Perfusion of tissues supported
Discharge planning/home care			• Review discharge instruction and checklist • Describe postpartum warning signs and when to call CNM/physician • Provide prescriptions. Gift pack given to woman • Arrangements made for baby pictures if desired • Postpartum visit scheduled • Newborn check scheduled ➤ **Expected Outcomes** Discharged with plan for follow-up healthcare and blood pressure monitoring Support network identified
Family involvement	• Assess woman's major concerns: eg, fear for fetus, relationship with other children, relationship with partner	• Encourage family member to stay with the woman as long as possible throughout labor and childbirth	• Family members urged to visit • Continue to involve support persons in teaching • Evidence of parental bonding behaviors apparent • Plans being made for providing support to mother following discharge. Support persons verbalize understanding of need for woman to rest, eat nutritionally, recover. ➤ **Expected Outcomes** Family able to participate as desired
Date			

*Interventions for a woman with a normal labor and birth and during the early postpartum period may be found in those appropriate clinical pathways.

Abbreviations used: BP, blood pressure; BRP, bathroom privileges; CBC, complete blood count; CNM/physician, certified nurse-midwife/physician; DTRs, deep tendon reflexes; Hct, hematocrit; Heparinlock, intravenous catheter that allows intermittent access; ICN, intensive care nursery; I&O, intake and output; IV, intravenous; NST, nonstress test; PRN, as needed or as desired; s/sx, signs and symptoms, TPR, temperature, pulse, respiration; VS, vital signs; WNL, within normal limits.

Table 20-6 • DEEP TENDON REFLEX RATING SCALE

Rating	Assessment
4+	Hyperactive; very brisk, jerky, or clonic response; abnormal
3+	Brisker than average; may not be abnormal
2+	Average response; normal
1+	Diminished response; low normal
0	No response; abnormal

tendons (Table 20–6 •). The patellar reflex is the easiest to assess. (See Procedure 20–1: Assessing Deep Tendon Reflexes and Clonus).

- *Clonus.* Clonus should also be assessed by vigorously dorsiflexing the woman's foot while her knee is held in a flexed position. Normally no clonus is present. If it is present, it is measured as one to four beats, or sustained, and is recorded as such.
- *Placental separation.* The woman should be assessed hourly for vaginal bleeding and/or uterine rigidity.
- *Headache.* The woman should be questioned about the existence and location of any headache.
- *Visual disturbance.* The woman should be questioned about any visual blurring or changes, including scotomata. The results of the daily funduscopic exam should be recorded on the chart.
- *Epigastric pain.* The woman should be asked about any epigastric pain. It is important to differentiate it from simple heartburn, which tends to be familiar and less intense. *Nausea and vomiting or right upper quadrant pain,* occasionally radiating to the back, are also of concern.
- *Laboratory blood tests.* Daily tests of hematocrit to measure hemoconcentration; BUN, creatinine, and uric acid levels to assess kidney function; clotting studies for any indication of thrombocytopenia or DIC; liver enzymes; and electrolyte levels for deficiencies are all indicated.
- *Level of consciousness.* The woman is observed for alertness, mood changes, and any signs of impending convulsion or coma.
- *Emotional response and level of understanding.* The woman's emotional response should be carefully assessed so that support and teaching can be planned accordingly.

In addition, the nurse continues to assess the effects of any medications administered. Because the administration of prescribed medications is an important aspect of care, the nurse is, of course, familiar with the more commonly used medications, their purpose, implications, and associated untoward or toxic effects.

Examples of nursing diagnoses that may apply for the pregnant woman with preeclampsia-eclampsia include the following:

- ***Fluid Volume Deficit*** related to fluid shift from the intravascular to extravascular space secondary to vasospasm and endothelial injury
- ***Risk of Injury*** to the woman related to convulsion secondary to cerebral edema
- ***Anxiety*** related to uncertain maternal and fetal status

Nursing Plan and Implementation

Community-Based Nursing Care

A woman with preeclampsia has several major concerns. She may fear losing the fetus. She may worry about her personal relationship with her other children and her personal and sexual relationship with her partner. She may be concerned about finances—health insurance does not always cover all the tests, prolonged hospitalization, and other expenses that may be associated with complications during pregnancy. Finally, the woman may be depressed or resentful about being left alone or may feel bored. If she has small children, she may have difficulty providing for their care. The woman who does not have children may worry that she never will.

The nurse should identify and discuss each of these areas with the woman and her partner. It is necessary to explain to them the reasons for bed rest. A woman with mild preeclampsia may feel very well and be unable to see the need for resting even a few hours a day. The nurse can refer the couple to many community resources, such as homemaking services, a support group for the partner, or a hotline. Arrangements may be made for the partner to attend childbirth classes if both are not able to, or a nurse may be found to teach the classes privately. In addition, childbirth classes can be accessed over the Internet, thereby enabling the couple to participate together even if the woman is limited to bed rest at home.

The woman needs to know which symptoms are significant and should be reported at once. Usually, the woman with mild preeclampsia is seen once or twice a week, but she may need to come in earlier if symptoms indicate the condition is progressing. She must understand her diet plan, which must match her culture, finances, and lifestyle.

Hospital-Based Nursing Care

The development of worsening preeclampsia is a cause for increased concern to the woman and her family. The most immediate concerns of the woman and her partner usually are about the prognosis for herself and the fetus. The nurse can offer honest, hopeful information. The nurse can also explain the plan of therapy and the reasons for procedures to the extent that the woman or her partner is interested. The nurse should keep the couple informed of the fetal status and should also take the time to discuss other concerns the couple may express. The nurse provides as much information as possible and seeks other sources of information or aid for the family as needed. Nurses can offer to contact a member of the clergy or counselor for additional support if the couple so chooses. In addition, the nurse can provide educational videos that help address the couple's educational needs and access other support services including social services, a nutritionist, and even a lactation consultant if the woman is hospitalized for an extended period of time.

Procedure 20–1

Assessing Deep Tendon Reflexes and Clonus

Preparation

1. Explain the procedure, indications for its use, and information that will be obtained.
2. Most nurses check the patellar reflex and one other such as the biceps, triceps, or brachioradialis.
   Rationale: DTRs are assessed to gain information about CNS irritability secondary to preeclampsia and to assess the effects of magnesium sulfate if the woman is receiving it.

Equipment and Supplies

- Percussion hammer

Procedure

1. Elicit reflexes.
   - Patellar reflex. Position the woman with her legs hanging over the edge of the bed (feet should not be touching the floor). (See Figure 20–7 •.) Briskly strike the patellar tendon, which is located just below the patella. Normal response is extension or a thrusting forward of the foot.
     Note: In an inpatient setting the patellar reflex is often assessed while the woman lies supine. Flex her knees slightly and support them.
   - Biceps reflex. Flex the woman's arm 45 degrees at the elbow and place your thumb on the biceps tendon. Allow your fingers to hold the biceps muscle. Strike your thumb in a slightly downward motion and assess the response. Normal response is flexion of the arm.
   - Triceps reflex. Flex the woman's arm up to 90 degrees and allow her hand to hang against the side of her body. Using the percussion hammer, strike the triceps tendon just above the elbow. Normal response is contraction of the muscle, which causes extension of the arm.
   - Brachioradialis reflex. Flex the woman's arm slightly and lay it on your forearm with her hand slightly pronated. Using the percussion hammer, strike the brachioradialis tendon, which is found about 1 to 2 inches above the wrist. Normal response is pronation of the forearm and flexion of the elbow.
     Rationale: The correct position causes the muscle to be slightly stretched. Then when the tendon is stretched, with a tap the muscle should contract. Correct positioning and technique are essential to elicit the reflex.

Clinical Tip

If a percussion hammer is not available, you may use the side of your hand to elicit DTRs.

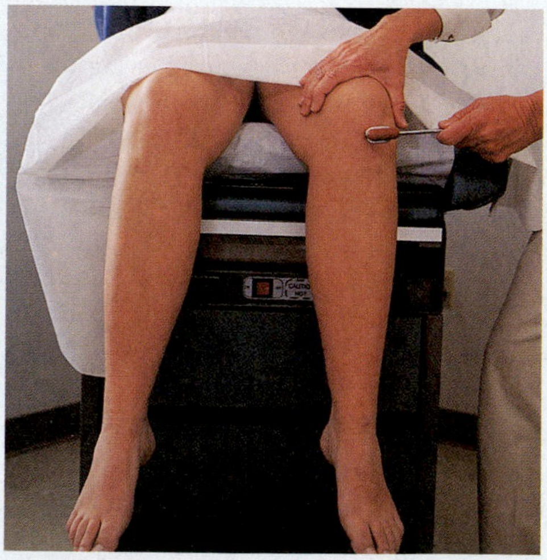

Figure 20–7 • Correct position for eliciting patellar reflex: sitting.

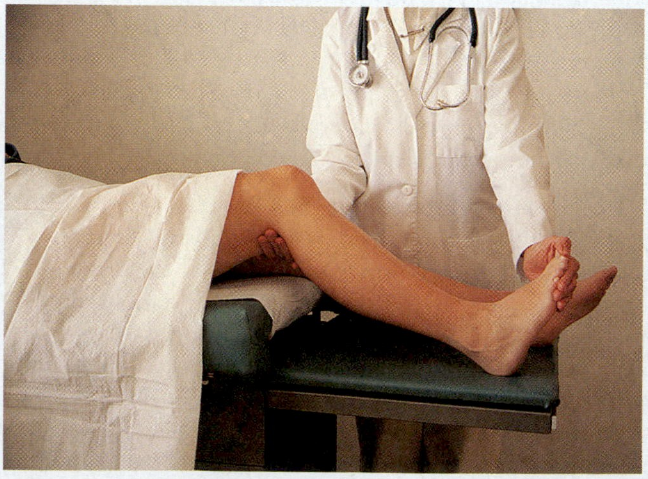

Figure 20–8 • To elicit clonus, sharply dorsiflex the foot.

Procedure 20–1 Assessing Deep Tendon Reflexes and Clonus *(continued)*

2. Grade reflexes. Reflexes are graded on a scale of 0 to 4+, as follows:
   - 4+ Hyperactive; very brisk, jerky, or clonic response; abnormal
   - 3+ Brisker than average; may not be abnormal
   - 2+ Average response; normal
   - 1+ Diminished response; low normal
   - 0 No response; abnormal

   Rationale: Normally reflexes are 1+ or 2+. With CNS irritation, hyperreflexia may be present; with high magnesium levels, reflexes may be diminished or absent.
3. Assess for clonus. With the woman's knee flexed and the leg supported, vigorously dorsiflex the foot, maintain the dorsiflexion momentarily, and then release (Figure 20–8 •). With a normal response, the foot returns to its normal position of plantar flexion. Clonus is present if the foot "jerks" or taps against the examiner's hand. If so, record the number of taps or beats of clonus.
   Rationale: Clonus occurs with more pronounced hyperreflexia and indicates CNS irritability.
4. Report and record findings. For example: DTRs 2+, no clonus or DTRs 4+, 2 beats clonus.

The nurse should maintain a quiet, low-stimulus environment for the woman. The woman should be placed in a private room in a quiet location where she can be watched closely. Visitors are limited to close family or main support persons. The woman should maintain the left lateral recumbent position most of the time, with side rails up for her protection. Unlimited phone calls are avoided because the phone ringing unexpectedly may be too jarring. To avoid a sense of isolation, however, some women find it preferable to limit calls to a certain time of the day rather than refusing all calls.

Nursing Management of Eclampsia

The occurrence of a convulsion is frightening to any family members who may be present, although the woman will not be able to recall it when she becomes conscious. Therefore, offering explanations to family members, and to the woman herself later, is essential.

When the tonic phase of the convulsion begins, the woman should be turned to her side (if she is not already in that position) to aid circulation to the placenta. Her head should be turned face down to allow saliva to drain from her mouth. Attempting to insert a padded tongue blade has been questioned, and in many facilities it is no longer advocated. In others, it is used if it can be done without force because it may prevent injury to the woman's mouth. The side rails should be padded or a pillow put between the woman and each side rail.

After 15 to 20 seconds, the clonic phase starts. When the thrashing subsides, intensive monitoring and therapy begin. An oral airway is inserted, the woman's nasopharnyx is suctioned, and oxygen administration is begun by nasal catheter. The attending physician and the anesthesiologist should be notified immediately. Fetal heart tones are monitored continuously. Maternal vital signs are monitored every 5 minutes until they are stable, then every 15 minutes.

Nursing Management During Labor and Birth

The plan of care for the woman with preeclampsia in labor depends on both maternal and fetal condition. The woman may have mild or severe preeclampsia, may become eclamptic during labor, or may have been eclamptic before the onset of labor. Therefore, careful monitoring of blood pressure and checking for edema and proteinuria are necessary for all women in labor. The prenatal record should be obtained so that current blood pressure readings may be compared with the baseline reading.

Clinical Tip *When caring for a woman with preeclampsia who is receiving IV magnesium sulfate, it is imperative that you follow protocols for monitoring blood levels of magnesium. You are probably already aware of the common signs of increasing magnesium levels, such as diminished reflexes and decreased respiratory rate. However, there are some subtle clues you can also watch for that may suggest either the therapeutic or toxic range. When a woman's magnesium level is in the therapeutic range, she usually has some slurring of speech, awkwardness of movement, and decreased appetite. If the woman begins to have difficulty swallowing and begins to drool, she may be approaching the toxic range.*

The woman with preeclampsia in labor is kept positioned on her side as much as possible. Both woman and fetus are monitored carefully throughout labor. Signs of progressing labor are noted. In addition, the nurse must be alert for indications of worsening preeclampsia, placental separation, pulmonary edema, circulatory renal failure, and fetal distress.

During the second stage of labor the woman is encouraged to push while lying on her side. If she is unable to do so comfortably or effectively, she can be helped to a semisitting position for pushing and resume the lateral position between each contraction. Birth is in the side-lying position if possible. If the lithotomy position is used, a wedge is placed under the woman's hip.

A family member is encouraged to stay with the woman as long as possible throughout labor and childbirth. This is especially needed if the woman has been transferred to a high-risk center from another facility. The woman in labor and the family member or support person should be oriented to the new surroundings and kept informed of progress and plan of care. When possible the woman should be cared for by the same nurses throughout her hospital stay.

Nursing Management During the Postpartal Period

MediaLink CASE STUDY: CLIENT WITH PREECLAMPSIA

The amount of postpartal vaginal bleeding should be noted carefully. Because the woman with preeclampsia is hypovolemic, even normal blood loss can be serious. Rising pulse rate and falling urine output are indications of excessive blood loss. The uterus should be palpated frequently and massaged when needed to keep it contracted.

Blood pressure and pulse are checked every 4 hours for 48 hours. Hematocrit, platelets, AST, and ALT may be measured daily. The woman is instructed to report any headache, visual disturbance, or epigastric pain. No ergot preparations, such as Methergine, are given because they have a hypertensive effect. Intake and output recordings are continued for 48 hours postpartum. Increased urinary output within 48 hours after birth is a highly favorable sign. With the diuresis, edema recedes and blood pressure returns to normal.

Postpartal depression can develop after the long ordeal of a difficult pregnancy. Family members are urged to visit, and as much mother-infant contact as possible should be allowed. There may be fears about a future pregnancy. The couple needs information about the chance of preeclampsia occurring again. They also should be given family-planning information. Combined oral contraceptives may be used if the woman's blood pressure has returned to normal by the time they are prescribed (usually 4 to 6 weeks postpartum). Progesterone-only pills may be prescribed regardless of hypertension and may be a good alternative for women with chronic hypertension or for those women who are breastfeeding.

Evaluation

Expected outcomes of nursing care include the following:

- The woman is able to explain preeclampsia, its implications for her pregnancy, the treatment regimen, and possible complications.
- The woman suffers no eclamptic seizures.
- The woman and her caregivers detect signs of increasing severity of the preeclampsia or possible complications early so that appropriate treatment measures can be instituted.
- The woman gives birth to a healthy newborn.

Chronic Hypertension

Chronic hypertension exists when the blood pressure is 140/90 or higher before pregnancy or before the 20th week of gestation or persists 42 days following childbirth. If the diastolic blood pressure is greater than 80 mm Hg during the second trimester, chronic hypertension should be suspected. For the majority of chronic hypertensive women, the disease is mild. One of the challenges the healthcare team faces is differentiating chronic hypertension from preeclampsia. This is even more difficult if a woman arrives for her first prenatal visit during the second trimester when blood pressure is generally lower and preexisting hypertension is more difficult to recognize.

Early prenatal care is important to determine accurately the gestational age and the severity of hypertension. At the time of the first visit, the woman should be counseled on several aspects of her pregnancy:

- **Nutrition.** Sodium is limited to about 2.4 g per day; the woman is advised about recommended weight gain.
- **Bed rest.** Frequent rest periods are advisable. At a minimum, the woman should rest twice a day for 1-hour periods of time.
- **Medication.** Studies have shown that women with mild chronic hypertension have outcomes similar to the general maternity population. Therefore, unless the blood pressure is over 150-160/100-110, antihypertensive medications are not used during pregnancy. Methyldopa is generally the first choice for use in pregnancy when medication is required.
- **Prenatal visits.** Counseling regarding the importance of frequent prenatal visits to reduce the incidence of adverse outcomes for mother or fetus is stressed.
- **Blood pressure monitoring.** The woman and her partner can be taught how to monitor blood pressure at home and maintain a record to be brought to each prenatal visit. Home monitoring is often more accurate because the woman is in a familiar environment and relaxed.
- **Fetal surveillance.** Starting at about 24 weeks, the woman should begin to keep fetal movement records and notify her care provider of any significant decrease in fetal movement. Serial ultrasonography to assess fetal growth and amniotic fluid volume is indicated. Antepartum fetal testing may begin as early as 26 weeks (Hallak, 1999).

During the first prenatal visit, the woman should have a thorough physical examination, which includes a funduscopic examination, blood pressure and pulses in all four extremities, and auscultation of chest and flanks. Laboratory work includes a urinalysis and culture; 24-hour urine for protein, creatinine clearance, sodium, and potassium; CBC; serum electrolytes; and a glucose tolerance test. The usual prenatal laboratory assessments and an ultrasound for confirming gestational age are also done if the woman is currently pregnant. Although essential hypertension is the most likely explanation for hypertension in early pregnancy, a thorough evaluation can rule out rare but serious causes of secondary hypertension such as pheochromocytoma or coarctation of the aorta.

A woman with chronic hypertension generally has more frequent prenatal visits. She should be seen every 2 to 3 weeks in the first two trimesters and then more frequently in the third trimester, depending on how she and the fetus are progressing. Twenty-four-hour urines, serum creatinine, uric acid, hematocrit, and ultrasound examinations are repeated at least once in the second and third trimesters.

Chronic Hypertension with Superimposed Preeclampsia

Preeclampsia develops in approximately 25% of women previously found to have chronic hypertension (NIH, 2000). When elevations of systolic blood pressure 30 mm Hg above the baseline or of diastolic blood pressure 15 mm Hg above the baseline are discovered on two occasions at least 6 hours apart, when proteinuria develops, or when edema occurs in the upper half of the body, the woman needs close monitoring and careful management. If the woman has underlying renal disease, it may be very difficult to confirm the diagnosis of superimposed preeclampsia. A rise in serum uric acid is helpful in identifying preeclampsia, which frequently occurs late in the second trimester or early in the third.

Gestational Hypertension

Gestational hypertension (also called *transient hypertension*) exists when transient elevation of blood pressure occurs for the first time after midpregnancy without proteinuria (NIH, 2000). The final determination that the woman has gestational hypertension is made in the postpartum period. If preeclampsia does not develop and blood pressure returns to normal by 12 weeks postpartum, the diagnosis of gestational hypertension may be assigned. If the blood pressure elevation persists after 12 weeks postpartum, the woman is diagnosed with chronic hypertension.

Care of the Woman at Risk for Rh Sensitization

Rh sensitization results from an antigen-antibody immunologic reaction within the body. Sensitization most commonly occurs when an Rh-negative woman carries an Rh-positive fetus, either to term or terminated by spontaneous or induced abortion. It can also occur if an Rh-negative nonpregnant woman receives an Rh-positive blood transfusion, experiences an Rh-positive tubal pregnancy, has an amniocentesis, or any other traumatic event that might allow Rh-positive fetal cells to enter the circulation of an Rh-negative woman.

A number of known red blood cell (RBC) antigens are involved in the Rh system, all of which are controlled by three pairs of genes: Cc, Dd, and Ee. Antigens in the D group are usually involved in incompatibility between the mother and fetus, although other RBC antigens can also cause isoimmunization.

Approximately 85% of white Americans, 92% to 93% of African Americans, and 99% of Asian populations are Rh positive (Weiner, 1999). Without treatment, an Rh-negative woman who gives birth to an Rh-positive infant has a 17% risk of becoming sensitized as a result of her pregnancy (ACOG, 1999c).

During a normal pregnancy, small amounts of fetal blood may cross the placenta. An Rh-negative mother whose fetus is Rh positive may develop anti-D antibodies in response to this exposure. During delivery of the placenta or as a result of trauma, even larger quantities of fetal blood can enter maternal circulation. After exposure to the Rh-positive antigen, the primary immune response is development of immunoglobulin M (IgM) antibodies. This primary response develops slowly over several weeks or months. IgM antibodies are large and do not cross the placenta. Once a woman develops these antibodies, she is immunized for life.

Following the primary response, the production of immunoglobulin G (IgG) anti-D antibodies develops rapidly. IgG is capable of crossing the placenta and coating the fetal Rh (D) positive red cells, causing hemolysis. A second exposure to a very small amount of Rh (D) positive cells produces a rapid secondary immune response, developing in a few days and stronger than the primary response (Figure 20–9 •). Thus although hemolysis is not generally a problem for the fetus during a first pregnancy, it may create problems during subsequent pregnancies.

The possibility also exists that an Rh-negative female fetus carried by an Rh-positive mother may become sensitized in utero. This female would not demonstrate signs of hemolytic disease, but because she would be sensitized before even becoming pregnant, she would have a positive antibody screen when receiving prenatal care with her first Rh-positive fetus.

Needle sharing among addicts poses a risk of sensitization because addicts draw some of their own blood up into the needle before injecting. Mismatched blood transfusion of Rh-positive blood to an Rh-negative person results in immunization in 55% to 80% of cases. Thus appropriate doses of Rh immune globulin must be given (Queenan, 1999).

Fetal-Neonatal Risks

The hemolysis caused by the maternal IgG antibodies in the fetus creates fetal anemia. The fetus responds by increasing red blood cell production. The presence of nucleated RBCs

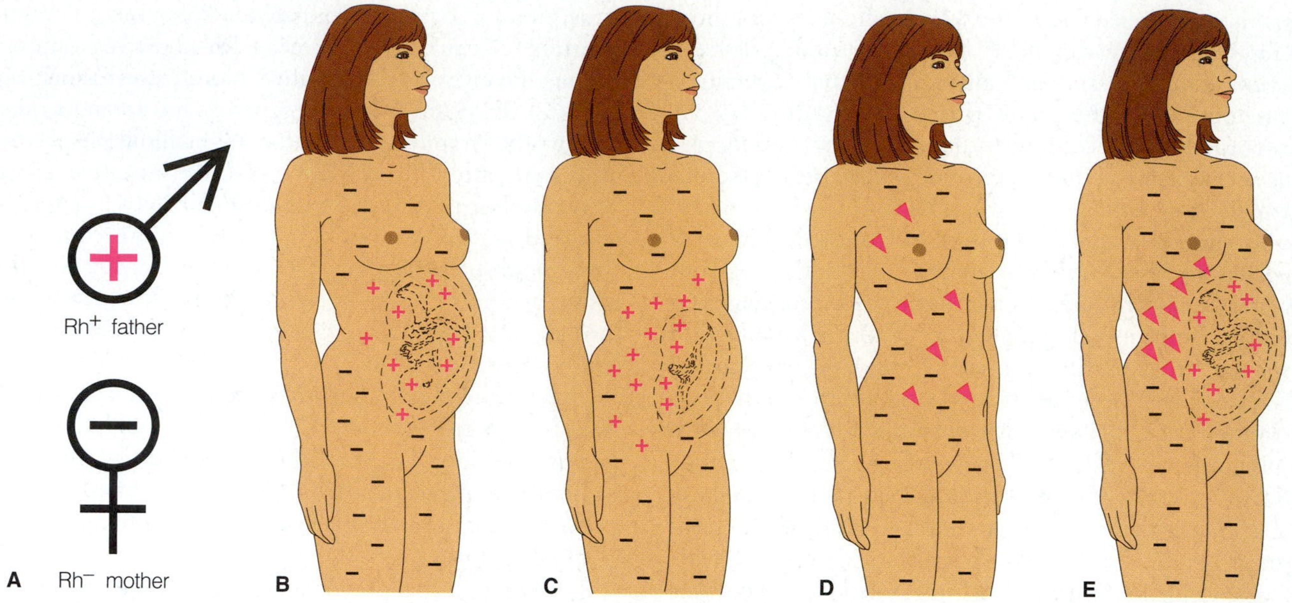

Figure 20–9 • Rh isoimmunization sequence. *A,* Rh-positive father and Rh-negative mother. *B,* Pregnancy with Rh-positive fetus. Some Rh-positive blood enters the mother's blood. *C,* As the placenta separates, the mother is further exposed to the Rh-positive blood. *D,* The mother is sensitized to the Rh-positive blood; anti-Rh-positive antibodies (triangles) are formed. *E,* In subsequent pregnancies with an Rh-positive fetus, Rh-positive red blood cells are attacked by the anti-Rh-positive maternal antibodies, causing hemolysis of red blood cells in the fetus.

(erythroblasts) is why the term **erythroblastosis fetalis** was coined for this severe hemolytic disease of the fetus and newborn. If treatment is not initiated, this anemia can also cause marked fetal edema, called **hydrops fetalis.** Congestive heart failure may result. Although maternal sensitization can now be prevented by appropriate administration of Rh immune globulin, infants still die of hemolytic disease secondary to Rh incompatibility.

Red blood cell destruction also leads to hyperbilirubinemia and jaundice (called *icterus gravis*), which can lead to neurologic damage (kernicterus).

Rh sensitization and the resultant hemolytic disease of the newborn are less common today because of the development of RhIgG. See Chapter 33 for further discussion of kernicterus and of treatment of the newborn affected by Rh sensitization.

Screening for Rh Incompatibility and Sensitization

At the first prenatal visit, (1) a history is taken of previous sensitization, abortions, blood transfusions, or children who developed jaundice or anemia during the neonatal period; (2) maternal blood type (ABO) and Rh factor are determined, and a routine Rh antibody screen is done; and (3) other medical complications, such as diabetes, infections, or hypertension, are identified. An antibody screen (*indirect Coombs' test*) is done to determine whether an Rh-negative woman is sensitized (has developed isoimmunity) to the Rh antigen. The indirect Coombs' test measures the number of antibodies in the maternal blood. If the Rh-negative woman is not D-isoimmunized, a repeat D antibody determination should be made at 28 weeks' gestation, and the expectant woman should receive 300 μg Rh immune globulin. Rh immune globulin is also administered after any amniocentesis, regardless of gestational age; after chorionic villi sampling, if there is an episode of bleeding during pregnancy; or if there has been maternal trauma such as injury resulting from a motor vehicle accident or from domestic violence. In addition, Rh immune globulin must be administered to any Rh-negative woman who experiences a first trimester spontaneous or induced abortion, or an ectopic pregnancy.

If the woman is Rh negative (dd), the father of the unborn child is asked to come into the clinic or physician's office to be assessed for his Rh factor and blood type. If he is homozygous for Rh positive (DD), all his offspring will be Rh positive. If he is heterozygous (Dd), 50% of his offspring will be Rh negative and 50% heterozygous for Rh positive. If the father is Rh negative, all their children will be Rh negative, and no Rh incompatibility with the mother will occur. If the father is Rh positive or the mother is known to have previously carried an Rh-positive fetus, further testing and careful management are needed.

In women who are isoimmunized, anti-D antibody titers should be determined every 2 to 4 weeks beginning at 16 to 18 weeks, biweekly during the third trimester, and the week before the due date. If the test shows a maternal antibody titer of 1:16 or greater, a delta optical density (ΔOD) analysis of the amniotic fluid is performed. (See later discussion.) If the titer is 1:16 or less late in pregnancy, birth at 38 weeks or spontaneous labor at term can be anticipated.

Negative antibody titers can consistently identify the fetus not at risk. However, the titers cannot reliably point out the fetus in danger because the level of the titer does not correlate with the severity of the disease. For instance, in a severely sensitized woman antibody titers may be moderately high and remain at the same level although the fetus is being more and more severely affected. Conversely, a woman sensitized by previous Rh-positive fetuses may show a high fixed antibody titer during a pregnancy in which the fetus is Rh negative. Fetal assessment includes percutaneous umbilical cord blood sampling (PUBS), amniocentesis, amniotic fluid analysis, and ultrasound. Previously, PUBS was the only direct method of assessing the Rh status of a fetus. This procedure requires a highly skilled physician and places the fetus at greater risk than does amniocentesis. It is now possible, however, to determine fetal Rh status from an amniotic fluid specimen using polymerase chain reaction (PCR).

Ultrasound should be done at 14 to 18 weeks to determine gestational age. Thereafter serial ultrasounds and amniotic fluid analysis should be done to follow fetal progress. The presence of ascites and subcutaneous edema are signs of severe fetal involvement (fetal hydrops). Other indicators of the fetal condition include an increase in fetal heart size, hydramnios, and placental thickness and texture. Ultrasound evaluation cannot distinguish mild from severe fetal anemia unless hydropic changes are present.

When red blood cells are hemolyzed, bilirubin is a breakdown product. If fetal RBCs are being hemolyzed because of isoimmunization, the fetus may excrete bilirubin in the amniotic fluid with voiding. Thus ΔOD analysis is done to determine the amount of bilirubin pigment found in the amniotic fluid. Normally the concentration of bilirubin pigments in the amniotic fluid declines during pregnancy. Elevated bilirubin levels are significant. Because the amount of bilirubin found in the amniotic fluid correlates roughly with the extent of the hemolysis, the ΔOD analysis serves as an indirect predictor of the severity of the fetal anemia (Cunningham et al, 2001). To determine the ΔOD level, amniotic fluid, obtained by transabdominal amniocentesis, is separated from its cellular components by centrifuge. The amount of bilirubin pigment from the degradation of red blood cells can then be measured by spectrophotometric analysis and plotted on a special chart called a Liley graph.

The ΔOD value and gestational age determine the plan of obstetric-pediatric management. If the spectrophotometric readings are in zone I (the lowest zone), a normal or mildly anemic newborn may be anticipated, and birth at term may be permitted. Prognosis for this newborn is good, but phototherapy or exchange transfusion may be necessary.

A reading in zone II (the middle zone) indicates a moderately anemic fetus who may be hydropic or stillborn if born at term. Fetuses with a ΔOD in the upper zone II need to be followed with a PUBS or repeat amniocentesis within the week. Once the fetus reaches viability, induced vaginal or cesarean birth is indicated. The exact timing of birth needs to be determined individually based on factors such as fetal well-being, lung maturity, and previous obstetric history. A fair prognosis and possible need for exchange transfusion are anticipated.

Readings within zone III (the highest zone) indicate a severely affected fetus who may require intrauterine transfusion every 1 to 2 weeks between weeks 26 and 32 until viability is reached, followed by birth, usually by cesarean. Neonatal exchange transfusion is anticipated. Prognosis is guarded. Fetal monitoring may identify the very ill fetus by documenting less movement or lack of movement. The appearance of sinusoidal pattern suggests fetal anemia and a deteriorating fetal condition (see Chapter 23).

Clinical Therapy

The goal of medical management is the birth of a mature fetus who has not developed severe hemolysis in utero. This requires early identification and treatment of maternal conditions that predispose the infant to hemolytic disease, coordinated obstetric-pediatric treatment for the seriously affected newborn, and prevention of Rh sensitization if none is present.

ANTEPARTUM MANAGEMENT

Two primary interventions are used by the physician to aid the fetus whose blood cells are being destroyed by maternal antibodies: early birth of the fetus and intrauterine transfusion, both of which carry risks. Ideally, birth should be delayed until fetal pulmonary maturity is confirmed at about 36 to 37 weeks. This is possible for most pregnancies with ΔOD readings in zones I and II. Severely sensitized fetuses may require birth at 32 to 34 weeks.

Intrauterine transfusion is done to correct the anemia produced by the red blood cell hemolysis and thereby improve fetal oxygenation. This may be done either intravascularly through PUBS or intraperitoneally as early as 18 weeks. In a fetus who shows no signs of hydrops, a fetal blood sample should be used to check for significant anemia (hematocrit >30%) prior to starting transfusion therapy.

Intravascular transfusion has greatly improved the outcome for severely affected fetuses. Under ultrasound visualization, the umbilical vein is entered, and the fetus is temporarily paralyzed with 0.1 mg/kg estimated fetal weight of pancuronium bromide. A fetal hematocrit is obtained; then leukocyte-poor Rh-negative packed red blood cells (PRBCs) are transfused. The volume of PRBCs is determined by a formula based on estimated normal blood volume, the pretransfusion hematocrit, the hematocrit of the blood to be transfused, and the desired hematocrit. Repeat transfusions can be scheduled as necessary until the fetus is sufficiently mature to tolerate birth. Prior to this technology, intrauterine transfusions were done by introducing the needle into the fetal abdomen and peritoneal cavity. Blood was transfused through a catheter into the peritoneal cavity, where diaphragmatic lymphatics absorbed the RBCs into fetal circulation.

About 80% to 90% of transfused fetuses survive. The procedure is hazardous to the fetus, however. Complications include fetal distress, fetal hematoma, fetal-maternal hemorrhage, fetal death, and chorioamnionitis. Birth is delayed until at least 32 weeks' gestation if possible. Premature newborns are generally more susceptible to damage from hemolytic disease. They often require exchange transfusion and usually require intensive nursery care.

POSTPARTUM MANAGEMENT

The goals of postpartum care are to prevent sensitization in the as-yet-unsensitized pregnant woman and to treat the isoimmune hemolytic disease in the newborn.

The Rh-negative mother who has no titer (indirect Coombs' negative, nonsensitized) and who has given birth to an Rh-positive fetus (direct Coombs' negative) is given an intramuscular injection of 300 μg RhIgG globulin—that is, **Rh immune globulin** (**RhoGAM,** HypRho-D)—within 72 hours so that she does not have time to produce antibodies to fetal cells that entered her bloodstream when the placenta separated. This protocol reduces the incidence of antenatal sensitization dramatically. Rh immune globulin works to destroy the fetal cells in the maternal circulation before sensitization occurs, thereby blocking maternal antibody production. This provides temporary passive immunity for the mother, which prevents the development of permanent active immunity (antibody formation).

The normal dose of Rh immune globulin should suppress the immune response to approximately 30 mL Rh-positive whole blood. However, if a larger fetomaternal bleed may have occurred, a Kleihauer-Betke test can be performed to obtain an estimate of its extent. Based on the findings, an additional 300 μg of Rh immune globulin is given for every 25 mL of fetal whole blood in the woman's circulation at a rate of 300 μg every 12 hours until the total necessary dose is given (Bowman, 1999).

When the woman is Rh negative and not sensitized and the father is Rh positive or unknown, Rh immune globulin is also given after each spontaneous or induced abortion, ectopic pregnancy, chorionic villus sampling, multifetal pregnancy reduction, amniocentesis, PUBS, antepartum hemorrhage, or external version. After any maternal trauma, a Kleihauer-Betke test can be performed to identify the need for Rh immune globulin administration. If abortion or ectopic pregnancy occurs in the first trimester, a smaller (50 μg) dose of Rh immune globulin (MICRhoGAM or Mini-Gamulin Rh) is used. A full dose is used following second trimester amniocentesis. Occasionally, sensitization can occur antepartally due to small transplacental bleeds. To prevent this from occurring, an antibody screen is performed on an Rh-negative woman at 28 weeks' gestation. If it is negative, 300 μg Rh immune globulin is administered prophylactically.

Rh immune globulin is not given to the newborn or the father. It is not effective for and should not be given to a previously sensitized woman. However, sometimes after childbirth or an abortion, the results of the blood test do not clearly show whether the mother is already sensitized to the Rh antigen. In such cases, Rh immune globulin should be given because it will cause no harm. Table 20–7 • summarizes the major considerations in caring for an Rh-negative woman. The treatment of the newborn with isoimmune hemolytic disease is discussed in Chapter 33.

Table 20–7 • RH SENSITIZATION

When trying to work through Rh problems, the nurse should remember the following:

- A potential problem exists when an Rh-negative mother and an Rh-positive father conceive a child who is Rh positive.
- In this situation, the mother may become sensitized or produce antibodies to her fetus's Rh-positive blood.

The following tests are used to detect sensitization:

- Indirect Coombs' tests—done on the mother's blood to measure the number of Rh-positive antibodies.
- Direct Coombs' test—done on the infant's blood to detect antibody-coated Rh-positive RBCs.

Based on the results of these tests, the following may be done:

- If the mother's indirect Coombs' test is negative and the infant's direct Coomb's test is negative (confirming that sensitization has not occurred), the mother is given Rh immune globulin within 72 hours of birth.
- If the mother's indirect Coombs' test is positive and her Rh-positive infant has a positive direct Coombs' test, Rh immune globulin is *not* given, in this case, the infant is carefully monitored for hemolytic disease.
- It is recommended that Rh immune globulin be given at 28 weeks antenatally to decrease possible transplacental bleeding concerns.
- Rh immune globulin is also administered after each abortion (spontaneous or therapeutic), antepartum hemorrhage mismatched blood transfusion, ectopic pregnancy, amniocentesis, chorionic villi sampling (CVS), percutaneous umbilical blood sampling (PUBS), fetal cephalic version, or maternal trauma.

NURSING CARE MANAGEMENT

Nursing Assessment and Diagnosis

As part of the initial prenatal history the nurse asks the mother whether she knows her blood type and Rh factor. Many women are aware that they are Rh negative and that this status has implications for pregnancy. If the woman knows she is Rh negative, the nurse can assess the woman's knowledge of what that means. The nurse can also ask the woman whether she ever received Rh immune globulin, whether she has had any previous pregnancies and their outcome, and whether she knows her partner's Rh factor. Should the partner be Rh negative, there is no risk to the fetus, who will also be Rh negative.

If the woman does not know what Rh immune type she is, intervention cannot begin until the initial laboratory data are obtained. If the woman is Rh negative, the father's blood type and zygosity, if he is Rh positive, are obtained. Once that is complete, the nurse plans intervention based on the findings.

If the woman becomes sensitized during her pregnancy, nursing assessment focuses on the knowledge level and coping skills of the woman and her family. The nurse also provides ongoing assessment during procedures to evaluate fetal well-being, such as ultrasound and amniocentesis.

Postpartally, the nurse reviews data about the Rh type of the fetus. If the fetus is Rh positive, the mother is Rh negative, and no sensitization has occurred, nursing assessment reveals the need to administer Rh immune globulin within 72 hours of birth.

Nursing diagnoses that might apply to the pregnant woman at risk for Rh sensitization include the following:

- ***Health-Seeking Behavior:*** Information about the purpose of RhIgG related to an expressed desire to understand the treatment of Rh incompatibility
- ***Ineffective Individual Coping*** related to depression secondary to the development of indications of the need for fetal exchange transfusion

I've been a nurse for over 35 years now. I remember when RhoGAM first started to be used—what a difference it made in the lives of so many women. Young women who are Rh negative today will hopefully never know the pain and tragedy the simple absence of a blood factor can mean. It is nothing short of miraculous!

Nursing Plan and Implementation

During the antepartal period, the nurse explains the mechanisms involved in isoimmunization and answers any questions the woman and her partner may have. It is imperative that the woman understand the importance of receiving Rh immune globulin after every spontaneous or therapeutic abortion or ectopic pregnancy if she is not already sensitized. The nurse also explains the purpose of the Rh immune globulin administered at 28 weeks if the woman is not sensitized.

If the woman is sensitized to the Rh factor, it poses a threat to any Rh-positive fetus she carries. The nurse provides emotional support to the family to help them deal with their grief and any feelings of guilt about the infant's condition. Should an intrauterine transfusion become necessary, the nurse continues to provide emotional support while also assuming responsibilities as part of the healthcare team.

During labor, the nurse caring for an Rh-negative woman who has not been sensitized ensures that the woman's blood is assessed for any antibodies and also has been crossmatched for Rh immune globulin. On the postpartum unit, the nurse generally is responsible for administering the Rh immune globulin (see Procedure 20–2: Administration of Rh Immune Globulin [Rho GAM, HypRho-D]).

Evaluation

Expected outcomes of nursing care include the following:

- The woman is able to explain the process of Rh sensitization and its implications for her unborn child and for subsequent pregnancies.
- If the woman has not been sensitized, she is able to explain the importance of receiving Rh immune globulin when necessary and cooperates with the recommended dosage schedule.
- The woman gives birth to a healthy newborn.
- If complications develop for the fetus (or newborn), they are detected quickly, and therapy is instituted.

Care of the Woman at Risk Due to ABO Incompatibility

ABO incompatibility is rather common (occurring in 20% to 25% of pregnancies) but rarely causes significant hemolysis. In most cases, ABO incompatibility is limited to type O mothers with a type A or B fetus. The group B fetus of a group A mother and the group A fetus of a group B mother are only occasionally affected. Group O infants, because they have no antigenic sites on the red blood cells, are never affected regardless of the mother's blood type. The incompatibility occurs as a result of the maternal antibodies present in her serum and interaction between the antigen sites on the fetal red blood cells.

Anti-A and anti-B antibodies are naturally occurring; that is, women are naturally exposed to the A and B antigens through the foods they eat and through exposure to infection by gram-negative bacteria. As a result, some women have high serum anti-A and anti-B titers before they become pregnant. Once the woman becomes pregnant, the maternal serum anti-A and anti-B antibodies cross the placenta and produce hemolysis of the fetal red blood cells. With ABO incompatibility, the first infant is frequently involved, and no relationship exists between the appearance of the disease and repeated sensitization from one pregnancy to the next.

Unlike the case of Rh incompatibility, treatment is never warranted antepartally. As part of the initial assessment, however, the nurse should note whether the potential for an ABO incompatibility exists. This alerts caregivers so that following birth the newborn can be assessed carefully for the development of hyperbilirubinemia (Chapter 33). Occasionally, affected fetuses require an exchange transfusion after birth (Queenan, 1999).

Care of the Woman Requiring Surgery During Pregnancy

Although elective surgery should be delayed until the postpartal period, essential surgery can generally be undertaken during pregnancy. Surgery does pose some risks. The incidence of spontaneous abortion is increased for women who have surgery in the first trimester. The risks to the pregnancy can be significantly reduced when surgery can be delayed until the second trimester or to the postpartum period. Surgery during the third trimester is difficult due to the enlarging uterus and an increased risk of preterm labor (Angelini, 1999; Mahomed, 1999).

Procedure 20-2 Administration of Rh Immune Globulin (RhoGAM, HypRho-D)

Preparation

1. Confirm that Rh immune globulin is indicated by checking the woman's prenatal or intrapartal record to verify that she is Rh negative. Then confirm that sensitization has not occurred—maternal indirect Coombs' negative. Postpartally, confirm that the baby is Rh positive but not sensitized (direct Coombs' negative) and that the mother's indirect Coombs' is negative. Rh immune globulin is *not* indicated if the infant is Rh negative, too.
   Rationale: Rh immune globulin is only indicated for Rh-negative, unsensitized women.
2. Confirm that the woman does not have a history of allergies to immune globulin preparations by checking entries on medication allergies in her chart and by asking her whether she has ever had any allergic reactions to medications, globulins, or blood products.
   Rationale: Rh immune globulin is made from the plasma portion of blood. Allergic reactions are possible.
3. Explain purpose and procedure. Have consent form signed if required by agency policy.
   Rationale: Many agencies require separate consent for the administration of Rh immune globulin because it is a blood product. The woman should clearly understand the purpose of the Rh immune globulin, its rationale, the administration procedure, and any related risks. Generally the primary side effects are redness and tenderness at the injection site and allergic responses.

Equipment and Supplies

- Rh immune globulin, which is obtained from the blood bank or pharmacy according to agency protocol. Lot numbers for the drug and the cross-match should be the same.
- Syringe and IM needle

Procedure

1. Confirm the woman's identity and administer one vial of 300 μg Rh immune globulin IM in the deltoid muscle.
2. An immune globulin microdose is used after miscarriage, elective abortion, ectopic pregnancy, or molar pregnancy occurring within the first 12 weeks' gestation. Antepartally, the Rh immune globulin is generally given within 3 hours but not longer than 72 hours of the event.
3. If a larger bleed is suspected at birth (as in cases of severe abruptio placentae), additional doses may be administered at one time using multiple sites at regular intervals as long as all doses are given within 72 hours of childbirth.
   Rationale: The normal 300-μg dose provides passive immunity following exposure of up to 15 mL of transfused RBCs or 30 mL of fetal blood.
4. Provide opportunities for the woman to ask questions and express concerns.
   Rationale: Many women, especially primigravidas, are not aware of the risks for an Rh-positive fetus of a sensitized Rh-negative mother. They need to understand the importance of receiving Rh immune globulin for each pregnancy to ensure continued protection.
5. Chart according to agency policy. Most agencies chart lot number, route, dose, and client education.

Clinical Tip

In most cases, Rh immune globulin is administered in the deltoid muscle. However, in an extremely thin woman, or in the cases of a larger-than-normal dose, consider administering the medication in the ventrogluteal or posterior gluteal site. You may also divide the dose into multiple injections.

Clinical Therapy

The most common nonpregnancy-related indications for surgical treatment are appendicitis, cholecystitis, and gastrointestinal obstruction. Although general preoperative and postoperative care are similar for pregnant and nonpregnant women, special considerations must be kept in mind whenever the surgical client is pregnant. The early second trimester is the best time to operate because there is less risk of causing spontaneous abortion or early labor, and the uterus is not so large as to impinge on the abdominal field.

The preoperative chest radiograph and electrocardiogram, which are routine for persons over age 40, should be done on the same basis for the pregnant woman. If a chest radiograph is done, the fetus should be shielded from the radiation. Because of decreased intestinal motility and decreased free gastric acid secretion during pregnancy, stomach emptying time is delayed, which increases risk of vomiting during induction of anesthesia and during the postoperative period. Therefore, a nasogastric tube is recommended prior to major surgery. An indwelling urinary catheter prevents bladder distention, decreases risk of injury to the bladder, and promotes ease of monitoring output. Support stockings during and after surgery help prevent venous stasis and the development of thrombophlebitis. Fetal heart tones must be monitored before, during, and after surgery.

Pregnancy causes increased secretions of the respiratory tract and engorgement of the nasal mucous membrane, often making breathing through the nose difficult. Because of this, pregnant women often need an endotracheal tube for respiratory support during surgery. Caregivers must guard against maternal hypoxia during surgery because uterine circulation will be decreased and fetal oxygenation can decline very quickly. During surgery and the recovery period, the woman is positioned to allow optimal uteroplacental–fetal circulation. A wedge is placed under her hip to tip the uterus and thereby avoid pressure by the fetus on the maternal vena cava.

Spinal or epidural anesthesia is preferred because local anesthetics are not associated with birth defects. Caution must be exercised because this type of anesthesia may produce hypotension and respiratory apnea in the pregnant woman. The frequency and degree of the hypotension increase with higher anesthetic levels. This can be prevented in many cases with a preanesthetic infusion of 900 to 1000 mL of fluid.

Blood loss during surgery is monitored carefully. Measurement of fetal heart tones gives the best indication of blood loss. Because of the normal increased blood volume of pregnancy, uterine blood flow may be reduced significantly before the maternal blood pressure begins to fall. Fluid replacement should be done with balanced electrolyte solution and, if needed, with whole blood.

NURSING CARE MANAGEMENT

Nursing Assessment and Diagnosis

During the preoperative period, the nurse assesses the pregnant woman's health status in the same way that any preoperative client is assessed. Is there any sign of respiratory infection, fever, urinary tract infection, or anemia? Are laboratory values all within normal limits for surgery (except in the case of emergency surgery, which may, of necessity, be done even with abnormal laboratory values)? Do the woman and her family understand the surgical procedure? Do they know what to expect postoperatively? Do they have any questions or concerns?

The nurse also considers the impact of surgery on the woman's pregnancy. Is the fetal heart rate normal? Does the woman understand the implications of surgery with regard to her pregnancy? How is she coping?

Intraoperatively, fetal heart rate is assessed if at all possible. Postoperatively, the nurse completes all necessary postoperative assessments and also continues to assess fetal status, primarily by monitoring the fetal heart rate.

Nursing diagnoses that might apply to the pregnant woman who requires surgery include the following:

- ***Altered Tissue Perfusion*** (fetal) related to the effects of general anesthesia on fetal oxygenation
- ***Anxiety*** related to lack of knowledge of preoperative and postoperative procedures
- ***Fear*** related to the possible effect of surgery on fetal outcome

Nursing Plan and Implementation

Much of the nurse's care during the preoperative period is directed toward the educational needs of the woman and her family. The nurse plans time to review the procedure and answer any questions the family may have. The nurse recognizes that the need for surgery during the woman's pregnancy is probably very distressing for the family. The nurse works to help decrease their anxiety by providing information and emotional support.

Postoperatively, the nurse is caring for two clients: the mother and her unborn child. In addition to monitoring the status of both, the nurse considers both in providing care. If surgery is done in the first trimester, the nurse should be aware of the potential teratogenic effect of any medications prescribed and should discuss the implications with the surgeon and obstetrician. During the third trimester, the nurse, recognizing the potential for vena caval syndrome if the woman lies flat on her back, helps the woman maintain a side-lying position. To avoid inadequate oxygenation, the nurse encourages the woman to turn, breathe deeply, and cough regularly and also to use any ventilation therapy, such as incentive spirometry, to avoid developing pneumonia. The pregnant woman is also at increased risk for thrombophlebitis, so the nurse applies antiembolism stockings, encourages leg exercises while the woman is confined to bed, and begins ambulation as soon as possible. In addition, the nurse encourages the woman to maintain or resume an adequate diet as soon as possible. If cultural factors influence the woman's dietary practices, the nurse and dietitian should work together to meet the woman's needs.

Discharge teaching is especially important. The woman and her family should have a clear understanding of what to expect regarding activity level, discomfort, diet, medications, and any special considerations. In addition, they ought to know any warning signs that they should report to their physician immediately.

Evaluation

Expected outcomes of nursing care include the following:

- The woman is able to explain the surgical procedure, its risks and benefits, and its implications for her pregnancy.
- Caregivers maintain adequate maternal oxygenation throughout surgery and postoperatively.
- Potential complications are avoided or detected early and treated successfully.
- The woman is able to describe any necessary postdischarge activities, limitations, and follow-up and agrees to cooperate with the recommended regimen.
- The woman maintains her pregnancy successfully.

Care of the Woman Suffering Trauma from an Accident

Accidents and injury are the leading causes of death in women of reproductive age. Estimates suggest that physical trauma complicates approximately 1 in 12 pregnancies and is the leading cause of nonobstetric maternal death. When the woman is critically injured, fetal death occurs at least 40% of the time (ACOG, 1998c; Bobrowski, 1999). Approximately two thirds of all trauma during pregnancy is the result of motor vehicle accidents (ACOG, 1998c). Falls and assault—including domestic violence—are the next most common causes of injury (Tillet & Hanson, 1999).

In early pregnancy, body changes increase the potential for injury through fatigue, fainting spells, and hyperventilation. Late in pregnancy, the woman has less balance and coordination and may fall. Her protruding abdomen is vulnerable to a variety of minor injuries. The fetus is usually well protected by the amniotic fluid, which distributes the force of a blow equally in all directions, and by the muscle layers of the uterus and abdominal wall. In early pregnancy, while the uterus is still in the pelvis, it is shielded from blows by the surrounding pelvic organs, muscles, and bony structures. Trauma that causes concern includes blunt trauma, from an automobile accident, for example; penetrating abdominal injuries, such as knife or gunshot wounds; and the complications that commonly accompany maternal trauma, such as shock, premature labor, and spontaneous abortion.

The normal physiologic changes of pregnancy have clinical implications for victims of trauma. Blood volume increases up to 50% and cardiac output increases about 40%. Generally, the pregnant woman has a greater volume of blood loss compared to a nonpregnant woman before evidence of shock is seen. The pregnant woman with significant volume loss is able to maintain hemodynamic stability temporarily by decreasing uteroplacental perfusion, thereby compromising fetal status. In the second and third trimesters, supine positioning can decrease blood return to the heart and cause overt hypotension and even loss of consciousness. During pregnancy, minute ventilation and oxygen consumption increase. This makes the gravid woman more susceptible to hypoxemia with apnea. Clotting factors normally increase in pregnancy, making it a hypercoagulable state. Thus, the risk of thrombosis after injury is increased. Disseminating intravascular coagulation (DIC) occurs commonly with severe trauma. Because the normal fibrinogen level in pregnancy is increased to between 350 and 400 mg/dL, normal nonpregnant values may indicate early DIC (Bobrowski, 1999; Gonik, 1999).

Maternal mortality most often occurs from head trauma or hemorrhage. Uterine rupture results from strong deceleration forces in an automobile accident in only 0.1% to 1% of pregnant women (ACOG, 1998c). All automobile passengers should wear seat belts. The small risk of uterine or placental injury from seat belt use is far outweighed by the fact that maternal death is the most common cause of fetal death. Traumatic separation of the placenta can occur even if the site of injury is remote from the abdomen. It results in a high rate of fetal mortality. Premature labor is another serious hazard to the fetus, often following rupture of membranes during an accident. Premature labor can ensue even if the woman is not injured.

Fractures of the pelvis can result in significant retroperitoneal hemorrhage. If there is an unstable or dislocated fracture of the pelvis, cesarean birth will probably be necessary, but with a slightly displaced pelvic fracture, vaginal birth may be attempted. Hematuria or difficulty placing a urinary catheter may be associated with injuries to the bladder or urethra.

Penetrating trauma includes gunshot wounds and stab wounds. The mother generally fares better than the fetus if the penetrating trauma involves the abdomen as the enlarged uterus is likely to protect the mother's bowel from injury. Unfortunately, the fetal injury rate is 59% to 80%.

Clinical Therapy

The goals of clinical therapy are to stabilize the injury and promote well-being for both mother and fetus. Thus clinical therapy initially focuses on ensuring airway adequacy, maintaining ventilation and adequate circulatory volume, controlling acute bleeding, and splinting fractures to prevent vascular or tissue injury. The Glasgow Coma Scale is useful in evaluating for neurologic deficit. Once the mother is stabilized, fetal status is assessed.

Care must be taken at the scene of the injury to avoid the development of supine hypotensive syndrome. A wedge is generally placed under the woman's right hip. A neck brace is used if a neck injury is suspected, or the woman is placed on a backboard and the entire board is tilted to displace the uterus. Prompt treatment of maternal hypotension or hypovolemia also averts poor fetal oxygenation. Obstetric consultation is necessary to ensure that the needs of both mother and fetus are met.

In cases of noncatastrophic trauma, that is, where the mother's life is not directly threatened, fetal monitoring for 4 hours should be sufficient if there is no vaginal bleeding, uterine tenderness, contractions, or leaking amniotic fluid. Abruptio placentae may occur following a blow to the abdomen as the flexible myometrium of the uterus sustains a contour-changing impact that the relatively inelastic placenta cannot match. The increased intrauterine pressure during the blow further shears the placenta from the underlying decidua basalis. Abruptio placentae may occur in up to 5% of women who sustain minor injuries and in up to 35% of women who sustain major abdominal trauma (Bobrowski, 1999). Increased uterine irritability in the first few hours following trauma helps identify women who may be at high risk for this potentially catastrophic complication. Of those women who contract every 10 minutes or more, 20% will have placental abruption. Ultrasonography does not seem to be as sensitive as fetal monitoring for diagnosing abruptio placentae. If the woman is bleeding, contracting, or has uterine tenderness or a nonreassuring fetal heart rate tracing, a 24- to 48-hour observation is recommended.

Fetomaternal hemorrhage occurs four to five times more often in pregnant women who have experienced trauma. A Kleihauer-Betke test may be useful in helping identify unsensitized Rh-negative women who have experienced fetal-maternal bleeds due to trauma. Rh immune globulin should be given to any unsensitized Rh-negative woman to be certain she is covered for small fetal hemorrhages that may be below the sensitivity of the Kleihauer-Betke test.

There has been controversy regarding the use of beta-adrenergic tocolytics in pregnant women following trauma because of the concerns regarding hemodynamic instability and the potential for masking uterine irritability or contractions that forewarn of abruptio placentae. Radiographic studies should be performed as needed to evaluate injuries regardless of fetal exposure.

When cardiopulmonary resuscitation (CPR) is performed on the pregnant woman late in gestation, perimortem cesarean birth is advocated if CPR is unsuccessful in the first 4 minutes. Chest compressions are less effective in the third trimester due to compression of the inferior vena cava by the gravid uterus. Cesarean birth alleviates this compression and improves resuscitation efforts in both the fetus and the mother.

NURSING CARE MANAGEMENT

Nursing Assessment and Diagnosis

Each individual must be assessed according to the type and extent of her injuries. As with all trauma victims, initial assessments focus on adequacy of the airway, evidence of breathing, existence of cardiovascular stability, extent of injury, and a brief neurologic assessment. When an injured woman is pregnant, it is necessary to assess fetal status as well in order to avoid fetal hypoxia. Frequent maternal blood gas determinations are indicated if respiratory function is compromised.

Ongoing assessments include evaluation of uterine tone, contractions and tenderness, fundal height, fetal heart rate, intake and output and other indicators of shock, normal postoperative evaluation in those women requiring surgery, determination of neurologic status, and assessment of mental outlook and anxiety level.

Nursing diagnoses that might apply to the pregnant woman suffering trauma include the following:

- ***Pain*** related to the effects of the trauma experienced
- ***Constipation*** related to immobility secondary to the effects of the accident
- ***Fear*** related to the effects of the trauma on fetal well-being

Nursing Plan and Implementation

As a member of the healthcare team the nurse is actively involved in the ongoing assessment of the status of the woman and fetus. The nurse also has a primary responsibility to assess the childbearing woman's emotional state. The trauma victim must be oriented to her situation and receive explanation and reinforcement as necessary to help her understand any interventions. Family members should be involved as appropriate. The nurse also gives the pregnant woman an opportunity to discuss her feelings and concerns.

Evaluation

Expected outcomes of nursing care include the following:

- The woman and her family are able to understand the effects of the trauma on her and on her unborn child.
- Adequate maternal oxygenation is maintained to ensure fetal well-being.
- The woman's pain is adequately relieved, and her trauma is treated.
- Potential complications are quickly identified, and appropriate interventions are instituted.
- The woman gives birth to a healthy newborn.
- If the trauma results in fetal demise, the woman is able to verbalize her feelings and begin working through the grief process.

Care of the Battered Pregnant Woman

The true extent of domestic violence during pregnancy is difficult to determine. Estimates suggest that violence during pregnancy affects up to 20% of women (ACOG, 1999a; Cokkinides, Coker, Sanderson, et al, 1999); however, these statistics are most likely understated because many victims are unwilling to disclose their experiences.

Battering may result in psychologic distress, loss of pregnancy, preterm labor, low-birth-weight infants, injury to the fetus, and fetal death. Complications such as poor maternal weight gain, infection, anemia, and second and third trimester bleeding are also seen more frequently among pregnant women who are abused. Women who are battered may also experience sexual abuse and are at increased risk of contracting sexually transmitted infections from their partner (Cokkinides et al, 1999).

This pattern of violence may escalate during pregnancy and may occur even more frequently in the postpartum period (ACOG, 1999a). The first step toward helping the battered woman is to identify her. She needs support, confidence in her decision making, and the recognition that she can help herself.

Chronic psychosomatic symptoms can be an indicator of abuse. The woman may have nonspecific or vague complaints. It is important to assess old scars around the head, chest, arms, abdomen, and genitalia. Any bruising or evidence of pain is also evaluated. The nurse should be especially alert for signs of bruising or injury to the woman's breasts, abdomen, or genitals because these areas are common targets of violence during pregnancy. Other indicators include a decrease in eye contact, silence when the partner is in the room, and a history of nervousness, insomnia, drug overdose, or alcohol problems. Frequent visits to the emergency department and a history of accidents without understandable causes are possible indicators of abuse.

The goals of treatment are to identify the woman at risk, increase her decision-making abilities to decrease the potential for further abuse, and provide a safe environment for her and her unborn child. Screening must be done in a private setting and by using direct questions. ACOG recommends that *all* women be screened for intimate partner violence. During pregnancy, women should be screened multiple times because they may not disclose abuse if they are asked only one time, or the abuse may begin later in pregnancy. The suggested schedule for screening is at the first prenatal visit, at least once per trimester, and at the postpartum visit. See Chapter 9 for discussion of specific screening questions.

Once domestic violence is identified, the next step is to determine the immediate safety of the woman. She needs to be aware of community resources available to her, such as emergency shelters; police, legal, and social services; and counseling. It is important to establish an exit plan in situations of ongoing violence. Pocket cards and resource materials can be handed to women or left in restrooms for them to pick up. Nurses need to recognize that, ultimately, it is the woman's decision either to seek assistance or to return to old patterns. For further information, see Chapter 9.

Care of the Woman with a Perinatal Infection Affecting the Fetus

Fetal infection may develop at any time during pregnancy. In general, perinatal infections are most likely to cause harm when the embryo is exposed during first trimester organ development. Infections later in pregnancy create various concerns such as growth restriction, nonimmune hydrops, and neurologic disturbances. The most commonly occurring viral and parasitic infections that may have an impact on the fetus if acquired during pregnancy include toxoplasmosis, rubella, cytomegalovirus, herpes simplex virus, group B streptococcus, and parvovirus B19.

Toxoplasmosis

Toxoplasmosis is caused by the protozoan *Toxoplasma gondii.* It is innocuous in most adults but can be devastating to the immunosuppressed person. When contracted in pregnancy, it can profoundly affect the fetus. The pregnant woman may contract the organism by eating raw or poorly cooked meat, by drinking unpasteurized goat's milk, or by contact with the feces of infected cats, either through the cat litter box or by gardening in areas frequented by cats. The most infectious organisms can live in warm, moist soil for up to a year (Gagne, 2001).

The percentage of childbearing women in North America who are seropositive for toxoplasmosis varies. In the United States, approximately 38% of pregnant women have antibodies to this organism (ACOG, 2000). Estimates suggest that about one out of every 1000 pregnant women becomes infected by toxoplasmosis, resulting in about 400 to 4000 cases of congenital toxoplasmosis each year (Soto, 2002). Toxoplasmosis is common in Western Europe. In Paris, for example, more than 80% of women of childbearing age have antibodies to this organism (Sison & Sever, 1999b).

FETAL-NEONATAL RISKS

Maternal infection during the first trimester is associated with the lowest incidence of fetal infection, but when it occurs, first trimester infection typically results in more severe fetal damage and often ends in a spontaneous abortion. The highest rate of fetal infection (65%) occurs when the mother contracts the infection in the third trimester, but almost 70% of infants are born without clinical signs of infection (Yankowitz & Pastorek, 1999).

In very mild cases, retinochoroiditis (inflammation of the retina and choroid layer of the eye) may be the only recognizable damage, and it and other manifestations may not appear until adolescence or young adulthood. Severe neonatal disorders associated with congenital infection include convulsions, coma, microcephaly, and hydrocephalus. The infant with a severe infection may die soon after birth. Survivors are often blind, deaf, and severely retarded. Treatment of the mother can reduce the incidence of fetal infection by 60% (ACOG, 2000).

CLINICAL THERAPY

The goal of medical treatment is to identify the woman at risk for toxoplasmosis and to treat the disease promptly if diagnosed. Diagnosis can be made by serologic testing, including the IgM and IgG fluorescent antibody tests. Elevated IgM titers are detectable 5 days after infection and may remain elevated for one year or more (ACOG, 2000). The indirect fluorescent Ab test (IFAT), the indirect hemagglutination test (IHAT), or the Sabin-Feldman dye test are also used to establish the diagnosis. Ultrasound can reveal findings suggestive of severe fetal infection such as ascites, ventriculomegaly, microcephaly, and growth restriction (ACOG, 2000). PCR testing of amniotic fluid or antibody testing of fetal blood is used in diagnosing congenital toxoplasmosis.

If fetal infection is documented by serologic and radiographic testing, the woman may be treated with sulfadiazine, leucovorin calcium, pyrimethamine, and spiramycin. Leucovorin calcium is included in this regimen to counteract the bone marrow suppression effects of pyrimethamine. This combination therapy should not be started until after 16 weeks' gestation because of the teratogenic effects of pyrimethamine (Soto, 2002). Sulfadiazine and erythromycin may be used during the first half of pregnancy.

NURSING CARE MANAGEMENT

Nursing Assessment and Diagnosis

The incubation period for the disease is 10 days. The woman with acute toxoplasmosis may be asymptomatic, or she may develop myalgia, malaise, rash, splenomegaly, fever, headache, and enlarged posterior cervical lymph nodes. Symptoms usually disappear in a few days or weeks.

Nursing diagnoses that might apply to the pregnant woman with toxoplasmosis include the following:

- ***Risk for Altered Health Maintenance*** related to lack of knowledge about ways in which a pregnant woman can contract toxoplasmosis
- ***Anticipatory Grieving*** related to potential effects on infant of maternal toxoplasmosis

Nursing Plan and Implementation

The nurse caring for women during the antepartal period has the primary opportunity to discuss methods of prevention of toxoplasmosis with the childbearing woman. The woman must understand the importance of avoiding poorly cooked or raw meat, especially pork, beef, lamb, and, in the arctic region, caribou. Fruits and vegetables should be washed. She should avoid contact with the cat litter box by having someone else clean it. In addition, because it takes approximately 48 hours for a cat's feces to become infectious, the litter should be cleaned frequently. The nurse should also discuss the importance of the woman's wearing gloves when gardening and of avoiding garden areas frequented by cats.

Evaluation

Expected outcomes of nursing care include the following:

- The woman is able to discuss toxoplasmosis, its method of transmission, the implications for her fetus, and measures she can take to avoid contracting it.
- The woman implements health measures to avoid contracting toxoplasmosis.
- The woman gives birth to a healthy newborn.

Rubella

Rubella is a mild illness in children and adults. In fact, up to 60% of the cases are subclinical (Signore, 2001). On the other hand, rubella infection in the fetus can have overwhelming consequences. In 1969, live, attenuated vaccines were licensed for use in the United States. In the following 20 years there was a 99.6% decrease in rubella and a 97.4% decrease in congenital rubella syndrome. From 1992 to 1996 the number of cases reported annually averaged 183 (Gibbs & Sweet, 1999). Yet, from 10% to 15% of US adults may remain seronegative (Grossman, 1999). These figures emphasize the need for routine immunization programs. Prepubertal girls and nonpregnant women of childbearing age who do not have antirubella antibodies should be immunized with the live attenuated rubella vaccine. Although no fetal infection has resulted from immunization of a pregnant woman, pregnancy should be avoided for 3 months after immunization (Signore, 2001). Nurses need to be aware of the importance of postpartum immunization of the nonimmune woman to decrease unnecessary perinatal transmission.

FETAL-NEONATAL RISKS

The period of greatest risk for the teratogenic effects of rubella on the fetus is during the first trimester, when over 80% of the fetuses exposed will be affected (Yankowitz & Pastorek, 1999). The most common clinical signs of rubella syndrome are congenital cataracts, sensorineural deafness, and congenital heart defects (particularly patent ductus arteriosus). Other abnormalities, such as mental retardation or cerebral palsy, may become evident in infancy. Diagnosis in the newborn can be conclusively made in the presence of these conditions and with an elevated rubella IgM antibody titer at birth.

Infants born with congenital rubella syndrome are infectious and should be isolated. These infants may continue to shed the virus for up to 12 months (Grossman, 1999).

CLINICAL THERAPY

The best therapy for rubella is prevention. Live attenuated vaccine is available and should be given to all children. Women of childbearing age should be tested for immunity and vaccinated if susceptible and if it is established that they are not pregnant. Health counseling in high school and in premarital clinic visits can stress the importance of screening prior to planning a pregnancy.

As part of the prenatal laboratory screen the woman is evaluated for rubella using hemagglutination inhibition (HAI), a serology test. The presence of a 1:18 titer or greater is evidence of immunity. A titer less than 1:8 indicates susceptibility to rubella.

Because the vaccine is made with attenuated virus, pregnant women are not vaccinated. However, it is considered safe for newly vaccinated children to have contact with pregnant women.

If a woman who is pregnant becomes infected during the first trimester, therapeutic abortion may be an alternative.

NURSING CARE MANAGEMENT

Nursing Assessment and Diagnosis

A woman who develops rubella during pregnancy may be asymptomatic or may show signs of a mild infection, including a maculopapular rash, lymphadenopathy, muscular achiness, and joint pain. The presence of IgM antirubella antibody is diagnostic of a recent infection. These titers remain elevated for approximately 1 month following infection.

Nursing diagnoses that may apply to the woman who develops rubella early in her pregnancy include:

- ***Ineffective Family Coping*** due to an inability to accept the possibility of fetal anomalies secondary to maternal rubella exposure
- ***Risk for Altered Health Maintenance*** related to lack of knowledge about the importance of rubella immunization prior to becoming pregnant

Nursing Plan and Implementation

Nursing support and understanding are vital for the couple contemplating abortion due to a diagnosis of rubella. Such a decision may initiate a crisis for the couple who have planned their pregnancy. They need objective data to understand the possible effects on their fetus and the prognosis for the offspring.

Evaluation

Expected outcomes of nursing care include the following:

- The woman is able to describe the implications of rubella exposure during the first trimester of pregnancy.
- If exposure occurs in a woman who is not immune, she is able to identify her options and make a decision about continuing her pregnancy that is acceptable to her and her partner.
- The nonimmune woman receives the rubella vaccine during the early postpartal period.
- The woman gives birth to a healthy infant.

Cytomegalovirus

Cytomegalovirus (CMV) belongs to the herpes simplex virus group and causes both congenital and acquired disorders. The significance of this virus in pregnancy is related to its ability to be transmitted by asymptomatic women across the placenta to the fetus or by the cervical route during birth.

CMV is the most common viral cause of intrauterine infection (Sison & Sever, 1999a). In the United States, 50% to 60% of middle-class women are seropositive; this increases to 70% to 80% in lower socioeconomic groups (Azam, Vial, Fawer, et al, 2001). The virus can be found in urine, saliva, cervical mucus, semen, and breast milk. It can be passed between humans by any close contact such as kissing, breastfeeding, and sexual intercourse. Asymptomatic CMV infection is particularly common in children and gravid women. It is a chronic, persistent infection in that the individual may shed the virus continually over many years. The cervix can harbor the virus, and an ascending infection can develop after birth. Although the virus is usually innocuous in adults and children, it may be fatal to the fetus.

Accurate diagnosis in the pregnant woman depends on the presence of CMV in the urine, a rise in IgM levels, and identification of the CMV antibodies within the serum IgM fraction; however, CMV IgM is detectable in only 80% of people with acute infection (Sison & Sever, 1999a). Advances in molecular biology have greatly contributed to prenatal diagnosis of congenital CMV. Tests can be performed on chorionic villus samples, amniotic fluid, and fetal blood samples. Ultrasound findings may include fetal hydrops, growth restriction, hydramnios, cardiomegaly, and fetal ascites (Sison & Sever, 1999a). At present no treatment exists for maternal CMV or for the congenital disease in the newborn.

FETAL-NEONATAL RISKS

The cytomegalovirus is the most frequent agent of viral infection in the human fetus. It infects 0.5% to 2.5% of newborns (Azam et al, 2001). Although 90% of infected fetuses will be asymptomatic at birth, the remaining 10% will have abnormalities of varying severity. There is a 20% to 30% mortality rate among the symptomatic infants, and 90% of the survivors have significant neurologic complications (Liesnard, Donner, Brancart, et al, 2000). Subclinical infections in the newborn are capable of producing mental retardation and auditory deficits, sometimes not recognized for several months, or learning disabilities not seen until childhood. CMV may be the most common cause of mental retardation.

For the fetus, this infection can result in extensive intrauterine tissue damage that leads to fetal death; in survival with microcephaly, hydrocephaly, cerebral palsy, or mental retardation; or in survival with no damage at all.

The infected neonate is often SGA. The principal tissues and organs affected are the blood, brain, and liver. However, virtually all organs are potentially at risk. Hemolysis leads to anemia and hyperbilirubinemia. Thrombocytopenia and hepatosplenomegaly may also develop.

Currently no effective therapy exists to manage this infection.

Herpes Simplex Virus

It has been estimated that more than 45 million people are infected with genital herpes in the United States (ACOG, 1999b). Herpes simplex virus (HSV-I or HSV-II) infection can cause painful lesions in the genital area. Lesions may also develop on the cervix. This condition and its implications for nonpregnant women are discussed in Chapter 6 ☍. However, because the presence of herpes lesions in the genital tract may profoundly affect the fetus, herpes infection as it relates to a pregnant woman is discussed here.

FETAL-NEONATAL RISKS

A primary herpes simplex infection can increase the risk of spontaneous abortion when infection occurs in the first trimester. Preterm labor, intrauterine growth restriction, and neonatal infection are greater risks if the primary infection occurs late in the second trimester or early in the third trimester. Following a primary infection with HSV-II, symptomatic and subclinical viral shedding from the lower genital tract occurs during the first 3 months after the lesions have healed (ACOG, 1999b). A local outbreak may occur weeks or months later. When the offending virus is HSV-II, recurrences occur more frequently than when the virus is HSV-I (Donahue, 2002).

The risk to the fetus varies with the route of birth and whether the lesion that is present at the time of birth is primary or recurrent. If a symptomatic *primary* lesion is present, the risk of transmission is 50% for a vaginal birth. Exposure of the newborn to a *recurrent* lesion drops the risk of transmission to between 0% and 3% (ACOG, 1999b). For a woman with either a primary or a secondary outbreak of genital herpes during labor, or symptoms that may indicate an impending outbreak, the preferred method of childbirth is cesarean birth. Although fetal transmission with recurrent outbreaks is low, a cesarean birth is warranted because of the serious nature of the disease in the newborn. Vaginal birth is appropriate for women with a history of HSV but no evidence of active genital disease at the time of childbirth (ACOG, 1999b).

The infected infant is often asymptomatic at birth but after an incubation period of 2 to 12 days develops symptoms of fever (or hypothermia), jaundice, seizures, and poor feeding. Approximately one half of infected infants develop the characteristic vesicular skin lesions. Vidarabine has been useful in decreasing serious effects from neonatal herpes, but no definitive treatment exists as yet. Some experts treat asymptomatic infants who were exposed to herpes simplex virus during birth with acyclovir. Positive herpes cultures taken 24 to 48 hours after birth should be obtained before treatment (Centers for Disease Control and Prevention [CDC], 2002).

CLINICAL THERAPY

Oral antiviral therapies are available, including acyclovir (Zovirax), famciclovir, and valacyclovir. At this time, acyclovir is the only drug for herpes that has been studied during pregnancy (Brown, 1999). Currently, there is no evidence that there are any adverse fetal effects related to exposure to any of these drugs during any trimester. The CDC does not recommend the routine use of acyclovir for recurrent infection during pregnancy but recognizes that the use of acyclovir near term may reduce the need for cesarean birth. The dosage is unchanged during pregnancy (Amstey, 1999).

NURSING CARE MANAGEMENT

Nursing Assessment and Diagnosis

During the initial prenatal visit, it is important to learn whether the woman or her partner have had previous herpes infections. If so, ongoing assessment is indicated as pregnancy progresses.

Nursing diagnoses that may apply to the pregnant woman with HSV include the following:

- ***Pain*** related to the presence of lesions secondary to herpes infection
- ***Sexual Dysfunction*** related to unwillingness to engage in sexual intercourse secondary to the presence of active herpes lesions
- ***Ineffective Individual Coping*** related to depression secondary to the risk to the fetus if herpes lesions are present at birth

Nursing Plan and Implementation

Nurses need to be particularly concerned with client education about this fast-spreading disease. Women should be informed about what herpes is, how it is spread, and preventive measures. Women should also receive information about the association of genital herpes with spontaneous abortion, neonatal mortality and morbidity, and the possibility of cesarean birth. A woman needs to inform her future healthcare providers of her infection. She also should know of the possible association of genital herpes with cervical cancer and the importance of a yearly Pap smear.

The woman who acquired HSV as an adolescent may be concerned by the possible risks as a mature young adult who wants to have a family. Clients may be helped by counseling that allows expression of the anger, shame, and depression so often experienced by women with herpes. Literature may be helpful and is available from Planned Parenthood and many public health agencies. The American Social Health Association has established the HELP program to provide information and the latest research results on genital herpes. The association has a quarterly journal, *The Helper*, for nurses and herpes clients.

Evaluation

Expected outcomes of nursing care include the following:

- The woman is able to describe her infection with regard to its method of spread, expected medical therapy, comfort measures, implications for her pregnancy, and long-term implications.
- The woman has appropriate cultures done as recommended throughout her pregnancy.
- The woman gives birth to a healthy infant.

Group B Streptococcal Infection

Group B streptococcus (GBS) infection is a bacterial infection found in the lower gastrointestinal or urogenital tracts. Women may transmit GBS to their fetus in utero or during childbirth. During the 1970s, GBS was recognized as the leading infectious cause of neonatal sepsis and mortality and remains so today (Watt, Schuchat, Erickson, et al, 2001). Fortunately, improved recognition and rapid treatment of infected infants has reduced morbidity and mortality rates considerably. Currently fewer than 10% of neonatal cases of GBS are fatal (Himmelberger, 2002).

Women who are carriers of GBS are often asymptomatic. Colonization may be intermittent, transient, or chronic. The reservoir for GBS is thought to be the intestinal tract. GBS can be recovered from the vagina or cervix in 10% to 40% of pregnant women at some time during gestation depending on population and culture technique (Dinsmoor, 1999). GBS can be recovered twice as frequently from rectal cultures (Sampson & Gravett, 1999).

In symptomatic women, GBS is also responsible for considerable maternal morbidity from infections such as amnionitis, postpartum endometritis, sepsis, wound infections, and stillbirths. Women with GBS are also more likely to have premature preterm rupture of the membranes and are also more likely to give birth prematurely.

It is estimated that in the United States, the cost of neonatal disease attributable to GBS is about $300 million annually (Brozanski, Jones, Krohn, et al, 2000). When costs of maternal disease are added to neonatal costs, it has been estimated to be over $700 million annually (Dinsmoor, 1999).

FETAL-NEONATAL RISKS

Newborns become infected either by vertical transmission from the mother as the fetus passes through the birth canal or from horizontal transmission from colonized nursery personnel or colonized infants. Between 40% and 70% of neonates who are born to colonized mothers will become colonized. The transmission rate is influenced by how heavily the mother is colonized, whether or not she is persistently culture-positive, and the site of colonization (rectal versus vaginal).

Risk factors for GBS neonatal sepsis include the following:

- Prematurity
- Maternal intrapartum fever
- Membranes ruptured for longer than 12 to 18 hours
- A previously infected infant with GBS disease
- GBS bacteriuria in the current pregnancy

GBS causes severe, invasive disease in infants. In newborns, the majority of cases occur within the first week of life and are thus designated as early-onset disease. Late-onset disease occurs one week or more after birth. Early-onset GBS is often characterized by signs of serious illness including respiratory distress or pneumonia, apnea, and shock. Infants with late-onset GBS often develop meningitis. Long-term neurologic complications are common in survivors of both types of GBS.

CLINICAL THERAPY

Guidelines for the detection of carriers and preventive treatment of newborns at risk were developed by the Centers for Disease Control and Prevention (CDC) with the American Academy of Pediatrics and the American College of Obstetricians and Gynecologists in 1996. These guidelines were updated in 2002. The CDC now recommends the following (Schrag, Gorwitz, Fultz-Butts, et al 2002):

- All pregnant women should be screened for both vaginal and rectal GBS colonization at 35 to 37 weeks' gestation.
- Women identified as GBS carriers should receive antibiotic prophylaxis at the onset of labor or the rupture of membranes.
- Women with GBS in their urine in any concentration should receive antibiotic prophylaxis intrapartally because such women typically have heavy colonization with GBS and thus have an increased risk of giving birth to a newborn with early-onset disease. These women do not need vaginal and rectal cultures at 35 to 37 weeks because therapy is already indicated.
- Women who have already given birth to a newborn with invasive GBS disease should receive intrapartum antibiotic prophylaxis. Culture-based screening is not necessary for them.
- If the results of GBS screening are not known when labor begins, prophylaxis is indicated for women with any of the following risk factors: gestation < 37 weeks, membranes ruptured ≥ 16 hours, temperature ≥ 100.4F (≥ 38.0C).

Figure 20–10 • provides an algorithm for assessing the need for intrapartum antibiotic prophylaxis.

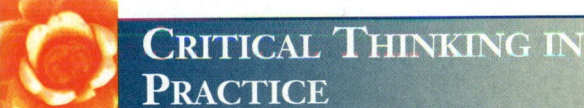

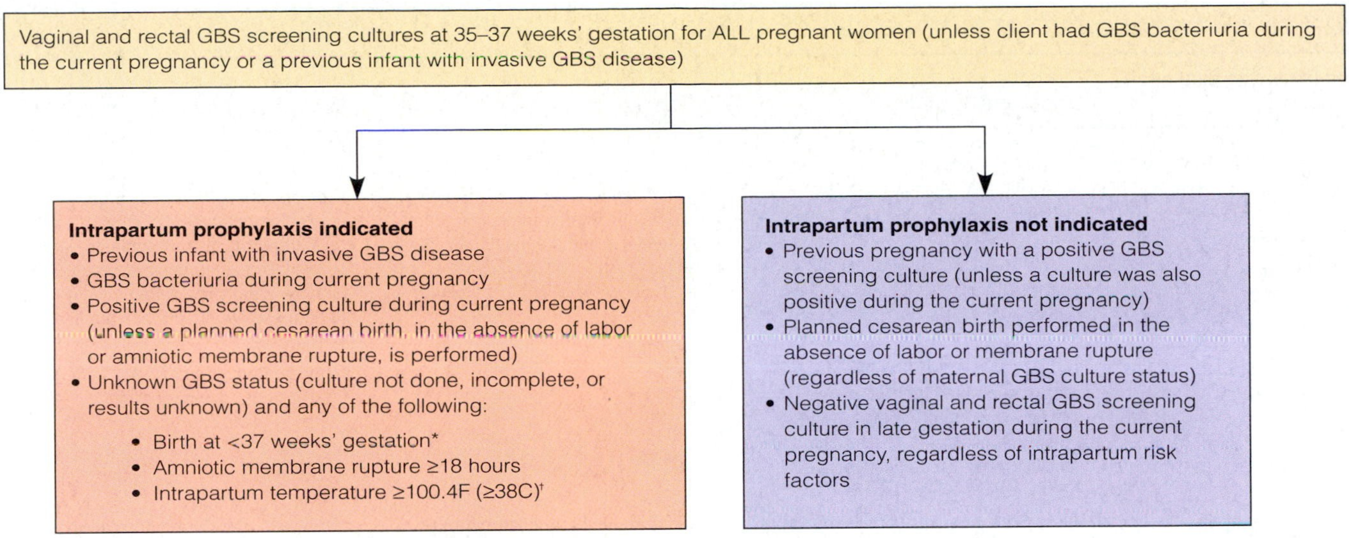

Vaginal and rectal GBS screening cultures at 35–37 weeks' gestation for ALL pregnant women (unless client had GBS bacteriuria during the current pregnancy or a previous infant with invasive GBS disease)
Intrapartum prophylaxis indicated
• Previous infant with invasive GBS disease
• GBS bacteriuria during current pregnancy
• Positive GBS screening culture during current pregnancy (unless a planned cesarean birth, in the absence of labor or amniotic membrane rupture, is performed)
• Unknown GBS status (culture not done, incomplete, or results unknown) and any of the following:
• Birth at <37 weeks' gestation*
• Amniotic membrane rupture ≥18 hours
• Intrapartum temperature ≥100.4F (≥38C)†
Intrapartum prophylaxis not indicated
• Previous pregnancy with a positive GBS screening culture (unless a culture was also positive during the current pregnancy)
• Planned cesarean birth performed in the absence of labor or membrane rupture (regardless of maternal GBS culture status)
• Negative vaginal and rectal GBS screening culture in late gestation during the current pregnancy, regardless of intrapartum risk factors

* If onset of labor or rupture of amniotic membrane occurs at <37 weeks' gestation and there is a significant risk for preterm birth (as assessed by the clinician)
† If amnionitis is suspected, broad-spectrum antibiotic therapy that includes an agent known to be active against GBS should replace GBS prophylaxis.

Figure 20–10 • Indications for intrapartum antibiotic prophylaxis to prevent perinatal GBS disease under a universal prenatal screening strategy based on combined vaginal and rectal cultures collected at 35 to 37 weeks' gestation from all pregnant women.
SOURCE: Centers for Disease Control and Prevention (CDC).

Intrapartum antibiotic therapy is recommended as follows: initial dose of penicillin G 5 million units intravenously (IV) followed by 2.5 million units IV every 4 hours until childbirth. Alternately, ampicillin 2 g initial dose IV followed by 1 g IV every 4 hours until childbirth may be used. Women at high risk for an anaphylactic reaction to penicillin because of marked allergy may be treated with clindamycin or erythromycin.

Additional information about GBS during pregnancy is available at the following Web sites:

- Group B Strep Association—www.groupbstrep.org
- Centers for Disease Control and Prevention—www.cdc.gov
- American College of Obstetricians and Gynecologists—www.acog.org
- American Academy of Pediatrics—www.aap.org
- March of Dimes—www.modimes.org

Human B19 Parvovirus

Human B19 parvovirus causes erythema infectiosum or fifth disease in children. It is a mild disease in adults that produces a characteristic "slapped cheek" rash. The risk to fetuses has received a lot of attention in the last 10 years. Although there is a low risk of fetal morbidity, transplacental transmission is reported to be as high as 33% (ACOG, 2000). Fetal infection is associated with spontaneous abortion, fetal hydrops, and stillbirth. Severe effects occur most frequently with maternal infection prior to 20 weeks' gestation. Hydrops may be seen up to 8 weeks after maternal infection. In fetuses who survive the infection, long-term development appears to be normal.

CRITICAL THINKING IN PRACTICE

Your friend Jena Yoo, G1P0, is 6 months pregnant and mentions to you that she is developing symptoms of a bladder infection. She has had several bladder infections over the past few years and feels she has warded off others by increasing her fluid intake and drinking acidic juices. Jena tells you that she plans to use the same approach this time because she just had her prenatal appointment last week. She assures you that if symptoms persist, she will discuss it with her caregiver at her next prenatal visit. What advice would you give her?

Answer can be found in Appendix I.

Other Infections in Pregnancy

Table 20–8 • summarizes other urinary tract, vaginal, and sexually transmitted infections that put pregnancy at risk. (These are described in detail in Chapter 6.) Spontaneous abortion is frequently the result of a severe maternal infection, and research links infection with prematurity. In addition, if the pregnancy is carried to term in the presence of infection, the risk of maternal and fetal morbidity and mortality increases. Thus it is essential to maternal and fetal health that infection be diagnosed and treated promptly.

Table 20–8 • INFECTIONS THAT PUT PREGNANCY AT RISK

Condition and Causative Organism	Signs and Symptoms	Treatment	Implications for Pregnancy
Urinary Tract Infections (UTI)			
Asymptomatic bacteriuria (ASB): *Escherichia, Klebsiella, Proteus* most common	Bacteria present in urine on culture with no accompanying symptoms.	Oral sulfonamides early in pregnancy, ampicillin and nitrofurantoin (Furadantin) in late pregnancy. Antibody sensitivity results will guide the selection of an appropriate antibiotic.	Women with ASB in early pregnancy may go on to develop cystitis or acute pyelonephritis by third trimester if not treated. Oral sulfonamides taken in the last few weeks of pregnancy may lead to neonatal hyperbilirubinemia and kernicterus.
Cystitis (lower UTI): Causative organisms same as for ASB	Dysuria, urgency, frequency; low-grade fever and hematuria may occur. Urine culture (clean catch) shows ↑ leukocytes. Presence of 10^5 (100,000) or more colonies bacteria per mL urine.	Same	If not treated, infection may ascend and lead to acute pyelonephritis.
Acute pyelonephritis: Causative organisms same as for ASB	Sudden onset. Chills, high fever, flank pain. Nausea, vomiting, malaise. May have decreased urine output, severe colicky pain, dehydration. Increased diastolic BP, positive fluorescent antibody (FA) test, low creatinine clearance. Marked bacteremia in urine culture, pyuria, WBC casts.	Hospitalization; IV antibiotic therapy. Other antibiotics safe during pregnancy include carbenicillin, methenamine, cephalosporins. Catheterization if output is ↓. Supportive therapy for comfort. Follow-up urine cultures are necessary.	Increased risk of premature birth and intrauterine growth restriction (IUGR). These antibiotics interfere with urinary estriol levels and can cause false interpretations of estriol levels during pregnancy.
Vaginal Infections			
Vulvovaginal candidiasis (yeast infections): *Candida albicans*	Often thick, white, curdy discharge, severe itching, dysuria, dyspareunia. Diagnosis based on presence of hyphae and spores in a wet-mount preparation of vaginal secretions.	Intravaginal insertion of miconazole butoconazole, or other topical azole preparation, clotrimazole suppositories at bedtime for 1 week. Cream may be prescribed for topical application to the vulva if necessary (CDC, 2002).	If the infection is present at birth and the fetus is born vaginally, the fetus may contract thrush.
Bacterial vaginosis: *Gardnerella vaginalis*	Thin, watery, yellow-gray discharge with foul odor often described as "fishy." Wet-mount preparation reveals "clue cells." Application of potassium hydroxide (KOH) to a specimen of vaginal secretions produces a pronounced fishy odor.	Metronidazole 250 mg PO TID × 7 days or clindamycin 800 mg PO BID × 7 days (CDC, 2002).	CDC (2002) reports that multiple studies have failed to demonstrate a teratogenic effect from metronidazole.
Trichomoniasis: *Trichomonas vaginalis*	Occasionally asymptomatic. May have frothy greenish gray vaginal discharge, pruritus, urinary symptoms. Strawberry patches may be visible on vaginal walls or cervix. Wet-mount preparation of vaginal secretions shows motile flagellated trichomonads.	Single 2-g dose of metronidazole orally (CDC, 2002).	Increased risk for PROM, preterm birth, and low birth weight.
Sexually Transmitted Infections			
Chlamydial infection: *Chlamydia trachomatis*	Women are often asymptomatic. Symptoms may include thin or purulent discharge, urinary burning and frequency, or lower abdominal pain. Lab test available to detect monoclonal antibodies specific for *Chlamydia*.	Although nonpregnant women are treated with tetracycline, it may permanently discolor fetal teeth. Thus, pregnant women are treated with erythromycin or amoxicillin followed by repeat culture in 3 weeks (CDC, 2002).	Infant of woman with untreated chlamydial infection may develop newborn conjunctivitis, which can be treated with erythromycin eye ointment (but not silver nitrate). Infant may also develop chlamydial pneumonia. May be responsible for premature labor and fetal death.
Syphilis: *Treponema pallidum,* a spirochete	Primary stage: chancre, slight fever, malaise. Chancre lasts about 4 weeks, then disappears. Secondary stage: occurs 6 weeks to 6 months after infection. Skin eruptions (condyloma latal) also symptoms of acute arthritis, liver enlargement, iritis, chronic sore throat with hoarseness. Diagnosed by blood tests such as VDRL, RPR, FTA, ABS. Dark-field examination or spirochetes may also be done.	For syphilis less than 1 year in duration: 2.4 million U benzathine penicillin G IM. For syphilis of more than 1 year's duration: 2.4 million U benzathine penicillin G once a week for 3 weeks. Sexual partners should also be screened and treated (CDC, 2002).	Syphilis can be passed transplacentally to the fetus. If untreated, one of the following can occur: second trimester abortion, stillborn infant at term, congenitally infected infant, uninfected live infant.

Table 20–8 • CONTINUED

Condition and Causative Organism	Signs and Symptoms	Treatment	Implications for Pregnancy
Gonorrhea: *Neisseria gonorrhoeae*	Majority of women asymptomatic; disease often diagnosed during routine prenatal cervical culture. If symptoms are present they may include purulent vaginal discharge, dysuria, urinary frequency, inflammation, and swelling of the vulva. Cervix may appear eroded.	Nonpregnant women are treated with cefixime orally or ceftriaxone IM plus doxycycline. Pregnant women are treated with ceftriaxone plus erythromycin (CDC, 2002). Some practitioners use azithromycin to treat possible co-infection with chlamydia. All sexual partners are also treated.	Infection at time of birth may cause ophthalmia neonatorum in the newborn.
Condyloma acuminata: caused by a papovavirus	Soft, grayish pink lesions on the vulva, vagina, cervix, or anus.	Podophyllin not used during pregnancy. Trichloroacetic acid, liquid nitrogen, or cryotherapy CO_2 laser therapy done under colposcopy is also successful (CDC, 2002).	Possible teratogenic effect of podophyllin. Large doses have been associated with fetal death.

CHAPTER REVIEW

EXPLOREMEDIALINK

NCLEX review questions, case studies, and other interactive resources for this chapter can be found on the Web site at http://www.prenhall.com/olds. Click on "Chapter 20" to select the activities for this chapter.

For tutorials including animations and videos, more NCLEX review questions, and an audio glossary, access the accompanying CD-ROM in this book.

Focus Your Study

- Several health problems associated with bleeding arise from the pregnancy itself, such as spontaneous abortion, ectopic pregnancy, and gestational trophoblastic disease. The nurse needs to be alert to early signs of these situations, to guard the woman against heavy bleeding and shock, to facilitate the medical treatment, and to provide educational and emotional support.
- Incompetent cervix, the premature dilatation of the cervix, is the most common cause of second trimester abortion. It is treated surgically with a Shirodkar or McDonald cerclage, which involves placing a suture in the cervix to keep it closed.
- Hyperemesis gravidarum, excessive vomiting during pregnancy, may cause fluid and electrolyte imbalance, dehydration, and signs of starvation in the mother and, if severe enough, death of the fetus. Treatment is aimed at controlling the vomiting, correcting fluid and electrolyte imbalance, correcting dehydration, and improving nutritional status.
- Premature rupture of the membranes and preterm labor both place the fetus at risk. Women with PROM and no signs of infection are managed conservatively with bed rest and careful monitoring of fetal well-being. Women with a history of preterm labor may be placed on home fetal monitoring programs. If preterm labor develops, tocolytics are often effective in delaying labor for 48 hours but do have associated side effects.
- Hypertension may exist prior to pregnancy or, more often, may develop during pregnancy. Preeclampsia can lead to growth retardation for the fetus and, if untreated, may lead to convulsions (eclampsia) and even death for the mother and fetus. A woman's understanding of the disease process helps motivate her to maintain the required rest periods in the left

lateral position. Antihypertensive or anticonvulsive drugs may be part of the therapy.

- Rh incompatibility can exist when an Rh-negative woman and an Rh-positive partner conceive a child who is Rh positive. The use of Rh immune globulin has greatly decreased the incidence of severe sequelae due to Rh incompatibility because the drug "tricks" the body into thinking antibodies have been produced in response to the Rh antigen.
- The impact of surgery or trauma on the pregnant woman and her fetus is related to timing in the pregnancy, seriousness of the situation, and other factors influencing the situation.
- Physical violence often begins or continues during pregnancy. The nurse needs to be alert for signs of abuse, including bruising or injury to the breasts, abdomen, and genitals. The nurse should provide the woman information about violence and about community resources available to assist her.
- Toxoplasmosis, rubella, cytomegalovirus, herpes, GBS, and other perinatal infections all pose a grave threat to the fetus. Prevention is the best therapy. There is no known treatment for rubella or CMV, but antimicrobial drugs are available for toxoplasmosis, herpes, and GBS.
- Universal screening for group B strep is now recommended for all pregnant women at 35 to 37 weeks' gestation.

References

Abramovici, D., & Sibai, B. M. (1999). Preeclampsia-eclampsia. In J. T. Queenan (Ed.), *Management of high-risk pregnancy* (4th ed.). Malden, MA: Blackwell Science.

American Academy of Pediatrics (AAP) & American College of Obstetricians and Gynecologists (ACOG). (1997). Obstetric complications. In *Guidelines for perinatal care* (4th ed., pp. 127–146). Elk Grove Village, IL: Author.

American College of Obstetricians and Gynecologists (ACOG). (1998a). *Antimicrobial therapy for obstetric patients* (ACOG Educational Bulletin No. 245). Washington, DC: Author.

American College of Obstetricians and Gynecologists (ACOG). (1998b). *Medical management of tubal pregnancy* (ACOG Practice Bulletin No. 3). Washington, DC: Author.

American College of Obstetricians and Gynecologists (ACOG). (1998c). *Obstetric aspects of trauma management* (ACOG Educational Bulletin No. 251). Washington, DC: Author.

American College of Obstetricians and Gynecologists (ACOG). (1999a). *Domestic violence* (ACOG Educational Bulletin No. 257). Washington, DC: Author.

American College of Obstetricians and Gynecologists (ACOG). (1999b). *Management of herpes in pregnancy* (ACOG Practice Bulletin No. 8). Washington, DC: Author.

American College of Obstetricians and Gynecologists (ACOG). (1999c). *Prevention of Rh D alloimmunization* (ACOG Practice Bulletin No. 4). Washington, DC: Author.

American College of Obstetricians and Gynecologists (ACOG). (2000). *Perinatal viral and parasitic infections* (ACOG Practice Bulletin No. 20). Washington, DC: Author.

American College of Obstetricians and Gynecologists (ACOG). (2001, February). *Management of recurrent early pregnancy loss* (ACOG Practice Bulletin No. 24). Washington, DC: Author.

Amstey, M. S. (1999). Herpes simplex infection. In J.T. Queenan (Ed.), *Management of high-risk pregnancy* (4th ed.). Malden, MA: Blackwell Science.

Ananth, C. V., Demissie, K., Smulian, J. C., & Vintzileos, A. M. (2001). Relationship among placenta previa, fetal growth restriction, and preterm delivery: A population based study. *Obstetrics & Gynecology, 98*(2), 299–306.

Andrews, W. W., Hauth, J. C., & Goldenberg, R. L. (2000). Infection and preterm birth. *American Journal of Perinatology, 17*(7), 357–365.

Angelini, D. J. (1999). Obstetric triage: Management of acute nonobstetric abdominal pain in pregnancy. *Journal of Nurse-Midwifery, 44*(6), 572–585.

Athey, J., & Spielvogel, A. M. (2000). Risk factors and interventions for psychological sequelae in women after miscarriage. *Primary Care Update for OB/GYNS,* 7(2), 64–69.

Azam, A., Vial, Y., Fawer, C., Zufferey, J., & Hohlfeld, P. (2001). Prenatal diagnosis of congenital cytomegalovirus infection. *Obstetrics & Gynecology,* 97(3), 443–448.

Bar, J., Maayan-Metsger, A., Hod, M., Rafael, Z. B., Orvieto, R., Shalev, Y., et al. (2000). Effect of antibiotic therapy in preterm premature rupture of the membranes on neonatal mortality and morbidity. *American Journal of Perinatology, 17*(5), 237–241.

Berman, M. L., Di Saia, M. J., & Brewster, W. R. (1999). Pelvic malignancies, gestational trophoblastic neoplasia, and nonpelvic malignancies. In R. K.Creasy & R. Resnik (Eds.), *Maternal fetal medicine* (4th ed.). Philadelphia: W.B. Saunders.

Blumenthal, M. (2000). *Herbal Medicine: Expanded Commission E Monographs.* Gusten, TX: American Botanical Council.

Bobrowski, R. (1999). Trauma in pregnancy. In D. K. James, P. J. Steer, C. P. Weiner, & B. Gonik (Eds.), *High risk pregnancy management options* (2nd ed.). Philadelphia: W. B. Saunders.

Bowman, J. M. (1999). Hemolytic disease (erythroblastosis fetalis). In R. K. Creasy & R. Resnik (Eds.), *Maternal fetal medicine* (4th ed.). Philadelphia: W.B. Saunders.

Brown, Z. A. (1999, January). Herpes simplex virus infection in pregnancy. *Contemporary OB/GYN, 44*(1), 27–34.

Brozanski, B. S., Jones, J. G., Krohn, M. A., & Sweet, R. L. (2000). Effect of a screening-based prevention policy on prevalence of early-onset group B streptococcal sepsis. *Obstetrics & Gynecology, 95*(4), 496–501.

Butler, E. L., Dashe, J. S., & Ramus, R. M. (2001). Association between maternal serum alpha-fetoprotein and adverse outcomes in pregnancies with placenta previa. *Obstetrics & Gynecology, 97*(1), 35–38.

Canterino, J. C., Verma, U., Visintainer, P. F., Elimian, A., Klein, S. A., & Tejani, N. (2001). Antenatal steroids and neonatal periventricular leukomalacia. *Obstetrics & Gynecology,* 97(1), 135–146.

Centers for Disease Control and Prevention (CDC). (2002). Sexually transmitted diseases treatment guidelines 2002. *Morbidity and Mortality Weekly Report, 51*(RR-6), 1–84.

Chien, L., Whyte, R., Aziz, K., Thiessen, P., Matthew, D., & Lee, S. K. (2001). Improved outcome of preterm infants when delivered in tertiary care centers. *Obstetrics & Gynecology, 98*(2), 247–252.

Cokkinides, V. E., Coker, A. L., Sanderson, M., Addy, C., & Bethea, L. (1999). Physical violence during pregnancy: Maternal complications and birth outcomes. *Obstetrics & Gynecology, 93*(5), 661–666.

Consider both the unborn child and the mother when treating hypertension in pregnancy. (2001) *Drug and Therapeutic Perspectives, 17*(18), 11–15. Retrieved Oct 8, 2001 from http://womenshealth.medscape.com/adis/DTP/2001/vn.n18/dtp17/. . . /mig-pmt dtp1718.03.htm

Creasy, R. K., & Iams, J. D. (1999). Preterm labor and delivery. In R. K. Creasy & R. Resnik (Eds.), *Maternal fetal medicine* (4th ed.). Philadelphia: W. B. Saunders.

Cunningham, F. G., Gant, N. F., Leveno, K. J., Gilstrap, L. C., III, Hauth, J. C., & Westrom, K. D. (2001). *Williams obstetrics* (21st ed.). New York: McGraw-Hill.

Dekker, G., & Sibai, B. (2001). Primary, secondary, and tertiary prevention of preeclampsia. *Lancet, 357*, 209–215.

Dinsmoor, M. J. (1999). Group B streptococcus infection. In J. T. Queenan (Ed.), *Management of high-risk pregnancy* (4th ed.). Malden, MA: Blackwell Science.

Donahue, D. B. (2002). Diagnosis and treatment of herpes simplex infection during pregnancy. *Journal of Obstetric, Gynecologic, and Neonatal Nursing, 31*(1), 99–106.

Edwards, R. K. (2000). Syphilis in women. *Primary Care Update for OB/GYNs*, 7(5), 186–191.

Edwards, R. K., Duff, P., & Ross, K. C. (2000). Amniotic fluid indices of fetal pulmonary maturity with preterm premature rupture of membranes. *Obstetrics & Gynecology, 96*(1), 102–105.

Edwards, R. K., Locksmith, G. J., & Duff, P. (2000). Expanded-spectrum antibiotics with preterm, premature rupture of membranes. *Obstetrics & Gynecology, 96*(1), 60–64.

Eliakim, R., Abulafia, O., & Sherer, D. M. (2000). Hyperemesis gravidarum: A current review. *American Journal of Perinatology, 17*(4), 207–218.

Feikin, D. R., Thorsen, P., Zywicki, S., Arip, M., Westergaard, J. G., & Schuchat, A. (2001). Association between colonization with group B streptococci during pregnancy and preterm delivery among Danish women. *American Journal of Obstetrics and Gynecology, 184*(3), 427–433.

Gagne, S. S. (2001). Toxoplasmosis. *Primary Care Update for OB/GYNs, 8*(3), 122–126.

Garite, T. J. (1999). Premature rupture of the membranes. In R. K. Creasy & R. Resnik (Eds.), *Maternal fetal medicine* (4th ed.). Philadelphia: W.B. Saunders.

Gibbs, R. S., & Sweet, R. L. (1999). Maternal and fetal infectious disorders. In R. K. Creasy & R. Resnik (Eds.), *Maternal fetal medicine* (4th ed.). Philadelphia: W.B. Saunders.

Giles, W., Bisits, A., Knox, M., Madsen, G., & Smith, R. (2000). The effect of fetal fibronectin testing on admissions to a tertiary maternal fetal medicine unit and cost savings. *American Journal of Obstetrics and Gynecology, 182*(2), 439–443.

Gonik, B. (1999). Intensive care monitoring of the critically ill pregnant patient. In R. K.Creasy & R. Resnik (Eds.), *Maternal fetal medicine* (4th ed.). Philadelphia: W.B. Saunders.

Gracia, C. R., & Barnhart, K. T. (2001). Diagnosing ectopic pregnancy: Decision analysis comparing six strategies. *Obstetrics & Gynecology, 97*(3), 464–470.

Grossman, J. H. (1999). Rubella. In J. T. Queenan (Ed.), *Management of high-risk pregnancy* (4th ed.). Malden, MA: Blackwell Science.

Hallak, M. (1999). Hypertensive disorders in pregnancy. In D. K. James, P. J. Steer, C. P. Weiner, & B. Gonik (Eds.), *High risk pregnancy management options* (2nd ed.). Philadelphia: W. B. Saunders.

Hassan, S. S., Romero, R., Maymon, E., Berry, S. M., Blackwell, S. C., Treadwell, M. C., et al. (2001). Does cervical cerclage prevent preterm delivery in patients with a short cervix? *American Journal of Obstetrics and Gynecology, 184*(7), 1325–1331.

Heaman, M. I., Sprague, A. E., & Stewart, P. J. (2000). Reducing the preterm birth rate: A population health strategy. *Journal of Obstetric, Gynecologic, and Neonatal Nursing, 30*(1), 20–29.

Helal, K. J., Gordon, M. C., Lightner, C. R., & Barth, W. H. (2000). Adrenal suppression induced by betamethasone in women at risk for premature delivery. *Obstetrics & Gynecology, 96*(2), 287–290.

Higgins, J. R., & de Swiet, M. (2001). Blood-pressure measurement and classification in pregnancy. *Lancet, 357*, 131–135.

Hill, J. A. (1999). Recurrent pregnancy loss. In R. K. Creasy & R. Resnik (Eds.), *Maternal fetal medicine* (4th ed.). Philadelphia: W.B. Saunders.

Himmelberger, S. A. (2002). Preventing group B strep in newborns. *AWHONN Lifelines, 6*(4), 339–342.

Iams, J. D. (1999). Cervical incompetence. In R. K. Creasy & R. Resnik (Eds.), *Maternal fetal medicine* (4th ed.). Philadelphia: W. B. Saunders.

Iams, J. D., Goldenberg, R. L., Mercer, B. M., Moawad, A. H., Meis, P. J., Das, A. F., et al. (2001). The preterm labor prediction study: Can low-risk women destined for spontaneous preterm birth be identified? *American Journal of Obstetrics and Gynecology, 184* (4), 652–655.

Isler, C. M., Barrilleaux, P. S., Magann, E. F., Bass, J. D., & Martin, J. N. (2001). A prospective, randomized trial comparing the efficacy of dexamethasone and betamethasone for the treatment of antepartum HELLP (hemolysis, elevated liver enzymes, and low platelet count) syndrome. *American Journal of Obstetrics and Gynecology, 184*(7), 1332–1339.

Knight, B., Mudge, C., Openshaw, S., White, A., & Hart, A. (2001). Effects of acupuncture on nausea of pregnancy: A randomized, controlled trial. *Obstetrics & Gynecology, 97*(2), 184–188.

Landy, H. J. (1999). The incompetent cervix. In J. T. Queenan (Ed.), *Management of high-risk pregnancy* (4th ed.). Malden, MA: Blackwell Science.

Liesnard, C., Donner, C., Brancart, F., Gosselin, F., Delforge, M., & Rodesch, F. (2000). Prenatal diagnosis of congenital cytomegalovirus infection: Prospective study of 237 pregnancies at risk. *Obstetrics & Gynecology, 95*(6) Part 1, 881–888.

Lipscomb, G. H., Stovall, T. G., & Ling, F. W. (2000). Nonsurgical treatment of ectopic pregnancy. *New England Journal of Medicine, 343*(18), 1325–1329.

MacKay, A. P., Berg, C. J., & Atrash, H. K. (2001). Pregnancy-related mortality from preeclampsia and eclampsia. *Obstetrics & Gynecology, 97*(4), 533–538.

Macones, G. A., Marder, S. J., Clothier, B., & Stamilio, D. M. (2001). The controversy surrounding indomethacin for tocolysis. *American Journal of Obstetrics and Gynecology, 184*(3), 264–72.

Magann, E. F., & Martin, J. N. (2000). Critical care of HELLP syndrome with corticosteroids. *American Journal of Perinatology*, 7(8), 417–422.

Magriples, U., Laifer, S., & Hayslett, J. P. (2001). Dilutional hyponatremia in preeclampsia with and without nephrotic syndrome. *American Journal of Obstetrics and Gynecology, 184*, 231–232.

Mahomed, K. (1999). Abdominal pain in pregnancy. In D. K. James, P. J. Steer, C.P. Weiner, & B. Gonik (Eds.), *High risk pregnancy management options* (2nd ed.). Philadelphia: W.B. Saunders.

Maloni, J. A., Brezinski-Tomasi, J. E., & Johnson, L. A. (2001). Antepartum bed rest: Effect upon the family. *Journal of Obstetric, Gynecologic, and Neonatal Nursing, 30*(2), 165–173.

Mashburn, J. (1999). Ectopic pregnancies: Triage do's and don'ts. *Journal of Nurse Midwifery, 44*(6), 549–557.

McGregor, J. A. (1999). Preterm premature rupture of membranes: Infection and inflammation. In J. T. Queenan (Ed.), *Management of high-risk pregnancy* (4th ed.). Malden, MA: Blackwell Science.

National Institutes of Health (NIH). (2000). *Working group report on high blood pressure in pregnancy.* Retrieved December 8, 2002 from www.nhibi.nih.gov/health/prof/heart/hbp/ hbp-preg.htm

National Institutes of Health (NIH) Consensus Development Panel. (2001). Antenatal corticosteroids revisited: Repeat courses—National Institutes of Health Consensus Development Conference Statement, August 17–18, 2000. *Obstetrics & Gynecology, 98*(1).

Nelen, W. L. D. M., Blom, H. J., Steegers, E. A. P., Den Heijer, M., Thomas, C. M. G., & Eskes, T. K. A. B. (2000). Homocysteine and folate levels as risk factors for recurrent early pregnancy loss. *Obstetrics & Gynecology, 95*(4), 519–524.

Nelson-Piercy, C., Fayers, P., & de Swiet, M. (2001). Randomised, double-blind, placebo controlled trial of corticosteroids for the treatment of hyperemesis gravidarum. *British Journal of Obstetrics and Gynaecology, 108,* 9–15.

Newman, R. B., Goldenberg, R. L., Moawad, A. H., Iams, J. D., Meis, P. J., Das, A., et al. (2001). Occupational fatigue and preterm rupture of membranes. *American Journal of Obstetrics and Gynecology, 184*(3), 438–447.

Ninia, J. G. (2000). Inherited coagulopathies in OB/GYN. *Primary Care Update for OB/GYNs,* 7(2), 70–73.

Norwitz, E. R. (2002). Emergency cerclage: What do the data *really* show? *Contemporary OB/GYN, 47*(10), 48–66.

Novy, M. J., Gupta, A., Wothe, D. D., Gupta, S., Kennedy, K. A., & Gravett, M. G. (2001). Cervical cerclage in the second trimester of pregnancy: A historical cohort study. *American Journal of Obstetrics and Gynecology, 184*(7), 1447–1456.

Parilla, B. V., Grobman, W. A., Holtzman, R. B., Thomas, H. A., & Dooley, S. L. (2000). Indomethacin tocolysis and risk of necrotizing enterocolitis. *Obstetrics & Gynecology, 96*(1), 120–123.

Pipkin, F. B. (2001). Risk factors for preeclampsia. *New England Journal of Medicine, 344*(12), 925–926.

Power, M. L., Holzman, G. B., & Schulkin, J. (2001). A survey on the management of nausea and vomiting in pregnancy by obstetrician/gynecologists. *Primary Care Update for OB/GYNS, 8(2),* 69–72.

Queenan, J. T. (1999). Rh and other blood group immunizations. In J. T. Queenan (Ed.), *Management of high-risk pregnancy,* (4th ed.). Malden, MA: Blackwell Science.

Roberts, J. M. (1999). Pregnancy-related hypertension. In R. K.Creasy & R. Resnik (Eds.), *Maternal fetal medicine* (4th ed.). Philadelphia: W. B. Saunders.

Roberts, J. M., & Cooper, D. W. (2001). Pathogenesis and genetics of pre-eclampsia. *Lancet, 357,* 53–56.

Rosevear, S. (1999). Bleeding in early pregnancy. In D. K. James, P. J. Steer, C. P. Weiner, & B. Gonik (Eds.), *High risk pregnancy management options* (2nd ed.). Philadelphia: W. B. Saunders.

Sampson, J. E., & Gravett, M. G. (1999). Other infectious conditions in pregnancy. In D. K. James, P. J. Steer, C. P. Weiner, & B. Gonik (Eds.), *High risk pregnancy management options* (2nd ed.). Philadelphia: W. B. Saunders.

Schrag, S., Gorwitz, R., Fultz-Butts, K. & Schuchat, A. (2002, August 16). Prevention of perinatal group B streptococcal disease: Revised guidelines from the CDC. *Morbidity and Mortality Weekly Report, 51,* (RR11), 1–22.

Scott, L. D. (1999). Gastrointestinal disease in pregnancy. In R. K. Creasy & R. Resnik (Eds.), *Maternal fetal medicine* (4th ed.). Philadelphia: W.B. Saunders.

Secki, M. J., Fisher, R. A., Salerno, G., Rees, H., Paradinas, F. J., Foskett, M., et al. (2000). Choriocarcinoma and partial hydatidiform moles. *Lancet, 356,* 36–39.

Shelton, S. D., Boggess, K. A., Murtha, A. P., Groff, A. O., & Herbert, W. N. (2001). Repeated fetal betamethasone treatment and birth weight and head circumference. *Obstetrics & Gynecology, 97*(2), 301–304.

Sheth, S., & Chalmers, I. (2002). Magnesium sulfate halves risk of eclampsia. *Lancet, 359,* 1877–1890.

Simpson, J. L., & Carson, S. A. (2002). Genetic and nongenetic causes of pregnancy loss. In J. J. Sciarra (Ed.), *Gynecology and obstetrics* (Vol. 5, chap. 48). Philadelphia: Lippincott Williams & Wilkins.

Signore, C. (2001). Rubella. *Primary Care Update for OB/GYNs, 8*(4), 133–137.

Sison, A. V., & Sever, J. L. (1999a). Cytomegalovirus infections. In J. T. Queenan (Ed.), *Management of high-risk pregnancy* (4th ed.). Malden, MA: Blackwell Science.

Sison, A. V., & Sever, J. L. (1999b). Toxoplasmosis. In J. T. Queenan (Ed.), *Management of high-risk pregnancy* (4th ed.). Malden, MA: Blackwell Science.

Skidmore-Roth, L. (2001). *Mosby's handbook of herbs and natural supplements.* St Louis, MO: Mosby.

Soto, C. (2002). Toxoplasmosis in pregnancy. *Clinician Reviews, 12*(6), 51–56.

Steele, N. M., French, J., Gatherer-Boyles, J., Newman, S., & Leclaire, S. (2001). Effects of acupressure by Sea-Bands on nausea and vomiting of pregnancy. *Journal of Obstetric, Gynecologic, and Neonatal Nursing, 30*(1), 61–70.

Suarez, R. D., Grobman, W. A., & Parilla, B. V. (2001). Indomethacin tocolysis and intraventricular hemorrhage. *Obstetrics & Gynecology, 97*(6), 921–925.

Svigos, J. M., Robinson, J. S., & Vigneswaran, R. (1999). Prelabor rupture of the membranes. In D. K. James, P. J. Steer, C. P. Weiner, & B. Gonik (Eds.), *High risk pregnancy management options* (2nd ed.). Philadelphia: W.B. Saunders.

Szulman, A. E. (2000). Choriocarcinoma after hydatidiform mole. [Letter to the editor]. *American Journal of Obstetrics and Gynecology, 183,* 257.

Tillet, J., & Hanson, L. (1999). Midwifery triage and management of trauma and second/third trimester bleeding. *Journal of Nurse-Midwifery, 44*(5), 439–448.

Towbin, J. A. (1999). Presentation and diagnosis of fetal infection. In D. K. James, P. J. Steer, C. P. Weiner, & B. Gonik (Eds.), *High risk pregnancy management options* (2nd ed.). Philadelphia: W.B. Saunders.

Tsatsaris, V., Papasonis, D., Goffinet, F., Dekker, G., & Carbonne, B. (2001). Tocolysis with nifedipine or beta-adrenergic agonists: A meta-analysis. *Obstetrics & Gynecology, 97*(5), 840–847.

Vutyavanich, T., Kraisarin, T., & Ruangsri, R. (2001). Ginger for nausea and vomiting in pregnancy: Randomized, double-masked, placebo-controlled trial. *Obstetrics & Gynecology,* 97(4), 577–582.

Watt, J. P., Schuchat, A., Erickson, K., Honig, J. E., Gibbs, R., & Schulkin, J. (2001). Group B streptococcal disease prevention practices of obstetrician-gynecologists. *Obstetrics & Gynecology, 98*(1), 7–13.

Weiner, C. P. (1999). Fetal hemolytic disease. In D. K. James, P. J. Steer, C.P. Weiner, & B. Gonik (Eds.), *High risk pregnancy management options* (2nd ed.). Philadelphia: W.B. Saunders.

Wong, L. C., Ngan, H. Y. S., Gheng, D. K. L., & Ng, T. Y. (2000). Methotrexate infusion in low-risk gestational trophoblastic disease. *American Journal of Obstetrics and Gynecology, 183*(6), 1579–1582.

Yankowitz, J., & Pastorek, J. G. (1999). Maternal and fetal viral infections including listeriosis and toxoplasmosis. In D. K. James, P. J. Steer, C. P. Weiner, & B. Gonik (Eds.), *High risk pregnancy management options* (2nd ed.). Philadelphia: W. B. Saunders.

Zhang, J., Klebanoff, M. A., & Roberts, J. M. (2001). Prediction of adverse outcomes by common definitions of hypertension in pregnancy. *Obstetrics & Gynecology,* 97(2), 261–267.

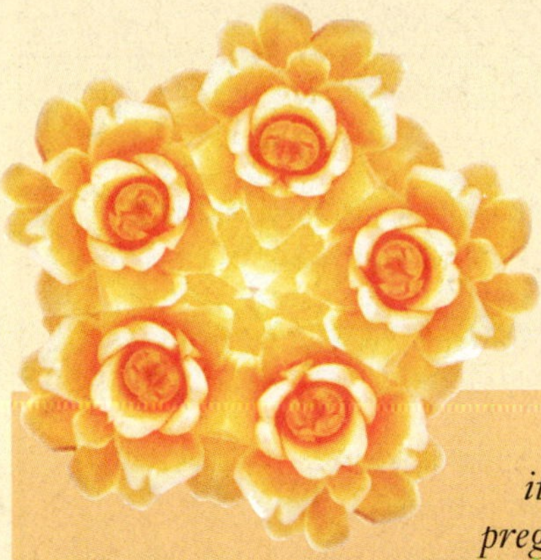

21 Assessment of Fetal Well-Being

My first pregnancy was so tenuous that I didn't know from one moment to the next how it would end. I hoped for our baby's safety, but in the end, our baby died. When I became pregnant again, I was very nervous. Being able to see the baby on ultrasound helped me so much. I knew our baby was alive and growing.

Objectives

- Describe the various psychologic responses to antenatal testing.
- Identify indications and interpret findings for ultrasound examinations performed in the first trimester.
- Describe the procedures used in the first trimester to confirm fetal viability.
- Delineate the use of ultrasound in the second trimester to assess fetal life, number, presentation, anatomy, age, and growth.
- Compare the indications and procedures for fetal movement awareness, the nonstress test, vibroacoustic stimulation, the contraction stress test, biophysical profile, and amniotic fluid index.
- Explain the purpose of maternal serum alpha-fetoprotein testing and the implications of abnormal values.
- Contrast the use of amniocentesis and chorionic villus sampling in detecting a fetus with a chromosomal disorder.
- Discuss fetal fibronectin and transvaginal measurement of cervical length as predictors of preterm labor.
- Discuss how the lecithin/sphingomyelin ratio of the amniotic fluid and phosphatidylglycerol (PG) can be used to assess fetal lung maturity.

Key Terms

Alpha-fetoprotein (AFP) 545
Amniocentesis 547
Amniotic fluid index (AFI) 534
Beta human chorionic gonadotropin (beta hCG) 530
Biophysical profile (BPP) 541
Cervical funneling 529
Chorionic villus sampling (CVS) 550
Contraction stress test (CST) 538
Fetal fibronectin (fFN) 552
Fetoscopy 552
Intrauterine growth restriction (IUGR) 544
Late decelerations 539
Lecithin/sphingomyelin (L/S) ratio 553
Macrosomia 544
Maternal serum alpha-fetoprotein (MSAFP) 546
Nonstress test (NST) 536
Oligohydramnios 540
Percutaneous umbilical blood sampling (PUBS) 552
Phosphatidylglycerol (PG) 553
Surfactant 553
Ultrasound 527
Vibroacoustic stimulation (VAS) 538

MediaLink

Additional resources for this content can be found on the Student CD-ROM and on the Companion Website at www.prenhall.com/olds. Click on "Chapter 21" to select the activities for this chapter.

CD-ROM
- Audio Glossary
- NCLEX Review

Companion Website
- Additional NCLEX Review
- Case Study: Client Undergoing Contraction Stress Test
- Care Plan Activity: Assessment of Fetal Well-Being

Every parent dreams of a perfectly healthy baby and indeed the vast majority of babies are born healthy. However, maternal conditions, genetics, and environmental influences continue to adversely affect a small percentage of babies. Although the antenatal fetal assessment techniques discussed in this chapter are designed to maximize the chances of identifying a fetus at risk, a perfect pregnancy outcome can never be predicted or guaranteed.

Although the United States spends a greater percentage of its gross national product on healthcare than any other country, it continues to have a higher infant mortality rate than many other industrialized countries (Dye, 2001). Reproductive technologies significantly raise the cost of healthcare. These technologic advances are not without risks; therefore, prevention of perinatal morbidity must always be a primary goal. The decision to use the tests discussed in this chapter is made by the childbearing family only after a careful analysis of their risks and costs compared to their possible benefit to the mother or her fetus. The nurse articulates the value of a particular test as well as its possible limitations at any point in pregnancy.

Psychologic Reactions to Antenatal Testing

Little has been written about the psychologic impact of antenatal diagnostic testing on childbearing families; however, several studies indicate that the need for testing usually provokes fear (Chandler & Smith, 1998; Chou, Lee, & Shih, 2001). Nurses often play a key role not only in teaching families about various testing procedures, but also in providing clarity and emotional support to the woman and her family undergoing antenatal testing. To decrease anxiety and alleviate fear for the woman and her partner, the nurse provides clear, concise explanations of the information expected to be obtained from the test, and potential options after the testing has been completed. See Table 21–1 • for sample nursing approaches to pretest teaching. Although the family may approach antenatal testing with a great deal of anxiety, the testing itself may assist in alleviating fears and decreasing anxiety.

Some tests, such as ultrasound, have become almost routine, and many couples view this antepartum test as an expected part of the prenatal care. The ultrasound may provide confirmation of a viable pregnancy through visualization of the fetal heartbeat, may identify the sex of the fetus, and may promote psychologic preparation for attachment after birth (Colucciello, 1998). However, when more invasive testing is recommended, it may evoke fear and anxiety in the woman and her partner as they consider the reason for the test, the risk to the fetus and woman during the test, and the implications of the test results.

Table 21-1 • SAMPLE NURSING APPROACHES TO PRETEST TEACHING

Assess whether the woman knows the reason the screening or diagnostic test is being recommended.

Examples:

"What has your doctor/nurse-midwife told you about this test?"

"Sometimes tests are done for many different reasons. Can you tell me why you are having this test?"

"What is your understanding about what the test will show?"

Provide an opportunity for questions.

Examples:

"What questions do you have about the test?"

"What things about the test are unclear to you?"

Explain the test procedure, paying particular attention to any preparation the woman needs to do prior to the test.

Example:

"The test that has been ordered for you is designed to . . ." (Add specific information about the particular test. Give the explanation in simple language.)

Validate the woman's understanding of the preparation.

Example:

"Tell me what you will have to do to get ready for this test."

Give permission for the woman to continue to ask questions if needed.

Example:

"I'll be with you during the test. If you have any questions at any time, please don't hesitate to ask."

NURSING CARE MANAGEMENT

Nurses in a variety of settings have an opportunity to provide care to families undergoing antenatal testing. Antenatal assessment tests are performed by perinatal nurse practitioners and/or nurses who have received additional specialized perinatal education and practice. The nurse, whatever the role, is a vital link between the woman and the physician or certified nurse-midwife. Nurses also need to provide easy to understand information to the mother and family. The nurse can encourage the family to ask questions, voice concerns and fears, and become actively involved in the antenatal testing process. Nurses are often responsible for the follow-up care that is needed as a result of test findings, such as arranging for additional testing, interpreting results, and answering questions the woman or her family may have.

Nursing Assessment and Diagnosis

Nursing assessment begins with a history of the present prenatal course and identifying possible indications for a particular diagnostic test. Examples may include identifying possible testing related to advanced maternal age, previous history of a child with a birth defect, or the presence of a particular maternal medical condition. The nurse assesses the woman and her partner's knowledge about the reason the test is being advised, the information that the woman and her support person have about the test, their questions and concerns, and the presence of any psychosociocultural factors that may influence the teaching or learning process. During the test and afterward, the nurse completes needed assessments to monitor the status of the woman and her fetus.

The primary nursing diagnoses are directed toward providing information about the diagnostic test and minimizing any risks to the woman and her unborn child. Examples of nursing diagnoses that may be applicable include:

- ***Health-Seeking Behavior:*** Information about the fetal assessment test related to an expressed desire to understand its purpose, benefits, risks, and alternatives
- ***Fear*** related to the risks of a specific test or possible unfavorable test results
- ***Disruption in Attachment*** due to high-risk label attached to the pregnancy

Nursing Plan and Implementation

The nursing plan of care is directed toward each specific nursing diagnosis. The nurse generally plays a vital role in providing needed and desired information about the diagnostic test. The nurse also functions as an advocate for the expectant woman by helping her clarify question areas and obtain needed information. The nurse frequently knows the areas of greatest concern for women and can anticipate many of their fears. When the woman is not able to verbalize questions, the nurse can assist by providing information that answers questions that other women have had. For example, many women undergoing an amniocentesis fear pain during the procedure. The nurse can inform the woman that she will feel pressure during the insertion of the needle and may feel subsequent cramping, which can last for several hours. The nurse can provide information about the procedure itself and follow-up monitoring to ensure fetal well-being.

It is important for the nurse to realize that women react differently to pregnancy. The nurse's role is to remain nonjudgmental and to offer support when needed. Establishing a trusting relationship increases the possibility that a woman will talk to the nurse and share her concerns and emotional needs. The nurse is often the one to coordinate services the woman may need such as community resources for financial, psychologic, or social support.

Nurses working in community clinics have an integral role in performing fetal surveillance tests throughout the antepartum period. Nurses may find themselves not only performing some of these tests, such as nonstress tests, but also performing comprehensive assessments of the woman's health, her family dynamics, and her living situation. Community health nurses often have a more accurate understanding of the woman's physical resources, such as the adequacy of living conditions, proximity to healthcare resources, and availability of public transportation. It is often the nurse who has the most contact with the pregnant woman. Because of this, the nurse is in an excellent position to provide anticipatory guidance, reiterate teaching provided by the woman's healthcare provider, and monitor her current plan of care. It is important for the nurse to be cognizant of the potential for any fetal surveillance testing to be emotionally charged for the pregnant woman and her family (Chou et al, 2001; Colucciello, 1998). The nurse should approach each encounter with calmness, compassion, and warranted reassurance.

Evaluation

The nurse evaluates the woman and her family's understanding of antepartum testing procedures. Determining if the family understands the need for follow-up testing is imperative. The nurse should also assess whether the teaching methods used are effective for that family. Evaluation should include both physical and psychologic factors. In addition, the nurse determines if adequate resources, such as social support and physical resources, are available for the pregnant woman. Women from different cultures may need additional support since they may encounter language and other cultural barriers.

Ultrasound

Ultrasound has become one of the most commonly used diagnostic and screening tools in pregnancy (Cunningham, Gant, Leveno, et al, 2001). For the last 20 years, it has played a critical role in the practice of obstetrics. Since ultrasound is used widely to assess fetal well-being in all three trimesters, it will also be discussed within this framework later in the chapter.

Ultrasound is a diagnostic procedure that uses high-frequency sound waves exceeding 20,000 cycles per second to produce an image that varies based on the density of the structure under the transducer. The reflected energy creates a small electrical voltage that is displayed on the screen. Very dense components, such as bone, appear white on the screen, whereas soft tissues appear gray and fluid appears black (Cunningham et al, 2001). Instruments used in ultrasonography operate at 2 to 10 megahertz (MHz). The higher the frequency of the sound, the shallower the depth of penetration but the better the resolution of the image produced. Ultrasound uses a device called a *transducer* to turn the sound waves into electrical signals. Transducers can be used either transabdominally (Figure 21–1 •), operating at 3.5 MHz, or transvaginally (Figure 21–2 •), operating at 5 to 7 MHz. These transducers and their use will be described fully later in the chapter.

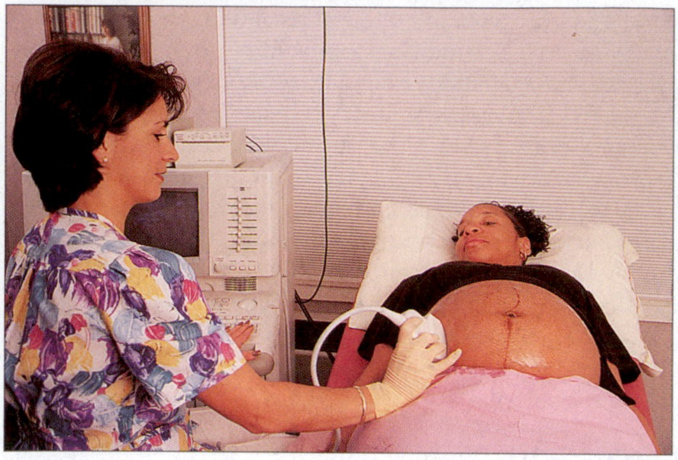

Figure 21–1 • Ultrasound scanning permits visualization of the fetus in utero.

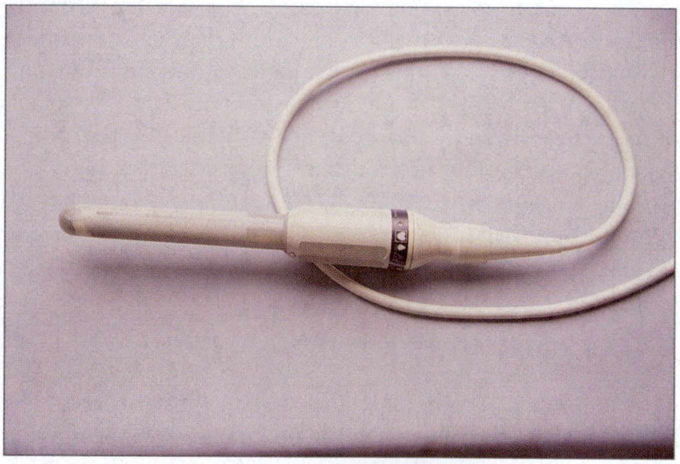

Figure 21–2 • Transvaginal ultrasound transducer.

Ultrasound can be used to produce images called *sonograms* in several different ways. In motion mode (M mode), the reflected echo generates a moving display. This is how fetal cardiac activity is seen. Brightness modulation (B mode) converts the signals into varying degrees of brightness and produces a two-dimensional image. Three-dimensional ultrasound uses algorithms to vary opacity, transparency, and depth to project an image. This allows curved structures such as the fetal face to be viewed (Figure 21–3 •).

Extent of Ultrasound Exams

An ultrasound exam may be either limited (identifying only certain components) or comprehensive (sometimes referred to as *basic*). A *limited sonogram* may be used to:

- Determine fetal presentation prior to or during labor.
- Locate the placenta.
- Confirm fetal viability.
- Determine the amniotic fluid index (AFI).

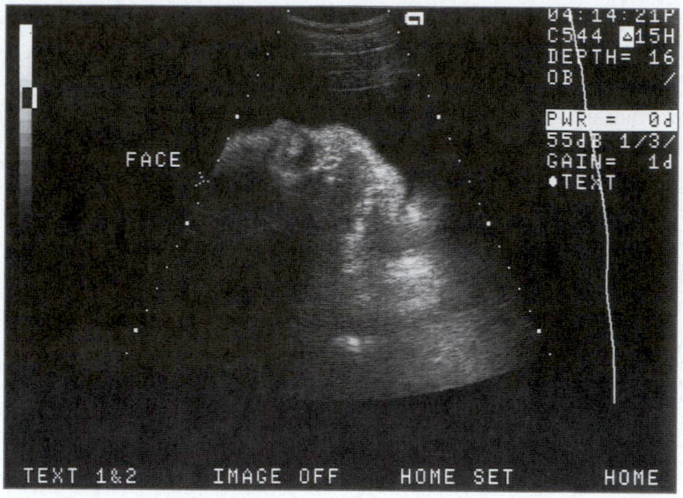

Figure 21–3 • Ultrasound of the fetal face.

- Diagnose multiple gestation.
- Guide amniocentesis.

A *comprehensive sonogram* provides the same information and also looks carefully at fetal anatomic structures and the placenta and notes maternal anatomic structures (Callen, 2000).

Methods of Ultrasound Scanning

The two most common methods of ultrasound scanning are *transabdominal* and *transvaginal* scanning.

TRANSABDOMINAL ULTRASOUND

In the transabdominal approach, a transducer is moved across the abdomen (see Figure 21–1). The woman is usually scanned with a full bladder, except when ultrasound is used to localize the placenta before amniocentesis. When the bladder is full, the examiner can assess other structures, especially the vagina and cervix, in relation to the bladder. This is particularly important when vaginal bleeding is noted and placenta previa is the suspected cause. It can also determine if vaginal bleeding is being caused by premature dilatation of the cervix. The woman is advised to drink 1 to 1.5 quarts of water approximately 2 hours before the examination, and she is asked to refrain from emptying her bladder. If the bladder is not sufficiently filled, she is asked to drink 3 to 4 (8 oz) glasses of water and is rescanned 30 to 45 minutes later.

Mineral oil or a transmission gel is generously spread over the woman's abdomen, and the sonographer slowly moves a transducer over the abdomen to obtain a picture of the contents of the uterus. Testing takes 20 to 30 minutes. The woman may feel discomfort from pressure applied over a full bladder. In some instances, the sonographer may advise the woman to urinate a small amount to relieve the discomfort. In addition, if the woman lies on her back during the test, shortness of breath can develop. This may be relieved by elevating her upper body during the test.

TRANSVAGINAL ULTRASOUND

The transvaginal (or endovaginal) method uses a probe inserted into the vagina (Figure 21–2). Once inserted, the endovaginal probe is close to the structures being imaged and so produces a better, clearer image. The improved images obtained by endovaginal ultrasound have enabled sonographers to identify structures and fetal characteristics earlier in pregnancy (Callen, 2000). Transvaginal ultrasound also allows better assessment of the cervix. It can identify potential preterm labor, shortened cervical length, and **cervical funneling** (a cone-shaped indentation in the cervical os), which is common in cases of cervical incompetence (Callen, 2000).

After the procedure is fully explained to the woman, she is prepared in the same manner as for a pelvic examination: in lithotomy position, with appropriate drapes to provide privacy, and a female attendant in the room. It is important that the woman's buttocks are at the end of the table so that, once inserted, the probe can be moved in various directions. The small, lightweight vaginal transducer is covered with a specially fitted sterile sheath, a condom, or one finger of a latex or vinyl glove. Ultrasound coupling gel is then applied to the covering, making insertion into the vagina easier and providing a medium for enhancing the ultrasound image. In addition to providing a clearer image than the transabdominal method, the transvaginal procedure can be accomplished with an empty bladder. Most women do not feel discomfort during the exam. The probe is smaller than a speculum, so insertion is usually completed with ease. The woman may feel some movement of the probe during the exam as various structures are imaged. Some women may want to insert the probe themselves to enhance their comfort; others may feel embarrassed even to be asked. The certified nurse-midwife, physician, or ultrasonographer offers the choice based on the clinician's comfort level and the rapport the clinician has established with the woman.

Safety of Ultrasound

In the last 20 years, the use of ultrasound as a diagnostic tool in pregnancy has increased exponentially. To date, studies show that infants exposed to ultrasound in utero have no significant differences in birth weight or length, childhood growth, cognitive function, acoustic or visual ability, or rates of neurologic deficits (Wagner & Calhoun, 1998). Experimental observations from animal studies suggest that high-intensity ultrasound, which is not used in obstetric ultrasounds, has definite and biologically harmful effects. Nevertheless, the Food and Drug Administration (FDA) has stated that obstetric sonograms fall within an acceptable level of safety because they use low-intensity ultrasound.

Is there such a category as "routine ultrasound" in pregnancy? Not necessarily, according to the American College of Obstetricians and Gynecologists (ACOG). In large studies, researchers compared several outcomes between a group of women who had ultrasound examinations performed and a group of women who did not. Outcomes included perinatal mortality, Apgar score, birth weight, maternal outcome, detections of multiple gestation and abnormalities, as well as cost-effectiveness (Fry, 2000). The group that had had ultrasound examinations had higher rates of detection of multiple gestations and abnormalities. There were no significant differences in outcomes related to the other factors. The National Institutes of Health (NIH), rather than suggesting routine use of sonograms in pregnancy, has established the following recommended indications for ultrasound. These indications have since been endorsed by ACOG:

- Estimation of gestational age for women with uncertain dates of conception
- Verification of dates for women who are to undergo scheduled elective repeat cesarean birth, indicated induction of labor, or elective termination of pregnancy
- Evaluation of fetal growth
- Evaluation of vaginal bleeding of undetermined cause in pregnancy
- Determination of fetal presentation
- Suspected multiple gestation
- Adjunct to amniocentesis
- Significant discrepancy between uterine size and date of conception
- Pelvic mass
- Suspected hydatidiform mole
- Adjunct to special procedures
- Adjunct to cervical cerclage placement
- Suspected fetal death
- Suspected ectopic pregnancy
- Suspected uterine anomaly
- Intrauterine device localization
- Biophysical profile for fetal well-being
- Observation of intrapartum events
- Suspected hydramnios or oligohydramnios
- Suspected abruptio placentae
- Adjunct to external version from breech to vertex presentation
- Estimation of fetal weight or presentation in premature rupture of membranes or premature labor
- Abnormal serum alpha-fetoprotein value to assess for neural tube defects or trisomy 18 or 21
- Follow-up observation of identified fetal anomaly
- Follow-up observation of placental location for identified "placenta previa"
- History of previous congenital anomaly
- Serial evaluation of fetal growth in multiple gestation
- Evaluation of fetal condition in late registrants for prenatal care

MEDIALINK ULTRASOUND IN OBSTETRICS

Who Should Perform Ultrasound Examinations?

The accuracy of ultrasound as a diagnostic tool is highly dependent on the knowledge, skills, and judgment of the person performing the exam. The risk of false-positive and false-negative results when performed by inexperienced or unprepared examiners must be considered as an important safety issue (Association of Women's Health, Obstetric, and Neonatal Nurses [AWHONN], 2001). Ultrasound is often used by members of the healthcare team to provide rapid assessment of the well-being of a pregnancy or fetus. However, it has been demonstrated that potential problems may be overlooked or false-positives may necessitate follow-up exams and cause anxiety to the mother and family (Callen, 2000). AWHONN has set guidelines and nursing practice competencies for experienced maternal-newborn nurses to perform limited ultrasound exams. The guidelines indicate that the nurse must complete an educational program that includes didactic presentations and a clinical practicum (AWHONN, 2001).

NURSING CARE MANAGEMENT

The nurse plays a key role in providing the mother and family with information related to the ultrasound procedure itself and expected outcomes. The nurse answers questions, and helps clarify ultrasound findings. Some women, especially those who lack insurance coverage, may worry about the cost of the test itself. The nurse can discuss the rationale for obtaining an ultrasound and what will be done with the information once it is obtained. The nurse provides support for the woman and her family, recognizing that some women may feel anxious or fearful.

Assessment of Fetal Well-Being in the First Trimester

The first trimester represents a crucial time for establishing fetal viability and determining an accurate gestational age. There are a variety of methods that the practitioner can use to determine fetal well-being in early pregnancy.

Viability

Viability, or the potential for the pregnancy to result in a live infant, is the first issue to consider in pregnancy. A positive urine pregnancy test does not confirm viability, only the presence of beta human chorionic gonadotropin (hCG) hormone. The developing embryo implants into the uterus approximately 14 days after conception has occurred (Callen, 2000). While about one third of pregnant women experience bleeding associated with this normal process, bleeding can also be associated with a nonviable pregnancy with an ultimate spontaneous abortion (miscarriage) or ectopic (tubal) pregnancy. Serial quantitative beta hCG testing, progesterone-level testing, and ultrasound can be used to distinguish a normally developing fetus from an ectopic pregnancy, which if undiagnosed, carries a high maternal morbidity.

QUANTITATIVE BETA HCG TESTING

Beta human chorionic gonadotropin (beta hCG) is a product of the trophoblast or placenta and is a very accurate marker of the presence of pregnancy and placental health. Beta hCG is detectable in the blood serum of approximately 5% of pregnant women by 8 days after conception, and in virtually all pregnancies by 11 days. The level in the serum approximately doubles every 2 days in the first 10 days of pregnancy, peaking at 60 to 90 days after conception (Cunningham et al, 2001) (Table 21–2 •). In early pregnancy, two quantitative beta hCG levels drawn 48 hours apart serve as an excellent test of the viability of the pregnancy. Conversely, if the beta hCG level remains stable or falls over 48 hours, a miscarriage or ectopic pregnancy should be suspected.

Although not routine in all pregnancies, serologic evaluation is indicated in women with a history of spontaneous abortion, ectopic pregnancy, or risk of ectopic pregnancy (intrauterine device in place, previous pelvic inflammatory disease, or reversal of a tubal sterilization). Women who are spotting should also have a beta hCG level drawn to ensure adequate levels. Many women who have conceived through assisted reproductive methods also have their beta hCG levels monitored to ensure the pregnancy is developing normally.

The 48 hours between the beta hCG tests can be an extremely anxious time for the couple. In order to offer effective counseling, the nurse must understand the information these tests provide, as well as their limitations. For example, the woman may not know why she must wait 48 hours for a repeat blood test. The nurse needs to allow time for the woman and her partner, if present, to express their anxiety and fears. False reassurances should not be offered. Instead, attention is directed toward helping them cope with the in-

Table 21–2 • APPROXIMATE BETA hCG VALUES IN PREGNANCY

Gestational Age (Weeks)	Beta hCG Values (mIU/mL)
1–2	16–156
2–3	101–4,870
3–4	1,110–31,500
4–5	2,560–82,300
5–6	23,100–151,000
6–7	27,300–233,000
7–11	20,900–291,000
11–16	6,140–103,000
16–21	4,720–80,100
21–39	2,700–78,100

herent uncertainty that occurs while the exams are being completed and until a definitive diagnosis can be made.

PROGESTERONE LEVEL TESTING

Progesterone is secreted in early pregnancy by the corpus luteum until approximately 8 weeks' gestation at which point the placenta begins to manufacture its own progesterone. Low levels of progesterone are associated with spontaneous abortions and ectopic pregnancies. Although progesterone levels are not routinely tested in early pregnancy, they can be assessed by performing a simple blood test when there is a history of spontaneous abortions or spotting in early pregnancy. Progesterone levels above 25 ng/mL are typically associated with normally developing intrauterine pregnancies. Progesterone levels that are below 5 ng/mL typically indicate a nonviable fetus. Levels between 5 ng/mL and 25 ng/mL are inconclusive. Approximately 10% of women have progesterone levels below 25 ng/mL. The nurse notifies the physician/certified nurse-midwife if levels are low. The physician/ certified nurse-midwife bases the decision of whether or not to supplement progesterone during early pregnancy on current progesterone levels, past history of spontaneous abortions, and presence of spotting or vaginal bleeding. Low progesterone levels can be treated by giving the woman progesterone either orally or via vaginal suppositories. This supplementation is warranted throughout the first trimester. After 12 gestational weeks, supplements are not needed since the placenta will make adequate progesterone levels.

ULTRASOUND

The sonographic landmarks (presence of gestational sac, cardiac motion, embryo development) of normal early pregnancy, detected by transvaginal ultrasound, are very predictable. Up to about 4½ to 5 weeks of gestation, prior to the appearance of a gestational sac, nothing can be seen in the uterus. The gestational sac at first appears empty and may be confused with the pseudogestational sac of ectopic pregnancy. A true gestational sac is associated with beta hCG levels of 1800 mIU/mL if the sonogram is being done transvaginally and 6500 mIU/mL if the sonogram is being done transabdominally. At approximately 5½ weeks the yolk sac, a small round structure sometimes resembling a "double ring," is visible within the gestational sac. It is an embryonic structure, so its appearance provides strong evidence supporting the presence of an intrauterine pregnancy (Callen, 2000). At 6 to 6½ weeks, the embryo itself becomes visible, and shortly thereafter cardiac activity is detectable (Callen, 2000). During the ultrasound examination, the gestational sac and embryo are measured to determine gestational age (Figure 21–4 •).

Gestational Age

Determination of an accurate expected date of birth (EDB) early in pregnancy is essential for evaluating well-being throughout the pregnancy. Labor contractions that may be perfectly normal at 37 weeks could be a problem if they occur at 34 weeks. Conversely, a 40-week pregnancy inadvertently thought to be 42 weeks may result in an unnecessary and risk-laden induction of labor. Much of the obstetrician or midwife's

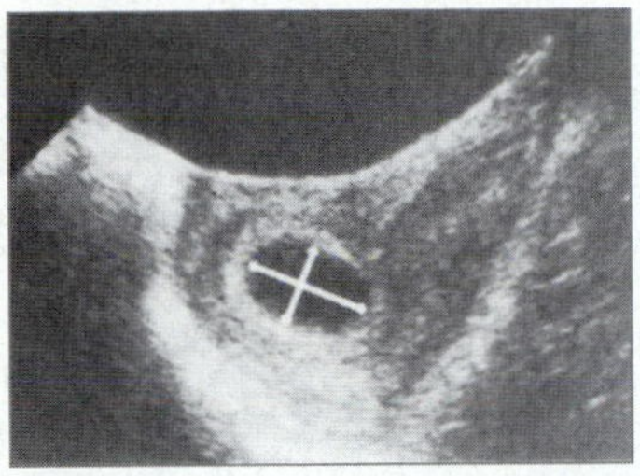

Figure 21–4 • Measurement of the gestational sac. The ultrasound shows the uterus; the blackened oval area is the gestational sac. The fluid in the gestational sac does not generate echoes from the ultrasound and thus appears dark in contrast to the uterine tissue surrounding it. The lines through the gestational sac represent measurements that are taken.
SOURCE: Callen, P. W. *Ultrasonography in obstetrics and gynecology* (2nd ed., p. 49). Copyright 1998, with permission from Elsevier Science.

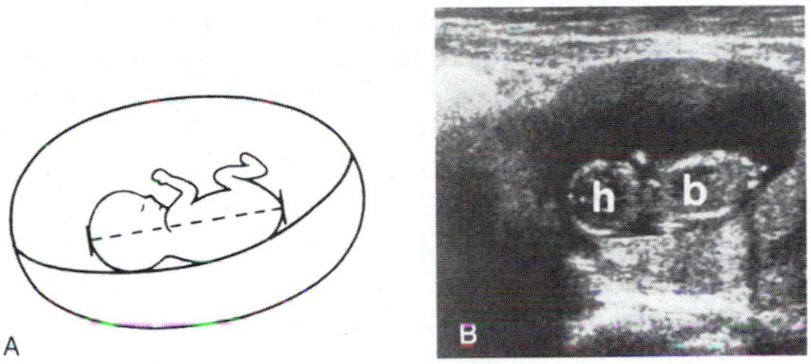

Figure 21–5 • Measurement of the crown-rump length. *A*, Schematic diagram. Dotted line shows the measurement from the top of the fetal crown (head) to the bottom of the rump (buttocks). *B*, Ultrasound scan of the pregnant uterus, showing the longest length of a 9-week fetus. The head (h) can be differentiated from the body (b), but the internal anatomy cannot be clearly distinguished.
SOURCE: Callen, P. W. *Ultrasonography in obstetrics and gynecology* (2nd ed., p. 50). Copyright 1998, with permission from Elsevier Science.

efforts are aimed at determining the most accurate EDB possible. Traditional means of establishing an EDB are documenting a reliable last menstrual period (LMP) from the woman, measuring uterine size, noting the date of the first audible fetal heart tones, and noting the date of quickening (the first recognized fetal movement). An accurate LMP established early in pregnancy is considered the most reliable indicator of an EDB (Smith & Wigton 2001). Problems occur if the woman cannot recall her LMP, if her menstrual cycles were extremely irregular, or if she had bleeding in early pregnancy.

An early transvaginal or abdominal sonogram is indicated when there is a need to establish an accurate gestational age. The crown-rump length is considered the most accurate sonographic measurement for gestational age if performed between 6 and 10 weeks' gestation. It is accurate to within plus or minus 3 to 5 days of the EDB based on the crown-rump length (Figure 21–5 •). This means that an ultrasound performed at 6 weeks would be accurate in predicting the EDB within either 3 to 5 days before or 3 to 5 days after the predicted EDB. Beyond 12 weeks, the fetus begins to curve and the crown-rump length

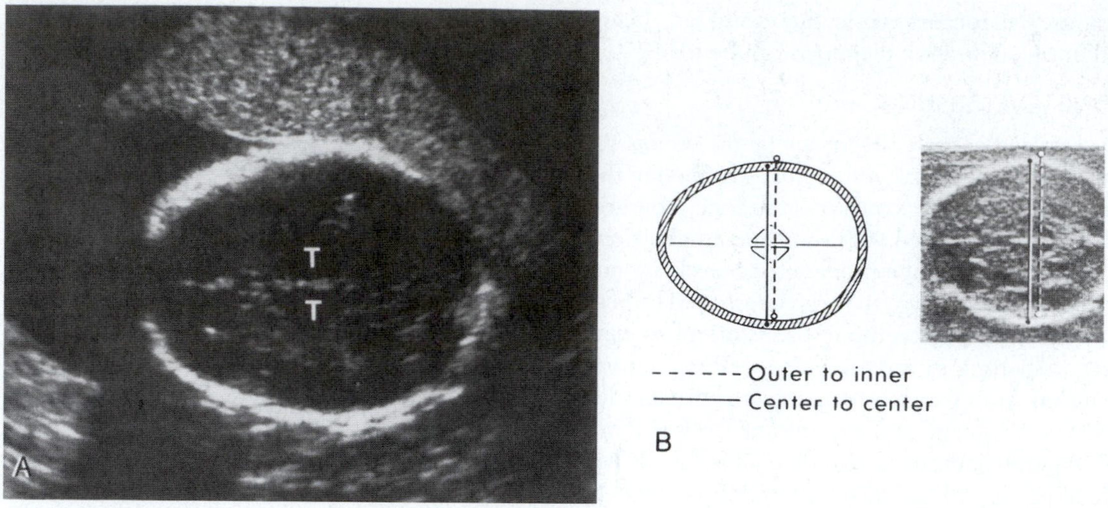

Figure 21–6 • Measurement of the biparietal diameter. *A,* Ultrasound transaxial image of the fetal head, taken with the thalami (T) imaged in the midline, equidistant from the temporoparietal tables of the calvarium. *B,* Diagram and image showing the leading edge (outer) to the leading edge (inner) measurements of the fetal head, taken at the level of the thalami.
SOURCE: Callen, P. W. *Ultrasonography in obstetrics and gynecology* (2nd ed., p. 51). Copyright 1998, with permission from Elsevier Science.

loses its accuracy. For example, if an EDB based on a 10-week sonogram is September 9, it is reasonable to expect that date is accurate from September 4 through September 14. After the first trimester, gestational age is obtained by a combination of measurements of femur length, abdominal circumference, and biparietal diameter (Figure 21–6 •). Gestational age is reliable in the second trimester to plus or minus 7 to 14 days. For example, if a due date of October 1 is given by a second trimester sonogram, the reasonable date of birth can be from September 16 through October 14. While practice may vary, most obstetricians and midwives do not change a due date based on the second trimester sonogram unless there is a discrepancy of greater than 11 to 14 days from the LMP. After 26 weeks, fetal growth rates are less uniform, making ultrasound an inappropriate means of determining gestational age. Specifically, during the third trimester, ultrasound can estimate an EDB with plus or minus 14 to 21 days of accuracy. See Table 21–3 •.

Determining an accurate EDB can be extremely important later in pregnancy if there is inadequate uterine or fetal growth. An accurate EDB based on a first trimester ultrasound can assist the physician/certified nurse-midwife in diagnosing intrauterine growth restriction (to be discussed later in this chapter).

Assessment of Fetal Well-Being in the Second Trimester

The second trimester is considered by many to be the most advantageous time for basic obstetric ultrasound for several reasons. First, the relative uniformity of fetal growth during the first 20 weeks allows biometric measurements that continue to provide an accurate estimation of gestational age. Second, the large volume of amniotic fluid relative to the fetal size allows for excellent images of fetal anatomy. Finally, fetal anatomy can be visualized in extreme detail, allowing confirmation of normal anatomy. The ideal time for the second trimester basic sonogram is 18 to 24 weeks. There is some evidence that sonograms done at 20 to 22 weeks may be easier to perform and less likely to require an additional scan than one done at 18 weeks (Schwarzler, Senat, Holden, et al, 1999).

A basic (comprehensive) second trimester sonogram provides the following information about the fetus, placenta, and uterine conditions:

- Fetal life
- Fetal number
- Fetal presentation
- Evaluation of fetal anatomy
- Gestational age and growth
- Amniotic fluid volume
- Placental localization
- Uterine anatomy

Fetal Life

Presence of cardiac motion confirms fetal life. If gestational age has already been established and fetal heart tones have been visualized with an ultrasound or heard with a Doppler, then absence of cardiac motion in the second trimester is consistent with fetal demise.

Fetal Number

The second trimester is an ideal time to identify multiple gestation or the number of fetuses in the uterus. The number of placentas and their location can also be noted at this point.

Fetal Presentation

Although an ultrasound in the second trimester can determine whether a fetus is in the breech, transverse, or vertex position, the large amount of amniotic fluid relative to the fetal size along with the lack of fetal engagement makes it highly likely that the

Table 21-3 • PARAMETERS FOR ESTIMATING GESTATIONAL AGE

Source of Evidence	When Obtained	Estimated Accuracy
In vitro fertilization	At conception	< 1 day
Ultrasound measurement of crown-rump length	6–10 weeks	3 days
Clinical measurement of normal uterus	<12 weeks	7 days
Ultrasound measurement of biparietal diameter	<20 weeks	7 days
Ultrasound measurement of biparietal diameter	20–26 weeks	10 days
Ultrasound measurement of biparietal diameter	26–30 weeks	14–21 days
Ultrasound measurement of biparietal diameter	> 30 weeks	21–28 days

noted presentation will change repeatedly prior to birth. Fetal presentation is commonly documented on a second trimester ultrasound, but it is not usually of any clinical significance.

Fetal Anatomy Survey

A systematic examination of the fetal parts is conducted to identify possible abnormalities. Components of this examination include the fetal parts discussed in the following sections.

HEAD

The skull should be symmetrical with the cranium ossified and intact. The ventricular system (passageways within the brain) is evaluated. The choroids should appear symmetrical. The choroid plexus are found within the ventricles of the brain and in the subarachnoid space around the brain and spinal cord. They produce cerebral spinal fluid. Choroid cysts, if noted, are usually benign but have been associated with chromosomal abnormalities in 1% of fetuses. The nuchal fold thickness should be measured because thickening of the nuchal fold, the skin at the base of the fetal skull, has also been associated with certain chromosomal abnormalities.

The most dramatic abnormality diagnosed by ultrasound is anencephaly (a neural tube defect in which a portion of the fetal brain is missing). It is abnormal not to see the bony structures of the skull above the orbits of the eye after 14 weeks' gestation. The skull is brightly echogenic (appearing white due to its increased density) and is easily visualized. Failure to see the skull should alert the experienced examiner to the possibility of anencephaly.

SPINE

The spine is examined both sagittally and coronally for the presence of a sac or an outward splaying of the vertebrae laminae. Either of these conditions may suggest a possible spinal cord defect such as spina bifida.

THORAX AND HEART

A transverse plane of the fetal thorax provides valuable information about the size, shape, and symmetry of the chest. The size, location, and axis of the heart are also evaluated. A four-chambered view of the heart should demonstrate ventricles and atria of approximately equal size and an intact intraventricular septum. The heart occupies one quarter to one third of the chest cavity on transverse image. The lungs should have a homogenous appearance. The diaphragm should be imaged. Chest size is correlated with lung size.

ABDOMEN

The bladder, stomach, and kidneys should all be visualized. The fetal stomach and bladder can be seen on ultrasound by 14 weeks. Persistent failure to visualize the fetal stomach can be due to various fetal abnormalities, the most common being esophageal atresia. Mild dilation of the renal pelvis of less than 10 mm is rarely progressive and usually physiologic. The abdominal wall should be visualized to be intact. A transverse image of the umbilical cord should reveal a three-vessel cord. Insertion site of the umbilical cord is also carefully inspected.

EXTREMITIES

The femur is the only bone routinely measured on the basic ultrasound. If length seems abnormal, a more comprehensive exam is performed to compare it with the lengths of the other long bones. The upper extremities and the presence of hands and feet are also documented.

Gestational Age and Growth

The Hadlock method uses an average of measures of the biparietal diameter, head circumference, abdominal circumference, and femur length to estimate gestational age (Figures 21–7 • to 21–10 •). Comparison of measures made at intervals to standardized measures can be used to estimate fetal growth.

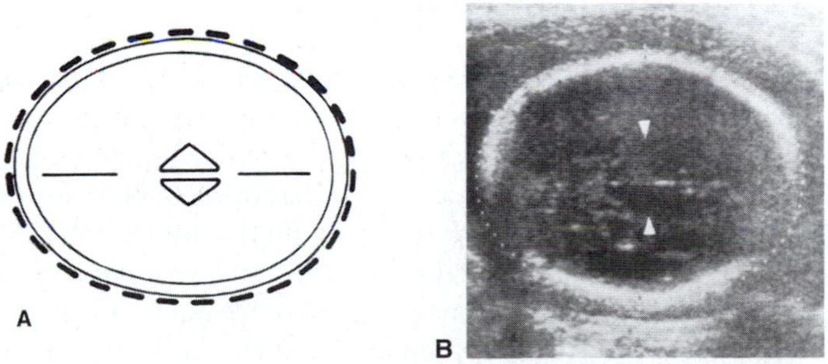

Figure 21-7 • Measurement of the head circumference. *A,* Diagram showing a dotted line outlining the head which indicates the correct place to make a circumference measurement. *B,* Ultrasound transaxial scan showing the thalami (arrowheads), positioned in midline. A dotted line created by the digitizer outlines the correct parameter, just outside of the hyperechoic calvarium to obtain a circumference measurement.
SOURCE: Callen, P. W. *Ultrasonography in obstetrics and gynecology* (2nd ed., p. 55). Copyright 1998, with permission from Elsevier Science.

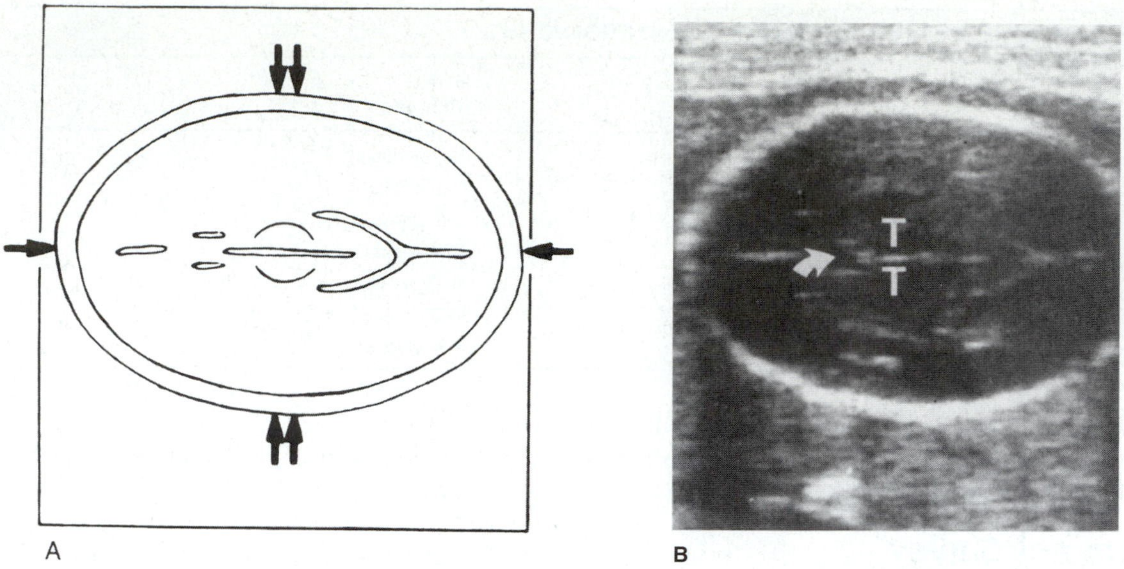

Figure 21-8 • Measurement of the cephalic index. *A,* The biparietal diameter (double arrows) and fronto-occipital diameter (single arrows) are both taken outer edge to outer edge. A ratio of the two gives the cephalic index. *B,* Ultrasound transaxial scan of the fetal head of the thalami (T) and cavum septi pellucidi (curved arrow).
SOURCE: Callen, P. W. *Ultrasonography in obstetrics and gynecology* (2nd ed., p. 53). Copyright 1998, with permission from Elsevier Science.

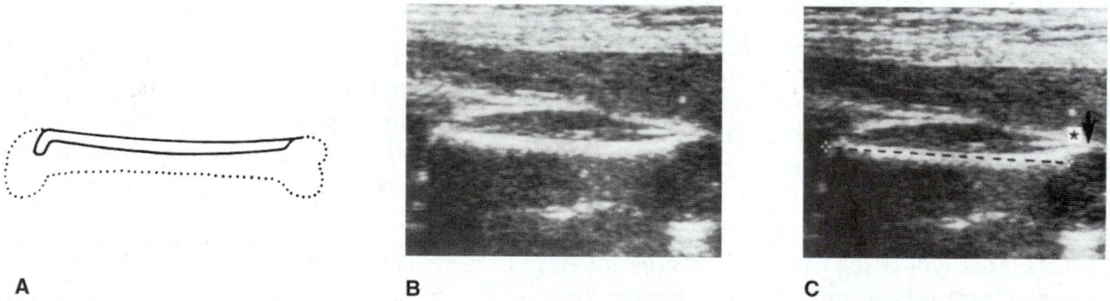

Figure 21-9 • Measurement of the femur length. *A,* Schematic diagram. *B,* Ultrasound image. The hyperechoic line is in the ossified lateral margin of the femoral diaphysis. The ends of the bone are the epiphyseal cartilages that have not yet calcified and are therefore hypoechoic. *C,* The hyperechoic diaphysis is measured from one end to the other, denoted by the cursors and a dotted line. The "distal femoral point" (* and arrow) is a nonossified extension of the distal epiphyseal cartilage. It should be included in the measurement.
SOURCE: Callen, P. W. *Ultrasonography in obstetrics and gynecology* (2nd ed., p.58). Copyright, 1998, with permission from Elsevier Science.

Amniotic Fluid Volume

Amniotic fluid volume changes with gestational age. In general, a subjective assessment of amniotic fluid volume as decreased, normal, or increased is adequate during the second trimester examination. However, the **amniotic fluid index (AFI)** is another method of reporting fluid volume. The AFI is calculated by dividing the maternal abdomen into four quadrants with the umbilicus as the reference point. Then, the deepest vertical pocket of fluid in each quadrant is measured, and these four measurements are summed to calculate the AFI.

Placenta Location

The placenta's appearance, location, and relationship to the cervical os should be evaluated. Placental position that is noted by sonogram in early pregnancy may not correlate well with the location at the time of birth. Factors such as the woman's position or overdistention of the bladder may give a false-positive diagnosis of placenta previa. Therefore, a possible low-lying placenta or placenta previa that is identified on a second trimester ultrasound must be confirmed by a follow-up sonogram in the third trimester.

Survey of Uterine Anatomy

The uterus is assessed to examine maternal anatomy and identify any uterine defects or abnormalities. Adnexal (ovarian) masses may be noted. Uterine myomas (fibroids) are common and must be noted and monitored because they may grow more quickly in pregnancy, affecting the growth and well-being of the fetus or causing overdistention of the uterus leading to preterm labor or birth. Ultrasound may also be used to measure both cervical length and dilatation of the in-

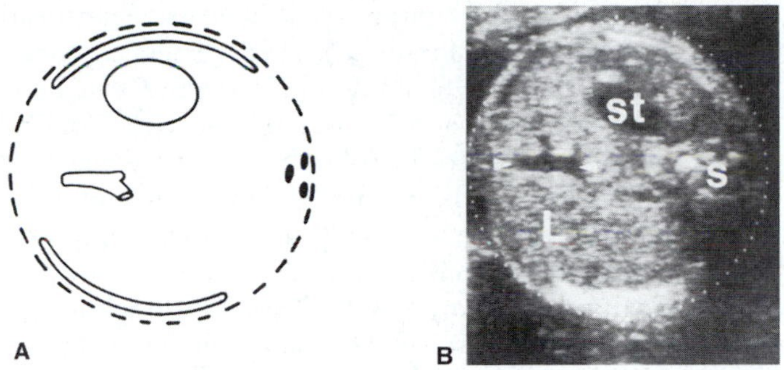

Figure 21–10 • Measurement of the abdominal circumference. *A,* Diagram showing the abdominal circumference as a dotted line traced at the outer margin of the abdomen. *B,* Ultrasound transaxial image showing the umbilical portion of the left portal vein (arrowheads) correctly positioned within the liver and equidistant from the lateral walls. (S, spine; L, liver; ST, stomach). A dotted line, created by a digitizer, outlines the outer margins of the abdomen, the correct place to obtain an abdominal circumference measurement.
SOURCE: Callen, P. W. *Ultrasonography in obstetrics and gynecology* (2nd ed., p. 57). Copyright, 1998, with permission from Elsevier Science.

ternal cervical os. A shortened cervix and a dilated internal os noted by ultrasound have been used to predict preterm birth. However, false-positive results using this technique may be common. Some obstetricians will schedule weekly transvaginal ultrasound to measure cervical length beginning at 20 weeks for their clients who have a history of preterm labor or cervical incompetence, and for women with cervical cerclage (a suture placed in the cervix) (see Chapter 20).

Assessment of Fetal Well-Being in the Third Trimester

Various maternal and prenatal conditions warrant antenatal testing during the third trimester. The type of testing performed is determined by the specific condition and the choice of the physician or certified nurse-midwife.

Conditions Warranting Fetal Surveillance

There are several indications for surveillance of fetal well-being in the third trimester. According to ACOG (2001), the following maternal and prenatal conditions require regular assessment:

Maternal conditions:

- Hypertensive disorders
- Type 1 diabetes mellitus
- Chronic renal disease
- Cyanotic heart disease
- Systemic lupus erythematosus
- Hyperthyroidism (poorly controlled)
- Antiphospholipid syndrome
- Hemoglobinopathies

Prenatal conditions:

- Preeclampsia
- Decreased fetal movement
- Oligohydramnios
- Hydramnios
- Intrauterine growth restriction
- Postterm pregnancy
- Isoimmunization (moderate to severe)
- Previous fetal demise
- Multiple gestation (with significant growth discrepancy)

Fetal Movement Assessment

Fetal movement assessment is considered an acceptable, noninvasive, cost-effective method of fetal surveillance in both high- and low-risk pregnancies. Monitoring fetal movement serves as an indirect measure of fetal central nervous system integrity and function. The coordination of whole-body movement in the fetus requires complex neurologic control. For this reason, clinicians generally agree that vigorous fetal movement provides reassurance of fetal well-being. A reduction in activity is often associated with complications of chronic rather than acute fetal distress as the compromised fetus decreases its oxygen requirements by reducing activity. Documented cessation of activity warns of impending death (Christensen & Rayburn, 1999). It is these observations that provide the rationale for utilizing fetal movement counting as a means of antepartum fetal surveillance.

Although there is considerable variation among individuals and according to the gestational age of the fetus, the average number of daily fetal movements during the third trimester is approximately 720 (or 30 gross fetal body movements per hour) (Druzin & Gabbe, 2001). Certain substances such as tobacco smoke, drugs, alcohol, and caffeine have been shown to affect fetal movements. Altered fetal movements will usually reverse after drug clearance. Contrary to earlier beliefs, maternal glucose levels are unrelated to fetal movement (Fisher, 1999).

Several methods are used to assess fetal movement perceived by the pregnant woman. The woman should be clearly instructed regarding the specific technique used and the importance of recognizing decreased fetal activity. Instruction is usually started at 28 weeks' gestation. Continued encouragement, education, and support by nurses within the office of the physician, midwife, or community clinic is important. The expectant woman should also be instructed to call the office if at any time she is concerned about a decrease in fetal movement from the fetus's usual daily pattern. The procedure for fetal movement assessment is discussed in Chapter 16.

Pregnant women need to understand that fetal movements are significant and that they change during pregnancy, both in number and strength. The expectant woman should be reassured that there are fetal rest-sleep states during which minimal or no movement may occur for an hour or so as the fetus rests. If less than the expected movements are perceived by the pregnant woman, further fetal surveillance tests, such as the nonstress test, may be used to assess fetal well-being. See Client Teaching: What to Tell the Pregnant Woman about Assessing Fetal Activity in Chapter 16.

> *In 1981, I visited the First International Peace Hospital in Shanghai. At the prenatal clinic, the mothers and fathers were given a jar that contained many small black stones. The couple was instructed to complete a fetal movement count each day by starting at a similar time and then placing a stone in the jar each time they felt the baby move. Toward the end of the pregnancy, the father was encouraged to place his hand on the expectant mother's abdomen and feel the movements. Then he was responsible for placing the stones in the jar. The mothers and fathers seemed so proud when they brought their recording of the movements back to the clinic for review.*
>
> *Since that visit, I have often wondered what it would have been like to hold my newborn in my arms and look at the jar of stones. A simple jar but so special.*
>
> ~SALLY

Nonstress Test

The **nonstress test (NST)** has become a widely accepted method of evaluating fetal status. This test involves using an electronic fetal monitor to obtain a tracing of the fetal heart rate (FHR) and observation of acceleration of the FHR with fetal movement. The test is based on the knowledge that the fetus is normally active throughout pregnancy and that fetal activity will result in acceleration of the fetal heart rate when the normal fetus moves. Accelerations of the FHR imply an intact central and autonomic nervous system that is not being affected by intrauterine hypoxia. Fetal heart rate acceleration in response to fetal movement is, therefore, an accepted sign of fetal health. It must be noted, however, that a nonreactive NST is not diagnostic of fetal compromise. In other words, failure to provide evidence of fetal health does not indicate that the fetus is in trouble.

The advantages of the NST are that it is relatively quick, inexpensive, and easy to interpret; it can be done in an outpatient setting and there are no known side effects. The disadvantages are that it is sometimes difficult to obtain a suitable tracing because the woman has to recline and be relatively still for 20 to 30 minutes, and the fetus may be in a sleep cycle at the time the test is performed resulting in a nonreactive test result.

Fetal age must be considered in the use and evaluation of NSTs. The central nervous system (parasympathetic and sympathetic nervous systems) of the fetus is not sufficiently mature to allow frequent accelerations of the heart rate when fetal movement occurs until 30 to 32 weeks of gestation. The National Institute of Child Health and Human Development fetal monitoring workshop (1997) defined acceleration based on gestational age. The acme of acceleration is 15 beats per minute or more above the baseline rate. The acceleration lasts 15 seconds or longer for less than 2 minutes in fetuses at or beyond 32 weeks (Figure 21–11 •). Before 32 weeks, accelerations are defined as having an acme of 10 beats per minute or more for 10 seconds or longer (Cunningham et al, 2001).

The NST can be used as an assessment tool in any pregnancy but is especially useful in the presence of diabetes, preeclampsia, intrauterine growth restriction, spontaneous rupture of membranes, multiple gestation, postdates, and other high-risk pregnancy conditions. These conditions can lead to a decline in uteroplacental functioning, which can result in decreased oxygenation to the fetus and eventual asphyxia. Testing intervals may vary, depending on the condition of the mother and fetus and recommendations of various ex-

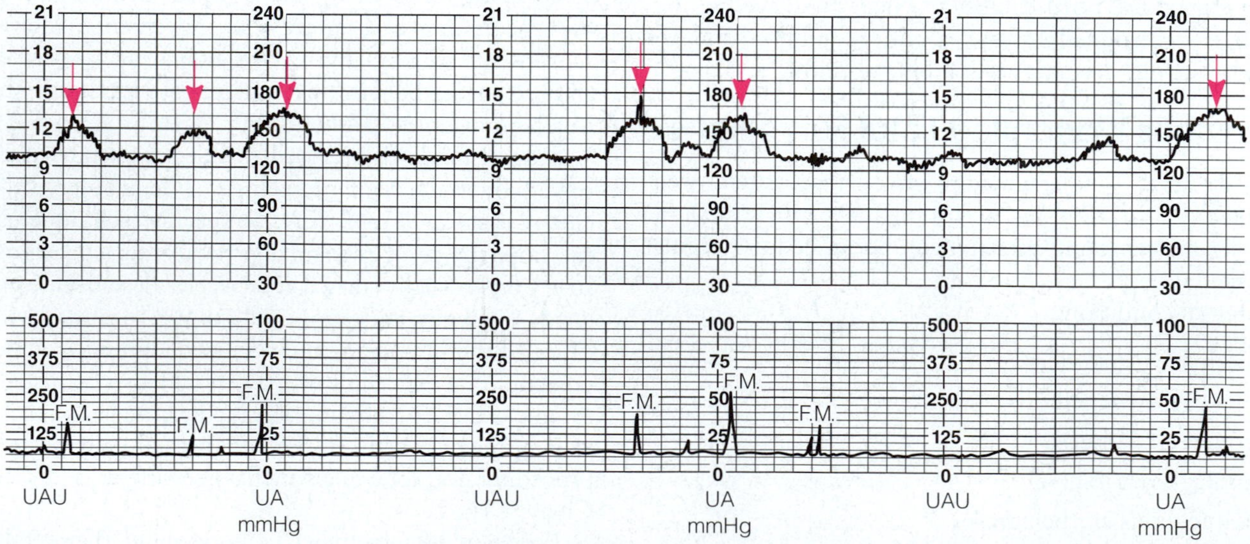

Figure 21–11 • Example of a reactive nonstress test (NST). Accelerations of 15 bpm lasting 15 seconds with each fetal movement (FM). Top of strip shows fetal heart rate (FHR); bottom of strip shows uterine activity tracing. Note that FHR increases (above the baseline) at least 15 beats and remains at that rate for at least 15 seconds before returning to the former baseline.

perts. Most clinicians test twice weekly for high-risk clients and once a week for other conditions (ACOG, 2001; Cunningham et al, 2001).

PROCEDURE FOR PERFORMING AN NST

The NST is usually scheduled during daytime hours. It may be performed either in the office or hospital setting. Women are requested to be nonfasting and to have refrained from recent cigarette smoking since this can adversely affect test results. The NST is performed with the woman in the semi-Fowler's position with a small pillow or blanket under the right hip to displace the uterus to the left. The fetal heart rate is monitored by the placement of an electronic fetal monitor (see discussion in Chapter 23). Either one or two belts are placed around the woman's abdomen. One belt holds the ultrasound transducer to record the fetal heart rate and the other holds a tocodynamometer that detects uterine or fetal movement. The fetal heart rate is usually monitored for 20 minutes, but monitoring may be extended to 40 minutes if it appears the fetus is in a sleep cycle. The woman is often requested to record each fetal movement by the use of self-operated markers. Under ideal conditions, a correlation of more than 90% between maternal perceived and actual fetal movements can be achieved; however, typically more than 50% of actual movements remain undetected by pregnant women (Devoe, 1999).

INTERPRETATION OF THE NST

NSTs are categorized as either reactive or nonreactive. The most common definition of a reactive (normal) test is that there are two or more fetal heart accelerations within a 20-minute period, with or without fetal movement discernible by the woman. The FHR acceleration must be at least 15 beats per minute above the baseline and last 15 seconds from baseline to baseline. A nonreactive (abnormal) NST is one that lacks sufficient fetal heart rate accelerations over a 40-minute period (Figure 21–12 •). Again, it is important to take into account the gestational age of the fetus. Both fetal movement and the amplitude of the fetal heart rate accelerations increase with gestational age.

Spontaneous decelerations of the FHR during the testing period must also be noted. Variable decelerations may be observed in up to 50% of NSTs. ACOG (2001) concluded that variable decelerations, if nonrepetitive and brief (less than 30 seconds), do not indicate fetal compromise nor the need for obstetric intervention. In contrast, repetitive variable decelerations (at least three in 20 minutes) even if mild, have been associated with an increased risk of cesarean birth for nonreassuring intrapartum fetal heart rate pattern. The prognosis for decelerations lasting 1 minute or longer is even more ominous (Cunningham et al, 2001). It is the responsibility of the nurse performing this test to consult the physician or nurse-midwife for further evaluation of fetal status if there is any question concerning the reactivity of the test or the presence of repetitive decelerations.

CLINICAL MANAGEMENT

The clinical management of a woman following a NST may vary. If the NST is reactive after 20 minutes, the test is concluded and the woman is rescheduled for further testing as indicated by the condition of, or risk factors present for, the mother and/or fetus. The interval between testing is typically one week if the maternal medical condition is stable. Testing may be performed twice weekly if warranted by maternal or fetal risk factors. Any significant deterioration in the maternal medical status requires fetal reevaluation regardless of the amount of time that has elapsed since the last test (ACOG, 2001).

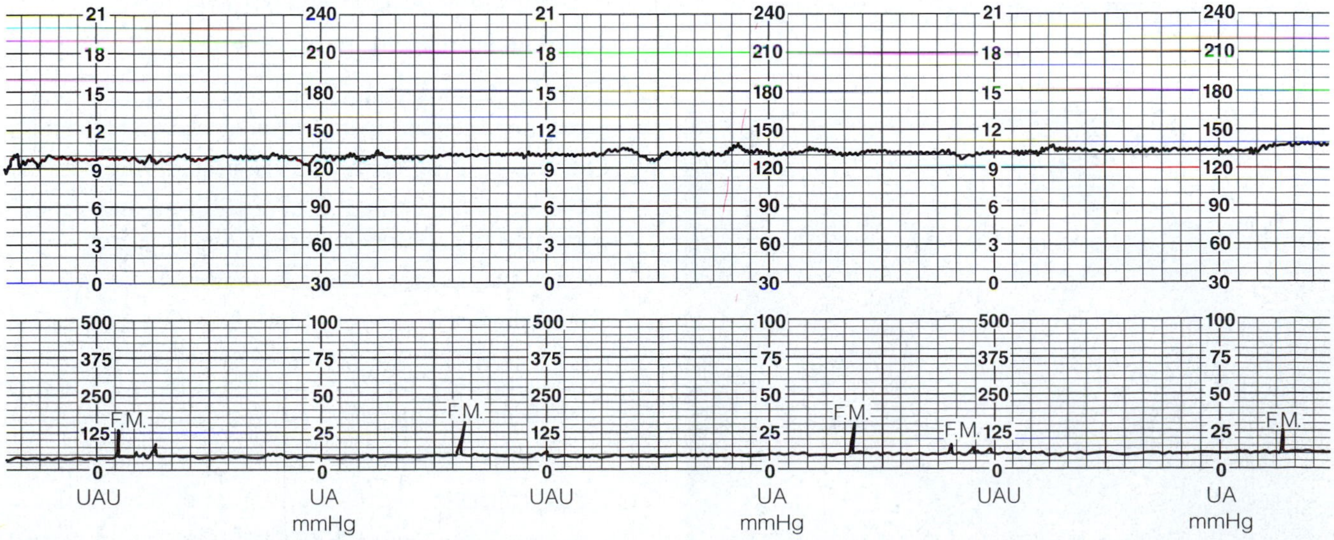

Figure 21–12 • Example of a nonreactive NST. There are no accelerations of FHR with fetal movement (FM). Baseline FHR is 130 bpm. The tracing of uterine activity is on the bottom of the strip.

NURSING CARE MANAGEMENT

The nurse first must ascertain the woman's understanding of the NST. The nurse then reviews the indications for the NST, the equipment being used, and the procedure prior to beginning the test. The nurse positions the woman and applies the electronic fetal monitor. Maternal blood pressure is monitored during the NST to determine whether hypotension is present. The nurse administers the NST, may or may not interpret the results, and reports the findings to the obstetrician or certified nurse-midwife and the client. The nurse uses this opportunity to assess learning needs concerning the importance of fetal movement and provides information and teaching.

Vibroacoustic Stimulation

Vibroacoustic stimulation (VAS), also called FAST for fetal acoustic stimulation test or VST for vibroacoustic stimulation test, is an application of sound and vibration to the mother's abdomen to stimulate movement in the fetus (Figure 21–13 •). A device is used that delivers 90 dB of sound for 1 to 3 seconds to the fetus with the purpose of changing the fetal behavioral state, thereby accelerating the fetal heart rate.

NSTs that are interpreted as nonreactive often depict the normal state of quiet sleep by the fetus, which can last for up to 70 minutes. In these cases, VAS can be used to facilitate the timely interpretation of the NST. The typical VAS response of a healthy term fetus shows a rise of at least 10 beats per minute in baseline, occurring within 10 seconds and lasting from 5 to 10 minutes. Gestational age influences the reliability and reproducibility of the fetal response. The purpose of the VAS is to improve the specificity and efficiency of interpretation of FHR monitoring patterns. While many obstetricians and certified nurse-midwives are enthusiastic about the VAS test because of its potential to minimize the need for more invasive follow-up testing, concerns for fetal hearing loss prevent universal use of this exam. Hearing loss has been demonstrated in newborns whose mothers were exposed to chronic levels of sound at 90 dB or more. Although there are no documented cases of newborn hearing loss related to VAS, some advocate judicious use of this exam. Others have advocated simply rescheduling the NST in 1 to 2 hours when the fetus is likely to have moved from the quiet sleep state that may have resulted in the first nonreactive test as an alternative to VAS.

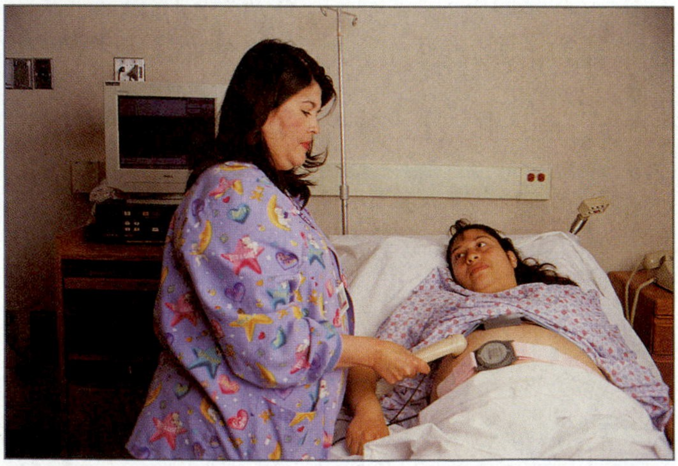

Figure 21–13 • Fetal acoustic stimulation testing.

Contraction Stress Test

The **contraction stress test (CST)** is a means of evaluating the respiratory function (oxygen and carbon dioxide exchange) of the placenta (ie, uteroplacental function). It enables the healthcare team to identify the fetus at risk for intrauterine asphyxia by observing the response of the FHR to the stress of uterine contractions (spontaneous or induced). During contractions, intrauterine pressure increases. Blood flow to the intervillous space of the placenta is reduced momentarily, thereby decreasing oxygen transport to the fetus. A healthy fetus usually tolerates this reduction well. If the placental reserve is insufficient, fetal hypoxia, depression of the myocardium, and a decrease in FHR occur.

INDICATIONS AND CONTRAINDICATIONS

The CST is indicated for pregnancies at risk for placental insufficiency or fetal compromise because of any of the following:

- Intrauterine growth restriction
- Diabetes mellitus
- Postdates (42 or more weeks' gestation)
- Nonreactive NST
- Abnormal or suspicious biophysical profile

Contraindications for the CST are the following:

- Third trimester bleeding (placenta previa, marginal abruptio placentae, or unexplained vaginal bleeding)
- Previous cesarean birth with classical uterine incision
- Instances in which the risk of possible preterm labor outweighs the advantage of the CST, including:
  a. Premature rupture of the membranes
  b. Incompetent cervix or Shirodkar-Barter operation (cerclage—surgical procedure in which an incompetent cervix is encircled with suture to prevent it from dilating before term) (See Chapter 20.)
  c. Multiple gestation

CST PROCEDURE

A necessary component of the CST is the presence of three uterine contractions of at least 40 seconds' duration in 10 minutes. The response of the fetal heart rate when contractions occur provides data on the fetal status. The contractions may occur spontaneously, or they may be induced by oxytocin or nipple stimulation. The most common method of stimulating uterine contractions for a CST has been intravenous administration of oxytocin (Pitocin), but many facilities now use breast self-stimulation to obtain a CST (see later discussion) (Curtis, Resnick, Evens, et al, 1999). This method is based on the fact that endogenous oxytocin is produced in response to stimulation of the breasts or nipples.

The CST is performed on an outpatient basis by qualified maternity nurses well acquainted with fetal monitoring and the interpretation of various FHR patterns. Most facilities require that the test be administered in or near the labor and birth unit so that treatment is available in the event that adverse reactions to oxytocin stimulation occur. The procedure, reasons for administering the test, equipment, and normal variations in monitoring that occur during the test should be clearly explained prior to the test to alleviate the woman's apprehension. A consent form may be signed.

During the test, the woman assumes a semi-Fowler's or side-lying position to avoid supine hypotension. The ultrasonic transducer (from the electronic fetal monitor) is placed on the woman's abdomen over the area of the fetal back or chest so that the FHR can be accurately recorded on the monitoring strip. (See Chapter 23 for further discussion of fetal monitoring.) To record uterine contractions, the tocodynamometer (pressure transducer) is placed over the area of the uterine fundus. For the first 15 to 20 minutes, the nurse records baseline measurements, including blood pressure, fetal activity, variations of the FHR during fetal movement, and spontaneous contractions. In addition, pertinent medical and obstetric information may be obtained from the woman to aid in her further management.

After the baseline recording is done, an intravenous oxytocin contraction stress test or breast self-stimulation test (BSST) is done.

Intravenous Oxytocin CST

In a CST using intravenous oxytocin, an electrolyte solution such as lactated Ringer's solution is started as a primary infusion. A piggyback infusion of oxytocin in a similar solution is attached. An infusion pump is used so that the amount of oxytocin being infused can be measured accurately. The administration procedure is the same as that for inducing labor through oxytocin administration (see Chapter 27). Oxytocin is administered until three uterine contractions lasting 40 to 60 seconds occur in a 10-minute period (called the 10-minute window). If late decelerations occur with all three contractions, the oxytocin infusion is discontinued. The woman's blood pressure and pulse are assessed every 15 minutes and recorded on the tracing.

CST with Breast Self-Stimulation Test (BSST)

A woman receiving a BSST is instructed to stimulate her nipples with her fingers, palms, or a warm, moist face cloth, either directly or through her clothing, for 2 minutes or until a contraction begins. Stimulation may also be done mechanically by the use of a breast pump (Curtis et al, 1999). Once the contraction begins, the woman is instructed to stop the stimulation, waiting to restart if another contraction has not followed by 5 minutes. It is important to monitor the frequency of contractions to avoid uterine hyperstimulation.

INTERPRETATION AND CLINICAL MANAGEMENT

A CST is usually not done prior to 28 weeks' gestation, primarily for two reasons. First, in light of a positive test, birth and extrauterine survival would be questionable at such an early gestational age. Second, sufficient research has not been done to determine whether the same test results apply to a fetus of this gestation. CST is usually done at 32 to 34 weeks' gestation.

Interpretation of CST Results

A CST can be interpreted once three moderately strong contractions of 40 to 60 seconds' duration have been noted in a 10-minute window of time. A CST can be interpreted as negative, positive, equivocal, or unsatisfactory (Table 21–4 •). Cunningham et al (2001) offered the following CST interpretations:

Negative —The absence of late or significant variable decelerations (the most common deceleration pattern noted during labor; attributed to umbilical cord compression or occlusion) is considered a reassuring sign that the fetus is receiving sufficient transfer of oxygen through the placenta (Figure 21–14 •).

Positive —The presence of **late decelerations** (a symmetrical decrease in fetal heart rate beginning at or after the peak of the contraction and returning to baseline only after the contraction has ended [ACOG, 2001] following 50% or more of contractions, even if the contraction frequency is fewer than three in 10 minutes) is a sign of

Table 21–4 • INTERPRETATION OF THE CONTRACTION STRESS TEST

Result	Interpretation
Negative	No late or significant variable decelerations.
Positive	Late decelerations following 50% or more of contractions (even if the contraction frequency is fewer than three in 10 minutes).
Equivocal	
Suspicious	Intermittent late decelerations or significant variable decelerations.
Hyperstimulatory	Fetal heart rate decelerations that occur in the presence of contractions more frequent than every 2 minutes or lasting longer than 90 seconds.
Unsatisfactory	Fewer than three contractions in 10 minutes or an uninterpretable tracing.

Source: ACOG Practice Bulletin No. 9, October 1999. *Clinical Management Guidelines for Obstetrician-Gynecologists*, pp. 2–3.

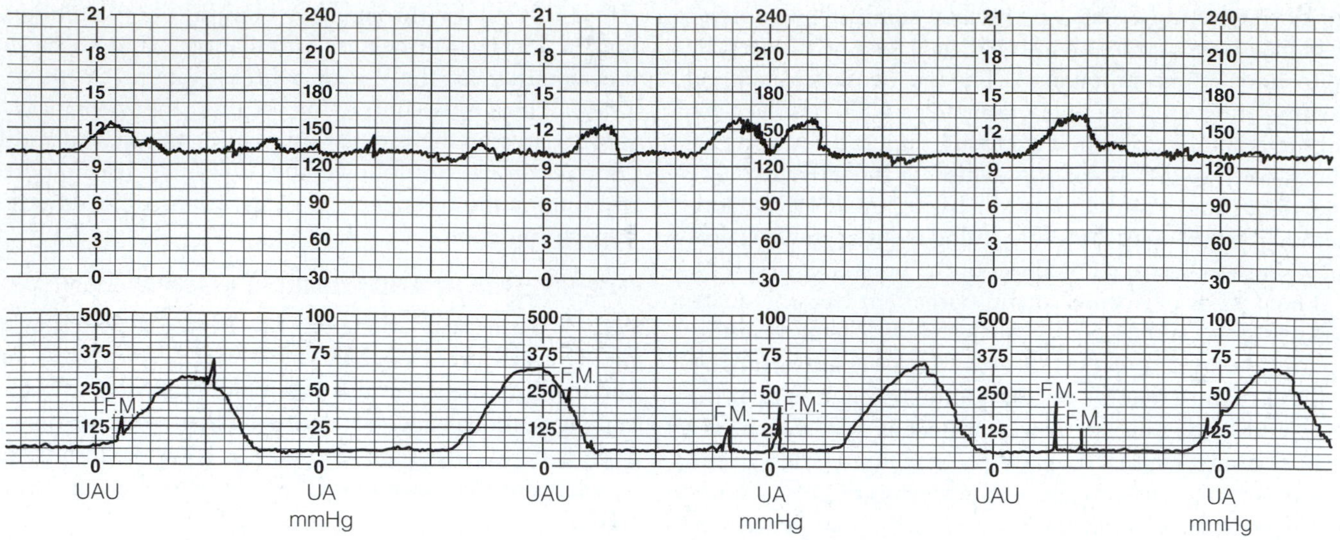

Figure 21–14 • Example of a negative CST (and reactive NST). The baseline FHR is 130 bpm with acceleration of FHR of at least 15 bpm lasting 15 seconds with each fetal movement (FM). Uterine contractions recorded on bottom half of strip indicate three contractions in 8 minutes.

MEDIALINK CASE STUDY: CLIENT UNDERGOING CONTRACTION STRESS TEST

uteroplacental insufficiency and may indicate that the fetus is not receiving adequate oxygenation (Figure 21–15 •).

Equivocal-suspicious —The presence of intermittent late decelerations or significant variable decelerations should be viewed as a suspicious finding that merits follow-up testing.

Equivocal-hyperstimulatory —Fetal heart rate decelerations may occur in the presence of contractions that occur more frequently than every 2 minutes or that last longer than 90 seconds. This test should be repeated after hyperstimulation has been rectified and the patient has been hydrated and allowed to rest.

Unsatisfactory —The CST cannot be interpreted if fewer than three contractions lasting 40 to 60 seconds occur in a 10-minute window of time.

Contraction stress test results are also evaluated for the presence of accelerations that would meet the criteria of the NST. Combining the CST assessment with NST results showing characteristics such as variability of the FHR baseline and the presence of other types of decelerations helps the clinician determine the best management plan for the fetus.

Clinical Management Based on CST Results

In most cases, a negative CST with a reactive NST is the desired result. The uteroplacental perfusion is sufficient at present to allow the fetus to withstand the stress of uterine contractions. Retesting would most likely be scheduled in 7 days. If the pregnant woman is diabetic, the CST schedule would remain the same, except an NST would be done in 3 to 4 days (Devoe, 1999). A negative CST with a nonreactive NST is more difficult. It should be assessed very carefully for subtle late decelerations. If there are none, a CST would be repeated in 7 days.

All equivocal tests should be repeated in 24 hours, especially in the presence of a postterm pregnancy (Devoe, 1999). If the gestation is less than 37 weeks, then other surveillance methods should be added.

A positive CST with a nonreactive NST presents evidence that the fetus would probably not withstand the stress of labor. If the gestation is 32 weeks or over, a cesarean birth should be scheduled (Devoe, 1999).

NURSING CARE MANAGEMENT

The nurse ascertains the woman's or couple's understanding of the CST prior to the procedure and the possible results. The nurse reviews the reasons for the CST and the procedure before beginning the test. The nurse then applies the external fetal monitor to the maternal abdomen. If oxytocin is to be used, the nurse inserts an intravenous line and begins the medication. If a BSST is being conducted, the nurse instructs the woman on self-stimulation of the breast or on the appropriate use of the breast pump. Continuous monitoring of the contraction pattern is warranted to ensure that hyperstimulation of the uterus or fetal compromise does not occur. The nurse then reports the findings to the physician/certified nurse-midwife and explains the results to the woman.

Amniotic Fluid Index

Assessment of amniotic fluid volume is based on the rationale that decreased uteroplacental perfusion may lead to diminished fetal renal blood flow, decreased urination, and ultimately, **oligohydramnios** (decreased amniotic fluid vol-

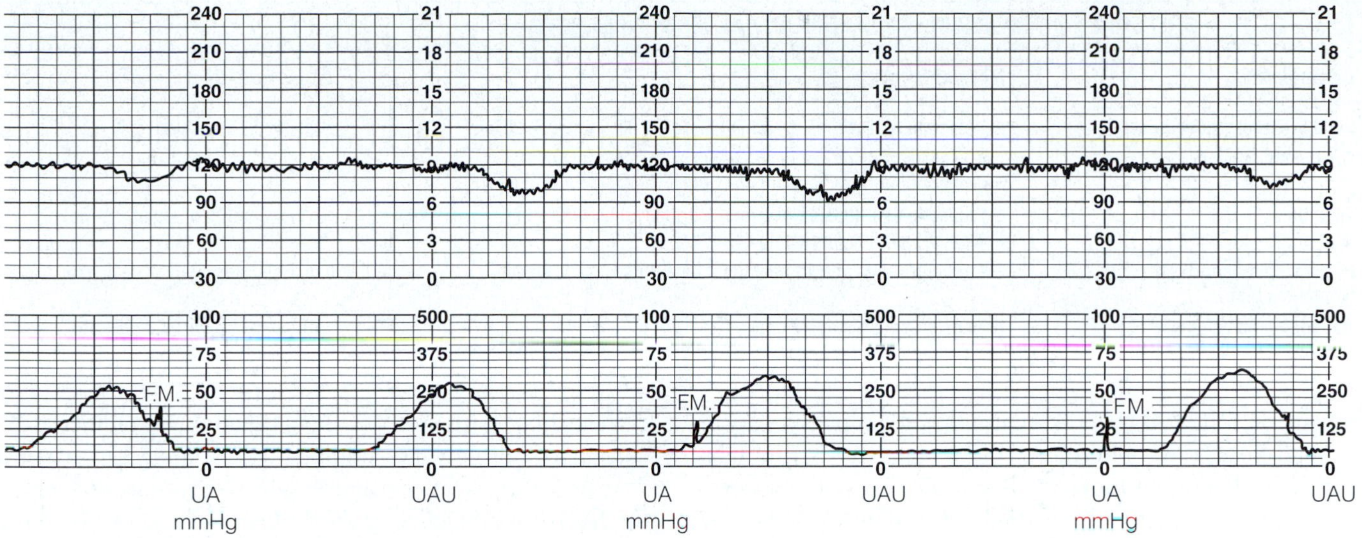

Figure 21–15 • Example of a positive contraction stress test (CST). Repetitive late decelerations occur with each contraction. Note that there are no accelerations of FHR with three fetal movements (FM). The baseline FHR is 120 bpm. Uterine contractions (bottom half of strip) occurred four times in 12 minutes.

ume). Fetal urine output and fetal swallowing are the major determinants of amniotic fluid volume. Oligohydramnios may be the result of diminished urinary output caused by fetal hypoxemia. The resulting placental insufficiency may cause hypoxia and hence oligohydramnios. Therefore, assessment of long-term uteroplacental function may be performed by evaluating amniotic fluid volume (Voxman, Tran, & Wing, 2002). Poor pregnancy outcomes, such as intrauterine growth restriction, postterm pregnancy, and fetal distress in labor, have been associated with abnormalities of amniotic fluid volume. The procedure for performing an amniotic fluid index (AFI) was discussed previously on p. 534.

An AFI value of 5 or less serves as a red flag that requires some type of further assessment or management decision (Voxman et al, 2002). The gestational age of the fetus and the composite maternal condition may influence management decisions, leading to additional testing, induction of labor, or cesarean birth (Magann & Martin, 1999).

Biophysical Profile

The **biophysical profile (BPP)** represents an assessment of five fetal biophysical variables:

- Fetal heart rate acceleration
- Fetal breathing
- Fetal movements
- Fetal tone
- Amniotic fluid volume

The first criterion is assessed with the nonstress test. The other variables are assessed by ultrasound scanning. By combining these five assessments, the BPP helps to identify the compromised fetus and confirm the healthy fetus. Average testing time is usually less than 8 minutes, with 90% of normal testing completed within the first 4 minutes (Manning, 1999). A time period of 30 minutes is selected for BPP testing (ultrasound components) to account for the average duration of sleep-wake cycles in the normal fetus, which are approximately 20 minutes.

Indications for the biophysical profile include those situations in which the NST and CST would be done. Assessment of these fetal biophysical activities is most useful in the evaluation of women who experience decreased fetal movement (who might subsequently have a nonreactive NST) and in the management of intrauterine growth restriction, preterm labor, gestational diabetes, postterm pregnancies, and premature rupture of the membranes (PROM) (Manning, 1999).

The two most important components of the BPP are the NST and the amniotic fluid volume index. The NST reflects the intactness of the nervous system and the AFI reflects kidney perfusion. A normal AFI indicates that shunting has not occurred and that the fetal kidneys are adequately functioning. Reactive NST and normal fluid therefore reflect fetal well-being.

Specific criteria for normal and abnormal assessments are delineated in Table 21–5 •. Normal variables are assigned a score of 2 each and abnormal variables a score of 0 (zero). Thus, the highest score possible for a normal fetus is 10.

Clinicians suggest that management not be based solely on BPP scores. Both Habek, Hodek, Herman, et al (2001) and Manning (1999) have noted that the biophysical activities of the fetus that develop first are the last to disappear when all activities are arrested due to asphyxia. Those that are the last to develop are the most sensitive to hypoxia, and their disappearance can be noted first. For example, fetal tone (exhibited by flexion of the extremities) is the first to develop and the last activity to cease during asphyxia. Other activities in the normal developmental sequence are fetal

Table 21-5 • CRITERIA FOR NORMAL AND ABNORMAL ASSESSMENTS

Component	Normal (score = 2)	Abnormal (score = 0)
Fetal breathing movements	≥ 1 episode of rhythmic breathing lasting ≥ 30 sec within 30 min	≤ 30 sec of breathing in 30 min
Gross body movements	≥ 3 discrete body or limb movements in 30 min (episodes of active continuous movement considered as single movement)	≤ 2 movements in 30 min
Fetal tone	≥ 1 episode of extension of a fetal extremity with return to flexion, or opening or closing of hand	No movements or extension/flexion
Reactive fetal heart rate Nonstress test	≥ 2 accelerations of ≥ 15 beats/min for ≥ 15 sec in 20–40 min	0 or 1 acceleration in 20–40 min
Amniotic fluid volume	Single vertical pocket > 2 cm	Largest single vertical pocket ≤ 2 cm

movement, followed by fetal breathing, and then reactivity of the fetal heart rate. Therefore, FHR reactivity is the most sensitive to hypoxia. One of the first indications of fetal compromise is a nonreactive NST. Table 21–6 • outlines BPP test interpretation and the recommended management (Cunningham et al, 2001; Manning, 1999).

Modified Biophysical Profile

The biophysical profile is labor intensive and expensive. It requires a trained person in ultrasonic visualization of the fetus. In addition, studies have shown that when the four dynamic ultrasound variables are normal, the probability of encountering an abnormal (nonreactive) NST is exceedingly small (Habek et al, 2001; Piazze, Anceschi, Ruozzi Berretta, et al, 2001). For these reasons, a modified BPP has been developed. This test consists of an NST and a measurement of the amniotic fluid index, which reflects long-term uteroplacental function. The functioning of the placenta is important since a poorly functioning placenta (placental dysfunction) may result in diminished fetal renal perfusion, leading to oligohydramnios. The amniotic fluid volume assessment can therefore be used to evaluate long-term uteroplacental function. A modified BPP is considered normal if the amniotic fluid volume is greater than 5 cm and if the NST is reactive. The test is abnormal if either the NST is nonreactive or the AFI is 5 or less. The frequency of this test is the same as with the standard BPP.

Doppler Flow Studies

Recent advances in ultrasound technology have made it possible to study noninvasively blood flow changes that occur in maternal and fetal circulations to assess placental function. An ultrasound beam, like that provided by the pocket Doppler (a handheld ultrasound device), is directed at the umbilical artery. The signal is reflected off the red blood cells moving within the vessels, and the subsequent "picture" (waveform) that is received looks like a series of waves. The highest velocity peak of the waves is the systolic measurement, and the lowest point is the diastolic velocity. The umbilical artery waveform can then be analyzed to provide information about velocity of blood flow in the vessel (Seyam, Al-Mahmeid, & Al-Tamimi, 2002). Examples of these waveforms are displayed in Figures 21–16 • and 21–17 •.

Table 21-6 • BPP TEST INTERPRETATION AND RECOMMENDED MANAGEMENT

Test Score	Interpretation	Perinatal Mortality Within 1 Week Without Intervention	Management
10/10	Normal nonasphyxiated fetus	<1/1000	No fetal indication for intervention; repeat test weekly except in client with diabetes and pregnancies that are postterm (twice weekly)
8/10 (normal fluid) 8/8 if no NST done	Risk of fetal asphyxia extremely rare	<1/1000	Same as above
8/10 (abnormal fluid)	Chronic fetal asphyxia suspected	89/1000	Induce birth
6/10	Possible fetal asphyxia	89/1000	If amniotic fluid volume abnormal, deliver If normal fluid at >36 weeks with favorable cervix, induce birth If repeat test ≤6 induce birth If repeat test >6, observe and repeat per protocol
4/10	Probable fetal asphyxia	91/1000	Repeat testing same day; if BPP score ≤6 deliver
2/10	Almost certain fetal asphyxia	125/1000	Induce birth
0/10	Certain fetal asphyxia	600/1000	Induce birth

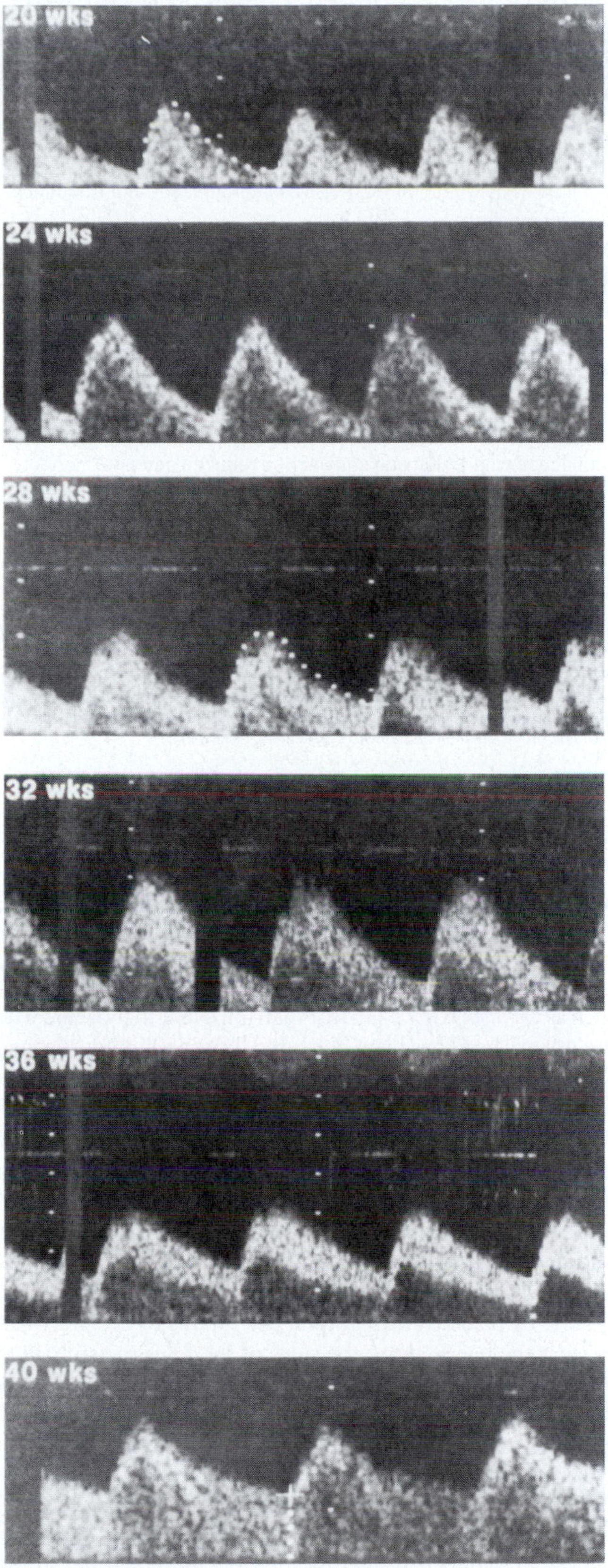

Figure 21–16 • Serial studies of the umbilical artery velocity waveforms in a normal pregnancy from one client.
SOURCE: AWHONN. (1990). Cundiff, J. L., Haybrich, K. L., & Hinzman, N. G. Umbilical artery Doppler flow studies during pregnancy. *Journal of Obstetric, Gynecologic, and Neonatal Nursing, 19*(4): 475–481. (Figure 3, p. 478). Washington, DC: Author. ©1990 by the Association of Women's Health, Obstetric and Neonatal Nurses. All rights reserved.

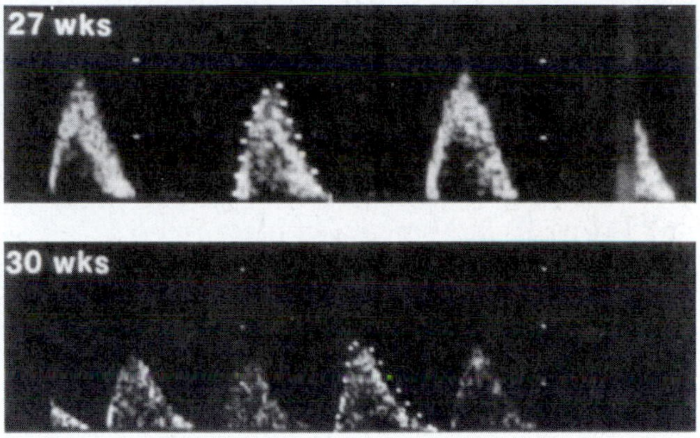

Figure 21–17 • Two examples of abnormal umbilical artery velocity waveforms taken from a client with intrauterine growth restriction.
SOURCE: AWHONN. (1990). Cundiff, J. L., Haybrich, K. L., & Hinzman, N. G. Umbilical artery Doppler flow studies during pregnancy. *Journal of Obstetric, Gynecologic, and Neonatal Nursing, 19*(4): 475–481. (Figure 4, p. 478). Washington, DC: Author. ©1990 by the Association of Women's Health, Obstetric and Neonatal Nurses. All rights reserved.

The most common evaluation of blood flow velocity is the systolic to diastolic (S/D) ratio. The S/D ratio normally decreases as the fetus nears term. This phenomenon reflects the decreasing resistance of placental and umbilical vasculature to allow for greater umbilical blood flow to meet the needs of a growing fetus. The S/D ratio is considered abnormal if elevated above the 95th percentile for gestational age or reversed after 18 to 20 weeks of gestation (Vergani, Roncaglia, Andreotti, et al, 2002). Absent or reversed end-diastolic flow signifies increased impedance and is uniquely associated with intrauterine growth restriction. It is also associated with a high perinatal mortality rate (Seyam et al, 2002; Vergani et al, 2002).

A decrease in fetal cardiac output or an increase in resistance of placental vessels will reduce umbilical artery blood flow. Doppler velocimetry is best used when intrauterine growth restriction is diagnosed, whether it occurs as an idiopathic process (cause unknown) or in the presence of hypertension or preeclampsia (Seyam et al, 2002). No benefit has been demonstrated for umbilical artery velocimetry for other conditions such as postterm pregnancy, diabetes, systemic lupus erythematosus, or antiphospholipid antibody syndrome. Also, it has not been shown to be of value as a screening test for detecting fetal compromise in the general obstetric population (Cunningham et al, 2001).

Evaluation of Placental Maturity

Placental maturity is evaluated by a grading process that uses ultrasound to measure the changes in the basal layer, chorionic plate, and intervening placental substance. A grade of 0 through III is assigned (grade III as the most mature, showing extensive calcifications) (Figure 21–18 •). Placentas with multiple calcifications are less likely to function as adequately as those with lower grades. Certain factors can cause a placenta to mature, including maternal smoking, postterm pregnancy, and certain maternal conditions, such as preeclampsia and gestational diabetes. Placental grade may

Evidence-Based Practice

Use of Doppler Ultrasound in High Risk Pregnancies

Clinical Question

Does the use of Doppler ultrasound in high risk pregnancies to investigate flow velocity waveforms in the umbilical artery (+/− uteroplacental artery) improve subsequent obstetric care and fetal outcome?

The Evidence

Because abnormal waveforms from Doppler ultrasound may indicate poor fetal prognosis, it is important to know if its use encourages inappropriate early birth. A systematic review of 11 studies involving nearly 7000 women was conducted. The use of Doppler ultrasound in high risk pregnancies to assess umbilical artery waveforms with or without uteroplacental studies was associated with a 29% reduction in overall perinatal mortality. This was especially true in pregnancies complicated by hypertension or impaired fetal growth. The use of Doppler ultrasound reduced the chances of admission to the hospital during pregnancy and of elective induction of labor and birth, without adverse effects. The procedure had little or no effect on fetal distress during labor and frequency of cesarean birth.

Best Practice

Recommendations for best practice are somewhat equivocal. Doppler ultrasound is a relatively new technique to be applied to the study of fetoplacental and/or uteroplacental circulatory dynamics. Although it has been rigorously evaluated and the trend is favorable, the numbers included in the research studies undercut the confidence with which one can ascribe reduced perinatal mortality to the use of Doppler ultrasound. Clinicians may conclude that best practice is the use of Doppler ultrasound in high risk pregnancies (especially those complicated by hypertension or presumed fetal growth restriction). At the same time, this practice should be examined within the context of any future definitive studies, which may shift best practice.

Reference: Neilson, J. P., & Alfirevic, Z. (2000). *Doppler ultrasound for fetal assessment in high risk pregnancies* [Systematic Review]. Cochrane Pregnancy and Childbirth Group, Cochrane Database of Systematic Reviews.

be used to correlate with other findings; however, placental grade alone does not dictate management of a pregnancy.

Estimation of Fetal Weight

Estimating the fetal weight in the third trimester of pregnancy is an important aspect of fetal assessment. Particularly, findings of the fetal weight at either end of the spectrum—inadequate fetal growth or excessive fetal growth—are critical risk factors for alterations in fetal well-being.

Intrauterine growth restriction (IUGR) is a term used to describe any fetus that falls below the 10th percentile in ultrasonic estimation of weight at a given gestational age. Other terms to describe the small fetus include *low birth weight, small for gestational age*, and *intrauterine growth restriction*. IUGR may or may not be associated with prematurity.

The etiology of IUGR can be separated into either fetoplacental or maternal origin. Fetoplacental etiologies would include infections, genetic abnormalities, and placental abnormalities. Maternal etiologies stem from reduced uteroplacental blood flow associated with hypertension, poor maternal weight gain, poor nutrition, substance use such as tobacco or medications, anemia, or chronic illness.

If a fetus is suspected to have IUGR, the management includes careful surveillance of the fetus with NSTs and BPPs and continuous assessment of growth through sonographic assessment. In addition to regular fetal surveillance, women with IUGR are instructed to do daily fetal movement assessments (previously discussed in this chapter) and to maintain bed rest. If growth ceases altogether or if other nonreassuring fetal factors occur (nonreassuring fetal heart rate patterns), delivery may be warranted.

Macrosomia is defined by ACOG as weight greater than 4000 to 4500 g (8 lb 13 oz to 9 lb 4 oz). If a fetus is suspected to be macrosomic, the management of the labor and birth is carefully evaluated to prevent birth-related complications such as *shoulder dystocia* (an intrapartum event that occurs when the infant's head has been delivered, but the shoulders remain wedged behind the mother's pubic bone, causing a difficult birth of the infant with potential for maternal or fetal injury).

The diagnosis of fetal macrosomia is imprecise. The accuracy of estimated fetal weight using ultrasound biometry is no better than that obtained with clinical palpation by the obstetrician or certified nurse-midwife (Weiner, Ben-Shoomo, Beck-Fruchter, et al, 2002). This clinical palpation of the fetus through the fetal abdomen by Leopold's maneuvers is done by placing two hands at the fundus of the uterus and moving the hands along the sides of the fetus to estimate the fetal size and position (see Chapter 23). The fundal height (measured in centimeters with a tape measure from the symphysis pubis to the fundus of the uterus) is another tool in estimating fetal growth. According to ACOG, these two primary methods for the clinical estimation of fetal weight should be combined to produce a more accurate measurement. Experienced providers may also ask the woman to provide her own estimate of the fetal weight if she has had a previous birth.

The greatest risk factor for macrosomic infants is birth trauma due to a shoulder dystocia. When macrosomia is present, a potential shoulder dystocia should be anticipated if the woman is giving birth vaginally. The woman should be

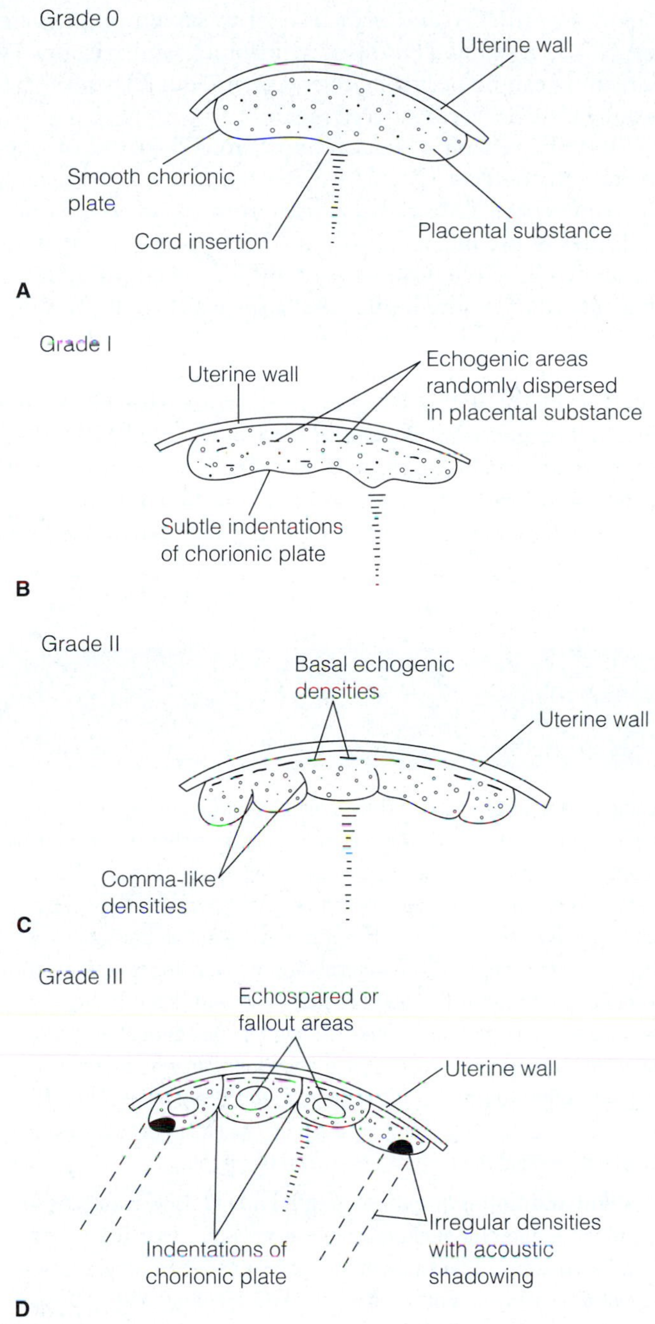

Figure 21–18 • Placental grading. *A,* Diagram showing the ultrasonic appearance of a grade 0 placenta. *B,* Diagram showing the ultrasonic appearance of a grade I placenta. *C,* Diagram showing the ultrasonic appearance of a grade II placenta. *D,* Diagram showing the ultrasonic appearance of a grade III placenta.

positioned in McRobert's position (legs flexed and pulled back toward the woman's shoulders) with the head of the bed lowered. A stool should be readily available in the event that suprapubic pressure is needed. If the physician/certified nurse-midwife requests suprapubic pressure, the nurse applies pressure directly over the symphysis pubis to aid in dislodging the fetal shoulder (see Chapter 26).

Women who are undergoing a trial of labor after a previous cesarean birth should be counseled on the risks of a shoulder dystocia when macrosomia is suspected. In addition, a macrosomic fetus may decrease the likelihood of a successful vaginal birth after cesarean (VBAC), especially if the previous cesarean birth was performed for cephalopelvic disproportion (see Chapter 26).

Other Diagnostic Tests

Birth defects, defined as structural abnormalities present at birth, are the leading cause of infant mortality and a major contributor to infant morbidity in the United States. Infant mortality due to birth defects has not declined as rapidly as overall infant mortality. It has been estimated that approximately 20% of all birth defects are due to gene mutations, and 5% to 10% are due to exposure to a teratogen such as drugs, chemicals, or radiation. About half of all birth defects remain unexplained (Iqbal, 2000).

Rapidly developing technologies of biochemical markers and ultrasonography aid in the prenatal diagnosis of fetal anomalies and genetic disorders. As discussed in Chapter 12, conditions that can be diagnosed prenatally include trisomies 21, 18, and 13, spina bifida and anencephaly, cystic fibrosis, and some familial conditions .

Alpha-Fetoprotein

Alpha-fetoprotein (AFP) is a fetal protein produced in the yolk sac during the first 6 weeks of gestation and then produced by the fetal liver. AFP is found in the amniotic fluid and the maternal serum. If the fetus has a neural tube defect (NTD), AFP levels are elevated.

The incidence of NTDs is 0.6% per 1000 births in the United States (Becske & Jallo, 2001) and range in severity from anencephaly (which is incompatible with extrauterine life) to spina bifida (which is associated with lower extremity paralysis, incontinence, and developmental delay). These lesions can be either open or closed. Because 90% of cases occur in families with no known risk factor (Becske & Jallo, 2001), universal screening should be offered to all pregnant women.

NTDs are the most common serious birth defect found in the United States. Although progress has been made in understanding NTDs, the etiology of most cases is unknown. High-risk groups include women with a past history of NTDs, maternal age of less than 20 or greater than 35 years, primiparity or grand multiparity, low socioeconomic status with nutritional deficiency, and English or Irish ancestry (DiGuiseppi, 2002). Research has shown that folate (folic acid), a B vitamin, plays a crucial role in the development of the central nervous system during the early weeks of gestation. Inadequate folate supply at this time in the embryonic development leads to failure of the primitive neural tube to close and differentiate normally, which results in an NTD. Therefore, the importance of adequate intake of folic acid in the weeks before conception and the first few weeks after cannot be stressed enough (see Chapter 18).

AFP levels can be used to determine if a fetus has an NTD. Amniotic fluid levels of AFP peak at about 15 weeks of gestation. The widest margin between normal and abnormal levels occurs between 16 and 18 weeks. Because concentrations vary at different gestational weeks, a particular level (called a *cutoff level*) has been established at each week of gestation. The accuracy of the testing varies between 56% up to 91% depending on which gestational week the test is performed. The most accurate results come from tests conducted during the 15th and 16th weeks of pregnancy.

Maternal Serum Alpha-Fetoprotein

Maternal serum alpha-fetoprotein (MSAFP) is a component of the screening test, the *"triple check"* that utilizes the multiple markers, including AFP, human chorionic gonadotropin (hCG), and urine estriol to screen pregnancies for NTD, trisomy 21 (Down syndrome), and trisomy 18. Screening can be performed between 15 and 22 weeks' gestation (15 to 18 is considered ideal).

MSAFP screening detects approximately 85% of open neural tube defects. The MSAFP is the first marker used in the triple check. Most laboratories use a cutoff of 2.0 to 2.5 multiples of the mean (MoM) of AFP to define a test as abnormally high. The lower the cutoff, the greater the detection rate but also the higher the false-positive rate. Using a cutoff of 2.5 MoM detects 85% of cases of open NTDs with a false-positive rate of 3% to 4% (DiGuiseppi, 2002). Elevated levels of MSAFP occur in up to 5% of all women tested. The majority of women with an elevated MSAFP do not have affected fetuses. In 90% to 95% of the group with an elevated MSAFP, the elevation is caused from other variables, such as incorrect gestational age, more than one fetus,

RESEARCH IN PRACTICE
Prenatal Screening: A Retrospective Study

What is this study about? Prenatal screening is widely used to determine fetal abnormalities that may result in a selective termination of the pregnancy by the parents. Little has been studied relative to the emotional implications of prenatal screening and the subsequent decisions that must be made about the pregnancy. This qualitative study explored the experience of women undergoing the quadruple test (a prenatal screen that detects the presence of several biochemical substances). The purpose of this research was to explore women's feelings and experiences during this screening process. The author also investigated the extent to which the threat of bad news influenced their recollections of their pregnancies.

How was this study done? This retrospective, exploratory study used a phenomenological framework to explore the experiences of women who screened high-risk to the quadruple test but subsequently gave birth to a normal baby. Seventy women who met the inclusion criteria were contacted and ten agreed to interviews. Interviews, which were conducted in the women's homes, were tape-recorded and transcribed. Content analysis was used to determine themes and sub-themes.

What were the results of the study? Four major categories were identified with associated themes and sub-themes. The four categories were the testing process, effects on the pregnancy, interpersonal skills of professionals, and present relationships/future decisions. In spite of written communications to the contrary, the majority of these women viewed the quadruple test as routine, and expected it to provide reassurance about the normalcy of their fetus. The method of notification that the test results indicated high risk–all ten learned of their results by telephone, one on an answering machine–upset and disturbed the mothers. Eight of the ten women were surprised that their baby had screened high risk. The mothers noted that the informational statistics they were given about being screened high risk made coping more difficult. It was clear these mothers struggled with the further choices involved, including those regarding amniocentesis and elective abortion. The high risk screening produced anxiety for these mothers, and these respondents felt that the professionals involved failed to demonstrate an understanding of their dilemma. A disconnection of the baby from the pregnancy was also described, as was a generally negative effect on their perceptions of the pregnancy. Although these mothers spoke universally about the trauma of the screening, six of the ten said they would choose testing again.

What additional questions might I have? How would these experiences differ for mothers who subsequently had a non-normal baby? How many of these mothers actually opted for amniocentesis? Would an amniocentesis disconfirming the abnormality change the pregnancy experience?

How can I use this study? Mothers who undergo prenatal testing need to be prepared for the possibility that they will be screened high-risk. Mothers should be discouraged from viewing the quadruple test as part of a routine testing procedure. Results of the test should be delivered personally whenever possible, so that support and information can be provided. Women should be made aware that false positive results are possible and may influence the mother's perception of her pregnancy experience. The nurse can help the mother understand the possible decisions that may need to be made as a result of the test and demonstrate compassion and understanding when high risk status has been determined.

Source: Robinson, J. (2001). Prenatal screening: A retrospective study. *British Journal of Midwifery, 9*(7): 412–417.

other fetal anomalies such as gastroschisis (a hole in the abdominal wall that allows the abdominal contents to protrude outside the body), and fetal death (DiGuiseppi, 2002). Women infected with HIV or those with decreased CD4 counts also have a higher chance of a false-positive result (Becske & Jallo, 2001).

The triple screen has also been used to screen for trisomy 21 (Down syndrome), which is the most common chromosomal abnormality found in live births, and for trisomy 18, which is less common, but usually results in death of the infant within the first year of life (see Chapter 12). Unlike NTDs, the risk of Down syndrome and trisomy 18 increases with increasing maternal age; thus genetic counseling and tests are usually offered to women who will be 35 years of age or older at their estimated date of birth.

Abnormal test results are generally defined as a calculated Down syndrome risk of 1 in 270 or 1 in 200 (depending on the laboratory). Women who have abnormal results are counseled about these risks and offered an amniocentesis. Unlike the MSAFP which is considered a screening test, the amniocentesis is a diagnostic test and considered to be greater than 99% accurate in the diagnosis of chromosomal anomalies.

Screening tests require client education and counseling to avoid confusion and undue stress. A key point for the nurse to understand and reinforce to the client is that the MSAFP and the triple check are screening tests, and are **not** diagnostic. The nurse has an important role in educating the woman about various aspects of these tests. The importance of an accurate gestational age determination prior to taking the test cannot be overstated. A miscalculated gestational age may result in the incorrect interpretation of the MSAFP level, causing extreme stress to the woman and her family. In addition, further testing is required. An elevation of the MSAFP requires recalculation with an accurate gestational age and repeat test, and a low MSAFP may require an amniocentesis. The nurse also educates the client on the importance of proper timing of the MSAFP. As stated earlier, the ideal time for screening is between 15 and 18 weeks. False positives can occur with tests done either prior to or after this window in the gestation.

All healthcare providers should be sensitive to the ethical issues these screening tests present to the childbearing family. What benefit would knowing the results of an abnormal MSAFP provide? If the fetus has an NTD, the family and healthcare provider can use this information prior to the birth to choose the appropriate birth site/ birth type. (An infant with an NTD would need to be born in a tertiary care center should immediate care need to be given to the infant.) Knowing an infant has Down syndrome would not necessarily change an obstetric decision about birth method or site, but it would give the family time for psychologic preparation, a chance to talk with social services and support groups, or the opportunity to opt for termination of the pregnancy.

Amniocentesis

Amniocentesis is a procedure used for genetic diagnosis. A sterile needle is inserted into the uterine cavity through the maternal abdomen so a small amount of amniotic fluid can be removed, and genetic testing is performed. Amniocentesis is performed between 15 and 20 weeks' gestation. Two large studies in the United States and Canada have confirmed the safety and the 99% diagnostic accuracy of this procedure (Cunningham et al, 2001).

Amniocentesis can make chromosomal and biochemical determinations (enzyme analysis, AFP measurement for neural tube defects, blood typing, or cytogenetic, metabolic, or other DNA testing) and can validate abnormalities detected by ultrasound. Later in pregnancy, from about 30 to 35 weeks' gestation, amniocentesis may be done for lung maturity studies, such as lecithin/sphingomyelin ratio and the presence of phosphatidylglycerol and phosphatidylcholine (see discussion on p.553).

INDICATIONS FOR AMNIOCENTESIS

The following conditions are commonly considered indications for amniocentesis:

- Pregnant women who will be 35 or older on their due date. The risk of having an infant with a chromosomal problem such as Down syndrome increases with the age of the woman (see Chapter 12).
- Couples who already have had a child with a birth defect or have a family history of certain birth defects.
- Pregnant women with other abnormal genetic test results.

PROCEDURE FOR PERFORMING AMNIOCENTESIS

Amniocentesis is done on an outpatient basis but needs to be performed near a birthing area in case acute fetal distress is encountered. The pregnant woman should have a left lateral tilt to prevent hypotension during the procedure.

The abdomen is scanned by ultrasound to locate the placenta, the fetus, and an adequate pocket of fluid. The needle insertion site is of the utmost importance because the fetus, placenta, umbilical cord, bladder, and uterine arteries must all be avoided (Figure 21–19 •). The importance of locating the placenta cannot be stressed enough, especially in cases of Rh isoimmunization, in which trauma to the placenta increases fetal–maternal transfusion and worsens the isoimmunization (see Chapter 20). If the amniocentesis is being performed in the last few weeks of pregnancy, the fetus may occupy what appears to be all the available space in the uterus, and there is a normal decrease in the amount of amniotic fluid, but with the aid of ultrasound, fluid can be located. The amniocentesis, or "tap," is then done before the fetus has the opportunity to move.

After the abdomen is scanned, the abdominal skin is cleansed with povidone-iodine (Betadine). The woman is given the option of a local anesthetic for the insertion site. A 22-gauge spinal needle is inserted into the uterine cavity.

MediaLink Amniocentesis

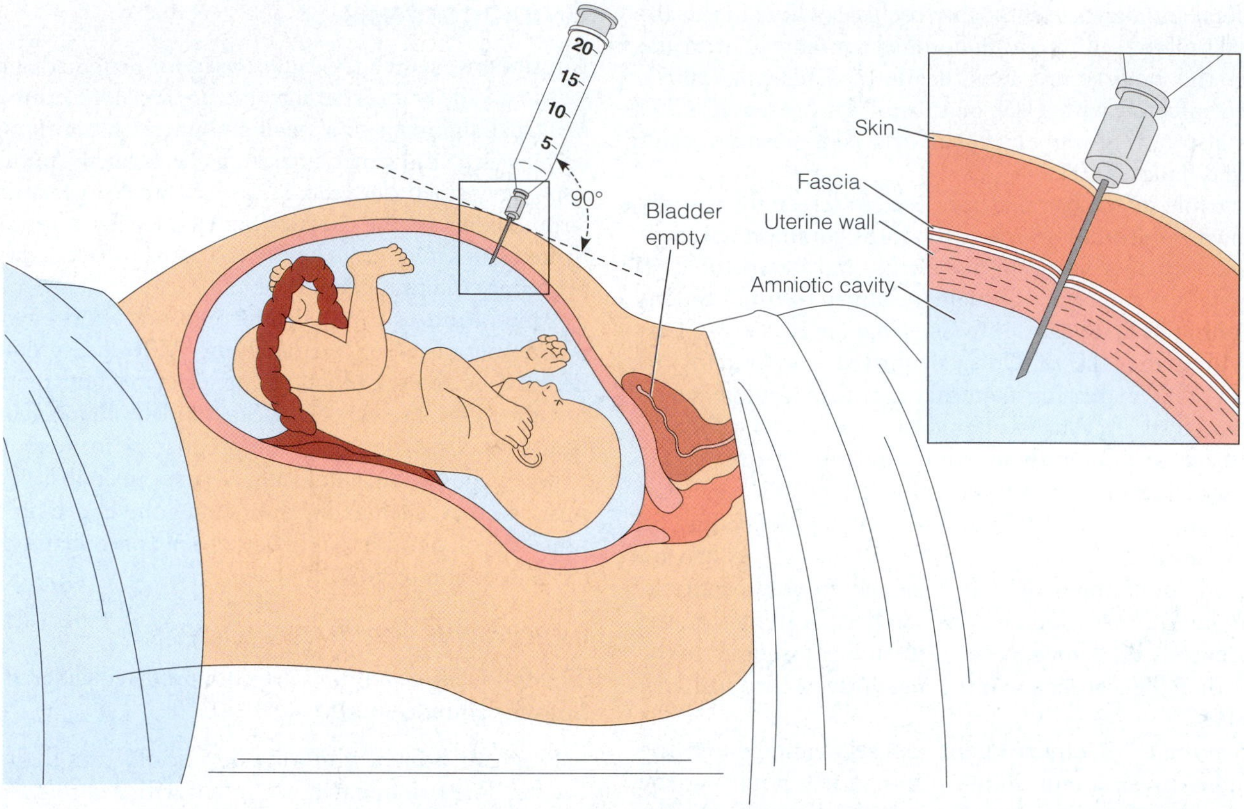

Figure 21–19 • Amniocentesis. The woman is usually scanned by ultrasound to determine the placental site and to locate a pocket of fluid. As the needle is inserted, three levels of resistance are felt when the needle penetrates the skin, fascia, and uterine wall. When the needle is placed within the amniotic cavity, amniotic fluid is withdrawn.

Generally, fluid immediately flows into the needle. The first few drops are discarded; a syringe is then attached to the needle, and the fluid is aspirated (Figure 21–20 •). From 15 to 20 mL of amniotic fluid are withdrawn, placed in brown-tinted test tubes (to shield the fluid from light to prevent breakdown of bilirubin and other pigments), and sent to the laboratory for analysis. The needle is withdrawn using ultrasound, and the insertion site is evaluated for streaming (movement of fluid), which would indicate bleeding into the amniotic fluid. The fetal heart rate (FHR) is monitored to assess fetal well-being. If the woman's vital signs and the FHR are normal, she is allowed to leave (see Procedure 21–1).

If the collected amniotic fluid is contaminated with blood, the fluid should be centrifuged immediately. The woman is observed for alterations in the FHR. The blood should be tested to determine whether it is maternal or fetal.

Rh-negative women are given Rh immune globulin after amniocentesis, provided that they are not already sensitized. If the amniotic fluid from these women is contaminated with blood, the sample should be tested to identify fetal cells. In this situation a larger dose of immune globulin is required.

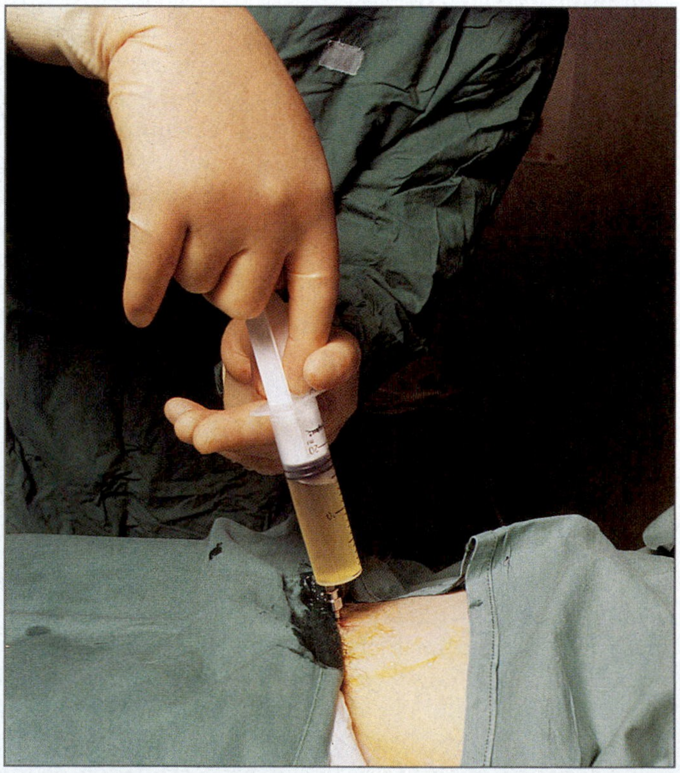

Figure 21–20 • During amniocentesis, amniotic fluid is aspirated into a syringe.

RISKS/SIDE EFFECTS

Minor complications are infrequent and may include transient vaginal spotting, cramping, or amniotic fluid leakage

Procedure 21-1 Assisting During Amniocentesis

Preparation

1. Explain the procedure and the indications for it and reassure the woman.
2. Determine whether an informed consent form has been signed. If not, verify that the woman's doctor has explained the procedure and ask her to sign a consent form.
   Rationale: It is the physician's responsibility to obtain informed consent. The woman's signature indicates her awareness of the risks and gives her consent to the procedure.

Equipment and Supplies

- 22-gauge spinal needle with stylet
- 10- and 20-mL syringes
- 1% lidocaine (Xylocaine)
- Povidone-iodine (Betadine)
- Three 10-mL test tubes with tops (amber colored or covered with tape)
  Rationale: Amniotic fluid must be protected from light to prevent breakdown of bilirubin.

Procedure: Sterile Gloves

1. Obtain baseline vital signs including maternal blood pressure (BP), pulse, respirations, temperature, and fetal heart rate (FHR) before procedure begins.
2. Monitor BP, pulse, respirations, and FHR every 15 minutes during procedure.
   Rationale: Baseline information is essential to detect any changes in maternal or fetal status that might be related to the procedure.
3. The physician uses real-time ultrasound to determine the location of the placenta and to locate a pocket of amniotic fluid. Provide gel for the ultrasound and assist with the procedure as needed.
4. Cleanse the woman's abdomen.
   Rationale: Cleansing the abdomen prior to needle insertion helps decrease the risk of infection.
5. The physician dons gloves, inserts the needle into the identified pocket of fluid (Figure 21-19) and withdraws a sample.
6. Obtain the test tubes from the physician. Label the tubes with the woman's correct identification and send to the lab with the appropriate lab slips.
7. Monitor the woman and reassess her vital signs.
   - Determine the woman's BP, pulse, respirations, and the FHR.
   - Palpate the woman's fundus to assess for uterine contractions.
   - Monitor her using an external fetal monitor for 20 to 30 minutes after the amniocentesis.
   - Determine a treatment course to counteract any supine hypotension and to increase venous return and cardiac output.

   Rationale: Monitoring maternal and fetal status postprocedure provides information about response to the procedure and helps detect any complications such as inadvertent fetal puncture.
8. Assess the woman's blood type and determine any need for Rh immune globulin.
9. Administer Rh immune globulin if indicated (see Procedure 20-2).
   Rationale: To prevent Rh sensitization in an Rh-negative woman, Rh immune globulin is administered prophylactically involving amniocentesis.

Clinical Tip

Have the woman lie on her left side to ensure adequate placental perfusion

(continued on next page)

Procedure 21-1 Assisting During Amniocentesis *(continued)*

10. Instruct the woman to report any of the following changes or symptoms to her primary caregiver:
    - Unusual fetal hyperactivity or, conversely, any lack of fetal movement
    - Vaginal discharge—either clear drainage or bleeding
    - Uterine contractions or abdominal pain
    - Fever or chills

    Rationale: These are signs of potential complications and require further evaluation.
11. Encourage the woman to engage only in light activities for 24 hours and to increase her fluid intake.

    Rationale: Decreased maternal activity helps decrease uterine irritability and increase uteroplacental circulation. Increased fluid intake helps replace amniotic fluid through the uteroplacental circulation.
12. Complete the client record. Record the type of procedure, the date and time, and the name of the physician who performed the procedure. Also record the maternal-fetal response, disposition of the specimen, and discharge teaching.

in 1% to 2% of cases performed. Chorioamnionitis may occur in fewer than 1 in 1000 cases. Needle injuries to the fetus are rare when ultrasound guidance is used. Fetal loss rate is less than 0.5% (1 in 200). When early amniocentesis is performed (11 to 14 weeks) there is a higher pregnancy loss and complication rate than with traditional amniocentesis (Cunningham et al, 2001). This is due to the lack of membrane fusion to the uterine wall, which makes the puncture of the sac difficult, and to the fact that there is less fluid to withdraw.

NURSING CARE MANAGEMENT

The nurse assists the physician during the amniocentesis (see Procedure 21–1: Assisting During Amniocentesis). In addition, the nurse supports the woman undergoing amniocentesis. Women are usually apprehensive about the procedure as well as about the information that will be obtained. The physician explains the procedure before the woman signs the consent form. As it is being performed, the woman may need additional emotional support. She may become anxious during the procedure. She may also become lightheaded, nauseated, and diaphoretic from lying on her back with a heavy uterus compressing the abdominal vessels, so it is important to have her in a lateral tilt with a wedge placed under her right hip. The nurse can provide support to the woman by further clarifying the physician's instructions or explanations, by relieving the woman's physical discomfort when possible, and by responding verbally and physically to the woman's need for reassurance.

Chorionic Villus Sampling

Much like amniocentesis, **chorionic villus sampling (CVS)** is a procedure that is used to detect genetic, metabolic, and DNA abnormalities. CVS involves obtaining a small sample (5 to 40 mg) of chorionic villi from the edge of the developing placenta. CVS is performed in some medical centers for first trimester diagnosis. Villi in the chorion frondosum, present from 8 to 12 weeks' gestation, are believed to reflect fetal chromosome, enzyme, and DNA content, thereby permitting earlier diagnosis than can be obtained by amniocentesis. CVS cannot detect neural tube defects, however.

RISKS AND BENEFITS OF CVS

The woman should be aware of the risks and benefits of CVS. An increased risk of spontaneous abortion is associated with CVS, and the pregnancy loss rate reported with CVS is higher than that associated with amniocentesis. There is also an incidence of 1 in 3000 births of fetal limb reduction defects (a portion of a finger or a toe is missing), especially when the CVS is performed before 9½ weeks' gestation. It is not recommended that CVS be performed before 10 weeks' gestation (ACOG, 1999).

Additional risks of CVS include failure to obtain tissue, rupture of membranes, leakage of amniotic fluid, bleeding, intrauterine infection, maternal tissue contamination of the specimen, and Rh isoimmunization. Rh-negative women are given Rh immune globulin to cover the risk of immunization from the procedure (Goldberg & Golbus, 1996).

Like amniocentesis, CVS can detect fetal karyotype, hemoglobinopathies (eg, sickle cell anemia and alpha and some beta thalassemias), phenylketonuria, alpha antitrypsin deficiency, Down syndrome, Duchenne muscular dystrophy, and factor IX deficiency. Early sex determination can be made so that pregnancies with a male fetus who would be affected in X-linked disorders can be identified. Because NTDs are not diagnosed by this test, all mothers undergoing CVS should be offered MSAFP screening at 15 to 20 weeks' gestation. A major disadvantage of the earlier testing (CVS) is that if a woman later has an abnormal MSAFP test indicating an increased risk of NTDs, she may then have to undergo an amniocentesis, thus again putting the fetus at risk with an additional invasive procedure.

One of the greatest advantages to a woman undergoing this procedure is earlier diagnosis and decreased waiting time for results. Whereas amniocentesis is not done until at least 16 weeks' gestation, CVS is performed between 10 and 12 weeks. The CVS results are obtained in 24 hours if the direct preparation method is used and in 7 to 10 days when tissue culture is used. Earlier diagnosis may relieve many of the personal, social, and psychologic concerns of families, particularly if therapeutic abortion is being considered. There may be less emotional stress involved with having an abortion at an earlier stage of gestation. First trimester abortions are also easier to perform, require less time, and are less costly.

PROCEDURE FOR CVS

Before CVS, an ultrasound is done to determine placental location, uterine position (retroverted or anteverted), and presence of intervening structures (ie, bowel, blood vessels). Various equipment can be used to aspirate chorionic villi from the placenta.

After counseling regarding diagnosis and procedure techniques, preliminary blood work may be obtained. The morning of the procedure, the woman is asked to drink fluids to fill her bladder because displacement of an anteverted uterus by a full bladder may aid in positioning the uterus for catheter insertion. Ultrasound is used to determine uterine position, cervical position, gestational sac size, and crown-rump length measurement and to identify the area of placental formation and cord insertion.

For the transcervical CVS the woman is placed in lithotomy position, the vulva is cleansed with povidone-iodine solution (Betadine), and a sterile speculum is inserted into the vagina. The vaginal vault and cervix are cleansed with the same solution to decrease contamination from the vagina into the uterus. The anterior lip of the cervix is sometimes grasped with a tenaculum to aid in straightening anteflexion of the uterus. The catheter (or cannula) is slowly inserted under ultrasound guidance through the endocervix to the sampling site at the extra-amniotic placental edge (outside the gestational sac). The obturator is withdrawn from the catheter. A 30-mL syringe, containing 3 to 4 mL of tissue culture medium with heparin, is attached, and a sample of villi is aspirated by using a pressure of 20 to 30 mL (Goldberg & Golbus, 1996). The contents of the syringe are flushed into a petri dish containing nutrient medium, and the villi are inspected microscopically and prepared for cell culture.

For the transabdominal sampling, the woman is placed in the supine position. After the skin is cleansed with Betadine and local anesthesia is given, an 18- or 20-gauge needle is inserted percutaneously through the maternal abdominal wall and uterine myometrium. The tip of the needle is advanced into the long axis of the chorion frondosum under ultrasound guidance. Chorionic villi are obtained by repeated, rapid aspirations of the syringe containing tissue culture medium and heparin.

A normal CVS in the first trimester does not ensure a healthy infant. Routine prenatal care and appropriate follow-up are needed. Follow-up ultrasound and lab evaluation of each pregnancy must be done after performance of this procedure to evaluate fetal status. Further neonatal follow-up studies are necessary to evaluate the long-term effects of this technique.

NURSING CARE MANAGEMENT

Before the test, the nurse ascertains the woman's understanding of the CVS, its uses, the procedure, and the possible results. The nurse provides opportunities for questions and acts as an advocate when additional questions or concerns are raised. The nurse completes assessments following the procedure including monitoring for vaginal bleeding or fluid leakage, excessive cramping, and basic maternal vital signs.

The nurse supports the woman or couple and encourages them to express any feelings and fears regarding the procedure and also regarding the decision-making process if abortion is being considered. That supportive role continues if abortion is chosen, even though the nurse may not be present for the procedure. It is important that support be provided following the procedure by the nurse who established a relationship with the couple previously.

Percutaneous Umbilical Blood Sampling

Percutaneous umbilical blood sampling (PUBS) (also called *cordocentesis*) is a technique used to obtain pure fetal blood from the umbilical cord while the fetus is in utero. This procedure has been used for diagnosis of hemophilias, hemoglobinopathies, fetal infections, chromosome abnormalities, nonimmune hydrops, and isoimmune hemolytic disorders, as well as assessment of fetal hemoglobin and hematocrit for calculation of transfusion requirements in the second and third trimesters (Capponi, Rizzo, Pasquini, et al, 1997). The indications for fetal blood sampling include the following:

- Rapid fetal karyotyping
- Diagnosis of fetal infection (cytomegalovirus, toxoplasmosis, parvovirus, rubella)
- Platelet disorders
- Fetal blood grouping
- Diagnosis and treatment of isoimmunization
- Assessment of fetal well-being (pH, Po_2)
- Fetal metabolic disorders

The woman is scanned with an ultrasound transducer with sterile probe cover. A 25-gauge spinal needle is inserted into her abdomen through the skin alongside the transducer and into the fetal umbilical vein approximately 1 to 2 cm from the insertion of the cord into the placenta. The stylet is removed from the needle, and fetal blood is aspirated into a syringe containing an anticoagulant. Red blood cell size is determined to distinguish fetal from maternal cells. A paralytic agent, such as pancuronium bromide (Pavulon), may be given to prevent fetal movement during the procedure. If the mother is given a medication to help her relax, care must be taken to avoid oversedating her and causing deep breathing. Deep chest/diaphragmatic respirations can interfere with accurate puncture of the umbilical vein.

Within the last 10 years, improvements in ultrasonographic technique have made PUBS a relatively safe procedure with overall fetal loss rate less than 2%. The complication rate after PUBS is less than 0.5%. Complications include failure to obtain a sample, bleeding from the sampling site, premature rupture of membranes, chorioamnionitis, and fetal bradycardia (Capponi et al, 1997). PUBS is used with less and less frequency since newer tests have replaced the need for a direct fetal sample.

NURSING CARE MANAGEMENT

The nurse collaborates with other members of the healthcare team to provide care for the woman for whom PUBS is recommended. Although a genetic counselor and/or obstetrician will have explained the risk for genetic defects and other disorders, the woman and her partner may need help to understand the procedure and its risks. They may need anticipatory guidance to help lessen their anxiety, as well as emotional support during the procedure and follow-up evaluation and testing. Support can come in many forms including encouraging relaxation, providing reassurance, and giving the woman information throughout the procedure. The nurse may need to assist with coordination of financial and social service resources. The nurse can help promote relaxation during the procedure by instructing the woman in shallow breathing techniques. The nurse completes assessments during and immediately following the procedure and in some cases performs a nonstress test following the procedure.

Fetoscopy

Fetoscopy is a procedure for directly observing the fetus and obtaining a sample of blood or skin. Popular during the 1970s and 1980s, this procedure has largely been replaced by amniocentesis, ultrasound, PUBS, and biochemical marker identification. It enables the physician to diagnose conditions such as fetal hemoglobinopathies, immunodeficient diseases, coagulation and metabolic disorders, first trimester varicella infection, chromosomal abnormalities, Rh isoimmunization, and serious skin defects.

Some surgical procedures are also performed through the fetoscope, including correcting problems such as abnormal blood flow between twin fetuses and a condition called *amniotic bands* that can cause deformed limbs and other structures in a fetus. However, surgical interventions with the fetoscope are primarily experimental, and carry significant risks to both the mother and the fetus. Fetoscope procedures are done in major medical centers with experienced physicians who specialize in this area of maternal-fetal medicine.

Fetal Fibronectin

Fetal fibronectin (fFN) is a glycoprotein produced by the trophoblast and other fetal tissues. The presence of cervicovaginal fetal fibronectin between 20 and 34 weeks' gestation has been shown to be a strong predictor of preterm delivery due to spontaneous preterm labor or premature rupture of membranes. Fetal fibonectin levels can be measured with an enzyme immunoassay.

Evaluation of Fetal Lung Maturity

In managing the woman and fetus at risk, the physician is constantly faced with the possibility of having to induce the birth of an infant prior to term and before the onset of labor. There are many indications for early termination of pregnancy, including repeat cesarean birth, premature rupture of membranes, diabetes, hypertensive conditions in the pregnant woman, and placental insufficiency. Unfortunately, the most common cause of perinatal mortality is prematurity, especially in infants weighing 1500 g or less and with particular complications arising from pulmonary immaturity (Cunningham et al, 2001). Birth of an infant with immature pulmonary function frequently results in respiratory distress syndrome (RDS), also known as hyaline membrane disease (Chapter 33).

Because gestational age, birth weight, and the rate of development of organ systems do not necessarily correspond, it may be necessary to determine the lung maturation of the fetus by amniotic fluid analysis before elective childbirth. In these cases, amniocentesis is performed, and concentrations of certain phospholipids in the amniotic fluid are measured. In many cases, birth of the infant can be delayed until the lungs show maturity.

L/S RATIO

The alveoli of the lungs are lined by a substance called **surfactant,** which is composed of phospholipids. Surfactant lowers the surface tension of the alveoli during extrauterine respiratory exhalation. By lowering the alveolar surface tension, surfactant stabilizes the alveoli, and a certain amount of air always remains in the alveoli during expiration. When a newborn with mature pulmonary function takes its first breath, a tremendously high pressure is needed to open the lungs. Upon breathing out, the lungs do not collapse, and about half the air in the alveoli is retained. An infant born too early, when synthesis of surfactant is incomplete, is unable to maintain lung stability, resulting in underinflation of the lungs and development of RDS.

Fetal lung maturity can be assessed by determining the ratio of two components of surfactant—**lecithin** and **sphingomyelin**. Early in pregnancy the lecithin concentration in amniotic fluid is less than that of sphingomyelin (0.5:1 at 20 weeks), resulting in a low **lecithin/sphingomyelin (L/S) ratio.** At about 30 to 32 weeks' gestation, the amounts of the two substances become equal (1:1). The concentration of lecithin begins to exceed that of sphingomyelin, and at 35 weeks the L/S ratio is 2:1. When at least two times as much lecithin as sphingomyelin is found in the amniotic fluid, RDS is very unlikely. Clinical outcomes, including respiratory distress and other respiratory disorders, should be correlated in individual institutions before specific ratios indicating pulmonary maturity are accepted. Infants of diabetic mothers (IDMs) are an exception to this finding and have a high incidence of false-positive results (ie, the L/S ratio is thought to indicate lung maturity, but after birth the baby develops RDS). Although the same ratios are used, it is important to remember that even when IDMs are term (greater than 37 weeks' gestational age), delayed lung maturation can occur because the high blood sugars interfere with biochemical development. A delay in lung maturation has also been found in babies whose mothers have nonhypertensive renal disease and isoimmunization (ACOG, 2001).

Some types of chronic intrauterine fetal stress cause an acceleration of lung maturation in the fetus. Prolonged rupture of membranes (over 24 hours) results in acceleration of lung maturation by approximately 1 week and therefore has a protective effect. Although the L/S ratio is the most universally used test for evaluating pulmonary maturity, the results are not accurate when blood or meconium contaminates the amniotic fluid.

The L/S ratio remains a cumbersome and labor-intensive test despite numerous changes to the original technique. Moreover, improper handling can affect results. For these reasons, many institutions are looking to other fetal lung maturity tests that are being developed.

PHOSPHATIDYLGLYCEROL

Phosphatidylglycerol (PG) is the second most abundant phospholipid in surfactant. PG appears at about 36 weeks' gestation and increases in amount until term. In instances of diabetes complicated by premature rupture of membranes, vascular disease, or severe preeclampsia, PG may be present before 35 weeks' gestation. PG is not measured in specific concentrations; rather, the mere presence of this substance is associated with very low risk of RDS, and the absence of PG is associated with the development of RDS.

PG determination is also useful in blood-contaminated specimens. Because PG is not present in blood or vaginal fluids, its presence in a vaginal specimen is reliable for indicating lung maturity.

In recent years lung maturity has been most frequently assessed by a combination of L/S ratio and PG. Lung maturity apparently can be confirmed in most pregnancies if PG is present in conjunction with an L/S ratio of 2:1.

NURSING CARE MANAGEMENT

In women whose amniotic membranes are prematurely ruptured, a vaginal specimen is obtained for analysis. The nurse assists the certified nurse-midwife/physician by gathering appropriate supplies. Typically, a sterile speculum, a light source, a syringe, and appropriate collection tubes are needed. The nurse positions the woman for the speculum exam while providing information about the collection process. The nurse places the woman in a lithotomy position and places her legs in stirrups. If stirrups are not available, the nurse can place a bedpan upside down and position the woman with her buttocks on the bedpan to facilitate collection of the vaginal fluid. The certified nurse-midwife/physician gathers vaginal secretions with a syringe and places the specimen in a collection tube.

In women undergoing early birth for medical indications (uncontrolled preeclampsia or eclampsia or uncontrolled diabetes) when the amniotic membranes are intact, evaluation of fetal lung maturity may be obtained through amniocentesis. See previous discussion on page 547 regarding nursing care management for the woman undergoing amniocentesis.

Chapter Review

EXPLOREMediaLink

NCLEX review questions, case studies, and other interactive resources for this chapter can be found on the Web site at http://www.prenhall.com/olds. Click on "Chapter 21" to select the activities for this chapter.

For tutorials including animations and videos, more NCLEX review questions, and an audio glossary, access the accompanying CD-ROM in this book.

Focus Your Study

- Nurses often play a key role not only in teaching families about various testing procedures, but also in providing clarity and emotional support to the woman and her family undergoing antenatal testing.
- Ultrasound offers a valuable means of assessing intrauterine fetal growth because the growth can be followed over a period of time. It is noninvasive and painless, allows the physician to study the gestation serially, is nonradiating to both the woman and her fetus, and to date has shown no known harmful effects.
- Using ultrasound, the gestational sac may be detected as early as 5 or 6 weeks after the last menstrual period. Measurement of the crown-rump length in early pregnancy is most useful for accurate dating of a pregnancy. The most important and frequently used ultrasound measurements are biparietal diameter, head circumference, abdominal circumference, and femur length.
- Maternal assessment of fetal activity is very useful as a screening procedure in evaluation of fetal status.
- A nonstress test (NST) measures fetal heart rate during fetal activity; FHR normally increases in response to fetal activity. The desired result is a reactive test.
- A contraction stress test (CST) provides a method for observing the response of the fetal heart rate to the stress of uterine contractions. The desired result is a negative test.
- A fetal biophysical profile (BPP) includes five fetal variables (breathing movement, body movement, tone, amniotic fluid volume, and FHR reactivity). It assesses the fetus at risk for intrauterine compromise.
- Triple screening of AFP, hCG, and estriol in maternal serum provides information about the possibility of open neural tube defects and chromosome abnormalities (trisomy 18 or 21) in the fetus.
- Amniocentesis can be used to obtain amniotic fluid for testing. A variety of tests is available to evaluate the presence of disease, genetic conditions, and fetal maturity.
- Chorionic villus sampling is a procedure that obtains fetal karyotype in the first trimester. It is used to diagnose hemoglobinopathies (eg, sickle cell anemia and alpha and some beta thalassemias), phenylketonuria, alpha antitrypsin deficiency, Down syndrome, Duchenne muscular dystrophy, and factor IX deficiency.
- Percutaneous umbilical blood sampling (PUBS) is a technique used in the second and third trimesters for fetal diagnosis, assessment, and therapy.
- The L/S ratio of the amniotic fluid can be used to assess fetal lung maturity. The presence of phosphatidylglycerol may also provide information about fetal lung maturity.

References

American College of Obstetricians and Gynecologists (ACOG). (1999). *Amniocentesis and chorionic villus sampling*. Washington, DC: Author.

American College of Obstetricians and Gynecologists (ACOG). (2001). *Compendium of selected publications, women's healthcare*. Washington, DC: Author.

Association of Women's Health, Obstetric, and Neonatal Nurses (AWHONN). (2001). *OB/GYN limited ultrasound series.* Davenport, IA: Kendall & Hunt.

Becske, T., & Jallo, G. (2001). *Neural tube defects.* Retrieved November 5, 2002, from www.emedicine.com/neuro/topic244.htm

Callen, P. W. (2000). *Ultrasonography in obstetrics and gynecology* (3rd ed.). Philadelphia: Saunders.

Capponi, A., Rizzo, G., Pasquini, L., Turri, E., Arduini, D., & Romanini, C. (1997). Indomethacin modifies the fetal hemodynamic response induced by percutaneous umbilical blood sampling. *American Journal of Obstetrics and Gynecology, 177*(4), 758–764.

Chandler, M., & Smith, A. (1998). Prenatal screening and women's perception of infant disability: A Sophie's Choice for every mother. *Nursing Inquiry, 5*(2), 71–76.

Chou, C., Lee, T., & Shih, F. (2001). The decision-making process of pregnant women with positive reaction to maternal serum screening for Down's syndrome when facing amniocentesis. *Journal of Nursing Research, 9*(1), 15–27.

Christensen, F. C., & Rayburn, W. F. (1999). Fetal movement counts. *Obstetrics and Gynecology Clinics, 26*(4), 607–621.

Colucciello, M. L. (1998). Pregnant adolescents' perceptions of their babies: Before and after realtime ultrasound. *Journal of Psychosocial Nursing, 36,* 12–19.

Cunningham, F. G., Gant, N. F., Leveno, K. J., Gilstrap, L. C., Hauth, J. C., & Wenstrom, K. D. (2001). *Williams obstetrics* (21st ed., chap. 40, pp. 1095–1109, chap. 31, pp. 813–826). Stamford, CT: Appleton & Lange.

Curtis, P., Resnick, J. C., Evens, S., & Thompson, C. J. (1999). A comparison of breast stimulation and intravenous oxytocin for the augmentation of labor. *Birth, 26*(2); 115–122.

Devoe, L. D. (1999). Nonstress testing and contraction stress testing. *Obstetrics and Gynecology Clinics, 26*(4), 535–556.

DiGuiseppi, C. (2002). *Guide for clinical services* (2nd ed.). Bethesda, MD: US Preventative Services Task Force.

Druzin, M. L., & Gabbe, S. G. (2001). Antepartum fetal evaluation. In S. G. Gabbe, J. R. Neibyl, & J. L. Simpson (Eds.), *Obstetrics: Normal and problem pregnancies* (4th ed.). New York: Churchill Livingstone.

Dye, T. R. (2001). *Understanding public policy* (10th ed.). Upper Saddle River, NJ: Prentice Hall.

Fisher, M. L. (1999). Fetal activity and maternal monitoring. *British Journal of Midwifery, 7(11), 705–710.*

Fry, L. R. (2000). Update in prenatal care. Prenatal screening. *Primary Care; Clinics in Office Practice, 27* (1), 55–67.

Goldberg, J. D., & Golbus, M. S. (1996). Chorionic villus sampling. In J. T. Queenan & J. C. Hobbins, (Eds.), *Protocols for high-risk pregnancies* (4th ed., pp. 115–119). Cambridge, MA: Blackwell.

Habek, D., Hodek, B., Herman, R., Maticevic, A., Jugovic, D., Habek, J. C., et al. (2001). Modified biophysical profile in the assessment of perinatal outcome. *Zentralblatt for Gynakologie, 123*(7); 411–414.

Iqbal, M. M. (2000). Prevention of neural tube defects by periconceptional use of folic acid. *Pediatrics in Review, 21*(2), 58–74.

Magann, E. F., & Martin, J. N. (1999). Amniotic fluid volume assessment in singleton and twin pregnancies. *Obstetrics and Gynecology Clinics, 26*(4), 579–593.

Manning, F. A. (1999). Fetal biophysical profile. *Obstetrics and Gynecology Clinics, 26*(4), 557–577.

National Institute of Child Health and Human Development. (1997). *Fetal monitoring workshop.* Bethesda, MD: Author.

Piazze, J. J., Anceschi, M. M., Ruozzi Berretta, A., Vitali, S., Maranghi, L., Amici, F., et al. (2001). The combination of computerized cardiotocography and amniotic fluid index for the prediction of fetal asphyxia at birth: A modified biophysical profile. *Journal of Maternal-Fetal Medicine, 10*(5), 323–327.

Pretorius, D. H., Borok, N. N., Coffler, M. S., & Nelson, T. R. (2001). Three-dimensional ultrasonography in obstetrics and gynecology. *Radiologic Clinics of North America, 39* (3).

Schwarzler, P., Senat, M. V., Holden, D., Bernard, J. P., Masroor, T., & Ville, Y. (1999). Feasibility of the second-trimester ultrasonography examination in an unselected population at 18, 20, or 22 weeks of pregnancy: A randomized trial. *Obstetrics & Gynecology, 14*(2), 92–97.

Seyam, Y. S., Al-Mahmeid, M. S., & Al-Tamimi, H. K. (2002). Umbilical artery Doppler flow velocimetry in intrauterine growth restriction and its relation to perinatal outcome. *International Journal of Gynaecology & Obstetrics,* 77(2), 131–137.

Siddiqi, T. A., Miodovnik, M., Meyer, R. A., & O'Brien W. D., Jr. (1999). In vivo ultrasonographic exposimetry: Human tissue-specific attenuation coefficients in the gynecologic examination. *American Journal of Obstetrics and Gynecology, 180* (4).

Smith, D. S., & Wigton, T. R. (2001). Rational use of screening for prenatal diagnosis. *Clinics in Family Practice, 3*(2), 183–201.

Smith, M., & French, L. (2001). Induction of labor for postdates pregnancy. *Clinics in Family Practice, 3* (2).

Vergani, P., Roncaglia, N., Andreotti, C., Andreotti, A., Teruzzi, M., Pezzullo, J. C., et al. (2002). Prognostic value of uterine Doppler velocimetry in growth-restricted fetuses delivered near term. *American Journal of Obstetrics and Gynecology, 187*(4); 932–936.

Voxman, E. G., Tran, S., & Wing, D. A. (2002). Low amniotic fluid index as a predictor of adverse perinatal outcome. *Journal of Perinatology, 22*(4), 282–285.

Wagner, R. K., & Calhoun, B. C. (1998). The routine obstetric ultrasound examination. *Obstetrics and Gynecology Clinics, 25*(3), 451–463.

Weiner, Z., Ben-Shoomo, I., Beck-Fruchter, R., Goldberg, Y., & Shaley, E. (2002). Clinical and ultrasonographic weight estimation in large for gestational age fetus. *European Journal of Obstetrics, Gynecology, & Reproductive Biology, 105*(1), 20.

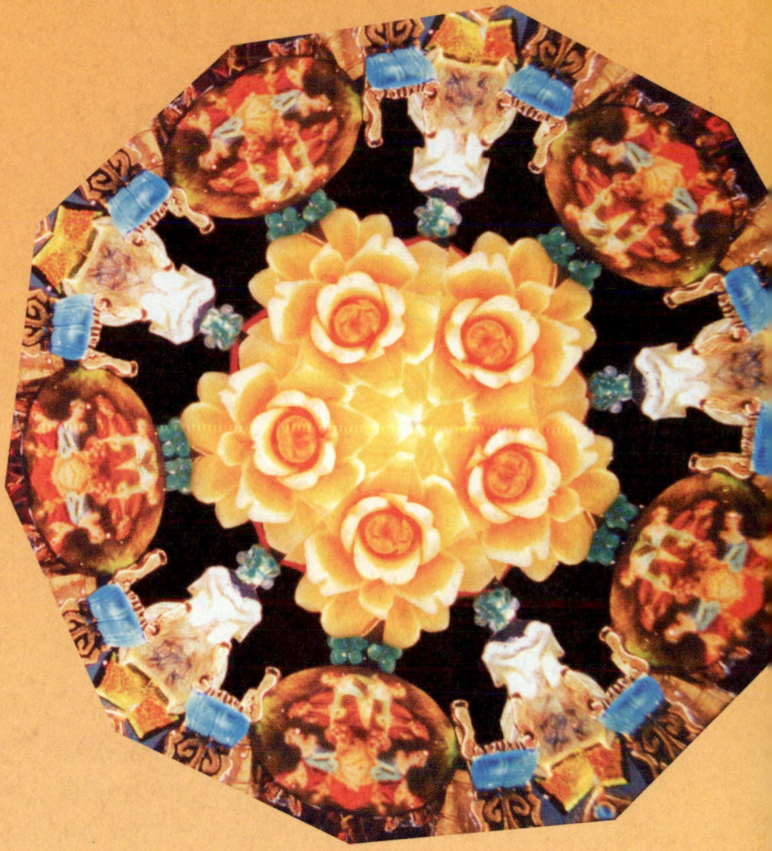

FIVE

Birth

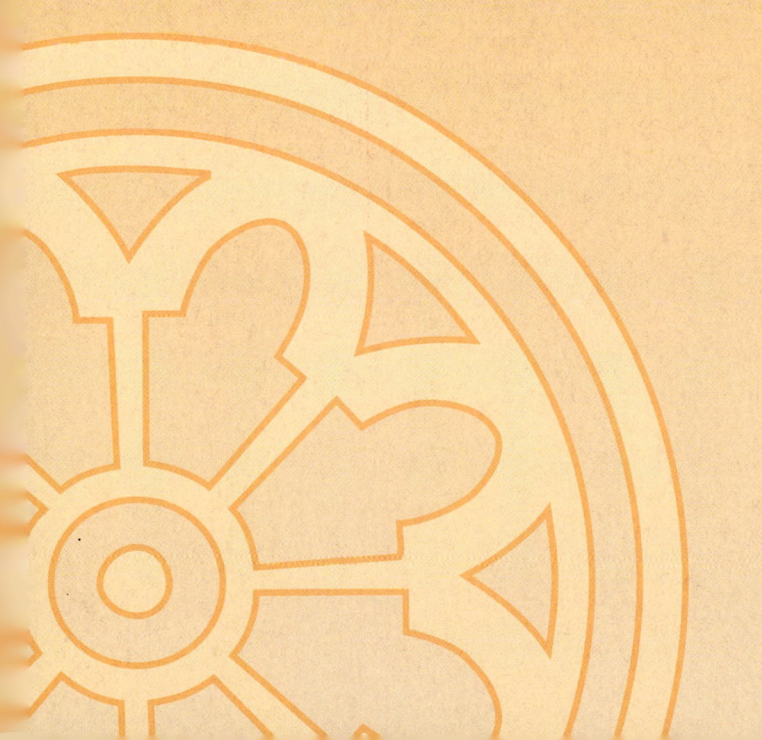

Processes and Stages of Labor and Birth

22

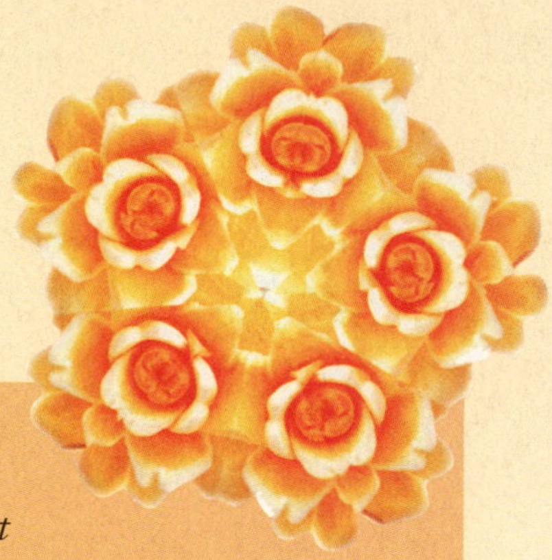

Birth usually feels like a steamy kitchen—similar to holiday preparations, except the smells are different. The smell of sweat is more acrid, there are some fetid odors, there is the smell and steam rising from blood. The air is thick, pungent, fertile. It is hard not to be reminded of fresh straw and night stars. There is near and heady promise.
-A Midwife's Story

Objectives

- Examine the five critical factors that influence labor.
- Describe the physiology of labor.
- Discuss premonitory signs of labor.
- Differentiate between false and true labor.
- Describe the physiologic and psychologic changes occurring in each of the stages of labor.
- Summarize maternal systemic responses to labor.
- Summarize fetal responses to labor.

Key Terms

Bloody show 569
Cardinal movements 572
Cervical dilatation 568
Crowning 572
Duration 566
Effacement 568
Engagement 563
Fetal attitude 560
Fetal lie 561
Fetal position 563
Fetal presentation 563
Fontanelles 560
Frequency 566
Intensity 566
Lightening 568
Malpresentations 561
Molding 559
Presenting part 561
Rupture of membranes (ROM) 569
Spontaneous rupture of membranes (SROM) 569
Station 563
Sutures 560

MediaLink

Additional resources for this content can be found on the Student CD-ROM and on the Companion Website at www.prenhall.com/olds. Click on "Chapter 22" to select the activities for this chapter.

CD-ROM
- Audio Glossary
- NCLEX Review
- Video: Fetal Lie
- Animation: Rupturing Membranes
- Videos: First Stage of Labor and Transition
- Video: Second Stage of Labor
- Videos: Third Stage of Labor
- Animation: Placental Delivery

Companion Website
- Additional NCLEX Review
- Case Study: Client in First Stage of Labor
- Care Plan Activity: Client in Uncomplicated Labor
- Care Plan Activity: Labor Progress

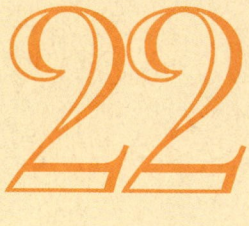

In the final weeks of pregnancy, both mother and baby begin to prepare for birth. The fetus develops and grows in readiness for life outside the womb. The expectant woman undergoes various physiologic and psychologic changes that gradually prepare her for childbirth and for the role of mother. The onset of labor begins a remarkable change in the relationship between the woman and her baby. During labor, particularly at the end, a woman instinctively knows she is engaging in one of the most important tasks she will ever do. A precious life is about to emerge. In those hours and moments the birth process may seem to carry all the power in the universe. The mother-to-be and her partner may be stretched beyond all of their normal limits of concentration, purpose, endurance, and pain. The dynamic nature of this experience is what makes the birth of a baby both a physiologic and a psychologic transition into parenthood.

Critical Factors in Labor

Five factors are important in the process of labor and birth: the birth passage, the fetus, the relationship between the maternal passage and the presenting part, the physiologic forces of labor, and the woman's psychosocial considerations (Table 22–1 •). The progress of labor is critically dependent on the complementary relationship of these five factors. Abnormalities that affect any component of these critical forces can alter the outcome of labor and jeopardize both the expectant woman and her baby. Complications during labor and birth are discussed in Chapter 26.

Table 22–1 • CRITICAL FACTORS IN LABOR

1. Birth passage
   a. Size of the maternal pelvis (diameters of the pelvic inlet, midpelvis, and outlet)
   b. Type of maternal pelvis (gynecoid, android, anthropoid, platypelloid, or a combination)
   c. Ability of the cervix to dilate and efface and ability of the vaginal canal and the external opening of the vagina (the introitus) to distend
2. Fetus
   a. Fetal head (size and presence of molding)
   b. Fetal attitude (flexion or extension of the fetal body and extremities)
   c. Fetal lie
   d. Fetal presentation (the body part of the fetus entering the pelvis in a single or multiple pregnancy)
3. The relationship between the passage and the fetus
   a. Engagement of the fetal presenting part
   b. Station (location of fetal presenting part in the maternal pelvis)
   c. Fetal position (relationship of the presenting part to one of the four quadrants of the maternal pelvis)
4. Physiologic forces of labor
   a. Frequency, duration, and intensity of uterine contractions as the fetus moves through the passage
   b. Effectiveness of the maternal pushing effort
5. Psychosocial considerations
   a. Mental and physical preparation for childbirth
   b. Sociocultural values and beliefs
   c. Previous childbirth experience
   d. Support from significant others
   e. Emotional status

Birth Passage

The true pelvis, which forms the bony canal through which the fetus must pass, is divided into three sections: the inlet, the pelvic cavity (midpelvis), and the outlet. (See Chapter 10 for a discussion of each part of the pelvis and Chapter 15 for techniques to assess the pelvis.)

The four classic types of pelvis are *gynecoid*, *android*, *anthropoid*, and *platypelloid*. Implications of each type for childbirth are described in Table 22–2 •.

Fetus

Several aspects of the fetus's body and position are critical to the outcome of labor. Primary among these are the size and the orientation of the fetal head.

FETAL HEAD

The fetal head is composed of bony parts, which can either hinder childbirth or make it easier. Once the head (the least compressible and largest part of the fetus) has been born, the birth of the rest of the body is rarely delayed.

The fetal skull has three major parts: the face, the base of the skull (cranium), and the vault of the cranium (roof). The bones of the face and cranial base are well fused and essentially fixed. The base of the cranium is composed of the two temporal bones, each with a sphenoid and ethmoid bone. The bones composing the vault are the two frontal bones, the two parietal bones, and the occipital bone (Figure 22–1 •). These bones are not fused, allowing this portion of the head to adjust in shape as the presenting part passes through the narrow portions of the pelvis. The cranial bones overlap under pressure of the powers of labor and the demands of the unyielding pelvis. This overlapping is called **molding.**

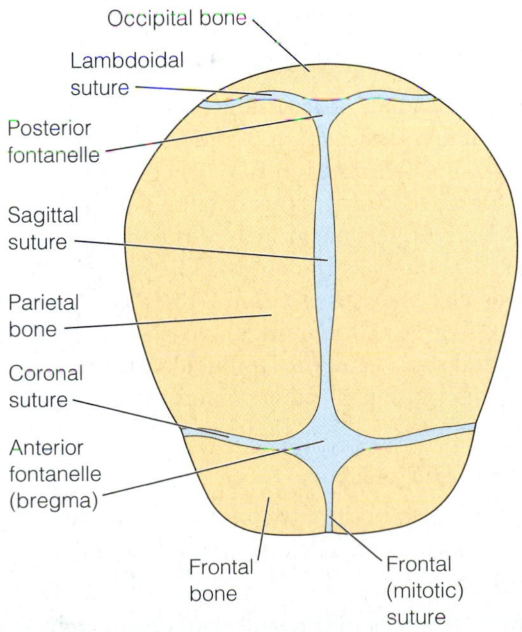

Figure 22–1 • Superior view of the fetal skull.

Table 22-2 • IMPLICATIONS OF PELVIC TYPE FOR LABOR AND BIRTH

Pelvic Type	Pertinent Characteristics	Implications for Birth
Gynecoid	Inlet rounded with all inlet diameters adequate Midpelvis diameters adequate with parallel side walls Outlet adequate	Favorable for vaginal birth
Android	Inlet heart-shaped with short posterior sagittal diameter Midpelvis diameters reduced Outlet capacity reduced	Not favorable for vaginal birth Descent into pelvis is slow Fetal head enters pelvis in transverse or posterior position with arrest of labor frequent
Anthropoid	Inlet oval in shape, with long anteroposterior diameter Midpelvis diameters adequate Outlet adequate	Favorable for vaginal birth
Platypelloid	Inlet oval in shape, with long transverse diameters Midpelvis diameters reduced Outlet capacity inadequate	Not favorable for vaginal birth Fetal head engages in transverse position Difficult descent through midpelvis Frequent delay of progress at outlet of pelvis

Note: Description of pelvic shape is exaggerated for easier comprehension.

The **sutures** of the fetal skull are membranous spaces between the cranial bones. The intersections of the cranial sutures are called **fontanelles.** These sutures allow for molding of the fetal head and help the clinician identify the position of the fetal head during vaginal examination. The important sutures of the cranial vault are as follows (Figure 22–1).

- **Frontal (mitotic) suture:** Located between the two frontal bones; becomes the anterior continuation of the sagittal suture
- **Sagittal suture:** Located between the parietal bones; divides the skull into left and right halves; runs anteroposteriorly, connecting the two fontanelles
- **Coronal sutures:** Located between the frontal and parietal bones; extend transversely left and right from the anterior fontanelle (bregma)
- **Lambdoidal suture:** Located between the two parietal bones and the occipital bone; extends transversely left and right from the posterior fontanelle

The anterior and posterior fontanelles are clinically useful in identifying the position of the fetal head in the pelvis and in assessing the status of the newborn after birth. The anterior fontanelle (bregma) is diamond shaped and measures 2 to 3 cm. It permits growth of the brain by remaining unossified for as long as 18 months. The posterior fontanelle is much smaller and closes within 8 to 12 weeks after birth. It is shaped like a small triangle and marks the meeting point of the sagittal suture and the lambdoidal suture.

Following are several other important landmarks of the fetal skull (Figure 22–2 •):

- **Mentum:** The fetal chin
- **Sinciput:** The anterior area known as the brow
- **Vertex:** The area between the anterior and posterior fontanelles
- **Occiput:** The area of the fetal skull occupied by the occipital bone, beneath the posterior fontanelle

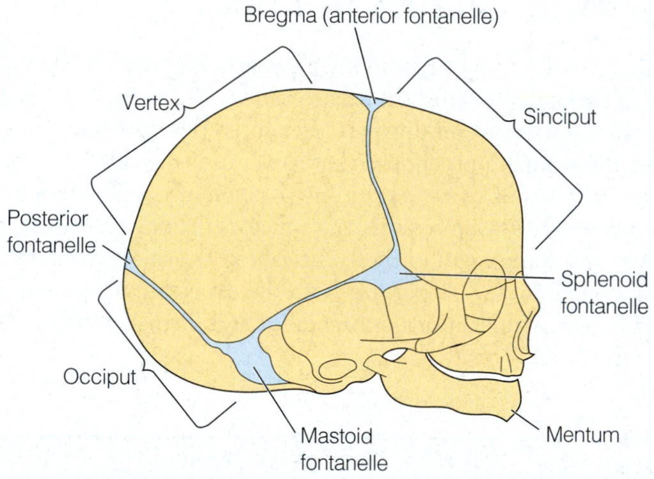

Figure 22–2 • Lateral view of the fetal skull identifying the landmarks that have significance during birth.

The diameters of the fetal skull vary considerably within normal limits. Some diameters shorten and others lengthen as the head is molded during labor. Fetal head diameters are measured between the various landmarks on the skull (Figure 22–3 •). For example, the suboccipitobregmatic diameter is the distance from the undersurface of the occiput to the center of the bregma (anterior fontanelle).

FETAL ATTITUDE

Fetal attitude refers to the relation of the fetal parts to one another. The normal attitude of the fetus is one of moderate flexion of the head, flexion of the arms onto the chest, and flexion of the legs onto the abdomen.

Changes in fetal attitude, particularly in the position of the head, cause the fetus to present larger diameters of the fetal head to the maternal pelvis. These deviations from a normal fetal attitude often contribute to a longer, more difficult labor (Figure 22–4 •).

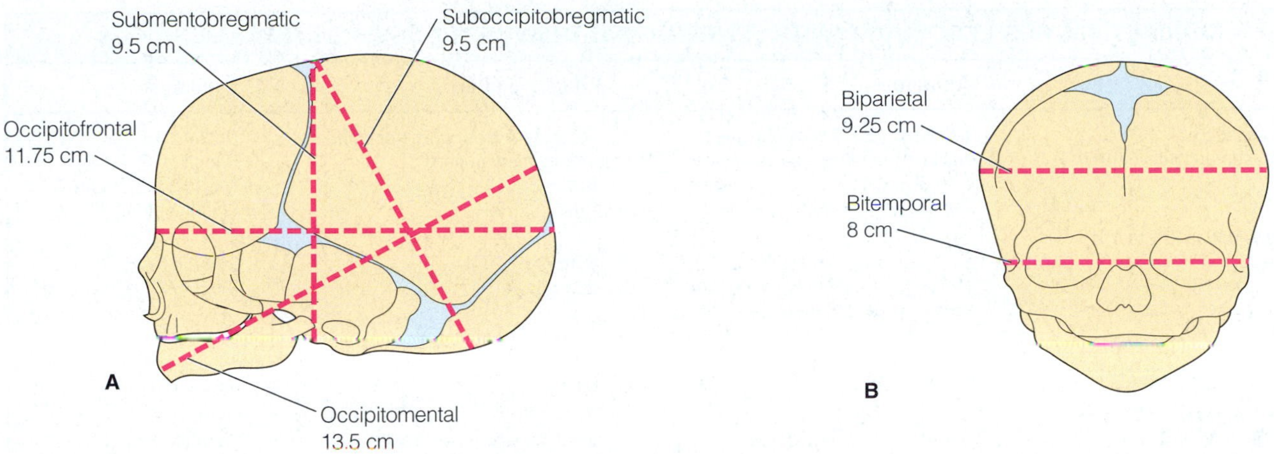

Figure 22–3 • *A,* Anteroposterior diameters of the fetal skull. When the vertex of the fetus presents and the fetal head is flexed with the chin on the chest, the smallest anteroposterior diameter (suboccipitobregmatic) enters the birth canal. *B,* Transverse diameters of the fetal skull.

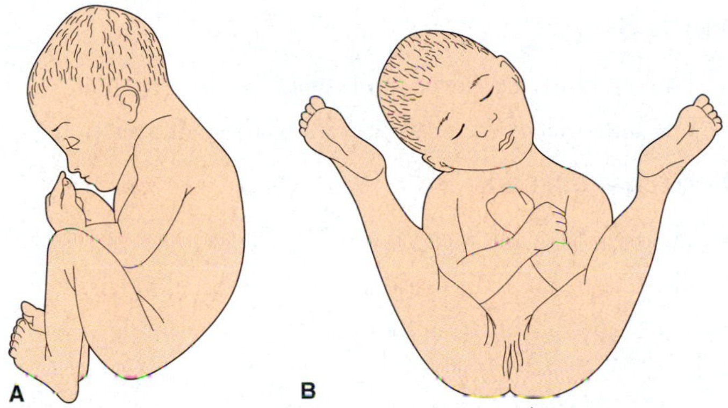

Figure 22–4 • Fetal attitude. *A,* The attitude (or relationship of body parts) of this fetus is normal. The head is flexed forward with the chin almost resting on the chest. The arms and legs are flexed. *B,* In this view, the head is tilted to the right. Although the arms are flexed, the legs are extended.

FETAL LIE

Fetal lie refers to the relationship of the cephalocaudal axis (spinal column) of the fetus to the cephalocaudal axis of the woman. The fetus may assume either a longitudinal or a transverse lie. A *longitudinal lie* occurs when the cephalocaudal axis of the fetus is parallel to the woman's spine. A *transverse lie* occurs when the cephalocaudal axis of the fetal spine is at right angles to the woman's spine. This type of fetal lie can lead to complications in the later stages of labor. A transverse lie is associated with a shoulder presentation, and is discussed in detail in Chapter 26. Table 22–3 • identifies the characteristics associated with a longitudinal versus transverse fetal lie.

FETAL PRESENTATION

Fetal presentation is determined by fetal lie and by the body part of the fetus that enters the maternal pelvis first. This portion of the fetus is referred to as the **presenting part.** Fetal presentation may be cephalic, breech, or shoulder.

The most common presentation is cephalic. When this presentation occurs, labor and birth are more likely to proceed normally. Breech and shoulder presentations are associated with difficulties during labor and do not proceed as normal; therefore, they are called **malpresentations.** (See Chapter 26 for discussion of malpresentations.)

Cephalic Presentation

The fetal head presents to the birth passage in approximately 97% of term births. The cephalic presentation can be further classified according to the degree of flexion or extension of the fetal head (attitude).

VERTEX PRESENTATION

- Vertex is the most common type of presentation.
- The fetal head is completely flexed onto the chest.
- The smallest diameter of the fetal head (suboccipitobregmatic) presents to the maternal pelvis (Figure 22–5, *A* •).
- The occiput is the presenting part.

MILITARY PRESENTATION

- The fetal head is neither flexed nor extended.
- The occipitofrontal diameter presents to the maternal pelvis (Figure 22–5, *B*).
- The top of the head is the presenting part.

BROW PRESENTATION

- The fetal head is partially extended.
- The occipitomental diameter, the largest anteroposterior diameter, is presented to the maternal pelvis (Figure 22–5, *C*).
- The sinciput (see Figure 22–2) is the presenting part.

FACE PRESENTATION

- The fetal head is hyperextended (complete extension).

MEDIALINK VIDEO: FETAL LIE

Table 22–3 • CHARACTERISTICS ASSOCIATED WITH LONGITUDINAL VERSUS TRANSVERSE FETAL LIE

Fetal Lie	Attitude	Presenting Part	Landmark
Longitudinal lie (99.5%)			
Cephalic presentation (96% to 97%)	Flexion of fetal head onto chest	Vertex (posterior part—occiput)	Occiput (O)
	Military (no flexion, no extension)	Vertex (median part)	Occiput (O)
	Partial extension	Brow	Forehead (frontum) (Fr)
	Complete extension of the head	Face	Chin (mentum) (M)
Breech presentation (3% to 4%)			
Complete	Flexed hips and knees	Buttocks	Sacrum (S)
Frank	Flexed hips, extended knees with legs against abdomen and chest	Buttocks	Sacrum (S)
Footling: single, double	Extended hips and at least one knee extended with foot in cervical canal	Feet (one or two)	Sacrum (S)
Kneeling: single, double	Extended hips, flexed knees	Knees	Sacrum (S)
Transverse or oblique lie (0.5%)			
Shoulder presentation	Variable	Shoulder, arm	Scapula (Sc or A)

- The submentobregmatic diameter presents to the maternal pelvis (Figure 22–5, *D*).
- The face is the presenting part.

Breech Presentation

A breech presentation indicates that the presenting part is the lower extremities or buttocks. Breech presentations occur in 3% of all term births (Cunningham, MacDonald, Gant, et al, 2001). These presentations are classified according to the attitude of the fetus's hips and knees. In all variations of the breech presentation the sacrum (the bone on the buttocks that is felt when palpating) is the landmark.

Complete Breech

- The fetal knees and hips are both flexed, the thighs are on the abdomen, and the calves are on the posterior aspect of the thighs.
- The buttocks and feet of the fetus present to the maternal pelvis.

Frank Breech

- The fetal hips are flexed, and the knees are extended.
- The buttocks of the fetus present to the maternal pelvis.

Footling Breech

- The fetal hips and legs are extended.
- The feet of the fetus present to the maternal pelvis.
- In a single footling one foot presents; in a double footling both feet present.

Shoulder Presentation

When the fetal shoulder is the presenting part, the fetus is in a transverse lie and the acromion process of the scapula is the landmark.

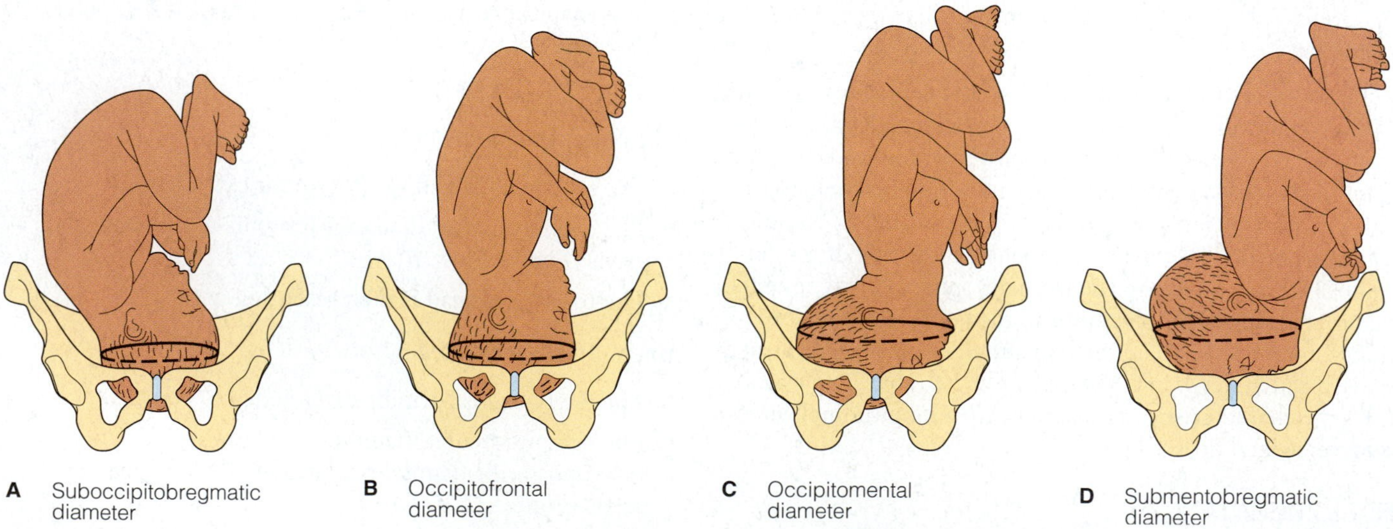

Figure 22–5 • Cephalic presentation. *A,* Vertex presentation. Complete flexion of the head allows the suboccipitobregmatic diameter to present to the pelvis. *B,* Military (median vertex) presentation with no flexion or extension. The occipitofrontal diameter presents to the pelvis. *C,* Brow presentation. The fetal head is in partial (halfway) extension. The occipitomental diameter, which is the largest diameter of the fetal head, presents to the pelvis. *D,* Face presentation. The fetal head is in complete extension, and the submentobregmatic diameter presents to the pelvis.

Relationship of Maternal Pelvis and Presenting Part

We have discussed the birth passage and the fetus, but the third critical factor is the relationship between these two. When assessing the relationship of the maternal pelvis and the presenting part of the fetal body, the nurse considers engagement, station, and fetal position.

ENGAGEMENT

Engagement of the presenting part occurs when the largest diameter of the presenting part reaches or passes through the pelvic inlet (Figure 22–6 •). When the fetal head is flexed, the biparietal diameter is the largest dimension of the fetal skull to pass through the pelvic inlet in a cephalic presentation. The intertrochanteric diameter (transverse diameter between the right and left trochanter) is the largest to pass through the inlet in a breech presentation.

Engagement can be determined by vaginal examination. In primigravidas engagement usually occurs 2 weeks before term. Multiparas, however, may experience engagement several weeks before the onset of labor or during the process of labor.

The presenting part is said to be *floating* (or *ballottable*) when it is freely movable above the inlet (Figure 22-6, *A*). When the presenting part begins to descend into the inlet, before engagement has truly occurred, it is said to be dipping into the pelvis (Figure 22-6, *B*).

STATION

Station refers to the relationship of the presenting part to an imaginary line drawn between the ischial spines of the maternal pelvis. In a normal pelvis the ischial spines mark the narrowest diameter through which the fetus must pass. These spines are not sharp protrusions but rather blunted prominences at the midpelvis. The ischial spines as a landmark have been designated as zero station (Figure 22–7 •). If the presenting part is higher than the ischial spines, a negative number is assigned, noting centimeters above zero station. Station −5 is at the inlet, and station +4 is at the outlet. If the presenting part can be seen at the woman's perineum, birth will occur momentarily. During labor the presenting part should move progressively from the negative stations to the midpelvis at zero station and into the positive stations. Failure of the presenting part to descend in the presence of strong contractions may be due to disproportion between the maternal pelvis and fetal presenting part.

FETAL POSITION

Fetal position refers to the relationship of the landmark on the presenting fetal part to the anterior, posterior, or sides

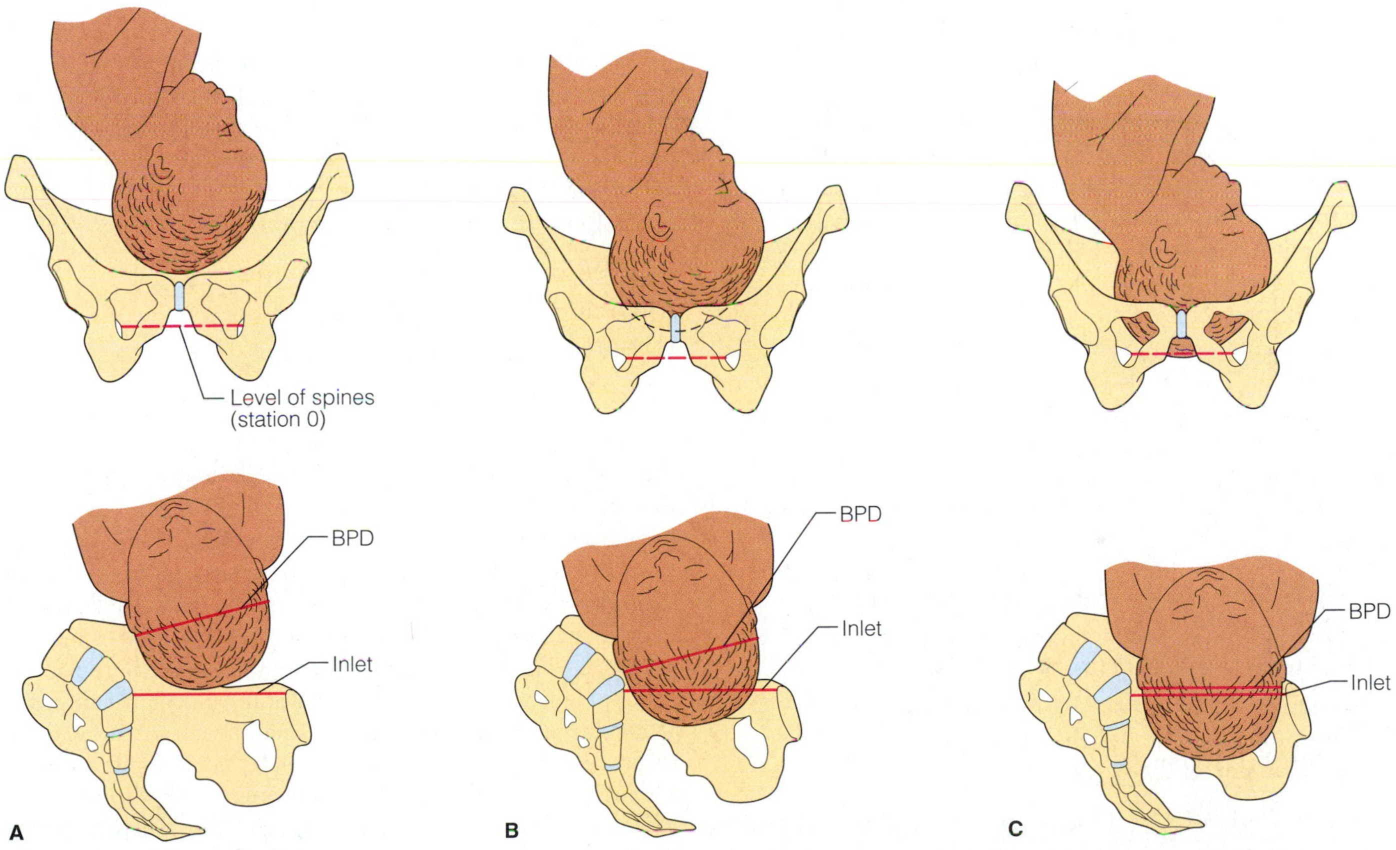

Figure 22–6 • Process of engagement in cephalic presentation. *A*, Floating. The fetal head is directed down toward the pelvis but can still easily move away from the inlet. *B*, Dipping. The fetal head dips into the inlet but can be moved away by exerting pressure on the fetus. *C*, Engaged. The biparietal diameter (BPD) of the fetal head is in the inlet of the pelvis. In most instances, the presenting part (occiput) will be at the level of the ischial spines (0 station).

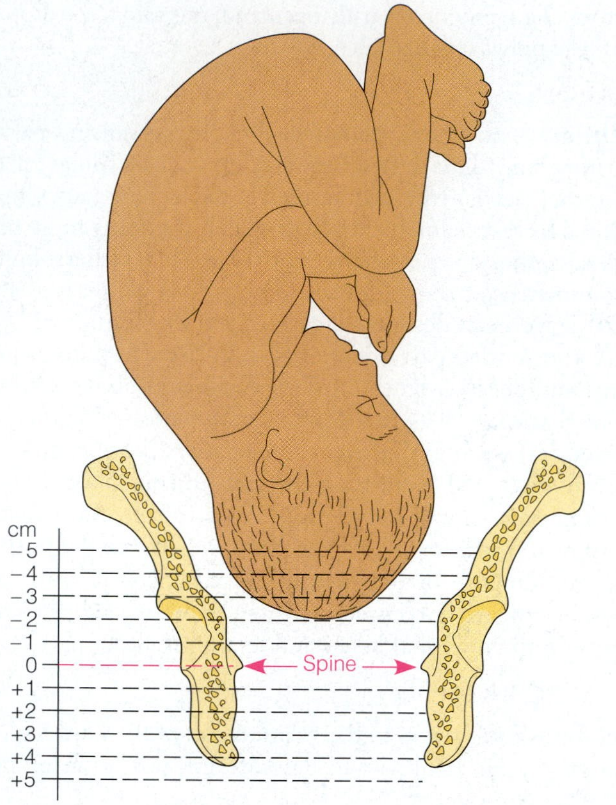

Figure 22–7 • Measuring the station of the fetal head while it is descending. In this view the station is − 2 / − 3.

(right or left) of the maternal pelvis. The landmark on the fetal presenting part is related to four imaginary quadrants of the maternal pelvis: left anterior, right anterior, left posterior, and right posterior. These quadrants designate where the presenting part is directed. If the landmark is directed toward the center of the side of the pelvis, fetal position is designated as transverse, rather than anterior or posterior.

The landmark chosen for vertex presentations is the occiput, and the landmark for face presentations is the mentum. In breech presentations the sacrum is the designated landmark, and the acromion process on the scapula is the landmark in shoulder presentations.

In summary, three notations are used to describe the fetal position:

1. Right (R) or left (L) side of the maternal pelvis
2. The landmark of the fetal presenting part: occiput (O), mentum (M), sacrum (S), or acromion process (A)
3. Anterior (A), posterior (P), or transverse (T), depending on whether the landmark is in the front, back, or side of the pelvis

The abbreviations of these notations help the healthcare team communicate the fetal position. Thus, when the fetal occiput is directed toward the back and to the left of the passage, the abbreviation used is LOP (left-occiput-posterior). Following is a list of positions for various fetal presentations, some of which are illustrated in Figure 22–8 •.

Positions in vertex presentation:

ROA Right-occiput-anterior
ROT Right-occiput-transverse
ROP Right-occiput-posterior
LOA Left-occiput-anterior
LOT Left-occiput-transverse
LOP Left-occiput-posterior

Positions in face presentation:

RMA Right-mentum-anterior
RMT Right-mentum-transverse
RMP Right-mentum-posterior
LMA Left-mentum-anterior
LMT Left-mentum-transverse
LMP Left-mentum-posterior

Positions in breech presentation:

RSA Right-sacrum-anterior
RST Right-sacrum-transverse
RSP Right-sacrum-posterior
LSA Left-sacrum-anterior
LST Left-sacrum-transverse
LSP Left-sacrum-posterior

The term *dorsal* (D) is added when denoting the fetal position in a shoulder presentation; it refers to the fetal back. Thus the abbreviation RADA indicates that the acromion process of the scapula is directed toward the woman's right, and the fetus's back is anterior.

Positions in shoulder presentation:

RADA Right-acromion-dorsal-anterior
RADP Right-acromion-dorsal-posterior
LADA Left-acromion-dorsal-anterior
LADP Left-acromion-dorsal-posterior

The fetal position influences labor and birth. For example, the fetal head presents a larger diameter in a posterior position than in an anterior position. A posterior position increases the pressure on the maternal sacral nerves, causing the laboring woman to experience backache and pelvic pressure. As a result, the woman may bear down or feel the urge to push earlier than needed. In addition, the second stage of labor may be prolonged when the fetal head remains in a posterior position.

The most common fetal position is occiput anterior. When this position occurs, the labor and birth are more likely to proceed normally. Positions other than occiput anterior are more frequently associated with problems during labor; therefore, they are called malpositions. (See Chapter 26 for discussion of malpositions and their management.)

Assessment techniques to determine fetal position include inspection and palpation of the maternal abdomen and vaginal examination. (See Chapter 23 for further discussion of assessment of fetal position.)

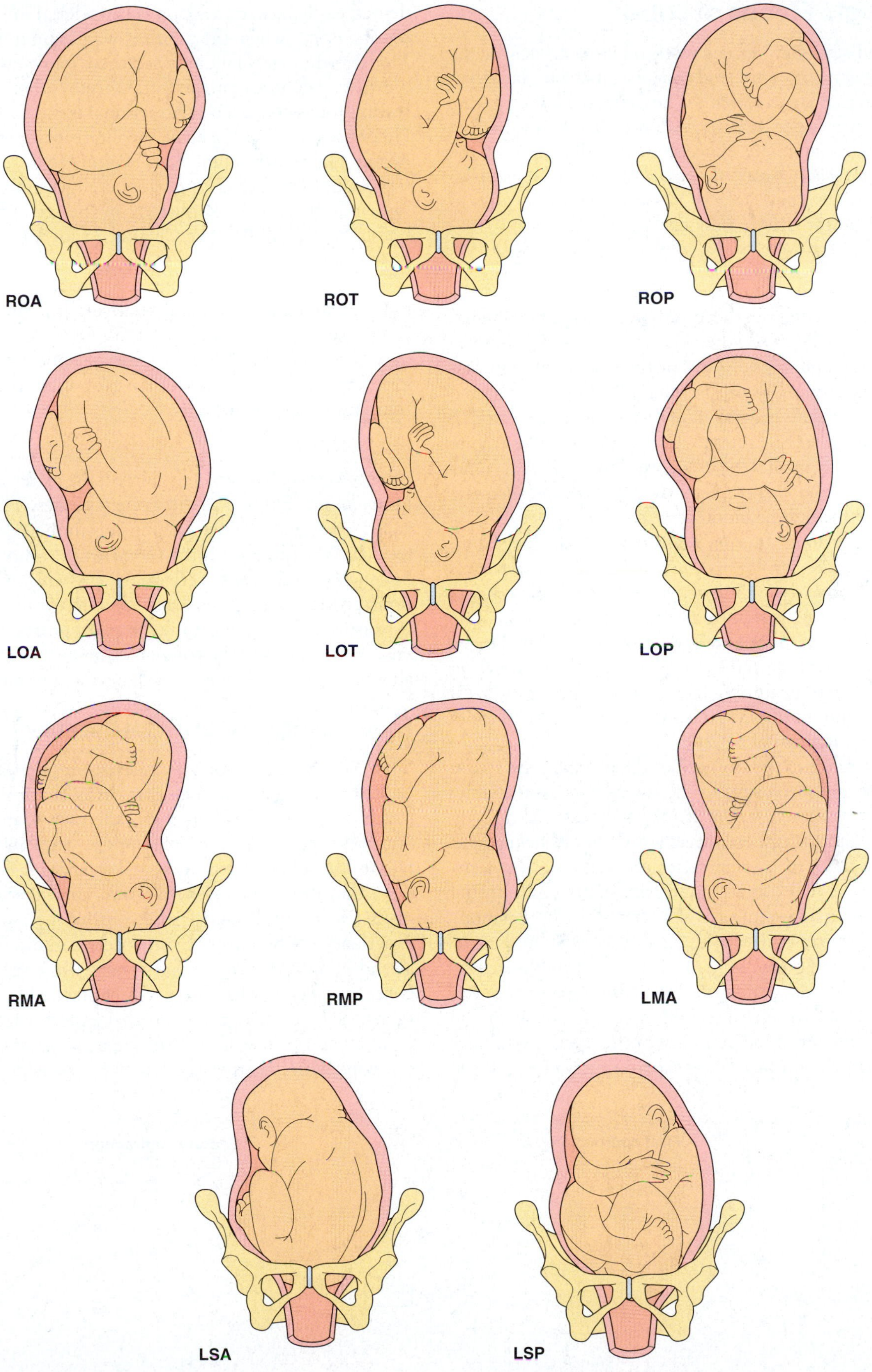

Figure 22–8 • Categories of presentation.
SOURCE: Courtesy of Ross Laboratories, Columbus, OH.

Physiologic Forces of Labor

Primary and secondary forces work together to deliver the fetus, the fetal membranes, and the placenta from the uterus into the external environment. The *primary force* is uterine muscular contractions, which cause the changes of the first stage of labor—complete effacement and dilatation of the cervix. The *secondary force* is the use of abdominal muscles to push during the second stage of labor. The pushing adds to the primary power after full dilatation.

CONTRACTIONS

Uterine contractions are rhythmic tightenings and shortenings of the uterine muscles during labor. Each contraction has three phases: (1) *increment*, the "building up" of the contraction (the longest phase); (2) *acme*, or the peak of the contraction; and (3) *decrement*, or the "letting up" of the contraction. Between contractions is a period of relaxation. This period of relaxation allows uterine muscles to rest and provides respite for the laboring woman. It also restores uteroplacental circulation, which is important to fetal oxygenation and adequate circulation in the uterine blood vessels.

When describing uterine contractions during labor, caregivers use the terms *frequency*, *duration*, and *intensity*. **Frequency** refers to the time between the beginning of one contraction and the beginning of the next contraction. The **duration** of each contraction is measured from the beginning of the contraction to the completion of the contraction (Figure 22–9 •). In beginning labor, the duration is 30 to 40 seconds. As labor continues, duration increases to 30 to 90 seconds (Cunningham et al, 2001).

Intensity refers to the strength of the uterine contraction during acme. In most instances the intensity is estimated by palpating the contraction, but it may be measured directly with an intrauterine catheter attached to an electronic fetal monitor. Intensity of uterine contractions cannot be accurately measured by external monitoring with an electronic fetal monitor, since several variables affect the external monitor, including maternal weight, specifically the amount of adipose tissue, and positioning of the monitor on the maternal abdomen. When estimating intensity by palpation, the nurse determines whether it is mild, moderate, or strong by judging the amount of indentability of the uterine wall during the acme of a contraction. If the uterine wall can be indented easily, the contraction is considered mild. Strong intensity exists when the uterine wall cannot be indented. Moderate intensity falls between these two ranges. When intensity is measured with an intrauterine catheter, the normal resting tonus (between contractions) is about 10 to 12 mm Hg of pressure. During acme the intensity ranges from 25 to 40 mm Hg in early labor, 50 to 70 mm Hg in active labor, 80 to 100 mm Hg during transition, and greater than 100 mm Hg while the woman is pushing in the second stage (Cunningham et al, 2001). (See Chapter 23 for further discussion of assessment techniques.)

At the beginning of labor the contractions are usually mild, of short duration, and relatively infrequent. As labor progresses, duration and intensity increase, and the frequency is every 2 to 3 minutes. Because the contractions are involuntary, the laboring woman cannot control their duration, frequency, or intensity.

BEARING DOWN

After the cervix is completely dilated, the maternal abdominal musculature contracts as the woman pushes. This pushing is called *bearing down*. The pushing aids in the expulsion of the fetus and the placenta. If the cervix is not completely dilated, bearing down can cause cervical edema (which retards dilatation), possible tearing and bruising of the cervix, and maternal exhaustion. The combined involuntary pressure of the uterine contractions and the voluntary muscle contractions of the abdomen forces the fetus toward the outlet so birth can occur.

Psychosocial Considerations

Thus far, the discussion has focused on physical influences on labor outcomes. But the final critical factor is the parents' psychosocial readiness, including their fears, anxieties, birth fantasies, and level of social support. Similar psychosocial factors affect both the mother and the father. Both are making a transition into a new role, and both have expectations of themselves and their partner during the labor and birth experience. Although many prospective mothers and fathers attend childbirth preparation classes, they still tend to be concerned about what labor will be like, whether they will each be able to perform the way they expect, whether the discomfort and pain will be more than the mother expects or can cope with, whether the father can provide helpful sup-

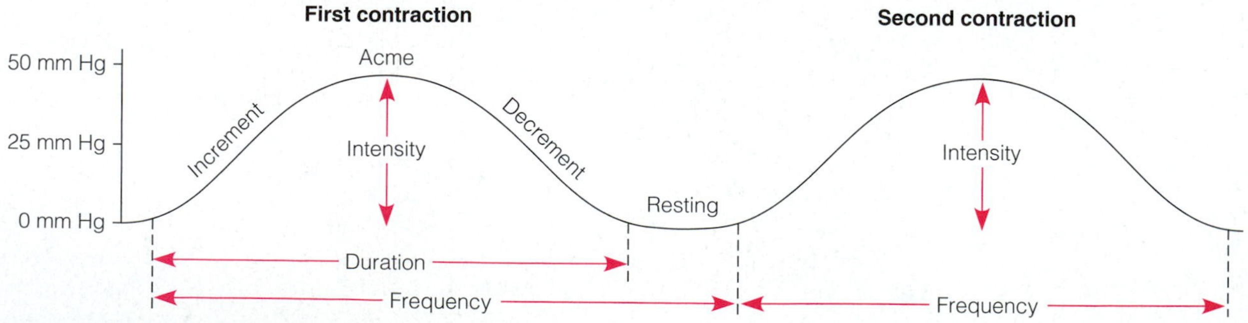

Figure 22-9 • Characteristics of uterine contractions.

port, and whether they can maintain a sense of control and be advocates for themselves (Mauger, 2000).

In addition, both partners face an irrevocable event—the birth of a new family member—and, consequently, disruption of lifestyle, relationships, and self-image (Gulland, 1998).

Many women have preconceived ideas about what birth should be like and some fear "losing control" of their body functions, emotions, or ability to handle the pain associated with labor. Women whose birth experiences do not meet their preconceived ideas may feel loss and disappointment. They may also feel that they have failed to live up to the expectations of friends, family, and peers.

Various factors influence a woman's reaction to labor and contribute to a positive birth experience (Table 22–4 •). Her accomplishment of the tasks of pregnancy, usual coping mechanisms in response to stressful life events, previous experiences, support system, preparation for childbirth, and cultural influences are all significant factors (Mullaly, 2000).

Many women have fantasies about their birth, their infant, and their early parenting experiences. A study by Sorenson and Schuelke (1999) examined the fantasies experienced by pregnant women. The authors found that fantasizing about the unborn baby was a developmental process of pregnancy. The nurse can encourage the woman to share her fantasies and use them as a tool to examine the woman's expectations, fears, and coping mechanisms. This can assist the woman in forming a maternal role and facilitate bonding with her fetus.

When a woman is facing labor, especially for the first time, she may worry about her ability to withstand the pain of contractions. Some women may place great emphasis on withstanding the pain of childbirth "stoically" without medication, crying, moaning, or making other sounds. The nurse's role is to help the childbearing family explore options and identify interventions to help each woman cope with the discomfort of labor in a way that is acceptable to her.

The laboring woman's support system may also influence the course of labor and birth. Although some women may prefer not to have a support person or family member with them, for many women the presence of the father and other significant persons (especially the nurse) tends to have a positive effect. A labor partner's presence at the bedside provides a means to enhance communication and to demonstrate feelings of love. Communication needs may include talking and the use of affectionate and understanding words from the partner. Showing love may take the form of holding hands, hugging, or touching (England & Horowitz, 1998).

How the woman views the birth experience in hindsight may have implications for mothering behaviors. A significant relationship exists between the birth experience and mothering behaviors. It appears that any activities by the expectant woman or by healthcare providers that enhance the birth experience will be beneficial to the mother-baby connection. The father's experience of childbirth and his opportunities for bonding may have important implications for fathering as well (England & Horowitz, 1998).

Table 22-4 • FACTORS ASSOCIATED WITH A POSITIVE BIRTH EXPERIENCE

Motivation for the pregnancy
Attendance at childbirth education classes
A sense of competence or mastery
Self-confidence and self-esteem
Positive relationship with mate
Maintaining control during labor
Support from mate or other person during labor
Not being left alone in labor
Trust in the medical/nursing staff
Having personal control of breathing patterns, comfort measures
Choosing a physician/certified nurse-midwife who has a similar philosophy of care
Receiving clear information regarding procedures

Physiology of Labor

In addition to considering the five critical factors affecting the progress of labor and birth, it is essential to explore the physiology of the normal labor experience.

Possible Causes of Labor Onset

Labor usually begins between the 38th and the 42nd week of gestation, when the fetus is mature and ready for birth. Despite medical advances, there is still no full understanding of the biochemical substances and interactions that stimulate labor and birth. Some important aspects have been identified. For example, estrogen is known to stimulate uterine muscle contractions to permit softening, stretching, and eventual thinning of the cervix. Collagen fibers in the cervix are broken down by the action of enzymes such as collagenase and elastase. As the collagen fibers change, their ability to bind is decreased because of increasing amounts of hyaluronic acid (which loosely binds collagen fibrils) and decreasing amounts of dermatan sulfate (which tightly binds collagen fibrils). There is also an increase in the water content of the cervix. All these changes result in a weakening and softening of the cervix which facilitates cervical stretching and effacement.

Hypotheses have also been formed about the roles of progesterone withdrawal, of prostaglandin, and of corticotropin-releasing hormone (Smith, 1999).

PROGESTERONE WITHDRAWAL HYPOTHESIS

Progesterone produced by the placenta relaxes uterine smooth muscle by interfering with conduction of impulses from one cell to the next. For this reason, the uterus is usually without coordinated contractions during pregnancy. Biochemical changes toward the end of gestation result in decreased availability of progesterone to myometrial cells. The decrease in availability may be associated with a yet-unknown antiprogestin that inhibits the relaxant effect on the uterus but allows other progesterone actions such as lactogenesis (Challis, 1999).

PROSTAGLANDIN HYPOTHESIS

Although the exact relationship between prostaglandin and the onset of labor is not yet established, the effect is clinically demonstrated by the successful induction of labor after vaginal application of prostaglandin E. In addition, preterm labor may be stopped by using an inhibitor of prostaglandin synthesis such as indomethacin (Challis, 1999).

The amnion and decidua are the focus of research on the source of prostaglandins. Once prostaglandin is produced, stimuli for its synthesis may include rising levels of estrogen, decreased availability of progesterone, increased levels of oxytocin or response to oxytocin, platelet-activating factor, and endothelin-1 (Challis, 1999).

CORTICOTROPIN-RELEASING HORMONE HYPOTHESIS

Corticotropin-releasing hormone (CRH) is also a focus for researchers. Its possible role in onset of labor is suggested by the fact that CRH concentration increases throughout pregnancy, with a sharp increase at term. Also, there is an increase in plasma CRH prior to preterm labor, and CRH levels are elevated in multiple gestations. Finally, CRH is known to stimulate the synthesis of prostaglandin F and prostaglandin E by amnion cells (Smith, 1999).

Myometrial Activity

In true labor the uterus divides into two portions. This division is known as the *physiologic retraction ring.* The upper portion, which is the contractile segment, becomes progressively thicker as labor advances. The lower portion, which includes the lower uterine segment and cervix, is passive. As labor continues, the lower uterine segment expands and thins out.

With each contraction, the muscles of the upper uterine segment shorten and exert a longitudinal traction on the cervix, causing effacement. **Effacement** is the taking up (or drawing up) of the internal os and the cervical canal into the uterine side walls. The cervix changes progressively from a long, thick structure to a structure that is tissue-paper thin (Figure 22–10 •). In primigravidas effacement usually precedes dilatation. The uterine muscle remains shorter and thicker and does not return to its original length. This phenomenon is known as *brachystasis.* The space in the uterine cavity decreases as a result of brachystasis, and this places downward pressure on the fetus (Cunningham et al, 2001).

The uterus elongates with each contraction, decreasing the horizontal diameter. This elongation causes a straightening of the fetal body, pressing the part of the fetus in the upper portion of the uterus against the fundus and thrusting the presenting part down toward the lower uterine segment and the cervix. The pressure exerted by the fetus is called *fetal axis pressure.* As the uterus elongates, the longitudinal muscle fibers are pulled upward over the presenting part. This action and the hydrostatic pressure of the fetal membranes cause **cervical dilatation.** The cervical os and cervical canal widen from less than 1 cm to approximately 10 cm, allowing birth of the fetus. When the cervix is completely dilated and retracted up into the lower uterine segment, it can no longer be palpated.

The round ligament pulls the fundus forward, aligning the fetus with the bony pelvis. This facilitates engagement of the presenting part. Pressure exerted on the cervix by the presenting part aids in both effacement and cervical dilatation.

Musculature Changes in the Pelvic Floor

The levator ani muscle and fascia of the pelvic floor draw the rectum and vagina upward and forward with each contraction, along the curve of the pelvic floor. As the fetal head descends to the pelvic floor, the pressure of the presenting part causes the perineal structure, which was once 5 cm in thickness, to change to a structure less than 1 cm thick. A normal physiologic anesthesia is produced as a result of the decreased blood supply to the area. The anus everts, exposing the interior rectal wall as the fetal head descends forward (Cunningham et al, 2001).

Premonitory Signs of Labor

Most primigravidas and many multiparas experience one or more of the following signs and symptoms of impending labor.

LIGHTENING

Lightening describes the effects that occur when the fetus begins to settle into the pelvic inlet (engagement). With fetal descent, the uterus moves downward, and the fundus no longer presses on the diaphragm, which eases breathing.

However, with increased downward pressure of the presenting part, the woman may notice the following (Wheeler, 2002):

- Leg cramps or pains due to pressure on the nerves that course through the obturator foramen in the pelvis
- Increased pelvic pressure
- Increased venous stasis leading to edema in the lower extremities
- Increased urinary frequency
- Increased vaginal secretions resulting from congestion of the vaginal mucous membranes

BRAXTON HICKS CONTRACTIONS

Prior to the onset of labor, *Braxton Hicks contractions*—the irregular, intermittent contractions that have been occurring throughout the pregnancy—may become uncomfortable. The pain seems to be in the abdomen and groin but may feel like the "drawing" sensations experienced by some women with dysmenorrhea. When these contractions are strong enough for the woman to believe she is in labor, she is said to be in false labor.

CERVICAL CHANGES

Considerable change occurs in the cervix during the prenatal and intrapartal period. At the beginning of pregnancy the cervix is rigid and firm, and it must soften so that it can stretch and dilate to allow fetal passage. This softening of the cervix, called *ripening,* is under the influence of hormonal factors discussed shortly.

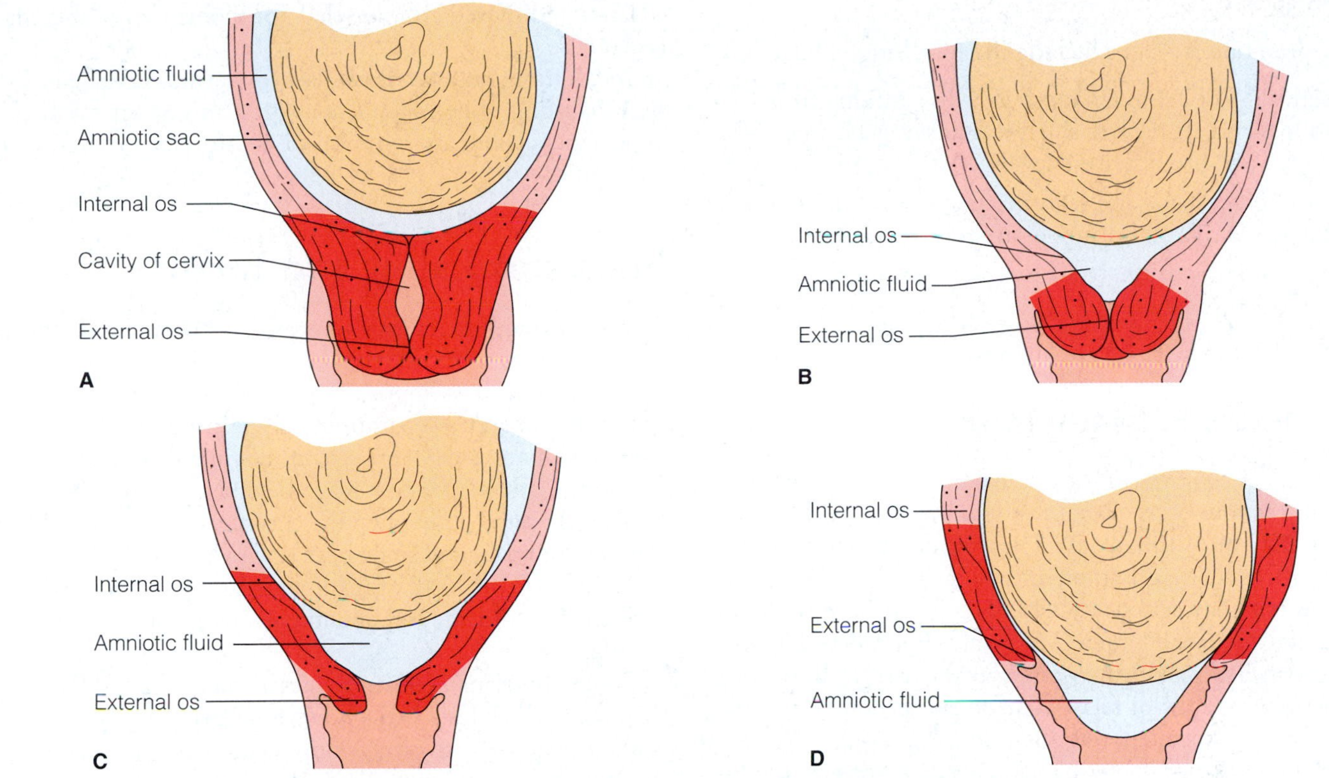

Figure 22–10 • Effacement of the cervix in the primigravida. *A,* At the beginning of labor, there is no cervical effacement or dilatation. The fetal head is cushioned by amniotic fluid. *B,* Beginning cervical effacement. As the cervix begins to efface, more amniotic fluid collects below the fetal head. *C,* Cervix is about one half (50%) effaced and slightly dilated. The increasing amount of amniotic fluid below the fetal head exerts hydrostatic pressure on the cervix. *D,* Complete effacement and dilatation.

BLOODY SHOW

During pregnancy, cervical secretions accumulate in the cervical canal to form a barrier called a *mucus plug*. With softening and effacement of the cervix, the mucus plug is often expelled, resulting in a small amount of blood loss from the exposed cervical capillaries. The resulting pink-tinged secretions are called **bloody show.**

Bloody show is considered a sign of impending labor, usually within 24 to 48 hours. Vaginal examination that includes manipulation of the cervix may also result in a blood-tinged discharge, which is sometimes confused with bloody show. However, this discharge is typically brownish in color and is not accompanied by the mucous plug.

RUPTURE OF MEMBRANES

In approximately 12% of women, the amniotic membranes rupture before the onset of labor. This is called **rupture of membranes (ROM).** After membranes rupture, 80% of women will experience spontaneous labor within 24 hours. If membranes rupture and labor does not begin spontaneously within 12 to 24 hours, labor may be induced to avoid infection (once the membranes have ruptured there is an open pathway into the uterine cavity). An induction of labor is done only if the pregnancy is near term.

At the beginning of labor, the amniotic membranes bulge through the cervix in the shape of a cone. When the membranes rupture, the amniotic fluid may be expelled in large amounts. **Spontaneous rupture of membranes (SROM)** generally occurs at the height of an intense contraction with a gush of the fluid out of the vagina. If engagement has not occurred, the danger exists that the umbilical cord may be expelled with the fluid (prolapsed cord). In addition, because of these potential problems, the woman is advised to notify her certified nurse-midwife/physician and proceed to the hospital/birthing center. In some instances the fluid is expelled in small amounts and may be confused with episodes of urinary incontinence associated with urinary urgency, coughing, or sneezing. The discharge should be checked to ascertain its source and to determine further action. (See Chapter 23 for assessment techniques.) In some instances, the membranes are ruptured by the certified nurse-midwife or physician, using an instrument called an amniohook. This procedure is called *amniotomy* or *artificial rupture of membranes (AROM)*, and is discussed in Chapter 27.

MEDIALINK ANIMATION: RUPTURING MEMBRANES

SUDDEN BURST OF ENERGY

Some women report a sudden burst of energy approximately 24 to 48 hours before labor. The cause of the energy spurt is unknown. In prenatal teaching the nurse should warn prospective mothers not to overexert themselves during this energy burst so that they will not be excessively tired when labor begins.

OTHER SIGNS

Other premonitory signs include the following:

- Weight loss of 2.2 to 6.6 kg (1 to 3 lb) resulting from fluid loss and electrolyte shifts produced by changes in estrogen and progesterone levels
- Increased backache and sacroiliac pressure from the influence of relaxin hormone on the pelvic joints
- Diarrhea, indigestion, or nausea and vomiting just prior to the onset of labor

The causes of these signs are unknown.

Differences Between True and False Labor

The contractions of true labor produce progressive dilatation and effacement of the cervix. They occur regularly and increase in frequency, duration, and intensity. The discomfort of true labor contractions usually starts in the back and radiates around to the abdomen. The pain is not relieved by ambulation (in fact, walking may intensify the pain) or by resting.

The contractions of false labor do not produce progressive cervical effacement and dilatation. Classically, they are irregular and do not increase in frequency, duration, and intensity. The contractions may be perceived as a hardening or "balling up" without discomfort, or discomfort may occur mainly in the lower abdomen and groin. The discomfort may be relieved by ambulation, changes of position, resting, or a hot bath or shower (King, 2002). A comparison between true and false labor is provided in Table 22–5 •.

NURSE'S RESPONSE TO FALSE LABOR

During the third trimester, the woman will find it helpful to learn the characteristics of true labor contractions as well as the premonitory signs of ensuing labor. The nurse informs the woman that false labor is common and many times cannot be distinguished from true labor except by vaginal examination. She must feel free to come in for accurate assessment of labor and should be counseled not to feel foolish if the labor is false.

In addition, false labor can last for several hours and can be exhausting. The nurse can suggest interventions to decrease the anxiety and physical discomforts associated with false labor.

Table 22-5 • COMPARISON OF TRUE AND FALSE LABOR

True Labor	False Labor
Contractions are at regular intervals.	Contractions are irregular.
Intervals between contractions gradually shorten.	Usually no change.
Contractions increase in duration and intensity.	Usually no change.
Discomfort begins in back and radiates around to abdomen.	Discomfort is usually in abdomen.
Intensity usually increases with walking.	Walking has no effect on or lessens contractions.
Cervical dilatation and effacement are progressive.	No change.
Contractions do not decrease with rest or warm tub bath.	Rest and warm tub baths lessen contractions.

Stages of Labor and Birth

To assist caregivers, common terms have been developed as benchmarks to subdivide the process of labor into *stages* and *phases* of labor. It is important to note, however, that these represent theoretic separations in the process. A laboring woman will not usually experience distinct differences from one to the other. The first stage begins with the beginning of true labor and ends when the cervix is completely dilated at 10 cm. The second stage begins with complete dilatation and ends with the birth of the infant. The third stage begins with the birth of the infant and ends with the expulsion of the placenta.

Some clinicians identify a fourth stage of labor. During this stage, which lasts 1 to 4 hours after expulsion of the placenta, the uterus effectively contracts to control bleeding at the placental site (Cunningham et al, 2001). Nursing care of the laboring woman is discussed in Chapter 24.

The following discussion characterizes the four stages and their accompanying phases.

First Stage

The first stage of labor is divided into the latent, active, and transition phases (Table 22–6 •). Each phase of labor is characterized by physical and psychologic changes.

LATENT PHASE

The latent phase begins with the onset of regular contractions. As the cervix begins to dilate it also effaces, although little or no fetal descent is evident. For a woman in her first labor (nullipara) the latent phase averages 8.6 hours but should not exceed 20 hours. The latent phase in multiparas averages 5.3 hours but should not exceed 14 hours (Cunningham et al, 2001).

Uterine contractions become established during the latent phase and increase in frequency, duration, and intensity. They may start as mild contractions lasting 20 to 40 seconds with a frequency of 3 to 30 minutes. They average 25 to 50 mm Hg by intrauterine pressure catheter (IUPC) at acme (Cunningham et al, 2001).

In the early or latent phase of the first stage of labor, contractions are usually mild. The woman feels able to cope with the discomfort. She may be relieved that labor has finally started. Although she may be anxious, she is able to recognize and express those feelings of anxiety. The woman is often talkative and smiling and is eager to talk about herself and answer questions. Excitement is high, and her partner or other support person is often as elated as she is.

Table 22-6 • CHARACTERISTICS OF LABOR

	First Stage			Second Stage
	Latent Phase	Active Phase	Transition Phase	
Nullipara	8.6 hr	4.6 hr	3.6 hr	Up to 3 hr
Multipara	5.3 hr	2.4 hr	Variable	0–30 min
Cervical dilatation	0–3 cm	4–7 cm	8–10 cm	
Contractions				
Frequency	Every 3–30 min	Every 2–5 min	Every 1 1/2–2 min	Every 1 1/2–2 min
Duration	20–40 sec	40–60 sec	60–90 sec	60–90 sec
Intensity	Begin as mild and progress to moderate; 25–40 mm Hg by intrauterine pressure catheter (IUPC)	Begin as moderate and progress to strong; 50–70 mm Hg by IUPC	Strong by palpation; 70–90 mm Hg by IUPC	Strong by palpation; 70–100 mm Hg by IUPC

ACTIVE PHASE

When the woman enters the early *active phase*, her anxiety tends to increase as she senses the intensification of contractions and pain. She begins to fear a loss of control and may use a variety of coping mechanisms. Some women exhibit a decreased ability to cope and a sense of helplessness. Women who have support persons and family available may experience greater satisfaction and less anxiety than those without support. During this phase the cervix dilates from about 4 to 7 cm. Fetal descent is progressive. The cervical dilatation should be at least 1.2 cm per hour in nulliparas and 1.5 cm per hour in multiparas (Cunningham et al, 2001).

TRANSITION PHASE

The transition phase is the last part of the first stage. When the woman enters the transition phase, she may demonstrate significant anxiety. She becomes acutely aware of the increasing force and intensity of the contractions. She may become restless, frequently changing position. By the time the woman enters the transition phase, she is often inner directed and tired. She may fear being left alone at the same time the support person may be feeling the need for a break. The nurse should reassure the woman that she will not be left alone. It is crucial that the nurse be available as a relief support at this time and keep the woman informed about where her labor support people are, if they leave the room (Ashe, 2000).

Cervical dilatation slows as it progresses from 8 to 10 cm and the rate of fetal descent increases. The average rate of descent is at least 1 cm per hour in nulliparas and 2 cm per hour in multiparas. The transition phase should not be longer than 3 hours for nulliparas and 1 hour for multiparas (Cunningham et al, 2001). The total duration of the first stage may be increased by approximately 1 hour if epidural anesthesia is used.

During the active and transition phases, contractions become more frequent, are longer in duration, and increase in intensity. At the beginning of the active phase the contractions have a frequency of 2 to 5 minutes, have a duration of 40 to 60 seconds, and are strong in intensity. During transition, contractions have a frequency of 1½ to 2 minutes, have a duration of 60 to 90 seconds, and are strong in intensity (Cunningham et al, 2001).

As dilatation approaches 10 cm, there may be increased rectal pressure and an uncontrollable urge to bear down, an increase in bloody show, and rupture of membranes (if this has not already occurred). The woman may also fear that she will be "torn open" or "split apart" by the force of the contractions. The woman may experience a sensation of pressure so great with the peak of a contraction that it seems to her that her abdomen will burst open. The woman should be informed that this is a normal sensation and reassured that such bursting will not happen.

During transition the woman will most likely withdraw into herself. Increasingly she may doubt her ability to cope with labor. The woman may become apprehensive and irritable. Although she may be terrified of being left alone, she may not want anyone to talk to her or touch her. However, with the next contraction she may ask for verbal and physical support. She may need help regaining focus. Other characteristics that may accompany this phase include the following:

- Hyperventilation, as the woman increases her breathing rate
- Restlessness
- Difficulty understanding directions
- A sense of bewilderment and anger at the contractions
- Generalized discomfort, including low back pain, shaking, and cramping in the legs
- Increased sensitivity to touch
- Increased need for partner's and/or nurse's presence or support
- Increased apprehension and irritability
- Statements that she "can't take it anymore"
- Requests for medication
- Hiccupping, belching, nausea, or vomiting
- Beads of perspiration on the upper lip
- Increasing rectal pressure
- Curling of her toes
- Loss of control
- Crying or yelling

MEDIALINK VIDEOS: FIRST STAGE OF LABOR AND TRANSITION

MEDIALINK CASE STUDY: CLIENT IN FIRST STAGE LABOR

MediaLink VIDEO: SECOND STAGE OF LABOR

The woman in this phase is anxious to "get it over with." She may be amnesic and sleep between her now-frequent contractions. Her support persons may start to feel helpless and may turn to the nurse for increased participation as their efforts to alleviate her discomfort seem less effective.

Second Stage

The second stage of labor begins when the cervix is completely dilated (10 cm) and ends with birth of the infant. The second stage is typically completed within 2 hours after the cervix becomes fully dilated for primigravidas (multiparas average 15 minutes). The use of epidural anesthesia may extend the duration of the second stage an additional hour. Contractions continue with a frequency of 1½ to 2 minutes, a duration of 60 to 90 seconds, and strong intensity. Descent of the fetal presenting part continues until it reaches the perineal floor.

As the fetal head descends, the woman has the urge to push because of pressure of the fetal head on the sacral and obturator nerves. As she pushes, intra-abdominal pressure is exerted from contraction of the maternal abdominal muscles. As the fetal head continues its descent, the perineum begins to bulge, flatten, and move anteriorly. The amount of bloody show may increase. The labia begin to part with each contraction. Between contractions, the fetal head appears to recede. With succeeding contractions and maternal pushing effort, the fetal head descends farther. **Crowning** occurs when the fetal head is encircled by the external opening of the vagina (introitus) and means birth is imminent. Some women feel acute, increasingly severe pain and a burning sensation as the perineum distends. The woman may continue to fear that she will tear apart. The nurse needs to instruct the woman to "push through the pain and burning."

Usually, a childbirth-prepared woman feels relieved that the acute pain she felt during the transition phase is over. She also may be relieved that the birth is near and she can now push. Some women feel a sense of control now that they can be actively involved. Others, particularly those without childbirth preparation, may become frightened. They tend to fight each contraction and any attempt of others to persuade them to push with contractions. The woman may feel she has lost control and become embarrassed and apologetic, or she may demonstrate extreme irritability toward the staff or her supporters in an attempt to regain control over external forces against which she feels helpless. Such behavior may be frightening and disconcerting to her support persons. The nurse needs to provide reassurance to the support person(s) that this is a common reaction.

SPONTANEOUS BIRTH (VERTEX PRESENTATION)

As the head distends the vulva with each contraction, the perineum becomes extremely thin, and the anus stretches and protrudes. As extension occurs under the symphysis pubis, the head is born. When the anterior shoulder meets the underside of the symphysis pubis, a gentle push by the mother aids in birth of the shoulders. The body then follows (Figure 22–11 •). Birth of infants in breech presentation is discussed in Chapter 26.

POSITIONAL CHANGES OF THE FETUS

For the fetus to pass through the birth canal, the fetal head and body must adjust to the maternal pelvis by certain positional changes. These changes, called **cardinal movements** or mechanisms of labor, are described in the order in which they occur (Figure 22–12 •).

Descent

Descent is thought to occur because of four forces: (1) pressure of the amniotic fluid, (2) direct pressure of the fundus of the uterus on the breech of the fetus, (3) contraction of the abdominal muscles, and (4) extension and straightening of the fetal body. The head enters the inlet in the occiput transverse or oblique position because the pelvic inlet is widest from side to side. The sagittal suture is an equal distance from the maternal symphysis pubis and sacral promontory.

Flexion

Flexion occurs as the fetal head descends and meets resistance from the soft tissues of the pelvis, the musculature of the pelvic floor, and the cervix. As a result of the resistance, the fetal chin flexes downward onto the chest.

Internal Rotation

The fetal head must rotate to fit the diameter of the pelvic cavity, which is widest in the anteroposterior diameter. As the occiput of the fetal head meets resistance from the levator ani muscles and their fascia, the occiput rotates from left to right, and the sagittal suture aligns in the anteroposterior pelvic diameter.

Extension

The resistance of the pelvic floor and the mechanical movement of the vulva opening anteriorly and forward assist with extension of the fetal head as it passes under the symphysis pubis. With this positional change the occiput, then brow and face, emerge from the vagina.

Restitution

The shoulders of the infant enter the pelvis obliquely and remain oblique when the head rotates to the anteroposterior diameter through internal rotation. Because of this rotation the neck becomes twisted. Once the head emerges and is free of pelvic resistance the neck untwists, turning the head to one side (restitution), and aligns with the position of the back in the birth canal.

External Rotation

As the shoulders rotate to the anteroposterior position in the pelvis, the head is turned farther to one side (external rotation).

Expulsion

After the external rotation and through expulsive efforts of the laboring woman, the anterior shoulder meets the undersurface of the symphysis pubis and slips under it. As lateral flex-

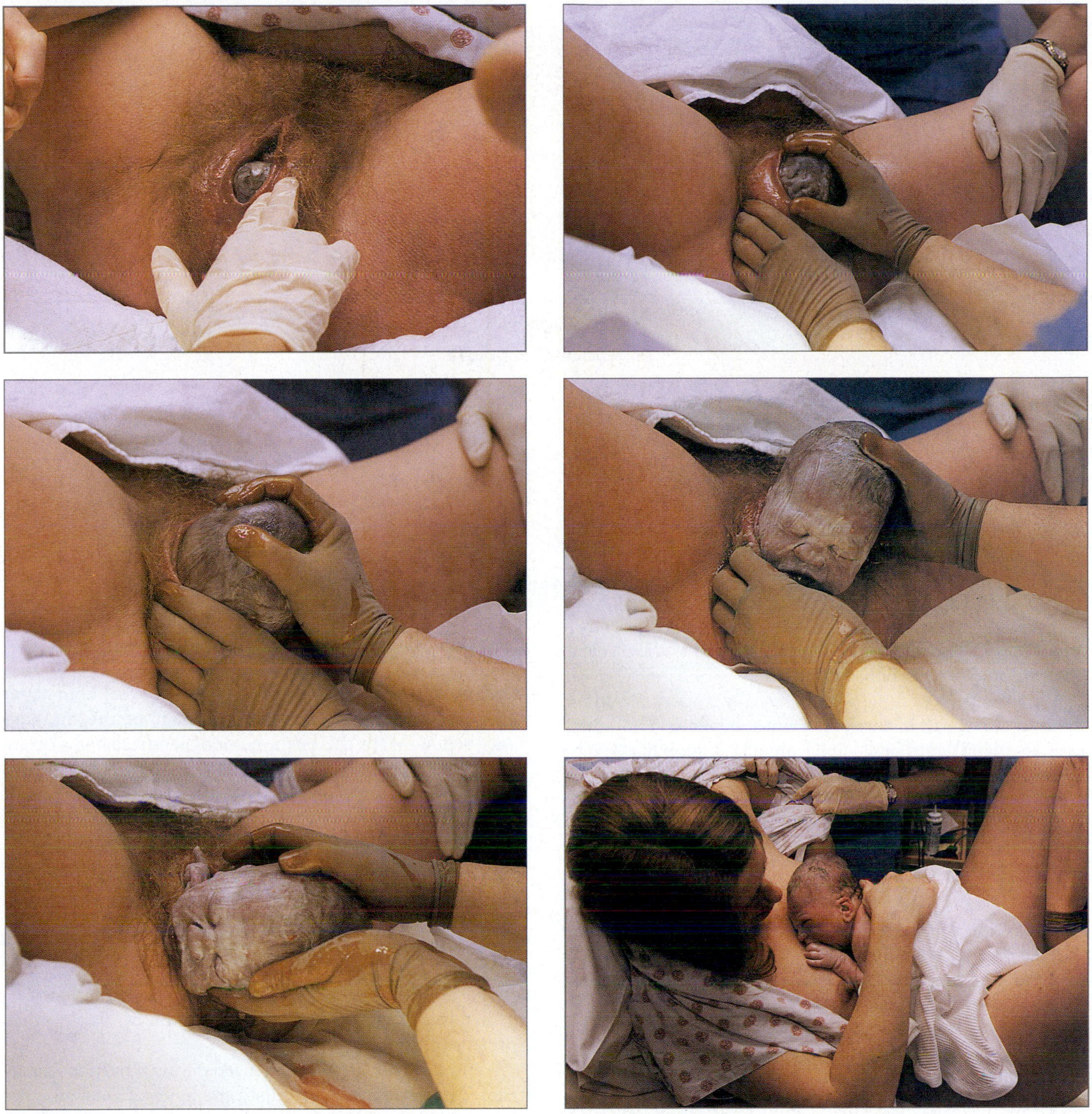

Figure 22–11 • The birth sequence.

MEDIALINK VIDEOS: THIRD STAGE OF LABOR

ion of the shoulder and head occurs, the anterior shoulder is born before the posterior shoulder. The body follows quickly.

Third Stage

The third stage of labor is defined as the period of time from the birth of the infant until the completed delivery of the placenta.

PLACENTAL SEPARATION

After the infant is born, the uterus contracts firmly, diminishing its capacity and the surface area of placental attachment. The placenta begins to separate because of this decrease in surface area. This separation is accompanied by bleeding, leading to the formation of a hematoma between the placental tissue and the remaining decidua. This hematoma accelerates the separation process. The membranes are the last to

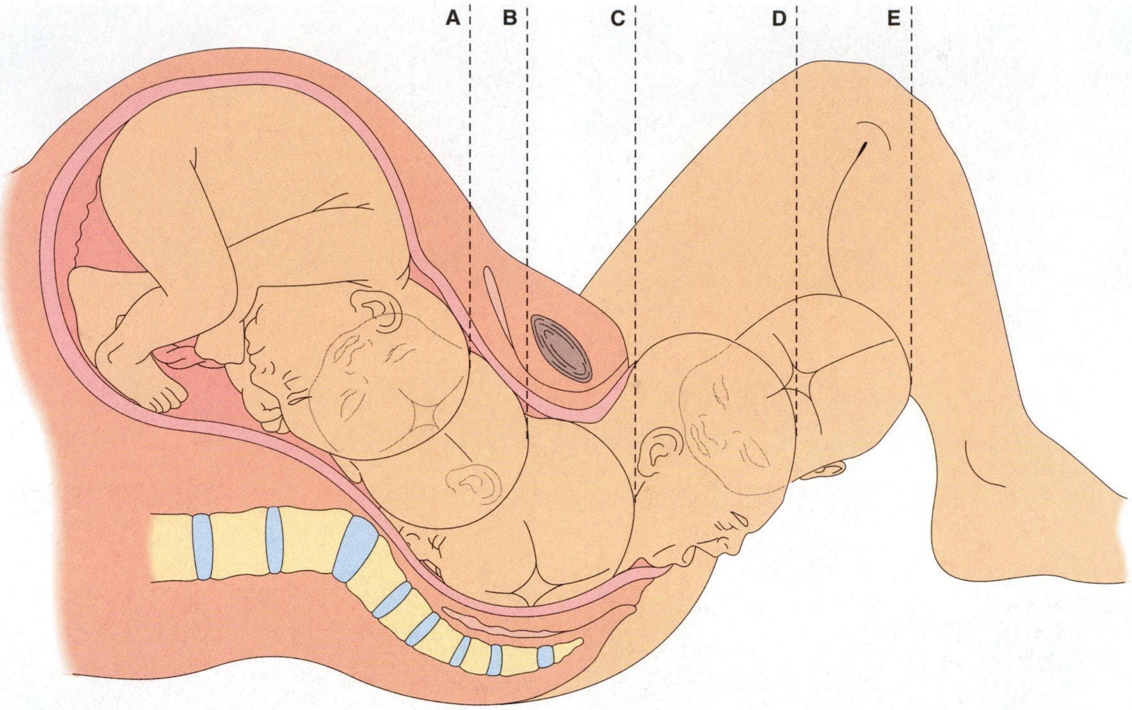

Figure 22–12 • Mechanisms of labor. *A, B,* Descent. *C,* Internal rotation. *D,* Extension. *E,* External rotation.

separate. They are peeled off the uterine wall as the placenta descends into the vagina.

Signs of placental separation usually appear around 5 minutes after birth of the infant, but can take up to 30 minutes to manifest. These signs are (1) a globular-shaped uterus, (2) a rise of the fundus in the abdomen, (3) a sudden gush or trickle of blood, and (4) further protrusion of the umbilical cord out of the vagina.

PLACENTAL DELIVERY

When the signs of placental separation appear, the woman may bear down to aid in placental expulsion. If this fails and the certified nurse-midwife/physician has ascertained that the fundus is firm, gentle traction may be applied to the cord while pressure is exerted on the fundus. The weight of the placenta as it is guided into the placental pan (a basin that holds the placenta once it is expelled) aids in the removal of the membranes from the uterine wall. A placenta is considered to be *retained* if more than 30 minutes have elapsed from completion of the second stage of labor.

If the placenta separates from the inside to the outer margins, it is expelled with the fetal (shiny) side presenting (Figure 22–13 •). This is known as the *Schultze mechanism* of placental delivery or more commonly *shiny Schultze*. If the placenta separates from the outer margins inward, it will roll up and present sideways with the maternal surface delivering first. This is known as the *Duncan mechanism* of placental delivery and is commonly called *dirty Duncan* because the placental surface is rough.

Nursing and medical interventions during the third stage of labor are discussed in Chapter 24.

MediaLink ANIMATION: PLACENTAL DELIVERY

Fourth Stage

The fourth stage of labor is the time from 1 to 4 hours after birth in which physiologic readjustment of the mother's body begins. With the birth, hemodynamic changes occur. Blood loss at birth ranges from 250 to 500 mL. With this blood loss and the easing of pressure exerted by the pregnant uterus on the surrounding vessels, blood is redistributed into venous beds. This results in a moderate drop in both systolic and diastolic blood pressure, increased pulse pressure, and moderate tachycardia (Cunningham et al, 2001).

The uterus remains contracted and is in the midline of the abdomen. The fundus is usually midway between the symphysis pubis and umbilicus. Its contracted state constricts the vessels at the site of placental implantation. Immediately after birth of the placenta, the cervix is widely spread and thick.

Nausea and vomiting experienced during transition usually cease. The woman may be thirsty and hungry. She may experience a shaking chill, which is thought to be associated with the ending of the physical exertion of labor. The bladder is often hypotonic due to trauma during the second stage and/or the administration of anesthetics that may decrease sensations. Hypotonic bladder leads to urinary retention. Nursing care during this stage is discussed in Chapter 24.

"I have had the privilege of practicing nursing in the birthing area for many years. In my head I know all the factors that must work together to bring this new life into the world. But it is in my heart and in working with and watching the laboring woman (and her partner if she has one), that I truly believe each labor and birth is

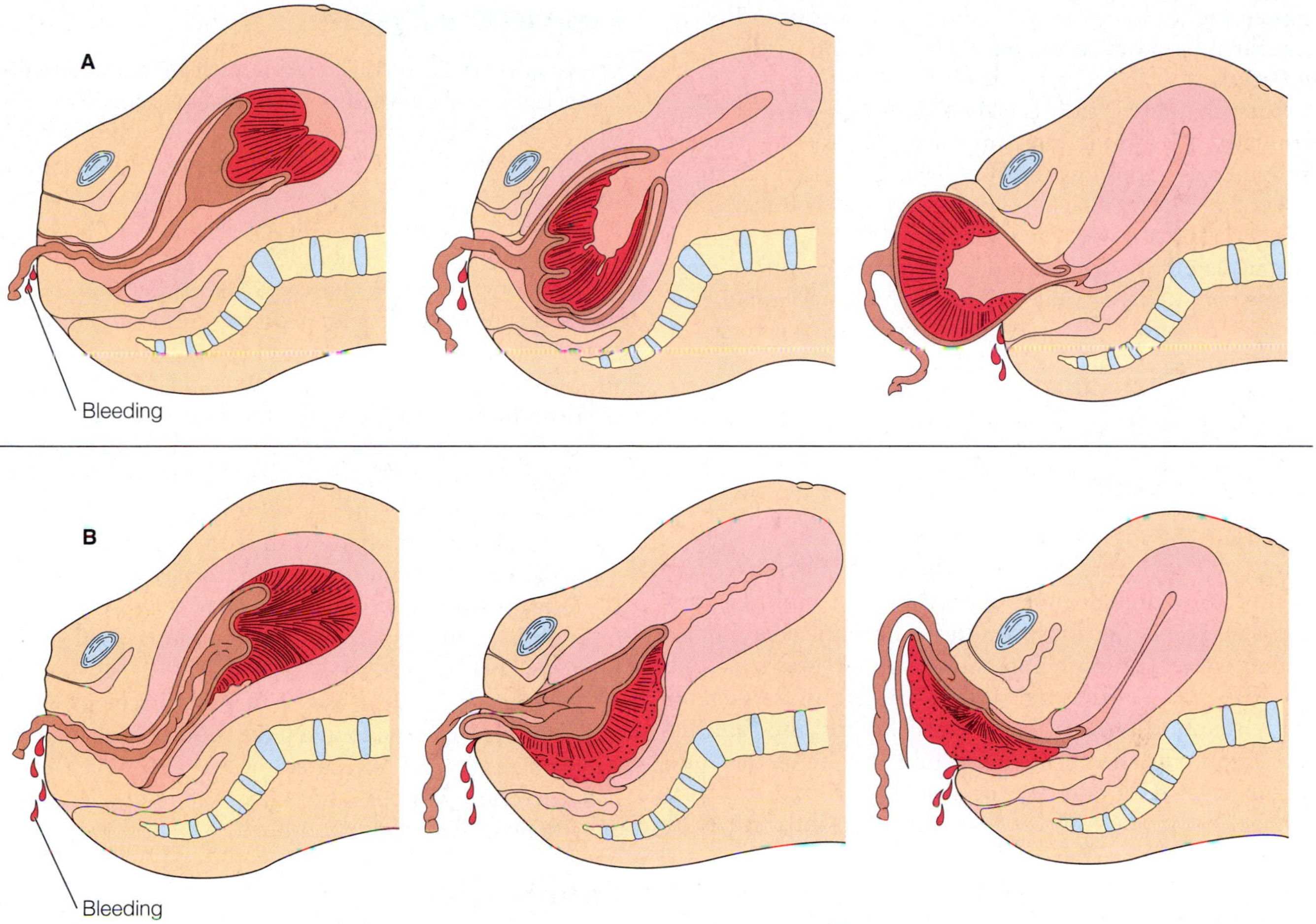

Figure 22–13 • Placental separation and expulsion. *A*, Schultze mechanism. *B*, Duncan mechanism.

a miracle. I, along with these parents, get to participate in a moment of time that will never occur again for any of us. I will never tire of this, will never get enough. ”

Maternal Systemic Response to Labor

The labor process affects nearly every major body system. Each system adapts to these changes through various compensation mechanisms.

Cardiovascular System

The woman's cardiovascular system is stressed both by the uterine contractions and by the pain, anxiety, and apprehension the woman experiences. In pregnancy, the resting pulse rate increases by 10 to 18 beats per minute (Chin, 2001). During labor there is a significant increase in cardiac output. Each strong contraction greatly decreases or completely stops the blood flow in the branches of the uterine artery that supply the intervillous space (in the placenta). This leads to a redistribution of about 300 to 500 mL of blood into the peripheral circulation and an increase in peripheral resistance, resulting in increased systolic and diastolic blood pressure, a slowing of the pulse rate, and an increase of about 30% in cardiac output (Chin, 2001; Cunningham et al, 2001).

Maternal position also affects cardiac output, blood pressure, and pulse. When the laboring woman turns to a side-lying position, cardiac output increases by about 22%, the pulse rate decreases by about 6 beats per minute, and stroke volume increases by 27%. When the woman is supine, cardiac output increases 25%, stroke volume increases 33%, pulse pressure increases more than 26%, blood pressure rises significantly, and pulse rate decreases by 15%.

There is an additional effect on hemodynamics during the bearing-down efforts in the second stage. When the laboring woman holds her breath and pushes against a closed glottis (Valsalva maneuver), intrathoracic pressure rises. As intrathoracic pressure increases, the venous return is interrupted, increasing venous pressure. In addition the blood in the lungs is forced into the left atrium, which leads to a transient increase in cardiac output, blood pressure, and pulse pressure, and causes bradycardia. As venous return to the lungs continues to be diminished while the breath is held, a decrease in blood pressure, pulse pressure, and cardiac output occurs.

When the next breath is taken (Valsalva maneuver is interrupted), the intrathoracic pressure is decreased. Venous return increases, refilling the pulmonary bed and resulting in recovery of the cardiac output and stroke volume. This process is repeated with each pushing effort.

Immediately after birth, cardiac output peaks with an 80% increase over prelabor values. Then in the first 10 minutes it decreases 20% to 25%. Cardiac output further decreases in the first hour after the birth. However, these decreases still leave the woman with an elevated cardiac output for at least 24 hours after the birth (Cunningham et al, 2001).

Blood Pressure

As a result of increased cardiac output, systolic blood pressure rises during uterine contractions. In the first stage, systolic pressure may increase by 35 mm Hg, and there may be further increases in the second stage during pushing efforts. Diastolic pressure also increases by about 25 mm Hg in the first stage and 65 mm Hg in the second stage. These increases begin just before the uterine contraction, with a return to baseline as soon as the contraction ends (Cunningham et al, 2001). Blood pressure may also rise as a result of fear, apprehension, and pain (Varney, 1997).

Blood pressure may drop precipitously when the woman lies in a supine position and experiences aortocaval compression. In addition to hypotension there is an increase in the pulse rate, diaphoresis, nausea, weakness, and air hunger. These changes are attributed to the decreased cardiac output and a subsequent drop in stroke volume.

Women with hydramnios, women with multiple gestation, and obese women have the highest risk of developing aortocaval compression. Other predisposing factors include hypovolemia, dehydration, hemorrhage, metabolic acidosis, administration of narcotics (which results in vasodilation and inhibits compensatory mechanisms), and administration of epidural anesthesia, which results in *sympathetic blockade* (blocking of the sympathetic nervous system, leading to vasodilation and hypotension).

Fluid and Electrolyte Balance

Profuse perspiration (diaphoresis) occurs during labor. Hyperventilation also occurs, altering electrolyte and fluid balance from insensible water loss. The muscle activity elevates the body temperature, which increases sweating and evaporation from the skin. As the woman responds to the work of labor, the rise in the respiratory rate increases the evaporative water volume because each breath of air must be warmed to the body temperature and humidified. With the increased evaporative water volume, maintaining adequate oral fluids/hydration is important. In some instances parenteral (IV) fluids are administered.

Respiratory System

Oxygen demand and consumption increase at the onset of labor because of the presence of uterine contractions. Approximately 50% of the increased oxygen is used by the placenta, the uterus, and the fetus (Chin, 2001). As anxiety and pain from uterine contractions increase, hyperventilation frequently occurs. With hyperventilation there is a fall in $PaCO_2$, and respiratory alkalosis results (Cunningham et al, 2001).

As labor progresses and contractions become more frequent, stronger, and prolonged, the workload, tension, and anxiety of the woman continue to change. A mild increase in the respiratory rate is normal in labor and is related to the increase in metabolism (Varney, 1997).

By the end of the first stage most women have developed a mild metabolic acidosis compensated by respiratory alkalosis. As she pushes in the second stage of labor, the woman's $PaCO_2$ levels may rise along with blood lactate levels (due to muscular activity), and mild respiratory acidosis occurs. By the time the baby is born (end of second stage), there is metabolic acidosis uncompensated by respiratory alkalosis (Cunningham et al, 2001).

The changes in acid-base status that occur in labor are quickly reversed in the fourth stage because of changes in the woman's respiratory rate. Acid-base levels return to pregnancy levels by 24 hours after birth, and nonpregnant values are attained a few weeks after birth.

Renal System

During labor there is an increase in maternal renin, plasma renin activity, and angiotensinogen. This elevation is thought to be important in the control of uteroplacental blood flow during birth and the early postpartal period (Cunningham et al, 2001).

Polyuria is common during labor. This results from the increase in cardiac output which causes an increase in the glomerular filtration rate and renal plasma flow. Slight proteinuria occurs in one half to one third of women in labor (Varney, 1997).

Structurally, the base of the bladder is pushed forward and upward when engagement occurs. The pressure from the presenting part may impair blood and lymph drainage from the base of the bladder, leading to edema of the tissues (Cunningham et al, 2001). Hematuria may be present as a result of trauma to the lower urinary tract.

Gastrointestinal System

During labor, gastric motility and absorption of solid food are reduced. Gastric emptying time is prolonged, and gastric volume (amount of contents that remain in the stomach) remains over 25 mL, regardless of the time the last meal was taken. This is even more marked in women who have received analgesia agents (Cunningham et al, 2001). These women may be at risk for aspiration should general anesthesia need to be used. During labor, anaerobic and aerobic carbohydrate metabolism rise due to an increase in skeletal muscle activity and maternal anxiety (Varney, 1997).

The fluid requirements of women in labor have not been clearly established. In some instances oral hydration is the primary goal. In other situations a saline lock may be inserted so that intravenous access is available if needed. If intravenous fluids are used, it is important to remember that when hypertonic glucose infusions are used, there is an increase in maternal blood glucose; this can lead to fetal hyperglycemia and hyperinsulinemia and to hypoglycemia in the newborn.

Immune System and Other Blood Values

The white blood cell (WBC) count increases to 25,000/mm^3 to 30,000/mm^3 during labor and early postpartum (Chin, 2001). The change in WBC count is due mostly to increased neutrophils resulting from a physiologic response to stress. The increased WBC count makes it difficult to identify the presence of an infectious process.

Maternal blood glucose levels decrease because glucose is used as an energy source during uterine contractions. The decreased blood glucose levels lead to a decrease in insulin requirements (Cunningham et al, 2001). Glucose levels can drop significantly during a prolonged or difficult labor.

Pain

Pain during labor comes from a complexity of physical causes. Each woman will experience and cope with pain differently. Multiple factors affect a woman's reaction to labor pain.

PAIN DURING LABOR

The pain associated with the first stage of labor is unique in that it accompanies a normal physiologic process. Even though perception of the pain is determined to some extent by cultural patterning, there is unquestionably a physiologic basis for pain during labor. Pain during the first stage of labor arises from (1) dilatation of the cervix, (2) hypoxia of the uterine muscle cells during contraction, (3) stretching of the lower uterine segment, and (4) pressure on adjacent structures. The primary source of pain is dilatation or stretching of the cervix. Nerve impulses travel through the uterine plexus, to the pelvic through hypogastric plexes, and then into the lumbar sympathetic chain (Figure 22–14 •). They enter the spinal cord through the posterior roots of the 10th through 12th thoracic and 1st lumbar nerves.

As with other visceral pain, pain from the uterus is also directly referred to the dermatomes supplied by the 10th through 12th thoracic nerves. The areas of referred pain include the lower abdominal wall and the areas over the lower lumbar region and the upper sacrum (Figure 22–15 •).

During the second stage of labor, pain is due to (1) hypoxia of the contracting uterine muscle cells, (2) distention of the vagina and perineum, and (3) pressure on adjacent structures including the lower back, buttocks, and thighs. The nerve impulses from the vagina and perineum are transmitted by way of the pudendal nerve plexus and enter the spinal cord through the posterior roots of the 2nd through 4th sacral nerves. The area of pain increases as shown in Figure 22–16 •.

Pain during the third stage results from uterine contractions and cervical dilatation as the placenta is expelled. Sensations of pain are felt above the symphysis pubis bone in the perineal area and in the lower back (Figure 22–17 •). The mechanism for the transmission of nerve impulses is the same as for the first stage of labor. The third stage of labor is short, and after this phase anesthesia is needed primarily for episiotomy repair.

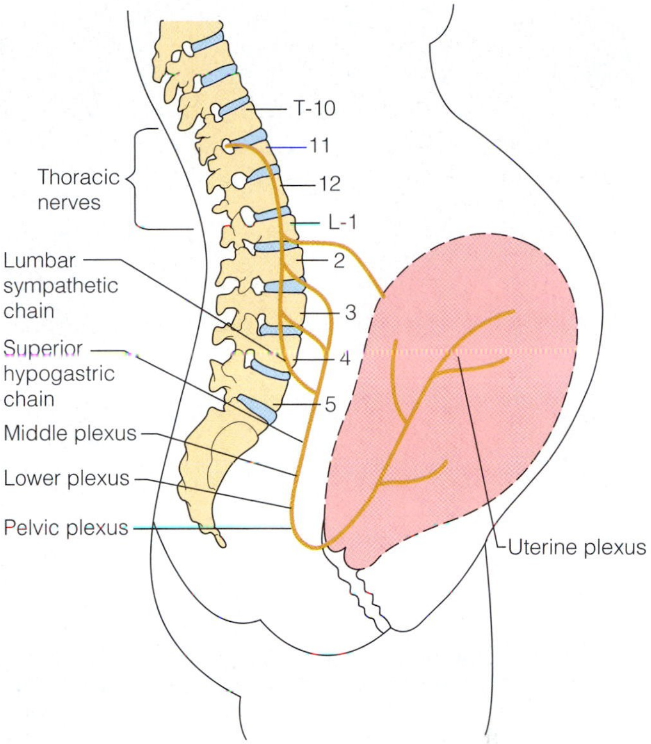

Figure 22–14 • Pain pathway from uterus to spinal cord. Nerve impulses travel through the uterine plexus; pelvic plexus; lower, middle, and superior hypogastric plexus; and lumbar sympathetic chain. They enter the neuroaxis through the 10th, 11th, and 12th thoracic and 1st lumbar spinal segments.

SOURCE: Modified from Bonica, J. J. (1972). *Principles and practice of obstetric analgesia and anesthesia* (p. 492). Philadelphia: Davis.

FACTORS AFFECTING RESPONSE TO PAIN

Many factors affect the individual's perception of pain impulses. Some psychologic and environmental influences particularly appropriate to labor are discussed here.

Preparation for childbirth has been shown to reduce the need for analgesia during labor. Preparing for labor and birth through reading, talking with others, or attending a childbirth preparation class frequently has positive effects for the laboring woman and her partner. The woman who knows what to expect and what techniques she may use to increase comfort tends to be less anxious during the labor. A tour of the birthing center and an opportunity to see and feel the environment also help reduce

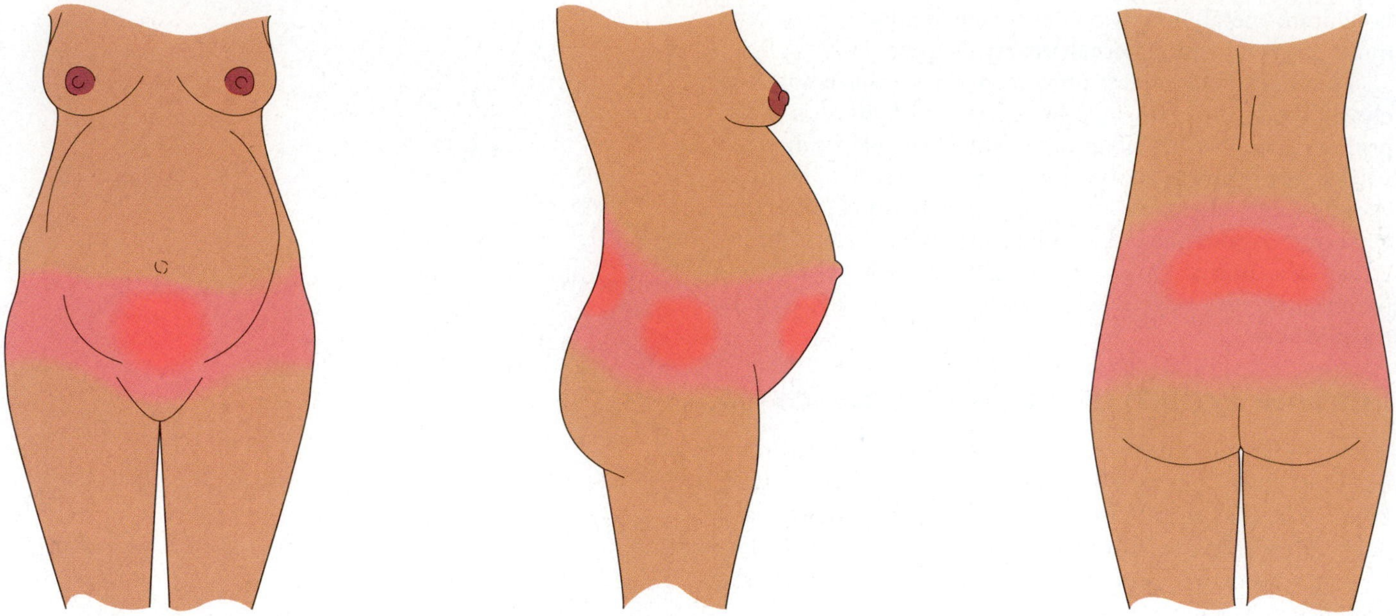

Figure 22–15 • Area of reference of labor pain during the first stage. Pain is most intense in the darker colored areas.
SOURCE: Bonica, J. J. (1972). *Principles and practice of obstetric analgesia and anesthesia* (p. 108). Philadelphia: Davis.

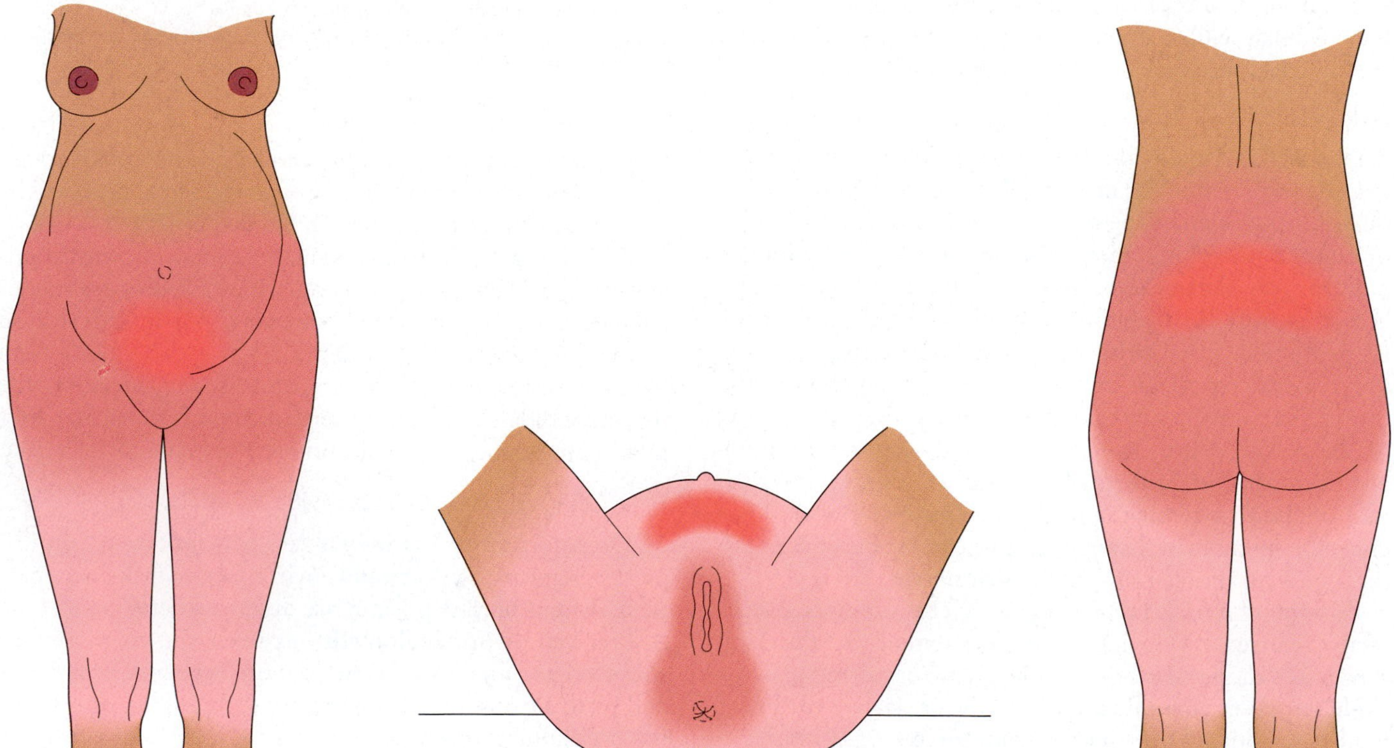

Figure 22–16 • Distribution of labor pain during the later phase of the first stage and early phase of the second stage. The darkest colored areas indicate the location of the most intense pain; moderate color, moderate pain; and light color, mild pain. The uterine contractions, which at this stage are very strong, produce intense pain.
SOURCE: Bonica, J. J. (1972). *Principles and practice of obstetric analgesia and anesthesia* (p. 109). Philadelphia: Davis.

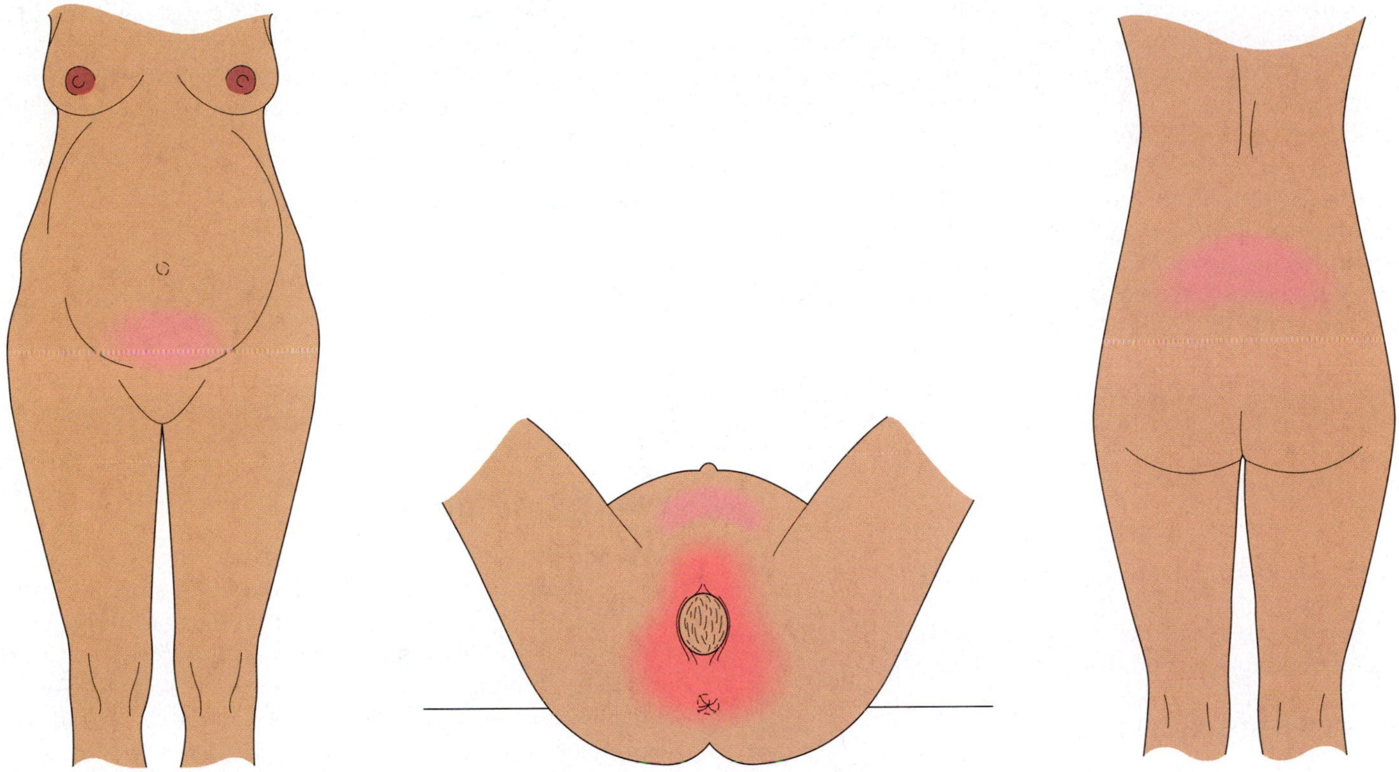

Figure 22–17 • Distribution of labor pain during the later phase of the second stage and actual birth. The perineal component is the primary cause of discomfort. Uterine contractions contribute much less.
SOURCE: Bonica, J. J. (1972). *Principles and practice of obstetric analgesia and anesthesia* (p. 109). Philadelphia: Davis.

anxiety because during admission (especially with the first child) many new things are happening and they seem to occur all at once. The more the woman and her partner learn during classes and through their own efforts, the more likely they will reduce some anxiety.

Individuals tend to respond to painful stimuli in the way that is acceptable in their culture. In some cultures, it is natural to communicate pain, no matter how mild, whereas members of other cultures stoically accept pain out of fear or because it is expected. Nurses need to be aware of cultural norms and demonstrate culturally sensitive care to women and their families in the intrapartum setting (Beckmann & Dysart, 2000).

Families will react to the healthcare system based on their own cultural beliefs. Nurses need to identify specific cultural norms with each individual family so appropriate care can be provided. Whenever possible, requests that include the family's cultural preferences should be incorporated into the woman's care. Nurses should avoid making generalizations about specific cultures. Instead, individual preferences and beliefs should be explored.

Another factor that may influence response to pain is *fatigue* and *sleep deprivation.* The fatigued woman has less energy and ability to use such strategies as distraction or imagination to deal with pain. As a result, she may lose her ability to cope with labor and choose analgesics or other medications to relieve the discomfort.

The woman's *previous experience* with pain also affects her ability to manage current and future pain. Those who have had experience with pain seem more sensitive to painful stimuli than those who have not.

Anxiety can affect a woman's response to pain. Unfamiliar surroundings and events can increase anxiety, as does separation from family and loved ones. The woman's anticipation of discomfort and concerns about whether she can cope with the contractions may also increase her anxiety level. It is not uncommon for laboring women to worry about their partner or other family members. Reassurance from family members that things are being "taken care of at home" can help.

Both attention and distraction have an influence on the perception of pain. When pain sensation is the focus of attention, the perceived intensity is greater. A sensory stimulus such as a backrub can be a distraction that focuses the woman's attention on the stimulus rather than the pain. The nurse can offer suggestions to support persons on interventions to initiate physical distractions for the laboring woman.

As part of the culture of healthcare, nursing and medical professionals have their own (collective and individual) expectations of the woman in labor and those who support her. In one setting, the woman may be expected to use a breathing technique and relaxation methods, whereas in another, most women receive an epidural block. Some nurses may believe that the woman and her

CARE PLAN: CLIENT IN UNCOMPLICATED LABOR
MEDIALINK

support persons should take care of themselves and ask for assistance only if really necessary; other nurses may believe that frequent interaction and support are essential as long as the woman and her support persons are comfortable with the interaction.

The healthcare professional is most likely to interpret pain according to the norms of the healthcare culture, although various other cultures have different ways of responding to pain. The absence of crying and moaning does not necessarily mean that pain is absent, nor does the presence of crying and moaning necessarily mean that pain relief is desired at that moment. It is very important for the nurse to accept and respect the fact that the pain is whatever the woman says it is and to assist her in coping with it.

Fetal Response to Labor

When the fetus is normal, the mechanical and hemodynamic changes of normal labor have no adverse effects.

Heart Rate Changes

CARE PLAN: LABOR PROGRESS
MEDIALINK

Fetal heart rate decelerations can occur with intracranial pressures of 40 to 55 mm Hg. The currently accepted explanation of this early deceleration is hypoxic depression of the central nervous system, which is under vagal control. The absence of these head compression decelerations (early decelerations) in some fetuses during labor is explained by the existence of a threshold that is reached more gradually in the presence of intact membranes and lack of maternal resistance. Early decelerations are harmless in the normal fetus.

Acid-Base Status in Labor

The blood flow to the fetus is slowed during the acme of the contraction, which leads to a slow decrease in the fetal pH. During the second stage, as uterine contractions become stronger and last longer and the woman pushes with each contraction, there is a more rapid decrease in fetal pH. There is also an increase in fetal base deficit and in Pa_{CO_2}, and a drop in fetal oxygen saturation. Persistent acid-base imbalance can lead to multiorgan dysfunction in the infant, including neurologic impairment.

Hemodynamic Changes

The adequate exchange of nutrients and gases in the fetal capillaries and intervillous spaces depends in part on the fetal blood pressure. Fetal blood pressure is a protective mechanism for the normal fetus during the anoxic periods caused by the contracting uterus during labor. The fetal and placental reserve is enough to see the fetus through these anoxic periods unharmed.

Behavioral States

The human fetus develops behavioral states between 36 and 38 weeks of gestation. The behavioral states seem to continue during labor even in the presence of uterine contractions. Two sleep states (quiet and active) are most prevalent, although quiet and active awake states are occasionally observed. A decrease in fetal heart rate variability accompanies the quiet sleep state, and there is also a decrease in fetal breathing movements and other general body activity. The quiet sleep state generally lasts less than 40 minutes.

Fetal Sensation

Beginning at about 37 or 38 weeks' gestation (full term) , the fetus is able to experience sensations of light, sound, and touch. The full-term fetus is able to hear music and the maternal voice. Even in utero, the fetus is sensitive to light and will move away from a bright light source. Additionally, the term baby is aware of pressure sensations during labor such as the touch of the caregiver during a vaginal exam or pressure on the head as a contraction occurs. Although the fetus may not be able to process this input, as the woman labors the fetus is experiencing the labor as well.

Chapter Review

EXPLOREMediaLink

NCLEX review questions, case studies, and other interactive resources for this chapter can be found on the Web site at http://www.prenhall.com/olds. Click on "Chapter 22" to select the activities for this chapter.

For tutorials including animations and videos, more NCLEX review questions, and an audio glossary, access the accompanying CD-ROM in this book.

Focus Your Study

- Five factors that continually interact during labor and birth are the birth passage, the fetus, the relationship between the passage and the fetus, the physiologic forces of labor, and factors associated with the woman's psychosocial status.
- Four types of pelves have been identified, and each has a different effect on labor. The diameters of gynecoid and anthropoid pelves are usually large enough for labor and birth to progress normally. In the android and platypelloid types, the pelvic diameters are diminished (smaller than in gynecoid and anthropoid). Labor is more likely to be difficult (longer) and a cesarean birth is more likely.
- Important dimensions of the maternal pelvis include the diameters of the pelvic inlet, pelvic cavity, and pelvic outlet.
- The fetal head contains bones in the top portion (cranial vault) that are not fused. This allows them to overlap somewhat in response to the pressures on the fetal head during labor. The pressure and overlapping of the sutures, which are membranous spaces between the cranial bones, result in a change in the shape of the head called molding.
- Fetal attitude refers to the relation of the fetal parts to one another. The head is usually held in midline and not to one side or the other, and the extremities are usually flexed and held close to the body because there is little extra room within the uterine cavity.
- Fetal lie refers to the relationship of the cephalocaudal (head to sacral area) axis of the fetus to the maternal spine. The fetal lie is either longitudinal (both the maternal and fetal spines are vertical) or transverse (the fetal spine is at a right angle to the maternal spine).
- Fetal presentation is determined by the body part lying closest to the inlet of the maternal pelvis. In a longitudinal lie the fetal presentation is usually cephalic (head first) but may also be breech (buttocks or one or both feet first). In a transverse lie the fetal shoulder is usually closest to the pelvic inlet.
- Engagement of the presenting part occurs when the largest diameter of the fetal presenting part reaches or passes through the pelvic inlet.
- Station refers to the relationship of the presenting part to an imaginary line drawn between the maternal ischial spines, which are in the midpoint of the pelvic cavity. The fetal presenting part enters the pelvic inlet at what is termed about a -5 and descends toward the ischial spines, where it is called a 0 (zero) station. Further descent from 0 to $+4$ occurs as the presenting part descends below the ischial spines toward the vaginal opening.
- Fetal position is the relationship of a specified landmark on the presenting fetal part to the sides, front, or back of the maternal pelvis. Once the position is known, the positions of the fetal head and back can be determined.
- Each uterine contraction has an increment, acme, and decrement.
- Contraction frequency is the time from the beginning of one contraction to the beginning of the next contraction.
- Duration of contractions refers to the period of time from the beginning to the end of one contraction.
- Intensity of contractions refers to the strength of the contraction during acme. Intensity of contractions is termed mild, moderate, or strong.
- Labor stresses the coping skills of women. Women with prenatal education about childbirth usually report more positive responses to labor.
- Women with support persons tend to use their coping skills more effectively than those who lack support.
- Premonitory signs of labor include lightening, Braxton Hicks contractions, cervical softening and effacement, bloody show, sudden burst of energy, weight loss, and sometimes rupture of membranes.
- True labor contractions occur regularly with an increase in frequency, duration, and intensity. The contractions usually start in the back and radiate around the abdomen. The discomfort is not relieved by ambulation, rest, or warm tub baths. False labor contractions do not produce progressive cervical effacement and dilatation. They are irregular and do not increase in intensity. The discomfort may be relieved by ambulation, rest, or warm tub baths.
- Possible causes of labor onset include the progesterone withdrawal hypothesis, the prostaglandin hypothesis, and the corticotropin-releasing hormone hypothesis.
- There are four stages of labor and birth. The first stage is from beginning of true labor to complete dilatation of the cervix. The second stage is from complete dilatation of the cervix to birth. The third stage is from birth to expulsion of the placenta. The fourth stage is from expulsion of the placenta to a period of 1 to 4 hours after.

- The fetus accommodates to the maternal pelvis in a series of movements called the cardinal movements of labor, which include descent, flexion, internal rotation, extension, restitution, external rotation, and expulsion.
- Placental separation is indicated by lengthening of the umbilical cord, a small spurt of blood, change in uterine shape, and a rise of the fundus in the abdomen.
- The placenta is expelled by Schultze or Duncan mechanism. This is determined by the way it separates from the uterine wall.
- Maternal systemic responses to labor involve the cardiovascular, respiratory, renal, gastrointestinal, and immune systems. Cardiac output and blood pressure increase, as do oxygen demand and consumption. Polyuria is common, and gastric motility and absorption are reduced. The white blood cell count increases, and blood glucose levels decrease.
- Factors that affect the response to labor pain include education, cultural beliefs, fatigue and sleep deprivation, personal significance of pain, previous experience, anxiety, and the availability of coping techniques.
- The fetus is usually able to tolerate the labor process with no untoward changes.

References

Ashe, D. (2000). From positive to parenthood. *Nursing Management, 31*(10), 30–32.

Beckmann, C. R. B., & Dysart, D. (2000). The challenge of multicultural medical care. *Contemporary OB/GYN, 45*(12), 12–33.

Challis, J. R. G. (1999). Characteristics of parturition. In R. Resnick, R. K. Creasy, L. Bralow, & R. Resnick (Eds.), *Maternal-fetal medicine* (4th ed., pp. 484–497). Philadelphia: Saunders.

Chin, H. G. (2001). *On call obstetrics and gynecology* (2nd ed.). Philadelphia: W. B. Saunders.

Cunningham, F. G., MacDonald, P. C., Gant, N. F., Leveno, K. J., & Gilstrap, L. C. (2001). *Williams obstetrics* (21st ed.). New York: McGraw-Hill.

England, P., & Horowitz, R. (1998). *Birthing from within.* Albuquerque, NM: Pantera Press.

Gulland, A. (1998, May 20–26). Life after birth . . . midwives should be teaching prospective parents about the psychological impact of having a child. *Nursing Times, 94*(20), 18.

King, T. (2002). Labor pain in the 21st century. *Journal of Midwifery and Women's Health, 47*(2), 67–69.

Liggins, G. C. (1997). Biology of parturition. In R. K. Creasy (Ed.), *Management of labor and delivery.* Malden, MA: Blackwell.

Mauger, B. (2000). *Reclaiming the spirituality of birth: Healing for mothers and babies.* Rochester, VT: Healing Arts Press.

Mullaly, L. M. (2000). Psychology of pregnancy. In S. Mattson & J. E. Smith (Eds.), *AWHONN: Maternal newborn nursing* (2nd ed., pp. 101–114). Philadelphia: Saunders.

Smith, R. (1999). Corticotrophin-releasing hormone and the fetoplacental clock: An Australian perspective. *American Journal of Obstetrics and Gynecology, 180,* 269–271.

Sorenson, D. S., & Schuelke, P. (1999). Fantasies of the unborn among pregnant women. *Journal of Maternal Child Nursing, 24*(2), 92–97.

Stamler, L. L. (1998). The participants' view of childbirth education: Is there congruency with an enablement framework for patient education? *Journal of Advanced Nursing, 28*(5) 939–947.

Stern, D. N., & Bruschweiler-Stern, N. (1998). *The birth of a mother.* New York: Perseus Books.

Varney, H. (1997). *Varney's midwifery* (3rd ed.). Subbury, MA: Jones & Bartlett.

Wheeler, L. (2002). *A practical guide to prenatal and postpartum care. Nurse-Midwifery Handbook* (2nd ed.). St. Louis: Lippincott, Williams & Wilkins.

23 Intrapartal Nursing Assessment

We knew that everything was going OK and that I was making progress, but it was so good to have our nurse come check me to see if I was dilating. It was not very comfortable, but he was as gentle as he could be, and when he told me that I had dilated another two centimeters, I felt that I could keep going on. It was nice for us to know that the birth was getting closer with every contraction.

Objectives

- Summarize intrapartal physical, psychosocial, and cultural assessments necessary for optimum maternal-fetal outcome.
- Define the outer limits of normal progress of each of the phases and stages of labor.
- Compare the various methods of monitoring fetal heart rate and contractions, giving advantages and disadvantages of each.
- Describe the procedure for performing Leopold's maneuvers and the information that can be obtained.
- Differentiate between baseline and periodic changes in the fetal heart rate.
- Outline the steps to be performed in the systematic evaluation of fetal heart rate tracings.
- List factors to consider in evaluation of abnormal findings on a fetal heart rate tracing.
- Identify the interventions that are indicated when a nonreassuring fetal heart rate pattern is identified.
- Delineate the indications for fetal blood sampling and guidelines for managing labor for related pH values.
- Discuss information to be taught to the woman and family when electronic fetal monitoring is used.
- Discuss the woman's and family's reactions to electronic fetal monitoring and the role of the nurse.

Key Terms

Accelerations 612
Baseline rate 607
Baseline variability 608
Combined decelerations 617
Decelerations 613
Early decelerations 613
Electronic fetal monitoring (EFM) 602
Fetal scalp blood sample 621
Intrauterine pressure catheter (IUPC) 597
Late decelerations 614
Leopold's maneuvers 598
Long-term variability (LTV) 608
Prolonged decelerations 617
Scalp stimulation 621
Short-term variability (STV) 612
Variable decelerations 615

MEDIALINK

Additional resources for this content can be found on the Student CD-ROM and on the Companion Website at www.prenhall.com/olds. Click on "Chapter 23" to select the activities for this chapter.

CD-ROM
- Audio Glossary
- NCLEX Review

Companion Website
- Additional NCLEX Review
- Case Study: Maternal Assessment During Labor
- Care Plan Activity: Client with Decelerations

The physiologic events that occur during labor call for many rapid adaptations by the mother and fetus; thus, accurate and frequent assessment is crucial. The nurse in the birth setting uses a wide variety of assessment skills including observation, palpation, and auscultation to provide care for two primary clients, the mother and her child. The expectant mother's partner or support person is also an important member of the birthing team, and assessments of the couple's coping, interactions, and teamwork are integral to the nurse's knowledge base. The nurse's physical presence with the laboring woman provides the best opportunity for ongoing assessment, even as the nurse quietly provides comfort measures and gently assists the "coach" in offering support.

In current practice, "hands-on" techniques can be augmented by the use of technology. For example, the nurse or clinician can use Doppler ultrasound to listen to the fetal heart rate (FHR) or an electronic fetal monitor to assist in recording contractions and the FHR. No matter what technology is used, however, it is important that the nurse remember that "the machine" or "the test" only provides information; it cannot replace the human interaction and support that is provided by the nurse. In the birth setting that provides "high touch" nursing care, the "high tech" assessments are easily integrated to provide comprehensive, high-quality care.

This chapter discusses the assessments that are an important part of nursing care in the birth setting.

Maternal Assessment

Assessment of the mother begins with a client history and screening for intrapartal risk factors.

History

The woman's physiologic history may be obtained in an abbreviated format when the woman is admitted to the labor and birth area. Each agency has its own admission form, but similar information is usually obtained. Relevant data include the following:

- Name and age
- Last menstrual period (LMP) and estimated date of birth (EDB)
- Attending physician or certified nurse-midwife (CNM)
- Personal data: blood type; Rh factor; results of serology testing; complete blood count (CBC); HIV testing, hepatitis testing, rubella titer; group B streptococcus (GBS) testing; maternal serum alpha-fetoprotein (MSAFP) testing; prepregnant and present weight; allergies to medications, foods, or substances; drug and alcohol consumption, and smoking during pregnancy
- History of previous illness, such as tuberculosis, heart disease, diabetes, convulsive disorders, thyroid disorders, asthma, sickle cell/Tay-Sachs and other inherited disorders
- Problems in the prenatal course, for example, elevated blood pressure, bleeding problems, recurrent urinary tract infection
- Pregnancy data: gravida, para, abortions, term and preterm infants, number of living children, neonatal deaths
- Method chosen for infant feeding
- Type of prenatal education (childbirth preparation classes)
- Woman's preferences regarding labor and birth, such as no episiotomy, no analgesics or anesthetics, or the presence/participation of the father or others at the birth
- History of special tests such as amniocentesis, nonstress test (NST), or ultrasound and reasons for test administration
- History of abnormal glucose screen indicating gestational diabetes
- History of elevated blood pressure
- Color and quantity of amniotic fluid
- History of any preterm labor requiring tocolytic therapy and/or corticosteroids
- Pediatrician/family practice physician
- Onset of labor
- Status of amniotic fluid membranes (intact or spontaneously ruptured); time of rupture is critical to GBS protocol (see chapter 20).
- Brief description of previous labor and birth and history of previous infant treated for neonatal infection (see group β streptococcus infection in Chapter 20).

Assessment of psychosocial history is a critical component of intrapartal nursing assessment. Because of the prevalence of physical and sexual assault against women in our society (see Chapter 9), the nurse needs to consider the possibility that the woman may have experienced such violence at some point in her life . If such is the case, she may be anxious about the labor process, or anxiety may arise during labor. Therefore, it is essential to review the woman's prenatal record and any other available records for information that may indicate abuse.

Psychologic disorders can also affect the intrapartum course. For example, the woman suffering from clinical depression may exhibit apathy, lack of energy, fear or hopelessness about the outcome of labor, or increased physical symptoms. The woman with a panic disorder may have short-lived, unpredictable episodes of intense anxiety, whereas the woman with a generalized anxiety disorder may experience continual and excessive anxiety or worrying. The woman with obsessive-compulsive disorder may have irrational impulses that are relieved only with performing a ritualistic behavior, such as repetitive handwashing. Psychosis is one of the most disabling psychiatric disorders, and the woman may experience hallucinations and delusions. Women with acute psychosis typically require inpatient hospitalization.

Pregnancy further complicates psychiatric disorders because many of the medications used to treat the symptoms are contraindicated in pregnancy. For these reasons, the woman with a psychologic disorder may require additional support from the nurse.

Intrapartal High-Risk Screening

Screening for intrapartal high-risk factors is an integral part of assessment of the normal laboring woman. While obtaining the history, the nurse notes the presence of any factors that may be associated with a high-risk condition. For example, the woman who reports a physical symptom such as intermittent bleeding needs further assessment to rule out abruptio placentae or placenta previa before the admission process continues. In addition to identifying the presence of a high-risk condition, the nurse must recognize the implications of the condition for the laboring woman and her fetus. For example, in the case of an abnormal fetal presentation, the nurse understands that the labor may be prolonged, prolapse of the umbilical cord may be more likely, and there is a greater possibility of a cesarean birth.

Although physical conditions are frequently listed as the major factors that increase risk in the intrapartal period, sociocultural variables such as poverty, nutrition, the amount of prenatal care, and cultural beliefs regarding pregnancy may also precipitate a high-risk situation in the intrapartal period. Recent research indicates that women who suffer from post-traumatic stress disorder (PTSD) may be at increased risk for some intrapartal complications (Kennedy & MacDonald, 2002). The nurse begins gathering data about sociocultural factors as the woman enters the birthing area.

Communication problems can also affect the course of labor, as well as the nurse's ability to provide support and education. Thus, the nurse observes the communication pattern between the woman and her support person(s) and their responses to admission questions and initial teaching. If the woman and her support persons are not fluent in English or are hearing impaired, the nurse must find some way to provide information in their primary language so that they can make informed decisions. If the nurse or other birthing room staff does not speak the woman's primary language, an appropriate interpreter should be obtained. (See further discussion in Appendices C, D, and E.) Communication may also be affected by cultural standards regarding when it is acceptable to speak, who should ask questions, or whether it is acceptable for the woman to let others know if she is experiencing discomfort (Austin, Gallop, McCay, et al, 1999).

The nurse should quickly review the prenatal record for number of prenatal visits, weight gain during pregnancy, progression of fundal height, assistance such as Medicaid and the Special Supplemental Food Program for Women, Infants, and Children (WIC), and exposure to environmental agents.

A partial list of intrapartal risk factors appears in Table 23–1 •. The factors precede the Intrapartal Assessment Guide because they must be kept in mind during the assessment.

Intrapartal Physical and Psychosociocultural Assessment

A physical examination is part of the admission procedure and part of the ongoing care of the client. Although the intrapartal physical assessment is not as complete and thorough as the initial prenatal physical examination (Chapter 15), it does involve assessment of some body systems and the actual labor process. The Intrapartal Assessment Guide on pages 587–593 provides a framework the maternity nurse can use when examining the laboring woman.

The physical assessment includes assessments performed immediately on admission as well as ongoing assessments. When labor is progressing very quickly, the nurse may not have time for a complete assessment. In this case, the critical physical assessments would include maternal vital signs, labor status, fetal status, and laboratory findings.

The cultural assessment provides a starting point for a plan that honors the values and beliefs of the laboring woman (Callister, 2001). Frequently, however, the nurse feels uncertain about what to ask or consider, perhaps because there has been no personal opportunity to become aware of varying cultural values and beliefs. This section of the assessment guide (see pages 590–591) should help.

The final section addresses psychosocial factors. The laboring woman's psychosocial status is an important part of the total assessment. The woman has previous ideas, knowledge, and fears about childbearing. By assessing her psychosocial status, the nurse can meet the woman's needs for information and support. The nurse can then support the woman and her partner; in the absence of a partner, the nurse may become the support person.

While performing the intrapartal assessment, it is imperative that the nurse follow the Centers for Disease Control and Prevention (CDC) guidelines for universal precautions to prevent exposure to body substances. The nurse can provide information in a factual manner regarding the precautions. Sharing information with the laboring woman and her support person(s) will promote a supportive, caring environment.

CRITICAL THINKING IN PRACTICE

You are the birthing center nurse and you have reason to suspect that Lynn Ling, who has just been admitted in labor, may be in an abusive relationship. How could you set up an interview so that the partner would leave the room (and take any accompanying children) without feeling that you are possibly increasing the risk to the woman? What communication techniques would you use to encourage Lynn to reveal if her partner is abusive?

Answers can be found in Appendix I.

Table 23–1 • INTRAPARTAL HIGH-RISK FACTORS

Factor	Maternal Implication	Fetal-Neonatal Implication
Abnormal presentation	↑ Incidence of cesarean birth ↑ Incidence of prolonged labor ↑ Incidence of fibroids	↑ Incidence of placenta previa Prematurity ↑ Risk of congenital abnormality Neonatal physical trauma ↑ Risk of intrauterine growth restriction
Multiple gestation	↑ Uterine distention → ↑ risk of postpartum hemorrhage ↑ Risk of cesarean birth ↑ Risk of preterm labor	Low birth weight Prematurity ↑ Risk of congenital anomalies Feto-fetal transfusion
Hydramnios	↑ Discomfort ↑ Dyspnea ↑ Risk of preterm labor Edema of lower extremities/varicosities	↑ Risk of esophageal or other high alimentary tract atresias ↑ Risk of CNS anomalies (myelocele) ↑ Risk of TORCH infections ↑ Risk of prolapse cord
Oligohydramnios	Maternal fear of "dry birth"	↑ Incidence of congenital anomalies ↑ Incidence of renal lesions ↑ Risk of intrauterine growth restriction ↑ Risk of fetal acidosis ↑ Risk of cord compression Postmaturity
Meconium staining of amniotic fluid	↑ Psychologic stress due to fear for baby	↑ Risk of fetal asphyxia ↑ Risk of meconium aspiration ↑ Risk of pneumonia due to aspiration of meconium
Premature rupture of membranes	↑ Risk of infection (chorioamnionitis) ↑ Risk of preterm labor ↑ Anxiety/fear for the baby Prolonged hospitalization ↑ Incidence of tocolytic therapy	↑ Perinatal morbidity Prematurity ↓ Birth weight ↑ Risk of respiratory distress syndrome Prolonged hospitalization
Induction of labor	↑ Risk of hypercontractility of uterus ↑ Risk of uterine rupture ↑ Length of labor if cervix not ready ↑ Anxiety	Prematurity if gestational age not assessed correctly Hypoxia if hyperstimulation occurs
Abruptio placentae/placenta previa	Hemorrhage Uterine atony ↑ Incidence of cesarean birth ↑ Maternal morbidity	Fetal hypoxia/acidosis Fetal exsanguination ↑ Perinatal mortality
Failure to progress in labor	Maternal exhaustion ↑ Incidence of augmentation of labor ↑ Incidence of cesarean birth	Fetal hypoxia/acidosis Intracranial birth injury
Precipitous labor (< 3 hours)	Perineal, vaginal, cervical lacerations ↑ Risk of postpartum hemorrhage	Tentorial tears
Prolapse of umbilical cord	↑ Fear for baby Cesarean birth → emergent	Acute fetal hypoxia/acidosis
Fetal heart aberrations	↑ Fear for baby ↑ Risk of cesarean birth, forceps, vacuum Continuous electronic monitoring and intervention in labor	Tachycardia, chronic asphyxic insult, bradycardia, Acute asphyxic insult Chronic hypoxia Congenital heart block
Uterine rupture	Hemorrhage Cesarean birth/hysterectomy ↑ Risk of morbidity/mortality	Fetal anoxia Fetal hemorrhage ↑ Neonatal morbidity and mortality
Postdates (> 42 weeks)	↑ Anxiety ↑ Incidence of induction of labor ↑ Incidence of cesarean birth ↑ Use of technology to monitor fetus ↑ Risk of shoulder dystocia	Postmaturity syndrome ↑ Risk of fetal-neonatal mortality and morbidity ↑ Risk of antepartum fetal death ↑ Incidence/risk of large baby
Diabetes	↑ Risk of hydramnios ↑ Risk of hypoglycemia or hyperglycemia ↑ Risk of preeclampsia	↑ Risk of malpresentation ↑ Risk of macrosomia ↑ Risk of intrauterine growth restriction ↑ Risk of respiratory distress syndrome ↑ Risk of congenital anomalies
Preeclampsia	↑ Abruptio placentae ↑ Risk of seizures ↑ Risk of stroke ↑ Risk of HELLP	↑ Risk of small-for-gestational-age baby ↑ Risk of preterm birth ↑ Risk of mortality
AIDS/STD	↑ Risk of additional infections	↑ Risk of transplacental transmission

ASSESSMENT GUIDE INTRAPARTAL—FIRST STAGE OF LABOR

PHYSICAL ASSESSMENT/ NORMAL FINDINGS	ALTERATIONS AND POSSIBLE CAUSES*	NURSING RESPONSES TO DATA†
➤ VITAL SIGNS		
Blood pressure (BP): ≤ 135 systolic and <85 diastolic in adult 18 years of age or older or no more than 15–20 mm Hg rise in systolic pressure over baseline BP during early pregnancy	High blood pressure (essential hypertension, preeclampsia, renal disease, apprehension, anxiety or pain) Low blood pressure (supine hypotension) Hemorrhage/hypovolemia Shock Drugs	Evaluate history of preexisting disorders and check for presence of other signs of preeclampsia. Do not assess during contractions; implement measures to decrease anxiety and reassess. Turn woman on her side and recheck BP. Provide quiet environment. Have O_2 available.
Pulse: 60–90 bpm	Increased pulse rate (excitement or anxiety, cardiac disorders, early shock, drug use)	Evaluate cause, reassess to see if rate continues; report to physician/CNM.
Respirations: 14–22/min (or pulse rate divided by 4)	Marked tachypnea (respiratory disease), hyperventilation in transition phase Decreased respirations (Narcotics)	Assess between contractions; if marked tachypnea continues, assess for signs of respiratory disease or respiratory distress.
	Hyperventilation (anxiety/pain)	Encourage slow breaths if woman is hyperventilating.
Pulse ox 95% or greater	< 90%: hypoxia, hypotension, hemorrhage	Apply O_2; notify physician/CNM.
Temperature: 36.2–37.6C (98–99.6F)	Elevated temperature (infection, dehydration, prolonged rupture of membranes, epidural regional block)	Assess for other signs of infection or dehydration.
➤ WEIGHT		
25–35 lb greater than prepregnant weight (ACOG, 1999)	Weight gain > 35 lb (fluid retention, obesity, large infant, diabetes mellitus, preeclampsia), weight gain < 15 lb (SGA, substance abuse, psychosocial problems)	Assess for signs of edema. Evaluate, OATA from prenatal record.
➤ LUNGS		
Normal breath sounds, clear and equal	Rales, rhonchi, friction rub (infection), pulmonary edema, asthma	Reassess; refer to physician.
➤ FUNDUS		
At 40 weeks' gestation located just below xiphoid process	Uterine size not compatible with estimated date of birth (SGA, large for gestational age [LGA], hydramnios, multiple pregnancy, placental/fetal anomolies, malpresentation)	Reevaluate history regarding pregnancy dating. Refer to physician for additional assessment.
➤ EDEMA		
Slight amount of dependent edema	Pitting edema of face, hands, legs, abdomen, sacral area (preeclampsia)	Check deep tendon reflexes for hyperactivity; check for clonus; refer to physician.
	*Possible causes of alterations are placed in parentheses.	†This column provides guidelines for further assessment and initial nursing intervention.

(continued on next page)

Assessment Guide: Intrapartal—First Stage of Labor *continued*

PHYSICAL ASSESSMENT/ NORMAL FINDINGS	ALTERATIONS AND POSSIBLE CAUSES*	NURSING RESPONSES TO DATA†
➤ HYDRATION		
Normal skin turgor, elastic	Poor skin turgor (dehydration)	Assess skin turgor; refer to physician for deviations. Provide fluids per physician/CNM orders.
➤ PERINEUM		
Tissues smooth, pink color (see Prenatal Initial Physical Assessment Guide, Chapter 15).	Varicose veins of vulva, herpes lesions/genital warts.	Note on client record need for follow-up in postpartal period; reassess after birth; refer to physician/CNM.
Clear mucus; may be blood tinged with earthy or human odor	Profuse, purulent, foul-smelling drainage	Suspected gonorrhea or chorioamnionitis; report to physician; initiate care to newborn's eyes; notify neonatal nursing staff and pediatrician.
Presence of small amount of bloody show that gradually increases with further cervical dilatation	Hemorrhage	Assess BP and pulse, pallor, diaphoresis; report any marked changes. Universal precautions.
➤ LABOR STATUS		
Uterine contractions: regular pattern	Failure to establish a regular pattern, prolonged latent phase Hypertonicity Hypotonicity Dehydration	Evaluate whether woman is in true labor; Ambulate if in early labor. Evaluate client status and contractile pattern. Obtain a 20-minute EFM strip. Notify physician or CNM. Provide hydration.
Cervical dilatation: progressive cervical dilatation from size of fingertip to 10 cm (Procedure 23–1)	Rigidity of cervix (frequent cervical infections, scar tissue, failure of presenting part to descend)	Evaluate contractions, fetal engagement, position, and cervical dilatation. Inform client of progress.
Cervical effacement: progressive thinning of cervix (Procedure 23–1)	Failure to efface (rigidity of cervix, failure of presenting part to engage); cervical edema (pushing effort by woman before cervix is fully dilated and effaced, trapped cervix)	Evaluate contractions, fetal engagement and position. Notify physician/CNM if cervix is becoming edematous; work with woman to prevent pushing until cervix is completely dilated. Keep vaginal exams to a minimum.
Fetal descent: progressive descent of fetal presenting part from station −5 to +4 (Figure 23–3 in Procedure 23–1)	Failure of descent (abnormal fetal position or presentation, macrosomic fetus, inadequate pelvic measurements)	Evaluate fetal position, presentation, and size.
Membranes: may rupture before or during labor	Rupture of membranes more than 12–24 hours before initiation of labor	Assess for ruptured membranes using Nitrazine test tape before doing vaginal exam. Follow universal precautions. Instruct woman with ruptured membranes to remain on bed rest if presenting part is not engaged and firmly down against the cervix. Keep vaginal exams to a minimum to prevent infection. When membranes rupture in the birth setting **immediately assess FHR** to detect changes associated with prolapse of umbilical cord (FHR slows).

*Possible causes of alterations are placed in parentheses.

†This column provides guidelines for further assessment and initial nursing intervention.

Assessment Guide: Intrapartal—First Stage of Labor *continued*

PHYSICAL ASSESSMENT/ NORMAL FINDINGS	ALTERATIONS AND POSSIBLE CAUSES*	NURSING RESPONSES TO DATA†
➤ LABOR STATUS *Continued*		
Findings on Nitrazine test tape: Membranes probably intact yellow pH 5.0 olive pH 5.5 olive green pH 6.0	False-positive results may be obtained if large amount of bloody show is present, previous vaginal examination has been done using lubricant, or tape is touched by nurse's fingers.	Assess fluid for consistency, amount, odor; assess FHR frequently. Assess fluid at regular intervals for presence of meconium staining. Follow universal precautions while assessing amniotic fluid.
Membranes probably ruptured blue-green pH 6.5 blue-gray pH 7.0 deep blue pH 7.5		Teach woman that amniotic fluid is continually produced (to allay fear of "dry birth"). Teach woman that she may feel amniotic fluid trickle or gush with contractions. Change Chux pads often.
Amniotic fluid clear, with earthy or human odor, no foul-smelling odor	Greenish amniotic fluid (fetal stress) Bloody fluid (vasoprevia abruptio placentae)	Assess FHR; do vaginal exam to evaluate for prolapsed cord; apply fetal monitor for continuous data; report to physician/CNM.
	Strong or foul odor (amnionitis)	Take woman's temperature and report to physician/CNM.
➤ FETAL STATUS		
FHR: 110–160 bpm	<110 or > 160 bpm (fetal stress); abnormal patterns on fetal monitor: decreased variability, late decelerations, variable decelerations, absence of accelerations with fetal movement	Initiate interventions based on particular FHR pattern.
Presentation: Cephalic, 97% Breech, 3%	Face, brow, breech, or shoulder presentation	Report to physician; after presentation is confirmed as face, brow, breech, or shoulder, woman may be prepared for cesarean birth.
Position: left-occiput-anterior (LOA) most common	Persistent occipital-posterior (OP) position; transverse arrest	Carefully monitor maternal and fetal status. Reposition mother side-lying or hands/knee to promote rotation of fetal head.
Activity: fetal movement	Hyperactivity (may precede fetal hypoxia)	Carefully evaluate FHR; apply fetal monitor.
	Complete lack of movement (fetal distress or fetal demise)	Carefully evaluate FHR; apply fetal monitor. Report to physician/CNM.
➤ LABORATORY EVALUATION		
Hematologic tests ***Hemoglobin:*** 12–16 g/dL	< 11 g/dL (anemia, hemorrhage, Sickle cell disorders, pernicious anemia)	Evaluate woman for problems due to decreased oxygen-carrying capacity caused by lowered hemoglobin.

*Possible causes of alterations are placed in parentheses.

†This column provides guidelines for further assessment and initial nursing intervention.

(continued on next page)

Assessment Guide: Intrapartal—First Stage of Labor *continued*

PHYSICAL ASSESSMENT/ NORMAL FINDINGS	ALTERATIONS AND POSSIBLE CAUSES*	NURSING RESPONSES TO DATA†
➤ **LABORATORY EVALUATION** *Continued*		
CBC ***Hematocrit:*** 38%–47% ***RBC:*** 4.2–5.4 million/mm^3 ***WBC:*** 4500–11,000/mm^3, although leukocytosis to 20,000/mm^3 is not unusual ***Platelets*** 150,000–400,000/mm^3	Presence of infection or blood dyscrasias, loss of blood (hemorrhage, disseminated intravascular coagulation [DIC])	Evaluate for other signs of infection or for petechiae, bruising, or unusual bleeding.
Serologic testing STS or VDRL test: nonreactive	Positive reaction (Chapter 15, Initial Prenatal Physical Assessment Guide)	For reactive test notify newborn nursery and pediatrician.
Rh	Rh-positive fetus in Rh-negative woman	Assess prenatal record for titer levels during pregnancy. Obtain cord blood for direct Coombs' at birth.
Urinalysis Glucose: negative	Glycosuria (low renal threshold for glucose, diabetes mellitus)	Assess blood glucose; test urine for ketones; ketonuria and glycosuria require further assessment of blood sugars.‡
Ketones: negative	Ketonuria (starvation ketosis)	
Proteins: negative	Proteinuria (urine specimen contaminated with vaginal secretions, fever, kidney disease); proteinuria of 2+ or greater found in uncontaminated urine may be a sign of ensuing preeclampsia	Instruct woman in collection technique; incidence of contamination from vaginal discharge is common. Report any increase in proteinuria to physician/CNM.
Red blood cells: negative	Blood in urine (calculi, cystitis, glomerulonephritis, neoplasm)	Assess collection technique (may be bloody show).
White blood cells: negative	Presence of white blood cells (infection in genitourinary tract)	Assess for signs of urinary tract infection.
Casts: none	Presence of casts (nephrotic syndrome)	

CULTURAL ASSESSMENT§	VARIATIONS TO CONSIDER	NURSING RESPONSES TO DATA†
Cultural influences determine customs and practices regarding intrapartal care.	Individual preferences may vary.	
Ask the following questions: Who would you like to remain with you during your labor and birth?	She may prefer only her coach to remain or may also want family and/or friends.	Provide support for her wishes by encouraging desired people to stay. Provide information to others (with the woman's permission) who are not in the room.

§ These are only a few suggestions. We do not mean to imply that this is a comprehensive cultural assessment; rather, it is a tool to encourage cultural sensitivity.

*Possible causes of alterations are placed in parentheses.

†This column provides guidelines for further assessment and initial nursing intervention.

‡Glycosuria should not be discounted. The presence of glycosuria necessitates follow-up.

➤

ASSESSMENT GUIDE: INTRAPARTAL—FIRST STAGE OF LABOR *continued*

CULTURAL ASSESSMENT[§]	VARIATIONS TO CONSIDER	NURSING RESPONSES TO DATA[†]
What would you like to wear during labor?	She may be more comfortable in her own clothes.	Offer supportive materials such as Chux if needed to protect her own clothing. Avoid subtle signals to the woman that she should not have chosen to remain in her own clothes. Have other clothing available if the woman desires. If her clothing becomes contaminated, it will be simple to place it in a plastic bag.
What activity would you like during labor?	She may want to ambulate most of the time, stand in the shower, sit in the jacuzzi, sit on a chair/stool/birthing ball, remain on the bed, and so forth.	Support the woman's wishes; provide encouragement and complete assessments in a manner so her activity and positional wishes are disturbed as little as possible.
What position would you like for the birth?	She may feel more comfortable in lithotomy with stirrups and her upper body elevated, or side-lying or sitting in birthing bed, or standing, or squatting, or on hands and knees.	Collect any supplies and equipment needed to support her in her chosen birthing position. Provide information to the coach regarding any changes that may be needed based on the chosen position.
Is there anything special you would like?	She may want the room darkened or to have curtains and windows open, music playing, a Leboyer birth, her coach to cut the umbilical cord, to save a portion of the umbilical cord, to save the placenta, to videotape the birth, and so forth.	Support requests, and communicate requests to any other nursing or medical personnel (so requests can continue to be supported and not questioned). If another nurse or physician does not honor the request, act as advocate for the woman by continuing to support her unless her desire is truly unsafe.
Ask the woman if she would like fluids, and ask what temperature she prefers.	She may prefer clear fluids other than water (tea, clear juice). She may prefer iced, room-temperature, or warmed fluids.	Provide fluids as desired.
Observe the woman's response when privacy is difficult to maintain and her body is exposed.	Some women do not seem to mind being exposed during an exam or procedure; others feel acute discomfort.	Maintain privacy and respect the woman's sense of privacy. If the woman is unable to provide specific information, the nurse may draw from general information regarding cultural variation: Southeast Asian women may not want any family member in the room during exam or procedures. Her partner may not be involved with coaching activities during labor or birth. Muslim women may need to remain covered during the labor and birth and avoid exposure of any body part. The husband may need to be in the room but remain behind a curtain or screen so he does not view his wife at this time.
If the woman is to breastfeed, ask if she would like to feed her baby immediately after birth.	She may want to feed her baby right away or may want to wait a little while.	

[§] These are only a few suggestions. We do not mean to imply that this is a comprehensive cultural assessment; rather, it is a tool to encourage cultural sensitivity.

[†]This column provides guidelines for further assessment and initial nursing intervention.

(continued on next page)

Assessment Guide: Intrapartal—First Stage of Labor *continued*

PSYCHOSOCIAL ASSESSMENT	VARIATIONS TO CONSIDER	NURSING RESPONSES TO DATA†
➤ PREPARATION FOR CHILDBIRTH		
Woman has some information regarding process of normal labor and birth.	Some women do not have any information regarding childbirth.	Add to present information base.
Woman has breathing and/or relaxation techniques to use during labor.	Some women do not have any method of relaxation or breathing to use, and some do not desire them.	Support breathing and relaxation techniques that client is using; provide information if needed.
Woman and support person have done extensive preparation for childbirth (Bradley Classes, Lamaze).	Some women have strong opinions regarding labor and birth preparation.	Support woman's wishes to participate her birth experience; support birth plan.
➤ RESPONSE TO LABOR		
Latent phase: relaxed, excited, anxious for labor to be well established	May feel unable to cope with contractions because of fear, anxiety, or lack of information	Provide support and encouragement; establish trusting relationship.
Active phase: becomes more intense, begins to tire ***Transitional phase:*** feels tired, may feel unable to cope, needs frequent coaching to maintain breathing patterns	May remain quiet and without any sign of discomfort or anxiety, may insist that she is unable to continue with the birthing process	Provide support and coaching if needed.
Coping mechanisms: Ability to cope with labor through use of support system, breathing, relaxation techniques, and comfort measures including frequent position changes in labor, warm water immersion, and massage.	May feel marked anxiety and apprehension, may not have coping mechanisms that can be brought into this experience, or may be unable to use them at this time	Support coping mechanisms if they are working for the woman; provide information and support if she exhibits anxiety or needs alternative to present coping methods.
	Survivors of sexual abuse may demonstrate fear of IVs or needles, may recoil when touched, may insist on a female caregiver, may be very sensitive to body fluids and cleanliness, and may be unable to labor lying down (Burrian, 1995)	Encourage participation of coach/significant other if a supportive relationship seems apparent. Establish rapport and a trusting relationship. Provide information that is true and offer your presence.
➤ ANXIETY		
Some anxiety and apprehension is within normal limits	May show anxiety through rapid breathing, nervous tremors, frowning, grimacing, clenching of teeth, thrashing movements, crying, increased pulse and blood pressure	Provide support, encouragement, and information. Teach relaxation techniques; support controlled breathing efforts. May need to provide a paper bag to breathe into if woman says her lips are tingling. Note FHR.
➤ SOUNDS DURING LABOR		
	Some women are very quiet; others moan or make a variety of noises.	Provide a supportive environment. Encourage woman to do what feels right for her.

†This column provides guidelines for further assessment and initial nursing intervention.

➤

ASSESSMENT GUIDE: INTRAPARTAL—FIRST STAGE OF LABOR *continued*

PSYCHOSOCIAL ASSESSMENT	VARIATIONS TO CONSIDER	NURSING RESPONSES TO DATA†
➤ SUPPORT SYSTEM		
Physical intimacy between mother and father (or mother and support person/doula) caretaking activities such as soothing conversation, touching	Some women would prefer no contact, others may show clinging behaviors.	Encourage caretaking activities that appear to comfort the woman; encourage support for the woman; if support is limited, the nurse may take a more active role.
Support person stays in close proximity	Limited interaction may come from a desire for quiet.	Encourage support person to stay close (if this seems appropriate).
Relationship between mother and father (or support person): involved interaction	The support person may seem to be detached and maintain little support, attention, or conversation.	Support interactions; if interaction is limited, the nurse may provide more information and support. Ensure that coach/significant other has short breaks, especially/prior to transition.

†This column provides guidelines for further assessment and initial nursing intervention.

Methods of Evaluating Labor Progress

In evaluating labor progress, the nurse assesses the progress of uterine contractions and the dilation and effacement of the cervix.

CONTRACTION ASSESSMENT

Uterine contractions may be assessed by palpation or continuous electronic monitoring.

Palpation

The nurse assesses contractions for frequency, duration, and intensity by placing one hand on the uterine fundus. The hand is kept relatively still because excessive movement may stimulate contractions or cause discomfort. The nurse determines the frequency of the contractions by noting the time from the beginning of one contraction to the beginning of the next. If contractions begin at 7:00, 7:04, and 7:08, for example, their frequency is every 4 minutes. To determine contraction duration, the nurse notes the time when tensing of the fundus is first felt (beginning of contraction) and again as relaxation occurs (end of contraction).

During the acme (peak) of the contraction, intensity can be evaluated by estimating the firmness of the fundus. Some nurses find it useful to compare the contraction to the firmness of a nose, chin, or forehead. For example, a contraction that can be indented as easily as a nose is a mild contraction, whereas strong contractions have the same firmness as a forehead. The nurse should assess at least three successive contractions to provide reliable data. Table 23–2 • compares contraction characteristics in different phases of labor.

This is also a good time to assess the laboring woman's perception of pain. What is her affect? Is this contraction more uncomfortable than the last one? Is the nurse's palpation of intensity congruent with the woman's perception? (For instance, the nurse might evaluate a contraction as mild in intensity while the laboring woman evaluates it as very strong.) The nurse can ask the laboring woman to use a pain scale (for example, a 1 to 10 scale) to evaluate her pain. A nurse's assessment is not complete unless the laboring woman's affect and response to the contractions are also noted and charted.

Table 23–2 • CONTRACTION AND LABOR PROGRESS CHARACTERISTICS

Contraction Characteristics	
Latent phase:	Every 10–30 min × 20–40 sec; mild, progressing to Every 5–7 min × 30–40 sec; moderate
Active phase:	Every 2–3 min × 40–60 sec; moderate to strong
Transition phase:	Every 1½–2 min × 60–90 sec; strong
Labor Progress Characteristics	
Primipara:	1.2 cm/hr dilatation 1 cm/hr descent <2 hr in second stage
Multipara:	1.5 cm/hr dilatation 2 cm/hr descent <1 hr in second stage

Procedure 23–1 Performing an Intrapartal Vaginal Examination

Preparation

Clinical Tip
Use nonlatex gloves if the woman has a latex allergy

1. Explain the procedure, the indications for the exam, what the exam may feel like, and that it may cause discomfort.
2. Assess for latex allergies.
3. Position the woman with her thighs flexed and abducted. Instruct her to put the heels of her feet together. Drape the woman with a sheet, leaving a flap to access the perineum.
   Rationale: This position provides access to the woman's perineum. The drape ensures privacy.
4. Encourage the woman to relax her muscles and legs.
   Rationale: Relaxation decreases muscle tension and increases comfort.
5. Inform the woman prior to touching her. Be gentle.

Equipment and Supplies

- Clean disposable gloves if membranes not ruptured.
- Sterile gloves if membranes ruptured.
- Lubricant
- Nitrazine test tape
- Slide
- Sterile cotton-tipped swab (Q-tip)

Before the Procedure: *Test for Fluid Leakage*

If fluid leakage has been reported or noted, use Nitrazine test tape and Q-tip with slide for fern test before performing the exam (see Procedure 23-2).

Procedure: *Clean Gloves (Sterile if membranes ruptured)*

Clinical Tip
Digital examination may be deferred if the woman has ruptured membranes but is not in active labor (AAP & ACOG, 2002).

1. Pull glove onto dominant hand.
   Rationale: Single glove is worn when membranes are intact. If a sterile exam is needed, both hands will be gloved with sterile gloves.
2. Using your gloved hand, position the hand with the wrist straight and the elbow tilted downward. Insert your well-lubricated second and index fingers of the gloved hand gently into the vagina until they touch the cervix. Use care when positioning your hand.
   Rationale: This position allows the fingertips to point toward the umbilicus and find the cervix.
3. If the woman verbalizes discomfort, acknowledge it and apologize. Pause for a moment and allow her to relax before progressing.
   Rationale: This validates the woman's discomfort and helps her feel more in control.
4. To determine the status of labor progress, perform the vaginal examination during and between contractions.
   Rationale: Cervical effacement, dilatation, and fetal station are affected by the presence of a contraction.
5. Palpate for the opening, or a depression, in the cervix. Estimate the diameter of the depression to identify the amount of dilatation (see Figure 23-1 •).
   Rationale: Allows determination of effacement and dilatation.
6. Determine the status of the fetal membranes by observing for leakage of amniotic fluid. If fluid is expressed, test for amniotic fluid.
7. Palpate the presenting part (see Figure 23-2 •).
   Rationale: Determine the presenting part is necessary to assess the position of the fetus and to evaluate fetal descent.
8. Assess the fetal descent (see Figure 23-3 •) and station by identifying the position of the posterior fontanelle.
9. Record findings on woman's chart and on fetal monitor strip if fetal monitor is being used.

Procedure 23-1 *(continued)*

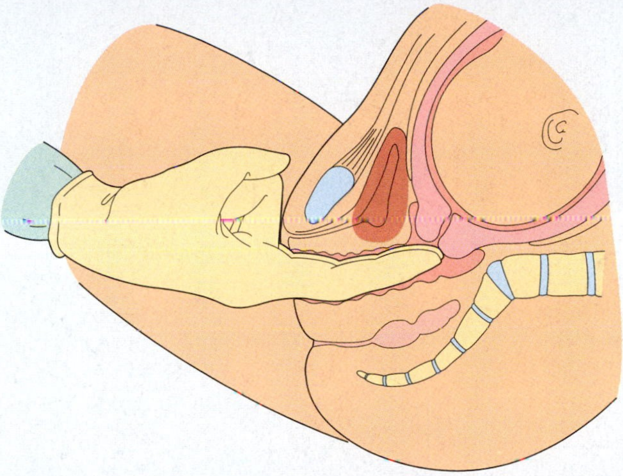

Figure 23–1 • To gauge cervical dilatation, the nurse places the index and middle fingers against the cervix and determines the size of the opening. Before labor begins, the cervix is long (approximately 2.5 cm), the sides feel thick, and the cervical canal is closed, so an examining finger cannot be inserted. During labor, the cervix begins to dilate, and the size of the opening progresses from 1 cm to 10 cm in diameter.

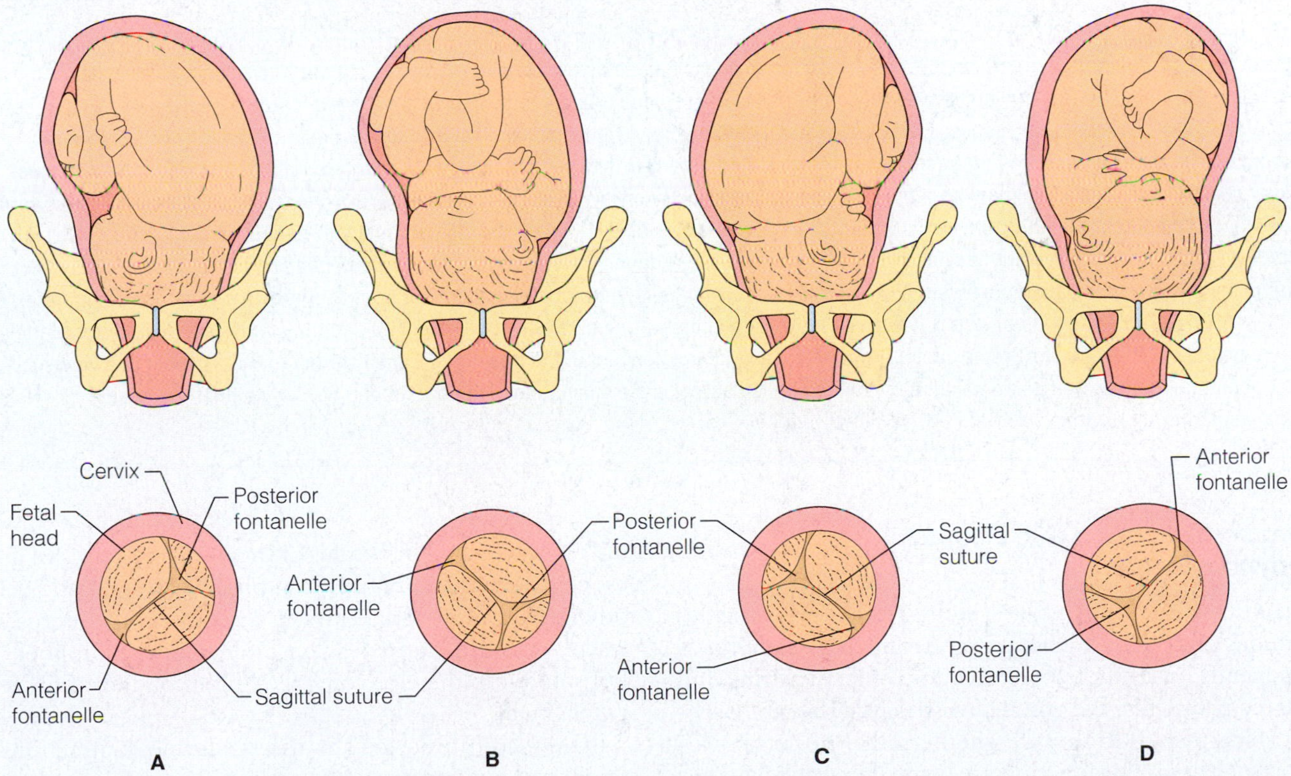

Figure 23–2 • Palpation of the presenting part (the portion of the fetus that enters the pelvis first). *A,* Left occiput anterior (LOA). The occiput (area over the occipital bone on the posterior part of the fetal head) is in the left anterior quadrant of the woman's pelvis. When the fetus is in LOA, the posterior fontanelles (located just above the occipital bone and triangular in shape) are in the upper left quadrant of the maternal pelvis. *B,* Left occiput posterior (LOP). The posterior fontanelle is in the lower left quadrant of the maternal pelvis. *C,* Right occiput anterior (ROA). The posterior fontanelle is in the upper right quadrant of the maternal pelvis. *D,* Right occiput posterior (ROP). The posterior fontanelle is in the lower right quadrant of the maternal pelvis. *Note:* The anterior fontanelle is diamond shaped. Because of the roundness of the fetal head, only a portion of the anterior fontanelle can be seen in each of the views, so it appears to be triangular in shape.

(continued on next page)

Procedure 23-1 Performing an Intrapartal Vaginal Examination (continued)

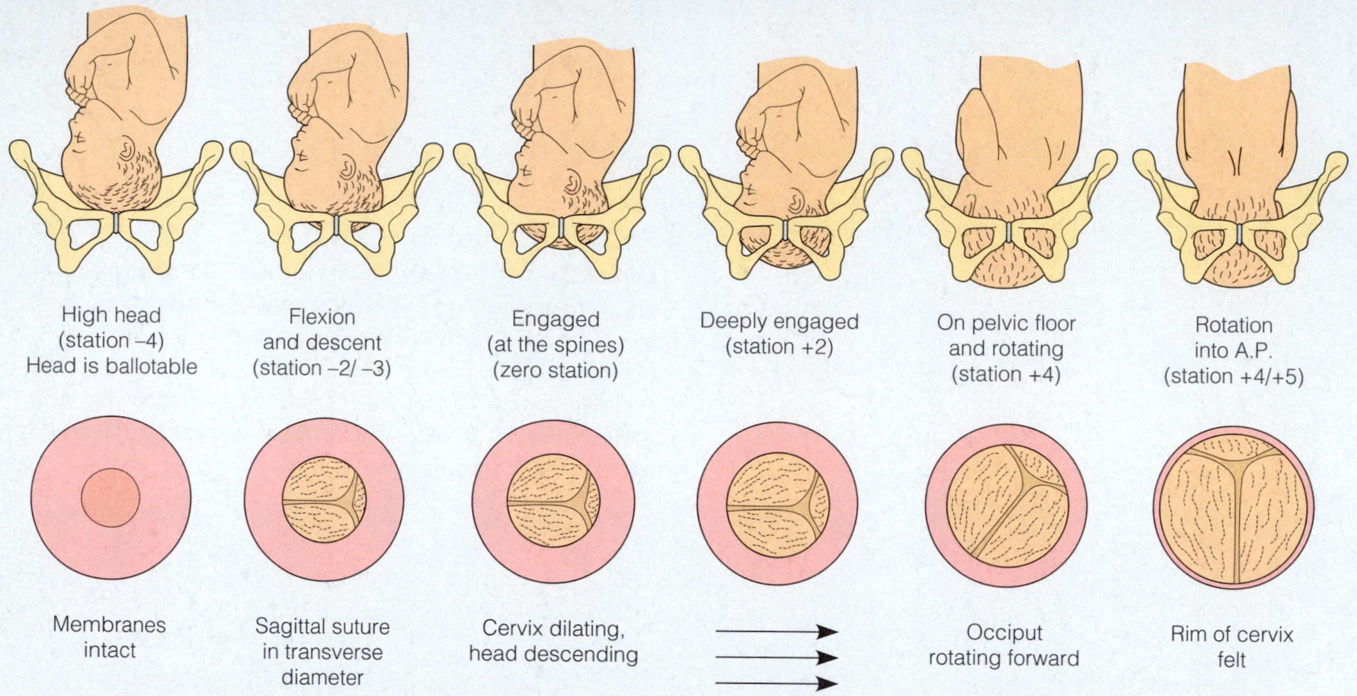

Figure 23–3 • Descent of the fetus through the maternal pelvis can be assessed by determining station (the relationship of the presenting part to an imaginary line between the maternal ischial spines). As the fetus moves downward, cardinal movements occur (see Chapter 22). The nurse assesses the station and identifies the cardinal movements by determining the position of the posterior fontanelle. The upper panels depict the fetal head progressing downward through the pelvis. From left to right, the first four views depict descent and flexion of the fetal chin onto the fetal chest. In the last two views, internal rotation occurs. Each view also depicts downward movement of the fetal head through the maternal pelvis as measured by the change in station. The lower panels depict the cervix, which is still rather thick (little effacement has occurred). The amniotic membranes are still intact over the fetal head. When the fetus is at −4 station, the fetal head is ballotable (when it is touched by the examining nurse's finger, the head floats upward and resettles downward). In the second view, note the thinner cervix (which indicates that more effacement has occurred). The sagittal suture and posterior fontanelle can be palpated. The next two views depict further effacement and descent of the fetal head from 0 station to +2. The last two views depict continuing effacement and position that would be felt on vaginal examination of the presenting part while the fetal head is completing internal rotation.

Electronic Monitoring with External Tocodynamometer

Electronic monitoring of uterine contractions provides continuous data. How much an electronic fetal monitor is used depends on many factors: the type of birth setting and associated protocols, the couple's wishes, whether the pregnancy is low risk or high risk, whether other obstetric procedures such as labor induction are being done, and whether other monitoring methods such as ultrasound can be used as a substitute.

Electronic monitoring may be done externally, with a device that is placed against the maternal abdomen, or internally, with an intrauterine pressure catheter. When monitoring by external means, the clinician places the portion of the monitoring equipment called the *tocodynamometer*, or "toco," against the fundus of the uterus (the area of greatest contractility) and holds it in place with an elastic belt or other adhesive material (Figure 23–4 •). As the uterus contracts, pressure exerted against the toco is amplified and transmitted to the electronic fetal monitor and recorded on graph paper.

The toco can be used to assess uterine contractions for frequency and duration, but not for intensity. The intensity (as displayed on the graph paper) is a reflection of how tightly the belt is applied around the maternal abdomen and/or maternal habitus. In thin women, the monitor may reflect a high level of pressure on the tracing even though the woman feels mild contractions. In contrast, a heavyset woman's tracing may reveal a low level of pressure on the monitoring strip although the woman notes strong contractions. When the belt

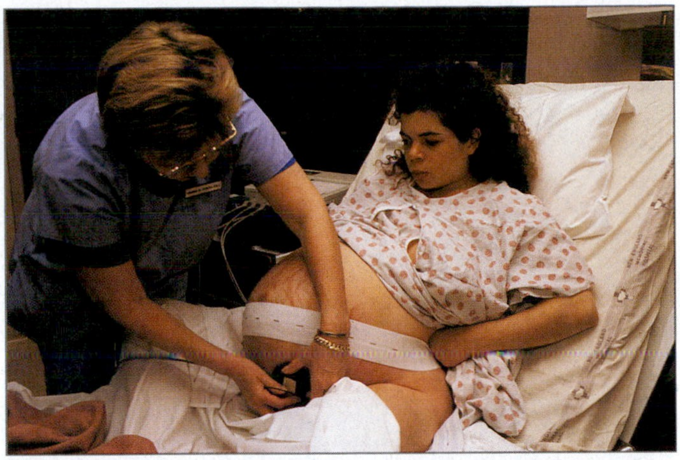

Figure 23–4 • Woman in labor with external monitor applied. The tocodynamometer placed on the uterine fundus is recording uterine contractions. The lower belt holds the ultrasonic device that monitors the fetal heart rate. The belts can be adjusted for comfort.

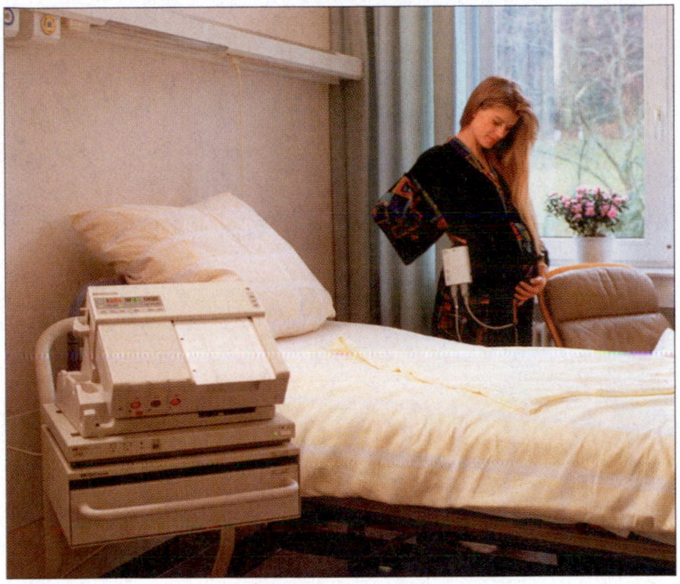

Figure 23–5 • The beltless tocodynamometer system features remote telemetry.
SOURCE: Courtesy of Hewlett-Packard Company.

is tight enough, the nurse should be able to note the beginning of contractions on the monitor just before or at the same time the woman begins to feel them.

The advantages to this method are that it may be used both prior to and following rupture of membranes and it provides a continuous recording of the duration and frequency of contractions. It is also noninvasive and can be used intermittently if the physician/CNM wants the woman to ambulate, or if the woman wishes to shower or use a whirlpool bath. The major disadvantage, as noted earlier, is that it cannot assess the intensity of contractions. Intensity of contractions must be assessed by palpation. Another disadvantage is that sometimes the belt bothers the woman because it must be snug to monitor uterine contractions accurately. The belt may require frequent readjustment as she changes position, or the woman may feel she needs to remain in one position so as not to disturb the belt.

A beltless tocodynamometer is available. This system consists of an adhesive transducer that is applied to the most prominent part of the woman's abdomen with a double-sided adhesive film. The nonbelted tocodynamometer tends to be preferred by the laboring woman because it allows more freedom of movement, is easily applied, needs readjustment only infrequently, and generally is more convenient (Figure 23–5 •). It enables upright positions, which promote fetal descent by gravity, as well as ambulation, which can shorten the labor course and increase comfort for the laboring woman.

It is of particular importance that the nurse evaluates the woman's labor status by means other than the fetal monitor. As with any type of technology, no machine is flawless, and the monitor cannot fill the role of the nurse. All too often, women are in active labor with adequate contractions that are regarded as being of "poor quality" because the monitor is not functioning properly. The nurse should routinely palpate the intensity of the contractions and the relaxation of the uterus between contractions and compare the assessment with data recorded by the monitor.

> *Trying to figure out if I was in labor was quite a task. Here I was, a birthing room nurse, and I couldn't decide if my contractions were the real thing. I timed them, and about the time I decided this was it, they would slow down. How exasperating not to know! It was so hard on me. But now I see that all women are in this spot. They want so much to be right, and we often treat them as if they should be able to sense when it's the real thing. I'd like birthing room nurses to remember this.*

Electronic Monitoring by Internal Pressure Catheter

If the amniotic membranes are ruptured, internal monitoring can be used. The **intrauterine pressure catheter (IUPC)** not only provides information regarding frequency and duration of uterine contractions, but also assesses intensity of uterine contractions. If the position of the placenta has been noted on a previous ultrasound, it can assist the physician/CNM in placing the IUPC in the correct position. Insertion of an IUPC with a low-lying placenta could result in placenta puncture, leading to hemorrhage and possible fetal distress.

One type of intrauterine catheter, called the INTRAN Plus, has a micropressure transducer (electronic sensor) at the tip. The catheter is slowly inserted through the cervical os into the uterine cavity, usually in the area where fetal small parts (arms or legs) are located. The catheter is advanced only as far as the black marking indicated on the catheter, which should be visualized at the opening to the vagina

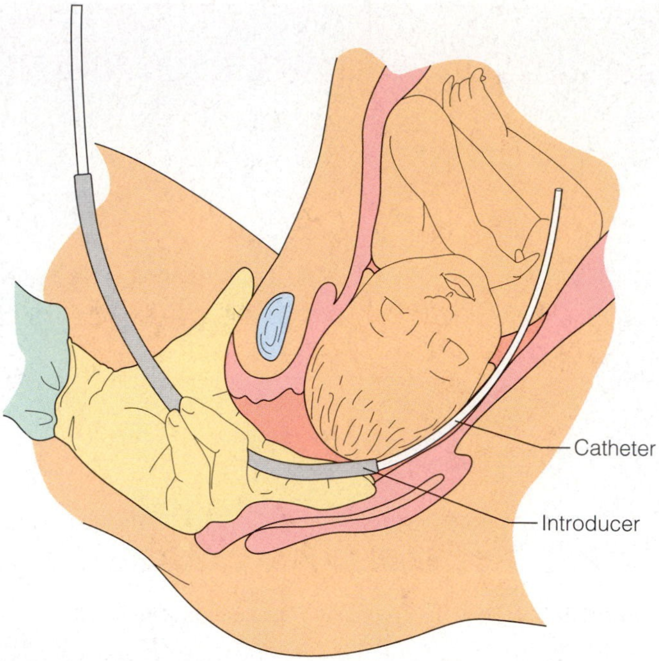

Figure 23–6 • Technique of inserting a uterine catheter. Note that the introducer (catheter guide) is inserted no farther than beyond the fingertips.

(Figure 23–6 •). The catheter is then connected by a cable to the electronic fetal monitor. This catheter incorporates a second lumen and a port for amnioinfusion (an infusion of fluid into the amniotic cavity to provide additional fluid or to dilute amniotic fluid that contains thick meconium). The second port permits amnioinfusion while simultaneously providing accurate monitoring of intrauterine pressure (Figure 23–7 •).

An IUPC is used when the provider needs closer uterine monitoring or amnioinfusion is indicated. It is particularly important to quantitate the intensity and frequency of contractions to avoid hyperstimulation and possible uterine rupture in women with a previous history of cesarean birth who are attempting a vaginal birth after cesarean (VBAC) and are receiving oxytocin. If the woman's labor is prolonged, internal monitoring can be used to accurately assess the frequency and strength of contractions and resultant FHR pattern response. When an intrauterine catheter is used, there is a 1% risk of infection, but this seems to depend on the duration of ruptured membranes and length of labor.

CERVICAL ASSESSMENT

Cervical dilatation and effacement are evaluated directly by vaginal examination (see Procedure 23–1: Performing an Intrapartal Vaginal Examination). The vaginal examination can also provide information regarding fetal position, station of the presenting part, and membrane status (intact or ruptured). To assist in evaluating membrane status, the nurse assesses for the presence of amniotic fluid (Procedure 23–2: Assessing for Amniotic Fluid).

MediaLink CASE STUDY: MATERNAL ASSESSMENT DURING LABOR

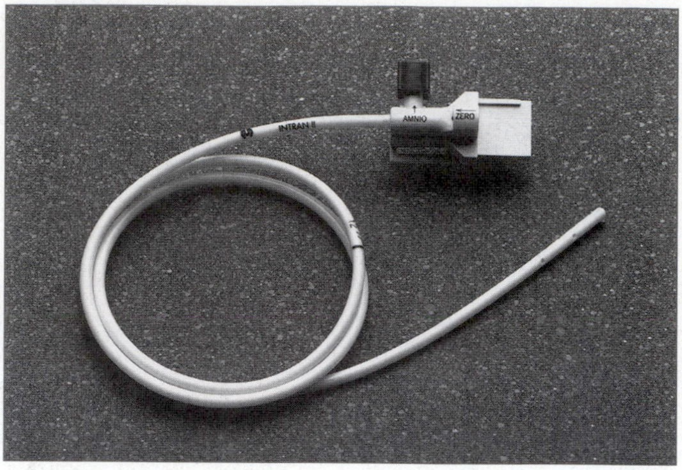

Figure 23–7 • INTRAN Plus intrauterine pressure catheter. There is a micropressure transducer (electronic sensor) located at the tip of the catheter and a port for amnioinfusion at the distal end of the catheter.

Fetal Assessment

A complete intrapartal fetal assessment requires determination of the fetal position and presentation, and evaluation of the fetal status.

Determination of Fetal Position and Presentation

Fetal position is determined in several ways, including the following:

- Inspection of the woman's abdomen
- Palpation of the woman's abdomen
- Vaginal examination to determine the presenting part
- Ultrasound

INSPECTION

The nurse should observe the woman's abdomen for size and shape. The lie of the fetus should be assessed by noting whether the uterus projects up and down (longitudinal lie) or left to right (transverse lie).

PALPATION: LEOPOLD'S MANEUVERS

Leopold's maneuvers are a systematic way to evaluate the maternal abdomen (Figure 23–8 •). Frequent practice increases the examiner's skill in determining fetal position by palpation. Leopold's maneuvers may be difficult to perform on an obese woman or on a woman who has excessive amniotic fluid (hydramnios).

Care should be taken to ensure the woman's comfort during Leopold's maneuvers. The woman should have recently emptied her bladder and should lie on her back with her abdomen uncovered. To aid in relaxation of the abdominal wall, the shoulders should be raised slightly on a pillow and the knees drawn up a little. The procedure should be completed between contractions. The examiner's hands should be warm.

Procedure 23–2 Assessing for Amniotic Fluid

Preparation

1. Explain the procedure, indications for the procedure, what the woman will feel, and information that may be obtained.
2. Determine whether she has noted the escape of any fluid from her vagina.

Equipment and Supplies

- Nitrazine test tape
- Sterile speculum
- A glass slide and a sterile cotton tipped swab (Q-tip)
- Sterile syringe
- Microscope

Procedure: *Sterile Gloves*

1. Complete this test before doing an examination that requires the use of lubricant.
2. Put on sterile gloves. With one gloved hand, spread the labia, and with the other gloved hand place a small section of nitrazine tape (approx. 2 in long) against the vaginal opening. Take care not to touch the tape with bare fingers prior to the test.
   Rationale: Contamination of the Nitrazine test tape with lubricant can make the test unreliable. Enough fluid needs to be placed on the test tape to make it wet.
3. Compare the color on the test tape to the guide on the back of the Nitrazine test tape container to determine test results.
   Rationale: Amniotic fluid is alkaline, and an alkaline fluid turns the Nitrazine test tape a dark blue. If the test tape remains a beige color, the test is negative for amniotic fluid.
4. Amniotic fluid may also be obtained by speculum exam. This is indicated in preterm premature rupture of membranes. If fluid is present in sufficient amount to draw some into a syringe, a small amount should be collected, or the pool of fluid in the posterior vagina can be obtained with a sterile cotton swab. A small amount of fluid is placed on a glass slide, allowed to dry, and then examined under the microscope. A ferning pattern confirms the presence of amniotic fluid. See figure 12–4 for an example of ferning.
   Rationale: Obtaining a specimen by speculum examination reduces the contamination of the fluid with other substances such as blood and cervical mucus and reduces the chance of infection for the woman who is not actively laboring.
5. Record the findings on the labor record.
   Rationale: Documentation of the status of membranes should include intact or ruptured. Other characteristics, such as color, odor, and amount of fluid present should also be recorded.

While inspecting and palpating the maternal abdomen, the nurse should consider the following questions:

- Is the fetal lie longitudinal or transverse?
- What is in the fundus? Am I feeling buttocks or head?
- Where is the fetal back?
- Where are the small parts or extremities?
- What is in the inlet? Does it confirm what I found in the fundus?
- Is the presenting part engaged, floating, or dipping into the inlet?
- Is there fetal movement?
- How large is the fetus (appropriate, large, or small for gestational age)?
- Is there one fetus or more than one?
- Is fundal height proportionate to the estimated gestational age?

First Maneuver

While facing the woman, the nurse palpates the upper abdomen with both hands (Figure 23–8, *A*). The nurse determines the shape, size, consistency, and mobility of the form that is found. The fetal head is firm, hard, and round and moves independently of the trunk. The breech feels softer and symmetric and has small bony prominences; it moves with the trunk.

Second Maneuver

After ascertaining whether the head or the buttocks occupies the fundus, the nurse tries to determine the location of the fetal back and notes whether it is on the right or left side of

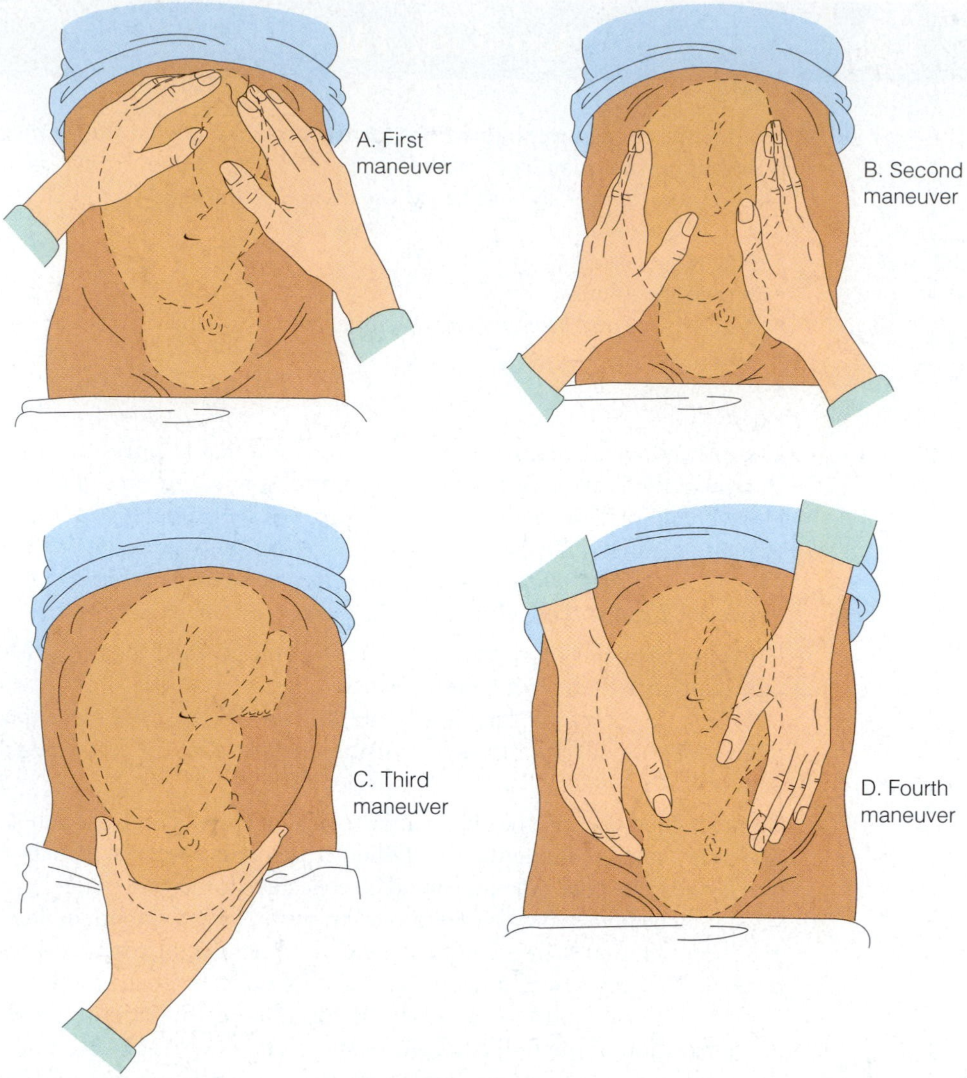

Figure 23–8 • Leopold's maneuvers for determining fetal position, presentation, and lie. *Note:* Many nurses do the fourth maneuver first to identify the part of the fetus in the pelvic inlet.

the maternal abdomen. Still facing the woman, the nurse palpates the abdomen with deep but gentle pressure, using the palms (Figure 23–8, *B*). The right hand should be steady while the left hand explores the right side of the uterus. The nurse then repeats the maneuver, probing with the right hand and steadying the uterus with the left hand. The fetal back should feel firm and smooth and should connect what was found in the fundus with a mass in the inlet. Once the back is located, the nurse validates the finding by palpating the fetal extremities (small irregularities and protrusions) on the opposite side of the abdomen.

Third Maneuver

Next the nurse should determine what fetal part is lying above the inlet by gently grasping the lower portion of the abdomen just above the symphysis pubis with the thumb and fingers of the right hand (Figure 23–8, *C*). This maneuver yields the opposite information from what was found in the fundus and validates the presenting part. If the head is presenting and is not engaged, it may be gently pushed back and forth.

Fourth Maneuver

For this portion of the examination, the nurse faces the woman's feet and attempts to locate the cephalic prominence or brow. Location of this landmark assists in assessing the descent of the presenting part into the pelvis. The fingers of both hands are moved gently down the sides of the uterus toward the pubis (Figure 23–8, *D*). The cephalic prominence (brow) is located on the side where there is greatest resistance to the descent of the fingers toward the pubis. It is located on the opposite side from the fetal back if the head is well flexed. However, when the fetal head is extended, the occiput is the first cephalic prominence felt, and it is located on the same side as the back. Therefore, when completing the fourth maneuver, if the first cephalic prominence palpated is on the same side as the back, the head is not flexed. If the first prominence found is opposite the back, the head is well flexed.

VAGINAL EXAMINATION

The vaginal examination reveals information regarding the fetus such as presentation, position, station, degree of flexion of the fetal head, and any swelling that might be present on the fetal scalp (caput succedaneum).

ULTRASOUND

Real-time ultrasound is frequently available in the birth setting. It may be used to assess fetal lie, presentation, and position; obtain measurements of biparietal diameter to estimate gestational age; assess for anomalies when a vaginal examination reveals suspicious findings; assess placement of the placenta; and sometimes confirm the presence of more than one fetus. (See Chapter 21 for further discussion of the use of ultrasound for fetal assessment.)

Auscultation of Fetal Heart Rate

The fetoscope or a handheld ultrasound device is used to auscultate the fetal heart rate (FHR) between, during, and immediately after uterine contractions (see Figure 23–9 •).

Before listening to the FHR the first time, the nurse may choose to perform Leopold's maneuvers to determine the probable location of the FHR. FHR is heard most clearly at the fetal back (Figure 23–10 •). Thus, in a cephalic presentation, FHR is best heard in the lower quadrant of the maternal abdomen. In a breech presentation it is heard at or above the level of the maternal umbilicus. In a transverse lie FHR may be heard best just above or just below the umbilicus. As the presenting part descends and rotates through the maternal pelvis during labor, FHR tends to descend and move toward the midline.

In some instances, the monitor may track the maternal heart rate instead of the fetal heart rate. However, the nurse can avoid the error by comparing the maternal pulse to the FHR.

After FHR is located, it is usually counted for 30 seconds and multiplied by 2 to obtain the number of beats per minute (bpm). The nurse should occasionally listen for 1 full minute, through and just after a contraction, to detect any abnormal heart rate, especially if the FHR is over 160 (tachycardia) or under 110 (bradycardia), or if irregular beats are heard. Listening through a contraction may be difficult because of maternal movement or a muffling of the FHR sounds. It is especially important to listen during and after the contraction to detect any deceleration that might occur. It is also important to listen immediately after each contraction when the woman is pushing during second stage because fetal bradycardia frequently occurs as pressure is exerted on the fetal head during descent. See

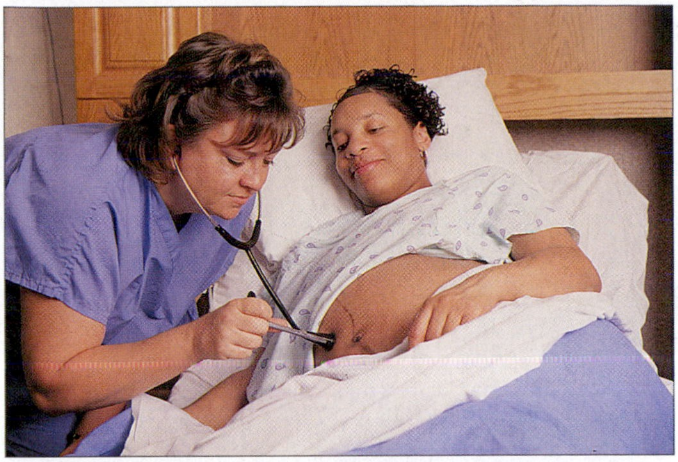

A

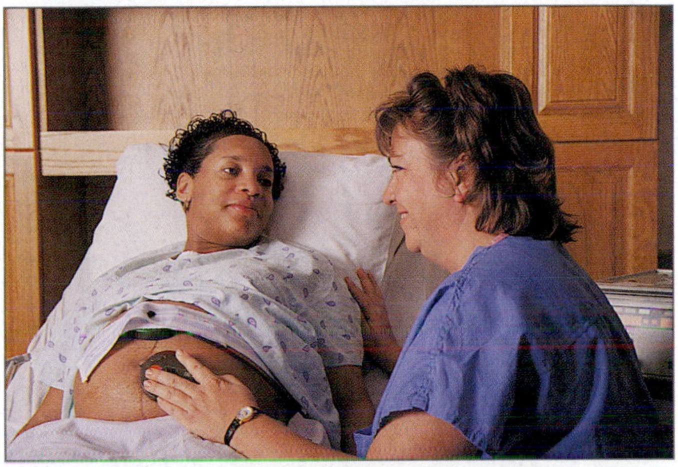

B

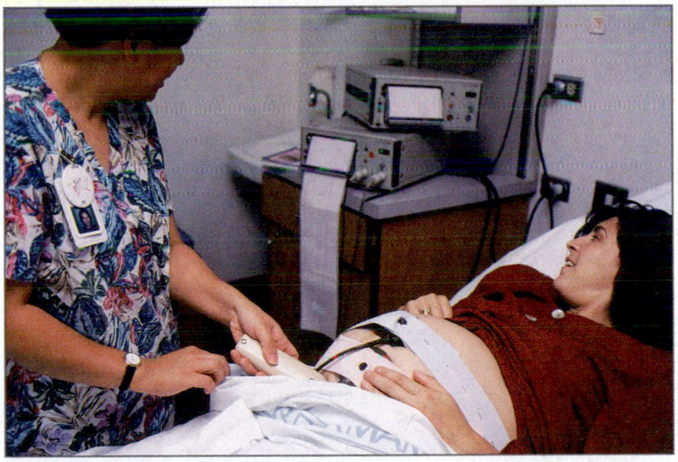

C

Figure 23–9 • *A,* The nurse holds the fetoscope as she places it against the maternal abdomen. *B,* When the fetal heart rate is picked up by the electronic monitor, the sound of the heartbeat can be heard by all persons in the room. *C,* The nurse uses a Doppler to assess the fetal heart rate. Doppler monitors can be used for intermittent labor monitoring or in the outpatient or community setting.
SOURCE: Michael Newman/PhotoEdit

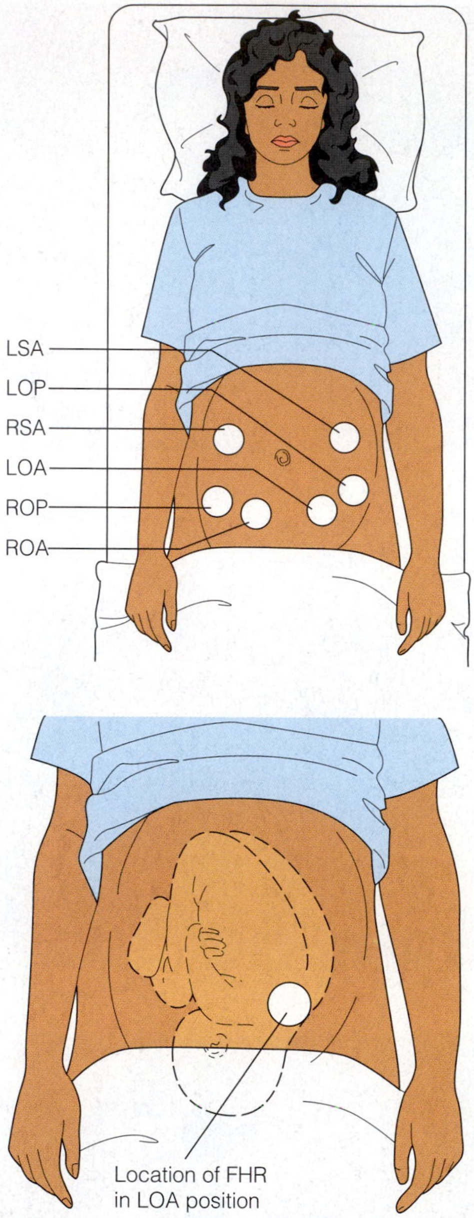

Figure 23–10 • Location of FHR in relation to the more commonly seen fetal positions. The fetal heart rate is heard more clearly over the fetal back.

Table 23–3 • FREQUENCY OF AUSCULTATION: ASSESSMENT AND DOCUMENTATION

Low-Risk Patients	High-Risk Patients
First stage of labor:	First stage of labor:
q1 hr in latent phase	q30 min in latent phase
q30 min in active phase	q15 min in active phase
Second stage of labor:	Second stage of labor:
q15 min	q5 min
Labor Events	
Assess FHR prior to:	
Initiation of labor-enhancing procedures (eg, artificial rupture of membranes)	
Periods of ambulation	
Administration of medications	
Administration or initiation of analgesia/anesthesia	
Assess FHR following:	
Rupture of membranes	
Recognition of abnormal uterine activity patterns, such as increased basal tone or tachysystole	
Evaluation of oxytocin (maintenance, increase, or decrease of dosage)	
Administration of medications (at time of peak action)	
Expulsion of enema	
Urinary catheterization	
Vaginal examination	
Periods of ambulation	
Evaluation of analgesia and/or anesthesia (maintenance, increase, or decrease of dosage)	

Source: Nurses' Association of the American College of Obstetricians and Gynecologists (NAACOG) (1990). *OGN nursing practice resource, fetal heart rate auscultation* (p. 5). Washington, DC: Author; Adapted from American Academy of Pediatrics (AAP), American College of Obstetricians and Gynecologists (ACOG) (1997). *Guidelines for perinatal care* (4th ed.). Washington, DC : Author.

Procedure 23–3: Auscultation of Fetal Heart Rate and Table 23–3 • for guidelines regarding how often to auscultate FHR.

Intermittent auscultation has been found to be as effective as electronic fetal monitoring (discussed next). A growing number of healthcare professionals, including obstetricians and labor and birth nurses, are beginning to question the widespread use of a technology that has not proven its overall worth (Feinstein, 2000).

Electronic Fetal Monitoring

Electronic fetal monitoring (EFM) provides a continuous tracing of the FHR, allowing many characteristics of the fetal heart rate to be observed and evaluated. (See Procedure 23–4: Electronic Fetal Monitoring.)

When the FHR is monitored electronically, the interval between two successive fetal heartbeats is continuously measured, and the rate is displayed as if the beats occurred at the same interval for 60 seconds. For example, if the interval between two beats is 0.5 second, the rate for 1 full minute would be 120 bpm.

INDICATIONS FOR ELECTRONIC FETAL MONITORING

The American College of Obstetricians and Gynecologists (ACOG) does not have a list of specific high-risk factors requiring EFM. Some physicians advocate monitoring only those women considered to be at risk or at high risk, whereas others require the procedure for all women in labor. Although there is no standardized list, Table 23–4 • identifies some common indications for EFM.

EXTERNAL MONITORING

External monitoring of the fetus is usually accomplished by ultrasound. A transducer, which emits continuous sound waves, is placed on the maternal abdomen. A water-soluble

Procedure 23–3 Auscultation of Fetal Heart Rate

Preparation

1. Explain the procedure, the indications for it, and the information that will be obtained.
2. Uncover the woman's abdomen.

Equipment and Supplies

- Doppler device
- Ultrasonic gel

Procedure

> **Clinical Tip**
> *The fetal heart rate (FHR) is heard most clearly through the fetal back. Locate the fetal back using Leopold's maneuvers.*

1. To use the Doppler:
   - Place ultrasonic gel on the diaphragm of the Doppler. Gel is used to maintain contact with the maternal abdomen and enhances conduction of sound.
   - Place the Doppler diaphragm on the woman's abdomen halfway between the umbilicus and symphysis and in the midline. You are most likely to hear the FHR in this area. Listen carefully for the sound of the fetal heartbeat.
2. Check the woman's pulse against the fetal sounds you hear. If the rates are the same, reposition the Doppler and try again.
   Rationale: If the rates are the same, you are probably hearing the maternal pulse and not the FHR.
3. If the rates are not similar, count the FHR for 1 full minute. Note that the FHR has a double rhythm and only one sound is counted.
4. If you do not locate the FHR, move the Doppler laterally (Figure 23–9, *B*).
5. Auscultate the FHR between, during, and for 30 seconds following a uterine contraction (UC).
6. Frequency recommendations:
   - Low-risk women: Every 1 hour in the latent phase, every 30 minutes in the active phase, and every 15 minutes in the second stage.
   - High-risk women: Every 30 minutes in the latent phase, every 15 minutes in the active phase, and every 5 minutes in the second stage.
   Rationale: This evaluation provides the opportunity to assess the fetal status and response to labor.
7. Document FHR data (rate and rhythm), characteristics of uterine activity, and any actions taken as a result of the FHR.

Sample Documentation

8-2-03 0730 FHR 136 by auscultation with slowing to 130 bpm noted during acme of UC and for 10 sec after the UC. STV present, LTV average. Client turned to left side. Maternal pulse 80, FHR 140, regular rhythm with no decrease during or following the next two UC. UC q3minX60 sec, strong. J.Smith, RN

The Fetoscope

The fetoscope is an older assessment tool; however, some clinicians prefer it because it is "natural" and does not rely on ultrasound.

To use the fetoscope:

- Place the fetoscope earpieces in your ears; use the handpiece to position the bell of the fetoscope on the mother's abdomen.
- Place the diaphragm halfway between the umbilicus and symphysis and in the midline. *You are most likely to hear the FHR in this area.*
- Without touching the fetoscope, listen carefully for the FHR (Figure 23–9, *A*)

Evidence-Based Practice

Clinical Outcomes between Continuous and Intermittent Fetal Monitoring in Labor

Clinical Question

What are the differences in outcomes between those women and infants who are continuously monitored with an electronic fetal monitor in labor compared to those who have intermittent fetal heart rate monitoring during labor?

The Evidence

Following a systematic review of published studies, nine random, controlled trials were analyzed. The primary outcome measures were: incidence of perinatal mortality, cerebral palsy, cesarean section births, presence of neonatal seizures, incidence of operative vaginal births (forceps-assisted births or vacuum-assisted births), low Apgar scores, and admission rates to special care nurseries. The following findings were identified:

- The use of continuous fetal monitoring does not reduce perinatal morbidity.
- The use of continuous electronic fetal monitoring does not reduce the incidence of cerebral palsy. There is a slight increase in cerebral palsy in infants who have been continuously monitored during labor.
- There is an increase incidence of cesarean birth in infants who are continuously monitored. The incidence of cesarean birth increased by 30%.
- There is a reduction in neonatal seizures in full term babies who have received continuous electronic monitoring. There is a direct correlation, however, in that these labors in which neonatal seizures occurred were those that were either induced or augmented with pitocin.
- There is an increase in operative vaginal delivery births by 30%.
- There are no differences between low (less than 7) or very low (less than 4) Apgar scores between the two groups.
- There are no differences in admission rates to special care nurseries between the two groups.

Best Practice

Routine continuous electronic fetal monitoring does not appear to improve outcomes, with the exception of a reduction in neonatal seizures, and may actually increase the incidence of operative vaginal births and cesarean births. Nurses should use continuous monitoring when warranted, but should strive to improve their skills on the use of appropriate intermittent monitoring. Low-risk women should be advised that intermittent fetal monitoring during labor is an option. Nurses should allow women to verbalize their own personal preferences for labor monitoring in the absence of maternal or fetal complications.

Reference: Thacker, S. B., & Stroup, D. F. (1999). Continuous electronic fetal monitoring verses intermittent auscultation for assessment during labour. (Cochrane Review). In *Cochrane Review Library*, Issue 3. Oxford: Update Software.

gel is applied to the underside of the transducer to aid in conduction of fetal heart sounds. When the transducer is placed correctly, the sound waves bounce off the fetal heart and are picked up by the electronic monitor. The actual moment-by-moment FHR is displayed simultaneously on a screen and on graph paper (Figure 23–11 •).

The transducer may inadvertently be directed toward a pulsating maternal vessel. In this case there will be a soft swooshing sound (uterine souffle), and the rate will be the same as the maternal pulse.

Disadvantages of monitoring FHR by external means are similar to those of external uterine contraction monitoring. In addition, the tracing may be poor if the fetus is quite active, if more than a normal amount of amniotic fluid is present (hydramnios), or if the woman is moving about frequently.

INTERNAL MONITORING

Internal monitoring of the fetus is accomplished through use of an internal spiral electrode, which is attached to the skin of the fetal head or buttocks (Figure 23–12 •). In order for the spiral electrode to be inserted, the cervix must be dilated at least 2 cm, the presenting fetal part must be accessible by vaginal examination, and the membranes must be ruptured. Even though it is not possible to apply the electrode and catheter under strict sterile conditions, the procedure should be performed as aseptically as possible. After determining

Procedure 23-4 Electronic Fetal Monitoring

Preparation

1. Explain the procedure, the indications for it, and the information that will be obtained.

Equipment and Supplies

- Monitor
- Two elastic monitor belts
- Tocodynamometer ("toco")
- Ultrasound transducer
- Ultrasound gel

Procedure

> **Clinical Tip**
> *Evaluating the FHR tracing provides information about fetal status and response to the stress of labor. The presence of reassuring characteristics is associated with good fetal outcomes. Rapid identification of nonreassuring charateristics allows prompt interventions and the opportunity to determine the fetal response to the interventions.*

1. Turn on the monitor.
2. Place the two elastic belts around the woman's abdomen.
3. Place the "toco" over the uterine fundus off the midline on the area palpated to be most firm during contractions. Secure it with one of the elastic belts.
   Rationale: The uterine fundus is the area of greatest contractility.
4. Note the UC tracing. The resting tone tracing (that is, without a UC) should be recording on the 10 or 15 mm Hg pressure line. Adjust the line to reflect that reading.
   Rationale: If the resting tone is set on the zero line, there often is a constant grinding noise.
5. Apply the ultrasonic gel to the diaphragm of the ultrasound transducer.
   Rationale: Ultrasonic gel is used to maintain contact with the maternal abdomen. The ultrasonic beam is directed toward the fetal heart.
6. Place the diaphragm on the maternal abdomen in the midline between the umbilicus and the symphysis pubis.
7. Listen for the FHR, which will have a whiplike sound. Move the diaphragm laterally if necessary to obtain a stronger sound (Figure 23–10).
8. When the FHR is located, attach the second elastic belt snugly to the transducer. See Figure 23–11
   Rationale: Firm contact is necessary to maintain a steazdy tracing.
9. Place the following information on the beginning of the fetal monitor paper: date, time, woman's name, gravida, para, membrane status, and name of physician or certified nurse-midwife
   Note: Each birthing unit may have specific guidelines about additional information to include.
10. Ongoing documentation should provide information about FHR including baseline rate in beats per minute (bpm), long-term variability (LTV), short-term variability (STV), response to uterine contractions (accelerations or decelerations), procedures performed, changes in position and the like, as well as any therapy initiated.
    Note: A full description of fetal monitoring analysis is beyond the scope of this manual. Refer to Maternal-Newborn and Child Nurisng for futher information.

Sample Documentation

Entry documenting reassuring FHR characteristics and response to UCs:

8-3-03 0700 FHR BL 135–140. STV and LTV present. Two accelerations of 20 bpm × 20 sec with fetal movement in 10 min. UC q3min × 50–60 sec of moderate intensity by palpation, resting tone soft. No decelerations noted. B Burch, RNC

(continued on next page)

Procedure 23–4 Electronic Fetal Monitoring *(continued)*

Entry documenting FHR, variability, response of FHR to UC, the intervention used, and subsequent positive fetal response to the intervention.

8-3-03 FHR BL 135–140. STV and LTV present. Late decelerations noted with
0730 decrease of FHR to 130 bpm for 20 sec. UC q3min × 50–60 sec of moderate intensity by palpation. Client turned to left side. No further deceleration with three subsequent UC. Two accelerations of 20 bpm × 20 sec noted with fetal movement Client instructed to remain on left side. B Burch, RNC

Table 23-4 • POSSIBLE INDICATIONS FOR ELECTRONIC FETAL MONITORING

Fetal Factors

- Decreased fetal movement
- Abnormal auscultory FHR
- Meconium passage
- Abnormal presentations/positions
- Intrauterine growth restriction (IUGR) or small-for-gestational-age (SGA) fetus
- Postdates (>41 weeks)
- Multiple gestation

Maternal Factors

- Fever
- Infections
- Preeclampsia
- Disease conditions (eg, hypertension, diabetes)
- Anemia
- Rh isoimmunization
- Previous perinatal death
- Grand multiparity
- Previous cesarean birth
- Borderline/contracted pelvis

Uterine Factors

- Dysfunctional labor
- Failure to progress in labor
- Oxytocin induction/augmentation
- Uterine anomalies

Complications of Pregnancy

- Prolonged rupture of membranes
- Premature rupture of membranes
- Preterm labor
- Marginal abruptio placentae
- Partial placenta previa
- Occult/frank prolapse of cord
- Amnionitis

Regional Anesthesia

Elective Monitoring

fetal position by vaginal examination, the examiner (physician or nurse) inserts the electrode, which is encased in a plastic guide, to the level of the internal cervical os and attaches it to the presenting part, being careful not to apply it to the face, suture lines, fontanelles, cervix, or perineum if the fetus is in a breech presentation. The electrode is rotated clockwise until it is attached to the presenting part and is then disengaged from the guide tube. The guide tube is removed, and the end wires are connected to a leg plate that is attached to the woman's thigh. The cable from the leg plate is connected to the monitor. Infections and injuries from internal electrodes and catheters are a small but actual risk. Although nurses in some facilities apply internal monitors, in many settings their application is limited to the physician or certified nurse-midwife (CNM).

Since the risk of transmission to the fetus is increased by the small puncture in the fetal scalp, use of internal scalp electrodes should be avoided if at all possible in the presence of known maternal infections such as HIV, hepatitis, or group B streptococcus. Also, women who have had internal monitors and subsequently give birth by cesarean are more likely to have postpartum infections (Garite, 2002). Fetal scalp monitors are also avoided in preterm infants because of the increased risk of ventricular hemorrhage.

The FHR tracing at the top of Figure 23–13 • was obtained by internal monitoring, and the uterine contraction tracing at the bottom by external monitoring. A comparison shows that the spiral electrode provides an instantaneous and continuous recording of FHR that is clearer than the data provided by external monitoring. Notice that the FHR is variable (the tracing moves up and down instead of in a straight line), ranging between about 140 to 155 bpm.

TELEMETRY

Fetal heart rate and uterine activity may also be monitored by a telemetry system. Equipment consists of ultrasound or fetal ECG transducers along with external uterine pressure transducers connected to a small battery-operated transmitter. Signals are transmitted to a receiver connected to a monitor which displays FHR and uterine activity data on an oscilloscope. A printout provides documentation. This system, which can be worn by means of a shoulder strap, allows the woman to ambulate, helping her to feel more comfortable and less confined during labor, yet provides for continuous monitoring. Telemetry provides for direct as well as

RESEARCH IN PRACTICE
Labor and Delivery Nurses' Attitudes Toward Intermittent Fetal Monitoring

What is this study about? Continuous electronic fetal monitoring (EFM) is used in the majority of births in the United States, despite recommendations of professional organizations and research findings that support the use of less-invasive intermittent auscultation for low-risk women. Continuous EFM has been associated with increased cesarean birth rates and decreased satisfaction with the birth process, while very little empirical evidence exists to show it reduces adverse outcomes. The reasons for the persistent use of routine continuous EFM for all women regardless of risk status has been linked to many factors, one of which is nurses' attitudes. This study had as its goal an exploration of labor and delivery nurses' attitudes about intermittent fetal monitoring as an alternative to continuous EFM.

How was the study done? Data were collected for this descriptive, correlational study using a questionnaire developed for this study. Demographic data were collected, followed by statements that assessed attitudes and beliefs about the use of intermittent and continuous fetal monitoring. Items were developed through a review of the literature and from expert opinions of experienced labor and delivery nurses. Statements were rated using a Likert scale. The instrument was pilot tested and evaluated for face and content validity. The survey was administered to a convenience sample of 150 hospital-based nurses who worked in the labor and birthing units of five large hospitals in metropolitan Detroit. Each hospital had similar policies guiding the application of intermittent fetal monitoring.

What were the results of the study? 72.4% of the nurses agreed that intermittent fetal monitoring should be the standard of care, and 87% expressed a willingness to use intermittent auscultation in their practice. However, 53.9% of the nurses responded that nurse/client ratio is a problem in providing intermittent monitoring. In addition, nearly 41% thought that current hospital guidelines for intermittent monitoring were unclear, and 59% indicated that their input is not used to develop hospital policy. 23% of the respondents were unaware that research on continuous EFM shows no clear benefits for low-risk women. Correlational analysis indicated an association between only one demographic–educational preparation–and nurse responses. Nurses with less than a baccalaureate degree were less supportive of intermittent auscultation than those with a baccalaureate degree or greater.

What additional questions might I have? Was the survey instrument tested for reliability and validity? Would nurses in hospitals with less access to technology have different attitudes? How might nurses' concerns about litigation affect their attitudes about intermittent monitoring? What impact did the client's expectations for monitoring have on these nurses' opinions?

How can I use this study? These findings show that nurses have a positive attitude toward intermittent fetal monitoring but may encounter obstacles to implementing this less invasive approach to evaluation of the fetus during labor. Nurses may perceive that they have little authority to change client-related procedures or may lack knowledge about the effects of each type of monitoring. Education can help change attitudes about using intermittent auscultation to ensure that evidence-based care is applied appropriately. Barriers to implementation of this less invasive method of monitoring must be examined and eliminated.

Source: Walker, D. S., Shunkwiler, S., Supanich, J., Williamsen, J., & Yensch, A. (2001). Labor and delivery nurses' attitudes toward intermittent fetal monitoring. *Journal of Midwifery & Women's Health, 46*(6): 374–380.

indirect monitoring of FHR, indirect monitoring of uterine pressure, and dual FHR monitoring of twins.

FETAL HEART RATE PATTERNS

Fetal heart rate is evaluated by assessing the baseline rate, the baseline variability, and the periodic changes that occur in response to the intermittent stress of uterine contractions. A compromised fetus may have a normal baseline heart rate but demonstrate decreased variability (the change in beat-to-beat FHR over a few seconds to a few minutes) and periodic changes indicative of intrauterine hypoxia.

Baseline Rate

The **baseline rate** refers to the range of FHR observed between contractions during a continuous 10-minute period of monitoring. The range does not include the rate during contractions. The normal baseline rate ranges from 110 to 160 bpm. Although these are the generally acceptable ranges of normal, some sources may use different parameters. Whereas Cunningham et al (2001) stated that 110 is the lower limit of normal, Youngkin and Davis (1998) described the lower limit of normal as 120. There are two abnormal variations of the baseline rate—those above 160 bpm (tachycardia) and those below 110 bpm (bradycardia). Variability (discussed shortly) also affects the baseline.

TACHYCARDIA. Fetal tachycardia is generally classified as mild or severe. Mild tachycardia is a baseline rate of 161 to 180 bpm, and severe tachycardia is a baseline of 181 or more (Cunningham et al, 2001). Possible causes of tachycardia include (Cunningham et al, 2001):

- Early fetal hypoxia (This leads to stimulation of the sympathetic nervous system as the fetus compensates for reduced blood flow.)
- Maternal fever (Metabolism of the fetus accelerates because of increased maternal temperature.)

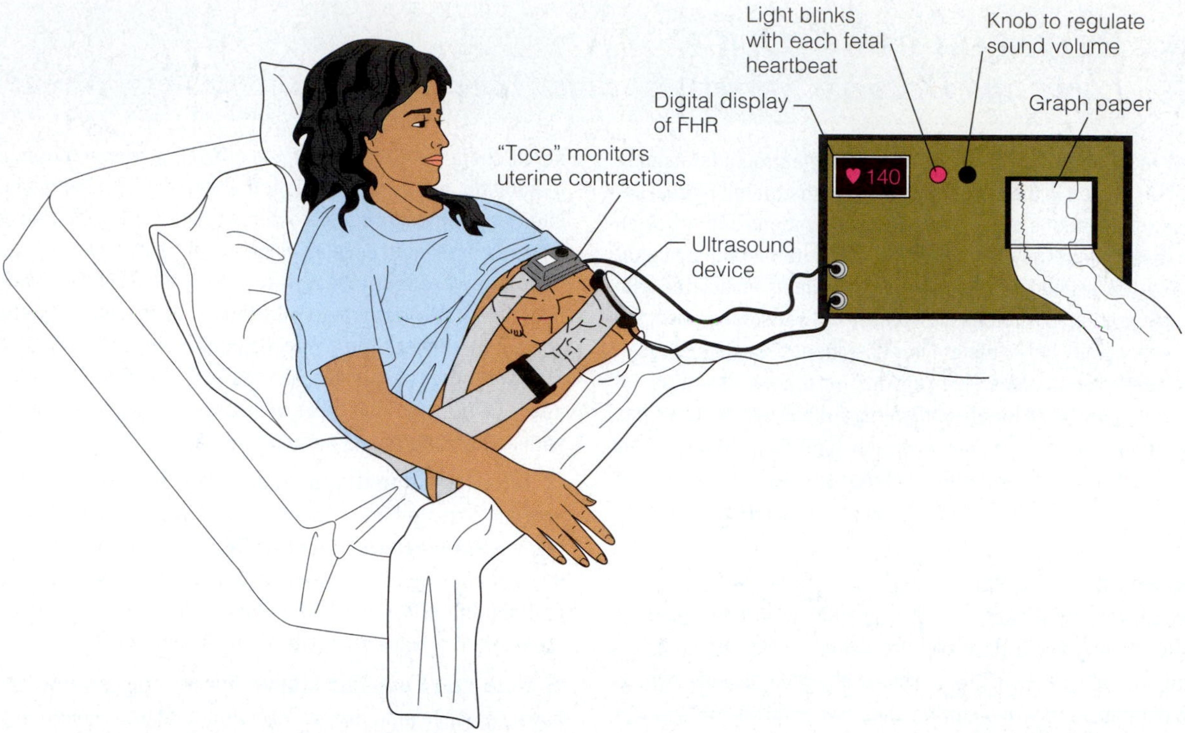

Figure 23–11 • Electronic fetal monitoring by external technique. The ultrasound device, placed over the fetal back, transmits information on the fetal heart rate. Information from both the tocodynamometer and ultrasound device is transmitted to the electronic fetal monitor. The fetal heart rate is indicated four ways: on the digital display, as a blinking light, by sound, and on special monitor paper. The uterine contractions are displayed on the graph paper.

- Betasympathomimetic drugs, such as ritodrine, terbutaline, atropine, and isoxsuprine (These drugs have a cardiac stimulant effect.)
- Maternal hyperthyroidism (Thyroid-stimulating hormones may cross the placenta and stimulate the fetal heart rate.)
- Fetal anemia (The heart rate increases as a compensatory mechanism to improve tissue perfusion.)
- Dehydration

Tachycardia is considered an ominous sign if it is accompanied by other FHR patterns such as late deceleration, severe variable decelerations, or decreased variability. If tachycardia is associated with maternal fever, treatment may consist of antipyretics, cooling measures, and antibiotics. Fetal arrhythmia needs to be ruled out. The pediatrician should be notified because tachycardia may cause heart failure in the newborn.

Bradycardia. Fetal *bradycardia* is defined as FHR of less than 110 to 120 bpm continuing for 10 minutes or more. Moderate bradycardia is defined as FHR of 80 to 110 bpm. Severe bradycardia is defined as FHR of less than 80 bpm for 2 to 3 minutes (Cunningham et al, 2001). Causes of fetal bradycardia include the following:

- Late (profound) fetal asphyxia (There is depression of myocardial activity.)
- Maternal hypotension (Maternal hypotension results in decreased blood flow to the fetus.)
- Prolonged umbilical cord compression (Fetal baroreceptors are activated by cord compression, which produces vagal stimulation, and in turn decreases FHR.)
- Fetal arrhythmia (This is associated with complete heart block in the fetus.)

Bradycardia may be a benign or ominous (preterminal) sign. If there is average variability present, the bradycardia is considered benign. When bradycardia is accompanied by decreased variability, late decelerations, or both, it is considered ominous and a sign of advanced fetal compromise (Cunningham et al, 2001).

Baseline Variability

One of the most important parameters of fetal well-being is noted in FHR variability. **Baseline variability** is a measure of the interplay (the "push-pull" effect) between the sympathetic nervous system (which acts to increase heart rate) and the parasympathetic nervous system (which acts to decrease heart rate). There are two major types of fetal heart variability—short term and long term (Figure 23–14 •).

Long-term variability (LTV) refers to the larger rhythmic fluctuations of the FHR that occur from 3 to 5 cycles per minute with a normal range of 6 to 10 bpm (Cunningham et al, 2001). The range refers to the difference between

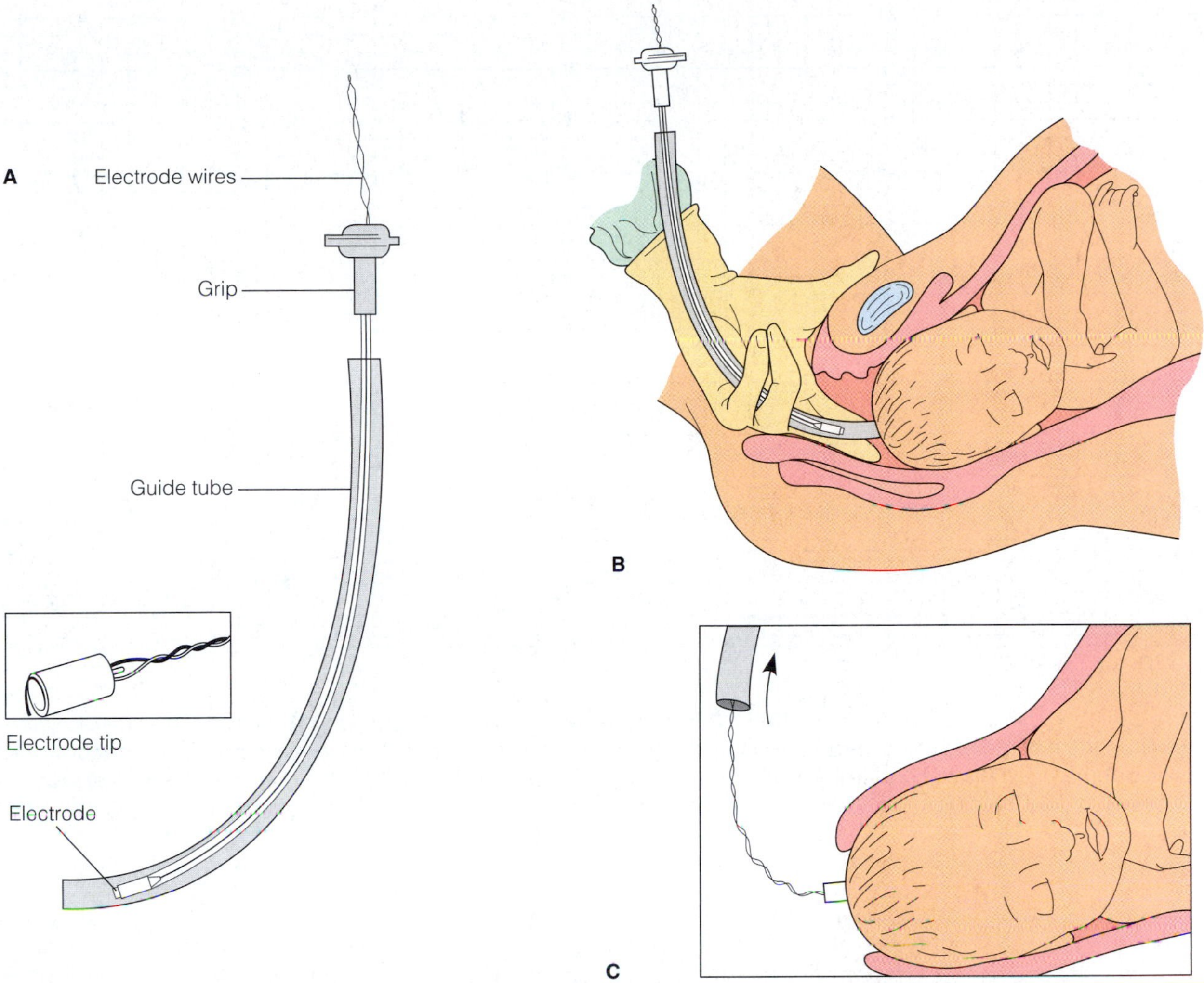

Figure 23–12 • Technique for internal fetal monitoring. *A,* Spiral electrode. *B,* Attaching the spiral electrode to the scalp. *C,* Attached spiral electrode with guide tube removed.

the lowest FHR and the highest FHR in each cycle within 1 minute. LTV is increased by fetal movement and decreased or absent when the fetus is in a sleep cycle. LTV has been classified as follows (Garite, 2002).

- Decreased/minimal variability 0–5 bpm
- Moderate/average variability 6–25 bpm
- Marked variability (saltatory) > 25 bpm

The *saltatory pattern* of marked or excessive variability is characterized by rapid variations in FHR that have a bizarre appearance. This type of LTV occurs with a cycle frequency of 2 to 5 per minute, and the amplitude is greater than 25 bpm (Figure 23–15 •). The etiologic origin of this pattern is uncertain. In the absence of other FHR concerns, saltatory patterns are not thought to indicate fetal compromise (Cunningham et al, 2001).

An unusual pattern referred to as *sinusoidal* is occasionally seen. It is characterized by an undulant sine wave that is equally distributed above and below the baseline. In a sinusoidal pattern, the FHR usually ranges between 120 and 160 bpm. This wavelike baseline FHR usually has amplitude of 5 to 15 bpm and appears to oscillate in a regular, uniform pattern of 2 to 5 cycles per minute (Kang & Boehm, 1999). Fetal activity may be minimal or absent, and there are no FHR accelerations. There is no beat-to-beat short-term variability (Figure 23–16 •). The pattern does not come and go with periods of normal variability. No fetal accelerations are present, even in response to fetal movement.

The sinusoidal pattern is associated with severe asphyxia, Rh isoimmunization, severe anemia, abruptio placentae, fetal-maternal hemorrhage, and severe fetal acidosis (Kang & Boehm, 1999). Pseudosinusoidal patterns have been reported secondary to administration of certain medications, such as analgesics. A transient sinusoidal pattern is also occasionally observed in a completely benign labor (Cunningham et al, 2001).

If a sinusoidal pattern is noted by external monitoring, internal fetal monitoring should be instituted, and cesarean birth should be considered if the pattern is confirmed. Fetal blood

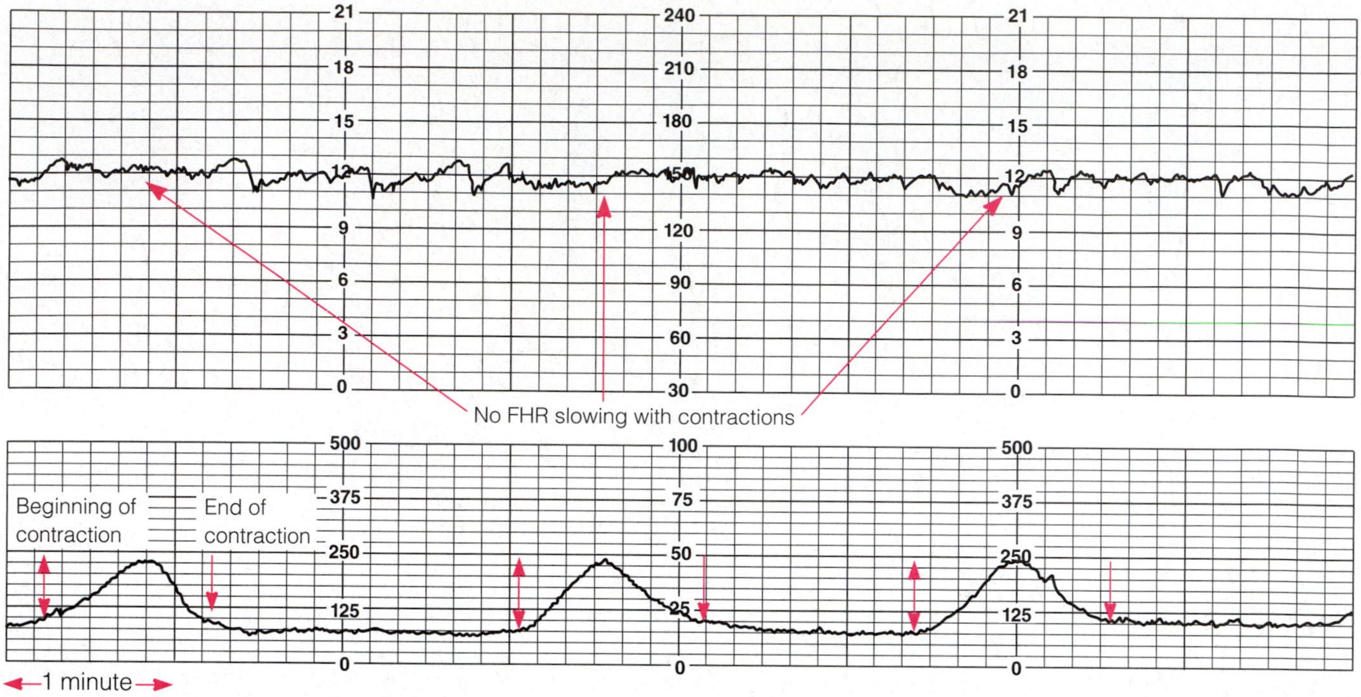

Figure 23–13 • Normal FHR range is from 110 to 160 beats per minute. The FHR tracing in the upper portion of the graph indicates an FHR range of 140 to 155 bpm. The bottom portion depicts uterine contractions. Each dark vertical line marks 1 minute, and each small rectangle represents 10 seconds. The contraction frequency is about every 3 minutes, and the duration of the contractions is 50 to 60 seconds.

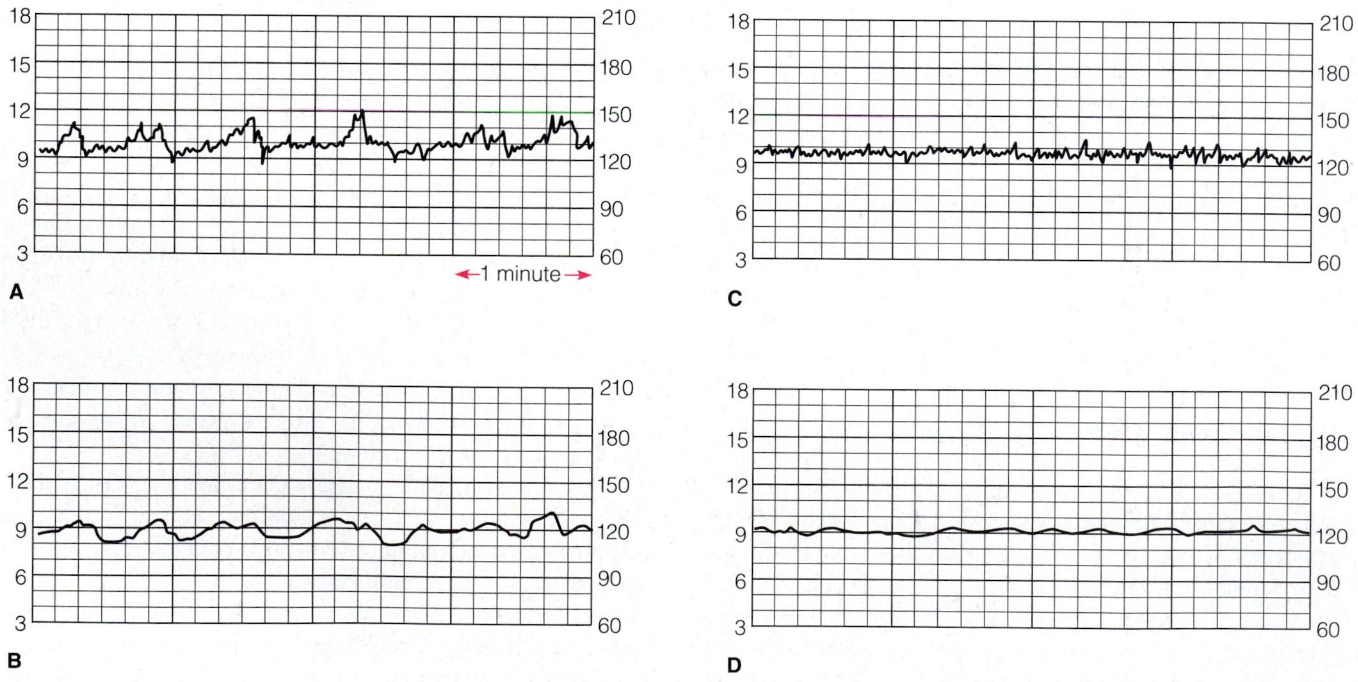

Figure 23–14 • Short- and long-term variability. *A,* Increased LTV; STV present. *B,* Average LTV; STV absent. *C,* Absent LTV; STV present. *D,* Absent LTV; STV absent.

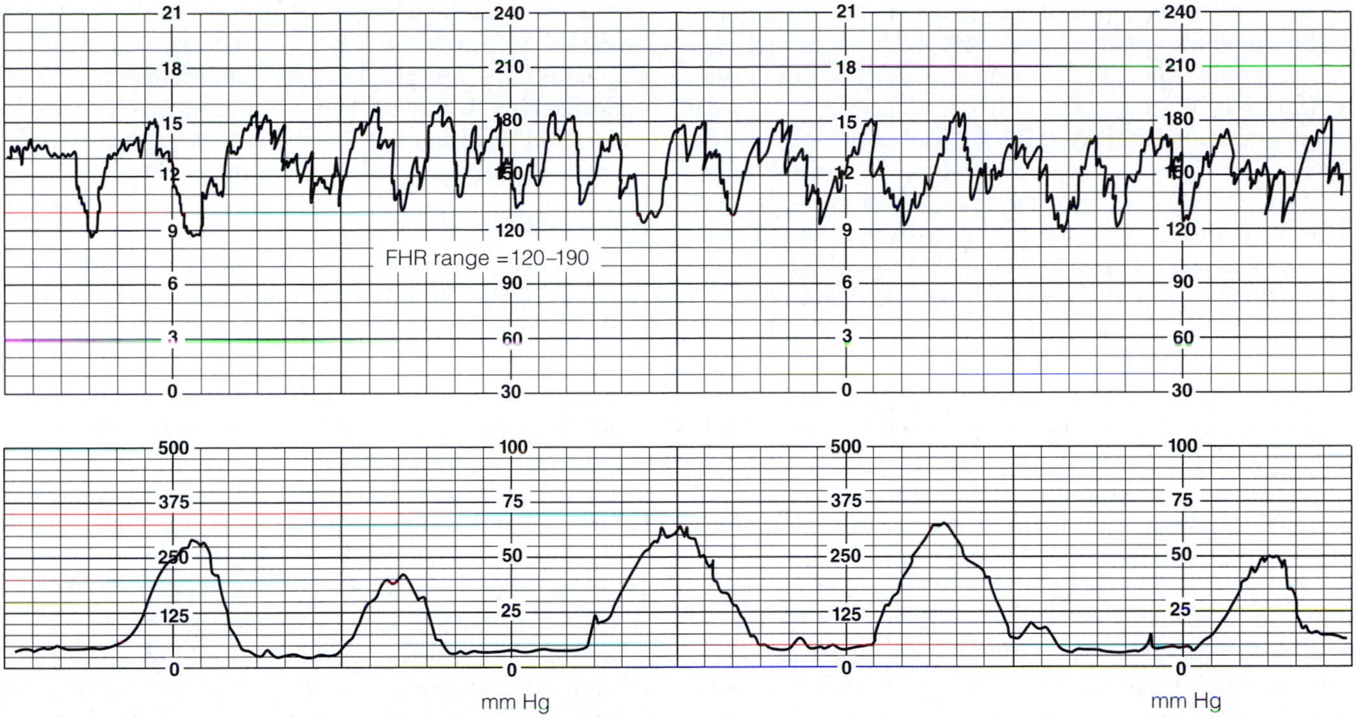

Figure 23–15 • Saltatory pattern. Note the pattern of marked LTV. FHR varies markedly between 120 and 190 beats per minute. With this type of pattern, it is not possible to determine an average baseline FHR because of the wide, marked variations. STV is present.

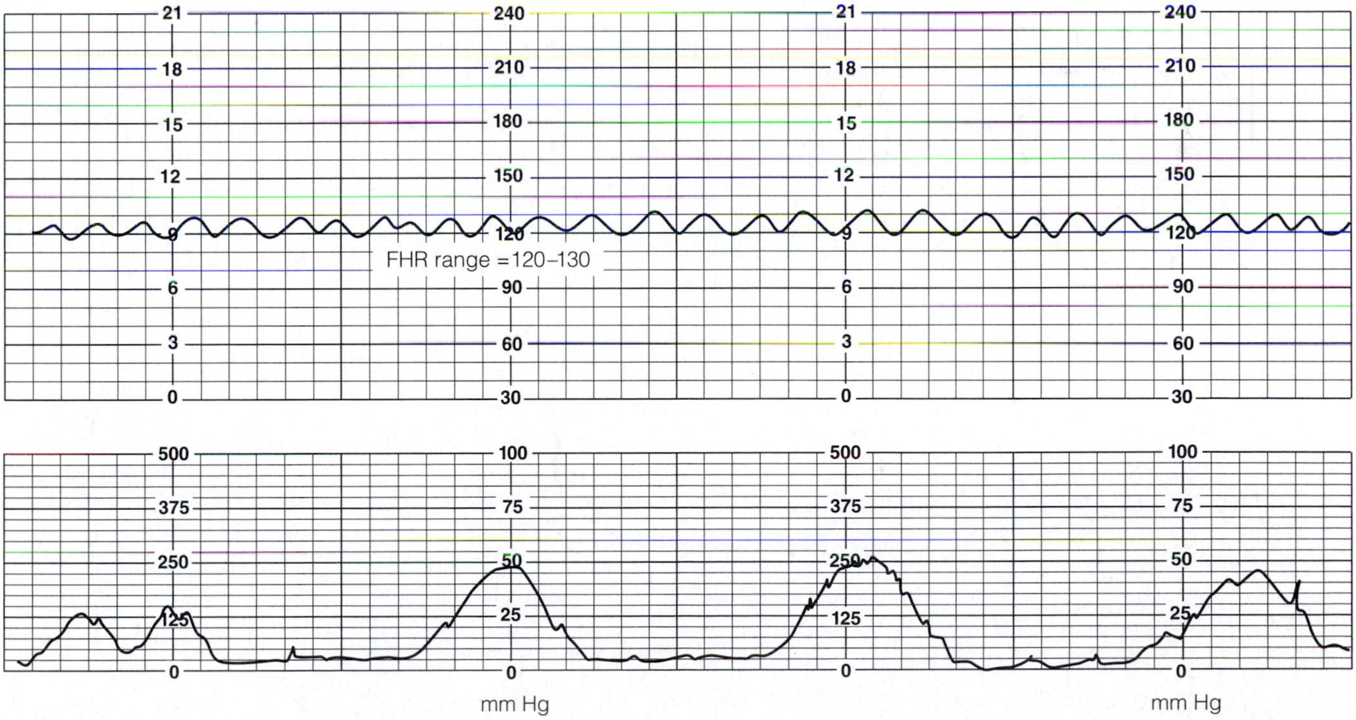

Figure 23–16 • Sinusoidal pattern. Note the undulating waveform evenly distributed between the 120 and 130 bpm baseline. There is no STV; accelerations or decelerations are not present.

sampling for determination of pH and hematocrit, ultrasound scan for signs of congestive heart failure and hydrops, and biophysical profile may aid in assessment, evaluation, and management of the fetus with this FHR pattern.

Short-term variability (STV) refers to the differences between successive heartbeats as measured by the R-R wave interval of the QRS cardiac cycle and therefore represents actual fluctuations from one heartbeat to the next. These tiny fluctuations average 2 to 3 bpm. STV is classified as either present or absent. STV can only be accurately measured with internal monitors.

Short-term variability indicates appropriate fetal central nervous system (CNS) function (previously described), so the presence of STV is reassuring. If there is an oxygen deficit in the CNS, the interplay is lost, and STV disappears. Thus, STV is a useful indicator of fetal oxygen reserve.

Variability should not be differentiated since short term and long term variability are visually determined as a unity. Rather than counting specific beats, the experienced nurse can usually look at the FHR variability and determine whether it is smooth (absent) or rough (present). Although increased variability is not well understood, decreased variability is associated with a variety of pathologic and nonpathologic conditions. For example, STV may be decreased in the presence of fetal tachycardia, prematurity, anomalies of the fetal heart and central nervous system, and fetal sleep. Factors that may decrease both LTV and STV include narcotics, tranquilizers, and epidural or spinal anesthetic agents administered to the laboring woman (NICHD Fetal Monitoring Workshop, 1997). Thus, when decreased variability is noted, the nurse must evaluate it carefully. Since STV can be evaluated only by internal monitoring, an appearance of decreased STV without a known medication-related cause warrants application of an internal electrode.

Accelerations

Accelerations are transient increases in the FHR (Figure 23–17 ●). Nonperiodic accelerations are normally caused by fetal movement. As the fetus moves in utero, the heart rate increases, as it does in adults when they exercise. When the fetus quiets down, the heart rate returns to normal. Spontaneous nonperiodic accelerations thus serve as the criterion for a reactive nonstress test (NST).

Periodic accelerations are ones that accompany contractions, and most likely result from fetal movement in response to pressure of the contracting uterine musculature. Accelerations of this type are thought to be a sign of fetal well-being and adequate oxygen reserve. Another explanation for periodic accelerations is that a mild compression of the umbilical cord with the contraction may occlude the umbilical vein. The resulting decrease in blood flow to the fetus causes a systemic decrease in blood pressure, which triggers a compensatory accelerative response in the fetal heart rate (Cunningham et al, 2001). This has implications for fetal assessment, as it may be an early warning sign of low amniotic fluid or cord compression.

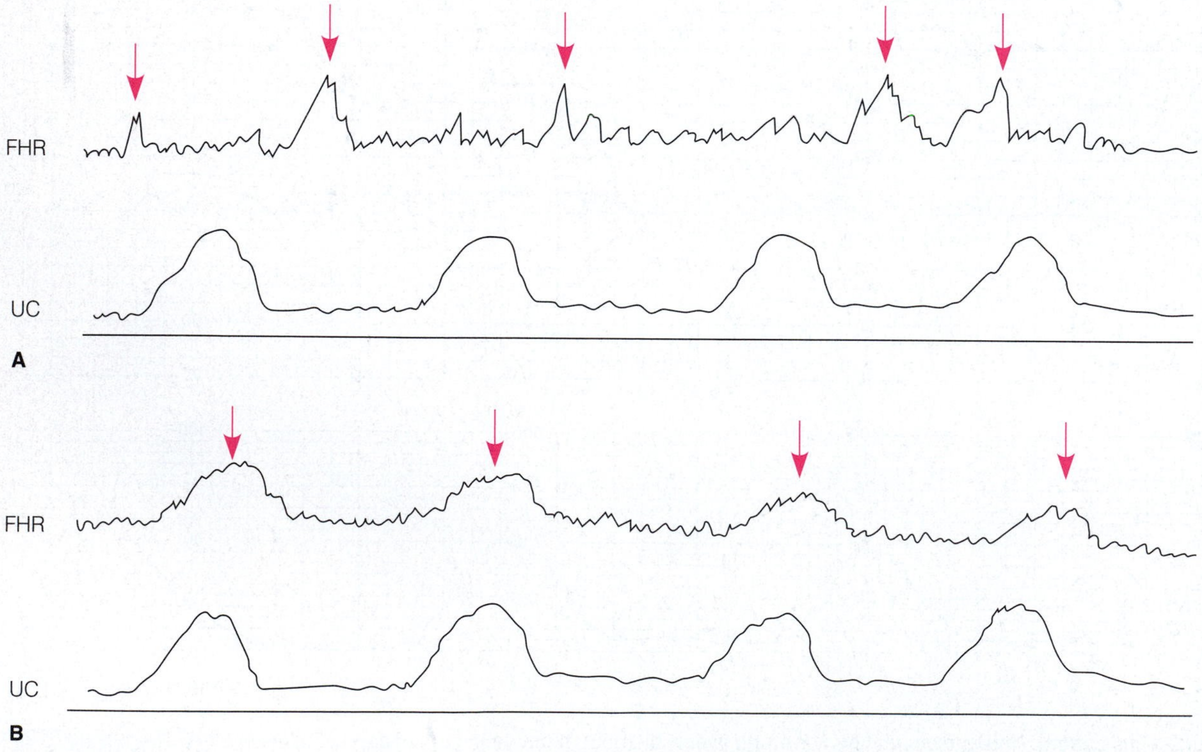

Figure 23–17 ● Types of accelerations. *A,* Nonperiodic accelerations. *B,* Periodic accelerations.

Decelerations

Decelerations are periodic decreases in FHR from the normal baseline. Hon and Quilligan (1967) categorized them as early, late, and variable, according to when they occur in the contraction cycle and to their waveform (Figure 23–18 •).

Early decelerations are due to pressure on the fetal head as it progresses down the birth canal. They have a uniform appearance that inversely mirrors that of the corresponding contraction. Early decelerations begin at the onset of the contraction and end as the contraction ends; the nadir (lowest point) occurs at the peak of the contraction. The nadir rarely falls below 100 to 110 bpm or 20 to 30 bpm below baseline (Cunningham et al, 2001) (Figure 23-19 •).

Early decelerations are generally benign and are usually seen in active labor when dilatation is 4 to 7 cm. Increased intracranial pressure stimulates the vagus nerve, which in turn slows heart rate (Figure 23–20 •). If this pattern occurs early in labor, it may be due to head compression from an unengaged presenting part, occiput posterior presentation, or cephalopelvic disproportion. A nurse must take great care in differentiating this type of deceleration from late decelerations. They look identical yet differ in time of onset.

Early decelerations are not associated with loss of variability, tachycardia, or other FHR changes or with fetal hypoxia, acidosis, or low Apgar scores. They are viewed as a reassuring FHR pattern unless seen with lack of descent of the fetal head.

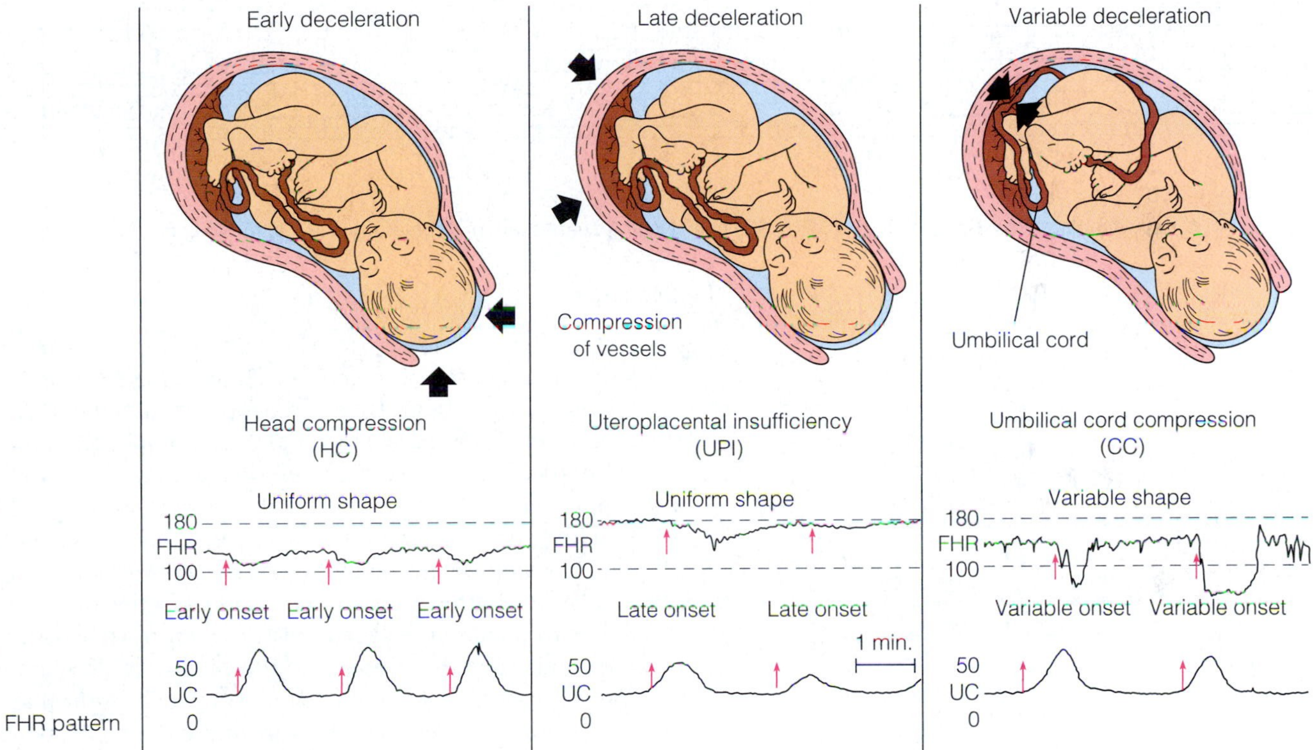

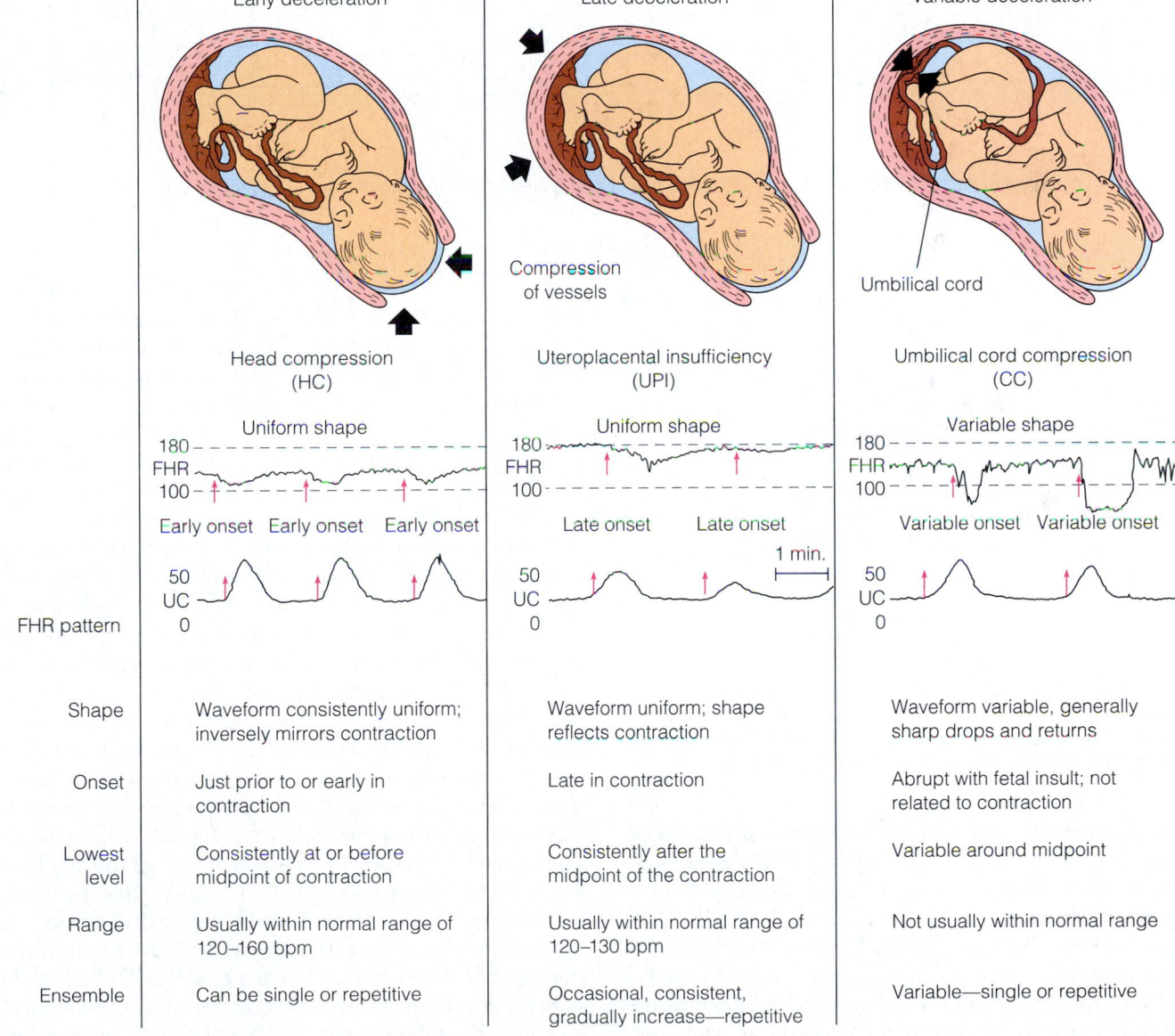

	Early deceleration	Late deceleration	Variable deceleration
Shape	Waveform consistently uniform; inversely mirrors contraction	Waveform uniform; shape reflects contraction	Waveform variable, generally sharp drops and returns
Onset	Just prior to or early in contraction	Late in contraction	Abrupt with fetal insult; not related to contraction
Lowest level	Consistently at or before midpoint of contraction	Consistently after the midpoint of the contraction	Variable around midpoint
Range	Usually within normal range of 120–160 bpm	Usually within normal range of 120–130 bpm	Not usually within normal range
Ensemble	Can be single or repetitive	Occasional, consistent, gradually increase—repetitive	Variable—single or repetitive

Figure 23–18 • Types and characteristics of early, late, and variable decelerations.
SOURCE: Hon, E. (1976). *An introduction to fetal heart rate monitoring,* (2nd ed., p. 29). Los Angeles: University of Southern California School of Medicine.

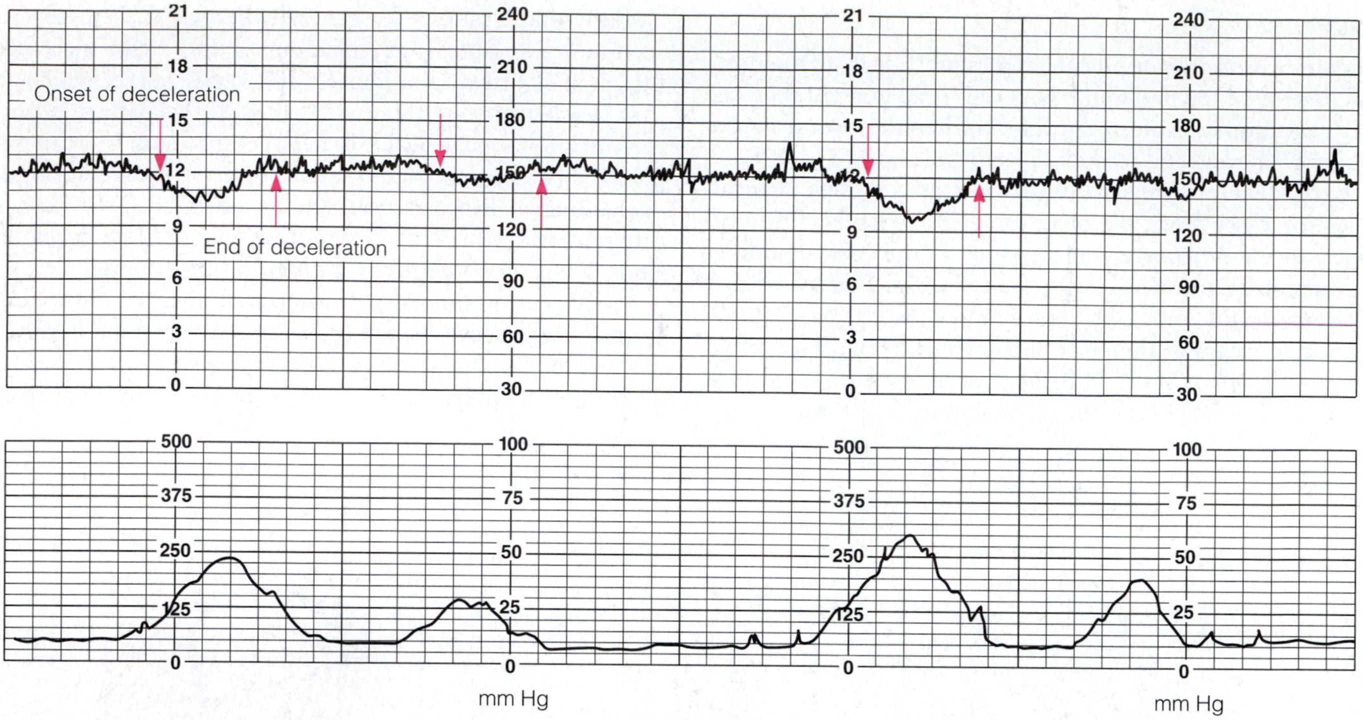

Figure 23–19 • Early decelerations. Baseline FHR is 150 to 155 bpm. Nadir (lowest point) of decelerations is 130 to 145 bpm. LTV is absent; STV is present.

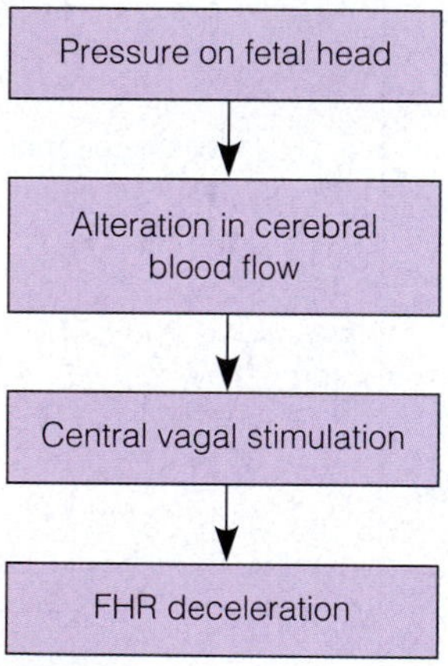

Figure 23–20 • Mechanism of early deceleration (head compression).

SOURCE: Adapted from Freeman, R. K., & Garite, T. J. (1981). The physiologic basis of fetal monitoring. In *Fetal heart rate monitoring* (p. 13). Baltimore, MD: Williams & Wilkins.

Late decelerations are due to uteroplacental insufficiency. They are the result of decreases in blood flow that impede oxygen transfer to the fetus through the intervillous space during uterine contractions, causing hypoxemia (Figure 23–21 •). Late decelerations have a smooth, uniform shape that inversely mirrors the contractions (as do early decelerations) and often reflect the strength of the contraction (indicated by the height of the recorded uterine contraction on the graph paper), but they are late in their onset and recovery. Late decelerations begin at or within a few seconds after the peak of the contraction; the nadir is noted near the end of the contraction. When uteroplacental reserve is adequate, the fetus normally tolerates the transient stress of repetitive contractions. If a decrease in uteroplacental blood flow (for example, from maternal hypotension or excessive uterine activity) leads to fetal hypoxia, late decelerations generally occur (Figure 23–22 •).

This pattern is always considered an ominous sign and requires prompt attention and intervention. Variability in the baseline is of utmost importance. The objective of intervention is to maintain oxygenation (variability) while assessing and eliminating the stressor as reflected by the deceleration. If this is not possible, immediate birth may be indicated.

Sometimes late decelerations are due to the supine position of the laboring woman. In this case, the decrease in uterine blood flow to the fetus may be alleviated by raising the woman's upper trunk or turning her to the side to displace pressure of the gravid uterus on the inferior vena cava. If the woman remains flat on her back, the fetus will continue to have decelerations due to oxygen compromise. Immediate nursing interventions include changing the maternal position, providing oxygen to the mother via face mask, and increasing the administration of intravenous fluids. If oxytocin (Pitocin) is being administered, the infusion should be stopped immediately until the FHR recovers or the physician/CNM has instructed that the infusion be resumed. The physician/CNM should be immediately notified in the event that late decelerations occur.

Late decelerations normally occur within the normal heart range (110 to 160 bpm) and may be quite obvious or very subtle and almost indistinguishable. Some fetuses at highest risk

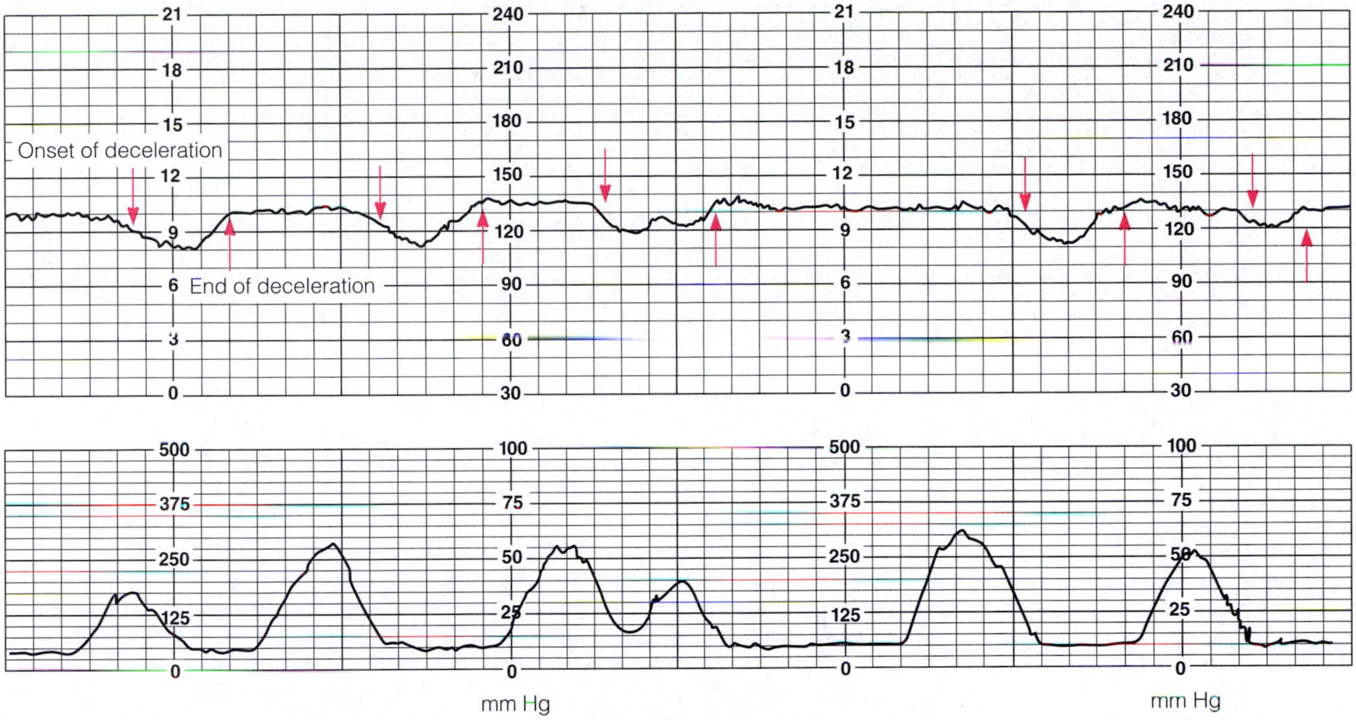

Figure 23–21 • Late decelerations. Baseline FHR is 130 to 148 bpm. Nadir (lowest point) of decelerations is 110 to 120 bpm. LTV and STV are absent.

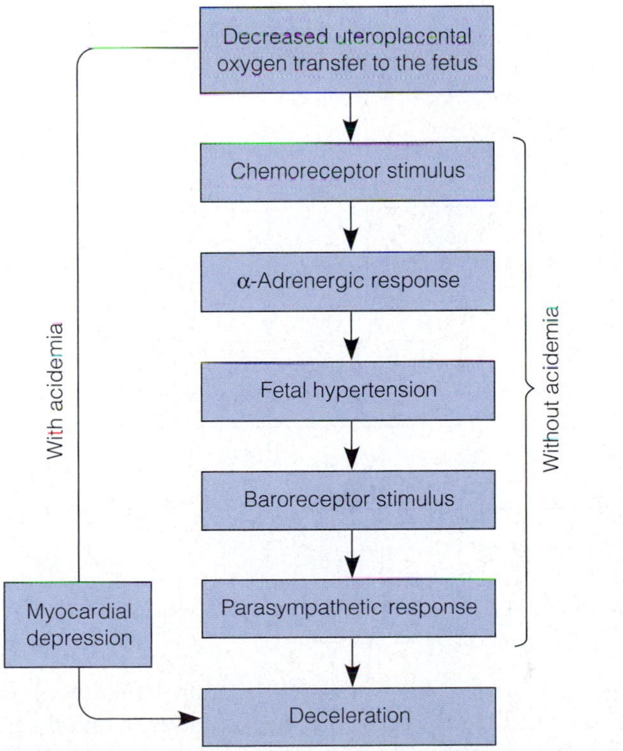

Figure 23–22 • Mechanism of late deceleration.
SOURCE: Freeman, R. K., & Garite, T. J. (1981). The physiologic basis of fetal monitoring. In *Fetal heart rate monitoring* (p. 15). Baltimore, MD: Williams & Wilkins.

demonstrate a flat FHR baseline with late decelerations that are barely noticeable. It must be kept in mind that the depth of the deceleration does not indicate the severity of the insult.

Variable decelerations, as the name suggests, vary in their onset, occurrence, duration, intensity, and waveform. They are diagnosed by a visually abrupt decrease in FHR. They are thought to be due to umbilical cord occlusion, which decreases the amount of blood flow (and therefore oxygen supply) to the fetus (Figure 23–23 •). For example, the fetus may squeeze the cord or roll over onto it, or the cord may be around the neck of the descending fetus. Thus, whereas an occasional or isolated variable deceleration is usually benign, variable decelerations that are repetitive and begin to worsen during the course of labor are a cause for concern. The mechanism of variable decelerations is depicted in Figure 23–24 •.

In addition to nuchal cord (umbilical cord around the neck), repetitive decelerations may indicate short cord or an occult prolapse of the cord in which the cord is compressed by the presenting part although a complete cord prolapse has not occurred. If they become evident early in labor, repetitive variable decelerations may subsequently demonstrate a gradual return to a lower baseline in response to repetitive stress. In all such cases, acid-base status of the fetus should be assessed because cesarean birth, forceps birth, or vacuum extraction might be indicated.

Variable decelerations are also seen in labor when the membranes are ruptured. This decreases protection to the

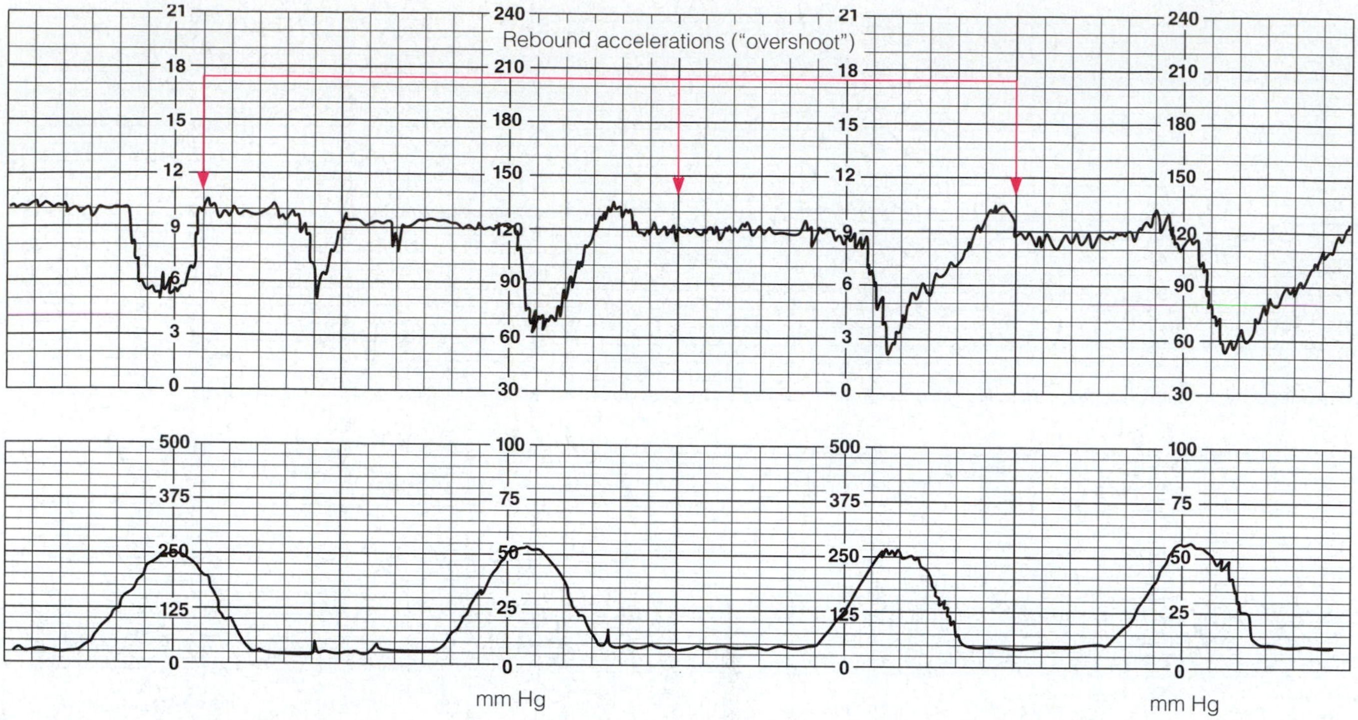

Figure 23–23 ● Variable decelerations with overshoot. The timing of the decelerations is variable, and most have a sharp decline. A rebound acceleration (overshoot) occurs after most of the decelerations. Baseline FHR is 115 to 130 bpm. Nadir of decelerations is 55 to 80 bpm. LTV is absent; STV is present.

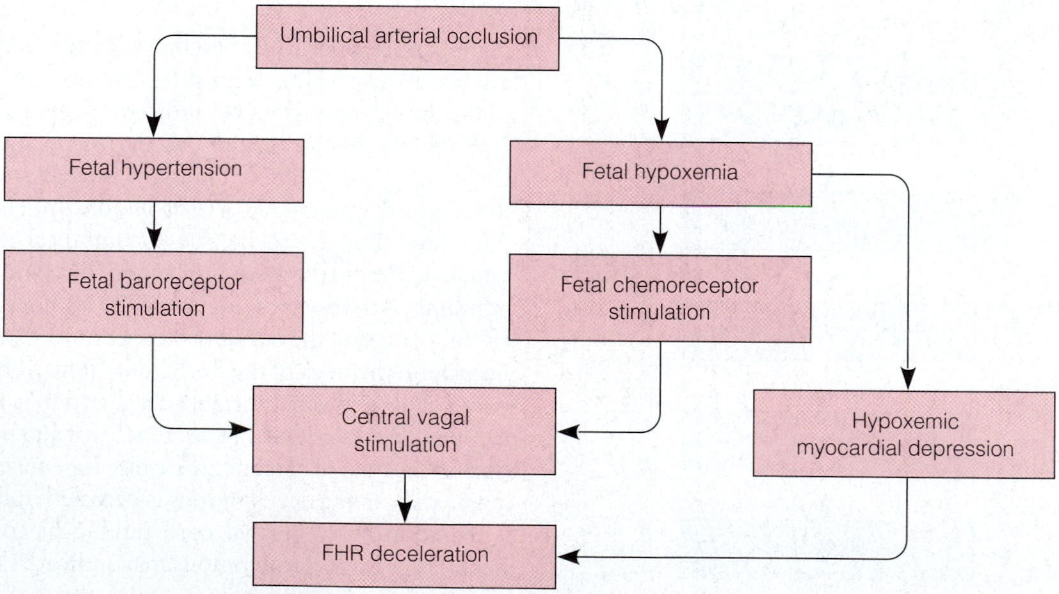

Figure 23–24 ● Mechanism of variable deceleration.
SOURCE: Adapted from Freeman, R. K., & Garite, T. J. (1981). The physiologic basis of fetal monitoring. In *Fetal heart rate monitoring* (p. 15). Baltimore, MD: Williams & Wilkins.

cord as the fetus descends through the birth canal. Repositioning the woman often corrects this type of pattern. If it does not, the clinician may attempt to alleviate it by inserting sterile saline via intrauterine catheter (amnioinfusion) to help take pressure off the umbilical cord.

Variable decelerations are usually innocuous. ACOG classifies variable decelerations as significant when they dip below 70 bpm and last longer than 60 seconds. In addition, Krebs, Petrie, and Dunn (1983) described various "atypical variable decelerations" that should be regarded as signs of fetal hypoxia (Figure 23–25 ●). The nurse should be able to recognize both severe and "atypical" variables. However, in the presence of normal variability of the FHR, these variables have not been found to be associated with fetal acidosis and poor outcome.

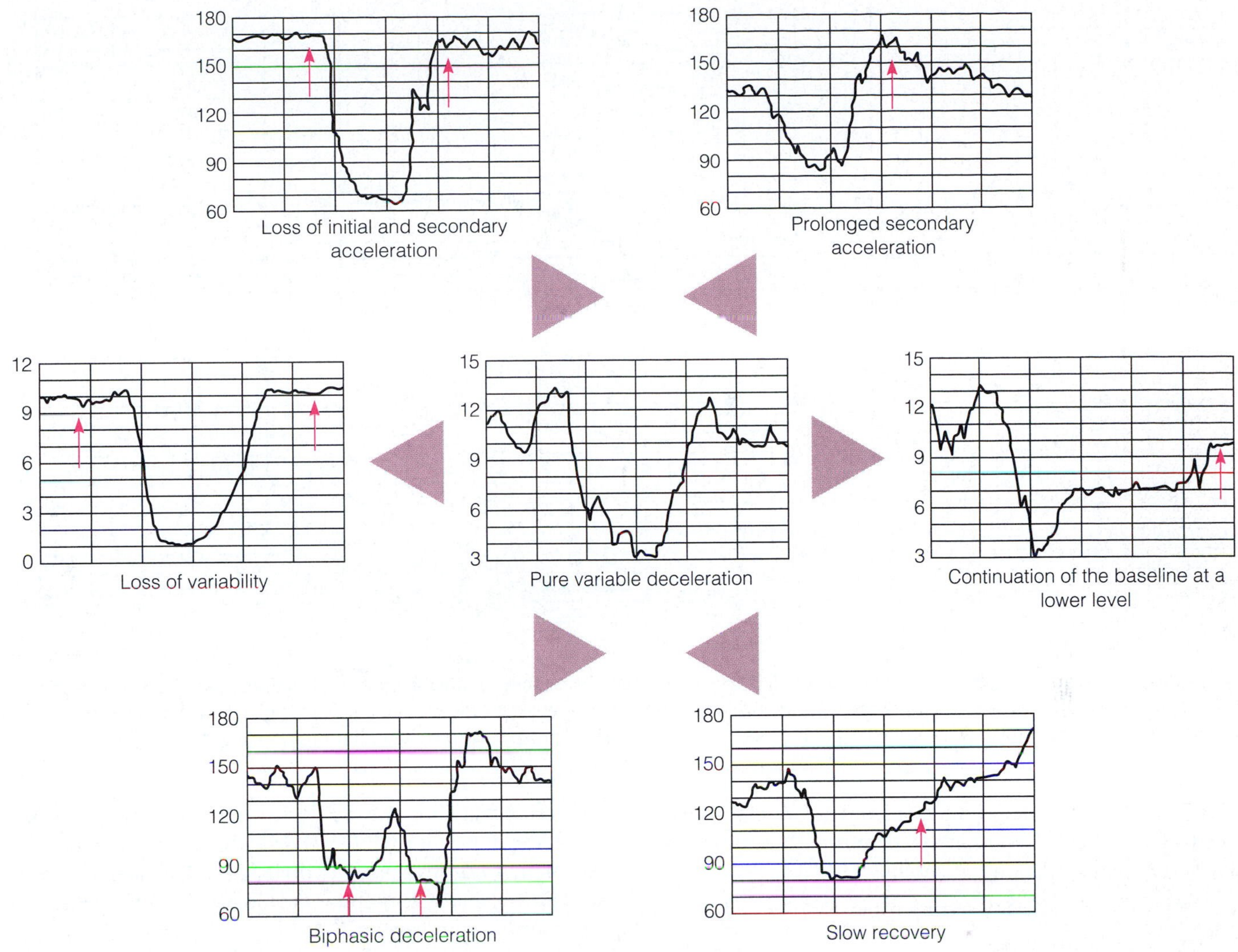

Figure 23–25 • Atypical variable decelerations. The presence of any of these types of variable decelerations strongly suggests fetal hypoxia, especially when variability is decreased.
SOURCE: Krebs, H. B., Petrie, R. E., & Dunn, L. J. (1983). Atypical variable decelerations. *American Journal of Obstetrics and Gynecology, 145*(3), 298.

Prolonged decelerations are those in which the FHR decreases from the baseline for 2 to 10 minutes (Figure 23–26 •). They may occur suddenly, and if the pattern is promptly corrected, FHR variability will remain good. Rebound tachycardia is an ominous sign implying that a state of hypoxia has occurred. Prolonged decelerations may often be seen with sudden occult or frank prolapse of the umbilical cord. They may also occur following administration of regional anesthesia in response to maternal hypotension. Other conditions that may result in a prolonged deceleration are extensive abruptio placentae, uterine hypertonus or hyperstimulus, drug reactions, terminal fetal conditions, maternal seizures, maternal death, or something as simple as a vagal response from a vaginal exam. The most important role of the nurse is to look for the cause or the stressor and correct the problem. Intervention may be as simple as a position change.

Combined decelerations may be seen occasionally when two different deceleration patterns occur together (for example, early/late, early/variable, or variable/late). The specific types of patterns must then be ascertained. For instance, variable decelerations with a slow return to baseline should be differentiated from a combined pattern of variable and late decelerations. The former is a sign that the compression of the umbilical cord is worsening; the latter is an indication of cord compression plus uteroplacental insufficiency. Initial management should be aimed at treatment of the most ominous pattern first.

EVALUATION OF FHR TRACINGS

The effective nurse uses a systematic approach in evaluating FHR tracings to avoid interpreting findings on the basis of inadequate or erroneous data. With a systematic approach, the nurse can make a more accurate and rapid assessment; easily communicate data to the woman, physician/CNM, and staff; and have a universal language for documenting the woman's record.

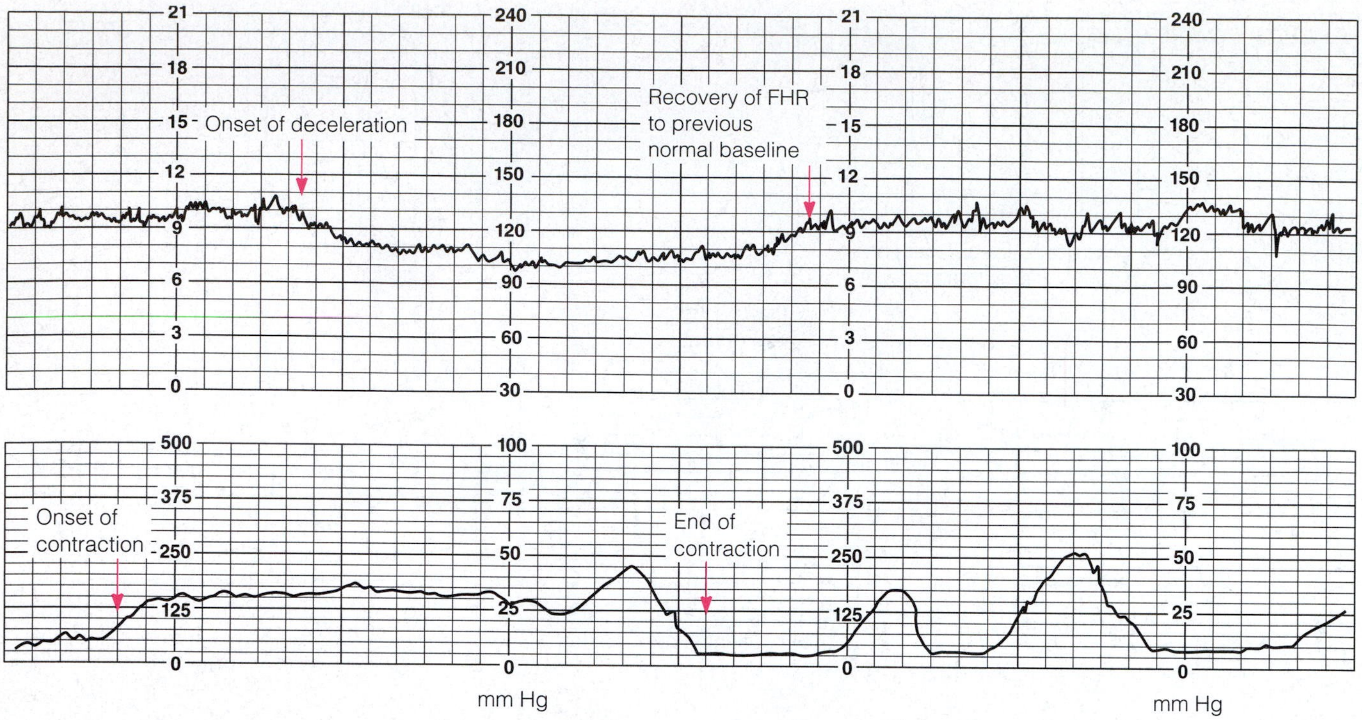

Figure 23–26 • The prolonged deceleration depicted lasts approximately 160 seconds. Note the prolonged contraction of 120 seconds. The deceleration begins after 80 seconds of uterine contraction. Note the beginning return of FHR 30 seconds after uterine tone returns to normal resting tone (contraction ends). An important aspect of this tracing is that STV is present despite the prolonged deceleration.

Evaluation of the electronic monitor tracing begins with a look at the uterine contraction pattern. To evaluate the contraction pattern, the nurse should:

1. Determine the uterine resting tone.
2. Assess the contractions:
   a. What is the frequency?
   b. What is the duration?
   c. What is the intensity (if internal monitoring)?

The next step is to evaluate the fetal heart rate tracing.

1. Determine the baseline:
   a. Is the baseline within normal range?
   b. Is there evidence of tachycardia?
   c. Is there evidence of bradycardia?
2. Determine FHR variability:
   a. Is short-term variability present or absent?
   b. Is long-term variability average, minimal, or marked?
3. Determine whether a sinusoidal pattern is present.
4. Determine whether there are periodic changes.
   a. Are accelerations present?
   b. Do they meet the criteria for a reactive NST?
   c. Are decelerations present?
   d. Are they uniform in shape? If so, determine if they are early or late decelerations.
   e. Are they nonuniform in shape? If so, determine if they are variable decelerations.

After evaluating the FHR tracing for the factors just listed, the nurse may further classify the tracing as reassuring (normal) or nonreassuring (worrisome). Reassuring patterns contain normal parameters and do not require additional treatment or intervention.

Characteristics of reassuring FHR patterns include the following:

- Baseline rate is 110 to 160 bpm.
- Short-term variability is present.
- Long-term variability ranges from three to five cycles per minute.
- Periodic patterns consist of accelerations with fetal movement, and early decelerations may be present.

Nonreassuring patterns indicate that the fetus is becoming stressed and intervention is needed. Characteristics of nonreassuring patterns include the following:

- Severe variable decelerations (FHR drops below 70 bpm for longer than 30 to 45 seconds and is accompanied by rising baseline or decreasing variability or slow return to baseline.)
- Late decelerations of any magnitude
- Absence of variability (No short-term or long-term variability is present.)
- Prolonged deceleration (Deceleration lasts 60 to 90 seconds or more.)
- Severe (marked) bradycardia (FHR baseline is 70 bpm or less.)

Table 23–5 • GUIDELINES FOR MANAGEMENT OF VARIABLE, LATE, AND PROLONGED DECELERATION PATTERNS

Pattern	Nursing Interventions
Variable decelerations Isolated or occasional Moderate	Report findings to physician/CNM and document in chart. Provide explanation to woman and partner. Change maternal position to one in which FHR pattern is most improved. Discontinue oxytocin if it is being administered and other interventions are unsuccessful. Perform vaginal examination to assess for prolapsed cord or change in labor progress. Monitor FHR continuously to assess current status and for further changes in FHR pattern.
Variable decelerations Severe and uncorrectable	Give oxygen if indicated. Report findings to physician/CNM and document in chart. Provide explanation to woman and partner. Prepare for probable cesarean birth. Follow interventions listed above. Prepare for vaginal birth unless baseline variability is decreasing or FHR is progressively rising—then cesarean, forceps, or vacuum birth is indicated. Assist physician with fetal scalp sampling if ordered. Prepare for cesarean birth if scalp pH shows acidosis or downward trend.
Late decelerations	Give oxygen if indicated. Report findings to physician/CNM and document in chart. Provide explanation to woman and partner. Monitor for further FHR changes. Maintain maternal position on left side. Maintain good hydration with IV fluids (normal saline or lactated Ringer's). Discontinue oxytocin if it is being administered and late decelerations persist despite other interventions. Administer oxygen by face mask at 7–10 L/min. Monitor maternal blood pressure and pulse for signs of hypotension; possibly increase flow rate of IV fluids to treat hypotension. Follow physician's orders for treatment for hypotension if present. Increase IV fluids to maintain volume and hydration (normal saline or lactated Ringer's). Assess labor progress (dilatation and station). Assist physician with fetal blood sampling: If pH stays above 7.25, physician will continue monitoring and resample; if pH shows downward trend (between 7.25 and 7.20) or is below 7.20, prepare for birth by most expeditious means.
Late decelerations with tachycardia or decreasing variability	Report findings to physician/CNM and document in chart. Maintain maternal position on left side. Administer oxygen by face mask at 7–10 L/min. Discontinue oxytocin if it is being administered. Assess maternal blood pressure and pulse. Increase IV fluids (normal saline or lactated Ringer's). Assess labor progress (dilatation and station). Prepare for immediate cesarean birth. Explain plan of treatment to woman and partner. Assist physician with fetal blood sampling (if ordered).
Prolonged decelerations	Perform vaginal examination to rule out prolapsed cord or to determine progress in labor status. Change maternal position as needed to try to alleviate decelerations. Discontinue oxytocin if it is being administered. Notify physician/CNM of findings/initial interventions and document in chart. Provide explanation to woman and partner. Increase IV fluids (normal saline or lactated Ringer's). Administer tocolytic if hypertonus noted and ordered by physician/CNM. Anticipate normal FHR recovery following deceleration if FHR previously normal. Anticipate intervention if FHR previously abnormal or deceleration lasts > 3 minutes.

Nonreassuring patterns may require continuous monitoring and more involved treatment and intervention.

It is important to provide information to the laboring woman regarding the FHR pattern and the interventions that will help her fetus. Sharing information with the laboring woman reassures her that a potential or actual problem has been identified and that she is an active participant in the interventions. Occasionally, a problem arises that requires immediate intervention. In that case, the nurse can say something like, "It is important for you to turn on your left side right now because the baby is having a little difficulty. I'll explain what is happening in just a few moments." This type of response lets the woman know that although an action needs to be accomplished rapidly, information will soon be provided. In the haste to act quickly, the nurse must not forget that it is the woman's body and her baby.

Labor and birth nurses must be skilled and competent in evaluating electronic FHR patterns and responding appropriately (Table 23–5 •). Competence can be maintained through frequent in-services, formal courses, and continuing education programs.

FAMILY'S RESPONSES TO ELECTRONIC FETAL MONITORING

Responses to electronic fetal monitoring can be as complex and varied among women and families as among practitioners in the nursing and medical community. Some women and families view the EFM as unneeded technology that interferes with a natural process; they feel that EFM should not be used unless there are clear indications. Such women who want minimal intervention during labor and birth may carefully develop a birth plan and hire a doula as an advocate (see Chapter 13) to help ensure that their wishes will be met once they arrive in the hospital birthing setting. Other women and families consider the monitor a normal part of the care surrounding birth and do not realize they may have some personal choice; therefore, they do not object. Still other women and families believe that technology such as EFM represents state-of-the-art practice and may demand it. They may perceive absence of an EFM as withholding of care, perhaps due to financial or other considerations (McConnell, 1998). Lastly, some women and families have a simple response to the EFM; they like it because hearing the fetal heartbeat provides a feeling of reassurance.

At times, even women who initially welcomed the monitor may begin to resent it. These feelings may be intensified when, for example, the nurse walks into the room and asks, "How are you doing?" while looking at the monitor instead of making eye contact with the woman. Such actions convey an attitude that the only important information emanates from the technologic device. The woman may be left feeling that she is not important and is not even a part of the process. Thus it is essential that the nurse relate primarily to the laboring woman, whose complex physical and emotional responses are not indicated on an EFM (Sandelowski, 1998).

MEDIALINK CARE PLAN: CLIENT WITH DECELERATIONS

NURSING CARE MANAGEMENT

As in all interactions with clients, nurses must always be aware of the healing presence that is theirs to bring to the process. The healing presence is more than just the presence of the nurse's physical body; rather, it is the result of the special focus of the nurse on the client's whole being and the unspoken willingness of both parties to enter into a special healing moment in which both will be changed.

Technology has been advancing at a rapid rate in the labor and birthing area, and each new development further challenges nurses to understand, incorporate, and balance the role of technology into holistic nursing practice. "The practice of nursing in a technological practice setting presents a contrast of strength and vulnerability" (Bernardo, 1998). A key strength of technology is its ability to explain and predict health patterns or problems with precision. For example, the EFM can reveal an ominous FHR pattern in precise detail. It would be difficult, if not impossible, for the nurse to obtain the same data with an auditory device such as a fetoscope. Another strength of some technologies is that they save time (eg, an ear thermometer can obtain a temperature in 1 to 3 seconds, in contrast to an oral mercury thermometer, now contraindicated for use, which must remain in place for 3 minutes). Still other technologic advances have led to more comfortable and less invasive procedures (eg, maternal blood gas levels may now be measured by pulse oximetry instead of requiring blood to be drawn).

Nursing's vulnerability in a technologic environment arises from technology's potential to dehumanize the nurse-client relationship (Bernardo, 1998). First, there is a tendency to allow technology to become the driving force in client care and therefore detach the nurse from meaningful interactions with the client. Second, technology may shift the nurse's focus away from the client's behavior as an indication of health status. Third, technology has the potential to focus attention on a problem or disease process rather than on the individual. Fourth, technology focuses on the tangible and visible rather than on the intuitive, personal nature of each nurse's practice. Lastly, the language used with technology can become contrived and removed from the client's understanding. This "special language" may act as a barrier, isolate the client, and deemphasize the client's experience. Use of technology can also be intimidating and stimulate fear and anxiety in some women. Women who desire minimum intervention should be provided with a detailed explanation if continuous monitoring or other technologic procedures are warranted.

Since the use of technology will continue to be an integral part of client care, questions arise about how it changes nursing practice. Experienced nurses recognize that technology can be a tremendously useful tool; however, they never lose sight of the client's perspective about her experiences. How does the nurse learn of the client's actual experience? Although several theories have been proposed, *nursing presence* seems to best describe the interaction between the nurse and the woman and family in the childbirth setting.

True presence in nursing comes from the "human becoming" theory, which emphasizes that the focus of care must clearly be from the person's perspective, not the nurse's. "The intent of the nurse in true presence is not to change, alter, or intervene but to bear witness to the person's experience in a nonjudgmental manner" (Bernardo, 1998).

> *As a nurse-midwife, I am grateful to be sharing in the miracle of birth with a family. I always place emphasis on the "high touch" aspect of care. While there is a place for "high tech" care, it never replaces the special bond that can be fostered when awaiting the arrival of a new family member.*

The nurse's awareness and active use of the healing presence help the woman and family develop trust. By sharing their perspectives and expectations, the nurse becomes better able to provide care that meets the needs of the woman and family and to advocate for them.

Client teaching is essential. Prior to applying the monitor, the nurse should fully explain to the woman the reason for using the EFM and the information that can be derived from its use. The nurse also explains how the monitor can help identify the beginning of contractions and thus aid in breathing during the various phases of labor. It is advantageous as well to provide education regarding the use of internal equipment, because the caregiver may quickly convert to this method as a result of examination findings. Women who are informed about the possibility of internal monitoring are better prepared if a quick decision must be made to apply an electrode or catheter.

After the monitor is applied, basic information should be recorded on the monitor strip. The data included are the date, time, woman's name, physician, hospital or agency number, age, gravida, para, estimated date of birth, membrane status, maternal vital signs, and current medical problems. As the monitor strip continues to run and care is provided, it is important that documentation be recorded not only in the nurse's notes on the woman's hospital record, but also on the fetal monitor tracing. The following information should be included on the tracing (American Academy of Pediatrics [AAP] & American College of Obstetricians and Gynecologists [ACOG], 2002):

1. Vaginal examinations (dilatation, effacement, station, and position)
2. Amniotomy or spontaneous rupture of membranes, color of amniotic fluid, presence and consistency of meconium
3. Maternal vital signs
4. Maternal position in bed and changes of position
5. Application of spiral electrode or intrauterine pressure catheter
6. Medications
7. Oxygen administration
8. Maternal behaviors (coughing, hiccupping)
9. Fetal scalp stimulation or fetal scalp blood sampling
10. Vomiting
11. Pushing
12. Administration of anesthesia blocks

In addition, if the monitor does not automatically add the time on the strip at specific intervals, the nurse should note the time when recording any information on the strip. If more than one nurse is adding information to the monitor strip, it is wise to initial each note. The tracing is considered a legal part of the woman's medical record and may be submitted as evidence in court.

It is important for the laboring woman to feel that what is happening to her is the central focus. The nurse can acknowledge this by always speaking to and looking at the woman when entering the room, before looking at the monitor.

Indirect Methods of Fetal Assessment

When there is a question regarding fetal status, indirect methods such as **scalp stimulation** (pressing on the fetal scalp with the examining fingers during a vaginal exam to elicit an acceleration of FHR), acoustic stimulation (using a sound device placed against the maternal abdomen to elicit an acceleration in FHR), or stimulation by maternal abdominal palpation (patting or shaking the abdomen) can be used before more invasive fetal blood sampling. When one of the indirect methods is used, the fetus that is not in any stress or distress responds with an acceleration of the FHR, described as a reactive response (acceleration of 15 bpm amplitude with a duration of 15 seconds). Whereas reactivity is associated with fetal well-being, the absence of acceleration does not diagnose acidemia or predict fetal compromise. Further observation and assessment measures are indicated.

Fetal Scalp Blood Sampling

When nonreassuring or confusing FHR patterns are noted, additional information about the acid-base status of the fetus must be sought. This may be accomplished by the physician/CNM obtaining a **fetal scalp blood sample.** Fetal pH is lower at the end of a contraction, so the sample is best collected before the beginning of a uterine contraction (Swaim & Creasy, 1997).

According to Swaim and Creasy (1997), the physician/CNM should consider fetal scalp blood sampling in two instances. The first instance is in the presence of equivocal FHR patterns. When these patterns are present, knowledge of fetal acid-base status can help care providers determine appropriate choices for managing labor. Examples of such situations may include the following (Swaim & Creasy, 1997):

- Fetal tachycardia with no known complications that does not respond to measures to reduce maternal temperature
- Decreased variability accompanied by a normal baseline for more than 60 minutes, or without periodic changes on admission
- Presence of a high-risk fetus with a normal baseline and no accelerations with scalp or vibroacoustic stimulation
- A premature fetus with FHR abnormality
- Decreased variability after drug administration and the presence of other concerns regarding the fetus
- An unusual FHR pattern
- Repetitive late decelerations that are unresponsive to fetal stimulation techniques
- Presence of severe variable decelerations

The second instance is the presence of a fetal heart rate pattern that is known to be compatible with the development of fetal acidosis, if the FHR pattern continues over time and the actual birth is close. In this case, knowledge of the fetal acid-base status provides information regarding fetal reserve. Although fetal scalp sampling is the ideal practice, it is used less frequently.

FETAL BLOOD SAMPLING PROCEDURE

Equipment needed for fetal blood sampling is available in sterile disposable kits. Items included are heparinized capillary tubes, a short capillary tube holder, a 2-mm micro scalpel on a long handle, a conical vaginal speculum that has an area fitted for placement of a light, clay sealant, silicone gel, and long sponge swabs. An extra overhead light source is needed. The woman's vulva and perineum are cleansed and sterile drapes arranged. The conical speculum is inserted into the vagina and through the cervix to visualize the fetal scalp and the site to be sampled (Figure 23–27 •). Working through the speculum, the physician cleanses the fetal site to remove vernix, blood, and amniotic fluid. Silicone gel is then applied to the site to enhance beading of the blood once the site is punctured. The site is punctured with the 2-mm micro scalpel in a stab rather than slash motion. A small amount (0.25 mL) of blood is then collected in a long heparinized capillary tube. Two samples should be collected during each procedure to confirm reliability of values. Determinations of pH and base deficit should be readily available in minutes for this procedure to be of value.

The clotting mechanism is compromised when pH is lowered; therefore, blood may ooze at the site for some time. Because loss of even minimal amounts of blood may be harmful to the fetus, pressure is applied to the puncture site throughout the next contraction. Pressure is continued if oozing is prolonged.

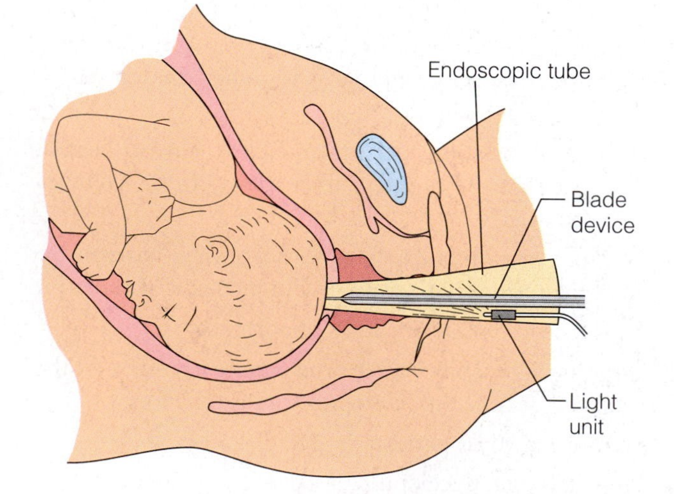

Figure 23–27 • Technique of obtaining fetal blood from the scalp during labor.

SOURCE: Creasy, R. K., & Parer, J. T. (1977). Prenatal care and diagnosis. In A. M. Rudolph (Ed.), *Pediatrics* (16th ed.). Englewood Cliffs, NJ: Appleton-Century-Crofts.

INTERPRETATION OF FETAL BLOOD SAMPLING RESULTS

A fetal blood pH of 7.25 or above is considered normal, and the physician will recommend that labor continue as long as the FHR pattern does not become worse. A result of 7.20 or lower is an indication for birth without delay. (For instance, if the fetal head is now visible and forceps criteria are met, a forceps-assisted birth is completed; if forceps criteria are not met, a cesarean is performed.) If the scalp pH is between 7.21 and 7.24, it is recommended that serial fetal blood sampling be done about every 20 minutes until the FHR pattern shows marked improvement or worsening (Swaim & Creasy, 1997).

Although not universally used at present, a pH electrode attached to the fetal scalp tissue can be used to monitor fetal pH continuously. This electrode does not measure fetal blood pH level per se, but rather the pH level of subcutaneous tissue. In hypoxia, alpha-adrenergic activity increases initially with accompanying fetal hypertension, causing acidosis to occur in peripheral tissue more rapidly than in the central circulation. Conversely, as hypoxia is corrected, there may be a recovery lag of about 5 minutes in the pH value in the peripheral tissue (Boylan & Parisi, 1994). A great deal of investigation is focused on obtaining continuous fetal O_2 saturation levels. Fetal oximetry monitoring is being tested and refined, and long-term newborn and perinatal outcomes are being studied.

Cord Blood Analysis at Birth

In cases where significant abnormal FHR patterns have been noted prior to birth, amniotic fluid is meconium stained, or the infant is depressed at birth, umbilical cord blood may be analyzed immediately after birth to assess the infant's respiratory status. The cord is usually clamped before the infant takes its first breath to provide an evaluation of blood gas status before the infant interacts with the extrauterine environment because values can change after only a few seconds of neonatal breathing.

An 8- to 10-inch segment of the umbilical cord is double-clamped and cut, and a small amount of blood is aspirated from one of the umbilical arteries (arterial blood seems to provide the most reliable indication of blood gas status and fetal tissue pH). Blood is collected in a heparinized syringe unless it is to be analyzed immediately; it should not be allowed to remain in the segment of cord longer than 30 minutes. Other clinicians may collect a segment of cord and send blood samples only if the Apgar score is below 7 at 5 minutes, as recommended by the AAP and ACOG (2002). In this instance, values might be used to clarify the cause of a low Apgar score while minimizing any medicolegal exposure and expense. Determination of pH and base deficit values can differentiate whether fetal acidemia is due to hypoperfusion of the placenta or cord compression.

CHAPTER REVIEW

EXPLOREMEDIALINK

NCLEX review questions, case studies, and other interactive resources for this chapter can be found on the Web site at http://www.prenhall.com/olds. Click on "Chapter 23" to select the activities for this chapter.

For tutorials including animations and videos, more NCLEX review questions, and an audio glossary, access the accompanying CD-ROM in this book.

Focus Your Study

- Intrapartal assessment includes attention to both physical and psychosociocultural parameters of the laboring woman, assessment of the fetus, and ongoing assessment for conditions that place the woman and her fetus at increased risk.
- Birthing room nurses have responsibilities in recognizing and interpreting fetal monitoring patterns, notifying the physician/CNM of problems, and initiating corrective and supportive measures when needed.
- Uterine contractions may be assessed by palpation or by an electronic monitor. The electronic monitor may be used for external or internal monitoring.
- A vaginal examination determines the status of cervical dilatation and effacement, and fetal presentation, position, and station.
- Fetal presentation and position may also be assessed by inspection, vaginal examination, or ultrasound.
- Leopold's maneuvers provide a systematic evaluation of fetal presentation and position.
- Indications for electronic monitoring include fetal, maternal, and uterine factors; presence of pregnancy complications; regional anesthesia; and elective monitoring.
- The fetal heart rate may be assessed by auscultation or electronic fetal monitoring.
- Electronic fetal monitoring is accomplished by indirect ultrasound or by direct methods that require the placement of a spiral electrode on the fetal presenting part.
- Short-term variability of the FHR can be assessed only by direct internal electronic monitoring.
- Baseline FHR refers to the range of FHR observed between contractions during a 10-minute period of monitoring.
- The normal range of FHR is 110 to 160 beats per minute.
- Baseline changes of the FHR include tachycardia, bradycardia, and variability.
- Tachycardia is defined as a rate of 160 beats per minute or more for a 10-minute segment of time.
- Bradycardia is defined as a rate of less than 110 beats per minute for a 10-minute segment of time.
- Baseline variability is an important parameter of fetal well-being. It includes both long- and short-term variability.
- Periodic changes are decelerations or accelerations of the FHR from the baseline in response to contractions. Accelerations are normally caused by fetal movement or early cord compression. Decelerations may be termed early, late, variable, or sinusoidal.
- Early decelerations are due to compression of the fetal head during contractions and are considered benign and require no intervention.
- Late decelerations are associated with uteroplacental insufficiency.
- Variable decelerations are associated with compression of the umbilical cord.
- Sinusoidal patterns are characterized by an undulant sine wave.
- Psychologic reactions to monitoring vary considerably but tend to reflect one of three

responses: (1) the belief that monitoring is invasive and only indicated if a medical reason exists; (2) the belief that monitoring is a necessary part of care; or (3) the belief that monitoring is state-of-the-art care and absolutely necessary.

- Fetal scalp stimulation can be used when there is a question regarding fetal status.
- Fetal acid-base status may be assessed by fetal blood sampling.

References

American Academy of Pediatrics (AAP) and the American College of Obstetricians and Gynecologists (ACOG). (2002). *Guidelines for perinatal care* (5th ed.). Washington, DC: Author.

American College of Obstetricians and Gynecologists (ACOG). (1999). *Nutrition during pregnancy.* Washington, DC: Author.

Austin, W., Gallop, R., McCay, E., Peternelj-Taylor, C., & Bayer, M. (1999). Culturally competent care for psychiatric clients who have a history of sexual abuse. *Clinical Nursing Research, 8,* 5–25.

Bernardo, A. (1998). Technology and true presence in nursing. *Holistic Nursing Practice, 12,* 40–49.

Boylan, P. C., & Parisi, V. M. (1994). Acid-base physiology in the fetus. In R. K. Creasy & R. Resnik (Eds.), *Maternal-fetal medicine: Principles and practice* (3rd ed.). Philadelphia: Saunders.

Burrian, J. (1995). Helping survivors of sexual abuse through labor. *Maternal-Child Nursing Journal, 20*(5), 252–255.

Callister, L. C. (2001). Culturally competent care of women and newborns: Knowledge, attitude and skills. *Journal of Obstetric, Gynecologic, & Neonatal Nursing, 30,* 209–215.

Creasy, R. K., & Parer, J. T. (1977). Prenatal care and diagnosis. In A. M. Rudolph (Ed.), *Pediatrics* (16th ed.). Englewood Cliffs, NJ: Appleton-Century-Crofts.

Cunningham, F. G., Gant, N. F., Leveno, K. J., Gilstrap, L. C. et al. (2001). *Williams obstetrics.* (21st ed.). New York: McGraw-Hill.

Feinstein, N. F. (2000). Fetal heart auscultation: Current and future practice. *Journal of Obstetric, Gynecologic & Neonatal Nursing, 29,* 306–315.

Freeman, R. K., & Garite, T. J. (1981). The physiologic basis of fetal monitoring. In *Fetal heart rate monitoring.* (p. 13). Baltimore, MD: Williams & Wilkins.

Garite, T. J. (2002). Intrapartum fetal evaluation. In S. G. Gabbe, J. R. Niebyl, & J. L. Simpson (Eds.). *Obstetrics: Normal and problem pregnancies.* (4th ed.). Churchill Livingstone.

Hon, E. (1976). *An introduction to fetal heart rate monitoring* (2nd ed.). Los Angeles: University of Southern California School of Medicine.

Hon, E., & Quilligan, E. J. (1967). The classification of fetal heart rate: II. A revised working classification. *Connecticut Medicine, 31,* 779.

Kang, A. H., & Boehm, F. H. (1999). The clinical significance of intermittent sinusoidal fetal heart rate. *American Journal of Obstetrics and Gynecology, 180,* 151–152.

Kennedy, H. P., & MacDonald, E. L. (2002). "Altered consciousness" during childbirth: Potential clues to posttraumatic stress disorder. *Journal of Midwifery & Women's Health, 45,* 380–382.

Krebs, H. B., Petrie, R. E., & Dunn, L. J. (1983). Atypical variable deceleration. *American Journal of Obstetrics and Gynecology, 145,* 298.

McConnell, E. A. (1998). The coalescence of technology and humanism in nursing practice: It doesn't just happen and it doesn't come easily. *Holistic Nursing Practice, 12,* 23–30.

National Institute of Child Health & Development (NICHD). (1997). NICHD Fetal Monitoring Workshop. Bethesda, MD: Author.

Nurse's Association of the American College of Obstetricians and Gynecologists (NAACOG). (1990, March). *Fetal heart rate auscultation* (OGN Nursing Practice Resource). Washington, DC: Author.

Sandelowski, M. (1998). Looking to care or caring to look? Technology and the rise of spectacular nursing. *Holistic Nursing Practice, 12,* 1–11.

Swaim, L. S., & Creasy, R. K. (1997). Fetal assessment and treatment during labor. In R. K. Creasy (Ed.), *Management of labor and delivery* (pp. 143–182). Malden, MA: Blackwell.

Youngkin, E. & Davis, M. S. (1998). *Women's health: A primary care clinical guide.* (2nd ed.). Upper Saddle River, N J: Prentice Hall.

24 The Family in Childbirth: Needs and Care

The moment our daughter was born, time seemed to stand still. We couldn't keep our eyes off of her. I remember vividly the first time I touched her tiny finger and stroked her cheek. Those moments together as a family are forever engraved in my memory.

Objectives

- Identify nursing diagnoses specific to the first, second, third, and fourth stages of labor.
- Describe factors that are assessed in the laboring woman during the admission process.
- Discuss the components of a social history and its role in caring for the laboring woman.
- Summarize the importance of incorporating family expectations and cultural beliefs into the nursing care plan.
- Discuss nursing interventions to meet the care needs of the laboring woman and her partner during each stage of labor.
- Describe nursing interventions for promoting the woman's comfort during each stage of labor.
- Summarize immediate nursing care of the newborn following birth.
- Discuss the components of care for the woman during the third stage of labor.
- Discuss initial measures to help the woman and family integrate the newborn into family life.
- Explore the nurse's role in providing sensitive care to adolescent parents.
- Delineate management of a nurse-managed precipitous birth.

Key Terms

MEDIALINK

Additional resources for this content can be found on the Student CD-ROM and on the Companion Website at www.prenhall.com/olds. Click on "Chapter 24" to select the activities for this chapter.

CD-ROM
- Audio Glossary
- NCLEX Review
- Videos: First Stage of Labor and Transition
- Video: Second Stage of Labor
- Videos: Third Stage of Labor
- Animation: Placental Delivery
- Video: Newborn Assessment
- Video: Fourth Stage of Labor

Companion Website
- Additional NCLEX Review
- Case Study: Labor and Birth
- Care Plan Activity: Presence of Extended Family

It is time for a child to be born. The waiting is over; labor has begun. The dreams and wishes of the past months fade as the expectant family faces the reality of the tasks of childbearing and childrearing that are ahead.

The couple is about to undergo one of the most meaningful and stressful events in their life together. Physical and psychologic resources, coping mechanisms, and support systems will all be challenged. Despite months of childbirth education classes, the laboring woman may question her ability to cope with labor and to meet her own expectations of herself. The partner may wonder whether he will be able to provide the support his partner and newborn will need. They may worry about the baby's health. Although they look forward to the birth of their baby, they are entering an unfamiliar landscape where, even with prenatal preparation, unknown possibilities await them.

Many childbearing families look to the nurse for support and guidance. Indeed, for laboring women who are admitted alone, the nurse may be their sole support. It is essential, therefore, to provide holistic care that addresses the client's or couple's physiologic, psychologic, and comfort needs throughout the challenging and emotional process of labor and birth.

The previous two chapters present information that lays the foundation for this chapter. Chapter 22 presents a database of information regarding physiologic and psychologic changes during labor and birth, and Chapter 23 discusses intrapartal assessment. This chapter discusses nursing care during labor and birth. The Clinical Pathway on pages 628–630 summarizes nursing care of the childbearing family in the first through fourth stages of labor and birth.

Nursing Diagnosis During Labor and Birth

In devising a plan of care for the intrapartal period, the nurse can develop a general plan that encompasses the whole process, from the beginning of labor through the fourth stage, or the nurse can develop a plan for each stage of labor and birth. An overall plan presents an overview of the whole process, but it is usually general in nature. A plan of care that identifies nursing diagnoses for (at least) each stage provides an opportunity to identify more specific nursing interventions.

In the first stage of labor, nursing diagnoses that may apply include the following:

- ***Fear/Anxiety*** related to discomfort of labor and unknown labor outcome
- ***Compromised Family Coping*** related to labor process
- ***Acute Pain*** related to uterine contractions, cervical dilatation, and fetal descent
- ***Deficient Knowledge*** related to lack of information about normal labor process and comfort measures
- ***Fear/Anxiety*** related to unknown birth outcome and anticipated discomfort

Nursing diagnoses for the second and third stages may include the following:

- ***Acute Pain*** related to uterine contractions, birth process, and/or perineal trauma from birth
- ***Deficient Knowledge*** related to lack of information about pushing methods
- ***Compromised Individual Coping*** related to birth process
- ***Fear/Anxiety*** related to outcome of birth process

In the fourth stage, possible nursing diagnoses include the following:

- ***Acute Pain*** related to perineal trauma
- ***Deficient Knowledge*** related to lack of information about involutional process and self-care needs
- ***Altered Family Processes*** related to incorporation of the newborn into the family

Nursing Care During Admission

Many families worry that they will not reach the birthing center in time for the birth or that cues indicating the onset of labor will be missed. Sometimes labor occurs so rapidly that birth is imminent upon admission. Usually, the family is advised to arrive at the birth setting at the beginning of the active phase of labor or when the following occur:

- Rupture of membranes (ROM)
- Decreased fetal movement
- Regular, frequent uterine contractions (nulliparas, about 5 minutes apart for 1 hour; multiparas, 6 to 8 minutes apart for 1 hour)
- Any vaginal bleeding

If time permits and the family is not familiar with what will occur during labor, the nurse can provide information on admission. (See Client Teaching: What to Expect During Labor.)

The family may be facing a number of unfamiliar procedures that are routine for healthcare providers. It is important to remember that each woman has the right to determine what happens to her body. Informed consent should be obtained prior to any procedure that involves touching the body.

Establishing a Positive Relationship

The initial interaction with the nurse and how it is perceived by the woman and her partner greatly influences the course of her hospital stay. For some women, the hospital environment itself can be perceived as cold, impersonal, and technical and can produce anxiety or emotional stress. If the family is greeted in a brusque, harried manner, they are less likely to look to the nurse for support. A calm, pleasant manner, in contrast, indicates to the family that they are important. It helps instill in the couple a sense of confidence in the staff's ability to provide quality care and ensure safety during this critical time.

It is important to establish rapport and to create an environment in which the family feels free to ask questions. The

CLIENT TEACHING — WHAT TO EXPECT DURING LABOR

Assessment As the woman is admitted into the birthing area, assess the woman's knowledge regarding the childbirth experience. Her knowledge base will be affected by previous births, attendance at childbirth education classes, and the amount of information she has been able to gather during her pregnancy by asking questions or reading. You may also assess the factors that affect communication and anxiety level. Assess labor progress to determine what to teach and the time available for teaching. If the woman is in early labor and she needs additional information, proceed with teaching.

Nursing Diagnosis The key nursing diagnosis will probably be ***Deficient Knowledge*** related to lack of information about nursing care during labor.

Nursing Plan and Implementation The teaching plan will focus on the assessments and support the woman will receive during labor.

Client Goals At the completion of teaching, the woman will be able to:

- Verbalize the assessments the nurse will complete during labor.
- Discuss the support and comfort measures that are available.

Teaching Plan

CONTENT	TEACHING METHOD
• Describe aspects of the admission process, including: • Taking an abbreviated history • Physical assessment (maternal vital signs [VS], fetal heart rate [FHR], contraction status, status of membranes) • Assessment of uterine contractions (frequency, duration, intensity) • Orientation to surroundings • Introductions to other support staff • Determination of woman's and family support person's expectations of the nurse	Provide information on the basic assessment and care activities. Allow time for questions and discussion as labor progress permits.
• Present aspects of ongoing physical care, such as when to expect assessment of material VS, FHR, and contractions.	
• If the electronic fetal monitor is used, describe how it works and the information it provides. Orient the woman to the sights and sounds of the monitor. Explain what "normal" data will look like and what characteristics are being watched for.	Demonstrate the fetal monitor.
• Be sure to note that assessments will increase as the labor progresses, especially during the transition phase (usually the time the woman would like to be left alone) to help keep the mother and baby safe by noting deviations from normal course.	
• Describe the vaginal examination and the information it elicits.	Use a cervical dilatation chart to illustrate the amount of dilatation.
• Review comfort techniques that may be used in labor and ascertain what the woman thinks will promote comfort.	Focus on open discussion.
• Review the breathing techniques the woman has learned so that you will be able to support her technique.	Ask the woman to demonstrate the techniques she has learned.
• Review comfort and support measures, such as positioning, backrub, effleurage, touch, distraction techniques, and ambulation.	Focus on open discussion.
• If the woman is in early labor, offer her a tour of the birthing area.	Provide a tour of birthing area, explaining equipment and routines. Include the woman's partner.

Evaluation

At the end of this teaching session, the woman will be able to describe the assessments that will occur during her labor and to discuss comfort and support measures that may be used.

CLINICAL PATHWAY FOR INTRAPARTAL STAGES

Category	First Stage	Second and Third Stage	Fourth Stage Birth to 1 Hour Past Birth
Referral	**Review prenatal record** **Advise CNM/physician of admission**	**Labor record for first stage**	**Report to recovery room nurse** **➤ Expected Outcomes** Appropriate resources identified and utilized
Assessments	Admission assessments: Ask about problems since last prenatal visit; labor status (contraction frequency and duration), membrane status (intact or ruptured); coping level; support; woman's desires during labor and birth; ability to verbalize needs; laboratory testing (blood and UA) Intrapartal assessments: Cervical assessment: from 1 to 10 cm dilatation; nullipara (1.2 cm/h), multipara (1.5 cm/h) Cervical effacement: from 0% to 100% Fetal descent: progressive descent from −4 to +4 Membrane assessment: intact or ruptured; when ruptured, Nitrazine positive, fluid clear, no foul odor Comfort level: woman states is able to cope with contractions Behavioral characteristics: facial expressions, tone of voice, and verbal expressions are consistent with comfort level and ability to cope Latent Phase: • BP, P, R q1h if in normal range (BP 90–140/60–90 or not >30 mm Hg systolic or 15 mm Hg diastolic over baseline; pulse 60–90; respirations 12–20/min, quiet, easy) • Temp q4h unless >37.6C (99.6F) or membranes ruptured then q2h • Uterine contractions q30min (contractions q5–10min, 15–40sec, mild intensity) • FHR q60min (for low-risk women) and q30min (for high-risk women) if reassuring (reassuring FHR has: baseline 110–160, STV present, LTV average, accelerations with fetal movement, no late nor variable decelerations); if nonreassuring, position on side, start O_2, assess for hypotension, monitor continuously, notify CNM/physician Active Phase: • BP, P, R, q1h if WNL • Temp as above • Uterine contractions q15–30min: contractions q2–3min, 60 sec, moderate to strong • FHR q30min (for low-risk women) and q15min (for high-risk women) if reassuring; if nonreassuring institute interventions Transition: • BP, P, R, q30min • Uterine contractions q15min: contractions q2min, 60–75 sec, strong • FHR q15 min if reassuring; if nonreassuring, see above	Second stage assessments: • BP, P, R q5–15min • Uterine contractions palpated continuously • FHR q15min (for low-risk women) and q5min (for high-risk women) if reassuring; if nonreassuring, monitor continuously Fetal descent: descent continues to birth Comfort level: woman states is able to cope with contractions and pushing Behavioral characteristics: response to pushing, facial expressions, verbalization Third stage assessments: • BP, P, R q5min • Uterine contractions, palpate occasionally until placenta is delivered, fundus maintains tone and contraction pattern continues to birth of placenta Newborn assessments: • Assess Apgar score of newborn • Respirations: 30–60, irregular • Apical pulse: 110–160 and somewhat irregular • Temperature: Skin temp above 36.5C (97.8F) • Umbilical cord: two arteries, one vein (if one artery, assess for anomalies and urine output) • Gestational age: 38–42 weeks	Immediate postbirth assessments of mother q15min for 1h: • BP: 90–140/60–90; should return to prelabor level • Pulse: slightly lower than in labor; range is 60–90 • Respirations: 12–20/min; easy; quiet • Temperature: 36.2–37.6C (98–99.6F) • Fundus firm, in midline, at the umbilicus • Lochia rubra; moderate amount; <1 pad/h; no free flow or passage of clots with massage • Perineum: sutures intact; no bulging or marked swelling; minimal bruising may be present; no c/o severe pain nor rectal pain • Bladder nondistended; spontaneous void of >100 mL clear, straw-colored urine; bladder nondistended following voiding • If hemorrhoids present, no tenseness or marked engorgement; <2 cm diameter Comfort level: <3 on scale of 1 to 10 Energy level: awake and able to hold newborn Newborn assessments if newborn remains with parents: • Respirations: 30–60; irregular • Apical pulse: 110–160 and somewhat irregular • Temperature: skin temp above 36.5C (97.8F); skin feels warm to touch • Skin color noncyanotic • Mucus: small amount, clear, easily suctioned with bulb syringe without skin color change • Behavioral: newborn opens eyes widely if room is slightly darkened • Movements rhythmic; no hand tremors present **➤ Expected Outcomes** Findings indicate normal progression with absence of complications

CLINICAL PATHWAY FOR INTRAPARTAL STAGES *CONTINUED*

Category	First Stage	Second and Third Stage	Fourth Stage Birth to 1 Hour Past Birth
Teaching/ psychosocial	Establish rapport Orient to environment, expected assessments, and procedures Answer questions and provide information Orient to EFM if used Teach relaxation, visualization, and breathing pattern if needed Explain comfort measures available Assume advocacy role for woman/family during labor and birth	Orient to expected assessments and procedures Answer questions and provide information Explain comfort measures available Continue advocacy role	Explain immediate assessments and care after this first hour Teach self-massage of fundus and expected findings Instruct to call for assistance if mother desires to get OOB Begin newborn teaching; bulb syringe, positioning, maintaining warmth Assist parents in exploring their newborn Assist with first breastfeeding experience ➤ **Expected Outcomes** Client and partner verbalize/demonstrate understanding of teaching
Nursing care management and report	Straight cath prn if bladder distended If regional block administered monitor BP, FHR, sensation per protocol Provide continuing status reports to CNM/physician Perform sterile vaginal examination as indicated	Straight cath prn if bladder distended Continue monitoring VS, FHR, and sensation if regional block has been given	Straight cath if bladder distended Monitor return of motor ability and sensation if regional block has been given Weigh perineal pads if lochia flow >1 saturated pad in 15 min, presence of boggy uterus and clots; ↓BP, ↑P ➤ **Expected Outcomes** • Maternal/fetal well-being maintained and supported • Mother and newborn experience safe labor and birth • Family participates in process as desired
Activity	Encourage ambulation unless contraindicated Maintain bed rest immediately after administration of IV pain medication, or following regional block Woman rests comfortably between contractions	Position comfortably for birth Woman rests comfortably between pushing efforts and while awaiting birth of placenta	Position of comfort ➤ **Expected Outcomes** • Activity maintained as desired unless contraindicated • Comfort enhanced by positioning/movement
Comfort	Institute comfort measures: ambulation, frequent position change, effleurage, focal point, patterned paced breathing, visualization, therapeutic touch, backrub, moist cloths to face, holding hand, words of encouragement, changing underpad, shower, whirlpool, staying with the woman/family, warmed blanket at back, sacral pressure Offer pain medication or administer if requested Assist with administration of regional block	Institute comfort measures: • Second stage: cool cloth to forehead, encouragement, coaching, help support legs while pushing, position of comfort for pushing and birth • Third stage: cool cloth to forehead, assist parents to see newborn, position mother to hold newborn, provide encouragement	Institute comfort measures: • Perineal discomfort: gently cleanse and apply ice pack; position to decrease pressure on perineum • Uterine discomfort: palpate fundus gently • Hemorrhoids: ice pack • General fatigue: position of comfort, encourage rest • Administer pain medication PRN ➤ **Expected Outcomes** • Optimal comfort level maintained • Active reduction of pain/discomfort achieved
Nutrition	Ice chips and clear fluids Evaluate for signs of dehydration	Ice chips and clear fluids	Regular diet if assessments are WNL Encourage fluids ➤ **Expected Outcomes** Nutritional needs met
Elimination	Voids at least q2h; urine clear, straw-colored, negative for protein Bladder nondistended May have bowel movement Monitor I & O with IVs	May void spontaneously with pushing May pass stool with pushing	Voids spontaneously ➤ **Expected Outcomes** Urinary bladder and bowel function unimpaired
Medications	Administer pain medication per woman's request	Local infiltration of anesthetic agent for birth by CNM/physician Pitocin 10 units IM, IVP per IV tubing, or added to IV fluids	Continue Pitocin infusion Administer pain medication PRN ➤ **Expected Outcomes** Comfort enhanced by pain-relieving techniques, administration of analgesia agent or an analgesic or anesthetic block

(continued on next page)

CLINICAL PATHWAY FOR INTRAPARTAL STAGES *CONTINUED*

Category	First Stage	Second and Third Stage	Fourth Stage Birth to 1 Hour Past Birth
Discharge planning	Evaluate knowledge of labor and birth process Evaluate support system and need for referral after birth		Provide information if mother to be moved from LDR room Provide opportunity for parents to ask questions regarding newborn Evaluate knowledge of normal postpartum, newborn care ➤ **Expected Outcomes** Mother and newborn transferred to low-risk postpartal and newborn care
Family involvement	Identify available support person(s) Recognize possible impact of culture on responses Observe interaction between woman and partner Create moment alone with woman to identify possible abuse Assess current parenting skills	Provide opportunities for woman and support person(s) to watch newborn assessments Perform newborn assessment on mother's abdomen/chest if possible	Provide opportunity for parents to be with baby Encourage skin-to-skin contact Darken room to encourage eye-to-eye contact Provide quiet time for new family Parenting: demonstrates early culturally expected parenting behaviors ➤ **Expected Outcomes** • Incorporation of newborn into family • Family verbalizes comfort with newborn care
Date			

CNM, certified nurse-midwife; BP, blood pressure; FHR, fetal heart rate; STV, short-term variability; LTV long-term variability; WNL, within normal limits; VS, vital signs; EFM, electronic fetal monitoring; IV, intravenous; I&O, intake & output; IM, intramuscularly; IVP, intravenous push; LDR, labor, delivery, and recovery; OOB, out of bed; UA, urinary analysis; PRN, as needed

support and encouragement of the nurse in maintaining a caring environment begins with the initial admission but needs to be attended to with all subsequent actions. Before completing assessments, the nurse may provide the opportunity for questions and may explain the environment and the procedures that will be a part of the labor and birthing care. In many hospitals, the admission process also includes signing an informed consent for treatment, and the client is given information on arranging advanced directives or instructions about her wishes if she were to become critically ill. In all cases, an identification bracelet and a bracelet that lists all known drug allergies are attached to her wrist.

Another important aspect of the initial contact is communicating in the woman and family's primary language. In addition to having interpreters available for Hispanic, Korean, Vietnamese, and other clients who do not speak English fluently, the nurse must consider the special needs of the deaf woman or family. There are more than 400,000 Americans who have a bilateral hearing loss, so there is a good chance that the nurse will work with a deaf expectant mother, father, grandparents, or siblings at some point. Table 24–1 • provides suggestions for communicating more effectively with a woman or support person who is deaf.

Labor Assessment

Following the initial greeting, the woman may either be taken into a labor assessment area (sometimes called a *triage area*) for evaluation or admitted directly into a birthing room. Some couples prefer to remain together during the admission process, and others prefer to have the partner or support person wait outside. The nurse should ask the woman's preference whenever possible. As the nurse helps the woman undress and get into a hospital gown, the nurse can begin to develop rapport and establish the nursing database. The labor and birth nurse can obtain essential information regarding the woman and her pregnancy. By doing an admission history, the nurse can initiate any immediate interventions needed and establish individualized priorities. The nurse is then able to make effective nursing decisions regarding intrapartal care:

- Is the woman in labor or is she a candidate to be sent home with a clear understanding of when to return?
- Are there factors that put the laboring woman or the fetus at risk?
- Should ambulation or bed rest be encouraged?
- Is more frequent monitoring needed?
- What does the woman and/or couple want during labor and birth?
- Who will be with the laboring woman for social support?

The woman is made comfortable. If she wants to rest in bed, a side-lying or semi-Fowler's position rather than a supine position is most comfortable and avoids supine hypotensive syndrome (vena caval syndrome).

After obtaining the essential information from the woman and her prenatal records from her certified nurse-

Table 24-1 • IMPROVING COMMUNICATION WITH A DEAF WOMAN OR SUPPORT PERSON

- Determine how the deaf individual prefers to communicate: speech reading (lip reading), sign language, pantomime, writing, or a combination of methods.
- If speech reading is used, face the person directly, speak with a natural tone and rhythm (exaggerated pronunciation may distort lip movements), and keep your hands away from your face. Do not chew gum.
- Use gestures and pantomime if necessary to enhance your speech.
- Do not assume written communication is the most effective approach. Writing carries a great potential for miscommunication and should not be forced unless the deaf person requests it.
- Most deaf individuals in the United States use American Sign Language (ASL). If the woman signs, call a professional ASL interpreter.
- Only use a family member as an interpreter until the professional interpreter arrives. Family members may not interpret all that is said or may add additional information. Professional ASL interpreters are bound by a code of ethics to maintain strict confidentiality, to transmit accurate messages, and to refrain from editing or adding information.
- Keep the woman's dominant hand and arm free for signing.
- Explain any procedures before they are needed.
- Look at the deaf individual, not the interpreter, when speaking.
- Be alert for signs of "smiling and nodding." Often, when a deaf person does not understand something, the person will simply smile and nod. If that occurs, assess the person's understanding by asking the person to repeat the information to you.

Source: Adapted from Shelp, S. G. (1997). Your patient is deaf, now what? *RN, 60*(2), 37–38, 40. Reprinted by permission of Medical Economics. Montvale, NJ.

midwife (CNM) or physician, the nurse begins the intrapartal assessment. (Chapter 23 considers intrapartal assessment in depth.)

As the assessments begin, the nurse auscultates the fetal heart rate (FHR). (Detailed information on monitoring FHR is presented in Chapter 21.) The woman's blood pressure, pulse, respirations, and oral temperature are assessed. Contraction status (frequency, duration, and intensity), cervical dilatation and effacement, and fetal presentation and station are determined. If the woman is a nullipara in the early latent phase (for example, contractions are 10 to 30 minutes apart, with mild intensity and very little discomfort; cervix is long and thick, with dilatation of 1 to 2 cm; membranes are intact) she may be sent home to ambulate and rest in her own surroundings or directed to remain in a birthing center area and ambulate. When further progress is documented, she is admitted. Women who are admitted in the latent phase are more likely to have a longer duration of labor, increased use of epidural analgesia for pain, and increased use of oxytocin to augment labor than women who are clearly in the active phase at admission.

After the vaginal examination, the nurse shares the findings with the couple. If there are signs of advanced labor (frequent contractions, advanced cervical dilatation and/or an urge to bear down), the physician/CNM is notified immediately, and actions are taken to prepare for the birth. If there are signs of excessive bleeding upon admission or if the woman reports episodes of painless bleeding in the last trimester, placenta previa may be present; in such cases, vaginal examination is not performed because it may stimulate copious bleeding.

Table 24-2 • INDICATORS OF NORMAL LABOR PROCESS ON ADMISSION

Indicator	Normal Characteristics
Uterine contractions	Frequency of not less than 2 minutes Duration of less than 75 seconds Uterine relaxation between contractions Most intense discomfort only with contractions (Some women, especially those with occiput posterior position, complain of less intense lower abdominal and/or back pain between contractions.)
Fetal heart rate	Rate 110–160 with average variability Absence of variable or late decelerations
Maternal vital signs	BP below +40/90 or less than +30/+15 above prepregnancy readings Pulse 60–100 Temperature between 97.8 and 99.6F (36.5 and 37.5C)
If membranes ruptured	Fluid clear without odor

Results of FHR assessment, uterine contraction evaluation, and the vaginal examination help determine whether the rest of the admission process can proceed at a more leisurely pace or whether additional interventions have higher priority. For example, an FHR of 100 beats per minute (bpm) on auscultation indicates that an electronic fetal monitor (EFM) should be applied immediately to obtain additional data. The woman's vital signs will then be assessed immediately (Table 24–2 •).

Depending on how rapidly labor is progressing, the nurse notifies the CNM or physician before or after completing the admission procedures. The report should include the following information: cervical dilatation and effacement, station, presenting part, status of the membranes, contraction pattern, FHR, vital signs that are not in the normal range, the woman's wishes, and her response to labor.

Collecting Laboratory Data

After admission data are obtained, multiple laboratory tests are performed to provide more extensive physiologic data that are used to determine appropriate care for the woman and her fetus. A clean-voided midstream urine specimen is usually collected. The woman with intact membranes may collect her specimen in the bathroom. The nurse can test the woman's urine for the presence of protein, ketones, glucose, and leukocytes by using a dipstick before sending the sample to the laboratory. This procedure is especially important if nondependent edema or elevated blood pressure is noted on admission. Proteinuria of +1 or more may be a sign of preeclampsia. Glycosuria is found frequently in pregnant women because of the increased glomerular filtration rate in the proximal tubules and the inability of these tubules to increase glucose reabsorption. However, it may also be associated with gestational diabetes and should not be discounted. Leukocytes can be found in the urine when bacteria is present. The presence of a urinary tract infection can contribute to uterine irritability, pelvic pressure, and back pain, all symptoms that can be mistaken for labor.

Laboratory tests can be performed in the outpatient setting prior to admission but are most commonly done at the time of admission in the birthing center. Hemoglobin and hematocrit values help determine the oxygen-carrying capacity of the circulatory system and the ability of the woman to withstand blood loss at birth. Elevation of the hematocrit indicates hemoconcentration of blood, which occurs with edema or dehydration. A low hemoglobin, in the absence of other evidence of bleeding, suggests anemia. Blood may be typed and cross-matched if the woman is in a high-risk category, has active bleeding, or has a history of blood disorders. A serology test for syphilis is obtained if one has not been done in the last 3 months or if an antepartal serology result was positive.

Social Assessment

Once initial physical assessments are performed, the nurse can then take a detailed social history that provides a comprehensive view of both the woman's social habits and psychologic factors that may affect her birth experience. The presence of certain risk factors—including family violence or sexual assault (see Chapter 9); use of drugs, alcohol, or tobacco; and presence of sexually transmitted infections—can influence a woman's labor, birth, and future childrearing choices. Since many women find questions about psychosocial risk factors embarrassing, the nurse should always ask such questions when the woman is alone, and should use a straightforward, nonjudgmental approach. For example, a question such as "How many times per week do you drink alcohol?" prompts the woman to be specific in her answer. If the woman reports that she does drink alcohol on a daily basis, the nurse then asks about the amount. Drug use can be assessed in a similar manner.

A social assessment should also include data about the woman's current living situation, availability of resources, preparedness for the infant, community resources, and the woman's social support network. This dialog provides an opportunity for the nurse to continue to build support, to provide information when requested, and to be direct yet supportive. Referrals to social services, the Special Supplemental Food Program for Women, Infants, and Children (WIC), and new parent support programs can be initiated. It is important to begin this dialog early in the admission process so that adequate resources can be obtained for the family.

Documentation of Admission

A nursing admission note is entered into the computer or the charting system. The admission note should include the reason for admission, the date and time and method of the woman's arrival, notification of the CNM/physician, the condition of the woman and her baby, labor and membrane status, and pertinent social assessment information. Her comfort level and support system should also be addressed.

Nursing Care During the First Stage of Labor

During the first stage of labor, the nurse is concerned about the physical safety of the laboring woman and her child, as well as the emotional well-being of the laboring couple and their support system. Therefore, the nurse continually assesses the effects of uterine contractions on the course of labor and the well-being of the fetus, and monitors the woman's vital signs, contraction pattern, cervical changes, and intake and output. Additionally, the nurse monitors the couple's and support system's responses to labor.

Labor support is a primary role for nurses who are caring for couples during the first stage of labor. Couples look to their nurse for information about labor progress, pain management, procedures, and examinations, and for assistance with pain management techniques such as breathing and relaxation. Couples need reassurance that labor is progressing in normal trajectory and explanations when it is not within normal limits. They also need praise for their accomplishments and support during labor. For most couples, the nurse's presence in the room is highly valued as labor advances; however, the nurse should assess the woman's individual preferences since some women may prefer privacy. Clinical research has established that laboring women have fewer complications and shorter labors when they perceive support from their nurse and/or friends and family members.

Integration of Family Expectations

Laboring families have certain expectations of the experience, of themselves, of the nurse, and of the physician or certified nurse-midwife (CNM). Some of these expectations may not be realistic. Unrealistic expectations can increase the anxiety level of both the laboring woman and her partner. The labor nurse should assess the family's expectations in order to integrate them into the labor plan and/or assist the family in reestablishing expectations that are realistic. Some families may present to the birthing center with a birth plan (discussed in Chapter 13). The plan should be reviewed and requests should be incorporated into the woman's nursing care plan whenever possible. Requests that cannot be met should be discussed and a clear rationale should be provided.

Laboring families' expectations of the nurse can range from wanting the nurse to be highly involved in the labor, to wanting the nurse to be minimally involved. The couple that desires high involvement expects the labor nurse to be in the room continuously and to provide direct labor support. The couple may view the labor nurse as the woman's primary labor coach. The couple that desires minimal involvement of the labor nurse prefers that the nurse is present only when assessments and interventions need to be done and when the couple requests the nurse's presence.

With the variety of expectations clients have of nurses, it becomes a challenge to provide individualized care. The

RESEARCH IN PRACTICE
Nursing Support During Labor

What is this study about? Technology has changed the way nurses provide care to laboring mothers. Support during labor involves providing more than technical support; support involves physical comfort measures, emotional support, information giving, and advocacy. Nursing support during labor has been linked to better outcomes, reduced requirements for invasive procedures, lower anxiety, and an increase in perceived control by women during childbirth. Interactions with healthcare providers during labor can have significant long-term influence on how mothers perceive the childbirth experience. This study examined the amount of support provided by nurses to women during childbirth and the factors that influence nurses' ability to provide support.

How was this study done? Data were collected at a Canadian teaching hospital that was staffed exclusively with RN's. This descriptive study used a work sampling procedure to quantify the amount of time the nurses spent providing supportive care. Observation periods were randomly selected over six day shifts in a three-week period. A total of 404 observations were recorded of the activities of 12 nurses. The nurses were observed for activity based on a structured observational checklist. Activities were coded and categorized as supportive care or "other." The list of supportive care activities was based on qualitative findings from interviews with postpartum women describing labor. Following the observation period, six interviews were used to collect data from the nurses regarding their perceptions of supportive care and the factors that influence the provision of supportive care. Data from the interviews were analyzed using content analysis.

What were the results of the study? Study findings suggest that nurses spend a minimal amount of time in supportive activities for laboring women. Nurses in the sample spent only 27.8% of their time in contact with laboring women, with 12.4% of their total time providing supportive care to laboring women. The most frequently observed category was informational support, comprising 70% of the support provided. During interview, the nurses described physical comfort measures, emotional support, and advocacy as other components of supportive nursing care, but identified short staffing as a major barrier to providing supportive care. Observation data, though, identified that this was an infrequent occurrence. The control that healthcare providers assume over the childbirth process was revealed as a barrier to providing supportive care. This control was in the form of adherence to procedures, the use of physicians to validate control, and the use of technology.

What additional questions might I have? How did the laboring mothers feel about control issues? Did they perceive that it interfered with supportive behaviors? How much supportive nursing care did these mothers desire? Why are nurses not providing the support that they describe in the interviews as being important?

How can I use this study? Given the benefits of intrapartum nursing support, it is important that birthing units facilitate its implementation. This can be accomplished by reducing barriers to the provision of supportive nursing care, including an emphasis on controlling behaviors and procedures. The environment must be conducive to the provision of supportive care during labor, and nurses should demonstrate their commitment to supportive care by increasing the amount of time spent in direct contact with laboring mothers.

Source: Gale, J., Fothergill-Bourbonnais, F., & Chamberlain, M. (2001). Measuring nursing support during childbirth. *The American Journal of Maternal/Child Nursing, 26*(5), 264–71.

nurse needs to assess and respond to the couple's needs and desires. To determine preferences, the nurse can look for cues. When the woman and her coach are admitted, do they seem to take control and know what is going to happen? Do they have a birth plan that they have already worked out, or do they seem hesitant and unsure of the process?

Although these two ends of the spectrum are obvious, they are a starting point. It would be fairly safe to assume that the "situation-is-in-control" couple would want a little less involvement, and the couple who is hesitant and asking questions will want more extensive involvement. The nurse can also gain more information by asking questions such as, "Other than the assessments that I will be making, what kind of involvement would you like from me? Would you like to call me when you need something or have me come in now and then, or would you be more comfortable if I stay in the room most of the time?" This gives the couple an opportunity to make their wishes known. It is also important that the couple knows that the nurse understands that their wishes may change during labor and that the nurse will be available for them throughout the process.

Integration of Cultural Beliefs

Values, customs, and practices of different cultures are as important during labor as they are in the prenatal period. Without this knowledge, a nurse is less likely to understand a family's behavior and may impose personal values and beliefs upon them. As cultural sensitivity increases, so does the likelihood of providing high-quality care (Callister, 2001).

The following sections briefly present a few possible cultural responses to labor. Additional information on culturally sensitive care is provided in Chapter 2. It is difficult to present such a limited discussion without appearing to advance stereotypes. No statement of a specific behavior can accurately reflect the preference of all people in a group. Within every culture, each person develops his or her own beliefs and value system. Nurses must regard general information about any culture or belief system as background information to help them determine the person's own needs and desires.

Clinical Tip *It is best not to assume that women of any culture have the information they desire regarding birth, self-care, and newborn care, regardless of the number of children they have had. An important aspect of nursing is to teach, so always offer culturally sensitive information. Most nurses are not knowledgeable regarding all cultural practices. So be sensitive, and ask what is important to the mother. For example, is there special clothing she wants the newborn to wear, or does she have any preference about how she wants the umbilical stump cared for? Remain aware that the information you learned in class or a text reflects primarily the nursing culture and the Western, chiefly European, culture. To believe that the healthcare practices of these two cultures are relevant to all people is an example of ethnocentrism. Strive to increase your understanding of other cultures as your clinical practice base grows.*

MODESTY

Modesty is an important consideration for women, regardless of the culture to which they belong. However, some women may be more uncomfortable than others with the degree of exposure needed for some procedures during the labor and the birth process. Some women may be particularly uncomfortable when men are present and feel more comfortable with women; others may be uncomfortable with exposure of personal body parts regardless of the gender of the examiner or person who assists them. The nurse needs to be observant of the woman's responses to examinations and procedures and to provide appropriate draping and privacy. It is more prudent to assume that embarrassment will occur with exposure and take measures to provide privacy than to assume that it will not matter to the woman.

For example, many Hispanic women may fear loss of privacy, so they labor at home as long as possible. Maintaining dignity for the couple is important (Murray & Zentner, 2001). Some Asian women are not accustomed to male physicians and attendants, and some Muslims forbid any male (other than the husband) to see a woman who is uncovered. The nurse should be aware that in the Muslim culture, the man is the primary source of information. It may be necessary to speak to the man before interacting with the woman. This communicates respect and shows cultural sensitivity. The nurse should ensure coverage of the woman whenever possible, even during vaginal exams and the second stage (Murray & Zentner, 2001).

PAIN EXPRESSION

Women's reactions to the discomfort of labor vary greatly. Some turn inward and remain very quiet during the whole process whereas others may be very vocal, with behaviors such as counting out loud, moaning quietly or loudly, crying, or cursing. They may also turn from side to side or change positions frequently. The nurse supports a woman's individual expression of pain, whatever it may be, in order to enhance the birthing experience for mother, baby, and family.

In the Korean culture it used to be important for the laboring woman to be silent so she would not bring shame on her family. However, today women are encouraged to be less passive. Vocalization is more common, although older in-laws or other family members may discourage shouting or outcries as aggressive behavior. Hmong women are frequently quiet during labor, although behavior varies from one individual to the next. European Americans demonstrate a wide variety of behaviors in response to pain. Some stay very quiet and seem to turn inward to "keep control"; others move about in bed, change positions frequently, moan, and cry. Especially in the transitional phase, some women want to squeeze their partner's (or the nurse's) hand, and some may be tempted to bite during the most intense part of the contraction.

EXAMPLES OF CULTURAL BELIEFS

Some differences between cultures are apparent with regard to specific practices related to position and food and drink during labor. In most non-European societies uninfluenced by Westernization, women assume an upright position in childbirth. For example, during birth some Native American women use meditation, self-control, or indigenous plants, and the father may be expected to avoid certain rituals such as eating meat. Some Native Americans may ask to take the placenta home for a ritualistic ceremony that involves returning the placenta to the earth.

For Hmong women from Laos, the beginning of labor signifies the beginning of a transition and entails certain dietary restrictions. The woman usually prefers only "hot" foods, tea made with loose tea leaves, and warm water to drink. The woman usually maintains self-control, and may wish to move about freely during the first stage of labor. She may smile even throughout intense contractions. The husband is frequently present and actively involved in providing comfort. Traditionally, the woman prefers that the amniotic membranes not be ruptured until just before birth. It is thought that the escape of fluid at this time makes the birth easier. She may choose to kneel or squat for the birth of her baby. As soon as the baby is born, a soft-boiled egg must be given to the mother to restore her energy. During the postpartum period, the mother prefers "warm" foods, such as chicken prepared with warm water and warm rice (Morrow, 1986). The newborn is protected from praise to prevent jealousy.

Latina women often want their partner to stay with them during labor and birth and to reassure them that everything will be all right. The women want the partner to show caring and love as they labor and to speak to them using affectionate words. Standing close to the woman and using touch are important roles for the partner (Murray & Zentner, 2001).

Muslim women may have their husband, a female friend or relative, or a male relative with them during childbirth. Family support may be particularly important but does not preclude the importance of the nurse's presence. The woman may want to retain her head covering (*khimar*), and two long-sleeved gowns can be offered. Examinations should be done by a female nurse, physician, or CNM whenever possible. Some Muslim women are not comfortable in the presence of a male physician or nurse. If a male physician is involved with their care, they may wish for their husband to remain in the room during all care by the physician. Male providers should only enter the room after receiving permission from the husband. Modesty needs vary, and each individual will need to be assessed. After the birth, Muslim fathers traditionally call praise to Allah (*adhan*) in the newborn's right ear and clean the newborn. It is helpful if the birthing room personnel are aware of these practices so that the family's expectations and wishes can be incorporated into care. Many Middle-Eastern clients also believe that compliments addressed to the parents about their new baby will bring on the evil eye. "The evil eye is a form of superstitious jealousy and mistrust of the admirer by the owner or the one being complimented" (Murray & Zentner, 2001, p. 28). Thus, the nurse should avoid directly complimenting the couple, but instead direct compliments to God (*Allah*).

> *I am in an area with a very small Muslim population, and one of the nursing students with me had the opportunity to work with a Muslim couple during labor, birth, and then in the postpartum area the following day. During labor, the woman's sister remained at her side, and her husband sat on the other side of a drawn curtain inside the labor room and close to the door. He requested that a sign be placed on the door indicating that no males were to enter the room. We took care to ensure that we asked for a female lab tech for blood drawing, and a female physician attended the birth. The labor and birth went smoothly, and the woman did not utter any sound, even during pushing. After the birth, the father was shown the child before his wife held the newborn boy. The father was very pleased and talked quietly to his son, with his head down beside the newborn's ear. The next day, the student was once again assigned to this family. The sign remained on the door, and at all times that day, the sister and father remained in the room, the father always sitting away from the bed, close to the door. This was the woman's fifth child, so at first the student thought that she would not want much self-care, newborn, or breastfeeding information. But she began to talk to the woman, with her husband interpreting all questions and giving answers, and as each topic was brought up, the mother indicated that she wanted more information. Building on the trust that they had established the previous day in labor, the father told the student to "give the instruction," and he left the room. The mother and sister were full of questions about their health and their bodies—questions they had had for years! The student was proud that she did not make assumptions and was able to share so much information with them. It was an experience that the student and I will always remember with great joy.*

Sometimes cultural norms are passed down from one generation to the next. African Americans, especially those whose ancestors are from Western Africa, may have beliefs rooted in traditional folk healing. A survey of African American adults found that 38% had a family member in the United States who still believed in traditional folk healing and 50% had a relative who told folk-healing stories (Parks, 1998). Some of these beliefs are centered around labor and childrearing. For example, it is widely believed that an infant born with a caul (a piece of the amniotic membrane covering the head at birth) will have the ability to communicate with spirits. This is viewed as a sign of good luck and is widely embraced within this culture.

In working with women from another culture, the nurse needs an awareness of their beliefs, values, and practices in order to understand their needs. The maternity nurse would do well to make it a priority to become acquainted with the beliefs and practices of the various cultures in the community. In the birthing situation, the nurse supports the family's cultural practices as long as it is safe to do so.

Provision of Care in the First Stage

Throughout the first stage, the nurse needs to evaluate physical parameters of the woman and her fetus. Maternal temperature is monitored every 4 hours unless the temperature is over 37.5C (99.6F); in such cases, it must be taken every hour. Once the amniotic fluid has ruptured, temperature should be monitored every 2 hours.

The nurse monitors blood pressure, pulse, and respirations every hour (Association of Women's Health, Obstetric, and Neonatal Nurses [AWHONN], 1999). If the woman's blood pressure is over 140/90 mm Hg or her pulse is more than 100, the CNM/physician must be notified. The blood pressure and pulse are then reevaluated more frequently. The nurse palpates uterine contractions for frequency, intensity, and duration.

Intrapartal vaginal exams are done to assess cervical changes, status of membranes, fetal position, and station. However, frequent vaginal exams increase the risk of infection and should be performed only when needed. Some providers advocate performing vaginal examinations only when a change of management will occur, such as prior to an epidural or to provide scalp stimulation.

The fetal heart rate (FHR) is auscultated every 60 minutes for low-risk women and every 30 minutes for high-risk women as long as it remains between 110 and 160 beats per minute (bpm) without the presence of decelerations. The FHR should be auscultated throughout one contraction and for about 15 seconds after the contraction to ensure that there are no decelerations. If the FHR is not in the 110 to 160 range and/or decelerations are heard, continuous electronic monitoring is recommended. Table 24–3 • summarizes nursing assessments in the first stage of labor. The nurse documents labor progress, status of fetus, and interventions in the woman's chart.

MEDIALINK VIDEOS: FIRST STAGE OF LABOR AND TRANSITION

Clinical Tip *If the monitor is no longer recording the fetal heart tracing, check that there is adequate gel under the transducer and reposition it before you assume there is a problem with the baby.*

Table 24-3 • NURSING ASSESSMENTS IN THE FIRST STAGE

Phase	Mother	Fetus
Latent	Blood pressure, respirations each hour if in normal range Temperature every 4 hours unless over 37.5C (99.6F) or membranes ruptured, then every hour Uterine contractions every 30 minutes	FHR every 60 minutes for low-risk women and every 30 minutes for high-risk women if normal characteristics present (average variability, baseline in the 110–160 bpm range, without late or variable decelerations). Note fetal activity. If electronic fetal monitor in place, assess for reactive NST.
Active	Blood pressure, pulse, respirations every hour if in normal range Uterine contractions palpated every 15 to 30 minutes	FHR every 30 minutes for low-risk women and every 15 minutes for high-risk women if normal characteristics are present (AWHONN, 1999).
Transition	Blood pressure, pulse, respirations every 30 minutes Contractions palpated at least every 15 minutes	FHR every 15 minutes if normal characteristics are present.

LATENT PHASE

If the laboring woman has not had childbirth education classes, the latent phase is a time when the nurse can give anticipatory guidance. Most women are not too uncomfortable with contractions at this time and are responsive to teaching about breathing and other techniques for coping with labor contractions. In fact, many women in the latent phase seek information about what to expect. The unprepared woman may hesitate to ask questions and thus can benefit even more from anticipatory guidance by the nurse.

As long as there are no contraindications (such as vaginal bleeding or rupture of membranes [ROM] with the fetus unengaged), the woman may be encouraged to ambulate, because upright positions shorten labor. A tour of the birthing facility can help decrease anxiety and distract her from her discomfort. Many women feel much more at ease and comfortable if they can move around and do not have to remain in bed. Ambulation also aids in fetal descent, increases the frequency and intensity of contractions, and provides the woman with a sense of control (Figure 24–1 •).

The nurse should offer fluids in the form of clear liquids or ice chips at frequent intervals. Because gastric emptying time is prolonged during labor, solid foods are usually avoided. Fasting during labor is the subject of some controversy. Some providers believe that eating and drinking in labor should be an option for women. Vomiting during labor occurs frequently due to the decreased gastric emptying time. It is not uncommon for women to vomit during first stage, especially during the transition phase. The nurse should reassure the woman and provide oral care.

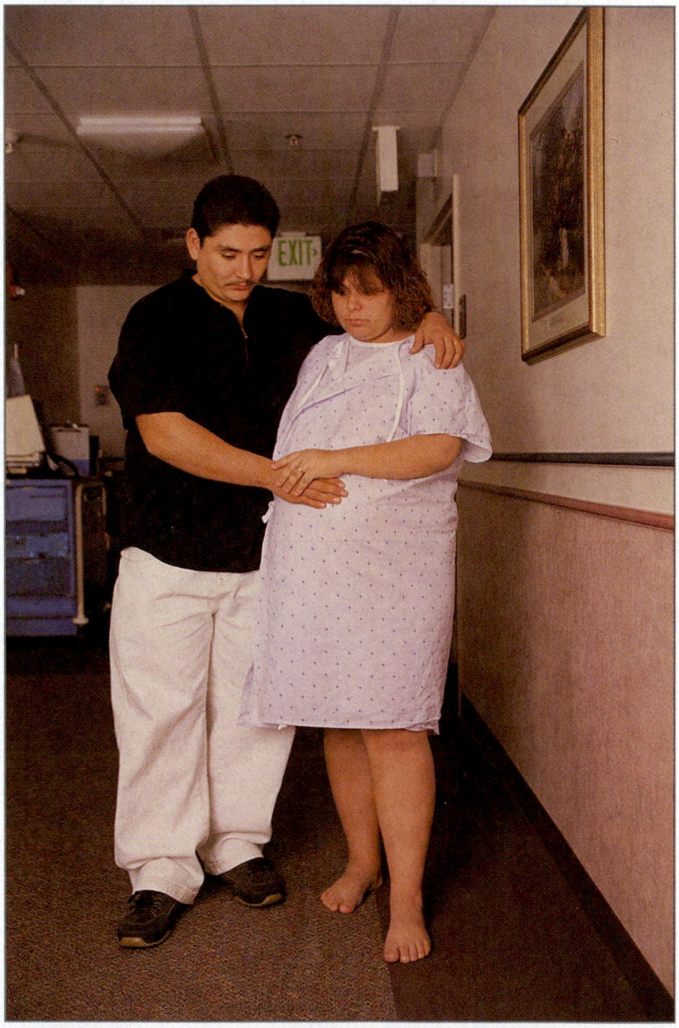

Figure 24–1 • Woman and her partner walking in the hospital during labor.

ACTIVE PHASE

During the active phase, the contractions have a frequency of 2 to 3 minutes, a duration of 50 to 60 seconds, and moderate intensity. Contractions need to be palpated every 15 to 30 minutes. As the contractions become more frequent and intense, intrapartal vaginal examination may be performed to assess cervical dilatation and effacement and fetal station and position. During the active phase, the cervix dilates from 4 to 7 cm, and vaginal discharge and bloody show increase. The woman should be encouraged to void because a full bladder can interfere with fetal descent. If the woman is unable to void, catheterization may be necessary. The FHR is auscultated every 30 minutes for low-risk women and every 15 minutes for high-risk women (AWHONN, 1999).

For the woman experiencing slow progress of labor or the inability to tolerate fluids, an intravenous electrolyte solution may be started to provide energy and prevent dehydration. If

A Day in the Life of a Nurse-Midwife

TO ME, PREGNANCY IS A WONDERFUL, normal experience—part of the cycle of life. That's why I love the fact that I can participate in all aspects of it, from pregnancy through birth and into the postpartal period. My practice enables me to ensure that a family's childbirth experience incorporates their personal beliefs and meets their expectations as much as possible. Come along with me for a day.

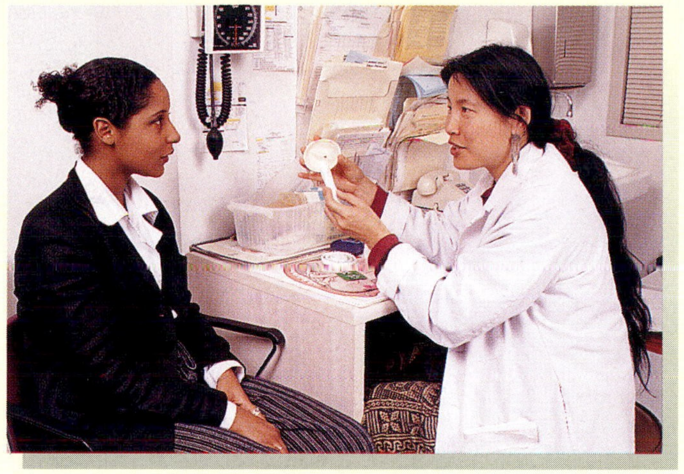

Cherrene has come for contraceptive information. I find it helpful to use models and examples during the discussion.

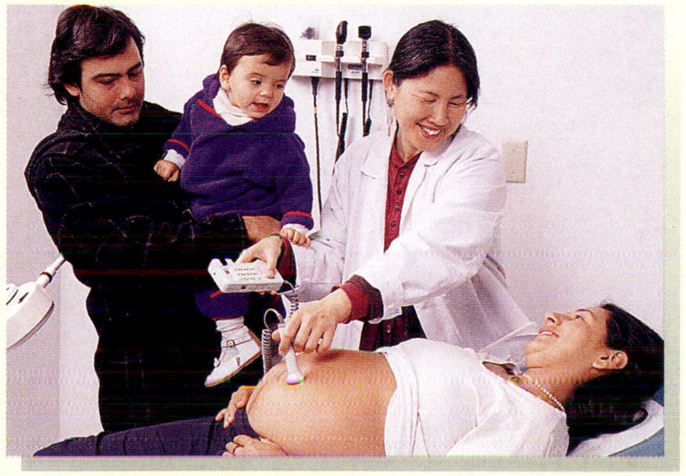

Dianne and her family come together for every appointment. We all enjoy listening to the fetal heartbeat.

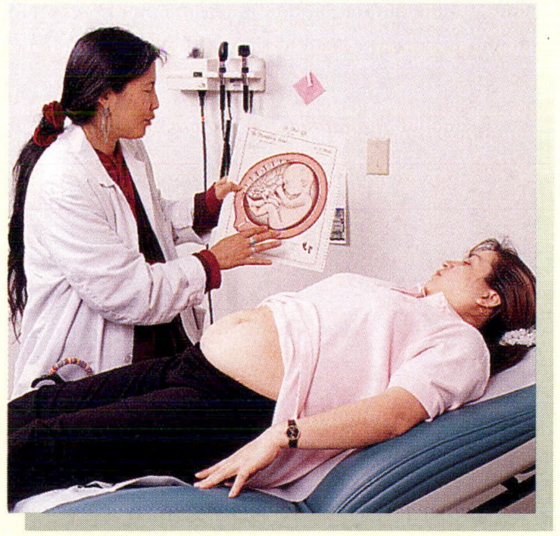

Gretchen's pregnancy is progressing well. She asks what her baby looks like now. I like to use a visual device as I talk with her about her baby's development.

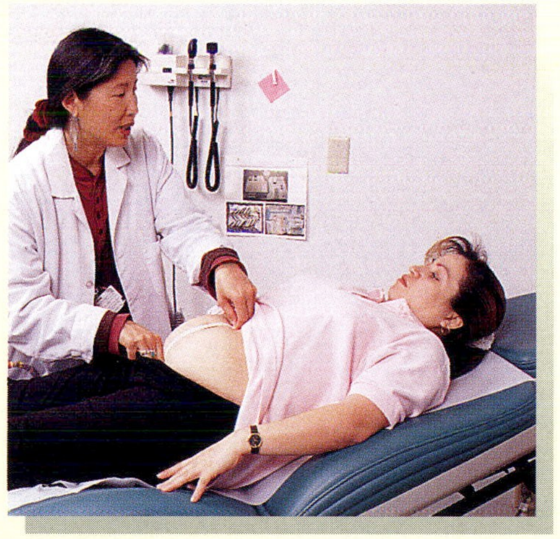

I measure the height of the fundus to determine if the baby is growing as expected. Gretchen and I talk about the impact of her nutrition, exercise, and healthy lifestyle habits on her baby and the outcome of her pregnancy.

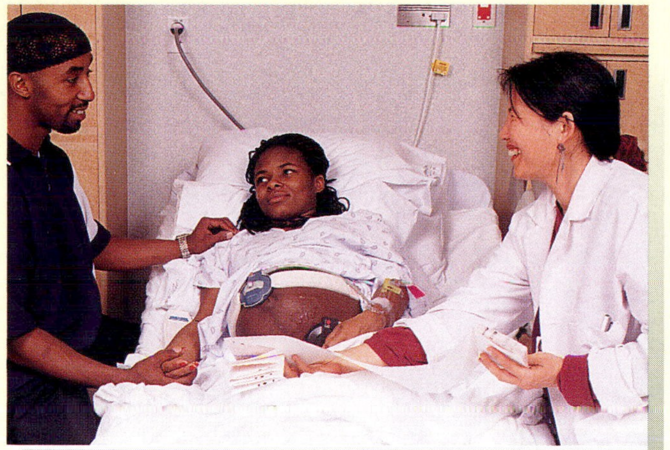

Darnell and Ayisha are expecting their first baby. Ayisha calls to tell me her labor has begun, and I meet them at the birth center. After the electronic fetal monitor is applied, we talk about the fetal heart tracing. I want to be sure they understand the monitor and have the opportunity to ask questions.

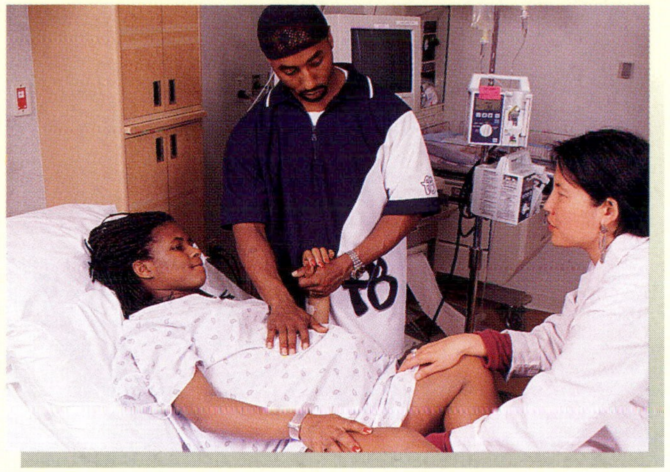

I do an exam to see how labor is progressing and share my findings with them.

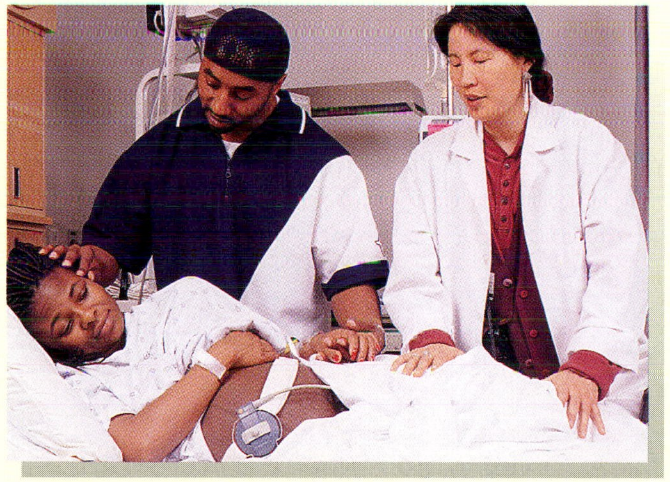

During the active phase of Ayisha's labor, Darnell lovingly provides comfort and support.

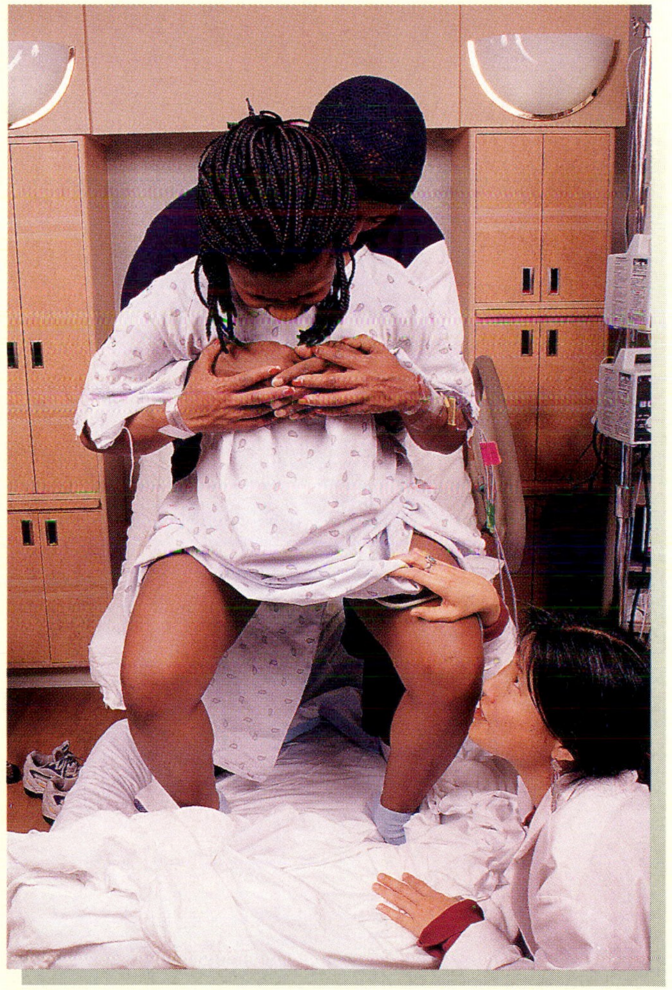

It's time to push. Ayisha wants to stand and is most comfortable on the bed. Darnell stands behind her and provides support. I continue to talk with them and provide encouragement. After an hour of pushing, baby Kinshasa is born.

MATERNAL-FETAL DEVELOPMENT

	0 CONCEPTION	1 4 WEEKS	2 8 WEEKS	3 12 WEEKS	4 16 WEEKS
FETAL DEVELOPMENT	*The sperm fertilizes the ovum, which then divides and burrows into the uterus.* 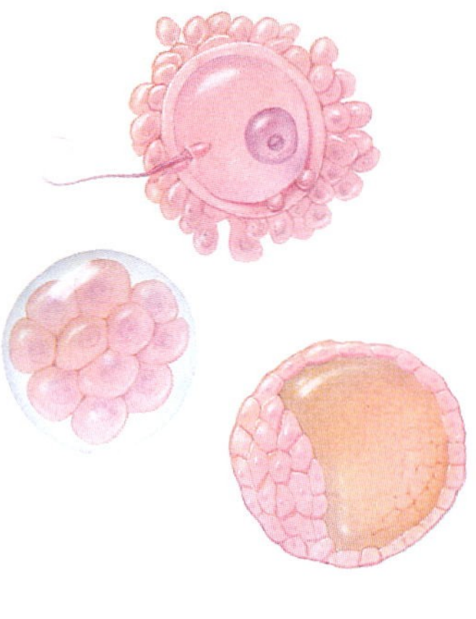	*From the embryonic disk (ectoderm, entoderm, mesoderm), the first body segments appear that will eventually become the spine, brain, and spinal cord. Heart, blood circulation, and digestive tract take shape. Embryo is less than a quarter-inch long.* 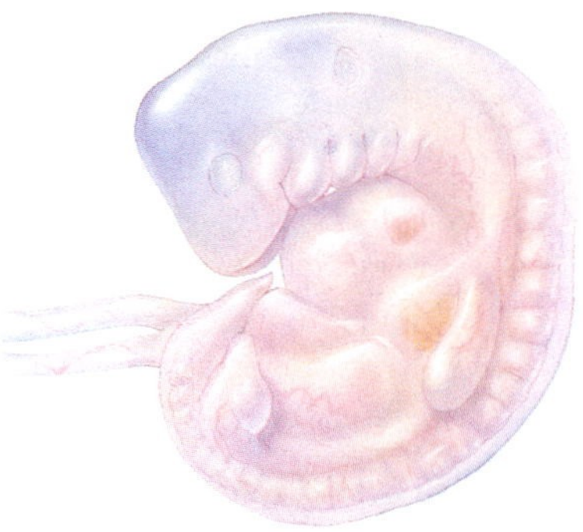	*Development is rapid; heart begins to pump blood; limb buds are well developed. Facial features and major divisions of the brain are discernible. Ears develop from skin folds; tiny bones and muscles are formed beneath the thin skin.* 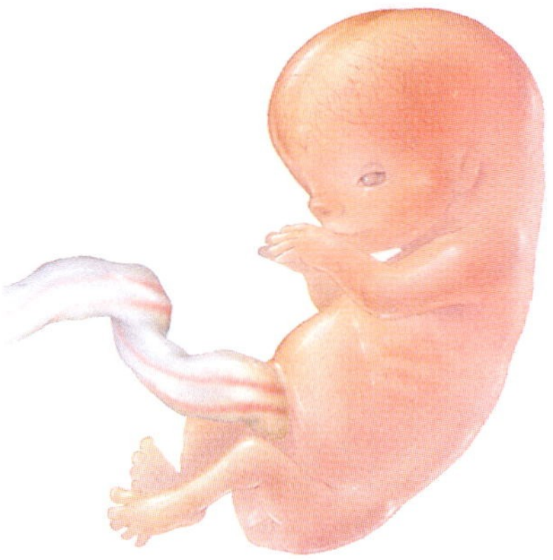	*Embryo becomes a fetus, its beating heart discernible by ultrasound. Assumes a more human shape as lower body develops. At week 12, first movements begin. Sex is determinable. Kidneys produce urine.* 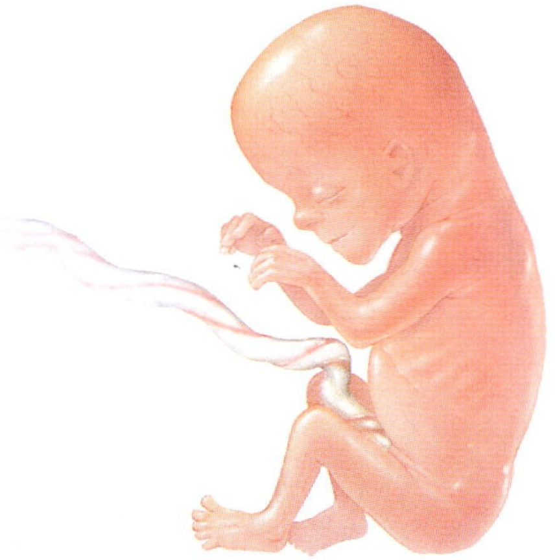	*Musculoskeletal system has matured; nervous system begins to exert control. Blood vessels rapidly develop. Fetal hands can grasp; legs kick actively. All organs begin to mature and grow. Fetus weighs about 7 oz (½ lb). FHT discernible with Doppler. Pancreas produces insulin.* 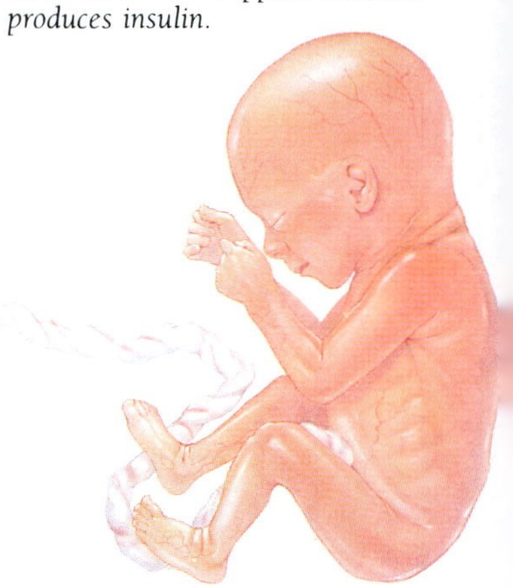
MATERNAL CHANGES	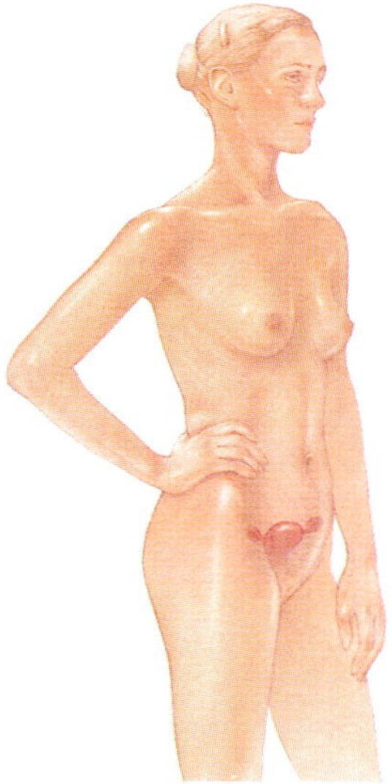	*Mother misses first period; breasts become tender, may enlarge. Chronic fatigue and urinary frequency begin, may persist for three or more months. hCG in urine and serum 9 days after conception.* 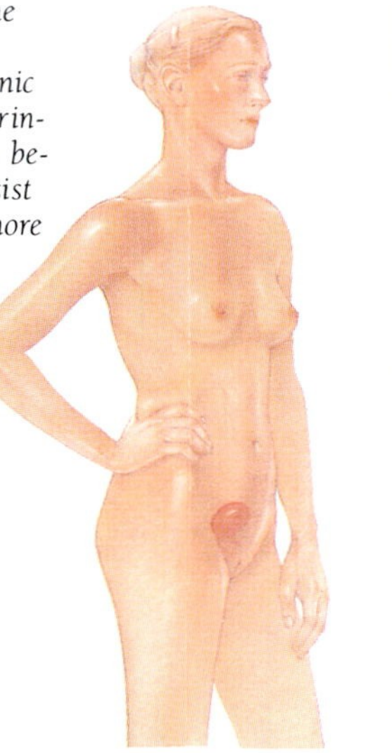	*Morning sickness, may persist to 12 weeks. Uterus changes from pear to globular shape. Hegar's, Goodell's and Piskacek's signs appear. Cervix flexes; leukorrhea increases. Surprise and ambivalence about pregnancy may occur. No noticeable weight gain.* 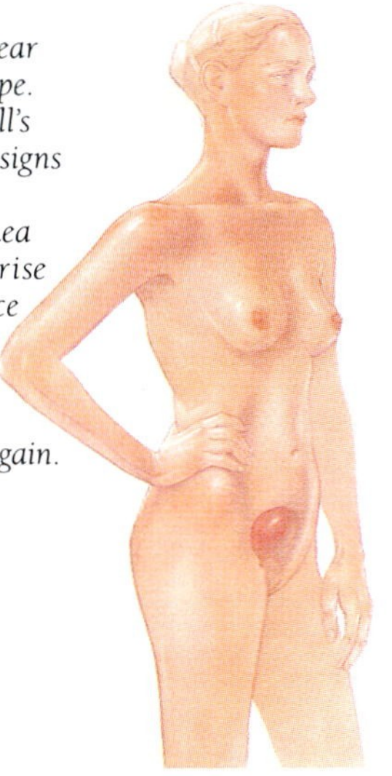	*Chadwick's sign appears. Uterus rises above pelvic brim by 12 weeks. Braxton Hicks contractions may begin and continue throughout pregnancy. Potential for urinary tract infection (UTI) increases and exists throughout pregnancy. Weight gain of about 2½ to 4 lb during first trimester.* *Placenta now fully functioning and producing hormones.* 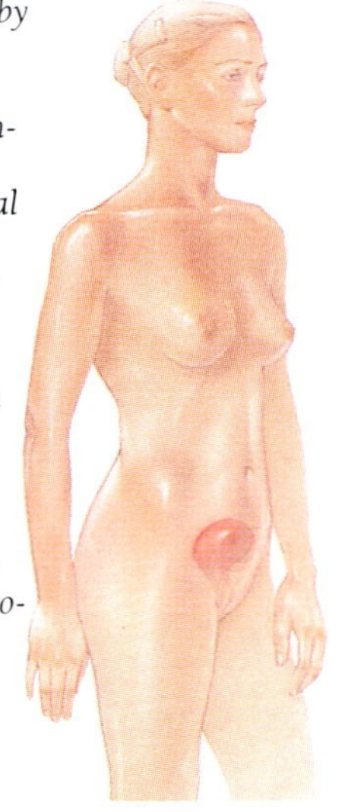	*Fundus halfway between symphysis and umbilicus. Woman gains slightly less than 1 lb per wk for remainder of pregnancy. May feel more energetic. BPD measurement on ultrasound. Vaginal secretions increase. Itching, irritation, malodor suggest infection. Woman may begin wearing maternity clothes. Pressure on bladder lessens and urinary frequency decreases.* 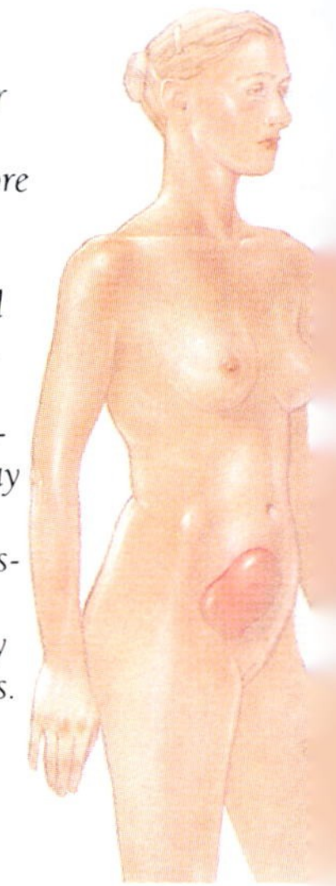
CLIENT TEACHING/ ANTICIPATORY GUIDANCE		*Supportive bra may ease discomfort. Increased rest and relaxation necessary now and throughout pregnancy. Increase fluids during the day; decrease fluid intake only at night to help prevent nocturia; sleep on side to decrease pressure on bladder. Avoid using any medications unless prescribed. Avoid use of social drugs; check with caregiver before using any OTC preparations.*	*Eat dry crackers before arising; try frequent small, dry, low-fat meals with fluids taken between meals. Avoid use of hot tubs, saunas, and steam rooms throughout pregnancy.* *Discuss attitudes toward pregnancy. Discuss value of early pregnancy classes that focus on what to expect during pregnancy. Provide information about childbirth preparation classes.*	*Adequate fluid intake and frequent voiding (every 2 hr while awake) help prevent UTI. Also helpful to void following intercourse. Wipe from front to rear.* *Discuss nutrition and appropriate weight gain. Stress value of regular physical exercise, especially nonweightbearing activities or walking. Discuss possible effects of pregnancy on sexual relationship.*	*Daily shower or bath and thorough drying of vulva helpful; avoid douching during pregnancy. Consult caregiver if infection suspected; use only prescribed medications.* *Review danger signs of pregnancy. Discuss infant feeding options; provide information on the value of breastfeeding. Provide information about clothing, shoes.*

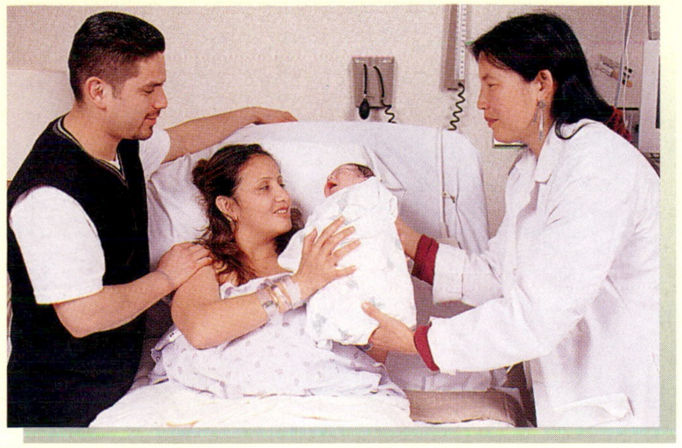

While I'm at the birth center, I check in on Alisa and Richard. Their baby, Lydia Rose, was born 6 hours ago. Alisa has asked for help with breast-feeding. Baby Lydia is a sleepy little one and needs encouragement to latch on and begin feeding.

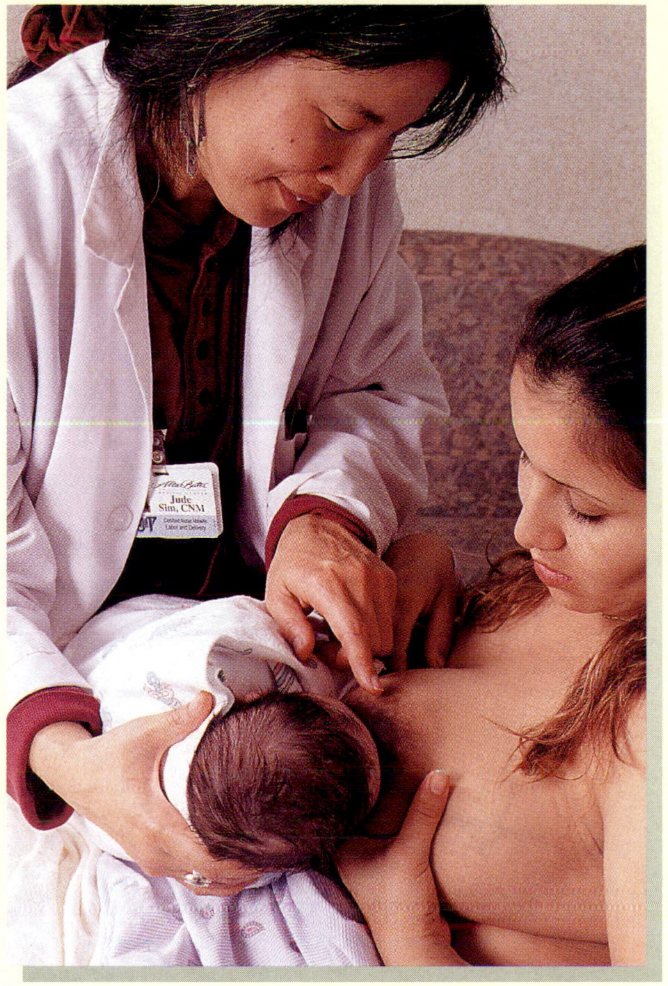

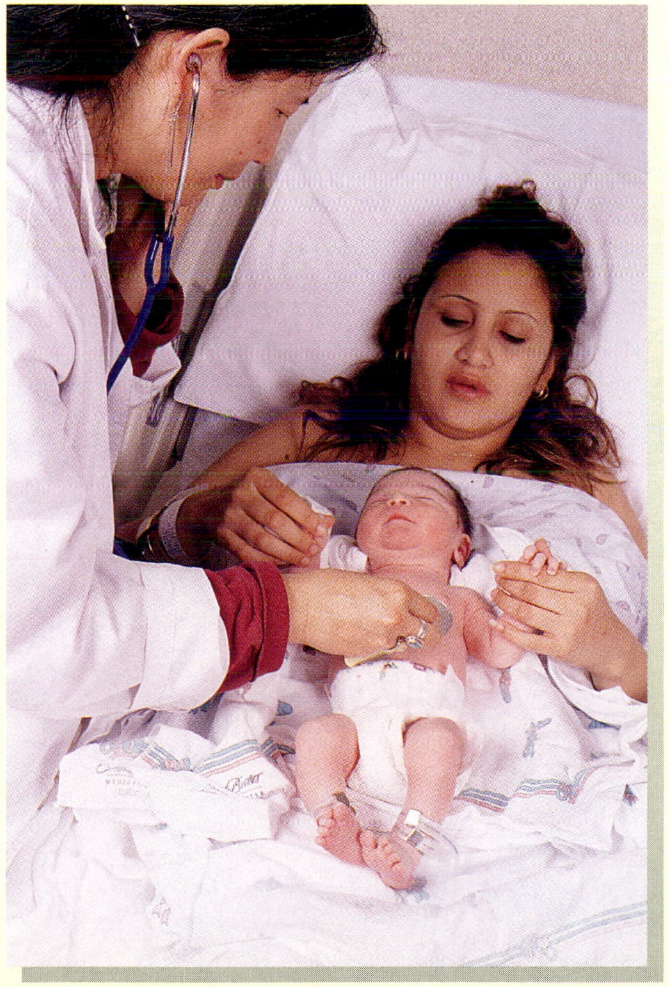

After baby Lydia has finished nursing, I do a physical assessment. I prefer to do an assessment in the room with the parents. It is such a wonderful opportunity for them to learn about their baby.

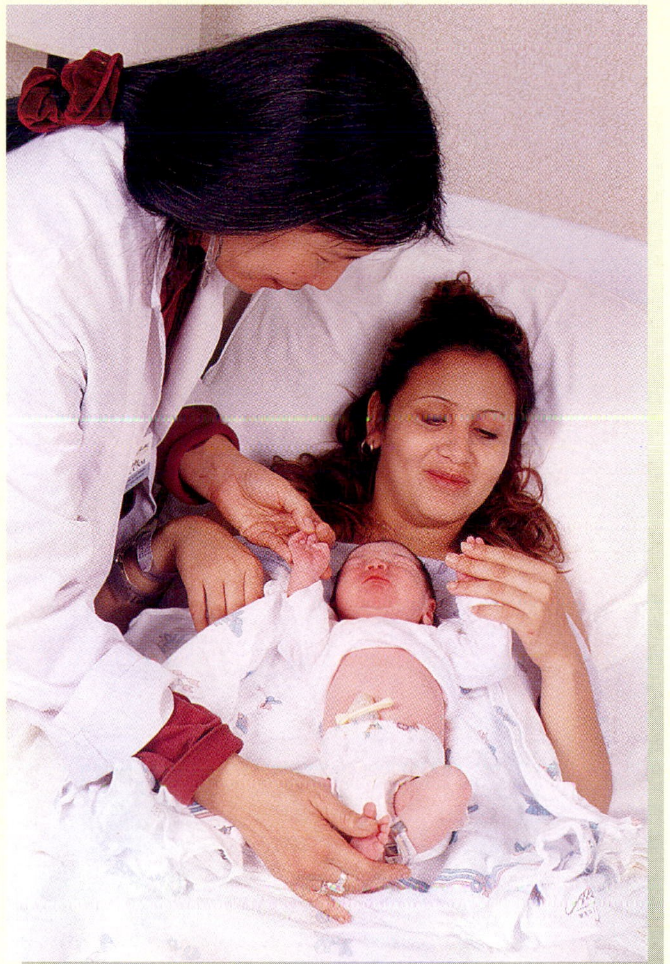

Alisa is fascinated with baby Lydia's tiny fingers and toes. I love being with parents as they explore their baby. Each new baby is such a wonder. . . such a miracle.

Now my attention turns to Alisa. As part of my assessment, I check the position and tone of her fundus. All is well. I head home after a busy, but rewarding, day.

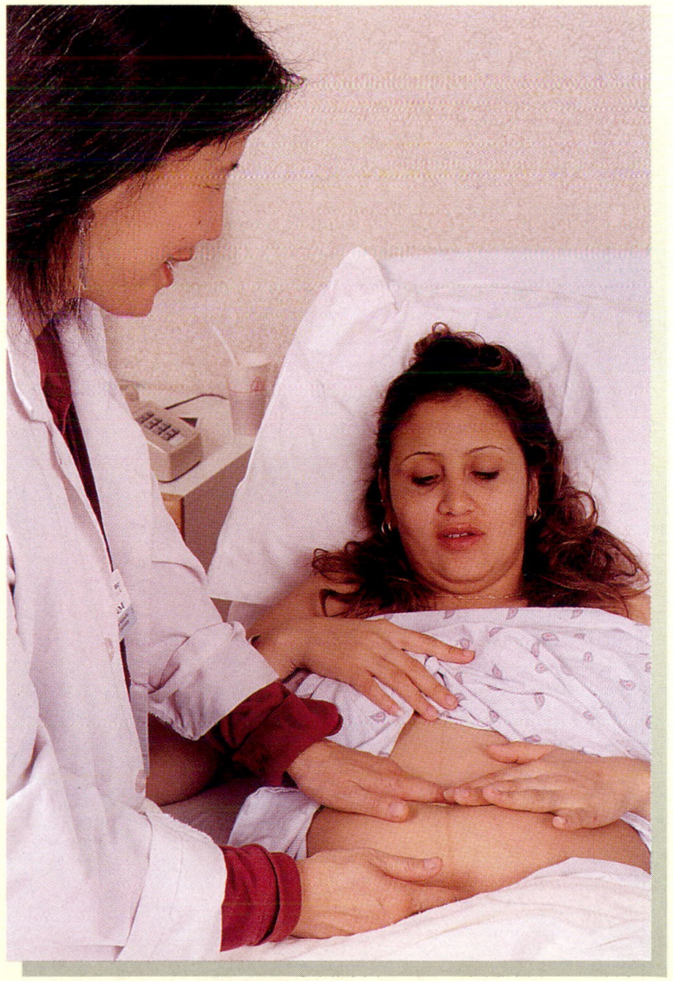

5 — 20 WEEKS

Vernix protects the body; fine hair (lanugo) covers the body and keeps the oil on the skin. Eyebrows, eyelashes, and head hair develop. Fetus develops a regular schedule of sleeping, sucking and kicking.

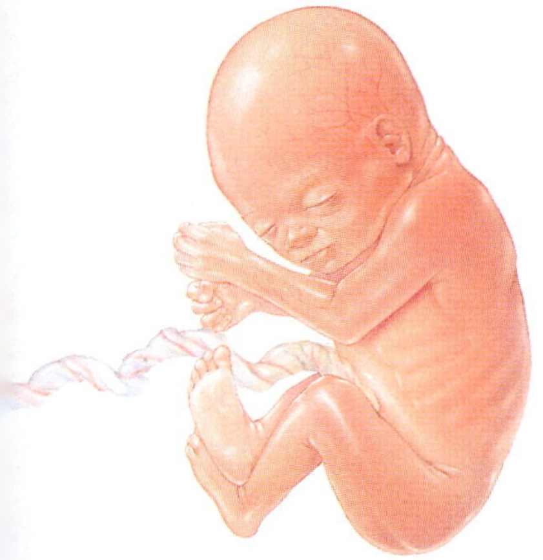

'undus reaches level f umbilicus. Breasts egin secreting co- strum. Amniotic ac holds about 00mL fluid. 'aintness and diz- iness may occur, specially with sud- en position changes. 'aricose veins may egin to develop. Voman experiences tal movement, and regnancy may sud- enly seem more eal." Areola arken. Nasal stuff- ess may develop. eg cramps may egin to occur. Con- ipation may evelop.

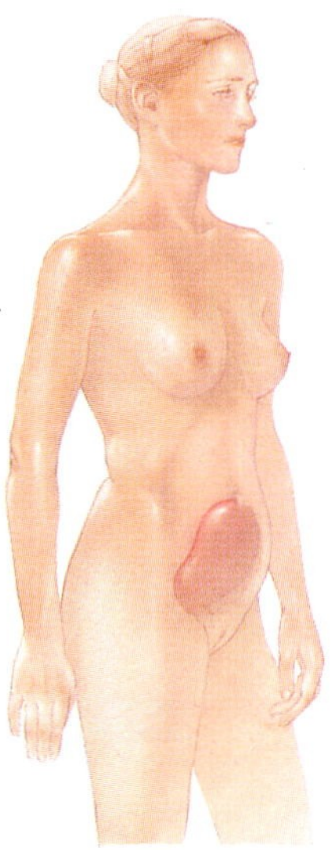

t with feet elevated when possible; se slowly and carefully. Avoid pres- re on lower thighs. Support stockings ay be helpful. Cool-air vaporizer ay help. Eat foods containing fiber, ch as raw fruits, vegetables, cereals ith bran; drink liquids and exercise equently.

iscuss breast care. Discuss dorsiflex- n of foot to relieve cramps; heat to fected muscle.

6 — 24 WEEKS

Skeleton develops rapidly as bone-forming cells increase activity. Respiratory movements begin. Fetus weighs about 1 lb, 10 oz.

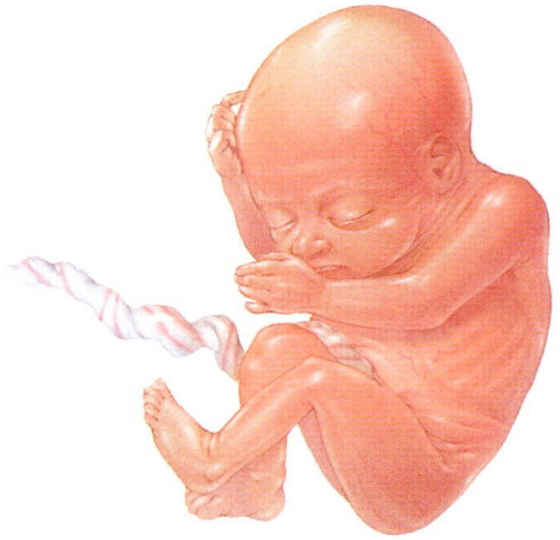

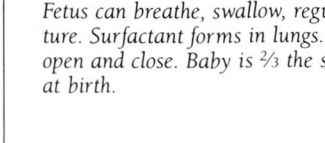

Fundus above umbilicus. Backache and leg cramps may begin. Skin changes can include striae gravidarum, chloasma, linea negra, acne, redness on palms of hands and soles of feet. Nosebleeds can occur. May experience abdominal itching as uterus enlarges; will continue until end of pregnancy.

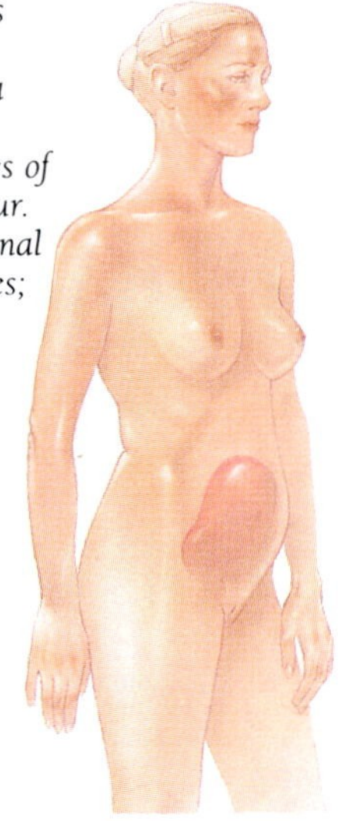

Assure woman that skin changes generally subside soon after birth. Discuss specific exercises such as pelvic tilt to help strengthen back and abdominal muscles, and stress importance of good body mechanics. Reiterate importance of avoiding medications, caffeine, alcohol and smoking.

Woman may choose to apply petroleum jelly in nostrils to relieve nosebleeds. Cool vaporizer may also help. Lanolin-based cream can relieve itching. Mild soap can remove excess oil associated with acne.

7 — 28 WEEKS

Fetus can breathe, swallow, regulate temperature. Surfactant forms in lungs. Eyes begin to open and close. Baby is ⅔ the size it will be at birth.

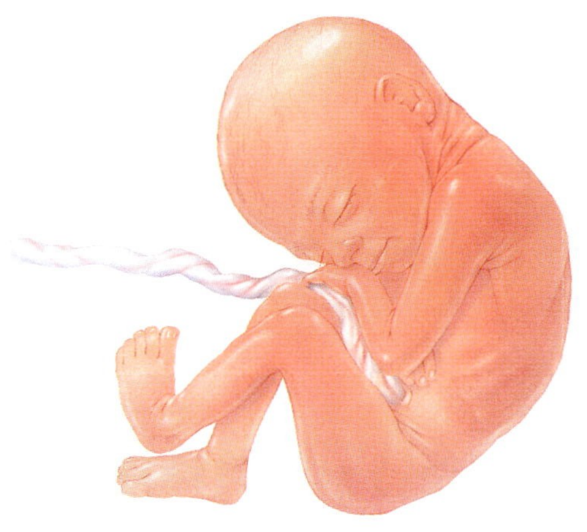

Fundus halfway between umbilicus and xyphoid process. May develop hemorrhoids. Thoracic breathing replaces abdominal breathing. Fetal outline palpable. May be tired of pregnancy and eager for the mothering role. Heartburn may begin to occur. May begin taking childbirth preparation classes with partner or support person.

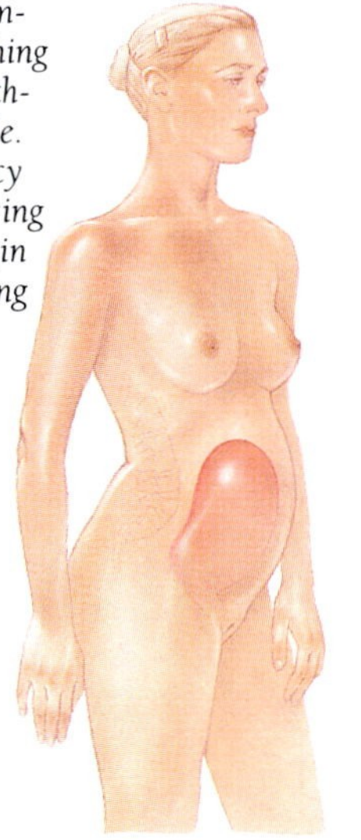

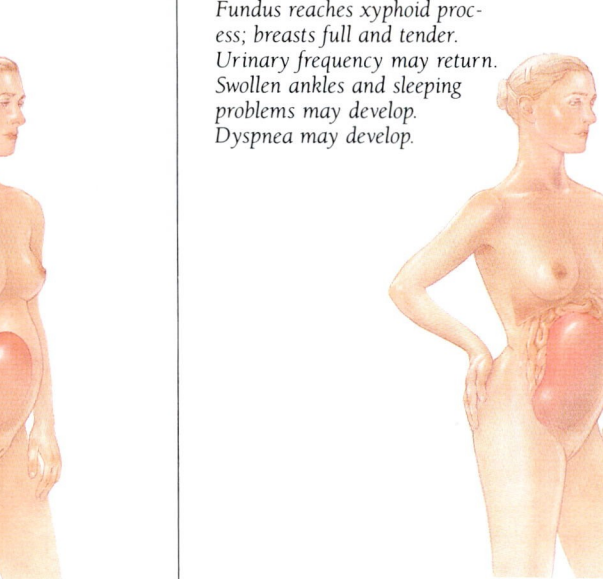

Avoid constipation; use sitz baths, gentle reinsertion of hemorrhoids with a fingertip as necessary. Topical anesthetic agents may offer relief of hemorrhoids. Stool softeners may be prescribed by caregiver. Elevate legs and assume sidelying position when resting. Eat small, more frequent meals; avoid fatty foods, lying down after eating. Maalox or mylanta may be helpful; Avoid sodium bicarbonate. Discuss expectations about labor and delivery, caring for an infant.

8 — 32 WEEKS

Brown fat deposits are developing beneath the skin to insulate the baby following birth. Baby has grown to about 15–17 in. Begins storing iron, calcium, and phosphorus.

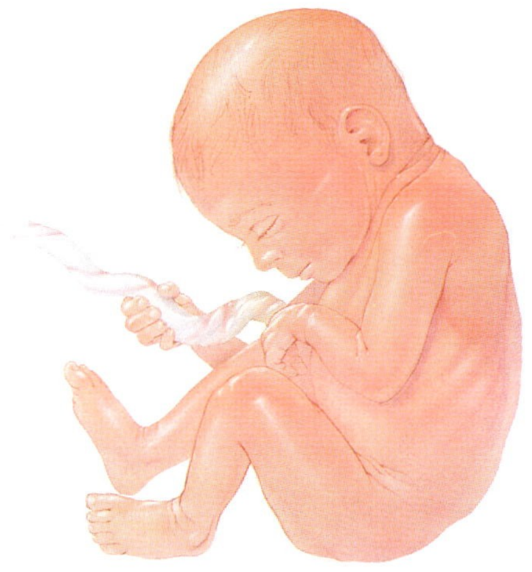

Fundus reaches xyphoid process; breasts full and tender. Urinary frequency may return. Swollen ankles and sleeping problems may develop. Dyspnea may develop.

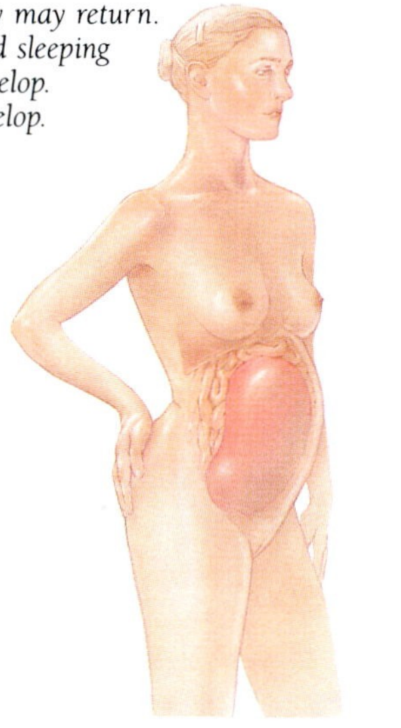

Wear well-fitting supportive bra. Elevate legs once or twice daily for an hour or so. Sleep on left side if possible. Use naturally occurring diuretics such as 2 tbsp lemon juice in 1 cup water or a generous serving of watermelon if available. Avoid most diuretics unless specifically prescribed. Maintain proper posture; use extra pillows at night for severe dyspnea. Following culture and personal preference, may begin preparing nursery now.

Review signs of labor. Discuss plans for other children (if any), transportation to agency.

9 — 38 WEEKS

The entire uterus is occupied by the baby, thus restricting its activity. Maternal antibodies are transferred to the baby. This provides immunity for about 6 months until the infant's own immune system can take over.

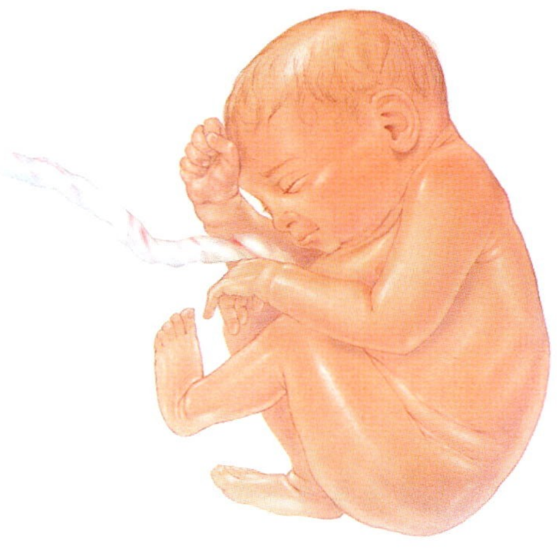

The fetus descends deeper into the mother's pelvis (lightening). The placenta is nearly 4 times as thick as it was 20 weeks ago, weighing nearly 20 oz. Mother is eager for birth, may have final burst of energy. Backaches, urinary frequency increase. Braxton Hicks contractions intensify as cervix and lower uterine segment prepare for labor. Couple may tour labor and delivery area.

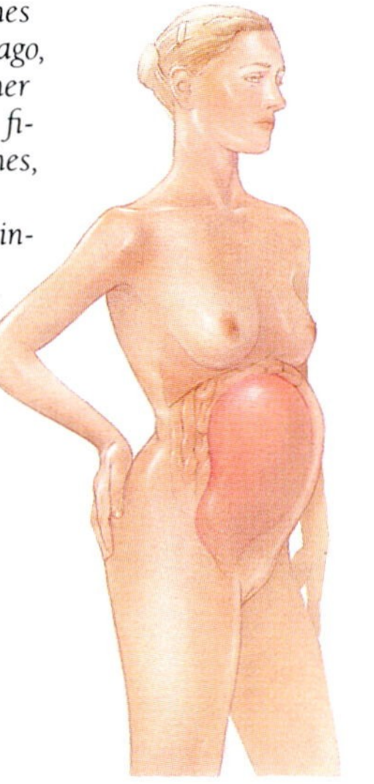

Continue pelvic tilt exercises. Wear low-heeled shoes or flats. Avoid heavy lifting. Sleep on side to relieve bladder pressure. Urinate frequently. Avoid all analgesics except acetominophen. Pack suitcase for delivery.

Discuss postpartum period including decisions such as circumcision, rooming-in. Discuss common postpartum discomforts; mention postpartum blues. Discuss family planning methods, infant care. Stress need for adequate rest postpartally. Provide support, especially if baby is overdue.

Prentice Hall Health
Upper Saddle River, New Jersey 07458
Illustrations by Charles W. Hoffman, MA, AMI

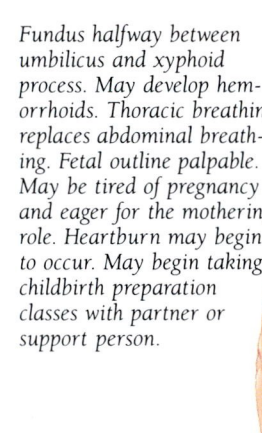

Clinical Tip *Catheterizing a woman during a contraction is uncomfortable for her and difficult to do because of the increased downward pressure. To avoid these problems, pass the catheter between contractions. If the baby's head is low in the pelvis, you will have to change the direction of the catheter. Visualize passing it up and over the baby's head rather than straight into the urethra.*

an IV is started, it becomes even more important to encourage voiding every 1 to 2 hours to prevent bladder distention.

If the amniotic membranes have not ruptured previously, the CNM/physician may do so during this phase. When the membranes rupture, the nurse notes the color and odor of the amniotic fluid and the time of rupture and immediately auscultates the FHR. The fluid should be clear with no odor. Meconium-stained amniotic fluid may be present when the fetus is in a breech presentation. In this case, meconium staining may not indicate any fetal stress. In a cephalic presentation, however, meconium staining may indicate fetal stress. Fetal stress relaxes the intestines and anal sphincter, leading to the release of meconium into the amniotic fluid. Meconium turns the fluid greenish brown. Whenever the nurse notes meconium-stained fluid, an electronic monitor is applied to continuously assess the FHR. The time of rupture is noted because the incidence of amnionitis increases with rupture over 24 hours. An additional concern is prolapse of the umbilical cord, which occurs when membranes rupture and the fetus is not engaged. The concern is that the amniotic fluid coming through the cervix will propel the umbilical cord through the cervix (prolapsed cord). Prolapsed cord is assessed by monitoring for signs of fetal distress and performing a vaginal examination with a sterile glove. The FHR is auscultated because a drop in the rate might indicate an undetected prolapsed cord. Immediate intervention is necessary to remove pressure on a prolapsed umbilical cord until a cesarean birth can be performed (Chapter 27). (See Table 24–4 • for additional deviations from normal.)

Table 24-4 • DEVIATIONS FROM NORMAL LABOR PROCESS REQUIRING IMMEDIATE INTERVENTION

Problem	Immediate Action
Woman admitted with vaginal bleeding or history of painless vaginal bleeding	Do not perform vaginal examination. Assess FHR. Evaluate amount of blood loss. Evaluate labor pattern. Notify physician/CNM immediately.
Presence of greenish or brownish amniotic fluid	Continuously monitor FHR. Evaluate dilatation of cervix and determine if umbilical cord is prolapsed. Evaluate presentation (vertex or breech). Maintain woman on complete bed rest on left side. Notify physician/CNM immediately.
Absence of FHR and fetal movement	Notify physician/CNM. Provide truthful information and emotional support to laboring couple. Remain with the couple.
Prolapse of umbilical cord	Relieve pressure on cord manually. Continuously monitor FHR; watch for changes in FHR pattern. Notify physician/CNM. Assist woman into knee-chest position or place in Trendelenburg position. Administer oxygen.
Woman admitted in advanced labor; birth imminent	Prepare for immediate birth. Obtain critical information: Estimated date of birth (EDB) History of bleeding problems History of medical or obstetric problems Past and/or present use/abuse of prescription/OTC/illicit drugs Problems with this pregnancy FHR and maternal vital signs Whether membranes are ruptured and how long since rupture Blood type and Rh Direct another person to contact physician/CNM. Do not leave woman alone. Provide support to couple. Put on gloves.

TRANSITION PHASE

During transition, the contraction frequency is every 2 to 3 minutes, duration is 60 to 90 seconds, and intensity is strong. Cervical dilatation increases from 8 to 10 cm, effacement is complete (100%), and a heavy amount of bloody show is usually present. Contractions are palpated at least every 15 minutes. Sterile vaginal examination can be done during this stage of labor to assess rapid changes in status. Maternal blood pressure, pulse, and respirations are taken at least every 30 minutes, and FHR is auscultated every 15 minutes.

Throughout labor the woman's center of focus gradually turns inward. She becomes less aware of what is going on around her and intensely aware of her uterine contractions. She experiences body boundary diffusion, which hampers her ability to know where her body ends and her external environment begins. Women during this time will reach out to others but may be uncomfortable with others touching them.

The woman's ability to speak in coherent sentences can be impaired during the transitional phase. This makes it difficult for the woman to communicate her needs to healthcare providers and her support team. The support person(s) and nurse need to follow the woman's cues and change interventions as needed.

The woman's mouth and lips can become dry due to her breathing being more rapid. The woman can be instructed to breathe in through her nose and out through her mouth. The nurse can also offer small spoons of ice chips to moisten the mouth and apply A and D ointment to the dry lips. If the woman vomits, the nurse should wipe her mouth and offer water to rinse her mouth.

The nurse should encourage the woman to rest between contractions by instructing the woman at the end of her contraction to take a deep breath and to let it out slowly while she relaxes her muscles. Helping to maintain a quiet room between contractions can also enhance the woman's ability to rest. The woman during this phase is present focused; thus, providing instruction between contractions should be kept to a minimum.

Some women have difficulty coping with the intensity of labor during this time and need assistance in performing breathing techniques. Either the support person or the nurse can breathe along with the woman during each contraction to help her maintain her pattern. It is helpful to encourage her and assure her that she is doing a good job. The woman will begin to feel increased rectal pressure as the fetal presenting part moves down the birth canal and sometimes a burning sensation as the tissues begin to stretch. The nurse encourages the woman to refrain from pushing until the cervix is completely dilated. For the woman who is unmedicated, the urge to push may seem unbearable. Specific instructions, such as encouraging the woman to "blow in short breaths like you are blowing out a candle" or "pant like a puppy" can help prevent the woman from involuntarily pushing. This measure also helps prevent cervical edema or lacerations.

The end of transition and beginning of the second stage may be indicated by involuntary passage of flatus or stool and the movement of the fetus from the side of the maternal abdomen to the midline. Other indications include a change in the woman's voice or the sounds she is making. As the fetus moves down and she feels increased pressure and a bearing-down sensation, her voice tends to deepen. A moan during a contraction takes on a more guttural quality. Labor nurses recognize this sound as a sign that the woman may have entered the second stage.

Promotion of Comfort in the First Stage

In labor, the more common pain reactions, such as increased pulse and respiratory rates, dilated pupils, increased blood pressure, and muscle tension, are transitory because the pain is intermittent. However, increased muscle tension may impede the progress of labor; therefore, the nurse encourages the woman to relax her skeletal muscles and avoid holding her breath.

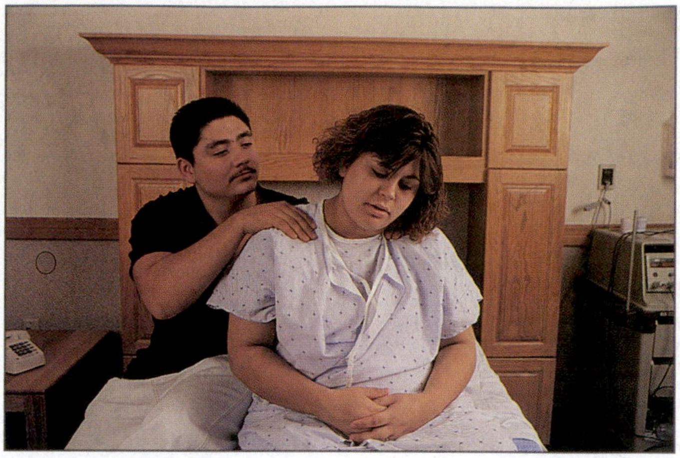

Figure 24–2 • The woman's partner provides support and encouragement during labor.

Sounds are an important part of the labor and birthing process. Some women naturally make sounds such as moans and grunts and feel that it helps them cope and do the work of labor; they are responding to what their body tells them to do. Others begin to make loud sounds (screams) only as they lose their ability to cope and feel they do not have any other options.

Some women may want physical contact during contractions (Figure 24–2 •). They may provide verbal and nonverbal signs, such as crying, moaning, and beseeching the coach or nurse to hold their hand or rub their back. They may look at the support person or reach out for help to indicate their anxiety. Touch may be used to convey support and enhance comfort for the woman. She may be soothed by a neck or back rub or by holding the hand of her partner or the nurse.

Evidence-Based Practice

Caregiver Support for Women During Labor

Clinical Question

Does continuous support during labor have a positive effect on mothers and infants?

The Evidence

A systematic review of 14 trials, involving more than 5000 women, examined the effect of continuous support provided by healthcare workers or laypeople. Continuous presence reduced the likelihood of medication for pain relief, operative vaginal birth, cesarean birth, and a 5-minute Apgar score less than 7, and slightly reduced the length of labor. Continuous support also favorably affected satisfaction, coping during pregnancy, and personal control during childbirth.

Best Practice

Continuous support during childbirth has a number of benefits for mother and infant and does not appear to produce any harmful effects. Every effort should be made to provide laboring women support from healthcare workers or laypeople. Effective support includes continuous presence, provision of hands-on comfort, and encouragement.

Reference: Hodnett, E. D. (2002). Caregiver support for women during childbirth (Cochrane Review). In: *The Cochrane Library*, Issue 3. Oxford: Update Software.

A woman generally wants touching and physical contact during the first part of labor, but when she moves into the transition phase, she may rebuff all efforts and pull away. Other women do not want to be touched at all, regardless of the phase of labor.

A decrease in the intensity of discomfort is one of the goals of nursing support during labor. Nursing measures to decrease pain include the following:

- Encouraging position changes
- Assisting with personal comfort measures
- Decreasing anxiety
- Providing information
- Using specific supportive relaxation techniques
- Encouraging paced breathing
- Administering pharmacologic agents as desired by the woman

POSITION CHANGES

As noted earlier, the woman is encouraged to ambulate if the fetal head is engaged and the electronic fetal monitor (EFM) has shown a reassuring FHR pattern. However, to avoid the risk of umbilical cord prolapse, the woman is generally instructed to remain in bed if membranes are ruptured and the presenting part is not engaged.

If she stays in bed, the woman is encouraged to assume any position that she finds comfortable (Figure 24–3 ●). A side-lying position is generally the most advantageous for the laboring woman. Care should be taken that all body parts are supported, with the joints slightly flexed. Pillows may be placed against her chest and under the uppermost arm. A pillow or folded bath blanket is placed between her knees to support the uppermost leg and relieve tension or muscle strain. A pillow (or warmed rolled blanket) placed at the woman's midback also helps provide support. If the woman is more comfortable on her back, the head of the bed should be elevated to relieve the pressure of the uterus on the vena cava and the uterus should be tilted by placing a towel or blanket under the woman's back. Pillows may be placed under each arm and under the knees to provide support. Because a pregnant woman is at increased risk for thrombophlebitis, excessive pressure behind the knee and calf should be avoided, and frequent assessment of pressure points needs to be made.

Frequent position changes (at least every hour) seem to achieve more efficient contractions, and contribute to comfort and relaxation. It is also helpful for the woman to sit up in a rocking chair or other comfortable chair, or in the shower.

PERSONAL COMFORT MEASURES

The use of hydrotherapy during labor promotes maternal relaxation and pain management and decreases the length of labor. Thus women can be encouraged to use a warm bath, shower, or whirlpool to increase comfort during labor.

Because vaginal discharge increases, the nurse needs to change the underpads frequently. Washing the perineum

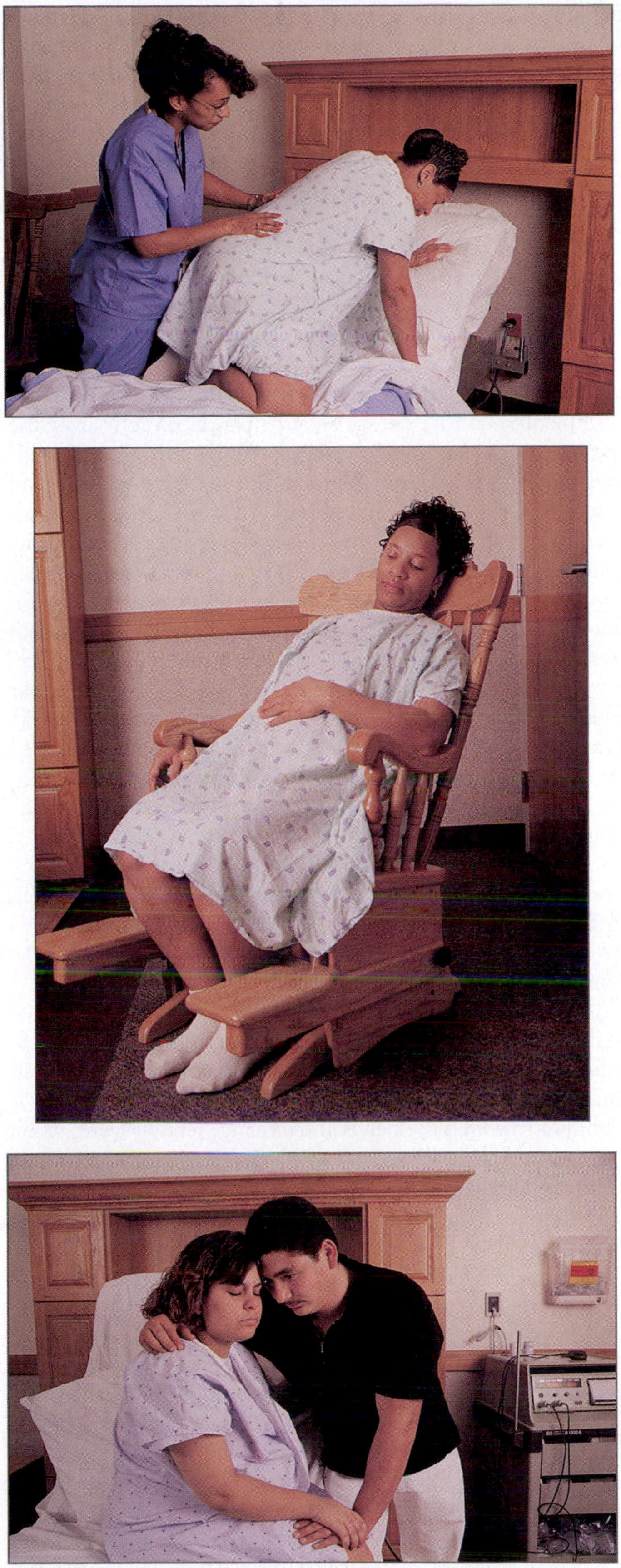

Figure 24–3 ● The laboring woman is encouraged to choose a position of comfort. The nurse modifies assessments and interventions as necessary.

MEDIALINK LABORING POSITIONS

with warm soap and water removes secretions and increases comfort. The nurse needs to use universal precautions to avoid exposure to vaginal secretions.

Diaphoresis and the constant leaking of amniotic fluid can dampen the woman's gown and bed linen. Fresh, smooth, dry bed linen promotes comfort. To avoid having to change the bottom sheet following ROM, the nurse may replace the underpads at frequent intervals (universal precautions need to be followed). The perineal area should be kept as clean and dry as possible to promote comfort.

A full bladder adds to the discomfort during a contraction and may prolong labor by interfering with the descent of the fetus. Even though the woman is voiding, urine may be retained because of the pressure of the fetal presenting part. A full bladder can be detected by palpation directly over the symphysis pubis. Some of the procedures for regional analgesia during labor contribute to the inability to void, and catheterization may be necessary. The woman should be encouraged to empty her bladder about every 1 to 2 hours. The nurse should offer the woman a bedpan prior to catheterization since some women are able to void despite anesthesia, and spontaneous voiding decreases the risk of infection that is associated with repeated catheterizations.

The woman may experience dryness of her mouth. Clear fluids and ice chips are usually offered unless a complication exists that makes cesarean birth a possibility. Some prepared childbirth programs advise the woman to bring lollipops to help combat the dryness that occurs with some of the breathing patterns.

Some women feel discomfort from cold feet. Wearing socks or slippers may increase their comfort. Some women may wish to wear their own nightgown, although they need to know that the gown will most likely be soiled and may be more difficult to move around in.

Birthing balls—large, heavy plastic balls that accommodate an adult's weight—are used by some laboring women to increase comfort (Figure 24–4 •). The woman sits on the ball and can roll it back and forth gently. The slow rock is thought to widen the pelvis and enhance fetal descent, while leaning forward on the knees with the head, arms, and chest over the ball simulates a hands-and-knees position and may facilitate rotation of an occiput-posterior. When a birthing ball is used, the nurse should remain close by the woman to help provide balance. Many balls come with aluminum frames to prevent falls.

Some family members or support persons can assist the woman with comfort measures. They may help with position changes, provide ice chips, walk with the laboring woman, and give effleurage or backrubs. If the family is not already involved in providing comfort measures and seems to want to be, the nurse can act as a role model while providing comfort measures and then invite the support person(s) to join in if they like.

Family members also need to be encouraged to maintain their own comfort. As their attention is directed toward the laboring woman, they may forget their own needs. The nurse may have to encourage them to take breaks, maintain food and fluid intake, and rest.

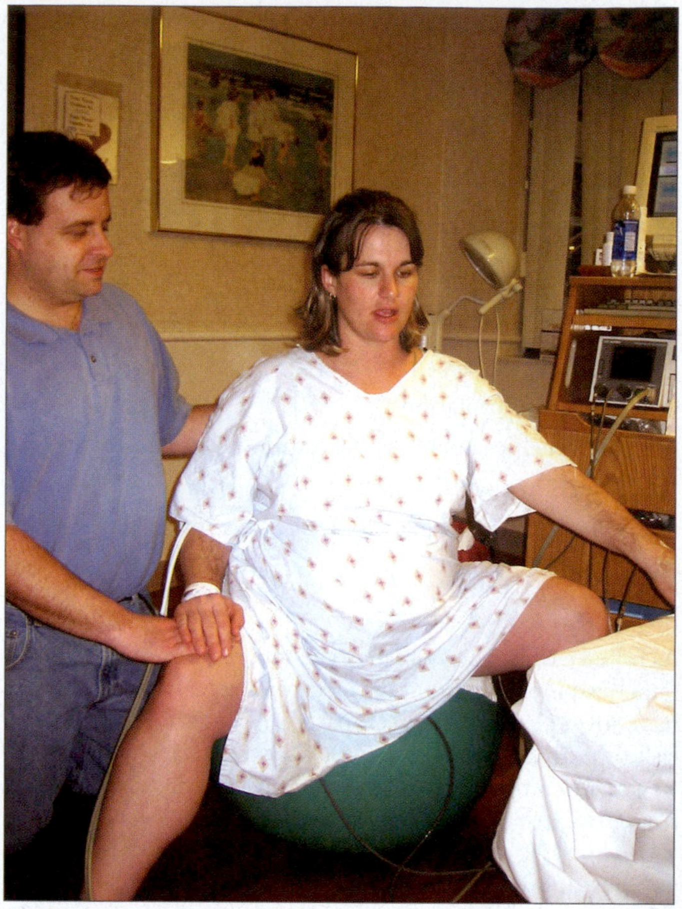

Figure 24–4 • A birthing ball is used to promote maternal comfort during labor. The birthing ball facilitates fetal descent and fetal rotation, and helps increase the diameter of the pelvis.

REDUCING ANXIETY

The anxiety experienced by women entering labor is related to a combination of factors inherent to the process. A moderate amount of anxiety enhances the ability to deal with the pain. But an excessive degree of anxiety decreases the woman's ability to cope with the pain.

To decrease anxiety that is not related to pain, the nurse can give information (which eases fear of the unknown), establish rapport with the couple (which helps them preserve their personal integrity), express confidence in the couple's ability to work with the labor process, and assist with breathing and relaxation techniques. In addition to being a good listener, the nurse needs to demonstrate genuine concern for the laboring woman. Remaining with the woman as much as possible conveys a caring attitude and dispels fear of abandonment. Praise for correct breathing, relaxation efforts, and pushing efforts not only encourages repetition of the behavior but also decreases anxiety about the ability to cope with labor.

The woman's partner and other members of her support team may also experience increasing anxiety as the woman advances through labor. Their anxiety can stem from watching their loved one in pain, feeling helpless about their ability to assist her in reducing the pain, a lack of knowledge or information about the labor experience, and lack of support from the labor nurse. Their anxiety may be reduced or kept at a minimum by keeping them informed about the progress of labor, reassuring them that the sounds and behaviors of the woman in labor are normal, explaining procedures and the use of equipment, and praising them for their assistance in supporting the woman through labor.

PROVIDING INFORMATION

Providing information about the nature of the discomfort that will occur during labor is important and is best achieved in the early portion of labor. Stressing the intermittent nature and maximum duration of the contractions can be most helpful. The woman can cope with pain better when she knows how far she has progressed and that a period of relief will follow. Describing the type of discomfort and specific sensations that will occur as labor progresses helps the woman recognize these sensations as normal and expected when she does experience them.

A thorough explanation of surroundings, procedures, and equipment being used also decreases anxiety, thereby reducing pain. For some clients, attachment to an electronic monitor can produce fear because equipment of this type is associated with critically ill people. For others, hearing their infant's heartbeat is reassuring. The nurse should explain the purpose of the monitor and the monitor strip, and show the woman and her support persons how the monitor can help them use controlled breathing techniques to relieve pain. The monitor may indicate the beginning of a contraction just seconds before the woman feels it. The woman and coach can learn how to read the tracing to identify the beginning of the contraction.

SUPPORTIVE RELAXATION TECHNIQUES

Tense muscles increase resistance to the descent of the fetus and contribute to maternal fatigue and anxiety. This fatigue increases pain perception and decreases the woman's ability to cope with the pain. Comfort measures, massage, techniques for decreasing anxiety, and client teaching can conserve energy. The laboring woman needs to be encouraged to use the periods between contractions to rest and relax her muscles.

Distraction is a method of increasing relaxation and coping with discomfort. During early labor, conversation or activities such as light reading, cards, or other games serve as distractions.

Touch is another type of distraction. Although some women regard touching as an invasion of privacy or threat to their independence, others want to touch and be touched during a painful experience. Nurses can make themselves available to the woman who desires touch. The nurse can place a hand on the side of the bed within the woman's reach. The person who needs touch will reach out for contact, and the nurse can pick up and follow through with this behavioral cue.

Mild to moderate abdominal discomfort during contractions may be relieved or lessened by effleurage. Back pain associated with labor may be relieved more effectively by firm pressure on the lower back or sacral area. To apply firm pressure, the nurse or a support person places a hand or a rolled, warmed towel or blanket in the small of the woman's back. Warm compresses can also provide relief.

Table 24–5 • SIMPLE VISUALIZATION METHOD
Direct a visualization by saying something like the following: "Think about a place you have been that has pleasant memories and feelings around it. A place that was relaxing, where all your stress disappeared. As you think about this place, take in a breath and remember the smells around it. If it was outside, feel the warmth of the sun or the way the breeze felt on your face. Sit in the place again in your mind. Let all your tension and tiredness leave your body as you feel the warmth and breezes."
Give the woman a few moments to think about her special place. Ask if she would like to share information about the setting. If the woman chooses to do this, add the information to help her with the visualization (for example, "Think about the mountain cabin and the warmth of the sun on your face as you sit in the rocking chair on the front porch.").
After the woman has a visualization set up, suggest thinking about it during contractions as a means of increasing relaxation and focusing concentration. You could say, "As each contraction begins, think about this special place for a moment, and let your body relax. Keep a picture of your place in your mind as you breathe with the contraction. When the contraction is over, let your body stay relaxed. Feel the comfort of this room and support of those around you."

Visualization techniques also enhance relaxation. For example, the nurse might encourage the woman to imagine herself floating in a warm pool of water, fully supported; to imagine the birth canal slowly opening up as the baby descends; or to visualize a rose opening its petals. Or the woman may simply wish to recall and concentrate on a pleasant experience she has had in the past. Table 24–5 • describes a simple visualization method.

In addition to these measures, the nurse can enhance the woman's relaxation by providing encouragement and support for controlled breathing techniques.

BREATHING TECHNIQUES

Breathing techniques may help the laboring woman. Breathing techniques increase the woman's pain threshold, encourage relaxation, provide distraction, enhance the ability to cope with uterine contractions, and allow the uterus to function more efficiently.

Many women learn breathing techniques during prenatal education classes. Patterned-paced breathing, which is commonly used in the Lamaze method, has three levels. The woman tends to begin with the first level and then proceed to the next when she feels the need. Regardless of the level of breathing used, a cleansing breath begins and ends each pattern. A cleansing breath involves only the chest. It consists of inhaling through the nose and exhaling through pursed lips (as if blowing on a spoonful of hot food). See Table 24–6 • for information regarding nursing support of patterned-paced breathing.

Other childbirth education models encourage different types of breathing exercises. Abdominal breathing, which is commonly used in the Bradley method, encourages the woman to move the abdominal wall upward as she inhales

Table 24–6 • NURSING SUPPORT OF PATTERNED-PACED BREATHING

Determine which breathing method the woman (couple) has learned. Provide encouragement as needed in maintaining breathing pattern. Provide support to the labor coach and assist as needed.

Lamaze Breathing Pattern Levels

First level (slow paced)

Pattern begins and ends with a cleansing breath (in through the nose and out through pursed lips as if cooling a spoonful of hot food). While inhaling through the nose and exhaling through pursed lips, slow breaths are taken, moving only the chest. The rate should be approximately 6–9/minute or 2 breaths/15 seconds. The coach or nurse may assist by reminding the woman to take a cleansing breath, and then the breaths could be counted out if needed to maintain pacing. The woman inhales as someone counts "one one thousand, two one thousand, three one thousand, four one thousand." Exhalation begins and continues through the same count.

First level for use during uterine contractions (The level begins and ends with a cleansing breath [CB]).

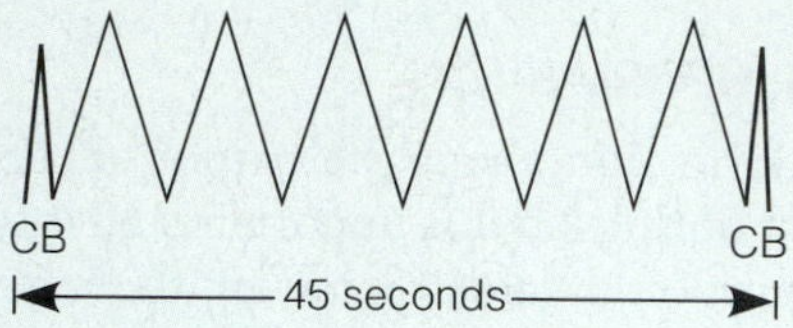

Second level (modified paced)

Pattern begins and ends with a cleansing breath. Breaths are then taken in and out silently through the mouth at approximately 4 breaths/5 seconds. The jaw and entire body need to be relaxed. The rate can be accelerated to 2–2 ½ breaths/second. The rhythm for the breaths can be counted out as "one and two and one and two and…" with the woman exhaling on the numbers and inhaling on "and."

Second level

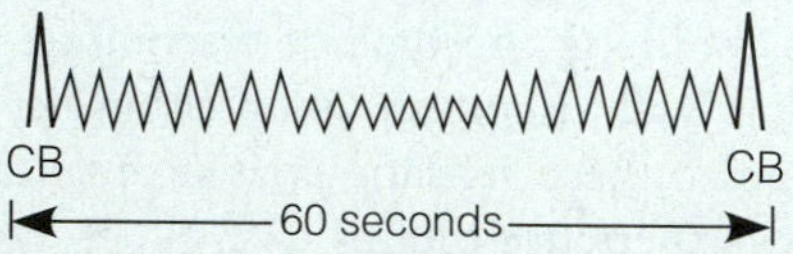

Third level (pattern paced)

Pattern begins and ends with a cleansing breath. All breaths are rhythmical, in and out through the mouth. Exhalations are accompanied by a "hee" or "hoo" sound in a varying pattern, 2:1, which begins as 3:1 (hee hee hee hoo) and can change to 2:1 (hee hee hoo) or 1:1 (hee hoo) as the intensity of the contraction changes. The rate should not be more rapid than 2–2 ½ breaths/second. The rhythm of the breaths would match a "one and two and …" count.

Third level (Darkened spike represents "hoo.")

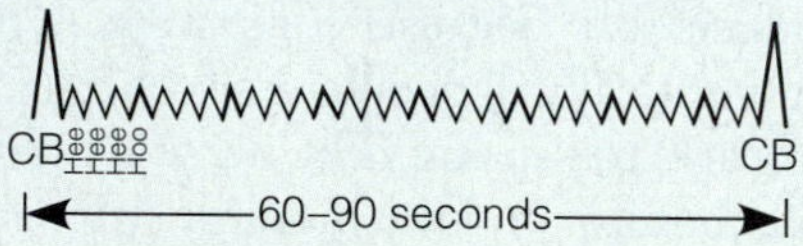

Abdominal Breathing Pattern Cues

The abdomen moves outward during inhalation and downward during exhalation. The rate remains slow with approximately 6–9 breaths/minute.

Breathing sequence for abdominal breathing

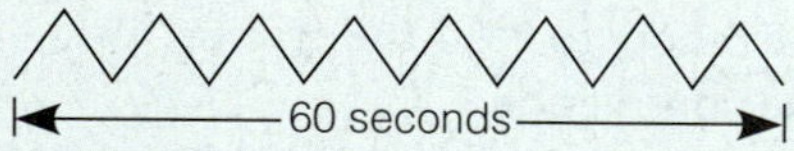

Quick Method

When the woman has not learned a particular method and is in active phase of labor, the nurse may teach her a combination of two patterns. Abdominal breathing may be used until labor is more advanced. Then a more rapid pattern consisting of two short blows from the mouth followed by a longer blow can be used. (This pattern is called "pant-pant-blow" even though all exhalations are a blowing motion.)

Pant-pant-blow breathing pattern

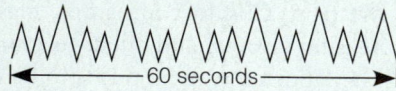

and downward as she exhales (see Table 24–6). This method tends to lift the abdominal wall off the contracting uterus and thus may provide some pain relief. The breathing is deep and rhythmic. If the woman has not been trained in a particular technique, teaching her the "quick method," which uses a pant-pant-blow breathing pattern, may help her from breathing too rapidly (see Table 24–6).

Hyperventilation may occur when a woman breathes very rapidly over a prolonged period of time. Hyperventilation is the result of an imbalance of oxygen and carbon dioxide (that is, too much carbon dioxide is exhaled, and too much oxygen remains in the body). The signs and symptoms of hyperventilation are tingling or numbness in the tip of nose, lips, fingers, or toes; dizziness; spots before the eyes; or spasms of the hands or feet (carpal-pedal spasms). If hyperventilation occurs, the woman should be encouraged to slow her breathing rate and to take shallow breaths. With instruction and encouragement, many women are able to change their breathing to correct the problem. Encouraging the woman to relax and counting out loud for her so she can pace her breathing during contractions are also helpful. If the signs and symptoms continue or become more severe (that is,

Table 24–7 • NORMAL PROGRESS, PSYCHOLOGIC CHARACTERISTICS, AND NURSING SUPPORT DURING FIRST AND SECOND STAGES OF LABOR

Phase	Cervical Dilatation	Uterine Contractions	Woman's Response	Support Measures
Stage 1				
Latent phase	1–4 cm	Every 10–20 minutes, 15–20 seconds' duration Mild intensity *progressing to* Every 5–7 minutes, 30–40 seconds' duration Moderate intensity	Usually happy, talkative, and eager to be in labor Exhibits need for independence by taking care of own bodily needs and seeking information	Establish rapport on admission and continue to build during care. Assess information base and learning needs. Be available to consult regarding breathing technique if needed; teach breathing technique if needed and in early labor. Orient family to room, equipment, monitors, and procedures. Encourage woman and partner to participate in care as desired. Provide needed information. Assist woman into position of comfort; encourage frequent change of position; encourage ambulation during early labor. Offer fluids/ice chips. Keep couple informed of progress. Encourage woman to void every 1 to 2 hours. Assess need for an interest in using visualization to enhance relaxation and teach if appropriate.
Active phase	4–7 cm	Every 2–3 minutes, 40–60 seconds' duration Moderate to strong intensity	May experience feelings of helplessness Exhibits increased fatigue and may begin to feel restless and anxious as contractions become stronger Expresses fear of abandonment Becomes more dependent as she is less able to meet her needs	Encourage woman to maintain breathing patterns. Provide quiet environment to reduce external stimuli. Provide reassurance, encouragement, support; keep couple informed of progress. Promote comfort by giving back rubs, sacral pressure, cool cloth on forehead, assistance with position changes, support with pillows, effleurage. Provide ice chips, ointment for dry mouth and lips. Encourage to void every 1 to 2 hours. Offer shower/whirlpool/warm bath if available.
Transition phase	8–10 cm	Every 2 minutes, 60–75 seconds' duration Strong intensity	Tires and may exhibit increased restlessness and irritability May feel she cannot keep up with labor process and is out of control Physical discomforts Fear of being left alone May fear tearing open or splitting apart with contractions	Encourage woman to rest between contractions. If she sleeps between contractions, wake her at beginning of contraction so she can begin breathing pattern (increases feeling of control). Provide support, encouragement, and praise for efforts. Keep couple informed of progress; encourage continued participation of support persons. Promote comfort as listed above but recognize many women do not want to be touched when in transition. Provide privacy. Provide ice chips, ointment for lips. Encourage to void every 1 to 2 hours.
Stage 2	Complete	Every 2 minutes	May feel out of control, helpless, panicky, or may be happy that she can take a more active role in pushing	Assist woman in pushing efforts. Encourage woman to assume position of comfort. Provide encouragement and praise for efforts. Keep couple informed of progress. Provide ice chips. Maintain privacy as woman desires.

if they progress from numbness to spasms), the woman can breathe into a paper surgical mask or into her hands until symptoms abate. Breathing into a mask or her hands causes rebreathing of carbon dioxide. The nurse should remain with the woman to reassure her.

As the woman uses her breathing technique, the nurse can assess and support the interaction between the woman and her coach or support person. In the absence of a coach, the nurse supports the laboring woman by helping to identify the beginning of each contraction and encouraging her as she breathes through it. Continued encouragement and support with each contraction through labor yield immeasurable benefits.

OTHER COMFORT MEASURES

In some instances, analgesic agents or regional anesthetic blocks may be used to enhance comfort and relaxation during labor. See Chapter 25 for a discussion of analgesia and anesthesia.

Table 24–7 • summarizes labor progress, possible responses of the laboring woman, and nursing care during the first stage of labor.

MediaLink VIDEO: SECOND STAGE OF LABOR

Nursing Care During the Second Stage of Labor

Nursing care in the second stage entails both physical and psychologic support, continual encouragement, and appropriate client teaching in order to facilitate birth.

Provision of Care in the Second Stage

The second stage begins when the cervix is completely dilated (10 cm). The uterine contractions continue as in the transition phase. Sterile vaginal examinations are performed to assess fetal descent. Maternal pulse, blood pressure, and fetal heart rate (FHR) are assessed every 5 to 15 minutes; some protocols recommend assessment after each contraction (AWHONN, 1999). Table 24–8 • summarizes nursing assessments in the second stage of labor.

As the woman pushes during the second stage, she may make a variety of sounds. At times, these sounds are disturbing for nurses and physicians, and they feel the need to help her or encourage her to be more quiet. Other nurses feel more comfortable with maternal sounds and use them as cues. For example, if the woman begins to feel she is losing control, her sound may change to a high-pitched cry or whimper, or she may even shriek in pain. The nurse stays sensitive to changes in the sounds for clues that the woman needs help coping with her pain. The nurse may encourage her to push harder and not let any breath out, or to put all her effort into the push and not into making noise. But the nurse needs to be aware that maternal sounds may be a coping mechanism for some women and may assist in their pain management.

Several nursing research studies have been conducted focusing on when a woman should push during the second stage of labor. A review article on research focusing on pushing during the second stage recommends that the woman be allowed to rest at the beginning of the second stage and to begin pushing when she feels the natural urge to bear down. There is a decrease in maternal fatigue levels and an increase in fetal oxygenation when women delay pushing until they feel the urge to push (Minato, 2000–2001).

When the woman reports feeling an uncontrollable urge to push (bear down), the nurse can help her greatly by letting her know that these new sensations are normal. This is because some women interpret the increased rectal pressure as a need to move her bowels. The instinctive response is to tighten muscles rather than bear down. The woman may also report that she fears she is "splitting apart" or that she feels a "ring of fire." The woman who expects these sensations and understands that bearing down contributes to progress at this stage is more likely to do so.

Table 24–8 • NURSING ASSESSMENTS IN THE SECOND STAGE

Mother	Fetus
Blood pressure, pulse, respirations every 5–15 minutes. Uterine contraction palpated continuously.	FHR every 15 minutes for low-risk women and every 5 minutes for high-risk women.

> *When I tried to push with the contractions, I felt as if I would tear apart. It hurt so badly that I was shaking. I knew it was time to push and my body was telling me, too, but it hurt so much. The nurse kept saying, "Just push and you will feel better." I wanted to scream at her. She had no idea what was happening to me.*

When the contraction begins, the nurse tells the woman to take two short breaths, then to take a third breath and hold it while pulling back on her knees and pushing down with her abdominal muscles (Figure 24–5 •). Some women prefer to exhale slightly (exhale breathing) while pushing to avoid the physiologic effects of the Valsalva maneuver. With this method the woman takes several deep breaths and then holds her breath for 5 to 6 seconds. Then, through slightly pursed lips, she exhales slowly every 5 to 6 seconds while continuing to hold her breath. The woman takes another breath and continues exhale breathing and pushing during the contraction.

> *I knew when I was completely dilated. I knew when to push and I did it without tearing. My body told me to listen. I knew what to do.*
>
> ~Harriette Hartigan, *Women in Birth*~

The woman is encouraged to rest between contractions. Although the laboring woman may appear exhausted at this time, most experience relief at being able to push with contractions. Perspiration increases with the pushing efforts, and a cold washcloth for forehead and face is most soothing. The birthing woman may also appreciate sips of fluid or ice chips at this time.

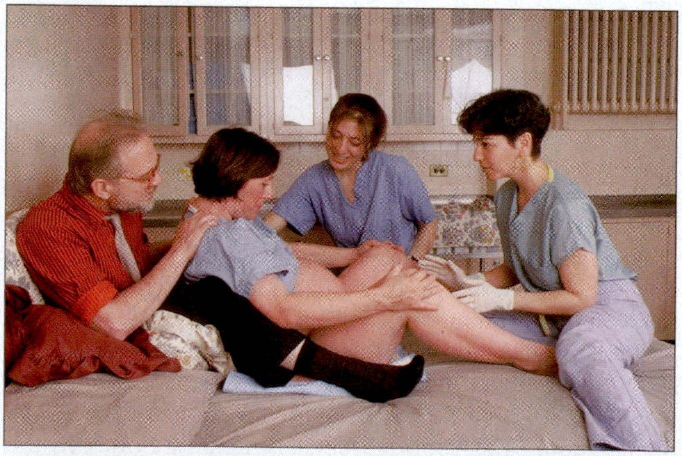

Figure 24–5 • The nurse provides encouragement and support during pushing efforts.
SOURCE: Margaret Miller/Photo Researchers, Inc.

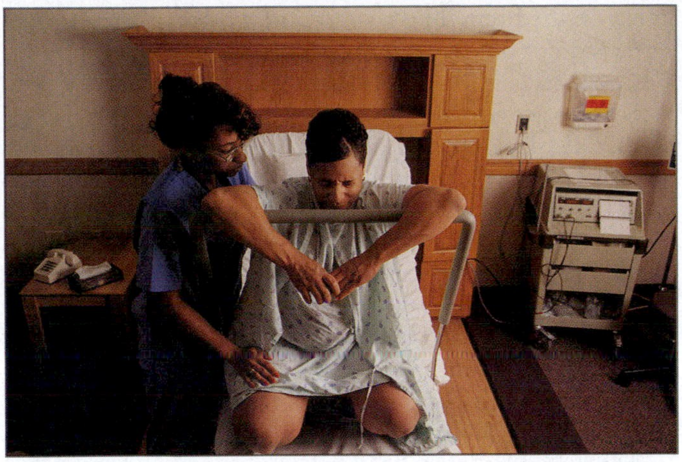

Figure 24–6 • Using a birthing bar.

> *When I began pushing, I felt in control because I could do something. . . . I could push the baby out. I knew he was ready to be born.*
>
> ~HARRIETTE HARTIGAN, *WOMEN IN BIRTH*~

The nurse and/or support person can assist the woman into a comfortable position for pushing. Maternal positions, such as standing, squatting while leaning back on a partner or on a birthing bar (Figure 24–6 •), lying in a lateral or Sims' position, or crouching on hands and knees, may increase comfort and effectiveness of pushing. Some women feel that sitting on a toilet seat is a comfortable position that assists their pushing efforts. This position may cause anxiety in the caregivers, however, for fear that the birth may occur quickly in this most inopportune place. Some women benefit from gripping the hands of the support person or nurse. This technique increases intra-abdominal pressure, which aids in the expulsion effort. Another variation of this technique, which can be quite effective, is to have the woman grip a towel while the support person or nurse pulls the towel in the opposite direction. Care should be taken that the nurse or support person does not suffer a back injury.

Additional comfort measures may be used during this stage. Warm perineal, abdominal, and back compresses may be used to increase muscle relaxation. Perineal massage and stretching with a lubricant (Lubafax) may relieve the tearing and burning sensation as the perineal tissue distends. Providing perineal massage prior to imminent crowning can result in considerable perineal edema. For this reason, some institutions may limit perineal massage to physicians and CNMs.

Visualization techniques may be helpful. The woman can be encouraged to envision the infant descending the birth canal and the vagina opening up. Phrases such as "Open to your baby" and "Let the baby come; don't try to hold back" can be useful and calming. Many women benefit from visualizing the descent of the fetus in a mirror. The nurse should ask the woman if she would like to watch in the mirror.

If anticipated progress is not made or the laboring woman wants to try other positions for pushing, the nurse should support her. Some nurses have their own preferences and may be more comfortable directing the laboring woman to use these preferred positions; however, it is important to remember that the nurse is there to support the birth, and that frequent changes in position may assist in the descent of the baby.

If the maternal pushing effort diminishes because of frustration or fatigue, many women benefit from short rest periods. Rest periods are appropriate if maternal and fetal assessments are stable. In addition, the physician or CNM should be informed of the actual time that has been spent pushing and not the time that has elapsed since the beginning of the second stage.

Throughout the second stage, it remains important to provide information regarding progress and what is happening in the labor. It is also imperative to address the woman's questions honestly, to acknowledge her concerns, and to continue to provide support.

A nullipara is usually prepared for birth when the perineum begins to bulge. A multipara usually progresses much more quickly, so she may be prepared for the birth when the cervix is dilated 7 to 8 cm.

The woman's blood pressure and the FHR are monitored between contractions, and the contractions are palpated until the birth. The nurse continues to assist the woman in her pushing efforts. Both the woman and the coach are kept informed of procedures and of progress, and both are supported throughout the birth.

In addition to assisting the woman and her partner, the nurse assists the physician or CNM in preparing for the birth. The physician/CNM usually dons a sterile gown and gloves and may place sterile drapes over the woman's abdomen and legs. Some providers may perform a sterile preparation prior to birth; others may not do so as part of their normal routine. While some physicians/CNMs may place the woman in stirrups for birth, others may opt to drop the foot of the bed lower than the upper portion and let the woman rest her feet on the bed to facilitate maternal comfort. An episiotomy may be done just before birth if there is a need for one or if the provider performs them on a routine basis. See the discussion of episiotomy in Chapter 27.

Promotion of Comfort in the Second Stage

Most of the comfort measures that have been used during the first stage remain appropriate at this time. Cool cloths to the face and forehead may help provide cooling as the woman is involved in the intense physical exertion of pushing. If she has been diaphoretic, a dry gown may be comforting. The woman may feel hot and want to remove some of the covering. Care still needs to be taken to provide privacy even though covers are removed. Some women may want to remove all of their clothing. Healthcare providers should allow the woman to give birth in a way that will promote her comfort. The woman can be encouraged to rest and "let all muscles go" during the period between contractions. The nurse and support person(s) can assist the woman into a pushing position with each contraction to further conserve energy. Sips of fluid or ice chips may be used to provide moisture and relieve dryness of the mouth. Constant reassurance is imperative.

Assisting the Couple and Physician/CNM During Birth

Shortly before the birth, the birthing room or delivery room is prepared with equipment and materials that may be needed. Family members do not need to change into other clothing if the birth occurs in a birthing room; they don a disposable scrub suit if the birth is to occur in a delivery room or surgery suite. Meticulous handwashing is required of the nurses and CNM/physician. Nurses who will be in direct contact with the mother at the time of birth need to wear protective clothing, such as an apron or gown with a splash apron, disposable gloves, and eye covering. The CNM/physician will also need to wear a gown with a splash apron or a plastic apron, eye covering, and sterile gloves.

Most facilities now use one room for labor, delivery, and recovery (LDR rooms). Use of a separate delivery room is rare. If the laboring woman is to give birth in a separate delivery room, she will be moved shortly before birth on her bed or a cart. It is important to preserve her privacy during the transfer, and safety must be provided by raising the side rails into a locked position. In the delivery room, the labor bed or transfer cart must be carefully supported against the delivery table; this ensures the woman's safety during the transfer.

If the woman is to be moved from one bed to another, it should be done between contractions. During the contraction, the woman feels increased discomfort and may be involved in pushing efforts. Perineal bulging may be occurring, which adds to the discomfort and difficulty in moving. All of these factors make moving the woman very uncomfortable. If birth seems imminent (within the next minute), it is safer for the woman to give birth in her labor bed or on the cart. Transfer to the delivery table is then delayed until after the baby is born and the cord has been clamped and cut.

Even though there are differences in the delivery room setting, the family can still be together during the birth. It is important to provide encouragement for family members to participate because the delivery room environment may be unfamiliar and seem less relaxed. The family member may be hesitant to continue to provide support for fear of interfering or being in the way.

MATERNAL BIRTHING POSITIONS

The woman is usually positioned for birth on a bed, birthing chair, or delivery table. In some instances, she may give birth standing at the side of the bed or on her hands and knees on the floor. The position the woman assumes is determined not only by her individual wishes but also by the CNM/physician.

Stirrups are not often used, but if they are, they are padded to alleviate pressure, and both legs should be lifted simultaneously to avoid strain on abdominal, back, and perineal muscles. The stirrups should be adjusted to fit the woman's legs. The feet are supported in the stirrup holders. The height and angle of the stirrups are adjusted so there is no pressure on the back of the knees or the calf, which might cause discomfort and postpartal vascular problems. This is particularly true of women with epidural anesthesia. The birthing bed is elevated 30 to 60 degrees to help the woman bear down, and handles are provided so she may pull back on them.

The upright posture for birth was considered normal in most societies until modern times. Alternatively, women selected squatting, kneeling, standing, and sitting for birth. Only within the last 200 years has the recumbent position become the norm in the Western world. Its use in this century has been reinforced because of the convenience it offers in applying new technology, and it has thus become the conventional manner in which North American women give birth in hospitals. In searching for alternative positions, consumers and professionals alike continue to refocus on the comfort of the laboring woman and the advantages of alternative positions rather than on the convenience of the CNM/physician (Table 24–9 •).

Recumbent Position

The recumbent (lithotomy) position for birth is used sometimes to enhance the maintenance of asepsis, assessment of FHR, and performance of episiotomy and repair. In contrast, when the comfort and well-being of the woman and fetus are considered, the following disadvantages have been noted:

- There is a decrease of as much as 30% in the blood pressure of 10% of women.
- Many women experience difficulty breathing because of pressure of the uterus on the diaphragm.
- The uterine axis is directed toward the symphysis pubis instead of the pelvic inlet.
- Aspiration of vomit is more likely.
- The woman may feel resentment at being forced to assume an "embarrassing" position.
- Tightening of the vagina and perineum as the thighs are flexed may increase the likelihood of an episiotomy or laceration.
- The position may interfere with the frequency and intensity of contractions.
- Stirrups cause excessive pressure on the legs.
- The woman works against gravity.

These disadvantages may be lessened slightly if the woman has her back elevated 30 to 40 degrees.

Table 24-9 • COMPARISON OF BIRTHING POSITIONS

Position	Advantages	Disadvantages	Nursing Actions
Recumbent	Enhances ability to maintain sterile field. May be easier to monitor FHR. Easier to perform episiotomy or laceration repair.	May decrease blood pressure. It is difficult for the woman to breathe due to pressure on the diaphragm. There is an increased risk of aspiration. May increase perineal presssure making laceration more likely. May interfere with uterine contractions.	Ensure that stirrups do not cause excess pressure on the legs. Assess legs for adequate circulation and support.
Left lateral Sims'	Does not compromise venous return from lower extremities. Increases perineal relaxation and decreases need for episiotomy. Appears to prevent rapid descent.	It is difficult for the woman to see the birth.	Adjust position so that the upper leg lies on the bed (scissor fashion) or is supported by the partner or on pillows.
Squatting	Size of pelvic outlet is increased. Gravity aids descent and expulsion of newborn. Second stage may be shortened (Sleep, Roberts, & Chalmers, 1989).	It may be difficult to maintain balance while squatting.	Help woman maintain balance. Use a birthing bar if available.
Semi-Fowler's	Does not compromise venous return from lower extremities. Women can view birth process.	If legs are positioned wide apart, relaxation of perineal tissues is decreased.	Assess that upper torso is evenly supported. Increase support of body by changing position of bed or using pillows as props.
Sitting in birthing bed	Gravity aids descent and expulsion of the fetus. Does not compromise venous return from lower extremities. Woman can view the birth process. Leg position may be changed at will.		Ensure that legs and feet have adequate support.
Sitting on birthing stool	Gravity aids descent and expulsion of infant. Does not compromise venous return from lower extremities. Woman can view birth process.	It is difficult to provide support for the woman's back.	Encourage woman to sit in a position that increases her comfort.
Hands and knees	Increases perineal relaxation and decreases need for episiotomy. Increases placental and umbilical blood flow and decreases fetal distress. Improves fetal rotation. Better able to assess perineum. Better access to fetal nose and mouth for suctioning at birth. Facilitates birth of infant with shoulder dystocia.	Woman cannot view birth. There is decreased contact with birth attendant. Caregivers cannot use instruments. There may be increased maternal fatigue.	Adjust birthing bed by dropping the foot down. Supply extra pillows for increased support.

Left Lateral Sims' Position

A common position favored by some women and birth attendants is the left lateral Sims' or side-lying position (Figure 24–7 •, *A*). In assuming this position for birth, the woman lies on her left side with her left leg extended and her right knee drawn against her abdomen or flexed by her side or with both legs bent at the knees. Those who favor this position find it increases overall comfort, does not compromise venous return from the lower extremities, puts less stress and pressure on the maternal neck, and diminishes the chances of aspiration should vomiting occur. Women also perceive the lateral Sims' as a more natural and comfortable position and less intrusive with no stirrups or overhead lights required. Birth attendants have found the position has a positive effect on the management of fetal shoulder dystocias. Fewer episiotomies are required in this position because the perineum tends to be more relaxed. The disadvantages cited relate to the difficulty of cutting and repairing large episiotomies and problems with difficult forceps births. These disadvantages, however, can be rectified by repositioning the woman if forceps are needed or if a repair is needed after the birth.

RESEARCH IN PRACTICE
Relationship of Birth Position and Type of Birth Attendant to Perineal Injury

What is this study about? Perineal injuries during birth can lead to adverse outcomes ranging from minor discomfort to more severe conditions such as infection and incontinence. The physical position of the mother during birth and type of birth attendant are two potentially important clinical factors affecting perineal injuries. Research is inconclusive regarding the effects of these two factors on perineal injuries, making it difficult to counsel mothers regarding their choices during the second stage of labor. This study investigated the relationship of maternal position and type of birth attendant to subsequent perineal injury.

How was this study done? This descriptive, quantitative study used a retrospective analysis of 2,891 consecutive normal vaginal births to evaluate the research question. The births occurred in a regional teaching hospital in Australia. Midwives or obstetricians attended the births. Demographic data and pregnancy history were collected, as well as labor history, birth position, perineal outcome, and baby Apgar score at 5 minutes. Descriptive statistics were generated, and cross-tabulations were generated to explore relationships between variables. Linear and logistic regression techniques were used to determine significant associations between birth position, attendant type, and perineal outcome.

What were the results of the study? The lateral position was associated with the most favorable perineal outcome, and the squatting position with the worst. Alternative positions (e.g., all fours, kneeling, and standing) did not perform better than the more traditional semi-recumbent position with respect to perineal outcome. Episiotomy rates of the obstetricians were five times those of the midwives; rates for tears requiring sutures were 5 to 7 percentage points higher for obstetricians than for midwives. Further analysis indicated that these results were not attributable to either parity of the mother or size of the neonate. For all mothers in the study, higher maternal parity was associated with a reduced probability of both episiotomy and tear requiring suture, and larger birth weights were associated with increased risk of perineal injury. A longer second stage of labor was positively associated with an increased rate of episiotomy.

What additional questions might I have? What impact did maternal requests of the obstetrician have on the outcome? Are these results applicable in populations other than Australia where midwives attend a significant number of women at birth? Would a randomized control trial demonstrate a cause-and-effect relationship, rather than describing an association? What specific interventions did the midwives use that were associated with these improved perineal outcomes?

How can I use this study? This study provides insight into the factors that are associated with an intact perineum after birth. These results can be used to counsel mothers about their choices regarding birth position and birth attendant.

Source: Shorten, A., Donsante, J., & Shorten, B. (2002). Birth position, accoucheur, and perineal outcomes: informing women about choices for vaginal birth. *Birth, 29* (1): 18–27.

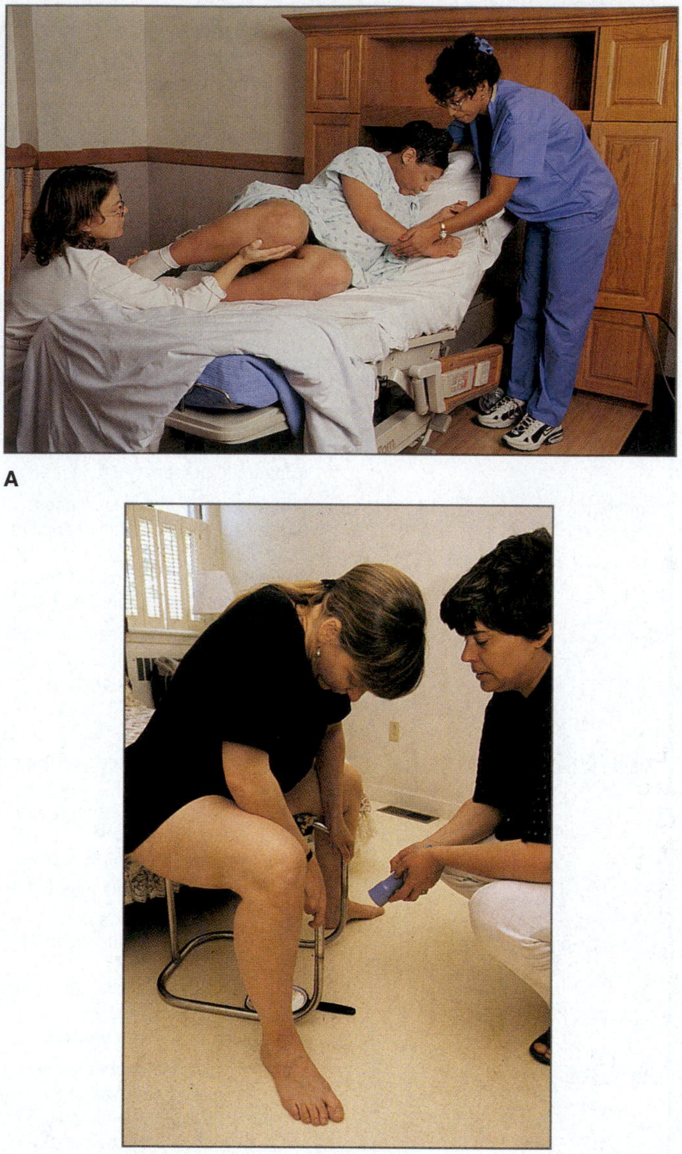

A

B

Figure 24–7 • Birthing positions. *A,* Side-lying (also known as left lateral Sims') position. *B,* Using a birthing stool.

Squatting Position

Squatting is favored by some women primarily for the positive use it makes of gravity. Squatting is thought to facilitate the entrance of the presenting part into the pelvic inlet, thus hastening engagement. A squatting bar (birthing bar) may be used across a bed or on the floor to increase the woman's balance and provide some support (see Figure 24–6). During the second stage of labor, squatting increases the size of the pelvic outlet and helps in the woman's pushing efforts. Some birth attendants object to this position because the perineum is relatively inaccessible, and it is difficult for them to control the birth process. Squatting also increases the difficulty of administering analgesia, using instruments, and monitoring fetal status. Perineal edema can also occur from prolonged squatting. Women with epidural anesthesia may be unable to assume this position due to the heaviness in their lower extremities.

Semi-Fowler's Position

Some care providers advocate a semi-Fowler's position as an appropriate middle ground between the recumbent and upright positions. This position enhances the effectiveness of the abdominal muscle efforts while the woman is pushing and thereby shortens the second stage of labor. Raising and supporting the torso helps the woman view the birth process. At the same time the birth attendant has access to the perineum. Supporting a woman in this position is not difficult with most birthing beds.

Sitting Position

The sitting position is becoming an option for more women with the increased availability of birthing chairs. The use of birthing chairs or stools can be traced back to ancient Egypt, and they were broadly used in ancient Greek, Roman, and Incan civilizations. In the wake of the 19th-century battle against puerperal fever, birthing chairs began to vanish on hygienic grounds. Birthing chairs are being used again during the second stage of labor and are perceived by some women as a positive way to participate in the birth process (Figure 24-7, *B*). A supported sitting position may also be achieved in a birthing bed.

The upright sitting position offers advantages similar to squatting. It has been postulated that the weight of a term fetus is sufficient force in itself to supply much of what is needed to bring the newborn into the world. Proponents of the birthing chair state that it makes possible spontaneous births that would have required operative assistance in the recumbent position. Women experiencing severe back pain have found that use of the chair can diminish or eliminate the pain. The woman can curl forward and grasp her knees and ankles during pushing efforts. She can usually see the birth without aid of mirrors, and following birth she can lift the baby up toward her face.

Duration of the second stage and fetal outcome are not significantly affected by use of the birthing chair. However, it may carry a potential for increased blood loss.

Hands and Knees Position

The hands and knees position is more comfortable for a woman experiencing back labor because there is less pressure on the maternal back from the fetus, and the fetus may be able to rotate more easily from the posterior position. The mother can be well supported by dropping the foot of the birthing bed and supplying extra pillows upon which she can rest her forearms. Because there is less pressure on the perineum, there is less need for an episiotomy, and the incidence of lacerations is less. The birth attendant is better able to assess the perineum for stretching and has good access to the fetal nose and mouth for suctioning at the time of birth. This position may also increase placental and umbilical blood flow during episodes of fetal distress. Lastly, the hands and knees position may increase the pelvic diameter and facilitate birth of the infant with shoulder dystocia. Disadvantages of this position include decreased eye contact between the mother and birth attendant, the inability to use instruments, and the potential necessity of repositioning the mother for perineal repair. Women may also become easily fatigued in this position.

CLEANSING THE PERINEUM

If a perineal prep is to be performed, the woman is positioned for the birth, and her vulvar and perineal area is cleansed to increase her comfort and to remove the bloody discharge that is present prior to the actual birth. An aseptic technique such as the one that follows is recommended.

After thorough handwashing, the nurse opens the sterile prep tray, dons sterile gloves, and cleans the vulva and perineum with the cleansing solution. Beginning with the mons pubis, the area is cleansed up to the lower abdomen. A second sponge is used to clean the inner groin and thigh of one leg, and a third is used to clean the other leg, moving upward to avoid carrying material from surrounding areas to the vaginal outlet. The last three sponges are used to clean the labia and vestibule with one downward sweep each. The used sponges are discarded. Once the cleansing is completed, the woman returns to the desired birthing position. Not all birthing facilities use such formalized cleansing procedures. Some facilities use a spray bottle with povidone-iodine (Betadine) or other cleansing agent and simply spray the perineal area. Since birth is not truly a "sterile procedure" some providers do not perform perineal cleansing techniques.

SUPPORTING THE COUPLE

The nurse assesses the woman's partner or other support person for comfort and knowledge and assists him/her in activities that will support the woman during the second stage. Some support persons will want to take an active role in coaching the woman through the birth process, whereas others will prefer simply to observe the birth process. The nurse assesses the roles the members of the support team desire and provides interventions that enhance these roles. It is important to keep the support team informed of the woman's progress, provide explanations of what is happening, and praise them for their supportive activities. A nurse who provides calm reassurance can help promote a positive experience.

ASSISTING WITH THE BIRTH OF THE INFANT

When the fetal head has distended the perineum, the clinician may perform a hand maneuver, such as supporting the perineum between the thumb and four fingers, which is believed to prevent undue trauma to the fetal head and maternal soft tissues. The woman may be asked to breathe rapidly, pant, or blow to avoid too rapid birth of the fetal head.

After the infant's head is born, the clinician palpates the neck for the presence of a cord, which can be slipped over the fetal head if it is loose. If the cord is tight, it is double-clamped and cut.

Restitution and external rotation occur after the head is born. The only assistance needed during this time is support of the maternal perineum. While awaiting completion of external rotation, the clinician suctions the newborn's nose and mouth to remove mucus. When the newborn's shoulder appears at the symphysis pubis, the clinician may use both hands to grasp the newborn's head gently and pull downward for release of the anterior shoulder. Gentle upward traction facilitates release of the posterior shoulder.

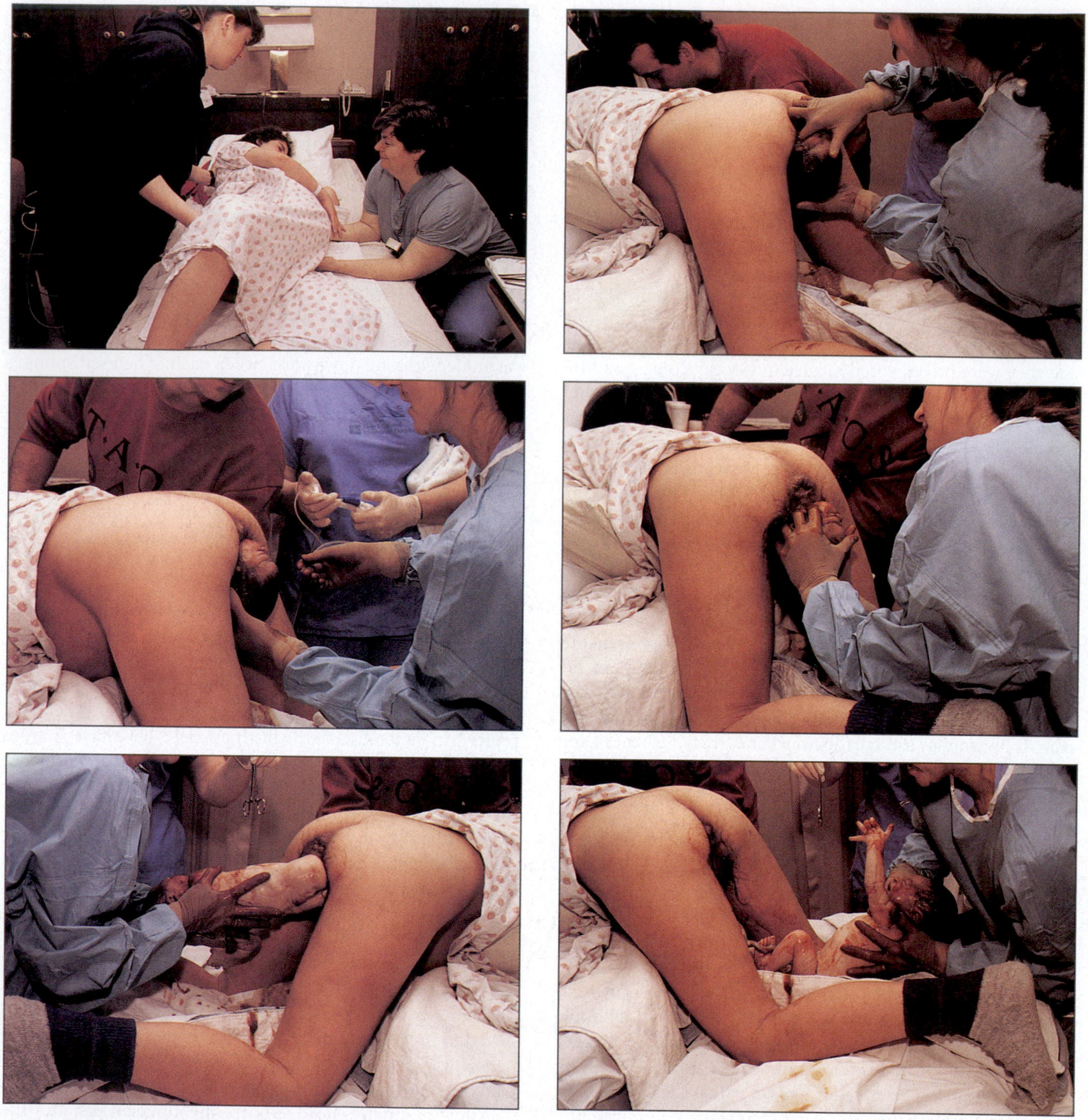

Figure 24–8 • A birthing sequence.

Birth of the newborn's body may be controlled by grasping the posterior shoulder with one hand, palm turned toward the perineum. The left hand may be used for this if the newborn is left occiput anterior (LOA). The right hand then follows along the infant's back, and the feet are grasped as they are expelled. The newborn's head is kept down and to the side as the feet, legs, and body are tucked under the clinician's left arm in a football hold. The clinician's right hand is then free for further care of the newborn, and the newborn is securely held. CNMs often place the newborn directly on the mother's abdomen. The nose and mouth are suctioned with a bulb syringe, and respiratory passages are cleared. Figure 24–8 • depicts an entire birthing experience.

ASSISTING WITH CLAMPING THE CORD

There is controversy about when to clamp and cut the cord. If the newborn is held at or below the vagina as cord clamping is delayed, as much as 50 to 100 mL of blood may be shifted from the placenta to the newborn. If the newborn is held 50 to 60 cm above the vagina, blood may be transferred

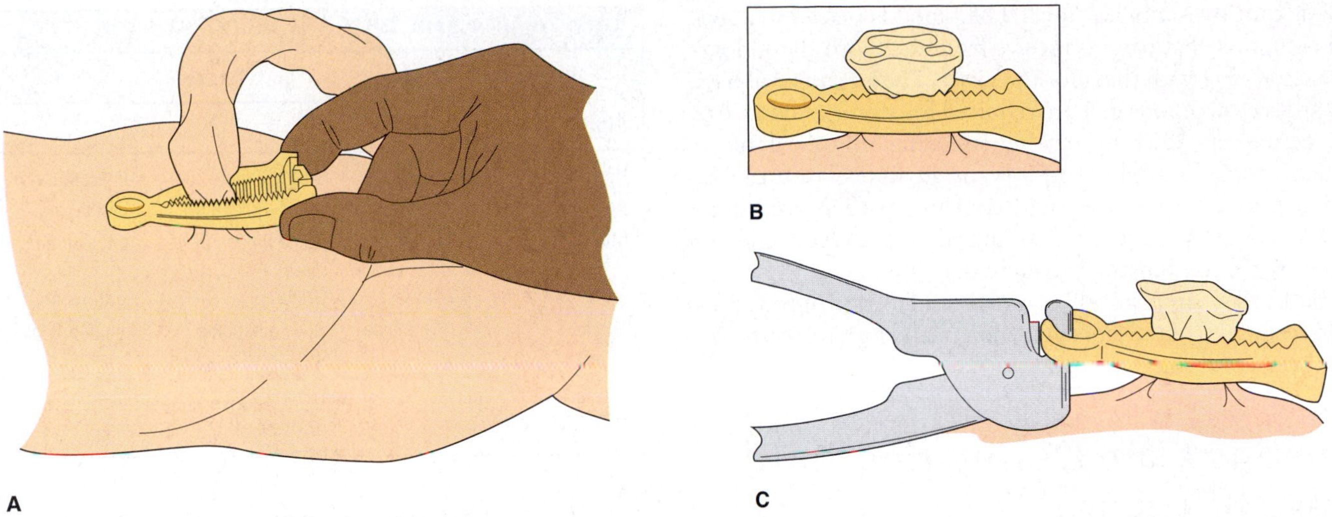

Figure 24–9 • Hollister cord clamp. *A,* Clamp is positioned 1/2 to 1 inch from the abdomen and then secured. *B,* Cut cord. The one vein and two arteries can be seen. *C,* Plastic device for removing clamp after cord has dried. After the cord is cut, the nurse grasps the Hollister clamp on either side of the cut area and gently separates it.

from the newborn to the placenta. The extra amount of blood added to the newborn's circulation by holding the newborn below the vagina may reduce the frequency of iron deficiency anemia, which can occur later in infancy. However, in some cases the circulatory overload may produce polycythemia and favor hyperbilirubinemia. The newborn is not elevated above the vagina. Some parents may specify a preference in their birth plan regarding exactly when the umbilical cord is to be cut. The pros and cons of early and late cord clamping can be discussed prior to the birth.

The cord is usually clamped with two Kelly clamps and cut between them. The father, other support person, or the mother may wish to cut the cord after it has been clamped by the physician/CNM.

The physician/CNM may double-clamp the cord so that a section can be made available for the collection of cord blood gases (discussed shortly). After the cord has been cut, cord blood is collected and sent to the lab as needed.

If the physician/CNM has not placed a cord clamp on the newborn's umbilical stump, it is the responsibility of the nurse to do so. Before applying the cord clamp, the nurse examines the cut end for the presence of two arteries and one vein. The umbilical vein is the largest vessel, and the arteries are smaller vessels. The presence of only one artery in the umbilical cord is associated with genitourinary abnormalities. The number of vessels is recorded on the birth and newborn records.

The cord is clamped approximately 1/2 to 1 inch from the abdomen to allow room between the abdomen and clamp as the cord dries (Figure 24–9 •). Abdominal skin must not be clamped because this will cause necrosis of the tissue. The clamp is removed in the newborn nursery approximately 24 hours after birth if the cord has dried. Some facilities now place an umbilical cord alarm with the cord clamp (Figure 24–10 •). This security measure triggers an alarm if the infant comes within a certain distance from the unit's exterior door. The alarm can only be removed with a special removal device.

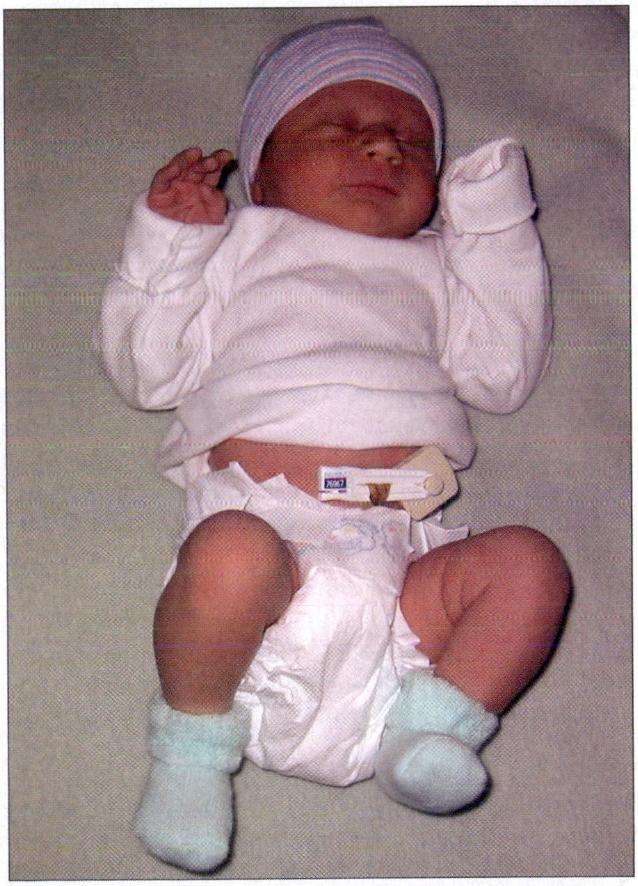

Figure 24–10 • Umbilical alarm in place on a newborn infant.

CORD BLOOD COLLECTION FOR BANKING

Growing numbers of parents are arranging for cord blood banking (see discussion in Chapter 1). Immediately after the newborn's umbilical cord is clamped and cut and prior to the placenta being expelled, the physician/CNM withdraws blood from the umbilical cord. The blood is placed in a special container that parents receive from the Cord Blood Registry and bring with them for the birth. The parents will have any special directions that are required for storage and care of the container. Current recommendations for cord blood banking include a family history of an illness that can be treated with fetal cells and children whose parents are from a nontraditional lineage, such as mixed race backgrounds or other ethnic combinations that are uncommon.

Table 24–7 on page 643 summarizes labor progress, possible responses of the laboring woman, and nursing care during the second stage of labor.

MEDIALINK VIDEOS: THIRD STAGE OF LABOR

Nursing Care During the Third Stage of Labor

Nursing care in the third stage focuses on providing initial newborn care and assisting with delivery of the placenta.

Provision of Initial Newborn Care

The physician or certified nurse-midwife (CNM) places the newborn on the mother's abdomen or in the radiant-heated unit to begin the initial care. If the newborn is not placed on the mother's abdomen, the radiant-heated unit is positioned so the parents can see the baby.

Because the first priority is to maintain respirations, the newborn is placed in a modified Trendelenburg position to aid drainage of mucus from the nasopharynx and trachea. The newborn is also suctioned with a bulb syringe or DeLee mucus trap as needed (Procedure 24–1: Performing Nasal Pharyngeal Suctioning).

The second priority is to provide and maintain warmth, so the newborn is dried immediately with warmed soft infant blankets. Wet blankets should be immediately removed to prevent heat loss. The nurse dries the newborn's head first to minimize heat loss. Warmth can be maintained by putting the newborn in skin-to-skin contact with the mother and placing warmed blankets over both of them. If the newborn is placed in a radiant-heated unit, he or she is dried, laid on a dry blanket, and left uncovered under the radiant heat. Because radiant heat warms the outer surface of objects, a newborn wrapped in blankets will receive no benefit. In many settings a stocking cap is placed on the newborn's head to conserve heat.

APGAR SCORING SYSTEM

The Apgar scoring system (Table 24–10 •) was designed in 1952 by Dr. Virginia Apgar, an anesthesiologist. The purpose of the **Apgar score** is to evaluate the physical condition of the newborn at birth and the immediate need for resuscitation. The newborn is rated 1 minute after birth and again at 5 minutes and receives a total score ranging from 0 to 10 based on the following criteria:

Table 24–10 • THE APGAR SCORING SYSTEM

Sign	Score 0	Score 1	Score 2
Heart rate	Absent	Slow—below 100	Above 100
Respiratory effort	Absent	Slow—irregular	Good crying
Muscle tone	Flaccid	Some flexion of extremities	Active motion
Reflex irritability	None	Grimace	Vigorous cry
Color	Pale blue	Body pink, blue extremities	Completely pink

Source: Apgar, V. (1966, August). The newborn (Apgar) scoring system, reflections and advice. *Pediatric Clinics of North America, 13,* 645.

1. The heart rate is auscultated or palpated at the junction of the umbilical cord and skin. This is the most important assessment. A newborn heart rate of less than 100 beats per minute (bpm) indicates the need for immediate resuscitation.
2. The respiratory effort is the second most important Apgar assessment. Complete absence of respirations is termed *apnea.* A vigorous cry indicates good respirations.
3. The muscle tone is determined by evaluating the degree of flexion and resistance to straightening of the extremities. A normal term newborn's elbows and hips are flexed, with the knees positioned up toward the abdomen.
4. The reflex irritability is evaluated as the newborn is dried or by lightly rubbing the soles of the feet. A cry is a score of 2. A grimace is 1 point, and no response is 0.
5. The skin color is inspected for cyanosis and pallor. Newborns generally have blue extremities, and the rest of the body is pink, which merits a score of 1. This condition, termed *acrocyanosis,* is present in 85% of normal newborns at 1 minute after birth. A completely pink newborn scores a 2, and a totally cyanotic, pale infant is scored 0. Newborns with darker skin pigmentation will not be pink. Their skin color is assessed for pallor and acrocyanosis, and a score is selected based on the assessment.

A score of 8 to 10 indicates a newborn in good condition and requires only nasopharyngeal suctioning and perhaps some oxygen near the face. An Apgar score between 4 and 7 indicates the need for stimulation; a score under 4 indicates the need for resuscitation. See the discussion in Chapter 33.

NEWBORN PHYSICAL ASSESSMENT BY THE NURSE

An abbreviated systematic physical assessment is performed by the nurse in the birthing area to detect any abnormalities (Table 24–11 •). First, the nurse notes the size of the newborn and the contour and size of the head in relationship to the rest of the body. The newborn's posture and movements indicate tone and neurologic functioning.

The skin is inspected for discoloration, presence of vernix caseosa and lanugo, and evidence of trauma and desquamation (peeling of skin). *Vernix caseosa* is a white, cheesy sub-

Procedure 24-1 Performing Nasal Pharyngeal Suctioning

Preparation

1. Suction equipment is always available in the birthing area to clear secretions from the newborn's nose or oropharynx if respirations are depressed or if amniotic fluid was meconium stained.
2. Tighten the lid on the DeLee mucus trap or other suction device collection bottle.
   Rationale: This avoids spillage of secretions and prevents air from leaking out of the lid.
3. Connect one end of the DeLee tubing to low suction.

Equipment and Supplies

- DeLee mucus trap or other suction device

Procedure: Clean Gloves

1. Don gloves.
2. Without applying suction, insert the free end of the DeLee tubing 3 to 5 inches into the newborn's nose or mouth (Figure 24–11 •).
   Rationale: Applying suction while passing the tube would interfere with smooth passage of the tube.
3. Place your thumb over the suction control and begin to apply suction. Continue to suction as you slowly remove the tube, rotating it slightly.
   Rationale: Suctioning during withdrawal removes fluid and avoids redepositing secretions in the newborn's nasopharynx.
4. Continue to reinsert the tube and provide suction for as long as fluid is aspirated.
   Note: Excessive suctioning can cause vagal stimulation, which decreases the heart rate.
5. If it is necessary to pass the tube into the newborn's stomach to remove meconium secretions that the newborn swallowed before birth, insert the tube through the mouth into the stomach. Apply suction and continue to suction as you withdraw the tube.
   Rationale: Because the newborn's nares are small and delicate, it is easier and faster to pass the suction tube through the mouth.
6. Document the completion of the procedure and the amount and type of secretions.
   Rationale: This documentation provides a record of the intervention and the status of the infant at birth.

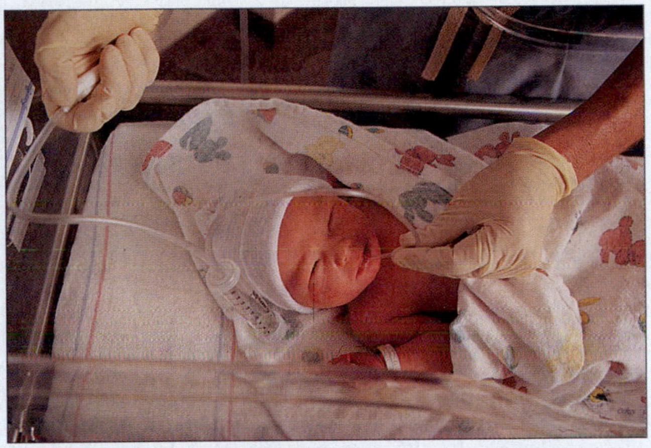

Figure 24-11 • A newborn infant being suctioned with a DeLee mucus trap to remove excess secretions from the mouth and nares.

MEDIALINK VIDEO: NEWBORN ASSESSMENT

stance normally found on newborns. It is absorbed within 24 hours after birth. Vernix is abundant on preterm infants and absent on postterm newborns. A large quantity of fine hair (*lanugo*) is often seen on preterm newborns, especially on their shoulders, foreheads, backs, and cheeks. Desquamation of the skin is seen in postterm newborns.

The nares are observed for flaring. As the newborn cries, the palate can be inspected for cleft palate. Mucus in the nose and mouth can be assessed and removed with the bulb syringe as needed. The chest is inspected for respiratory rate and the presence of retractions. If retractions are present, the newborn is assessed for grunting or stridor. A normal respiratory

Table 24-11 • INITIAL NEWBORN EVALUATION

Assess	Normal Findings
Respirations	Rate 30–60, irregular No retractions, no grunting
Apical pulse	Rate 110–160 and somewhat irregular
Temperature	Skin temp above 36.5C (97.8F)
Skin color	Body pink with bluish extremities
Umbilical cord	Two arteries and one vein
Gestational age	Should be 38–42 weeks to remain with parents for extended time
Sole creases	Sole creases that involve the heel

In general, expect scant amount of vernix on upper back, axilla, groin; lanugo only on upper back; ears with incurving of upper ⅔ of pinnae and thin cartilage that springs back from folding; male genitals—testes palpated in upper or lower scrotum; female genitals—labia majora larger; clitoris nearly covered

In the following situations, newborns should generally be stabilized rather than remaining with parents in the birth area for an extended period of time:

- Apgar less than 8 at 1 minute and less than 9 at 5 minutes or baby requires resuscitation measures (other than whiffs of oxygen)
- Respirations below 30 or above 60, with retractions and/or grunting
- Apical pulse below 110 or above 160 with marked irregularities
- Skin temperature below 36.5C (97.8F)
- Skin color pale blue or circumoral pallor
- Baby less than 38 or more than 42 weeks' gestation
- Baby very small or very large for gestational age
- Congenital anomalies involving open areas in the skin (meningomyelocele)

rate is 30 to 60 per minute. The lungs may be auscultated bilaterally for breath sounds. Absence of breath sounds on one side may indicate pneumothorax. Rales may be heard immediately after birth because a small amount of fluid may remain in the lungs; this fluid will be absorbed. Rhonchi indicate aspiration of oral secretions.

The elimination of urine or meconium is noted and recorded on the newborn record.

NEWBORN IDENTIFICATION

To ensure correct identification, the nurse gives the mother and the newborn identification bands with identical codes in the birthing or delivery room. One bracelet is placed on the mother's wrist and sometimes on the wrist of her partner or a support person whom she designates. Two bracelets are placed on the newborn—one on the wrist and one on the ankle. The newborn bands must be applied snugly to prevent their loss. Infants should not be removed from the room until these identification bands have been placed.

Some hospitals footprint the newborn and fingerprint the mother for further identification purposes. To prepare the newborn for footprinting, the nurse wipes the soles of both the newborn's feet to remove any vernix caseosa.

INITIATION OF ATTACHMENT

The birth of the baby is usually an emotionally charged time for all members of the family. The sight of the new baby and the sounds of the first cry may fill the parents with utter amazement. As the baby is placed on the mother's abdomen or chest, she frequently reaches out to touch and stroke her baby. When the newborn is placed in this position, the father also has a very clear, close view and can also reach out to touch his baby.

When the parents feel comfortable in the environment, they may talk to the newborn, and some mothers talk to their babies in a high-pitched voice, which seems to soothe newborns. Some couples verbally express amazement and pride when they see they have produced a beautiful, healthy baby. Their verbalization enhances feelings of accomplishment and ecstasy.

If lights in the birthing area can be dimmed, the newborn will probably open his or her eyes wide and gaze at the surroundings. In this first hour after birth, the newborn is usually quiet and continues to gaze. This is a wonderful opportunity for eye contact with the parents, and many parents are content to gaze quietly at their newborn.

Even though the baby is on the mother's abdomen or chest, the nurse can complete any needed assessments or interventions such as footprinting and applying an identification bracelet to the child. As soon as possible the nurse can assist the mother to a more comfortable position for holding the newborn. Breastfeeding can be encouraged if the mother and baby desire. When the baby is held close to the breast, the baby will seek out the nipple. Even if the newborn does not actively nurse, she or he can lick, taste, and smell the mother's skin. This activity stimulates the maternal release of prolactin, which promotes the onset of lactation.

The initial parental-newborn attachment period can be enhanced if the care providers keep routine investigations to a minimum, delay instillation of ophthalmic antibiotic for the first hour, keep the room slightly darkened, avoid loud noises, talk in quiet tones, and provide privacy. Both parents need to be encouraged to do whatever they feel most comfortable doing. Parents may have differing wishes concerning contact with their newborn. Some want immediate and unlimited time; some prefer to wait until all birth-related activities are completed (the placenta is expelled and episiotomy repair is completed); others prefer limited contact immediately after birth and quiet time later. Although immediate contact may be important for attachment and initiation of breastfeeding, the parents' wishes need to be supported.

Parents can be encouraged to delay phone calls and visits from friends until after the first hour of birth since it is a time when the baby is the most alert. Most facilities have policies in place where the newborn is taken to the nursery for assessment and bathing after an initial visit with the parents. This is an excellent time for phone calls and visits with family and friends. It enables the new family to spend valuable time together and facilitates bonding.

> *I was hungry for the baby as he was born. I wanted to see, hold him. It was hours before I realized or even thought love in relation to him.*
>
> ~Harriette Hartigan, *Women in Birth*~

GLOBAL PERSPECTIVES

In Malaysia, 75% of all births are attended by a *dukun* (midwife). In many parts of the country, especially in rural areas, a home setting is preferred over a hospital setting for birth. It is believed that the baby's first cry is symbolic of loyalty to the parents and should be heard at home. The birth itself is a social event in which many women sit with the laboring woman. It is customary for the woman in labor and her female company to chew red-staining betel nuts. At the time of birth, either the mother or a female relative is given the honor of cutting the umbilical cord.

Delivery of the Placenta

After the cord has been clamped and cut, the physician/CNM observes for the following signs of placental separation:

1. The uterus rises upward in the abdomen because the placenta settles downward into the lower uterine segment.
2. As the placenta proceeds downward, the umbilical cord lengthens.
3. A sudden trickle or spurt of blood appears.
4. The uterus changes from a discoid to a globular shape.

While waiting for these signs, the nurse gently palpates the uterus to check for ballooning caused by uterine relaxation and subsequent bleeding into the uterine cavity.

After the placenta has separated, it may be expelled by various techniques such as maternal bearing-down effort, controlled cord traction, and fundal pressure. Maternal effort allows the placenta to be expelled spontaneously and is best accomplished in an upright position. When the mother is in a dorsal recumbent or lithotomy position, she or the nurse can help the process by splinting or supporting her abdominal muscles. The mother or nurse can place her palms over the lower abdomen, or the mother can flex her thighs over her abdomen. The mother then bears down to expel the placenta.

To help the woman expel her placenta, the physician/CNM first ensures that separation has occurred and then places one hand above the symphysis pubis with the palm against the anterior surface of the uterus. The uterus is displaced upward and backward as the mother is asked to relax her abdominal muscles and breathe through an open mouth. The elevation of the uterus straightens out the birth canal and facilitates expulsion of the placenta, as well as protecting the uterus from inversion. Gentle traction is exerted on the umbilical cord. Excessive pulling may increase the risk of uterine involution, snapping off of the cord, and subsequent hemorrhage. During this procedure, the nurse encourages the mother to continue breathing through an open mouth and to relax her abdominal muscles.

Fundal pressure is not a method of choice because it is very uncomfortable for the mother, may damage uterine supports, and may invert the uterus. If this method is needed, the mother is asked to relax her abdominal muscles, and then the hand of the physician/CNM is placed behind the uterus with the fingers directed downward toward the maternal spine. With a quick "scooping" motion, the contracted uterus is pressed downward in an arc. This motion is different from direct downward pressure, which folds the uterus over the lower segment and does not enhance movement of the placenta. During the procedure, the nurse provides continued encouragement to maintain abdominal relaxation. This is very difficult due to the discomfort of the procedure.

After expulsion of the placenta, the physician/CNM inspects the placental membranes to make sure they are intact and that all cotyledons are present. This inspection is especially important with placentas expelled via the Duncan mechanism (the chance of tearing off a portion of a cotyledon is greatest with this mechanism of placental separation). If there is a defect or a part missing from the placenta, a digital uterine examination is done. The time and mechanism (Schultze or Duncan) of expulsion of the placenta are noted on the birth record (see Chapter 22). The vagina and cervix are inspected for lacerations, and any necessary repairs are made. An episiotomy or laceration may be repaired now if it has not been done previously. (See further discussion of episiotomy in Chapter 27.) The fundus of the uterus is palpated; normal position is at the midline and below the umbilicus. If the fundus is displaced, it may be because of a full bladder or a collection of blood in the uterus.

MEDIALINK ANIMATION: PLACENTAL DELIVERY

The medical-nursing culture tends to refer to the placenta as the "afterbirth" and considers that its value is fulfilled once it is expelled and examined. Disposal of the placenta is prescribed by the hospital or birth center, and no more thought is given to it. However, many cultures have other beliefs regarding the placenta. Some clients will have specific beliefs about disposal of the placenta and will ask to take it home with them. Labor nurses will need to review hospital policies for disposal of the placenta before giving the placenta to the woman or family members.

Use of Oxytocics

Some CNMs and physicians advocate the use of an oxytocic drug (Pitocin) to stimulate uterine contractions after birth and to reduce the incidence of third-stage hemorrhage.

The physician/CNM may request that 10 units of oxytocin be given intramuscularly to the woman when the anterior shoulder of the infant appears at the vaginal opening. Some practitioners believe this procedure facilitates the expulsion of the placenta. Others question whether this method increases the incidence of neonatal hyperviscosity because an additional bolus of blood may be infused into the fetus when the uterus contracts in response to the oxytocin. At other times 10 units of oxytocin may be administered intramuscularly at the time of placental expulsion. Both techniques are thought to prevent uterine atony and excessive bleeding.

Some prefer to add 10 to 20 units of oxytocin to intravenous fluids administered over a period of hours. Additional information and associated nursing implications are presented in the Drug Guide: Oxytocin (Pitocin) in Chapter 27.

Nursing Care During the Fourth Stage of Labor

The period immediately following expulsion of the placenta is referred to as the fourth stage of labor and birth. Actually, the label is misleading because labor and birth are completed with delivery of the placenta, and the next few hours are actually the immediate recovery phase. The fourth stage is usually defined as lasting from 1 to 4 hours after the birth or until vital signs are stable. Nursing care in this phase involves the basics of postpartum nursing care.

Immediately after the placenta is expelled, the episiotomy or vaginal lacerations are repaired. The uterus is palpated at frequent intervals, usually every 15 minutes for an hour until bleeding is within normal limits, to ensure that it remains firmly contracted. Although labor is completed, the uterus is sensitive to touch. Palpation of the uterine fundus will be uncomfortable for the woman. If the mother has not held her baby, immediate newborn care should be completed at her side and within her reach so that she can touch her baby during this time. As soon as immediate care is completed, the new mother is usually eager to cuddle and explore her baby. If she plans to breastfeed and the baby is interested, she should be encouraged and helped to do so right after birth while the baby is awake and alert. Care should be taken not to try to force an uninterested baby to breastfeed because it will just lead to frustration for both mother and baby.

MediaLink VIDEO: FOURTH STAGE OF LABOR

Behavioral characteristics of the mother vary, according to such factors as the length of labor, level of fatigue, extent of interruption in normal sleep patterns, and cultural norms. After the initial excitement of becoming acquainted with their new baby and notifying others of the birth, many new mothers are very tired and want to rest. Others are wide awake, eager to talk about their labor and satisfy basic body needs, such as hunger and thirst.

Provision of Care in the Fourth Stage

As soon as the CNM/physician completes the repair of any perineal lacerations or an episiotomy, drapes (if used) are removed. If the mother is to remain in the birthing bed, the nurse places clean absorbent pads beneath her and applies maternity pads. A cold pack may be placed directly on the perineum if perineal edema is present or an episiotomy has been done. If a mother prefers to shower immediately after birth, the nurse can assist her as needed and change the bed linens while the mother is up.

If stirrups were used, her perineum is cleansed and maternity pads applied before her legs are removed from the stirrups. In order to avoid muscle strain, both legs are removed from the stirrups at the same time. The legs may be held together and gently pushed toward the woman's abdomen, back to a neutral position and then gently lowered toward her right side and then the left side to promote circulation return. If the woman has given birth on a delivery table she is transferred to a recovery room bed. If the mother has not had a chance to hold her infant, she may do so before she is transferred from the birthing room. The nurse ensures that the mother and father or support person and newborn are given time to begin the attachment process.

In addition to encouraging family celebration of the birth, the immediate recovery period involves assessing both maternal bleeding and newborn stabilization. The most significant source of bleeding is from the site where the placenta was implanted and where uterine vessels previously provided pooling of maternal blood to nourish the fetus. It is therefore critical that the fundus stay well contracted to clamp off these uterine vessels and prevent hemorrhage. It is the nurse's responsibility to assess the mother's blood pressure, pulse, firmness and position of fundus, and amount and character of vaginal blood flow every 15 minutes for the first 1 or 2 hours. Deviations from the normal ranges require more frequent checking. Table 24–12 • summarizes maternal changes following birth. Blood pressure should return to the prelabor level, and pulse rate should be slightly lower than it was in labor. The return of the blood pressure is due to an increased volume of blood returning to the maternal circulation from the uteroplacental shunt. Baroreceptors cause a vagal response, which slows the pulse. The physiologic slowing may be offset by excitement, increased temperature, or dehydration. A rise in the blood pressure may be a response to oxytocic drugs or may be caused by preeclampsia. Blood loss may be reflected by a lowered blood pressure and a rising pulse rate.

The fundus should be firm at the umbilicus or lower and in the midline. The uterus should be palpated but not massaged unless boggy (atonic) (Procedure 24–2). When the uterus becomes boggy, pooling of blood occurs within it, resulting in the formation of clots. Anything left in the uterus prevents it from contracting effectively. Thus if it becomes boggy or appears to rise in the abdomen, the fundus should be massaged until firm. The uterus at this time is very tender, and palpation and massage cause discomfort. All palpation and massage should be done as gently as possible.

Table 24–12 • MATERNAL ADAPTATIONS FOLLOWING BIRTH

Characteristic	Normal Finding
Blood pressure	Returns to prelabor level
Pulse	Slightly lower than in labor
Uterine fundus	In the midline at the umbilicus or 1–2 fingerbreadths below the umbilicus
Lochia	Red (rubra), small to moderate amount (from spotting on pads to ¼ – ½ of pad covered in 15 minutes) Doesn't exceed saturation of one pad in first hour
Bladder	Nonpalpable
Perineum	Smooth, pink, without bruising or edema
Emotional state	Wide variation, including excited, exhilarated, smiling, crying, fatigued, verbal, quiet, pensive, and sleepy

Procedure 24–2 Assessing the Uterine Fundus Following Vaginal Birth

Preparation

1. Explain the procedure, the information it provides, and what it might feel like.
2. Ask the woman to void.
   Rationale: A full bladder can cause uterine atony.
3. Have the woman lie flat in bed with her head on a pillow. If the procedure is uncomfortable, she may find that it helps to flex her legs.
   Rationale: The supine position prevents falsely high assessment of fundal height. Flexing the legs relaxes the abdominal muscles.

Equipment and Supplies

- A clean perineal pad

Procedure: Clean Gloves

1. Gently place one hand on the lower segment of the uterus. Using the side of the other hand, palpate the abdomen until you locate the top of the fundus.
   Rationale: One hand stabilizes the uterus while the other hand locates the top of the fundus.
2. Determine whether the fundus is firm. If it is, it will feel like a hard round object in the abdomen. If it is not firm, massage the abdomen lightly until the fundus is firm.
   Rationale: A firm fundus indicates that the uterine muscles are contracted and bleeding will not occur.
3. Measure the top of the fundus in fingerbreadths above, below, or at the fundus. See Figure 24–12 •.
   Rationale: Fundal height gives information about the progress of involution.
4. Determine the position of the fundus in relation to the midline of the body. If it is not in the midline, locate it and then evaluate the bladder for distention.
   Rationale: The fundus may deviate from the midline when the bladder is full because the enlarged bladder pushes the uterus aside.
5. If the bladder is distended, use nursing measures to help the woman void. If she is not able to void after a specified period of time, catheterization may be necessary.
6. Measure urine output for the next few hours until normal elimination is established.
   Rationale: During the postpartum as diuresis occurs, the bladder may fill far more rapidly than normal, putting the woman at risk for uterine atony and hemorrhage.
7. Assess the lochia. (Leugenbiehl et al. 1990).

Clinical Tip

Gloves may be put on before assessing the abdomen and fundus or when you are ready to assess the perineum and lochia.

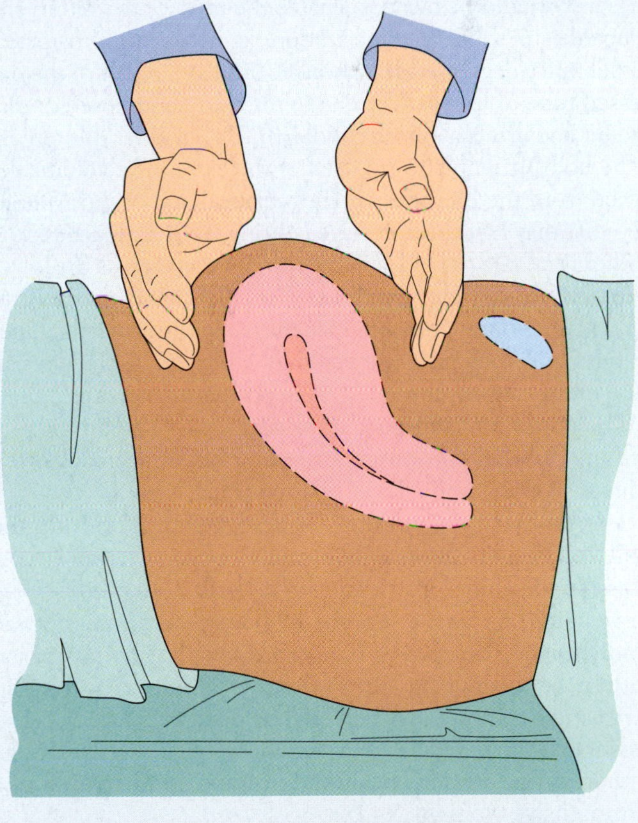

Figure 24–12 • Suggested method of palpating the fundus of the uterus during the fourth stage. The left hand is placed just above the symphysis pubis, and gentle downward pressure is exerted. The right hand is cupped around the uterine fundus.

A boggy uterus feels very soft instead of firm and hard. The uterus may have relaxed so much that it cannot be found when the nurse attempts to palpate it. In this case the nurse places a hand in the midline of the abdomen at the level of the umbilicus and begins to make kneading motions. This motion stimulates the uterine fundus to contract, and the nurse will feel the fundus tighten to a firm, hard object.

The nurse inspects the bloody vaginal discharge, called *lochia*, for amount and charts it as minimal, moderate, or heavy (see Chapter 34). It should be bright red. Because different brands of maternity pads absorb varying amounts of blood, it may be necessary to weigh the maternity pad to determine actual blood loss. A gram scale is used, and 1 g is equivalent to approximately 1 mL of blood. If the perineal pad becomes soaked in a 15-minute period or if blood pools under the buttocks, continuous observation is necessary. As long as the woman remains in bed during the first hour, bleeding should not exceed saturation of one pad. Laceration of the vagina, cervix, or an unligated vessel in the episiotomy may be indicated by a continuous trickle of blood even though the fundus remains firm. (See Procedure 34–2: Evaluating Lochia, in Chapter 34.)

If the fundus rises and displaces to the right, the nurse palpates the bladder to determine whether it is distended. All measures should be taken to enable the mother to void. If she is unable to void, catheterization is necessary. Postpartal women have decreased sensations to void as a result of the decreased tone of the bladder due to the trauma imposed on the bladder and urethra during childbirth. The bladder fills rapidly as the body attempts to rid itself of the extra fluid volume returned from the uteroplacental circulation and of intravenous fluid that may have been received during labor and birth. If the mother is unable to void, a warm towel placed across the lower abdomen, warm water poured over the perineum, or spirits of peppermint poured into a bedpan may help the urinary sphincter relax and thus facilitate voiding. A distended bladder can cause uterine atony, thus increasing postpartal bleeding.

The perineum is inspected for edema and hematoma formation. With an episiotomy or laceration, an ice pack often reduces swelling and alleviates discomfort.

The following conditions should be reported to the CNM/physician: hypotension, tachycardia, uterine atony, excessive bleeding, or a temperature over 38C (100F). The nurse should be aware that the blood pressure may not fall rapidly in the presence of dangerous bleeding in postpartal mothers because of the extra systemic volume. However, an increasing pulse rate may be noted before a decrease in blood pressure is detected. A normal blood pressure with the mother in the Fowler's position is a good confirmation of a normotensive woman.

Promotion of Comfort in the Fourth Stage

Women frequently have tremors in the immediate postpartal period. It has been proposed that this shivering response is caused by a difference in internal and external body temperatures (higher temperature inside the body than on the outside). Another theory is that the woman is reacting to the fetal cells that have entered the maternal circulation at the placental site. A heated bath blanket placed next to the woman and perhaps a warm drink tend to alleviate the problem.

The couple may be tired, hungry, and thirsty. Some hospitals serve the couple a meal. The tired mother will probably drift off into a welcome sleep. The partner should also be encouraged to rest because his supporting role is physically and mentally tiring. The mother is usually transferred from the birthing unit to the postpartal unit after 2 hours or more, depending on agency policy and whether the following criteria are met: stable vital signs, stable lochia, nondistended bladder, firm fundus, and sensations fully recovered from any anesthetic agent received during childbirth.

Nursing Care of the Adolescent

Each adolescent in labor is different. The nurse must assess what each client brings to the experience by asking the following questions:

- Has the young woman received prenatal care?
- What are her attitudes and feelings about the pregnancy?
- How does her developmental stage influence her behavior, and how are her specific needs different?
- Who will support her during the birth, and what is the person's relationship to her?
- What preparation has she had for the experience?
- What are her expectations and fears regarding labor and birth?
- How has her culture influenced her?
- What are her usual coping mechanisms?
- Does she have adequate social support?
- Does she plan to keep the newborn? If so, does she need to learn parenting skills?
- Will the father of the baby be involved in the labor and birth experience?

Adolescents are at highest risk for pregnancy and labor complications and must be assessed carefully. Any adolescent who has not had prenatal care requires especially close observation during labor. The status of the fetus is monitored to ensure its well-being. The young woman's prenatal record is carefully reviewed for risks. The adolescent is more likely to have preeclampsia, cephalopelvic disproportion (CPD), anemia, drugs ingested during pregnancy, sexually transmitted infections, and size-date discrepancies (gestation appears to be less than dates indicate because of minimal weight gain).

The nurse's support role depends on the young woman's support system during labor. When the client is not accompanied by someone who will stay with her during childbirth, it is even more important for the nurse to establish a trusting relationship with her. In this way, the nurse can help her cope with labor and understand what is happening to her. Establishing rapport without recrimination will provide emotional support and encouragement. The adolescent who is given positive reinforcement for "work well done" will leave the experience with increased self-esteem, despite the emotional stress and difficulty of giving birth at such a young age.

The adolescent who has taken childbirth education classes is generally better prepared than the adolescent who has had no preparation. The nurse must keep in mind, however, that the younger the adolescent, the less she may be able to participate actively in the process.

Age-Related Responses to Labor and Birth

The very young adolescent (under age 14) has fewer coping mechanisms and less experience to draw on than her older counterparts have. Because her cognitive development is incomplete, the younger adolescent may have fewer problem-solving capabilities. Her ego integrity may be more threatened by the experience, and she may be more vulnerable to stress and discomfort.

The very young woman needs someone to rely on at all times during labor. She may be more childlike and dependent than older teens. The nurse must be sure that instructions and explanations are simple and concrete. During the transition phase, the young teenager may become withdrawn and unable to express her need to be nurtured. Touch, soothing encouragement, and measures to promote her comfort help her maintain control and meet her needs for dependence. During the second stage of labor, the young adolescent may feel as if she is losing control and may reach out to those around her. By remaining calm and giving directions, the nurse helps her control feelings of helplessness.

> *One of the most memorable expectant mothers I cared for during my nursing course was Cara, a 13-year-old. I met her each week as she came into the OB clinic at our hospital and stayed with her as she waited for her appointment and was then seen by the medical student. I noticed that with each passing visit, she became more and more anxious. I did my best to determine the source of her anxiety, provided general teaching, and tried to answer all of her questions. I consulted with my professor, and she sat in with me during some visits. But Cara became more and more anxious. Near term, she began asking if she could just have the baby cut out. Whatever was she afraid of? Finally, in the 38th week, after 2 1/2 months of building trust, she told me she was afraid because her baby had gotten too big, and it would never be able to come out through her belly button. I was speechless for a moment. For 2 1/2 months, I had answered questions and felt so proud of my support and teaching, and for all this time, she had not been able to ask the most important question of all—the question that paralyzed her with fear. I was finally able to provide specific information, made drawings on a paper towel, had the medical student talk with her, and best of all, was able to be on call and be with her in labor and during birth. The beautiful smile on her face as her baby daughter was born was unbelievable. Cara wasn't afraid! It's been 39 years since then, and I still remember her.*

The middle adolescent (ages 14 to 16 years) often attempts to remain calm and unflinching during labor. If unable to break through the teenager's stoic barrier, the nurse needs to rise above frustration and realize that a caring attitude will still positively affect the young woman.

Many older adolescents feel that they "know it all," but they may be no more prepared for childbirth than their younger counterparts. The nurse's reinforcement and nonjudgmental manner will help them save face. If the adolescent has not taken classes, she may require preparation and explanations. The older teenager's response to the stresses of labor is similar to that of the adult woman.

The Adolescent Father

Consideration of the adolescent father is a very important aspect of labor and birthing care. Nurses need to be aware that this is a stressful time for the young father. There are some specific interventions that increase comfort, enhance education, and perhaps decrease stress. In the early part of labor, the nurse can talk with the father about his expectations for parenting the newborn and what resources are available in the community. Many adolescents are reluctant to ask questions, but an accepting attitude may help in establishing rapport and gaining trust.

The teen father may need encouragement to provide supportive care and to know what actions are acceptable in the birthing area. He may be encouraged to hold the mother's hand, to sit on the bed beside her, to give a back massage, or to stroke her forehead. He may need assistance in how to give a shoulder rub or back rub; he can watch the nurse first and then perform the action himself with the encouragement of the nurse. He may need more encouragement than the older father to share a Jacuzzi or shower or to support the mother in changing positions and ambulating. It is important for the nurse to speak in lay terms and to anticipate questions, to answer all vocalized questions honestly, and to provide opportunities for the parents to ask for further information.

Other Members of the Support Team

In addition to the adolescent's partner, the mother may want her parents or friends with her as members of her support team. Some teens may want their mother as their primary support person whereas others may strive to prove their independence and "do this on their own." Still other young women may look to friends for advice and support. The nurse includes parents and friends of the adolescent mother in the client teaching and other aspects of the mother's care.

Teaching the Adolescent Mother

During the latent phase of labor, the nurse can explain to the young woman what changes in body sensations and emotional reactions she might anticipate as labor and birth progress. The adolescent also needs teaching about what possible medical procedures (such as electronic fetal monitoring, etc) might be used, as well as what nursing care measures are available. Some

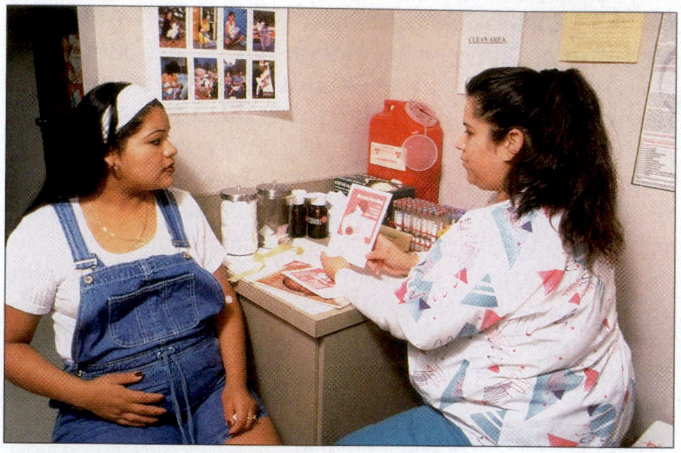

Figure 24–13 • An adolescent mother receives breastfeeding assistance in the immediate postpartum period.
SOURCE: Amy Etra/PhotoEdit

adolescents might not realize that they can request the nurse's presence, touch, or advice, unless the nurse specifically informs them that these options are available.

Adolescents are oriented to the present time and may not adequately predict future needs for themselves or their infant. The nurse should assess to make sure adequate resources are available including infant and postpartum supplies, transportation to and from follow-up visits, and child care, if the adolescent mother is planning on returning to school or work.

Young mothers may need more information on infant care and feeding choices than older women. Some adolescents may be reluctant to breastfeed due to embarrassment or lack of information. The nurse can assist the young woman to explore her feelings related to breastfeeding and provide information (Figure 24–13 •). The nurse should provide encouragement and support the young mother's decision. Sometimes, young women feel "pressured" to breastfeed their infants when they truly do not feel comfortable with this feeding choice. The nurse should give the young mother permission to make her own decision. Young women who choose to use formula should be given clear instructions on the importance of mixing the formula per the manufacturer's directions since overdiluting or underdiluting can cause adverse side effects for the baby.

Although more rare than in previous decades, some adolescents may choose to relinquish their newborns. In these situations, the nurse informs the adolescent that seeing the infant can facilitate the grieving process, but lets her know that seeing the newborn is her choice. (See Chapter 35 for further discussion of the relinquishing mother and the adolescent parent.)

Nursing Care During Precipitous Birth

Occasionally, labor progresses so rapidly that the nurse is faced with the task of managing the birth of the baby. This is called a **precipitous birth.** The attending nurse has the primary responsibility for providing a physically and psychologically safe experience for the woman and her baby.

A woman whose physician or CNM is not present may feel disappointed, frightened, and abandoned, especially if she is not prepared through childbirth education. The nurse can support the woman by keeping her informed about the labor progress and assuring her that the nurse will stay with her. If birth is imminent, the nurse must not leave the mother alone. Auxiliary personnel can be directed to contact the attending physician or CNM, or other physicians/CNMs who are in the facility. The auxiliary personnel should also retrieve the emergency pack ("precip pack"), which should be readily accessible to the birthing/labor rooms. A typical pack contains the following items: a small drape that can be placed under the woman's buttocks to provide a sterile field, a bulb syringe to clear mucus from the newborn's mouth, two sterile clamps (Kelly or Rochester) to clamp the umbilical cord before applying a cord clamp, sterile scissors to cut the umbilical cord, a sterile umbilical cord clamp, a baby blanket to wrap the newborn in after birth, and a package of sterile gloves.

As the materials are being gathered, the nurse must remain calm. The woman is reassured by the nurse's composure and feels that the nurse is competent. The primary goal of nursing care is the safe birth of the infant.

Birth of Infant

The nurse manages precipitous birth in the hospital by encouraging the woman to assume a comfortable position. If time permits, the nurse scrubs both hands with soap and water and puts on sterile gloves. Sterile drapes are placed under the woman's buttocks.

At all times during the birth, the nurse gives clear instructions to the woman, supports her efforts, and provides reassurance. The nurse needs to remain calm and proceed in a slow, confident manner.

Most infants will be born in vertex presentation. When the infant's head crowns, the nurse instructs the woman to either blow or pant, which decreases her urge to push. The nurse checks whether the amniotic sac is intact. If it is, the nurse tears the sac with a clamp so that the newborn will not breathe in amniotic fluid with the first breath.

The nurse may place an index finger inside the lower portion of the vagina and the thumb on the outer portion of the perineum and gently massage the area to aid in stretching of perineal tissues and to help prevent perineal lacerations. This is called "ironing the perineum."

With one hand, the nurse applies gentle pressure against the fetal head to maintain flexion and prevent it from popping out rapidly. The nurse does not hold the head back forcibly. Rapid birth of the head may tear the woman's perineal tissues. The rapid change in pressure within the fetal head may cause subdural or dural tears. The nurse supports the perineum with the other hand and allows the head to be delivered between contractions.

As the woman continues to blow or pant, the nurse inserts one or two fingers along the back of the fetal head to check for the umbilical cord. If the cord is around the neck, the nurse bends her fingers like a fish hook, grasps the cord, and pulls it over the baby's head, loosens it, or slips it down over the shoulders. It is important to check that the cord is not wrapped around more than one time. If the cord is tightly looped and cannot be slipped over the baby's head, the nurse places two clamps on the cord, cuts it between the clamps, and unwinds the cord. Because this ceases oxygenation to the baby, all efforts should be made to reduce (remove) the cord over the head whenever possible. The head typically rotates (restitutes) to the left or right. The nurse needs to let the head rotate (restitute) to the side before attempting delivery of the head.

Immediately after birth of the head, the nurse suctions first the mouth, throat, and then the nasal passages. The nurse places a hand on each side of the head and instructs the woman to push gently so that the rest of the body can be expelled quickly. The newborn must be supported as it emerges.

Breech vaginal births are quite rare since the incidence of breech presentations is only 3%, most breech presentations are scheduled for cesarean births, and women are advised to come to the hospital immediately if labor does begin spontaneously. Since the primary concern in a breech birth is to prevent the entrapment of the head in the cervix, intervention is avoided until the buttocks are born. The nurse then pulls down a loop of cord (to avoid stress on its point of insertion) and supports the breech in both hands. The infant's body is lifted slightly upward for birth of the posterior shoulder and arm. The newborn may then be lowered, and the anterior shoulder and arm will pass under the symphysis pubis. Suprapubic pressure should be applied to maintain the normal flexion of the baby's head and should be continued until the baby is born. The nape of the neck pivots under the symphysis, and the rest of the head is born over the perineum by a movement of flexion.

Regardless of the presentation at birth, the newborn is held at the level of the uterus to facilitate blood flow through the umbilical cord immediately after birth. The combination of amniotic fluid and vernix makes the newborn very slippery, so the nurse must be careful to avoid dropping the baby. Placing the woman in stirrups is not recommended for this reason; instead, the foot of the bed can be lowered. The nurse suctions the nose and mouth of the newborn again, using a bulb syringe. The nurse then dries the newborn quickly to prevent heat loss. Wet blankets should be removed and replaced with warmed, dry blankets.

As soon as the nurse determines that the newborn's respirations are adequate, the infant can be placed on the mother's abdomen. The newborn's head should be slightly lower than the body to aid drainage of fluid and mucus. The weight of the newborn on the mother's abdomen stimulates uterine contractions, which aid in placental separation. The umbilical cord should not be pulled. The Apgar score is assessed at 1 and 5 minutes.

The nurse is alert for signs of placental separation. When these signs are present, the nurse places one hand just above the symphysis pubis to guard the uterus and uses the other hand to maintain gentle downward traction on the cord while instructing the mother to push so that the placenta can be expelled. In some instances the mother can squat, and this usually helps expel the placenta. The nurse inspects the placenta to determine whether it is intact. Since the physician/CNM is usually en route, delivery of the placenta can be delayed until the practitioner arrives. Traction should not be applied since this can result in hemorrhage or detaching the umbilical cord from the placenta.

The nurse checks the firmness of the uterus. Palpation of the uterus should not be performed prior to separation of the placenta. The fundus may be gently massaged to stimulate contractions and decrease bleeding. Putting the newborn to breast also stimulates uterine contractions through release of oxytocin from the pituitary gland.

The umbilical cord may now be cut. Two sterile clamps are placed approximately 2 to 4 inches from the newborn's abdomen. The cord is cut between them with sterile scissors. A sterile cord clamp (Hollister or Hesseltine) can be placed adjacent to the clamp on the newborn's cord, between the clamp and the newborn's abdomen. The clamp must not be placed snugly against the abdomen because the cord will dry and shrink.

The area under the mother's buttocks is cleaned, and her perineum is inspected for lacerations. Bleeding from lacerations may be controlled by pressing a clean perineal pad against the perineum and instructing the woman to keep her thighs together. Further evaluation by the CNM/physician will be needed to determine if lacerations are present that need to be repaired.

If the arrival of the physician or CNM is delayed or if the newborn is having respiratory distress, the newborn should be transported immediately to the nursery. The newborn must be properly identified before he or she leaves the birthing area.

Record Keeping

The nurse notes and places on the record the following information:

1. Position of fetus at birth
2. Presence of cord around neck or shoulder (nuchal cord)
3. Time of birth
4. Apgar scores at 1 and 5 minutes after birth
5. Gender of newborn
6. Time of expulsion of placenta
7. Method of placental expulsion
8. Appearance and intactness of placenta
9. Mother's condition
10. Any medications that were given to mother or newborn (per agency protocol)

Postbirth Interventions

Postbirth interventions are the same as those listed under Nursing Care During the Third Stage of Labor.

Evaluation

Evaluation provides an opportunity to determine the effectiveness of nursing care. As a result of comprehensive nursing care during the intrapartal period, the following outcomes may be anticipated:

- The mother's physical needs and the psychologic well-being of the family have been maintained and supported.
- The baby's physical and psychologic well-being has been protected and supported.
- The family has had input into the birth process, and members have participated as much as they desired.
- The birth was safe and promoted family cohesiveness.

Chapter Review

ExploreMediaLink

NCLEX review questions, case studies, and other interactive resources for this chapter can be found on the Web site at http://www.prenhall.com/olds. Click on "Chapter 24" to select the activities for this chapter.

For tutorials including animations and videos, more NCLEX review questions, and an audio glossary, access the accompanying CD-ROM in this book.

Focus your study

- Admission to the birth setting involves assessment of many physiologic, psychologic, and social factors. The information gained helps the nurse establish priorities of care.
- Before initiating care, the nurse explains what will be done, the reasons, potential benefits and risks, and possible alternatives if appropriate. This helps the woman determine what happens to her body and is a critical element in the process of obtaining informed consent.
- Behavioral responses to labor vary with the phase of labor, the woman's preparation and previous experience, cultural beliefs, and developmental level.
- Each woman's cultural beliefs affect her need for privacy, her expression of discomfort, her expectations for the birth, and the role she wishes the father to play in the birth event.
- The laboring woman's comfort may be increased by general comfort measures, supportive relaxation techniques, methods of handling anxiety, controlled breathing, and support by a caring person.
- The laboring woman fears being alone during labor. Even though there is a support person available, the woman's anxiety may be decreased when the nurse remains with her.
- Maternal birthing positions include a wide variety of possibilities, such as recumbent, side-lying, sitting, squatting, and crouching on hands and knees.
- Immediate assessments of the newborn include evaluation of the Apgar score and an abbreviated physical assessment. These early assessments help determine whether there is a need for resuscitation and whether the newborn's adaptation to extrauterine life is progressing normally. The newborn who is not experiencing problems may remain with the parents for an extended period of time following birth.
- Immediate care of the newborn following birth also includes maintaining respirations, promoting warmth, preventing infection, and accurate identification.
- The new parents and their baby are given time together as soon as possible after birth.
- Nursing assessments continue after the birth and are important to ensure that normal physiologic adaptations are taking place.
- The adolescent has special needs in the birth setting. Her developmental needs require specialized nursing care.
- Nurse-assisted births are sometimes performed in the absence of the CNM/physician when birth is imminent.

References

Association of Women's Health, Obstetric, and Neonatal Nurses (AWHONN). (1999). Guidelines for fetal monitoring. In L.K. Mandeville & N.H. Troiano (Eds.), *High risk and critical care intrapartum nursing.* Philadelphia: Lippincott.

Calhoun, M. A. (1986). The Vietnamese woman: Health/illness attitudes and behaviors. In P. N. Stern (Ed.), *Women, health and culture.* Washington, DC: Hemisphere.

Callister, L. C. (2001). Culturally competent care of women and newborns: Knowledge, attitude, and skills. *Journal of Obstetric, Gynecologic, and Neonatal Nursing, 30*(2), 209–215.

dePaula, T., Lagana, K., & Gonzalez-Ramirez, L. (1996). Mexican Americans. In J. G. Lipson, S. L. Dibble, & P. A. Minarik (Eds.), *Culture and nursing care: A pocket guide* (chap. 20, pp. 203–221). San Francisco: UCSF Nursing Press.

Hutchinson, M. K., & Baqi-Aziz, M. (1994). Nursing care of the childbearing Muslim family. *Journal of Obstetric, Gynecologic, and Neonatal Nursing, 23,* 67.

Johnson, S. (1996). Hmong. In J. G. Lipson, S. L. Dibble, & P. A. Minarik (Eds.), *Culture and nursing care: A pocket guide* (chap. 16, pp. 161–168). San Francisco: UCSF Nursing Press.

Kramer, J. (1996). American Indians. In J. G. Lipson, S. L. Dibble, & P. A. Minarik (Eds.), *Culture and nursing care: A pocket guide* (chap. 3, pp. 11–22). San Francisco: UCSF Nursing Press.

LaDu, E. B. (1985). Childbirth care for Hmong families. *Maternal-Child Nursing Journal, 10,* 382.

Leugenbiehl, D. L., Brophy, G. H., Artigue, G. S., Phillips, K. E., & Flak, R. J. (1990). Standardized assessment of blood loss. *Maternal-Child Nursing Journal, 15*(4), 241–244.

Minato, J. (2000–2001). Is it time to push? *AWHONN Lifelines, 4*(6), 20–23.

Morrow, K. (1986). Transcultural midwifery: Adapting to Hmong birthing customs in California. *Journal of Nurse-Midwifery, 31,* 285.

Murray, R. B., & Zentner, J. P. (2001). *Health promotion strategies through the life span* (7th ed.). Upper Saddle River, NJ: Prentice Hall.

Parks, F. M. (1998). Models of helping and coping: A transgenerational theory of African-American traditional healing. *Interamerican Society of Psychology, 32,* 95–110.

Shelp, S. G. (1997). Your patient is deaf, now what? *RN, 60*(2), 37–38, 40.

Pain Management During Labor

25

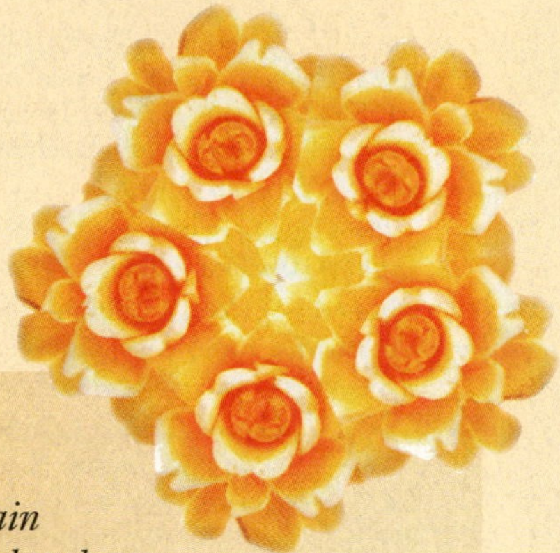

We had attended childbirth classes and practiced through the last few weeks, and I had hoped to go through all of labor and birth without medication. But when the contractions really came on strong, I just wasn't ready for the amount and the kind of pain that I felt. I've always been able to tolerate pain well, but this was different. My husband and I talked about it and he reassured me that, if I felt I needed something, it was okay with him. My nurse was also very supportive. She helped me feel I was making a good decision and wasn't failing somehow.

Objectives

- Discuss the nurse's role in supporting pharmaceutical pain relief measures in labor.
- Describe the use of systemic analgesics to promote pain relief during labor.
- Compare the major types of regional analgesia and anesthesia, including area affected, advantages, disadvantages, techniques, and nursing implications.
- Summarize possible complications of regional anesthesia.
- Describe the major inhalation and intravenous anesthetics used to provide general anesthesia.
- Delineate the major complications of general anesthesia.
- Identify contraindications to specific types of analgesia and anesthesia for high-risk mothers.

MediaLink

Additional resources for this content can be found on the Student CD-ROM and on the Companion Website at www.prenhall.com/olds. Click on "Chapter 25" to select the activities for this chapter.

CD-ROM

- Audio Glossary
- NCLEX Review
- Epidural Placement Video

Companion Website

- Additional NCLEX Review
- Case Study: Pain Management in Labor
- Care Plan Activity: Pain in a Laboring Woman

Key Terms

Epidural block 674
General anesthesia 687
Local anesthesia 686
Pudendal block 686
Regional analgesia 671
Regional anesthesia 671
Spinal block 682

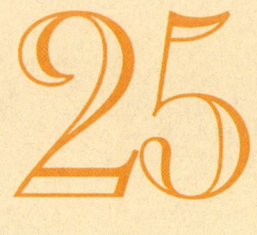

When a childbearing woman experiences discomfort during labor and birth, the nurse can assist her to have a positive birth experience by providing effective comfort measures. Nursing interventions directed toward pain relief begin with the nonpharmacologic measures described in Chapter 24, such as providing information, encouragement, backrubs, and clean linens. Many women need no further interventions.

For other women, the progression of labor brings increasing levels of pain that interfere with their ability to cope effectively. For these women, pharmacologic agents may be used to decrease discomfort, increase relaxation, and reestablish the ability to participate more actively in the labor and birth experience. In addition to systemic analgesics, regional nerve blocks (epidural, spinal, and combined epidural-spinal) and local anesthetic blocks (pudendal and perineal) are available. The methods are not mutually exclusive, and may be used in combination with nonpharmacologic comfort measures.

Nurses need to recognize that the decision to have an unmedicated or a medicated birth involves many factors and reflects a great deal of thought and planning for most women and their families. Some of these factors include client and caregiver preferences, availability of anesthesia and analgesia, fear of risks and complications, and cultural influences.

Each year in the United States, over 4 million infants are born. Of these births, 40% to 45% of all women will receive epidural anesthesia while another 35% to 40% will receive some form of analgesia (American Society of Anesthesiologists [ASA], 1999; Goldberg, Cohen, & Lieberman, 1999).

Many couples who have had childbirth education approach their birth experience confident that the techniques they have learned will enable them to cope with the pain of labor. Nurses should respect these couples' choices and provide support to help them meet their goals. Analgesics and anesthetics do affect the fetus and can be accompanied by maternal side effects. Following an unmedicated birth, women commonly report a quicker postpartum recovery. Many are able to ambulate, urinate, shower, and eat within an hour of giving birth. Additionally, many women feel an enormous sense of empowerment after successfully having an unmedicated birth.

For the woman who has advised the nursing staff that she wants no pharmacologic remedies, the nurse should offer alternative comfort measures. All nurses in the intrapartum setting need to be familar with various nonpharmacologic techniques available to help women cope with the pain they may experience. The nurse should avoid offering these women pain medication unless they specifically ask for them or for information about pharmacologic options.

On the other hand, many women are simply unprepared for the intense pain of active labor and may request medication. They may begin labor undecided about whether or not to use medication, then request pain relief as contractions intensify. Frequently, feelings of inadequacy and guilt accompany such decisions. The nurse plays a special role in assisting the woman and her partner to explore their options for pain relief realistically. The nurse can explain to the couple that, while pharmacologic agents do affect the fetus, so do the pain and stress

CRITICAL THINKING IN PRACTICE

Luisa Silva, a 33-year-old G1P0, is 32 weeks pregnant. She is trying to decide whether she should accept any analgesia during her labor. She has finished childbirth education classes and wants an unmedicated labor and birth. She says, "I want to do this on my own, but I'm afraid it may be too much. Will it be OK if I need to take something?" What will you tell her?

Answers can be found in Appendix I.

MEDIALINK PAIN RELIEF

experienced by the laboring mother. In response to stress, the woman's ventilation and oxygen consumption increase, which decreases the amount of oxygen available to the fetus. In addition, pain and stress can lead to metabolic acidosis and the release of catecholamines, causing the maternal blood vessels to constrict. This in turn decreases oxygen and nutrient supply to the fetus (ASA, 1999). Thus, if the woman's pain and anxiety are more than she can cope with, the adverse physiologic effects on the fetus may be as great as would occur with the administration of a small amount of an analgesic agent. The nurse should reassure the woman and her partner that accepting medication for pain is not a failure. The emphasis should be on the goal of a healthy, satisfying outcome for the family.

Systemic Analgesia

The goal of systemic analgesia during labor is to provide maximal pain relief with minimal risk for the woman and fetus.

Multiple factors must be considered in the use of analgesic agents:

- Effects on the woman
- Effects on the fetus
- Effects on the labor contractions
- Medical status of the woman
- Progress of labor

The effects on the mother are of primary importance because the well-being of the fetus depends on adequate functioning of the maternal cardiopulmonary system. Any alteration of function that disturbs the woman's homeostatic mechanism affects the fetal environment. Maintaining the maternal respiratory rate and blood pressure within normal range is thus of prime importance. The use of electronic fetal monitoring (EFM) provides a means of accurately assessing the effects of pharmacologic agents on uterine contractions.

All systemic analgesics can cross the placental barrier by simple diffusion, with some agents crossing more readily than others. Drug action in the body depends on the rate at which the substance is metabolized by liver enzymes and excreted by the kidneys. The fetal liver enzymes and renal systems are inadequate to metabolize analgesic agents, so high doses remain active in fetal circulation for a prolonged period of time. The percentage of blood volume flowing to the brain increases during intrauterine stress, so the hypoxic fetus receives an even larger amount of a depressant drug. The blood-brain barrier is more permeable at the time of birth, a factor that also increases the amount of drug carried to the central nervous system (Chestnut, 1999).

Administration of Analgesic Agents

The optimal time for administering analgesia is determined after a complete assessment of many factors. In general, an analgesic agent is administered to nulliparas when the active phase of labor is well established (cervix has dilated to 5 or 6 cm) and to multiparas when the cervix has reached 3 or 4 cm dilatation. This is only a generalization, however; the character of each labor must be taken into account. There is debate on the ideal timing of medication administration; however, both the American College of Obstetricians and Gynecologists (ACOG) and the American Society of Anesthesiologists (ASA) agree that a woman's request for pain medications is ample reason to administer them (ASA, 1999; Goetzl, 2002). Analgesia given too early may prolong labor and depress the fetus. Analgesia given too late is of no value to the woman and may cause neonatal respiratory depression. In many institutions, the nurse decides when to give the analgesic agent prescribed by the physician, certified nurse-midwife (CNM), or certified registered nurse-anesthetist (CRNA). The nurse observes the woman for cues that indicate she would benefit from the administration of analgesics. The nurse performs needed assessments (as discussed in the next section) and then notifies the CNM/physician. The decision to administer pain medication is based on a complete assessment of the woman and the progress of labor. The CNM/physician may evaluate the woman at the bedside or may rely on the nurse's assessment and instruct the nurse to administer the medications. In most institutions, the CRNA is available to monitor analgesia-related complications and provide ongoing monitoring for women who later receive an epidural. Some facilities may have anesthesiologists (physicians who specialize in administering anesthesia) provide these services.

MATERNAL ASSESSMENT

The following maternal assessments are critical prior to administering systemic analgesics:

- The woman is willing to receive medication after being advised about it.
- Vital signs are stable.
- Contraindications (such as drug allergies, respiratory compromise, or current drug dependence) are not present.

FETAL ASSESSMENT

The following assessments of the fetus are also required:

- The fetal heart rate (FHR) is between 110 and 160 beats per minute, reactive nonstress test (NST) (accelerations of FHR are present with fetal movement), short-term variability is present, long-term variability is average, and periodic late decelerations or nonperiodic (variable) decelerations are absent.
- The fetus is at term.
- Meconium staining is not present.

ASSESSMENT OF LABOR

The following assessment parameters must also be present:

- The contraction pattern is well established.
- The cervix is dilated at least 4 to 5 cm in nulliparas and 3 to 4 cm in multiparas.
- The fetal presenting part is engaged.
- There is progressive descent of the fetal presenting part.
- No complications that would preclude administering an analgesic agent are present.

If normal parameters are absent or if nonreassuring maternal or fetal factors are present, the nurse may need to complete further assessments with the physician/CNM.

Prior to administering the medication, the nurse once again ascertains whether the woman has a history of any drug reactions or allergies and provides information regarding the medication (Table 25–1 •). After giving the medication, the nurse records the drug name, dose, route, site, and the woman's blood pressure and pulse (before and after) on the EFM strip and on the woman's record. If the woman is alone, the nurse raises the side rails to provide safety and assesses the FHR for possible side effects of the medication.

Oral analgesics are not used because they are poorly absorbed and gastric emptying time is prolonged during labor. The intramuscular (IM), intravenous (IV), or subcutaneous (SC) routes are used instead. For IM administration, the needle must be of sufficient length to penetrate the muscle and the subcutaneous fat. The IV route is preferred because it results in prompt, smooth, and more predictable action with a smaller total dose required than the IM route. When an agent is given intravenously, it is suggested that the injection be given with the onset of a contraction, when the blood flow to the uterus and the fetus is normally decreased.

When an analgesic medication is administered by IM or SC route, it takes a few minutes for the effect to be felt. The nurse can continue with other supportive measures to en-

Table 25–1 • WHAT WOMEN NEED TO KNOW ABOUT PAIN RELIEF MEDICATIONS

Before receiving medications, the woman should understand the following:

- Type of medication administered
- Route of administration
- Expected effects of medication
- Implications for fetus/newborn
- Safety measures needed (for example, remain in bed with side rails up)
- Side effects/complications

hance comfort until the effect of the medication is perceived. When the medication begins to take effect, the woman may be able to sleep between contractions. This short period of rest can restore her energy. When an IV route is prescribed, the woman feels the effect of the drug within a minute or two, so if any change of position is necessary or if the woman needs to void, the nurse may suggest that these activities be completed before the drug is administered. Some women may be so uncomfortable that they do not want anything except the medication. Administering the medication first is more helpful for these women. As in all cases when there is a possibility of coming into contact with body fluids, the nurse should use universal precautions when epidural or spinal anesthesia is being placed. Consistent handwashing before and after procedures along with wearing disposable gloves can reduce the risk of blood or body fluid exposure. Sometimes analgesics are administered via IV and IM routes simultaneously. The benefit of this technique is that the woman receives a rapid onset from the IV route as well as the longer duration of pain control that is achieved with the IM route.

Narcotic Analgesics

Narcotic analgesic agents that are injected into the circulation have their primary action at sites in the brain. Specifically, a narcotic that diffuses out of cerebral capillaries and reaches the periventricular/periaqueductal gray matter of the brain activates the neurons that descend to the spinal cord and inhibits the transmission of pain impulses in the substantia gelatinosa. Nausea and vomiting are produced by stimulation of the medullary chemoreceptor trigger zone.

A brief discussion of some selected narcotic analgesic agents follows. The drugs are summarized in Table 25–2 ●.

BUTORPHANOL TARTRATE (STADOL)

Butorphanol tartrate (Stadol) is a mixed agonist-antagonist agent. The analgesic potency is 30 to 40 times that of meperidine and 7 times that of morphine (*Nurse Practitioner's Prescribing Reference*, 2002). Administration of butorphanol reverses the analgesic effect of other opioids or narcotics in the woman's body and precipitates withdrawal in drug-dependent individuals. For this reason, it is important to assess each woman's history of drug use during the admission assessment; if she has been using drugs, she should not receive butorphanol.

For the woman in labor, butorphanol is most frequently given by the IV route; however, it can also be given by IM injection. When administered intravenously, the recommended dose is 1 to 2 mg (the smaller dose is most frequently used). The onset of action is rapid, peak analgesia occurs in 30 to 60 minutes (*Nurse Practitioner's Prescribing Reference*, 2002), and duration is 3 to 4 hours (Karch, 1999). If given by IM route, the recommended dose is 1 to 2 mg, although 2 mg is the most usual dose. Onset of action occurs in 10 to 15 minutes, peak analgesia occurs in 30 to 60 minutes (*Nurse Practitioner's Prescribing Reference*, 2002), and duration is 3 to 4 hours (Karch, 1999).

Respiratory depression of both the mother and fetus/newborn can occur. The effects of butorphanol (Stadol) can be reversed with naloxone (Narcan). Although not a common side effect, urinary retention can occur. The nurse should frequently assess the woman's bladder for distention. The nurse may need to perform an in-and-out catheterization using sterile technique to alleviate bladder distention.

NURSING CARE MANAGEMENT

Administering butorphanol with other central nervous system depressants, such as sedatives, phenothiazides, other tranquilizers, hypnotic agents, and general anesthetics, can exacerbate respiratory depression and cause other effects. For this reason, the nurse should evaluate the woman's respiratory and cardiac status by careful observation of vital signs and pulse oximetry. The woman's level of consciousness is also checked frequently. Continuous electronic monitoring of the FHR pattern is recommended. Respiratory depression in the mother or fetus/newborn can be reversed by naloxone (Narcan), which is a specific antagonist for this agent. The nurse ensures that naloxone is readily available should respiratory depression occur. A slightly depressed newborn is not likely to experience prolonged drowsiness or sluggishness, however, because the metabolites of butorphanol are inactive.

NALBUPHINE HYDROCHLORIDE (NUBAIN)

Like butorphanol, nalbuphine hydrochloride (Nubain) is a synthetic agonist-antagonist narcotic analgesic and may precipitate drug withdrawal if the woman is physically dependent on narcotics (*Nurse Practitioner's Prescribing Reference*, 2002). Nalbuphine crosses the placenta to the fetus and can cause fetal distress and neonatal respiratory depression (Deglin & Vallerand, 2002). Nalbuphine may be given by the IM, SC, or IV route. It is most frequently given by the IV route in the birth setting. The usual dose for adults is 10 mg/70 kg. If given intravenously, onset of action occurs in 2 to 3 minutes, peak of action occurs in 15 to 20 minutes, and duration is 3 to 6 hours. When given by the IM or SC route, the onset of action occurs in less than 15 minutes, peak of action occurs in 30 to 60 minutes, and duration is 3 to 6 hours. When given by the IV route, nalbuphine may be given directly into the tubing of a running IV infusion; 10 mg should be administered over 3 to 5 minutes (Deglin & Vallerand, 2002). Adverse effects in the woman include respiratory depression, drowsiness, dizziness, crying, blurred vision, nausea, diaphoresis, and urinary urgency (Deglin & Vallerand, 2002). See Drug Guide: Nalbuphine Hydrochloride (Nubain).

Table 25-2 • ANALGESICS USED IN LABOR

Drug/Class	Dosage, Route, Frequency	Common Side Effects	Life-Threatening Reactions	Contraindications
Stadol (butorphanol tartrate): CNS agent, analgesic, narcotic agonest/antagonist	IM 1–4 mg every 3–4 hours IV 0.5–2 mg every 6–8 hours. Intranasal: 1 mg (1 puff) may repeat in 90 seconds (max dose every 3–4 hours)	Sedation	Respiratory depression	Narcotic dependency, breastfeeding
Nubain (nalbuphine hydrochloride): CNS agent, analgesic, narcotic agonist, antagonist	10–20 mg every 3–6 hours prn SC/IM/IV	Sedation; sweaty, clammy skin; nausea and vomiting	Respiratory depression	Hypersensitivity to the drug
Demerol (meperidine hydrochloride): CNS agent, analgesic, narcotic agonist	IV 2.5–15 mg every 4 hours IM/SC 5–20 mg every 4 hours	Pruritus, dizziness, sedation, nausea, constipation	Respiratory depression, convulsions, cardiovascular collapse, cardiac arrest, respiratory depression in newborn, bronchoconstriction	Hypersensitivity to the drug, convulsive disorders, breastfeeding, undiagnosed acute abdomen
Morphine (morphine sulfate): CNS agent, analgesic, narcotic, agonist	IV 2.5–15 mg every 4 hours IM/SC 5–20 mg every 4 hours	Pruritus, constipation, nausea	Anaphylactic reaction, respiratory depression; overdose; respiratory arrest, cardiac arrest	Hypersensitivity to opiates, increased intracranial pressure, convulsive disorders, acute alcoholism, acute asthma, chronic pulmonary diseases, decreased respirations, pulmonary edema, biliary tract surgery, anastomosis, pancreatitis, acute ulcerative colitis, liver/renal insufficiency, Addison disease, hypothyriodism
Phenergan (promethazine hydrochloride): GI agent, antiemetic, antivertigo agent, phenothiazine	25–50 mg every 3–4 hours po/pr/IM/IV	Sedation, drowsiness, dry mouth, blurred vision	Respiratory depression, agranulocytosis	Hypersensitivity to phehothiazines, glaucoma, peptic ulcer, pyloroduodenal obstruction, bladder neck obstruction, epilepsy, bone marrow depression, and breastfeeding
Vistaril (hydroxyzine pamoate): antihistamine, antianxiety, sedative, antipruritic, antiemetic	25–100 mg po/IM every 6 hours	Sedation, dizziness, dry mouth, nausea, headache	Seizures	Hypersensitivity to drug, use with caution in glaucoma, urinary retention
Benadryl (diphenhydramine hydrochloride): antihistamine, antiemetic, antivertigo, antitussive, sedative-hypnotic	25–50 mg every 6 hours po/IM/IV	Drowsiness, sedation, dry mouth, hypotension, nausea and vomiting, GI symptoms	Anaphylaxis, seizures, coma, respiratory depression	Hypersensitivity to drug, use during an acute asthma attack, use with caution in glaucoma, bladder obstruction, hypertension, hypothyriodism, renal disease

NURSING CARE MANAGEMENT

The nurse assesses the woman's history to identify contraindications to use of nalbuphine, such as the possibility of current narcotic drug dependence, sensitivity to sulfites, and history of asthma (*Nurse Practitioner's Prescribing Reference*, 2002). If no contraindications exist, the IV route is frequently used during labor. The woman's respiratory rate, quality of respirations, and characteristics of the FHR must be carefully assessed. Anticipation of urinary urgency is important. Because the woman may experience dizziness and sedation, use of a bedpan may be necessary.

OPIATE ANTAGONIST: NALOXONE (NARCAN)

Because naloxone (Narcan) is an antagonist with little or no agonistic effect, it exhibits little pharmacologic activity in the absence of narcotic agents. Naloxone can be used to reverse the mild respiratory depression, sedation, and hypotension following small doses of opiates (Deglin & Vallerand, 2002). Naloxone (Narcan) exerts its effect by competing for opiate receptors and taking the place of the opiate on the receptor.

DRUG GUIDE NALBUPHINE HYDROCHLORIDE (NUBAIN)

• Overview of Action

Nubain is a synthetic narcotic analgesic with agonist and weak antagonist properties. Analgesic properties are equal to that produced by morphine. Nubain's potency is 3 to 4 times greater than pentazocine. The incidence of respiratory depression that occurs is equivalent to morphine.

• Dosage Route

Nubain is indicated for moderate to severe pain. Adults: 10–20 mg every 3–6 hours prn SC/IM/IV.

• Maternal Contraindications

Hypersensitivity or allergy to nalbuphine hydrochloride.

• Maternal Side Effects

Sedation; clammy, sweaty skin; dry mouth; bitter taste in mouth; nausea and vomiting; dizziness; vertigo; nervousness; restlessness; depression; crying; euphoria; dysphoria; confusion; hallucinations; unusual dreams; distortion of body image; numbness; tingling sensations; headache; miosis; hypertension; hypotension; bradycardia; tachycardia; flushing; abdominal cramps; dyspnea; asthma; speech difficulty; and urinary urgency.

• Nursing Considerations

Assess client's sensitivity to narcotics on admission.

Inform woman of potential side effects.

Monitor and evaluate analgesic effect. Ask client about comfort level and notify anesthesiologist of inadequate pain relief.

Observe for symptoms of hypersensitivity: pruritus, urticaria, and/or burning sensation.

May produce an allergic response in clients with sulfite sensitivity.

If allergic reaction (urticaria, edema, or respiratory difficulties) occurs, administer naloxone or diphenhydramine per physician order.

Assess respiratory rate prior to administration. Notify healthcare provider if respirations less than 12 per minute.

Monitor urinary output and assess bladder for distention. Assist client to void.

Assist client with ambulation after administration.

Counsel client that use with alcohol or other central nervous system depressants may increase medication effects.

Prolonged use with abrupt discontinuation can result in symptoms consistent with narcotic withdrawal.

In this manner, naloxone blocks or reverses the action of the narcotic analgesic (*Nurse Practitioner's Prescribing Reference*, 2002). The drug is useful for respiratory depression caused by butorphanol (Stadol) and nalbuphine (Nubain) (Deglin & Vallerand, 2002). *Naloxone is the drug of choice when the depressant is unknown because it will cause no further depression.* Naloxone's duration of action is less than that of most narcotic analgesics; however, respiratory depression may return as the antagonistic effect of naloxone wears off.

The expected action is reversal of narcotic-induced respiratory depression. Adverse actions include nausea and vomiting, sweating, and hypertension due to reversal of the narcotic depression. When used postoperatively, excessive dosages of naloxone may cause ventricular tachycardia and fibrillation, hypotension or hypertension, and pulmonary edema (Deglin & Vallerand, 2002; *Nurse Practitioner's Prescribing Reference*, 2002).

For reversal of respiratory depression in the laboring woman, initial recommended dosage is 0.4 mg to 2 mg intravenously; if necessary, the dose may be repeated at 2- to 3-minute intervals (Deglin & Vallerand, 2002). If no response is obtained after a total of 10 mg has been administered, diagnosis of narcotic-induced depression should be questioned. When naloxone is administered intravenously, onset of action occurs in 2 minutes, peak effect occurs in 5 to 15 minutes, and the duration of action varies depending on the dose but may be as short as 45 minutes (*Nurse Practitioner's Prescribing Reference*, 2002) or as long as 4 to 6 hours (Deglin & Vallerand, 2002). If the expectant mother is very young or of low weight, the appropriate dosage may need to be calculated on the basis of milligrams per kilogram of weight. When the age or size of the laboring mother raises questions, the nurse should calculate the expected dosage and compare it to the physician-prescribed dosage. If the prescribed dosage exceeds the mg/kg dose, the nurse must consult with the physician prior to administering the medication.

Naloxone may also be administered to the newborn immediately after birth if needed (see Drug Guide: Naloxone [Narcan] in Chapter 33 for discussion of neonatal dosages). After naloxone administration, the newborn should be observed for at least 4 hours in a special care area (such as an admission nursery) before transfer to regular care so the respiratory status can be monitored since respiratory depression can reoccur as Narcan wears off.

NURSING CARE MANAGEMENT

When naloxone is administered to the laboring mother or to the newborn just after birth, resuscitative measures and trained personnel should be readily available in the event that additional respiratory support is needed. When administered to the laboring mother, naloxone may be injected undiluted at a rate of 0.4 mg over 15 seconds into the tubing of a running IV infusion. Naloxone may also be diluted in an IV infusion of 5% dextrose or normal saline for a titrated dose. Titrated doses of naloxone are more likely to be used in a postoperative setting, when epidural analgesia has been given with a cesarean birth. After the direct IV administration, maternal vital signs should be obtained at 5-minute intervals until the respiratory rate has been stabilized and then every 30 minutes (Deglin & Vallerand, 2002). The duration of the drug is shorter (minutes to hours) than the analgesic drug it is acting as an antagonist for, so the nurse must be alert to the return of respiratory depression and the need for repeated doses. Naloxone should be given with caution in women with known or suspected opiate dependence because it may precipitate severe withdrawal symptoms in the mother and the newborn.

Sedatives

In current labor and birth practice, sedatives are used primarily in the early latent phase of labor, when the cervix is long, closed, and thick, and rest is prescribed for the expectant woman. Sedatives promote relaxation and allow the woman to sleep for a few hours. Upon the woman's awakening, contractions have either ceased (ie, the woman was in false labor) or contractions return and take on a regular pattern that promotes changes in cervical dilatation and effacement. Sedatives should not be given when a woman is in active labor because they can cause respiratory depression in the infant. Sedatives have minimal analgesic properties and can actually increase the reaction to painful stimuli. They should only be administered to decrease anxiety and promote sleep (Faucher & Brucker, 2000).

BARBITURATES

The most common barbiturate used in labor is secobarbital (Seconal). Seconal is fast acting, usually providing effects in 10 to 15 minutes with a duration of 3 to 4 hours. It is administered orally and is well tolerated. Its primary role is to treat false labor and produce a sedation effect. It can be used in latent labor to promote rest and relaxation and thereby prevent maternal exhaustion. Hypnotic effects also occur with many drugs in this category. A barbiturate should not be administered to women in active labor because it can cause fetal depression, and in fact is rarely used at anytime during true labor.

BENZODIAZEPINES

Benzodiazepines, such as diazepam (Valium), are simular to barbiturates in their mechanism of action. They are primarily used to treat anxiety. They can also be used for their anticonvulsant action. They have a rapid onset of action and are absorbed quite easily when ingested orally. Although this class of drugs can be used to decrease anxiety, some have an amnestic effect which may not be desirable for childbearing women. Fetal side effects have been reported but are usually mild. These include a decrease in beat-to-beat variability of the FHR. Midazolam (Versed), which is commonly used during operative procedures, has been associated with low Apgar scores when administered 5 minutes or less prior to birth. Because of this side effect, it is not advisable to use midazolam for childbearing women (Faucher & Brucker, 2000). Flumazenil, the drug used to reverse benzodiazepine sedative effects, should be kept on hand in case of accidental overdose.

H_1-RECEPTOR ANTAGONISTS

H_1-receptor antagonists block the action of histamines at the receptor sites. These drugs cross the blood-brain barrier and inhibit N-methyltransferase, which is a by-product of histamine. It is this mechanism that leads to the sedative effects of this class of drugs. In addition, these drugs also have anti-Parkinson and antiemetic effects. There are seven subtypes of H_1-receptor antagonists. These drugs cause drowsiness and are frequently used in early labor to promote sleep and decrease anxiety. The degree of drowsiness experienced depends on which drug is administered. Common H_1-receptor antagonists used in labor include promethazine (Phenergan), hydroxyzine (Vistaril), and diphenhydramine (Benadryl) (Hawkins, Chestnut & Gibbs, 2002).

Promethazine (Phenergan), which is a phenothiazine, results in marked sedation and is often combined with opiates because it potentiates their effects. It also has strong antiemetic effects and can be combined with opiates to relieve nausea and vomiting, which can be a side effect of certain drugs, like meperidine (Demerol). All phenothiazines cross the placental barrier and can result in decreased beat-to-beat variability. Promethazine has not, however, resulted in lower Apgar scores. Phenothiazines can also bind to bilirubin binding sites in newborns whose mothers are exposed to the drug at term. This can result in an increased incidence of neonatal hyperbilirubinemia and jaundice (Hawkins et al, 2002).

Hydroxyzine (Vistaril) is a piperazine subtype. It can be given in early or prodromal labor to decrease anxiety and nausea. It also results in sedation so the mother can rest. This drug is administered intramuscularly in a large muscle. Women in false labor are able to rest and frequently will awaken to find that their uterine contractions have dissipated. Commonly, women who receive this drug in early or prodromal labor are able to rest and frequently enter active labor.

Diphenhydramine (Benadryl) is an ethanolamine subtype of the H_1 antagonists. Most commonly, this over-the-counter medication is used to treat allergic rhinitis and urticaria; however, it also possesses sedative and antiemetic properties which can be used to treat women in early labor. The drug has a relatively short half-life (1 to 4 hours) and can last up to 6 to 8 hours. Nurses can advise women to use this drug at home if medically indicated since it is readily available. It should be noted that this drug causes agitation in some women. If this side effect occurs, women should discontinue the medication.

NURSING CARE MANAGEMENT

The nurse should carefully assess the woman prior to administration of analgesic agents. Common indications for various medications are summarized in Table 25–3 •. Since they are not indicated for women in active labor, the nurse needs to determine the stage of labor. The nurse should evaluate the woman to determine the frequency, duration, and intensity of her contractions. A vaginal exam is performed to determine if cervical change has occurred. Fetal well-being is established by obtaining electronic fetal monitoring and ensuring a reactive fetal heart tracing. The nurse should explain the desired effects of the medication and possible side effects. Since drowsiness can occur, the nurse needs to ensure the woman has a safe form of transportation home. If the woman is not in active labor, she can be given the medication and be advised to return home and rest. Nurses need to review the symptoms of active labor and warning signs and advise the woman to call her healthcare provider should they occur.

Regional Analgesia and Anesthesia

Regional anesthesia is the temporary and reversible loss of sensation produced by injecting an anesthetic agent (called a local anesthetic) into an area that will bring the agent into direct contact with nervous tissue. Loss of sensation occurs because the local agents stabilize the cell membrane, which prevents initiation and transmission of nerve impulses. The regional anesthetic blocks most commonly used in childbearing include epidural, spinal, or combined epidural-spinal. Epidural blocks may be used for analgesia during labor and vaginal birth and for anesthesia during cesarean birth. A combined epidural-spinal block may also be used. With this approach, the epidural is used to provide analgesia for labor, and the spinal provides anesthesia for birth or analgesia following birth.

Table 25-3 • COMMON INDICATIONS FOR MEDICATIONS IN LABOR

Drug	Pain Relief	Anxiety or Apprehension	Sedation	Antiemetic
Demerol (meperidine)	X		X	
Nubain (nalbuphine)	X		X	
Phenergan (promethazine)		X	X	X
Stadol (butorphanol)	X		X	
Vistaril (hydroxyzine)		X	X	
Seconal (secobarbital)		X	X	X
Benadryl (diphenhydramine hydrochloride)		X	X	X

GLOBAL PERSPECTIVES

In the former Soviet Union, pain medication typically is not given to laboring women. While some complementary pain relief methods, such as massage and water therapy, are used, traditional customs are also incorporated. These include tying and untying knots, locking and unlocking doors, and placing the father's clothing under the laboring woman.

An epidural relieves pain associated with the first stage of labor by blocking the sensory nerves supplying the uterus. Pain associated with the second stage of labor and with birth can be alleviated with epidural, combined epidural-spinal, and pudendal blocks (Figure 25–1 • and Table 25–4 •).

Until fairly recently, the same anesthetic agents used for regional epidural anesthesia were also used to produce **regional analgesia** (pain relief) during labor. This approach was somewhat problematic because anesthetic agents alter the transmission of impulses to the bladder, making voiding difficult. The agents also interfere with the woman's ability to maintain her blood pressure and move her lower extremities. In addition, the descent of the fetus may be slowed because the agents also decrease the woman's ability to push effectively during the second stage of labor (Fraser, Cayer, Soeder, et al, 2002). To address these problems, regional analgesia is now obtained by injecting a narcotic agent such as fentanyl along with only a small amount of a local anesthetic agent. This approach yields effective pain relief without the troubling side effects of epidural anesthesia. The woman's pain is relieved, her blood pressure remains stable, and, because there is no motor blockage, she is able to move about freely and ambulate. Urinary retention can still occur, but it can be treated with the placement of an indwelling Foley catheter or an in-and-out catheter (Cunningham, MacDonald, Gant, et al, 2001). Urinary retention is usually a short-term complication that resolves on its own after the anesthesia has completely worn off.

The intrathecal injection of narcotics results in another type of regional analgesia. In this case, the narcotic is injected into the subarachnoid space. Fentanyl citrate and preservative-free morphine are the most frequently used narcotic agents. The woman's pain is usually relieved; however, she may experience urinary retention. Delayed respiratory depression may also occur and seems to be more frequent with the use of morphine (Deglin & Vallerand, 2002).

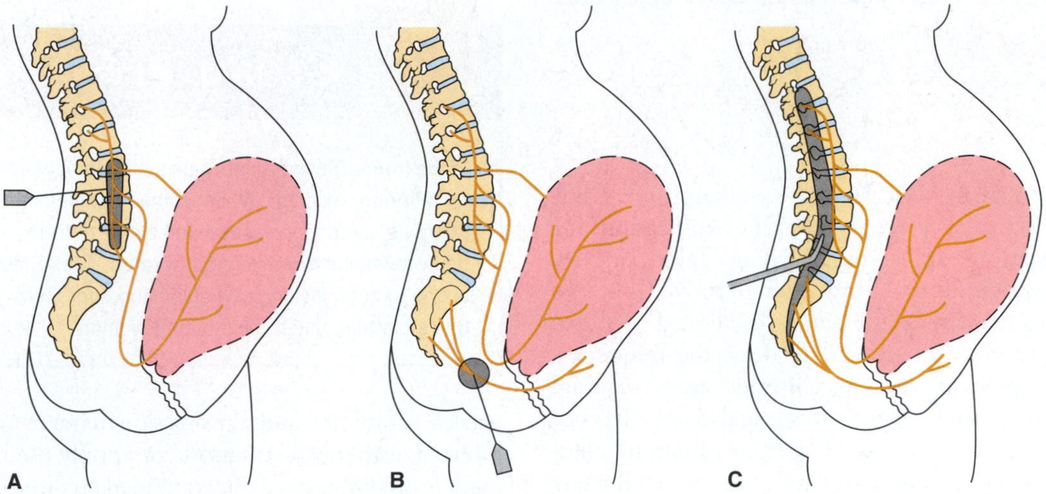

Figure 25–1 • Schematic diagram showing pain pathways and sites of interruption. *A,* Lumbar sympathetic (spinal) block: relief of uterine pain only. *B,* Pudendal block: relief of perineal pain. *C,* Lumbar epidural block: Dark area demonstrates peridural (epidural) space and nerves affected, and the gray tube represents a continuous plastic catheter.
SOURCE: Bonica, J. J. (1972). *Principles and practice of obstetric analgesia and anesthesia* (pp. 492, 512, 521, 614). Philadelphia: Davis.

It is important for the laboring woman to have information about the regional analgesia or anesthesia that is to be administered. As with other procedures, the woman needs to know how the block is given, the expected effect on her and the fetus, advantages and disadvantages, and possible risks. Many women discuss possible analgesic and anesthetic blocks with their physician or certified nurse-midwife (CNM) during the pregnancy. If they have not, they should have an opportunity to ask questions and obtain information prior to receiving any regional analgesia or anesthesia while in labor. The nurse should answer questions and address concerns in early labor prior to the onset of acute pain. This ensures that the woman fully understands the information and can make an informed choice. Informed consent is obtained in writing prior to the administration of the medication.

Action and Absorption of Anesthetic Agents

Local anesthetic agents block nerve conduction by impairing propagation of the action potential in axons. The agents interact directly with specific receptors on the sodium channel, inhibiting sodium ion influx (Russell & Reynolds, 1997). The types of nerve fibers are differentially sensitive

Table 25–4 • SUMMARY OF COMMONLY USED REGIONAL BLOCKS

Type of Block	Areas Affected	Use During Labor and Birth	Nursing Actions
Lumbar epidural	Uterus, cervix, vagina, and perineum	Given in first stage and second stage of labor.	Assess woman's knowledge regarding the block. Act as advocate to help her obtain further information if needed. Monitor maternal blood pressure to detect the major side effect, which is hypotension. Provide support and comfort. See Clinical Pathway for Epidural Anesthesia for further nursing actions.
Combined spinal epidural	Uterus, cervix, vagina, and perineum	Spinal analgesia may be given in latent phase for pain relief. Epidural is given when active labor begins.	Assess woman's knowledge regarding the block. Monitor maternal vital signs and FHR status. Provide comfort measures.
Pudendal	Perineum and lower vagina	Given in the second stage just prior to birth to provide anesthesia for episiotomy or for low forceps birth.	Assess woman's knowledge regarding the block. Act as advocate to help her obtain further information if needed.
Local infiltration	Perineum	Administered just before birth to provide anesthesia for episiotomy.	Assess woman's knowledge regarding the block. Provide information as needed. Provide comfort and support. Observe perineum for bruising or other discoloration in the recovery period.
Spinal	Uterus, cervix, vagina, and perineum	Given during first stage for pain relief. Provides immediate onset of anesthesia.	Assess woman's knowledge regarding the block. Monitor maternal vital signs and FHR status.

to the various anesthetic agents. In general, the smaller the fiber, the more sensitive it is to local agents. For example, it is possible to block the small C and A delta fibers, which transmit pain, touch, and temperature, without blocking the larger A alpha, A beta, and A gamma fibers, which continue to maintain a sense of pressure, muscle tone, position sense, and motor function (Russell & Reynolds, 1997).

Absorption of local anesthetic agents depends primarily on the vascularity of the area of injection. The agents also increase blood flow by causing vasodilation. Higher concentrations cause greater vasodilation. Good maternal physical condition or a high metabolic rate aids absorption. Malnutrition, dehydration, electrolyte imbalance, and cardiovascular and pulmonary problems increase the potential for toxic effects. The pH of tissues affects the rate of absorption, which has implications for fetal complications, such as acidosis. The addition of vasoconstrictors, such as epinephrine, delays absorption and prolongs the anesthetic effect. Epinephrine decreases uteroplacental blood flow, making it an undesirable additive in many situations. The breakdown of local anesthetics in the body is accomplished by the liver and plasma esterase, and the resulting substance is eliminated by the kidneys. It is important to use the weakest concentration and the smallest amount necessary to produce the desired results.

Types of Local Anesthetic Agents

Three types of local anesthetic agents are currently available—esters, amides, and opiates. The ester type includes procaine hydrochloride (Novocain), chloroprocaine hydrochloride (Nesacaine), and tetracaine hydrochloride (Pontocaine). Esters are rapidly metabolized; therefore, toxic maternal levels are not as likely to be reached, and placental transfer to the fetus is prevented.

Amide types include bupivacaine hydrochloride (Marcaine), mepivacaine hydrochloride (Carbocaine), and lidocaine hydrochloride (Xylocaine). Amide types are more powerful and longer acting agents. They readily cross the placenta, can be measured in the fetal circulation, and affect the fetus for a prolonged period.

Opioids are used with epidural blocks to produce analgesia for labor. Some of the agents used include morphine, fentanyl, butorphanol, and meperidine. When only opioids are used epidurally, the amount of pain relief is not as great. A combination of opioids and a low dose of a local anesthetic agent achieve better pain control with reduced motor impairment. There does appear to be a higher incidence of pruritus (itching) when this combination method is used. There are no differences in the occurrence of nausea, hypotension, duration of labor, and neonatal outcomes when epidural local anesthesia and epidural local anesthetics combined with opiates are compared (American Society of Anesthesiologists [ASA], 1999).

A variety of anesthetic agents and a wide range of doses have been used for epidural anesthesia with varying results. The most commonly used agents are lidocaine 2% with epinephrine 1:200,000, bupivacaine 0.5%, and 2-chloroprocaine 3%. Each agent provides adequate anesthesia with 15 to 20 mL of the solution, but each has been associated with side effects. The pharmacology of each drug must be understood before it is used.

Adverse Maternal Reactions to Anesthetic Agents

Reactions to local anesthetic agents range from mild symptoms to cardiovascular collapse. Mild reactions include palpitations, vertigo, tinnitus, apprehension, confusion, headache, and a metallic taste in the mouth. Common side effects include pruritus, vertigo, dizziness, and urinary retention. Moderate reactions include more severe degrees of the mild symptoms plus nausea and vomiting, hypotension, and muscle twitching, which may progress to convulsions and loss of consciousness. Severe reactions are sudden loss of consciousness, coma, severe hypotension, bradycardia, respiratory depression, and cardiac arrest. High concentrations of the agents may also cause local toxic effects on tissues. It is important to remember that when the mother experiences an adverse reaction, the fetus is also affected.

Systemic toxic reactions most commonly occur with an excessive dose because of too great a concentration or too large a volume. Accidental intravenous injection that suddenly increases the amount of the drug in maternal circulation results in depression of vasomotor, respiratory, and other medullary centers of the brain. It also depresses the heart and peripheral vascular bed. A massive intravascular dose can result in sudden circulatory collapse within 1 minute. Reactions to subcutaneous and extradural injection occur in 5 to 40 minutes. The short-acting agent procaine can produce toxic reactions in 10 to 15 minutes, and the long-acting agent mepivacaine in 20 to 40 minutes (Deglin & Vallerand, 2002). It is imperative that the woman is under close supervision by knowledgeable personnel throughout the time that an agent is being used and that an intravenous line is in place.

MEDIALINK LOCAL ANESTHESIA

If epinephrine has been added to the anesthetic agent to prolong the anesthesia, it is necessary to differentiate between reaction to the anesthetic agent and to the epinephrine. Reaction to epinephrine is characterized by pallor, perspiration, dyspnea, and a greater increase in blood pressure and pulse than occurs with reactions to anesthetic agents.

Psychogenic reactions such as severe anxiety, hallucinations, inability to move or speak, or catatonic appearance can also occur, with symptoms similar to those occurring with systemic toxic reactions. This phenomenon may occur as the procedure is begun and prior to the injection of the anesthetic agent. Regardless of the cause, the symptoms must be treated.

Allergic reactions to anesthetic agents may also occur. The manifestations of the antigen-antibody reaction include urticaria, laryngeal edema, joint pain, swelling of the tongue, and bronchospasm.

TREATMENT OF SYSTEMIC TOXICITY

Preferred treatment of mild toxicity involves the administration of oxygen by mask and intravenous injection of a short-acting barbiturate to decrease anxiety. The clinician should anticipate the possibility of convulsions or cardiovascular collapse and make appropriate preparations to treat them.

Specific nursing interventions in the treatment of systemic toxicity are included in the Clinical Pathway Epidural Anesthesia on pages 675 to 677.

TREATMENT OF CONVULSIONS

The best treatment for convulsions is to establish the airway and administer 100% oxygen. Thiopental or diazepam may be administered to stop convulsions. Small doses are adequate and help avoid cardiorespiratory depression.

TREATMENT OF SUDDEN CARDIOVASCULAR COLLAPSE

In sudden cardiovascular collapse, an airway must be established as cardiopulmonary resuscitation begins. Intravenous fluids are increased, and emergency cesarean birth may be started immediately.

Lumbar Epidural Block

A lumbar **epidural block** involves injection of a local anesthetic agent into the epidural space. The epidural space is a potential space between the dura mater and the ligamentum flavum extending from the base of the skull to the end of the sacral canal (Figure 25–2 •). It contains areolar tissue, fat, lymphatics, and the internal vertebral venous plexus. This space is accessed through the lumbar area. The technique is most often used as a continuous block to provide analgesia and anesthesia from active labor through the birth and episiotomy repair. Complete pain relief is achieved for 85% of women. Another 12% experience partial relief, while only 3% of women report no relief at all (Cunningham et al, 2001).

Lumbar epidural block has become fairly common during labor and birth. In the United States, epidural blocks (41%) and spinal blocks (43%) are far more common for cesarean births than general anesthesia, which is used for only 16% of all cesareans (ASA, 1999).

Use of epidural blocks in Great Britain averages around 10%. Green, Coupland, and Kitzinger (1998) conducted a study in England that examined women's preferences for pain medication in labor. A majority of the women (80%) preferred not to have an epidural. In the United States, on the other hand, 51% of women receive epidural anesthesia for pain management during labor. This high rate is partially related to the 24-hour availability of anesthesia services. The varying use of epidural block raises questions regarding how and to whom the procedure is offered. In the United States, regrettably, there have been some cases in which a third-party payer or managed care company deemed a woman ineligible for an epidural block. The American College of Obstetricians and Gynecologists (ACOG) has stated, "There is no other circumstance where it is considered acceptable for a person to experience severe pain, amenable to safe intervention, while under a physician's care" (ACOG, 2000, p. 1). ACOG supports the woman's request as sufficient justification for providing an epidural (ACOG, 2000; ASA, 2000).

Epidural blocks can be administered in a number of ways. To provide analgesia and anesthesia during labor, the block

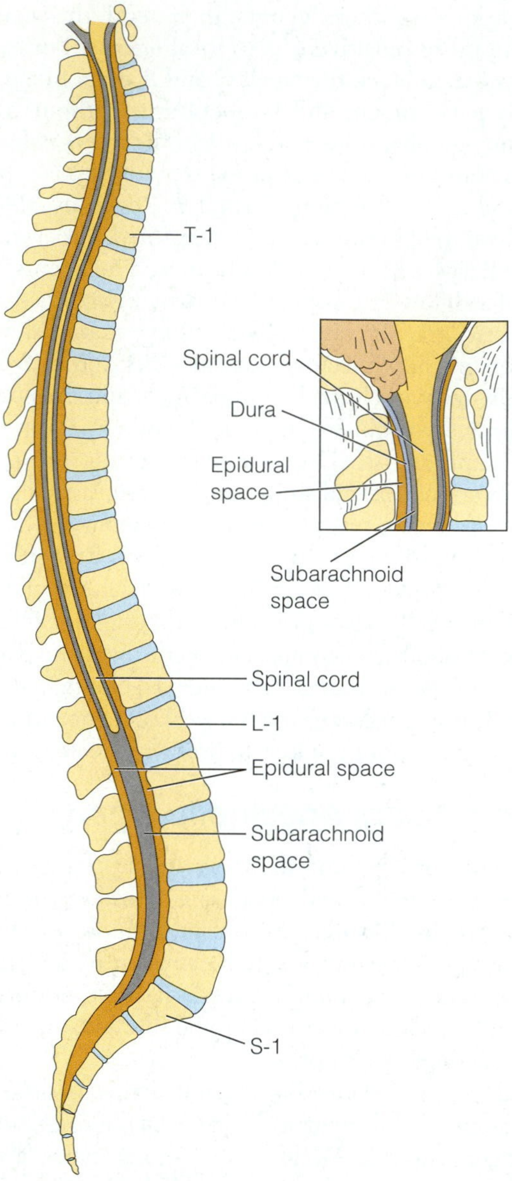

Figure 25–2 • The epidural space lies between the dura mater and the ligamentum flavum, extending from the base of the skull to the end of the sacral canal.

can be administered as a single dose with an epidural needle, as a single dose through an epidural catheter with additional doses (called "top-ups" or "top-offs") given as needed, or as a continuous epidural. Some procedures require that the woman remain in bed, whereas others—called "walking," "ambulatory," or "mobile" epidurals—are given with analgesic agents, anesthetic agents, or both that leave the woman with sufficient motor control to be out of bed (Mayberry & Clemmens, 2002). When an epidural block is used for cesarean birth, an epidural catheter is inserted and a single dose is usually given. The catheter provides access to the epidural space, so that additional anesthetic agents and opioids may be administered if needed and so that opioids may be given to provide pain relief for the 24 hours following birth.

CLINICAL PATHWAY FOR EPIDURAL ANESTHESIA

Category	First Stage	Second and Third Stage	Fourth Stage Birth to 1 Hour Past Birth
Referral	**Review prenatal record** **Advise CNM/physician of admission**	**Labor record for first stage**	**Report to recovery room nurse** ➤ **Expected Outcomes** Appropriate resources identified and utilized
Assessments	Admission assessments: Ask about problems since last prenatal visit; labor status (contraction frequency and duration, cervical dilatation, and effacement), membrane status; coping level; support; woman's desires during labor and birth; ability to verbalize needs; laboratory testing (blood and UA) Woman's request for epidural Intrapartal assessment: timing *Latent Phase:* • BP, P, R, q1h if in normal range (BP 90–140/60–90 or no increase >30 mm Hg systolic or 15 mm Hg diastolic over baseline; pulse 60–90; respirations 12–20/min, quiet, easy) • Temp q4h unless >37.6C (99.6F) or membranes ruptured; then q2h. Uterine contractions q30min: contractions q5–10min, 15–40 sec, mild intensity) • FHR q60min (for low-risk women) and q30min for high-risk women if reassuring (FHR baseline 110–160, STV present, LTV average, accelerations with fetal movement, no late nor variable decelerations); if nonreassuring, position on side, start O_2, assess for hypotension, monitor continuously, notify CNM/physician *Active Phase:* • BP, P, R, q1h if WNL • Temp as above • Uterine contractions assessed q 15–30 min • FHR assessed continuously per EFM • Pulse ox >95% *Transition Phase:* • BP, P, R, q30min if in normal range • Uterine contractions q15–30min • FHR q30min (for low-risk women) and q15min (for high-risk women) if reassuring: if nonreassuring, see above • Pulse ox >95% Cervical assessment: from 1–10 cm dilatation; nullipara (1.2 cm/h), multipara (1.5 cm/h) Cervical effacement: from 0% to 100% Fetal descent: progressive descent from −4 to +4 Membrane assessment: when ruptured, Nitrazine positive, fluid clear, no foul odor Behavioral characteristics: response to labor process, facial expressions, verbalizations, tone of voice, changes in behavior during contractions, body movement	Second stage assessments: • BP, P, R q5–15min • Uterine contractions palpated continuously • FHR q15min (for low-risk women) and q5min (for high-risk women) if reassuring; if nonreassuring, monitor continuously Fetal descent: descent continues to birth Behavioral characteristics: response to pushing, facial expressions, verbalization Third stage assessments: • BP, P, R q5min • Uterine contractions, palpate occasionally until placenta is delivered, fundus maintains tone and contraction pattern continues to birth of placenta Newborn assessments: • Assess Apgar score of newborn • Respirations: 30–60, irregular • Apical pulse: 110–160 and somewhat irregular • Temperature: skin temp above 36.5C (97.8F) • Umbilical cord: 2 arteries, 1 vein (if 1 artery, assess for anomalies and urine output) • Gestational age: 38 to 42 weeks	Immediate postbirth assessments q15 min for one hour • BP: 90–140/60–90; should return to prelabor level • Pulse: slightly lower than in labor; range is 60–90 • Respirations: 12–20/min; easy; quiet • Temperature: 36.2–37.6C (98-99.6F) • Fundus firm, in midline, at the umbilicus or 1–2 fingerbreadths below the umbilicus • Lochia rubra; moderate amount; <1 pad/h; no free flow or passage of clots with massage • Perineum: sutures intact; no bulging or marked swelling; minimal bruising may be present; no c/o severe pain nor rectal pain • Bladder nondistended; spontaneous void of >100 mL clear, straw-colored urine; bladder nondistended following voiding (catheterize if necessary) • If hemorrhoids present, no tenseness or marked engorgement; <2 cm diameter Comfort level: <3 on scale of 1 to 10 Energy level: awake and able to hold newborn Newborn assessments if newborn remains with parents: • Respirations: 30–60; irregular • Apical pulse: 110–160 and somewhat irregular • Temperature: skin temp above 36.5C (97.8F); skin feels warm to touch • Skin color noncyanotic • Mucus: small amount, clear, easily suctioned with bulb syringe without skin color change • Behavioral: newborn opens eyes widely if room is slightly darkened • Movements rhythmic; no hand tremors present ➤ **Expected Outcomes** Assessment findings indicate labor is progressing WNL, maternal vital signs stable and within established parameters, and reassuring fetal heart rate Maternal/fetal well-being unimpaired

(continued on next page)

CLINICAL PATHWAY FOR EPIDURAL ANESTHESIA *CONTINUED*

Category	First Stage	Second and Third Stage	Fourth Stage Birth to 1 Hour Past Birth
Teaching/ psychosocial	Establish rapport Orient to environment, expected assessments and procedures Answer questions and provide information/give emotional support Orient to EFM Teach relaxation, visualization, and breathing pattern if needed Explain comfort measures available. Provide information regarding the reason for the block, possible side effects, and nursing care that may be expected Assume advocacy role for woman/family during labor and birth Explain possible delayed effects of anesthetic agents on fetus	Orient to expected assessments and procedures Answer questions and provide information Continue advocacy role Instruct woman to maintain bed rest until full function of lower extremities returns	Explain immediate assessments and care after this first hour Teach self-massage of fundus and expected findings Instruct to call for assistance if mother desires to get OOB Begin newborn teaching; bulb syringe, positioning, maintaining warmth Assist with first breastfeeding experience ➤ **Expected Outcomes** Woman verbalizes/demonstrates understanding of teaching
Nursing care management and reports	Straight cath PRN if bladder distended If regional block administered monitor BP, FHR, sensation per protocol and obtain consent for procedure Provide continuing status reports Perineal clip per woman's request Small enema per woman's request Perform sterile vaginal examination as indicated Position woman correctly for regional block Assess maternal status: • Obtain baseline vital signs before any anesthetic agent is given • Monitor blood pressure q1–2min for 10 min and then q5–15min following administration of anesthetic agent • Monitor pulse and respiration • Monitor FHR continuously Observe, record, and report complications of anesthesia, including hypotension, fetal stress, respiratory paralysis, changes in uterine contractility, decrease in voluntary muscle effort, trauma to extremities, nausea and vomiting, and loss of bladder tone Observe, record, and report symptoms of hypotension, including systolic pressure $<$ 100 mm Hg or a 20–30% fall in systolic pressure, apprehension, restlessness, dizziness, tinnitus, headache Initiate treatment measures: • Place woman in left lateral position or position as directed with the foot of the bed elevated • Increase IV fluid rate • Administer oxygen by face mask at 7–10 L/min as needed • Administer vasopressors as ordered (usually ephedrine 5–15 mg IV) • Manually displace uterus laterally to left • Keep woman supine (semireclining) for 5–10 min following administration of block to allow drug to diffuse bilaterally. After 5–10 min position woman on side Observe, record, and report fetal bradycardia (FHR $<$110 bpm) and loss of beat-to-beat variability	Straight cath PRN if bladder distended Continue monitoring VS, FHR, and sensation Assess for potential problems of epidural infusion: sedation, nausea, vomiting, pruritus, hypotension, and "breakthrough pain"	Straight cath if bladder distended Monitor return of motor ability and sensation if regional block has been given Weigh perineal pads if lochia flow $>$1 saturated pad in 1 h; presence of boggy uterus and clots; decreased BP, increased P ➤ **Expected Outcomes** Mother and fetus experience safe labor and birth Actual/potential complication identified and minimized Woman and family actively participate in decision making and plan of care

➤

CLINICAL PATHWAY FOR EPIDURAL ANESTHESIA *CONTINUED*

Category	First Stage	Second and Third Stage	Fourth Stage Birth to 1 Hour Past Birth
Activity	Encourage ambulation unless contraindicated Maintain bed rest immediately after administration of IV pain medication, or following regional block Encourage woman to rest between contractions	Position comfortably for birth Encourage woman to rest between pushing efforts, and while awaiting birth of placenta	Position of comfort ➤ **Expected Outcomes** Activity maintained per protocol. Comfort and uterine perfusion enhanced by position/movement
Comfort	Woman states that she desires regional anesthesia Assist with administration of epidural block	Second stage: assess and inform woman of progress of labor. Provide reassurance throughout labor. Assist with "sitting dose" reinjection for birth. Encouragement, coaching, help support legs while pushing, position of comfort for pushing and birth. Third stage: cool cloth to forehead, assist parents to see newborn, position mother to hold newborn, provide encouragement	Institute comfort measures. Perineal discomfort: gently cleanse and apply ice pack; position to decrease pressure on perineum Uterine discomfort: palpate fundus gently Hemorrhoids: ice pack General fatigue: position of comfort, encourage rest Administer pain medication ➤ **Expected Outcomes** Optimal comfort maintained
Nutrition	Ice chips and clear fluids Evaluate for signs of dehydration	Ice chips and clear fluids	Regular diet if assessments are WNL Encourage fluids ➤ **Expected Outcomes** Nutrition and hydration needs met
Elimination	Voids at least q2h; urine clear, straw-colored, negative for protein Bladder nondistended; empty before regional block administered May have bowel movement Monitor I & O with IVs	Monitor bladder at frequent intervals	Monitor bladder status with each assessment ➤ **Expected Outcomes** Intake and output WNL
Medications	Hydrate the woman receiving an epidural block with 500–1000 mL fluid prior to procedure (dextrose-free solution is recommended)	Local infiltration of anesthetic agent for birth by CNM/physician Pitocin 10 units IM, IVP per IV tubing, or added to IV fluids	Continue Pitocin infusion Administer pain medication ➤ **Expected Outcomes** Perfusion and hydration supported Uterine hemorrhage prevented or successfully treated
Discharge planning/ home care	Evaluate knowledge of labor and birth process Evaluate support system and need for referral after birth		Provide information if mother to be moved from LDR room Provide opportunity for parents to ask questions regarding newborn Evaluate knowledge of normal postpartum, newborn care ➤ **Expected Outcomes** Individualized discharge teaching completed
Family involvement	Identify available support person(s) Recognize possible impact of culture on responses Observe interaction between woman and partner Create moment alone with woman to identify possible abuse Assess current parenting skills	Provide opportunities for woman and support person(s) to watch newborn assessments Perform newborn assessment on mother's abdomen/chest if possible	Provide opportunity for parents to be with baby Encourage skin-to-skin contact Darken room to encourage eye-to-eye contact Provide quiet time for new family ➤ **Expected Outcomes** Family demonstrates support of family members Parenting: demonstrates early culturally expected parenting behaviors Family able to identify supportive resources in the community
Date			

BP, P, R, blood pressure, pulse, respirations; CNM certified nurse-midwife; EFM, electronic fetal monitor; FHR, fetal heart rate; IV, intravenous; IVP, intravenous push; LDR, labor, delivery, recovery; LTV long-term variability; PRN, as needed or as desired; O_2, oxygen; OOB, out of bed; STV, short-term variability; temp, temperature; VS, vital signs; WNL, within normal limits; c/o, complaints of.

When used during labor, the block may be administered as soon as active labor is established (nullipara is 5 to 6 cm dilated, multipara is 3 to 4 cm) and the fetal vertex is engaged (zero station) (Holt, Diehl, & Wright, 1999).

Although ACOG has recommended postponing epidural administration until active labor is established, the ASA is not in agreement. While earlier literature indicated there was a slight risk of cesarean birth (2%) with early epidural placement, current practice that involves using a low dose of bupivacaine does not increase the risk of cesarean (Santos, 2000).

ADVANTAGES

The lumbar epidural block produces good analgesia that alters maternal physiologic responses to pain. The woman is fully awake during labor and birth. The continuous technique allows different blocking for each stage of labor so that internal rotation of the fetus can be accomplished. In many cases, the dose of anesthetic agent can be adjusted to preserve the woman's reflex urge to bear down.

DISADVANTAGES

The most common complication of an epidural block is maternal hypotension. This is generally prevented by preloading with a rapid infusion of intravenous fluids, then providing intravenous fluids continuously. Kemmerly, Lambard, and Russell (1999) conducted a study that evaluated complications of epidurals and found that the incidence of hypotension requiring ephedrine was low (1.53%). Other serious complications, although rare, have been reported including postdural puncture seizures, meningitis, cardiorespiratory arrest, and vertigo (vestibulocochlear dysfunction) (Jackson, Henry, Van Denkerhof, et al, 2000). Another disadvantage is that the onset of analgesia may not occur for up to 30 minutes. Epidural block requires skilled personnel for administration and close observation of the woman and her fetus. The anesthesiologist must be careful while administering the block to avoid perforating the dura mater, which would place the needle in the subarachnoid space; if the error is not recognized, the anesthetic agent would be injected into the spinal canal. Skilled nurses are also required to maintain close observation of the laboring woman and her fetus. Variability of the fetal heart rate (FHR) may decrease, and late decelerations may occur if maternal hypotension develops.

Some women with epidurals may have decreased sensation and movement, or may have essentially no control over movement in the anesthetized region. Thus, some clinicians believe that epidural blocks lengthen the first and second stage of labor and increase the incidence of cesarean birth; however, this belief is controversial as several studies fail to document delays (Halpern et al, 1998; Thompson, Thorp, Mayer, et al, 1998; Yancey, Pierce, Schweitzer, et al, 1999). Other studies have demonstrated that epidural use prolonged the first stage of labor and contributed to the need to augment labors with oxytocin (Alexander et al, 1998; Lieberman, & O'donoghue, 2002). On the other hand, many healthcare providers assert that epidural analgesia may shorten the active and transition phases because of the pain relief. Howell (2002) reviewed 11 research studies that included 3157 women and found that although epidural anesthesia was associated with greater pain relief, it prolonged both the first and second stages of labor. Epidurals also increased the incidence of fetal malposition and the use of oxytocin. Other studies have shown a relationship between epidural use and the need for instrument-assisted births (Howell, 2002; Lieberman & O'donoghue, 2002) which increases the risk of perineal trauma (Robinson, Norwitz, Cohen, et al, 1999).

CONTRAINDICATIONS

The absolute contraindications for epidural block are maternal refusal, local or systemic infection, coagulation disorders, actual or anticipated maternal hemorrhage, low platelet counts (below 100,000 μL), hypovolemia, allergy to a specific class of local anesthetic agents, suspicion of neurologic disease, and lack of trained staff (Cunningham et al, 2001).

TECHNIQUE FOR CONTINUOUS LUMBAR EPIDURAL BLOCK

In administering a continuous lumbar epidural block the following actions are taken:

1. Maternal and fetal status and labor progress are assessed. Because maternal blood pressure and pulse will be taken frequently, an automatic blood pressure device may be useful. FHR is continuously monitored by an electronic fetal monitor.
2. Oxygen and resuscitative equipment is readied.
3. An intravenous infusion is begun, and a preload of 500 to 1000 mL of balanced salt solution (eg, 0.45% normal saline) is given over approximately 15 to 30 minutes.
4. The woman is positioned on her left or right side, at the edge of the bed (the mattress is firmer and provides more support), with her legs slightly flexed, or she is asked to sit on the edge of the bed. She is advised to drop her shoulders, round out the small of her back, and place her chin on her chest. It may be helpful to advise the woman to "arch her back like a cat" to achieve the proper position. This position is especially effective for positioning obese women. The spinal column is not kept convex, as it is for a spinal block, because the convex position reduces the peridural space to a greater degree and stretches the dura mater, making it more susceptible to puncture. The epidural space is decreased during pregnancy because of venous engorgement. It is also smaller in obese and short individuals (Cunningham et al, 2001). A small pillow may be placed under the woman's head and in front of her chest to provide support for her arms (Figure 25–3 ●).
5. The skin is prepared with an antiseptic agent.
6. A skin wheal is made to anesthetize the supraspinous and interspinous ligaments.
7. A short, beveled 16- to 18-gauge needle with stylet is passed to the ligamentum flavum in the widest

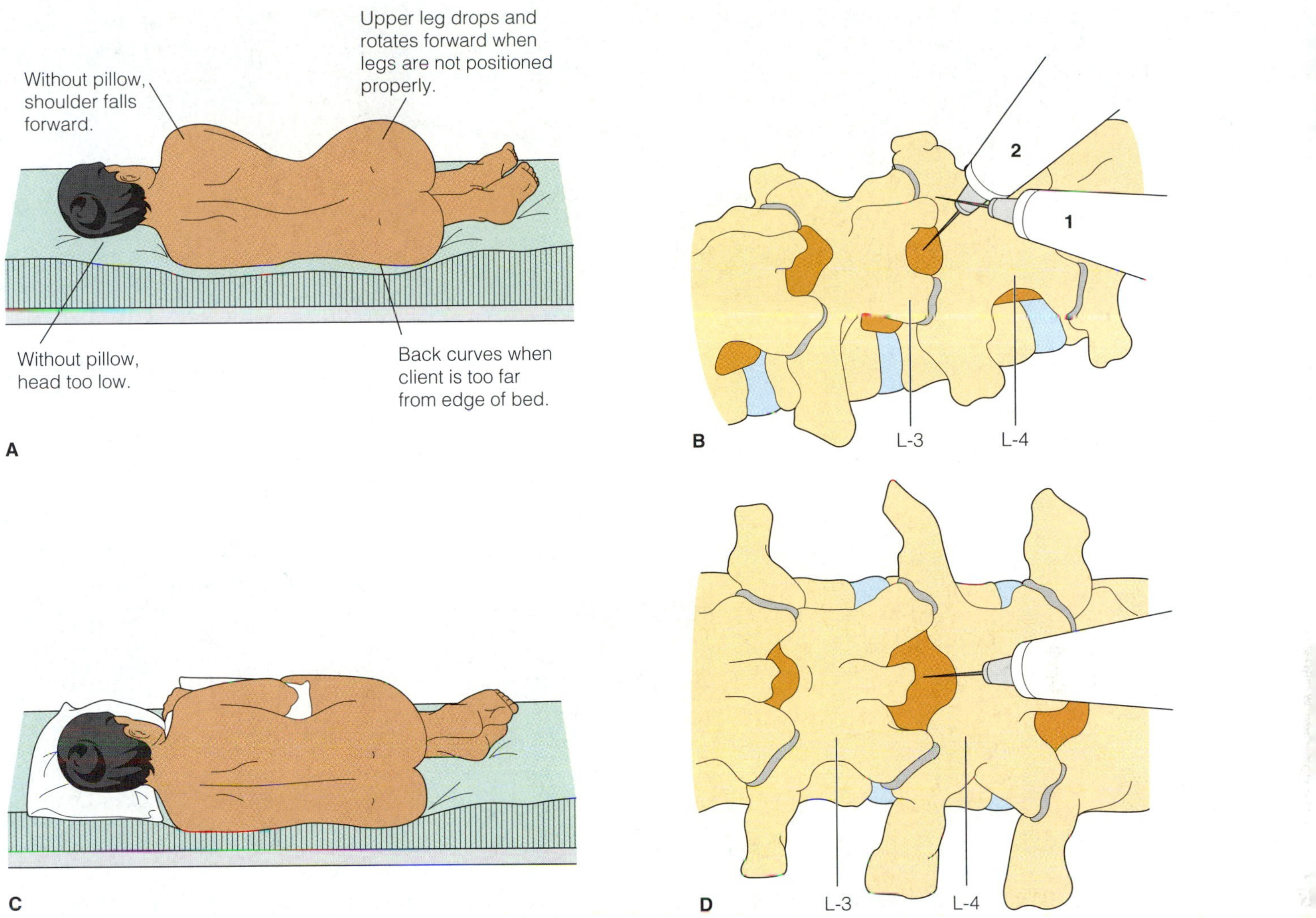
Upper leg drops and rotates forward when legs are not positioned properly.
Without pillow, shoulder falls forward.
Without pillow, head too low.
Back curves when client is too far from edge of bed.
A
2
1
B
L-3
L-4
C
D
L-3
L-4

Figure 25–3 • Positioning woman for epidural anesthesia block. *A,* Incorrect maternal positioning for placing subarachnoid or epidural block. The upper shoulder has fallen forward, upper leg has rotated forward, and the client is positioned on the center of the bed so that there is no support from the edge and the back can curve. *B,* Vertebral position with client in incorrect position. The vertebrae rotate forward and, if the needle is inserted in the usual way (needle 1), the apophyseal joints are encountered. Needle 2 shows the proper insertion of the needle entering the epidural space. *C,* Correct maternal positioning. The back is straight and vertical, the shoulders are square, and the upper leg is prevented from rolling forward. *D,* Vertebral position with the woman correctly positioned.
SOURCE: Shnider, S. M., & Levinson, G. (1993) *Anesthesia for obstetrics* (3rd ed., figs. 9.0, 9.10, 9.11, 9.12). Baltimore, MD: Williams & Wilkins.

interspace below the second lumbar vertebra (usually in the third or fourth lumbar interspace) (Figure 25–4 •). The ligamentum flavum is identified by its resistance to injection of saline or air (called loss of resistance technique). Resistance disappears as the peridural space is entered.

8. Five mL of preservative-free saline is injected in order to pass the catheter into the epidural space more easily.
9. The catheter is inserted approximately 1 to 2 cm into the epidural space. The needle is removed. Aspiration for blood (indicating that a vessel has been inadvertently entered) or cerebrospinal fluid (indicating the dura mater has been punctured) is attempted.
10. If aspiration tests are negative, a test dose of local anesthetic agent containing 1.5% lidocaine with epinephrine 1:200,000 concentration or 3 mL of 0.25% bupivacaine with 1:200,000 concentration of epinephrine is injected. The anesthesiologist usually injects the medication after aspiration and after a uterine contraction to minimize the risk of tachycardia that can occur if the drug is directly injected into a vessel (Chestnut, 1999). If the subarachnoid space has been entered, sensory and motor changes occur in the woman's extremities. If there are no untoward effects, additional anesthetic agent is injected. The catheter is securely taped so that its placement will not be disturbed. Pain relief should occur within 15 to 20 minutes after administration (Cunningham et al, 2001).
11. The woman is placed in a semireclining position with left lateral tilt of her uterus for 10 minutes to allow for

MEDIALINK EPIDURAL PLACEMENT VIDEO

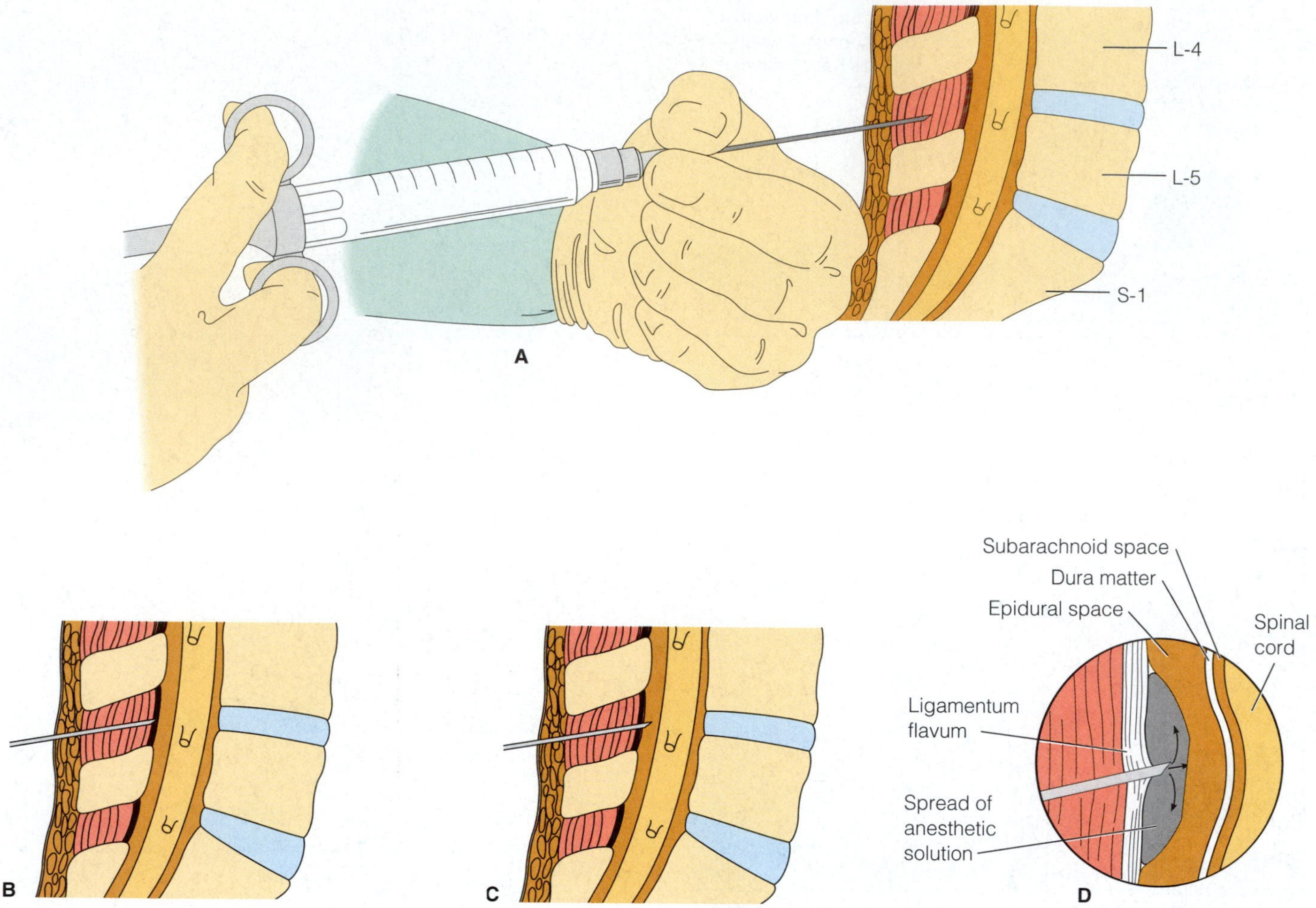

Figure 25–4 • Technique for lumbar epidural block. *A,* Proper position of insertion. *B,* Needle in the ligamentum flavum. *C,* Tip of needle in epidural space. *D,* Force of injection pushing dura away from tip of needle.
SOURCE: Bonica, J.J. (1972). *Principles and practice of obstetric analgesia and anesthesia* (p. 631). Philadelphia: Davis.

distribution of the block. This also prevents aortocaval compression (see Chapter 14). She is then maintained in a side-lying position to maximize uteroplacental perfusion. If she needs to be turned to a supine position for fetal blood sampling or other procedures, the nurse turns the woman as quickly as possible and repositions her on her side.

12. The maternal blood pressure is monitored every 1 to 2 minutes for the first 10 minutes past the injection and then every 5 to 15 minutes until the block wears off. Maternal vital signs are evaluated against baseline readings obtained just prior to the beginning of the procedure.
13. The woman must be attended by a nurse, anesthesiologist, or both for the first 20 minutes following the initial dose and after administration of any additional dose.
14. If hypotension (a 20% to 30% fall in systolic pressure or a drop to below 100 mm Hg) occurs, the nurse ensures that left lateral displacement of the uterus is maintained, and the intravenous fluids are infused more rapidly. Oxygen is delivered by a face mask to ensure proper oxygenation of the fetus. A 10- to 20-degree Trendelenburg position may be used. If the blood pressure is not restored within 1 to 2 minutes, a vasopressor such as ephedrine, 5 to 15 mg, may be administered intravenously (Macarthur, 2002).
15. The maternal blood pressure and pulse and the FHR continue to be monitored.
16. If the epidural is not being administered by continuous pump, the anesthesiologist aspirates the catheter prior to administering subsequent doses.

TECHNIQUE FOR SINGLE-DOSE LUMBAR EPIDURAL BLOCK

The procedure of a single-dose lumbar epidural block is the same as for the lumbar block just described, except that instead of injecting 5 mL of saline, the anesthesiologist injects a test dose of 2 to 3 mL of anesthetic agent to make sure the dura mater has not been penetrated. After checking again to confirm the dura mater has not been perforated, the clinician injects a single dose of 10 to 12 mL to provide anesthesia for birth. Subsequent care continues as for the procedure just described, from step 11 (Chestnut, 1999).

PROBLEMS AND ADVERSE EFFECTS

The major adverse effect of epidural anesthesia is maternal hypotension caused by a spinal blockade, which lowers peripheral resistance, decreases venous return to the heart, and subsequently lessens cardiac output and lowers blood pressure. The risk of hypotension can be minimized by hydrating the vascular system with 500 to 1000 mL of IV solution (Kemmerly, Lambard, & Russell, 1999) prior to the procedure and changing the woman's position and/or increasing the IV rate afterward.

A potentially distressing maternal problem is an inadequate block, unilateral block, or block failure. Epidural anesthesia has a higher failure rate than spinal anesthesia because the catheter must be properly placed to produce adequate anesthesia. A one-sided block is fairly common and can be overcome by having the woman lie on the unanesthetized side and injecting more of the local anesthetic agent. If the woman has a continuous epidural block, she should turn from side to side every hour to avoid a one-sided block. A block may be effective except for a "spot" or "window" of pain in the inguinal or suprapubic area. Breakthrough pain may occur at any time during the epidural infusion. It usually occurs when the continuous infusion rate of the anesthetic agent is below the recommended rate for a therapeutic dose. It may also occur when the infusion pump rate is altered or the integrity of the epidural line is broken.

Pruritus may occur at any time during the epidural infusion. It usually appears first on the face, neck, or torso and is generally the result of the agent used in the epidural infusion.

Maternal temperature may be elevated to 37.8C or higher with the use of epidural anesthesia. A meta-analysis revealed this increase in temperature may be due to a prolonged first stage of labor that can occur with epidural anesthesia (Sharma, 2000). In addition, sympathetic blockade may decrease sweat production and, in turn, diminish heat loss. It has also been suggested that heat loss may result from a failure of the central nervous system to regulate temperature (Sharma, 2000). Headaches, migraine headaches, neckaches, and tingling of the hands and fingers have also been reported (Cunningham et al, 2001).

Short-term localized tenderness at the needle puncture site occurs in about 40% of women during the first week after birth. Backache is fairly common and is thought to result from inadvertently maintaining stressed positions during periods of muscle relaxation and pain relief from the epidural block. Long-term back pain is uncommon. Other problems or adverse effects include urinary retention, shivering, nausea, and vomiting.

COMPLICATIONS

One of the most serious complications of regional anesthesia, systemic toxic reaction, has been discussed in Adverse Maternal Reactions to Anesthetic Agents on p. 673. Toxic reactions following a lumbar epidural block may be caused by unintentional placement of the drug in the arachnoid or subarachnoid space, excessive amount of the drug in the epidural space (massive epidural), or accidental intravascular injection. Because large quantities of anesthetic agent are used for epidural block, the likelihood of toxic reactions is higher than with some of the other regional procedures. The incidence of drug reactions is relatively low, but the possibility is always present.

Pain during cesarean birth with epidural anesthesia has been reported by a growing number of women. In light of this, some anesthesiologists use both temperature and pinprick tests to assess sensory loss. Bourne, de Melo, Bastianpillai, et al (1997) recommend that all dermatomes from T_4 to S_3 be tested for sensory loss before beginning a cesarean. The method of assessment and the results should be documented in the anesthesia record.

NURSING CARE MANAGEMENT

The nurse assesses the maternal vital signs and the FHR for baseline information and to ensure that both maternal and fetal vital signs are within normal limits. (*Note:* All information regarding assessments, procedures, and other activities are recorded on the fetal electronic monitor strip as well as in the nursing notes.) Labor progress is also assessed. The procedure and expected results are explained, and the woman's questions are answered. The nurse acts as an advocate and arranges for consultation with the anesthesiologist if questions arise. Informed consent for the epidural should be obtained.

The nurse starts an IV infusion, if one is not already in place. The nurse preloads at a rapid infusion rate to increase both blood volume and cardiac output per physician's order or agency protocol. It is recommended that dextrose-free solutions be used because dextrose can cause fetal hyperglycemia with rebound hypoglycemia the first few hours after birth. It is helpful to provide an opportunity for the woman to void just before administering the block because her urge to urinate will be decreased. The nurse assists the woman with positioning on either side or in a sitting position on the side of the bed or stretcher. The nurse provides emotional support throughout the procedure.

After the epidural block is given, the woman may be positioned in a semireclining position (head at 25 degrees) with lateral uterine tilt to provide equal distribution of the block; then she is turned to a side-lying position. If she is supine for procedures such as sterile vaginal examinations or fetal scalp blood sampling, the nurse places a wedge under her right hip to help eliminate aortocaval compression. The nurse takes maternal blood pressure and pulse every 5 minutes for at least 30 minutes and then at least every 30 minutes thereafter while the block is present (Chestnut, 1999). The FHR is monitored and assessed by continuous electronic fetal monitor.

If hypotension (systolic blood pressure below 100 mm Hg) occurs, the nurse assists with corrective measures such as positioning the woman in a left side-lying position, increasing the flow rate of the intravenous infusion, and placing the bed in a 10- to 20-degree Trendelenburg position. If maternal blood pressure does not increase within 1 to 2 minutes, 5 to 15 mg of ephedrine may be administered intravenously per physician or protocol order. These measures are usually sufficient; however, if hypotension persists, oxygen by mask at 7 to 10 L/min and additional vasopressors may be needed (Cunningham et al, 2001). Nausea and vomiting may be associated with hypotension. An antiemetic may be ordered to increase the woman's comfort. With severe or prolonged hypotension, added treatment includes elevating the woman's legs for 2 or 3 minutes to increase blood return from the extremities.

If additional local anesthetic agents are injected, the regimen of assessing maternal blood pressure and initial surveillance should be repeated each time the epidural catheter is reinjected. If the woman's legs have been in stirrups during a vaginal birth, her blood pressure should be assessed as soon as her legs are taken out of the stirrups. While the legs were elevated, circulating blood volume in the trunk increased. Restoring circulation to the legs decreases the overall blood volume and may precipitate hypotension.

Additional nursing care following the block includes frequent assessment of the bladder to avoid bladder distention. Catheterization may be necessary because most women are unable to void; however, the nurse should first offer the woman a bedpan since catheterization increases the risk of urinary tract infections.

Shivering may be caused by heat loss from increased peripheral blood flow or alteration of thermal input to the central nervous system when warm but not cold sensations have been suppressed. Applying warmed blankets and reassuring the woman may make her feel more comfortable.

The nurse assesses the woman's level of pain relief. The nurse can promote equal distribution of the anesthetic agent by assessing the temperature of the woman's feet. If one foot warms more quickly than the other, the woman should be positioned with the cooler side dependent (Russell & Reynolds, 1997). It is important for the woman to turn from side to side every hour to promote equal distribution of the anesthetic agent. If positioning changes do not help and the woman has inadequate pain relief, the anesthesiologist needs to be notified. During a continuous epidural block, the anesthesiologist should titrate the infusion to maintain a sensory level of T_{10}, and the presence of motor block and height of sensory block should be documented at least hourly (Russell & Reynolds, 1997).

Respiratory rate and quality of the respirations should be assessed at least every 15 to 30 minutes. The nurse should notify the anesthetist of any significant decreases in respiratory rate or respiratory pattern changes. If the respiratory rate falls below 14 respirations per minute, naloxone (Narcan) may be given to remove the effect of the anesthetic agent; respirations will then return to a normal rate.

The nurse asks the woman if she is experiencing pruritus (itching) and is alert for signs of scratching, especially on the face, neck, and torso. If present, it is usually treated with diphenhydramine (Benadryl), 25 mg administered intravenously or 50 mg intramuscularly per physician's order.

During the second stage of labor, the woman may require assistance with pushing because she may not feel her contractions or experience the urge to push. She may also need assistance holding or controlling her legs in order to push. After birth, return of complete sensation and the ability to control the legs are essential before ambulation is attempted. This may take several hours, depending on the agent and the total dose. The woman must also be able to maintain blood pressure in a sitting and then standing position. For further discussion of nursing care, see Clinical Pathway for Epidural Anesthesia on pages 675 to 677.

MediaLink CARE PLAN: CLIENT WITH AN EPIDURAL

Epidural Analgesia after Birth

To provide analgesia for approximately 24 hours after the birth, the anesthesiologist may inject an opioid, such as morphine (Duramorph) 5.0 mg or 7.5 mg, into the epidural space immediately following the birth. The analgesic effect of Duramorph begins approximately 30 to 60 minutes after the injection. The side effects include pruritus, nausea and vomiting, and urinary retention (*Nurse Practitioner's Prescribing Reference*, 2002). See Drug Guide: Postbirth Epidural Morphine in Chapter 35.

Other agents are being examined that offer equal or better pain control with fewer side effects. Meperidine (Demerol) may be injected during an epidural block for birth, and then continued through use of patient-controlled epidural analgesia (PCEA). Epidural meperidine is associated with fewer side effects than epidural morphine and does not cause hemodynamic changes (Macarthur, 2002). Epidural fentanyl and lidocaine have also been used. The addition of lidocaine has been associated with a more rapid onset of sensory block without the increased side effects (Cherng, Wong, & Ho, 2001).

Spinal Block

In a **spinal block,** a local anesthetic agent is injected directly into the spinal fluid in the subarachnoid space to provide anesthesia for cesarean birth. The subarachnoid space is the fluid-filled area between the dura mater and the spinal cord. During pregnancy, the space decreases because of the distention of the epidural veins. Thus a specific dose of anesthetic produces a much higher level of anesthesia in the pregnant woman than in the nonpregnant woman. When a spinal block is properly administered, failure rate is low. Cesarean birth requires anesthetic blockade to the T_8 dermatome (Figure 25–5 •).

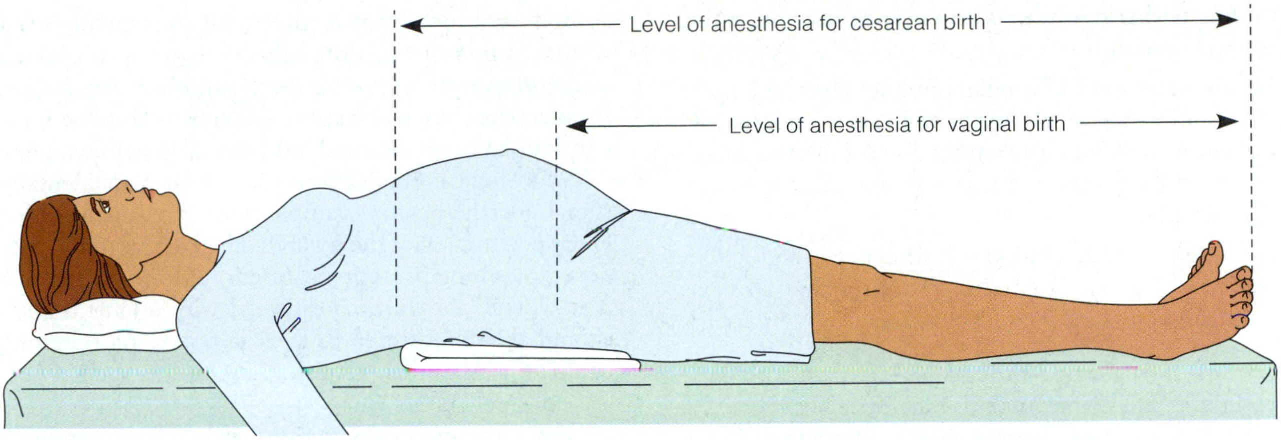

Figure 25–5 • Levels of anesthesia for vaginal and cesarean births.
SOURCE: Reprinted with permission of Ross Laboratories, Columbus, OH. From Clinical Education Aid No. 17.

ADVANTAGES

The advantages of spinal block are immediate onset of anesthesia, relative ease of administration, a smaller drug volume, and maternal compartmentalization of the drug.

DISADVANTAGES

The primary disadvantage of spinal block is intense blockade of sympathetic fibers, resulting in a high incidence of hypotension. This leads to a greater potential for fetal hypoxia. In addition, uterine tone is maintained, which makes intrauterine manipulation difficult.

CONTRAINDICATIONS

Spinal anesthesia is contraindicated for women with severe hypovolemia, regardless of cause; central nervous system disease; infection over the site of puncture; maternal coagulation problems; and allergy to local anesthetic agents. Sepsis and active genital herpes may be considered relative rather than absolute contraindications. Spinal block is also contraindicated for women who do not wish to have spinal procedures (Cunningham et al, 2001).

TECHNIQUE

The following steps are followed in administering a subarachnoid block:

1. The nurse assists the woman into a sitting or left lateral position.
2. Intravenous infusion is checked for patency.
3. The woman places her arms between her knees, bows her head, and arches her back to widen the intervertebral space.
4. The anesthesiologist prepares the skin carefully, maintaining sterility before initiating the procedure.
5. A skin wheal is made over L3 or L4.
6. An 18- or 19-gauge needle is introduced through the skin and into the interspinous ligament. Then, a 24- to 27-gauge pencil-point needle is introduced inside the larger needle and inserted into the ligamentum flavum, the epidural space through the dura mater, and into the subarachnoid space (Figure 25–6 •).
7. The appropriate amount of anesthetic agent is injected slowly, and both needles are removed.
8. Upon removal, a drop of cerebrospinal fluid can be seen in the hub of the needle if the subarachnoid space has been entered.

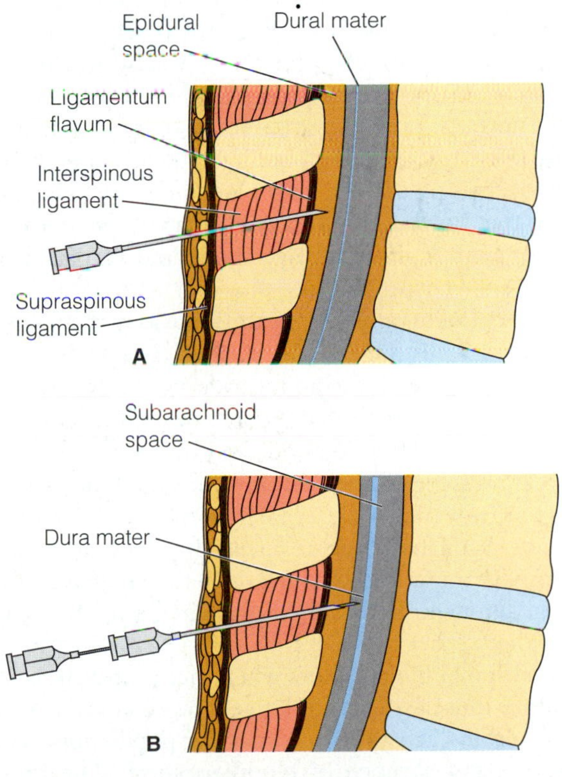

Figure 25–6 • Double-needle technique for spinal injection. *A,* Large needle in epidural space. *B,* 25-gauge needle in larger needle entering the subarachnoid space.
SOURCE: Bonica, J. J. (1972). *Principles and practice of obstetric analgesia and anesthesia* (p. 563). Philadelphia: Davis.

9. With hyperbaric solutions, the woman remains sitting up for 45 seconds.
10. The nurse assists the woman onto her back with a pillow under her head. Position changes can alter the dermatome level if done within 3 to 5 minutes. After 10 minutes, a position change will not affect the level of anesthesia.
11. The nurse monitors blood pressure, pulse, and respirations every 1 to 2 minutes for the first 10 minutes, then every 5 to 10 minutes.

The nurse provides encouragement and support during the procedure. The nurse informs the physician when a contraction is beginning so the anesthetic agent will not be injected at that time.

In the absence of maternal hypotension or toxic reaction, a spinal block exerts no direct effect on the fetus. The amount of anesthetic used is too small to reach fetal circulation in a quantity that might cause fetal depression. Spinal anesthesia has been shown to be well tolerated by a healthy fetus when a maternal IV fluid preload in excess of 500 to 1000 mL precedes the administration of the spinal.

COMPLICATIONS

The complications of spinal anesthesia include hypotension, drug reaction, total spinal neurologic sequelae, and spinal headache. The side effects include nausea, shivering, and urinary retention.

Hypotension can be minimized by prehydrating with 500 to 1000 mL of non-dextrose-containing fluids and displacing the uterus to the left. The practice of placing an already hypotensive woman in a sitting position following injection to prevent upward spread of hyperbaric solution is dangerous because it will cause venous pooling in the lower extremities, further decreasing the maternal blood pressure. The normal curve of the thoracic spine prevents cranial spread of an intrathecal agent. A pillow is placed under the woman's head to exaggerate the curve.

Treatment of hypotension is the same as with an epidural block: positioning the woman in a left lateral, head-down position and rapidly infusing intravenous fluids. Preventing cardiovascular collapse requires early detection, supplemental oxygen, assisted ventilation, and measures to maintain the blood pressure. The extent to which the fetus is affected relates to the degree of maternal hypotension. When maternal hypotension has been reversed, it is best to delay the birth for 4 to 5 minutes to allow the fetus to recover. Resuscitative equipment and trained personnel must be available to treat the mother and baby.

A total spinal block occurs when there is paralysis of the respiratory muscles. It is a relatively rare but critical event. The symptoms are apnea, dilation of pupils, loss of consciousness, and absence of blood pressure. The onset of symptoms usually occurs within minutes of the injection but can occur in a span of time ranging from 30 seconds to 45 minutes. Resuscitative treatment, airway control, and support of blood pressure must begin immediately. If this complication occurs, it is important to remember that this woman is not asleep; although she may be paralyzed, she is aware of everything going on around her. She requires assurance that her respiration is being maintained and will continue to be maintained until she can breathe on her own.

Neurologic complications may occur coincidentally with spinal anesthesia, for example, with preexisting disease or faulty positioning of the woman. Hypotension and apnea can occur, requiring prompt treatment to prevent cardiac arrest. The woman should be positioned with a left tilt and fluids should be administered to treat hypotension (Cunningham et al, 2001). Genuine neurologic sequelae, such as paralysis, are extremely rare.

Although much less serious than other complications, headache may be an unpleasant aftermath of spinal anesthesia. It is the most frequent complication with an incidence of about 2% (Russell & Reynolds, 1997). Leakage of spinal fluid at the site of dural puncture is thought to be the cause. Several techniques have been suggested to decrease the possibility of headache. The use of a narrow-gauge pencil-point anesthesia needle (24- to 27-gauge) reduces the incidence of spinal headache to less than 1.5% (Cunningham et al, 2001). Hyperhydration and keeping the woman flat in bed for 6 to 12 hours after birth have been recommended as preventive measures, but there is no evidence that these procedures are effective. An abdominal binder may provide some relief. In severe cases, a blood patch can be performed. A few milliliters of the woman's blood is drawn and, before coagulation occurs, is injected into the epidural space at the site of the puncture. This technique generally results in immediate pain relief.

NURSING CARE MANAGEMENT

The nurse should assist in positioning the woman, provide oxygen via nasal cannula or mask, assess and record baseline vital signs of the mother and fetus, and start an intravenous infusion prior to administration of the block. After the block is instilled, the nurse should continue to monitor maternal blood pressure, pulse, and respiration until the anesthesiologist takes over. The nurse monitors the FHR at least every 5 minutes until it is no longer accessible because the abdominal surgical prep is begun. The anesthesiologist is responsible for assessing and recording the level of the spinal block.

The nurse positions the woman as described earlier, and supports her in this position. The nurse palpates the woman's uterus to detect the beginning of a contraction. Intrathecal agents are not administered during a contraction because the increased pressure could cause a higher level of anesthesia than desired. After the agent has been administered, the woman is supported upright for the length of time determined by the anesthesiologist and is then assisted to the supine position with a wedge under her right hip to displace the uterus; a pillow is placed under her head. The nurse monitors blood pressure, pulse, and respirations every 5 minutes until the birth. Some physicians administer oxygen as a prophylactic measure. The woman should be kept informed of everything that is going on in the birthing area, particularly if she is receiving mask oxygen. Placing her legs in stirrups facilitates venous return from the extremities. Both legs should be raised at the same time to avoid undue tension and possible injury to back muscles.

If hypotension should occur, the intravenous fluids should be increased and the uterus displaced manually to the left. If the woman reports that she is having difficulty breathing, she needs to be assessed very carefully. Total spinal block rarely occurs, but the possibility must always be kept in mind. The woman should be observed for apnea, unconsciousness, pupil dilation, and unobtainable blood pressure. Prompt treatment, which may include the use of a vasopressor (such as ephedrine), may avert maternal or fetal death. It is essential to establish an airway and give oxygen with positive pressure until the woman can be intubated and other emergency measures instituted.

Following the birth, the woman is typically kept flat. Although the effectiveness of the supine position to avoid headache following a spinal is controversial, the physician's orders may include lying flat for 6 to 12 hours.

Combined Spinal-Epidural Block

Spinal anesthesia may be combined with an epidural block. The combined spinal-epidural (CSE) can be used for labor analgesia and for cesarean birth. The anesthetic and analgesic agents used differ according to the purpose of the CSE. A CSE is accomplished by inserting an epidural needle into the epidural space. A narrow-gauge pencil-point anesthesia needle (24- to 27-gauge) is inserted through the epidural needle, through the dura, and into the cerebral spinal fluid. A small amount of local anesthetic agent, opioid, or both, is injected, and the needle is withdrawn. An epidural catheter is then threaded through the epidural needle into the epidural space. The epidural needle is removed and the epidural catheter is securely placed against the woman.

An advantage of CSE is that the spinal agent will have a faster onset than medications that are injected into the epidural space. A CSE is versatile in that medication can be added to increase the effectiveness. Additional medication can also be added if an instrument-assisted birth or cesarean is needed (Harris, 1998). CSE also preserves motor functioning. Most drugs are used in low dose, so spinal analgesia may be given in early labor to assist with labor pain. When CSE is used, there does appear to be a higher incidence of nausea and pruritus. There are no reports of increased risks of fetal or neonatal complications.

Research in Practice: *Women's Evaluation of Nonpharmacologic Pain Relief During Labor*

What is this study about? Pain in labor is acute, increases quickly, and provokes considerable emotion and anxiety for the laboring mother. The laboring mother may seek comforting contact through therapeutic massage to manage pain and associated anxiety. This study used a scientific experimental method to determine if therapeutic massage has an effect on pain and anxiety during labor.

How was this study done? Subjects for this study were 60 primiparous women giving birth in a hospital in Taiwan. Only mothers with uncomplicated, normal vaginal births were included in the study. The subjects were randomly assigned to either an experimental group or a control group. The experimental group received 30 minutes of a specific massage procedure during each phase of labor. Subjects in the control group received standard nursing care and 30 minutes of individual nursing attention during each phase. A nurse-rated scale was used to assess behavioral manifestations of pain. The subjects used a visual analogue scale to report anxiety. After childbirth, all subjects were asked to subjectively rate satisfaction with the childbirth experience, support levels from their partners, and assistance levels from nurses. Intensity of pain and anxiety were compared statistically between the experimental and control groups for each phase of labor.

What were the results of the study? Pain intensity and anxiety showed a steady increase through each phase of labor for both groups. The massage group had significantly lower pain behavioral intensity scores at all three phases of labor. The massage group also had a lower anxiety score but only in phase 1; massage had no effect on anxiety during phases 2 and 3. Subjects reported a sense of satisfaction from massage, and 87% of the experimental group reported that massage was of more than moderate helpfulness in managing the pain and anxiety of labor. There was no difference between groups in their perceptions of helpfulness of the caregiver or partner, so differences between groups cannot be attributed to these two effects.

What additional questions might I have? Would the differences be even greater if the partner were trained to administer the massage? Would longer or more frequent periods of massage reduce the pain level even more?

How can I use this study? Massage can be a simple, nonpharmacologic, and safe method of support and relief for women during childbirth. The effects on pain, as well as the beneficial effects on anxiety early in labor, make this an effective intervention to implement with laboring mothers.

Source: Chang, M., Wang, S., & Chen, C. (2002). Effects of massage on pain and anxiety during labour: A randomized controlled trial in Taiwan. *Journal of Advanced Nursing, 38*(1): 68–73.

Pudendal Block

The **pudendal block** technique provides perineal anesthesia for the second stage of labor, birth, and episiotomy repair. An anesthetic agent is injected below the pudendal plexus, as shown in Figure 25–1. The pudendal plexus arises from the anterior division of the second and third sacral nerves and the entire fourth sacral nerve. Below the plexus, the branches converge into the pudendal nerve which crosses the sacrosciatic notch and passes the tip of the ischial spine, where it divides into the perineal, dorsal, and inferior hemorrhoidal nerves of the pudendal plexus. The perineal nerve, which is the largest branch of the pudendal plexus, supplies the skin of the vulvar area, the perineal muscles, and the urethral sphincter. The dorsal nerve supplies the clitoris, and the inferior hemorrhoidal nerve supplies the skin and muscles of the perineal region as well as the internal anal sphincter. Pudendal block provides relief of pain from perineal distention but does not relieve pain of uterine contractions (Figure 25–7 •).

ADVANTAGES AND DISADVANTAGES

The advantages of pudendal block are ease of administration and absence of maternal hypotension. It also allows the use of low forceps or vacuum extraction for birth.

A moderate dose of anesthetic agent (10 mL per side) has minimal ill effects on the woman and the course of labor. The urge to bear down during the second stage of labor may be decreased, but the woman is able to do so with appropriate coaching. There is usually little effect on the uncompromised fetus unless overly rapid or intravascular injection occurs. The block may be done by a transvaginal or transperineal approach. Transvaginal injection is simpler, safer, and more direct, making it the procedure of choice.

COMPLICATIONS

A systemic toxic reaction can occur from accidental vascular injection. Other possible maternal complications specific to pudendal block include broad ligament hematoma, perforation of the rectum, and trauma to the sciatic nerve.

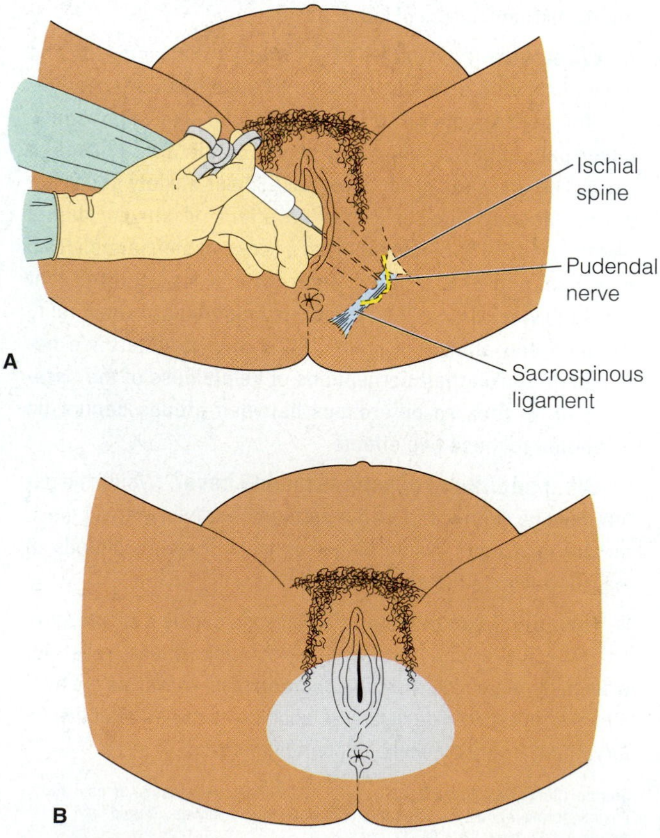

Figure 25–7 • *A,* Pudendal block by the transvaginal approach. *B,* Area of perineum affected by pudendal block.

NURSING CARE MANAGEMENT

The nurse explains the procedure and the expected effect and answers any questions. Pudendal block does not alter maternal vital signs or FHR, so assessments in addition to the expected ones are not necessary.

Local Infiltration Anesthesia

Local anesthesia is accomplished by injecting an anesthetic agent into the intracutaneous, subcutaneous, and intramuscular areas of the perineum (Figure 25–8 •). It is generally used at the time of birth for episiotomy and repair and is especially useful for women giving birth without previous pharmacologic interventions. The procedure is essentially free from complications.

ADVANTAGES

The major advantage of the local block is that it involves the use of the least amount of anesthetic agent. It can be done if an episiotomy is needed just prior to the birth. It can also be used when a laceration has occurred and a repair is needed.

DISADVANTAGES

The major disadvantage is that large amounts of solution must be used. Although any local anesthetic may be used, chloroprocaine (Nesacaine), lidocaine (Xylocaine), and mepivacaine (Carbocaine) are the agents of choice in local infiltration because of their capacity for diffusion.

NURSING CARE MANAGEMENT

The nurse explains the procedure and the expected effect and answers any questions. Local anesthetic agents have no effect on maternal vital signs or FHR, so additional assessments are unnecessary.

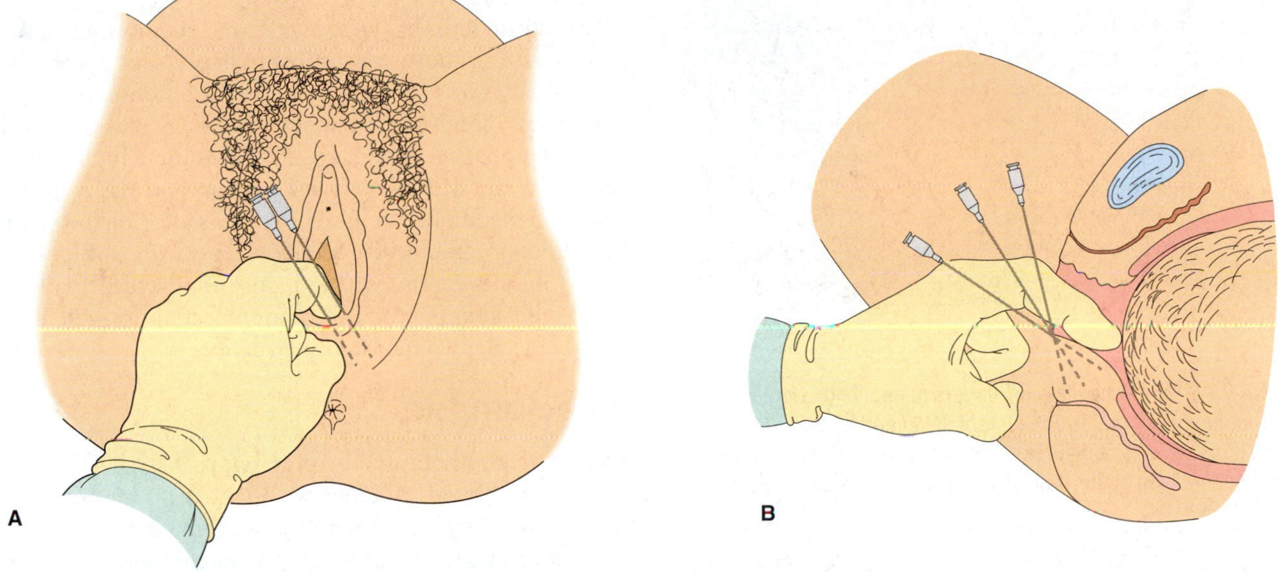

Figure 25–8 • Local infiltration anesthesia. *A,* Technique of local infiltration for episiotomy and repair. *B,* Technique of local infiltration showing fan pattern for the fascial planes.
SOURCE: Bonica, J. J. (1972). *Principles and practice of obstetric analgesia and anesthesia* (p. 505). Philadelphia: Davis.

General Anesthesia

General anesthesia (induced unconsciousness) may be needed for cesarean birth and surgical intervention with some obstetric complications. The method used to achieve general anesthesia may be intravenous injection, inhalation of anesthetic agents, or a combination of both methods.

Intravenous Anesthetics

Sodium thiopental (Pentothal) is an ultra-short-acting barbiturate, which means that it exerts its effect rapidly and has a brief duration of action. Sodium thiopental produces narcosis within 30 seconds after intravenous administration. Introduction and emergence from its effects are smooth and pleasant, with little incidence of nausea and vomiting. Sodium thiopental is most frequently used for initiating unconsciousness and as an adjunct to other more potent anesthetics. Ketamine is an intermediate-acting barbiturate that is used for anesthesia induction. The effects typically last 20 to 60 minutes. Hypersalivation can occur but can be treated with an anticholinergic drug to decrease this side effect. The drug is contraindicated in women with preeclampsia or chronic hypertension.

Complications of General Anesthesia

A primary danger of general anesthesia is fetal depression. Most general anesthetic agents reach the fetus in about 2 minutes. The depression of the fetus is directly proportional to the depth and duration of the anesthesia. The long-term significance of fetal depression in a normal birth has not been determined. The poor fetal metabolism of general anesthetic agents is similar to that of analgesic agents administered during labor. General anesthesia is not advocated when the fetus is considered to be at high risk, particularly in preterm birth.

Most general anesthetic agents cause some degree of uterine relaxation. They may also cause vomiting and aspiration.

Pregnancy results in decreased gastric motility, and the onset of labor halts the process almost entirely. Food eaten hours earlier may remain undigested in the stomach. Even when food and fluids have been withheld, the gastric juice produced during fasting is highly acidic and can produce chemical pneumonitis if aspirated. This pneumonitis is known as Mendelson syndrome. The signs and symptoms are chest pain, respiratory distress, cyanosis, fever, and tachycardia. Women undergoing emergency cesarean births appear to be at considerable risk for adverse events. The leading cause of maternal deaths in women who have had general anesthesia is the failure to establish a patent airway (Crawford, 2002).

Care During General Anesthesia

Prophylactic antacid therapy is given to reduce the acidic content of the stomach before general anesthesia. Administration of a nonparticulate antacid (such as Bicitra) may be used. Cimetidine (Tagamet) may also be used (Cunningham et al, 2001).

Before the induction to anesthesia, the woman should have a wedge placed under her right hip to displace the uterus and avoid vena caval compression in the supine position. She should also be preoxygenated with 3 to 5 minutes of 100% oxygen. Intravenous fluids should be started so that access to the intravascular space is immediately available.

During the process of rapid induction of anesthesia, the nurse applies cricoid pressure. This is accomplished by

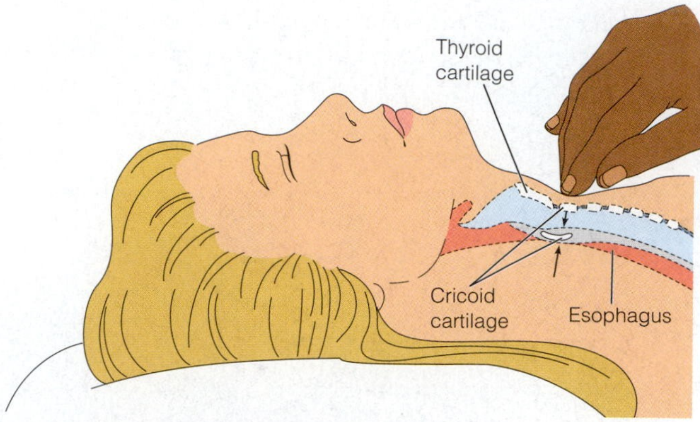

Figure 25–9 • Proper position for fingers in applying cricoid pressure until a cuffed endotracheal tube is placed by the anesthesiologist or certified nurse-anesthetist. The cricoid cartilage is depressed 2 to 3 cm posteriorly so that the esophagus is occluded.

depressing the cricoid cartilage 2 to 3 cm posteriorly so that the esophagus is occluded. Cricoid pressure is continued until the anesthesiologist has placed the cuffed endotracheal tube and indicates that the pressure can be released. Figure 25–9 • shows the appropriate technique. The woman's neck should be supported by the nurse's other hand.

Neonatal Neurobehavioral Effects of Anesthesia and Analgesia

Studies have focused on the neurobehavioral effects on the newborn of pharmacologic agents used during labor and birth. Although analgesic and anesthetic agents may alter the behavioral and adaptive function of the newborn, physiologic factors such as hunger, degree of hydration, and time within the sleep-wake cycle may also exert an influence (Chestnut, 1999). The long-range importance of these findings has not been well established.

Analgesic and Anesthetic Considerations for the High-Risk Mother and Fetus

Up to this point the discussion of obstetric analgesia and anesthesia has dealt with the healthy woman and healthy fetus. Pain relief for high-risk women during labor and birth requires skill in decision making, close observation, and awareness of potential threats to the woman and fetus. Safety for all involved requires the close cooperation of obstetrician, anesthesiologist, pediatrician, and labor nurse. The pathophysiologic changes that accompany maternal disorders have a direct influence on the choice of agent or technique. It is difficult to separate maternal and fetal complications because whatever alters the woman's response will also affect the fetus. The effects on the woman cannot be considered without the potential effects on the fetus.

Preterm Labor

The preterm fetus has special risks and requirements. An immature fetus is more susceptible to depressant drugs because he or she has less protein available for binding; has a poorly developed blood-brain barrier, which increases the likelihood that pharmacologic agents will attain a higher concentration in the central nervous system; and has a decreased ability to metabolize and excrete drugs after birth. Analgesia during labor should be avoided whenever possible. If it becomes necessary, the smallest dose that will provide relief should be administered. Emotional support will be very valuable to the woman in this situation.

Preeclampsia

Pregnancies complicated by preeclampsia are high-risk situations, as indicated in Chapter 20 . The potential for chronic placental insufficiency or preterm birth is also present. The woman with mild preeclampsia usually may have the analgesia or anesthesia of choice, although the incidence of hypotension with epidural anesthesia is increased. If hypotension occurs with the epidural block, it provides further stress on an already compromised cardiovascular system. Hypotension can usually be managed with judicial fluid increase and positioning.

The woman with severe preeclampsia poses a real challenge. Regional anesthesia seems to be the preferred method as long as hypotension can be avoided. Raising the central venous pressure by 3 to 4 cm H_2O with intravenous fluids helps avoid hypotension, but it must be remembered that this woman is already threatened with heart failure. The effect of fluid intake can be monitored with a central venous pressure (CVP) line or pulmonary catheter. Although pulmonary artery catheterization can be safely used in obstetric clients, placement should be considered on a case by case basis (ASA, 1999). It is important to monitor and record the fluid intake and output. Some physicians use vasopressors; others avoid them because of the possible decrease in uterine blood flow to an already compromised fetus and the threat of a maternal cerebral vascular accident. Spinal anesthesia is rarely used because of the greater potential for hypotension.

The use of general anesthesia poses a risk of aggravating maternal hypertension. In general, the safest method for general anesthesia is intubation, but because it may cause a hypertensive episode, it is avoided if possible.

Diabetes Mellitus

The fetus of a mother with diabetes mellitus may have a reduction in placenta blood flow. Hypotension, which can result during regional anesthesia, can deplete this blood flow even further. If labor can be managed without fetal distress, small doses of intravenous narcotics with pudendal block at birth or the continuous epidural technique may be undertaken. If fetal distress occurs, cesarean birth may be necessary.

Anesthesia for cesarean birth requires special consideration in this case. The diabetic woman is more likely to experience cardiovascular depression during a regional block because of higher sympathetic blockade. If a regional block is selected, it is recommended that acute hydration (preload) be provided by administering dextrose-free solution. In addition, left uterine displacement is initiated prior to the administration of the block and maintained throughout the surgery. Hypotension is treated promptly.

Cardiac Disease

Pregnancy imposes significant risks for the woman with cardiac disease. With mild mitral stenosis, the preferred anesthetic is continual epidural anesthesia with low forceps birth. This method avoids the cardiovascular changes associated with contractions and the Valsalva maneuver during bearing down in the second stage of labor. Hypotension can be avoided with carefully controlled intravenous fluids and measuring CVP to avoid overload. Epidural block or general anesthesia may be used in cesarean birth. Ketamine should be avoided because it produces tachycardia.

Bleeding Complications

The current trend in treating bleeding complications during labor is to schedule cesarean birth when possible. When the maternal cardiovascular system is stable and there is no evidence of fetal distress, an epidural may be given for birth. However, when either of these conditions results in active bleeding, the threat of hypovolemia must be treated immediately. Maternal hypovolemia and shock produce fetal hypoxia, acidosis, and possible fetal death.

Regional blocks are contraindicated during active bleeding because the sympathetic block causes vasodilation and further reduction of the vascular volume. General anesthesia is recommended for these cases. Sodium thiopental may be used, but it is a cardiac depressant and vasodilator, and ketamine may be a more appropriate choice for induction. Following birth of the infant and placenta, oxytocin should not be given as an intravenous bolus to contract the uterus because it causes vasodilation, which in turn causes a decrease in blood pressure and in total peripheral resistance. Oxytocin should be given as a dilute infusion to gain an oxytocic effect to treat uterine atony (relaxation) and to control postpartum bleeding. Resources that should be on hand to handle hemorrhagic emergencies include large-bore intravenous catheters, a fluid warmer, a forced-air body warmer, the woman's specific blood type or O negative blood, and equipment to infuse blood products rapidly (ASA, 1999).

Chapter Review

EXPLOREMEDIALINK

NCLEX review questions, case studies, and other interactive resources for this chapter can be found on the Web site at http://www.prenhall.com/olds. Click on "Chapter 25" to select the activities for this chapter.

For tutorials including animations and videos, more NCLEX review questions, and an audio glossary, access the accompanying CD-ROM in this book.

Focus Your Study

- Pain relief during labor may be enhanced by nonpharmacologic methods and administration of analgesic agents and regional anesthesia blocks.
- The goal of pharmacologic analgesia during labor is to provide maximal pain relief with minimal risk for the woman and fetus.
- The optimal time for administering analgesia is determined after a complete assessment of many factors. An analgesic agent is generally administered to nulliparas when the cervix has dilated 5 to 6 cm and to multiparas when the cervix has reached 3 to 4 cm dilatation.
- Two common analgesic agents are butorphanol (Stadol) and nalbuphine (Nubain).
- Opiate antagonists, such as naloxone (Narcan), counteract the respiratory depressant effect of the opiate narcotics by acting at specific receptor sites in the central nervous system.
- Regional anesthesia is achieved by injecting local anesthetic agents into an area that will bring the agent into direct contact with nerve tissue. Methods most commonly used in childbearing include lumbar epidural, spinal block, pudendal block, and local infiltration.

- Three types of local anesthetic agents used in regional blocks are amides, esters, and opiates. The amides are absorbed quickly and can be found in maternal blood within minutes after administration. The esters are metabolized more rapidly and have only limited placental transfer. Opiates act on specific opiate receptors in the spinal cord and have a greater analgesic effect when combined with a low dose of local anesthetic.
- New agents in use for epidural and spinal routes include the opioids morphine and fentanyl. Adverse reactions of the woman to local anesthetic agents range from mild symptoms, such as palpitations, to cardiovascular collapse.
- Pudendal blocks provide perineal anesthesia during the second stage of labor, birth, episiotomies, or laceration repair.
- The goal of general anesthesia is to provide maximal pain relief with minimal side effects to the woman and her fetus.
- Complications of general anesthesia include fetal depression, uterine relaxation, vomiting, and aspiration.
- The choice of analgesia and anesthesia for the high-risk woman and fetus requires careful evaluation.

References

Alexander, J. M., Lucas, M. J., Ramin, S. M., et al. (1998). The course of labor with and without epidural analgesia. *American Journal of Obstetrics and Gynecology, 178*(3), 516–520.

American College of Obstetricians and Gynecologists (ACOG). (1996). *Pain relief during labor* (ACOG Committee Opinion No. 118). Washington, DC: Author.

American College of Obstetricians and Gynecologists (ACOG). (2000). *American College of Obstetricians and Gynecologists Task Force on Cesarean Delivery Rates.* Washington, DC: Author.

American Society of Anesthesiologists (ASA). (1999). *New guidelines to promote safer anesthesia care for women in labor.* Washington, DC: Author.

American Society of Anesthesiologists (ASA). (2000). *Statement on pain relief for labor.* Washington, DC: Author.

Bourne, T. M., de Melo, A. E., Bastianpillai, B. A., & May, A. E. (1997). A survey of how British obstetric anesthetists test regional anaesthesia before Caesarean section. *Anaesthesia, 52*, 896–913.

Cherng, C. H., Wong, C. S., & Ho, S. T. (2001). Epidural fentanyl speeds the onset of sensory block during epidural lidocaine anesthesia. *Regional Anesthesia and Pain Relief, 26*(6), 523–526.

Chestnut, D. H. (1999). *Obstetric anesthesia: Principles and practice* (2nd ed.). St. Louis, MO: Mosby-Yearbook.

Crawford, K. (2002). The AANA Foundation closed malpractice claims study: Obstetric anesthesia. *American Association of Nurse Anesthetists Journal, 70*(2), 97–104.

Cunningham, F. G., MacDonald, P. C., Gant, N. F., Leveno, K. J., et al. (2001). *Williams Obstetrics* (21st ed.). New York: McGraw-Hill.

Deglin, J. H., & Vallerand, A. H. (2002). *Davis's drug guide for nurses* (8th ed.). Philadelphia: F. A. Davis.

Faucher, M. A., & Brucker, M. A. (2000). Intrapartum pain: Pharmacologic management. *Journal of Obstetric, Gynecologic, and Neonatal Nursing, 29*(2), 169–180.

Fraser, W. D., Cayer, M., Soeder, B. M., Turcot, L., & Marcoux, S. (2002). Risk factors for difficult delivery in nulliparas with epidural analgesia in second stage. *Obstetrics & Gynecology, 99*, 409–418.

Goetzl, L. M. (2002). ACOG practice bulletin. Obstetric analgesia and anesthesia. *Obstetrics & Gynecology, 100*, 177–191.

Goldberg, A., Cohen, A. B. A., & Lieberman, E. (1999). Nulliparas' preferences for epidural analgesia: Their effects on actual use in labor. *Birth, 26*(3), 139–143.

Green, J. M., Coupland, V. A., & Kitzinger, J. V. (1998). *A prospective study of women's expectations and experiences of childbirth.* Chesire, England: Books for Midwives Press.

Halpern, D., Jensen, D. E., & Grotberg, J. B. (1998). A theoretical study of surfactant and liquid delivery into the lung. *Journal of Applied Physiology, 85*(1), 333–352.

Harris, L. G. (1998). Spinal and combined epidural techniques for labor analgesia: Clinical application in a small hospital. American *Association of Nurse Anesthetists Journal, 66*(6), 587–594.

Hawkins, J. L., Chestnut, D. H., & Gibbs, C. P. (2002). Obstetric anesthesia. In S. G. Gabbe, J. R. Niebyl, & J. L. Simpson (Eds.). *Obstetrics: Normal and problem pregnancies* (4th ed.). New York: Churchill Livingstone, 431–472.

Holt, R. O., Diehl, S. J., & Wright, J. W. (1999). Station and cervical dilation at epidural placement in predicting cesarean risk. *Obstetrics & Gynecology, 93*, 281–284.

Howell, C. J. (2002). Epidural versus non-epidural analgesia for pain relief in labour. The Cochrane Library (Oxford) 1 (CD000331). (1).

Jackson, A., Henry, R., Van Denkerhof, E., et al. (2000). Informed consent for labour epidurals: What labouring women want to know. *Canadian Journal of Anasthesia, 47*(11), 1068–1073.

Karch, S. (1999). The problem with methamphetamine toxicity. *Western Journal of Medicine, 170*(2), 232.

Kemmerly, J. R., Lambard, W. W., & Russell, R. C. (1999). Epidural analgesia provided during labor by obstetricians: Outcome analysis. *Southern Medical Association Journal, 92*(11), 1075–1078.

Knaw, K. S., Kee, W. D., & Critchey, L. A. (2000). Epidural meperidine does not cause hemodynamic changes in the term parturient. *Canadian Journal of Anaesthesia, 47*(2), 155–159.

Lieberman, E., & O'donoghue, C. (2002). Unintended effects of epidural analgesia during labor: A systematic review. *American Journal of Obstetrics and Gynecology, 186*(Suppl. 5 Nature)S:31–68.

Macarthur, A. (2002). Solving the problem of spinal-induced hypotension in obstetric anesthesia. *Canadian Journal of Anaesthesia, 49*(6), 536–539.

Mayberry, L. J., & Clemmens, D. D. A. (2002). Epidural anesthesia side effects, co-interventions, and care of women during childbirth: A systematic review. *American Joural of Obstetrics and Gynecology, 186* (5 Suppl Nature): S81–93.

Nurse practitioner's prescribing reference. (2002, Spring). New York: Prescribing Reference.

Robinson, J. N., Norwitz, E. R., Cohen, A. P., Mcelrath, T. F., & Lieberman, E. S. (1999). Epidural anesthesia and third or fourth degree lacerations in nulliparas. *Obstetrics & Gynecology, 94*, 256–259.

Russell, R., & Reynolds, F. (1997). Pain relief and anesthesia during labor. In R. K. Creasy (Ed.), *Management of labor and delivery* (pp. 183–222). Malden, MA: Blackwell.

Santos, A. C. (2000, October). Society for obstetric anesthesia and perinatology: A new life. *American Society of Anesthesiology Newsletter, 64*, 10. Retrieved July 19, 2002 from www.asahq.org/NEWSLETTERS/2000/10_00/Santos.htm

Sharma, S. K. (2000). Epidural analgesia during labor and maternal fever. *Current Opinions in Anesthesiology, 13*, 257.

Task Force on Obstetric Anesthesia. (1999). *Practice guidelines for obstetric anesthesia.* Washington, DC: American Society of Anesthesiologists.

Thompson, T. T., Thorp, J. M., Mayer, D., Kuller, J. A., & Bowes, W. A. (1998). Does epidural analgesia cause dystocia? *Journal of Clinical Anesthesia, 10*, 58.

Yancey, M. K., Pierce, B., Schweitzer, D., & Daniels, D. (1999). Observations on labor epidural analgesia and operative delivery rates. *American Journal of Obstetrics and Gynecology, 180*, 353.

Childbirth at Risk: The Intrapartal Period

26

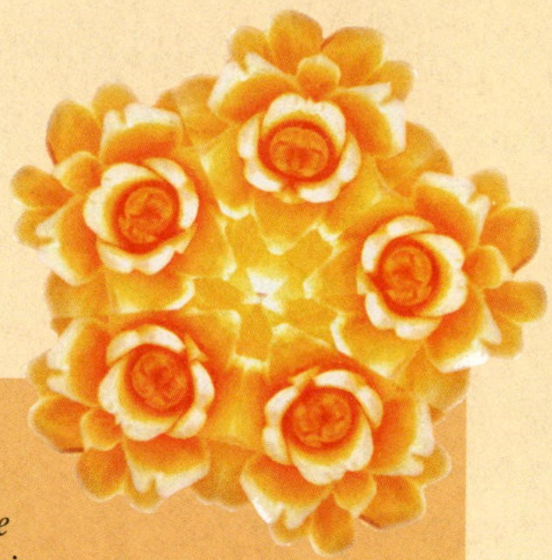

I couldn't wait to begin labor. I wasn't afraid. We had wonderful plans for our labor and birth. My nurse helped me with my breathing as I entered transition. Everything was going so well. Suddenly, the baby began having decelerations. The nurse assisted me onto my side and called for assistance. Time seemed to stand still as the once rapidly beating heart suddenly sounded so slow. It seemed like it took forever to return to its previous rapid pace. For an instant, I was terrified, but after that one episode, there were no further problems.

Objectives

- Describe psychologic disorders that may contribute to difficulty in coping during labor and birth.
- Discuss dysfunctional labor patterns.
- Identify the potential maternal risks of precipitous labor and birth.
- Describe the impact of postterm pregnancy on the childbearing family.
- Summarize various types of fetal malposition and malpresentation and possible associated problems.
- Discuss the implications of macrosomia and hydrocephalus on the woman and the fetus.
- Identify maternal and fetal risks associated with multiple gestations.
- Compare abruptio placentae and placenta previa.
- Identify variations that may occur in the umbilical cord and insertion into the placenta.
- Discuss the identification, management, and nursing care of women with amniotic fluid embolus, hydramnios, and oligohydramnios.
- Delineate the effects of pelvic contractures on labor and birth.
- Discuss complications of the third and fourth stages of labor.
- Discuss intrauterine fetal death, including etiology, diagnosis, management, and the nurse's role in assisting the family.

Key Terms

Abruptio placentae 719
Active management of labor (AMOL) 698
Amniotic fluid embolism 730
Cephalopelvic disproportion (CPD) 731
Dystocia 693
Hydramnios 730
Macrosomia 710
Oligohydramnios 731
Persistent occiput-posterior (OP) position 702
Placenta accreta 733
Placenta increta 733
Placenta percreta 733
Placenta previa 721
Postterm pregnancy 700
Precipitous labor and birth 699
Prolapsed umbilical cord 726
Psychologic disorders 693
Retained placenta 733
Vasa previa 723

MediaLink

Additional resources for this content can be found on the Student CD-ROM and on the Companion Website at www.prenhall.com/olds. Click on "Chapter 26" to select the activities for this chapter.

CD-ROM
- Audio Glossary
- NCLEX Review

Companion Website
- Additional NCLEX Review
- Case Study: Client with Placental Problems
- Care Plan Activity: Prevention of Cord Prolapse

The successful completion of the 40-week gestational period requires the harmonious functioning of the five critical factors we discussed in Chapter 22: the birth passage, the fetus, the relationship between the passage and fetus, forces of labor, and psychosocial considerations. Disruptions in any of these components may result in **dystocia** (at-risk or difficult labor). Some of the most common at-risk conditions are discussed in this chapter.

Care of the Woman at Risk Due to Psychologic Disorders

Anxiety and fear are common emotions in many women in labor. The onset of labor is a time of mixed emotions. Joy, happiness, excitement, fear of the unknown, and anxiety related to pain sensations may all occur. Even women who are well prepared can experience anxious feelings. Although these reactions are expected in the woman with normal coping mechanisms and adequate social support, women with psychologic disorders may face additional emotional challenges and need additional nursing care and support in the intrapartum period.

The prevalence of psychologic disorders of adults in the United States is 22.1% (Table 26–1 •). **Psychologic disorders** are characterized by alterations in thinking, mood, or behavior (US Department of Health and Human Services [DHHS], 1999). Although there are many different types of psychologic disorders, only the most common are presented here. Since an in-depth description is beyond the scope of this text, we focus on the impact of these disorders on labor and birth (Table 26–2 •). Postpartal psychologic disorders are discussed in Chapter 37.

Depression affects millions of Americans annually. More women are affected than men (Dorland, 2001). Depression is believed to be caused by a central nervous system (CNS) imbalance in serotonin and other neurotransmitters. The hormonal changes associated with pregnancy can directly impact a woman with a previous history of depression. Individuals with depression may have persistent sad mood, physical slowing, agitation, energy loss, feelings of worthlessness, difficulty thinking or concentrating, and sleep disturbances (National Institute of Mental Health [NIMH], 2001).

Depression can affect the labor process in a variety of ways. The woman may be unable to concentrate or process information being provided by healthcare team members. Since

Table 26–2 • PSYCHOLOGIC DISORDERS THAT CAN AFFECT LABOR AND BIRTH

Anxiety Disorders
Generalized anxiety disorder (GAD)
Social anxiety disorder
Obsessive-compulsive disorder (OCD)
Post-traumatic stress disorder (PTSD)
Specific phobias
Depression
Major depression
Bipolar depression
Personality Disorders
Antisocial personality
Avoidant personality
Borderline personality
Narcisisstic personality
Dissociative Identity Disorder
Schizophrenia

Source: Adapted from National Institute of Mental Health (NIMH). *Do you suffer from a mental disorder?* (2002). Rockville, MD: Author.

Table 26–1 • PREVALENCE OF PSYCHOLOGICAL DISORDERS

Disorder	US Prevalence	Prevalence in Women/Men	Maternal Implication
Generalized anxiety disorder	4 million (2.8%)	Two times higher in women	Anxiety related to the birth process or medical interventions
Bipolar disorder	2.3 million (1.2%)	Women and men equally affected	Depressive or manic symptoms during labor
Depression	9.9 million (5%)	Two times higher in women	Withdrawn behavior, physical fatigue due to insomnia, crying spells, sadness, hopelessness
Obsessive-compulsive disorder	3.3 million (2.3%)	Equal in men and women	Ritualistic behaviors or thoughts, difficulty focusing on directions
Panic disorder	2.4 million (1.7%)	Two times higher in women	Intense fear or sense of panic related to birth process
Phobias	5.3 million (3.6%)	Higher in women	May have specific fear related to an individual(s) or a procedure or place
Posttraumatic stress disorder (PTSD)	5.2 million (3.6%)	Higher in women	Repressed memories may be triggered during labor causing intense anxiety, fear, and emotional distress
Schizophrenia	2.2 million (1.1%)	Affects men and women equally	May have hallucinations or delusions, lack of sense of present events

Source: Adapted from National Institute of Mental Health (NIMH). *Do you suffer from a mental disorder?* (2002). Rockville, MD: Author.

depression often causes difficulty sleeping, she may begin labor fatigued or sleep deprived. The labor process may overwhelm her physically and emotionally, since she has no energy "reserves" on which to draw. She may feel unworthy of motherhood or experience hopelessness about the outcome of her labor. However, she may not be able to articulate any of these feelings, and may instead appear irritable or withdrawn.

Individuals with *bipolar disorder* can have depressive symptoms that alternate with episodes of mania. Although a complete discussion of bipolar disorder is beyond the scope of this text, students should refer to a psychiatric nursing text for a more complete discussion. Individuals with bipolar disorder experience the same symptoms as depression (previously discussed) during the depressive phase. Mania is characterized by expansiveness, elation, agitation, hyperactivity, and increased speed of thought and ideas (Dorland, 2001). During manic phases, individuals commonly exhibit poor judgment and hyperexcitability. A pregnant woman experiencing a manic episode may engage in behaviors that are dangerous for herself or her fetus including alcohol or drug use, fast driving, driving without a seat belt, or engaging in unprotected intercourse with individuals at high risk for sexually transmitted infections (see Chapter 6). There is also a higher risk of suicide in individuals with mood disorders (Zuspan & Quilligan, 1998). Women with a previous diagnosis of bipolar depression have a 25% risk of developing a manic episode postpartum (Zuspan & Quilligan, 1998). Although postpartum psychosis is a rare disorder (see Chapter 37), it is more common in women with bipolar disorder.

Anxiety disorders include a cluster of diagnoses, such as panic disorder, obsessive-compulsive disorder (OCD), post-traumatic stress disorder (PTSD), generalized anxiety disorder, social phobia, and other specific phobias. These disorders can cause a wide range of symptoms in laboring women. Specifically, women with panic attacks can experience intense feelings of terror without warning that result in physical symptoms (chest pain, shortness of breath, weakness, faintness, or dizziness) and/or psychologic symptoms (fear, terror, or anxiety). Other serious medical conditions need to be excluded (eg, amniotic fluid embolism, cardiac complications, asthma attack). Women with OCD may need to repeat specific rituals as a means of coping in labor. Ritualistic activities that are safe for the mother and the fetus can be used to reduce anxiety. Women who have a history of rape or sexual abuse may suffer from PTSD. The events of labor may trigger flashbacks, avoidance behaviors, or anxiety symptoms. Generalized anxiety disorder, while not acutely disabling, may make the woman very uncomfortable as she enters labor. She may have a vague sense of something being "wrong" with her labor progress or her fetus, and may need repeated reassurances that she and her baby are "doing just fine." A woman with social phobia may feel overwhelmed or embarrassed, especially if excessive numbers of staff are needed to care for her or her newborn. These women may also exhibit symptoms that mimic more serious medical conditions. Women with specific phobias may exhibit fears that seem irrational to healthcare providers, such as fear of needles or of their own contractions. Such phobias may be difficult to manage intrapartally, and may require pharmacologic intervention.

Schizophrenia is the most disabling psychologic disorder. It is often difficult to treat schizophrenia in pregnant women because many of the medications are contraindicated since they are teratogenic. Women with uncontrolled schizophrenia may have difficulty managing emotions, interacting with the healthcare team, or thinking clearly. The woman's behavior may be dramatically inappropriate or she may simply be withdrawn.

> "*As a nurse-midwife, all of the women I care for are special, but Karen was one person I will never forget. Karen was diagnosed with bipolar disorder with psychotic episodes that became uncontrolled in pregnancy as a result of discontinuing her medication. In labor, she arrived in a manic state. Her speech was excessively fast-paced and she rocked in her bed violently throughout the labor. We ensured her physical safety throughout the labor, monitored her contractions and the baby as infrequently as possible, and provided continuous encouragement. At one point, Karen was adamant everyone must "get low" and sit on the floor to facilitate fetal descent. Although it did not seem rational to us, we did sit on the floor. Remarkably, her anxiety dramatically decreased and the sense of control she felt enabled her to focus and 15 minutes later, she pushed her baby out. At her 6-week postpartum visit, Karen was back on medication and enjoying her new role as a mother.*"

In general, women with psychologic disorders tend to exhibit somewhat exaggerated behaviors during labor. They may need absolute control of everything that happens and refuse to participate until they feel secure. Although responses vary with different disorders, the woman may not be able to articulate her fears or needs, may not respond to supportive nursing measures, may be unaware of what will happen in labor and birth, may be unable to understand what is happening, or may be suddenly overwhelmed by terrifying memories.

> "*One young woman I'll call Cheryl Ann was in preterm labor. I was evaluating her, and she was cooperative but anxious. Then the on-call physician began the vaginal exam. Suddenly, Cheryl Ann's face changed, and she began screaming over and over: "Don't hurt me, I'll do anything you want. No, keep the fire away, please, please, please." She was not with us in the room, she was in another event in her life, and she was terrified! I didn't know what to do. I stayed right beside her and kept talking softly. "It's all right, Cheryl Ann, you are here in the birth center. I'm your nurse. I will stay with you, and I won't let anyone hurt you. There is no fire here. Can you look at me? Hold my hand. You are safe here." She held my hand and in a few moments was able to look at me. She became less anxious and finally was able to be present in her experience.*"

Clinical Therapy

The goal of clinical therapy is to provide support that will help decrease the woman's anxiety, keep her oriented to reality, and promote optimal functioning while in labor. The physician or certified nurse-midwife (CNM) may prescribe a sedative as needed to help with symptoms and may seek the assistance of the on-call psychiatrist to assess and talk with the woman. The physician/CNM may also provide written orders for analgesic medications since relieving the pain may decrease the psychologic symptoms.

NURSING CARE MANAGEMENT

Nursing Assessment and Diagnosis

Unless birth is imminent or severe complications exist, the nurse begins the assessment by reviewing the woman's background. Factors such as age, parity, family support, culture, past and present experiences, and knowledge of the labor process affect the woman's psychologic response to labor. Past or current history of psychologic disorders should be evaluated. Current and past treatment can also yield helpful information.

As labor progresses, the nurse remains alert for the woman's verbal and nonverbal behavioral responses to the pain and anxiety of labor. The woman who is agitated and seems uncooperative or too quiet and compliant may require further appraisal for psychologic symptoms. Questions such as, "Is everything okay?" or "What's going on?" usually indicate some degree of anxiety and concern. Some women may be irritable, require frequent explanations, or repeat the same questions. The nurse further observes for nonverbal cues, including a tense posture, clenched hands, or pain out of context to the stage of labor (Roberts, Reardon, & Rosenfeld, 1999). Recognizing the impact of fatigue on pain and anxiety is another important nursing responsibility. Women with sudden physical complaints need extensive evaluation to determine if the etiology is physical or psychologic. The nurse should assess what coping mechanisms have been effective for the woman in the past.

Nursing diagnoses that may apply to the woman with a psychologic disorder include the following:

- ***Potential Ineffective Individual Coping*** related to increased anxiety and stress
- ***Ineffective Family Coping*** related to anxiety associated with labor and birth
- ***Fear*** related to invasive medical procedures and unknown outcome of birth process
- ***Anxiety*** related to unfamiliar surroundings and care by unknown medical personnel
- ***Sensory/Perceptual Alteration*** related to reactivation of traumatic memories
- ***Impaired Adjustment*** related to delayed developmental tasks of pregnancy

Nursing Plan and Implementation

Primary nursing interventions center on supporting the laboring woman and her family and support persons. If the woman begins to lose her ability to cope or her orientation to reality, the nurse may be able to help her regain control and orientation by:

- Ensuring that the woman's external environment is free from excessive stimuli.
- Maintaining consistency in care providers to the extent possible.
- Encouraging her to identify and to use coping mechanisms that work well for her.
- Identifying and reducing the source of distress if possible.
- Acknowledging the woman's fears, pain, and other symptoms.
- Repeatedly orienting the woman to person, place, and time by statements such as "Janine, I am Tony Martinez and I am your nurse. It is Tuesday and you are in the birthing center because you are in labor now."
- Offering methods to promote relaxation and comfort (see Chapter 24).
- Providing clear but succinct information about the labor process, medical procedures, the environment, simple breathing exercises, and relaxation techniques.
- Employing a calm, caring, confident, and nonjudgmental approach.
- Providing frequent attention and therapeutic interaction.

Although providing emotional support and comfort measures is imperative, some women with severe uncontrolled psychologic disorders may continue to have excessive symptoms throughout labor and birth. Care for these women should focus on maintaining a safe environment and ensuring maternal and fetal well-being. Pharmacologic interventions may be needed to control excessive symptoms.

Evaluation

Expected outcomes of nursing care include the following:

- The woman experiences a decrease in physiologic and psychologic stress and an increase in physiologic and psychologic comfort.
- The woman remains oriented to person, place, and time.
- The woman uses effective coping mechanisms to manage her stress and anxiety in labor.
- The woman's and the family's fear is decreased.
- The woman verbalizes feelings about her labor.

Care of the Woman Experiencing Dystocia Related to Dysfunctional Uterine Contractions

MediaLink DYSTOCIA

Dystocia encompasses many problems in labor, the most common of which is dysfunctional (or uncoordinated) uterine contractions that result in a prolongation of labor. This form of dystocia is the most common indication for cesarean birth in nulliparous women, accounting for 50% of cesarean births in this group. In contrast, dystocia accounts for less than 5% of cesareans in multiparous women (American College of Obstetricians and Gynecologists [ACOG], 2000a).

Contractions associated with normal progress in labor tend to occur regularly, at 3 to 5 contractions per 10 minutes with a mean amplitude of 35 mm Hg in early labor. Later in a normal labor, the contractions progress to 4 to 5 in 10 minutes with a mean amplitude of 40 to 50 mm Hg (ACOG, 2000a). In contrast, dysfunctional uterine contractions typically are irregular, are of low amplitude, and result in a poor pattern of cervical change (less than 1 cm dilatation per hour). Alternatively, cervical dilatation may be arrested; that is, contractions continue but cervical dilatation progresses to a certain point and then remains the same. Figure 26–1 • depicts normal and hypotonic uterine contraction patterns.

Hypertonic Labor Patterns

In hypertonic labor patterns, ineffectual uterine contractions of poor quality occur in the latent phase of labor, and the resting tone of the myometrium increases. Contractions usually become more frequent. Although the contractions are painful, they are ineffective in dilating and effacing the cervix, and a prolonged latent phase may result.

Maternal risks of hypertonic labor include the following:

- Increased discomfort due to uterine muscle cell anoxia
- Fatigue as the pattern continues and no labor progress results
- Stress on coping abilities
- Dehydration and increased incidence of infection if labor is prolonged

Fetal-neonatal risks include the following:

- Fetal distress because contractions and increased resting tone interfere with the uteroplacental exchange
- Prolonged pressure on the fetal head, which may result in cephalhematoma, caput succedaneum, or excessive molding

CLINICAL THERAPY

Management of hypertonic labor may include bed rest and sedation to promote relaxation and reduce pain. If the hypertonic pattern continues and develops into a prolonged latent phase, oxytocin infusion or amniotomy may be considered (see Chapter 27). These methods are instituted only after cephalopelvic disproportion (CPD) and fetal malrepresentation have been ruled out. CPD is a disparity between the size of the maternal pelvis and the size of the presenting fetal head due to position, presentation, or increased fetal weight that precludes a vaginal birth. When an oxytocin infusion is used to stimulate uterine contractions, the physician or certified nurse-midwife (CNM) needs to assess whether vaginal birth is possible (ie, whether the maternal pelvis is large enough for the fetus to pass through). If the maternal pelvis diameters are less than average, or if the fetus is particularly large or is in

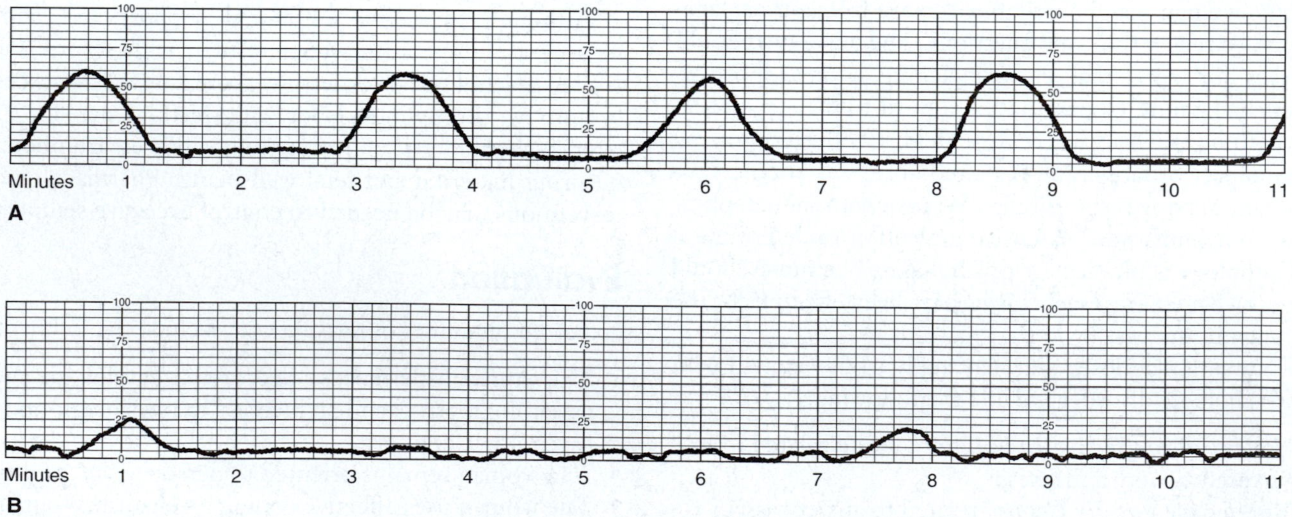

Figure 26–1 • Comparison of labor patterns. *A,* Normal uterine contraction pattern. Note that the contraction frequency is every 3 minutes; duration is 60 seconds. The baseline resting tone is below 10 mm Hg. *B,* Hypotonic uterine contraction pattern. Note in this example that the contraction frequency is every 7 minutes with some uterine activity between contractions, duration is 50 seconds, and intensity increases approximately 25 mm Hg during contractions.

a malpresentation or malposition, CPD is said to be present. In the presence of true CPD, labor is not stimulated because vaginal birth is not possible.

NURSING CARE MANAGEMENT

Nursing Assessment and Diagnosis

As part of the labor assessment, the nurse should evaluate the relationship between the intensity of the pain being experienced and the degree to which the cervix is dilating and effacing. The nurse should also note whether anxiety is negatively affecting labor progress. Evidence of increasing frustration and discouragement on the part of the mother and her partner may indicate that the nurse needs to provide some additional information or assurance.

Nursing diagnoses that may apply to the woman in hypertonic labor include the following:

- ***Pain*** related to the woman's inability to relax secondary to hypertonic uterine contractions
- ***Ineffective Individual Coping*** related to ineffectiveness of breathing techniques to relieve discomfort
- ***Anxiety*** related to slow labor progress

Nursing Plan and Implementation

A key nursing responsibility is to provide comfort and support to the laboring woman and her partner. The woman experiencing a hypertonic labor pattern will probably be very uncomfortable because of the increased force of contractions. Her anxiety level and that of her partner may be high. The nurse attempts to reduce the woman's discomfort and promote a more effective labor pattern.

The nurse may suggest supportive measures such as a change of position: left lateral side-lying, high Fowler's, rocking in a rocking chair, sitting up, or walking. Soothing measures include a warm shower, whirlpool, quiet environment, backrub, therapeutic touch, and visualization. Mouth care, change of linens, effleurage, and relaxation exercises may provide comfort. If sedation is ordered, the nurse ensures that the environment is conducive to relaxation. The labor partner may also need assistance in helping the woman cope. A calm, understanding approach by the nurse offers the woman and her partner further support. Providing information about the cause of the hypertonic labor pattern and assuring the woman that she is not overreacting to the situation are important nursing actions.

Client education is key for the woman experiencing hypertonic labor. She needs information about the dysfunctional labor pattern and the possible implications for herself and her baby. Information will help relieve anxiety and thereby increase relaxation and comfort. The nurse needs to explain treatment options and offer opportunities to ask questions.

Evaluation

Anticipated outcomes of nursing care include the following:

- The woman has increased comfort and decreased anxiety.
- The woman and her partner are able to cope with the labor.
- The woman experiences a more effective labor pattern.

Hypotonic Labor Patterns

The specific cause of hypotonic contractions is unknown; however, genetic factors may control the normal physiologic processes of labor. Cesarean birth and operative vaginal birth (use of forceps or vacuum extractor), for example, tend to run in families. Some research suggests there is a relationship between uterine dysfunction and advancing maternal age. Thus age over 25 is sometimes cited as a risk factor for uterine dysfunction (ACOG, 2000a).

The familial tendencies for difficult labor give rise to the theory that genetic processes control normal labor. It is hypothesized that there may be an inheritable tendency toward poor uterine contractions and/or soft-tissue relaxation (Dizon-Townson & Ward, 1997). In one study, nulliparas who underwent cesarean birth because of prolonged labor had a "significantly higher concentration of collagen, with a decrease in solubility, in the uterine isthmus and cervix" (Dizon-Townson & Ward, 1997). Further research may establish additional evidence of a familial alteration in collagen composition.

> ***Clinical Tip*** *As you know, normal cervical dilatation in a first-time mother—commonly known as a "primip"— is just over 1.0 cm per hour, and dilatation in a "multip" is about 1.5 cm per hour. If your assessments reveal that this expected pattern is not occurring, consider that a problem may be developing. The most likely causes of the problem are related to either the contractions or to fetal position or size.*

CLINICAL THERAPY

When uterine contractions are irregular and of low amplitude and there is commonly less than 1 cm cervical dilatation per hour (called protracted labor) or there has been no change of cervical dilatation for 2 hours (arrest of progress), the physician/CNM evaluates the woman for the presence of any factor that would preclude the use of oxytocin (Pitocin) augmentation. The physician/CNM evaluates the size of the maternal pelvis, the position and presentation of the fetus, and fetal weight. The physician/CNM carefully considers the possibility of CPD. Station is a key component when evaluating for CPD. If the presenting part is not engaged ("out of the pelvis"), especially in a nulliparous woman, it is possible that CPD is present. The physician/CNM may attempt to push the presenting part into the pelvis with fundal pressure to assess if CPD exists. If CPD exists, oxytocin (Pitocin) augmentation should not be used.

When CPD is ruled out, an amniotomy (artificial rupture of membranes [AROM]) can be performed if membranes are intact. Studies of the effectiveness of amniotomy have not demonstrated conclusive results. Amniotomy should not be performed if the presenting part is not well applied to the cervix since this increases the risk of cord prolapse (discussed later in the chapter). However, it is an accepted procedure with the diagnosis of dystocia secondary to uterine hypocontractility (ACOG, 1995). Oxytocin (Pitocin) augmentation can be implemented if adequate contractions do not occur. (See Drug Guide: Oxytocin in Chapter 27.)

ACOG has outlined two regimens of oxytocin administration: a low-dose regimen and a high-dose regimen. (See complete discussion in Chapter 27.) Low-dose regimens in which the frequency of increases are less help prevent uterine hyperstimulation. High-dose regimens are said to shorten the length of labor, decrease the incidence of chorioamnionitis, and decrease the incidence of cesarean births related to dystocia (ACOG, 1999a). Continuous electronic fetal monitoring (EFM) is used to provide ongoing information regarding fetal response to the augmentation. With augmentation of labor, the contraction pattern and progressive cervical dilatation pattern should improve, and fetal descent (measured by station) should occur. If there is no improvement in these areas, cesarean birth may be necessary.

Some practitioners support the use of **active management of labor (AMOL).** This method of labor management of nulliparous women has four components: (1) standardized criteria for diagnosis of labor, (2) standardized method of labor management, (3) one-to-one nursing care throughout the course of labor, and (4) prenatal education to teach women about the protocol (ACOG, 2000a). In this process labor is managed from the beginning with amniotomy, timed cervical examinations, and augmentation of labor with intravenous oxytocin if adequate progress is not made. Supporters of AMOL contend that it is preventive treatment that reduces the potential for protracted labor or arrest of progress. AMOL begins with careful assessment of the laboring woman, AROM (if the membranes are still intact) within 1 hour of diagnosis of the presence of actual labor, and hourly cervical examinations for the first 3 hours. Thereafter cervical examinations are performed every 2 hours, and at least 1 additional centimeter of dilatation is expected at each examination. If cervical dilatation is less than expected, augmentation with an intravenous oxytocin infusion is begun. AMOL also incorporates a strong one-to-one nursing care program, in which the nurse remains with the woman. This permits ongoing assessment and provides the beneficial aspect of constant nursing support (Lopez-Zeno, 1997). Proponents of AMOL believe that its use can avoid dysfunctional labor patterns, instrument-assisted birth, and cesarean birth.

Those who oppose AMOL, in contrast, contend that labor needs to be considered a normal process and allowed to progress without automatic intervention. Frequent examinations can increase the risk of maternal fever, intrauterine infection, and fetal compromise. Although some women may not strictly adhere to the expected normal time limits of labor, many will go on to give birth without complications if given an opportunity to progress through labor at their own pace. Just as all women do not have the same emotional reactions to labor, all women do not go through labor at the same pace and speed. Only if problems occur should the labor be augmented.

NURSING CARE MANAGEMENT

Nursing Assessment and Diagnosis

Assessing maternal vital signs, contractions, cervical dilatation, fetal descent, and fetal heart rate characteristics provides the nurse with data to evaluate maternal-fetal status. The nurse also assesses for signs and symptoms of infection and dehydration. During the vaginal examination, the fetal presenting part (usually vertex) is assessed for the development of a caput. If the fetal vertex presses down on the cervix during contractions without further descent, a *caput succedaneum* may occur. As hypotonic labor continues, the caput increases in size; it seems that the head is descending, but it is not (Figure 26–2 •).

Because labor progress is slow, the nurse assesses the woman's stress and coping, noting whether anxiety is having a deleterious effect on labor progress. Evidence of increasing frustration and discouragement on the part of the mother and her partner may become apparent as labor continues.

Nursing diagnoses that may apply to the woman experiencing dysfunctional labor include the following:

- ***Pain*** related to the woman's difficulty in relaxing secondary to uterine contractions
- ***Risk for Ineffective Individual Coping*** related to ineffectiveness of breathing techniques to relieve discomfort
- ***Anxiety*** related to slow labor progress

Nursing Plan and Implementation

Nursing measures are aimed at promoting maternal and fetal well-being. The nurse frequently monitors maternal

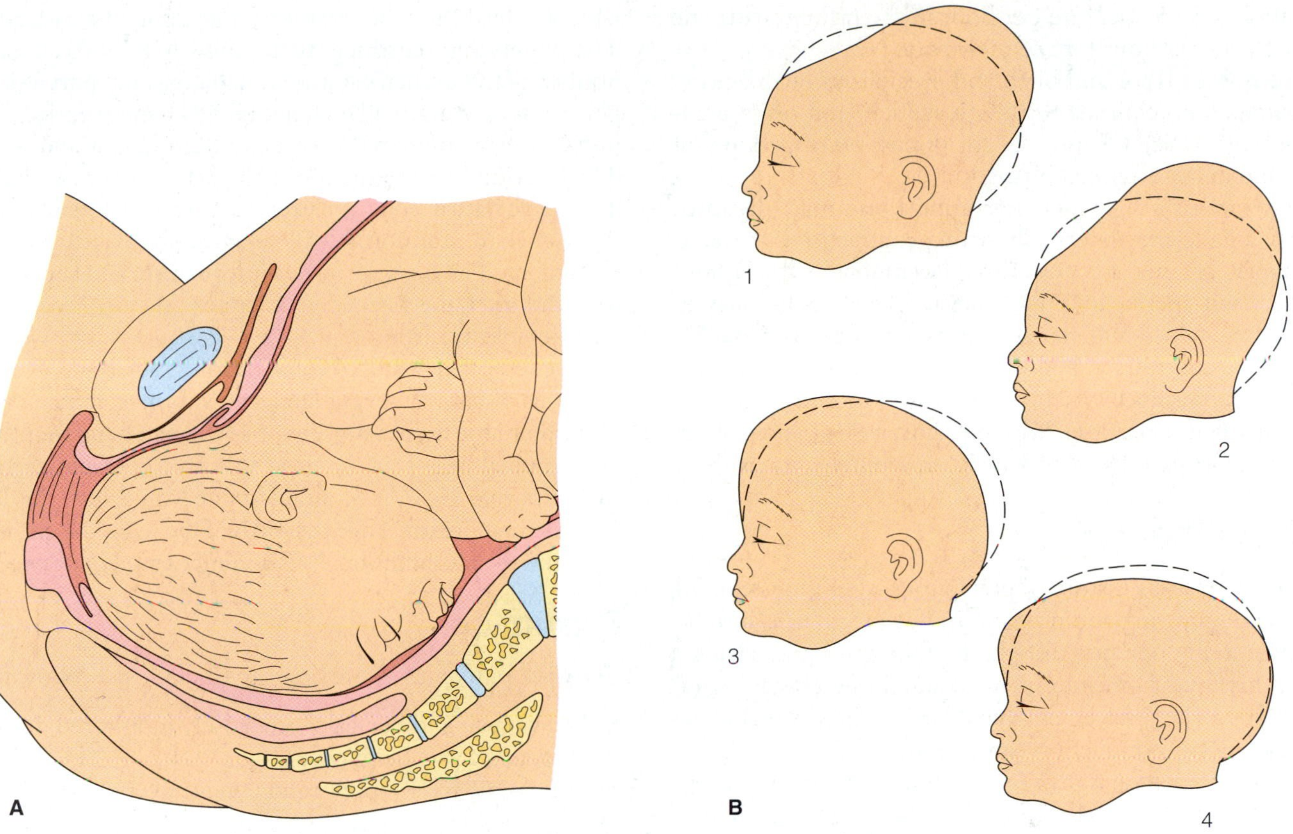

Figure 26–2 • Effects of labor on the fetal head. *A,* Caput succedaneum formation. The presenting portion of the scalp area is encircled by the cervix during labor, causing swelling of the soft tissue. *B,* Molding of the fetal head in cephalic presentations: (1) occiput anterior, (2) occiput posterior, (3) brow, (4) face.

vital signs; notes the frequency, duration, and strength of contractions; and assesses the fetal heart rate. Once the amniotic membranes are ruptured, the nurse assesses the amount of fluid and the presence of blood or meconium (dark green or black stool present in the large intestine of the fetus). Since meconium can be associated with fetal stress, ongoing observation of the amniotic fluid is critical. Maternal hydration status can be monitored by recording intake and output. The nurse assesses the bladder every 2 hours for distention; an in-and-out catheterization can be performed for women unable to void on their own.

Ongoing evaluation for symptoms of infection should be performed, especially for prolonged labors. These symptoms include fever, chills, foul-smelling amniotic fluid, and fetal tachycardia. Vaginal examinations should be kept to a minimum to reduce the incidence of infections.

The laboring woman needs information about the hypotonic labor pattern and the possible implications for herself and her baby. It is particularly important to address the couple's concerns and questions with clear, accurate information. They need to be informed of progress and possible treatment measures. Disadvantages and treatment alternatives also need to be discussed and understood by the woman and her support person.

Evaluation

Expected outcomes of nursing care include the following:

- The woman and her partner understand the labor pattern and its possible implications.
- The woman and her partner are able to cope with the labor.
- The woman's comfort increases and her anxiety decreases.
- The woman experiences a more effective labor pattern.

Care of the Woman and Fetus at Risk for Precipitous Labor and Birth

Precipitous labor and birth occurs when the entire process of labor and birth occurs within 3 hours. The most common causes are abnormally low resistance in maternal soft tissues, which allows for rapid cervical dilatation and fetal descent, and abnormally strong uterine contractions (Cunningham, MacDonald, Gant, et al, 2001). In precipitous labor, cervical dilatation is 5 cm or more per hour in the primigravida and up to 10 cm per hour for the multipara.

Precipitous labor and birth and precipitous birth are not the same. A precipitous birth is a sudden, and often unattended, birth. See Chapter 24 for discussion of precipitous birth and nurse-attended births.

Maternal risks may include abruptio placentae (discussed shortly) due to the abnormally strong contractions. If maternal tissues are not soft, extensive lacerations of the cervix, vagina, and perineum may occur. Fetal risks include meconium-stained fluid that may be aspirated at birth, low Apgar scores, and intracranial trauma resulting from the rapid birth and resistance of the birth canal to the fetal head (Cunningham et al, 2001). Women who have had a precipitous labor and birth are also at risk for postpartum hemorrhage.

Clinical Therapy

Any woman with a history of precipitous labor requires close medical monitoring and preparation for precipitous birth to facilitate a safe outcome for the mother and fetus. Women with a history of precipitous birth should be closely monitored for cervical effacement and dilatation in the final weeks of pregnancy. An induction can be scheduled to control the birth environment and prevent complications that can occur with an unattended birth. Drugs such as magnesium sulfate or a tocolytic agent such as terbutaline may be used to slow the uterine contractions (Cunningham et al, 2001). (See Drug Guide: Magnesium Sulfate in Chapter 20.)

NURSING CARE MANAGEMENT

Nursing Assessment and Diagnosis

During the intrapartal nursing assessment, the nurse can identify a woman at increased risk of precipitous labor. (For example, a previous history of precipitate or short labor places a woman at risk.) During the labor, accelerated cervical dilatation and fetal descent and intense contractions with little uterine relaxation between contractions are indicative of precipitous labor.

Nursing diagnoses that may apply to the woman with precipitous labor include the following:

- ***Risk for Injury*** related to rapid labor and birth
- ***Pain*** related to rapid labor process

Nursing Plan and Implementation

If the woman has a history of precipitous labor, it is imperative that the nurse establish rapport quickly because the nurse and woman may be involved in another precipitous labor and birth, and the situation has the potential to be tense. The physician or certified nurse-midwife (CNM) should be notified of the woman's status immediately. Rapport and support from the nurse will enhance all other interventions. The nurse closely monitors the woman's contractions and cervical dilatation, and an emergency birth pack is kept near the bed. The nurse stays in constant attendance if at all possible, assists the woman to a comfortable position, and provides a quiet environment. The nurse provides information and support before and after the birth. See Chapter 24, for discussion of nurse-managed birth.

The fetus is monitored for signs of hypoxia and other indications of nonreassuring fetal status. If meconium staining of the amniotic fluid is present, the fetal nares and mouth will be suctioned just after the head is born to prevent the baby from drawing more meconium-stained fluid into the lungs with the first breath. After the birth of the baby, the cords will be visualized and additional suctioning carried out as needed.

Evaluation

Expected outcomes of nursing care include the following:

- The woman and her baby are closely monitored during labor, and a safe birth occurs.
- The couple feels support and enhanced comfort during labor and birth.

Care of the Woman with Postterm Pregnancy

Postterm pregnancy is one that extends more than 294 days or 42 completed weeks past the first day of the last menstrual period. It is important to understand the phrase "42 completed weeks." "Pregnancies between 41 weeks 1 day and 41 weeks 6 days, although in the 42nd week, do not complete 42 weeks until the 7th day has elapsed" (Cunningham et al, 2001, p. 730). The incidence of postterm pregnancy is approximately 3% to 7% of all pregnancies in the United States. Postterm pregnancy occurs more frequently in primigravidas and women over 35.

The most frequent cause of postterm pregnancy is error in determining the time of ovulation and conception according to the first day of the last menstrual period. This error can be corrected by performing ultrasound scans between 14 and 22 weeks. The scan reveals the biparietal diameter of the fetal head, which is then compared to conventional dating tables. The cause of true postterm pregnancy is unknown.

Maternal Risks

Although postterm pregnancy does not pose any significant risk to the woman during the pregnancy, the labor and birth process may be affected. In many instances, labor is induced. Because postterm pregnancy is associated with an increased incidence of large-for-gestational-age (LGA) or macrosomic (weight in excess of 4500 g) fetuses, vaginal birth is frequently associated with the use of forceps or vacuum extractor. Maternal hemorrhage may occur. Cesarean birth may also be necessary. Many women experience anxiety and are emotionally fatigued as their estimated date of birth (EDB) passes. Normal discomforts associated with late pregnancy persist which can lead to irritability and loss of sleep.

> *When I went over my due date, I felt so anxious and overwhelmed. I was mentally prepared to carry my baby until a certain date, but once that date was reached, I felt unable to deal with all of the discomforts of pregnancy. I couldn't sleep well. I was uncomfortable eating, walking, even putting on my shoes. Well-wishing friends and family would call and say "Haven't you had that baby yet?" The calls just made it worse. I can't tell you how relieved I was when labor started and I knew I would soon meet my new baby.*

Fetal-Neonatal Risks

True postterm pregnancies are frequently associated with placental changes that cause a decrease in the uterine-placental-fetal circulation. This decrease reduces the blood supply, oxygen, and nutrition for the fetus. Oligohydramnios (decreased amount of amniotic fluid) is frequently present and may increase the risk of umbilical cord compression (because the cord does not have as much fluid to float in). In such cases, the fetus is more likely to be small-for-gestational-age (SGA) due to decreased nutrition associated with decreased utero-placental-fetal circulation. If utero-placental-fetal circulation is not compromised, the fetus continues to gain weight until the 42nd week; therefore, the fetus is often LGA and macrosomic. The LGA or macrosomic fetus has a higher incidence of birth trauma or shoulder dystocia (difficulty or inability to deliver the baby's shoulders) (Cunningham et al, 2001). During labor, the postterm fetus may have meconium staining of the amniotic fluid which can lead to fetal stress and meconium aspiration at birth (Cunningham et al, 2001). Perinatal mortality is slightly increased.

Clinical Therapy

When the 40th week of gestation is completed and birth has not occurred, most practitioners begin using the nonstress test (NST), biophysical profile (BPP) (especially the amniotic fluid volume portion of the BPP), and Doppler flow studies as assessment tools. According to ACOG, there is not consensus on the frequency of antenatal surveillance. No evidence exists that indicates more favorable outcomes between 40 and 42 completed weeks (ACOG, 1999a). Any time that tests indicate fetal problems or there is decreased amniotic fluid volume, induction of labor is recommended (Cunningham et al, 2001).

NURSING CARE MANAGEMENT

Nursing Assessment and Diagnosis

When the woman is admitted into the birthing area, it is important to establish the EDB and ascertain the type of antenatal testing that has been completed. During labor, ongoing assessments of the fetal heart rate (FHR) by continuous electronic fetal monitoring (EFM) are important to identify reassuring characteristics (presence of short-term and long-term variability, accelerations with fetal movement) and to determine the presence of nonperiodic variable decelerations so that corrective actions may be taken. When amniotic membranes rupture, the nurse assesses the fluid for the presence of meconium. Ongoing assessments of labor progress (contractions, progressive cervical dilatation and effacement, and fetal descent) may provide clues to the presence of a macrosomic fetus because labor may be lengthened and fetal descent may not occur.

Possible nursing diagnoses for the woman with postterm pregnancy include the following:

- ***Fear*** related to the unknown outcome for the baby
- ***Risk for Ineffective Individual Coping*** or ***Ineffective Family Coping*** related to concern regarding the status of the baby

Nursing Plan and Implementation

Community-Based Nursing Care

If the woman has not been assessing fetal activity every day, the nurse teaches her how to do it so that she can identify inadequate fetal movement and contact her healthcare provider (see Chapter 21 for further discussion of techniques to detect fetal movement). The nurse encourages the woman to keep all appointments for BPPs and other testing and provides information regarding the postterm pregnancy and the antenatal testing that will be indicated. In addition, the nurse addresses the implications and associated risks for the baby, as well as possible treatment plans, and provides the woman and her partner opportunities to ask questions and clarify information.

Hospital-Based Nursing Care

In the birth setting, the response of the fetus during labor is assessed carefully. Continuous electronic monitoring of FHR is important to determine whether reassuring characteristics are present and to detect variable decelerations, especially if oligohydramnios is present. If variable decelerations are present, the laboring woman's position is changed to attempt to take pressure off the umbilical cord, and FHR is reevaluated. When an amnioinfusion is performed to increase the volume of fluid or to dilute meconium-stained fluid, the nurse assists with the procedure and monitors the infusion and the response of the FHR. (See Chapter 27 for further discussion.)

Evaluation

Expected outcomes of nursing care include the following:

- The woman is able to explain the implications of the postterm pregnancy.
- The woman and her partner and family feel supported and able to cope with the labor and birth.
- Fetal problems are identified quickly.

Care of the Woman and Fetus at Risk Due to Fetal Malposition

Persistent occiput-posterior (OP) position of the fetus is the most common fetal malposition, occurring in approximately 25% of pregnancies at term (Cunningham et al, 2001). This position may be normal in some races, particularly those whose women tend to have a small pelvis. For a fetus in an OP position to rotate to an occiput-anterior (OA) position, it must rotate 135 degrees (ROP to ROT to ROA to OA), and in most cases this rotation is accomplished. In others, however, it is not. Labor progress may cease or the fetus may be born in a posterior position.

Maternal-Fetal-Neonatal Risks

The woman usually experiences intense pain in the small of her back throughout the labor, unless the baby rotates. At birth, if the fetus remains in a posterior position, the woman may suffer a third- or fourth-degree perineal laceration or extension of a midline episiotomy. There is no increased risk of fetal mortality due to the OP position unless labor is protracted or an operative birth is performed.

Clinical Therapy

Medical treatment focuses on close monitoring of both maternal and fetal status and labor progress to determine whether vaginal or cesarean birth is the safer method. According to Cunningham et al (2001), vaginal birth is possible via:

1. Spontaneous birth
2. Forceps-assisted birth with the occiput directly posterior
3. Forceps rotation of the occiput to the anterior position and birth (Scanzoni maneuver; Figure 26–3 •)
4. Manual rotation to the anterior position followed by forceps-assisted birth (Figure 26–4 •)

If the pelvis has larger diameters and the perineal muscles are relaxed, as found in grandmultiparity, the fetus may have no particular problem emerging spontaneously in the OP position. If, however, the perineum is rigid, the second stage of labor may be prolonged. A prolonged second stage is one that lasts over an hour in multiparas and 2 hours or more in nulliparas.

In the event of a prolonged second stage with arrest of descent due to OP position, a midforceps or manual rotation may be done if no cephalopelvic disproportion (CPD) is present. In cases of CPD, cesarean birth is the preferred treatment.

NURSING CARE MANAGEMENT

Nursing Assessment and Diagnosis

The first sign of occiput-posterior position is intense back pain in the first stage of labor. The back pain is

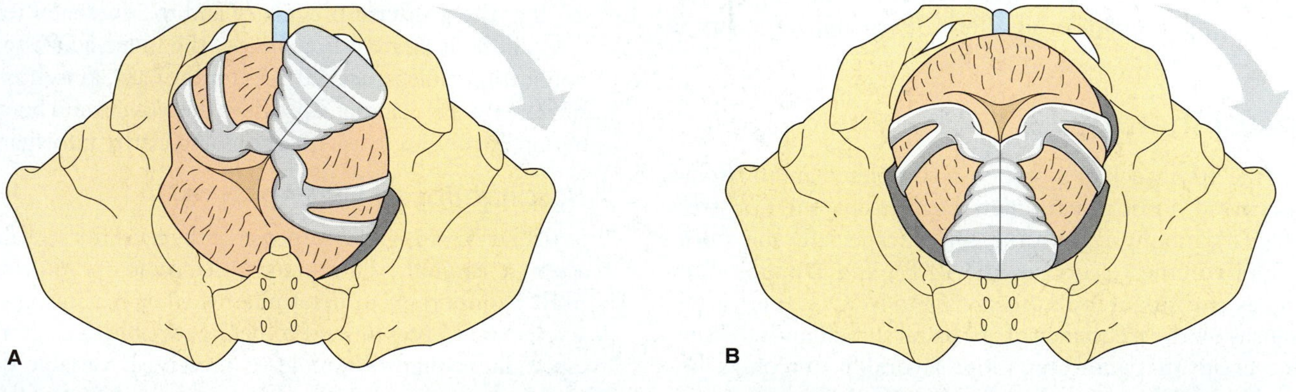

Figure 26–3 • Scanzoni maneuver, anterior rotation. *A,* Forceps are applied to the fetal head, which is in ROP position. Fetal head is then rotated 45 degrees to ROT, then another 45 degrees to ROA, then a final 45 degrees to OA. *B,* The fetal position has now changed from ROP to OA for a total rotation of 135 degrees. The forceps are now upside down, so they are removed and reapplied to provide the traction necessary for a forceps-assisted birth.

SOURCE: Oxorn, H., and Foote, W. (1986). *Human labor and birth* (5th ed., p. 401). Norwalk, CT: Appleton & Lange. Reproduced with permission of The McGraw-Hill Companies.

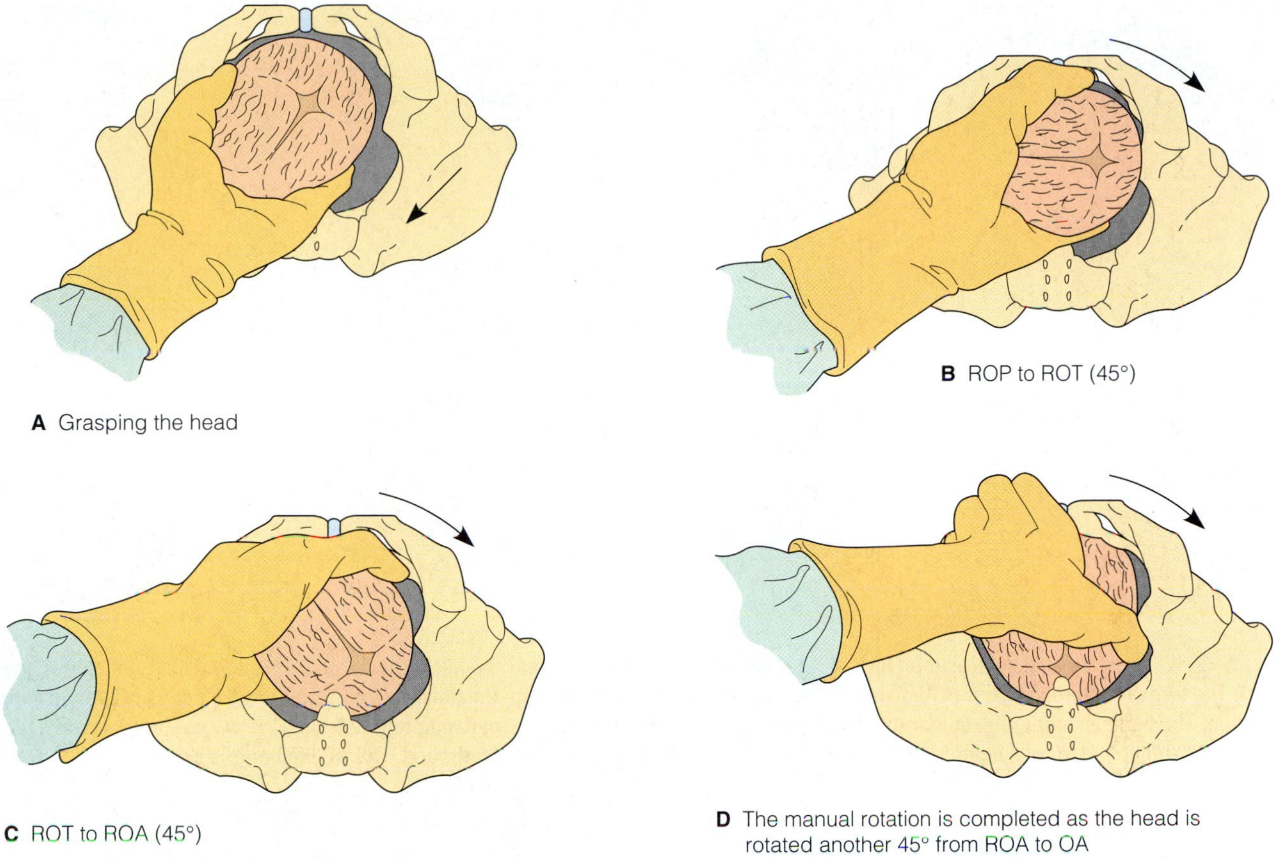
A Grasping the head
B ROP to ROT (45°)
C ROT to ROA (45°)
D The manual rotation is completed as the head is rotated another 45° from ROA to OA

Figure 26–4 • Manual rotation of ROP to OA. *A,* The physician's left hand is inserted into the vagina and the back of the fetal head is grasped. *B,* The head is flexed and then rotated 45 degrees to ROT. *C,* The head is rotated another 45 degrees to ROA. *D,* The manual rotation is completed as the head is rotated another 45 degrees from ROA to OA. During the manual rotation, the physician's other hand is placed on the maternal abdomen, and the body is turned in the same direction as the head by applying pressure to the fetal breech or shoulders.

caused by the fetal occiput compressing the sacral nerves. Other signs and symptoms may include a dysfunctional labor pattern, a prolonged active phase, secondary arrest of dilatation, or arrest of descent. Further assessment may reveal a depression in the maternal abdomen above the symphysis pubis (because the fetal face, rather than the back of its head, is turned up against the symphysis). Fetal heart rate may be heard far laterally on the maternal abdomen, and on vaginal examination the nurse will find the wide diamond-shaped anterior fontanelle in the anterior portion of the pelvis. This fontanelle may be difficult to feel because of molding of the fetal head.

Nursing diagnoses that may apply to women with persistent OP position include the following:

- ***Pain*** related to back discomfort secondary to occiput-posterior position
- ***Ineffective Individual Coping*** related to persistent back pain

Nursing Plan and Implementation

Changing maternal posture has been used for many years to enhance rotation of OP or OT to OA. The woman may be placed on one side and then asked to move to the other side as the fetus begins to rotate. This side-lying position may promote rotation; it also enables the support person to apply counterpressure on the sacral area to decrease discomfort. A knee-chest position provides a downward slant to the vaginal canal, directing the fetal head downward on descent and is often effective in rotating the fetus. In addition to maintaining a hands-and-knees position on the bed, the woman may do pelvic rocking, and the support person may perform firm stroking motions on the abdomen. The stroking begins over the fetal back and swings around to the other side of the abdomen. After the fetus has rotated, the woman lies in Sims' position on the side opposite the fetal back. In addition to assuming these positions, the woman may want to sit on the toilet, walk around the room, stand beside the bed and lean forward with her hands on the bed and do the pelvic rock, rest in a whirlpool, or lie on her side in the bed.

Evaluation

Expected outcomes of nursing care include the following:

- The woman's discomfort is decreased.
- The woman and her partner apply comfort measures and position changes that assist her.

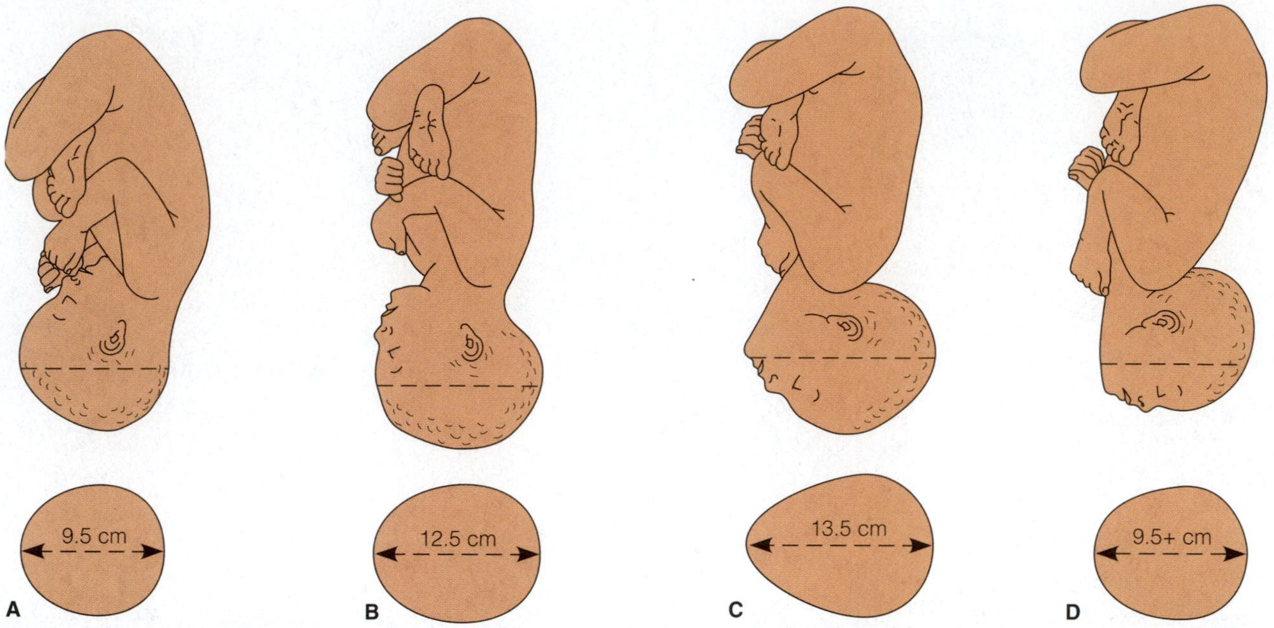

Figure 26–5 • Types of cephalic presentations. *A,* The occiput is the presenting part because the head is flexed and the fetal chin is against the chest. The largest anteroposterior (AP) diameter that presents and passes through the pelvis is approximately 9.5 cm. *B,* Military (sinciput) presentation. The head is neither flexed nor extended. The presenting AP diameter is approximately 12.5 cm. *C,* Brow presentation. The largest diameter of the fetal head (approximately 13.5 cm) presents in this situation. *D,* Face presentation. The AP diameter is 9.5 cm.
SOURCE: Danforth, D. N., & Scott, J. R. (Eds.). (1990). *Obstetrics and gynecology* (5th ed., p. 170, fig. 8–9). New York: Lippincott.

- The woman's coping abilities are strengthened.
- The woman and her partner state that they feel supported and encouraged.

Care of the Woman and Fetus at Risk Due to Fetal Malpresentation

In a normal cephalic presentation, the occiput is the presenting part (Figure 26–5, *A* •). Three cephalic presentations are classified as abnormal presentations: military (sinciput), brow, and face (Figure 26–5, *B–D*). The fetal body straightens out in these malpresentations from the classic fetal position to an S-shaped position. Of these, the military presentation is probably the least difficult for the woman and fetus. In most cases, as soon as the head reaches the pelvic floor, flexion occurs and a vaginal birth results. Thus, of the cephalic malpresentations, only brow and face are discussed here.

In addition to the cephalic malpresentations, the breech, shoulder (transverse lie), and compound presentations can cause significant difficulty during labor. These malpresentations are also discussed in this chapter.

Brow Presentation

Brow presentations are the least common of all presentations with an incidence of 1 in 1500 births to 1 in 3543 births (Parker & Napolitano, 2001). In a brow presentation, the forehead of the fetus becomes the presenting part. The fetal head is slightly extended instead of flexed, with the result that the fetal head enters the birth canal with the widest diameter of the head (occipitomental) foremost (Figure 26–5, *C*). Although no specific cause can be identified, proposed causes include high parity, placenta previa, uterine anomaly, hydramnios, fetal anomaly, low birth weight, and large fetus.

Cesarean birth is preferred in the presence of cephalopelvic disproportion (CPD) or failure of a brow presentation to convert to a normal vertex or face presentation. If a vaginal birth is attempted, the woman will probably have an episiotomy and may require extension of the episiotomy at the moment of birth.

Fetal mortality is increased because of injuries received during the birth. Trauma during the birth process can include cerebral and neck compression, and damage to the trachea and larynx.

CLINICAL THERAPY

Active medical intervention is not necessary as long as cervical dilatation and fetal descent are occurring. If labor progress is slow, clinical pelvimetry findings and ultrasound to determine the presence of fetal anomalies are important. Oxytocin may be used with caution to correct an inadequate labor pattern, as 30% to 50% of these labors are prolonged. Use of forceps or manual conversion is contraindicated (Parker & Napolitano, 2001). If problems occur, cesarean birth is indicated.

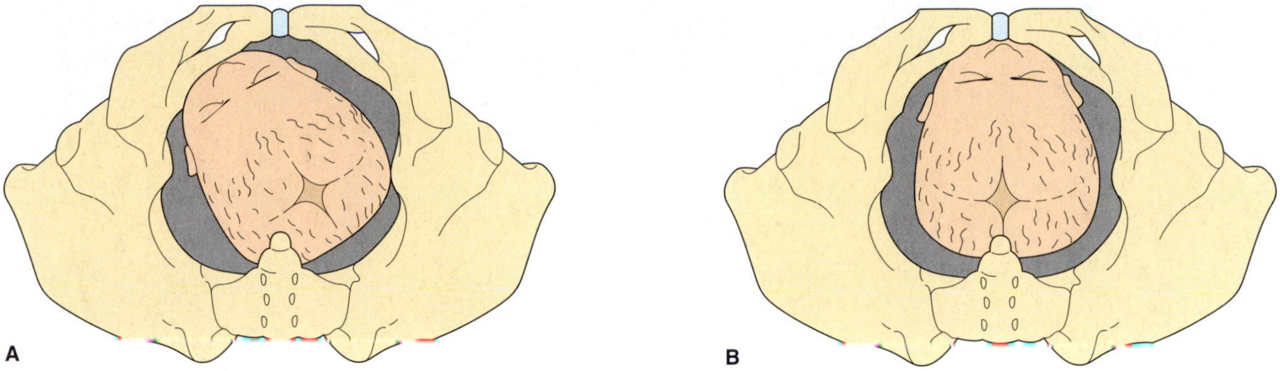

Figure 26–6 • Brow presentation. *A,* Descent. *B,* Internal rotation in the pelvic cavity.
SOURCE: Oxorn, H., and Foote, W. (1986). *Human labor and birth* (5th ed., p. 211). Norwalk, CT: Appleton & Lange. Reproduced with permission of The McGraw-Hill Companies.

NURSING CARE MANAGEMENT

Nursing Assessment and Diagnosis

Leopold's maneuvers suggest a brow presentation when both the chin and occiput are palpable. A brow presentation may be detected on vaginal examination by palpation of the diamond-shaped anterior fontanelle and orbital ridges (Figure 26–6 •).

Nursing diagnoses that may apply to brow presentation include the following:

- ***Anxiety*** or ***Fear*** related to outcome for fetus
- ***Deficient Knowledge*** related to lack of information about possible maternal-fetal effects of brow presentation
- ***Risk for Injury*** to the fetus related to pressure on fetal structures secondary to brow presentation

Nursing Plan and Implementation

Nursing management of the brow presentation includes close observation of the woman for labor aberrations and of the fetus for signs of nonreassuring fetal status. The fetus should be observed closely during labor for signs of hypoxia as evidenced by periodic (late) decelerations.

The nurse may need to explain the position of the fetus to the laboring couple or to interpret what the physician or certified nurse-midwife (CNM) has told them. The nurse should stay close at hand to reassure the couple, inform them of any changes, and assist them with labor-coping techniques.

In both brow and face presentation, the appearance of the newborn may be affected. The couple may need help in beginning the attachment process because of the newborn's facial appearance. After the infant is inspected for gross abnormalities, the pediatrician and nurse can assure the couple that the facial edema and excessive molding are only temporary and will subside in a few days.

Evaluation

Expected outcomes of nursing care include the following:

- The woman and her partner understand the implications and associated problems of brow presentation.
- The mother and her baby have a safe labor and birth.

Face Presentation

In a face presentation, the face of the fetus is the presenting part. The fetal head is hyperextended even more than in the brow presentation. Face presentation occurs most frequently in multiparous, in preterm birth, and in the presence of anencephaly. The incidence of face presentation is about 1 in 500 births overall or 0.2% of all births (Parker & Napolitano, 2001).

The risks of CPD and prolonged labor are increased with face presentation. As with any prolonged labor, the chance of infection is increased.

The fetus may develop edema, making vaginal examination for placement of heart rate electrodes difficult. After birth the edema gives the newborn an unusual appearance. As with the brow presentation, the neck and internal structures may swell as a result of trauma received during descent. Petechiae and ecchymoses are often seen in the superficial layers of the facial skin because of the birth trauma.

CLINICAL THERAPY

If no CPD is present, the mentum (chin) is anterior, and the labor pattern is effective, the objective of medical treatment is a vaginal birth (Figure 26–7 •). Mentum posteriors can become wedged on the anterior surface of the sacrum (Figure 26–8 •). In this case as well as in the presence of CPD, cesarean is the preferred method of birth.

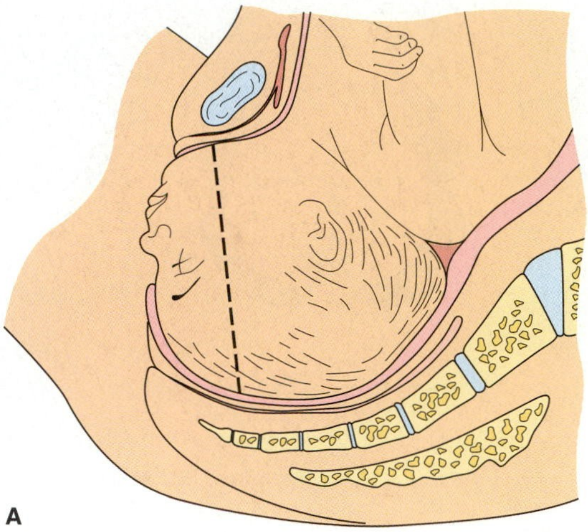

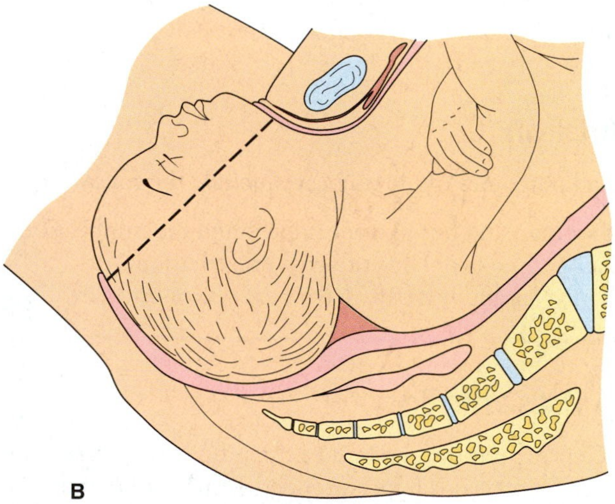

Figure 26–7 • Face presentation. Mechanism of birth in mentoanterior position. *A,* The submentobregmatic diameter at the outlet. *B,* The fetal head is born by movement of flexion.

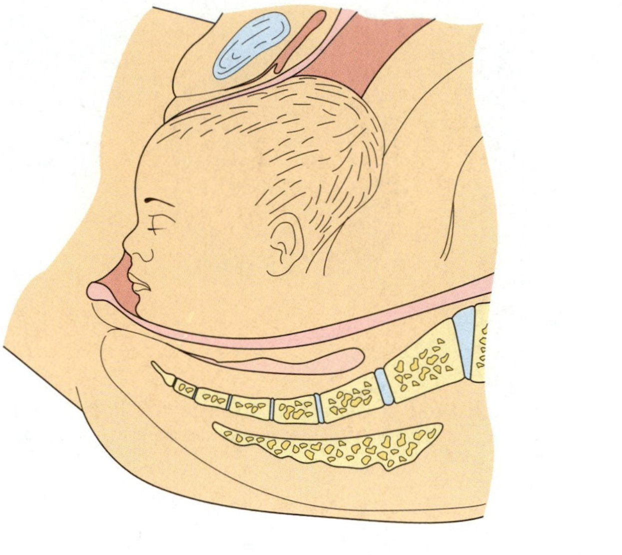

Figure 26–8 • Face presentation. Mechanism of birth in mentoposterior position. Fetal head is unable to extend farther. The face becomes impacted.

NURSING CARE MANAGEMENT

Nursing Assessment and Diagnosis

When performing Leopold's maneuvers, the nurse finds that the back of the fetus is difficult to outline, and a deep furrow can be palpated between the hard occiput and the fetal back (Figure 26–9 •). Fetal heart tones can be heard on the side where the fetal feet are palpated. It may be difficult to determine by vaginal examination whether a breech or a face is presenting, especially if facial edema is already present. During the vaginal examination, palpation of the saddle of the nose and the gums should be attempted. When assessing engagement, the nurse needs to remember that the face has to be deep within the pelvis before the biparietal diameter has entered the inlet.

Nursing diagnoses that may apply to the woman with a fetus in face presentation include the following:

- ***Fear*** related to unknown outcome of the labor and appearance of the baby
- ***Risk for Injury*** to the newborn's face related to edema secondary to the birth process

Nursing Plan and Implementation

Nursing interventions are the same as for the brow presentation.

Evaluation

Expected outcomes of nursing care include the following:

- The woman and her partner understand the implications and problems of face presentation.
- The mother and her baby have a safe labor and birth.

Breech Presentation

Breech presentation is the most common malpresentation, with an overall incidence of approximately 4% of births. The incidence of breech presentation is directly related to gestational age: at 25 to 26 weeks' gestation, the incidence is about 25%, but by 34 weeks, the incidence has decreased to 3% to 4% (Toth & Juthivijayarani, 2001).

Frank breech is the most common type of breech (especially at term) and occurs in about 65% of breech births (Figure 26–10, *A* •). Single or double footling breech (incomplete breech) accounts for about 25% of breech births

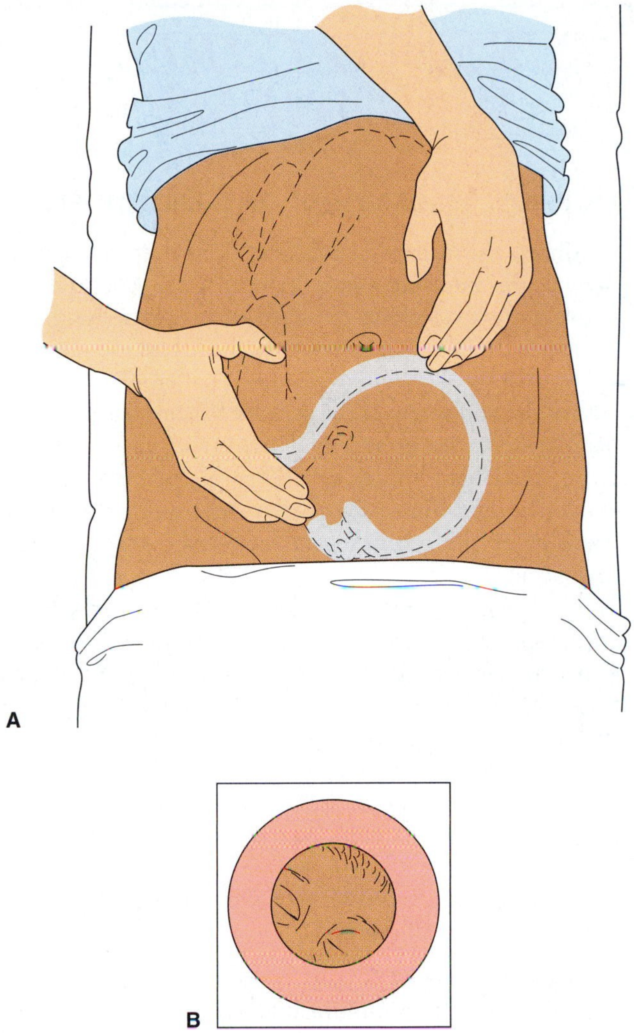

Figure 26–9 • Face presentation. *A,* Palpation of the maternal abdomen with the fetus in right mentum posterior (RMP). *B,* Vaginal examination may permit palpation of facial features of the fetus.

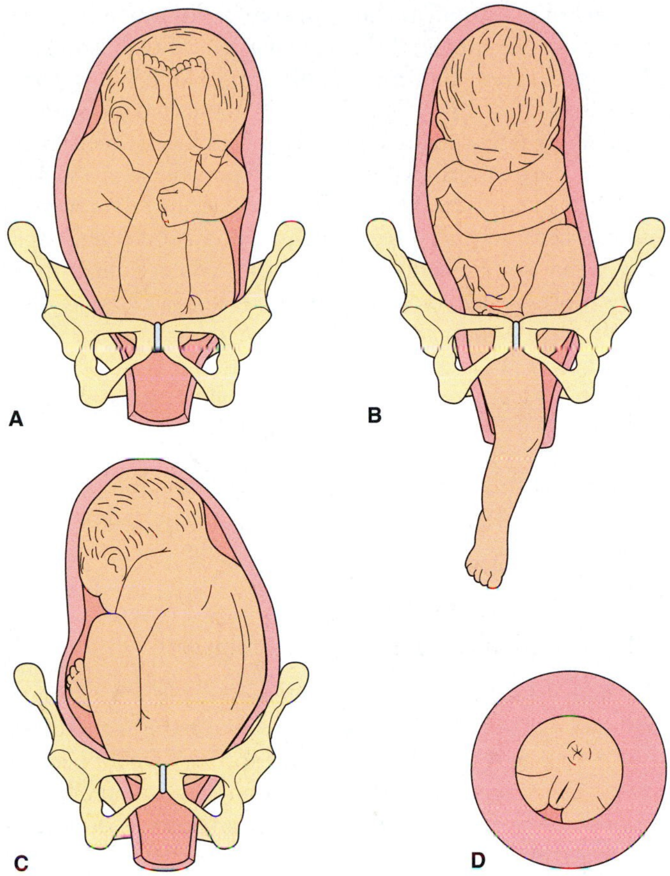

Figure 26–10 • Breech presentation. *A,* Frank breech. *B,* Incomplete (footling) breech. *C,* Complete breech in left sacral anterior (LSA) position. *D,* On vaginal examination, the nurse may feel the anal sphincter. The tissue of the fetal buttocks feels soft.

(Figure 26–10, *B*) and occurs more frequently in preterm fetuses. The remaining 5% of breech presentations are complete breech presentations (Figure 26–10, *C*).

Breech presentation is most frequently associated with placenta previa, implantation of the placenta in either cornual area, hydramnios, multiple gestation, and fetal anomalies (Toth & Juthivijayarani, 2001). Because the presenting part does not completely fill the space in the lower uterine segment, once membranes rupture, cord prolapse is more likely. The incidence of cord prolapse is approximately 4% as compared to an incidence of 0.5% with cephalic presentations at term (Toth & Juthivijayarani, 2001). Fetal anomalies are three times more likely to be present in a breech versus a cephalic presentation. Major congenital malformations have been reported in 17% of preterm breech fetuses, in 9% of term breech fetuses, and in 50% of term breech babies who die just before birth, at birth, or within 28 days after birth (Toth & Juthivijayarani, 2001).

Head trauma during vaginal birth is more likely in breech presentation because it does not allow for the slow molding that occurs in a cephalic presentation as the fetal head moves through the birth canal. The head is the largest and least resilient part of the fetal body. It is the last to come through the maternal pelvis in breech presentations; thus molding does not occur. In the case of a preterm breech, a single or double footling and the torso may emerge through a cervix that is not completely dilated, leaving the larger head entrapped by the cervix. Entrapment may also occur with cesarean birth if the incision is inadequate or uterine relaxation is less than optimum.

A recent multicenter trial demonstrated that planned cesarean births of breech fetuses had a lower risk of perinatal morbidity and mortality than planned vaginal births (Hannah, Hannah, & Hewson, 2001).

CLINICAL THERAPY

An external cephalic version (ECV) is usually attempted at 37 to 38 weeks' gestation. The ECV can reduce breech presentation by 50% to 60% (ACOG, 2000b). Complementary alternative therapies have also been used with some success. *Moxibustion* is a technique in which certain herbs are burned to stimulate an acupressure point at the outside of the fifth toenail (see Complementary and Alternative Therapies: Moxibustion).

This technique stimulates the pressure point, much like acupressure or acupuncture. One study that used moxibustion had a 75% success rate in turning fetuses from a breech to a vertex presentation (Cardini & Weixin, 1999). If the version is unsuccessful or the fetus spontaneously turns back into a breech presentation, the physician will evaluate the possibility of a vaginal birth or plan a cesarean birth. Many physicians recommend a cesarean birth when a breech presentation is detected, especially if the woman is nulliparous because breech births have higher mortality and morbidity rates as well as an increased incidence of cord prolapse, birth trauma, and fetal cervical spinal cord injuries due to hyperextension of the head (Kayem, Goffinet, Clement, et al, 2002). Contraindications for labor and vaginal birth include the following:

- Fetal weight less than 1500 g or more than 3800 g
- Hyperextension of the fetal neck of more than 90 degrees
- Extension of the fetal arms over the head
- Anomalies, such as hydrocephalus
- Diminished maternal pelvic measurements

If a vaginal birth is being attempted, narcotic agents or an epidural block may be used for pain relief. Epidural anesthesia may be advantageous during the latter portion of labor because it will help prevent the pushing sensation the woman may feel prior to complete dilatation. If the woman pushes before cervical dilatation is complete, the fetal body may be expelled and the head entrapped. At the time of birth the physician may have an assistant available in case forceps are needed. Once the fetal body is born, an assistant supports the fetal body as the physician applies Piper forceps to assist in birth of the fetal head (called the *aftercoming head*) (Toth & Juthivijayarani, 2001).

Complementary and Alternative Therapies

Moxibustion to Promote Version in Breech Presentation

Traditional Chinese medicine (TCM) uses the herb mugwort in the form of moxa to promote version in a breech presentation. *Moxa* is a system of treatment, often combined with acupuncture, in which an herb is dried, rolled into cones (like incense cones), and placed on certain meridian parts of the body. The moxa is then lit and allowed to burn close to the skin, hence the *-bustion* component of the name. The heat and pungency of mugwort stimulates the point, and energy moves through. It is believed that the effect of moxibustion increases fetal activity.

The meridian point used in moxibustion to promote version in breech presentations is acupoint BL67, located beside the outer corner of the fifth toenail (Cardini & Weixin, 1998). Treatment may take from 7 days to 2 weeks. In two recent clinical trials, moxibustion was found to be an effective modality in the management of breech presentations (Cardini & Weixin, 1998).

NURSING CARE MANAGEMENT

Nursing Assessment and Diagnosis

At times, the nurse is the first person to recognize a breech presentation. On palpation using Leopold's maneuvers, the nurse feels the hard vertex in the fundus and can perform ballottement of the head independently of the fetal body. The wider sacrum is palpated in the lower part of the abdomen. If the sacrum has not descended, on ballottement the entire fetal body will move. Furthermore, fetal heart tones (FHTs) are usually auscultated above the umbilicus. Passage of meconium from compression of the infant's intestinal tract during descent may occur.

The nurse is particularly alert for a prolapsed umbilical cord, especially in single or double footling breeches, because there is space between the cervix and presenting part through which the cord can slip. If the infant is small and the membranes rupture, the danger is even greater. This is one reason why any woman admitted to the birthing area with a history of ruptured membranes should not ambulate until a full assessment, including vaginal examination, is performed.

Nursing diagnoses that may apply to breech presentation include the following:

- ***Risk for Impaired Gas Exchange*** in the fetus related to interruption in umbilical blood flow secondary to compression of the cord
- ***Health-Seeking Behavior:*** information about breech presentation related to an expressed desire to understand the implications of the procedure.

Nursing Plan and Implementation

During labor, the fetus is at increased risk for prolapse of the cord. Some agency protocols may therefore call for continuous fetal monitoring even though there are no current research studies to support the use of an electronic fetal monitor (EFM). Ongoing assessments of contractions, cervical dilatation, effacement, and fetal descent are also important to monitor labor progress. Emotional support and sharing of information are critical to the childbearing woman and her support person. They need to be kept apprised of the labor's current status as well as the possible treatment plans so they can continue to make informed choices.

During a vaginal birth, the nurse continues to assess the fetal heart rate (FHR) and to provide encouragement and support for the couple. Piper forceps need to be readily available to the physician; the nurse may assist the physician if the forceps are needed for the birth.

Evaluation

Expected outcomes of nursing care include the following:

- The woman and her partner can describe the implications and associated problems with breech presentation.
- The mother and baby have a safe labor and birth.
- Major complications are recognized early, and corrective measures are instituted.

Shoulder Presentation (Transverse Lie) of a Single Fetus

It is not uncommon in multiple gestations for one or more of the fetuses to be in a transverse lie. An incidence of transverse lie of a single fetus is approximately 1 in 300 term births (Cunningham et al, 2001). The infant's long axis lies across the woman's abdomen, and on inspection the contour of the maternal abdomen appears widest from side to side (Figure 26–11 •).

Maternal conditions associated with a transverse lie are grandmultiparity with lax uterine musculature (the most common cause); obstructions such as bony dystocia, placenta previa, neoplasms, and fetal anomalies; hydramnios; and preterm fetus.

Vaginal birth is impossible with a transverse lie. Labor should not be allowed to continue, and a cesarean birth is done quickly. Frequently a vertical incision is made in the uterus because the fetal head and fetal feet lie in the upper portion of the uterus; a low transverse incision may lead to difficulties in extracting the fetus (Cunningham et al, 2001).

If labor is allowed to continue, the fetal shoulder will be forced down into the pelvis and the fetus will become impacted. With no relief, uterine rupture may occur (Cunningham et al, 2001).

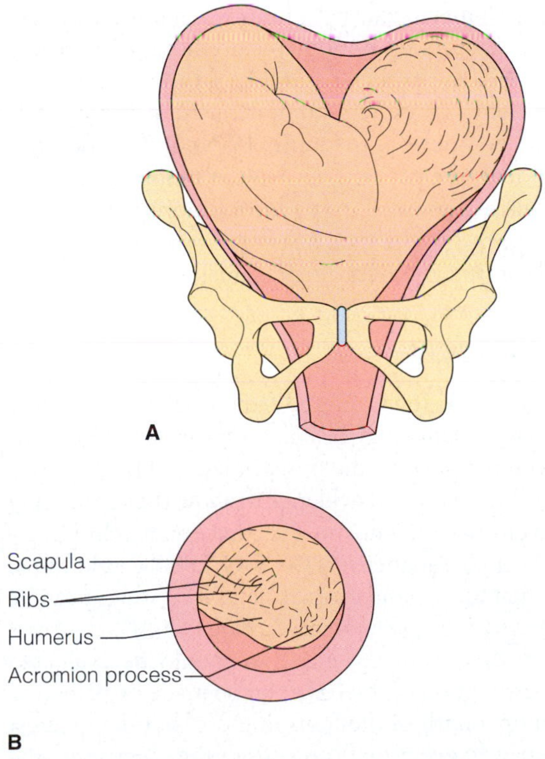

Figure 26–11 • Transverse lie. *A,* Shoulder presentation. *B,* On vaginal examination, the nurse may feel the acromion process as the fetal presenting part.

CLINICAL THERAPY

Transverse lie may be diagnosed using Leopold's maneuvers and can then be confirmed by ultrasound. At the time of the ultrasound examination, it is important to confirm fetal position, fetal biparietal diameters (to confirm gestational age), and location of the placenta and to carry out an examination for the presence of fetal anomalies and structural abnormalities of the uterus such as leiomyoma (fibroid tumor) or adnexal tumors.

Management varies, depending on the length of gestation, because many transverse lies convert to either cephalic or breech presentation by term (38 weeks). If the fetus is still in a transverse lie at term, an ECV may be done if (1) there is no contraindication to vaginal birth (for example, a fetal anomaly, complete placenta previa, or a structural problem in the uterus); and (2) fetal pulmonary lung maturity is confirmed either by ultrasound measurements or by amniocentesis for assessment of phospholipids (2:1 lecithin/sphingomyelin [L/S] ratio and the presence of phosphatidylglycerol). An ECV is most likely to be successful close to term. Spontaneous version will likely occur by 37 weeks. The use of tocolytics for the procedure may be helpful for nulliparas. The fetus is assessed with a nonstress test or biophysical profile prior to the procedure. If the version is successful, the woman may be induced if she is at term and her cervix is favorable. However, scientific studies do not support immediate induction as a routine to minimize the chance the fetus will return to the original position (ACOG, 1997).

NURSING CARE MANAGEMENT

Nursing Assessment and Diagnosis

The nurse can identify a transverse lie by inspection and palpation of the abdomen, by auscultation of FHTs in the midline of the abdomen (not conclusive), and by vaginal examination.

On palpation, no fetal part is felt in the fundal portion of the uterus or above the symphysis pubis. The head may be palpated on one side and the breech on the other. FHTs are usually auscultated just below the midline of the umbilicus. On vaginal examination, if a presenting part is palpated, it is the ridged thorax or possibly an arm that is compressed against the chest. Women with a transverse lie may report less shortness of breath, pelvic pressure, and urinary frequency than other women since pressure is not exerted on the diaphragm and the bladder.

Nursing diagnoses that may apply when transverse lie is present include the following:

- ***Risk for Impaired Gas Exchange*** in the fetus related to decrease in blood flow secondary to cord compression associated with prolapsed cord
- ***Risk for Ineffective Individual Coping*** or ***Ineffective Family Coping*** related to unknown outcome
- ***Fear*** related to unknown outcome of birth

Nursing Plan and Implementation

The primary nursing actions are to help evaluate the fetal presentation and to provide information and support to the couple. If an ECV has been accomplished and an induction is started, the nurse completes all interventions related to the induction. (See discussion in Chapter 27.) If transverse lie is discovered when the woman is admitted to the birthing unit in labor, the nurse provides information regarding the need for either an ECV or a cesarean birth and assists with preparation for the birth. If an ECV is not performed or is unsuccessful, a cesarean birth will be performed. Prior to the cesarean, the nurse watches for rupture of membranes and the possibility of prolapse of the umbilical cord. (See Chapter 27 for further information regarding teaching with cesarean birth.)

Evaluation

Expected outcomes of nursing care include the following:

- The transverse lie is recognized promptly, and crucial assessments are completed.
- Measures to perform an ECV or a cesarean birth are completed.
- The mother and baby have a safe birth.
- The couple can describe the implications and associated problems of transverse lie.

Compound Presentation

A compound presentation is one in which there are two presenting parts. It can occur when the pelvic inlet is not totally occluded by the primary presenting part. If the prolapsed part is a hand, the birth is generally not difficult. Sometimes the hand slips back, and occasionally it is born alongside the head. This may increase the chance of laceration. Cesarean birth is indicated in the presence of uterine dysfunction or fetal distress (Cunningham et al, 2001).

Care of the Woman and Fetus at Risk Due to Macrosomia

Fetal **macrosomia** is defined as weight of more than 4500 g. It is important to remember that the mean birth weight varies throughout the world. For instance, mean birth weight in Sweden is 3490 g, whereas in Pakistan the mean birth weight is 2770 g. In Latino cultures, "fat" babies are more desirable and are viewed as more healthy. Nurses working with Latino women may encounter resistance if counseling is focused on preventing a large baby. Instead, nurses should stress the importance of the baby's health status (Ulijaszek, Johnston, & Preece, 1998). The definition of macrosomia will thus differ according to the ethnic group being discussed.

A woman who is obese is 3 to 4 times more likely to have a macrosomic fetus (> 4500 g) (ACOG, 2000b). Obesity has been defined a number of ways. For a complete discussion on maternal obesity, see Chapter 18. There is also an association between macrosomia and both pregestational and gestational diabetes. Increased maternal glucose levels have also been shown to increase fetal weight to more than 4500 g (ACOG, 2000b). Other risk factors include postterm pregnancy, multiparity, previous macrosomic infant, previous shoulder dystocia, male sex, excessive weight gain, and maternal birth weight.

A woman's pelvis that is adequate for an average-sized fetus may be disproportionately small for an oversized fetus. Distention of the uterus causes overstretching of the myometrial fibers, which may lead to dysfunctional labor and an increased incidence of postpartal hemorrhage. If the oversized fetus is not able to descend, the chance of uterine rupture during labor increases. Vaginal birth poses an increased risk of perineal lacerations and extensions of an episiotomy. The mother is also at risk for postpartum hemorrhage and puerperal infection. The incidence of vacuum and forceps birth increases with fetal size.

The most significant complication in macrosomia is *shoulder dystocia*, which is an obstetric emergency. However, shoulder dystocia may occur with fetuses weighing less than 4000 g, and risk factors are not reliable predictors. Following birth of the head, the anterior shoulder of the macrosomic fetus may not emerge either spontaneously or with gentle traction (Wagner, Nielson, & Gonik, 1999). If shoulder dystocia is not managed correctly, permanent injury to the baby may result. Brachial plexus injury (due to improper or excessive traction applied to the fetal head) and fractured clavicles may occur. Asphyxia and neurologic damage can also occur.

Clinical Therapy

The occurrence of the maternal and fetal problems associated with macrosomic infants may be somewhat lessened by identifying macrosomia prior to the onset of labor. The diagnosis is not precise. There is good evidence to show that estimating fetal size with ultrasound is no more accurate than a clinical estimate from Leopold's maneuvers (ACOG, 2000b). Additional studies show that ultrasound estimation of fetal weight can be in error of 300 to 550 g (Zamorski & Biggs, 2001). If a large fetus is suspected, the maternal pelvis should be evaluated carefully. An estimation of fetal size can be made by palpating the crown-rump length of the fetus in utero, but the greatest errors in estimation occur on both ends of the spectrum—the macrosomic fetus and the very small fetus. Several studies have shown that clinical estimation can be in error as well. The mean error is 300 g (Zamorski & Biggs, 2001). Whenever the uterus appears excessively large, hydramnios, an oversized fetus, or a multiple pregnancy must be considered.

Labor and vaginal birth for a fetus up to 5000 grams is not contraindicated in women without a history of diabetes (ACOG, 2000b). If difficulty extracting the shoulders occurs during the birth, the obstetrician or certified nurse-midwife (CNM) may direct the woman to sharply flex her thighs up against her abdomen (McRoberts maneuver). This position is thought to change the maternal pelvic angle and therefore reduce the force needed to extract the shoulders thereby decreasing the incidence of brachial plexus stretching and clavicular fracture (Figure 26–12 •) (Wagner et al, 1999). McRoberts maneuver has a high success rate. The maternal head should be lowered and the nurse applies suprapubic pressure directly over the symphysis pubis to aid release of the anterior shoulder. Fundal pressure (pressure exerted at the top of the maternal fundus) should not be performed since this can further wedge the shoulder against the suprapubic bone.

In addition, the obstetrician/CNM may incorporate other interventions, such as checking the placement of the shoulder, performing an episiotomy, and using the Woods Screw maneuver (which consists of rotating the anterior shoulder 180 degrees to the posterior position). In cases where these interventions fail, the obstetrician/CNM may electively break the clavicle to facilitate extraction of the shoulders.

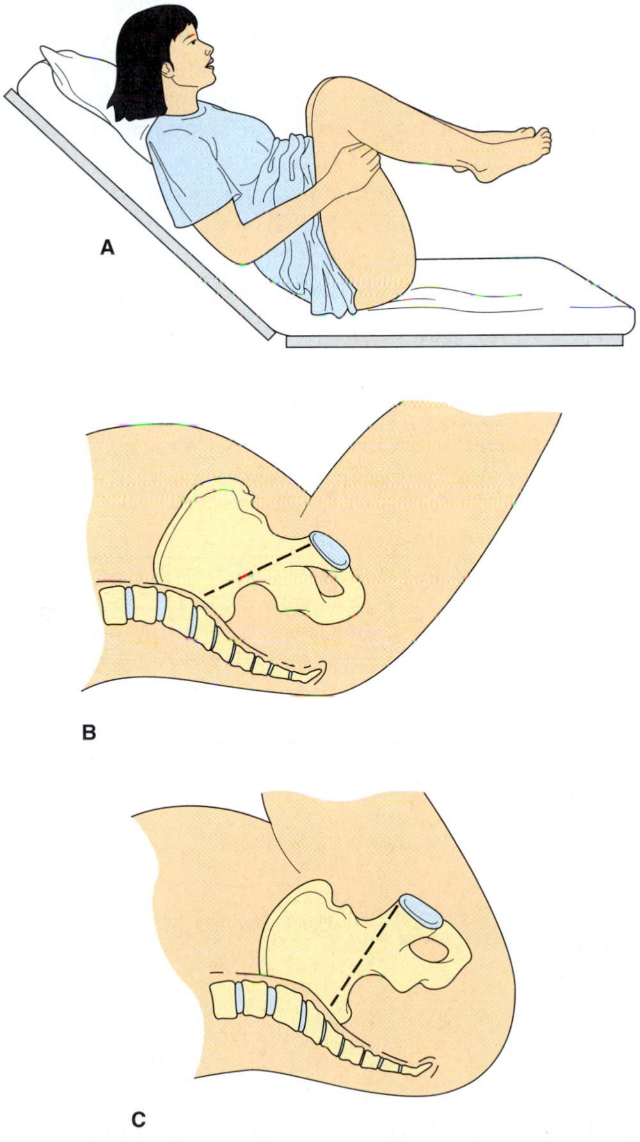

Figure 26–12 • McRoberts maneuver. *A,* The woman flexes her thighs up onto her abdomen. *B,* The angle of the maternal pelvis prior to McRoberts maneuver. *C,* The angle of the pelvis with McRoberts maneuver.

NURSING CARE MANAGEMENT

Nursing Assessment and Diagnosis

The nurse assists in identifying factors associated with macrosomic infants. During the intrapartum period, the risk factors include slow descent of the fetus and prolonged second stage. Because women with these risk factors are prime candidates for dystocia and its complications, the nurse frequently assesses the fetal heart rate (FHR) for nonreassuring heart rate patterns which may indicate fetal stress, evaluates the rate of cervical dilatation, and assesses fetal descent.

Nursing diagnoses that may apply to the woman with a macrosomic fetus include the following:

- ***Risk for Injury*** to the fetus related to trauma during the birth process
- ***Risk for Infection*** related to traumatized tissue secondary to maternal tissue damage during birth

Nursing Plan and Implementation

The nurse monitors labor closely for a dysfunctional pattern, assessing FHR and reporting any sign of labor dysfunction or nonreassuring heart rate patterns to the physician/CNM. The nurse notes any arrest of descent, excessive molding of the fetal head, or the presence of caput succedaneum, which can also indicate a large fetus or cephalopelvic disproportion (CPD).

The nurse provides support for the laboring woman and her partner and information regarding the implications and possible associated problems. The nurse can provide the couple with directions for proper positioning at the time of birth to facilitate extraction of the shoulders. If the nurse anticipates a possible shoulder dystocia, additional staff should be notified and appropriate support personnel for the newborn should be informed. During the birth, the nurse continues to provide support and encouragement to the couple. Informing the woman that possible suprapubic pressure may be needed can help reduce anxiety for the couple.

After the birth, the nurse inspects the newborn for cephalhematoma, Erb palsy (caused by overstretching of the brachial plexus and damage to C5, C6, C7), and fractured clavicles (exhibited by nonmovement of one arm) and informs the admission nursery of any problems. The newborn will need to be observed closely for cerebral and neurologic damage.

Postpartally, the nurse checks the uterus for potential atony and the maternal vital signs for deviations suggesting hypovolemic shock. Frequent fundal checks should be performed to evaluate the woman for postpartum bleeding.

Evaluation

Expected outcomes of nursing care include the following:

- The woman and her partner can describe the implications of macrosomia and possible associated problems.
- The mother and baby have a safe labor and birth.

Care of the Woman with a Multiple Gestation

The incidence of naturally occurring twins in the United States is 3% of all pregnancies; however with advances in reproductive technologies, the incidence is increasing (Cunningham et al, 2001). It is estimated that pregnancies resulting from assisted technologies have a 25% to 30% incidence of twins and a 5% incidence of triplets. Higher order multiple gestations (four or more fetuses) account for only 0.5% to 1% of all births (ACOG, 1998a). Because twin birth is by far the most common multiple birth, the discussion focuses on this type. The chapter also identifies specific variations for triplets and higher order multiple gestations as appropriate.

Embryology of Multiple Gestation

Terminology related to various types of twins is presented in Table 26–3 •. Twins can develop from either the fertilization of two separate ova or from the division of one fertilized ovum. Twins that occur from two separate ova are called *dizygotic* (two zygotes, also referred to as fraternal twins). In this type, the fetuses may be the same sex or different sexes and there are two complete amnions and two chorions. The fetuses are no more closely related genetically than any other siblings.

In contrast, 33% of twins are *monozygotic* (also referred to as identical twins); that is, they develop from one fertilized ovum (Moses, 2001). These twins are genetically identical, and thus always of the same sex (Table 26–3). If the zygote divides within the first 72 hours past fertilization, the twins will be diamniotic and dichorionic. If the division occurs from the fourth to the eighth day past fertilization, the embryos will develop with two separate amnions and one chorion. If the division happens after the eighth day, the two fetuses will share both a common amniotic sac and chorion. The terminology is important because the perinatal morbidity and mortality rates differ greatly among different types of twins (Chasen & Chervenak, 1998; Keith, Papiernik & Oleszczuk, 1998). For example, monozygotic twins have a high incidence of cord entrapment, twin-to-twin transfusion, and fetal demise (Moses, 2001).

Pregnancy Loss in Multiple Gestation

The development of sensitive human chorionic gonadotropin (hCG) assays and increasingly sensitive ultrasound tech-

Table 26–3 • CHARACTERISTICS OF TWIN PREGNANCY

Type	Time of Division	Characteristics	Frequency	Mortality Rate
Dizygotic (Two separate ova) Fraternal twins Dichorionic-diamniotic twins	Develop from two ova released at the same time.	Each twin has own placenta, chorion, amnion. Dizygotic twins are called fraternal twins. They may be the same or different sex.	67% of all twins	11.5%
Monozygotic (Single ovum) Identical twins			33% of all twins	
Dichorionic-diamniotic twins	Division occurs within 72 hours past fertilization.* Inner cell mass not yet developed.	Each twin has own chorion, amnion, placenta.	30% of monozygotic twins	9%
Monochorionic-diamniotic twins	Division occurs at blastocyst stage, 4 to 8 days after fertilization.* Inner cell mass divides in two.	Placenta has one chorion and two amnions. Each twin lies in own sac.	68% of monozygotic twins	25%
Monochorionic-monoamniotic twins	Division occurs in primitive germ disk, 9 to 13 days past fertilization.*	Twins lie in the same amniotic sac. Increased risk of umbilical cords becoming tangled or knotted.	2% of monozygotic twins	>50%

*Chasen, S. T., & Chervenak, F. A. (1998). What is the relationship between the universal use of ultrasound, the rate of detection of twins, and outcome differences? *Clinical Obstetrics and Gynecology, 41,* 67–77.

RESEARCH IN PRACTICE
Specialized Care for Twin Gestations

What is this study about? The management of twin gestations can be a challenge for care providers. Maternal complications and preterm births are more common for twin pregnancies. This study compared newborn outcomes and costs of hospital stays for mothers using a specialized twin clinic and those receiving standard prenatal care.

How was this study done? This was a retrospective cohort design comparing the outcomes of 30 women who received care in a specialized twin clinic with those of 41 women who gave birth one year before following standard prenatal care. The women either qualified for Medicaid or were uninsured and were considered economically disadvantaged. In the specialized twin clinic, care was provided by a nurse practitioner following an evidence-based protocol in collaboration with a perinatologist. A home visit was a routine part of prenatal care, as were more frequent clinic visits. A nutritionist, social worker, and genetic counselor were available. Outcome measures included birth weight and gestational age, hospital charges for labor, birth and postpartum care, and lengths of stay for newborns. Differences between groups were assessed using standard statistical techniques.

What were the results of the study? No differences were found between the groups in the number of maternal gestational complications or surgical complications from cesarean birth. The twins born of the specialized clinic group weighed on average 249 grams more than the standard prenatal care group. There were no births before 30 weeks and fewer births at less than 36 weeks in the specialized clinic group compared to the standard prenatal group. Fewer very low birth weight neonates were born in the clinic group. With respect to resources, the twin clinic group had substantially lower length of stay (10.5 versus 18) and neonatal intensive care unit days (7.8 versus 17.) Hospital charges were $30,000 less per infant in the clinic group.

What additional questions might I have? Would the outcome be different if the experimental and control groups were measured concurrently? Are these findings applicable to groups that are not economically disadvantaged?

How can I use this study? This study showed reduced costs and improved outcomes for twins that had specialized prenatal care. An advanced practice nurse can address issues with twin gestations effectively using specialized protocols. The development and application of evidence-based protocols can improve the outcomes for high-risk twin gestations.

Source: Ruiz, R., Brown, C., Peters, M., & Johnson, A. (2001). Specialized care for twin gestations: Improving newborn outcomes and reducing costs. *Journal of Obstetric, Gynecologic, and Neonatal Nursing, 30*(1): 52–59.

niques has made it possible to determine more accurately the early pregnancy loss rate of twins, including both complete pregnancy loss and spontaneous resorption of one twin (called the "vanishing twin" phenomenon). Evidence suggests that 75% of twin pregnancies are lost before the end of the first trimester (Grobman & Peaceman, 1998). Causative factors in the loss of both twins in the first trimester include environmental factors, infectious organisms, trophoblast dysfunction, poor embryo quality, or a lower concentration of placentally produced substances. Although loss of one twin can occur at any time during the pregnancy, it more commonly occurs in the first trimester. Only 50% of pregnancies diagnosed with twins during the first trimester result in the birth of two live infants (ACOG, 1998a). Marginal and velamentous cord insertions (to be discussed shortly) are more likely to be present when there is a vanishing twin, and the presence of a monochorionic placenta is more likely to result in either a singleton gestation (because of a vanishing twin) or complete pregnancy loss (Grobman & Peaceman, 1998).

Pregnancy loss of twins in the second trimester is associated with congenital anomalies, growth restriction, chromosomal abnormalities, and cervical incompetence. In a monochorionic placenta, there may be a vascular anastomosis that leads to twin-to-twin transfusion syndrome. When this syndrome is present, blood is chronically drained from one fetus to the other. The donor fetus becomes growth restricted, and oligohydramnios develops. The recipient fetus becomes polycythemic and hydropic, and hydramnios develops. If the fetuses become severely affected during the second trimester, untreated mortality may be 100% (Grobman & Peaceman, 1998).

The incidence of preterm birth is also higher in multiple gestations. Preterm birth is 5.9 times more likely in twins than in singletons, and 10.7 times more likely in triplets (Keith et al, 1998). In singletons, the perinatal mortality is at the lowest point at 40 weeks' gestation; for twins, the perinatal mortality rate decreases until 38 weeks and then increases steadily from 39 to 42 weeks (Keith et al, 1998). A woman pregnant with twins who has not spontaneously begun labor by 40 gestational weeks is typically induced at her due date.

Implications

Women with a multiple gestation are more likely to develop complications, which include the following (Senat, Ancel, Bouvier-Colle, et al, 1998; Keith et al, 1998; ACOG, 1998a):

- Spontaneous abortions are more common, as previously discussed.
- Hypertension is the major maternal complication. The risk of developing severe hypertension or preeclampsia is two to three times greater.
- Maternal anemia occurs because of demands of the multiple gestation. The hemoglobin averages 10 g/dL

from the 20th week on. Anemia is indicated by hemoglobin levels below 11 g/dL in the first or third trimester or below 10.5 g/dL in the second trimester. When decreased hemoglobin is accompanied by serum ferritin concentration of less than 12 mg/dL, iron deficiency anemia is diagnosed.

- Hydramnios may be due to increased renal perfusion from cross-vessel anastomosis of monozygotic twins.
- Premature rupture of membranes, incompetent cervix, and intrauterine growth restriction occur more commonly.
- Rare complications associated with twins include twin-to-twin transfusion (previously discussed), conjoined (Siamese) twins, and *acardia* (twin reversed arterial perfusion sequence).
- Complications during labor include preterm labor, uterine dysfunction due to an overstretched myometrium, abnormal fetal presentations, instrumental or cesarean birth, and postpartum hemorrhage.

The woman with a multiple gestation may experience more physical discomfort during her pregnancy, such as shortness of breath, dyspnea on exertion, backaches, round ligament pain, heartburn, pelvic or suprapubic pressure, and pedal edema, because of the oversized uterus.

Clinical Therapy

The goals of medical care are to promote normal fetal development to prevent maternal complications, to prevent preterm birth, and to diminish fetal trauma during labor.

Ultrasound examinations play a crucial role in the care and treatment of multiple gestations. Ultrasound assists with identifying the presence of more than one fetus early in the pregnancy, providing accurate dating of the pregnancy, and detecting fetal anomalies. Because the incidence of perinatal mortality and morbidity is increased in twins, use of ultrasound in the first and second trimester can be particularly helpful. Evidence supports the use of ultrasound for accurately determining chorionicity and amnionicity in multiple pregnancies (Devlieger, et al, 2001). Knowledge of chorionicity is essential in differentiating twin-to-twin transfusion from fetal growth restriction secondary to abnormal placental blood flow. Knowledge of chorionicity is also important in determining the management of a multiple pregnancy in which one twin is sonographically abnormal. If the twins are dichorionic/diamniotic (DC/DA), then selective termination could be considered. Determination of amnionicity is based on ultrasound visualization or the lack of visualization of an intertwin membrane. Visualization of this membrane becomes more difficult as the gestation advances because of progressive thinning of the intertwin membrane, fetal crowding, and an increasing incidence of oligohydramnios. Knowledge regarding the presence of one amnion is crucial, because management of monochorionic/monoamniotic (MC/MA) twins requires more intensive surveillance and earlier birth, usually by cesarean (Chasen & Chervenak, 1998). Women with MC/MA twins are frequently cared for by perinatologists in a facility that has high-risk services available.

Preventing preterm labor is a major goal. The rate of preterm birth for twins increased from 40.9% in 1981 to 55% in 1997. Similarly, among twins, low-birth-weight infants increased from 51% to 54% and preterm small-for-gestational-age (SGA) infants increased from 11.9% to 14.1% in that same period (Kogan, Alexander, Kotelchuck, et al, 2000). Prenatal care should begin early, and more frequent visits are usually scheduled. Many practitioners perform vaginal examinations at each visit after 28 weeks to identify cervical changes, such as cervical shortening, effacement, or dilatation, or the beginning of bulging membranes. An ultrasound vaginal probe may be used to measure the dimensions of the cervix and changes in the lower uterine segment. Roberts and Morrison (1998) demonstrated that the dimensions of the cervix were different when the woman was reclining as opposed to standing. In the standing position, the cervix was shorter and wider. These changes may be associated with the suggestion that prolonged standing is a high-risk factor for preterm labor (Manning, 1999).

According to the Society of Obstetricians and Gynecologists of Canada, there is evidence to support routine cervical measurements for preterm prevention. There is insufficient evidence, however, to support policies for routine cervical cerclage, reduced activity and work, and prophylactic bed rest (Watson-Blasiolie, 2001). A systematic review of studies of hospitalization and bed rest for multiple pregnancy showed insufficient evidence to support routine bed rest (Cochrane Review, 2001).

Home monitors have been helpful in identifying uterine hyperactivity and the presence of contractions. Early detection of contractions can provide an opportunity for the woman to seek assistance more quickly (Roberts & Morrison, 1998).

Some areas offer twin clinics, which provide many advantages for the woman with multiple gestation. These advantages include consistent evaluation, intensive prenatal education, counseling, and support from the same healthcare providers.

Intrapartal management and assessment require careful attention to maternal and fetal status. The mother should have an intravenous infusion in place with a large-bore needle. Anesthesia and cross-matched blood should be readily available. The twins are monitored by dual electronic fetal monitoring. The labor may progress very slowly or very quickly.

The decision about method of birth may not be made until labor occurs, and the method depends on a variety of factors. The presence of maternal complications such as placenta previa, abruptio placentae, or severe preeclampsia usually indicates the need for cesarean birth. Fetal factors such as severe intrauterine growth restriction (IUGR), preterm birth, fetal anomalies, fetal stress, or unfavorable fetal position or presentation also require cesarean birth. Typically, a cesarean birth is performed if the presenting twin is in a presenting position other than vertex and cannot be turned to a vertex presentation.

Birth of three or more fetuses is best accomplished by cesarean because of the risk of fetal insult due to decreased placental perfusion and hemorrhage from the separating placenta during the intrapartal period (Cunningham et al, 2001). Complicated obstetric maneuvers such as breech extraction and podalic version, the risk of prolapse of the cord, and an increase in fetal collision provide additional reasons for cesarean birth.

Any combination of presentations and positions can occur with twins (Figure 26–13 •). Approximately 50% of twins are born by cesarean, which is chosen in the hope of reducing complications for the twins, especially birth asphyxia (Cunningham et al, 2001).

The placentas are examined after the birth. If the twins are of the same sex, the placentas are sent to the pathology laboratory for examination to determine whether they are monozygotic or dizygotic twins.

NURSING CARE MANAGEMENT

Nursing Assessment and Diagnosis

When obtaining a maternal history at the beginning of antenatal care, the nurse should identify any family history of twinning. Equally important is a history of medication taken to enhance fertility. These facts should be noted on the antepartal record.

At each antepartal clinic visit, the nurse should measure the fundal height. During the prenatal period, a fundal height greater than expected for the weeks of gestation and auscultation of two heartbeats that differ by at least 10 beats per minute are the most likely clues of twin pregnancy. Some women experience severe nausea and vomiting and develop severe anemia despite the intake of multiple-vitamin therapy. The α-fetoprotein level may be elevated (ACOG, 1998a).

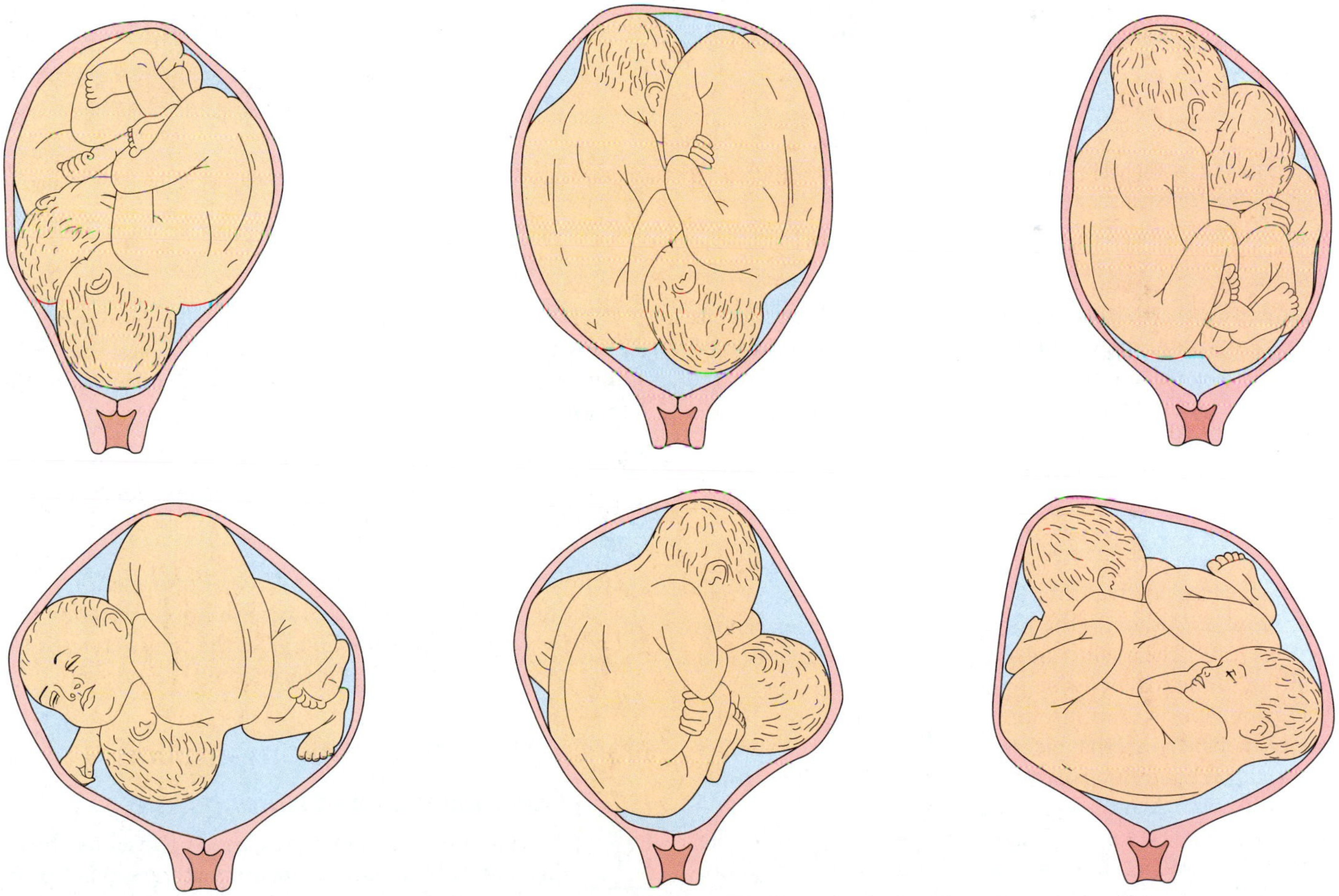

Figure 26–13 • Twins may be in any of these presentations while in utero.

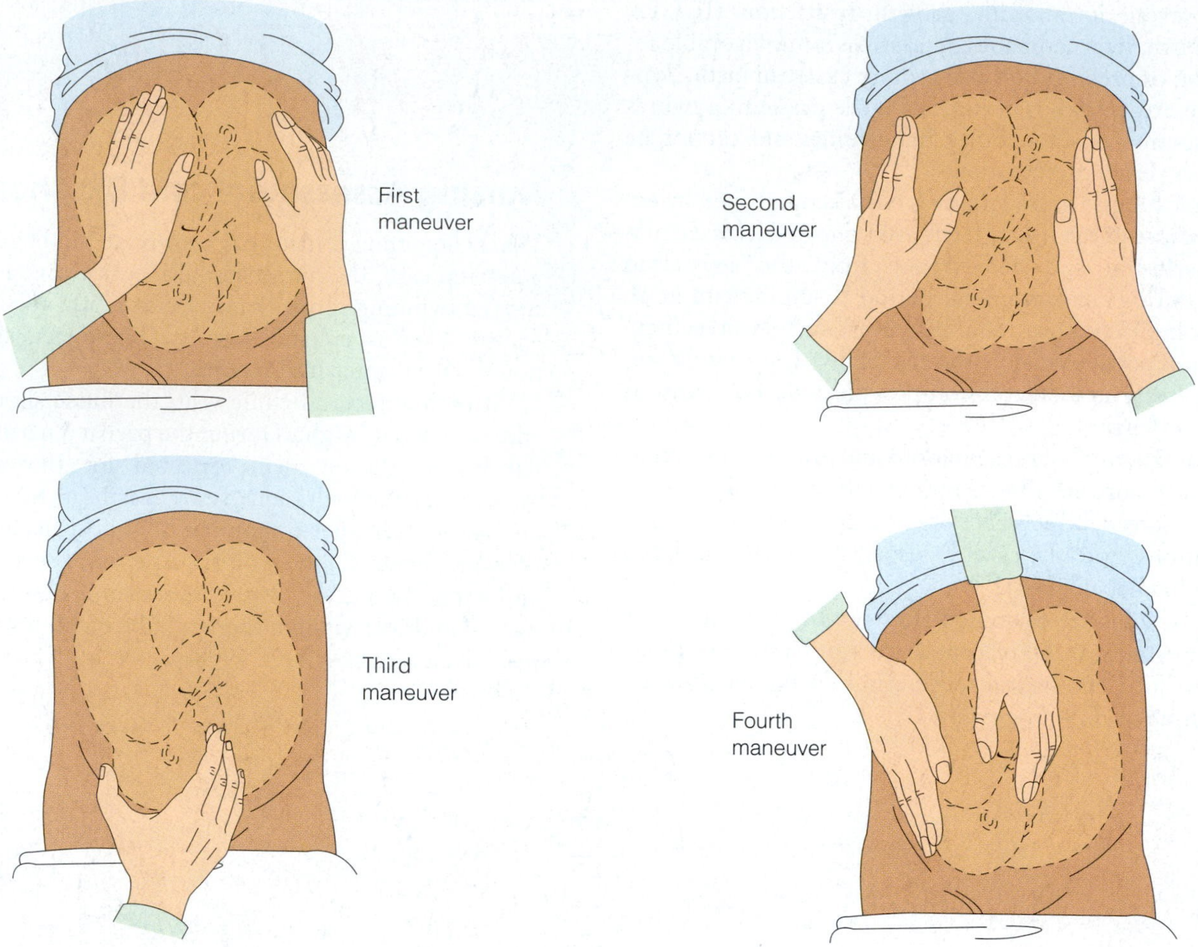

Figure 26–14 ● Leopold's maneuvers in twin pregnancy. The fetus on the mother's right side is in cephalic presentation, and the fetus on the left is in breech presentation.

Any growth, fetal movement, or heart tone auscultation out of proportion to gestational age by dates is indicative of twins. During palpation, the nurse may feel many small parts on all sides of the abdomen (Figure 26–14 ●). If twins are suspected, the nurse should attempt to auscultate two separate heartbeats in different quadrants of the maternal abdomen. Use of the Doppler device may be helpful. Conclusive evidence of twins is found on sonography.

During the prenatal visits the nurse should determine the family's level of preparation for integrating more than one new member. Although the thought of having twins can be very exciting, the reality of attaching to two infants and adapting to the parental role may be trying.

During labor it is important to monitor each fetus. In the case of twins, an external electronic monitor can be applied to both, or if conditions permit, the internal monitor can be applied to twin A and the external monitor to twin B. The heart rates may be auscultated on different quadrants of the maternal abdomen, but continuous monitoring is more beneficial. Signs of nonreassuring heart rate patterns should be reported to the certified nurse-midwife (CNM) or obstetrician.

After a multiple birth, the mother is closely monitored for postpartal hemorrhage. Nursing diagnoses that may apply to a woman with a multiple gestation include the following:

- ***Fear*** related to unknown outcome of the birth process
- ***Ineffective Individual Coping*** or ***Ineffective Family Coping*** related to uncertainty about the labor and birth plan
- ***Deficient Knowledge*** related to lack of information about the problems associated with multiple gestation
- ***Risk for Impaired Gas Exchange*** in the fetuses related to decreased oxygenation secondary to cord compression

Nursing Plan and Implementation

Community-Based Nursing Care

Antepartally, the woman may need counseling about diet and daily activities. The nurse can help her plan meals to meet her increased needs. A daily intake of 4000 kcal (minimum) and 135 g of protein is recommended for optimal weight gain and fetal growth. A prenatal vitamin and 1 mg of folic acid and iron should also be taken daily. A weight gain of 35 to 45 lb is recommended.

Maternal hypertension is treated with bed rest in the lateral position to increase uterine and kidney perfusion. Back discomfort can be alleviated by pelvic rocking, good posture, and good body mechanics. The nurse can help the woman schedule frequent periods of rest during the day. Family members or friends may be willing to care for the woman's other children periodically to allow her time to get rest. Community support systems, such as neighbors or church members, may be available to assist the family with meals, grocery shopping, and household chores. Many communities now have support groups specifically designed for mothers of multiples. Members provide invaluable peer support throughout pregnancy and the postpartum period. Teaching regarding prevention and recognition of preterm labor is very important. For further discussion see Chapter 20.

Hospital-Based Nursing Care

The nurse needs to prepare to receive multiple newborns. This means a multiplication of resuscitation equipment and newborn identification papers and bracelets. The newborns may be placed in individual radiant warmers or in the same one once identification bands have been applied. Additional staff members should be available for newborn resuscitation, monitoring, and newborn care. Special precautions should be observed to ensure correct identification of the newborns. The first born is usually tagged Baby A; the second, Baby B; and so on.

Evaluation

Expected outcomes of nursing care include the following:

- The woman is able to discuss the implications and problems associated with multiple gestation.
- The woman feels she is able to cope with the pregnancy and birth.
- The woman understands the treatment plan and how to gain further information.
- The mother, father, and babies have a safe prenatal course, labor, and birth and a safe postpartal and newborn course.

Care of the Woman and Fetus in the Presence of Nonreassuring Fetal Status

When the oxygen supply is insufficient to meet the physiologic demands of the fetus, a nonreassuring fetal status may result. *Nonreassuring fetal status* is the term used to identify data describing the fetal status. Previously, the term *fetal distress* was used; however, its use implied an ill fetus despite the fact that the condition is often transient, not chronic.

A variety of factors may contribute to a nonreassuring fetal status. The most common are related to cord compression and uteroplacental insufficiency associated with placental abnormalities and preexisting maternal or fetal disease. If the resultant hypoxia persists and metabolic acidosis follows, the situation can be life threatening to the fetus.

The most common initial signs of nonreassuring fetal status are meconium-stained amniotic fluid (in a vertex presentation) and changes in the fetal heart rate (FHR). The presence of ominous FHR patterns, such as late or severe variable decelerations, decrease in or lack of variability, and progressive acceleration in the FHR baseline, are indicative of hypoxia. Fetal scalp blood samples demonstrating a pH value of 7.20 or less provide a more sophisticated indication of fetal problems and are generally obtained when questions about fetal status arise. (See also Chapter 23.)

Clinical Therapy

When there is evidence of possible fetal stress, treatment centers on relieving the hypoxia and minimizing the effects of anoxia on the fetus. Initial interventions include changing the mother's position, increasing infusion rates of intravenous fluids, and administering oxygen by mask at 6 to 10 L per minute. If electronic fetal monitoring (EFM) has not yet been used, it is usually instituted at this time. If oxytocin is in use, it should be discontinued. Fetal scalp stimulation can be performed. Fetal scalp blood samples can be taken. If EFM is ineffective, the certified nurse-midwife (CNM) or physician may utilize internal monitoring devices to more accurately assess FHR changes. Figure 26–15 • depicts intrapartal management of nonreassuring fetal status heart rate patterns.

NURSING CARE MANAGEMENT

Nursing Assessment and Diagnosis

The nurse reviews the woman's prenatal history to anticipate the possibility of nonreassuring fetal status. When the membranes rupture, it is important to assess FHR and to observe for meconium staining. As labor progresses, the nurse is particularly alert for even subtle changes in the FHR pattern and the fetal scalp pH, if available. Reports by the mother of increased or greatly decreased fetal activity may also be associated with nonreassuring fetal status. For further discussion of FHR patterns and characteristics, see evaluation of fetal status during labor in Chapter 23.

Nursing diagnoses that may apply in the presence of nonreassuring fetal status include the following:

- ***Decreased Cardiac Output*** in fetus related to decreased uteroplacental perfusion secondary to maternal hypotension, decreased blood volume, or vasoconstriction with preeclampsia
- ***Anxiety*** related to knowledge of fetal stress

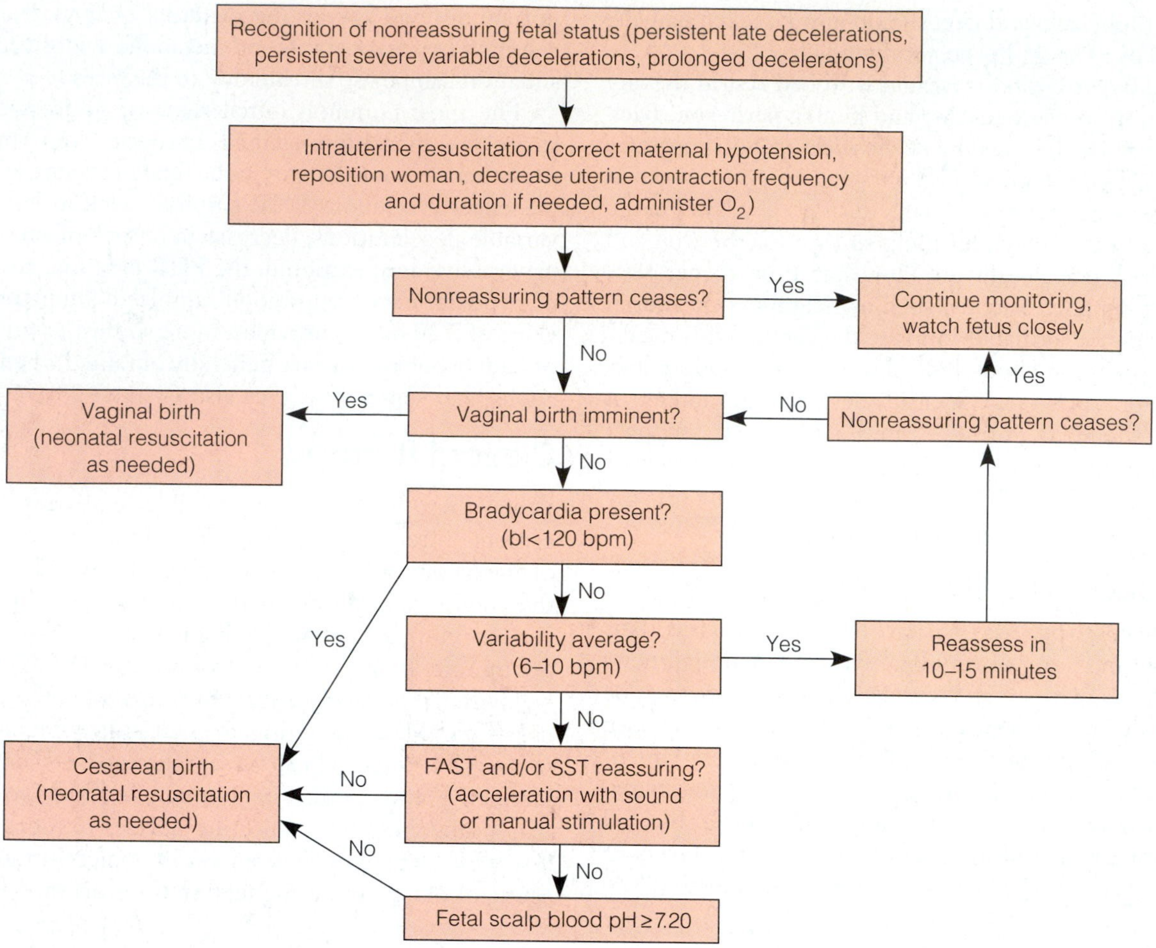

Figure 26–15 • Intrapartal management of nonreassuring fetal status. Note: bl = baseline; FAST = fetal acoustic stimulation test; SST = scalp stimulation test.
SOURCE: From Zuspan, F. P., & Quilligan, E. J. *Handbook of obstetrics, gynecology, and primary care.* Copyright 1998, Mosby reprinted with permission from Elsevier Science.

CRITICAL THINKING IN PRACTICE

A fetal heart tracing demonstrates the following: baseline heart rate of 140 with variability of 6 to 10 bpm. When you compare the FHR with the uterine contractions, you note that there is a slowing of the FHR at the time of the contraction and that the FHR tracing looks like the contraction curve, but it is upside down. Based on this tracing, what would you do?

Answers can be found in Appendix I.

Nursing Plan and Implementation

Staff members may become so involved in assessing fetal status and initiating corrective measures that they fail to give explanations and emotional support to the woman, her partner, and other family members. It is imperative that the nurse provide both full explanations of the problem and comfort to the couple. In many instances, if birth is not imminent, the woman must undergo cesarean birth. Anticipation of this surgery may cause fear and frustration for the couple, especially if they were committed to a shared, prepared birth experience.

Evaluation

Expected outcomes of nursing care include the following:

- The woman and her family become less anxious and more able to cope with their situation.
- The fetal heart rate remains in normal range, or, alternatively, supportive measures maintain the FHR as normal as possible.

Care of the Woman and Fetus at Risk Due to Placental Problems

Maintaining placental function is paramount to ensuring fetal well-being and continuation of the pregnancy. Because the placenta is highly vascular, problems that develop are usually associated with maternal and possibly fetal hemorrhage. Causes and sources of hemorrhage are reviewed in Table 26–4 •.

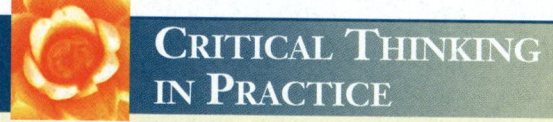

Table 26–4 • CAUSES AND SOURCES OF HEMORRHAGE

Causes and Sources	Signs and Symptoms
Antepartal period	
Abortion	Vaginal bleeding Intermittent uterine contractions Rupture of membranes
Placenta previa	Painless vaginal bleeding after seventh month
Abruptio placentae	
Partial	Vaginal bleeding; no increase in uterine pain
Severe	Vaginal bleeding may or not be present Extreme tenderness of abdominal area Rigid, boardlike abdomen Increase in size of abdomen
Intrapartal period	
Placenta previa	Bright red vaginal bleeding
Abruptio placentae	Same signs and symptoms listed above
Uterine atony in stage III	Bright red vaginal bleeding Ineffectual contractility
Postpartal Period	
Uterine atony	Boggy uterus Dark vaginal bleeding Presence of clots
Retained placental fragments	Boggy uterus Dark vaginal bleeding Presence of clots
Lacerations of cervix or vagina	Firm uterus Bright red blood

Abruptio Placentae

Abruptio placentae is the premature separation of a normally implanted placenta from the uterine wall. The incidence of abruptio placentae is 1 in 120 births but accounts for 15% of perinatal mortality (Gaufberg, 2001). It is more frequent in pregnancies complicated by cocaine abuse (Cunningham et al, 2001). The risk of recurrence is much higher than for the general population, varying between 5% and 17%. In the woman with a history of two previous abruptions, the chance of recurrence is 25% (Cunningham et al, 2001).

The cause of abruptio placentae is largely unknown. Theories have been proposed relating its occurrence to decreased blood flow to the placenta through the sinuses during the last trimester. It is estimated that maternal hypertension is the most common cause (44%) with maternal trauma accounting for 2% to 10% of the cases. Cigarette smoking, presence of fibroids, advanced maternal age, alcohol consumption, cocaine use, a short umbilical cord, and high parity also contribute. Abruptions also appear to be more common in certain ethnic groups. Caucasian and African American women have higher incidences of abruptions than Asian and Latin American women (Cunningham et al, 2001). Classification of abruption is based on the extent of separation (Table 26–5 •).

Table 26–5 • CLASSIFICATION OF ABRUPTION

Class 0	Asymptomatic; diagnosed after birth
Class I	Mild; most common, occurring in 48% of cases
Class II	Moderate; both mother and fetus show signs of distress; 27% of cases
Class III	Severe; maternal shock and fetal death likely; 24% of cases

Source: Used with permission from Gaufberg, S. A. *Abrupto Placenta eMedicine Journal* [serial online]. Available at: http:www.emedicine.com/emerg/topic12.htm

PATHOPHYSIOLOGY

Premature separation of the placenta may be divided into three types (Figure 26–16 •):

1. *Marginal.* The blood passes between the fetal membranes and the uterine wall and escapes vaginally. Separation begins at the periphery of the placenta; this marginal sinus rupture may or may not become more severe.
2. *Central.* The placenta separates centrally, and the blood is trapped between the placenta and the uterine wall. Entrapment of the blood results in concealed bleeding.
3. *Complete.* Massive vaginal bleeding is seen in the presence of almost total separation.

In severe cases of central abruptio placentae, a blood clot forms behind the placenta. With no place to escape, the blood invades the myometrial tissues between the muscle fibers. This occurrence accounts for the uterine irritability that is a significant sign of premature separation of the placenta. If hemorrhage continues, eventually the uterus turns entirely blue in color. After the baby is born, the uterus contracts only with difficulty. This syndrome is known as a *Couvelaire uterus* and frequently necessitates hysterectomy.

As a result of the damage to the uterine wall and the retroplacental clotting with covert abruption, large amounts of thromboplastin are released into the maternal blood supply, which in turn triggers the development of disseminated intravascular coagulation (DIC) and the resultant hypofibrinogenemia. Fibrinogen levels, which are ordinarily elevated in pregnancy, may drop to incoagulable amounts within a matter of minutes as a result of rapidly developing premature separation of the placenta. Additional information on DIC may be found in a medical-surgical nursing textbook.

MATERNAL RISKS

Maternal mortality is now uncommon, although maternal morbidity is still common (Cunningham et al, 2001). Problems following the birth depend in large part on the severity of the intrapartal bleeding, coagulation defects (DIC), hypofibrinogenemia, and length of time between separation and the birth. Moderate to severe hemorrhage results in hemorrhagic shock, which ultimately may prove fatal to the mother if not reversed. In the postpartal period, women who have

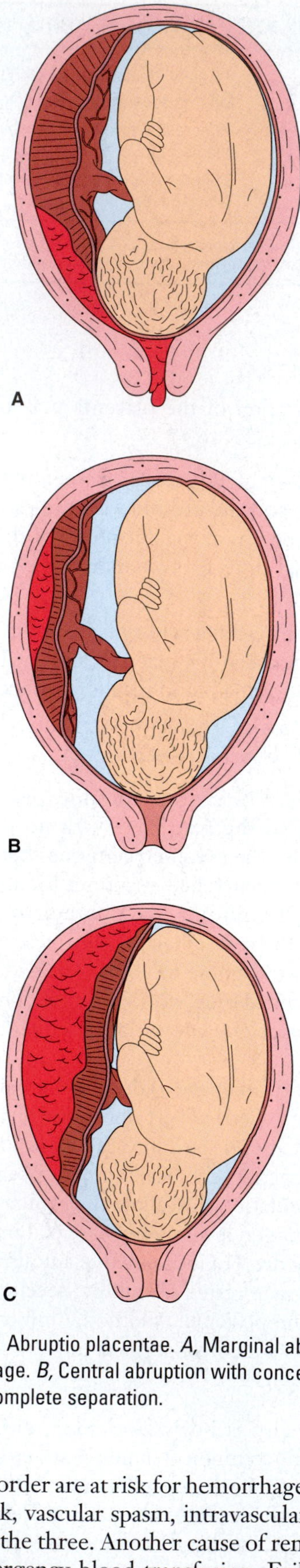

Figure 26–16 • Abruptio placentae. *A,* Marginal abruption with external hemorrhage. *B,* Central abruption with concealed hemorrhage. *C,* Complete separation.

suffered this disorder are at risk for hemorrhage and renal failure due to shock, vascular spasm, intravascular clotting, or a combination of the three. Another cause of renal failure is incompatible emergency blood transfusion. Failure is directly proportional to the number of units transfused. In some cases, hysterectomy is performed if bleeding cannot be controlled.

FETAL-NEONATAL RISKS

Perinatal mortality associated with abruptio placentae is approximately 25% (Cunningham et al, 2001). In severe cases in which separation occurs to approximately 50% of the placenta, infant mortality is 100%. In less severe separation, fetal outcome depends on the level of maturity. The most serious complications in the newborn arise from preterm labor, anemia, and hypoxia. If fetal hypoxia progresses unchecked, irreversible brain damage or fetal demise may result. Neurologic defects within the first year of life occur in approximately 14% of infants who survive (Cunningham et al, 2001). With thorough assessment and prompt action on the part of the healthcare team, fetal and maternal outcome can be optimized.

CLINICAL THERAPY

Because of the risk of DIC, evaluating the results of coagulation tests is imperative. In DIC, fibrinogen levels and platelet counts are usually decreased; prothrombin times (PT) and partial thromboplastin times (PTT) are normal to prolonged. If the values are not markedly abnormal, serial testing may be helpful in establishing an abnormal trend that is indicative of coagulopathy. Another very sensitive test determines fibrin degradation products; these levels rise with DIC.

After the diagnosis is established, emphasis is placed on maintaining the cardiovascular status of the mother and developing a plan for effecting the birth of the fetus. Intravenous access with a large-gauge cannula is warranted along with continuous EFM. Which birth method is selected depends on the condition of the woman and fetus; in many circumstances cesarean birth may be the safest option.

If the separation is mild and gestation is near term, labor may be induced, and the fetus may be born vaginally with as little trauma as possible. If rupture of membranes and oxytocin infusion by pump do not initiate labor within a short time, a cesarean birth is usually done. A longer delay would increase the risk of hemorrhage, with resulting hypofibrinogenemia. Supportive treatment to decrease risk of DIC includes typing and cross-matching for blood transfusions (at least three units), clotting mechanism evaluation, and intravenous fluids.

In cases of moderate to severe placental separation, a cesarean birth is done after hypofibrinogenemia has been treated by intravenous infusion of cryoprecipitate or fresh frozen plasma (FFP). Vaginal birth is impossible in the event of a Couvelaire uterus because it could not contract properly in labor. Cesarean birth is necessary in the face of severe hemorrhage to allow an immediate hysterectomy to save both woman and fetus.

The hypovolemia that accompanies severe abruptio placentae is life threatening and must be combated with whole blood. If the fetus is alive but experiencing stress, emergency cesarean birth is the method of choice. With a stillborn fetus, vaginal birth is preferable unless shock from hemorrhage is uncontrollable. Intravenous fluids of a balanced salt solution such as lactated Ringer's solution are given through a 16- or 18-gauge cannula (Cunningham et al, 2001). Central venous pressure (CVP) monitoring may be needed to evaluate intravenous fluid replacement. Hemodynamic monitoring is an essential aspect of nursing care for the woman with abruption. If there is any evidence of hypovolemia, two venous lines should be started. Urine output should be monitored with an indwelling catheter. If the output drops below 30 mL per hour with adequate fluid replacement, CVP should be used to assess for hypovolemia. CVP will be the guide to fluid replacement. An absolute level is not as significant as the response to fluid replacement. Pulmonary artery catheter measurement, such as with a Swan-Ganz catheter, may be necessary to manage the hemodynamic changes. However, a significant abruption may preclude placing a catheter in the jugular or subclavian vein because the DIC is causing bleeding from multiple sites. The CVP is evaluated hourly, and results are communicated to the physician. Elevations of CVP may indicate fluid overload and pulmonary edema. The hematocrit is maintained at 30% through the administration of packed red cells, whole blood, or both (Cunningham et al, 2001).

Laboratory testing is ordered to provide ongoing data regarding hemoglobin, hematocrit, and coagulation status. A clot observation test may be done at the bedside to evaluate coagulation status. A red top glass tube containing 5 mL of maternal blood is inverted four to five times. If a clot fails to form in 6 minutes, a fibrinogen level of less than 150 mg/dL is suspected. If a clot is not formed in 30 minutes, the fibrinogen level may well be less than 100 mg/dL. A clot observation test may be completed by a physician or a nurse.

Measures are taken to stimulate labor to effect vaginal birth as indicated by the condition of the mother and fetus. The birth may be hastened by performing an amniotomy and by oxytocin stimulation. Previously, birth within 6 hours of the diagnosis of severe placental abruption was recommended to reduce maternal mortality and morbidity. Currently, changing medical practice directed to ensuring adequate fluid replacement, especially blood, appears to accomplish the same outcome (Cunningham et al, 2001).

NURSING CARE MANAGEMENT

Nursing Assessment and Diagnosis

Electronic monitoring of the uterine contractions and resting tone between contractions provides information regarding the labor pattern and effectiveness of the oxytocin induction. Because uterine resting tone is frequently increased with abruptio placentae, it must be evaluated frequently for further increase. Abdominal girth measurements may be ordered hourly and are obtained by placing a tape measure around the maternal abdomen at the level of the umbilicus. Another method of evaluating uterine size, which increases as more bleeding occurs at the site of abruption, is to place a mark at the top of the uterine fundus. The distance from the symphysis pubis to the mark may be evaluated hourly.

Nursing diagnoses that may apply to the woman with abruptio placentae include the following:

- ***Fluid Volume Deficit*** related to hypovolemia secondary to excessive blood loss
- ***Risk for Altered Tissue Perfusion*** related to blood loss secondary to uterine atony following birth
- ***Anxiety*** related to concern for personal status and the baby's safety
- ***Risk for Impaired Gas Exchange*** in the fetus related to decreased blood volume and hypotension

Nursing Plan and Implementation

The psychologic aspects of nursing care are very important. Maternal apprehension increases as the clinical picture changes. Factual reassurance and an explanation of the procedures and what is happening are essential for the emotional well-being of the expectant couple. The nurse can reinforce positive aspects of the woman's condition, such as normal FHR, normal vital signs, and decreased evidence of bleeding.

Other nursing care measures are addressed in the Clinical Pathway for Hemorrhage in Third Trimester and at Birth on pages 722 to 723.

Evaluation

Expected outcomes of nursing care include the following:

- The woman and her baby have a safe labor and birth without further complications for the mother or child.
- The woman and family verbalize understanding of reasons for medical therapy and risks.

Placenta Previa

In **placenta previa,** the placenta is improperly implanted in the lower uterine segment. This implantation may be on a portion of the lower segment or over the internal os (Figure 26–17 •). As the lower uterine segment contracts and dilates in the later weeks of pregnancy, the placental villi are torn from the uterine wall, thus exposing the uterine sinuses at the placental site. Bleeding begins, but because the amount depends on the number of sinuses exposed, it may initially be either scanty or profuse.

The cause of placenta previa is unknown. Statistically, it occurs in about 1 in 200 pregnancies (Cunningham et al, 2001). Factors associated with placenta previa are multiparity, increasing age, placenta accreta (discussed shortly), defective development of blood vessels in the decidua, prior cesarean birth, smoking, a recent spontaneous or induced abortion, and a large placenta (Cunningham et al, 2001).

CLINICAL PATHWAY FOR HEMORRHAGE IN THIRD TRIMESTER AND AT BIRTH

Category	Immediate Care	Outcomes
Referral	Perinatologist Neonatologist	➤ **Expected Outcomes** Appropriate resources identified and utilized
Assessments	Obtain history to identify if any factors are present predisposing to hemorrhage: • Presence of preeclampsia-eclampsia • Overdistention of the uterus; multiple pregnancy; hydramnios • Grandmultiparity • Advanced age • Uterine contractile problems: hypotonicity; hypertonicity • Painless vaginal bleeding after seventh month • Presence of hypertension • Presence of diabetes • History of previous hemorrhage or bleeding problems, blood coagulation defects, abortion • Retention of placental fragments • Cervical and/or vaginal lacerations Determine religious preference to establish whether client will permit a blood transfusion	➤ **Expected Outcomes** • Potential/actual hemorrhage identified • Related complications minimized
Teaching/ psychosocial	Keep woman informed of present status Provide accurate information Provide opportunities for questions Establish a trusting relationship with client Encourage the woman to participate in decision making if at all possible Instruct client to keep bladder empty Notify RN if vag bleeding or leaking noted, decreased fetal movement, abdominal pain/discomfort or uterine contractions Report saturation $>$ 1 pad within 1 h or less	➤ **Expected Outcomes** Woman verbalizes/demonstrates understanding of teaching
Nursing care management and reports	Observe, record, and report blood loss Evaluate using the following parameters: • Monitor rate and quality of respirations frequently • Measure pulse rate • Assess pulse quality by direct palpation • Determine pulse deficit by comparing apical-radial rates • Compare present BP with woman's baseline BP; note pulse pressure • Inspect skin for presence of pallor and cyanosis, coldness, and clamminess • Evaluate state of consciousness frequently • Measure CVP: normal CVP is 5–10 cm H_2O • Assess amount of blood loss: • Count pads • Weigh pads and Chux (1 g = approximately 1 mL blood) • Record amount in a specific amount of time (eg, 50 mL bright red blood on pad in 20 min) Relieve decreased blood pressure by administering whole blood per physician order While waiting for whole blood to be available, infuse isotonic fluids, plasma, plasma expanders, or serum albumin, per physician order If marginal abruptio placentae is present: • Evaluate blood loss • Assess uterine contractile pattern, tenderness, and height • Start continuous monitoring of uterine contractions by EFM • Monitor maternal vital signs • Assess fetal status per continuous EFM • Assess cervical dilatation and effacement to determine labor progress if uterine contractions are present • Rule out placenta previa • Assist with amniotomy, and begin oxytocin infusion per physician order if labor does not start immediately or is ineffective • Review and evaluate diagnostic lab tests (hemoglobin, hematocrit, PT, PTT, fibrin split products, fibrinogen, platelets)	➤ **Expected Outcomes** • Blood loss reduced, controlled, or halted • Perfusion and oxygenation supported

Placenta previa is classified in four degrees:

1. *Total placenta previa.* Internal os is covered completely by the placenta.
2. *Partial placenta previa.* Internal os is partially covered by the placenta.
3. *Marginal placenta previa.* Edge of the placenta is at the margin of the internal os.
4. *Low-lying placenta.* Placenta is implanted in the lower segment but does not reach the os although it is in close proximity of it (Cunningham et al, 2001).

CLINICAL PATHWAY FOR HEMORRHAGE IN THIRD TRIMESTER AND AT BIRTH *CONTINUED*

Category	Immediate Care	Outcomes
Nursing care management and reports *continued*	If central abruptio placentae with severe blood loss is present: • Perform same assessments as for marginal abruptio placentae • Monitor CVP • Replace blood loss • Observe for signs and symptoms of disseminated intravascular coagulation (DIC) Woman is at risk for uterine atony following birth: • Assess contractility of uterus and amount of vaginal bleeding • Assess uterus q15min × 1, q30min × 2, q60min × 2–4. Evaluate more frequently if uterus is boggy or not in the midline. Administer oxytocin per protocol or physician order.	
Activity	Complete bed rest Diversional activity	➤ **Expected Outcomes** No exacerbation of hemorrhage occurs
Comfort	Assess comfort of woman	➤ **Expected Outcomes** Woman's comfort maintained
Nutrition	IV fluids infusing NPO	➤ **Expected Outcomes** Optimal hydration and blood volume maintained
Elimination	Monitor urine output (decrease to less than 30 mL/h is sign of shock): • Insert Foley catheter • Measure output hourly • Measure specific gravity to determine concentration of urine	➤ **Expected Outcomes** Urinary output maintained
Medications	IV—lactated Ringer's at 150 mL/h If premature—Betamethasone O_2 as indicated	➤ **Expected Outcomes** Circulation and perfusion maintained
Discharge planning/ home care	Determine need for assistance in the home Provide information regarding community resources	➤ **Expected Outcomes** Woman is discharged with plan for follow-up care related to fatigue and blood loss
Family involvement	Establish a trusting relationship with family	➤ **Expected Outcomes** Family development and newborn attachment unimpaired
Date		

BP, blood pressure; CVP, central venous pressure; EFM, electronic fetal monitor; NPO, nothing by mouth

Another condition, **vasa previa,** occurs when the fetal vessels course through the amniotic membranes and are present at the cervical os. Although this is a rare cause of antepartum bleeding, it is associated with a high rate of fetal death (Cunningham et al, 2001).

CLINICAL THERAPY

Women who present with vaginal bleeding should be questioned regarding any history of abnormal placenta placement that was diagnosed during the pregnancy. When possible, prenatal records should be reviewed. Women who have not had a routine ultrasound examination and have no history of bleeding during the pregnancy may have an undiagnosed placenta previa. The goal of medical care is to identify the cause of bleeding and to provide treatment that will ensure birth of a mature newborn. It must be determined whether the cause of the bleeding is placenta previa or advanced labor with copious bloody show (which is normal). Indirect diagnosis is made by localizing the placenta via tests that require no vaginal examination. The most commonly employed diagnostic test is the transabdominal ultrasound scan. Abdominal or transvaginal sonography is used to identify the presence of placenta previa. If placenta previa is ruled out, a vaginal examination can be performed with a speculum to determine the cause of bleeding (such as cervical lesions or polyps).

Direct diagnosis of placenta previa can be made only by feeling the placenta inside the cervical os. However, such an examination may cause profuse bleeding due to tearing of tissue in the cotyledons of the placenta. Because of the danger of bleeding, a vaginal examination is generally contraindicated and is performed only if ultrasound is not available, the pregnancy is near term, and there is already profuse vaginal bleeding. The examination is done by a physician using a double setup procedure; that is, the delivery room is set up for the vaginal examination and normal vaginal birth and for a cesarean birth should placenta previa be present and the examination precipitate brisk bleeding. Adequate personnel must be present to respond to treatment decisions.

The differential diagnosis of placental or cervical bleeding takes careful consideration. Table 26–6 • provides a comparison of the signs and symptoms of placenta previa and abruptio placentae. Partial separation of the placenta may

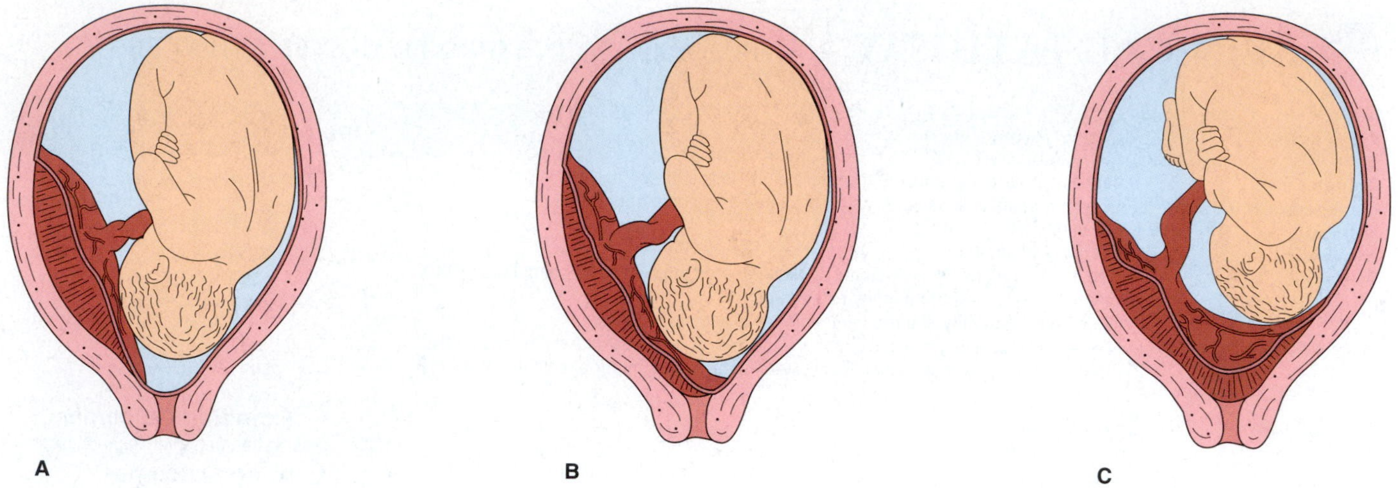

Figure 26–17 • Placenta previa. *A,* Low placental implantation. *B,* Partial placenta previa. *C,* Total placenta previa.

also present with painless bleeding, and a true placenta previa may not demonstrate overt bleeding until labor begins, thus confusing the diagnosis. In fact, the causes of slight to moderate antepartal bleeding episodes in 20% to 25% of women are never accurately diagnosed.

Care of the woman with painless late gestational bleeding depends on (1) the week of gestation during which the first bleeding episode occurs and (2) the amount of bleeding (Figure 26–18 •). If the pregnancy is less than 37 weeks' gestation, expectant management is employed to delay birth until about 37 weeks' gestation to allow the fetus to mature. Expectant management involves stringent compliance with the following:

1. Bed rest with bathroom privileges only as long as the woman is not bleeding
2. No vaginal examinations
3. Monitoring of blood loss, pain, and uterine contractility
4. Evaluation of FHRs with external monitor
5. Monitoring of maternal vital signs
6. Complete laboratory evaluation: hemoglobin, hematocrit, Rh factor, and urinalysis
7. Administration of intravenous fluid (lactated Ringer's solution) with drip rate monitored
8. Availability of two units of cross-matched blood for possible transfusion
9. Administration of betamethasone to facilitate fetal lung maturity

If frequent, recurrent, or profuse bleeding persists or if fetal well-being appears threatened, a cesarean birth needs to be performed.

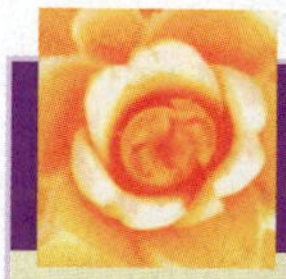

EVIDENCE-BASED PRACTICE:

RISK FACTORS RELATED TO PLACENTA PREVIA

Clinical Question

Do clients with previous cesarean birth, spontaneous abortion, or induced abortion experience an increased risk of placenta previa?

The Evidence

From 36 high-quality research studies, the reported incidence of placenta previa was approximately 1 in 200 pregnancies. Women who had previous cesarean births showed an increased risk of placenta previa; the risk of placenta previa increased with the number of previous cesarean births. There was also an increased risk of placenta previa for women who had previous spontaneous abortion and an increased risk of placenta previa for women who had previous induced abortion.

Best Practice

Best practice would include accurate assessment of a woman's obstetric history. Women who have had a previous cesarean birth or a spontaneous or induced abortion have a greater risk of developing placenta previa. The risk increases with the number of previous cesarean births or abortions. Women with any of these factors should be carefully monitored for placenta previa.

Reference: Ananth, C. V., Smulian, J. C., & Vintzileos, A. M. (1997). The association of placenta previa with history of cesarean delivery and abortion: A metaanalysis. *American Journal of Obstetrics and Gynecology, 177,* 1071–1078.

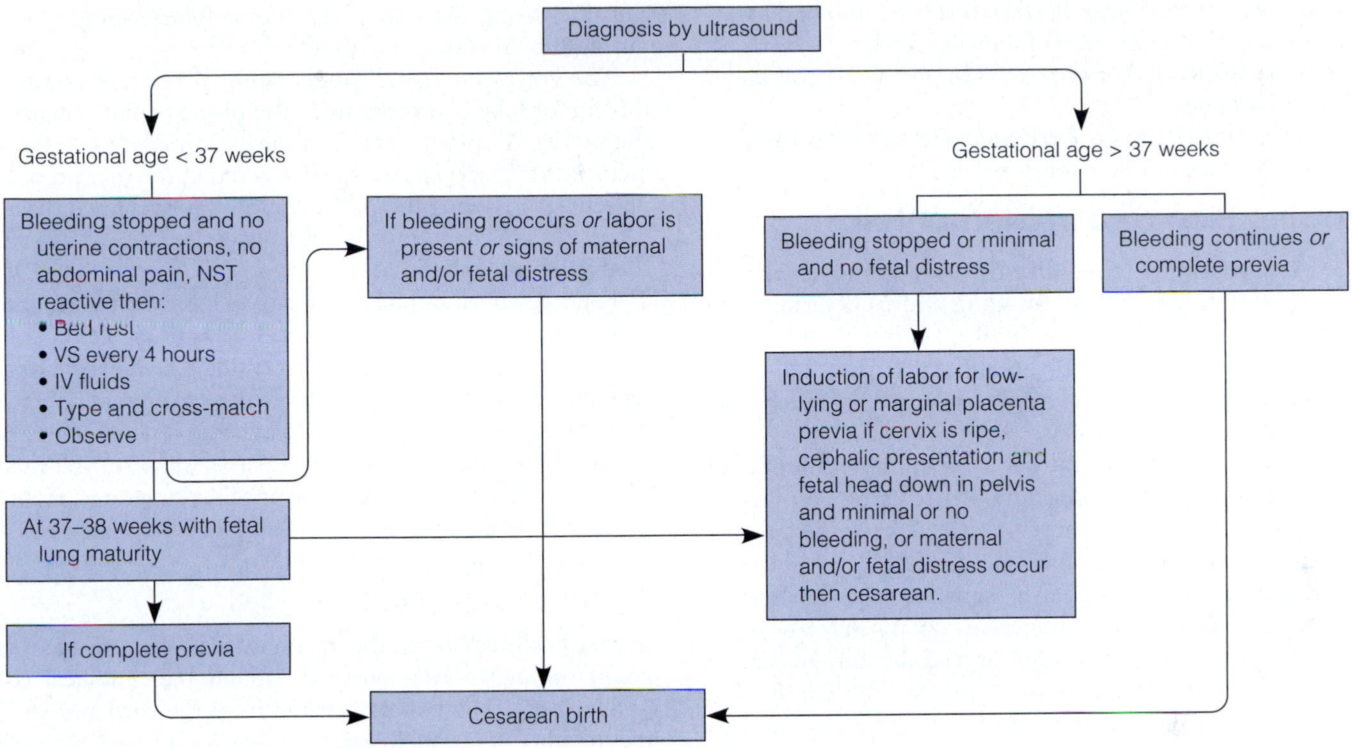

Figure 26–18 • Management of placenta previa.
SOURCE: Zuspan, F. P., & Quilligan, E. J. *Handbook of obstetrics, gynecology, and primary care.* Copyright 1998, with permission from Elsevier Science.

NURSING CARE MANAGEMENT

Nursing Assessment and Diagnosis

Assessment of the woman with placenta previa must be ongoing to prevent or treat complications that are potentially lethal to the mother and fetus. Painless, bright red vaginal bleeding is the best diagnostic sign of placenta previa. If this sign should develop during the last 3 months of a pregnancy, placenta previa should always be considered until ruled out by ultrasound examination. The first bleeding episode is generally scanty. If no vaginal examinations are performed, it often subsides spontaneously. However, each subsequent hemorrhage is more profuse.

The uterus remains soft, and if labor begins, it relaxes fully between contractions. The FHR usually remains stable unless profuse hemorrhage and maternal shock occur. As a result of the placement of the placenta, the fetal presenting part is often unengaged, and transverse lie is common.

The nurse appraises blood loss, pain, and uterine contractility from both subjective and objective perspectives. Maternal vital signs and the results of blood and urine tests provide the nurse with additional data about the woman's condition. FHR is evaluated with an external fetal monitor. Another nursing responsibility is observing and verifying the family's ability to cope with the anxiety associated with an unknown outcome.

Table 26–6 • **DIFFERENTIAL SIGNS AND SYMPTOMS OF PLACENTA PREVIA AND ABRUPTIO PLACENTAE**

	Placenta Previa	Abruptio Placentae
Onset	Quiet and sneaky	Sudden and stormy
Bleeding	External	External or concealed
Color of blood	Bright red	Dark venous
Anemia	= Blood loss	> Apparent blood loss
Shock	= Blood loss	> Apparent blood loss
Toxemia	Absent	May be present
Pain	Only labor	Severe and steady
Uterine tenderness	Absent	Present
Uterine tone	Soft and relaxed	Firm to stony hard
Uterine contour	Normal	May enlarge and change shape
Fetal heart tones	Usually present	Present or absent
Engagement	Absent	May be present
Presentation	May be abnormal	No relationship

Source: Oxorn, H (1986). *Human labor and birth,* (5th ed., p. 507). Norwalk, CT: Appleton & Lange.

Nursing diagnoses that may apply to the woman experiencing placenta previa are as follows:

- ***Fluid Volume Deficit*** related to hypovolemia secondary to excessive blood loss

- ***Risk for Altered Tissue Perfusion*** related to blood loss secondary to uterine atony following birth
- ***Anxiety*** related to concern for own personal status and the baby's safety
- ***Risk for Impaired Gas Exchange*** related to decreased blood volume and hypotension

Nursing Plan and Implementation

The nurse continues to monitor the woman and her fetus to determine the status of the bleeding and to determine the mother's and baby's responses. Vital signs, intake and output, and other pertinent assessments must be made frequently. The nurse evaluates the electronic monitor tracing to evaluate the fetal status.

Emotional support for the family is an important nursing care goal. When active bleeding is occurring, the assessments and management must be directed toward physical support. However, emotional aspects need to be addressed simultaneously. The nurse can explain the assessments being completed and the treatment measures that need to be done. Time can be provided for questions, and the nurse can act as an advocate in obtaining information for the family. The nurse can also offer emotional support by staying with the family and by the use of touch.

The newborn's hemoglobin, cell volume, and erythrocyte count should be checked immediately after birth and then monitored closely. The newborn may require oxygen and administration of blood and admission into a neonatal intensive care unit.

Additional information regarding nursing care is addressed in the Clinical Pathway for Hemorrhage in Third Trimester and at Birth.

Evaluation

Expected outcomes of nursing care include the following:

- The cause of hemorrhage is recognized promptly, and corrective measures are taken.
- The woman's vital signs remain in the normal range.
- The woman and her baby have a safe labor and birth.
- The family understands what has happened and the implications and associated problems of placenta previa.

MEDIALINK CASE STUDY: CLIENT WITH PLACENTAL PROBLEMS

Other Placental Problems

Other problems of the placenta can be divided into those that are developmental and those that are degenerative. Developmental problems of the placenta include placental lesions, succenturiate placenta, circumvallate placenta, and battledore placenta (Table 26–7 •). Degenerative changes include infarcts and placental calcification.

SUCCENTURIATE PLACENTA

In *succenturiate placenta,* one or more accessory lobes of fetal villi have developed on the placenta, with vascular connections of fetal origin (see Table 26–7). Vessels from the major to the minor lobe(s) are supported only by the membranes, thus increasing the risk of the minor lobe's being retained during the third stage of labor.

The gravest maternal danger is postpartal hemorrhage if this minor lobe is severed from the placenta and remains in the uterus. All placentas should be examined closely for intactness. If vessels appear to be severed at the margin of the placenta, the uterus should be explored for retained placental tissue. This condition is not usually diagnosed until after the birth of the placenta.

Fetal/newborn implications can be life threatening if the vascular connections rupture between the placenta lobes since a fatal fetal hemorrhage can result. Examination of the fetal membrane following birth may reveal a small hole with vessels running toward it. This is another indication of a retained lobe (Cunningham et al, 2001). At birth, the infant should be inspected for pallor, cyanosis, retractions, tachypnea, tachycardia, and feeble pulse. The infant's cry will be weak and the muscle tone flaccid.

CIRCUMVALLATE PLACENTA

In *circumvallate placenta,* the fetal surface of the placenta is exposed through a ring opening around the umbilical cord (Table 26–7). The vessels descend from the cord and end at the margin of the ring instead of coursing through the entire surface area of the placenta. The ring is composed of a double fold of amnion and chorion with some degenerative decidua and fibrin between. The cause of this condition is unknown. Maternal-fetal problems include an increased incidence of late abortion or fetal death, antepartal hemorrhage, prematurity, and abnormal maternal bleeding during or following the third stage of labor, resulting from improper placental separation or shearing of membranes from the placenta.

BATTLEDORE PLACENTA

In *battledore placenta,* the umbilical cord is inserted at or near the placental margin (Table 26–7). As a result, all fetal vessels transverse the placental surface in the same direction. The chances of preterm labor are high because of interference with fetal circulation and nutrition. Fetal distress or bleeding during labor is also likely because of cord compression or vessel rupture.

PLACENTAL INFARCTS AND CALCIFICATIONS

As the placenta grade matures (previously discussed in Chapter 21), the placenta may develop infarcts and calcifications. They become significant if they cover a large enough area to interfere with the uterine-placental-fetal exchange. Altered exchange can also occur with certain maternal disease processes, such as hypertension. Infarcts are most often seen in cases of severe preeclampsia and in women who smoke.

Care of the Woman and Fetus at Risk Due to Problems Associated with the Umbilical Cord

Prolapsed Umbilical Cord

An umbilical cord that precedes the fetal presenting part is known as a **prolapsed umbilical cord.** It occurs when the cord

Table 26-7 • PLACENTAL AND UMBILICAL CORD VARIATIONS

Placental Variation	Maternal Implications	Fetal-Neonatal Implications	
Succenturiate placenta One or more accessory lobes of fetal villi will develop on the placenta.	Postpartal hemorrhage from retained lobe	None, as long as all parts of the placenta remain attached until after birth of the fetus	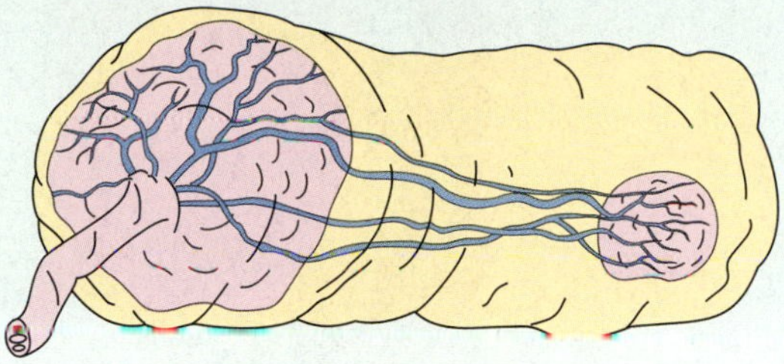
Circumvallate placenta A double fold of chorion and amnion form a ring around the umbilical cord, on the fetal side of the placenta.	Increased incidence of late abortion, antepartal hemorrhage, and preterm labor	Intrauterine growth restriction, prematurity, fetal death	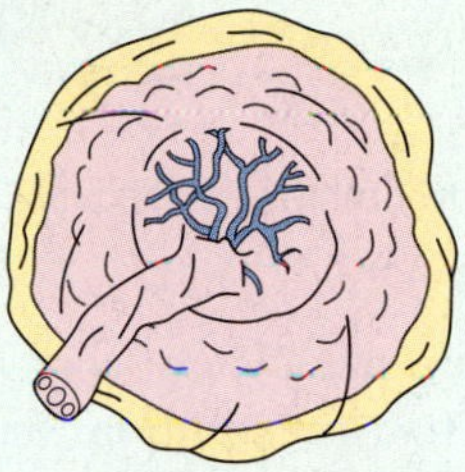
Battledore placenta The umbilical cord is inserted at or near the placental margin.	Increased incidence of preterm labor and bleeding	Prematurity, fetal stress	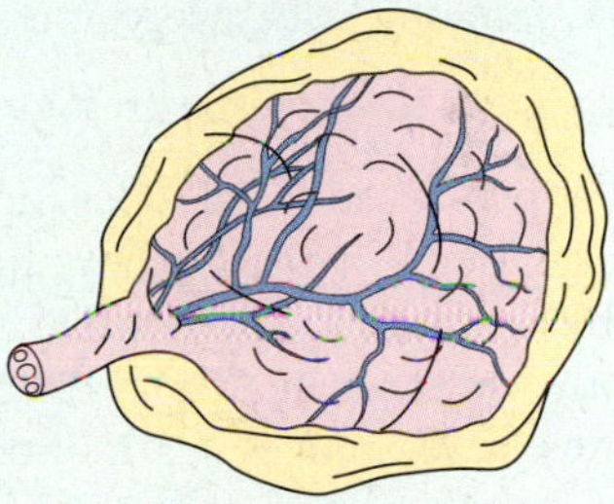
Velamentous insertion of the umbilical cord The vessels of the umbilical cord divide some distance from the placenta in the placental membranes.	Hemorrhage if one of the vessels is torn	Fetal stress, hemorrhage	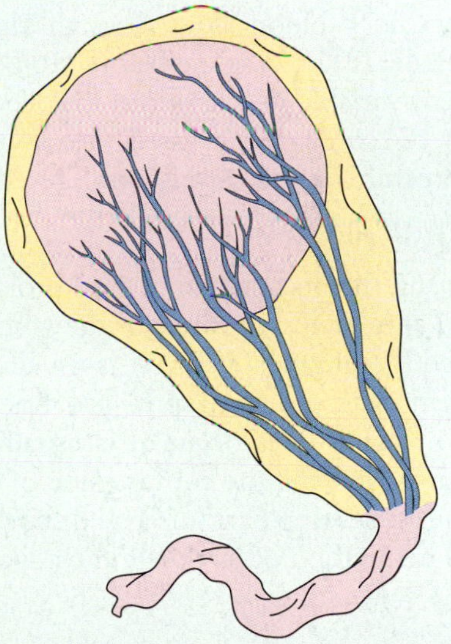

falls or is washed down through the cervix into the vagina and becomes trapped between the presenting part and the maternal pelvis. Because of this entrapment, the vessels carrying blood to and from the fetus are compressed. In rare circumstances a prolapsed cord may be visible at the lower edge of the vagina. In other cases, the umbilical cord lies beside or just ahead of the fetal head; this is called *occult cord prolapse.*

Any time that the pelvic inlet is not completely filled by the fetus or the presenting part is not firmly against the cervix, and the membranes rupture, the umbilical cord can be washed down into the birth canal in front of the presenting part (Figure 26–19 •). The incidence of prolapse of the cord is 20 times greater with abnormal axis lie (Gabbe, 1996)—especially footling breech and shoulder presentations—low birth weight, a multipara with more than five previous births, multiple gestation, obstetric manipulation (amniotomy), and the presence of a long cord (longer than 80 cm). Approximately 50% of cord prolapses occur in the second stage of

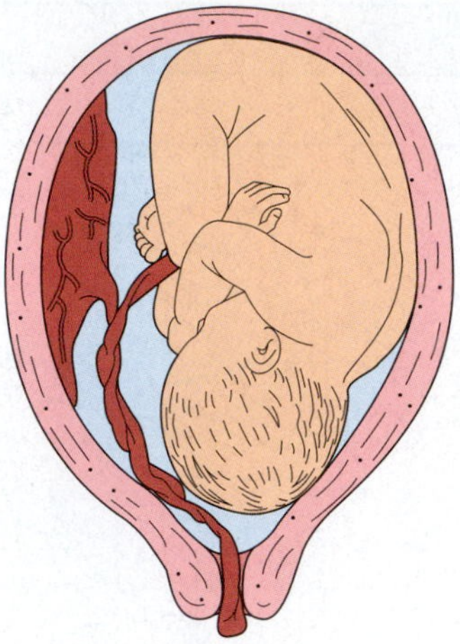

Figure 26–19 • Prolapse of the umbilical cord.

MediaLink CARE PLAN: PREVENTION OF CORD PROLAPSE

labor. An additional 47% of cord prolapses occur as a result of some obstetric intervention, such as amniotomy, application of fetal scalp electrode, intrapressure catheter, or external cephalic version (Usta, Mercer, & Sibai, 1999).

MATERNAL-FETAL-NEONATAL RISKS

Although a prolapsed cord does not directly precipitate physical alterations in the woman, her immediate concern for the baby creates enormous stress. The woman may need to deal with some unusual interventions, a cesarean birth, and in some circumstances death of the fetus.

The fetus is affected because compression of the umbilical cord occludes blood flow through the umbilical vessels. Bradycardia (FHR baseline below 110 beats per minute) and persistent variable decelerations may develop. If labor is occurring, the cord is compressed further with each contraction. If the pressure on the cord is not relieved, the fetus will die.

CLINICAL THERAPY

Preventing the occurrence of cord prolapse is the preferred medical approach. For all laboring women with a history of ruptured membranes, bed rest is usually indicated until engagement with no cord prolapse has been documented. When prolapse does occur, it is usually discovered by the nurse, and relieving the compression of the cord by pushing back the presenting part (discussed shortly) is critical for the fetus. The method of birth will most likely be cesarean.

NURSING CARE MANAGEMENT

Nursing Assessment and Diagnosis

In the intrapartal area, the nurse reviews the nursing history and ascertains whether the woman is likely to be at risk for prolapse of the cord. Particularly when the presenting part is not engaged and spontaneous or artificial rupture of the membranes occurs, the nurse observes the perineum and assesses the FHR for bradycardia and severe, recurrent, variable decelerations.

Nursing diagnoses that may apply to the woman with a prolapsed cord include the following:

- ***Risk for Impaired Gas Exchange*** in the fetus related to decreased blood flow secondary to compression of the umbilical cord
- ***Fear*** related to unknown outcome

Nursing Plan and Implementation

Because there are few outward signs of cord prolapse, each pregnant woman is advised to call her physician or certified nurse-midwife (CNM) when the membranes rupture and to go immediately to the office, clinic, or birthing facility. A sterile vaginal examination determines whether there is danger of cord prolapse. If the presenting part is well engaged, the risk is minimal and ambulation may be encouraged. If the presenting part is not well engaged, bed rest is recommended to prevent cord prolapse. Maintaining bed rest after rupture of membranes can lead to conflict if the laboring woman and her partner do not hold the same beliefs. The nurse can ease this situation by helping communication between the physician/CNM and the couple.

If membranes have not yet ruptured when the woman arrives at the facility, at the time of spontaneous rupture or amniotomy the FHR should be monitored by electronic fetal monitoring or auscultated for at least a full minute and again at the end of a contraction and after a few contractions. In the presence of cord prolapse, EFM tracings show baseline bradycardia or severe, moderate, or prolonged nonperiodic decelerations. If these patterns are found, the nurse performs a vaginal examination.

If a loop of cord is discovered, the nurse's gloved fingers are left in the vagina, and the presenting part is pushed upward to lift the fetal part off the cord and relieve cord compression until the physician/CNM arrives. This is a life saving measure. Oxygen is administered, and FHR is monitored by EFM to see if the cord compression is adequately relieved (baseline will rise above 110 beats per minute, and variable decelerations are lessened or relieved). The nurse may also feel pulsation in the cord; however, in some instances a pulsation cannot be felt, and FHR can be detected only by EFM. A large-gauge intravenous cannula is inserted and intravenous fluids should be initiated. Anesthesia and neonatology services should be notified of impending birth.

In some cases, another nurse may insert an indwelling bladder catheter and, using a sterile asepto syringe or infusion device, fill the bladder with approximately 350 to 500 mL of warmed, sterile normal saline. The filled bladder lifts the fetal head upward and relieves pressure on the umbilical cord (Griese & Prickett, 1993). Filling her bladder and maintaining the woman in a side-lying position may be all that is needed to relieve the pressure on the cord. If the bladder is not filled, the force of gravity can be incorporated. In this instance, the nurse maintains pressure on the presenting part and instructs the woman to bring her knees to her chest or adjusts the bed to the Trendelenburg position. The nurse maintains pressure on the presenting part while the woman is transported to the birthing or operating room in this position. The nurse maintains this position until the fetus is born via cesarean birth.

Evaluation

Expected outcomes of nursing care include the following:

- The FHR remains in normal range with supportive measures.
- The fetus is born safely.
- The woman and her partner feel supported.
- The woman and her partner understand the problem and the corrective measures that are undertaken.

Umbilical Cord Abnormalities

Umbilical cord abnormalities include congenital absence of an umbilical artery, insertion variations, cord length variations, and knots and loops of the cord. Insertion variations include velamentous insertion and vasa previa, and cord length problems include long and short cords.

CONGENITAL ABSENCE OF UMBILICAL ARTERY

Absence of an umbilical artery may have serious fetal implications. The incidence of all types of fetal anomalies is 25% in infants born with two-vessel cords.

Immediately after the umbilical cord is cut, it should be inspected to determine whether the correct number of vessels is present. If an artery is absent, the nurse should examine the newborn closely for anomalies and gestational age problems and alert the attending pediatrician.

INSERTION VARIATIONS

In a *velamentous insertion*, the vessels of the umbilical cord divide some distance from the placenta in the placental membranes (see Table 26–7). Velamentous insertions occur more frequently in multiple gestations than in singletons. Other placental anomalies, such as succenturiate placenta, often accompany this condition. The velamentous insertion is more easily compressed or kinked during pregnancy or labor because of the lack of Wharton's jelly to protect it. If the vessels become torn during labor, fetal hemorrhage can occur, and the blood can escape from the vagina. When fetal hemorrhage occurs, it results in FHR abnormalities.

When the vessels of a velamentous insertion transverse the internal os and appear in front of the fetus, a vasa previa has occurred. Fetal hemorrhage with asphyxia is likely to result because as the fetal blood escapes out of the vagina the hemorrhage will probably be diagnosed as maternal.

CORD LENGTH VARIATIONS

The average length of the umbilical cord is 55 cm. Although short cords rarely cause complications directly, they have been associated with umbilical hernias in the fetus, abruptio placentae, and cord rupture. Long cords tend to twist and tangle around the fetus, causing transient variable decelerations. A long cord rarely causes fetal death, however, because it is generally not pulled tight until descent at the time of birth. With a long cord and an active fetus, one or more true knots can result. Again, these knots usually are not pulled tight enough to cause fetal stress until the infant has been born, and the cord can then be clamped and cut.

CLINICAL THERAPY

The goals of medical treatment are to prevent serious fetal complications and to examine the newborn for anomalies that coexist with umbilical cord abnormalities.

Any vaginal bleeding during labor warrants continuous monitoring of the fetus, preferably with an external electronic monitor. Any signs of nonreassuring heart rate patterns should be reported immediately. In the presence of bleeding, laboratory tests may be used to differentiate fetal from maternal red blood cells. Fetal hemorrhage is resolved by terminating the pregnancy vaginally or through cesarean birth and by correcting neonatal anemia. Expediting the birth, whether vaginally or surgically, is paramount when a severe nonreassuring heart rate pattern is apparent. Following the birth, the pediatric team identifies and treats any neonatal complications or anomalies.

NURSING CARE MANAGEMENT

Nursing Assessment and Diagnosis

Umbilical abnormalities may not become evident until the birth of the fetus. During labor the nurse should observe for signs of nonreassuring fetal status and excessive bleeding (with velamentous insertion and vasa previa). Nursing diagnoses that may apply include the following:

- ***Risk for Impaired Gas Exchange*** in the fetus related to decreased blood flow secondary to placental abnormalities
- ***Health-Seeking Behavior:*** information about of placental abnormalities related to an expressed desire to understand the implications of the finding.

Nursing Plan and Implementation

The nurse is alert for an unusual amount of bleeding during the labor and birth. Following the birth, the placenta is inspected for abnormalities. Examination of the placenta by a pathologist may be indicated.

Often any mild or moderate variable deceleration can be successfully managed by the nurse. Repositioning of the woman often alleviates pressure on the cord if this is the reason for the deceleration.

Evaluation

Expected outcomes of nursing care include the following:

- The mother and baby have a safe labor and birth.
- The woman's bleeding is assessed quickly, and corrective measures are taken.
- The family is able to cope successfully with fetal or neonatal anomalies, if they exist.

Care of the Woman and Fetus at Risk Due to Amniotic Fluid-Related Complications

MediaLink AMNIOTIC FLUID PROBLEMS

Complications related to amniotic fluid include amniotic fluid embolism, hydramnios, and oligohydramnios.

Amniotic Fluid Embolism

Amniotic fluid embolism occurs when a bolus of amniotic fluid enters the maternal circulation and then the maternal lungs. The cause of this obstetric emergency is unknown. It is the second leading cause of maternal deaths, resulting in 100 to 150 per year in the United States (Benson, Kobayashi, Silver, et al, 2001). Because amniotic fluid embolism is a rare complication, a national registry was initiated in 1988 to collect retrospective data for analysis. The first findings from this registry were published in 1995 and showed that 78% of the women who had an amniotic fluid embolism had ruptured membranes (Locksmith, 1999).

Hydramnios

Hydramnios (also called *polyhydramnios*) occurs when there is over 2000 mL of amniotic fluid. It typically occurs in 1% of all pregnancies (Cunningham et al, 2001). The exact cause of hydramnios is unknown; however, it often occurs in cases of major congenital anomalies. It is postulated that a major source of amniotic fluid is found in special amnion cells that lie over the placenta (Cunningham et al, 2001). In cases of hydramnios, no pathology has been found in this amniotic epithelium. However, during the second half of the pregnancy, the fetus normally begins to swallow and inspire amniotic fluid and to urinate, which contributes to the amount present. Fetal malformations that affect this swallowing mechanism—as well as neurologic disorders in which the fetal meninges are exposed in the amniotic cavity—can result in hydramnios.

This condition is also found in cases of anencephaly, in which the fetus is thought to urinate excessively due to overstimulation of the cerebrospinal centers. When a monozygotic twin manifests hydramnios, it is possible that the twin with the increased blood volume urinates excessively. The weight of the placenta has been found to be increased in some cases of hydramnios, indicating that increased functioning of the placental tissue may contribute to the problem.

There are two types of hydramnios: chronic and acute. The chronic type, in which the fluid volume gradually increases, is a problem of the third trimester. Most cases are of this variety. In acute cases, the volume increases rapidly over a period of a few days. The acute type is usually diagnosed between 20 and 24 weeks' gestation.

When the amount of amniotic fluid is over 3000 mL, the woman experiences shortness of breath and edema in the lower extremities from compression of the vena cava. If hydramnios is severe enough, she can experience intense pain. The acute form of hydramnios tends to be more severe. Milder forms of hydramnios occur more frequently and are associated with minimal symptoms. Hydramnios is associated with such maternal disorders as diabetes and Rh sensitization. It can also occur as a result of infections such as syphilis, toxoplasmosis, cytomegalovirus, herpes, and rubella.

Fetal malformations and preterm birth are common with hydramnios; thus there is a fairly high rate of perinatal mortality. Prolapsed umbilical cord can occur when the membranes rupture, which adds a further complication for the fetus. The incidence of malpresentations is also increased.

CLINICAL THERAPY

Hydramnios is managed with supportive treatment unless the intensity of the woman's distress and symptoms dictate otherwise.

If the accumulation of amniotic fluid is severe enough to cause maternal dyspnea and pain, hospitalization and removal of the excessive fluid are required. This can be done vaginally by artificial rupture of membranes (AROM) or by amniocentesis. The dangers of performing AROM vaginally are prolapsed cord and the inability to remove the fluid slowly. A *needle amniotomy* may be preferred since this releases the fluid at a slower rate and allows the presenting part to descend gradually. A needle amniotomy is performed by the CNM/physician. A needle or a fetal scalp electrode is used to make a small puncture in the amniotic sac. There is a risk that the force of the fluid could make a larger hole in the amniotic sac, thus increasing the risk of a prolapsed cord. If amniocentesis is performed, it should be done with the aid of sonography to prevent inadvertent damage to the fetus and placenta.

A prostaglandin synthesis inhibitor (indomethacin) is often used to treat hydramnios. Indomethacin has been shown to decrease amniotic fluid volume by decreasing fetal urine output (Cunningham et al, 2001).

NURSING CARE MANAGEMENT

Nursing Assessment and Diagnosis

Hydramnios should be suspected when the fundal height increases out of proportion to the gestational age.

With increased fluid, the nurse may have difficulty palpating the fetus and auscultating the FHR. In more severe cases the maternal abdomen appears extremely tense and tight on inspection. On sonography large spaces can be identified between the fetus and the uterine wall.

Nursing diagnoses that may apply for a woman with hydramnios include the following:

- ***Risk for Impaired Gas Exchange*** related to pressure on the diaphragm secondary to hydramnios
- ***Fear*** related to unknown outcome of the pregnancy

Nursing Plan and Implementation

When amniocentesis is performed, sterile technique is used to prevent infection. The nurse can offer support to the couple by explaining the procedure to them.

If the fetus has been diagnosed with a congenital defect in utero or is born with the defect, psychologic support is needed to assist the family. Often the nurse collaborates with social services to offer the family this additional help. The nurse can also offer to contact chaplain services at the family's request.

Evaluation

Expected outcomes of nursing care include the following:

- The woman and her partner can discuss the procedure, implications, risks, and characteristics that need to be reported to the caregiver.

Oligohydramnios

Oligohydramnios is defined as a less than normal amount of amniotic fluid (approximately 500 mL is considered normal). Although no exact amount of fluid has been definitively identified as diagnostic of this condition oligohydramnios is diagnosed when the largest vertical pocket of amniotic fluid visible on ultrasound examination is 5 cm or less (Cunningham et al, 2001). The exact cause of oligohydramnios is unknown. It is found in cases of postmaturity, with intrauterine growth restriction (IUGR) secondary to placental insufficiency, and in fetal conditions associated with major renal malformations, including renal aplasia with dysplastic kidneys and obstructive lesions of the lower urinary tract. If oligohydramnios occurs in the first part of pregnancy, there is a danger of fetal adhesions (one part of the fetus may adhere to another part).

During the gestational period, fetal skin and skeletal abnormalities may occur because fetal movement is impaired as a result of inadequate amniotic fluid volume. Because there is less fluid available for the fetus to use during fetal breathing movements, pulmonary hypoplasia may develop. During the labor and birth, the lessened amounts of fluid reduce the cushioning effect for the umbilical cord, and cord compression is more likely to occur.

CLINICAL THERAPY

During the antepartum period, oligohydramnios may be suspected when the uterus does not increase in size in accordance with established gestational dating, the fetus is easily palpated and outlined by the examiner, and the fetus is not ballottable. The fetus can be assessed by biophysical profiles, nonstress tests, and serial ultrasounds. During labor the fetus will be monitored by continuous electronic fetal monitoring to detect cord compression, which will be indicated by nonperiodic decelerations. Amnioinfusion can replace some fluid volume and remove pressure on the umbilical cord (see Chapter 27).

NURSING CARE MANAGEMENT

Continuous electronic fetal monitoring is an important part of assessment during the labor and birth. The nurse evaluates the EFM tracing for the presence of nonperiodic decelerations or other nonreassuring signs (such as increasing or decreasing baseline, decreased variability, or presence of periodic decelerations). If nonperiodic decelerations are noted, the nurse can change the woman's position (to relieve pressure on the umbilical cord) and must then notify the physician/CNM. If position changes are insufficient to relieve the pattern, an amnioinfusion may be performed. After the birth, the newborn is evaluated for signs of congenital anomalies, pulmonary hypoplasia, or postmaturity.

Care of the Woman with Cephalopelvic Disproportion

The birth passage includes the maternal bony pelvis, beginning at the pelvic inlet and ending at the pelvic outlet, and the maternal soft tissues within these anatomic areas. A contracture (narrowing) in any of the described areas can result in **cephalopelvic disproportion (CPD).** Abnormal fetal presentations and positions occur in CPD as the fetus moves to accommodate passage through the maternal pelvis.

The gynecoid and anthropoid pelvic types are usually adequate for vertex birth, but the android and platypelloid types predispose to CPD. Certain combinations of types also can result in pelvic diameters inadequate for vertex birth. (See Chapter 10 for a description of the types of pelves and their implications for childbirth.) Clues that may lead to suspicion of contractures of the maternal pelvis are presented in Table 26–8 •. Women with a history of pelvic fractures may also be at risk for CPD.

MEDIALINK CEPHALOPELVIC DISPROPORTION

Types of Contractures

CONTRACTURES OF THE INLET

The pelvic inlet is contracted if the shortest anterior-posterior diameter is less than 10 cm or the greatest transverse diameter

Table 26–8 • CLUES TO CONTRACTURES OF MATERNAL PELVIS
Diagonal conjugate <11.5 cm (contracture of inlet), outlet <8 cm (contracture of outlet)
Unengaged fetal head in early labor in primigravidas (consider contracture of inlet, malpresentation, or malposition)
Hypotonic uterine contraction pattern (consider contracted pelvis)
Deflexion of fetal head (fetal head not flexed on fetal chest; may be associated with occiput posterior)
Uncontrollable pushing prior to complete dilatation of cervix (may be associated with occiput posterior)
Failure of fetal descent (consider contracture of inlet, midpelvis, or outlet)
Edema of anterior portion (lip) of cervix (consider obstructed labor at the inlet)

is less than 12 cm. The anterior-posterior diameter may be approximated by measuring the diagonal conjugate, which in the contracted inlet is less than 11.5 cm. Clinical and x-ray pelvimetry are used to determine the smallest anterior-posterior diameter through which the fetal head must pass.

The treatment goal is to allow the natural forces of labor to push the biparietal diameter of the fetal head beyond the potential interspinous obstruction. Although forceps may be used, they cause difficulty because pulling on the head destroys flexion and because they further diminish the available space. A bulging perineum and crowning indicate that the obstruction has been passed.

CONTRACTURES OF THE OUTLET

An interischial tuberous diameter of less than 8 cm constitutes an outlet contracture. Outlet and midpelvic contractures frequently occur simultaneously. Whether vaginal birth can occur depends on the woman's interischial tuberous diameters and the fetal posterosagittal diameter.

Implications of Pelvic Contractures

Labor is prolonged and protracted in the presence of CPD, and premature rupture of the membranes (PROM) can result from the force of the unequally distributed contractions being exerted on the fetal membranes. In obstructed labor (the fetus is not able to pass through the birth canal) uterine rupture can also occur. With delayed descent, necrosis of maternal soft tissues can result from pressure exerted by the fetal head. Eventually, necrosis can cause fistulas from the vagina to other nearby structures. Difficult forceps-assisted births can also result in damage to maternal soft tissue.

If the membranes rupture and the fetal head has not entered the inlet, there is a danger of cord prolapse. Extreme molding of the fetal head can result. Traumatic forceps-assisted births can damage the fetal skull and central nervous system.

Clinical Therapy

Fetopelvic relationships can be assessed by comparing the estimated weight of the fetus as obtained by ultrasound measurements to pelvic measurements obtained by a manual examination prior to labor and by computed tomography (CT). Occasionally, in high-risk centers magnetic resonance imaging (MRI) is used to identify adequacy of pelvic diameters.

When the pelvic diameters are borderline or questionable, a trial of labor (TOL) may be advised. In this process the woman continues to labor, and careful assessments of uterine contractions, cervical dilatation, and fetal descent are made by the CNM/physician and nurse. As long as there is continued progress, the TOL continues. If progress ceases, the decision for a cesarean birth is made.

NURSING CARE MANAGEMENT

Nursing Assessment and Diagnosis

The adequacy of the maternal pelvis for a vaginal birth should be assessed intrapartally as well as antepartally. During the intrapartal assessment, the size of the fetus and its presentation, position, and lie must also be considered. (See Chapter 23 for intrapartal assessment techniques.)

The nurse should suspect CPD when labor is prolonged, cervical dilatation and effacement are slow, and engagement of the presenting part is delayed or lack of fetal descent occurs.

Nursing diagnoses that may apply include the following:

- ***Deficient Knowledge*** related to lack of information about implications of CPD
- ***Fear*** related to unknown outcome of labor

Nursing Plan and Implementation

Nursing actions during the TOL are similar to care during any labor, with the exception that the assessments of cervical dilatation and fetal descent are done more frequently. Contractions should be monitored and the labor progress charted. The fetus should also be monitored frequently. Any signs of fetal stress are reported to the physician/CNM immediately.

The woman may be positioned in a variety of ways to increase the pelvic diameters. Sitting or squatting increases the outer diameters and may be effective in instances where there is failure of or slow fetal descent. Changing from one side to the other or maintaining a hands-and-knees position may assist the fetus in occiput-posterior position to change to an occiput-anterior position. The woman may instinctively want to assume one of these positions. If not, the nurse may encourage a change of position. Women with an epidural may use position changes with adequate support.

A couple may need help in coping with the stresses of complicated labor. The nurse should keep the couple informed of what is happening and explain the procedures that are being used. This should reassure the couple that measures are being taken to resolve the problem.

Evaluation

Expected outcomes of nursing care include the following:

- The woman's fear is lessened.
- The woman has additional knowledge regarding the problems, implications, and treatment plans.

Care of the Woman at Risk Due to Complications of Third and Fourth Stages of Labor

Common complications of the third and fourth stages of labor include retained placenta, lacerations, and placenta accreta.

Retained Placenta

Retention of the placenta beyond 30 minutes after birth is termed **retained placenta.** It occurs in 2% to 3% of all vaginal births. Bleeding as a result of a retained placenta can be excessive. If placenta expulsion does not occur, a manual removal of the placenta by physician/CNM is attempted. In women who do not have an epidural in place, intravenous sedation may be required because of the discomfort caused by the procedure. Retained placenta may be a symptom of an accreta, increta, or percreta. Failure to retrieve the placenta via manual removal usually necessitates surgical removal by curettage. If the woman does not have an epidural in place, the procedure can be performed under general anesthesia.

Lacerations

Lacerations of the cervix or vagina may be present when bright red vaginal bleeding persists in the presence of a well-contracted uterus. The incidence of lacerations is higher among childbearing women who are young, are nulliparous, have an epidural block, undergo forceps-assisted or vacuum-assisted birth, or undergo an episiotomy. Vaginal and perineal lacerations are often categorized in terms of degree:

- First-degree laceration is limited to the fourchette, perineal skin, and vaginal mucous membrane.
- Second-degree laceration involves the perineal skin, vaginal mucous membrane, underlying fascia, and muscles of the perineal body; it may extend upward on one or both sides of the vagina.
- Third-degree laceration extends through the perineal skin, vaginal mucous membranes, and perineal body and involves the anal sphincter; it may extend up the anterior wall of the rectum.
- Fourth-degree laceration is the same as the third degree but extends through the rectal mucosa to the lumen of the rectum; it may be called a third-degree laceration with a rectal wall extension.

Placenta Accreta

In **placenta accreta,** the chorionic villi attach directly to the myometrium of the uterus. Two other types of placental adherence are **placenta increta,** in which the myometrium is invaded, and **placenta percreta,** in which the myometrium is penetrated. These placenta adherent disorders can be life threatening. The adherence itself may be total, partial, or focal, depending on the amount of placental involvement. The incidence of placenta accreta is 1 in 2500 births (Cunningham et al, 2001). Placenta accreta is the most common type of adherent placenta.

The primary complication of placenta accreta is maternal hemorrhage and failure of the placenta to separate following birth of the infant. An abdominal hysterectomy may be the necessary treatment, depending on the amount and depth of involvement. Chapter 37 discusses hemorrhage following birth.

Care of the Family at Risk Due to Intrauterine Fetal Death

Fetal death, often referred to as fetal demise, accounts for one half of perinatal mortality after 20 weeks' gestation. Recent evidence shows an association between higher maternal age and an increased risk for perinatal loss, including fetal demise (Anderson, Wolfhardt, Christens, et al, 2000). Intrauterine fetal death (IUFD) results from unknown causes or a number of physiologic maladaptations, including preeclampsia, abruptio placentae, placenta previa, diabetes, infection, congenital anomalies, and isoimmune disease.

Prolonged retention of the dead fetus may lead to the development of disseminated intravascular coagulation (DIC), also referred to as consumption coagulopathy. After the release of thromboplastin from the degenerating fetal tissues into the maternal bloodstream, the extrinsic clotting system is activated, triggering the formation of multiple tiny blood clots. Fibrinogen and factors V and VII are subsequently depleted, and the woman begins to display symptoms of DIC. Fibrinogen levels begin a linear descent 3 to 4 weeks after the death of the fetus and continue to decrease without appropriate medical intervention.

Clinical Therapy

Abdominal ultrasound may reveal Spalding's sign (an overriding of the fetal cranial bones). Diagnosis of IUFD is confirmed by absence of heart action on ultrasonography. In addition, maternal estriol levels fall.

Most women have spontaneous labor within 2 weeks of fetal death. If other complications are not present, some physicians wait for labor to begin spontaneously (Cunningham et al, 2001). Many women will elect to undergo an induction of labor to facilitate birth. Women undergoing an induction for IUFD will need uterine monitoring to prevent hyperstimulation. Pain and anxiety medications can be given as needed.

NURSING CARE MANAGEMENT

Nursing Assessment and Diagnosis

Cessation of fetal movement reported by the mother to the nurse is frequently the first indication of fetal death. It is followed by a gradual decrease in the signs and symptoms of pregnancy. Fetal heart tones are absent, and fetal movement is no longer palpable. Once fetal demise is established by the CNM/physician, ongoing support and communication become even more important. Open communication among the mother, her partner, and the healthcare team members contributes to a more realistic understanding of the medical condition and its associated treatments. The nurse may discuss prior experiences the family has had with stress and what they feel were their coping abilities at that time. Determining the family's social supports and resources is also important.

> *Birth and death together. It's confusing and frightening enough for adults, but how are young children to understand it? For them the baby never really existed, or lived only briefly. What does this mean for them? Why are the parents so distraught? Too often, children's feelings about these issues are ignored or misunderstood. When parents are struggling to deal with their own feelings, they find it even harder to respond to the emotional needs of their other children.*
>
> ~When Pregnancy Fails~

Nursing diagnoses that may apply to the woman experiencing intrauterine fetal death include the following:

- ***Grieving*** related to the death of the anticipated baby
- ***Altered Family Processes*** related to loss of a family member
- ***Ineffective Individual Coping*** related to depression in response to loss of child

> *A friend asked if we had named our stillborn baby. After telling her the name, we both began referring to the baby by her name, Sarah. It felt good to call her a name.*
>
> ~When Pregnancy Fails~

Nursing Plan and Implementation

The parents of a stillborn infant suffer a devastating experience, precipitating an intense emotional trauma. During the pregnancy, the couple has already begun the attachment process, which now must be terminated through the grieving process. The behaviors that couples exhibit while mourning may be associated with the five stages of grieving described by Kübler-Ross (1969). Often, the first stage is *denial* of the death of the fetus. Even when the initial healthcare provider suspects fetal demise, the couple is hoping that a second opinion will be different. Some couples may not be convinced of the death until they view and hold the stillborn infant. The second stage is *anger*, resulting from the feelings of loss, loneliness, and perhaps guilt. The anger may be projected at significant others and healthcare team members, or it may be absent when the death of the fetus is sudden and unexpected. *Bargaining*, the third stage, may or may not be present, depending on the couple's preparation for the death of the fetus. If the death is unanticipated, the couple may have no time for bargaining. In the fourth stage, *depression* is evidenced by preoccupation, weeping, and withdrawal. Physiologic postpartal depression appearing 24 to 48 hours after the stillbirth may compound the depression associated with grief. The final stage is *acceptance*, which involves the process of resolution. This is a highly individualized process that may take months or years to complete.

In some facilities, a checklist is used to make sure important aspects of working with the parents are addressed. The checklist becomes a communication tool between staff members to share information particular to this couple. Such a checklist might include the following items:

- When the fetal death is known before admission, inform the admission department and nursing staff so that inappropriate remarks are not made.
- A symbol—such as flowers or commonly a card with a leaf—is placed on the mother's door to inform staff of the family's status.
- Allow the woman and her partner and other family members to remain together as much as they wish. Provide privacy by assigning them to a private room.
- Discuss preferences with the couple to assess if they prefer time alone or continuous support/presence from the nurse.
- As much as possible, have the same nurse provide care to increase the support for the couple. Develop a care plan to provide for continuity of care. Encourage family members to visit support persons.
- Have the most experienced labor and birth nurse auscultate for fetal heart tones. This avoids the searching that a more inexperienced nurse might feel compelled to do. Avoid the temptation to listen again "to make sure." An ultrasound should be performed by the physician/CNM to verify the absence of fetal heart tones.
- Listen to the couple; do not offer explanations. They require solace without minimizing the situation.

- Avoid inappropriate comments such as "this was for the best" or "it wasn't meant to be."
- Facilitate the woman's and her partner's participation in the labor and birth process. When possible, allow them to make decisions about who will be present and what ritual will occur during the birth process. Allow the woman to make the decision regarding whether to have sedation during labor and birth. Provide a quiet supportive environment; ideally, the labor and birth should occur in a labor room or possibly a birthing room rather than the delivery room.
- Give parents accurate information regarding plans for labor and birth.
- Allow the couple to develop a birth plan: placement of infant on maternal abdomen, opportunity for father to cut the cord, who will hold the infant, and so on.
- Provide ongoing opportunities for the couple to ask questions.
- Arrange for the woman to be assigned to a room that is away from new mothers and babies if she requests it. It is important to let the woman decide whether she wants to be on another unit. If early discharge is an option, allow the family to make that selection.
- Encourage the couple to experience the grief that they feel. Accept the weeping and depression. A couple may have intense feelings that they are unable to share with each other. Encourage them to talk together, and allow emotions to flow freely. Help them understand that they may each experience different feelings.
- Give the couple and family an opportunity to see and hold the stillborn infant in a private, quiet location. (Advocates of seeing the stillborn believe that viewing assists in dispelling denial and enables the couple to progress to the next step in the grieving process.) If they choose to see their stillborn infant, prepare the couple for what they will see, including cold skin temperature, blue color, bruising, and fetal defects.
- Some families may elect to bathe or dress their stillborn; support them in their choice.
- Offer to call a chaplain, clergy, or other religious persons to provide support. Notify parents of chaplain services available within the facility.
- Take a photograph of the infant, and let the family know it is available if they want it now or some time in the future.
- Offer a card with footprints, crib card, ID band, hat, blanket, and possibly a lock of hair to the parents. These items may be kept with the photo if the parents do not want them at this time.
- If available, coordinate the facility's social worker for client evaluation prior to discharge. Counseling services may be needed for some couples.
- Prepare the couple for returning home. If there are siblings, each will usually progress through age-appropriate grieving. Provide the parents with information about normal mourning reactions, both psychologic and physiologic.
- Furnish the mother with educational materials that discuss the changes she will experience in returning to the nonpregnant state.
- Provide information about community support groups, including group name, contact person if possible, and phone number. Use materials such as the book *When Hello Means Goodbye* by Schwiebert and Kirk (1985).
- Remember it is not so important to "say the right words." Caring support can be conveyed through silence and your presence.
- Discuss further care of the stillborn baby (dress, rituals).
- Provide information regarding burial and cremation services when appropriate. Many funeral homes offer minimal or no-charge services for grieving parents. Provide resources for the parents.

The nurse experiences many of the same grief reactions as the parents of a stillborn infant. Support persons and colleagues should be available for counseling and support. Recent studies further support the importance of the caregiver's role for the woman who has a perinatal death. Caregivers should acknowledge past losses as well and the effect that has on the current pregnancy (Chambers & Chan, 2000).

Evaluation

Expected outcomes of nursing care include the following:

- The family members express their feelings about the death of their baby.
- The family participates in decisions regarding whether to see their baby and in other decisions regarding the baby.
- The family knows what community resources are available and has names and phone numbers to use if they choose.
- The family moves into and through the grieving process.

I knew something was wrong just by the way everyone was scurrying around in the delivery room and by that terrible silence. Then we knew the baby was dead. The doctor's only comment was, "It must be congenital," as if to say it certainly must be my fault, not his. Then a nurse said: "It would be worse if you had a five-year-old that died." I suppose she was right, but it certainly didn't make me feel any better. Later, the doctor said, "You're young, you'll have lots more kids." I was appalled—I was thirty-three already. Where do they learn all these stupid comments?

~WHEN PREGNANCY FAILS~

Chapter Review

ExploreMediaLink

NCLEX review questions, case studies, and other interactive resources for this chapter can be found on the Web site at http://www.prenhall.com/olds. Click on "Chapter 26" to select the activities for this chapter.

For tutorials including animations and videos, more NCLEX review questions, and an audio glossary, access the accompanying CD-ROM in this book.

Focus Your Study

- Intense anxiety; fear; loss of orientation to person, place, or time; or other inappropriate behaviors may be associated with an underlying psychologic disorder that results in difficulties with coping.
- Hypotonic labor patterns begin normally and then progress to infrequent, less intense contractions. If there are no contraindications, oxytocin is administered intravenously as treatment.
- Precipitous labor and birth is extremely rapid labor and birth that lasts less than 3 hours. It is associated with an increased risk to the mother and newborn infant.
- Postterm pregnancy is one that extends more than 294 days, or 42 weeks, past the first day of the last menstrual period.
- The occiput-posterior position of the fetus prolongs the labor process, causes severe back discomfort in the laboring woman, and predisposes her to vaginal and perineal trauma and lacerations during birth.
- The types of fetal malpresentations include face, brow, breech, and shoulder.
- A fetus or newborn weighing more than 4500 g is termed *macrosomic*. Macrosomia may lead to problems during labor and birth, and in the early neonatal period.
- In multiple gestation, preventing and treating problems that infringe on the development and birth of normal fetuses are significant medical-nursing activities.
- Major bleeding problems in the intrapartal period are abruptio placentae and placenta previa.
- Abruptio placentae is the separation of the placenta from the side of the uterus prior to birth of the infant. Abruptio placentae may be central, marginal, or complete.
- Placenta previa occurs when the placenta implants low in the uterus near or over the cervix. A low-lying or marginal placenta is one that lies near the cervix. In partial placenta previa, part of the placenta lies over the cervix. In complete placenta previa, the cervix is completely covered.
- Prolapsed umbilical cord results when the umbilical cord precedes the fetal presenting part. When this occurs, pressure is placed on the umbilical cord, and blood flow to the fetus is diminished.
- Amniotic fluid embolism occurs when a bolus of amniotic fluid enters the maternal circulation and then enters the maternal lungs. Maternal mortality is very high with this complication.
- Hydramnios (also called polyhydramnios) is the presence of over 2000 mL of amniotic fluid contained within the amniotic membranes. Hydramnios can be associated with fetal malformations that affect fetal swallowing and with maternal diabetes mellitus, Rh sensitization, and multiple gestations.
- Oligohydramnios is a severely reduced volume of amniotic fluid. Oligohydramnios is associated with intrauterine growth restriction, postterm pregnancy, and fetal renal or urinary malfunctions. The fetus is more likely to experience variable decelerations because the amniotic fluid is insufficient to keep pressure off the umbilical cord.
- Cephalopelvic disproportion occurs when there is a narrowed diameter in the maternal pelvis. The narrowed diameter is called a contracture, and it may occur in the pelvic inlet, midpelvis, or outlet. If pelvic measurements are borderline, a trial of labor may be attempted. Failure of cervical dilatation or fetal descent would then necessitate a cesarean birth.

- Third- and fourth-stage complications usually involve a hemorrhage. Causes of hemorrhage include lacerations of the birth canal or cervix, retained placenta, and placenta accreta.
- Nonreassuring fetal status is indicated by persistent late decelerations, persistent severe variable decelerations, and prolonged decelerations. If fetal stress is recognized and treated appropriately, the fetus may be spared any permanent damage.
- Intrauterine fetal death poses a major nursing challenge to provide support and care for the parents.

References

American College of Obstetricians and Gynecologists. (ACOG). (1995). *Dystocia and the augmentation of labor.* (Technical Bulletin No. 218). Washington, DC: Author.

American College of Obstetricians and Gynecologists. (ACOG). (1997). *Management of post-term pregnancy.* (Practice Pattern No. 6). Washington, DC: Author.

American College of Obstetricians and Gynecologists. (ACOG). (1998a). *Special problems with multiple gestation.* (Education Bulletin No. 253). Washington, DC: Author.

American College of Obstetricians and Gynecologists. (ACOG). (1998b). *Inappropriate use of the terms fetal distress and birth asyphyxia.* (Committee Opinion No. 197). Washington, DC: Author.

American College of Obstetricians and Gynecologists. (ACOG). (1999a). *Induction of labor.* (Practice Bulletin No. 10). Washington, DC: Author.

American College of Obstetricians and Gynecologists. (ACOG). (1999b). *Antepartum fetal surveillance.* (Practice Bulletin No. 9). Washington, DC: Author.

American College of Obstetricians and Gynecologists. (ACOG). (2000a). *Evaluation of cesarean delivery.* Washington, DC: Author.

American College of Obstetricians and Gynecologists. (ACOG). (2000b). *Macrosomia.* (Practice Bulletin No. 22). Washington, DC: Author.

Anderson, N., Wolfhardt, J., Christens, P., Olsen, J., & Melbye, M. (2000). Maternal age and fetal loss. *British Medical Journal, 320,* 1708–1712.

Benson, M. D., Kobayashi, H., Silver, R. K., Oi, H., Greenberger, P. A., & Terao, T. (2001). Immunologic studies in presumed amniotic fluid embolism. *Obstetrics & Gynecology, 97*(4), 510–514.

Cardini, F., & Weixin, H. (1998). Moxibustion for correction of breech presentation: A randomized controlled trial. *Obstetrical and Gynecological Survey, 54*(5), 291–292.

Chambers, H. M., & Chan, F. Y. (2000). Support for women/families after perinatal death. *Cochrane Database of Systematic Reviews. (2)*: CD000452.

Chasen, S. T., & Chervenak, F. A. (1998). What is the relationship between the universal use of ultrasound, the rate of detection of twins, and outcome differences? *Clinical Obstetrics and Gynecology, 41,* 67–77.

Cochrane Review. (2001). Bedrest and hospitalization for multiple pregnancy. *Cochrane Library,* Issue 4.

Cunningham, F. G., MacDonald, P. C., Gant, N. F., Leveno, K. J., Gilstrap, L. C., Hankins, G. D. V., et al. (2001). *Williams obstetrics* (21st ed.). Stamford, CT: Appleton & Lange.

Devlieger, R., Demeyere, T., Deprest, J., VanSchoubroeck, D., Witters, I., Timmerman, D., et al. (2001). Ultrasound determination of chronicity in twin pregnancy: Accuracy and operator experience. *Twin Research, 4*(4) 223–226.

Dizon-Townson, D., & Ward, K. (1997). The genetics of labor. *Clinical Obstetrics and Gynecology, 40,* 479–484.

Dorland's pocket medical dictionary (2001). (26th ed.). Philadelphia: W.B. Saunders.

Gabbe, S. G. (1996). Diabetes mellitus. In J. T. Queenan & J. C. Hobbins (Eds.), *Protocols for high-risk pregnancies* (3rd ed., pp. 253–263). Cambridge, MA: Blackwell.

Gaufberg, S. (2001, March 15). Abruptio placenta. *Emedicine Journal, 2*(3).

Gillogley, K. (1991). Abnormal labor and delivery. In K. R. Niswander (Ed.), *Manual of obstetrics.* Boston: Little, Brown.

Griese, M. E., & Prickett, S. A. (1993). Nursing management of umbilical cord prolapse. *Journal of Obstetric, Gynecologic, and Neonatal Nursing, 22,* 311.

Grobman, W. A., & Peaceman, A. M. (1998). What are the rates and mechanisms of first and second trimester pregnancy loss in twins? *Clinical Obstetrics and Gynecology, 41,* 37–45.

Hannah, M., Hannah, W., & Hewson, S. (2001). Planned cesarean section vs vaginal birth for breech presentation at term: A randomized multicenter trial. *Lancet, 356,* 1375–1383.

Kayem, G., Goffinet, F., Clement, D., Hessabi, M., & Cabrol, D. (2002). Breech presentation at term: Morbidity and mortality according to the type of delivery at Port Royal Maternity hospital from 1993 through 1999. *European Journal of Obstetrics, Gynecology, & Reproductive Biology, 102*(2), 137–142.

Keith, L., Papiernik, E., & Oleszczuk, J. J. (1998). How should the efficacy of prenatal care be tested in twin gestations? *Clinical Obstetrics and Gynecology, 41,* 85–93.

Kogan, M., Alexander, G., Kotelchuck, M., MacDorman, M. F., Buekens, P., Martin, J. A., et al. (2000). Trends in twin birth outcomes and prenatal care utilization in the US 1981-1997. *Journal of the American Medical Association, 284*(3), 335–341.

Kübler-Ross, E. (1969). *On death and dying.* New York: Macmillan.

Locksmith, G. (1999). Amniotic fluid embolism. *Obstetric and Gynecology Clinics of North America, 26,* (3).

Lopez-Zeno, J. A. (1997). Active management of labor: The American experience. *Clinical Obstetrics and Gynecology, 40,* 510–515.

Manning, F. A. (1999). General principles and applications of ultrasonography. In R. K. Creasy & R. Resnik (Eds.), *Maternal-fetal medicine* (4th ed., pp. 169–206). Philadelphia: Saunders.

Moses, S. (2001). *Twin pregnancy.* Family Practice Notebook. Retrieved July 30, 2002 from www.Fpnotebook.com

Naiden, T., & Despande, P. (2001). Using active management of labor and vaginal birth after previous cesarean delivery to lower cesarean delivery rates: A 10 year experience. *American Journal of Obstetrics and Gynecology, 184*(7), 1535–1543.

National Institute of Mental Health, (NIMH) (2001). *Depression research at the National Institute of Mental Health* (NIH Publication No. 00-4501). Rockville, MD: Author.

Oxorn, H. (1986). *Oxorn-Foote human labor and birth* (5th ed.). Norwalk, CT: Appleton & Lange.

Papiernik, E., Keith, L., Oleszczuk, J. J., & Cervantes, A. (1998). What interventions are useful in reducing the rate of preterm delivery in twins? *Clinical Obstetrics and Gynecology, 41,* 13–23.

Parker, J., & Napolitano, P. (2001). Brow presentation. *Emedicine Journal, 2*(6). Retrieved July 10, 2002 from www.emedicine.com/med/topic

Roberts, S. J., Reardon, K. M., & Rosenfeld, S. (1999). Childhood sexual abuse: Surveying its impact on primary care. *AWHONN Lifelines, 3*(2), 39–45.

Roberts, W. E., & Morrison, J. C. (1998). How has the use of home monitors, fetal fibronectin, and measurement of cervical length helped predict labor and/or prevent preterm delivery in twins? *Clinical Obstetrics and Gynecology, 41*, 95–102.

Schwiebert, P., & Kirk, P. (1985). *When hello means goodbye.* Eugene: Oregon Health Sciences University.

Senat, M. V., Ancel, P. Y., Bouvier-Colle, M. H., & Breart, G. (1998). How does multiple pregnancy affect maternal mortality and morbidity? *Clinical Obstetrics and Gynecology, 41*, 79–83.

Toth, P., & Juthivijayarani M. (2001). *University of Iowa family practice handbook* (3rd ed.). Retrieved July 10, 2002 from www.vh.org/Providers/ClinRef/FPHandbook

Ulijaszek, S. J., Johnston, F. E., & Preece, M. A. (Eds.). (1998). *The Cambridge encyclopedia of human growth & development.* Cambridge, England: Cambridge University Press.

U.S. Department of Health and Human Services (DHHS). (1999). *Mental health: A report of the Surgeon General.* Rockville, MD: US DHHS, Substance Abuse and Mental Health Services. Administration Center for Mental Health Services, Betnesda, MD: NIH, NIMH.

Usta, I., Mercer, B. M., & Sibai, B. M. (1999). Current obstetrical practice and umbilical cord prolapse. *American Journal of Perinatology, 16*(9), 479–484.

Wagner, R., Nielson, P., & Gonik, B. (1999). Shoulder dystocia. *Obstetrics and Gynecology Clinics of North America, 26*(2), 371–383.

Watson-Blasiolie, J. (2001). Double take. AWHONN. *Lifelines, 5*(2), 35–42.

Zamorski, M. A., & Biggs, W. S. (2001). Management of suspected fetal macrosomia. *American Family Physician, 63*(2), 302–306.

Zuspan, F. P., & Quilligan, E. J. (1998). Handbook of obstetrics, gynecology, and primary care. St. Louis, MO: Mosby.

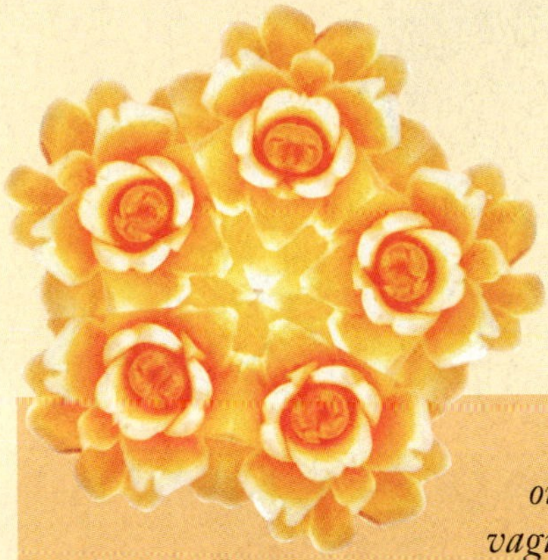

27 Birth-Related Procedures

With our first baby I suddenly had to have a cesarean. Everything happened so fast, but our son was OK, and that's all that mattered. With our second baby I wanted to try for a vaginal birth but nevertheless I was afraid. I don't know what I would have done without my nurse. She stayed with me the whole time I labored and kept giving me support. She explained everything, so I knew what was happening. I felt safe. I had a beautiful baby girl after 8 hours of labor. Everything went well postpartally, and I am so glad I was able to avoid another cesarean. We don't plan to have another baby, but if we did, I wouldn't be so afraid.

Objectives

- Describe the impact of selected procedures on the childbearing woman and her family or support system.
- Contrast the methods of external cephalic version and internal version and the related nursing management.
- Discuss the use of amniotomy in current maternal-newborn care.
- Compare methods for inducing labor, explaining their advantages and disadvantages.
- Discuss the use of transcervical intrapartum amnioinfusion.
- Describe the types of episiotomies performed, the rationale for each, and the associated nursing interventions.
- Summarize the indications for forceps-assisted birth, types of forceps that may be used, complications, and related interventions.
- Discuss the use of vacuum extraction, including indications, procedure, complications, and related nursing management.
- Explain the indications for cesarean birth, impact on the family unit, preparation and teaching needs, and associated nursing management.
- Discuss vaginal birth following cesarean birth.

Key Terms

Amnioinfusion 752
Amniotomy 751
Cesarean birth 760
Cervical ripening 743
Episiotomy 753
External cephalic version (ECV) 740
Forceps-assisted birth 755
Labor induction 744
Podalic version 740
Vacuum extraction 759
Vaginal birth after cesarean (VBAC) 763

MEDIALINK

Additional resources for this content can be found on the Student CD-ROM and on the Companion Website at www.prenhall.com/olds. Click on "Chapter 27" to select the activities for this chapter.

CD-ROM

- Audio Glossary
- NCLEX Review
- Video: Vacuum Extractor
- Cesarean Birth Videos:
  - Types of Incisions
  - Epidural Placement
  - Delivery of Infant
  - Assessment of Infant
  - Delivery of Placenta
  - Bonding
  - Suturing of Uterus
  - Scrub and Circulating Nurse Roles

Companion Website

- Additional NCLEX Review
- Case Study: Undergoing Labor Induction
- Care Plan Activity: Client With Pitocin for Labor Augmentation

Most births occur without the need for operative obstetric intervention. In some instances, however, obstetric procedures are necessary to maintain the safety of the woman and the fetus. The most common obstetric procedures are amniotomy, induction of labor, episiotomy, cesarean birth, and vaginal birth following a previous cesarean birth.

Generally, women are aware of the possible need for an obstetric procedure during their labor and birth, and many women accept whatever procedure is recommended based on the belief that the caregiver knows what is needed and that it is in the baby's best interest. However, some women expect to have a "natural" birth experience and do not desire or anticipate any medical intervention. These women may feel disappointed or even guilty when an unanticipated obstetric procedure is needed. This conflict between expectation and the need for intervention presents a challenge to maternity nurses. The nurse can provide information regarding any procedure to enhance the woman's and her partner's understanding of what is proposed, the anticipated benefits and possible risks, and any possible alternative treatments. The nurse must provide emotional support to the woman and her family to assist them in accepting the unanticipated procedure.

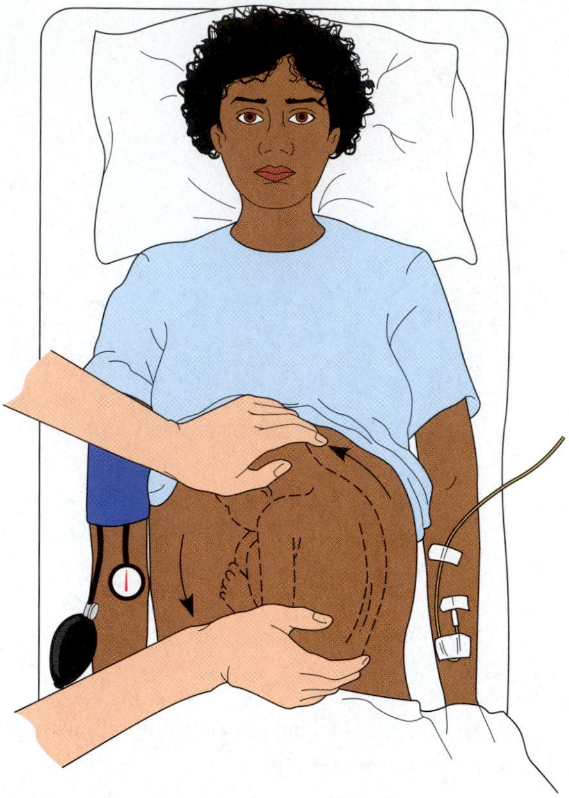

Figure 27–1 • External (or cephalic) version of the fetus. A new technique involves applying pressure to the fetal head and buttocks so that the fetus completes a "backward flip" or "forward roll."

Care of the Woman During Version

Version, or turning the fetus, is a procedure used to change the fetal presentation by abdominal or intrauterine manipulation. The most common type of version is **external cephalic version (ECV)** in which the fetus is changed from a breech, transverse, or oblique lie to a cephalic presentation by external manipulation of the maternal abdomen (Figure 27–1 •). The success rates for version are the highest for transverse presentations. Successful ECVs decrease the chances of nonvertex and cesarean births (Hofmeyr & Kulier, 2002).

The other type of version, called a **podalic version,** is used only with the second twin during a vaginal birth. In an internal version, the obstetrician places a hand inside the uterus, grabs the fetus's feet, and then turns the fetus from a transverse or cephalic presentation to a breech presentation (Figure 27–2 •). The fetus is then born in a breech presentation. This maneuver is used only when the second twin is not in a cephalic position. It is considered superior to an external cephalic version because it causes less fetal stress (Cunningham, MacDonald, Gant, et al, 2001). Some obstetricians may elect to have the second twin give birth by cesarean if the twin is not in a cephalic presentation.

External Cephalic Version

If breech or shoulder presentation (transverse lie) is detected in the later weeks of pregnancy, an ECV may be attempted. The version is usually done after 36 to 37 weeks' gestation because most fetuses still in breech presentation at this time will not spontaneously change back to a vertex presentation. In addition, if complications arise from the procedure, the risk of prematurity is eliminated. The overall success rate for ECV is 68% (Coco & Silverman, 1998); however, it varies based on the experience of the clinical practitioner, components of the procedure (eg, whether a tocolytic agent such as terbutaline is used), and factors associated with the woman, fetus, and pregnancy. Lau, Lo, and Rogers (1997) reported that nine factors can serve as predictors of a successful external version: parity, maternal weight, placental site, type of breech or presentation, position of fetal spine, amniotic fluid volume, engagement, station, and estimated fetal weight. Other factors associated with higher failure rates include nulliparity, advanced dilatation, fetal weight less than 2500 g, anterior placenta, and a low station (American College of Obstetricians and Gynecologists [ACOG], 2000).

Criteria for External Version

The following criteria should be met prior to performing ECV (Lau, Lo, & Rogers, 1997; Hofmeyr & Kulier, 2002):

- A single fetus (also called a singleton) must be present. If a multiple gestation exists, a variety of concerns preclude an external version. For example, a cesarean rather than

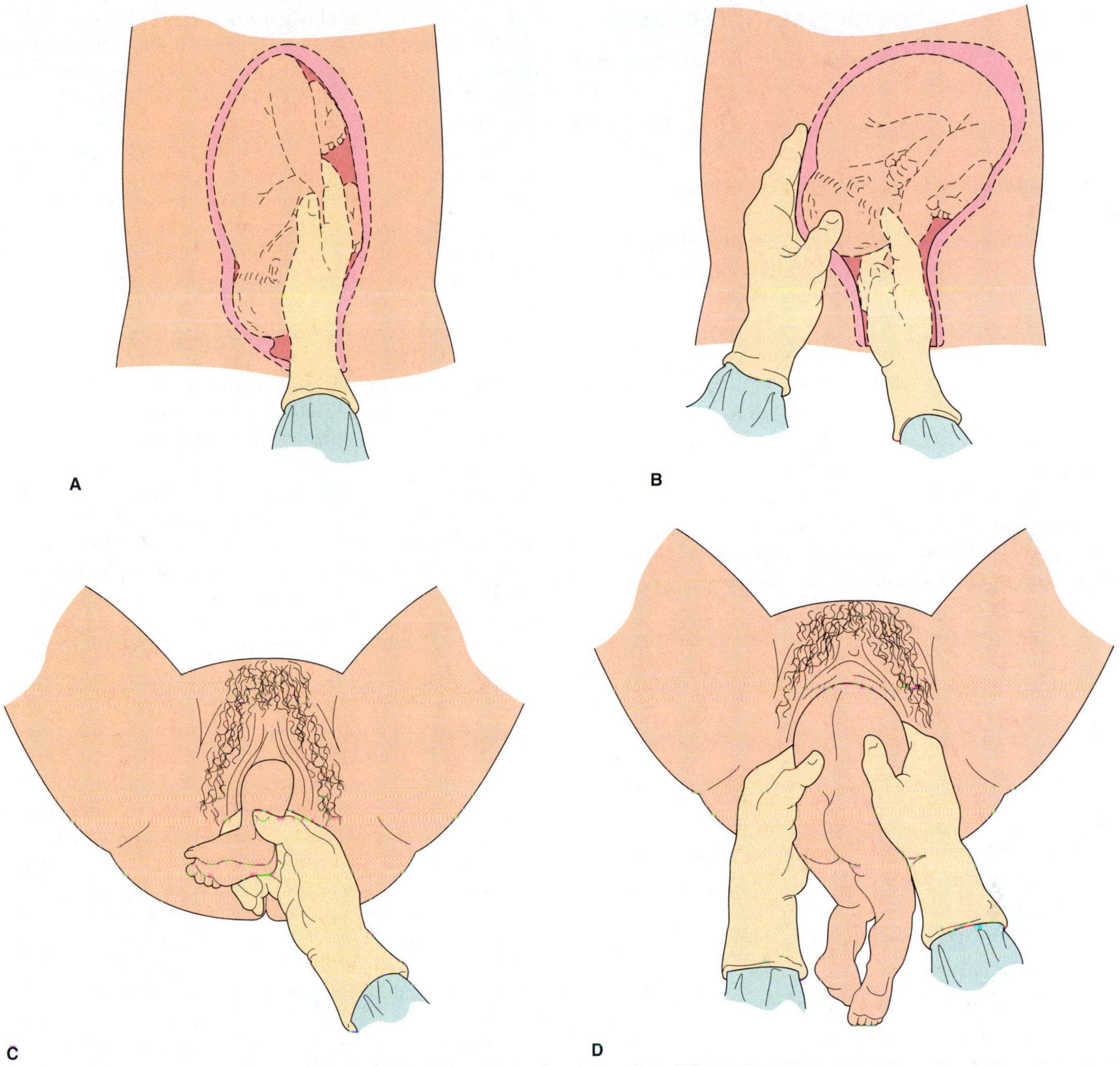

Figure 27–2 • Use of podalic version and extraction of the fetus to assist in the vaginal birth of the second twin. *A,* The physician reaches into the uterus and grasps a foot. Although a vertex birth is always preferred in a singleton birth, in this instance of assisting in the birth of a second twin it is not possible to grasp any other fetal part. The fetal head would be too large to grasp and pull downward, and grasping the fetal arm would result in a transverse lie and make vaginal birth impossible. *B,* While applying pressure on the outside of the abdomen to push the baby's head up toward the top of the uterus with one hand, the physician pulls the baby's foot down toward the cervix. *C,* Both feet have been pulled through the cervix and vagina. *D,* The physician now grasps the baby's trunk and continues to pull downward on the baby to assist the birth.

vaginal birth may need to be considered, and the fetuses might become entangled during a version.

- The fetal breech is not engaged. Once the presenting part is engaged, it is difficult if not impossible to do a version.
- An adequate amount of amniotic fluid must exist. The amniotic fluid helps ease movement of the fetus and provides adequate room for the umbilical cord to float without being compressed.
- A reactive nonstress test (NST) should be obtained immediately prior to performing the version. A reactive NST indicates fetal well-being.
- The fetus must be 36 to 37 or more weeks' gestation. A version may be accompanied by complications that require immediate birth by cesarean. If gestation is less than 37 weeks, a preterm birth would result. (*Note:* Occasionally, a physician may do an external version while the woman is in labor.)

Contraindications for External Version

Absolute contraindications to ECV include the following (ACOG, 1998; Bowes, 1999):

- **Suspected intrauterine growth restriction.** The fetus has been stressed and amniotic fluid may be decreased.
- **Fetal anomalies.** This category includes major abnormalities.
- **Presence of an abnormal fetal heart rate (FHR) tracing.** A nonreassuring FHR pattern might indicate that the fetus is already stressed and other action needs to be taken.
- **Rupture of the membranes.** Rupture of the membranes would result in an inadequate amount of amniotic fluid.
- **Cesarean birth indicated anyway.** For example, if a complete previa is present, birth will be by cesarean. If a marginal previa or low-lying placenta is present, the manipulation during the version may precipitate bleeding.
- **Maternal problems** such as gestational diabetes that has required insulin, uncontrolled chronic hypertension, preeclampsia, or maternal cardiac disease.
- **Amniotic fluid abnormalities.** Oligohydramnios (amniotic fluid index < 5 cm) makes the fetus difficult to maneuver and increases risk of umbilical cord compression. Hydramnios (amniotic fluid index > 25 cm) stretches the uterine walls, increasing pressure and decreasing the chance the fetus will remain in a cephalic presentation.

Relative contraindications to ECV include the following:

- Previous lower uterine segment cesarean birth. Prior scarring of the uterus may increase the risk of uterine tearing or uterine rupture.
- Nuchal cord. A nuchal cord may tighten around the fetal neck and decrease circulation to the fetus.
- Multiple gestation
- Evidence of uteroplacental insufficiency
- Significant third trimester bleeding
- Uterine malformation

External Version Procedure

The external version is accomplished in a birthing unit, rather than an outpatient setting, in case further intervention (such as emergency cesarean birth) is necessary. The risk of major complications resulting from an ECV has been reported as 1% to 2% since 1979. There have been no reported fetal deaths from the procedure since 1980 (Coco & Silverman, 1998). The woman is instructed to fast for 8 hours preceding the version in case a cesarean birth needs to be performed due to complications. The physician uses ultrasound to confirm the presence of a single fetus, the amount of amniotic fluid, the location of the placenta, the position of the umbilical cord, and that a breech presentation still exists. Maternal vital signs are assessed, and continuous electronic fetal monitoring is done to evaluate the FHR, to obtain a reactive NST, and to evaluate the presence of uterine contractions or uterine wall tenseness. Blood work is drawn including a complete blood count (CBC), and a blood type and antibody screen. The physician explains the procedure and the client signs a consent form.

An intravenous line is established for medication administration and in case of difficulties. A beta-mimetic agent (a subcutaneous dose of terbutaline) or intravenous infusion of magnesium sulfate (if a beta-mimetic agent is contraindicated because of a medical condition) is administered to achieve uterine relaxation. Occasionally, some physicians do not use a beta-mimetic agent during the version. However, it greatly enhances the comfort of the woman (Theron & Theron, 2002).

The woman is placed in a supine or slight Trendelenburg position. Once uterine relaxation is achieved, the maternal abdomen is copiously covered with warmed ultrasound gel to decrease excessive manipulation and friction, and the physician grasps the fetal breech between the index finger and the thumb. First the presenting part is gently pushed upward or lifted out of the maternal pelvis by exerting pressure over the skin on the maternal abdomen. If the fetal breech can be lifted out, then the breech and head are rotated or moved out in opposite directions. In most cases, a direction similar to a forward roll is attempted initially. If that is not successful, a roll in the opposite direction is attempted. The procedure should be concluded when any of the following occur: the fetal head is moved to a head-down position; repeated failures have occurred; the woman has indicated that the procedure has become too painful or stressful; or signs of maternal or fetal problems occur, including a nonreassuring FHR pattern (Coco & Silverman, 1998). The intravenous tocolytic agent is discontinued, and frequently the fetus is held in the new presentation by either the physician or the nurse until the uterus regains tone. In the event of a failed version, a repeat attempt can be made within a week if the procedure was well tolerated by the woman and her fetus. If the woman is Rh negative, an adequate amount of Rh immune globulin must always be administered after the version since there is a 4.1% risk of maternal-fetal hemorrhage (Coco & Silverman, 1998) (see Chapter 20). A vaginal examination and ultrasound are done to evaluate cervical dilatation and to confirm position and fetal descent. The risk of spontaneous reversion is approximately 7% (Coco & Silverman, 1998).

NURSING CARE MANAGEMENT

The nurse begins by ensuring that the expectant woman understands the procedure, knows that the procedure may be uncomfortable or very painful, and realizes that she can tell the physician to stop if the pain is too great.

The possibility of failure of the ECV and the slight risk of a cesarean birth if the fetus becomes stressed or exhibits a nonreassuring fetal status should also be discussed. Explaining what will occur in either of these circumstances better prepares the woman and partner if intervention becomes necessary. Prior to the version, the nurse completes initial maternal and fetal assessments, provides ongoing evaluation of FHR, performs the NST, and obtains blood work. The nurse provides psychologic support throughout the procedure through reassurance. The nurse also provides continuous explanations about the procedure while the version is being performed and answers any questions. The nurse continues to monitor maternal blood pressure and pulse about every 2 minutes throughout the period of time the betamimetic agent is used and for about 30 minutes after. The FHR is monitored for approximately 1 to 2 hours following the ECV. The nurse also assesses the maternal-fetal response to the tocolytic agent. The nurse continues to provide information by reiterating aftercare instructions, such as monitoring for uterine contractions, being aware of fetal movement (fetal kick counts), and recognizing signs of reversion (excessive movement or a sensation described as the fetus "turning around").

Care of the Woman During Cervical Ripening

Prostaglandin E_2 (PGE_2) gel for **cervical ripening** (softening and effacing the cervix) may be used for the pregnant woman at or near term when there is a medical or obstetric indication for induction of labor. The two most commonly used types of gel are Prepidil and Cervidil. Prepidil gel contains 0.5 mg dinoprostone (a form of prostaglandin E_2 for intracervical application) and is placed intracervically. Cervidil is packaged in an intravaginal insert that resembles a 2-cm-square piece of cardboardlike material. It is placed in the posterior vagina and is left in place to provide a slow release of 10 mg dinoprostone at a rate of 0.3 mg/hr over 12 hours.

Advantages and Disadvantages of Prostaglandin Administration

The advantage of Cervidil is that it can be easily removed if uterine hyperstimulation occurs (Deglin & Vallerand, 2002). Both preparations have been demonstrated to cause cervical ripening, shorter labor, and lower requirements for oxytocin

DRUG GUIDE Dinoprostone (Cervidil) Vaginal Insert

• Pregnancy Risk Category: C

• Overview of Maternal-Fetal Action

Dinoprostone is a naturally occurring form of prostaglandin E_2. Dinoprostone can be used at term to ripen the cervix and can stimulate the smooth muscle of the uterus to enhance uterine contractions. A single vaginal insert may be used to ripen the cervix and then oxytocin can be administered 30 minutes later. (Forrest Pharmaceuticals, 1995).

• Route, Dosage, Frequency

The vaginal insert contains 10 mg of dinoprostone. The insert is placed transversely in the posterior fornix of the vagina, and the client is kept supine for 2 hours but then may ambulate. The dinoprostone is released at approximately 0.3 mg/hr over a 12-hour period. The vaginal insert should be removed by pulling on the retrieval string upon onset of uterine contractions or after 12 hours (Forrest Pharmaceuticals, 1995).

• Contraindications

- Client with known sensitivity to prostaglandins
- Presence of fetal distress
- Unexplained bleeding during pregnancy
- Strong suspicion of cephalopelvic disproportion
- Client already receiving oxytocin
- Client with 6 or more previous term pregnancies
- Client who is not anticipated to be able to give birth vaginally

Dinoprostone vaginal insert should be used with CAUTION in clients with ruptured membranes, a fetus in breech presentation, presence of glaucoma, or history of asthma (Forrest Pharmaceuticals, 1995).

• Maternal Side Effects

Uterine hyperstimulation with or without fetal distress has occurred in a very small number (2.8%–4.7%) of clients. Fewer than 1% of clients have experienced fever, nausea, vomiting, diarrhea, or abdominal pain (Forrest Pharmaceuticals, 1995).

• Effects on Fetus/Newborn

Nonreassuring fetal heart rate patterns

• Nursing Considerations

- Assess for presence of contraindications.
- Monitor maternal vital signs, cervical dilatation, and effacement carefully.
- Monitor fetal status for presence of reassuring fetal heart rate pattern (baseline 110–160 bpm, presence of short-term variability, average variability presence of accelerations with fetal movement, absence of late or variable decelerations).
- Remove vaginal insert if uterine hyperstimulation, sustained uterine contractions, fetal distress, or any other maternal adverse actions occur.

Table 27–1 • ABSOLUTE CONTRAINDICATIONS TO LABOR INDUCTION
• Complete placenta previa
• Vasa previa
• Abruptio placentae
• Prolapsed umbilical cord
• Fetal bradycardia
• Acute fetal distress
• Previous classic uterine incision or transfundal uterine surgery
• Previous myomectomy
• Vaginal bleeding with unknown cause
• Pelvic structure abnormality
• Active genital herpes (HSV) infection
• Invasive cervical cancer
Source: Adapted from American College of Obstetricians and Gynecologists. *Induction of Labor.* (Practice Bulletin No. 10). Washington, DC: © ACOG, November 1999.

during labor induction. Vaginal birth is achieved within 24 hours for most women.

Risks of prostaglandin administration include uterine hyperstimulation, nonreassuring fetal status, and a higher incidence of postpartum hemorrhage (Deglin & Vallerand, 2002). Contraindications to the use of PGE_2 gel are found in Table 27–1 •. Prostaglandin should be used with caution in women with compromised cardiovascular, hepatic, or renal function and in women with asthma or glaucoma (Cunningham et al, 2001).

Prostaglandin Agent Insertion Procedure

It is recommended that prostaglandin gel be used only in a hospital birthing unit and that an obstetrician be readily available in case an emergency cesarean birth is needed. The use of PGE in outpatient settings and birth centers is currently under study. When Prepidil is used, it is introduced by means of a prefilled syringe with a catheter attached to the hub. The catheter is inserted through the vagina and into the endocervix, where the gel is injected. The catheter has a small shield at the top so that the gel cannot be deposited above the internal os. Dinoprostone is available as a gel that may be placed in a diaphragm and applied to the cervix, and as a suppository that is placed in the posterior fornix of the vagina.

NURSING CARE MANAGEMENT

Physicians, certified nurse-midwives (CNMs), and birthing room nurses who have had special education and training may administer PGE products. Maternal vital signs are assessed for a baseline, and an electronic fetal monitor is applied for at least 30 minutes to obtain an external tracing of uterine activity, fetal heart rate (FHR) pattern, and a reactive nonstress test. If a nonreactive test is obtained, consultation with the physician/CNM is required. After the gel is inserted, the woman is instructed to remain lying down with a rolled blanket or hip wedge under her right hip to tip the uterus slightly to the left for the first 30 to 60 minutes to minimize leakage of the gel from the endocervix. The nurse monitors the woman for uterine hyperstimulation and FHR abnormalities (changes in baseline rate, variability, and presence of decelerations) for 30 minutes to 2 hours (Deglin & Vallerand, 2002). If tachysystole (hyperstimulation) of the uterus greater than five contractions in 10 minutes occurs, the woman is positioned on her left side and oxygen is administered if fetal stress is noted. The administration of a tocolytic agent (such as a subcutaneous injection of 0.25 mg terbutaline) should be considered if the uterine hyperstimulation pattern continues. The gel may be removed if hyperstimulation, severe nausea, vomiting, or tachysystole develops (ACOG, 1999b). Treatment with antiemetics, antipyretics, and antidiarrheal agents usually is not indicated.

Care of the Woman During Induction of Labor

The American College of Obstetricians and Gynecologists defines **labor induction** as the stimulation of uterine contractions before the spontaneous onset of labor, with or without ruptured fetal membranes, for the purpose of accomplishing birth (ACOG, 1999b). Induction may be indicated in the presence of the following:

- Diabetes mellitus
- Renal disease
- Preeclampsia
- Premature rupture of membranes (PROM)
- Chorioamnionitis
- Fetal demise
- Postterm gestation
- Intrauterine growth restriction (IUGR)
- Isoimmunization
- History of rapid labor (precipitous labor and birth) to prevent an unattended birth
- Mild abruptio placentae, no fetal stress or unreassuring fetal heart rate
- Nonreassuring antepartal testing (poor biophysical profile score)
- Severe oligohydramnios
- Macrosomia

Table 27-2 • RELATIVE CONTRAINDICATIONS TO LABOR INDUCTION

- Abnormal fetal heart rate patterns
- Breech presentation
- Unknown fetal presentation
- Multiple gestation
- Polyhydramnios
- Presenting fetal part above the maternal pelvic inlet
- Severe hypertension
- Maternal heart disease

Source: Adapted from American College of Obstetricians and Gynecologists. *Induction of Labor* (Practice Bulletin No. 10). Washington, DC: © ACOG, November 1999.

Contraindications of Labor Induction

All contraindications to spontaneous labor and vaginal birth are contraindications to the induction of labor (see Table 27-1). Relative maternal contraindications are included in Table 27–2 •.

Before induction is attempted, appropriate assessment must indicate that both the woman and fetus are ready for the onset of labor. This includes evaluation of fetal maturity and cervical readiness.

The gestational age of the fetus is best evaluated by accurate menstrual dating, ultrasound visualization of the gestational sac between 5 and 6 weeks' gestation, and quickening at 18 to 20 weeks. Serial ultrasounds are helpful in validating gestational age. When needed, amniotic fluid studies for lecithin/sphingomyelin (L/S) ratio and phosphatidylglycerol are also beneficial in assessing fetal lung maturity (see Chapter 21).

The findings on vaginal examination will help determine whether cervical changes favorable for induction have occurred. Bishop (1964) developed a prelabor scoring system that is still helpful in predicting the inducibility of women (Table 27–3 •). Components evaluated are cervical dilatation, effacement, consistency, and position, as well as the station of the fetal presenting part. A score of 0, 1, 2, or 3 is given to each assessed characteristic. The higher the total score for all the criteria, the more likely that labor will occur. The lower the total score, the higher the failure rate. A favorable cervix is the most important criterion for a successful induction (Cunningham et al, 2001). The presence of a cervix that is anterior, soft, 50% effaced, and dilated at least 2 cm, with the fetal head at +1 station or lower (Bishop score of 9), is favorable for successful induction (Bishop, 1964). Low Bishop scores have been correlated with prolonged labors and a higher incidence of cesarean births (Cunningham et al, 2001).

Fetal fibronectin assay (fFN) has been suggested as a biochemical marker for predicting impending term labor and successful labor induction (Rozenberg, Goffinet, & Hessabi, 2000). The presence of fetal fibronectin in the cervicovaginal secretions has been associated with successful induction of labor (Kiss, Ahner, Hohlagschwandtner, et al, 2000). Currently, the high cost of fFN testing has limited its use to the detection of preterm births (see Chapter 21).

Table 27-3 • PRELABOR STATUS EVALUATION SCORING SYSTEM

	Assigned Value			
Factor	**0**	**1**	**2**	**3**
Cervical dilatation	Closed	1–2 cm	3–4 cm	5 cm or more
Cervical effacement	0% to 30%	40% to 50%	60% to 70%	80% or more
Fetal station	−3	−2	−1, 0	+1, or lower
Cervical consistency	Firm	Moderate	Soft	
Cervical position	Posterior	Midposition	Anterior	

Source: Bishop, E.H. (1964). Pelvic scoring for elective inductions. *Obstetrics & Gynecology, 24,* 266.

Methods of Inducing Labor

When the cervix is favorable, the most frequently used methods of induction are stripping the amniotic membranes, amniotomy, intravenous oxytocin (Pitocin) infusion, and complementary methods. Amniotomy is discussed later in this section.

STRIPPING THE MEMBRANES

A nonpharmacologic method of induction frequently used by physicians and CNMs is called *stripping* (or *sweeping*) *the amniotic membranes.* This is usually done in the office of the physician or CNM during a prenatal visit at term (38 through 42 weeks' gestation). The CNM or physician inserts a gloved finger as far as possible into the internal cervical os and rotates the finger 360 degrees, twice. This motion separates the amniotic membranes that are lying against the lower uterine segment and internal os from the distal part of the lower uterine segment. The stripping or sweeping is thought to release $PGF_{2\alpha}$ from the amniotic membranes or PGE_2 from the cervix. The efficiency of the procedure, although widely practiced, has not been statistically proven in scientific studies (Boulvain, Stan, & Irion, 2002). Women should be advised that this procedure can cause discomfort. In addition, uterine contractions, cramping, and a bloody discharge can occur after the procedure is performed. Although the procedure is not 100% effective as a labor induction method, if labor is initiated, it typically begins within 24 to 48 hours.

OXYTOCIN INFUSION

Intravenous administration of oxytocin is an effective method of initiating uterine contractions to induce labor. The goal is to achieve three uterine contractions with a duration of 40 to 60 seconds in 10 minutes with good uterine relaxation and return to the baseline tone between contractions (Medifocus, 2002).

A primary bottle of intravenous fluid is prepared and used to start and maintain the infusion. This avoids the risk of infusing a large dose of oxytocin as the line is begun and provides additional fluids while the oxytocin solution is being kept at a low infusion rate. After the infusion is started, the oxytocin solution is piggybacked into the primary tubing port closest to the catheter insertion. This allows only a small amount of oxytocin to backflow into the tubing and ensures greater dosage accuracy. The oxytocin should be administered with a device that permits precise control of the flow rate. Oxytocin should not be administered intramuscularly or without the aid of an intravenous electric pump. Over the past few years, differences in opinion regarding oxytocin dosage have surfaced.

Ten units of oxytocin (Pitocin) are added to 1 L of a secondary line of intravenous fluid (usually 5% dextrose in balanced saline solution—for example, 5% dextrose in lactated Ringer's solution). The resulting mixture will contain 10 mU of oxytocin per milliliter (1 mU/min, or 6 mL/hr), and the prescribed dose can be calculated easily. Some facilities are now using 30 units of oxytocin (Pitocin) per 500 mL of intravenous fluid to reduce the risk of pulmonary edema in the postpartum period. Other dilutions can also be used. Other dosage concentrations are presented in the Drug Guide: Oxytocin (Pitocin) on page 747–748.

ACOG (1999b) recommends a low-dose or a high-dose regimen. The low-dose regimen utilizes a starting dose of 0.5 to 2 mU/min with increases of 1 to 2 mU/min every 15 to 40 minutes until an adequate labor pattern is established. The high-dose regimen has a starting dose of up to 6 mU/min with incremental increases of 1 to 6 mU/min every 20 to 40 minutes. However, some studies suggest that smaller dose regimens are as effective as previous larger dose regimens and that adverse effects of oxytocin are dose related (Cunningham et al, 2001).

Oxytocin induction is not without some associated risks: hyperstimulation of the uterus, resulting in uterine contractions that are too frequent (more often than every 2 minutes), uterine contractions that are too intense, or an increased uterine resting tone. Other risks include uterine rupture and water intoxication. Nonreassuring fetal heart rate patterns have also been observed (Deglin & Vallerand, 2002).

Researchers continue to investigate a new method of labor induction with pulsatile oxytocin administration by a computer-controlled pump.

COMPLEMENTARY METHODS

In addition to the allopathic cervical ripening and induction methods previously discussed, there are a variety of more "natural" and noninvasive methods that CNMs tend to suggest or administer either in the home setting or in tertiary care centers. These methods include the following (Allaire, 2001): sexual intercourse/lovemaking; self or partner stimulation of the woman's nipples and breasts; the use of herbs, such as blue/black cohosh, evening primrose oil, and red raspberry leaves; the use of homeopathic solutions, such as caulophyllum or pulsatilla; castor oil; enemas; and acupressure/acupuncture. Mechanical dilation of the cervix with balloon catheters is another technique used.

Although not widely described in nursing and medical textbooks, the use of complementary and alternative medicine (CAM) has risen dramatically. It is estimated that 48.9% of women use some type of CAM therapy and that 90% of nurse-midwives recommend CAM for labor stimulation or relaxation (Allaire, 2001). Natural methods are very effective and are frequently the preferred choice of many CNMs and their clients. It is important for nursing students, nurses, and consumers to be aware of all aspects of pregnancy care.

Sexual intercourse is a logical method of stimulating cervical ripening and uterine contractions; female orgasm stimulates uterine contractions, and the male ejaculate contains a rich source of natural prostaglandins. Breast and nipple stimulation are also a frequent part of lovemaking, and this stimulates the release of endogenous oxytocin, which in turn stimulates the uterus to contract. Until recently, most literature about sexual intercourse and lovemaking during pregnancy has focused on the possible harmful effects that may arise; however, more current research is dispelling the older beliefs (Summers, 1997).

Nipple stimulation for cervical ripening may be done at term. The woman gently massages her breasts with a warm washcloth for 30 to 60 minutes, three times a day. Alternatively, a breast pump can be used 10 minutes on and 10 minutes off until a regular contraction pattern is established. In one study, nipple stimulation increased most women's Bishop score, and some women went into labor (Summers, 1997). Women can also use breast and nipple stimulation as a means of induction or augmentation.

Herbal preparations such as blue and black cohosh, evening primrose oil, and red raspberry leaf teas are used for both cervical ripening and induction of labor. Although extensive scientific data are not available, they have been widely used to promote uterine contractions and stimulate labor (Allaire, 2001; McFarlin, Gibson, O'Rear, et al, 1999).

Homeopathic solutions, such as caulophyllum, cimicifuga, pulsatilla, and others, are used for cervical ripening and induction of labor. The midwife/physician needs thorough personal knowledge of homeopathic remedies or ongoing consultation with a homeopathic physician.

Castor oil has been used for many years but has not frequently been studied as a method of labor induction. The method by which castor oil stimulates uterine contractions is not understood. Few studies have documented its effectiveness in labor stimulation. Other studies have reported a rapid onset of labor, precipitous birth, and meconium-stained amniotic fluid (McFarlin et al, 1999).

Acupressure and acupuncture are not as accepted in the United States as in other countries. However, the rising interest in and use of holistic practices and alternative

DRUG GUIDE Oxytocin (Pitocin)

• Overview of Obstetric Action

Oxytocin (Pitocin) exerts a selective stimulatory effect on the smooth muscle of the uterus and blood vessels. Oxytocin affects the myometrial cells of the uterus by increasing the excitability of the muscle cell, increasing the strength of the muscle contraction, and supporting propagation of the contraction (movement of the contraction from one myometrial cell to the next). Its effect on the uterine contraction depends on the dosage used and on the excitability of the myometrial cells. During the first half of gestation, there is little excitability of the myometrium, and the uterus is fairly resistant to the effects of oxytocin. However, from midgestation on, the uterus responds increasingly to exogenous intravenous oxytocin. Cautious use of diluted oxytocin administered intravenously at term results in a slow rise of uterine activity.

The circulatory half-life of oxytocin is 3 to 5 minutes. It takes approximately 40 minutes for a particular dose of oxytocin to reach a steady-state plasma concentration (Skidmore-Roth, 2003).

The effects of oxytocin on the cardiovascular system can be pronounced. Blood pressure initially may decrease but after prolonged administration increase by 30% above the baseline. Cardiac output and stroke volume increase. With doses of 20 mU/min or above, oxytocin exerts an antidiuretic effect decreasing free water exchange in the kidney and markedly decreasing urine output.

Oxytocin is used to induce labor at term and to augment uterine contractions in the first and second stages of labor. Oxytocin may also be used immediately after birth to stimulate uterine contraction and thereby control uterine atony.

• Route, Dosage, Frequency

For induction of labor: Add 10 units of Pitocin (1 mL) to 1000 mL of intravenous solution. (The resulting concentration is 10 mU oxytocin per 1 mL of intravenous fluid.) Using an infusion pump, administer IV, starting at 0.5–1 mU/min and increase by 1–2 mU/min every 40–60 minutes. Alternatively, start at 1–2 mU/min and increase by 1 mU/min every 15 minutes until a good contraction pattern (every 2–3 minutes and lasting 40–60 seconds) is achieved.

• Maternal Contraindications

- Severe preeclampsia-eclampsia
- Predisposition to uterine rupture (in nullipara over 35 years of age, multigravida 4 or more, overdistention of the uterus, previous major surgery of the cervix or uterus)
- Cephalopelvic disproportion
- Malpresentation or malposition of the fetus, cord prolapse
- Preterm infant
- Rigid, unripe cervix; total placenta previa
- Presence of nonreassuring fetal status

• Maternal Side Effects

Hyperstimulation of the uterus results in hypercontractility, which in turn may cause the following:

- Abruptio placentae
- Impaired uterine blood flow, leading to fetal hypoxia
- Rapid labor, leading to cervical lacerations
- Rapid labor and birth, leading to lacerations of cervix, vagina, or perineum, uterine atony; fetal trauma
- Uterine rupture
- Water intoxication (nausea, vomiting, hypotension, tachycardia, cardiac arrhythmia) if oxytocin is given in electrolyte-free solution or at a rate exceeding 20 mU/min; hypotension with rapid IV bolus administration postpartum

• Effect on Fetus-Newborn

- Fetal effects are primarily associated with the presence of hypercontractility of the maternal uterus. Hypercontractility decreases the oxygen supply to the fetus, which is reflected by irregularities or decrease in fetal heart rate (FHR).
- Hyperbilirubinemia (Skidmore-Roth, 2003)
- Trauma from rapid birth

• Nursing Considerations

- Explain induction or augmentation procedure to client.
- Apply fetal monitor, and obtain 15- to 20-minute tracing and nonstress test (NST) to assess FHR before starting IV oxytocin.
- For induction or augmentation of labor, start with primary IV, and piggyback secondary IV with oxytocin and infusion pump.
- Ensure continuous monitoring of the fetus and uterine contractions.
- The maximum rate is 40 mU/min (ACOG, 1995). Not all protocols recommend a maximum dose. When indicated, the maximum dose is generally between 16 and 40 mU/min. Decrease oxytocin by similar increments once labor has progressed to 5–6 cm dilatation. Protocols may vary from one agency to another.

0.5 mU/min = 3 mL/hr
1.0 mU/min = 6 mL/hr
1.5 mU/min = 9 mL/hr
2 mU/min = 12 mL/hr
4 mU/min = 24 mL/hr
6 mU/min = 36 mL/hr
8 mU/min = 48 mL/hr
10 mU/min = 60 mL/hr
12 mU/min = 72 mL/hr
15 mU/min = 90 mL/hr
18 mU/min = 108 mL/hr
20 mU/min = 120 mL/hr

(continued on next page)

DRUG GUIDE Oxytocin (Pitocin)—Continued

- Assess FHR, maternal blood pressure, pulse, frequency and duration of uterine contractions, and uterine resting tone before each increase in the oxytocin infusion rate.
- Record all assessments and IV rate on monitor strip and on client's chart.
- Record oxytocin infusion rate in mU/min and mL/hr (eg, 0.5 mU/min [3 mL/hr]).
- Record on monitor strip all client activities (such as change of position, vomiting), procedures done (amniotomy, sterile vaginal examination), and administration of analgesic agents to allow for interpretation and evaluation of tracing.
- Assess cervical dilatation as needed.
- Apply nursing comfort measures.
- Discontinue IV oxytocin infusion and infuse primary solution when (1) nonreassuring fetal status is noted (bradycardia, late or variable decelerations; (2) uterine contractions are more frequent than every 2 minutes; (3) duration of contractions exceeds more than 60 seconds; or (4) insufficient relaxation of the uterus between contractions or a steady increase in resting tone are noted (ACOG, 1995). In addition to discontinuing IV oxytocin infusion, turn client to side, and if fetal distress is present, administer oxygen by tight face mask at 7–10 L/min; notify physician.
- Maintain intake and output record.

For augmentation of labor:

Prepare and administer IV Pitocin as for labor induction. Increase rate until labor contractions are of good quality. The flow rate is gradually increased at no less than every 30 minutes to a maximum of 10 mU/min (Cunningham et al, 2001). In some settings or in a situation when limited fluids may be administered, a more concentrated solution may be used. When 10 U Pitocin are added to 500 mL IV solution, the resulting concentration is 1 mU/min = 3 mL/hr. If 10 U Pitocin are added to 250 mL IV solution, the concentration is 1 mU/min = 1.5 mL/hr.

For administration after expulsion of placenta:

- One dose of 10 units of Pitocin (1 mL) is given intramuscularly or added to IV fluids for continuous infusion.
- Assess FHR, maternal blood pressure, pulse, frequency and duration of uterine contractions, and uterine resting tone before each increase in oxytocin infusion rate.
- Record all assessments and IV rate on monitor strip and on client's chart. Record oxytocin infusion rate in mU/min and mL/hr (eg, 0.5 mU/min [3 mL/hr]).
- Record on monitor strip all client activities (such as change of position, vomiting), procedures done (amniotomy, sterile vaginal examination), and administration of analgesic agents to allow for interpretation and evaluation of tracing.
- Assess cervical dilatation as needed.
- Apply nursing comfort measures.
- Discontinue IV oxytocin infusion and infuse primary solution when (1) fetal stress is noted (tachycardia or bradycardia, late or variable decelerations), (2) uterine contractions are more frequent than every 2 minutes, (3) duration of contractions exceeds 60 seconds, or (4) insufficient relaxation of the uterus between contractions or a steady increase in resting tone are noted (ACOG, 1995). In addition to discontinuing IV oxytocin infusion, turn client to side, and if fetal distress is present, administer oxygen by tight face mask at 7–10 L/min; notify physician.
- Maintain intake and output record. Assess intake and output every hour.

medicine is prompting a closer look at acupuncture as a method of inducing labor and relieving labor pain (Allaire, 2001). Although acupuncture requires extensive education and training, some CNMs can work with an acupressurist/acupuncturist to learn manual massage of acupuncture and acupressure points, shiatsu, and other touch techniques.

Balloon catheters have been used for cervical ripening for many years. Currently, a Foley catheter with a 25-mL to 50-mL balloon is passed through the undilated cervix and then inflated. The weighted balloon applies pressure on the internal os of the cervix and acts to ripen the cervix. One study examined cervical ripening after Foley catheter insertion and compared it with intracervical dinoprostone (Sciscione, McCullough, Manley, et al, 1999). The group that received the Foley catheter had higher Bishop scores than the women who received dinoprostone. Balloon catheter use is primarily an option in developing countries.

MediaLink CARE PLAN: CLIENT WITH PITOCIN

NURSING CARE MANAGEMENT

No matter which induction method is used, close observation and accurate assessments are mandatory to provide safe, optimal care for both woman and fetus. The nurse obtains maternal vital signs (temperature, pulse, respirations, and blood pressure) before beginning an oxytocin infusion. Induction protocols also recommend obtaining a 20- to 30-minute electronic fetal monitor recording demonstrating a reassuring fetal heart rate (FHR) and a reactive nonstress test and contraction status before the infusion is started. Client teaching includes the purpose and procedure for the induction, as

COMPLEMENTARY AND ALTERNATIVE THERAPIES

Evening primrose oil is a natural substance that is extracted from the plant's seeds. It has been widely used for centuries by midwives as a means of softening the cervix, vagina, and perineum to facilitate the onset of labor. Evening primrose oil contains a fatty acid called gamma linolinic acid, which is converted into a prostaglandin compound. Prostaglandins play a key role in ripening the cervix so labor can begin. Women can be advised to begin evening primrose oil supplementation during the 36th week of pregnancy. The recommended dose is 2500 mg per day taken either orally or vaginally until birth. Side effects are rare but can include headaches, nausea, or skin rashes. Women who experience side effects should be counseled to discontinue the supplement unless advised otherwise by their CNM/physician (Midwifery Today E-News, 2002).

well as a review of the care that will be provided, including assessments and comfort measures.

During the oxytocin infusion, an obstetrician should be readily accessible to manage any complication that occurs. A fetal monitor is used to provide continuous data. Women may ambulate if a portable or walking monitor is available.

Before each advancement of the infusion rate, assessments of the following should be made:

- Maternal blood pressure and pulse
- Uterine contraction status, including frequency, duration, intensity, resting tone between contractions, and maternal response to the contractions
- FHR baseline, variability (short term and long term), presence of accelerations with fetal movement, and periodic or nonperiodic decelerations

As contractions are established, vaginal examinations are performed to evaluate cervical dilatation, effacement, and station. The frequency of vaginal examinations depends primarily on the woman's parity and on characteristics of contractions. For example, a nullipara with contractions every 5 to 7 minutes, each lasting 30 seconds, who does not perceive her contractions does not usually require a vaginal examination. But when her contractions occur every 2 to 3 minutes, lasting 50 to 60 seconds with good intensity, a vaginal examination may be needed to evaluate her progress.

When evaluating the need for analgesia, a vaginal examination should be performed to avoid giving the medication too early and increasing the risk of prolonging labor and to identify advanced dilatation and imminent birth. Women who complain of rectal pressure or an urge to push should be assessed for advanced dilatation or rapid descent of the presenting part.

For additional information regarding nursing interventions during the use of oxytocin, see the Drug Guide: Oxytocin (Pitocin) on pages 747–748 and the Clinical Pathway for Induction of Labor on pages 750-751.

Women who are undergoing alternative methods of induction also need continous assessment and nursing support. For women who have entered labor after stripping of the amniotic membranes, a normal labor pattern should ensue. Intermittent external fetal monitoring can be used if the fetus is reactive and the maternal vital signs are within normal parameters. Women should be advised that they may continue to have a blood-tinged discharge from the procedure. The nurse continues to assess the contraction pattern, including the frequency, intensity, and duration of the contractions.

Women who choose to use nipple stimulation as a means of inducing labor should be continously monitored with the external fetal monitor while the electric breast pump is in use. Release of oxytocin stimulated by breast pumping can result in surges of oxytocin release which can lead to nonreassuring fetal status. Some fetuses who are unable to tolerate the release of oxytocin from breast pumping may react without stress to intravenous oxytocin administration since this results in a small amount of oxytocin being released in a controlled manner.

Women undergoing induction via balloon catheters do not need continous fetal monitoring. The nurse can perform intermittent monitoring along with the maternal vital signs. The nurse should also assess the location of the catheter to ensure the catheter has not become displaced. This can be achieved by marking the catheter tubing at the introitus and noting whether movement has occurred. After the catheter is inserted, the woman should remain in a recumbent position. Vaginal examinations should not be performed. A bedpan should be used since ambulation should be avoided.

In cases where homeopathic or herbal remedies have been used to induce labor, normal intermittent monitoring and assessment of maternal vital signs can be performed. If oxytocin is to be administered, the nurse should inform the physician or CNM of what has been given, the dose, the last time administered, and the immediate effects that were achieved. An assessment is performed prior to administration of pharmacologic substances.

CRITICAL THINKING IN PRACTICE

You are a birthing center nurse caring for Wendy Johnson, G2P1, during an oxytocin infusion to induce her labor. Wendy has been receiving the medication via infusion pump for 4 hours and currently is receiving 6 mU/min (36 mL/hr). You have just completed your assessments and found the following: BP 120/80, pulse 80, respirations 16; contractions every 3 minutes lasting 60 seconds and of strong intensity; the FHR baseline is 144–150 with average long-term variability; and cervical dilatation is 6 cm. Will you continue the same infusion rate, increase the rate, or decrease the rate?

Answers can be found in Appendix I.

MEDIALINK CASE STUDY: CLIENT UNDERGOING LABOR INDUCTION

CLINICAL PATHWAY FOR INDUCTION OF LABOR

Category	Immediate Care	Outomes
Referral	Review prenatal record Advise CNM/physician of admission Anesthesia	➤ **Expected Outcomes** Appropriate resources identified and utilized
Assessments	Previous pregnancies, present pregnancy, and childbirth preparation Estimated gestational age of the fetus Assess woman's feelings regarding induction as well as knowledge base regarding the induction process Assess knowledge of breathing techniques. If woman does not have a method to use, teach breathing techniques before starting oxytocin infusion.	➤ **Expected Outcomes** Potential/actual complications identified
Teaching/ psychosocial	Provide emotional support through teaching and answering all questions	➤ **Expected Outcomes** Woman verbalizes/demonstrates understanding of information given
Nursing care management and reports	Examination of pregnant uterus (Leopold's maneuvers to determine fetal size and position) Vaginal examination to evaluate cervical readiness: • Ripe cervix feels soft to the examining finger, is located in a medial to anterior position, is more than 50% effaced, and is 2–3 cm dilated • Unripe cervix feels firm to the examining finger, is long and thick, is perhaps in a posterior position, and is dilated little or not at all Presence of contractions Membranes intact or ruptured Maternal vital signs and a 20 min baseline fetal monitoring strip prior to induction to determine fetal well-being Diagnostic studies: • Fetal maturity tests (L/S ratio, creatinine concentrations, ultrasonography), NST, CST, BPP • Maternal blood studies (CBC, hemoglobin, hematocrit, blood type, Rh factor) • Urinalysis Monitor for nausea, vomiting, hypotension, tachycardia, cardiac arrhythmias, headache, mental confusion, decreased urinary output Monitor FHR by continuous electronic fetal monitoring. Do not start infusion or advance rate (if induction has already begun) if FHR is not in range of 110–160 bpm, if decelerations are present, or if variability decreases. Evaluate and document maternal BP and pulse before beginning induction and then before each increase in infusion rate. Do not advance infusion rate in presence of maternal hypertension or hypotension or radical changes in pulse rate. If the woman becomes hypotensive: • Keep her on her side. May change to other side. • Discontinue oxytocin infusion • Increase rate of primary IV • Monitor FHR • Notify physician • Assess for cause of hypotension Evaluate and document contraction frequency, duration, and intensity prior to each increase in infusion rate Discontinue oxytocin infusion if: • Contractions are more frequent than q2min • Contraction duration exceeds 90 sec • Uterus does not relax between contractions Increase oxytocin IV infusion rate q20min until adequate contractions are achieved. Do not exceed an infusion rate of 20–40 mL/min. (Note: Protocols directing how often oxytocin is increased may vary from 15–60 min. See ACOG 1995 guidelines and institutional protocol.) Check infusion pump to assure oxytocin is infusing. Check whether pump is on, chamber refills and empties, level of fluid in IV bottle becomes lower. If problem is found, correct and restart infusion at beginning dose. Check main IV site frequently. Check piggyback connection to primary tubing to assure solution is not leaking. Evaluate cervical dilatation by vaginal examination as indicated.	➤ **Expected Outcomes** • Progression of labor and birth without difficulty • Potential/actual complications minimized

Expected outcomes of nursing care include the following:

- The woman and family understand the induction process and are able to relate the advantages, disadvantages, risks and possible outcomes.
- The woman's labor is successfully induced.
- The labor and birth process are within normal limits, and the woman and her baby do not experience any complications.

CLINICAL PATHWAY FOR INDUCTION OF LABOR *CONTINUED*

Category	Immediate Care	Outomes
Nursing care management and reports continued	Monitor FHR continuously (normal range is 110–160 bpm). In episodes of bradycardia (<110 bpm) lasting for more than 30 sec, administer oxygen by face mask at 7–10 L/min. Stop oxytocin infusion. Position woman on left side if quick recovery of FHR does not occur. Carefully evaluate fetal tachycardia (>160 bpm). Sustained tachycardia may necessitate discontinuation of oxytocin infusion. Assess for presence of meconium staining. Notify physician.	
Activity	Ambulate until 5–10 cm then bed rest Position woman in left lateral or semi-Fowler's position Encourage her to avoid supine position	➤ **Expected Outcomes** Activity individualized for woman
Comfort	Provide support to woman as she uses breathing techniques Encourage use of effluerage, backrub, and other supportive measures Assess need for analgesia or anesthesia	➤ **Expected Outcomes** Optimal comfort level maintained
Nutrition	IV/lactated Ringer's Ice chips, clear fluids	➤ **Expected Outcomes** Nutritional and hydration needs met
Elimination	Encourage voiding q2h. Monitor and record I/O.	➤ **Expected Outcomes** Intake and output WNL
Medications	Start primary IV as ordered Administer oxytocin in electrolyte solution (Piggyback oxytocin onto primary IV at closest site to IV needle insertion.) Pain meds PRN	➤ **Expected Outcomes** Induction/augmentation of labor occurs within expected parameters
Discharge planning/home care	Photo packet Birth certificate worksheet Sibling visitation Car seat	➤ **Expected Outcomes** Individualized discharge teaching completed
Family involvement	Family visitation policy per institutional protocol Encourage significant other to stay close and assist with breathing of woman	➤ **Expected Outcomes** Family/support person involvement maximized
Date		

BP, blood presure; bpm, beats per minute; BPP, biophysical profile; CBC, complete blood count; CST, contraction stress test; FHR, fetal heart rate; I&O, intake and output; IV, intravenous; NST, nonstress test; PRN, as needed; WNL, within normal limits

Care of the Woman During an Amniotomy

Amniotomy is the artificial rupture of the amniotic membranes (AROM). It is probably the most common procedure performed in obstetrics. Because the amniotomy requires that an instrument be inserted through the cervix, at least 2 cm of cervical dilatation must be present. The amniotomy may be performed as a method of induction of labor (to stimulate the beginning of labor), or it may be done at any time during the first stage of labor to accelerate the labor. If an amniotomy is done after 3 cm of cervical dilatation, the labor will probably be shortened by 1 to 2 hours (Fraser, Turcot, Krauss, et al, 2000). Amniotomy may also be performed during labor to allow access to the fetus in order to apply an internal fetal heart monitoring electrode to the scalp, to insert an intrauterine pressure catheter, or to obtain a fetal scalp blood sample for acid-base determination.

Advantages and Disadvantages of Amniotomy

Amniotomy as a method of labor induction has the following advantages:

1. The contractions elicited are similar to those of spontaneous labor.
2. There is usually no risk of hypertonus or rupture of the uterus, as with intravenous oxytocin induction.
3. The woman does not require the same intensive monitoring as with intravenous oxytocin induction.
4. Electronic Fetal Monitoring (EFM) is facilitated because, once the membranes are ruptured, a fetal scalp electrode may be applied, an intrauterine catheter may be inserted, and scalp blood sampling for pH determinations may be done to assist in evaluating a fetal heart rate pattern.
5. The color and composition of amniotic fluid can be evaluated.

The disadvantages of amniotomy are as follows:

1. Once an amniotomy is done, birth should occur within 24 hours because microorganisms can now invade the intrauterine cavity and cause amnionitis.
2. The danger of a prolapsed cord is increased once the membranes have ruptured, especially if the fetal presenting part is not firmly pressed down against the cervix.

3. Compression and molding of the fetal head are increased due to loss of the cushioning effect of the amniotic fluid for the fetal head during uterine contractions.

Amniotomy Procedure

Before an amniotomy is performed, the fetus is assessed for presentation, position, station, and fetal heart rate (FHR). Unless the fetal head is well engaged in the pelvis, some practitioners do not advocate an amniotomy because of the danger of prolapsed cord (refer to Chapter 26 for discussion of prolapsed cord). Other risks are abruptio placentae (due to rapid decompression of the uterus with the rapid loss of amniotic fluid), infection (due to the introduction of organisms into the cervix and intrauterine cavity), and amniotic fluid embolus (due to rapid decompression of the uterus and small amounts of fluid entering the maternal vascular system from under the edge of the placenta). These complications may also be associated with spontaneous rupture of membranes.

While performing a sterile vaginal examination, the physician or certified nurse-midwife (CNM) introduces an amnihook (or other rupturing device) into the vagina, through the cervix, and against the amniotic membrane which is in front of the fetal presenting part. A small tear is made in the amniotic membrane. Following rupture of the membranes, amniotic fluid is allowed to escape slowly.

NURSING CARE MANAGEMENT

The nurse explains the procedure to the woman. The fetal presentation, position, and station are assessed because amniotomy is usually delayed until engagement has occurred (to decrease the risk of a prolapsed cord when the fluid is expelled). The woman is positioned in a semireclining position and draped to provide privacy. Disposable underpads and/or towels are placed under the woman's buttocks to absorb the amniotic fluid. The FHR is assessed just prior to and immediately after the amniotomy, and the two FHR assessments are compared. If there are marked changes, the nurse should check for prolapse of the cord. The amniotic fluid is inspected for amount, color, odor, and the presence of meconium or blood. While wearing disposable gloves, the nurse cleanses and dries the perineal area and changes the disposable underpads. The nurse advises the woman that fluid will continue to be expelled from her vagina. Frequent pericare and pad changes should be done to increase client comfort. Because there is now an open pathway for organisms to ascend into the uterus, strict sterile technique must be observed during vaginal examinations. In addition, the number of vaginal examinations must be kept to a minimum to reduce the chance of introducing an infection, and the woman's temperature should be monitored every 2 hours. Bed rest is maintained unless the presenting part is engaged and is firmly against the cervix (to decrease the risk of prolapsed cord). The nurse needs to provide information about the amniotomy and the expected effects. Some couples may worry that all the amniotic fluid will be gone and that they will experience a "dry birth." It is important for them to know that amniotic fluid is constantly produced.

Care of the Woman During Amnioinfusion

Amnioinfusion (AI) is a technique by which a volume of warmed, sterile, normal saline or Ringer's lactate solution is introduced into the uterus through the use of an intrauterine pressure catheter (IUPC). Amnioinfusion can be used intrapartally to increase the volume of fluid when oligohydramnios is present and the physician either wants to prevent the possibility of variable decelerations by increasing the volume of amniotic fluid or wants to treat nonperiodic decelerations that are already occurring. The AI increases the volume of fluid, relieving pressure on the umbilical cord and promoting increased perfusion to the fetus. When AI is used for this indication or for prolonged decelerations in FHR patterns, the abnormal FHR pattern is usually relieved in 20 to 30 minutes (Medifocus, 2002). Amnioinfusion used for meconium dilution in the presence of medium to heavy meconium staining has resulted in a significant decrease of meconium below the newborn's vocal cords (when viewed with a laryngoscope) after birth and a decrease in meconium aspiration. It is not known whether the decreased incidence is due to dilution of the meconium in the amniotic fluid or to the decreased incidence of variable decelerations; however, use of AI decreases cesarean births and fetal morbidity (Hofmeyr, 2002; Rather, Singh, Ramji, et al, 2002). AI is also indicated for preterm labor with premature rupture of membranes. Contraindications include amnionitis, hydramnios, uterine hypertonus, multiple gestation, known fetal anomaly, uterine anomaly, nonreassuring fetal status requiring immediate birth, nonvertex presentation, scalp pH below 7.20, placenta previa, vasa previa, or abruptio placentae (Hofmeyr, 2002).

There is no one accepted protocol for AI. However, most procedures involve infusing from 250 to 500 mL of warmed normal saline through an intrauterine catheter using an infusion pump over 20 to 30 minutes.

NURSING CARE MANAGEMENT

The nurse is frequently the first person to detect changes in FHR associated with cord compression or to observe thick, meconium-stained amniotic fluid. When cord compression is suspected, the immediate intervention is to assist the laboring woman to another position in an effort to relieve the compression and to apply O_2 via face mask (see Chapter 26 for further discussion). If this intervention is not successful, an AI will be considered. The nurse helps with the AI and monitors the woman's vital signs (blood pressure, pulse, and respiration) and contraction status (frequency, duration, intensity, resting tone, and associated maternal discomfort). FHR is monitored by continuous EFM. The nurse should provide ongoing information to the laboring woman and her partner and answer questions as they arise. Comfort measures and positioning are very important because AI requires the woman to be on bed rest.

The amnioinfusion should not cause pain or discomfort for the laboring woman other than the need for bed rest. The nurse needs to ensure that the fluid infused is being expelled from the woman's vagina. This is achieved with frequent examination of the woman's sanitary pad or an absorbent pad that is placed beneath her buttocks. The woman should be advised that fluid will leak from her vagina. The nurse should change absorbent pads and provide pericare on a regular basis.

Care of the Woman During an Episiotomy

An **episiotomy** is a surgical incision of the perineal body. Traditionally some physicians and CNMs performed episiotomies in order to prevent damage to the periurethra, perineum, anal sphincter, and rectum from lacerations during the birth; to prevent damage to the posterior wall of the vagina; to prevent jagged tears from lacerations; to reduce mechanical and metabolic risk to the fetus/newborn; to protect the maternal bladder; and to prevent future perineal relaxation. However, new research indicates that routine episiotomy is now typically performed because of time pressures, conventional education practices, birth setting, malpractice concerns, lack of experience with perineal stretching techniques, and interventionist practice patterns (Eason & Feldman, 2000; Webb & Culhane, 2002).

Although the incidence of episiotomies in the United States has declined from 57% in 1989 to 35.2% in 1999 (Popovic, 2001), it is still the most common surgical procedure performed on women in the United States (Webb & Culhane, 2002). In 1999, it is estimated that 1 million episiotomies were performed in the United States (National Center for Health Statistics, 2001). In Canada, the incidence is approximately 37.8%, which reflects a decline of 29.1% since the early 1980s (Graham & Graham, 1997). Typically, nurse-midwives tend to perform fewer episiotomies than physicians (Davidson, 2002).

Even though the procedure is very common, its routine use has been questioned. Research suggests that, rather than protecting the perineum from lacerations, the presence of an episiotomy makes it more likely that the woman will have deep perineal tears. It has also been suggested that perineal lacerations heal more quickly in the absence of episiotomy. Major perineal trauma (extension to or through the anal sphincter) is *more* likely to occur if a midline episiotomy is performed (Angiolo, Gommez-Marin, Cantuaria, et al, 2000). Additional complications associated with an episiotomy are blood loss, infection, pain, and perineal discomfort that may continue for days or weeks past birth, including dyspareunia (painful intercourse) (Myers-Helfgott & Helfgott, 1999). Flatal incontinence (uncontrollable passage of gas) has also been reported (Eason, Labrecque, Marcoux, et al, 2002). There are no scientific data to support the beliefs that episiotomies yield a shorter second stage, improved Apgar scores, or a decrease in perinatal asphyxia (Myers-Helfgott & Helfgott, 1999). In light of the debate over the value of episiotomy, it is now suggested that the procedure be used selectively to facilitate birth in the presence of maternal or fetal stress or when a shoulder dystocia is anticipated. There is debate on whether episiotomies should be performed to create more room in the presence of a breech presentation, multiple gestation, or a large-for-gestational-age infant (> 4000 g), or for the use of an instrument (forceps or vacuum extractor) to assist birth. Some researchers argue that midline episiotomy and vacuum-assisted birth should be avoided when a large baby is anticipated. Although many practitioners perform episiotomies when an instrument is being used to assist birth, new research suggests this may result in more third and fourth-degree extensions (Angiolo et al, 2000).

Risk Factors that Predispose Women to Episiotomy

Overall factors that place a woman at increased risk for an episiotomy are primigravid status, large or macrosomic fetus, occiput-posterior position, use of forceps or vacuum extractor, shoulder dystocia, and white race (Goldberg, Holtz, Hyslop, et al, 2002). Other factors that predispose a woman to episiotomy may be mitigated by nurses and physicians/CNMs. These include the following (Maier & Maloni, 1997):

- Use of lithotomy position or other recumbent position (causes excessive perineal stretching)
- Encouraging or requiring sustained breath holding during second-stage pushing (causes excessive perineal stretching, can adversely affect blood flow in mother and fetus, and encourages woman to be responsive to caregiver directions rather than to her own urges to push spontaneously)
- Arbitrary time limit placed by the physician/CNM on the length of the second stage

Nursing advocacy is needed to promote selective rather than routine episiotomies. The nurse can begin by encouraging pregnant women to read about prenatal perineal preparation and to talk with the physician or CNM about their personal beliefs and the incidence of episiotomy in their practice. Nurses can share current research with nursing colleagues through staff meetings and explore and strongly encourage nursing care interventions that avoid the lithotomy position. The woman should be encouraged to respond to her body's urges to push during the second stage. Just as clients ask physicians and CNMs about their episiotomy philosophy and incidence, clients may at some time in the future ask labor and birthing nurses to provide information about their actions to help decrease episiotomy rates. It is imperative that each nurse continue to stay current about new information and research in order to maintain current practice standards.

Episiotomy Procedure

The episiotomy is performed with a sharp scissors that has rounded points, just before birth, when approximately 3 to 4 cm of the fetal head is visible during a contraction (Cunningham et al, 2001). There are two types of episiotomy: midline and mediolateral (Figure 27–3 •). A midline episiotomy is performed along the median raphe of the perineum. It extends down from the vaginal orifice to the fibers of the rectal sphincter. This type of episiotomy avoids muscle fibers and major blood vessels because it divides the insertions of the superficial perineal muscles. A midline episiotomy is preferred if the perineum is of adequate length and no difficulty is anticipated during the birth because it entails less blood loss, is easy to repair, and heals with less discomfort for the mother. The major disadvantage is that a tear of the midline incision may extend through the anal sphincter and rectum.

In the presence of a short perineum, macrosomia, and instrument-assisted birth (use of forceps or vacuum extractor), a mediolateral episiotomy provides more room and decreases the possibility of a traumatic extension into the rectum. The mediolateral episiotomy begins in the midline of the posterior fourchette (to avoid incision into the Bartholin's gland) and extends at a 45-degree angle downward to the right or left (the direction depending on the handedness of the clinician). The mediolateral episiotomy may be complicated by greater blood loss, a longer healing period, and more postpartal discomfort.

The episiotomy is usually performed with regional or local anesthesia but may be performed without anesthesia in emergency situations. It is generally suggested that as crowning occurs, the distention of the tissues causes numbing. Adequate anesthesia must be given for the repair.

Repair of the episiotomy (episiorrhaphy) and any lacerations is performed either during the period between birth of the baby and before expulsion of the placenta or after expulsion of the placenta. Many providers wait until after expulsion of the placenta in case a manual removal of the placenta or a uterine exploration is indicated.

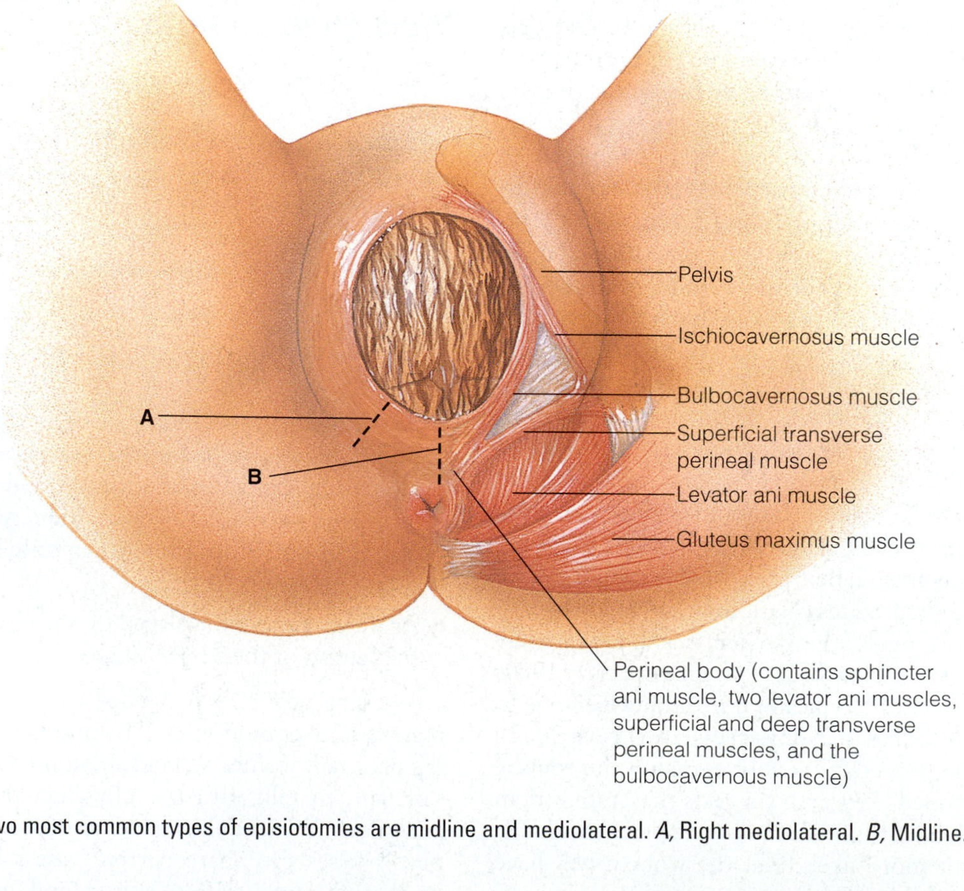

Figure 27–3 • The two most common types of episiotomies are midline and mediolateral. *A,* Right mediolateral. *B,* Midline.

NURSING CARE MANAGEMENT

The woman needs to be supported during the episiotomy and the repair because she may feel some pressure sensations. It is not uncommon for the woman to feel a "pulling" or "tugging" sensation. In the absence of adequate anesthesia, she may feel pain. Placing a hand on her shoulder and talking with her can provide comfort and distraction from the repair process. If the woman is having more discomfort than she can comfortably handle, the nurse needs to act as an advocate in communicating the woman's needs to the physician/CNM. At all times, the woman needs to be the one who decides whether the amount of discomfort is tolerable, and she should never be told, "This doesn't hurt." She is the person experiencing the discomfort, and her evaluation needs to be respected. If there are just a few (three to five) stitches left, she may choose to forgo more local anesthesia, but she should be given the choice. For women with severe pain or anxiety, intravenous medication such as Demerol or Nubain can be administered for both pain and anxiety control.

The nurse notes the type of episiotomy on the birth record. This information should also be included in a report to the postpartum nurse so that adequate assessments can be made and relief measures can be instituted if necessary.

Pain relief measures may begin immediately after birth with application of an ice pack to the perineum. For optimal effect, the ice pack should be applied for 20 to 30 minutes and removed for at least 20 minutes before being reapplied. This is advisable because the ice causes vasoconstriction; however, if the ice pack is left in place more than 30 minutes, vasodilation and subsequent edema may occur. The perineal tissues should be assessed frequently to prevent injury from the ice pack. The episiotomy site is inspected every 15 minutes during the first hour after the birth for redness, swelling, tenderness, and hematomas. As a part of postpartal care, the mother will need instruction in perineal hygiene care and comfort measures. (See Chapter 35 for additional discussion of relief measures for the immediate postpartum period.)

It is important for nurses to recognize that perineal pain continues for a period of time. Women who experience prolonged pain tend to have other problems, such as breastfeeding difficulties and depression, and are more reluctant to reestablish sexual activity. Risk factors for subsequent lacerations include use of repeat episiotomy and instrument-assisted births (Peleg et al, 1999).

Care of the Woman During Forceps-Assisted Birth

Forceps are designed to assist the birth of a fetus by providing traction or by providing the means to rotate the fetal head to an occiput-anterior position. In medical literature and practice, **forceps-assisted birth** is also known as *instrumental delivery, operative delivery, or operative vaginal delivery.* There are many different types of forceps, each with special functions. For example, Piper forceps are designed to be used with a breech presentation (buttocks as presenting part); they are applied after the birth of the body, when the fetal head is still in the birth canal and assistance is needed. In conversational language, Piper forceps are said to be applied to the aftercoming head. All other forceps are used in situations when the fetus is in a cephalic (head down) presentation. In such situations, the forceps are applied to the sides of the head. The type of forceps used is determined by the physician assisting with the birth.

MEDIALINK FORCEPS DELIVERY

Criteria for Forceps Application

The American College of Obstetricians and Gynecologists (ACOG, 2000) has classified the definitions of forceps applications into three categories: outlet, low, and midforceps. Criteria for *outlet forceps* application are as follows:

1. Forceps are applied when the fetal skull has reached the pelvic floor and is at or on the perineum. (There is bulging of the perineum.)
2. The scalp is visible between contractions without separating the labia. (Earlier in labor, as the woman pushes during the contraction, the fetal scalp may be visible, but when the pushing effort ceases, the scalp recedes and is no longer visible. This criterion indicates that the scalp remains visible even when the woman is not pushing.)
3. The sagittal suture is not more than 45 degrees from the midline. The sagittal suture is the anterior-posterior suture on the top of the fetal head. At this point in a spontaneous birth, extension has almost been completed, external rotation is beginning, and the sagittal suture is between the midline and 45 degrees from the midline. (For example, think of a clock face. If 12:00 is the maternal symphysis pubis and the fetus is in LOA, the sagittal suture and the occiput are between 12:00 and 1:30.) (See Chapter 22). The important aspect of this criterion is that with outlet forceps, the fetal head is moving naturally from extension to external rotation, and the forceps are being used to guide or lift the head out.

The criterion for *low forceps* application is that the leading edge (presenting part) of the fetal skull must be at a station of + 2 or below (for example, + 3) but not on the pelvic

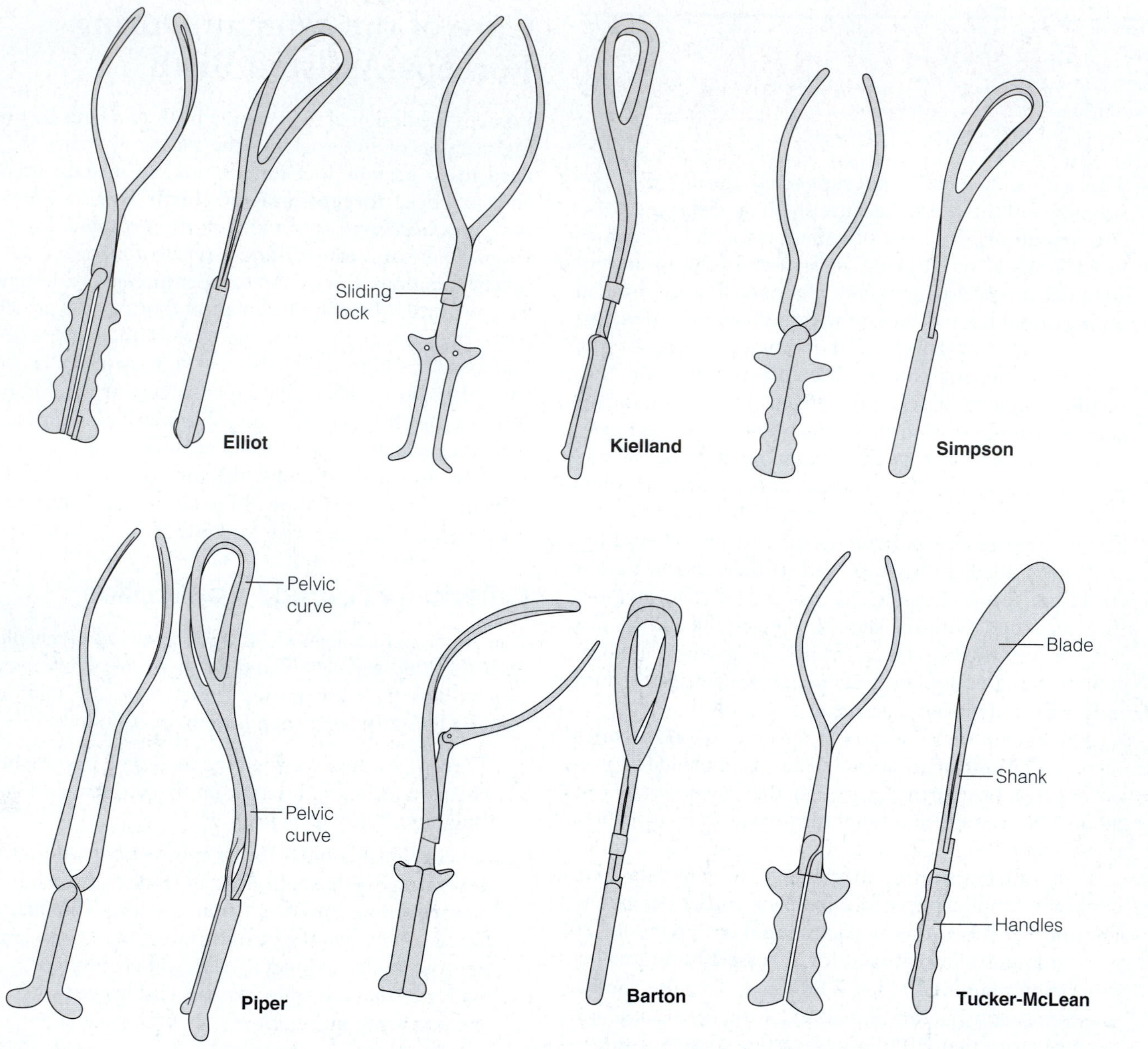

Figure 27–4 • Forceps are composed of a blade, shank, and handle and may have a cephalic and pelvic curve. (Note labels on Piper and Tucker-McLean forceps.) The blades may be fenestrated (open) or solid. The front and lateral views of these forceps illustrate differences in blades, open and closed shanks, and cephalic and pelvic curves. Elliot, Simpson, and Tucker-McLean forceps are used as outlet forceps. Kielland and Barton forceps are used for midforceps rotations. Piper forceps are used to provide traction and flexion of the aftercoming head (the head comes after the body) of a fetus in breech presentation.

floor. The rotation (internal rotation, which is part of the cardinal movements) of the fetal head is less than 45 degrees (right or left occiput anterior to occiput anterior, or right or left occiput posterior to occiput posterior) (ACOG, 2000).

The criterion for *midforceps* application is that the fetal head must be engaged (largest diameter of the head reaches or passes through the pelvic inlet), but the leading edge (presenting part) of the fetal skull is above a + 2 station (for example + 1, 0, − 1, − 2). When midforceps are used, the goal is to apply traction, and, frequently, to rotate the head and facilitate the vaginal birth.

High forceps are not indicated in current obstetric practice. A woman whose fetus is at a station of −3 or is above the pelvic inlet should give birth by cesarean. Types of forceps are depicted in Figure 27–4 •.

Indications for Use of Forceps

Indications for the use of forceps include the presence of any condition that threatens the mother or fetus and that can be relieved by birth. Conditions that put the woman at risk include heart disease, acute pulmonary edema, intrapartal infection, or exhaustion. Fetal conditions include premature placental separation and nonreassuring fetal status. Forceps may be used electively to shorten the second stage of labor and spare the woman's pushing effort (when exhaustion or heart disease is present) or when regional anesthesia has affected the woman's motor innervation and she cannot push effectively. In the past, outlet forceps have been used to protect the head of a preterm infant during birth; however, the advantages of this practice are now being questioned (Cunningham et al, 2001).

Risk factors for a forceps- or vacuum-assisted birth (discussion to follow) are as follows (Kabiru, Jamieson, Graves, et al, 2001):

- Nulliparity
- Maternal age (35 and over)
- Maternal height of less than 150 cm (4 ft 11 in)
- Pregnancy weight gain of more than 15 kg (33 lb)
- Postdate gestation (41 weeks or more)
- Epidural anesthesia
- Infant presentation other than occipitoanterior
- Presence of dystocia
- Presence of a midline episiotomy
- Abnormal fetal heart rate tracing

Neonatal and Maternal Risks

Some newborns may develop a small area of ecchymosis, edema, or both along the sides of the face as a result of forceps application. Caput succedaneum or cephalhematoma (and subsequent hyperbilirubinemia) may occur as well as transient facial paralysis. Other reported complications include low Apgar scores, retinal hemorrhage, corneal abrasions, ocular trauma, other trauma (Erb's palsy, fractured clavicle), elevated neonatal bilirubin levels, and prolonged infant hospital stay (ACOG, 2000; Cunningham et al, 2001).

Maternal risks may include trauma such as lacerations of the birth canal, periurethral lacerations, and extensions of a median episiotomy into the anus, resulting in increased bleeding, bruising, hematomas, and pelvic floor injuries (ACOG, 2000). Women who give birth with the assistance of forceps report more perineal pain and sexual problems in the postpartum period (Thompson, Roberts, Currie, et al, 2002). In addition, an increase in postpartum infections, cervical lacerations, and prolonged hospital stays has been reported (Kabiru et al, 2001). Women who have given birth with forceps may also experience intra-anal pressure and a weakening of the pelvic floor (Meyer, Hohlreld, Achtar, et al, 2000).

Prerequisites for Forceps Application and Birth

It is very important that all of the prerequisites be met before the forceps procedure is attempted. The prerequisites are as follows (Cunningham et al, 2001):

- The physician must be knowledgeable about the advantages and disadvantages of different types of forceps and their use.
- The cervix must be completely dilated.
- The fetal head must be engaged, and the station, presentation, and exact position of the head must be known. The fetus should be in a vertex or a face presentation with the chin anterior.
- Amniotic membranes must be ruptured to allow a firm grasp on the fetal head.
- The type of pelvis should be identified, because certain pelvic types do not permit rotation. In addition, there must be no disproportion between the fetal head and the maternal pelvis.
- Maternal bladder should be empty.
- There must be no obstructions to the birth below the fetal head, such as an incurving coccyx that will not allow the fetus to pass or a disproportion between the size of the head and the outlet or the midpelvis.
- Adequate anesthesia must be given for the type of forceps procedure that is anticipated. For instance, low forceps may be done with a pudendal block; however, midforceps or a rotation of more than 45 degrees requires an epidural, spinal-epidural, or general anesthesia.

Trial or Failed Forceps Procedure

ACOG (2000) advocates for the use of forceps or vacuum when the clinician believes a successful outcome can occur. In a trial forceps procedure, the physician attempts to use forceps with the knowledge that there could be a degree of cephalopelvic disproportion. A complete setup for immediate cesarean birth needs to be available before the forceps are applied. If a good application cannot be obtained or if no descent occurs with the application, a vacuum technique can be attempted. If this yields no descent, then a cesarean birth is the method of choice.

NURSING CARE MANAGEMENT

The nurse directs nursing care measures toward the variable(s) that may be positively affected by specific nursing interventions. For instance, dystocia may be corrected by changing maternal position, ambulation, rocking, frequent bladder emptying, and so on. Fetal heart rate (FHR) abnormalities may be affected by utero-placental-fetal circulation, so the nurse could support ambulation (if not contraindicated), frequent position changes, intake of adequate fluids, and monitoring to detect early FHR changes.

If a forceps-assisted birth is required, the nurse explains the procedure briefly to the woman. With adequate regional anesthesia, the woman should feel some pressure but no pain. The nurse encourages her to avoid pushing during application of the forceps (Figure 27–5 • depicts

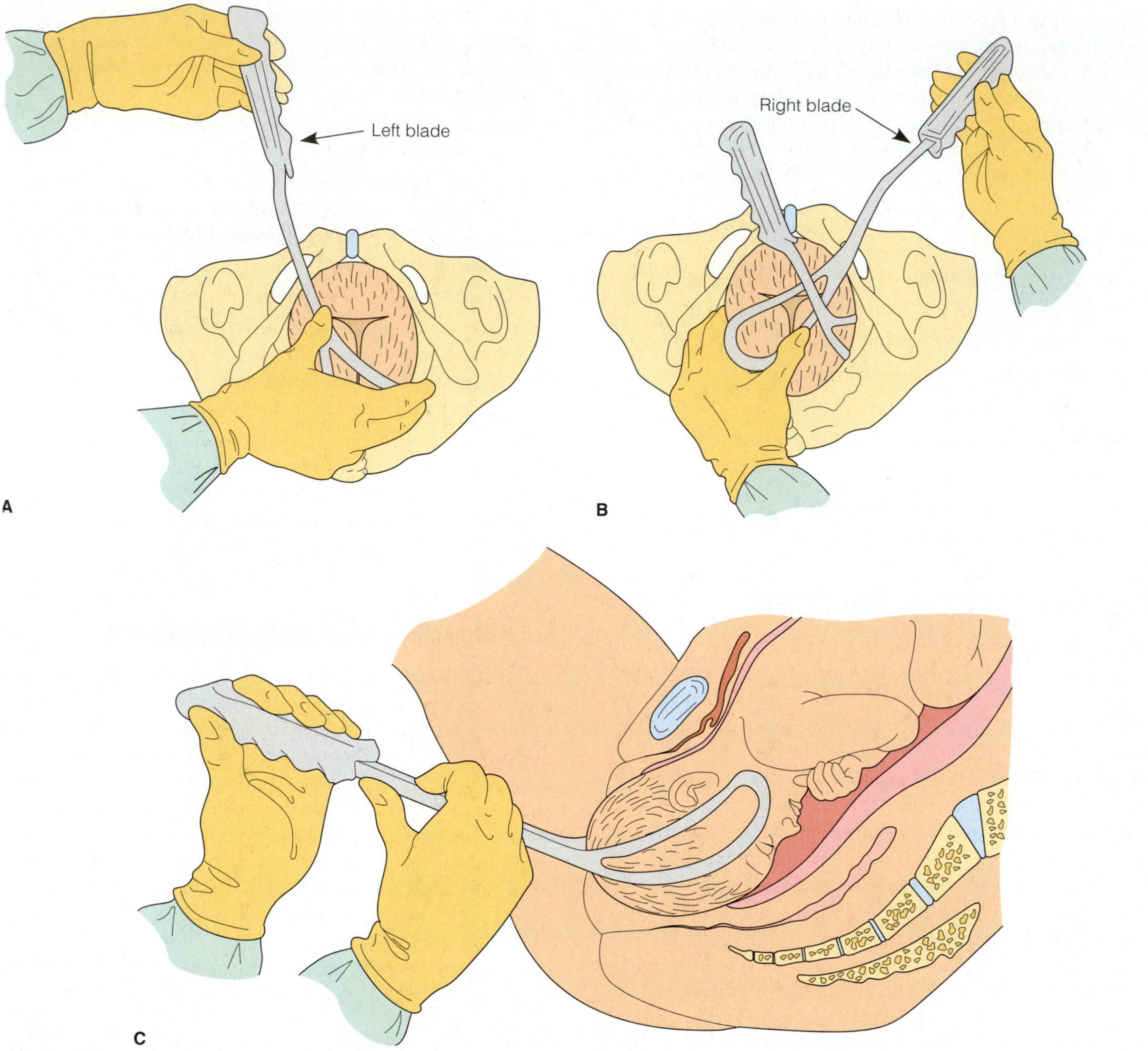

Figure 27–5 • Application of forceps in occiput anterior (OA) position. *A,* The left blade is inserted along the left side wall of the pelvis over the parietal bone. *B,* The right blade is inserted along the right side wall of the pelvis over the parietal bone. *C,* With correct placement of the blades, the handles lock easily. During uterine contractions, traction is applied to the forceps in a downward and outward direction to follow the birth canal.

the application). The nurse monitors contractions and advises the physician when one is present because traction is applied only with a contraction. During the contraction, as the forceps are applied, the nurse again advises the woman to avoid pushing. With each contraction, *after the forceps are in place,* the physician provides traction on the forceps as the woman pushes. It is not uncommon to observe mild bradycardia as traction is applied to the forceps. This bradycardia results from head compression and is transient.

Following birth, the newborn is assessed for facial edema, bruising, caput succedaneum, cephalhematoma, and any sign of cerebral edema. In the fourth stage, the nurse assesses the woman for perineal swelling, bruising, hematoma, excessive bleeding, and hemorrhage. In the postpartum period it is important to assess for signs of infection if lacerations occurred during the procedure.

The nurse answers questions and reiterates explanations provided, reviews nursing assessments of the woman and her newborn, and provides opportunities for the woman and family to ask further questions. Some women may feel a sense of loss or failure as a result of needing forceps for birth. The nurse provides reassurance to the woman and her family.

MediaLink VIDEO: VACUUM EXTRACTOR

Care of the Woman During Vacuum Extraction

Vacuum extraction is an obstetric procedure used to assist the birth of a fetus by applying suction to the fetal head. The vacuum extractor is composed of a soft suction cup attached to a suction bottle (pump) by tubing. The suction cup, which comes in various sizes, is placed against the occiput of the fetal head. Care must be taken to ensure that no cervical or vaginal tissue is trapped under the cup. The pump is used to create negative pressure (suction) of approximately 50 to 60 mm Hg. An artificial caput ("chignon") is formed as the fetal scalp is pulled into the cup. The physician or CNM then applies traction in coordination with uterine contractions. The fetal head should descend with each contraction until it emerges from the vagina (Figure 27–6 •).

Research indicates that negative suction applied for more than 10 minutes is associated with a greater incidence of scalp injury. The longer the duration of suction, the more likely the newborn will have scalp injury. Although there are no data on the duration of use, ACOG advises a 30-minute time limit (ACOG, 1998). Many practitioners limit the time to 20 minutes (Perez, 1999). While there are no specifications on the number of attempts, failure to descend with multiple attempts is an indicator that a cesarean birth may be needed. In addition, if more than three "pop-offs" occur (the suction cup pops off the fetal head), the procedure should be discontinued (Perez, 1999).

The most common indication for the use of the vacuum extractor is a prolonged second stage of labor or nonreassuring heart rate pattern. Vacuum extraction is also used to relieve the woman of pushing effort, or when analgesia or fatigue interfere with her ability to push effectively, or in cases of nonreassuring fetal status when prompt birth is indicated. The vacuum extractor is preferred to forceps in cases of borderline cephalopelvic disproportion (CPD), when successful passage of the fetal head requires all potential space inside the vaginal canal. True CPD is an absolute contraindication to vacuum extraction. Other contraindications include nonvertex presentations, maternal or suspected fetal coagulation defects, known or suspected hydrocephalus, and fetal scalp trauma (Perez, 1999). Relative contraindications include suspected fetal macrosomia, high fetal station, face or breech presentation, gestation less than 35 weeks, incompletely dilated cervix, and previous fetal scalp blood sampling (Cunningham et al, 2001).

Neonatal complications include scalp lacerations, bruising, subdural hematomas, cephalhematomas, intracranial hemorrhages, subconjunctival hemorrhages, neonatal jaundice, fractured clavicle, Erb's palsy, damage to the sixth and seventh cranial nerves, retinal hemorrhage, and fetal death (Cunningham et al, 2001). In addition, there is an increased incidence of shoulder dystocia in infants weighing more than 4500 g (Perez, 1999). There appear to be more neonatal complications and injuries with use of a metal suction cup device than with soft cup devices (ACOG, 2000). In the presence of a preterm gestation, risk of periventricular-intraventricular

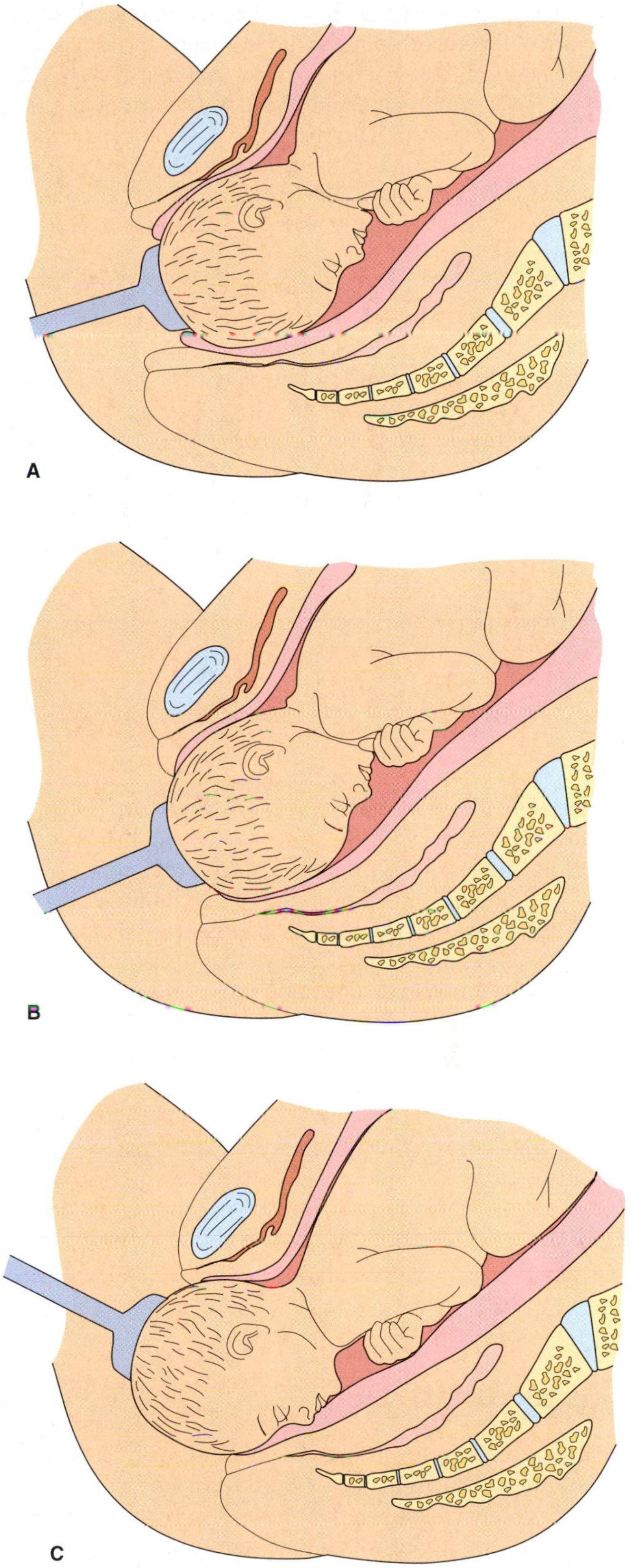

Figure 27–6 • Vacuum extractor traction. *A*, The cup is placed on the fetal occiput creating suction. Traction is applied in a downward and outward direction. *B*, Traction continues in a downward direction as the fetal head begins to emerge from the vagina. *C*, Traction is maintained to lift the fetal head out of the vagina.

hemorrhage (PV-IVH) has been a concern, and some studies provide conflicting recommendations. Maternal complications include perineal trauma, edema, third- and fourth-degree lacerations, postpartum pain, and infection (Kabiru et al, 2001). Women who give birth with the aid of a vacuum extractor report more sexual difficulties in the postpartum period (Thompson et al, 2002). Maternal genital tract and anal sphincter injuries occur less frequently with the vacuum extractor than with forceps (Vacca, 2002).

In 1998, the US Food and Drug Administration (FDA) released a health advisory statement that vacuum extraction can cause serious or fatal complications. Twelve deaths and nine serious injuries occurred between 1994 and 1998. The FDA recommended caution in using rocking movements when using the device. They also recommended that pediatricians be alerted when a vacuum-assisted birth occurred so the infant could be closely monitored for related injuries (Center for Devices & Radiological Health, 1998).

NURSING CARE MANAGEMENT

There are different types of vacuum extractors. The nurse must be familiar with the types used within the birthing setting and learn the pressure limits of each type.

The nurse should inform the woman about what is happening during the procedure. If adequate regional anesthesia has been administered, the woman feels only pressure during the procedure. The nurse pumps the vacuum to the appropriate level to provide suction by the physician or CNM. The FHR is auscultated at least every 5 minutes or assessed by continuous electronic fetal monitoring. The parents need to be informed that the caput (chignon) on the baby's head will disappear within 2 to 3 days.

The nurse continues to assess the newborn for cephalhematomas, intracranial hemorrhage, and retinal hemorrhages (Sachs, Kobelin, Castro, et al, 1999).

Care of the Family During Cesarean Birth

Cesarean birth is the birth of the infant through an abdominal and uterine incision. Cesarean birth is one of the oldest surgical procedures known. Until the 20th century, cesareans were primarily equated with an attempt to save the fetus of a dying woman. As the maternal and perinatal morbidity and mortality rates associated with cesarean birth steadily decreased throughout the 20th century, the rate of cesarean births increased. In 1970, cesarean births comprised 5.5% of all births and progressed to a high of 24.7% in 1988 (Sachs et al, 1999). Then, as a result of concern about the high rates and about the associated increase in healthcare costs, the rates decreased to 21% in 2001. In some countries, the incidence has been much lower throughout the 20th century. England, Scotland, Sweden, Denmark, and Saudi Arabia have rates of approximately 10% to 14%, although the rates in New Zealand and Mexico are higher than in the United States (Mesleh, Asiri, & Al-Naim, 2000; Buist, Brown, & McNamara, 1999; Rasmussen, Pedersen, Wilken-Jensen et al, 2000; Juarez Ocana, Fajardo Gutierrez, Perez Palacios, et al, 1999).

Many factors affect the cesarean birth rate, and they need to be considered in discussions about decreasing the current rate in the United States. These factors include changing philosophies regarding the best method of birth with a breech presentation, interpretations of EFM tracings, changing practice related to vaginal birth after cesarean birth, increased use of epidural anesthesia, physician convenience, and type of provider (Sachs et al, 1999).

Indications

Cesarean births are performed in the presence of a variety of maternal and fetal conditions. Commonly accepted indications include complete placenta previa, CPD, placental abruption, active genital herpes, umbilical cord prolapse, failure to progress in labor, proven nonreassuring fetal status, and benign and malignant tumors that obstruct the birth canal. Indications that are more controversial include breech presentation, previous cesarean birth, major congenital anomalies, cervical cerclage, and severe Rh isoimmunization.

Maternal Mortality and Morbidity

Cesarean births have a higher maternal mortality rate than vaginal births. Approximately 5.8 women per 100,000 live births die, and about half of the deaths are attributed to the operation and a coexisting medical condition (Bowes, 1999). Perinatal morbidity is primarily associated with infection, reactions to anesthesia agents, blood clots, and bleeding.

Surgical Techniques

Cesarean birth requires both a skin and a uterine incision, which are not necessarily the same type of incision.

SKIN INCISIONS

The skin incision for a cesarean birth is either transverse (Pfannenstiel) or vertical and is not indicative of the type of incision made into the uterus. The type of skin incision is determined by time factor, client preference, or physician preference.

The transverse incision is made across the lowest and narrowest part of the abdomen. Because the incision is made just below the pubic hair line, it is almost invisible after healing. Other advantages of this type of incision include less bleeding and better healing. The limitations of this type of skin incision are that it does not allow for extension of the incision if needed. Because it usually requires more time, this incision is used when time is not of the essence (eg, with failure to progress and no fetal or maternal stress).

The vertical (infraumbilical midline) incision is made between the navel and the symphysis pubis. This incision is quicker and is therefore preferred in cases of nonreassuring fetal status when rapid birth is indicated, with preterm or macrosomic infants, or when the woman is obese (Cunningham et al, 2001).

UTERINE INCISIONS

The type of uterine incision depends on the need for the cesarean. The choice of incision affects the woman's opportunity for a subsequent vaginal birth and her risks of a ruptured uterine scar with a subsequent pregnancy.

The two major locations of uterine incisions are the lower uterine segment and the upper segment of the uterine corpus.

The most common lower uterine segment incision is a transverse incision (Figure 27–7 •, *A*), which is preferred for the following reasons (Cunningham et al, 2001):

1. The lower segment is the thinnest portion of the uterus and involves less blood loss.
2. It requires only moderate dissection of the bladder from underlying myometrium.
3. It is easier to repair, although repair takes longer.
4. The site is less likely to rupture during subsequent pregnancies.
5. There is a decreased chance of adherence of bowel or omentum to the incision line.

The disadvantages include the following:

1. It takes longer to make a transverse incision.
2. It is limited in size because of the presence of major blood vessels on either side of the uterus.
3. It has a greater tendency to extend laterally into the uterine vessels.
4. The incision may stretch and become a thin window, but it usually does not create problems clinically until subsequent labor ensues.

The lower uterine segment vertical incision is preferred for multiple gestation, abnormal presentation, placenta previa, nonreassuring fetal status, and preterm and macrosomic fetuses (Figure 27–7, *B*).

Disadvantages of this incision are as follows:

1. The incision may extend downward into the cervix.
2. More extensive dissection of the bladder is needed to keep the incision in the lower uterine segment.
3. If the incision extends upward into the upper segment, hemostasis and closure are more difficult.
4. The vertical incision carries a higher risk of rupture with subsequent labor. Consequently, once a vertical incision is performed, future births need to be via cesarean.

One other incision, the classic incision, was the method of choice for many years but is used infrequently now

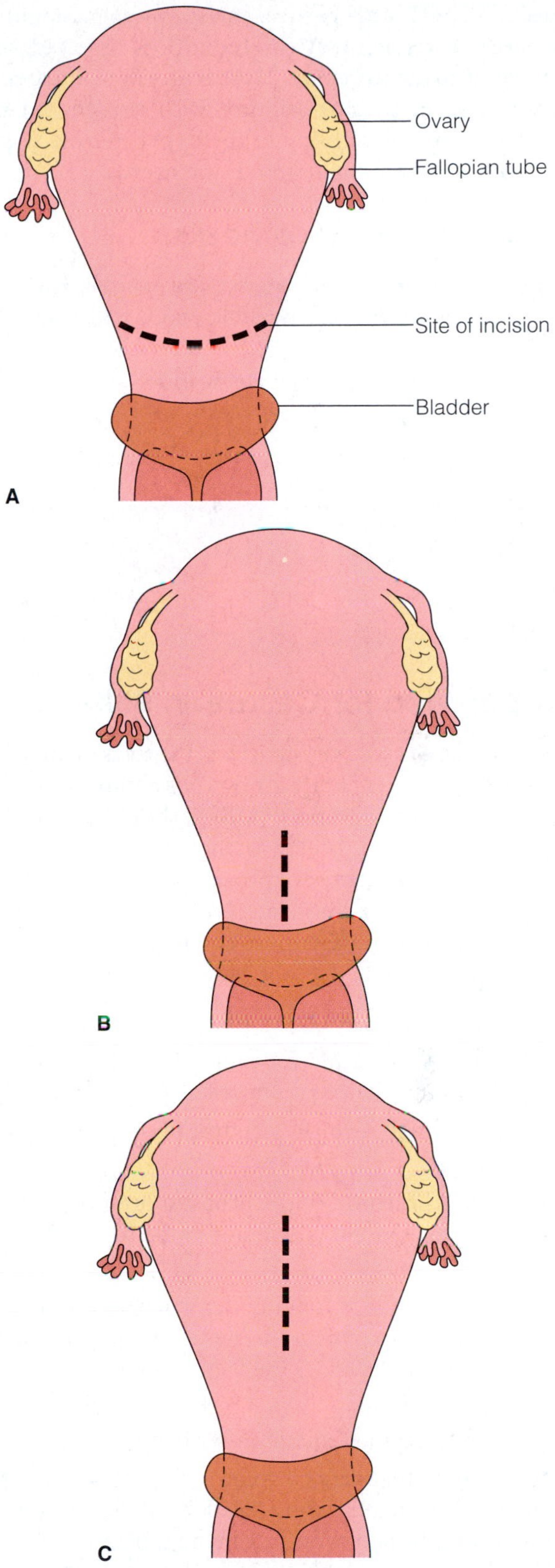

Figure 27–7 • Uterine incisions for a cesarean birth. *A,* This transverse incision in the lower uterine segment is called a Kerr incision. *B,* The Sellheim incision is a vertical incision in the lower uterine segment. *C,* This view illustrates the classic uterine incision that is done in the body (corpus) of the uterus. The classic incision was commonly done in the past and is associated with increased risk of uterine rupture in subsequent pregnancies and labor.

MEDIALINK VIDEO: TYPES OF INCISIONS

MediaLink VIDEO: EPIDURAL PLACEMENT

(Figure 27–7, *C*). This vertical incision was made into the upper uterine segment. More blood loss resulted, and it was more difficult to repair. Most important, it carried an increased risk of uterine rupture with subsequent pregnancy, labor, and birth because the upper uterine segment is the most contractile portion of the uterus.

Analgesia and Anesthesia

There is no perfect anesthesia for cesarean birth. Each has its advantages, disadvantages, possible risks, and side effects. Goals for analgesia and anesthesia administration include safety, comfort, and emotional satisfaction for the client. See Chapter 25.

NURSING CARE MANAGEMENT

Preparation for Cesarean Birth

Because one out of every five births is a cesarean, preparing the woman and family for this possibility is an integral part of prenatal education. Nurses should encourage all pregnant women and their partners to discuss with their obstetrician/CNM what approach would be taken in the event of a cesarean. They can also discuss their needs and desires as a couple under those circumstances. Their preferences may include the following:

- Participating in the choice of anesthetic
- Presence of the father (or significant other) during the procedures in the recovery or postpartum room
- Audio or video recording and/or photographing of the birth
- Delayed instillation of eye drops to promote eye contact between parent and infant in the first hours after birth
- Physical contact or holding the newborn while on the operating room table or in the recovery room (If the mother cannot hold the newborn, the father can hold the baby for her.)
- Breastfeeding immediately after birth
- Preparation that may be done, such as abdominal prep, insertion of an indwelling bladder catheter, and starting an intravenous infusion and epidural placement
- Description or viewing of the delivery room
- Types of anesthesia for birth and analgesia available postpartum
- Sensations that may be experienced
- Roles of significant others
- Interaction with newborn
- Immediate recovery phase
- Postpartal phase

Preparing the woman for surgery involves more than the procedures of establishing intravenous lines and a urinary indwelling catheter or doing an abdominal prep. As discussed previously, good communication skills are essential in assisting the couple. Therapeutic use of touch and eye contact (if culturally acceptable and possible) do much to maintain reality orientation and control. These measures reduce anxiety for the woman during the stressful preparatory period.

If the cesarean birth is scheduled and not an emergency, the nurse has ample time for preoperative teaching. The woman needs to practice her turning, coughing, and deep breathing. It is helpful if she is taught to splint her abdominal muscles when she coughs. An informed consent for surgery needs to be signed.

To prepare the woman for the surgery, she is given nothing by mouth. To reduce the likelihood of serious pulmonary damage should aspiration of gastric contents occur, antacids may be administered within 30 minutes of surgery. If epidural anesthesia is used, the nurse may assist with the procedure, monitor the woman's blood pressure and response, and continue EFM. An abdominal and perineal prep is done, and an indwelling catheter is inserted to prevent bladder distention. For women receiving epidural anesthesia, it may be more comfortable to place the Foley catheter after the epidural has been placed. An intravenous line is started with a needle of adequate size to permit blood administration, and preoperative medication may be ordered. The pediatrician, neonatologist, or neonatal intensive care unit should be notified and adequate preparation made to receive the infant. The nurse should make sure that the infant warmer is functional and that appropriate resuscitation equipment is available.

The nurse assists in positioning the woman on the operating table. Fetal heart rate should be ascertained before surgery and during preparation because fetal hypoxia can result from aortocaval compression. The operating table may be adjusted so it slants slightly to one side, or a wedge (folded blanket or towels) may be placed under the right hip. The uterus should be displaced about 15 degrees from the midline. This helps relieve the pressure of the heavy uterus on the vena cava and lessens the incidence of vena caval compression and supine maternal hypotension. The suction should be in working order, and the urine collection bag should be positioned under the operating table to ensure proper urinary drainage. Auscultation or electronic monitoring of the fetal heart rate needs to continue until immediately prior to the surgery. A last-minute check is done to ensure that the fetal scalp electrode has been removed if the fetus was internally monitored.

The nurse should continue to provide reassurance and describe the various procedures being performed along with a rationale to ease anxiety and give the woman a sense of control.

Preparation for Repeat Cesarean Birth

When a couple is anticipating a repeat cesarean birth, they have time to reflect on their past experiences, analyze and synthesize the new information they are given, and prepare for the experience. Couples who have had previous negative experiences need an opportunity to describe what they felt contributed to these events. They should be encouraged to identify what they would like to have altered and to list interventions that would make the experience more positive. Those who have had positive experiences need reassurance that their needs and desires will be met in the same manner. In addition, the nurse should provide an opportunity for the couple to discuss any fears or anxieties.

Preparation for Emergency Cesarean Birth

The period preceding surgery must be used to its greatest advantage. The couple needs some time for privacy to assimilate the information given to them and to ask for additional information. It is imperative that caregivers use their most effective communication skills. The nurse must address what the couple may anticipate during the next few hours. Asking the couple, "What questions do you have about the decision?" gives the couple an opportunity for further clarification. The nurse can prepare the woman in stages, giving her information and the rationale for each procedure before commencing. Before carrying out a procedure, it is essential to tell the woman (1) what is going to happen, (2) why it is being done, and (3) what sensations she may experience. This allows the woman to be informed and to consent to the procedure. The woman experiences a sense of control and therefore less helplessness and powerlessness.

Supporting the Father/Partner

Every effort should be made to include the father/partner or support person in the cesarean birth experience. When the father or support person attends the cesarean birth, he or she must scrub and wear a surgical gown and mask as do others in the operating suite. The father or support person can sit on a stool placed beside the woman's head to provide physical touch, visual contact, and verbal reassurance to his partner.

Many support persons worry about their own reactions to the operative procedure. A sterile drape is placed between the woman's head and the sterile field. The nurse can advise the support person that this can be used as a partition if he or she does not wish to view the procedure itself. The nurse should encourage support persons to eat if possible prior to the surgery. Most fathers or support persons who fear "fainting" or "feeling queasy" do not have difficulties in the operating room and frequently forget these fears as they are swept away in the excitement of the birth.

Other measures, such as the following, can be taken to promote the participation of the father or partner who chooses not to be present in the delivery room:

1. Allowing the father or partner to be near the delivery/operating room, where he can hear the newborn's first cry
2. Encouraging the father/partner to carry or accompany the infant to the nursery for the initial assessment
3. Involving the father/partner in postpartal care in the recovery room

Immediate Postpartal Recovery Period

After birth, the nurse assesses the Apgar score and completes the initial assessment and identification procedures as after a vaginal birth. Every effort must be made to assist the parents in bonding with the infant. If the mother is awake, one of her arms should be freed to enable her to touch and stroke the infant. The baby can be given to the father to hold until she or he must be taken to the nursery.

The nurse caring for the postpartal woman should check her vital signs every 5 minutes until they are stable, then every 15 minutes for an hour, then every 30 minutes until she is discharged to the postpartal unit. The nurse should remain with the woman until she is stable.

The dressing and perineal pad must be checked every 15 minutes for at least an hour, and the fundus should be gently palpated to determine whether it is remaining firm. The fundus may be palpated by placing a hand to support the incision. Intravenous oxytocin is usually administered to promote the contractility of the uterine musculature. If the woman has had general anesthesia, she should be positioned on her side to facilitate drainage of secretions, turned, and assisted with coughing and deep breathing every 2 hours for at least 24 hours. If she has received a spinal or epidural anesthetic, the level of anesthesia should be checked every 15 minutes. It is important to monitor intake and output and to observe the urine for bloody tinge, which could mean surgical trauma to the bladder. The physician prescribes medication to relieve the mother's pain and nausea, and this should be administered as needed. Some physicians use a single dose of epidural morphine (5 to 7.5 mg) for postsurgical pain relief. Facilitation of parent-infant interaction following birth and postpartal care is discussed in Chapter 35. Pertinent areas of nursing care are addressed in the Cesarean Birth Clinical Pathway in Chapter 35.

Care of the Woman Undergoing Vaginal Birth After Cesarean

In the late 1990s there was an increasing trend to have a trial of labor and **vaginal birth after cesarean (VBAC)** birth in cases of nonrecurring indications for a cesarean (for example, twins, umbilical cord accident, placenta previa, fetal distress). This trend was influenced by consumer demand and studies that support VBAC as a viable and safe alternative. Recent media reports have reintroduced the debate regarding the safety of VBACs.

The 1999 ACOG guidelines state that the following aspects need to be considered for VBAC:

- A woman with one previous cesarean birth and a low transverse uterine incision should be counseled and encouraged to attempt VBAC.

- A woman with two or more previous cesareans may attempt VBAC.
- A physician who is able to do a cesarean needs to be available throughout active labor.

Contraindications include previous T-incision or classic incision, previous transfundal uterine surgery (myomectomy), contracted pelvis, medical or obstetric complications that preclude a vaginal birth, and inadequate facility or staff if a cesarean birth is required.

The most common risks associated with VBAC are hemorrhage and uterine scar separation (uterine rupture). The risk of uterine rupture is approximately 1% (Sachs et al, 1999) and is primarily dependent on the location and type of previous uterine incision. The most common type, a low transverse uterine incision, has a 0.2% to 1.5% risk of rupture (ACOG, 1999a). Although the risk of rupture is relatively low, concerns over malpractice issues have resulted in an upward trend in repeat cesarean births. More studies are needed to establish maternal and fetal safety for women who choose VBAC.

Success rates for VBAC have been encouraging. Women whose previous cesarean was performed because of nonrecurring indications have been reported to have approximately a 60% to 80% chance of success with VBAC (ACOG, 1999a). Women whose previous cesarean was performed for dystocia have lower success rates (50% to 70%) (ACOG, 1999a).

NURSING CARE MANAGEMENT

The nursing care of a woman undergoing VBAC varies according to institutional protocols. Generally, if the woman is at very low risk (has had one previous cesarean with a lower uterine segment incision), her blood count, type, and screen are obtained on admission; a heparin lock is inserted for intravenous access if needed; continuous EFM is used; and clear fluids may be taken. If the woman is at higher risk, NPO status should be maintained and, in addition to the care listed, an intrauterine catheter may be inserted to monitor intrauterine pressures during labor.

Supportive and comfort measures are very important. The woman may be excited about this opportunity to experience labor and vaginal birth, or she may be hesitant and frightened about the possibility of complications. The nurse provides information and encouragement for the laboring woman and her partner.

Chapter Review

EXPLOREMediaLink

NCLEX review questions, case studies, and other interactive resources for this chapter can be found on the Web site at http://www.prenhall.com/olds. Click on "Chapter 27" to select the activities for this chapter.

For tutorials including animations and videos, more NCLEX review questions, and an audio glossary, access the accompanying CD-ROM in this book.

Focus Your Study

- An external (or cephalic) version may be done after 37 weeks' gestation to change a breech presentation to a cephalic presentation, thereby making a lower risk vaginal birth more possible.
- The version is accomplished with the use of tocolytic agents to relax the uterus. An internal (podalic) version is used only when needed during the vaginal birth of a second twin.
- Amniotomy (AROM) is performed to hasten labor. The risks are prolapse of the umbilical cord and infection.
- Prostaglandin E_2 may be used before an induction of labor to soften the cervix (called cervical ripening). The gel is inserted into the vagina and may be held in place with a diaphragm.
- Labor is induced for many reasons. The methods include amniotomy, stripping of the membranes, intravenous oxytocin infusion, and alternative and complementary methods. Nursing responsibilities are heightened during an induced labor.
- Amnioinfusions are used in cases of oligohydramnios or nonperiodic decelerations to increase the volume of amniotic fluid which relieves cord compression and promotes perfusion to the fetus.
- An episiotomy may be performed just before birth of the fetus. Although it is still prevalent in the

United States, it is becoming somewhat controversial.

- Forceps-assisted birth can be accomplished using outlet forceps, low forceps, or midforceps. Outlet forceps are the most common and are associated with few maternal-fetal complications. Midforceps are associated with more complications but, when needed, are an important aid to birth.
- A vacuum extractor is a soft, pliable cup attached to suction that can be applied to the fetal head and used in much the same way as forceps.
- At least one in five births is accomplished by cesarean. The nurse has a vital role in providing information, support, and encouragement to the couple participating in a cesarean birth.
- Vaginal birth after cesarean (VBAC) carries a low risk of uterine rupture; however, many physicians perform repeat cesarean births out of fear of malpractice issues. Overcoming the old fears of uterine rupture is a high priority for both the parents and the medical and nursing community.

References

Adair, C. D., Weeks, J. W., Barrilleaux, S., Edwards, M., Burlison, K., & Lewis, D. F. (1998). Oral or vaginal misoprostol administration for induction of labor: A randomized, double blind trial. *Obstetrics & Gynecology, 92*, 810.

Allaire, A. D. (2001). Complementary and alternative medicine in the labor and delivery suite. *Clinical Obstetrics and Gynecology, 44*(4), 681–691.

American College of Obstetricians & Gynecologists (ACOG). (1995). *Dystocia and the augmentation of Labor.* (Technical Bulletin No. 218). Washington, D.C.: Author.

American College of Obstetricians and Gynecologists (ACOG). (1998). *Delivery by vacuum extraction* (ACOG Committee Opinion No. 208). Washington, DC: Author.

American College of Obstetricians and Gynecologists (ACOG). (1999a). *Guidelines for vaginal birth after previous cesarean birth* (ACOG Practice Bulletin No. 5). Washington, DC: Author.

American College of Obstetricians and Gynecologists (ACOG). (1999b). *Induction of labor* (ACOG Practice Bulletin No. 10). Washington, DC: Author.

American College of Obstetricians and Gynecologists (ACOG). (2000). *Operative vaginal delivery* (ACOG Practice Bulletin No. 17). Washington, DC: Author.

Angiolo, R., Gommez-Marin, O., Cantuaria, G., & O'sullivan, M. J. (2000). Severe perineal laceration during vaginal delivery: The University of Miami experience. *American Journal of Obstetrics and Gynecology, 182*(5), 1083–1085.

Bishop, E. H. (1964). Pelvic scoring for elective induction. *Obstetrics & Gynecology, 24*, 266.

Boulvain, M., Stan, C., & Irion, O. (2002). Membrane sweeping for induction of labour. *Cochrane Library*, Issue 3. Oxford.

Bowes, W. A. (1999). Clinical aspects of normal and abnormal labor. In R. K. Creasy & R. Resnik (Eds.), *Maternal-fetal medicine* (4th ed., pp. 541–568). Philadelphia: Saunders.

Buist, R., Brown, J., & McNamara, T. (1999). For whom is caesarean section rate high? *New Zealand Medical Journal, 112*(1101), 469–471.

Center for Devices & Radiological Health. (1998). *FDA Public Health Advisory: Need for caution when using vacuum assisted delivery devices.* Retrieved June 8, 2002 from at http://www.fda.gov/cdrh/fetal/598.htm

Coco, A. S., & Silverman, S. D. (1998). External cephalic version. *American Family Physician, 58*(3), 731–738, 742–744.

Cunningham, F. G., MacDonald, P. C., Gant, N. F., Leveno, L. J., Gilstrap, L. C., Hankins, G. V., et al. (2001). *Williams obstetrics* (21st ed.). Norwalk, CT: Appleton & Lange.

Davidson, M. R. (2002). Outcomes of high-risk women cared for by certified nurse midwives. *Journal of Midwifery & Women's Health, 47*(1), 46–49.

Deglin, J. H., & Vallerand, A. H. (2002). *Davis's drug guide for nurses* (8th ed.). Philadelphia: F. A. Davis.

Eason, E., & Feldman, P. (2000). Much ado about a little cut: Is episiotomy worthwhile? *Obstetrics & Gynecology, 95*(4), 616–618.

Eason, E., Labrecque, M., Marcoux, S., & Mondour, M. (2002). Anal incontinence after childbirth. *Canadian Medical Association Journal, 166*(3), 326–330.

Forrest Pharmaceuticals. (1995). *Cervidil dinoprostone 10 mg vaginal insert.* St. Louis, MO: UAB Laboratories.

Fraser, W. D., Turcot, L., Krauss, I., & Brisson-Carrol, G. (2000). Amniotomy for shortening spontaneous labor. *Cochrane Database Systematic Review, 2000*(2), CD000015.

Goldberg, J., Holtz, D., Hsylop, T., Tolosa, J. E. (2002). Has the use of routine episiotomy decreased? Examination of episiotomy rates from 1983 to 2000. *Obstetrics & Gynecology, 99*(3), 395–400.

Graham, I. D., & Graham, D. F. (1997). Episiotomy counts: Trends and prevalence in Canada, 1981/1982 to 1993/1994. *Birth, 24*, 141–147.

Hofmeyr, G. J. (2002). Amnioinfusion for meconium-stained liquor in labour. [Update of *Cochrane Database Systematic Review, 2000*(2), CD000014;10796085.]

Hofmeyr, G. J., & Kulier, R. (2002). External cephalic version for breech presentation at term. *Cochrane Library* (Oxford) 1 (CD000083), (1).

Juarez Ocana, S. J., Fajardo Gutierrez, A., Perez Palacios, G., Guerrero Morales, R. G., & Gomez Delgado, A. (1999). The trend in pregnancies terminated by cesarean operation in Mexico during 1991-1995. *Gynecology & Obstetrics Mexico, 67*, 308–318.

Kabiru, W. N., Jamieson, D., Graves, W., & Lindsay, M. (2001). Trends in operative vaginal delivery rates and associated maternal complication rates in inner city hospital. *American Journal of Obstetrics and Gynecology, 184*(6), 1112–1114.

Kiss, H., Ahner, R., Hohlagschwandtner, M., Leitch, H., & Huslein, P. (2000). Fetal fibronectin as a predictor of term labor. *Acta Obstetricia et Gynecologica Scandinavica, 79*(1), 3–7.

Lau, T. K., Lo, L. W. K., & Rogers, M. S. (1997). Pregnancy outcome after successful external cephalic version for breech presentation at term. *American Journal of Obstetrics and Gynaecology, 176*, 218–223.

Lau, T. K., Lo, L. W. K., Wan, D., & Rogers, M. S. (1997). Predictors of successful external cephalic version at term: A prospective study. *British Journal of Obstetrics and Gynaecology, 104*, 798–802.

Low, L. K., Seng, J. S., Murtland, T. L., & Oakley, D. (2000). Clinician specific episiotomy rates: Impact on perineal outcomes. *Journal of Midwifery and Women's Health, 45*(2), 87–93.

Maier, J. S., & Maloni, J. A. (1997). Nurse advocacy for selective versus routine episiotomy. *Journal of Obstetric, Gynecologic, and Neonatal Nursing, 26*, 155–161.

McFarlin, B. L., Gibson, M. H., O'Rear, J., & Harman, P. (1999). A national survey of herbal preparation use by nurse midwives for labor stimulation. *Journal of Nurse Midwifery, 44*(3), 205–216.

Medifocus. (2002). *Electronic fetal monitoring.* Silver Spring, MD: Author.

Mesleh, R. A., Asiri, F., & Al-Naim, M. F. (2000). Cesarean section in the primigravid. *Saudi Medical Journal, 21*(10), 957–959.

Meyer, S., Hohlreld, P., Achtar, C., Russolo, A., & Degrandi, P. (2000). Birth trauma: Short and long term effects of forceps delivery complications and spontaneous delivery on various pelvic floor parameters. *British Journal of Obstetrics and Gynaecology, 107*(11), 1360–1365.

Midwifery Today E-News. (2002). Herbs. *Midwifery Today Forums, 1*, 44. Retrieved on December 20, 2002 at www.midwiferytoday.com/enews

Myers-Helfgott, M. G., & Helfgott, A. W. (1999). Routine use of episiotomy in modern obstetrics: Should it be performed? *Obstetrics and Gynecology Clinics of North America, 26*(2), 305–325.

National Center for Health Statistics. (2001). *Obstetrical Procedures.* Washington, D.C.: Author.

Peleg, D., Kennedy, C. M., Merrill, D., & Zlatnik, F. J. (1999). Risk of repetition of a severe perineal laceration. *Obstetrics & Gynecology, 93*, 1021–1024.

Perez, A. (1999, March). Cutting your legal risk with vacuum assisted deliveries. *American Family Physician*, 22–35.

Popovic, J. R. (2001). 1999 national hospital discharge survey: Annual summary with detailed diagnosis and procedure data. *Vital and Health Statistics Series, 13*(151). Hyattsville, MD: National Center for Health Statistics.

Rasmussen, O. B., Pedersen, B. L., Wilken-Jensen, C., & Vejerslev, L. O. (2000). Stratified rates of cesarean section and spontaneous vaginal deliveries: Data from five labor wards in Denmark. *Acta Obstetricia et Gynecologica Scandinavica, 79*(2), 227–231.

Rather, A. M., Singh, R., Ramji, S., & Tripathi, R. (2002). Randomized trial of amnioinfusion during labour with meconium-stained amniotic fluid. *British Journal of Obstetrics and Gynaecology, 109*(1), 17–20.

Rozenberg, P., Goffinet, F., & Hessabi, M. (2000). Comparison of the Bishop score, ultrasonographically measured cervical length, and fetal fibronectin assay in predicting time until delivery and type of delivery at term. *American Journal of Obstetrics and Gynecology, 182*(1, Pt. 1), 108–113.

Sachs, B. P., Kobelin, C., Castro, M. A., & Frigoletto, F. (1999). Sounding board: The risks of lowering the cesarean-delivery rate. *New England Journal of Medicine, 340*, 54–57.

Sciscione, A. C., McCullough, H., Manley, J. S., Shlossman, P. A., Pollock, M., & Colmorgen, G. H. C. (1999). A prospective, randomized comparison of Foley catheter insertion versus intracervical prostaglandin E_2 gel for preinduction cervical ripening. *American Journal of Obstetrics and Gynecology, 180*, 55.

Skidmore-Roth, L. (2003). *2003 Mosby's drug reference.* St. Louis: Mosby.

Summers, L. (1997). Methods of cervical ripening and labor induction. *Journal of Nurse-Midwifery, 42*, 71–82.

Theron, G. B., & Theron, A. M. (2002). Routine external version by physicians in training for abnormal presentation. *International Journal of Gynaecology & Obstetrics, 76*(2), 173–174.

Thompson, J. F., Roberts, C. L., Currie, M., & Ellwood, D. A. (2002). Prevalence and persistence of health problems after childbirth: Associations with parity and method of birth. *Birth, 29*(2), 83–94.

Vacca, A. (2002). Vacuum-assisted delivery. *Best Practice & Research in Clinical Obstetrics & Gynaecology, 16*(1), 17–30.

Webb, D. A., & Culhane, J. (2002). Hospital variation in episiotomy use and the risk of perineal trauma during childbirth. *Birth, 29*(2), 132–136.

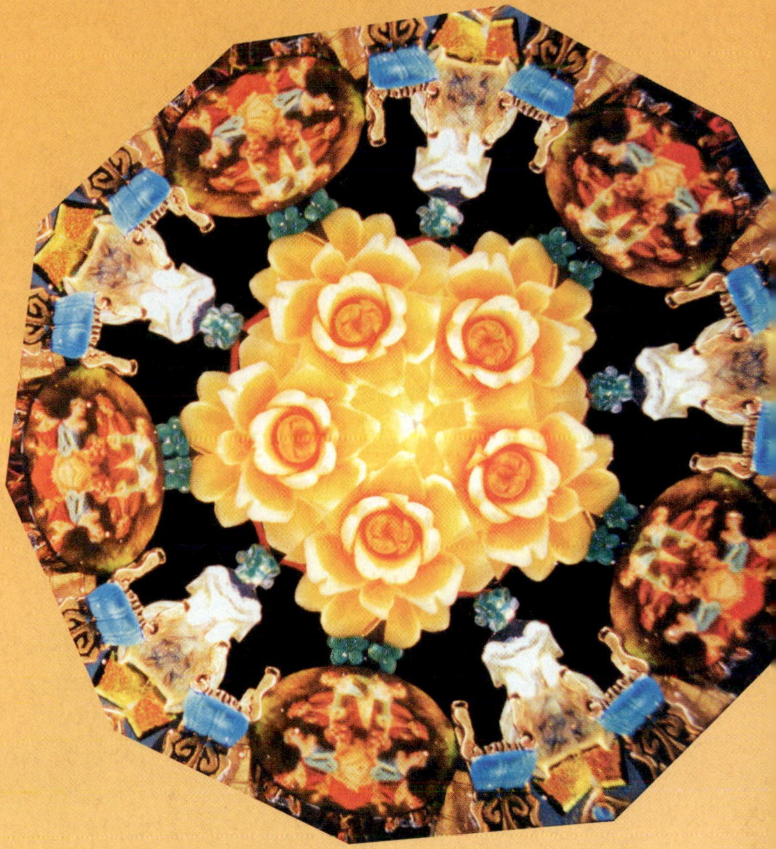

SIX

The Newborn

Physiologic Responses of the Newborn to Birth

28

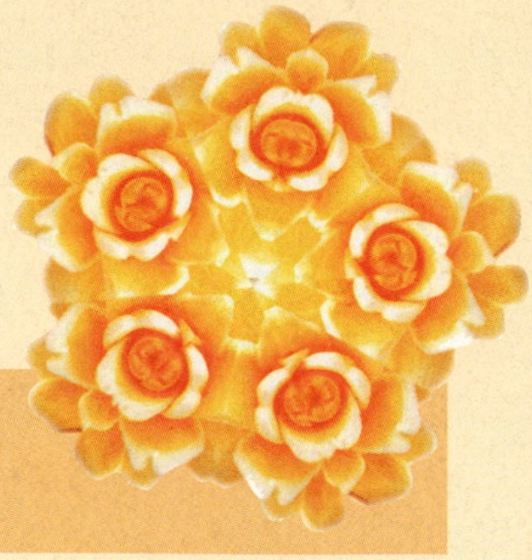

The incredible attributes of the newborn have a major purpose. They prepare the baby for interaction with the family and for life in the world.
~The Amazing Newborn ~

Objectives

- Summarize the respiratory and cardiovascular changes that occur during the transition to extrauterine life.
- Describe how various factors affect the newborn's blood values.
- Correlate the major mechanisms of heat loss in the newborn to the process of thermogenesis in the newborn.
- Explain the steps involved in conjugation and excretion of bilirubin in the newborn.
- Discuss the reasons why the newborn may develop jaundice.
- Delineate the functional abilities of the newborn's gastrointestinal tract and liver.
- Identify the reasons the newborn's kidneys have difficulty maintaining fluid and electrolyte balance.
- List the immunologic responses available to the newborn.
- Explain the physiologic and behavioral responses of newborns during the periods of reactivity, and identify possible interventions.
- Describe the normal sensory/perceptual abilities and behavioral states present in the newborn period.

Key Terms

Active acquired immunity 787
Brown adipose tissue (BAT) 780
Cardiopulmonary adaptation 772
Conduction 780
Convection 779
Evaporation 780
Habituation 790
Meconium 786
Neonatal transition 769
Neutral thermal environment (NTE) 777
Orientation 790
Passive acquired immunity 787
Periodic breathing 773
Periods of reactivity 788
Physiologic anemia of infancy 777
Physiologic jaundice 782
Radiation 779
Self-quieting ability 790
Surfactant 769
Total serum bilirubin 782

MediaLink

Additional resources for this content can be found on the Student CD-ROM and on the Companion Website at www.prenhall.com/olds. Click on "Chapter 28" to select the activities for this chapter.

CD-ROM
- Audio Glossary
- NCLEX Review

Companion Website
- Additional NCLEX Review
- Case Study: Newborn Responses to Birth

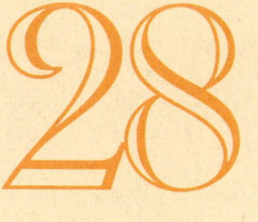

The newborn period is the time from birth through the first 28 days of life. During this period, the newborn adjusts from intrauterine to extrauterine life. The nurse needs to be knowledgeable about a newborn's normal physiologic and behavioral adaptations and be able to recognize alterations from normal. The first few hours of life, in which the newborn stabilizes respiratory and circulatory functions, are called **neonatal transition.** All other newborn body systems change their level of functioning or become established over a longer period of time during the neonatal period.

Respiratory Adaptations

To begin life as a separate being, the baby must immediately establish respiratory gas exchange, which occurs in conjunction with marked circulatory changes. These radical and rapid changes are crucial to the maintenance of extrauterine life.

Intrauterine Factors Supporting Respiratory Function

Although the significant respiratory events occur at birth, certain intrauterine factors also enhance the newborn's ability to breathe.

FETAL LUNG DEVELOPMENT

The respiratory system is in a continuous state of development during fetal life, and lung development continues into early childhood. During the first 20 weeks of gestation, lung development is limited to the differentiation of pulmonary, vascular, and lymphatic structures. At 20 to 24 weeks, alveolar ducts begin to appear, followed by primitive alveoli at 24 to 28 weeks. During this time, the alveolar epithelial cells begin to differentiate into type I cells (structures necessary for respiratory gas exchange) and type II cells (structures that provide for the synthesis and storage of surfactant). **Surfactant** is composed of a group of surface-active phospholipids (lecithin and sphingomyelin), which are critical for alveolar stability.

At 28 to 32 weeks of gestation, the number of type II cells increases further, and surfactant is produced by a choline pathway within them. Surfactant production by this pathway peaks at about 35 weeks of gestation and remains high until term, paralleling late fetal lung development. At this time, the lungs are structurally developed enough to maintain good lung expansion and adequate exchange of gases.

Clinically, the peak production of lecithin—one component of surfactant—corresponds closely to the marked decrease in incidence of idiopathic respiratory distress syndrome for babies born after 35 weeks' gestation. Production of sphingomyelin—the other component—remains constant during gestation. The newborn born before the lecithin/sphingomyelin (L/S) ratio is 2:1 will have varying degrees of respiratory distress. (See discussion of L/S ratio in Chapters 21 and 33.)

FETAL BREATHING MOVEMENTS

The newborn's ability to breathe immediately on exposure to air in the extrauterine environment appears to be the consequence of weeks of intrauterine practice. In this respect, breathing can be regarded as a continuation of an intrauterine process in which the lungs convert from fluid-filled to gas-filled organs. Fetal breathing movements (FBM) occur as early as 11 weeks' gestation (see Chapter 21 for discussion). These breathing movements are essential for developing the chest wall muscles and the diaphragm and, to a lesser extent, for regulating lung fluid volume and resultant lung growth.

Initiation of Breathing

To maintain life, the lungs must function immediately after birth. Two radical changes must take place for the lungs to function:

1. Pulmonary ventilation must be established through lung expansion following birth.
2. A marked increase in the pulmonary circulation must occur.

The first breath of life—the gasp in response to mechanical, chemical, thermal, and sensory changes associated with birth—initiates the serial opening of the alveoli. So begins the transition from a fluid-filled environment to an air-breathing, independent, extrauterine life. Figure 28–1 • summarizes the initiation of respiration.

MECHANICAL EVENTS

During the latter half of gestation, the fetal lungs continuously produce fluid. This fluid production expands the lungs almost completely, filling the air spaces. Some of the lung fluid moves up into the trachea and into the amniotic fluid. The amniotic fluid is then swallowed by the fetus.

Production of lung fluid diminishes 2 to 4 days before onset of labor. However, approximately 80 to 110 mL of fluid remains in the respiratory passages of a normal term fetus at the time of birth. This fluid must be removed from the lungs to permit adequate movement of air.

The primary mechanical events that initiate respiration involve removal of fluid from the lungs as the fetus passes through the birth canal. During the birth process the fetal chest is compressed, increasing intrathoracic pressure, and approximately one third of the fluid is squeezed out of the lungs. After the birth of the newborn's trunk, the chest wall recoils. This chest recoil creates negative intrathoracic pressure, which is thought to produce a small, passive inspiration of air that replaces the fluid that was squeezed out.

After this first inspiration, the newborn exhales, with crying, against a partially closed glottis, creating a positive intrathoracic pressure. The high positive intrathoracic pressure distributes the inspired air throughout the alveoli and begins the establishment of *functional residual capacity (FRC)*, the air left in the lungs at the end of a normal expiration. The higher intrathoracic pressure also increases absorption of lung fluid via the capillaries and lymphatic system. The negative intrathoracic pressure

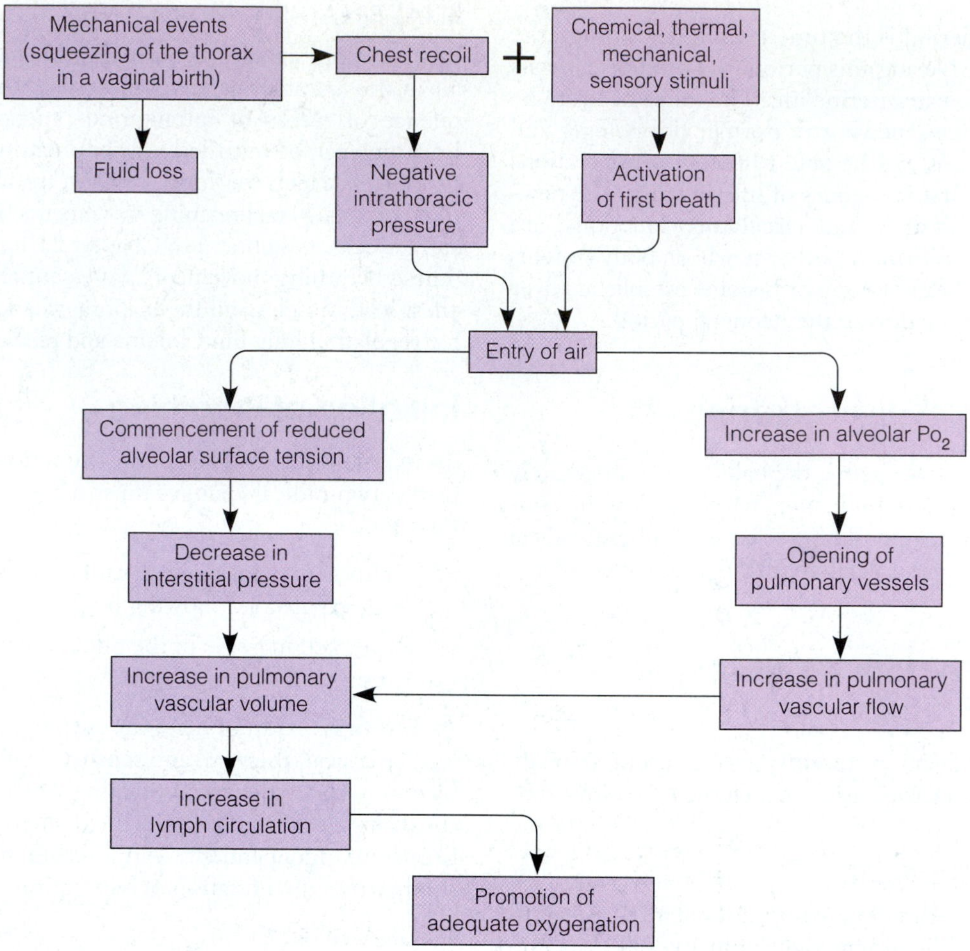

Figure 28–1 • Initiation of respiration in the newborn.

resulting from downward movement of the diaphragm with inspiration causes lung fluid to flow from the alveoli across the alveolar membranes into the pulmonary interstitial tissue.

With each succeeding breath, the lungs expand, stretching the alveolar walls and increasing the alveolar volume. Because the protein concentration is higher in the pulmonary capillaries, oncotic pressure draws the interstitial fluid into the capillaries and lymphatic tissue. The expansion of the lung facilitates movement of the remaining lung fluid into the interstitial tissue. As pulmonary vascular resistance decreases, pulmonary blood flow increases, and more interstitial fluid is absorbed into the bloodstream. In the normal term newborn, lung fluid moves rapidly into the interstitial tissue but may take several hours to move into the lymph and blood vessels. Figure 28–2 • depicts the changes in fetal lung fluid with the first and subsequent breaths. About 80% of the fluid is reabsorbed within 2 hours after birth, and it is completely absorbed within 12 to 24 hours after birth.

Although the initial chest compression and recoil should clear the airways of accumulated fluid and permit further inspiration, most clinicians feel it is wise to suction mucus and fluid from the newborn's mouth and oropharynx. They use a mucus trap attached to suction as soon as the newborn's head and shoulders are born and again as the newborn adapts to extrauterine life and stabilizes (see Procedure 24–1, and Chapter 24).

Problems associated with lung fluid clearance or initiation of respiratory activity may be caused by a variety of factors. The lymphatic system may be underdeveloped, thus decreasing the rate at which the fluid is absorbed from the lungs. Complications that occur antenatally or during labor and birth can interfere with adequate lung expansion, causing failure to decrease pulmonary vascular resistance, resulting in decreased pulmonary blood flow. These complications include inadequate compression of the chest wall in a very small newborn, the absence of the chest wall compression in the newborn born by cesarean birth, respiratory depression secondary to maternal anesthesia, or aspiration of amniotic fluid or meconium.

CHEMICAL STIMULI

An important chemical stimulator that contributes to the onset of breathing is transitory asphyxia of the fetus and newborn. The first breath is really an inspiratory gasp triggered by the elevation in P_{CO_2} and decrease in pH and P_{O_2}, which are the natural result of normal vaginal birth with cessation of placental gas exchange when the cord is clamped. These changes, present in all newborns to some degree, stimulate the aortic and carotid chemoreceptors, initiating impulses

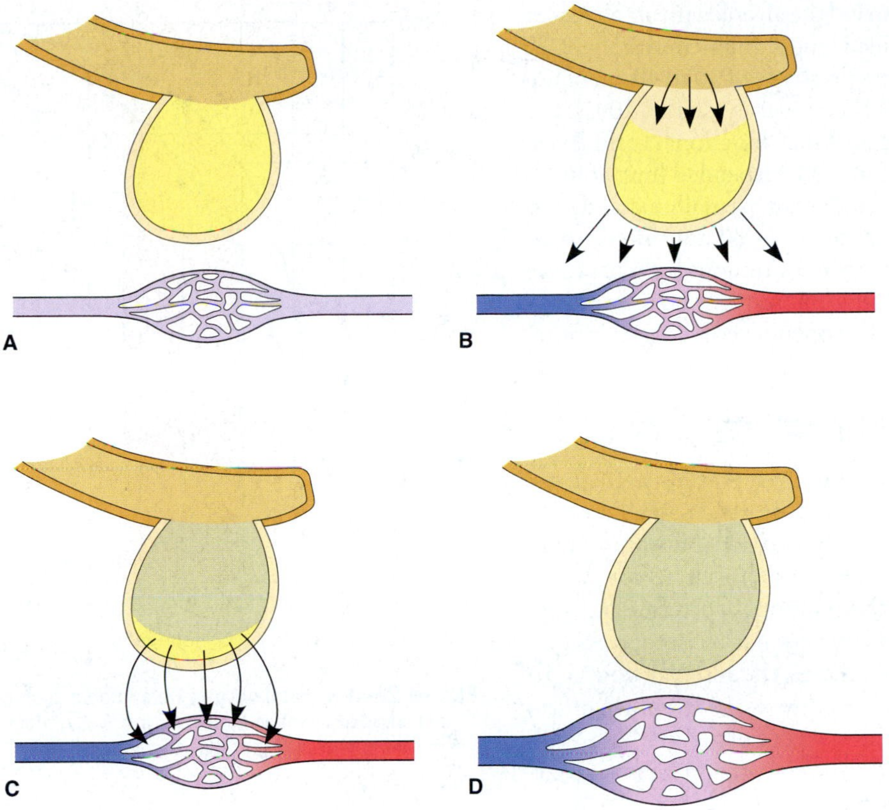

Figure 28–2 • Process of absorption of fetal lung fluid during breathing after birth. *A,* Fetal alveoli filled to functional residual capacity with fetal lung fluid. Fetal lung fluid is produced by the alveoli, fills the airways, and eventually enters the amniotic fluid. *B,* After fetal chest compression, one third of the fetal lung fluid is squeezed out, allowing air to enter passively as the chest recoils. *C,* With each subsequent breath, the lungs expand, facilitating the movement of the remaining fetal lung fluid into the capillaries and lymphatic system. Pulmonary blood flow is increasing. *D,* Normal alveoli after removal of fetal lung fluid and dilatation of pulmonary arteries. Surfactant has lined the inside of the alveoli to prevent collapse.

that trigger the medulla's respiratory center. Although this brief period of asphyxia is a significant stimulator, prolonged asphyxia is abnormal and acts as a central nervous system (CNS) respiratory depressant.

THERMAL STIMULI

A significant decrease in ambient temperature after birth—from 37C to 21 to 23.9C (98.6F to 70 to 75F)—also stimulates the initiation of breathing. The cold stimulates nerve endings of the skin, and the newborn responds with rhythmic respirations. Normal temperature changes that occur at birth are apparently within acceptable physiologic limits. Excessive cooling, however, may result in profound respiratory depression and evidence of cold stress (see Chapter 33 for discussion of cold stress).

SENSORY STIMULI

As the fetus moves from a familiar, comfortable environment, a number of sensory and physical influences help initiate respiration. They include the numerous tactile, auditory, and visual stimuli of birth. During intrauterine life, the fetus is in a dark, sound-dampened, fluid-filled environment and is nearly weightless. After birth the newborn experiences light, sounds, and the effects of gravity for the first time. Joint movement results in enhanced proprioceptor stimulation to the respiratory center to sustain respirations. Historically, vigorous stimulation was provided by slapping the buttocks or heels of the newborn, but today greater emphasis is placed on gentle physical contact. Thoroughly drying the newborn and placing it in skin-to-skin contact with the mother's chest and abdomen provides stimulation in a far more comforting way and also decreases heat loss.

Factors Opposing the First Breath

Three major factors may oppose the initiation of respiratory activity: (1) alveolar surface tension, (2) viscosity of lung fluid within the respiratory tract, and (3) degree of lung compliance.

The contracting force between the moist surfaces of the alveoli is called *alveolar surface tension.* This tension, which is necessary for healthy respiratory function, would nevertheless cause the small airways and alveoli to collapse after each inspiration were it not for the presence of surfactant. By reducing the attracting force between alveoli, surfactant prevents the alveoli from completely collapsing with each expiration and thus promotes lung expansion. Similarly, surfactant promotes lung compliance, the ability of the lung to fill with air easily. When surfactant is decreased, compliance is also decreased, and the pressure needed to expand the alveoli with air increases. Resistive forces of the fluid-filled lung combined with the small radii of the airways necessitates pressures of 30 to 40 cm of water to open the lung initially (Niermeyer & Clarke, 2002).

The first breath usually establishes functional residual capacity that is 30% to 40% of the fully expanded lung volume. This FRC allows alveolar sacs to remain partially expanded on expiration. Thus the air that remains in the lung after expiration (FRC) decreases the need for continuous high pressures for each of the following breaths. Subsequent breaths require only 6 to 8 cm H_2O pressure to open alveoli during inspiration. Thus, the first breath of life is usually the most difficult.

Cardiopulmonary Physiology

The onset of respiration stimulates in the cardiovascular system changes that are necessary for the successful transition to extrauterine life, hence the term **cardiopulmonary adaptation.** As air enters the lungs, Po_2 rises in the alveoli, which stimulates the relaxation of the pulmonary arteries and triggers a decrease in the pulmonary vascular resistance. As pulmonary vascular resistance decreases, the vascular flow in the lung increases very rapidly and achieves 100% normal flow volume at 24 hours of life. This delivery of greater blood volume to the lungs contributes to the conversion from fetal circulation to newborn circulation.

After pulmonary circulation is established, blood is distributed throughout the lung, although the alveoli may or may not be fully open. For adequate oxygenation to occur, sufficient blood must be delivered by the heart to the functioning open alveoli. Shunting of blood is common in the early newborn period. Bidirectional blood flow, or right-to-left shunting through the ductus arteriosus, may divert a significant amount of blood away from the lungs, depending on the pressure changes of respiration, crying, and the cardiac cycle. This shunting in the newborn period is also responsible for the unstable transitional period in cardiopulmonary function.

Oxygen Transport

The transportation of oxygen to the peripheral tissues depends on the type of hemoglobin in the red blood cell. In the fetus and newborn, a variety of hemoglobins exists, the most significant being fetal hemoglobin (HbF) and adult hemoglobin (HbA). Approximately 70% to 90% of hemoglobin in the fetus and newborn is fetal hemoglobin. The greatest difference between HbF and HbA is related to the transport of oxygen.

The oxygen-carrying capacity of fetal hemoglobin is lower than that of adult hemoglobin. Although each gram of fetal hemoglobin carries less oxygen, it has a greater affinity for the oxygen molecules it carries. At any given arterial oxygen level, fetal hemoglobin has a greater oxygen saturation than adult hemoglobin. Thus the oxygen-hemoglobin dissociation curve for fetal hemoglobin lies to the left of that for adult hemoglobin (Figure 28–3 ●). Fetal hemoglobin's greater affinity for oxygen benefits the fetus and newborn because it facilitates oxygen transfer across

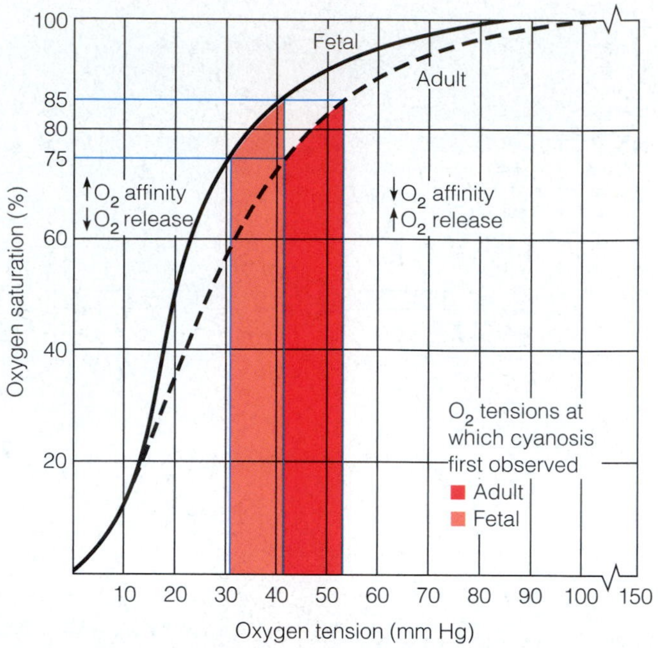

Figure 28–3 ● Fetal oxygen-hemoglobin dissociation curve.
SOURCE: Modified from Klaus, M., & Fanaroff, A. A. *Care of the high risk infant* (3rd ed., p. 234). Copyright 1986, with permission from Elsevier Science.

the placenta and into the newborn's tissues. In utero, the fetus has an arterial oxygen tension (Pao_2) between 30 and 40 mm Hg. Because of the nature of the fetal hemoglobin as depicted in the curve, small changes in fetal Pao_2 result in a great amount of oxygen loading in the placenta or unloading to the tissues as compared to the adult. Fetal hemoglobin's greater affinity for oxygen also requires that a lower tissue oxygen level exist prior to oxygen unloading than required by adult hemoglobin. Due to this phenomenon, the newborn will have both a lower arterial oxygen level and lower oxygen saturation than the adult before cyanosis becomes clinically apparent.

In addition to the specific characteristics of fetal hemoglobin, other conditions affect the transport of oxygen. Alkalosis and hypothermia result in increased oxygen affinity and thus less oxygen availability to the tissues; acidosis, hypercarbia, and hyperthermia result in decreased oxygen affinity, resulting in greater oxygen release to the tissues. Therefore, as blood is perfusing active tissues that are producing acids and carbon dioxide, hemoglobin's affinity for oxygen decreases, allowing oxygen unloading and carbon dioxide and acid uptake. This blood is then transferred to the placenta or the lungs, where its lower carbon dioxide and acid content results in uploading of these waste products from hemoglobin and the uptake of oxygen to be transferred to the tissues.

Other factors that regulate oxygen delivery to the tissues are oxygen-carrying capacity and cardiac output. The oxygen-carrying capacity of blood is defined as the product of the hemoglobin concentration and the maximum amount of oxygen that 1 g of hemoglobin can hold when it is fully saturated. The amount of oxygen bound to hemoglobin divided by the oxygen-carrying capacity yields a percentage that signifies oxygen saturation. Oxygen saturation usually reaches a value between 96% and 98% after several hours of life. Although fetal hemoglobin can hold only 1.26 mL of oxygen per gram of hemoglobin, compared to 1.34 mL of oxygen per gram of adult hemoglobin, the newborn's hemoglobin level at birth (17 g/dL) is substantially greater than in adults (13 g/dL). Therefore, the absolute oxygen-carrying capacity of fetal blood (21.42 vol%) is greater than in adult blood (17.42 vol%) and allows the fetus to tolerate the relatively hypoxic intrauterine environment.

A significant reduction in the oxygen-carrying capacity results in an increased cardiac output to compensate for hemoglobin's decreased oxygen concentration. Lastly, cardiac output of the fetus and newborn is relatively greater per body weight than in the adult, which contributes to the rapid delivery of oxygenated blood to tissues with high metabolic demands.

CRITICAL THINKING IN PRACTICE

Thomas and David Smith are monoamniotic, monochorionic twins born by cesarean birth to a 29-year-old, G1P0, woman at 36 weeks' gestation. Shortly after birth, Thomas, whose birth weight was 2750 g, is noted to have acrocyanosis and has a respiratory rate of 62. His hemoglobin is 20 g/dL; his hematocrit is 59%; the oxygen saturation monitor is reading 93%. David, whose birth weight was 2670 g, is pale and has a respiratory rate of 88. David's hemoglobin is 11 g/dL; his hematocrit is 32%; his oxygen saturation monitor is reading 100%. Which of these two infants is at greater risk for developing tissue hypoxia?

Answers can be found in Appendix I .

Maintaining Respiratory Function

The lungs' ability to maintain oxygen and carbon dioxide exchange (ventilation) is influenced by such factors as lung compliance and airway resistance. Lung compliance is influenced by the elastic recoil of the lung tissue and by anatomic differences in the newborn. The newborn has a relatively large heart as well as mediastinal structures that reduce available lung space. Also, the newborn chest is equipped with weak intercostal muscles, a rib cage with horizontal ribs, and a high diaphragm that restricts the space available for lung expansion. The large abdomen further encroaches on the high diaphragm to decrease lung space. Another factor that limits ventilation is airway resistance, which depends on the radii, length, and number of airways. Airway resistance is increased in the newborn when compared to adults.

Characteristics of Newborn Respiration

The normal newborn respiratory rate is 30 to 60 breaths per minute. Initial respirations may be largely diaphragmatic, shallow, and irregular in depth and rhythm. The abdomen's movements are synchronous with chest movements. When the breathing pattern is characterized by pauses lasting 5 to 15 seconds, **periodic breathing** is occurring. Periodic breathing is rarely associated with differences in skin color or heart rate changes, and it has no prognostic significance. Tactile or other sensory stimulation stimulates the respiratory center and converts periodic breathing patterns to normal breathing patterns during neonatal transition. With deep sleep, the pattern is reasonably regular. Periodic breathing occurs with rapid eye movement (REM) sleep, and grossly irregular breathing is evident with motor activity, sucking, and crying. Cessation of breathing lasting more than 20 seconds is defined as apnea and is abnormal in term newborns. Apnea may or may not be associated with changes in skin color or heart rate (drop below 100 beats per minute). Apnea always needs to be further evaluated.

The newborn is an obligatory nose breather, and any obstruction will cause respiratory distress, so it is important to keep the throat and nose clear. Immediately after birth and for about 2 hours after birth, respiratory rates of 60 to 70 breaths per minute are normal. Some cyanosis and acrocyanosis are normal for several hours; thereafter, a steady improvement in color occurs. If respirations drop below 30 or exceed 60 per minute when the baby is at rest, or if dyspnea, cyanosis, or nasal flaring and expiratory grunting occur, the clinician should be notified. Any increased use of the intercostal muscle (retracting) may indicate respiratory distress. (See Chapter 33 and Table 33–1 for signs of respiratory distress .)

Cardiovascular Adaptations

As described earlier, the onset of respiration triggers increased pulmonary blood flow after birth, which contributes to the transition from fetal to neonatal circulation.

Fetal-Newborn Transitional Physiology

During fetal life, blood with the highest oxygen content is directed to the heart and brain. Blood in the descending aorta is less oxygenated and supplies the kidneys and intestinal tract before it is returned to the placenta. Limited amounts of blood, pumped from the right ventricle toward the lungs, enter the pulmonary vessels. In the fetus, increased pulmonary resistance forces most of the blood through the ductus arteriosus into the descending aorta (Table 28–1 •).

Marked changes occur in the cardiovascular system at birth. Expansion of the lungs with the first breath decreases the pulmonary vascular resistance and increases pulmonary blood flow. Pressure in the left atrium increases as blood returns from the pulmonary veins. Pressure in the right atrium drops, and systemic vascular resistance increases as umbilical venous flow is halted when the cord is clamped.

These physiologic mechanisms mark the beginning of transition from fetal to neonatal circulation and show the

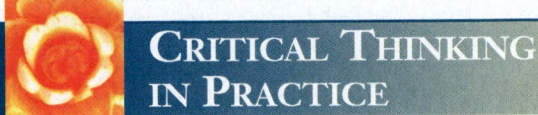

Table 28–1 • FETAL AND NEONATAL CIRCULATION

System	Fetal	Neonatal
Pulmonary blood vessels	Constricted with very little blood flow; lungs not expanded	Vasodilation and increased blood flow; lungs expanded; increased oxygen stimulates vasodilation.
Systemic blood vessels	Dilated with low resistance; blood mostly in placenta	Arterial pressure rises due to loss of placenta; increased systemic blood volume and resistance.
Ductus arteriosus	Large with no tone; blood flow from pulmonary artery to aorta	Reversal of blood flow. Now from aorta to pulmonary artery because of increased left atrial pressure. Ductus is sensitive to increased oxygen and body chemicals and begins to constrict.
Foramen ovale	Patent with large blood flow from right atrium to left atrium	Increased pressure in left atrium attempts to reverse blood flow and shuts one-way valve.

interplay of the cardiovascular and respiratory systems (Figure 28–4 •).

There are five major areas of change in cardiopulmonary adaptation (Figure 28–5 •):

1. *Increased aortic pressure and decreased venous pressure.* Clamping of the umbilical cord eliminates the placental vascular bed and reduces the intravascular space. Consequently, aortic (systemic) blood pressure increases. At the same time, blood return via the inferior vena cava decreases, resulting in decreased right atrial pressure and a small decrease in pressure within the venous circulation.
2. *Increased systemic pressure and decreased pulmonary artery pressure.* With the loss of the low-resistance placenta, systemic resistance increases, resulting in greater systemic pressure. At the same time, lung expansion increases pulmonary blood flow, and the increased blood PO_2 associated with initiation of respirations dilates pulmonary blood vessels. The combination of vasodilation and increased pulmonary blood flow decreases pulmonary artery resistance. As the pulmonary vascular beds open, the systemic vascular pressure increases, enhancing perfusion of the other body systems.
3. *Closure of the foramen ovale.* Closure of the foramen ovale is a function of changing atrial pressures. In utero, pressure is greater in the right atrium, and the foramen ovale is open after birth. Decreased pulmonary resistance and increased pulmonary blood flow increase pulmonary venous return into the left atrium, thereby increasing left atrial pressure slightly. The decreased pulmonary vascular resistance and the decreased umbilical venous return to the right atrium also cause a decrease in right atrial pressure. The pressure gradients across the atria are now reversed, with left atrial pressure

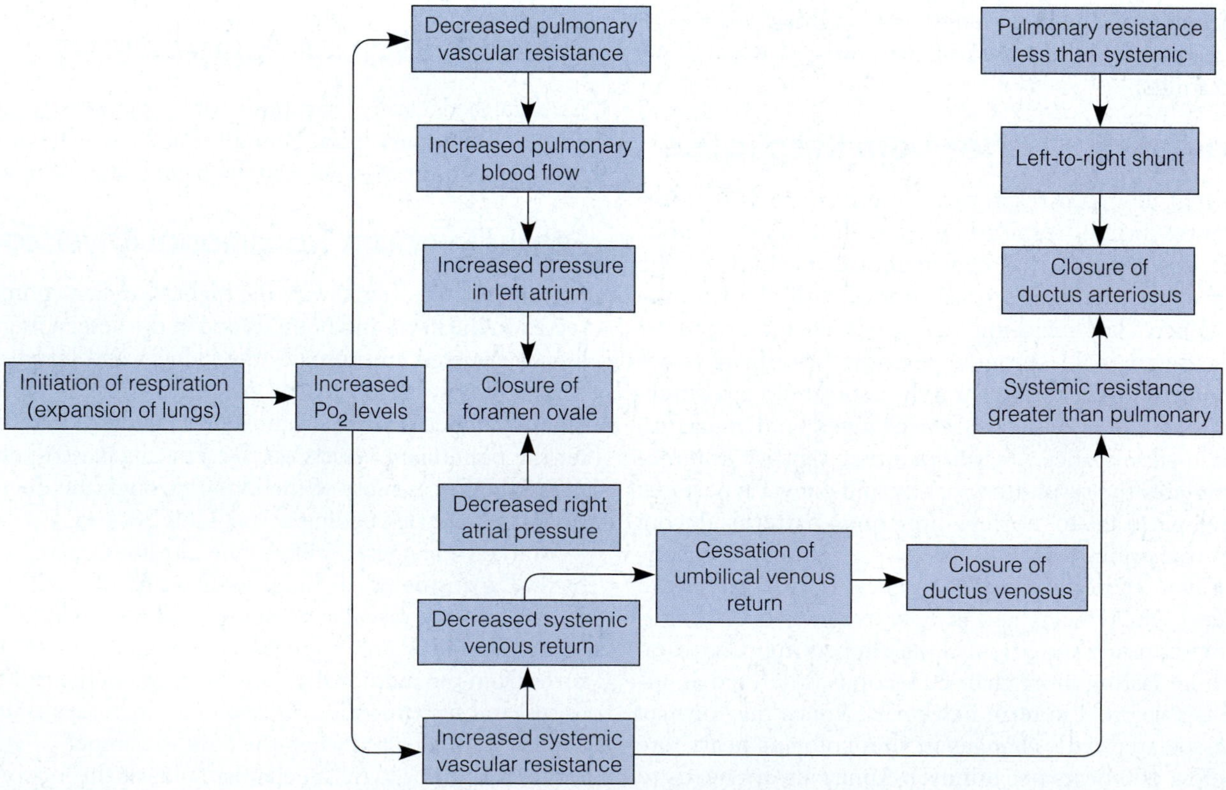

Figure 28–4 • Transitional circulation: conversion from fetal to neonatal circulation.

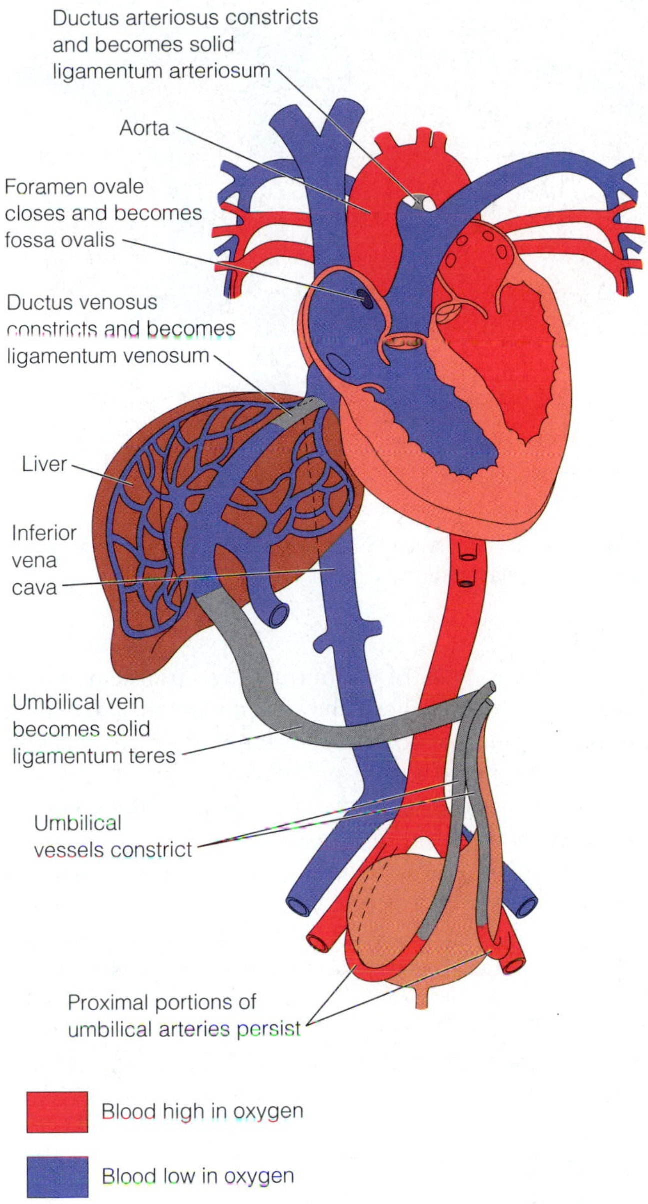

Figure 28–5 • Major changes that occur in the newborn's circulatory system.
SOURCE: Hole, J. W. (1990). *Human anatomy and physiology,* (5th ed.). Dubuque, IA: William C Brown. All rights reserved.

greater, and the foramen ovale is functionally closed 1 to 2 hours after birth. However, a slight right-to-left shunting may occur in the early neonatal period. Any increase in pulmonary resistance or right atrial pressure, such as occurs in crying, acidosis, cold stress, or induced hypoxia, may cause the foramen ovale to reopen, causing a right-to-left shunt. Permanent closure of the foramen ovale occurs within 6 months.

4. *Closure of the ductus arteriosus.* Initial elevation of the systemic vascular pressure above the pulmonary vascular pressure increases pulmonary blood flow by reversing the flow through the ductus arteriosus. Blood now flows from the aorta into the pulmonary artery. Furthermore, although the presence of oxygen causes the pulmonary arterioles to dilate, an increase in blood Po_2 triggers the opposite response in the ductus arteriosus—it constricts.

   In utero the placenta produces prostaglandin E_2 (PGE_2), which causes ductus vasodilation. With the loss of the placenta and increased pulmonary blood flow, PGE_2 levels drop, leaving the active constriction by Po_2 unopposed. If the lungs fail to expand or if Po_2 levels drop, the ductus remains patent. Functional closure is accomplished within 15 hours of birth, and fibrosis of the ductus occurs within 3 weeks after birth (Blackburn, 2003).

5. *Closure of the ductus venosus.* Although the mechanism of initiating closure of the ductus venosus is not known, it appears to be related to mechanical pressure changes that result from severing of the cord, redistribution of blood, and cardiac output. Closure of the ductus venosus forces perfusion of the liver. Fibrotic closure occurs within 2 months. Figure 28–6 • depicts the changes in blood flow and oxygenation as the fetal cardiopulmonary circulation adapts to extrauterine life.

Characteristics of Cardiac Function

Evaluation of the newborn's heart rate, blood pressure, heart sounds, and cardiac workload provides data for evaluating cardiac function.

HEART RATE

Shortly after the first cry and the start of changes in cardiopulmonary circulation, the newborn heart rate accelerates to 175 to 180 beats per minute (bpm). The average resting heart rate in the first week of life is 110 to 150 bpm in a quiet, full-term newborn but may vary significantly during deep sleep or active awake states (Lissauer, 2002). In full-term newborns, the heart rate may drop to a low of 85 bpm during sleep.

Apical pulse rates should be obtained by auscultation for a full minute, preferably when the newborn is asleep. The heart rate should be evaluated for abnormal rhythms or beats. Peripheral pulses of all extremities should also be evaluated to detect any lags or unusual characteristics. Peripheral radial pulses are difficult to palpate in the newborn. They can be assessed when blood pressure is measured if blood pressure readings are taken on all four extremities.

BLOOD PRESSURE

The blood pressure tends to be highest immediately after birth, and then it descends to its lowest level at about 3 hours of age. By 4 to 6 days of life, the blood pressure rises and plateaus at a level approximately the same as the initial level. Blood pressure is sensitive to the changes in blood volume that occur in the transition to newborn circulation. Figure 28–7 • diagrams this response. Peripheral perfusion pressure is a particularly sensitive indicator of the newborn's ability to compensate for alterations in blood volume prior to changes in blood pressure. Capillary refill should be less than 2 to 3 seconds when the skin is blanched.

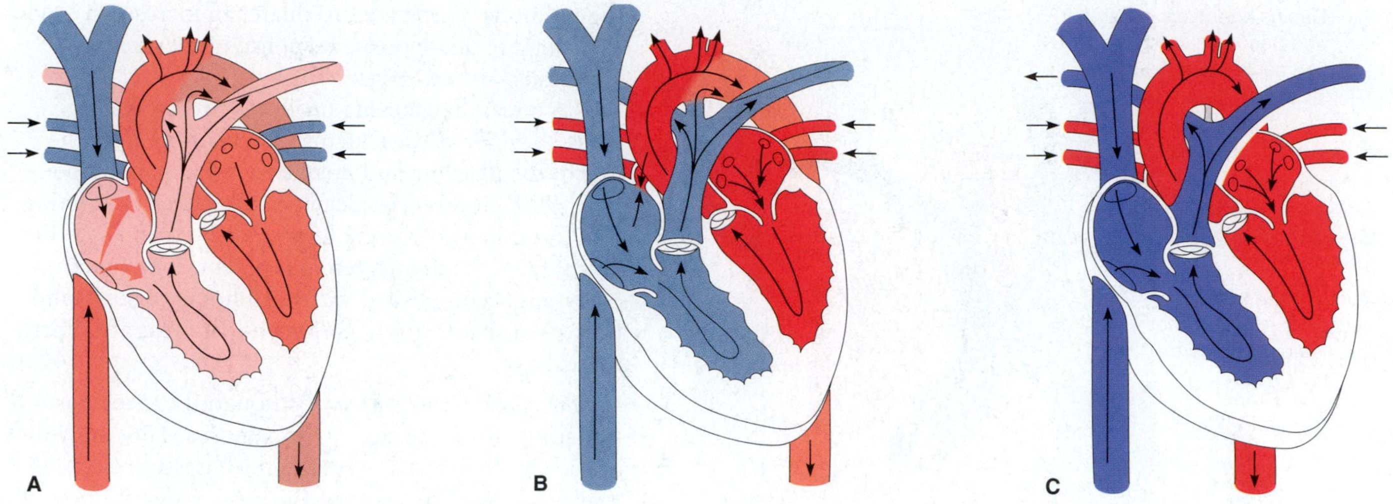

Figure 28–6 • Fetal-neonatal circulation. *A,* Pattern of blood flow and oxygenation in fetal circulation. *B,* Pattern of blood flow and oxygenation in transitional circulation of the newborn. *C,* Pattern of blood flow and oxygenation in neonatal circulation.

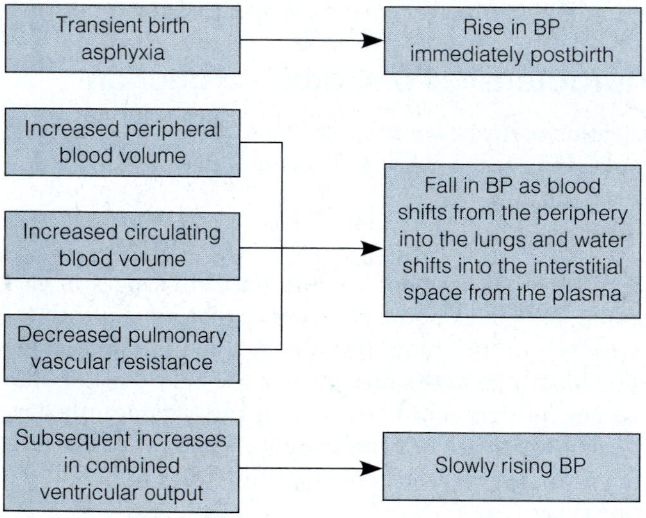

Figure 28–7 • Response of blood pressure (BP) to changes in neonatal blood volume.

Blood pressure values during the first 12 hours of life vary with the birth weight. In the full-term resting newborn, the average blood pressure is 72/47 mm Hg. In the preterm newborn, the average blood pressure varies according to weight. Crying may cause an elevation of 20 mm Hg in both the systolic and diastolic blood pressure; thus accuracy is more likely in the quiet newborn. The measurement of blood pressure is best accomplished by using the Doppler technique or a 1- to 2-inch cuff and a stethoscope over the brachial artery.

HEART MURMURS

Murmurs are usually produced by turbulent blood flow. Murmurs may be heard when blood flows across an abnormal valve or across a stenosed valve, when there is an atrial septal or ventricular septal defect, or when there is increased flow across a normal valve.

In newborns, 90% of all murmurs are transient and not associated with anomalies. They usually involve incomplete closure of the ductus arteriosus or foramen ovale. Soft murmurs may be heard as the pulmonary branch arteries increase their blood flow from 7% to 50% of the combined ventricular output during transition, causing a physiologic peripheral pulmonary stenosis. Clicks may normally be heard at the lower left sternal border as the great vessels dilate to accommodate systolic blood flow in the first few hours of life. Because of the current practice of early discharge, murmurs associated with ventricular septal defect and patent ductus arteriosus are often not detected until the first well-baby checkup at 4 to 6 weeks of age. Murmurs are sometimes absent in seriously malformed hearts (Zahka & Lane, 2002).

CARDIAC WORKLOAD

In the first 2 hours after birth, when the ductus arteriosus remains mostly patent, about one third of the left ventricular output is returned to the pulmonary circulation. As a result, the left ventricle has a significantly greater volume load than the right ventricle after birth. In the adult, right and left ventricular outputs are equal; in the newborn, right ventricular output reflects systemic venous return, and left ventricular output reflects pulmonary venous return. Systemic blood volume and pulmonary blood volume are not equal in the newborn. The newborn's combined cardiac output (left and right ventricular) is greater per unit of body weight than it will be in later childhood.

Before birth, the right ventricle does approximately two thirds of the cardiac work, resulting in increased size and thickness of the right ventricle at birth. After birth, the left ventricle must assume a larger share of the cardiac workload, and it progressively increases in size and thickness. This may explain why right-sided heart defects are better tolerated than left-sided lesions and why left-sided heart defects rapidly become symptomatic after birth.

Hematopoietic Adaptations

Fetal blood flowing through the umbilical vein in utero is 50% oxygen saturated; this relative hypoxia causes increased amounts of erythropoietin to be secreted, resulting in active erythropoiesis (an increase in nucleated red blood cells and reticulocytes). After birth, the increases in oxygen saturation and arterial oxygen levels shut off the production of erythropoietin. In the first days of life, hemoglobin concentration may rise 1 to 2 g/dL above fetal levels as a result of placental transfusion, low oral fluid intake, and diminished extracellular fluid volume. By 1 week postnatally, peripheral hemoglobin is comparable to fetal blood counts. The hemoglobin level declines progressively thereafter during the first 2 to 3 months after birth (Polin & Fox, 1998). This initial decline in hemoglobin creates a phenomenon known as **physiologic anemia of infancy.** A factor that influences the degree of physiologic anemia is the nutritional status of the newborn. Supplies of vitamin E, folic acid, and iron may be inadequate given the amount of growth in the later part of the first year of life. Hemoglobin values fall, mainly from a decrease in red cell mass rather than from the dilutional effect of increasing plasma volume. The fact that red cell survival is lower in newborns than in adults, and that red cell production is less, also contributes to this anemia. Neonatal red blood cells have a lifespan of 80 to 100 days, approximately two thirds of an adult's red blood cell lifespan. About 5% of neonatal red blood cells retain their nucleus.

Leukocytosis is a normal finding because the stress of birth stimulates increased production of neutrophils during the first few days of life. Neutrophils then decrease to 35% of the total leukocyte count by 2 weeks of age. Lymphocytes play a role in antibody formation and eventually become the predominant type of leukocyte, and the total white blood count falls. Also, megakaryocytes appear in the liver and spleen as platelets at about 11 weeks' gestation and approach adult values by 30 weeks' gestation.

Blood volume of the term infant is estimated to be 80 to 85 mL/kg of body weight. For example, a 3.6 kg (8 lb) newborn has a blood volume of 290 to 309 mL. Blood volume varies according to the amount of placental transfusion received during the expulsion of the placenta as well as other factors, including the following:

1. *Delayed cord clamping and the normal shift of plasma to the extravascular spaces.* Newborn hemoglobin and hematocrit values are higher when a placental transfusion occurs at birth. Placental vessels contain about 100 mL of blood at term, most of which can be transfused into the newborn through the umbilical vein by holding the newborn below the level of the placenta and by delaying clamping of the cord (Figure 28–8 •). Blood volume increases by 50% with delayed cord clamping (Polin & Fox, 1998). The increase is reflected by a rise in hemoglobin level and an increase in the hematocrit to about 65% after birth (compared with 48% when the cord is clamped immediately). For greatest accuracy, the initial hemoglobin and hematocrit levels should be measured in the cord blood, although this is not a routine practice.
2. *Gestational age.* There appears to be a positive association between gestational age, red blood cell numbers, and hemoglobin concentration.
3. *Prenatal or perinatal hemorrhage.* Significant prenatal or perinatal bleeding decreases the hematocrit level and causes hypovolemia.
4. *Site of the blood sample.* Hemoglobin and hematocrit levels taken simultaneously are significantly higher in capillary blood than in venous blood. Sluggish peripheral blood flow creates stasis of red blood cells, thereby increasing their concentration in the capillaries. Because of this, blood samples taken from venous blood sites are more accurate.

The concentration of serum electrolytes in the blood indicates the fluid and electrolyte status of the newborn. See Table 28–2 • for normal electrolyte and blood values of the full-term newborn.

Temperature Regulation

Temperature regulation is the maintenance of balance between the loss of heat to the environment and the production of heat. Newborns are *homeothermic;* they attempt to stabilize their internal (core) body temperatures within a narrow range in spite of significant temperature variations in their environment. At birth, the fetus moves from a warm intrauterine environment to the relatively colder extrauterine environment. The newborn's temperature may fall 2C to 3C after birth mainly because of evaporative losses; this triggers cold-induced metabolic responses and heat production. Term newborns can increase their metabolic rate by 100% by 15 to 30 minutes after birth.

Thermoregulation in the newborn is closely related to the rate of metabolism and oxygen consumption. Within a specific environmental range called the **neutral thermal environment (NTE),** the rates of oxygen consumption and metabolism are minimal, and internal body temperature is maintained because of thermal balance (Table 28–3 •) (LeBlanc, 2002). For an unclothed full-term newborn, the NTE range is an ambient environmental temperature of 32C to 34C (89.6F to 93.2F). The limits for an adult are 26C to 28C (78.8F to 82.4F) (Polin & Fox, 1998). Thus the normal newborn requires higher environmental temperatures to maintain a neutral thermal environment.

Several newborn characteristics affect establishment of the NTE. The newborn has less subcutaneous fat than an adult and a thin epidermis. Blood vessels of the newborn are closer to the skin than those of an adult. Therefore, the circulating blood is influenced by changes in environmental temperature and in turn influences the hypothalamic temperature-regulating center.

MediaLink: Neonatal Thermoregulation

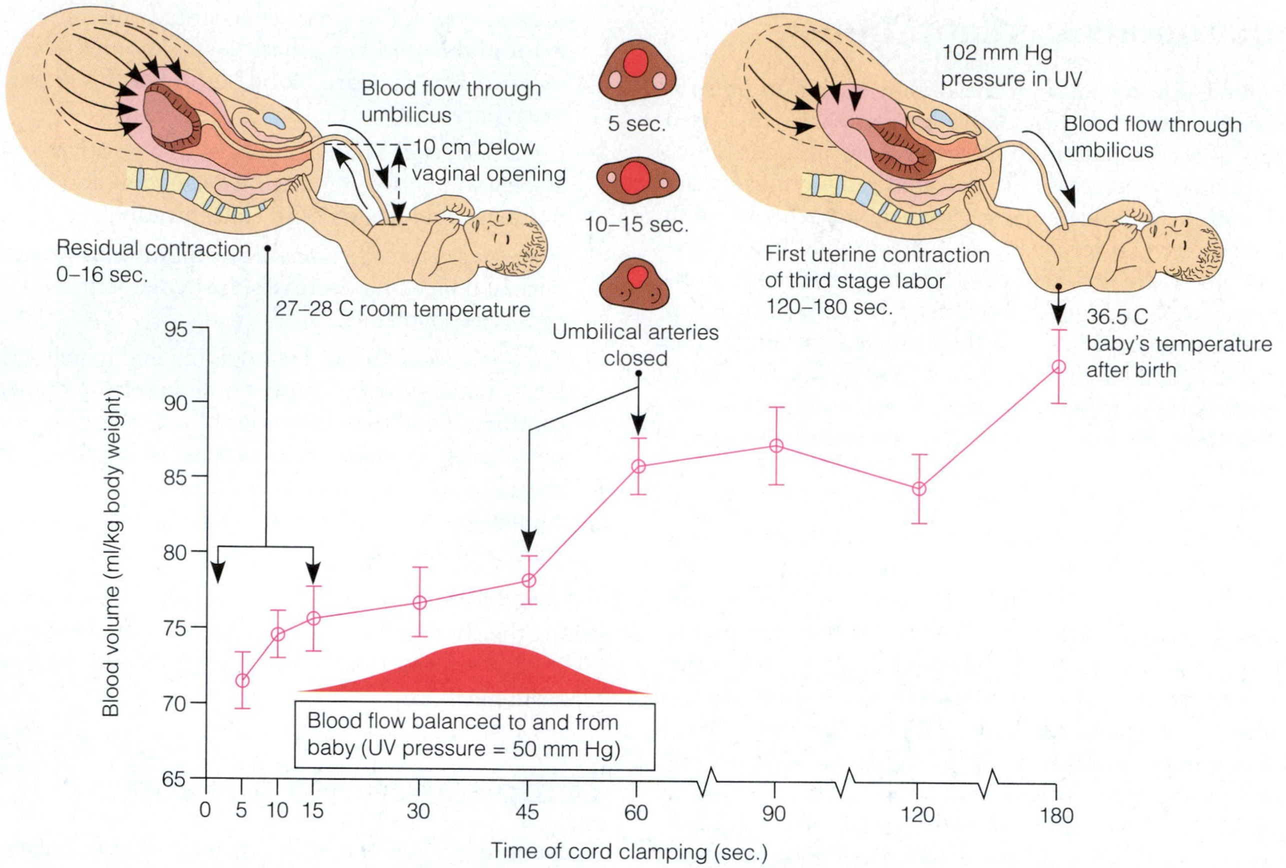

Figure 28–8 • Schematic illustration of the mechanisms in placental transfusion (normal term births) through the umbilical vein. The mean neonatal blood volume at 30 minutes is plotted against the time of cord clamping after birth (mean + 1 SE, data from 114 full-term infants). Note episodic, stepwise increments in blood volume at 10, 60, and 180 seconds.
SOURCE: Yao, A. C., & Lind, J. (1982). *Placental transfusion: A clinical and physiological study.* Springfield, IL: Charles C Thomas.

Table 28–2 • NORMAL TERM NEWBORN CORD BLOOD VALUES

Laboratory Data	Normal Range
Hemoglobin	14–20 g/dL
Hematocrit	43%–63%
WBC	10,000–30,000/mm^3
Neutrophils	40%–80%
Platelets	150,000–350,000/mm^3
Reticulocytes	3%–7%
Blood volume	82.3 mL/kg (third day after early cord clamping) 92.6 mL/kg (third day after delayed cord clamping)
Sodium	126–166 mEq/L
Potassium	5.6–12.0 mEq/L
Chloride	98–110 mEq/L
Calcium	8.2–11.1 mg/dL
Glucose	45–96 mg/dL

Source: Fanaroff, A. A., & Martin, R. J. (Eds.). (2002). *Neonatal-perinatal medicine* (7th ed., pp.1651, 1661). St. Louis, MO: Mosby.

The flexed posture of the term infant decreases the surface area exposed to the environment, thereby reducing heat loss. Other newborn characteristics such as size, ratio of surface area to body weight, and age may also affect establishment of the NTE. The preterm small-for-gestational-age (SGA) newborn has less adipose tissue and is hypoflexed, and therefore requires higher environmental temperatures to achieve a thermal neutral environment. A larger, well-insulated newborn may be able to cope with lower environmental temperatures. If the environmental temperature falls below the lower limits of the NTE, the newborn responds with increased oxygen consumption and raised metabolism, which results in greater heat production. Prolonged exposure to the cold may result in depleted glycogen stores and acidosis. Oxygen consumption also increases if the environmental temperature is above the NTE.

Heat Loss

A newborn is at a distinct disadvantage in maintaining a normal temperature. With a large body surface in relation

Table 28–3 • NEUTRAL THERMAL ENVIRONMENTAL TEMPERATURES

Age and Weight*	Range of Temperature (C)
0–6 Hours	
Under 1200 g	34.0–35.4
1200–1500 g	33.9–34.4
1501–2500 g	32.8–33.8
Over 2500 (and >36 weeks)	32.0–33.8
6–12 Hours	
Under 1200 g	34.0–35.4
1200–1500 g	33.5–34.4
1501–2500 g	32.2–33.8
Over 2500 (and >36 weeks)	31.4–33.8
12–24 Hours	
Under 1200 g	34.0–35.4
1200–1500 g	33.3–34.3
1501–2500 g	31.8–33.8
Over 2500 (and >36 weeks)	31.0–33.7
24–36 Hours	
Under 1200 g	34.0–35.0
1200–1500 g	33.1–34.2
1501–2500 g	31.6–33.6
Over 2500 (and >36 weeks)	30.7–33.5
36–48 Hours	
Under 1200 g	34.0–35.0
1200–1500 g	33.0–34.1
1501–2500 g	31.4–33.5
Over 2500 (and >36 weeks)	30.5–33.3
48–72 Hours	
Under 1200 g	34.0–35.0
1200–1500 g	33.0–34.0
1501–2500 g	31.2–33.4
Over 2500 (and >36 weeks)	30.1–33.2
72–96 Hours	
Under 1200 g	34.0–35.0
1200–1500 g	33.0–34.0
1501–2500 g	31.1–33.2
Over 2500 (and >36 weeks)	29.8–32.8
4–12 Days	
Under 1500 g	33.0–34.0
1501–2500 g	31.0–33.2
Over 2500 (and >36 weeks)	
4–5 days	29.5–32.6
5–6 days	29.4–32.3
6–8 days	29.0–32.2
8–10 days	29.0–31.8
10–12 days	29.0–31.4
12–14 Days	
Under 1500 g	32.6–34.0
1500–2500 g	31.0–33.2
Over 2500 (and >36 weeks)	29.0–30.8
2–3 Weeks	
Under 1500 g	32.2–34.0
1500–2500 g	30.5–33.0
3–4 Weeks	
Under 1500 g	31.6–33.6
1500–2500 g	30.0–32.7
4–5 Weeks	
Under 1500 g	31.2–33.0
1500–2500 g	29.5–32.2
5–6 Weeks	
Under 1500 g	30.6–32.3
1500–2500 g	29.0–31.8

*Generally speaking, the smaller infants in each weight group will require a temperature in the higher portion of the temperature range. Within each time range, the younger the infant, the higher the temperature required.

Source: Adapted from Scopes and Ahmed (1966) (For his table Scopes had the walls of the incubator 1 to 2 degrees warmer than the ambient air temperatures.) Reproduced, with permission, from Klaus, M. H., & Fanaroff, A. A. (1986). *Care of the high-risk neonate,* (3rd ed., p. 103). Philadelphia: Saunders.

to mass and a limited amount of insulating subcutaneous fat, the full-term newborn loses about four times as much heat as an adult. The newborn's poor thermal stability is due primarily to excessive heat loss rather than to impaired heat production. Because of the risk of hypothermia and possible cold stress, minimizing heat loss in the newborn after birth is essential. (See Chapters 24 and 30 for nursing measures).

Two major routes of heat loss are from the internal core of the body to the body surface and from the external body surface to the environment. Usually the core temperature is higher than the skin temperature, resulting in continuous transfer or conduction of heat to the surface (LeBlanc, 2002). The greater the difference in temperatures between core and skin, the more rapid the transfer. The transfer is accomplished through an increase in oxygen consumption, depletion of glycogen stores, and metabolizing of brown fat.

Heat loss from the body surface to the environment takes place by four avenues—convection, radiation, evaporation, and conduction (Figure 28–9 •).

- **Convection** is the loss of heat from the warm body surface to the cooler air currents. Air-conditioned rooms, air currents with a temperature below the infant's skin temperature, oxygen by mask, and removal of the infant from an incubator for procedures increase convective heat loss of the newborn.
- **Radiation** losses occur when body heat rises to cooler surfaces and objects not in direct contact with the body. The walls of a room or of an incubator are potential causes of heat loss by radiation, even if the ambient temperature of the incubator is within the neutral thermal range for the infant. Placing cold objects (such as ice for blood gases) onto the incubator or near the infant in the radiant warmer will increase radiant heat losses.

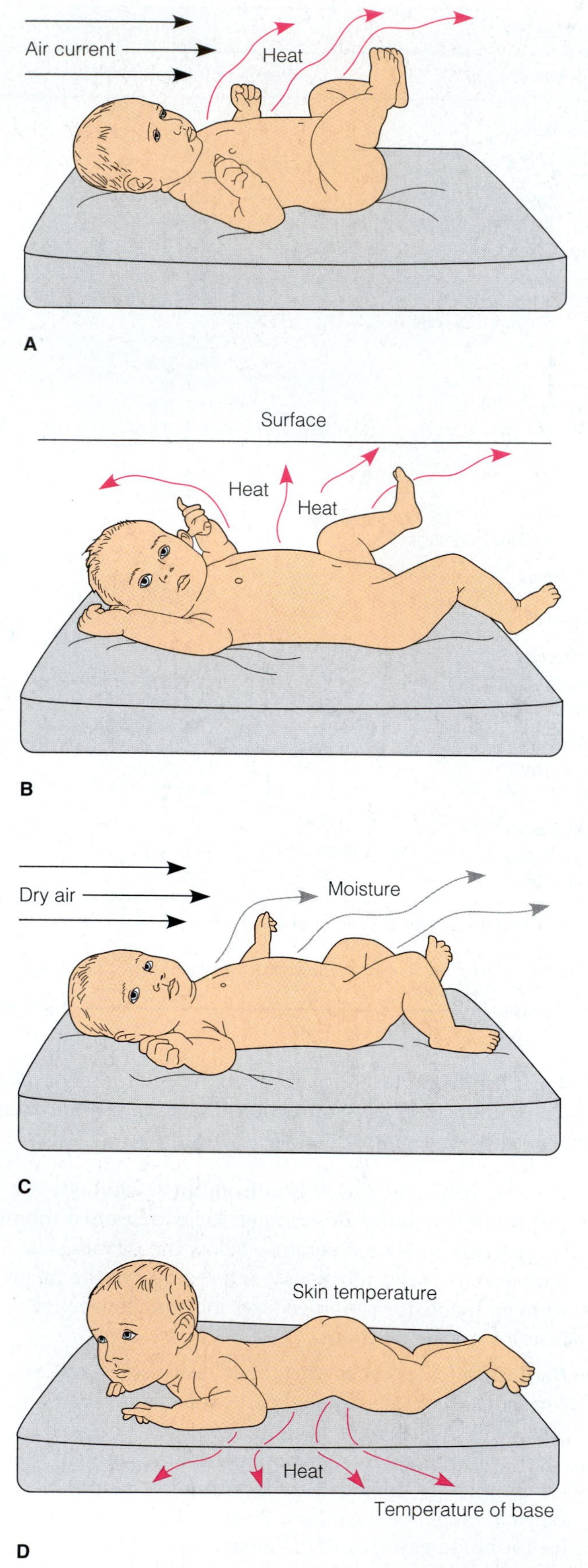

Figure 28-9 • Methods of heat loss. *A,* Convection. *B,* Radiation. *C,* Evaporation. *D,* Conduction.

- **Evaporation** is the loss of heat incurred when water is converted to a vapor. The newborn is particularly prone to heat loss by evaporation immediately after birth, when the baby is wet with amniotic fluid, and during baths; thus drying the newborn is critical.
- **Conduction** is the loss of heat to a cooler surface by direct skin contact. Chilled hands, cool scales, cold examination tables, and cold stethoscopes can cause heat loss by conduction. Even if objects are warmed to the incubator temperature, there still may be a significant temperature difference between the infant's core temperature and the ambient temperature. This results in heat transfer.

Once the infant has been dried after birth, the highest losses of heat generally result from radiation and convection because of the newborn's large ratio of body surface to weight, and from thermal conduction because of the marked difference between core temperature and skin temperature. The newborn can respond to the cooler environmental temperature with adequate peripheral vasoconstriction, but this mechanism is less effective because of the minimal amount of fat insulation present, the large body surface, and ongoing thermal conduction. Because of these factors, minimizing the baby's heat loss and preventing hypothermia are imperative. Nursing measures for preventing hypothermia are described in Chapter 30.

Heat Production (Thermogenesis)

When exposed to a cool environment, the newborn requires additional heat. The newborn has several physiologic mechanisms that increase heat production, or *thermogenesis.* These include increased basal metabolic rate, muscular activity, and chemical thermogenesis (also called *nonshivering thermogenesis [NST]*) (LeBlanc, 2002).

Nonshivering thermogenesis, an important mechanism of heat production, is unique to the newborn. NST occurs when skin receptors perceive a drop in environmental temperature and transmit sensations to the central nervous system, which in turn stimulates the sympathetic nervous system to metabolize the newborn's stores of **brown adipose tissue (BAT)** (also called *brown fat*) for heat. This is triggered by release of norepinephrine by the adrenal gland and at abundant local nerve endings in the brown fat, which in turn causes the BAT triglycerides to be metabolized into glycerol and fatty acids. The oxidation of fatty acids is highly exothermic (heat producing). In addition, brown fat possesses a rich blood supply to enhance distribution of heat throughout the body, including to the periphery.

Thus, BAT is the primary source of heat in the cold-stressed newborn. It first appears in the fetus at 26 to 30 weeks' gestation and continues to increase until 2 to 5 weeks after the birth of a term infant, unless it is depleted by cold stress. Brown fat is deposited in the midscapular area, around the neck, and in the axillas, with deeper placement around the trachea, esophagus, abdominal aorta, kidneys, and adre-

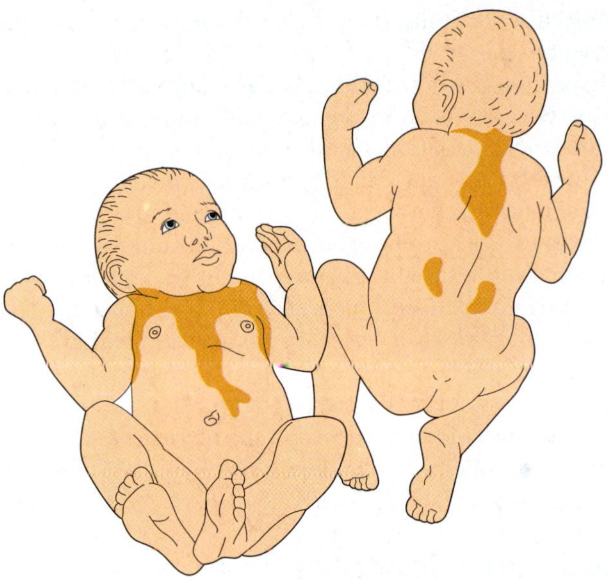

Figure 28–10 • The distribution of brown adipose tissue (brown fat) in the newborn.
SOURCE: Adapted from Davis, V. (1980). Structure and function of brown adipose tissue in the neonate. *Journal of Obstetric, Gynecologic, and Neonatal Nursing, 9,* 364.

nal glands (Figure 28–10 •). BAT constitutes 2% to 6% of the newborn's total body weight. Brown fat receives its name from its dark color, which is due to its enriched blood supply, dense cellular content, and abundant nerve endings.

Shivering, a form of muscular activity common in the cold adult, is rarely seen in the newborn, although it has been observed at ambient temperatures of 15C (59F) or less (Polin & Fox, 1998). If the newborn does shiver, it means the newborn's metabolic rate has already doubled. The extra muscular activity does little to produce needed heat.

Thermographic studies of newborns exposed to cold show an increase in the skin heat over the brown fat deposits in the newborn between 1 and 14 days of age. If the brown fat supply has been depleted, the metabolic response to cold will be limited or lacking. An increase in basal metabolism as a result of hypothermia results in an increase in oxygen consumption. A decrease in the environmental temperature of 2C, from 33C to 31C, is a drop sufficient to double the oxygen consumption of a term newborn. Keeping the normal newborn warm promotes normal oxygen requirements, whereas chilling can cause the newborn to show signs of respiratory distress.

When exposed to cold, the normal term newborn is usually able to cope with the increase in oxygen requirements, but the preterm newborn may be unable to increase ventilation to the necessary level of oxygen consumption. (See Chapter 33 for discussion of cold stress.) Because oxidation of fatty acids depends on the availability of oxygen, glucose, and adenosine triphosphate (ATP), the newborn's ability to generate heat can be altered by pathologic events such as hypoxia, acidosis, and hypoglycemia or by medications that block the release of norepinephrine. The effect of certain drugs such as meperidine (Demerol) may also prevent metabolism of brown fat. Meperidine given to the laboring woman leads to a greater fall in the newborn's body temperature during the neonatal period. Neonatal hypothermia prolongs as well as potentiates the effects of many analgesic and anesthetic drugs in the newborn.

GLOBAL PERSPECTIVES

In Jordan, the birth of a male infant is a much celebrated event. The newborn is bathed daily during the first week of life. During the final bath, salt is added to the water to help the newborn's skin adjust to the external environment and protect it from changes in the weather.

Response to Heat

Sweating is the usual initial response of the term newborn to hyperthermia. The newborn has six times as many sweat glands as the adult, but the capacity of the sweat gland is one third that of the adult. The glands have limited function until after the fourth week of extrauterine life. Heat is dissipated by peripheral vasodilation and evaporation of insensible water loss. In term SGA infants, the onset of sweating is delayed; it is virtually nonexistent in preterm infants of less than 30 weeks' gestation because of the underdevelopment of the sweat glands. Oxygen consumption and metabolic rate also increase in response to hyperthermia. Severe hyperthermia can lead to death or to gross brain damage if the baby survives.

Hepatic Adaptations

In the newborn, the liver is frequently palpable 2 to 3 cm below the right costal margin. It is relatively large and occupies about 40% of the abdominal cavity. The neonatal liver plays a significant role in iron storage, carbohydrate metabolism, conjugation of bilirubin, and coagulation.

Iron Storage and Red Blood Cell Production

As red blood cells (RBCs) are destroyed after birth, their iron content is stored in the liver until needed for new RBC production. Newborn iron stores are determined by total body hemoglobin content and length of gestation. The term newborn has about 270 mg of iron at birth, and about 140 to 170 mg of this amount is in the hemoglobin. If the mother's iron intake has been adequate, enough iron will be stored to last until 5 months of age. After about 6 months of age, foods containing iron or iron supplements must be given to prevent anemia.

Carbohydrate Metabolism

At term, the newborn's cord blood glucose is 70% to 80% of the maternal blood glucose level (Cornblath, Hawdon, Williams, et al., 2000). Neonatal carbohydrate reserves are relatively low. One third of this reserve is in the form of liver glycogen. Neonatal glycogen stores are twice that of the adult.

The newborn enters an energy crunch at the time of birth with the removal of the maternal glucose supply and the increased energy expenditure associated with the birth process and extrauterine life. Fuel sources are consumed at a faster rate because of the work of breathing, loss of heat when exposed to cold, activity, and activation of muscle tone. Glucose is the main source of energy in the first 4 to 6 hours after birth. During the first 2 hours of life, the serum blood glucose level declines, then rises, and finally reaches a steady state 2 to 3 hours after birth (Cornblath et al, 2000)

Glucose level is assessed by using a Chemstrip method on the infant's admission to the neonatal nursery and at 4 hours of age. As stores of liver and muscle glycogen and blood glucose decrease, the newborn compensates by changing from a predominantly carbohydrate metabolism to fat metabolism. Energy is derived from fat and protein as well as from carbohydrates. The amount and availability of each of these "fuel substrates" depends on the ability of immature metabolic pathways (ie, lacking specific enzymes or hormones) to function in the first few days of life.

Conjugation of Bilirubin

Conjugation of bilirubin is the conversion of yellow lipid-soluble pigment into water-soluble pigment. Unconjugated (indirect) bilirubin is a breakdown product derived from hemoglobin that is released primarily from destroyed red blood cells. Unconjugated bilirubin is not in an excretable form and is a potential toxin. **Total serum bilirubin** is the sum of conjugated (direct) and unconjugated (indirect) bilirubin.

MediaLink Neonatal Jaundice

Fetal unconjugated bilirubin crosses the placenta to be excreted, so the fetus doesn't need to conjugate bilirubin. Total bilirubin at birth is less than 3 mg/dL unless an abnormal hemolytic process has been present. After birth, the newborn's liver must begin to conjugate bilirubin. This produces a rise in serum bilirubin in the first few days of life. The newborn liver has relatively less metabolic and enzymatic activity at birth and in the first few weeks of life than an adult liver. This reduction in hepatic activity, along with a relatively large bilirubin load, decreases the liver's ability to conjugate bilirubin and increases susceptibility to jaundice.

The bilirubin formed after RBCs are destroyed is transported in the blood bound to albumin. The bilirubin is transferred into the hepatocytes and bound to intracellular proteins. These proteins determine the amount of bilirubin that is held in the liver cells for processing and consequently determine the amount of bilirubin uptake into the liver. The activity of uridine diphosphoglucuronosyl transferase (UDPGT) enzyme results in the attachment of unconjugated bilirubin to glucuronic acid (a product of liver glycogen), producing bilirubin glucuronides (conjugated, direct bilirubin). Direct bilirubin is excreted into the tiny bile ducts, then into the common duct and duodenum. The (direct) conjugated bilirubin then progresses down the intestines, where bacteria transform it into urobilinogen (urine bilirubin) and stercobilinogen. Stercobilinogen is not reabsorbed but is excreted as a yellow-brown pigment in the stools.

Even after the bilirubin has been conjugated and bound, it can be changed back to unconjugated bilirubin via the enterohepatic circulation. In the intestines, β-glucuronidase enzyme acts to split off (deconjugate) the bilirubin from bilirubin glucuronides if it is not first acted upon by gut bacteria to produce urobilinogen; the free bilirubin is reabsorbed through the intestinal wall and brought back to the liver via portal vein circulation. This recycling of the bilirubin and decreased ability to clear bilirubin from the system are prevalent in babies who have very high β-D-glucuronidase activity levels as well as delayed bacterial colonization of the gut (such as with the use of antibiotics) and further increases the newborn's susceptibility to jaundice. Conjugation of bilirubin in newborns is depicted in Figure 28–11 ●.

Physiologic Jaundice

Physiologic jaundice is caused by accelerated destruction of fetal RBCs, impaired conjugation of bilirubin, and increased bilirubin reabsorption from the intestinal tract. This condition does not have a pathologic basis, but rather is a normal biologic response of the newborn.

Halamek & Stevenson, (2002) describes six factors—several of which can also be related to pathologic events—whose interactions may give rise to physiologic jaundice:

1. *Increased amounts of bilirubin delivered to the liver.* The increased blood volume due to delayed cord clamping combined with faster RBC destruction in the newborn leads to an increased bilirubin level in the blood. A proportionately larger amount of nonerythrocyte bilirubin is formed in the newborn. Therefore, newborns have two to three times greater production or breakdown of bilirubin. The use of forceps, which sometimes causes facial bruising or cephalhematoma (entrapped hemorrhage), can increase the amount of bilirubin to be handled by the liver.
2. *Defective uptake of bilirubin from the plasma.* If the newborn does not ingest adequate calories, the formation of hepatic intracellular binding proteins diminishes, resulting in higher levels of bilirubin remaining in the plasma.
3. *Defective conjugation of the bilirubin.* Decreased uridine diphosphoglucuronosyl activity as in hypothyroidism, or inadequate caloric intake causes the intracellular binding proteins to remain saturated and results in greater unconjugated bilirubin levels in the blood. The fatty acids in maternal breast milk compete with bilirubin for albumin binding sites; this process is thought to impede bilirubin processing.
4. *Defect in bilirubin excretion.* Delay in introduction of bacterial flora and decreased intestinal motility can also delay excretion and increase enterohepatic circulation of bilirubin. Also a congenital infection may cause impaired excretion of conjugated bilirubin.

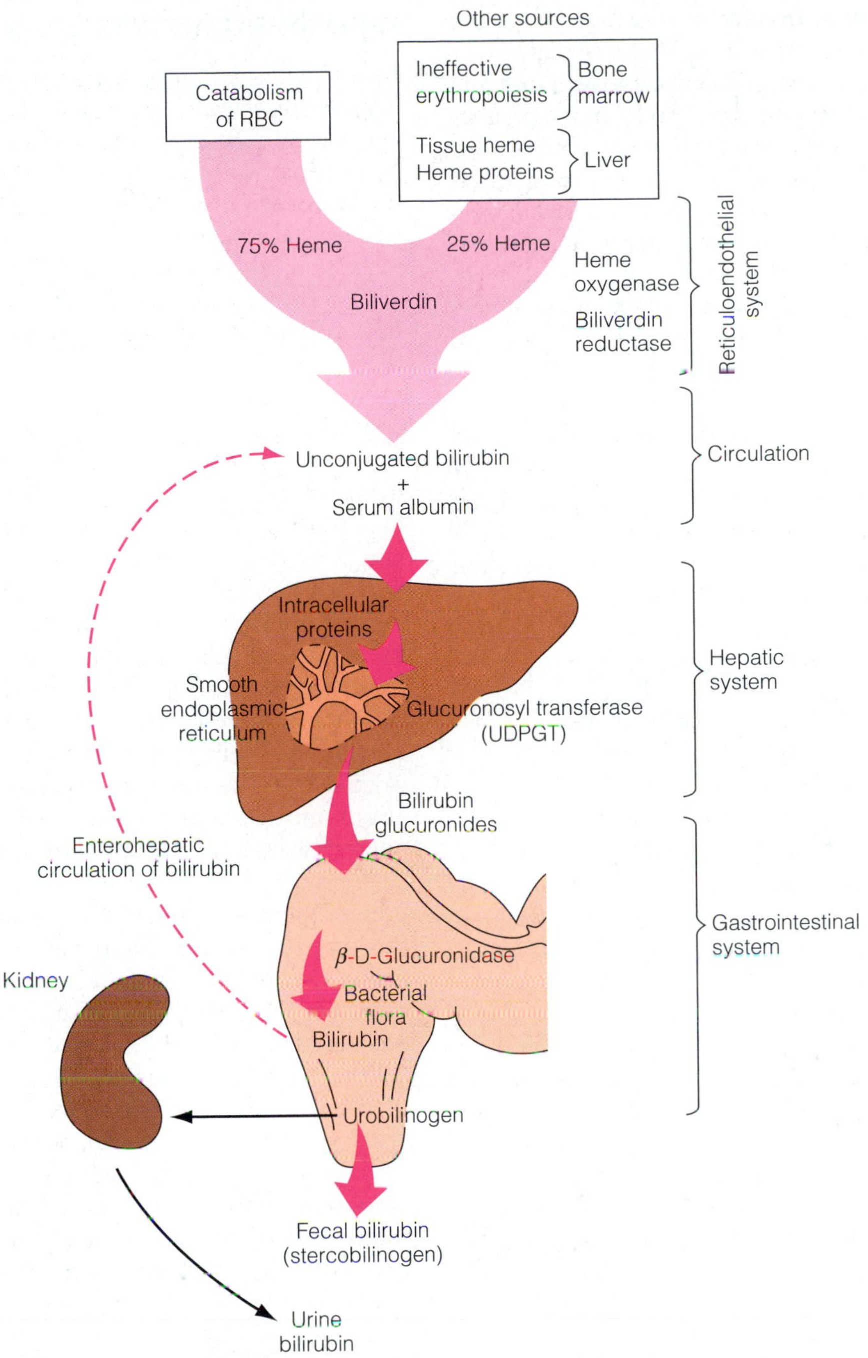

Figure 28–11 • Conjugation of bilirubin in newborns.
SOURCE: Adapted from Avery, G. B., Fletcher, M. A., & MacDonald, M. G. (1999). *Neonatology: Pathophysiology and management of the newborn* (5th ed., p. 767, 38–5). Philadelphia: Lippincott. Williams & Wilkins.

5. *Inadequate hepatic circulation.* Decreased oxygen supplies to the liver associated with neonatal hypoxia or congenital heart disease lead to a rise in the bilirubin level.
6. *Increased reabsorption of bilirubin from the intestine.* Reduced bowel motility, intestinal obstruction, or delayed passage of meconium increases the circulation of bilirubin in the enterohepatic pathway, thereby resulting in higher bilirubin values.

About 50% of full-term and 80% of preterm newborns exhibit physiologic jaundice on about the second or third day after birth. The characteristic yellow color results from increased levels of unconjugated bilirubin, which are a normal product of RBC breakdown and reflect a temporary inability of the body to eliminate bilirubin. Serum levels of bilirubin are about 4 to 6 mg/dL before yellow coloration of the skin and sclera appears. The signs of physiologic jaundice appear *after* the first 24 hours postnatally. This differentiates physiologic jaundice from pathologic jaundice (Chapter 33), which is clinically seen at birth or within the first 24 hours of postnatal life.

Peak bilirubin levels are reached between days 3 and 5 in the full-term infant and between days 5 and 7 in the preterm infant. These values are established for European and American Caucasian newborns. Chinese, Japanese, Korean, and Native American newborns have considerably higher bilirubin levels that are not as apparent and that persist for longer periods with no apparent ill effects (Halamek & Stevenson, 2002).

The nursery or postpartum room environment, including lighting, can hinder the early detection of the degree and type of jaundice. Pink walls and artificial lights mask the beginning of jaundice in newborns. Daylight assists the observer in early recognition by eliminating distortions caused by artificial light.

If jaundice is suspected, the nurse can quickly assess the newborn's coloring by pressing the skin, generally on the forehead or nose, with a finger. As blanching occurs, the nurse can observe the icterus (yellow coloring).

There are several newborn care procedures designed to decrease the probability of high bilirubin levels:

- Maintain the newborn's skin temperature at 36.5C (97.8F) or above, because cold stress results in acidosis. Acidosis in turn decreases available serum albumin-binding sites, weakens albumin-binding powers, and causes elevated unconjugated bilirubin levels.
- Monitor stool for amount and characteristics. Bilirubin is eliminated in the feces; inadequate stooling may result in reabsorption and recycling of bilirubin. Encourage early breastfeeding because the laxative effect of colostrum increases excretion of stool.
- Encourage early feedings to promote intestinal elimination and bacterial colonization and to provide caloric and protein intake necessary for the formation of hepatic binding proteins.

MediaLink Breastfeeding and Jaundice

If jaundice becomes apparent, nursing care is directed toward keeping the newborn well hydrated and promoting intestinal elimination. For specific nursing management and therapies, see the Clinical Pathway for care of a Newborn with Hyperbilirubinemia in Chapter 33.

Physiologic jaundice may be very upsetting to parents; they require emotional support and thorough explanation of the condition. If the baby is placed under phototherapy, a few additional days of hospitalization may be required. This may also be disturbing to parents. They should be encouraged to provide for the emotional needs of their newborn by continuing to feed, hold, and caress the infant. If the mother is discharged, the parents should be encouraged to return for feedings and feel free to telephone or visit whenever possible. In many instances the mother, especially if she is breastfeeding, may elect to remain hospitalized with her newborn; this decision should be supported. As an alternative to continued hospitalization, some newborns are treated in home phototherapy programs.

Breastfeeding and Breast Milk Jaundice

Breastfeeding is implicated in jaundice in some newborns. *Breastfeeding jaundice* occurs in the first days of life in breastfed newborns. It appears to be associated with poor feeding practices and not with any abnormality in milk composition. Prevention of early breastfeeding jaundice includes encouraging frequent (every 2 to 3 hours) breastfeeding, avoiding supplementation, and accessing maternal lactation counseling.

In *breast milk jaundice*, the bilirubin begins to rise after the first week of life, when physiologic jaundice is waning after the mother's milk has come in. The level peaks at 5 to 10 mg/dL at 2 to 3 weeks of age and declines over the first several months of life (Halamek & Stevenson, 2002).

In contrast to breastfeeding jaundice, breast milk jaundice is related to milk composition. Some women's breast milk may contain several times the normal concentration of certain free fatty acids. These free fatty acids may compete with bilirubin for binding sites on albumin and inhibit the conjugation of bilirubin or increase lipase activity, which disrupts the red blood cell membrane. Increased lipase activity enhances absorption of bile across the gastrointestinal tract membrane, thereby increasing the enterohepatic circulation of bilirubin. In the past it was thought that the breast milk of women whose newborns have breast milk jaundice contained an enzyme that inhibited glucuronyl transferase, but this hypothesis is no longer believed to be true.

Newborns with breast milk jaundice appear well, and at present there is an absence of documented kernicterus with this type of jaundice. Temporary cessation of breastfeeding may be advised if bilirubin reaches presumed toxic levels of approximately 20 mg/dL or if the interruption is necessary to establish the cause of the hyperbilirubinemia. Most physicians believe that breastfeeding may be resumed once other causes of jaundice have been ruled out. Within 24 to 36 hours after breastfeeding is discontinued, the newborn's serum bilirubin levels begin to fall dramatically (Halamek & Stevenson, 2002).

With resumption of breastfeeding, the bilirubin concentration may show a slight rise of 2 to 3 mg/dL with a subsequent decline. Breastfeeding mothers need encouragement and support in their desire to breastfeed their infants, assistance and instruction regarding pumping and expressing milk during the interrupted breastfeeding period, and reassurance that nothing is wrong with their milk or their mothering abilities. Table 28–4 • summarizes key factors in physiologic and breast milk jaundice.

Coagulation

The liver plays an important part in blood coagulation during fetal life and continues this function following birth. Coagulation factors II, VII, IX, and X (synthesized in the liver) are activated under the influence of vitamin K and therefore are considered vitamin K dependent. The absence of normal intestinal flora needed to synthesize vitamin K in the newborn gut results in low levels of vitamin K and creates a transient blood coagulation alteration between the second and

Table 28-4 • JAUNDICE

Physiologic Jaundice

Physiologic jaundice occurs after the first 24 hours of life.

During the first week of life, bilirubin should not exceed 13 mg/dL. Some pediatricians allow levels up to 15 mg/dL.

Bilirubin levels peak at 3 to 5 days in term infants.

Breast Milk Jaundice

Bilirubin levels begin to rise about the fourth day after mature breast milk comes in.

Peak of 5–10 mg/dL is reached at 2 to 3 weeks of age.

It may be necessary to interrupt breastfeeding for a short period when bilirubin reaches 20 mg/dL.

fifth day of life. From a low point at about 2 to 3 days after birth, these coagulation factors rise slowly but do not approach adult levels until 9 months of age or later. Other coagulation factors with low cord blood levels are XI, XII, and XIII. Fibrinogen and factors V and VII are near adult ranges.

Although newborn bleeding problems are rare, an injection of vitamin K (AquaMEPHYTON) is given prophylactically on the day of birth to combat potential clinical bleeding problems. (Hemorrhagic disease of the newborn is discussed in more depth in Chapter 33.)

Platelet counts at birth are in the same range as for older children, but newborns may manifest mild transient difficulty in platelet aggregation functioning. This platelet problem is accentuated by phototherapy. Prenatal maternal therapy with phenytoin sodium (Dilantin) or phenobarbital also causes abnormal clotting studies and newborn bleeding in the first 24 hours after birth. Infants born to mothers receiving warfarin (Coumadin) compounds may bleed because these agents cross the placenta and accentuate existing vitamin K-dependent factor deficiencies. Transient neonatal thrombocytopenia may occur in infants born to mothers with severe hypertension or HELLP syndrome (hemolysis, elevated liver enzymes, and low platelet count) and in infants born to mothers who have idiopathic isoimmune thrombocytopenic purpura.

Gastrointestinal Adaptations

By 36 to 38 weeks of fetal life, the gastrointestinal tract is adequately mature, with the presence of enzymatic activity and the ability to transport nutrients. The term newborn has adequate intestinal and pancreatic enzymes to digest most simple carbohydrates, fat, and proteins.

The carbohydrates requiring digestion in the newborn are usually disaccharides (lactose, maltose, sucrose), which are split into monosaccharides (galactose, fructose, and glucose) by the enzymes of the intestinal mucosa. Lactose is the primary carbohydrate in the breastfeeding newborn and is generally easily digested and well absorbed. The only enzyme lacking at birth is pancreatic amylase, which remains relatively deficient during the first few months of life. Newborns have trouble digesting starches (changing more complex carbohydrates into maltose). Therefore, starches should not be introduced into the diet until after the first few months of life.

Although proteins require more digestion than carbohydrates, they are well digested and absorbed from the newborn intestine. The newborn digests and absorbs fats less efficiently because of the minimal activity of pancreatic lipase. The newborn excretes 10% to 20% of the dietary fat intake, compared with 10% for the adult. The fat in breast milk is absorbed more completely by the newborn than is the fat in cow's milk because it consists of more medium-chain triglycerides and contains lipase. (See Chapter 31 for a more detailed discussion of infant nutrition.)

By birth, the newborn has experienced swallowing, gastric emptying, and intestinal propulsion. In utero, swallowing is accompanied by gastric emptying and peristalsis of the fetal intestinal tract. By the end of gestation, peristalsis becomes much more active in preparation for extrauterine life. Fetal peristalsis is also stimulated by anoxia, causing the expulsion of meconium into the amniotic fluid in more mature fetuses.

Air enters the stomach immediately after birth. The small intestine is air filled within 2 to 12 hours, and the large bowel within 24 hours. The salivary glands are immature at birth, and little saliva is manufactured until the infant is about 3 months old. The newborn's stomach has a capacity of 50 to 60 mL. It empties intermittently, starting within a few minutes of the beginning of a feeding and ending between 2 and 4 hours after feeding. Bowel sounds are present within the first 30 to 60 minutes of birth and the newborn can successfully feed during this time (Gardner, Johnson, & Lubchenco, 2002). The newborn's gastric pH becomes less acidic about a week after birth and remains less acidic than that of adults for the next 2 to 3 months.

The cardiac sphincter is immature, as is neural control of the stomach, so some regurgitation may be noted in the neonatal period. Regurgitation of the first few feedings during the first day or two of life can usually be lessened by avoiding overfeeding and by burping the newborn well during and after the feeding.

When no other signs and symptoms are evident, vomiting is limited and ceases within the first few days of life. Continuous vomiting or regurgitation should be monitored closely. If the newborn has swallowed bloody or purulent amniotic fluid, lavage of the stomach may be indicated in the term newborn to relieve the problem. Bilious vomiting is abnormal and must be evaluated thoroughly because it might represent a condition that warrants prompt surgical intervention.

Adequate digestion and absorption are essential for newborn growth and development. If optimal nutritional support is available, postnatal growth ideally should parallel intrauterine growth; that is, after 30 weeks of gestation the fetus gains 30 g per day and adds 1.2 cm to body length daily. To gain weight at the intrauterine rate, the term newborn requires 120 kcal/kg/day. Following birth, caloric intake is often insufficient for weight gain until the newborn is 5 to 10 days old. During this time there may be a weight loss of 5% to 10% in term newborns. Shift of intracellular water to extracellular space and insensible water loss account for the

5% to 10% weight loss. Thus failure to lose weight when caloric intake is limited may indicate fluid retention.

Term newborns normally pass **meconium** within 8 to 24 hours of life—and almost always within 48 hours. Meconium is formed in utero from the amniotic fluid and its constituents, with intestinal secretions and shed mucosal cells. It is recognized by its thick, tarry, black (or dark green) appearance. Transitional (thinner brown to green) stools consisting of part meconium and part fecal material are passed for the next day or two, after which the stools become entirely fecal. Generally, the stools of a breastfed newborn are pale yellow (but may be pasty green); they are more liquid and more frequent than those of formula-fed newborns, whose stools are paler (Figure 28–12 •). Frequency of bowel movement varies but initially ranges from one every 2 to 3 days to as many as ten daily. Totally breastfed infants often progress to stools that occur every 5 to 7 days. Mothers should be counseled that this is not constipation as long as the bowel movement remains soft. Table 28–5 • describes the progression of stools and other physiologic adaptations to extrauterine life.

> *When the nurse took my first child and put him to my breast his tiny mouth opened and reached for me as if he had known forever what to do.*
>
> ~Leslie Kenton, *All I Ever Wanted Was a Baby* ~

Urinary Adaptations

Kidney Development and Function

Certain physiologic features of the newborn's kidneys may affect the newborn's ability to handle body fluids and excrete urine:

1. The term newborn's kidneys have a full complement of functioning nephrons by 34 to 36 weeks of gestation.

Table 28–5 • PHYSIOLOGIC ADAPTATIONS TO EXTRAUTERINE LIFE

Periodic breathing may be present.
Desired skin temperature 36C–36.5C (96.8F–97.7F), stabilizes 4 to 6 hours after birth.
Desired blood glucose level reaches 60–70 mg/dL by third postnatal day.
Stools (progress from):
Meconium (thick, tarry, black)
Transitional stools (thin, brown to green)
Breastfed infants (yellow gold, soft, or mushy)
Formula-fed infants (pale yellow, formed, and pasty)

2. The glomerular filtration rate of the newborn's kidneys is low in comparison with the adult rate. Because of this physiologic decrease in kidney glomerular filtration, the newborn's kidneys are unable to dispose of water rapidly when necessary.
3. The juxtamedullary portion of the nephron has limited capacity to reabsorb HCO_3 and H^+ and concentrate urine (reabsorb water back into the blood). The limitation of tubular reabsorption can lead to inappropriate loss of substances present in the glomerular filtrate, such as amino acids, bicarbonate, glucose, and sodium.

Full-term newborns are less able than adults to concentrate urine because the tubules are short and narrow. Also, the reduced ability to concentrate urine is caused by the limited tubular reabsorption of water and limited excretion of solutes (principally sodium, potassium, chloride, bicarbonate, urea, and phosphate) in the growing newborn. The ability to concentrate urine fully is attained by 3 months of age. Feeding practices may affect the osmolarity of the urine but have limited effect on concentration of the urine.

Because the newborn has difficulty concentrating urine, the effect of excessive insensible water loss or restricted fluid intake is unpredictable. The newborn kidney is also limited

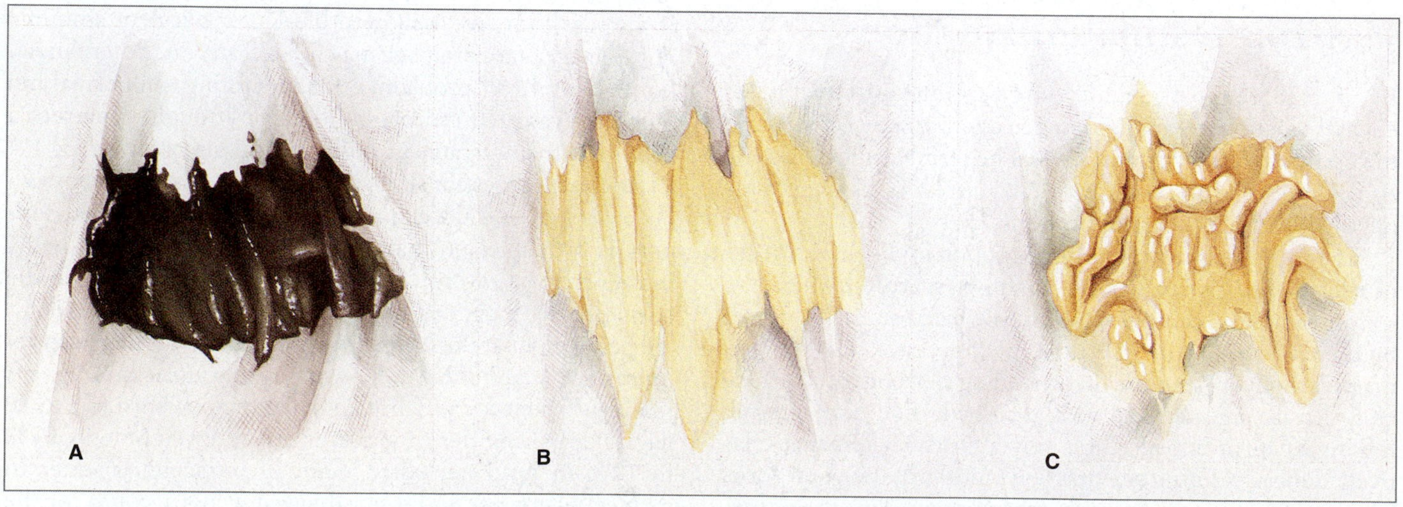

Figure 28–12 • Newborn stool samples. *A,* Meconium stool. *B,* Breast milk stool. *C,* Cow's milk stool.

Table 28-6 • NEWBORN URINALYSIS VALUES

Protein < 5–10 mg/dL
WBC <2–3/hpf
RBC 0
Casts 0
Bacteria 0
Color pale yellow

in its dilutional capabilities. Concentrating and dilutional limitations of renal function are important considerations in monitoring fluid therapy to avoid dehydration and overhydration (Vogt & Avner, 2002).

Characteristics of Newborn Urinary Function

Many newborns void immediately after birth, and the voiding frequently goes unnoticed. Among normal newborns, 92% void by 24 hours after birth, and 99% void by 48 hours (Swinford, Bonilla-Felix, Cerda, et al, 2002). A newborn who has not voided by 48 hours should be assessed for adequacy of fluid intake, bladder distention, restlessness, and symptoms of pain. The appropriate clinical personnel should be notified if indicated.

The initial bladder volume is 6 to 44 mL of urine. Unless edema is present, normal urinary output is often limited, and the voidings are scanty until fluid intake increases. (The fluid of edema is eliminated by the kidneys, so infants with edema have a much higher urinary output.) The first 2 days postnatally the newborn may void two to six times daily, with a urine output of 15 mL/kg/day. The newborn subsequently voids 5 to 25 times every 24 hours, with a volume of 25 mL/kg/day.

Following the first voiding, the newborn's urine frequently appears cloudy (due to mucus content) and has a high specific gravity, which decreases as fluid intake increases. Occasionally, pink stains ("brick dust spots") appear on the diaper. These are caused by urates and are innocuous. Blood may occasionally be observed on the diapers of female infants. This *pseudomenstruation* is related to the withdrawal of maternal hormones. Males may have bloody spotting from a circumcision. In the absence of apparent causes for bleeding, the clinician should be notified. During early infancy, normal urine is straw colored and almost odorless, although odor occurs when there is a metabolic disorder or when infection is present. Table 28–6 • summarizes urinalysis values of the normal newborn.

Immunologic Adaptations

The newborn possesses varying degrees of impairment of the nonspecific and specific immune responses. The inflammatory response and phagocytosis are altered in newborns primarily because functional limitations of their polymorphonuclear neutrophils (PMNs) affect leukocyte metabolic activities, mobilization, chemotaxis, opsonization, phagocytic activity, and intracellular killing. Newborns, particularly preterm infants, have decreased serum opsonization activity (the process of coating invasive bacteria to prepare them for phagocytic ingestion), resulting from low levels of immunoglobins and complement components. These limitations in the newborn's inflammatory response result in failure to recognize, localize, and destroy invasive bacteria. Thus the signs and symptoms of infection are often subtle and nonspecific in the newborn. The newborn also has a poor hypothalamic response to pyrogens; therefore, fever is not a reliable indicator of infection. In the neonatal period, hypothermia is a more reliable sign of infection.

Of the three major types of immunoglobulins primarily involved in immunity—IgG, IgA, and IgM—only IgG crosses the placenta. The pregnant woman forms antibodies in response to illness or immunization. This process is called **active acquired immunity.** When IgG antibodies are transferred to the fetus in utero, **passive acquired immunity** results because the fetus does not produce the antibodies itself. IgG is very active against bacterial toxins.

Because the maternal immunoglobin is transferred primarily during the third trimester, preterm newborns (especially those born prior to 34 weeks) may be more susceptible to infection. In general, newborns have maternally induced immunity to tetanus, diphtheria, smallpox, measles, mumps, poliomyelitis, and a variety of other bacterial and viral diseases. The period of resistance varies: Immunity against common viral infections such as measles may last 4 to 8 months, whereas immunity to certain bacteria may disappear within 4 to 8 weeks.

The normal newborn does produce antibodies in response to an antigen, but not as effectively as an older child would. It is customary to begin immunization at 2 months of age so the infant can develop active acquired immunity.

IgM immunoglobulins are produced in response to blood group antigens, gram-negative enteric organisms, and some viruses in the expectant mother. Because IgM does not normally cross the placenta, most or all is produced by the fetus beginning at 10 to 15 weeks' gestation. Elevated levels of IgM at birth may indicate placental leaks or, more commonly, fetal antigenic stimulation in utero. Consequently, elevations suggest that the infant was exposed to an intrauterine infection such as syphilis, toxoplasmosis, rubella, cytomegalovirus, or herpes virus hominis type 2 infection. (For in-depth discussion, see Chapter 20 and Table 33–5.) The lack of available maternal IgM in the newborn also accounts for the infant's susceptibility to gram-negative enteric organisms such as *Escherichia coli.*

The functions of IgA immunoglobins are not fully understood. IgA appears to provide protection mainly on secreting surfaces such as the respiratory tract, gastrointestinal tract, and eyes. Serum IgA does not cross the placenta and is not normally produced by the fetus in utero. Unlike the other immunoglobins, IgA is not affected by gastric action. Colostrum, the forerunner of breast milk, is very high in the secretory form of IgA. Consequently, it may be of significance in providing some passive immunity to the infant of a breastfeeding mother. Newborns begin to produce secretory IgA in their intestinal mucosa at about 4 weeks after birth.

Neurologic and Sensory/ Perceptual Functioning

The newborn's brain is about one quarter the size of an adult's, and myelination of nerve fibers is incomplete. Unlike the cardiovascular or respiratory systems, which undergo tremendous changes at birth, the nervous system is minimally influenced by the actual birth process.

Because many biochemical and histologic changes have yet to occur in the newborn's brain, the postnatal period is considered a time of risk in regard to the development of the brain and nervous system. For neurologic development—including development of intellect—to proceed, the brain and other nervous system structures must mature in an orderly, unhampered fashion. For discussion of cranial nerves, see Chapter 29.

Intrauterine Factors Influencing Newborn Behavior

Newborns respond to and interact with the environment in a predictable pattern of behavior that is shaped somewhat by their intrauterine experience. This intrauterine experience is affected by intrinsic factors such as maternal nutrition and external factors such as the mother's physical environment. Depending on the newborn's intrauterine experience and individual temperament, newborn behavioral responses to different stresses vary. Some newborns react quietly to stimulation, others become overreactive and tense, and some may exhibit a combination of the two.

MediaLink Infant Abilities

Factors such as exposure to intense auditory stimuli in utero can eventually be manifested in the behavior of the newborn. For example, the fetal heart rate (FHR) initially increases when the pregnant woman is exposed to an auditory stimuli, but repetition of the stimuli leads to decreased FHR. Thus the newborn who was exposed to intense noise during fetal life is significantly less reactive to loud sounds postnatally.

Characteristics of Newborn Neurologic Function

Partially flexed extremities with the legs near the abdomen is the usual position of the normal newborn. When awake, the newborn may exhibit purposeless, uncoordinated bilateral movements of the extremities. The organization and intensity of the newborn's motor activity are influenced by a number of factors, including the following (Brazelton, 1984): (1) sleep-wake states; (2) presence of environmental stimuli, such as heat, light, cold, and noise; (3) conditions causing a chemical imbalance, such as hypoglycemia; (4) hydration status; (5) state of health; and (6) recovery from the stress of labor and birth.

Eye movements are observable during the first few days of life. An alert newborn is able to fixate on faces and geometric objects or patterns such as black and white stripes. A bright light shining in the newborn's eyes elicits the blinking reflex.

The cry of the newborn should be lusty and vigorous. High-pitched cries, weak cries, or no cries are all causes for concern.

Growth of the newborn's body progresses in a cephalocaudal (head-to-toe), proximal-distal fashion. The newborn is somewhat hypertonic; that is, there is resistance to extending the elbow and knee joints. Muscle tone should be symmetric. Diminished muscle tone and flaccidity may indicate neurologic dysfunction.

Specific symmetric deep tendon reflexes can be elicited in the newborn. The knee jerk is brisk; a normal ankle clonus may involve three or four beats. Plantar flexion is present. Other reflexes, including the Moro, grasping, rooting, Babinski, and sucking reflexes, are characteristics of neurologic integrity. (For further discussion, see Chapter 29.)

Performance of complex behavioral patterns reflects the newborn's neurologic maturation and integration. The newborn who can bring a hand to the mouth is demonstrating motor coordination as well as a self-quieting technique, thus increasing the complexity of the behavioral response. Newborns also possess complex organized defensive motor patterns as exhibited by the ability to remove an obstruction, such as a cloth across the face.

Periods of Reactivity

The baby usually shows a predictable pattern of behavior during the first several hours after birth, characterized by two **periods of reactivity** separated by a sleep phase.

FIRST PERIOD OF REACTIVITY

The first period of reactivity lasts approximately 30 minutes after birth. During this period the newborn is awake and active and may appear hungry and have a strong sucking reflex. This is a natural opportunity to initiate breastfeeding if the mother has chosen it (Figure 28–13 •). Bursts of random, diffuse movements alternating with relative immobility may occur. Respirations are rapid, as high as 80 breaths per minute,

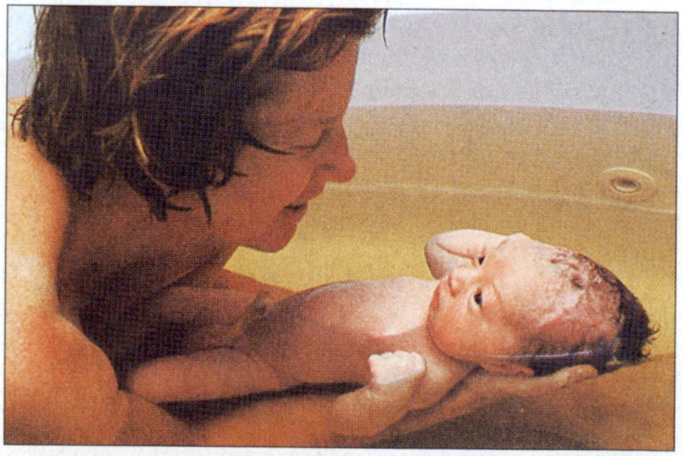

Figure 28–13 • Mother and baby gaze at each other. This quiet alert state is the optimal state for interaction.

and there may be retraction of the chest, transient flaring of the nares, and grunting. The heart rate is rapid, and rhythm may be irregular. Bowel sounds are usually absent.

PERIOD OF INACTIVITY TO SLEEP PHASE

After approximately half an hour, the newborn's activity gradually diminishes, and the heart rate and respirations decrease as the newborn enters the sleep phase. The sleep phase may last from a few minutes to 2 to 4 hours. During this period the newborn will be difficult to awaken and will show no interest in sucking. Bowel sounds become audible, and cardiac and respiratory rates return to baseline values.

SECOND PERIOD OF REACTIVITY

During the second period of reactivity, the newborn is again awake and alert. This period lasts 4 to 6 hours in the normal newborn. Physiologic responses are variable during this stage. The heart and respiratory rates increase; however, the nurse must be alert for apneic periods, which may cause a drop in the heart rate. The newborn is stimulated to continue breathing during such times. The newborn may develop rapid color changes and become mildly cyanotic or mottled during these fluctuations. Production of respiratory and gastric mucus increases, and the newborn responds by gagging, choking, and regurgitating.

Continued close observation and intervention may be required to maintain a clear airway during this period of reactivity. The gastrointestinal tract becomes more active. The first meconium stool is frequently passed during this second active stage, and the initial voiding may also occur at this time. The newborn will indicate readiness for feeding by such behaviors as sucking, rooting, and swallowing. If feeding was not initiated in the first period of reactivity, it is done at this time. See Chapter 31 for further discussion of this first feeding.

Behavioral States of the Newborn

The behavior of the newborn can be divided into two categories: the sleep state and the alert state (Brazelton, 1999). These postnatal behavioral states are similar to those that have been identified during pregnancy. Subcategories are identified under each major category.

SLEEP STATES

The sleep states are as follows:

1. *Deep or quiet sleep.* Deep sleep is characterized by closed eyes with no eye movements, regular even breathing, and jerky motion or startles at regular intervals. Behavioral responses to external stimuli are likely to be delayed. Startles are rapidly suppressed, and changes in state are not likely to occur. Heart rate may range from 100 to 120 beats per minute.
2. *Active REM.* Irregular respirations, eyes closed with REM, irregular sucking motions, minimal activity, and irregular but smooth movement of the extremities can be observed in active REM sleep. Environmental and internal stimuli initiate a startle reaction and a change of state.

Sleep cycles in the newborn have been recognized and defined according to duration. The length of the cycle depends on the age of the newborn. At term, REM active sleep and quiet sleep occur in intervals of 50 to 60 minutes (Gardner & Goldson, 2002). About 45% to 50% of the total sleep of the newborn is active sleep, 35% to 45% is quiet (deep) sleep, and 10% of sleep is transitional between these two periods. Growth hormone secretion depends on regular sleep patterns. Any disturbance of the sleep-wake cycle can result in irregular spikes of growth hormone. REM sleep stimulates the highest peaks of growth hormone and the growth of the neural system. Over a period of time, the newborn's sleep-wake patterns become diurnal; that is, the newborn sleeps at night and stays awake during the day. (See Chapter 29 for in-depth discussion of assessment of neonatal states.)

MediaLink NEWBORN SLEEP

ALERT STATES

In the first 30 to 60 minutes after birth, many newborns display a quiet alert state, characteristic of the first period of reactivity. Nurses should use these alert states to encourage bonding and breastfeeding. These periods of alertness tend to be short the first 2 days after birth to allow the baby to recover from the birth process. Subsequently, alert states are of choice or of necessity (Brazelton, 1999). Increasing choice of wakefulness by the newborn indicates a maturing capacity to achieve and maintain consciousness. Heat, cold, and hunger are but a few of the stimuli that can cause wakefulness by necessity. Once the disturbing stimuli are removed, sleep tends to recur.

The following are subcategories of the alert state (Brazelton, 1999):

1. *Drowsy or semidozing.* The behaviors common to the drowsy state are open or closed eyes, fluttering eyelids, semidozing appearance, and slow, regular movements of the extremities. Mild startles may be noted from time to time. Although the reaction to a sensory stimulus is delayed, a change of state often results.
2. *Wide awake.* In the wide awake state, the newborn is alert and follows and fixates on attractive objects, faces, or auditory stimuli. Motor activity is minimal, and the response to external stimuli is delayed.
3. *Active awake.* The eyes are open, and motor activity is quite intense, with thrusting movements of the extremities in the active awake state. Environmental stimuli increase startles or motor activity, but discrete reactions are difficult to distinguish because of generalized high activity level.
4. *Crying.* Intense crying is accompanied by jerky motor movements. Crying serves several purposes for the newborn. It may be used as a distraction from disturbing stimuli such as hunger and pain. Fussiness often allows the newborn to discharge energy and reorganize behavior. Most important, crying elicits an appropriate response of help from the parents.

Behavioral and Sensory Capacities of the Newborn

The newborn has several behavioral capacities that assist in adaptation to extrauterine life. For example, **self-quieting ability** is the ability of newborns to use their own resources to quiet and comfort themselves. Their repertoire includes hand-to-mouth movements, sucking on a fist or tongue, and attending to external stimuli. Neurologically impaired newborns are unable to use self-quieting activities and require more frequent comforting from caregivers when stimulated. For example, drug-positive newborns often exhibit abnormal sleep and feeding patterns and irritability.

Habituation is the newborn's ability to process and respond to complex stimulation. For example, when a bright light is flashed into the newborn's eyes, the initial response is blinking, constriction of the pupil, and perhaps a slight startle reaction. However, with repeated stimulation the newborn's response repertoire gradually diminishes and disappears. The capacity to ignore repetitious disturbing stimuli is a neonatal defense mechanism readily apparent in the noisy, well-lighted nursery.

Sensory abilities include visual, auditory, olfactory, taste, and tactile capacities.

VISUAL CAPACITY

Orientation is the newborn's ability to be alert to, to follow, and to fixate on complex visual stimuli that have a particular appeal and attraction. The newborn prefers the human face and eyes and bright shiny objects. As the face or object is brought into the line of vision, the newborn responds with bright, wide eyes, still limbs, and fixed staring. This intense visual involvement may last several minutes, during which time the newborn is able to follow the stimulus from side to side. Figure 28–14 • illustrates this response. The newborn uses this sensory capacity to become familiar with family, friends, and surroundings.

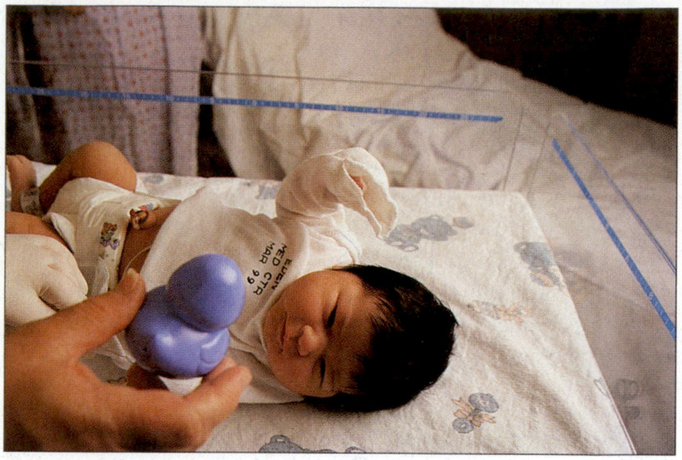

Figure 28–14 • Head turning to follow an object.

AUDITORY CAPACITY

The newborn responds to auditory stimulation with a definite, organized behavior repertoire. The stimulus used to assess auditory response should be selected to match the state of the newborn. A rattle is appropriate for light sleep, a voice for an awake state, and a clap for deep sleep. As the newborn hears the sound, the cardiac rate rises, and a minimal startle reflex may be seen. If the sound is appealing, the newborn will become alert and search for the site of the auditory stimulus.

OLFACTORY CAPACITY

Newborns are apparently able to select people by smell. In one study, newborns were able to distinguish their mothers' breast pads from those of other mothers at just 1 week postnatally (Gardner & Goldson, 2002).

TASTE AND SUCKING

The newborn responds differently to varying tastes. Sugar, for example, increases sucking. Sucking pattern variations also exist in newborns fed with a rubber nipple versus the breast. When breastfeeding, the newborn sucks in bursts with frequent regular pauses. The bottle-fed newborn tends to suck at a regular rate with infrequent pauses.

When awake and hungry, the newborn displays rapid searching motions in response to the rooting reflex. Once feeding begins, the newborn establishes a sucking pattern according to the method of feeding. Finger sucking is present not only postnatally, but also in utero. The newborn frequently uses nonnutritive sucking as a self-quieting activity, which assists in the development of self-regulation. Nonnutritive sucking with a pacifier should not be discouraged if the infant is bottle-fed. Pacifiers should be offered to breastfed infants only after breastfeeding is well established. If the pacifier is offered too soon, a phenomenon called "nipple confusion" may occur in which the breastfed infant has difficulty learning to suck from the breast. (See Chapter 31 for a more in-depth discussion).

TACTILE CAPACITY

The newborn is very sensitive to being touched, cuddled, and held. Often a mother's first response to an upset or crying newborn is touching or holding. Swaddling, placing a hand on the abdomen, or holding the arms to prevent a startle reflex are other methods of soothing the newborn. The settled newborn is then able to attend to and interact with the environment.

MEDIALINK CASE STUDY: NEWBORN RESPONSES TO BIRTH

CHAPTER REVIEW

EXPLOREMEDIALINK

NCLEX review questions, case studies, and other interactive resources for this chapter can be found on the Web site at http://www.prenhall.com/olds. Click on "Chapter 28" to select the activities for this chapter.

For tutorials including animations and videos, more NCLEX review questions, and an audio glossary, access the accompanying CD-ROM in this book.

Focus Your Study

- Newborn respiration is initiated primarily by chemical and mechanical events in association with thermal and sensory stimulation.
- The production of surfactant is crucial to keeping the lungs expanded during expiration by reducing alveolar surface tension.
- The newborn is an obligatory nose breather. Respirations move from being primarily shallow, irregular, and diaphragmatic to synchronous abdominal and chest breathing.
- Normal respiratory rate is 30 to 60 breaths per minute.
- Periodic breathing is normal, and newborn sleep states affect breathing patterns.
- The status of the cardiopulmonary system may be measured by evaluating the heart rate, blood pressure, and presence or absence of murmurs. The normal heart rate is 120 to 160 bpm.
- Oxygen transport in the newborn is significantly affected by the presence of greater amounts of HbF (fetal hemoglobin) than HbA (adult hemoglobin). HbF holds oxygen more efficiently but releases it to the body tissues only at low Po_2 levels.
- Blood values in the newborn are modified by several factors, such as site of the blood sample, gestational age, prenatal or perinatal hemorrhage, and the timing of the clamping of the umbilical cord.
- The newborn is considered to have established thermoregulation when oxygen consumption and metabolic activity are minimal.
- Evaporation is the primary heat loss mechanism in newborns who are wet from amniotic fluid or a bath. In addition, excessive heat loss occurs from radiation and convection because of the newborn's larger surface area compared to weight and from thermal conduction because of the marked difference between core temperature and skin temperature.
- The primary source of heat in the cold-stressed newborn is brown adipose tissue.
- Blood glucose levels should reach a steady state by 3 hours of age.
- The newborn's liver plays a crucial role in iron storage, carbohydrate metabolism, conjugation of bilirubin, and coagulation.
- Controversy continues about the relationship of breastfeeding and the development of prolonged jaundice.
- The normal newborn possesses the ability to digest and absorb nutrients necessary for newborn growth and development.
- The newborn's stools change from meconium (thick, tarry, black) to transitional stools (thinner, brown to green) and then to the distinct forms for either breastfed newborns (yellow-gold, soft, or mushy) or formula-fed newborns (pale yellow, formed, and pasty). Most newborns pass their first stool within 48 hours of birth.
- The newborn's kidneys are characterized by a decreased rate of glomerular flow, limited tubular reabsorption, limited excretion of solutes, and limited ability to concentrate urine. Most newborns void within 48 hours of birth.
- The immune system in the newborn is not fully activated until sometime after birth, but the newborn does possess some immunologic abilities.
- Neurologic and sensory perceptual functioning in the newborn is evident from the newborn's

interaction with the environment, presence of synchronized motor activity, and well-developed sensory capacities.

- The first period of reactivity lasts for 30 minutes after birth. The newborn is alert and hungry at this time, making this a natural opportunity to promote attachment.
- The second period of reactivity requires close monitoring by the nurse because apnea, decreased heart rate, gagging, choking, and regurgitation are likely to occur and require nursing intervention.
- Behavioral states in the newborn can be divided into sleep states and alert states.
- Sensory development proceeds in a specific order: tactile/vestibular, olfactory/gustatory, and auditory/visual.

References

Blackburn, S. T. (2003) *Maternal, fetal, & neonatal physiology: A clinical perspective.* (2nd ed.,) St. Louis, MO: Saunders.

Brazelton, T. B. (1984). *Neonatal behavioral assessment scale* (2nd ed.). London: Heineman.

Brazelton, T. B. (1999). Behavioral competence. In G. B. Avery, M. A. Fletcher, & M. G. MacDonald (Eds.), *Neonatology: Pathophysiology and management of the newborn* (5th ed., pp. 321–332). Philadelphia: Lippincott.

Cornblath, M., Hawdon, J. M., Williams, A. F., Aynseley-Green, A., Ward-Platt, M. P., Schwartz, R., et al. (2000). Controversies regarding definition of neonatal hypoglycemia: Suggested operational thresholds. *Pediatrics, 105*(5), 1141–1145.

Gardner, S. L., & Goldson, E. (2002). The neonate and the environment: Impact on development. In G. B. Merenstein & S. L. Gardner (Eds.), *Handbook of neonatal intensive care* (5th ed., pp. 219–282). St. Louis, MO: Mosby.

Gardner, S. L., Johnson, J. L., & Lubchenco, L. (2002). Initial nursery care. In G. B. Merenstein & S. L. Gardner (Eds.), *Handbook of neonatal intensive care* (5th ed., pp. 70–101). St. Louis, MO: Mosby.

Halamek, L. P., & Stevenson, D. K. (2002). Neonatal jaundice and liver disease. In A. A. Fanaroff & R. J. Martin (Eds.), *Neonatal-perinatal medicine* (7th ed., pp. 1309–1350). St. Louis, MO: Mosby.

LeBlanc, M. H. (2002). The physical environment. In A. A. Fanaroff & R. J. Martin (Eds.), *Neonatal-perinatal medicine* (7th ed., pp. 512–530). St. Louis, MO: Mosby.

Lissauer, T. (2002). Physical examination of the newborn. In A. A. Fanaroff & R. J. Martin (Eds.), *Neonatal-perinatal medicine* (7th ed., pp. 444–450). St. Louis, MO: Mosby.

Niermeyer, S., & Clarke, S. B. (2002). Delivery room care. In G. B. Merenstein & S. L. Gardner (Eds.), *Handbook of neonatal intensive care* (5th ed., pp. 46–69). St. Louis, MO: Mosby.

Polin, R. A., & Fox, W. W. (1998). *Fetal and neonatal physiology* (2nd ed.). Philadelphia: Saunders.

Swinford, R. D., Bonilla-Felix, M., Cerda, R. D., & Portman, R. J. (2002). Neonatal nephrology. In G. B. Merenstein & S. L. Gardner (Eds.), *Handbook of neonatal intensive care* (5th ed., pp. 609–643). St. Louis, MO: Mosby.

Vogt, B. A., & Avner, E. D. (2002). The kidney and urinary tract. In A. A. Fanaroff & R. J. Martin (Eds.), *Neonatal-perinatal medicine* (7th ed., pp. 1517–1536). St. Louis, MO: Mosby.

Zahka, K. G., & Lane, J. R. (2002). Approach to the neonate with cardiovascular disease. In A. A. Fanaroff & R. J. Martin (Eds.), *Neonatal-perinatal medicine* (7th ed., pp. 1112–1120). St. Louis, MO: Mosby.

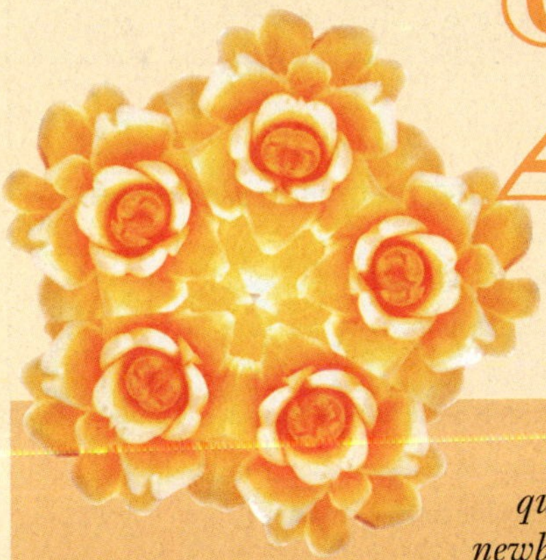

29 Nursing Assessment of the Newborn

Something very special occurs within the first hour after birth. If the environment is quiet, the birthing without complications, the lights lowered, the handling diminished, newborn infants—aside from all the physiological adaptations they must make—begin in a uniquely human way to adapt to the new experience of being in the world.

~ The Amazing Newborn ~

Objectives

- Describe the normal physical and behavioral characteristics of the newborn.
- Summarize the components of a complete newborn assessment and the significance of normal variations and abnormal findings.
- Explain the various components of the gestational age assessment.
- Discuss the neurologic and neuromuscular characteristics of the newborn and the reflexes that may be present at birth.
- Describe the categories of the newborn behavioral assessment.

Key Terms

Acrocyanosis 806
Babinski reflex (plantar reflex) 819
Barlow maneuver 818
Brazelton's Neonatal Behavioral Assessment Scale 821
Caput succedaneum 810
Cephalhematoma 809
Chemical conjunctivitis 811
Epstein's pearls 812
Erb-Duchenne paralysis (Erb's palsy) 816
Erythema toxicum 807
Forceps marks 807
Gestational age assessment tools 795
Grasping reflex 819
Harlequin sign 807
Jaundice 807
Milia 807
Molding 808
Mongolian spots 808
Moro reflex 819
Mottling 807
Nevus flammeus (port wine stain) 808
Nevus vasculosus (strawberry mark) 808
Ortolani maneuver 817
Pseudomenstruation 816
Rooting reflex 819
Skin turgor 807
Subconjunctival hemorrhage 811
Sucking reflex 819
Telangiectatic nevi (stork bites) 807
Thrush 812
Tonic neck reflex 819
Trunk incurvation (Galant reflex) 819
Vernix caseosa 807

MEDIALINK

Additional resources for this content can be found on the Student CD-ROM and on the Companion Website at www.prenhall.com/olds. Click on "Chapter 29" to select the activities for this chapter.

CD-ROM
- Audio Glossary
- NCLEX Review

Companion Website
- Additional NCLEX Review
- Case Study: Newborn Maturity Assessment
- Care Plan Activity: Assessment of the Newborn

Unlike adults, newborns communicate their needs primarily by behavior. Because nurses are the most consistent observers of the newborn, they must be able to interpret this behavior to gain information about the newborn's condition and to respond with appropriate nursing interventions. This chapter focuses on the assessment of the newborn and interpretation of findings.

Assessment of the newborn is a continuous process used to evaluate development and adjustments to extrauterine life. In the birthing area, Apgar scoring (see Chapter 24 for discussion) and careful observation of the newborn form the basis of the assessment and are correlated with information such as the following:

- Maternal prenatal care history
- Birthing history
- Maternal analgesia and anesthesia
- Complications of labor or birth
- Treatment instituted in birthing room, in conjunction with determination of clinical gestational age
- Consideration of the newborn's classification by weight and gestational age and by neonatal mortality risk
- Physical examination of the newborn

MEDIALINK NORMAL NEWBORN HEALTH ASSESSMENT

The nurse incorporates data from these sources with the assessment findings during the first 1 to 4 hours after birth to formulate a plan for nursing intervention.

The various newborn assessments and the data obtained from them are only as effective as the degree to which the findings are shared with the parents. The parents must be included in the assessment process from the moment of their child's birth. The Apgar score and its meaning should be explained immediately to the family. As soon as possible, the parents should be a part of the physical and behavioral assessments, as well.

The nurse encourages the parents to identify the unique behavioral characteristics of their newborn and to learn nurturing activities. Attachment is promoted when parents have the opportunity to explore their newborn in private, identifying individual physical and behavioral characteristics. The nurse's supportive responses to the parents' questions and observations are essential throughout the assessment process. The newborn physical examination therefore is the beginning of newborn health surveillance and health education for the newborn's family that continues into the community.

Timing of Newborn Assessments

The first 24 hours of life are significant because during this period the newborn makes the critical transition from intrauterine to extrauterine life. The risk of mortality and morbidity is statistically high during this period. Assessment of the newborn is essential to ensure that the transition is proceeding successfully (Rinehart, Terrone, & Magann, 2000).

Table 29–1 • TIMING AND TYPES OF NEWBORN ASSESSMENTS

Assess immediately after birth:
Need for resuscitation
If newborn is stable and can be placed with parents to initiate early attachment/bonding
Assessments within 1 to 4 hours after birth:
Progress of newborn's adaptation to extrauterine life
Determination of gestational age
Ongoing assessment for high-risk problems
Assessment procedures within first 24 hours or prior to discharge:
Complete physical examination (Depending on agency protocol, the nurse may complete some components independently with the certified nurse-midwife/ physician/nurse practitioner completing the exam prior to discharge.)
Nutritional status and ability to formula-feed or breastfeed satisfactorily
Behavioral state organization abilities

There are three major time frames for assessing newborns while they are in the birth facility. The first assessment is done in the birthing area immediately after birth to determine the need for resuscitation or other interventions. The newborn who is stable can stay with the family after birth to initiate early attachment. The newborn who has complications is usually taken to the nursery for further evaluation and intervention.

A second assessment is done in the first 1 to 4 hours after birth as part of the routine admission procedures. During this assessment, the nurse carries out a brief physical examination to evaluate the newborn's adaptation to extrauterine life and to estimate gestational age. The accuracy of gestational age assessment decreases when performed more than 24 hours after birth. No later than 2 hours after birth, the admitting nursery nurse should evaluate the newborn's status and any problems that place the newborn at risk (American Academy of Pediatrics [AAP] & the American College of Obstetricians and Gynecologists [ACOG], 2002).

Prior to discharge, a certified nurse-midwife, physician, or nurse practitioner carries out a behavioral assessment and a complete physical examination to detect any emerging or potential problems. A general assessment is also done at this time (Table 29–1 •).

This chapter presents the procedures for estimating gestational age and performing the complete physical examination and behavioral assessment. Chapter 24 discusses the immediate postbirth assessment. Chapter 30 describes the brief assessment performed during the first 4 hours of life.

Estimation of Gestational Age

The nurse must establish the newborn's gestational age in the first 4 hours after birth so that careful attention can be given to age-related problems. Traditionally, a newborn's gestational age was determined from the date of the pregnant woman's last menstrual period. This method was accurate only 75% to 85% of the time. Because of the problems that develop with the newborn who is preterm or whose weight is inappropriate for gestational age, a more accurate system was developed to evaluate the newborn. Once learned, the procedure can be done in a few minutes. *It is essential that the nurse wear gloves when assessing the newborn in these early hours after birth prior to the first bath.*

Clinical **gestational age assessment tools** have two components: external physical characteristics and neurologic or neuromuscular development evaluations. Both components will be discussed in detail shortly.

Physical characteristics generally include sole creases, amount of breast tissue, amount of lanugo, cartilaginous development of the ear, testicular descent, and scrotal rugae or labial development. These objective clinical criteria are not influenced by labor and birth and do not change significantly within the first 24 hours after birth.

During the first 24 hours of life, the newborn's nervous system is unstable; thus neurologic evaluation findings based on reflexes or assessments dependent on the higher brain centers may not be reliable. If the neurologic findings drastically deviate from the gestational age derived by evaluation of the external characteristics, a second assessment is done in 24 hours.

The neurologic assessment components (excluding reflexes) are especially helpful in assessing the gestational age of newborns of less than 34 weeks' gestation. This is because between 26 and 34 weeks, neurologic changes are significant, whereas significant physical changes are less evident. The most important of these neurologic changes is replacement of extensor tone by flexor tone in a caudocephalad (tail-to-head) progression.

The *estimation of gestational age by maturity rating* by Ballard, Khoury, Wedig, et al (1991) is a simplified version of the well-researched Dubowitz tool. The Ballard tool omits some of the neuromuscular tone assessments, such as head lag, ventral suspension (which is difficult to assess in very ill newborns or those on respirators), and leg recoil. In Ballard's tool, each physical and neuromuscular finding is given a value, and the total score is matched to a gestational age (Figure 29–1 •). The maximum score on the Ballard tool is 50, which corresponds to a gestational age of 44 weeks.

For example, on completing a gestational assessment of a 1-hour-old newborn, the nurse gives a score of 3 to all the physical characteristics, for a total of 18, and gives a score of 3 to all the neuromuscular assessments, for a total neurologic score of 18. The physical characteristics score of 18 is added to the neurologic score of 18 for a total score of 36, which correlates with 38+ weeks' gestation. Because all newborns vary slightly in the development of physical characteristics and maturation of neurologic function, scores will usually vary instead of all being 3, as in the example.

Postnatal gestational age assessment tools can overestimate preterm gestational age and underestimate postterm gestational age. The tools have been shown to lose accuracy when newborns of fewer than 28 weeks' or more than 43 weeks' gestation are assessed. Ballard et al (1991) added criteria for more accurate assessment of the gestational age of newborns between 20 and 28 weeks' gestation and less than 1500 g. They suggest that the assessment be made within 12 hours of birth to optimize accuracy, especially in infants of less than 26 weeks' gestational age.

In carrying out gestational age assessments, the nurse keeps in mind that some maternal conditions, such as preeclampsia, diabetes, and maternal analgesia and anesthesia, may affect certain gestational assessment components and warrant further study. Maternal diabetes, although it appears to accelerate fetal physical growth, seems to retard maturation. Maternal hypertension states, which retard fetal physical growth, seem to speed maturation.

Newborns of women with preeclampsia have a poor correlation with the criteria involving active muscle tone and edema. Maternal analgesia and anesthesia may cause the baby to have respiratory depression. Babies with respiratory distress syndrome (RDS) tend to be flaccid and edematous and to assume a "froglike" posture. These characteristics affect the scoring of the neuromuscular components of the assessment tool used.

Assessment of Physical Maturity Characteristics

The nurse first evaluates observable characteristics without disturbing the baby (Rinehart et al, 2000). Selected physical characteristics common to the Dubowitz and Ballard gestational assessment tools are presented here in the order in which they might be evaluated most effectively:

1. *Resting posture*, although a neuromuscular component, should be assessed as the baby lies undisturbed on a flat surface (Figure 29–2 •).
2. *Skin* in the preterm newborn appears thin and transparent, with veins prominent over the abdomen early in gestation. As term approaches, the skin appears opaque because of increased subcutaneous tissue. Disappearance of the protective vernix caseosa promotes skin desquamation and is commonly seen in postmature infants (infants of more than 42 weeks' gestational age and showing signs of placental insufficiency; see Chapter 32).
3. *Lanugo*, a fine hair covering, decreases as gestational age increases. The amount of lanugo is greatest at 28 to 30 weeks and then disappears, first from the face, then from the trunk and extremities.
4. *Sole (plantar) creases* are reliable indicators of gestational age in the first 12 hours of life. After this the skin of the foot begins drying, and superficial creases appear. Development of sole creases begins at the top (anterior) portion of the sole and, as gestation progresses, proceeds to the heel (Figure 29–3 •). Peeling may also occur. Plantar creases vary with race. In newborns of African descent, sole creases may be less developed at term.

MEDIALINK CASE STUDY: NEWBORN MATURITY ASSESSMENT

NEWBORN MATURITY RATING & CLASSIFICATION

ESTIMATION OF GESTATIONAL AGE BY MATURITY RATING

Symbols: X - 1st Exam O - 2nd Exam

NEUROMUSCULAR MATURITY

	−1	0	1	2	3	4	5
Posture							
Square Window (wrist)	>90°	90°	60°	45°	30°	0°	
Arm Recoil		180°	140°–180°	110°–140°	90°–110°	<90°	
Popliteal Angle	180°	160°	140°	120°	100°	90°	<90°
Scarf Sign							
Heel to Ear							

Gestation by Dates ____________ wks

Birth Date ____________ Hour ____________ am pm

APGAR ____________ 1 min ____________ 5 min

MATURITY RATING

score	weeks
−10	20
−5	22
0	24
5	26
10	28
15	30
20	32
25	34
30	36
35	38
40	40
45	42
50	44

PHYSICAL MATURITY

Skin	sticky friable transparent	gelatinous red, translucent	smooth pink, visible veins	superficial peeling &/or rash, few veins	cracking pale areas rare veins	parchment deep cracking no vessels	leathery cracked wrinkled
Lanugo	none	sparse	abundant	thinning	bald areas	mostly bald	
Plantar Surface	heel-toe 40–50 mm:−1 <40 mm:−2	>50 mm no crease	faint red marks	anterior transverse crease only	creases ant. 2/3	creases over entire sole	
Breast	imperceptible	barely perceptible	flat areola no bud	stippled areola 1–2 mm bud	raised areola 3–4 mm bud	full areola 5–10 mm bud	
Eye/Ear	lids fused loosely:−1 tightly:−2	lids open pinna flat stays folded	sl. curved pinna; soft; slow recoil	well curved pinna; soft but ready recoil	formed & firm instant recoil	thick cartilage ear stiff	
Genitals male	scrotum flat, smooth	scrotum empty faint rugae	testes in upper canal rare rugae	testes descending few rugae	testes down good rugae	testes pendulous deep rugae	
Genitals female	clitoris prominent labia flat	prominent clitoris small labia minora	prominent clitoris enlarging minora	majora & minora equally prominent	majora large minora small	majora cover clitoris & minora	

SCORING SECTION

	1st Exam = X	2nd Exam = 0
Estimating Gest Age by Maturity Rating	______Weeks	______Weeks
Time of Exam	Date ______ Hour ______ am pm	Date ______ Hour ______ am pm
Age at Exam	______ Hours	______ Hours
Signature of Examiner	______ M.D.	______ M.D.

Figure 29–1 • Newborn maturity rating and classification. If a 1-hour-old newborn is given a score of 3 for each of the physical characteristics and neuromuscular assessments, the newborn's total score would be 36. A total score of 36 correlates with 38 or more weeks' gestation.
SOURCE: Ballard, J. L., et al. (1991). New Ballard score, expanded to include extremely premature infants. *Journal of Pediatrics, 119,* 417.

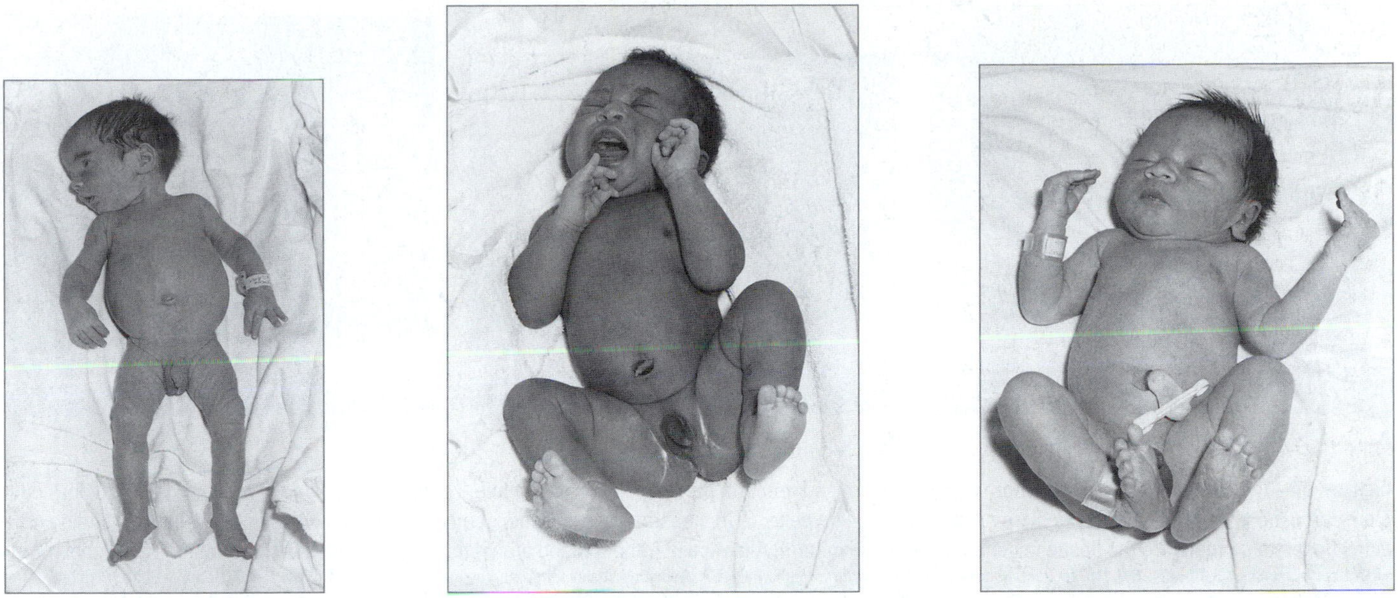

A B C

Figure 29–2 • Resting posture. *A,* Infant exhibits beginning of flexion of the thigh. The gestational age is approximately 31 weeks. Note the extension of the upper extremities. *B,* Infant exhibits stronger flexion of the arms, hips, and thighs. The gestational age is approximately 35 weeks. *C,* The full-term infant exhibits hypertonic flexion of all extremities.

SOURCE: Dubowitz, L., & Dubowitz, V. (1977). *The gestational age of the newborn.* Menlo Park, CA: Addison-Wesley. Reprinted by permission of V. Dubowitz, MD, Hammersmith Hospital, London, England.

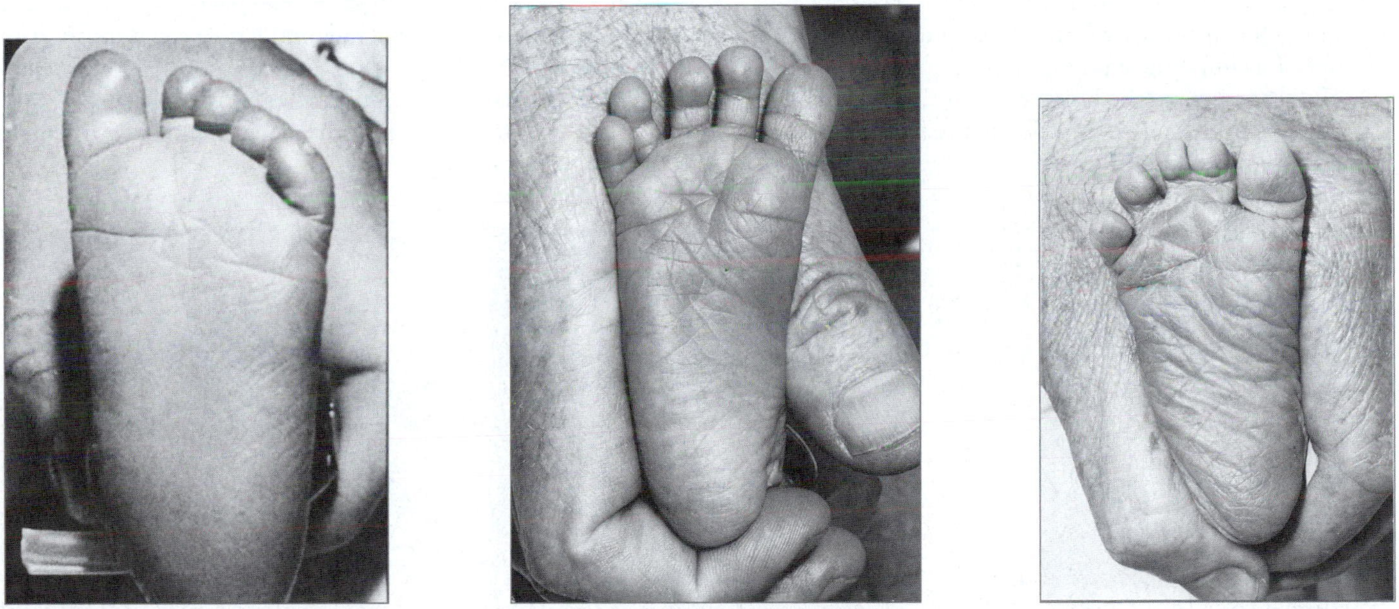

A B C

Figure 29–3 • Sole creases. *A,* Infant has a few sole creases on the anterior portion of the foot. Note the slick heel. The gestational age is approximately 35 weeks. *B,* Infant has a deeper network of sole creases on the anterior two thirds of the sole. Note the slick heel. The gestational age is approximately 37 weeks. *C,* The full-term infant has deep sole creases down to and including the heel as the skin loses fluid and dries after birth. Sole (plantar) creases can be seen even in preterm newborns.

SOURCE: Dubowitz, L., & Dubowitz, V. (1977). *Gestational age of the newborn.* Menlo Park, CA: Addison-Wesley. Reprinted by permission of V. Dubowitz, MD, Hammersmith Hospital, London, England.

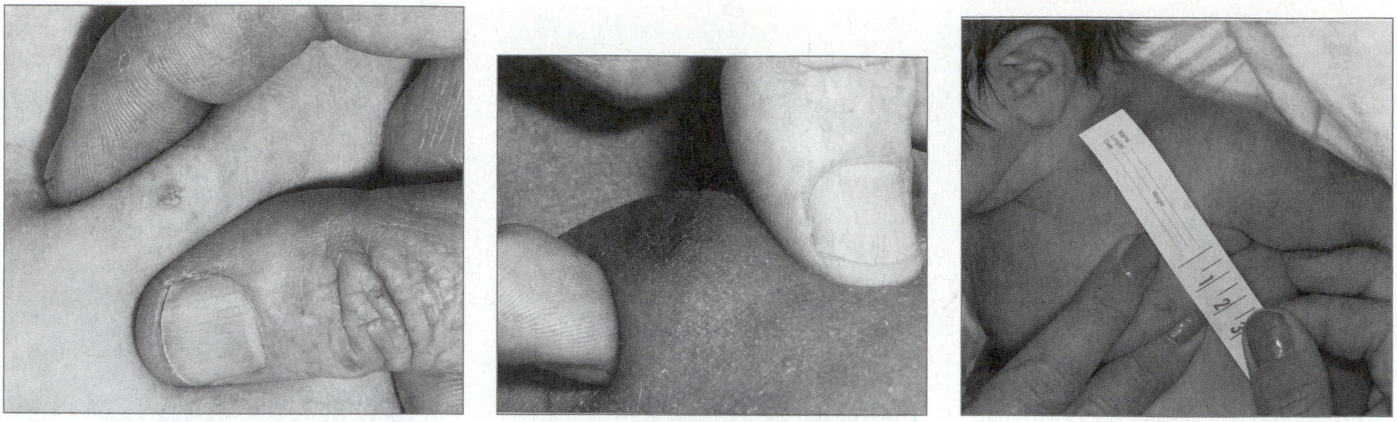

A B C

Figure 29–4 • Breast tissue. *A,* Newborn has a visible raised area. On palpation the area is 4 mm. The gestational age is 38 weeks. *B,* Newborn has a breast tissue area of 10 mm. The gestational age is 40 to 44 weeks. *C,* To measure breast tissue, gently compress the tissue between the middle and index fingers, and measure the tissue in centimeters or millimeters. Absence of or decreased breast tissue often indicates premature or SGA newborn.
SOURCE: Dubowitz, L., & Dubowitz, V. (1977). *Gestational age of the newborn.* Menlo Park, CA: Addison-Wesley. Reprinted by permission of V. Dubowitz, MD, Hammersmith Hospital, London, England.

5. The nurse inspects the *areola* and gently palpates the breast bud tissue by applying the forefinger and middle finger to the breast area and measuring the tissue between them in centimeters or millimeters (Figure 29–4 •). At term gestation, the tissue will measure between 0.5 and 1 cm (5 to 10 mm). During the assessment, the nipple should not be grasped firmly because skin and subcutaneous tissue will prevent accurate estimation of size. The nurse must do this procedure gently to avoid causing trauma to the breast tissue.

As gestation progresses, the breast tissue mass and areola enlarge. However, a large breast tissue mass can occur as a result of conditions other than advanced gestational age or the effects of maternal hormones on the baby. In the large-for-gestational-age infant of a diabetic mother, accelerated development of breast tissue is a reflection of subcutaneous fat deposits. Small-for-gestational-age term or postterm newborns may have used subcutaneous fat (which would have been deposited as breast tissue) to survive in utero; as a result their lack of breast tissue may indicate a gestational age of 34 to 35 weeks, even though other factors indicate a term or postterm newborn.

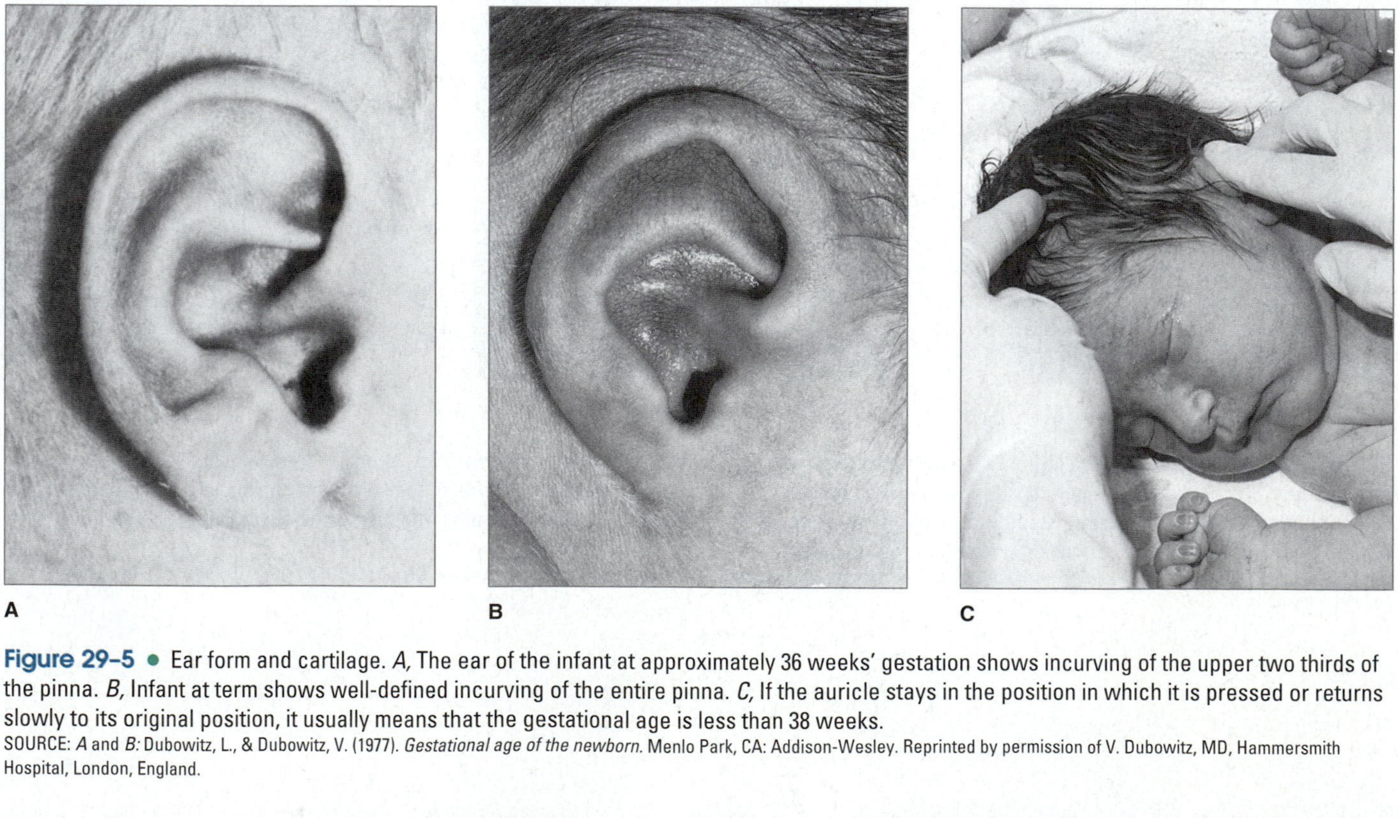

A B C

Figure 29–5 • Ear form and cartilage. *A,* The ear of the infant at approximately 36 weeks' gestation shows incurving of the upper two thirds of the pinna. *B,* Infant at term shows well-defined incurving of the entire pinna. *C,* If the auricle stays in the position in which it is pressed or returns slowly to its original position, it usually means that the gestational age is less than 38 weeks.
SOURCE: *A* and *B:* Dubowitz, L., & Dubowitz, V. (1977). *Gestational age of the newborn.* Menlo Park, CA: Addison-Wesley. Reprinted by permission of V. Dubowitz, MD, Hammersmith Hospital, London, England.

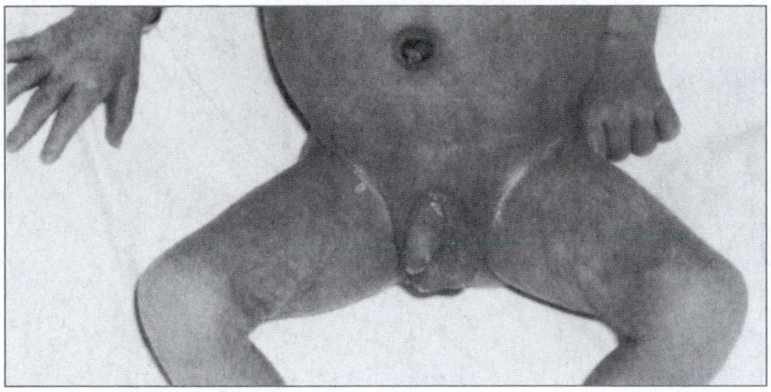

A

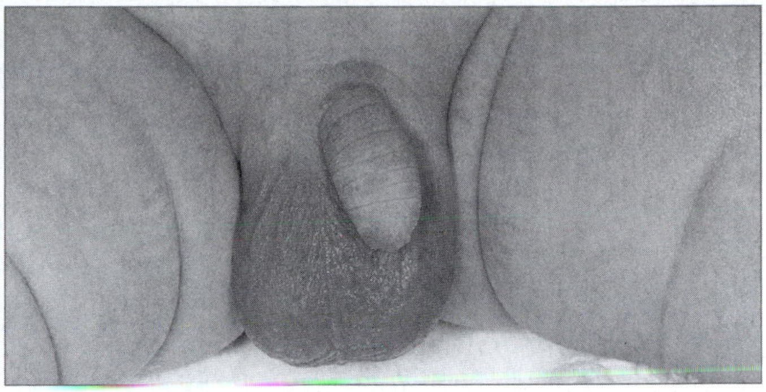

B

Figure 29–6 • Male genitals. *A,* Preterm infant's testes are not within the scrotum. The scrotal surface has few rugae. *B,* Term infant's testes are generally fully descended. The entire surface of the scrotum is covered by rugae.
SOURCE: Dubowitz, L., & Dubowitz, V. (1977). *Gestational age of the newborn.* Menlo Park, CA: Addison-Wesley. Reprinted by permission of V. Dubowitz, MD, Hammersmith Hospital, London, England.

6. *Ear form and cartilage distribution* develop with gestational age. The cartilage gives the ear its shape and substance (Figure 29–5 •). In a newborn of less than 34 weeks' gestation, the ear is relatively shapeless and flat; it has little cartilage, so the ear folds over on itself and remains folded. By approximately 36 weeks' gestation, some cartilage and slight incurving of the upper pinna are present, and the pinna springs back slowly when folded. (The nurse tests this response by holding the top and bottom of the pinna together with the forefinger and thumb and then releasing it, or by folding the pinna of the ear forward against the side of the head and releasing it, and observing the response.) By term, the newborn's pinna is firm, stands away from the head, and springs back quickly from the folding.
7. *Male genitals* are evaluated for size of the scrotal sac, the presence of rugae, and descent of the testes (Figure 29–6 •). Prior to 36 weeks, the small scrotum has few rugae, and the testes are palpable in the inguinal canal. By 36 to 38 weeks, the testes are in the upper scrotum, and rugae have developed over the anterior portion of the scrotum. By term, the testes are generally in the lower scrotum, which is pendulous and covered with rugae.
8. The appearance of the *female genitals* depends in part on subcutaneous fat deposition and therefore relates to fetal nutritional status (Figure 29–7 •). The clitoris varies in size and occasionally is so large that it is difficult to identify the sex of the newborn. This may be caused by adrenogenital syndrome, which causes the adrenals to secrete excessive amounts of androgen and other hormones. At 30 to 32 weeks' gestation, the clitoris is prominent, and the labia majora are small and widely separated. As gestational age increases, the labia majora increase in size. At 36 to 40 weeks, they nearly cover the clitoris. At 40 weeks and beyond, the labia majora cover the labia minora and clitoris.

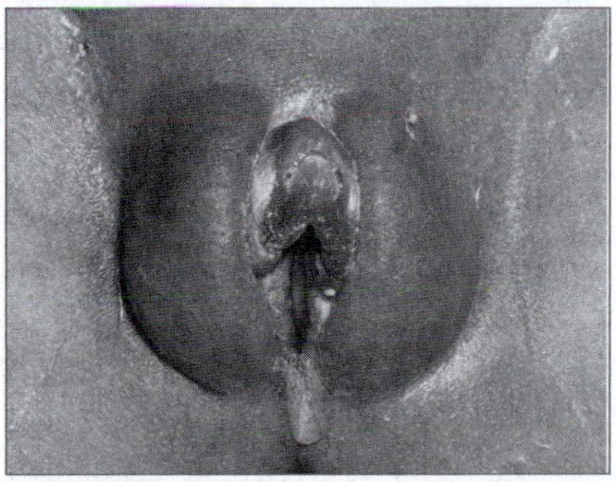

A

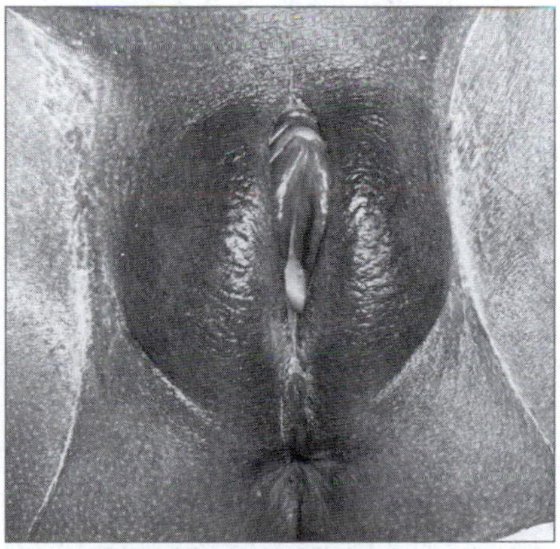

B

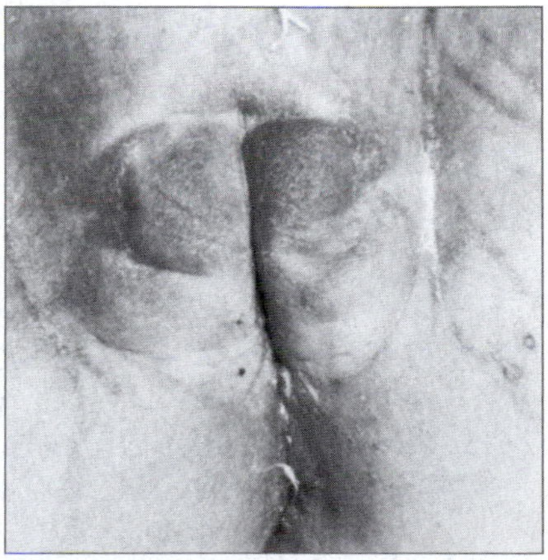

C

Figure 29–7 • Female genitals. *A,* Infant has a prominent clitoris. The labia majora are widely separated, and the labia minora, viewed laterally, would protrude beyond the labia majora. The gestational age is 30 to 36 weeks. *B,* The clitoris is still visible. The labia minora are now covered by the larger labia majora. The gestational age is 36 to 40 weeks. *C,* The term infant has well-developed, large labia majora that cover both clitoris and labia minora.
SOURCE: Dubowitz, L., & Dubowitz, V. (1977). *Gestational age of the newborn.* Menlo Park, CA: Addison-Wesley. Reprinted by permission of V. Dubowitz, MD, Hammersmith Hospital, London, England.

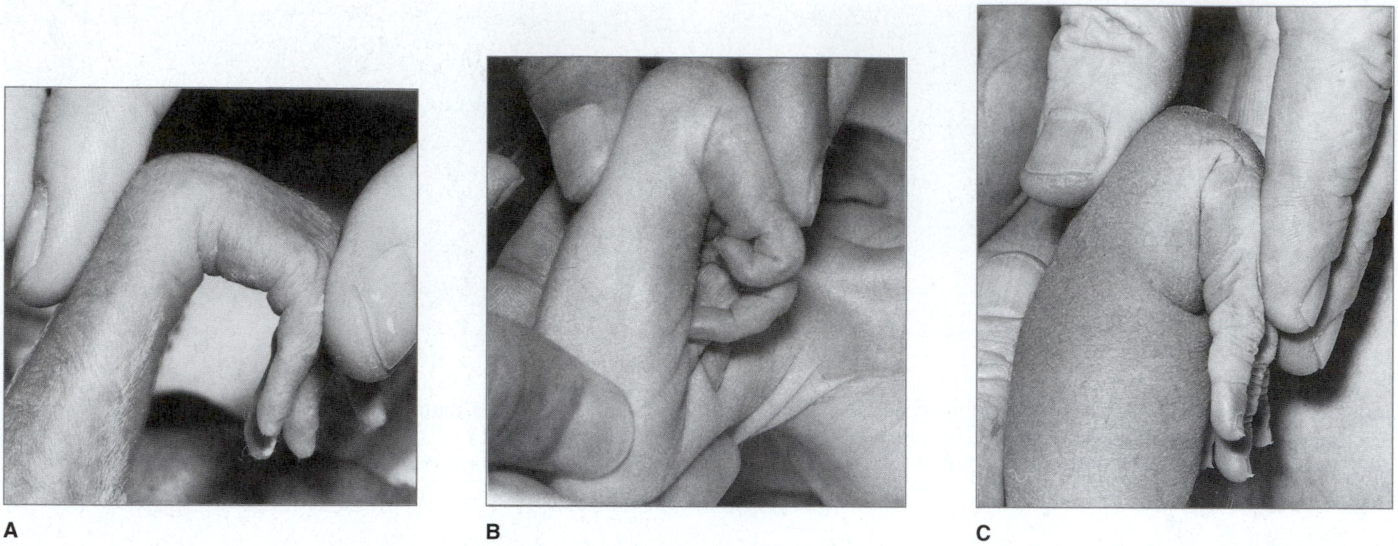

Figure 29–8 • Square window sign. *A,* This angle is 90 degrees and suggests an immature newborn of 28 to 32 weeks' gestation. *B,* A 30-degree angle is commonly found in newborns from 38 to 40 weeks' gestation. *C,* A 0-degree angle occurs in newborns from 40 to 42 weeks' gestation.
SOURCE: Dubowitz, L., & Dubowitz, V. (1977). *Gestational age of the newborn.* Menlo Park, CA: Addison-Wesley. Reprinted by permission of V. Dubowitz, MD, Hammersmith Hospital, London, England.

Other physical characteristics assessed by some gestational age scoring tools include the following:

1. *Vernix* covers the preterm newborn. The postterm newborn has no vernix. After noting vernix distribution, the birthing area nurse (wearing gloves) dries the newborn to prevent evaporative heat loss, thus disturbing the vernix and potentially altering this gestational age criterion. The birthing area nurse must communicate to the neonatal nurse the amount of vernix and the areas of vernix coverage.
2. *Hair* of the preterm newborn has the consistency of matted wool or fur and lies in bunches rather than in the silky, single strands of the term newborn's hair.
3. *Skull firmness* increases as the fetus matures. In a term newborn, the bones are hard, and the sutures are not easily displaced. The nurse should not attempt to displace the sutures forcibly.
4. *Nails* appear and cover the nail bed at about 20 weeks' gestation. Nails extending beyond the fingertips may indicate a postterm newborn.

Assessment of Neuromuscular Maturity Characteristics

The central nervous system of the human fetus matures at a fairly constant rate. Tests have been designed to evaluate neurologic status as manifested by development of neuromuscular tone. As noted earlier, in the fetus, neuromuscular

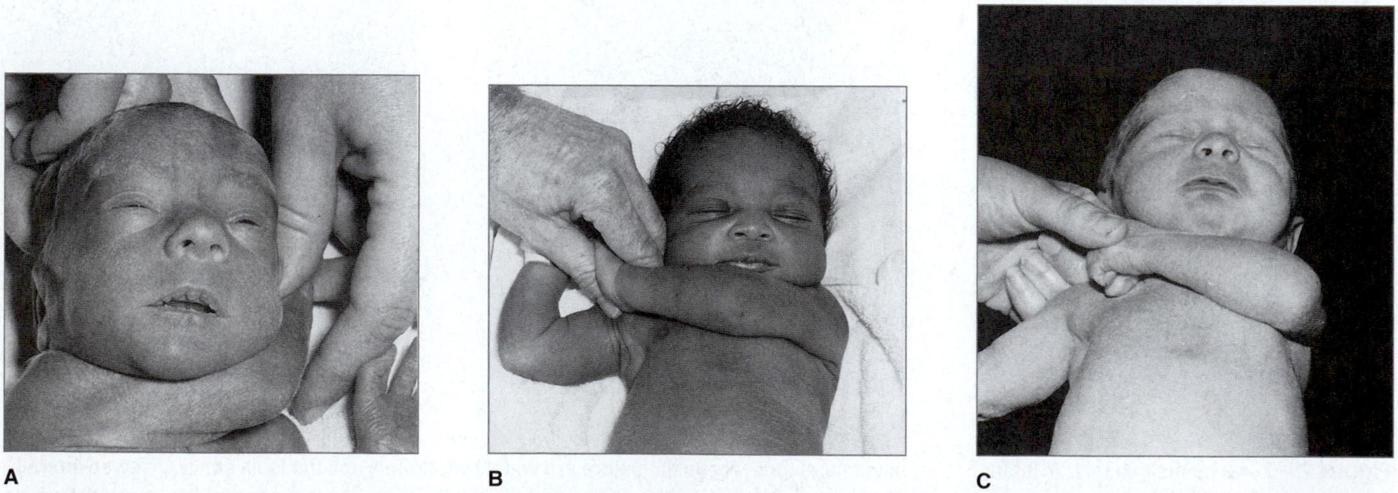

Figure 29–9 • Scarf sign. *A,* No resistance is noted until after 30 weeks' gestation. The elbow can be readily moved past the midline. *B,* The elbow is at midline at 36 to 40 weeks' gestation. *C,* Beyond 40 weeks' gestation, the elbow will not reach the midline.
SOURCE: Dubowitz, L., & Dubowitz, V. (1977). *Gestational age of the newborn.* Menlo Park, CA: Addison-Wesley. Reprinted by permission of V. Dubowitz, MD, Hammersmith Hospital, London, England.

tone develops in a caudocephalic direction, from the lower to the upper extremities.

Because the neurologic evaluation requires more manipulation and disturbances than the physical evaluation of the newborn, it is best performed when the infant has stabilized. The following characteristics are evaluated (Figure 29–1):

1. The *square window sign* is elicited by flexing the baby's hand toward the ventral forearm until resistance is felt. The angle formed at the wrist is measured (Figure 29–8 •).
2. *Recoil* is a test of flexion development. Because flexion first develops in the lower extremities, recoil is first tested in the legs. The newborn is placed on its back on a flat surface. With a hand on the newborn's knees and while manipulating the hip joint, the nurse places the baby's legs in flexion, then extends them parallel to each other and flat on the surface. The response to this maneuver is recoil of the newborn's legs. According to gestational age, they may not move, or they may return slowly or quickly to the flexed position. Preterm infants have less muscle tone than term infants, so preterm infants have less recoil.

   Arm recoil is tested by flexion at the elbow and extension of the arms at the newborn's side. While the baby is in the supine position, the nurse completely flexes both elbows, holds them in this position for 5 seconds, extends the arms at the baby's side, and releases them. Upon release, the elbows of a full-term newborn form an angle of less than 90 degrees and rapidly recoil back to flexed position. The elbows of preterm newborns have slower recoil time and form a greater than 90-degree angle. Arm recoil is also slower in healthy but fatigued newborns after birth; therefore, arm recoil is best elicited after the first hour of birth, when the baby has had time to recover from the stress of birth. The deep sleep state also decreases the arm recoil response. Assessment of arm recoil should be bilateral to rule out brachial palsy.
3. The *popliteal angle* (degree of knee flexion) is determined with the newborn flat on its back. The thigh is flexed on the abdomen and chest, and the nurse places the index finger of the other hand behind the newborn's ankle to extend the lower leg until resistance is met. The angle formed is then measured. Results vary from no resistance in the very immature newborn to an 80-degree angle in the term newborn.
4. The *scarf sign* is elicited by placing the newborn supine and drawing an arm across the chest toward the newborn's opposite shoulder until resistance is met. The location of the elbow is then noted in relation to the midline of the chest (Figure 29–9 •).
5. The *heel-to-ear extension* is performed by placing the newborn in a supine position and then gently drawing the foot toward the ear on the same side until resistance is felt. The nurse should allow the knee to bend during the test. It is important to hold the buttocks down to keep from rolling the baby. Both the proximity of foot to ear and degree of knee extension are assessed. A preterm, immature newborn's leg will remain straight, and its foot will go to the ear or beyond. With advancing gestational age, the newborn demonstrates increasing resistance to this maneuver. Maneuvers involving the lower extremities of newborns who had frank breech presentation should be delayed to allow for resolution of leg positioning.
6. *Ankle dorsiflexion* is determined by flexing the ankle on the shin. The examiner uses a thumb to push on the sole of the newborn's foot while the fingers support the back of the leg. Then the angle formed by the foot and the interior leg is measured (Figure 29–10 •). This sign can be influenced by intrauterine position and congenital deformities.
7. *Head lag* (neck flexors) is measured by pulling the baby to a sitting position and noting the degree of head lag. Total lag is common in infants up to 34 weeks' gestation, whereas the postmature newborn (42+ weeks) will hold the head in front of the body line. Full-term newborns are able to support their heads momentarily.

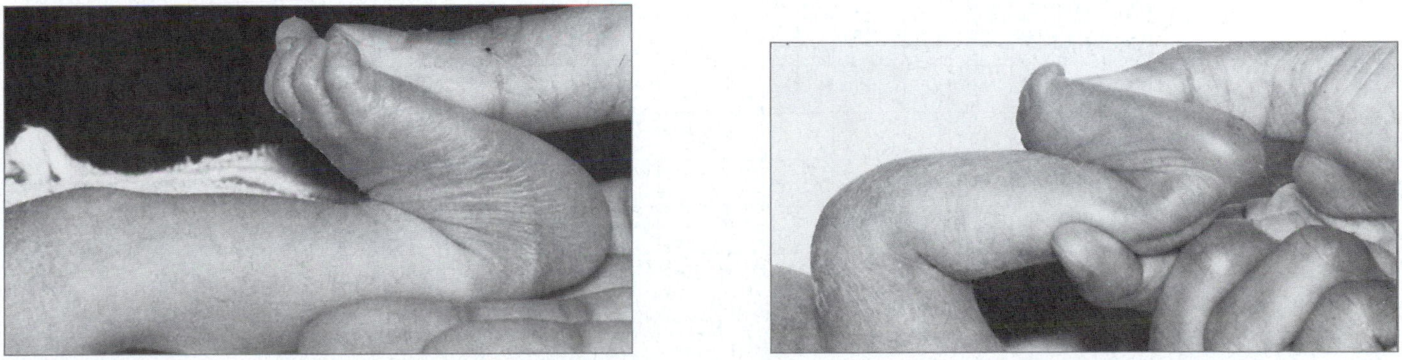

A B

Figure 29–10 • Ankle dorsiflexion. *A,* A 45-degree angle indicates 32 to 36 weeks' gestation. A 20-degree angle indicates 36 to 40 weeks' gestation. *B,* A 0-degree angle is common at gestational age of 40 weeks or more.

SOURCE: Dubowitz, L., & Dubowitz, V. (1977). *Gestational age of the newborn.* Menlo Park, CA: Addison-Wesley. Reprinted by permission of V. Dubowitz, MD, Hammersmith Hospital, London, England.

8. *Ventral suspension* (horizontal position) is evaluated by holding the newborn prone on the examiner's hand. The position of head and back and degree of flexion in the arms and legs are then noted. Some flexion of arms and legs indicates 36 to 38 weeks' gestation; fully flexed extremities, with head and back even, are characteristic of a term newborn.
9. Major reflexes such as sucking, rooting, grasping, Moro, tonic neck, Babinski, and others are also evaluated during the newborn exam. These are discussed later in the chapter.

A supplementary method for estimating gestational age (done by the physician or nurse practitioner) is to view the vascular network of the cornea with an ophthalmoscope. The amount of vascularity present over the surface of the lens has excellent correlation with infants of 27 through 34 weeks' gestational age. In babies of less than 27 weeks' gestation, the cornea is cloudy, and the vascular network is not visible; after 34 weeks' gestation the vascular network has generally disappeared completely.

When the gestational age determination and birth weight are considered together, the newborn can be identified as one whose *growth is below the 10th percentile*, or *small for gestational age (SGA); appropriate for gestational age (AGA);* or *above the 90th percentile*, or *large for gestational age (LGA)* (Figure 29–11 •). This determination enables the nurse to anticipate possible physiologic problems. This information is used in conjunction with a complete physical examination to establish a plan of care appropriate for the individual newborn. For example, an SGA newborn often requires frequent glucose monitoring and early feedings. See Chapter 32 for discussion of these categories and their potential problems.

The nurse also plots the gestational age against the newborn's length, head circumference, and weight on the appropriate growth chart to determine whether these measurements fall within the average range—the 10th to 90th percentile for the corresponding gestational age (Figure 29–12 •). These

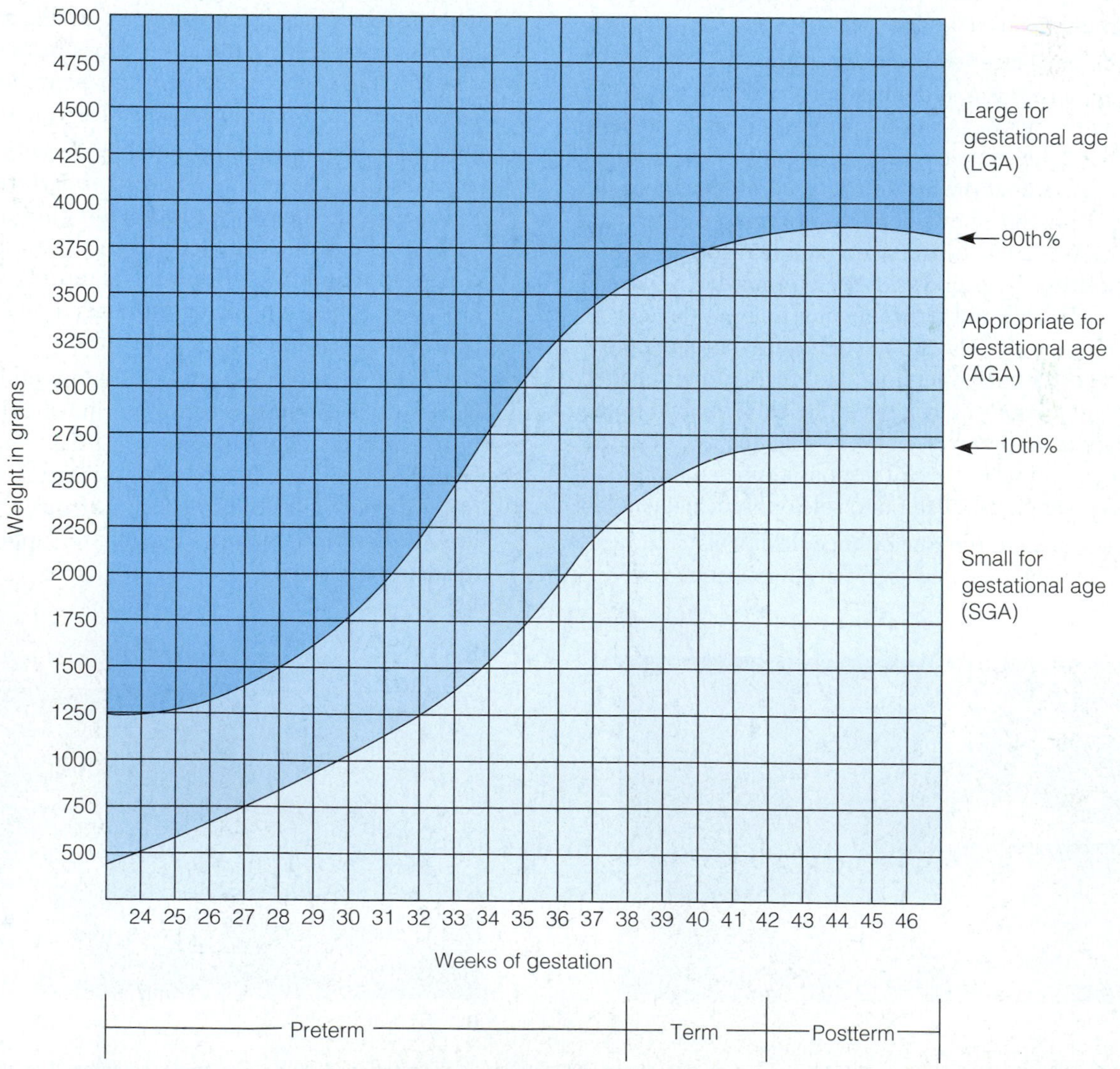

Figure 29–11 • Classification of newborns by birth weight and gestational age. The newborn's birth weight and gestational age are placed on the graph. The newborn is then classified as large for gestational age (LGA), appropriate for gestational age (AGA), or small for gestational age (SGA).
SOURCE: Battaglia, F. C., & Lubchenco, L. O. (1967). A practical classification of newborn infants by weight and gestational age. *Journal of Pediatrics, 71*, 161.

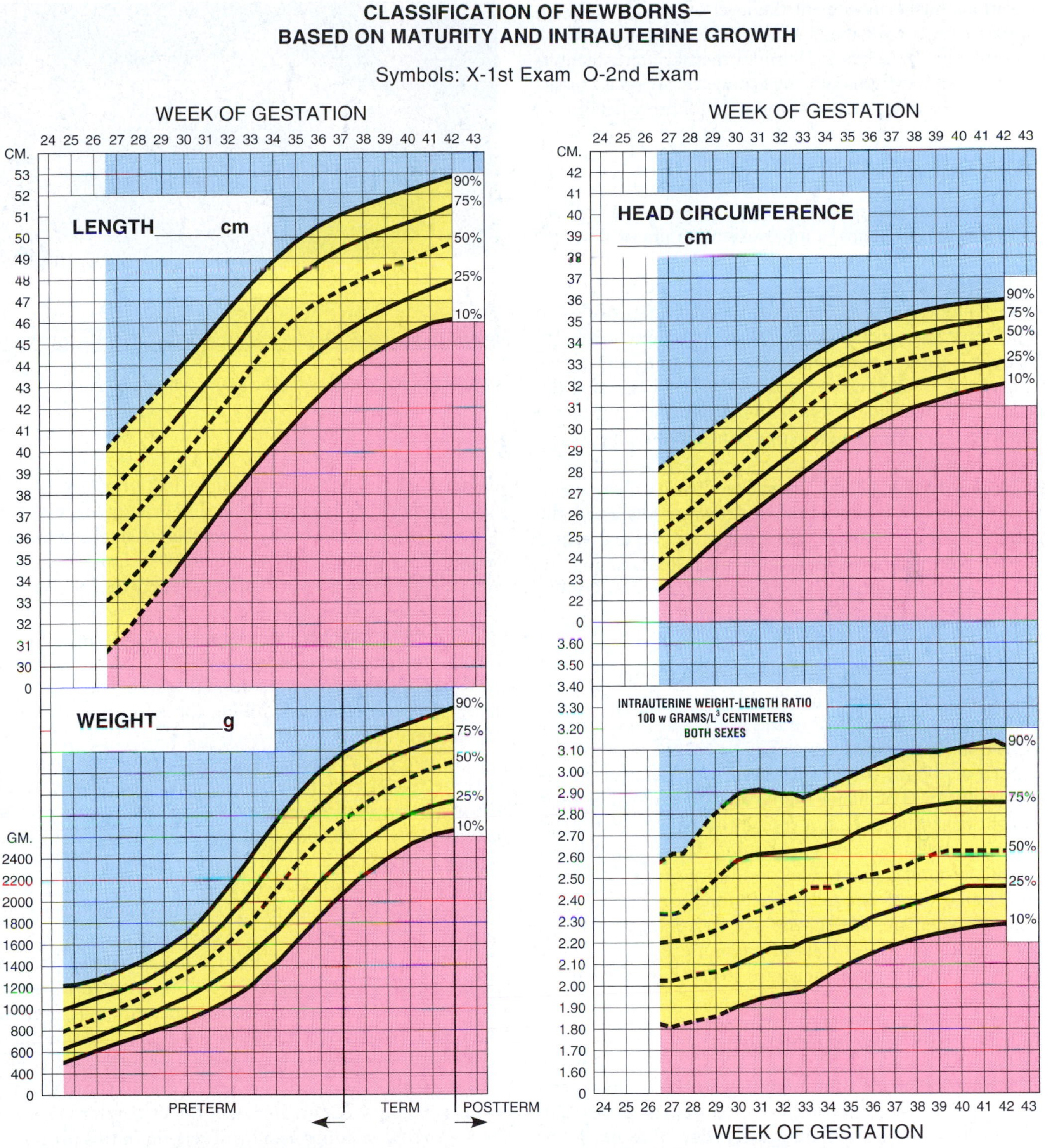

	1st Exam (X)	2nd Exam (O)
LARGE FOR GESTATIONAL AGE **(LGA)**		
APPROPRIATE FOR GESTATIONAL AGE **(AGA)**		
SMALL FOR GESTATIONAL AGE **(SGA)**		
Age at Exam	hrs	hrs
Signature of Examiner	M.D.	M.D.

Figure 29–12 ● Classification of newborns based on maturity and intrauterine growth.

SOURCE: Adapted from Lubchenco, L.O., Hansman, C., & Boyd, E. (1966). *Pediatrics, 37,* 404, Figure 1. Reprinted with permission from the American Academy of Pediatrics. Battaglia, F. C., & Lubchenco, L. O. (1967). A practical classification of newborn infants by weight and gestational age. *Journal of Pediatrics, 71,* 161.

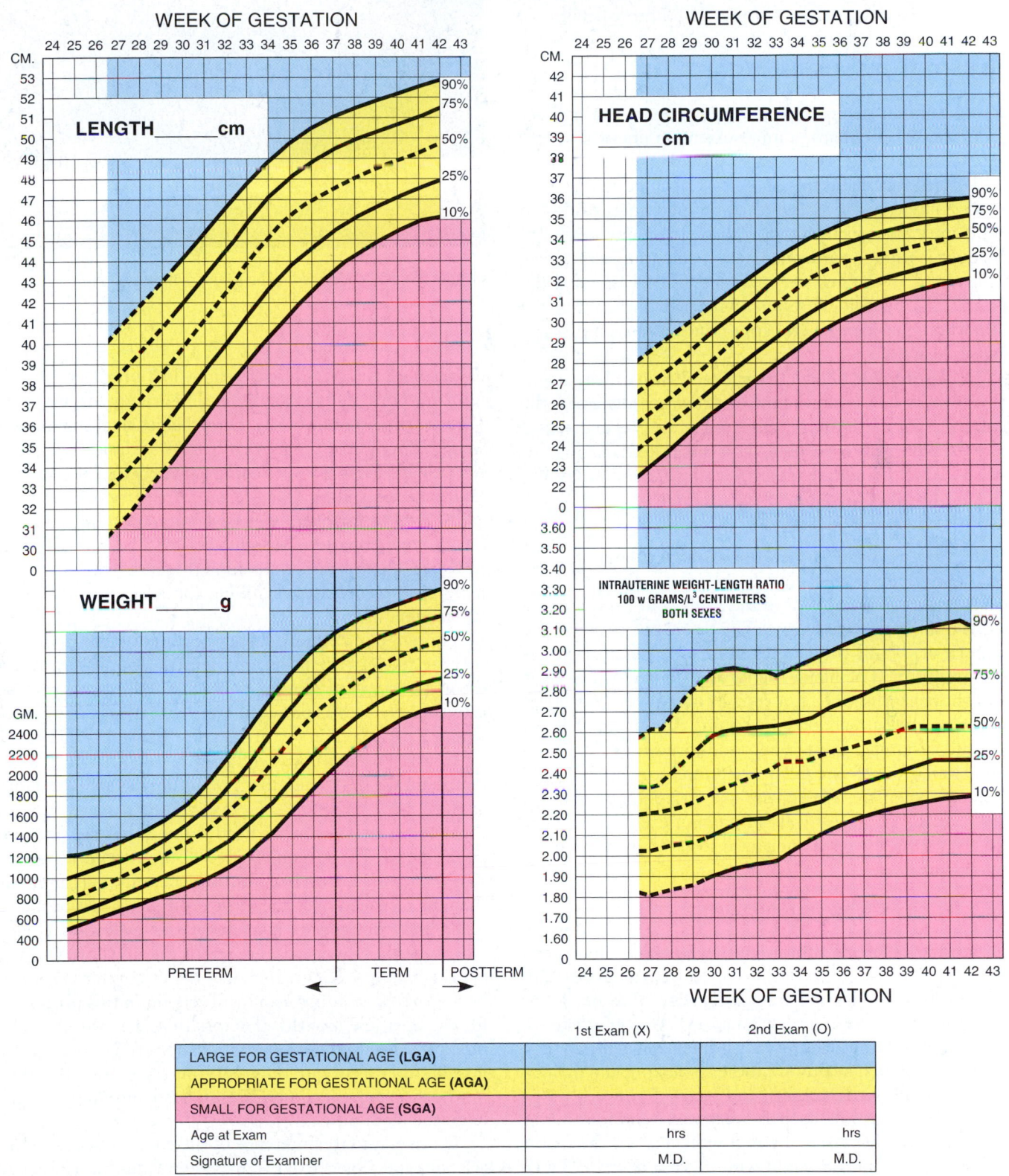

correlations further document the level of maturity and appropriate category for the newborn. The comparison of the newborn's ratio of weight to length further facilitates identification of SGA newborns as being symmetrically or asymmetrically growth restricted. See Chapter 32 for more detail.

Physical Assessment

After the initial determination of gestational age and related potential problems, a more extensive physical assessment is carried out. The nurse should choose a warm, well-lighted area that is free of drafts. Completing the physical assessment in the presence of the parents provides an opportunity to acquaint them with their unique newborn. The examination is performed in a systematic, head-to-toe manner, and all findings are recorded. When assessing the physical and neurologic status of the newborn, the nurse should first consider general appearance and then proceed to specific areas.

The Assessment Guide: Newborn Physical Assessment on pages 822–835 outlines how to systematically assess the newborn. Normal findings, alterations, and related causes are presented and correlated with suggested nursing responses. The findings are typical for a full-term newborn.

General Appearance

The newborn's head is disproportionately large for the body. The center of the baby's body is the umbilicus rather than the symphysis pubis, as in the adult. The body appears long and the extremities short. The flexed position that the newborn maintains contributes to the short appearance of the extremities. The hands are tightly clenched. The neck looks short because the chin rests on the chest. Newborns have a prominent abdomen, sloping shoulders, narrow hips, and a rounded chest. They tend to stay in a flexed position similar to the one maintained in utero and will offer resistance when the extremities are straightened. After a breech birth, the feet are usually dorsiflexed, and it may take several weeks for the newborn to assume typical newborn posture.

Weight and Measurements

The normal full-term Caucasian newborn has an average birth weight of 3405 g (7 lb, 8 oz). Newborns of African, Asian, or Mexican descent are usually somewhat smaller at term (Overpeck, Hediger, Zhang, et al, 1999; Wu & Daniel, 2001). Other factors that influence weight are age and size of parents, health of mother (smoking and malnutrition decrease birth weight), and interval between pregnancies (short intervals, such as every year, tend to result in lower birth weight). After the first week and for the first 6 months, the newborn's weight will increase about 198 g (7 oz) weekly.

Approximately 70% to 75% of the newborn's body weight is water. During the initial newborn period (the first 3 or 4 days), there is a physiologic weight loss of 5% to 10% for term newborns due to fluid shifts. This weight loss may reach 15% for preterm newborns. Large babies tend to lose more weight. If weight loss is greater than 10%, clinical reappraisal is necessary. Factors contributing to weight loss include small fluid intake resulting from delayed breastfeeding or a slow adjustment to formula, increased volume of meconium excreted, and urination. Weight loss may be marked in the presence of temperature elevation (because of associated dehydration) or consistent chilling (because of nonshivering thermogenesis).

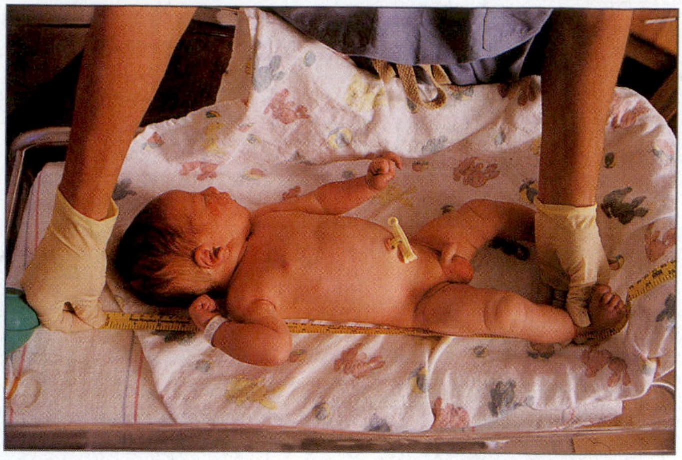

Figure 29–13 ● Measuring the length of the newborn.

The length of the normal newborn is difficult to measure because the legs are flexed and tensed. To measure length, the nurse should place newborns flat on their backs with legs extended as much as possible (Figure 29–13 ●). The average length is 50 cm (20 in), with the range being 48 to 52 cm (18 to 22 in). The newborn will grow approximately 1 inch a month for the next 6 months. This is the period of most rapid growth.

At birth, the newborn's head is one third the size of an adult's head. The circumference of the newborn's head is 32 to 37 cm (12.5 to 14.5 in). For accurate measurement, the tape is placed over the most prominent part of the occiput and brought to just above the eyebrows (Figure 29–14, *A* ●). The circumference of the newborn's head is approximately 2 cm greater than the circumference of the newborn's chest at birth and will remain in this proportion for the next few months. (Factors that alter this measurement are discussed under the Head section.) It is best to take another head circumference on the second day if the newborn experienced significant head molding or caput from the birth process.

The average circumference of the chest at birth is 32 cm (12.5 in) and ranges from 30 to 35 cm. Chest measurements should be taken with the tape measure at the lower edge of the scapulas and brought around anteriorly directly over the nipple line (Figure 29–14, *B* and Table 29–2 ●). The abdom-

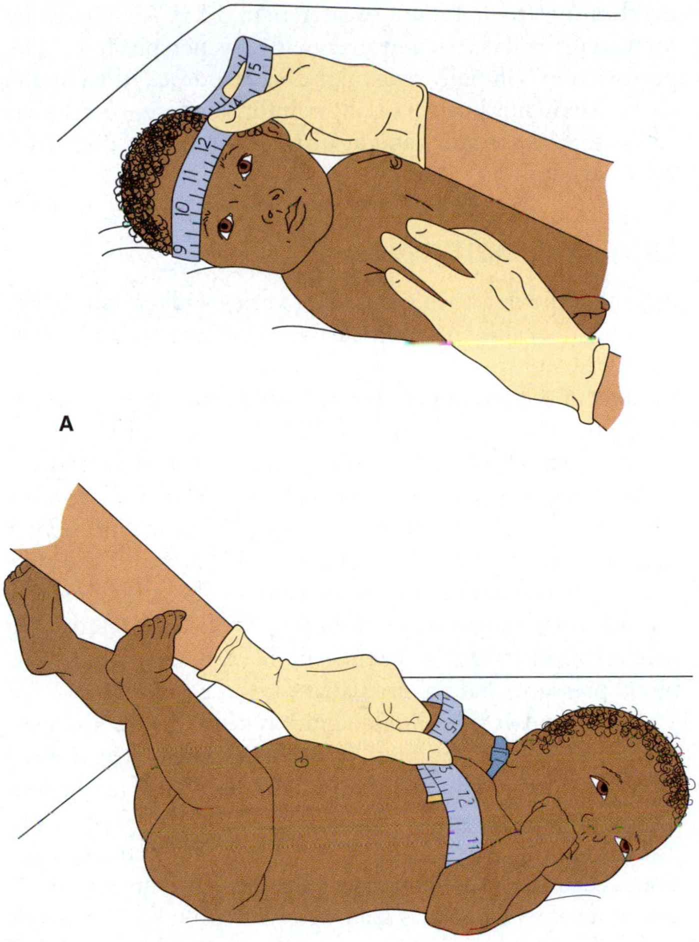

Figure 29–14 • *A*, Measuring the head circumference of the newborn. *B*, Measuring the chest circumference of the newborn.

Table 29–2 • NEWBORN MEASUREMENTS

Weight	
Average: 3405 g (7 lb, 8 oz)	
Range: 2500–4000 g (5 lb, 8 oz–8 lb, 13 oz)	
Weight is influenced by racial origin and maternal age and size.	
Physiologic weight loss: 5%–10% for term newborns, up to 15% for preterm newborns	
Growth: 198 g (7 oz) per week for first 6 months	
Length	
Average: 50 cm (20 in)	
Range: 48–52 cm (18–22 in)	
Growth: 2.5 cm (1 in) per month for first 6 months	
Head Circumference	
32–37 cm (12.5–14.5 in)	
Approximately 2 cm larger than chest circumference	
Chest Circumference	
Average: 32 cm (12.5 in)	
Range: 30–35 cm (12–14 in)	

inal circumference or girth may also be measured at this time by placing the tape around the newborn's abdomen at the level of the umbilicus, with the bottom edge of the tape at the top edge of the umbilicus.

Temperature

Initial assessment of the newborn's temperature is critical. In utero, the temperature of the fetus is about the same as or slightly higher than the expectant mother's. When babies enter the outside world, their temperatures can suddenly drop as a result of exposure to cold drafts and the skin's heat loss mechanisms.

If no heat conservation measures are started, the normal term newborn's deep body temperature falls 0.1C (0.2F) per minute; skin temperature lowers 0.3C (0.5F) per minute. Skin temperature markedly decreases within 10 minutes after exposure to room air. The temperature should stabilize within 8 to 12 hours. Temperature should be monitored when the newborn is admitted to the nursery and at least every 30 minutes until the newborn's status has remained stable for 2 hours. Thereafter the nurse should assess temperature at least once every 8 hours or according to institutional policy (AAP & ACOG, 2002). (See Chapter 28 for a discussion of the physiology of temperature regulation).

Temperature can be assessed by the axillary skin method, a continuous skin probe, the rectal route, or a tympanic thermometer. Axillary temperature reflects body (core) temperature and the body's compensatory response to the thermal environment. Axillary temperatures are the preferred method and are considered to be a close estimation of the rectal temperature. In preterm and term newborns there is less than 0.1C (0.2F) difference between temperatures taken by the axillary and rectal route. If the axillary method is used, the thermometer must remain in place at least 3 minutes, unless an electronic thermometer is used (Figure 29–15 •). Axillary temperature ranges from

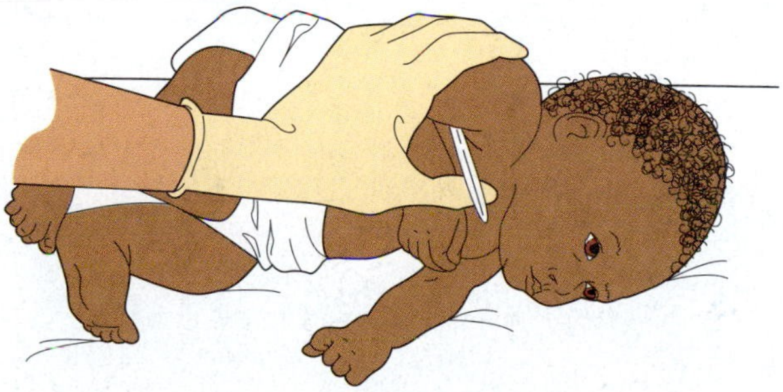

Figure 29–15 • Axillary temperature measurement. The axillary temperature should be taken for 3 minutes. The newborn's arm should be tightly but gently pressed against the thermometer and the newborn's side, as illustrated.

36.5C to 37.0C (97.7F to 98.6F). Keep in mind that axillary temperatures can be misleading because the friction caused by apposition of the inner arm skin and upper chest wall and the nearness of brown fat to the probe may elevate the temperature.

Skin temperature is measured most accurately by continuous skin probe, especially for small newborns or newborns maintained in incubators or under radiant warmers. Normal skin temperature is 36C to 36.5C (96.8F to 97.7F). Assessing skin temperature allows time for interventions to be initiated before a more serious fall in core temperature occurs (Figure 29–16 •).

Rectal temperature is assumed to be the closest approximation to core temperature, but the accuracy of this method depends on the depth to which the thermometer is inserted. Normal rectal temperature is 36.6C to 37.2C (97.8F to 99F). The rectal route is not recommended as a routine method because it may predispose to rectal mucosal irritation and increase chances of perforation. Many institutions use tympanic thermometers. These are portable sensor probes with disposable covers that are placed in the auditory canal. The probe uses infrared technology to measure the temperature of the internal carotid artery blood flow within several seconds. Research suggests that tympanic and digital thermometer axillary temperatures provide accurate estimations of body temperature in *healthy* newborns (Blackburn, 2003). Current research still questions the accuracy of tympanic thermometer readings from sick or potentially ill newborns (Blackburn, 2003).

Temperature instability, a deviation of more than 1C (2F) from one reading to the next, or a subnormal temperature may indicate an infection. In contrast with an elevated temperature in older children, an increased temperature in a newborn may indicate reactions to too many coverings, too hot a room, or dehydration. Dehydration, which tends to increase body temperature, occurs in newborns whose feedings have been delayed for any reason. Newborns respond to overheating (temperature greater than 37.5C or 99.5F) by increased restlessness and eventually by perspiration. The perspiration is initially seen on the head and face, then on the chest. Many newborns initially cannot perspire, so they increase their respiratory and heart rates, which increases oxygen consumption.

Skin Characteristics

Although the newborn's skin color varies with genetic background, all healthy newborns have a pink tinge to their skin. The ruddy hue results from increased red blood cell concentrations in the blood vessels and from limited subcutaneous fat deposits.

Skin pigmentation is slight in the newborn period, so color changes may be seen even in darker skinned babies. A newborn who is cyanotic at rest and pink only with crying may have choanal atresia (congenital blockage of the passageway between the nose and pharynx). If crying increases the cyanosis, heart or lung problems may be suspected. Very pale newborns may be anemic or have hypovolemia (low blood pressure) and are evaluated for these problems.

Acrocyanosis (bluish discoloration of the hands and feet) may be present in the first 2 to 6 hours after birth (Figure 29–17 •). This condition is due to poor peripheral circulation, which results in vasomotor instability and capillary stasis, especially when the baby is exposed to cold. If the central circulation is adequate, the blood supply should return quickly to the extremity after the skin is blanched with a finger. Blue hands and nails are a poor indicator of oxygenation in a newborn. The face and mucous membranes should be assessed for pinkness reflecting adequate oxygenation.

Mottling (lacy pattern of dilated blood vessels under the skin) occurs as a result of general circulation fluctuations. It may last several hours to several weeks or may come and go periodically. Mottling may be related to chilling or prolonged apnea.

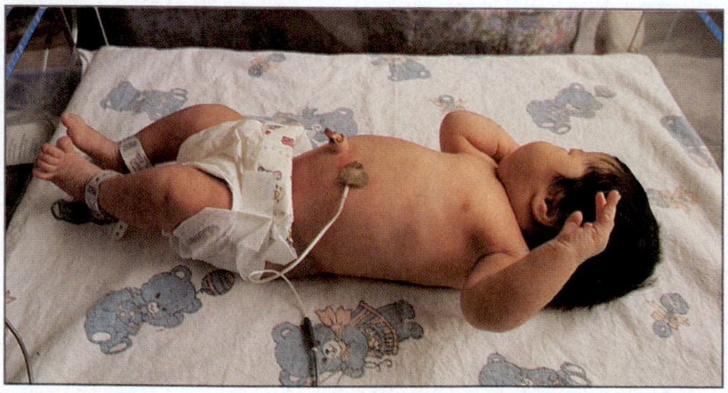

Figure 29–16 • Temperature monitoring for the newborn. A skin thermal sensor is placed on the newborn's abdomen, upper thigh, or arm and secured with porous tape or a foil-covered foam pad.

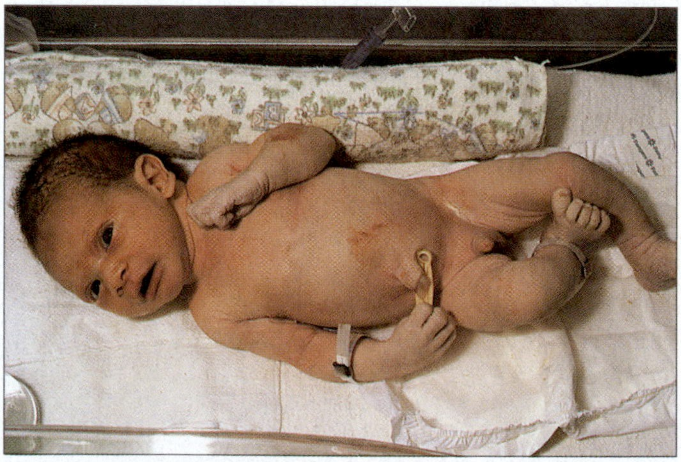

Figure 29–17 • Acrocyanosis.

Harlequin sign (clown) color change is occasionally noted. A deep color develops over one side of the newborn's body while the other side remains pale, so that the skin resembles a clown's suit. This color change results from a vasomotor disturbance in which blood vessels on one side dilate while the vessels on the other side constrict. It usually lasts from 1 to 20 minutes. Affected newborns may have single or multiple episodes, but they are transient and not of clinical significance.

Jaundice is first detectable on the face (where skin overlies cartilage) and the mucous membranes of the mouth. It is evaluated by blanching the tip of the nose, the forehead, or the gum line. This procedure must be carried out in appropriate lighting. If jaundice is present, the area will appear yellowish immediately after blanching. Another area to assess for jaundice is the sclera. Jaundice must be evaluated and its cause determined immediately to prevent possibly serious sequelae. The jaundice may be related to breastfeeding (in a few cases), hematomas, immature liver function, or bruises from forceps, or it may be caused by blood incompatibility, oxytocin (Pitocin) augmentation or induction, or severe hemolytic process. Any jaundice noted before 24 hours of age should be reported to the physician or nurse practitioner. For a detailed discussion of the causes and assessment of jaundice, see Chapter 33.

Erythema toxicum is a perifollicular eruption of lesions that are firm, vary in size from 1 to 3 mm, and consist of a white or pale yellow papule or pustule with an erythematous base. It is often called "newborn rash" or "flea bite" dermatitis. The rash may appear suddenly, usually over the trunk and diaper area, and is frequently widespread (Figure 29–18 •). The lesions do not appear on the palms of the hands or the soles of the feet. The peak incidence is at 24 to 48 hours of life. The condition rarely presents at birth or after 5 days of life. The cause is unknown and no treatment is necessary. Some clinicians feel it may be caused by irritation from clothing. The lesions disappear in a few hours or days.

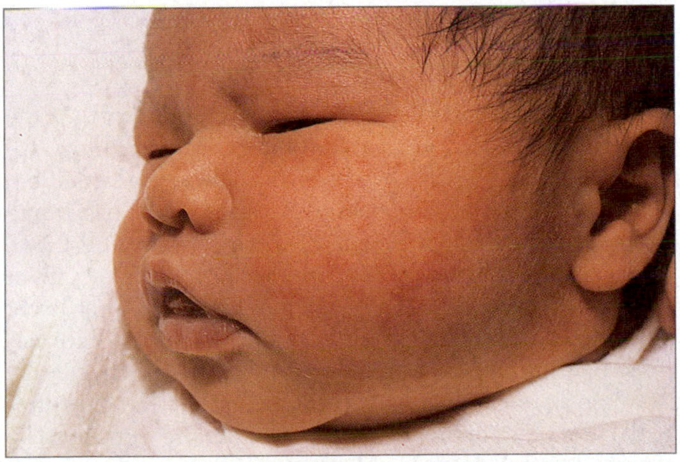

Figure 29–18 • Erythema toxicum.

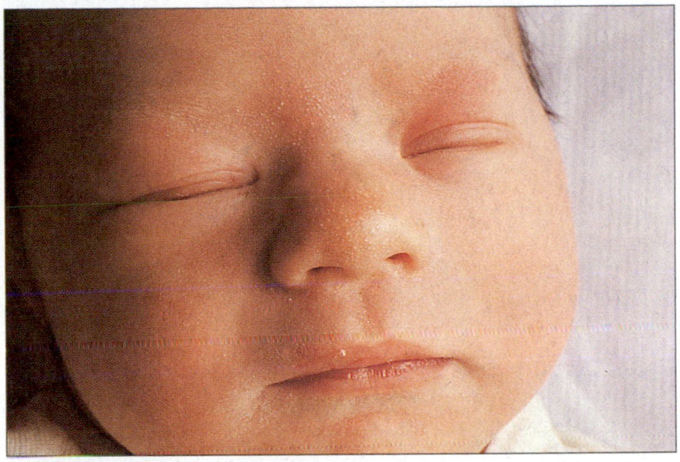

Figure 29–19 • Facial milia.

Should a maculopapular rash (eruption consisting of both macules and papules) appear, a smear of the aspirated papule will show numerous eosinophils on staining; no bacteria will be cultured.

Milia, which are exposed sebaceous glands, appear as raised white spots on the face, especially across the nose (Figure 29–19 •). No treatment is necessary, because they will clear up spontaneously within the first month. Infants of African heritage have a similar condition called transient neonatal pustular melanosis (Drolet & Esterly, 2002).

Skin turgor is assessed to determine hydration status, the need to initiate early feedings, and the presence of any infectious processes. The usual place to assess skin turgor is over the abdomen or the thigh. Skin should be elastic and should return rapidly to its original shape.

Vernix caseosa, a whitish cheeselike substance, covers the fetus while in utero and lubricates the skin of the newborn. The skin of the term or postterm newborn has less vernix and is frequently dry; peeling is common, especially on the hands and feet.

Forceps marks may be present after a difficult forceps birth. The newborn may have reddened areas over the cheeks and jaws. It is important to reassure the parents that these will disappear, usually within 1 or 2 days. Transient facial paralysis resulting from the forceps pressure is a rare complication. Suction marks on the vertex of the scalp are often seen when vacuum extractors are used to assist with the birth. These are benign and do not indicate any underlying brain lesions.

Birthmarks

Telangiectatic nevi (stork bites) appear as pale pink or red spots and are frequently found on the eyelids, nose, lower occipital bone, and nape of the neck (Figure 29–20 •). These

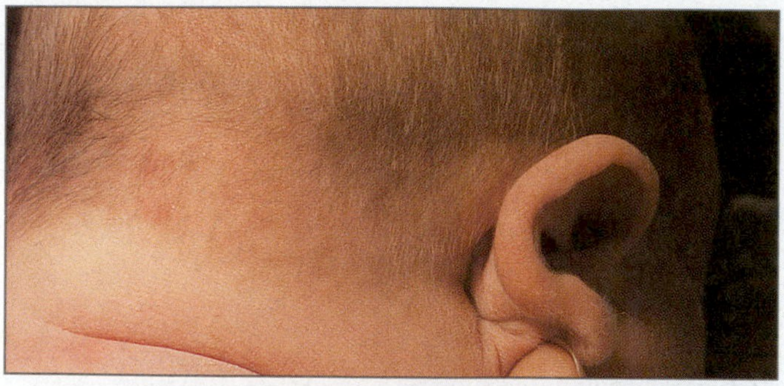

Figure 29–20 • Stork bites.

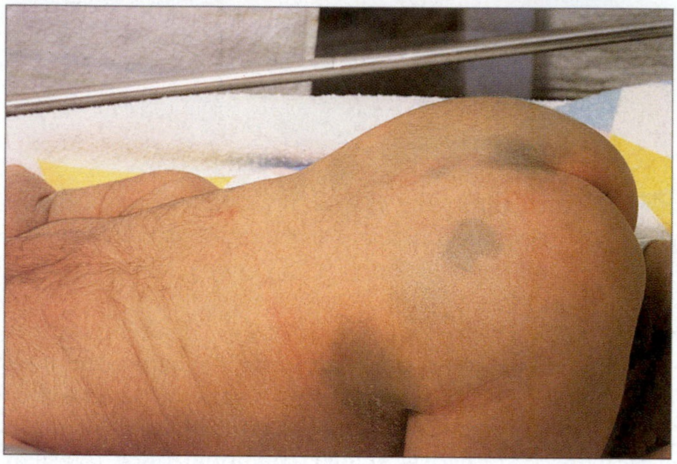

Figure 29–21 • Mongolian spots.

lesions are common in light-complexioned newborns and are more noticeable during periods of crying. These areas have no clinical significance and usually fade by the second birthday.

Mongolian spots are macular areas of bluish black or gray-blue pigmentation found on the dorsal area and the buttocks (Figure 29–21 •). They are common in newborns of Asian and African descent and other dark-skinned races. They gradually fade during the first or second year of life. They may be mistaken for bruises and should be documented in the newborn's chart.

Nevus flammeus (port wine stain) is a capillary angioma directly below the epidermis. It is a nonelevated, sharply demarcated, red to purple area of dense capillaries (Figure 29–22 •). In infants of African descent it may appear as a purple-black stain. The size and shape varies, but it commonly appears on the face. It does not grow in size, does not fade with time, and does not blanch as a rule. The birthmark may be concealed by an opaque cosmetic cream. If convulsions and other neurologic problems accompany the nevus flammeus, the clinical picture is suggestive of Sturge-Weber syndrome with involvement of the fifth cranial nerve (the ophthalmic branch of the trigeminal nerve).

Nevus vasculosus (strawberry mark) is a capillary hemangioma. It consists of newly formed and enlarged capillaries in the dermal and subdermal layers. It is a raised,

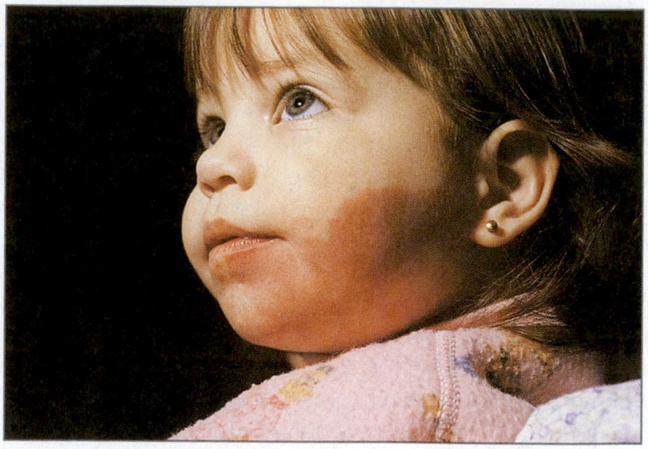

Figure 29–22 • Port wine stain.

clearly delineated, dark red, rough-surfaced birthmark commonly found in the head region. Such marks usually begin to grow (often rapidly) during the second or third week of life and may not reach their full size for 1 to 3 months (Rinehart et al, 2000). They begin to shrink and start to resolve spontaneously several weeks to months after they reach peak growth. Parents can be told that resolution is heralded by a pale purple or gray spot on the surface of the hemangioma. The best cosmetic effect is achieved when the lesions are allowed to resolve spontaneously.

Birthmarks are frequently a cause of concern for the parents. The mother may be especially anxious, fearing that she is to blame. ("Is my baby marked because of something I did?") Guilt feelings are common in the presence of misconceptions about the cause. Birthmarks should be identified and explained to the parents. By providing appropriate information about the cause and course of birthmarks, the nurse frequently relieves the fears and anxieties of the family. The nurse should note any bruises, abrasions, or birthmarks seen on the newborn's admission to the nursery.

Head

GENERAL APPEARANCE

The newborn's head is large (approximately one fourth of the body size), with soft, pliable skull bones. The head may appear asymmetric in the newborn of a vertex presentation. This asymmetry, called **molding,** is caused by the overriding of the cranial bones during labor and birth (Figure 29–23 •). The degree of molding varies with the amount and length of pressure exerted on the head. Within a few days after birth, the overriding usually diminishes, and the suture lines become palpable. Because head measurements are affected by molding, a second measurement is indicated a few days after birth. The heads of breech-born newborns and those born by elective cesarean birth are characteristically round and well shaped because pressure was not exerted on them during birth. Any extreme differences in head size may indicate microcephaly or hydrocephalus. Variations in the shape, size, or

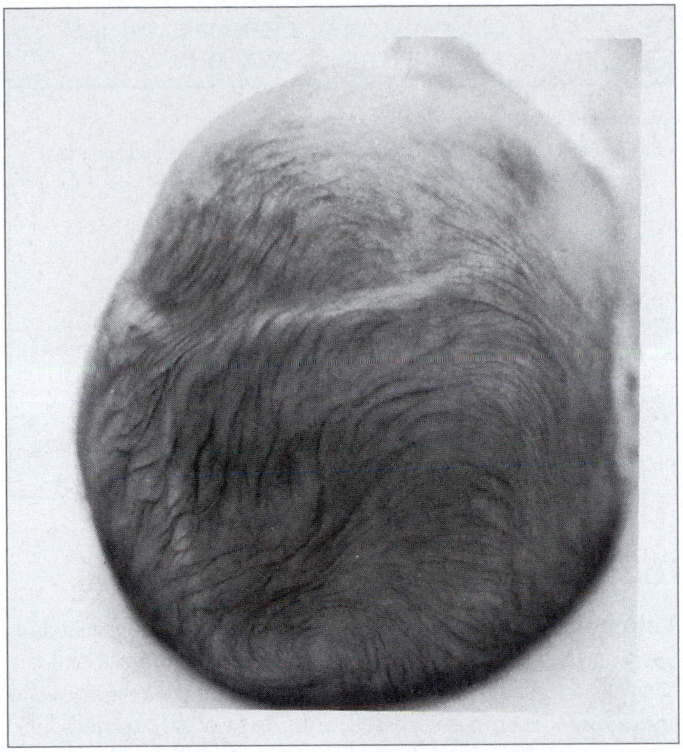

Figure 29–23 • Overlapped cranial bones produce a visible ridge in a small premature infant. Easily visible overlapping does not occur often in term infants.
SOURCE: Korones, S. B. *High-risk newborn infants* (4th ed.). Copyright 1986, with permission from Elsevier Science.

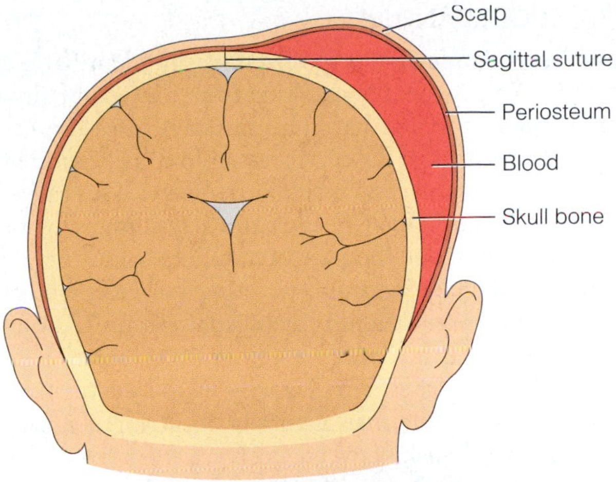

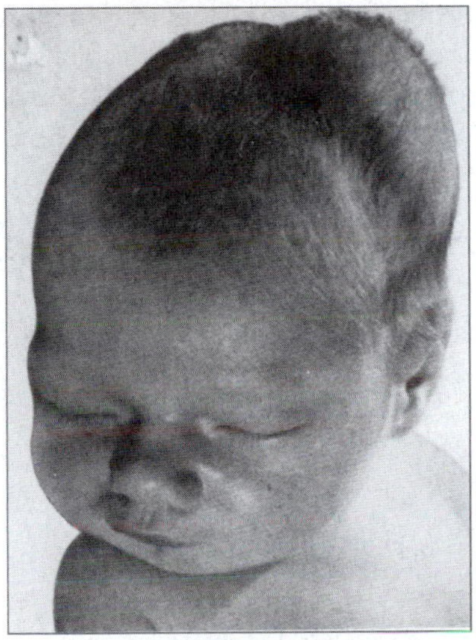

Figure 29–24 • Cephalhematoma is a collection of blood between the surface of a cranial bone and the periosteal membrane. This is a cephalhematoma over the left parietal bone.
SOURCE: Photo reproduced with permission from Potter, E. L., & Craig, J. M. *Pathology of the fetus and infant* (3rd ed.). Copyright 1975, with permission from Elsevier Science.

appearance of the head may be due to *craniostenosis* (premature closure of the cranial sutures), which is corrected through surgery to allow brain growth, or *plagiocephaly* (asymmetry caused by pressure on the fetal head during gestation).

Two *fontanelles* ("soft spots") may be palpated on the newborn's head. Fontanelles, which are openings at the juncture of the cranial bones, can be measured with the fingers. Accurate measurement necessitates that the examiner's finger be measured in centimeters. The assessment should be carried out with the newborn in sitting position and not crying. The diamond-shaped *anterior fontanelle* is 3 to 4 cm long by 2 to 3 cm wide. It is located at the juncture of the frontal and parietal bones. The *posterior fontanelle*, smaller and triangular, is formed by the parietal bones and the occipital bone and is 0.5 cm by 1 cm. Because of molding, the fontanelles tend to be smaller immediately after birth than several days later. The anterior fontanelle closes within 18 months, whereas the posterior fontanelle closes within 8 to 12 weeks.

The fontanelles are a useful indicator of the newborn's condition. The anterior fontanelle may swell when the newborn cries or passes a stool or may pulsate with the heartbeat, which is normal. A bulging fontanelle usually signifies increased intracranial pressure, and a depressed fontanelle indicates dehydration.

The sutures between the cranial bones should be palpated for amount of overlap. In growth-retarded newborns, the sutures may be wider than normal, and the fontanelle may also be larger because of impaired fetal growth of the cranial bones. In addition to being inspected for degree of molding and size, the head should be evaluated for soft-tissue edema and bruising.

CEPHALHEMATOMA

Cephalhematoma is a collection of blood resulting from ruptured blood vessels between the surface of a cranial bone (usually parietal) and the periosteal membrane (Figure 29–24 •). The scalp in these areas feels loose and slightly edematous. These areas emerge as defined hematomas between the first and second day. Although external pressure may cause the mass to fluctuate, it does not increase in size when the newborn cries. Cephalhematomas may be unilateral or bilateral and do not cross suture lines. They are relatively common in vertex births and may disappear within 2 to 3 weeks or slowly over subsequent months. They may be associated with physiologic jaundice, because there are extra red blood cells being destroyed within the cephalhematoma.

CAPUT SUCCEDANEUM

Caput succedaneum is a localized, easily identifiable soft area of the scalp, generally resulting from a long and difficult labor or vacuum extraction. The sustained pressure of the presenting part against the cervix results in compression of local blood vessels, and venous return is slowed. This causes an increase in tissue fluids, an edematous swelling, and occasional bleeding under the periosteum. The caput may vary from a small area to a large area covering a severely elongated head. The fluid in the caput is reabsorbed within 12 hours to a few days after birth. Caputs resulting from vacuum extractors are sharply outlined, circular areas up to 2 cm thick. They disappear more slowly than naturally occurring edema. It is possible to distinguish between a cephalhematoma and a caput because the caput overrides suture lines (Figure 29–25 •), whereas the cephalhematoma, because of its location, never crosses a suture line (Table 29–3 •). Caput succedaneum is present at birth, whereas cephalhematoma generally is not.

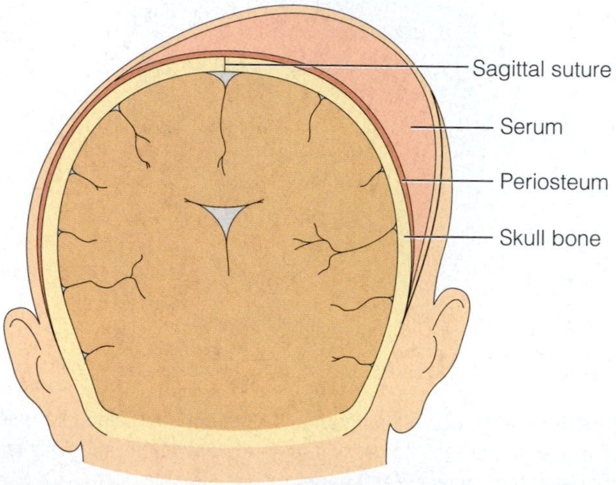

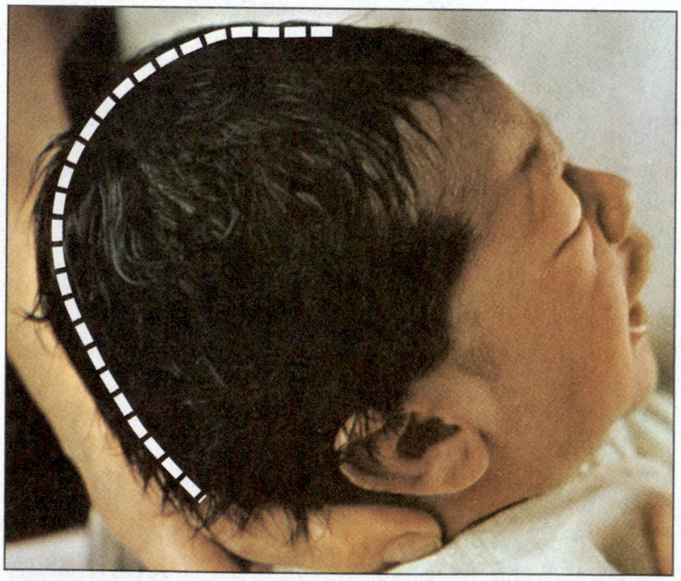

Figure 29–25 • Caput succedaneum is a collection of fluid (serum) under the scalp.
SOURCE: Photo courtesy of Mead Johnson Nutritionals, Evansville, IN.

Table 29–3 • COMPARISON OF CEPHALHEMATOMA AND CAPUT SUCCEDANEUM

Cephalhematoma
Collection of blood between cranial (usually parietal) bone and periosteal membrane
Does not cross suture lines
Does not increase in size with crying
Appears on first and second day
Disappears after 2 to 3 weeks or may take months
Caput Succedaneum
Collection of fluid, edematous swelling of the scalp
Crosses suture lines
Present at birth or shortly thereafter
Reabsorbed within 12 hours or a few days after birth

Face

The newborn's face is well designed to help the infant suckle. Sucking (fat) pads are located in the cheeks, and a labial tubercle (sucking callus) is frequently found in the center of the upper lip. The chin is recessed, and the nose is flattened. The lips are sensitive to touch, and the sucking reflex is easily initiated.

Symmetry of the eyes, nose, and ears is evaluated. See the Assessment Guide: Newborn Physical Assessment for deviations in symmetry and variations in size, shape, and spacing of facial features. Facial movement symmetry should be assessed to determine the presence of facial palsy.

Facial paralysis appears when the newborn cries; the affected side is immobile, and the palpebral (eyelid) fissure widens (Figure 29–26 •). Paralysis may result from forceps-

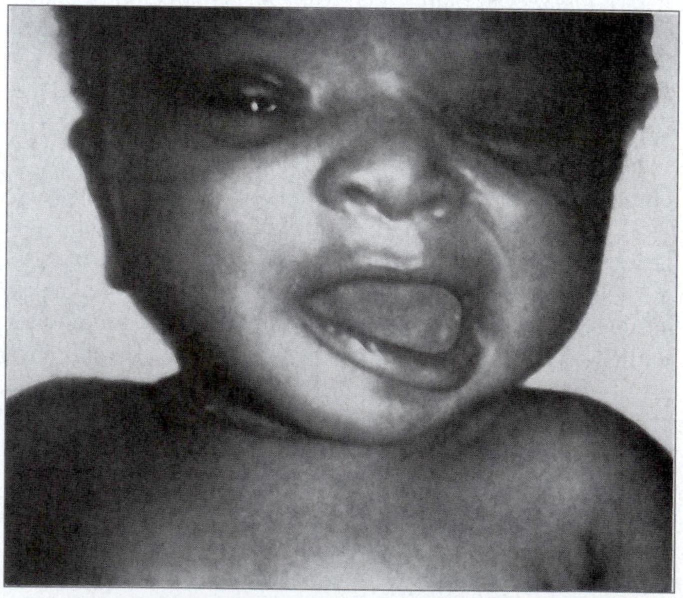

Figure 29–26 • Paralysis of the right side of the face from an injury to the right facial nerve.
SOURCE: Potter, E.L., & Craig, J.M. *Pathology of the fetus and infant* (3rd ed.). Copyright 1975, with permission from Elsevier Science. Courtesy of Dr. Ralph Platow.

assisted birth or pressure on the facial nerve from the maternal pelvis during birth. Facial paralysis usually disappears within a few days to 3 weeks, although in some cases it may be permanent.

EYES

The eyes of newborns of northern European descent are a blue or slate blue-gray. Scleral color tends to be white to bluish white because of its relative thinness. A blue sclera is associated with osteogenesis imperfecta (Cooperman & Thompson, 2002). The infant's eye color is usually established at approximately 3 months, but it may change any time up to 1 year. Dark-skinned newborns tend to have dark eyes at birth.

The eyes should be checked for size, equality of pupil size, reaction of pupils to light, blink reflex to light, and edema and inflammation of the eyelids. The eyelids can be edematous during the first few days of life because of the pressure associated with birth. Erythromycin and tetracycline are now frequently used prophylactically instead of silver nitrate and usually don't cause chemical irritation of the eye. The instillation of silver nitrate drops in the newborn's eyes may cause edema and **chemical conjunctivitis,** which may appear a few hours after instillation and disappear in 1 to 2 days. If infectious conjunctivitis exists, the newborn has the same purulent (greenish yellow) discharge as in chemical conjunctivitis, but it is caused by gonococcus, *Chlamydia*, staphylococci, or a variety of gram-negative bacteria and requires treatment with ophthalmic antibiotics. Onset is usually after the second day. Edema of the orbits or eyelids may persist for several days until the newborn's kidneys can evacuate the fluid.

Small **subconjunctival hemorrhages** appear in about 10% of newborns and are commonly found on the sclera. These hemorrhages are caused by the changes in vascular tension or ocular pressure during birth. They will remain for a few weeks and are of no pathologic significance. Parents need reassurance that the infant is not bleeding from within the eye and that vision will not be impaired.

The newborn may demonstrate transient strabismus (pseudostrabismus) or squinting caused by neuromuscular control of eye muscles (Figure 29–27 •). It gradually regresses in 3 to 4 months. The "doll's eye" phenomenon is also present for about 10 days after birth. As the newborn's head position is changed to the left and then to the right, the eyes move to the opposite direction. "Doll's eye" results from underdeveloped integration of head-eye coordination.

The nurse should observe the newborn's pupils for opacities or whiteness and for the absence of a normal red retinal reflex. Red retinal reflex is a red-orange flash of color observed when an ophthalmoscope light reflects off the retina. In a newborn with dark skin color, the retina may appear paler or more grayish. Absence of red reflex occurs with cataracts. Congenital cataracts should be suspected in infants of mothers with a prenatal history of rubella, cytomegalic inclusion disease, or syphilis.

The cry of the newborn is commonly tearless because the lacrimal structures are immature at birth and are not usually fully functional until the second month of life. However, some babies may produce tears during the newborn period. Poor oculomotor coordination and absence of accommodation limit visual abilities, but newborns do have peripheral vision and can fixate on near objects (8 to 10 in) in front of their faces for short periods, can accommodate to large objects (3 in tall by 3 in wide), and can seek out high-contrast geometric shapes. Newborns can perceive faces, shapes, and colors and begin to show visual preferences early. Visual acuity has been reported to be 20/140 (Gardner & Goldson, 2002). Newborns generally blink in response to bright lights, to a tap on the bridge of the nose (glabellar reflex), or to a light touch on the eyelids. Pupillary light reflex is also present. The eye is best examined by rocking the newborn from an upright position to the horizontal a few times or by other methods, such as diminishing overhead lights, which will elicit an opened-eye response.

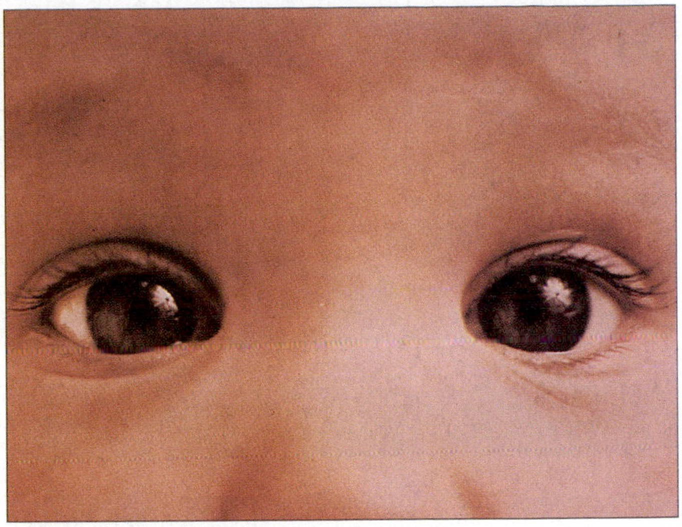

Figure 29–27 • Transient strabismus in the newborn may be due to poor neuromuscular control.
SOURCE: Courtesy of Mead Johnson Nutritionals, Evansville, IN.

NOSE

The newborn's nose is small and narrow. Infants are characteristically nose breathers for the first few months of life. The newborn generally removes obstructions by sneezing. Nasal patency is assured if the baby breathes easily with mouth closed. If respiratory difficulty occurs, the nurse checks for choanal atresia (congenital blockage of the passageway between nose and pharynx).

The newborn has the ability to smell after the nasal passages are cleared of amniotic fluid and mucus. This ability is demonstrated by the search for milk. Newborns will turn their heads toward the milk source, whether bottle or breast. Newborns react to strong odors, such as alcohol, by turning their heads away or blinking.

MOUTH

The lips of the newborn should be pink, and a touch on the lips should produce sucking motions. Saliva is normally scant. The taste buds are developed prior to birth, and the newborn can easily discriminate between sweet and bitter flavors.

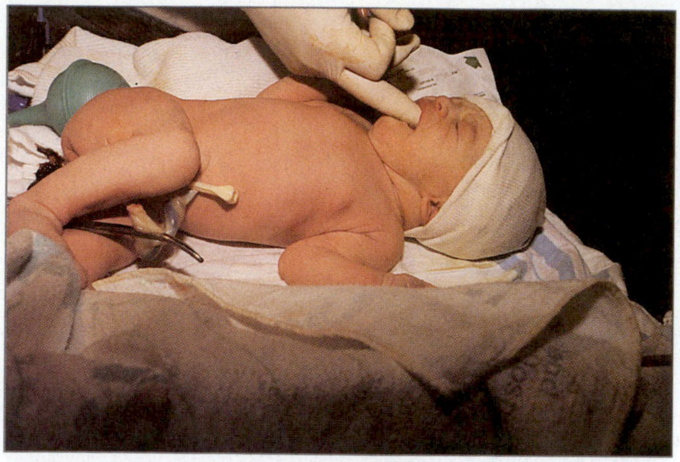

Figure 29–28 • The nurse inserts the index finger into the newborn's mouth and feels for any openings along the hard and soft palates. Note that gloves are worn to examine the palate.

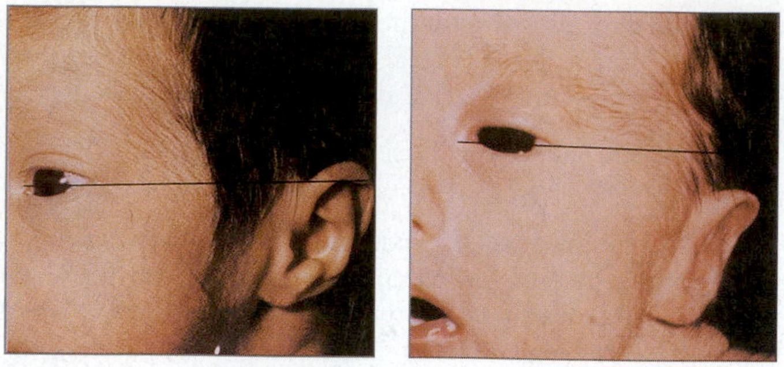

Figure 29–29 • The position of the external ear may be assessed by drawing a line across the inner and outer canthus of the eye to the insertion of the ear. *A*, Normal position. *B*, True low-set position.
SOURCE: Courtesy of Mead Johnson Nutritionals, Evansville, IN.

The easiest way to examine the mouth completely is to stimulate infants gently to cry by depressing their tongue, thereby causing them to open the mouth fully. It is extremely important to observe the entire mouth to look for a cleft palate, which can be present even in the absence of a cleft lip. The examiner moves a gloved index finger along the hard and soft palate to feel for any openings (Figure 29–28 •). Glove powder should always be removed before examining the newborn's mouth.

Occasionally, an examination of the gums will reveal precocious teeth on the lower central incisor. If they appear loose, they should be removed to prevent aspiration. Gray-white lesions (inclusion cysts) on the gums may be confused with teeth. On the hard palate and gum margins, **Epstein's pearls,** small glistening white specks (keratin-containing cysts) that feel hard to the touch are often present. These usually disappear in a few weeks and are of no significance. **Thrush** may appear as white patches that look like milk curds adhering to the mucous membranes and cause bleeding when removed. Thrush is caused by *Candida albicans,* often acquired from an infected vaginal tract during birth or if the mother uses poor handwashing when handling her newborn. Thrush is treated with a preparation of nystatin (Mycostatin).

A newborn who is tongue-tied has a ridge of frenulum tissue attached to the underside of the tongue at varying lengths from its base, causing a heart shape at the tip of the tongue. "Clipping the tongue," or cutting the ridge of tissue, is not recommended. This ridge does not affect speech or eating, but cutting does create an entry for infection.

Transient nerve paralysis resulting from birth trauma may be manifested by asymmetric mouth movements when the newborn cries or by difficulty with sucking and feeding.

EARS

The ears of the newborn should be soft and pliable and should recoil readily when folded and released. In the normal newborn, the top of the ear (pinna) should be parallel to the outer and inner canthus of the eye. The ears should be inspected for shape, size, position, and firmness of ear cartilage.

Low-set ears are characteristic of many syndromes and may indicate chromosomal abnormalities (especially trisomies 13 and 18), mental retardation, or internal organ abnormalities, especially bilateral renal agenesis as a result of embryologic developmental deviations (Figure 29–29 •). A preauricular skin tag may be present just in front of the ear. *Preauricular tags* are ligated at the base and allowed to slough off.

Visualization of the tympanic membranes is not usually done soon after birth because blood and vernix block the ear canal.

Following the first cry, the newborn's hearing becomes acute as mucus from the middle ear is absorbed, the eustachian tube is aerated, and the tympanic membrane becomes visible.

The newborn's hearing initially can be evaluated by response to loud or moderately loud noises unaccompanied by vibrations. The sleeping newborn should stir or awaken in response to the nearby sounds. (This is not a very accurate test, but it may help to alert the examiner to possible problems.) The newborn can discriminate the individual characteristics of the human voice and is especially sensitive to sound levels within the normal conversation range (Gardner & Goldson, 2002). The newborn in a noisy nursery may be able to habituate to the sounds and not stir unless the sound is sudden or much louder.

The AAP has endorsed universal newborn hearing screening (UNHS) in birthing units as the standard of care (Johnson, 2002). The current goal is to screen all infants by 1 month of age, confirm hearing loss with audiologic examination by 3 months of age, and treat with comprehensive early intervention services before 6 months of age (AAP & ACOG, 2002).

Risk factors (AAP & ACOG, 2002; Gardner & Goldson, 2002) associated with potential hearing loss include the following:

- The presence of familial hearing loss
- Serum bilirubin level greater than 20 mg/dL for the full-term newborn or hyperbilirubinemia with a level exceeding indications for exchange transfusion due to toxic drugs
- Prolonged mechanical ventilation of more than 5 days

- Congenital infection with rubella, herpes, cytomegalovirus, toxoplasmosis, or syphilis
- Bacterial meningitis or sepsis
- Congenital defects of the ear, nose, or throat
- Small preterm newborns, particularly less than 1500 g at birth
- Perinatal asphyxia
- Ototoxic medications

If congenital hearing loss risk factors exist, two types of tests are commonly used: otoacoustic emissions (OAEs) and auditory brainstem response (ABR). Typically, screening programs use a two-stage screening approach (OAE repeated twice, OAE followed by ABR, or automated ABR repeated twice) (US Preventive Services Task Force, 2001). Families need to be educated about appropriate interpretation of screening test results and appropriate steps for follow-up.

Neck

A short neck, creased with skin folds, is characteristic of the normal newborn. Because muscle tone is not well developed, the neck cannot support the full weight of the head, which rotates freely. The head lags considerably when the newborn is pulled up from a supine to a sitting position, but the prone newborn is able to raise the head slightly. The neck is palpated for masses and presence of lymph nodes and is inspected for webbing. Adequacy of range of motion and neck muscle function is determined by fully extending the head in all directions. Injury to the sternocleidomastoid muscle (congenital torticollis) must be considered in the presence of neck rigidity.

The clavicles are evaluated for evidence of fractures, which occasionally occur during difficult births or in newborns with broad shoulders. The normal clavicle is straight. If fractured, a lump and a grating sensation (crepitus) during movements may be palpated along the course of the side of the break. The Moro reflex (page 819) is also elicited to evaluate bilateral equal movement of the arms. If the clavicle is fractured, this response will be demonstrated only on the unaffected side.

Chest

The thorax is cylindrical and symmetric at birth, and the ribs are flexible. The general appearance of the chest should be assessed. A protrusion at the lower end of the sternum, called the xiphoid cartilage, is frequently seen. It is under the skin and will become less apparent after several weeks as the infant accumulates adipose tissue.

Engorged breasts occur frequently in both male and female newborns. This condition, which appears by the third day, is a result of maternal hormonal influences and may last up to 2 weeks (Figure 29–30 •). A whitish secretion from the nipples may also be noted. The infant's breast should not be massaged or squeezed because this practice may cause a breast abscess. Extra nipples or supernumerary nipples are occasionally noted below and medial to the true nipples. These harmless pink or brown (in darker skinned newborns) spots vary in size and do not contain glandular tissue. Accessory nipples can be differentiated from a pigmented nevus (mole) by placing the fingertips alongside the accessory nipple and pulling the adjacent tissue laterally. The accessory nipple will appear dimpled. At puberty the accessory nipple may darken.

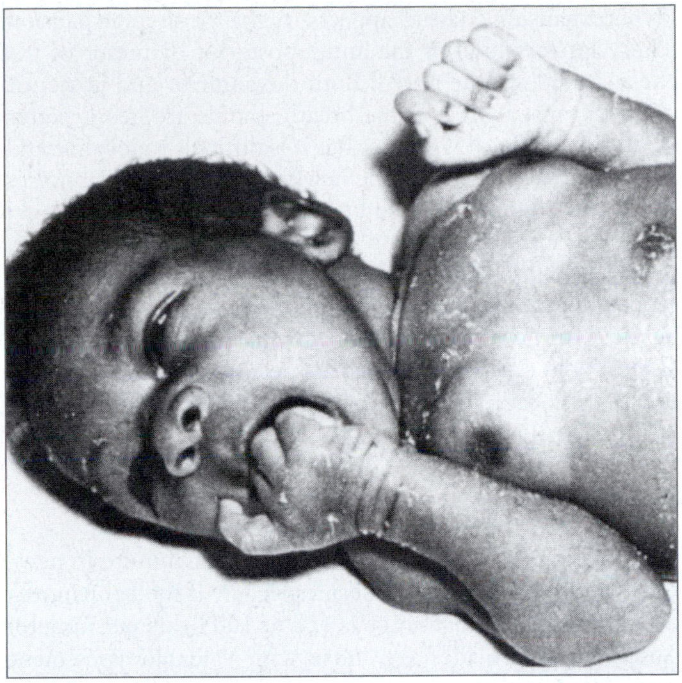

Figure 29–30 • Breast hypertrophy.
SOURCE: Korones, S. B. *High-risk newborn infants* (4th ed.). Copyright 1986, with permission from Elsevier Science.

Cry

The newborn's cry should be strong, lusty, and of medium pitch. A high-pitched, shrill cry is abnormal and may indicate neurologic disorders or hypoglycemia. Periods of crying vary in length after consoling measures are used. A baby's cries are an important method of communication and alert caregivers to changes in the baby's condition and needs.

> **Clinical Tip** *Vital sign assessments are most accurate if the newborn is at rest, so measure pulse and respirations first if the baby is quiet. To soothe a crying baby, try placing your moistened gloved finger in the baby's mouth, and then complete your assessment while the baby suckles.*

Respiration

Normal breathing for a term newborn is 30 to 60 respirations per minute and predominantly diaphragmatic, with associated rising and falling of the abdomen during inspiration and expiration. Any signs of respiratory distress, nasal flaring, intercostal or xiphoid retractions, expiratory grunting or sighing, seesaw respirations, or tachypnea (sustained or greater than 60 respirations per minute) should be noted.

Hyperexpansion (chest appears high) or hypoexpansion (chest appears low) of the anteroposterior diameter of the chest should also be noted. Both the anterior and posterior chest are auscultated. Some breath sounds are heard better when the newborn is crying, but it is difficult to localize and identify breath sounds in the newborn. Upper airway noises and bowel sounds may also be heard over the chest wall and make auscultation difficult. Because sounds may be transmitted from the unaffected lung to the affected lung, the absence of breath sounds may not be diagnosed. Air entry may be noisy in the first couple of hours until lung fluid resolves, especially in cesarean births. Brief periods of apnea (episodic breathing) occur, but no color or heart rate changes occur in healthy, term newborns.

Heart

Heart rates can be as rapid as 180 beats per minute in newborns and fluctuate a great deal, especially if the baby moves or is startled. Normal range is 120 to 160 beats per minute. Auscultation provides the nurse with valuable assessment data. The heart is examined for rate and rhythm, position of the apical impulse, and heart sound intensity. Dysrhythmias should be reassessed by a physician.

The pulse rate is variable and is influenced by physical activity, crying, state of wakefulness, and body temperature. Auscultation is performed over the entire heart region (precordium), below the left axilla, and below the scapula. Apical pulse rates are obtained by auscultation for a full minute, preferably when the newborn is asleep.

The placement of the heart in the chest should be determined when the newborn is in a quiet state. The heart is relatively large at birth and is located high in the chest, with its apex somewhere between the fourth and fifth intercostal spaces.

A shift of heart tones in the mediastinal area to either side may indicate pneumothorax, dextrocardia (heart placement on the right side of the chest), or a diaphragmatic hernia. The experienced nurse can diagnose these and many other problems early with a stethoscope. Normally, the heartbeat has a "toc tic" sound. A slur or slushing sound (usually after the first sound) may indicate a murmur. Although 90% of all murmurs are transient and are considered normal, they should be monitored closely by a physician. Many murmurs are related to a patent ductus arteriosus, which closes in about 1 to 2 days.

In newborns, a low-pitched, musical murmur heard just to the right of the apex of the heart is fairly common. Occasionally, significant murmurs will be heard, including the murmur of a patent ductus arteriosus, aortic or pulmonary stenosis, or small ventricular septal defect. See Chapter 32 for a discussion of congenital heart defects.

Peripheral pulses (brachial, femoral, pedal) are also evaluated to detect any lags or unusual characteristics. Brachial pulses are palpated bilaterally for equality and compared with the femoral pulses. Femoral pulses are palpated by applying gentle pressure with the middle finger over the femoral canal (Figure 29–31 ●). Decreased or absent femoral pulses indicate coarctation of the aorta and require additional investigation. A wide difference in blood pressure between the upper and lower extremities also indicates coarctation. The measurement of blood pressure is best accomplished by using the Doppler technique or a 1- to 2-inch cuff and a stethoscope over the brachial artery (Figure 29–32 ●). If a Doppler device is used, the newborn's extremities must be immobilized during the assessment, and the cuff should cover two thirds of the upper arm or upper leg. Movement, crying, and inappropriate cuff size can give inaccurate measurements of the blood pressure.

Blood pressure may not be measured routinely on healthy newborns but is an essential measurement on newborns who are having distress, are premature, or are suspected of cardiac anomaly. Infants who have birth asphyxia and are on ventilators have significantly lower systolic and diastolic blood pressures than healthy infants. If cardiac anomaly is

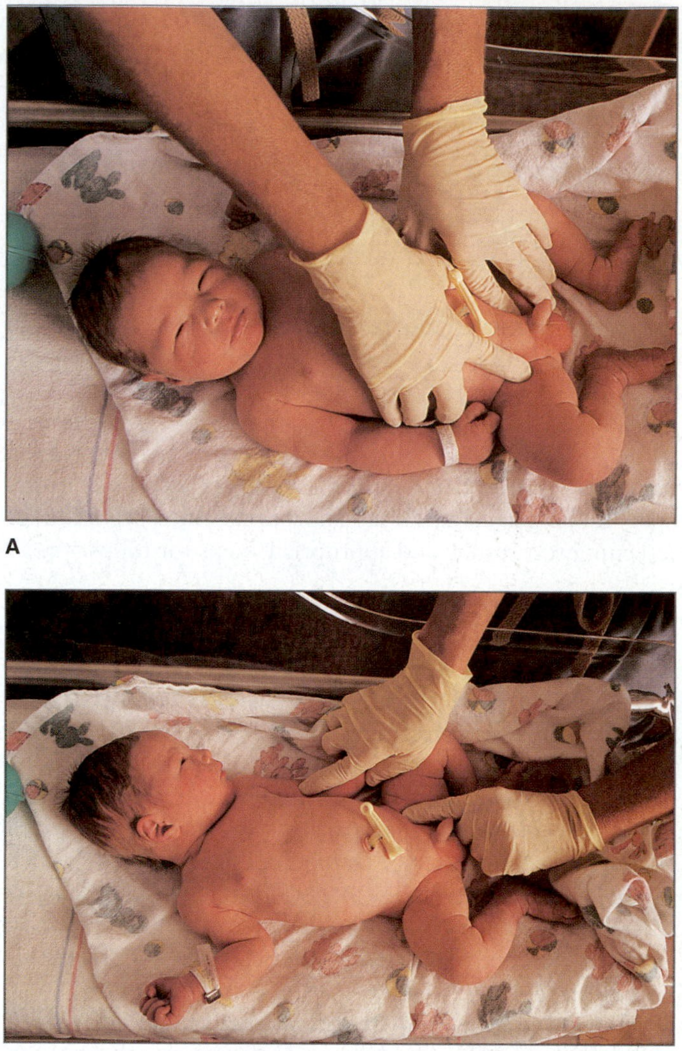

A

B

Figure 29–31 ● *A,* Bilaterally palpate the femoral arteries for rate and intensity of the pulses. Press fingertip gently at the groin as shown. *B,* Compare the femoral pulses to the brachial pulses by palpating the pulses simultaneously for comparison of rate and intensity.

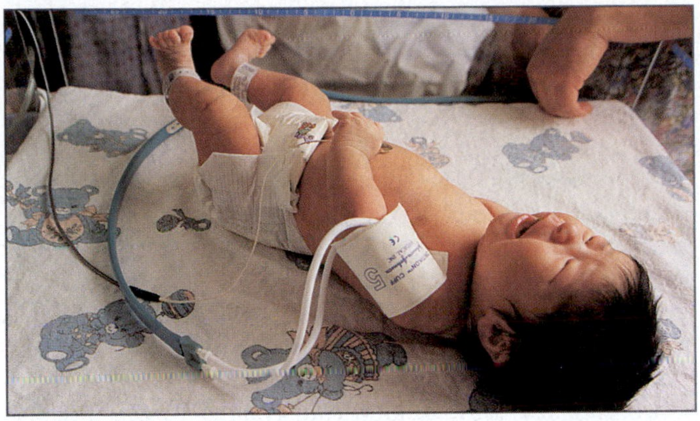

Figure 29–32 • Blood pressure measurement using the Dinemapp and Doppler devices. The cuff can be applied to either the newborn's upper arm or the thigh.

Table 29–4 • NEWBORN VITAL SIGNS

Pulse 120–160 bpm During sleep as low as 100 bpm; if crying, up to 180 bpm Apical pulse counted for 1 full minute **Respirations** 30–60 respirations/minute Predominantly diaphragmatic but synchronous with abdominal movements Respirations are counted for 1 full minute	**Blood Pressure** 80–60/45–40 mm Hg at birth 100/50 mm Hg at day 10 **Temperature** Normal range: 36.5C–37.5C (97.7F–99.4F) Axillary: 36.4C–37.2C (97.5F–99F) Skin: 36C–36.5C (96.8F–97.7F) Rectal: 36.6C–37.2C (97.8F–99F)

suspected, blood pressure is palpated in all four extremities (Table 29–4 •). At birth, systolic values usually range from 80 to 45 mm Hg and diastolic values from 60 to 40 mm Hg. By the tenth day of life, blood pressure rises to 100/50 mm Hg.

Abdomen

The nurse can learn a great deal about the newborn's abdomen without disturbing the infant. The abdomen should be cylindrical, protrude slightly, and move with respiration. A certain amount of laxness of the abdominal muscles is normal. A scaphoid (hollow-shaped) appearance suggests the absence of abdominal contents. No cyanosis should be present, and few if any blood vessels should be apparent to the eye. There should be no gross distention or bulging. The more distended the abdomen, the tighter the skin becomes, and engorged vessels appear. Distention is the first sign of many of the abnormalities found in the gastrointestinal tract.

Before palpation of the abdomen, the nurse should auscultate the presence or absence of bowel sounds in all four quadrants. Bowel sounds should be present by 1 hour after birth. Palpation can cause a transient decrease in bowel sound intensity.

Abdominal palpation should be carried out systematically. The nurse palpates each of the four abdominal quadrants, moving in a clockwise direction, checking for softness, tenderness, and the presence of masses. When palpating the abdomen, the nurse may feel for the liver. The newborn's liver is large in proportion to the rest of the body and can usually be felt between 1 and 2 cm below the right costal margin. Depending on institutional protocol, palpation of the kidney may be performed by the staff nurse. Kidneys are more difficult to feel but can be more easily examined within 4 to 6 hours after birth, before the intestines become distended with air and feedings are initiated. By placing a finger at the posterior flank and pushing upward while pressing downward with the opposite hand, each kidney may be palpated as a firm oval mass between the examiner's finger and hand. The lower pole of the kidney is usually found 1 to 2 cm above the umbilicus. The spleen tip may be palpated in the lateral aspect of the left upper quadrant in the normal newborn.

Umbilical Cord

Initially, the umbilical cord is white and gelatinous in appearance, with the two umbilical arteries and one umbilical vein readily apparent. Because a single umbilical artery is frequently associated with congenital anomalies, the vessels should be counted as part of the newborn assessment. The cord begins drying within 1 or 2 hours after birth and is shriveled and blackened by the second or third day. Within 7 to 10 days it sloughs off, although a granulated area may remain for a few days longer.

Cord bleeding is abnormal and may result because the cord was inadvertently pulled or because the cord clamp was loosened. Foul-smelling drainage is also abnormal and is generally caused by infection, which requires immediate treatment to prevent septicemia. If the newborn has a patent urachus (abnormal connection between the umbilicus and bladder), moistness or draining urine may be apparent at the base of the cord. Another umbilical cord anomaly that must be assessed for is umbilical cord hernia and associated patent omphalomesenteric duct.

Serous or serosanguineous drainage that continues after the cord falls off may indicate a granuloma. It appears as a small, red button deep in the umbilicus. Treatment involves cauterization by a physician with a silver nitrate stick.

GLOBAL PERSPECTIVES

In the Woodland Indian tribe, upon birth, the umbilical cord is tied and a small piece is saved. This section of the umbilical cord is sewn into a deerskin diamond-shaped pocket. The pocket is hung over the infant's crib to provide protection for the infant.

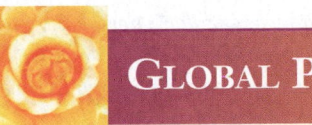

Genitals

FEMALE INFANTS

The nurse examines the labia majora, labia minora, and clitoris, noting the size of each as appropriate for gestational age. A vaginal tag or hymenal tag is often evident and will usually disappear in a few weeks. During the first week of life, the newborn may have a vaginal discharge composed of thick whitish mucus. This discharge, which can become tinged with blood, is referred to as **pseudomenstruation** and is caused by the withdrawal of maternal hormones. *Smegma*, a white cheeselike substance, is often present between the labia. Removing it may traumatize tender tissue.

MALE INFANTS

The penis is inspected to determine whether the urinary orifice is correctly positioned. *Hypospadias* occurs when the urinary meatus is located on the ventral surface of the penis. It occurs most commonly among Western Europeans in the United States. *Phimosis* is a condition occurring in newborn males in which the opening of the foreskin (prepuce) is small, and the foreskin cannot be pulled back over the glans at all. This condition may interfere with urination, so the adequacy of the urinary stream should be evaluated.

The scrotum is inspected for size and symmetry and should be palpated to verify the presence of both testes and to rule out *cryptorchidism* (failure of testes to descend). The testes are palpated separately between the thumb and forefinger, with the thumb and forefinger of the other hand placed together over the inguinal canal. Scrotal edema and discoloration are common in breech births. *Hydrocele* (a collection of fluid surrounding the testes in the scrotum) is common in newborns and should be identified. It usually resolves without intervention. The presence of a discolored or dusky scrotum and solid testis should raise the suspicion of testicular torsion (Juretschke, 2000).

Anus

The anal area is inspected to verify that it is patent and has no fissure. Imperforate anus and rectal atresia may be ruled out by observation. A digital examination, if necessary, is done by a physician. The passage of the first meconium stool is also noted. Atresia of the gastrointestinal tract or meconium ileus with resultant obstruction must be considered if the newborn does not pass meconium in the first 24 hours of life.

> ***Clinical Tip*** *Always examine more closely any infant who is reluctant to move an extremity. Fractures are often asymptomatic in the newborn: paralytic injuries are characterized by immobility of an extremity.*

Extremities

Extremities are examined for gross deformities, extra digits or webbing, clubfoot, and range of motion. Normal newborn extremities appear short, are generally flexible, and move symmetrically.

ARMS AND HANDS

Nails extend beyond the fingertips in term newborns. Fingers and toes should be counted. *Polydactyly* is the presence of extra digits on either the hands or the feet. *Syndactyly* refers to fusion (webbing) of fingers or toes. Hands should be inspected for normal palmar creases. A single palmar crease, called simian line (see also Figure 12–19), is frequently present in children with Down syndrome.

Brachial palsy, which is partial or complete paralysis of portions of the arm, results from trauma to the brachial plexus during a difficult birth. It occurs most commonly when strong traction is exerted on the head of the newborn in an attempt to deliver a shoulder lodged behind the symphysis pubis in the presence of shoulder dystocia. Brachial palsy may also occur during a breech birth if an arm becomes trapped over the head and traction is exerted.

The portion of the arm affected is determined by the nerves damaged. **Erb-Duchenne paralysis (Erb's palsy)** involves damage to the upper arm (fifth and sixth cervical nerves) and is the most common type. Injury to the eighth cervical and first thoracic nerve roots and the lower portion of the plexus produces the relatively rare *lower arm injury.* The *whole arm type* results from damage to the entire plexus.

With Erb-Duchenne paralysis, the newborn's arm lies limply at the side (Figure 29–33 •). The elbow is held in ex-

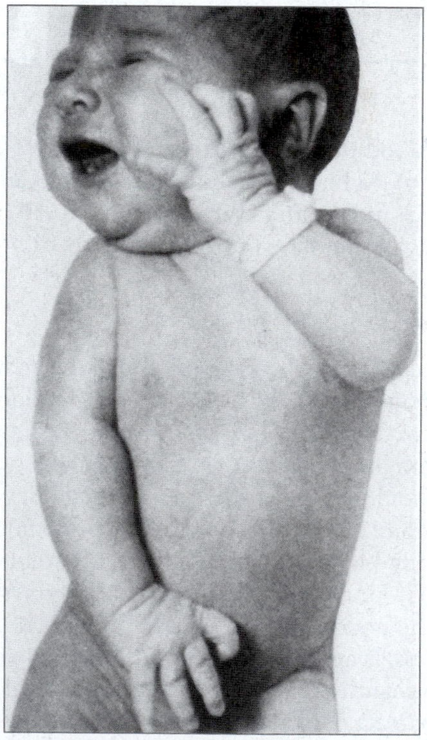

Figure 29–33 • Right Erb's palsy resulting from injury to the fifth and sixth cervical roots of brachial plexus.

SOURCE: Potter, E. L., & Craig, J. M. *Pathology of the fetus and infant* (3rd ed.). Copyright 1975, with permission from Elsevier Science.

tension, with the forearm pronated. The newborn is unable to elevate the arm, and therefore the Moro reflex cannot be elicited on the affected side. When lower arm injury occurs, paralysis of the hand and wrist results; complete paralysis of the limb occurs with the whole arm type.

The nurse carefully instructs the parents in the correct method of performing passive range-of-motion exercises (to prevent muscle contractures and restore function) and arranges supervised practice sessions. In more severe cases, splinting of the arm is indicated until the edema decreases. The arm is held in a position of abduction and external rotation with the elbow flexed 90 degrees, often called the "Statue of Liberty" position. The "Statue of Liberty" splint is commonly used, although similar results are obtained by attaching a strip of muslin to the head of the crib and tying the other end around the wrist, thereby holding the arm up.

Prognosis is related to the degree of nerve damage resulting from trauma and hemorrhage within the nerve sheath. Complete recovery occurs within a few months with minimal trauma. Moderate trauma may result in some partial paralysis. Recovery is unlikely with severe trauma, and muscle wasting may develop.

LEGS AND FEET

The legs of the newborn should be of equal length, with symmetric skin folds. However, they may assume a "fetal posture" secondary to position in utero, and it may take several days for the legs to relax into normal position.

To evaluate for hip dislocation or hip instability, the Ortolani and Barlow maneuvers are performed (Figure 29–34 •). The nurse performs the **Ortolani maneuver** to rule out the possibility of congenital hip dysplasia (hip dislocatability). With the newborn relaxed and quiet on a firm surface, the

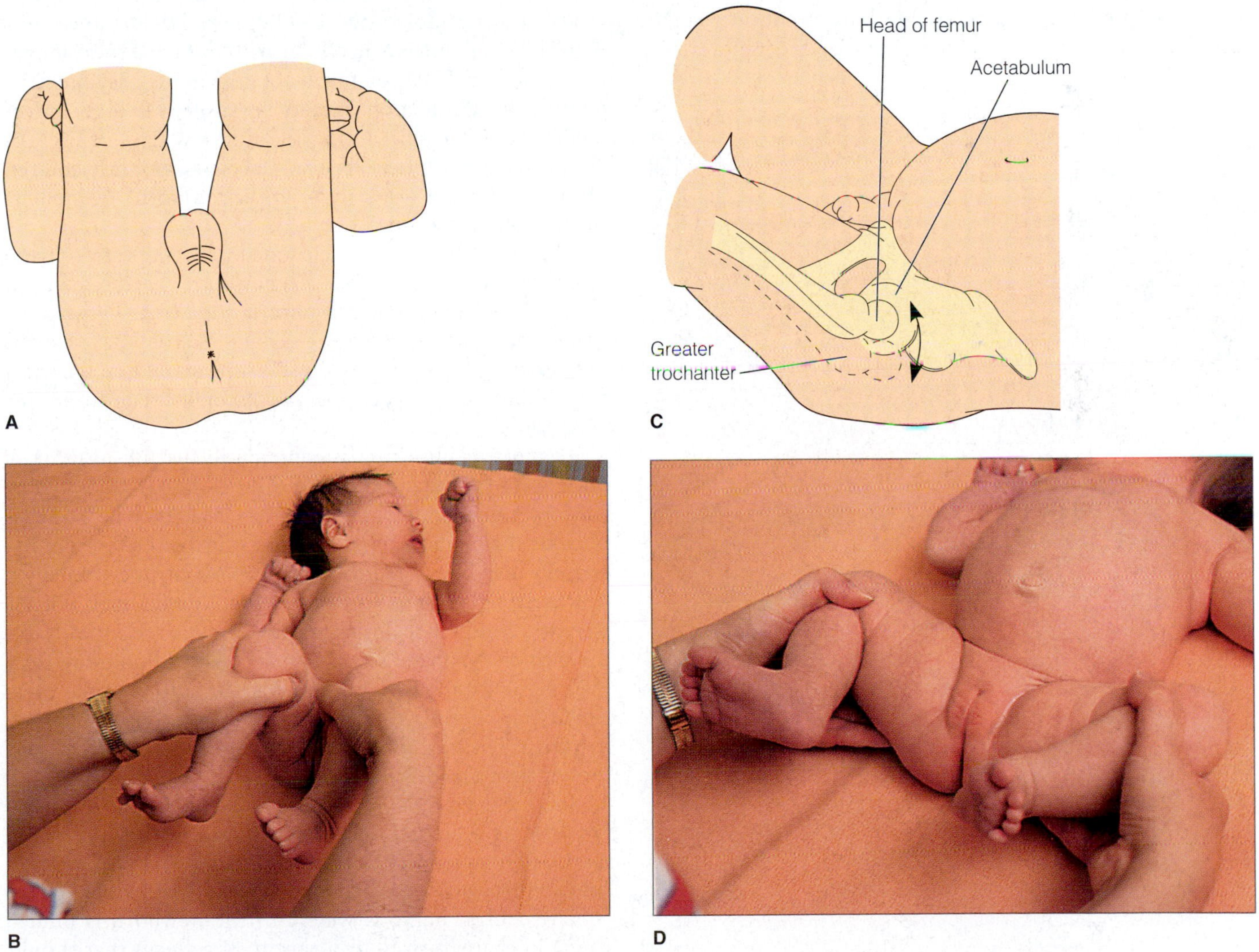

Figure 29–34 • *A,* Congenitally dislocated right hip in a young infant as seen on gross inspection. *B,* Barlow (dislocation) maneuver. Baby's thigh is grasped and adducted (placed together) with gentle downward pressure. *C,* Dislocation is palpable as femoral head slips out of acetabulum. *D,* Ortolani maneuver puts downward pressure on the hip and then inward rotation. If the hip is dislocated, this maneuver will force the femoral head back into the acetabular rim with a noticeable "clunk."

hips and knees flexed at a 90-degree angle, the nurse grasps the infant's thigh with the middle finger over the greater trochanter and lifts the thigh to bring the femoral head from its posterior position toward the acetabulum. With gentle abduction of the thigh, the femoral head is returned to the acetabulum and the examiner feels a sense of reduction or a "clunk." This reduction is palpable and cannot be heard. With the **Barlow maneuver,** the nurse grasps and adducts the infant's thigh and applies gentle downward pressure. Dislocation is felt as the femoral head slips out of the acetabulum. The femoral head is then returned to the acetabulum using the Ortolani maneuver, confirming the diagnosis of an unstable or dislocatable hip.

The feet are then examined for evidence of a talipes deformity (clubfoot). Intrauterine position frequently causes the feet to appear to turn inward (Figure 29–35 •); this is termed a "positional" clubfoot. If the feet can easily be returned to midline by manipulation, no treatment is indicated. Range-of-motion exercises can be taught to the family. Further investigation is indicated when the foot will not turn to the midline position or align readily. This is considered the most severe type of "true clubfoot," or talipes equinovarus.

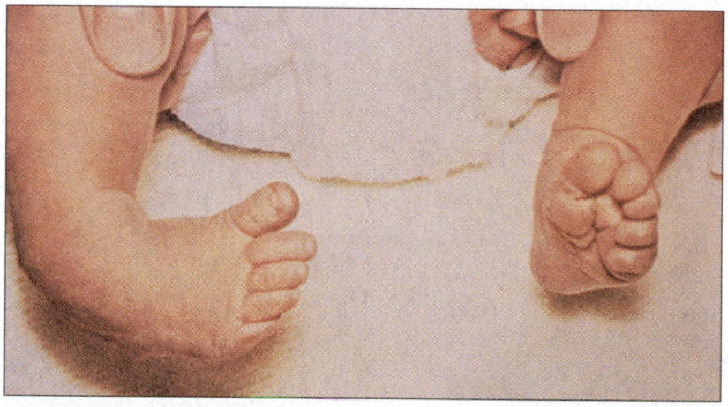

A

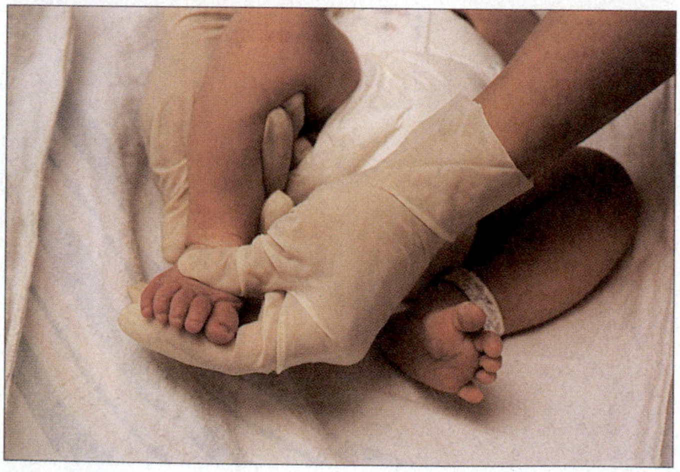

B

Figure 29–35 • *A,* Unilateral talipes equinovarus (clubfoot). *B,* To determine the presence of clubfoot, the nurse moves the foot to the midline. Resistance indicates true clubfoot.

Back

With the baby prone, the nurse examines the back. The spine should appear straight and flat because the lumbar and sacral curves do not develop until the infant begins to sit. The base of the spine is then examined for a dermal sinus. The nevus pilosus ("hairy nevus") is only occasionally found at the base of the spine in newborns, but it is significant because it is frequently associated with spina bifida. A pilonidal dimple should be examined to ascertain that there is no connection to the spinal canal.

Assessment of Neurologic Status

The nurse should begin the neurologic examination with a period of observation, noting the general physical characteristics and behavior of the newborn. Important behaviors to assess are the *state of alertness, resting posture, cry,* and *quality of muscle tone* and *motor activity.*

The usual position of the newborn is with partially flexed extremities with the legs abducted to the abdomen. When awake, the newborn may exhibit purposeless, uncoordinated bilateral movements of the extremities. If these movements are absent, minimal, or obviously asymmetric, neurologic dysfunction should be suspected. Eye movements are observable during the first few days of life. An alert newborn is able to fixate on faces and brightly colored objects. Shining a bright light in the newborn's eyes elicits the blinking response.

The nurse evaluates muscle tone by moving various parts of the newborn's body while the newborn's head remains in a neutral position. The newborn is somewhat hypertonic; that is, the newborn resists the examiner's attempts to extend the elbow and knee joints. Muscle tone should be symmetric. Diminished muscle tone and flaccidity require further evaluation.

Tremors or jitteriness is common in the full-term newborn and must be evaluated to differentiate it from a convulsion. A fine jumping of the muscle is likely to be a central nervous system disorder and requires further evaluation. Jitteriness may be related to hypoglycemia, hypocalcemia, or substance withdrawal. Environmental stimuli may initiate tremors. Holding or flexing the involved extremity will stop the tremor. Neonatal seizures may consist of no more than chewing or swallowing movements, deviations of the eyes, rigidity, or flaccidity because of central nervous system immaturity. Seizures are not usually initiated by stimuli, and cannot be stopped by holding.

Specific deep tendon reflexes can be elicited in the newborn but have limited value unless they are obviously asymmetric. The knee jerk is brisk; a normal ankle clonus may involve three or four beats. Plantar flexion is present.

The central nervous system of the newborn is immature and characterized by a variety of reflexes that should be carefully assessed. Because the movements of newborns are uncoordinated, their methods of communication are limited, and their ability to control their body functions is drastically limited, their reflexes serve a variety of purposes in promoting their well-being. Some are protective (blink, gag, sneeze); some aid in feeding (rooting, sucking) and may not be very active if the infant has eaten recently; and some stimulate human interaction (grasping).

The most common reflexes found in the normal newborn are the following:

- The **tonic neck reflex** (fencer position) is elicited when the newborn is supine and the head is turned to one side. In response, the extremities on the same side straighten, whereas on the opposite side they flex (Figure 29–36 •). This reflex may not be seen during the early newborn period, but once it appears, it persists until about the third month.
- The **grasping reflex** is elicited by stimulating the newborn's palm with a finger or object. The newborn will grasp and hold the object or finger firmly enough to be lifted momentarily from the crib (Figure 29–37 •).
- The **Moro reflex** is elicited when the newborn is startled by a loud noise or is lifted slightly above the crib and then suddenly lowered. In response the newborn straightens arms and hands outward while the knees flex. Slowly, the arms return to the chest, as in an embrace. The fingers spread, forming a C, and the newborn may cry (Figure 29–38 •). This reflex may persist until about 6 months of age.
- The **rooting reflex** is elicited when the side of the newborn's mouth or cheek is touched. In response the newborn turns toward that side and opens the lips to suck (if not fed recently) (Figure 29–39 •).
- The **sucking reflex** is elicited when an object is placed in the newborn's mouth or anything touches the lips. Newborns suck even while sleeping; this is called nonnutritive sucking, and it can have a quieting effect on the baby.
- The **Babinski reflex (plantar reflex)**, or fanning and hyperextension of all toes, occurs when the lateral aspect of the sole is stroked from the heel upward across the ball of the foot. In adults, by contrast, the toes flex (Figure 29–40 •).
- **Trunk incurvation (Galant reflex)** is seen when the newborn is prone. Stroking the spine causes the pelvis to turn to the stimulated side.

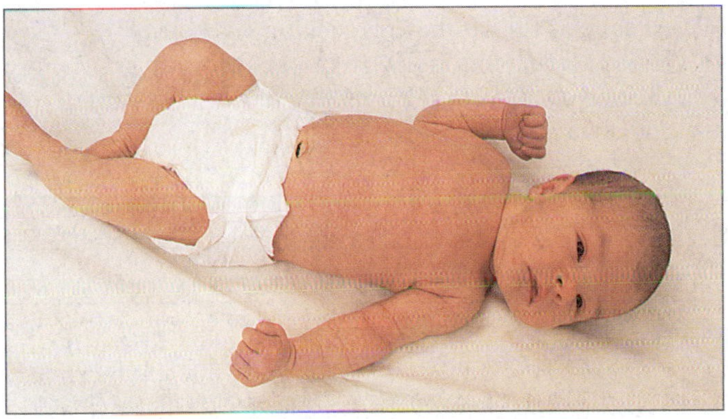

Figure 29–36 • Tonic neck reflex.

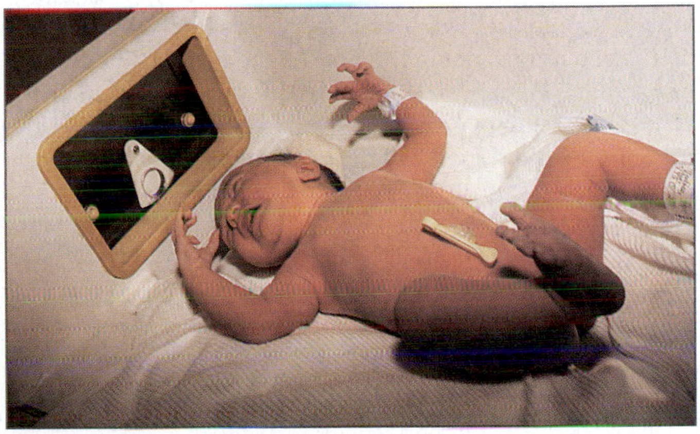

Figure 29–38 • Moro reflex.

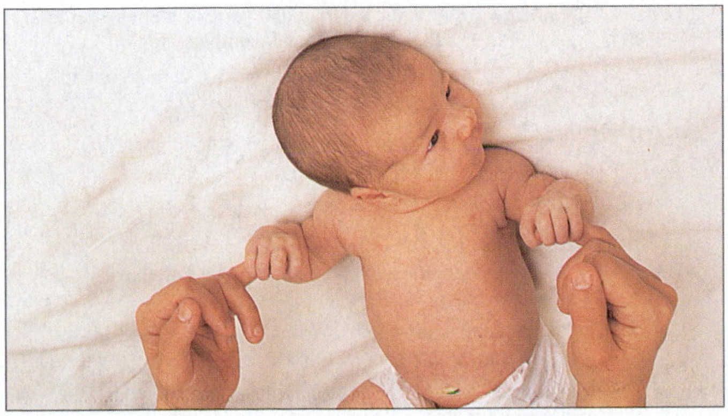

Figure 29–37 • Grasping reflex.

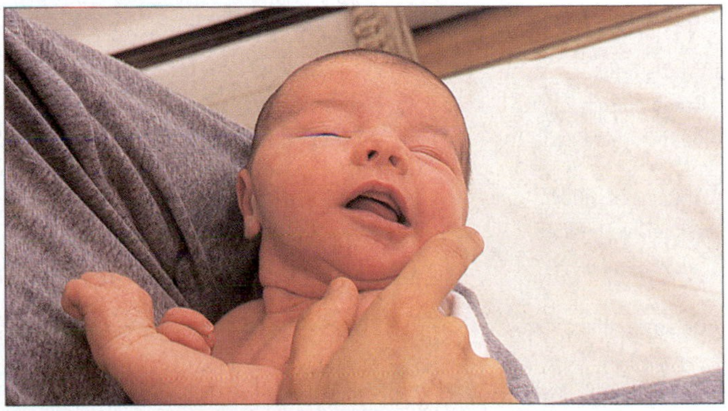

Figure 29–39 • Rooting reflex.

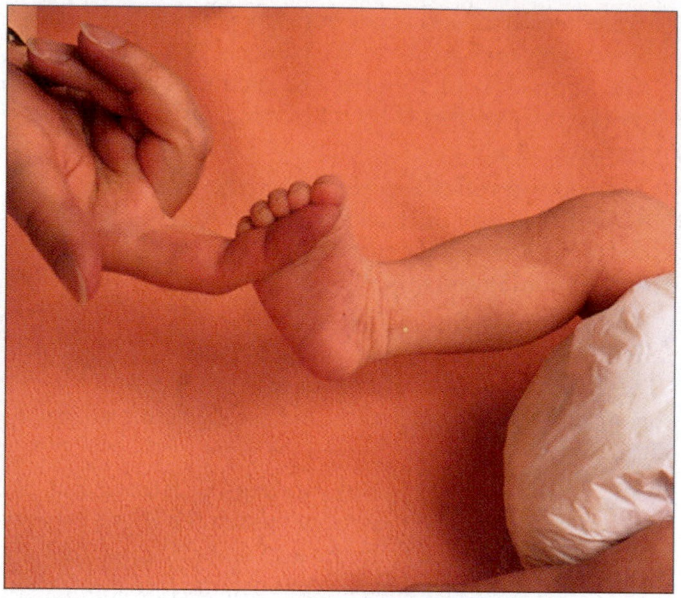

Figure 29–40 • The Babinski (or plantar) reflex.

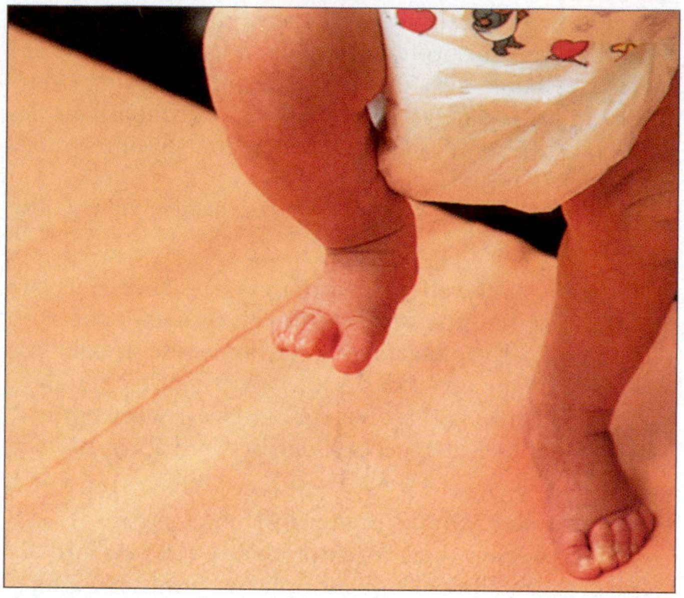

Figure 29–41 • The stepping reflex disappears between 4 and 8 weeks.

In addition to these reflexes, newborns can *blink*, *yawn*, *cough*, *sneeze*, and draw back from pain (protective reflexes). They can even move a little on their own. When placed on their stomachs, they push up and try to crawl (prone crawl). When held upright with one foot touching a flat surface, the newborn puts one foot in front of the other and "walks" (stepping reflex) (Figure 29–41 •). This reflex is more pronounced at birth and is lost in 4 to 8 weeks. Table 29–5 • summarizes the stimulus for and response of the common newborn reflexes.

Brazelton (1984) recommends the following steps as a means of assessing central nervous system integration:

1. Insert a gloved finger into the newborn's mouth to elicit a sucking reflex.
2. As soon as the newborn is sucking vigorously, assess hearing and vision responses by noting sucking changes in the presence of a light, a rattle, and a voice.

Table 29–5 • COMMON REFLEXES OF THE NEWBORN

Reflex Name	Evoking Stimulus	Response
Blinking reflex	Light flash	Eyelids close.
Pupillary reflex	Light flash	Pupil constricts.
Rooting reflex	Light touch of finger on cheek close to mouth	Head rotates toward stimulation; mouth opens and attempts to suck finger. Disappears by about 4 months of age.
Sucking reflex	Finger (or nipple) inserted into mouth	Rhythmic sucking occurs.
Moro reflex	Infant lying on back: slightly raised head suddenly released; infant held horizontally, lowered quickly about 6 in, and stopped abruptly	Arms are extended, head is thrown back, fingers are spread wide; arms are then brought back to center convulsively with hands clenched; spine and lower extremities are extended. Disappears by about 6 months of age.
Startle reflex	Loud noise	Similar to Moro reflex flexion in arms; fists are clenched.
Grasping reflex	Finger placed in palm of hand	Infant's fingers close around and grasp object.
Tonic neck reflex	Head turned to one side while infant lies on back	Arm and leg are extended on the side the infant faces. Opposite arm and leg are flexed.
Abdominal reflex	Tactile stimulation or tickling	Abdominal muscles contract.
Withdrawal reflex	Slight pinprick to the sole of the infant's foot	Leg flexes.
Walking reflex	Infant supported in an upright position with feet lightly touching a flat surface	Rhythmic stepping movement. Disappears at about 4 to 8 weeks of age.
Babinski reflex	Gentle stroking on the sole of each foot	Fanning and extension of the toes (adults respond to this stimulation with flexion of toes).
Plantar, or toe-grasping, reflex	Pressure applied with the finger against the balls of the infant's feet	A plantar flexion of all toes. Disappears by the end of the first year of life.

Source: Adapted from Mott, S. R., James, S. R., & Sperhac, A. M. (1990). *Nursing care of children and families: A holistic approach* (2nd ed.). Menlo Park, CA: Addison-Wesley Nursing.

Table 29–6 • POTENTIAL BIRTH INJURIES

Classification	Examples*
Soft-tissue injuries	Lacerations, abrasions, bruising, fat necrosis
Skull injuries	Cephalhematoma,* fractures
Scalp laceration	Fetal scalp electrode
Scalp abscess	Fetal scalp electrode
Intracranial hemorrhage	Subdural, subarachnoid
Eye injuries	Subconjunctival* and retinal hemorrhages
Fractures	Clavicle,* facial bones, humerus, femur
Dislocations	
Torticollis	Sternocleidomastoid muscle
Nerve injuries	Facial nerve*, brachial plexus*, phrenic nerve, recurrent laryngeal nerve (vocal cord paralysis), Horner syndrome
Spinal cord injuries	
Visceral rupture	Liver, spleen

*Most common birth injuries seen in newborns.

Critical Thinking in Practice

Maria Reyes, a 19-year-old G2P2 mother, gave birth to a 40-week-old female infant 24 hours ago. The newborn exam was normal. Mrs Reyes asks about the newborn's exam. She says she has noticed that the baby cries more than her first child and seems to require holding for longer periods of time after feeding before "quieting down." She is concerned that she is doing something wrong and wants to know when her newborn will start to act like her first baby. What should you discuss with her about newborn behavior?

Answers can be found in Appendix I.

3. The newborn should respond with a brief cessation of sucking followed by continuous sucking with repeated stimulation.

This examination demonstrates auditory and visual integrity as well as complex behavioral interactions.

As healthcare providers carry out the newborn physical and neurologic assessment, they are always on the alert to recognize possible alterations and possible injuries related to the birth process that require further investigation and intervention. (See Table 29–6 • for potential birth injuries.)

Newborn Physical Assessment Guide

Following is a guide for systematically assessing the newborn. Normal findings, alterations, and related causes are presented in correlation with suggested nursing responses. The findings are typical for a full-term newborn.

Newborn Behavioral Assessment

Two conflicting forces influence parents' perceptions of their newborn. One is the parents' preconceptions, based on hopes and fears, of what their newborn will be like. The other is their initial reaction to their baby's temperament, behaviors, and physical appearance. Nurses can assist parents in identifying their baby's specific behaviors.

> *One of the newborn's first responses is to move into a quiet but alert state of consciousness. The baby is still; his body molds to yours; his hands touch your skin; his eyes open wide and are bright and shiny. He looks directly at you.*
>
> *This special alert state, this innate ability to communicate, may be the initial preparation for becoming attached to other human beings. One feels awed by the intensity and appealing power of this little bud of humanity meeting the world for the first time.*
>
> ~ The Amazing Newborn ~

Brazelton's Neonatal Behavioral Assessment Scale provides valuable guidelines for assessing the newborn's state changes, temperament, and individual behavior patterns. It furnishes a means by which the healthcare provider, in conjunction with the parents (primary caregivers), can identify and understand the individual newborn's states and capabilities. Families learn which responses, interventions, or activities best meet the special needs of their newborn, and this understanding fosters positive attachment experiences.

The assessment tool attempts to identify the newborn's repertoire of behavioral responses to the environment and also documents the newborn's neurologic adequacy and capabilities. The examination usually takes 20 to 30 minutes and involves about 30 tests. Some items are scored according to the newborn's response to specific stimuli. Others, such as consolability and alertness, are scored as a result of continuous behavioral observations throughout the assessment.

Because the first few days after birth are a period of behavioral disorganization, the complete assessment should be done on the third day after birth. The nurse should make every effort to elicit the best response. This may be accomplished by repeating tests at different times or by testing during situations that facilitate the best possible response, such as when parents are holding, cuddling, rocking, and singing to their baby.

The assessment of the newborn should be carried out initially in a quiet, dimly or softly lighted room, if possible. The nurse should determine the newborn's state of consciousness, because scoring and introduction of the test items correlate with the sleep or awake state. The newborn's state depends on physiologic variables, such as the amount of time from the last feeding, positioning, environmental temperature, and health status; presence of such external stimuli as noises and bright lights; and the sleep-wake cycle of the infant. An important characteristic of the neonatal period is the pattern of states, as

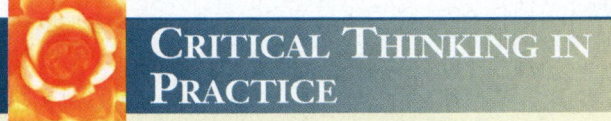

Assessment Guide — Newborn Physical Assessment

Physical Assessment/ Normal Findings	Alterations and Possible Causes*	Nursing Responses to Data†
➤ VITAL SIGNS		
Blood pressure (BP) At birth: 80–60/45–40 mm Hg Day 10: 100/50 mm Hg (may be unable to measure diastolic pressure with standard sphygmomanometer)	Low BP (hypovolemia, shock)	Monitor BP in all cases of distress, prematurity, or suspected anomaly. Low BP: Refer to physician immediately so measures to improve circulation are begun.
Pulse 120–160 bpm (if asleep 100 bpm; if crying, up to 180 bpm)	Weak pulse (decreased cardiac output)	Assess skin perfusion by blanching (capillary refill test).
	Bradycardia (severe asphyxia, arrhythmia)	Correlate finding with BP assessments; refer to physician.
	Tachycardia (over 160 bpm at rest) (infection, central nervous system problems, arrhythmia)	Carry out neurologic and thermoregulation assessments.
Respirations 30–60 breaths/minute Synchronization of chest and abdominal movements Diaphragmatic and abdominal breathing	Tachypnea (pneumonia, respiratory distress syndrome [RDS]) Rapid, shallow breathing (hypermagnesemia due to large doses given to mothers with preeclampsia) Respirations below 30 breaths/minute (maternal anesthesia or analgesia)	Identify sleep-wake state; correlate with respiratory pattern. Evaluate for all signs of respiratory distress; report findings to physician.
Transient tachypnea	Expiratory grunting, subcostal and substernal retractions; flaring of nares (respiratory distress); apnea (cold stress, respiratory disorder)	Evaluate for cold stress. Report findings to physician/nurse practitioner.
Crying Strong and lusty Moderate tone and pitch Cries vary in length from 3 to 7 minutes after consoling measures are used	High pitched, shrill (neurologic disorder, hypoglycemia) Weak or absent (CNS disorder, laryngeal problem)	Discuss newborn's use of cry for communication. Assess and record abnormal cries. Reduce environmental noises.
Temperature Axilla 36.4–37.2C (97.5–99F) Rectal 36.6–37.2C (97.8–99F); 36.8C (98.8F) desired Heavier newborns tend to have higher body temperatures	Elevated temperature (room too warm, too much clothing or covers, dehydration, sepsis, brain damage) Subnormal temperature (brainstem involvement, cold, sepsis) Swings of more than 2F from one reading to next or subnormal temperature (infection)	Notify physician of elevation or drop. Counsel parents on possible causes of elevated or low temperatures, appropriate home-care measures, when to call physician. Teach parents how to take rectal and/or axillary temperature; assess parents, information regarding use of thermometer; provide teaching as needed.
Weight 2500–4000 g (5 lb, 8 oz–8 lb, 13 oz)	< 2748 g (< 6 lb) = SGA or preterm infant > 4050 g(> 9 lb) = LGA or infants of diabetic mothers	Plot weight and gestational age on growth chart to identify high-risk infants. Ascertain body build of parents. Counsel parents regarding appropriate caloric intake.

*Possible causes of alterations are placed in parentheses.

†This column provides guidelines for further assessment and initial nursing interventions.

➤

Assessment Guide: Newborn Physical Assessment *continued*

PHYSICAL ASSESSMENT/ NORMAL FINDINGS	ALTERATIONS AND POSSIBLE CAUSES*	NURSING RESPONSES TO DATA†
➤ VITAL SIGNS *Continued*		
Within first 3 to 4 days, normal weight loss of 5%–10% Large babies tend to lose more due to greater fluid loss in proportion to birth weight except infants of diabetic mother	Loss greater than 15% (small fluid intake, loss of meconium and urine, feeding difficulties)	Notify physician of net losses or gains. Calculate fluid intake and losses from all sources (insensible water loss, radiant warmers, and phototherapy lights).
Length 48–52 cm (18–22 in) Grows 10 cm (3 in) during first 3 months	Less than 45 cm (congenital dwarf) Short/long bones proximally (achondroplasia) Short/long bones distally (Ellis-van Creveld syndrome)	Assess for other signs of dwarfism. Determine other signs of skeletal system adequacy. Plot progress at subsequent well-baby visits.
➤ POSTURE		
Body usually flexed, hands may be tightly clenched, neck appears short as chin rests on chest In breech births feet are usually dorsiflexed	Only extension noted, inability to move from midline (trauma, hypoxia, immaturity) Constant motion (maternal caffeine intake)	Record spontaneity of motor activity and symmetry of movements. If parents express concern about newborn's movement patterns, reassure and evaluate further if appropriate.
➤ SKIN		
Color Color consistent with genetic background Newborns of European descent: pink-tinged or ruddy color over face, trunk, extremities Newborns of African or Native American descent: pale pink with yellow or red tinge Newborns of Asian descent: pink or rosy red to yellow tinge	Pallor of face, conjunctiva (anemia, hypothermia, anoxia) Beefy red (hypoglycemia, immature vasomotor reflexes, polycythemia)	Discuss with parents common skin color variations to allay fears. Document extent and time of occurrence of color change.
Common variations: acrocyanosis, circumoral cyanosis, or harlequin color change	Meconium staining (fetal distress) Jaundice (hemolytic reaction from blood incompatibility within first 24 hours, sepsis)	Obtain hemiglobin and hematocrit values, obtain bilirubin levels. Assess for respiratory difficulty. Differentiate between physiologic and pathologic jaundice.
Mottled when undressed	Cyanosis (choanal atresia, CNS damage or trauma, respiratory or cardiac problem, cold stress)	Assess degree of (central or peripheral) cyanosis and possible causes; refer to physician.
Minor bruising over buttocks in breech presentation and over eyes and forehead in facial presentations		Discuss with parents cause and course of minor bruising related to labor and birth.
Texture Smooth, soft, flexible, may have dry, peeling hands and feet	Generalized cracked or peeling skin (SGA or postterm; blood incompatibility; metabolic, kidney dysfunction) Seborrheic-dermatitis (cradle cap) Absence of vernix (postmature) Yellow vernix (bilirubin staining)	Report to physician. Instruct parents to shampoo the scalp and anterior fontanelle areas daily with soap; rinse well; avoid use of oil.
	*Possible causes of alterations are placed in parentheses.	†This column provides guidelines for further assessment and initial nursing interventions.

(continued on next page)

Assessment Guide: NEWBORN PHYSICAL ASSESSMENT *continued*

PHYSICAL ASSESSMENT/ NORMAL FINDINGS	ALTERATIONS AND POSSIBLE CAUSES*	NURSING RESPONSES TO DATA†
➤ **SKIN** *Continued*		
Turgor Elastic, returns to normal shape after pinching	Maintains tent shape (dehydration)	Assess for other signs and symptoms of dehydration.
Pigmentation Clear; milia across bridge of nose, forehead, or chin will disappear within a few weeks		Advise parents not to pinch or prick these pimplelike areas.
Café-au-lait spots (one or two)	Six or more (neurologic disorder such as von Recklinghausen disease, cutaneous neurofibromatosis)	If there are six or more café-au-lait spots, refer for genetic and neurologic consult.
Mongolian spots common over dorsal area and buttocks in dark-skinned infants		Assure parents of normalcy of this pigmentation; it will fade in first year or two.
Erythema toxicum	Impetigo (group A β-hemolytic streptococcus or *Staphylococcus aureus* infection)	If impetigo occurs, instruct parents about handwashing and linen precautions during home care.
Telangiectatic nevi	Hemangiomas: Nevus flammeus (port wine stain) Nevus vascularis (strawberry hemangioma) Cavernous hemangiomas	Collaborate with physician. Counsel parents about birthmark's progression to allay misconceptions. Record size and shape of hemangiomas. Refer for follow-up at well-baby clinic.
Rashes	Rashes (infection)	Assess location and type of rash (macular, papular, vesicular). Obtain history of onset, prenatal history, and related signs and symptoms.
Petechiae of head or neck (breech presentation, cord around neck)	Generalized petechiae (clotting abnormalities)	Determine cause; advise parents if further healthcare is needed.
➤ **HEAD**		
General appearance, size, movement Round, symmetric, and moves easily from left to right and up and down; soft and pliable	Asymmetric, flattened occiput on either side of the head (plagiocephaly) Head held at angle (torticollis)	Instruct parents to change infant's sleeping positions frequently.
	Unable to move head side to side (neurologic trauma)	Determine adequacy of all neurologic signs.
Circumference 32–37 cm (12.5–14.5 in); 2 cm greater than chest circumference Head one fourth of body size	Extreme differences in size may be microencephaly (Cornelia de Lange syndrome, cytomegalic inclusion disease [CID], rubella, toxoplasmosis, chromosome abnormalities), hydrocephalus (meningomyelocele, achondroplasia), anencephaly (neural tube defect) Head is 3 cm or more larger than chest circumference (preterm, hydrocephalus)	Measure circumference from occiput to frontal area using metal or paper tape. Measure chest circumference using metal or paper tape and compare to head circumference. Record measurements on growth chart. Reevaluate at well-baby visits.

*Possible causes of alterations are placed in parentheses.

†This column provides guidelines for further assessment and initial nursing interventions.

ASSESSMENT GUIDE: NEWBORN PHYSICAL ASSESSMENT *continued*

PHYSICAL ASSESSMENT/ NORMAL FINDINGS	ALTERATIONS AND POSSIBLE CAUSES*	NURSING RESPONSES TO DATA†
➤ HEAD *Continued*		
Common variations Molding Breech and cesarean newborns' heads are round and well shaped	Cephalhematoma (trauma during birth, persists up to 3 weeks) Caput succedaneum (long labor and birth; disappears in 1 week)	Evaluate neurologic response. Observe for hyperbilirubinemia. Reassure parents regarding common manifestations due to birth process and when they should disappear.
Fontanelles Palpation of juncture of cranial bones Anterior fontanelle: 3–4 cm long by 2–3 cm wide, diamond shaped Posterior fontanelle: 1–2 cm at birth, triangle shaped	Overlapping of anterior fontanelle (malnourished or preterm newborn) Premature closure of sutures (craniostenosis) Late closure (hydrocephalus)	Discuss normal closure times with parents and care of "soft spots" to allay misconceptions. Refer to physician. Observe for signs and symptoms of hydrocephalus.
Slight pulsation	Moderate to severe pulsation (vascular problems)	Refer to physician.
Moderate bulging noted with crying, stooling, or pulsations with heartbeat	Bulging (increased intracranial pressure, meningitis) Sunken (dehydration)	Evaluate hydration status. Evaluate neurologic status. Report to physician.
➤ HAIR		
Texture Smooth with fine texture variations (Note: Variations depend on ethnic background.)	Coarse, brittle, dry hair (hypothyroidism) White forelock (Waardenburg syndrome)	Instruct parents regarding routine care of hair and scalp.
Distribution Scalp hair high over eyebrows (Spanish-Mexican hairline begins mid-forehead and extends down back of neck.)	Low forehead and posterior hairlines may indicate chromosomal disorders.	Assess for other signs of chromosomal aberrations. Refer to physician.
➤ FACE		
Symmetric movement of all facial features, normal hairline, eyebrows and eyelashes present		Assess and record symmetry of all parts, shape, regularity of features, sameness or differences in features.
Spacing of features Eyes at same level, nostrils equal size, cheeks full, and sucking pads present	Eyes wide apart—ocular hypertelorism (Apert syndrome, cri-du-chat, Turner syndrome)	Observe for other signs and symptoms indicative of disease states or chromosomal aberrations.
Lips equal on both sides of midline	Abnormal face (Down syndrome, cretinism, gargoylism)	
Chin recedes when compared to other bones of face	Abnormally small jaw—micrognathia (Pierre Robin syndrome, Treacher Collins syndrome)	Maintain airway; do not position supine. Initiate surgical consultation and referral.
	*Possible causes of alterations are placed in parentheses.	†This column provides guidelines for further assessment and initial nursing interventions.

(continued on next page)

ASSESSMENT GUIDE: NEWBORN PHYSICAL ASSESSMENT *continued*

PHYSICAL ASSESSMENT/ NORMAL FINDINGS	ALTERATIONS AND POSSIBLE CAUSES*	NURSING RESPONSES TO DATA†
➤ **FACE** *Continued*		
Movement Makes facial grimaces	Inability to suck, grimace, and close eyelids (cranial nerve injury)	Initiate neurologic assessment and consultation.
Symmetric when resting and crying	Asymmetry (paralysis of facial cranial nerve)	Assess and record symmetry of all parts, shape, regularity of features, and sameness or differences in features.
➤ **EYES**		
General placement and appearance Bright and clear; even placement; slight nystagmus (involuntary cyclical eye movements)	Gross nystagmus (damage to third, fourth, and sixth cranial nerves)	
Concomitant strabismus	Constant and fixed strabismus	Reassure parents that strabismus is considered normal up to 6 months.
Move in all directions		
Blue or slate blue-gray	Lack of pigmentation (albinism) Brushfield spots may indicate Down syndrome (a light or white speckling of the outer two thirds of the iris)	Discuss with parents any necessary eye precautions. Assess for other signs of Down syndrome.
Brown color at birth in dark-skinned infants		Discuss with parents that permanent eye color is usually established by 3 months of age.
Eyelids Position: above pupils but within iris, no drooping	Elevation or retraction of upper lid (hyperthyroidism)	Assess for other signs of hydrocephalus and hyperthyroidism.
	"Sunset sign" lid retraction and downward gaze (hydrocephalus), ptosis (congenital or paralysis of oculomotor muscle)	Evaluate interference with vision in subsequent well-baby visits.
Eyes on parallel plane	Upward slant in non-Asians (Down syndrome)	Assess for other signs of Down syndrome.
Epicanthal folds in Asians and 20% of newborns of northern European descent	Epicanthal folds (Down syndrome, cri-du-chat syndrome)	
Movement Blink reflex in response to light stimulus	Blink absent (CNS injury)	Evaluate neurologic status.
Eyes open wide in dimly lighted room		Refer to physician.
Inspection Edematous for first few days of life, resulting from birth and instillation of silver nitrate (chemical conjunctivitis); no lumps or redness	Purulent drainage (infection); infectious conjunctivitis (gonococcus, chlamydia, staphylococcus, or gram-negative organisms) Marginal blepharitis (lid edges red, crusted, scaly)	Initiate good handwashing. Refer to physician. Evaluate infant for seborrheic dermatitis; scales can be removed easily.

*Possible causes of alterations are placed in parentheses.

†This column provides guidelines for further assessment and initial nursing interventions.

Assessment Guide: Newborn Physical Assessment *continued*

PHYSICAL ASSESSMENT/ NORMAL FINDINGS	ALTERATIONS AND POSSIBLE CAUSES*	NURSING RESPONSES TO DATA†
➤ EYES *Continued*		
Cornea Clear Corneal reflex present	Ulceration (herpes infection); large cornea or corneas of unequal size (congenital glaucoma) Clouding, opacity of lens (cataract)	Refer to ophthalmologist. Assess for other manifestations of congenital herpes; insititute nursing care measures.
Sclera May appear bluich in newborn, then white; slightly brownish color frequent in newborns of African descent	True blue sclera (osteogenesis imperfecta)	Refer to physician.
Pupils Pupils equal in size, round, and react to light by accommodation	Anisocoria—unequal pupils (CNS damage) Dilation or constriction (intracranial damage, retinoblastoma, glaucoma) Pupils nonreactive to light or accommodation (brain injury)	Refer for neurologic examination.
Slight nystagmus in newborn who has not learned to focus Pupil light reflex demonstrated at birth or by 3 weeks of age	Nystagmus (labyrinthine disturbance, CNS disorder)	
Conjunctiva Chemical conjunctivitis Subconjunctival hemorrhage	Pale color (anemia)	Obtain hematocrit and hemoglobin. Reassure parents that chemical conjunctivitis will subside in 1 to 2 days and subconjunctival hemorrhage disappears in a few weeks.
Palpebral conjunctiva (red but not hyperemic)	Inflammation or edema (infection, blocked tear duct)	
Vision 20/150 Tracks moving object to midline Fixed focus on objects at a distance of about 10–20 in; may be difficult to evaluate in newborn Prefers faces, geometric designs, and black and white to colors	Cataracts (congenital infection)	Record any questions about visual acuity, and initiate follow-up evaluation at first well-baby checkup.
Lashes and lacrimal glands Presence of lashes (lashes may be absent in preterm newborns)	No lashes on inner two thirds of lid (Treacher Collins syndrome); bushy lashes (Hurler syndrome); long lashes (Cornelia de Lange syndrome)	
Cry commonly tearless	Excessive tearing (plugged lacrimal duct, natal narcotic withdrawal), glaucoma	Demonstrate to parents how to milk blocked tear duct. Refer to ophthalmologist if tearing is excessive before third month of life.

*Possible causes of alterations are placed in parentheses.

†This column provides guidelines for further assessment and initial nursing interventions.

(continued on next page)

ASSESSMENT GUIDE: NEWBORN PHYSICAL ASSESSMENT *continued*

PHYSICAL ASSESSMENT/ NORMAL FINDINGS	ALTERATIONS AND POSSIBLE CAUSES*	NURSING RESPONSES TO DATA†
➤ NOSE		
Appearance of external nasal aspects May appear flattened as a result of birth process	Continued flat or broad bridge of nose (Down syndrome)	Arrange consultation with specialist.
Small and narrow in midline, even placement in relationship to eyes and mouth	Low bridge of nose, beaklike nose (Apert syndrome, Treacher Collins syndrome) Upturned (Cornelia de Lange syndrome)	Initiate evaluation of chromosomal abnormalities.
Patent nares bilaterally (nose breathers)	Blockage of nares (mucus and/or secretions), choanal atresia	Inspect for obstruction of nares.
Sneezing common to clear nasal passages	Flaring nares (respiratory distress)	Maintain oral airway until surgical correction is made.
Responds to odors, may smell breast milk	No response to stimulating odors	Inspect for obstruction of nares.
➤ MOUTH		
Function of facial, hypoglossal, glossopharyngeal, and vagus nerves Symmetry of movement and strength	Mouth draws to one side (transient seventh cranial nerve paralysis due to pressure in utero or trauma during birth, congenital paralysis) Fishlike shape (Treacher Collins syndrome)	Initiate neurologic consultation. Administer eye care if eye on affected side of face is unable to close.
Presence of gag, swallowing, coordinated with sucking reflexes Adequate salivation	Suppressed or absent reflexes	Evaluate other neurologic functions of these nerves.
Palate (soft and hard) Hard palate dome-shaped Uvula midline with symmetrical movement of soft palate	High-steepled palate (Treacher Collins syndrome), bifid uvula (congenital anomaly)	Assess for other congenital anomalies.
Palate intact, sucks well when stimulated	Clefts in either hard or soft palate (polygenic disorder)	Initiate a surgical consultation referral.
Epithelial (Epstein's) pearls appear on mucosa		Assure parents that these are normal and will disappear at 2 or 3 months of age.
Esophagus patent, some drooling common in newborn	Excessive drooling or bubbling (esophageal atresia)	Test for patency of esophagus.
Tongue Free moving in all directions, midline	Lack of movement or asymmetric movement (neurologic damage) Tongue-tied	Further assess neurologic functions. Test reflex elevation of tongue when depressed with tongue blade.
	Deviations from midline (cranial nerve damage)	Check for signs of weakness or deviation.
Pink color, smooth to rough texture, noncoated	White cheesy coating (thrush) Tongue has deep ridges	Differentiate between thrush and milk curds. Reassure parents that tongue pattern may change from day to day.

*Possible causes of alterations are placed in parentheses.

†This column provides guidelines for further assessment and initial nursing interventions.

➤

Assessment Guide: NEWBORN PHYSICAL ASSESSMENT *continued*

PHYSICAL ASSESSMENT/ NORMAL FINDINGS	ALTERATIONS AND POSSIBLE CAUSES*	NURSING RESPONSES TO DATA†
➤ MOUTH *Continued*		
Tongue proportional to mouth	Large tongue with short frenulum (cretinism, Down syndrome, other syndromes)	Evaluate in well-baby clinic to assess development delays. Initiate referrals.
➤ EARS		
External ear Without lesions, cysts, or nodules	Nodules, cysts, or sinus tracts in front of ear	Evaluate characteristics of lesions.
	Adherent earlobes Low set	Counsel parents to clean external ear with washcloth only; discourage use of cotton-tip applicators.
	Preauricular skin tags	Refer to physician for ligation.
Hearing Eustachian tubes are cleared with first cry Absence of all risk factors	Presence of one or more risk factors	Assess history of risk factors for hearing loss.
Attends to sounds; sudden or loud noise elicits Moro reflex	No response to sound stimuli (deafness)	Test for Moro reflex.
➤ NECK		
Appearance Short, straight, creased with skin folds	Abnormally short neck (Turner syndrome) Arching or inability to flex neck (meningitis, congenital anomaly)	Report findings to physician.
Posterior neck lacks loose extra folds of skin	Webbing of neck (Turner syndrome, Down syndrome, trisomy 18)	Assess for other signs of the syndromes.
Clavicles Straight and intact	Knot or lump on clavicle (fracture during difficult birth)	Obtain detailed labor and birth history; apply figure-8 bandage.
Moro reflex elicitable	Unilateral Moro reflex response on unaffected side (fracture of clavicle, brachial palsy, Erb-Duchenne paralysis)	Collaborate with physician.
Symmetric shoulders	Hypoplasia	
➤ CHEST		
Appearance and size Circumference: 32.5 cm, 1–2 cm less than head Wider than it is long		Measure at level of nipples after exhalation.
Normal shape without depressed or prominent sternum Lower end of sternum (xiphoid cartilage) may be protruding; is less apparent after several weeks Sternum 8 cm long	Funnel chest (congenital or associated with Marfan syndrome) Continued protrusion of xiphoid cartilage (Marfan syndrome, "pigeon chest") Barrel chest	Determine adequacy of other respiratory and circulatory signs. Assess for other signs and symptoms of various syndromes.

*Possible causes of alterations are placed in parentheses.

†This column provides guidelines for further assessment and initial nursing interventions.

(continued on next page)

Assessment Guide: Newborn Physical Assessment *continued*

PHYSICAL ASSESSMENT/ NORMAL FINDINGS	ALTERATIONS AND POSSIBLE CAUSES*	NURSING RESPONSES TO DATA†
➤ CHEST *Continued*		
Expansion and retraction Bilateral expansion	Unequal chest expansion (pneumonia, pneumothorax, respiratory distress)	Assess respiratory effort regularity, flaring of nares, difficulty on both inspiration and expiration.
No intercostal, subcostal, or supracostal retractions	Retractions (respiratory distress) See-saw respirations (respiratory distress)	Record and consult physician.
Auscultation Breath sounds are louder in infants	Decreased breath sounds (decreased respiratory activity, atelectasis, pneumothorax)	Perform assessment and report to physician any positive findings.
Chest and axilia clear on crying	Increased breath sounds (resolving pneumonia or in cesarean births)	
Bronchial breath sounds (heard where trachea and bronchi closest to chest wall, above sternum and between scapulae): Bronchial sounds bilaterally Air entry clear Rales may indicate normal newborn atelectasis Cough reflex absent at birth, appears in 2 or more days	Adventitious or abnormal sounds (respiratory disease or distress)	Evaluate color for pallor or cyanosis. Report to physician.
Breasts Flat with symmetric nipples Breast tissue diameter 5 cm or more at term Distance between nipples 8 cm	Lack of breast tissue (preterm or SGA) Discharge	Evaluate for infection.
Breast engorgement occurs on third day of life; liquid discharge may be expressed in term newborns	Enlargement Breast abscesses	Reassure parents of normality of breast engorgement.
Nipples	Supernumerary nipples Dark-colored nipples	No intervention is necessary.
➤ HEART		
Auscultation Location: lies horizontally, with left border extending to left of midclavicle Regular rhythm and rate	Arrhythmia (anoxia), tachycardia, bradycardia	Refer all arrhythmia and gallop rhythms. Initiate cardiac evaluation.
Determination of point of maximal impulse (PMI) Usually lateral to midclavicular line at third or fourth intercostal space	Malpositioning (enlargement, abnormal placement, pneumothorax, dextrocardia, diaphragmatic hernia)	
Functional murmurs No thrills	Location of murmurs (possible congenital cardiac anomaly)	Evaluate murmur: location, timing, and duration; observe for accompanying cardiac pathology symptoms; ascertain family history.
Horizontal groove at diaphragm shows flaring of rib cage to mild degree	Marked rib flaring (vitamin D deficiency) Inadequacy of respiratory movement	Initiate cardiopulmonary evaluation; assess pulses and blood pressures in all four extremities for equality and quality.

*Possible causes of alterations are placed in parentheses.

†This column provides guidelines for further assessment and initial nursing interventions.

Assessment Guide: Newborn Physical Assessment *continued*

PHYSICAL ASSESSMENT/ NORMAL FINDINGS	ALTERATIONS AND POSSIBLE CAUSES*	NURSING RESPONSES TO DATA†
➤ ABDOMEN		
Appearance Cylindrical with some protrusion, appears large in relation to pelvis, some laxness of abdominal muscles No cyanosis, few vessels seen Diastasis recti—common in infants of African descent	Distention, shiny abdomen with engorged vessels (gastrointestinal abnormalities, infection, congenital megacolon) Scaphoid abdominal appearance (diaphragmatic hernia) Increased or decreased peristalsis (duodenal stenosis, small bowel obstruction) Localized flank bulging (enlarged kidneys, ascites, or absent abdominal muscles)	Examine abdomen thoroughly for mass or organomegaly. Measure abdominal girth. Report deviations of abdominal size. Assess other signs and symptoms of obstruction. Refer to physician.
Umbilicus No protrusion of umbilicus (protrusion of umbilicus common in infants of African descent) Bluish white color Cutis navel (umbilical cord projects), granulation tissue present in navel	Umbilical hernia Patent urachus (congenital malformation) Gastroschisis Omphalocele Redness or exudate around cord (infection) Yellow discoloration (hemolytic disease, meconium staining)	Measure umbilical hernia by palpating the opening and record; it should close by 1 year of age; if not, refer to physician. Cover omphalocele with sterile, moist dressing. Instruct parents on cord care and hygiene.
Two arteries and one vein apparent Begins drying 1 to 2 hours after birth No bleeding	Single umbilical artery (congenital anomalies) Discharge or oozing of blood from the cord	Refer anomalies to physician.
Auscultation and percussion	Bowel sounds in chest (diaphragmatic hernia)	Collaborate with physician.
Soft bowel sounds heard shortly after birth every 10–30 seconds	Absence of bowel sounds Hyperperistalsis (intestinal obstruction)	Assess for other signs of dehydration and/or infection.
Femoral pulses Palpable, equal bilateral	Absent or diminished femoral pulses (coarctation of aorta)	Monitor blood pressure in upper and lower extremities.
Inguinal area No bulges along inguinal area No inguinal lymph nodes felt	Inguinal hernia	Initiate referral. Continue follow-up in well-baby clinic.
Bladder Percusses 1–4 cm above symphysis Emptied about 3 hours after birth; if not, at time of birth Urine—inoffensive, mild odor	Failure to void within 24–48 hours after birth Exposure of bladder mucosa (exstrophy of bladder) Foul odor (infection)	Check whether baby voided at birth. Consult with specialist. Obtain urine specimen if infection is suspected.
➤ GENITALS		
Gender clearly delineated	Ambiguous genitals	Refer for genetic consultation.

*Possible causes of alterations are placed in parentheses.

†This column provides guidelines for further assessment and initial nursing interventions.

(continued on next page)

Assessment Guide: Newborn Physical Assessment *continued*

PHYSICAL ASSESSMENT/ NORMAL FINDINGS	ALTERATIONS AND POSSIBLE CAUSES*	NURSING RESPONSES TO DATA†
➤ MALE		
Penis Slender in appearance, about 2.5 cm long, 1 cm wide at birth Normal urinary orifice, urethral meatus at tip of penis	Micropenis (congenital anomaly) Meatal atresia Hypospadias, epispadias	Observe and record first voiding. Collaborate with physician in presence of abnormality. Delay circumcision.
Noninflamed urethral opening	Urethritis (infection)	Palpate for enlarged inguinal lymph nodes and record painful urination.
Foreskin adheres to glans	Ulceration of meatal opening (infection, inflammation)	Evaluate whether ulcer is due to diaper rash; counsel regarding care.
Uncircumcised foreskin tight for 2 to 3 months	Phimosis—if still tight after 3 months	Instruct parents on how to care for uncircumcised penis.
Circumcised		Teach parents how to care for circumcision.
Erectile tissue present		
Scrotum Skin loose and hanging or tight and small; extensive rugae and normal size Normal skin color Scrotal discoloration common in breech	Large scrotum containing fluid (hydrocele) Red, shiny scrotal skin (orchitis) Minimal rugae, small scrotum	Shine a light through scrotum (transilluminate) to verify diagnosis. Assess for prematurity.
Testes Descended by birth; not consistently found in scrotum	Undescended testes (cryptorchidism)	If testes cannot be felt in scrotum, gently palpate femoral, inguinal, perineal, and abdominal areas for presence.
Testes size 1.5–2 cm at birth	Enlarged testes (tumor) Small testes (Klinefelter syndrome or adrenal hyperplasia)	Refer and collaborate with physician for further diagnostic studies.
➤ FEMALE		
Mons Normal skin color, area pigmented in dark-skinned infants Labia majora cover labia minora in term and postterm newborns; symmetric size appropriate for gestational age	Hematoma, lesions (trauma) Labia minora prominent	Evaluate for recent trauma. Assess for prematurity.
Clitoris Normally large in newborn Edema and bruising in breech birth	Hypertrophy (hermaphroditism)	Refer for genetic work-up.
Vagina Urinary meatus and vaginal orifice visible (0.5 cm circumference) Vaginal tag or hymenal tag disappears in a few weeks	Inflammation; erythema and discharge (urethritis) Congenital absence of vagina	Collect urine specimen for laboratory examination. Refer to physician.
Discharge; smegma under labia	Foul-smelling discharge (infection)	Collect data and further evaluate reason for discharge.
Bloody or mucoid discharge	Excessive vaginal bleeding (blood coagulation defect)	

*Possible causes of alterations are placed in parentheses.

†This column provides guidelines for further assessment and initial nursing interventions.

Assessment Guide: Newborn Physical Assessment *continued*

PHYSICAL ASSESSMENT/ NORMAL FINDINGS	ALTERATIONS AND POSSIBLE CAUSES*	NURSING RESPONSES TO DATA†
➤ BUTTOCKS AND ANUS		
Buttocks symmetric	Pilonidal dimple	Examine for possible sinus. Instruct parents about cleansing this area.
Anus patent and passage of meconium within 24–48 hours after birth	Imperforate anus, rectal atresia (congenital gastrointestinal defect)	Evaluate extent of problems. Initiate surgical consultation. Perform digital examination to ascertain patency if patency uncertain.
No fissures, tears, or skin tags	Fissures	
➤ EXTREMITIES AND TRUNK		
Short and generally flexed, extremities move symmetrically through range of motion but lack full extension	Unilateral or absence of movement (spinal cord involvement) Fetal position continued or limp (anoxia, CNS problems, hypoglycemia)	Review birth record to assess possible cause.
All joints move spontaneously; good muscle tone, of flexor type, birth to 2 months	Spasticity when infant begins using extensors (cerebral palsy, lack of muscle tone, "floppy baby" syndrome) Hypotonia (Down syndrome)	Collaborate with physician.
Arms Equal in length Bilateral movement Flexed when quiet	Brachial palsy (difficult birth) Erb-Duchenne paralysis Muscle weakness, fractured clavicle Absence of limb or change of size (phocomelia, amelia)	Report to clinician.
Hands Normal number of fingers	Polydactyly (Ellis-van Creveld syndrome) Syndactyly—one limb (developmental anomaly) Syndactyly—both limbs (genetic component)	Report to clinician.
Normal palmar crease	Simian line on palm (Down syndrome)	Refer for genetic work-up.
Normal size hands	Short fingers and broad hand (Hurler syndrome)	
Nails present and extend beyond fingertips in term newborn	Cyanosis and clubbing (cardiac anomalies) Nails long or yellow stained (postterm)	Evaluate for history of distress in utero.
Spine C-shaped spine Flat and straight when prone Slight lumbar lordosis Easily flexed and intact when palpated At least half of back devoid of lanugo Full-term infant in ventral suspension should hold head at 45-degree angle, back straight	Spina bifida occulta (nevus pilosus) Dermal sinus Myelomeningocele Head lag, limp, floppy trunk (neurologic problems)	Evaluate extent of neurologic damage; initiate care of spinal opening.
Hips No sign of instability Hips abduct to more than 60 degrees	Sensation of abnormal movement, jerk, or snap of hip dislocation	Examine all newborn infants for dislocated hip prior to discharge from birthing center. If this is suspected, refer to orthopedist for further evaluation. Reassess at well-baby visits.

*Possible causes of alterations are placed in parentheses.

†This column provides guidelines for further assessment and initial nursing interventions.

(continued on next page)

Assessment Guide: Newborn Physical Assessment *continued*

PHYSICAL ASSESSMENT/ NORMAL FINDINGS	ALTERATIONS AND POSSIBLE CAUSES*	NURSING RESPONSES TO DATA†
➤ EXTREMITIES AND TRUNK *Continued*		
Inguinal and buttock skin creases	Asymmetry (dislocated hips) Symmetric inguinal and buttock creases	Refer to orthopedist for evaluation. Counsel parents regarding symptoms of concern, and discuss therapy.
Legs Legs equal in length Legs shorter than arms at birth	Shortened leg (dislocated hips) Lack of leg movement (fractures, spinal defects)	Refer to orthopedist for evaluation. Counsel parents regarding symptoms of concern, and discuss therapy.
Feet Foot is in straight line Positional clubfoot—based on position in utero	Talipes equinovarus (true clubfoot)	Discuss differences between positional and true clubfoot with parents. Teach parents passive manipulation of foot.
Fat pads and creases on soles of feet	Incomplete sole creases in first 24 hours of life (premature)	Refer to orthopedist if not corrected by 3 months of age.
Talipes planus (flat feet) normal under 3 years of age		Reassure parents that flat feet are normal in infants.
➤ NEUROMUSCULAR		
Motor function Symmetric movement and strength in all extremities	Limp, flaccid, or hypertonic (CNS disorders, infection, dehydration, fracture)	Appraise newborn's posture and motor functions by observing activities and motor characteristics.
May be jerky or have brief twitchings	Tremors (hypoglycemia, hypocalcemia, infection, neurologic damage)	Evaluate electrolyte imbalance, hypoglycemia, and neurologic functioning.
Head lag not over 45 degrees	Delayed or abnormal development (preterm, neurologic involvement)	
Neck control adequate to maintain head erect briefly	Asymmetry of tone or strength (neurologic damage)	Refer for genetic evaluation.
➤ REFLEXES		
Blink Stimulated by flash of light; response is closure of eyelids	Lack of blink response (damage to cranial nerve, CNS injury)	Assess neurologic status.
Pupillary reflex Stimulated by flash of light; response is constriction of pupil	Lack of reflex (damage to cranial nerve, CNS injury)	
Moro Response to sudden movement or loud noise should be one of symmetric extension and abduction of arms with fingers extended; then return to normal relaxed flexion Infant lying on back: slightly raised head suddenly released; infant held horizontally, lowered quickly about 6 in, and stopped abruptly Fingers form a C Present at birth; disappears by 6 months of age	Asymmetry of body response (fractured clavicle, injury to brachial plexus) Consistent absence (brain damage)	Discuss normality of this reflex in response to loud noises and/or sudden movements. Absence of reflex requires neurologic evaluation.

*Possible causes of alterations are placed in parentheses.

†This column provides guidelines for further assessment and initial nursing interventions.

ASSESSMENT GUIDE: NEWBORN PHYSICAL ASSESSMENT *continued*

PHYSICAL ASSESSMENT/ NORMAL FINDINGS	ALTERATIONS AND POSSIBLE CAUSES*	NURSING RESPONSES TO DATA†
➤ **REFLEXES** *Continued*		
Rooting and sucking Turns in direction of stimulus to cheek or mouth; opens mouth and begins to suck rhythmically when finger or nipple is inserted into mouth; difficult to elicit after feeding; disappears by 4 to 7 months of age Sucking is adequate for nutritional intake and meeting oral stimulation needs; disappears by 12 months	Poor sucking or easily fatigable (preterm, breastfed infants of barbiturate-addicted mothers, possible cardiac problem) Absence of response (preterm, neurologic involvement, depressed newborns)	Evaluate strength and coordination of sucking. Observe newborn during feeding, and counsel parents about mutuality of feeding experience and newborn's responses.
Palmar grasp Fingers grasp adult finger when palm is stimulated and held momentarily; lessens at 3 to 4 months of age	Asymmetry of response (neurologic problems)	Evaluate other reflexes and general neurologic functioning.
Plantar grasp Toes curl downward when sole of foot is stimulated; lessens by 8 months	Absent (defects of lower spinal column)	Assess for other lower extremity neurologic problems.
Stepping When held upright and one foot touching a flat surface, will step alternately; disappears at 4 to 5 months of age	Asymmetry of stepping (neurologic abnormality)	Evaluate muscle tone and function on each side of body. Refer to specialist.
Babinski Fanning and extension of all toes when one side of sole is stroked from heel upward across ball of foot; disappears at about 12 months	Absence of response (low spinal cord defects)	Refer for further neurologic evaluation.
Tonic neck Fencer position—when head is turned to one side, extremities on same side extend and on opposite side flex; this reflex may not be evident during early neonatal period; disappears at 3 to 4 months of age Response often more dominant in leg than in arm	Absent after 1 month of age or persistent asymmetry (cerebral lesion)	Assess neurologic functioning.
Prone crawl While on abdomen, newborn pushes up and tries to crawl	Absence or variance of response (preterm, weak, or depressed newborns)	Evaluate motor functioning. Refer to specialist.
Trunk incurvation (Galant) In prone position, stroking of spine causes pelvis to turn to stimulated side	Failure to rotate to stimulated side (neurologic damage)	

*Possible causes of alterations are placed in parentheses.

†This column provides guidelines for further assessment and initial nursing interventions.

well as the transitions from one state to another. The pattern of states is a predictor of the newborn's receptivity and ability to respond to stimuli in a cognitive manner. Babies learn best in a quiet, alert state and in an environment that is supportive and protective and that provides appropriate stimuli.

The nurse should observe the newborn's sleep-wake patterns (as discussed in Chapter 28) and the rapidity with which the newborn moves from one state to another, the newborn's ability to be consoled, and the newborn's ability to diminish the impact of disturbing stimuli. The following questions may provide the nurse with a framework for assessment:

- Does the newborn's response style and ability to adapt to stimuli indicate a need for parental interventions that will alert the newborn to the environment so that the baby can grow socially and cognitively?
- Are parental interventions necessary to lessen the outside stimuli, as in the case of the baby who responds to sensory input with intensity?
- Can the baby control the amount of sensory input to be dealt with?

The behaviors and the sleep-wake states in which they are assessed are categorized as follows:

- *Habituation.* The newborn's ability to diminish or shut down innate responses to specific repeated stimuli, such as a rattle, bell, light, or pinprick to heel.
- *Orientation to inanimate and animate visual and auditory assessment stimuli.* How often and where the newborn attends to auditory and visual stimuli are observed. Orientation to the environment is determined by an ability to respond to cues given by others and by a natural ability to fix on and to follow a visual object horizontally and vertically. This capacity and parental appreciation of it are important for positive communication between infant and parents; the parents' visual (*en face*) and auditory (soft, continuous voice) presence stimulates their infant to orient to them. Inability or lack of response may indicate visual or auditory problems. It is important for parents to know that their newborn can turn to voices usually soon after birth or by 3 days of age and can become alert at different times with a varying degree of intensity in response to sounds.
- *Motor activity.* Several components are evaluated. Motor tone of the newborn is assessed in the most characteristic state of responsiveness. This summary assessment includes overall use of tone as the newborn responds to being handled—whether during spontaneous activity, prone placement, or horizontal holding—and overall assessment of body tone as the newborn reacts to all stimuli.
- *Variations.* Frequency of alert states, state changes, color changes (throughout all states as examination progresses), activity, and peaks of excitement are assessed.
- *Self-quieting activity.* Assessment is based on how often, how quickly, and how effectively newborns can use their resources to quiet and console themselves when upset or distressed. Considered in this assessment are such self-consolatory activities as putting hand to mouth, sucking on a fist or the tongue, and attuning to an object or sound. The newborn's need for outside consolation must also be considered—for example, seeing a face; being rocked, held, or dressed; using a pacifier; and being swaddled.
- *Cuddliness or social behaviors.* This area encompasses the infant's need for and response to being held. Also considered is how often the newborn smiles. These behaviors influence the parents' self-esteem and feelings of acceptance or rejection. Cuddling also appears to be an indicator of personality. Cuddlers appear to enjoy, accept, and seek physical contact; are easier to placate; sleep more; and form earlier and more intense attachments. Noncuddlers are active, are restless, have accelerated motor development, and are intolerant of physical restraint. Smiling, even as a grimace reflex, greatly influences parent-infant feedback.
Parents identify this response as positive.

MediaLink CARE PLAN: ASSESSMENT OF THE NEWBORN

Chapter Review

ExploreMediaLink

NCLEX review questions, case studies, and other interactive resources for this chapter can be found on the Web site at http://www.prenhall.com/olds. Click on "Chapter 29" to select the activities for this chapter.

For tutorials including animations and videos, more NCLEX review questions, and an audio glossary, access the accompanying CD-ROM in this book.

Focus Your Study

- A perinatal history, determination of gestational age, physical examination, and behavioral assessment form the basis for complete newborn assessment.
- The common physical characteristics included in the gestational age assessment are skin, lanugo, sole (plantar) creases, breast tissue and size, ear form and cartilage, and genitals.
- The neuromuscular components of gestational age scoring tools are usually posture, square window sign, popliteal angle, arm recoil, heel-to-ear extension, and scarf sign.
- By assessing the physical and neuromuscular components specified in a gestational age tool, the nurse can determine the gestational age of the newborn.
- After determining the gestational age of the baby, the nurse can assess how the newborn will make the transition to extrauterine life and can anticipate potential physiologic problems.
- The nurse identifies the newborn as small for gestational age (SGA), appropriate for gestational age (AGA), or large for gestational age (LGA), and prioritizes individual needs.
- Normal ranges for vital signs assessed in newborns are heart rate of 120 to 160 beats per minute; respiratory rate of 30 to 60 respirations per minute; axillary temperature of 36.4C to 37.2C (97.5F to 99F); skin temperature of 36C to 36.5C (96.8F to 97.7F); rectal temperature of 36.6C to 37.2C (97.8F to 99F); and blood pressure of 80/45 to 60/40 mm Hg (at birth).
- Normal newborn measurements include weight from 2500 to 4000 g (5 lb, 8 oz to 8 lb, 13 oz), with weight dependent on maternal size and age; length from 48 to 52 cm (18 to 22 in); and head circumference from 32 to 37 cm (12.5 to 14.5 in). Head circumference is approximately 2 cm larger than the chest circumference.
- Commonly elicited newborn reflexes are tonic neck, Moro, grasping, rooting, sucking, and blink.
- Newborn behavioral abilities include habituation, orientation to visual and auditory stimuli, motor activity, cuddliness, and self-quieting activity.
- An important role of the nurse during the physical and behavioral assessments of the newborn is to teach parents about their newborn and involve them in their baby's care. This facilitates the parents' identification of their newborn's uniqueness and allays their concerns.

References

American Academy of Pediatrics (AAP) Committee on Fetus and Newborn & American College of Obstetricians and Gynecologists (ACOG) Committee on Obstetrics (2002). *Guidelines for perinatal care* (5th ed.). Evanston, IL: Author.

Ballard, J. L., Khoury, J. C., Wedig, K., Wang, L., Eilers-Walsman, B. L., & Lipp, R. (1991). New Ballard score, expanded to include extremely premature infants. *Journal of Pediatrics, 119*(3), 417–423.

Blackburn, S. T. (2003). *Maternal, fetal, and neonatal physiology: A clinical perspective.* St. Louis, MO: Saunders.

Brazelton, T. (1984). Neonatal behavior and its significance. In M. E. Avery & H. W. Taeusch, Jr. (Eds.), *Schaffer's diseases of the newborn.* Philadelphia: Saunders.

Brazelton, T. B., & Nugent, J. K. (1995). *The neonatal behavioral assessment scale* (3rd ed.). London: MacKeith.

Cooperman, D. R., & Thompson, G. H. (2002). Neonatal orthopedics. In A. A. Fanaroff & R. J. Martin (Eds.), *Neonatal-perinatal medicine* (7th ed., pp. 1603–1632). St. Louis, MO: Mosby.

Drolet, B. A., & Esterly, N. B. (2002). The skin. In A. A. Fanaroff & R. J. Martin (Eds.), *Neonatal-perinatal medicine* (7th ed., pp. 1537–1567). St. Louis, MO: Mosby.

Gardner, S. L., & Goldson, E. (2002). The neonate and the environment: Impact on development. In G. B. Merenstein & S. L. Gardner (Eds.), *Handbook of neonatal intensive care.* (5th ed.). St. Louis, MO: Mosby.

Johnson, A. N. (2002). Update on newborn hearing screening programs. *Pediatric Nursing, 22*(3), 267–270.

Juretschke, L. J. (2000). Unilateral neonatal testicular torsion. *Journal of Obstetrics, Gynecologic, and Neonatal Nursing, 29*(5), 451–456.

Overpeck, M. D., Hediger, M. L., Zhang, J., Trumble, A. C., & Klbanoff, M. A. (1999). Birth weight for gestational age of Mexican American infants born in the United States. *Obstetrics & Gynecology, 93*(6), 943–947.

Rinehart, T. T., Terrone, D. A., & Magann, E. (2000). The normal neonate: Assessment of early physical findings. In J. J. Sciarri & T. J. Watkins (Eds.), *Gynecology and obstetrics* (Vol. 2, chap. 97, pp. 1–15). Philadelphia: Lippincott, Williams & Wilkins.

US Preventive Services Task Force. (2001). Newborn hearing screening: Recommendations and rationale. *American Family Physician, 64*(12), 1995–1999.

Wu, Tsu-Yin, & Daniel, L. (2001). Growth of immigrant Chinese infants in the first year of life. *American Journal of Maternal Child Nursing, 26*(4), 202–207.

The Normal Newborn: Needs and Care

30

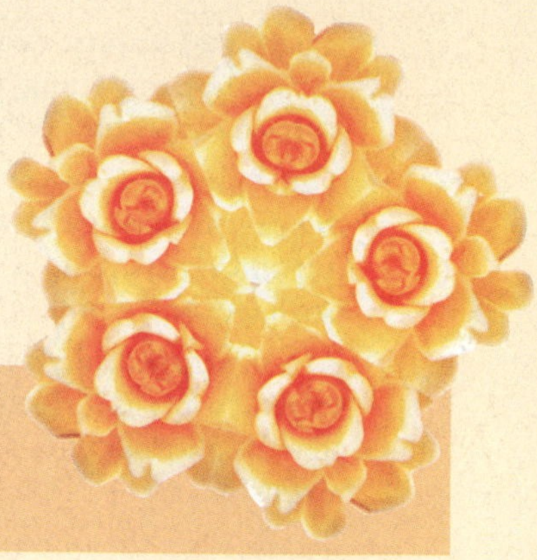

This moment of meeting seemed to be a birth time for both of us; her first and my second life. Nothing, I knew, could ever be the same again.
~*Laurie Lee*, Two Women~

Objectives

- Summarize the essential areas of information to be obtained about a newborn's birth experience and immediate postnatal period.
- Relate the physiologic and behavioral responses of newborns to possible interventions needed.
- Discuss the major nursing considerations and activities to be carried out during the first 4 hours after birth (admission and transitional period) and subsequent daily care.
- Identify activities that should be included in a daily care plan for a normal newborn.
- Determine common concerns of families regarding their newborns.
- Describe topics and related content to be included in parent teaching on newborn and infant care.
- Identify opportunities to individualize parent teaching and enhance each parent's abilities and confidence while providing infant care in the birthing unit.
- Delineate the information to be included in discharge planning with the newborn's family.

Key Terms

Circumcision 850
Newborn screening tests 860
Parent-newborn attachment 848

MediaLink

Additional resources for this content can be found on the Student CD-ROM and on the Companion Website at www.prenhall.com/olds. Click on "Chapter 30" to select the activities for this chapter.

CD-ROM
- Audio Glossary
- NCLEX Review
- Video: Newborn Care

Companion Website
- Additional NCLEX Review
- Case Study: Newborn Care
- Care Plan Activity: Initial Newborn Care
- Care Plan Activity: Infant Care During Transition

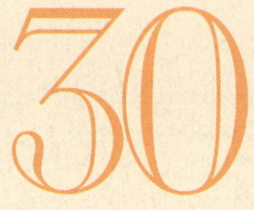

At the moment of birth, numerous physiologic adaptations begin to take place in the newborn's body. Because of these dramatic changes, newborns require close observation to determine how smoothly they are making the transition to extrauterine life. Newborns also require special care that enhances their chances of making the transition successfully.

The two broad goals of nursing care during this period are (1) to promote the physical well-being of the newborn, and (2) to support the establishment of a well-functioning family unit. The first goal is met by providing comprehensive care to newborns while in the mother-baby unit, and the second by teaching the baby's family how to care for their newborn and by supporting their parenting efforts as they gain competence and confidence. Empowered with knowledge about the healthcare needs of the newborn, as well as about family adjustments that need to be made, the parents can return home confident in their ability to care for their newborn and adjust to their new roles.

The previous two chapters discussed physiologic and behavioral changes occurring in the newborn and the pertinent nursing assessments that are needed. This chapter discusses nursing care management while the newborn is in the birthing unit. The Clinical Pathway for Newborn Care starts on page 840.

Nursing Care During Admission and the First Four Hours of Life

Immediately after birth, the baby is formally admitted to the healthcare facility.

Nursing Assessment and Diagnosis

During the first 4 hours after birth, the nurse carries out a preliminary physical examination, including an assessment of the newborn's physiologic adaptations. In many facilities, the nurse performs and documents the initial head-to-toe physical assessment during the first hour of transition. The nurse is responsible for notifying the physician or nurse practitioner of any deviations from normal. A complete physical examination is also performed later by the physician or nurse practitioner, within the first 24 hours after birth and within 24 hours before discharge. This can be accomplished with one physical examination (American Academy of Pediatrics [AAP] & the American College of Obstetricians and Gynecologists [ACOG], 2002) (see Chapter 29 and Table 29–1).

Nursing diagnoses are based on an analysis of the assessment findings. Physiologic alterations of the newborn form the basis of many nursing diagnoses, as does the family's incorporation of them in caring for their new baby. Nursing diagnoses that may apply to the newborn include the following:

- ***Ineffective Airway Clearance*** related to presence of mucus and retained lung fluid
- ***Risk for Altered Body Temperature*** related to evaporative, radiant, conductive, and convective heat losses
- ***Altered Peripheral Tissue Perfusion*** related to ineffective thermoregulation
- ***Acute Pain*** related to vitamin K injection or heel sticks for glucose or hematocrit

Many of these nursing diagnoses and associated interventions must be identified and implemented in a very short period of time. As discussed in Chapter 28, the newborn's physiologic adaptation to extrauterine life occurs rapidly and affects all body systems . The newborn requires close monitoring during the first few hours of life to immediately identify any deviation from normal and begin appropriate interventions.

Nursing Plan and Implementation

The nurse initiates newborn admission procedures and evaluates the newborn's need to remain under observation. This evaluation may take place in a special transition area or at the mother's bedside. It includes the following:

- Maternal and birth history
- Airway clearance
- Vital signs
- Body temperature
- Neurologic status
- Ability to feed
- Evidence of complications

If the evaluation is normal, the baby is successfully making the transition to extrauterine life and may need less frequent observations. In some settings, this may also be a time for moving the mother and baby to another care unit.

INITIATION OF ADMISSION PROCEDURES

Although the admission procedure varies somewhat among healthcare facilities, it typically includes a review of prenatal and birth information for possible risk factors, a gestational age assessment, and an assessment to ensure that the newborn's adaptation to extrauterine life is proceeding normally. This evaluation for risk factors and the status of the newborn must be done no later than 2 hours after birth (AAP & ACOG, 2002).

If the initial assessment indicates that the newborn is not at risk physiologically, the nurse performs many of the routine admission procedures in the presence of the parents and others in the birthing area. Some care measures indicated by the assessment findings may be performed by the nurse or by family members under the guidance of the nurse in an effort to educate and support the family. Other interventions might best be delayed if the newborn must be transferred to an observational nursery.

The nurse responsible for the newborn first checks and confirms the newborn's identification with the mother's

CLINICAL PATHWAY NEWBORN CARE

Category	First 4 Hours	4–8 Hours Past Birth	8–24 Hours Past Birth
Referral	Review labor/birth record Review transitional nursing record Check ID bands Consult prn: orthopedics, genetics, infectious disease	Check ID bands Transfer to mother-baby care at 4–6 hours of age if stable As parents desire, obtain circumcision permit after their discussion with physician Lactation consult prn	Check ID bands q shift **➤ Expected Outcomes** Mother/baby ID bands correlate at time of discharge; consults completed prn
Assessments	Continue assessments begun first hour after birth Vital sign: TPR, BP prn, q1h × 4 (skin temp 97.8–98.6F, resp may be irregular but within 30–60 per min) **➤ Newborn Assessments** • Respiratory status with resp distress scale × 1 then prn. If resp distress, assess q 5–15 min • Cord: bluish white color, clamp in place • Color: skin, mucous membranes, extremities, trunk pink with slight acrocyanosis of hands and feet • Wt (5 lb, 8 oz–8 lb, 13 oz), length (18–22 in), HC (12.5–14.5 in), CC (32.5 cm, 1–2 cm less than head) • Extremity movement—may be jerky or brief twitches • Gestational age classification—term AGA • Anomalies (cong. anomalies can interfere with normal extrauterine adaptation)	Assess newborn's progress through periods of reactivity Vital signs: TPR q8h and prn, BP prn **➤ Newborn Assessments** • Skin color q4h prn (circulatory system stabilizing, acrocyanosis decreased) • Eyes for drainage, redness, hemorrhage • Ausculate lungs q4h (noisy, wet resp normal) • Increased mucus production (normal in 2nd period of reactivity) • Check apical pulse q4h • Umbilical cord base for redness, drainage, foul odor, drying, damp in place • Externity movements q4h • Check for expected reflexes (suck, rooting, Moro, grasp, blink, yawn, sneeze, tonic neck, Babinski) • Note common normal variations • Assess suck and swallow during feeding • Note behavioral characteristics • Temp before and after admission bath	VS q8h; normal ranges: T, 97.5–99F; P, 120–160; R, 30–60; BP, 80–60/45-40 mm Hg **➤ Continue Newborn Assessments** • Skin color q4h • Signs of drying or infection in cord area • Check out clamp in place until removed before discharge • Check circ for bleeding after procedure, then q30min × 2, then q4h and prn **➤ Expected Outcomes** Vital signs medically acceptable, color pink, assessments WNL, circ site without s/s infection, cord site without s/s of infection and clamp removed; newborn behavior WNL
Teaching/ psychosocial	Admission activities performed at mother's bedside if possible, orient to nursery prn, handwashing, assess teaching needs Teach parents use of bulb syringe, signs of choking, positioning, and when to call for assistance Teach reasons for use of radiant warmer, infant hat, and warmed blankets when out of warmer Discuss/teach infant security, identification	Reinforce teaching about choking, bulb syringe use, positioning, temperature maintenance with clothing and blankets Teach infant positioning to facilitate breathing and digestion Teach new parents holding and feeding skills Teach parents soothing and calming techniques	Final discharge teaching: diapering, normal void and stool patterns, bathing, nail and cord care, circumcision/ uncircumcised penis/genital care and normal characteristics, rashes, jaundice, sleep-wake cycles, soothing activities, taking temperatures, thermometer reading Explain s/s of illness and when to call healthcare provider Infant safety: car seats, immunizations, metabolic screening **➤ Expected Outcomes** Mother/family verbalize comprehension of teaching; demonstrate care capabilities
Nursing care management and reports	Place under radiant warmer Place hat on newborn (decreases convection heat loss) Suction nares/mouth with bulb syringe prn Keep bulb syringe with infant Attach security sensor Obtain lab tests: blood glucose; as needed Obtain blood type, Rh, Coombs on cord blood, HSV culture if parental hx Notify physician's office of infant's birth and any change in status Maintain Standard Precautions	Wean from radiant warmer (T 98F axillary) Chemstrips prn; BP prn Oxygen saturation prn Bathe infant if temp > 97.8F Position on side Suction nares prn (esp during 2nd period of reactivity) Obtain peripheral Hct per protocol Cord care per protocol Fold diaper below cord (for plastic diapers, turn plastic layer away from skin)	Check for hearing test results Weigh before discharge Cord care q shift DC cord clamp before discharge Perform newborn metabolic screening blood tests before discharge Circumcision if indicated; circumcision care: change diaper prn, noting ability to void; follow policy for circumcision damp or Plastibell care **➤ Expected Outcomes** Newborn maintains temp, lab test WNL, cord dry without s/s infection and clamp removed, screening tests accomplished, circ site without s/s infection or bleeding

CLINICAL PATHWAY NEWBORN CARE *CONTINUED*

Category	First 4 Hours	4–8 Hours Past Birth	8–24 Hours Past Birth
Activity and comfort	Place under radiant warmer or wrap in prewarmed blankets until stable Soothe baby as needed with voice, touch, cuddling, nesting in warmer	Leave in warmer until stable, then swaddle Position on side after each feeding	Place in open crib Swaddle to allow movement of extremities in blanket, including hands to face ➤ **Expected Outcomes** Infant maintains temp WNL in open crib; infant attempts self-calming
Nutrition	Assist newborn to breastfeed as soon as mother/baby condition allows Supplement breast only when medically indicated or per agency policy Initiate formula-feeding within first hour Gavage feed if necessary to prevent hypoglycemia	Breastfeed on demand, at least q3-4h Teach positions, observe/assist with feeding, breast/nipple care, establishing milk supply, breaking suction, feeding cues, latching-on techniques, nutritive suck, burping Formula-feed on demand, at least q3-6h Determine readiness to feed and feeding tolerance	Continue breastfeeding or formula feeding pattern Assess feeding tolerance q4h Discuss normal feeding requirements, signs of hunger and satiation, handling feeding problems, and when to seek help ➤ **Expected Outcomes** Mother verbalizes knowledge of feeding information; breastfeeds on demand without supplement; bottle—tolerates formula feeding, nipples without problems
Elimination	Note first void and stool if not noted at birth	Note all voids, amount and color of stools q4h	Evaluate all voids and stool color q8h ➤ **Expected Outcomes** Voids qs; stools qs without difficulty; stool character WNL diaper area without s/s of skin breakdown or rashes
Medication	Prophylactic ophthalmic ointment OU after baby makes eye contact with parents within 1 hr after birth Administer AquaMEPHYTON IM, dosage according to infant weight per MD/NP order	Hepatitis B injection as ordered by physician after consent signed by parents	Hepatitis B vaccine before discharge ➤ **Expected Outcomes** Baby has received ophthalmic ointment and vitamin K injection; baby has received first Hep B vaccine if ordered and parental permission received
Discharge planning/home care	Hepatitis B consent signed Hearing screen consent signed Plan discharge call with parent or guardian in 24 hr to 2 days Assess parents' discharge plans, needs, and support systems	Review/reinforce teaching with mother and significant other Review home preparedness Present birth certificate instructions	Initial newborn screening tests (hearing, blood tests, metabolic screen; ie, PKU) before discharge Bath and feeding classes, videos, or written information given Give written copy of discharge instructions Newborn photographs Set up appointment for follow-up PKU test Have car seat available before discharge All discharge referrals made, follow-up appt. scheduled ➤ **Expected Outcomes** Infant discharged home with family; mother verbalizes follow-up appt. time/date
Family involvement	Facilitate early investigation of baby's physical characteristics (maintain temp during unwrapping), hold infant *en face* Dim lights to help infant keep eyes open	Assess parents' knowledge of newborn behaviors, such as alertness, suck and rooting, attention to human voice, response to calming techniques	Assess mother-baby bonding/interaction Incorporate father and siblings in care Enhance parent-infant interaction by sharing characteristics and behavioral assessment Support positive parenting behaviors Identify community referral needs and refer to community agencies ➤ **Expected Outcome** Demonstrates caring and family incorporation of infant
Date			

AGA, average for gestational age; Appt, appointment; CC, chest circumference; cong, congenital; esp, especially; HC, head circumference; Hct, hematocrit; Hx, history; ID, identification; OU, both eyes; s/s, signs and symptoms; temp, temperature; TPR, temperature, pulse, respirations; VS, vital signs; WNL, within normal limits.

identification and then obtains and records all significant information. The essential data to be recorded as part of the newborn's chart include the following:

1. *Condition of the newborn.* Pertinent information includes the newborn's Apgar scores at 1 and 5 minutes, resuscitative measures required in the birthing area, physical examination, vital signs, voidings, and passing of meconium. Complications to be noted include excessive mucus, delayed spontaneous respirations or responsiveness, abnormal number of cord vessels, and obvious physical abnormalities.
2. *Labor and birth record.* A copy of the labor and birth record should be placed in the newborn's chart or be accessible on computer. The record contains all the significant data about the birth, for example, duration, course, and status of mother and fetus throughout labor and birth and any analgesia or anesthesia administered to the mother. Particular care is taken to note any variation or difficulties such as prolonged rupture of membranes, abnormal fetal position, meconium-stained amniotic fluid, signs of fetal distress during labor, nuchal cord (cord around the newborn's neck at birth), precipitous birth, use of forceps, vacuum extraction, maternal analgesia and anesthesia received within 1 hour of birth, and administration of antibiotics during labor.
3. *Antepartal history.* Any maternal problems that may have compromised the fetus in utero—such as preeclampsia, spotting, illness, recent infections, rubella status, serology results, hepatitis B screen results, exposure to group B streptococci, or a history of maternal substance abuse—are of immediate concern in newborn assessment. The chart should also include information about maternal age, estimated date of birth (EDB), previous pregnancies, and presence of any congenital anomalies. A human immunodeficiency virus (HIV) test result, if obtained, is also relevant. State statutes vary as to who may have access to this information (AAP & ACOG, 2002).
4. *Parent-newborn interaction information.* The nurse notes parents' interactions with their newborn and their desires regarding care, such as rooming-in, circumcision, and type of feeding. Information about other children in the home, available support systems, and patterns of interaction within each family unit assists the nurse in providing comprehensive care.

Table 30–1 • summarizes normal findings for the newborn during transition.

As part of the admission procedure, the nurse weighs the newborn in both grams and pounds. In the United States, parents understand weights best when stated in pounds and ounces (Figure 30–1 •). The nurse cleans and covers the scales each time a newborn is weighed to prevent cross-infection and heat loss from conduction.

Table 30–1 • SIGNS OF NEWBORN TRANSITION

Normal findings for the newborn during the first few days of life include the following:

Pulse: 120–160 beats/minute
- During sleep as low as 100 beats/minute
- If crying, up to 180 beats/minute
- Apical pulse is counted for 1 full minute because rate may fluctuate

Respirations: 30–60 respirations/minute
- Predominantly diaphragmatic but synchronous with abdominal movements
- Brief periods of apnea (5–10 seconds) with no color or heart rate changes

Temperature: axillary: 36.5C–37C (97.5F–98.6F)

Skin: 36C–36.5C (96.8F–97.7F)

Blood pressure: 80–60/45–40 mm Hg at birth; 100/50 mm Hg at day 10

Blood glucose: greater than or equal to 40 mg%

Hematocrit: less than 65%–70% central venous sample

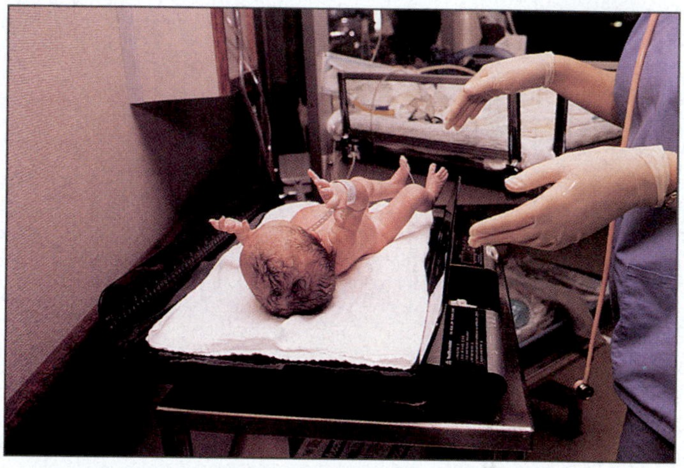

Figure 30–1 • Weighing a newborn. The scale is balanced before each weighing, with the protective pad in place. The caregiver's hand is poised above the infant as a safety measure.

The nurse then measures the newborn, recording the measurements in both centimeters and inches. Three routine measurements are length, circumference of the head, and circumference of the chest. In some facilities, abdominal girth may also be measured. The nurse rapidly assesses the baby's color, muscle tone, alertness, and general state. Remember that the first period of reactivity may have concluded, and the baby may be in the sleep-inactive phase, which makes the infant hard to arouse. The nurse does basic assessments for estimating gestational age and completes the physical assessment. (For more discussion of the process of newborn assessment, see Chapter 29).

In addition to obtaining vital signs, the nurse performs hematocrit and blood glucose evaluations on at-risk newborns or as clinically indicated (such as for small-for-gestational-age [SGA] or large-for-gestational-age [LGA] infants or if the newborn is jittery). These procedures may be

CRITICAL THINKING IN PRACTICE

You overhear Mr. Johannson speaking to his mother on the phone. He is telling her about the "cute little noises" his 30-minute-old baby makes. The infant is in the room with the mother. What is your best course of action?

Answers can be found in Appendix I .

done on admission or within the first 2 hours after birth (AAP & ACOG, 2002). (See Procedure 33–1).

MAINTENANCE OF A CLEAR AIRWAY AND STABLE VITAL SIGNS

Free-flow oxygen should be readily available. The nurse positions the newborn on his or her back (or side, if the infant has copious secretions). If necessary, a bulb syringe or DeLee wall suction (Procedure 24–1) is used to remove mucus from the nasal passages and oral cavity . A DeLee catheter attached to suction may be used to remove mucus from the stomach to help prevent possible aspiration. When possible, this procedure should be delayed for 10 to 15 minutes after birth, reducing the potential for severe vasovagal reflex apnea (Beers & Berdow, 2000).

In the absence of any newborn distress, the nurse continues with the admission by taking the newborn's vital signs. The initial temperature is taken by the axillary method. A wider range of normal exists for axillary temperature, specifically 36.5C to 37.0C (97.7F to 98.6F).

Once the initial temperature is taken, the nurse monitors the core temperature either by obtaining axillary temperatures at intervals or by placing a skin sensor on the newborn for continuous reading. The usual skin sensor placement site is on the newborn's abdomen, but placement on the upper thigh or arm can give a reading closely correlated with the mean body temperature. The vital signs for a healthy term newborn should be monitored at least every 30 minutes until the newborn's condition has remained stable for 2 hours (AAP & ACOG, 2002). The newborn's respirations may be irregular yet still be normal. Brief periods of apnea, lasting only 5 to 10 seconds with no color or heart rate changes, are considered normal. The normal pulse range is 120 to 160 beats per minute (bpm), and the normal respiratory range is 30 to 60 respirations per minute.

MAINTENANCE OF A NEUTRAL THERMAL ENVIRONMENT

A neutral thermal environment is essential to minimize the newborn's need for increased oxygen consumption and use of calories to maintain body heat in the optimal range of 36.5C to 37.0C (97.7F to 98.6F). If the newborn becomes hypothermic, the body's response can lead to metabolic acidosis, hypoxia, and shock.

The nurse can best achieve a neutral thermal environment by performing the assessment and interventions with a newborn unclothed and under a radiant warmer. The radiant warmer's thermostat is controlled by the thermal skin sensor taped to the newborn's abdomen, upper thigh, or arm. The sensor indicates when the newborn's temperature exceeds or falls below the acceptable temperature range. The nurse should be aware that leaning over the newborn may block the radiant heat waves from reaching the newborn. It is common practice in some institutions to cover the newborn's head with a cap made of wool lined with gauze and cotton, Thinsulate, or cotton and polyester terry cloth to prevent further heat loss in addition to placing the baby under a radiant warmer (Blackburn, 2003).

Clinical Tip *A cap can be fashioned from a piece of stockinette to help reduce heat loss from the head.*

When the newborn's temperature is normal and vital signs are stable (about 2 to 4 hours after birth), the baby may be given a sponge bath. However, this admission bath may be postponed for some hours if the newborn's condition dictates or the parents wish to give the first bath. In light of early discharge practices (12 to 48 hours), healthy term infants can be safely bathed immediately after the admission assessment is completed (Behring, Vezeau, & Fink, 2003). The baby is bathed while still under the radiant warmer. This may be done in the parents' room. Bathing the newborn offers an excellent opportunity for teaching and welcoming parent involvement in the care of their baby.

The nurse rechecks the temperature after the bath, and if it is stable, dresses the newborn in a shirt, diaper, and cap; wraps the baby; and places the baby in an open crib at room temperature. If the baby's axillary temperature is below 36.5C (97.7F), the nurse returns the baby to the radiant warmer. The rewarming process should be gradual to prevent the possibility of hyperthermia. In an isolette, gradual warming may be accomplished by maintaining a difference between the ambient temperature and the infant's skin temperature of less than 1.5C (3F) (Blackburn, 2003). When this new skin temperature is reached, the nurse increases the air temperature in hourly increments of 1.0C until the desired skin temperature is reached and the infant's temperature is stable. Once the newborn is rewarmed, the nurse implements measures to prevent further neonatal heat loss, such as keeping the newborn dry, swaddled in one or two blankets with hat on, and away from cool surfaces or instruments. The nurse also protects the newborn from drafts, open windows or doors, and air conditioners. Blankets and clothing are stored in a warm place. See Temperature Regulation in Chapter 29 and Procedure 30–1 .

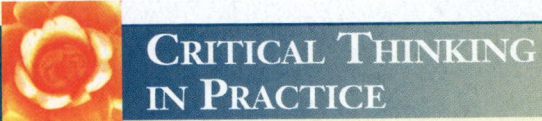

Procedure 30-1 Thermoregulation of the Newborn

Preparation

1. Prewarm the incubator or radiant warmer. Make sure warm towels and/or lightweight blankets are available.
2. Maintain the temperature of the birthing room at 22C (71F), with a relative humidity of 60% to 65%.
   Rationale: The change from a warm, moist intrauterine environment to a cool, dry, drafty environment stresses the newborn's immature thermoregulation system.

Equipment and Supplies

- Prewarmed towels or blankets
- Infant stocking cap
- Servocontrol probe
- Infant T-shirt and diaper
- Open crib

Procedure: *Clean Gloves*

1. Don gloves.
   Rationale: Gloves are worn whenever there is the possibility of contact with body fluids—in this case, a newborn wet with amniotic fluid, vernix, and maternal blood.
2. Place the newborn under the radiant warmer. Wipe the newborn free of blood, fluid, and excess vernix, especially from the head, using prewarmed towels.
   Rationale: The radiant warmer creates a heat-gaining environment. Drying is important to prevent the loss of body heat through evaporation.
3. If the newborn is stable, wrap him or her in a prewarmed blanket, apply a stocking cap, and carry the newborn to the mother. The mother and her support person can hold and enjoy the newborn together. Alternatively, carry the newborn wrapped to the mother, loosen the blanket, and place the infant skin to skin on the mother's chest under a warmed blanket.
   Rationale: Use of a prewarmed blanket reduces convection heat loss and facilitates maternal-newborn contact without compromising the newborn's thermoregulation. Skin-to-skin contact with the mother or father helps maintain the newborn's temperature.
4. After the newborn has spent time with the parents, return him or her to the radiant warmer and apply a diaper. Leave the newborn uncovered (except for the cap and diaper) under the radiant warmer.
   Rationale: Radiant heat warms the outer skin surface, so the skin needs to be exposed.
5. Tape a servocontrol probe on the newborn's anterior abdominal wall, with the metal side next to the skin. Do not place it over the ribs. Secure the probe with porous tape or a foil-covered aluminum heat deflector patch. Figure 30-2 • shows a newborn with a skin probe. Note that in this picture the newborn is no longer wearing a stocking cap.

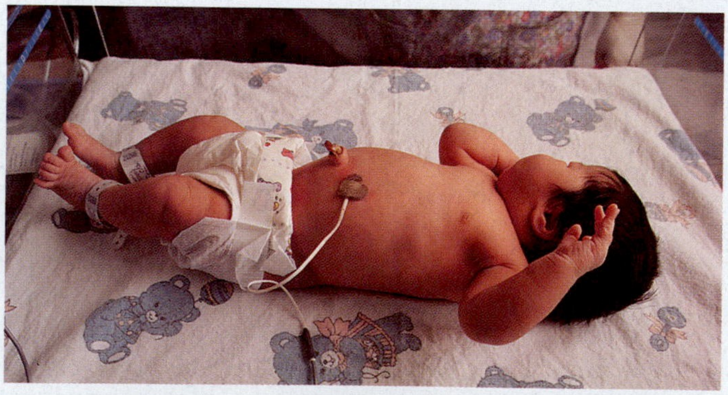

Figure 30-2 • Temperature monitoring for the newborn. A skin thermal sensor is placed on the newborn's abdomen, upper thigh, or arm and secured with porous tape or a foil-covered foam pad.

Procedure 30-1 (continued)

Clinical Tip

Take action to help the newborn maintain a stable temperature:

- Keep the newborn's clothing and bedding dry.
- Double-wrap the newborn and put a stocking cap on him or her.
- Use the radiant warmer during procedures.
- Reduce the newborn's exposure to drafts.
- Warm objects that will be in contact with the newborn (eg, stethoscopes).
- Encourage the mother to snuggle with the newborn under blankets or to breast-feed the newborn with hat and light cover on.

6. Turn the heater to servocontrol mode so that the abdominal skin is maintained at 36.5C to 37C (97.7F to 98.6F).
7. Monitor the newborn's axillary and skin probe temperatures per agency protocol.
   Rationale: The temperature indicator on the radiant warmer continually displays the newborn's probe temperature. The axillary temperature is checked to ensure that the machine is accurately recording the newborn's temperature.
8. When the newborn's temperature reaches 37C (98.6F), add a T shirt, double wrap the infant (two blankets), and place the newborn in an open crib.
9. Recheck the newborn's temperature in 1 hour and regularly thereafter according to agency policy.
   Rationale: It is important to monitor the newborn's ability to maintain his or her own thermoregulation.
10. If the newborn's temperature drops below 36.1C (97F), rewarm the infant gradually. Place the infant (unclothed except for a diaper) under the radiant warmer with a servocontrol probe on the anterior abdominal wall.
    Rationale: Rapid heating can lead to hyperthermia, which is associated with apnea, insensible water loss, and increased metabolic rate.
11. Recheck the newborn's temperature in 30 minutes, then hourly.
12. When the temperature reaches 37C (98.6F), dress the newborn, remove him or her from the radiant warmer, double-wrap, and place in an open crib. Check the temperature hourly until stable, then regularly according to agency policy.

PREVENTION OF COMPLICATIONS OF HEMORRHAGIC DISEASE OF NEWBORN

A prophylactic injection of vitamin K_1 (AquaMEPHYTON) is given to prevent hemorrhage, which can occur due to low prothrombin levels in the first few days of life (see the Drug Guide: Vitamin K_1 Phytonadione [AquaMEPHYTON]). The potential for hemorrhage results from the absence of gut bacterial flora, which influences the production of vitamin K in the newborn. (See Chapter 33 for further discussion.) Controversy exists over whether the administration of vitamin K may predispose the newborn to significant hyperbilirubinemia. All newborns should receive a single parenteral dose of 0.5 to 1.0 mg of natural vitamin K_1 oxide (phytonadione) parenterally (preferred) or subcutaneously within 1 hour of birth (AAP & ACOG, 2002). Some people have questioned the need to give vitamin K to newborns who have had a nontraumatic birth.

Vitamin K injection is given intramuscularly in the middle third of the vastus lateralis muscle located in the lateral aspect of the thigh (Figure 30–3 •). Before injecting, the nurse must clean the newborn's skin site for the injection thoroughly with

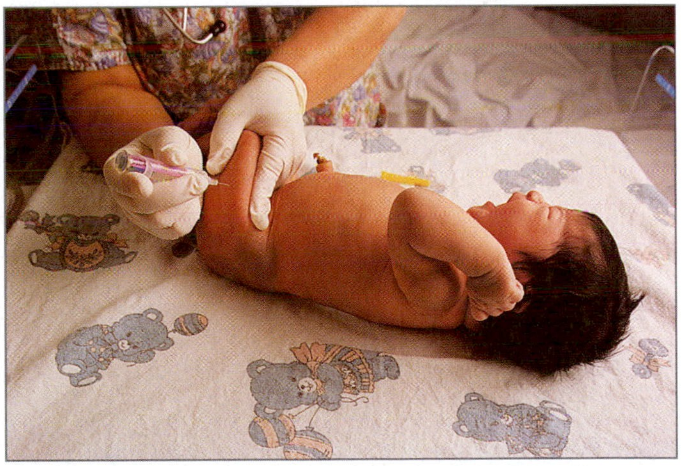

Figure 30–3 • Procedure for vitamin K injection. Cleanse area thoroughly with alcohol swab, and allow skin to dry. Bunch the tissue of the upper thigh (vastus lateralis muscle) and quickly insert a 25-gauge 5/8-inch needle at a 90-degree angle to the thigh. Aspirate, then slowly inject the solution to distribute the medication evenly and minimize the baby's discomfort. Remove the needle and massage the site with an alcohol swab.

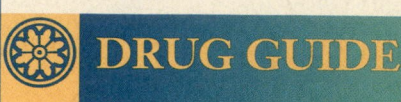

DRUG GUIDE: Vitamin K_1 Phytonadione (AquaMEPHYTON)

• Overview of Neonatal Action

Phytonadione is used in prophylaxis and treatment of hemorrhagic disease of the newborn. It promotes liver formation of the clotting factors II, VII, IX, and X. At birth, the newborn does not have the bacteria in the colon that are necessary for synthesizing fat-soluble vitamin K_1. Therefore, the newborn may have decreased levels of prothrombin during the first 5 to 8 days of life, reflected by a prolongation of prothrombin time.

• Route, Dosage, Frequency

Intramuscular injection is given in the vastus lateralis thigh muscle. A one-time-only prophylactic dose of 0.5 to 1 mg is given intramuscularly in the birthing area or within 1 hour of birth (AAP & ACOG, 2002).

If the mother received anticoagulants during pregnancy, an additional dose may be ordered by the physician and is given 6 to 8 hours after the first injection. IM/SC concentration: 1 mg/0.5 mL (neonatal strength); can use 10 mg/mL concentration to minimize volume injected.

• Neonatal Side Effects

Pain and edema may occur at injection site. Allergic reactions, such as rash and urticaria, may also occur.

• Nursing Considerations

- Observe for bleeding (usually occurs on second or third day). Bleeding may be seen as generalized ecchymoses or bleeding from umbilical cord, circumcision site, nose, or gastrointestinal tract. Results of serial prothrombin time (PT) and partial thromboplastin time (PTT) should be assessed.
- Observe for jaundice and kernicterus, especially in preterm infants.
- Observe for signs of local inflammation.
- Protect drug from light.
- Give vitamin K_1 before circumcision procedure.

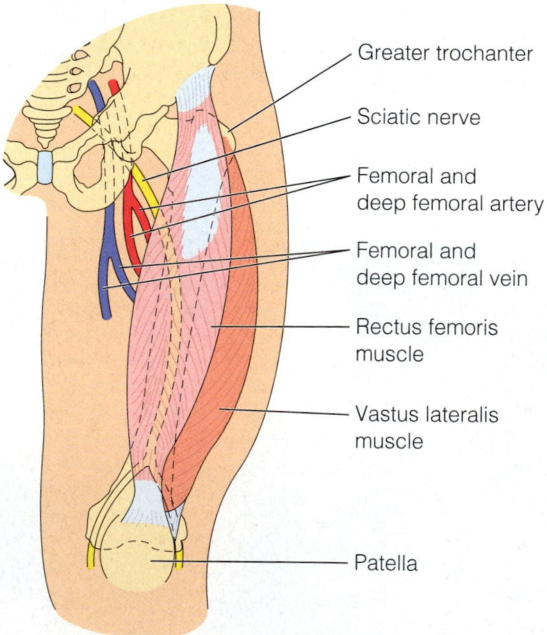

Figure 30–4 • Injection sites. The middle third of the vastus lateralis muscle is the preferred site for intramuscular injection in the newborn. The middle third of the rectus femoris is an alternative site, but its proximity to major vessels and the sciatic nerve necessitates caution in using this site for injection.

MEDIALINK VIDEO: NEWBORN CARE

a small alcohol swab. The nurse uses a 25-gauge, 5/8-inch needle for the injection. An alternative site is the rectus femoris muscle in the anterior aspect of the thigh. However, this site is near the sciatic nerve and femoral artery and should be used with caution (Figure 30–4 •).

PREVENTION OF EYE INFECTION

The nurse is also responsible for giving the legally required prophylactic eye treatment for *Neisseria gonorrhoeae*, which may have infected the newborn of an infected mother during the birth process. A variety of topical agents appear to be equally effective. Ophthalmic ointments that are used include 0.5% erythromycin (Ilotycin Ophthalmic) (see the Drug Guide: Erythromycin [Ilotycin Ophthalmic], 1% tetracycline and opthalmic solution of povidone-iodine (2.5%). All are also effective against chlamydia, which has a higher incidence than gonorrhea.

Successful eye prophylaxis requires that the medication be instilled into the lower conjunctival sac of each eye (Figure 30–5 •). The nurse massages the eyelid gently to distribute the ointment. Instillation may be delayed up to 1 hour after birth to allow eye contact during parent-newborn bonding.

Eye prophylaxis medication can cause chemical conjunctivitis, which gives the newborn some discomfort and may interfere with the baby's ability to focus on the parents' faces. The resulting edema, inflammation, and discharge may cause concern if the parents have not been informed that the side effects will clear in 24 to 48 hours and that this prophylactic eye treatment is necessary for the newborn's well-being.

EARLY ASSESSMENT OF NEONATAL DISTRESS

During the first 24 hours of life, nurses are constantly alert for signs of distress. If the newborn is with the parents during this period, the nurse must take extra care to teach them how to maintain their newborn's temperature, recognize the hallmarks of newborn distress, and respond im-

DRUG GUIDE ERYTHROMYCIN OPHTHALMIC OINTMENT (ILOTYCIN OPHTHALMIC)

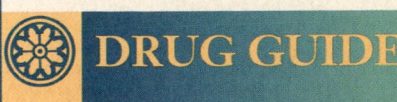

• Overview of Neonatal Action

Erythromycin (Ilotycin Ophthalmic) is used as prophylactic treatment of ophthalmia neonatorum, which is caused by the bacteria *Neisseria gonorrhoeae.* Preventive treatment of gonorrhea in the newborn is required by law. Erythromycin is also effective against ophthalmic chlamydial infections. It is either bacteriostatic or bactericidal, depending on the organisms involved and the concentration of drug.

• Route, Dosage, Frequency

Ophthalmic ointment (0.5%) is instilled as a narrow ribbon or strand, 1/4 inch long, along the lower conjunctival surface of each eye, starting at the inner canthus. It is instilled only once in each eye. The ointment may be administered in the birthing area or, alternatively, later in the nursery so that eye contact between infant and parent is facilitated and the bonding process immediately after birth is not interrupted. After administration, gently close eye and manipulate to ensure spread of ointment.

• Neonatal Side Effects

Sensitivity reaction; may interfere with ability to focus and may cause edema and inflammation. Side effects usually disappear in 24 to 48 hours.

• Nursing Considerations

- Wash hands immediately prior to instillation to prevent introduction of bacteria.
- Do not irrigate the eyes after instillation. Use new tube or single-use container for ophthalmic ointment administration shortly after birth. May wipe away excess after 1 minute.
- Observe for hypersensitivity.
- Teach parents about need for eye prophylaxis. Educate them regarding side effects and signs that need to be reported to the healthcare provider.

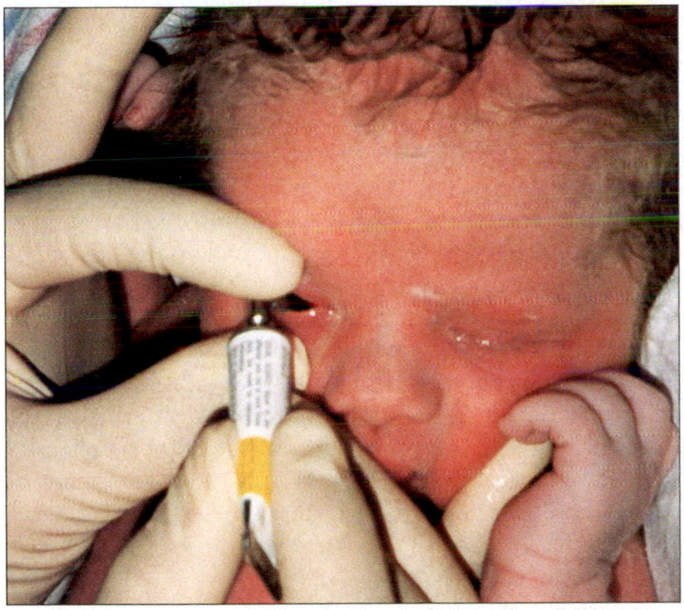

Figure 30–5 • Ophthalmic ointment. Retract lower eyelid outward to instill a 1/4-inch strand of ointment from a single-dose ampule along the lower conjunctival surface.

Table 30–2 • SIGNS OF NEONATAL DISTRESS

Increased respiratory rate (more than 60/minute) or difficult respirations
Sternal retractions
Nasal flaring
Grunting
Excessive mucus
Facial grimacing
Cyanosis (central: skin, lips, tongue)
Abdominal distention or mass
Vomiting of bile-stained material
Absence of meconium elimination within 24 hours of birth
Absence of urine elimination within 24 hours of birth
Jaundice of the skin within 24 hours of birth or due to hemolytic process
Temperature instability (hypothermia or hyperthermia)
Jitteriness or glucose less than 40 mg%

Source: Adapted from Tappero, E. P. & Honeyfield, M. E. (1996). *Physical assessment of the newborn* (2nd ed.). Petaluma, CA: NICU Ink.

mediately to signs of respiratory problems. The parents should learn to observe the newborn for changes in color or activity, grunting or "sighing" sounds with breathing, rapid breathing with chest retractions, nasal flaring, changes in skin color, or facial grimacing. Their interventions should include nasal and oral suctioning with bulb syringe, positioning, and vigorous fingertip stroking of the newborn's spine to stimulate respiratory activity if necessary. The nurse must be immediately available to provide appropriate interventions should the newborn develop distress (Table 30–2 •).

A common cause of neonatal distress is early-onset group B streptococcal (GBS) disease. Infected mothers transmit GBS infection to their infants during labor and birth; thus it is recommended that at-risk mothers receive intrapartum antimicrobial prophylaxis (IAP) for GBS disease. All infants of mothers identified as at risk should be assessed and observed for signs and symptoms of sepsis.

INITIATION OF FIRST FEEDING

The timing of the first feeding varies, depending on whether the newborn is to be breastfed or formula-fed and whether there were any complications during pregnancy or birth, such as maternal diabetes, intrauterine growth restriction (IUGR), and so forth. Mothers who choose to breastfeed their newborns should be encouraged to put their baby to breast during the first period of reactivity. This practice should be encouraged because successful, long-term breastfeeding during infancy appears to be related to beginning breast feedings in the first few hours of life. Sleep-wake states affect feeding behavior and need to be considered when evaluating the newborn's sucking ability (MacMullen & Dulski, 2000). Formula-fed newborns usually begin the first feedings by 5 hours of age, during the second period of reactivity, when they awaken and appear hungry.

Signs indicating newborn readiness for the first feeding are active bowel sounds, absence of abdominal distention, and a lusty cry that quiets with rooting and sucking behaviors when a stimulus is placed near the lips.

FACILITATION OF PARENT-NEWBORN ATTACHMENT

To facilitate **parent-newborn attachment,** eye-to-eye contact between parents and their newborn is extremely important during the early hours after birth, when the newborn is in the first period of reactivity. The newborn is alert during this time, the eyes are wide open, and direct eye contact is made with human faces within optimal range for visual acuity (7 to 8 in). It is theorized that this eye contact is an important foundation in establishing attachment in human relationships (Klaus & Klaus, 1985). Consequently, the prophylactic eye medication is often delayed, but no more than 1 hour, to provide an opportunity for this period of eye contact between parents and their newborn, thus facilitating the attachment process (AAP & ACOG, 2002). Parents who cannot be with their newborns in this first period due to maternal or infant distress may need reassurance that the bonding process can proceed normally as soon as both mother and baby are stable. Other situations, such as the newborn's bath, can be used to promote attachment. The newborn becomes an active participant and parents are drawn into an interaction with their newborn. The nurse can interpret the infant's behavior, model ways to respond to the behavior, and support parental strategies for doing so (Karl, 1999).

> *Now I believe in love at first sight!*
>
> ~A NEW MOTHER HOLDING HER INFANT FOR THE FIRST TIME

Evaluation

When evaluating the nursing care provided during the period immediately after birth, the nurse may anticipate the following outcomes:

- The newborn baby's adaptation to extrauterine life is supported and complete.
- The baby's physiologic and psychologic integrity is supported.

Nursing Care of Newborn Following Transition

Nursing Diagnosis

Examples of nursing diagnoses that may apply during daily care of the newborn include the following:

- ***Risk for Ineffective Breathing Pattern*** related to periodic breathing
- ***Altered Nutrition: Less than Body Requirements*** related to limited nutritional or fluid intake and increased caloric expenditure
- ***Altered Urinary Elimination*** related to meatal edema secondary to circumcision
- ***Risk for Infection*** related to umbilical cord healing, circumcision site, immature immune system, or potential birth trauma (forceps or vacuum extraction delivery)
- ***Health-Seeking Behaviors*** related to lack of information about basic baby care, male circumcision, and breast- and/or formula-feeding
- ***Altered Family Processes*** related to integration of newborn into family unit or demands of newborn care and feeding

Nursing Plan and Implementation

MAINTENANCE OF CARDIOPULMONARY FUNCTION

The nurse assesses vital signs every 6 to 8 hours or more, depending on the newborn's status. The newborn should be placed on its back (supine) for sleeping. A bulb syringe is kept within easy reach should the baby need oral-nasal suctioning. If the newborn has respiratory difficulty, the airway is cleared. Vigorous fingertip stroking of the baby's spine will frequently stimulate respiratory activity. A cardiorespiratory monitor can be used on newborns who are not being observed at all times and are at risk for decreased respiratory or cardiac function. Indicators of risk are pallor, cyanosis, ruddy color, apnea, or other signs of instability. Changes in skin color may indicate the need for closer assessment of temperature, cardiopulmonary status, hematocrit, glucose, and bilirubin levels.

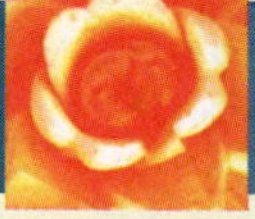

CRITICAL THINKING IN PRACTICE

Aisha Khan gave birth to a healthy girl 2 hours ago. Now she calls you to her room. She sounds frightened and says her baby can't breathe. You find Aisha cradling her newborn in her arms. The baby is mildly cyanotic, waving her arms, and has mucus coming from her nose and mouth. What would you do?

Answers can be found in Appendix I.

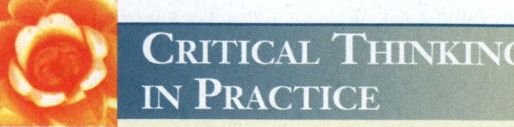

MAINTENANCE OF A NEUTRAL THERMAL ENVIRONMENT

The nurse makes every effort to maintain the newborn's temperature within the normal range. The nurse must make certain the newborn is dressed and exposed to the air as little as possible. A head covering should be used initially, and continued with the small newborn, who has less subcutaneous fat to act as insulation in maintaining body heat. Ambient temperature of the room where the newborn is kept should be monitored to prevent excessive cooling. Parents may be advised to dress the newborn in one more layer of clothing than is necessary for an adult to maintain thermal comfort. The use of layering allows for flexibility as the infant is moved from one area to another.

A newborn whose temperature falls below optimal levels will use calories to maintain body heat rather than for growth. Chilling also decreases the affinity of serum albumin for bilirubin, thereby increasing the likelihood of newborn jaundice. It also increases oxygen use and may cause respiratory distress.

An overheated newborn will increase activity and respiratory rate in an attempt to cool the body. Both measures deplete caloric reserves. In addition, the increased respiratory rate leads to increased insensible fluid loss (Blackburn, 2003).

PROMOTION OF ADEQUATE HYDRATION AND NUTRITION

Newborn nutrition is addressed in depth in Chapter 31. The nurse records the newborn's caloric and fluid intake and enhances adequate hydration by maintaining a neutral thermal environment and offering early and frequent feedings. Early feedings promote gastric emptying and increase peristalsis, thereby decreasing the degree of hyperbilirubinemia by limiting the amount of time fecal material is in contact with the enzyme β-glucuronidase in the small intestine. This enzyme acts to free the bilirubin from the stool, allowing bilirubin to be reabsorbed into the vascular system. The nurse records voiding and stooling patterns. The first voiding should occur within 24 hours and passage of stool within 48 hours. When they do not occur, the nurse continues the normal observation routine while assessing for abdominal distention, bowel sounds, hydration, fluid intake, voiding pattern, and temperature stability.

The newborn should be weighed at the same time each day for accurate comparisons and must be kept warm during the weighing. A weight loss of up to 10% for term newborns is considered within normal limits during the first week of life. This is the result of limited intake, loss of excess extracellular fluid, and passage of meconium. Parents should be told about the expected weight loss, the reason for it, and the expectations for regaining the birth weight. Birth weight should be regained by 2 weeks if feedings are adequate.

Excessive handling of the newborn can cause an increase in the newborn's metabolic rate and calorie use and cause fatigue. The nurse should be alert to the baby's subtle cues of fatigue. These include a decrease in muscle tension and activity in the extremities and neck and loss of eye contact, which may be manifested by fluttering or closing the eyelids or turning the head away. The nurse quickly ceases stimulation when signs of fatigue appear. The nurse's care should demonstrate to the parents the need to be aware of newborn cues of fatigue and to wait for periods of alertness in the baby for contact and stimulation. The nurse is also responsible for assessing the woman's comfort and latching-on techniques in breastfeeding or bottle-feeding.

PROMOTION OF SKIN INTEGRITY

Newborn skin care, including bathing, is important for the health and appearance of the individual newborn and for infection control within the nursery. Ongoing skin care involves cleansing the buttock and perianal areas with fresh water and cotton, or with a mild soap and water, with diaper changes. If commercial baby wipes are used, those without alcohol should be selected. Wipes that are perfume- and latex-free are also available.

The umbilical cord is assessed for signs of bleeding or infection. Removal of the cord clamp within 24 hours of birth reduces the chance of tension injury to the area. Keeping the umbilical stump clean and dry can reduce the chance for infection. Many types of routine cord care are practiced, including the use of triple-dye or an antimicrobial agent such as bacitracin and application of 70% alcohol to the cord stump. These practices are largely based on tradition rather than current research findings. The skin absorption and toxicity of triple-dye agents in newborns have not been carefully studied (AAP & ACOG, 2002). Recent studies have shown that alcohol may not be helpful in promoting drying or preventing infection. Folding the diaper down to prevent coverage of the cord stump can prevent contamination of the area and promote drying (AWHONN, 2001). The nurse is responsible for cord care per agency policy. It is also the nurse's responsibility to instruct parents in caring for the cord and observing for signs and symptoms of infection after discharge, such as foul smell, redness and drainage, localized heat and tenderness, or bleeding.

PREVENTION OF COMPLICATIONS AND PROMOTION OF SAFETY

Newborns are at continued risk for the complications of hemorrhage, late-onset cardiac symptoms, and infection. Pallor may be an early sign of hemorrhage and must be reported to the physician. The newborn is placed on a cardiorespiratory monitor to permit continuous assessment. Several newborn conditions or procedures such as circumcision put the newborn at risk for bleeding. Cyanosis that is not relieved by oxygen administration requires emergency intervention, may indicate a congenital cardiac condition or shock, and requires ongoing assessment.

Infection in the nursery is best prevented by requiring that all personnel having direct contact with newborns scrub for 2 to 3 minutes from fingertips to and including elbows at the beginning of each shift. The hands must be washed with soap and rubbed vigorously for 15 seconds before and after contact with every newborn or after

MediaLink Care Plan: Infant Care During Transition

RESEARCH IN PRACTICE
Neonatal Skin Care

What is this study about? Newborns require skin care practices that preserve skin integrity, prevent toxicity from antiseptics, and minimize chemical exposure. Even normal bathing with soap can be irritating and drying to an infant's sensitive skin. The use of alcohol on the umbilical cord, the application of antimicrobial ointments, and the use of adhesives may further compromise skin integrity. The Association of Women's Health, Obstetric and Neonatal Nurses (AWHONN) and the National Association of Neonatal Nurses (NANN) developed an evidence-based protocol for neonatal skin care. The Neonatal Skin Care Project was initiated to test the outcomes of the protocol for nurses and newborns. This study reported the effects of the project on nursing care practices and neonatal skin outcomes.

How was this study done? This descriptive study was conducted in neonatal intensive care units, special-care nurseries, and well-baby nurseries in 51 US hospitals. Data were collected about typical skin care practices and nursing knowledge of neonatal skin care at each site. Baseline assessment of the existing skin condition of newborns at each site was also collected. Nurses were formally trained regarding the guideline for skin care. The training involved review of the physiologic differences between adult and newborn skin, and guideline-based principles of infant skin care. A skin assessment tool was used twice weekly to assess neonatal skin condition.

What were the results of the study? Typical skin care practices showed variation between sites. The units reported 111 different products used on newborn skin. After training, nurses used more emollients, less antibiotic ointment, and more positioning devices and bedding, all recommendations in the guidelines. The use of isopropyl alcohol as a skin disinfectant, discouraged in the guideline, decreased from 80% of units to less than 45%. Themes reported by the sites included the benefits of an evidence-based guideline and improved skin integrity in newborns as a result. Less frequent bathing, better skin assessment, and the use of emollients were also seen as positive changes.

What additional questions might I have? What were the difficulties encountered in attempting to change nursing practice? How long did the changes take to be fully implemented? Were there any negative effects for the skin of newborns when the new protocol was implemented? Are there increases in costs of care relative to the guideline?

How can I use this study? Research-based practices in the well-baby setting help nurses give optimal care to newborns and teach parents about appropriate skin care. Using training to help nurses understand effective skin care can result in changes in nursing practice and improvements in newborn skin integrity.

Source: Lund, C., Kuller, J., Lane, A., Lott, J., Raines, D., & Thomas, K. (2001). Neonatal skin care: Evaluation of the AWHONN/NANN research-based practice project on knowledge and skin care practices. *Journal of Obstetric, Gynecologic, and Neonatal Nursing, 30*(1), 30–40.

touching any soiled surface, such as the floor or one's hair or face. Parents are instructed to practice good handwashing and/or use of an antiseptic hand cleaner before touching the baby. They are also instructed that anyone holding the baby should wash their hands as well, even after the family returns to their home. In some clinical settings family members are requested to wear a gown (preferably disposable) over their street clothes during contact with infants. These are good opportunities for the nurse to reinforce the efficacy of handwashing in preventing the spread of infection.

Safety of the newborn is paramount. It is essential that the nurse and other caregivers verify the identity of the newborn by comparing the numbers and names on the identification bracelets of mother and newborn before giving a baby to a parent. Another form of identification band has a built-in sensor unit that sounds an alarm if the baby is transported beyond set birthing unit boundaries. Individual birthing units should practice safety measures to prevent infant abduction and provide information to parents regarding their role in this area (Carroll, 2000). Parental measures to prevent abduction include the following:

- Checking that identification bands are in place as they care for their infant and, if missing, asking that they be replaced immediately
- Allowing only people with proper birthing unit identification to remove their baby from their room
- Returning baby to nursery or having baby accompany the parent when leaving the room
- Reporting the presence of any suspicious people on the birthing unit

CIRCUMCISION

Circumcision is a surgical procedure in which the prepuce, an epithelial layer covering the tip of the penis, is separated from the glans penis and excised. This permits exposure of the glans for easier cleaning.

Circumcision was originally a religious rite practiced by Jews and Muslims. The practice gained widespread cultural acceptance in the United States but is done infrequently in many European countries. Many parents choose circumcision because they want the male child to have a physical appearance similar to that of the father or the majority of other children, or they may feel that it is expected by society. Another commonly cited reason for circumcising newborn males is to prevent the need for anesthesia, hospitalization, pain, and trauma should the procedure be needed later in life (AAP & ACOG, 2002). During the prenatal period, the nurse ensures that parents have clear and current information regarding the risks and benefits of circumcision.

Families make the decision about circumcision for their newborn male child. In most cases, the choice is based on cultural, social, and family tradition. To ensure informed consent, parents should be informed about possible long-term medical effects of circumcision and noncircumcision during the prenatal period.

Evidence-Based Practice

Umbilical Cord Care

Clinical Question

Are topical agents for umbilical cord care effective for preventing cord infection, illness, and death in newborn infants?

The Evidence

Ten randomized controlled trials were conducted in developing countries. The studies were conducted on newborns of all gestational ages whose cord care involved single or multiple applications to the cord of any of the following: topical antiseptics (alcohol, triple dye, silver sulfadiazine, acriflavine, iodine, chlorhexidine, or gentian violet); antibiotics (bacitracin, nitrofurazone, or tetracycline); or powders with or without antiseptics. In the study population, no systemic bacterial infections or deaths were reported. The studies' findings included the following:

- Antiseptics did not reduce cord and other skin infections, as compared to no care.
- Antiseptics prolonged the time to cord separation (7 days for powder, 8 days for no intervention, 10 days for alcohol, 12 days for antibiotics, 8 to 16 days for triple dye, and 11 to 14 days for silver sulfadiazine).
- Use of antiseptics reduced maternal concern about the cord.

Best Practice

In full-term infants born in developing countries, simply keeping the cord clean appears to be as effective and safe as using antibiotics or antiseptics (James & Dinulos, 2000; Zupan & Garner, 2001). Parental education regarding the perceived advantages of use of alcohol should be part of best practice (Zupan & Garner, 2001).

References: James, G., & Dinulos, L. (2000). Neonatal skin care. *Pediatric Clinics of North America, 47*(4), 757–782;

Zupan, J., & Garner, P. (2001). Topical umbilical cord care at birth (Cochrane Review). In *The Cochrane Library,* Issue 2. Oxford: Update Software.

Current Recommendations

In the past, recommendations regarding circumcision have varied. The 1999 AAP policy statement does not recommend routine circumcision but acknowledges that medical indications for circumcision still exist. The policy recommends that analgesia (eg, EMULA cream, dorsal penile nerve block [DPNB], or subcutaneous ring block) be used during circumcision to decrease procedural pain (Kaufman, Clark, & Castro, 2001). If a circumcision is to be performed it should be done using the least painful method.

Circumcision should not be performed if the newborn is premature or compromised, has a known bleeding problem, or is born with a genitourinary defect, such as hypospadias or epispadias, that may necessitate the use of the foreskin in future surgical repairs (Beers & Berdow, 2000).

Nurse's Role

The nurse plays an essential role in providing parents with current information regarding the medical, social, and psychologic aspects of newborn circumcision. A knowledgeable nurse can allay parents' anxiety, answer questions, and provide an opportunity for parents to express their concerns. In order for parents to make a truly informed decision, they must be knowledgeable about the potential risks and outcomes of circumcision. Hemorrhage, infection, difficulty in voiding, separation of the edges of the circumcision, pain, and restlessness are early potential problems. Later there is the risk that the glans and urethral meatus can become irritated and inflamed from contact with ammonia from urine. Ulcerations and progressive stenosis may develop. Adhesions, entrapment of the penis, and damage to the urethra are all potential complications that could require surgical correction (AAP & ACOG, 2002).

The parents of an uncircumcised male infant require information from the nurse about good hygiene practices. They should be told that the foreskin and glans are two similar layers of cells that separate from each other. The separation process begins prenatally and is normally completed at between 3 and 5 years of age. In the process of separation, sterile sloughed cells build up between the layers. This buildup looks similar to the smegma secreted after puberty, and it is harmless. Occasionally during the daily bath, the parents can gently test for retraction. If retraction has occurred, daily gentle washing of the glans with soap and water is sufficient to maintain adequate cleanliness. The parents should teach the child to incorporate this practice into his daily self-care activities. Most uncircumcised males have no difficulty doing so.

If circumcision is desired, the procedure should be performed after the newborn is well stabilized and has received his initial physical examination by a healthcare provider. The parents may also choose to have the circumcision done after discharge. However, they need to be advised that if the baby is older than 1 month, the current practice is to hospitalize him for the procedure.

Prior to a circumcision, the nurse ascertains that the physician has explained the procedure, determines whether the parents have any further questions about the procedure, and checks that the circumcision permit is signed. The nurse gathers the equipment and prepares the newborn by removing the diaper and placing him on a circumcision board or some other type of restraint, but restraining only the legs. In Jewish circumcision

MediaLink Circumcision Resources

MEDIALINK CASE STUDY: NEWBORN CARE

ceremonies, the infant is held by the father or grandfather and given wine before the procedure (Reynolds, 1996).

There are a variety of techniques for circumcision (Figures 30–6 • and 30–7 •), and all produce minimal bleeding. Therefore the nurse should make special note of infants with family history of bleeding disorders or with mothers who took anticoagulants, including aspirin, prenatally. During the procedure, the nurse assesses the newborn's response. One important consideration is pain experienced by the newborn. A DPNB using 1% lidocaine without epinephrine significantly minimizes the pain and the shifts in behavioral patterns, such as crying, irritability, and erratic sleep cycles associated with circumcision. Other studies are investigating the use of topical anesthetic applied 60 to 90 minutes prior to prepuce removal, acetaminophen, and cryoanalgesia (Taddio, Pollock, Gilbert-MacLeod, et al, 2000).

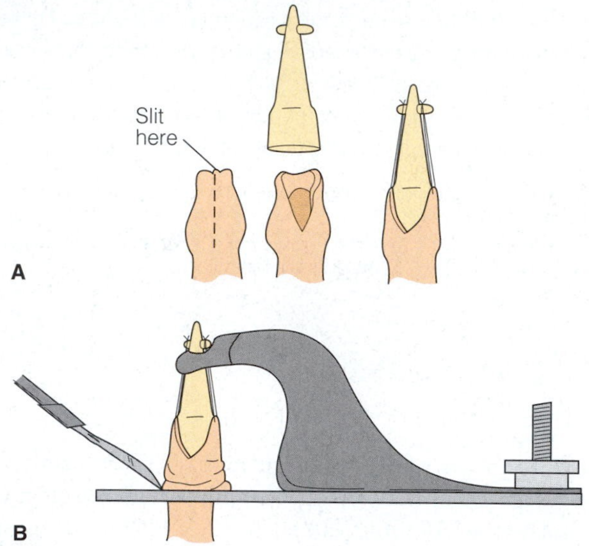

Figure 30–6 • Circumcision using the Yellen or Gomco clamp. *A,* The prepuce is drawn over the cone. *B,* The clamp is applied. Pressure is maintained for 3 to 4 minutes, and then excess prepuce is cut away.

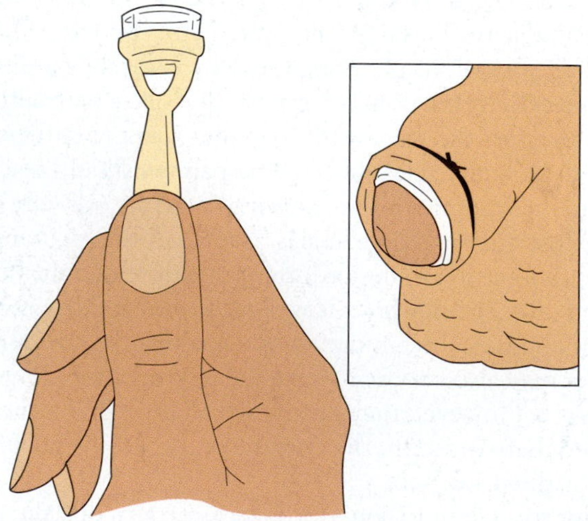

Figure 30–7 • Circumcision using the Plastibell. The bell is fitted over the glans. A suture is tied around the bell's rim, and the excess prepuce is cut away. The plastic rim remains in place for 3 to 4 days until healing occurs. The bell may be allowed to fall off; it is removed if still in place after 8 days.

During the procedure, the nurse can provide comfort measures such as lightly stroking the baby's head, providing a pacifier, and talking to him. Following the circumcision, the infant should be held and comforted by a family member or the nurse. The nurse must be alert to any cues that these measures are overstimulating the newborn instead of comforting him. Such cues include turning away of the head, increased generalized body movement, skin color changes, hyperalertness, and hiccuping.

Ideally, the circumcision should be assessed for signs of hemorrhage and infection every 30 minutes for at least 2 hours following the procedure (Kaufman et al, 2001). It is important to observe for the first voiding after a circumcision to evaluate for urinary obstruction related to penile injury and/or edema. Petroleum and gauze are applied to the site immediately following the procedure to help prevent bleeding and can be used to protect the healing tissue afterward.

The nurse must also teach family members how to assess for unusual bleeding, how to respond if it is present, and how to care for the newly circumcised penis. Parents of babies circumcised with a method other than Plastibell should receive the following information:

- Apply petroleum and gauze immediately following the procedure and for the next few diaper changes to help prevent further bleeding.
- If bleeding does occur, apply light pressure with a sterile gauze pad to stop the bleeding within a short time. If this is not effective, contact the physician immediately, or take the baby to the caregiver's office.
- The glans normally has granulation tissue (a yellowish film) on it during healing. Continued application of a petroleum ointment (or ointment suggested by the healthcare provider) can help protect the granulation tissue that forms as the glans heals.
- Report to the care provider any signs or symptoms of infection, such as increasing swelling, pus drainage, and cessation of urination.
- When diapering, ensure that the diaper is not loose enough to cause rubbing with movement, or tight enough to cause pain.
- If the infant's care provider recommends oral analgesics, follow instructions for proper measuring and administration.

If the Plastibell is used, parents should receive information about normal appearance and how to observe for infection. The parents are informed that the Plastibell should fall off

Evidence-Based Practice

Pain Management of Newborns During Painful Procedures

Clinical Question

Does sucrose offer effective and safe pain reduction in newborns during common medical procedures?

The Evidence

A meta-analysis of five blind randomized-control trials used sucrose as the pain intervention with term and preterm newborns in one of the following procedures: heel stick, venipuncture, and circumcision. Analyzed was the percentage of time spent crying during a 3-minute period after the painful procedure began or ended and its relationship to the amount of sucrose given.

The proportion of time spent crying after sucrose dosages ranging from 0.24 to 1.0 g was lower than the proportion of time spent crying after 0.18 g sucrose or plain water. There was no difference in the proportion of time spent crying after being given dosages of 0.24 g versus 0.50 g or 1.0 g. No differences were found between term and preterm newborn infants, and no adverse effects were reported in any study.

Best Practice

Provision of sucrose reduces the proportion of time spent crying during heel sticks, venipunctures, and circumcisions in newborn infants. The lowest concentration of sucrose should always be used. Newborns should be monitored for situations in which sucrose may be contraindicated.

Reference: Stevens, B., Taddio, A., Ohlsson, A., Einarson, T. (1997). The efficacy of sucrose for relieving procedural pain in neonates—a systematic review and meta-analysis. *Acta Paediatrica, 86,* 837–842.

within 8 days. If it remains after 8 days, they should consult with their physician. Though no ointments or creams should be used while the bell remains, use of petroleum to protect granulation tissue may be useful afterward.

ENHANCEMENT OF PARENT-NEWBORN ATTACHMENT

Parent-newborn attachment is promoted by encouraging all family members to be involved with the new member of the family. Some specific interventions are examined in Chapters 24 and 35 and the accompanying Client Teaching: Enhancing Attachment. Infant massage is a common child care practice in many parts of the world, especially Africa and Asia, and has recently gained attention in the United States. Parents can be taught to use infant message as a method to facilitate the bonding process and to reduce the stress and pain associated with teething, inoculations, constipation, and colic. Infant massage not only induces relaxation for the infant, but also provides a calming and "feel good" interaction for the parents that fosters the development of warm, positive relationships.

The nurse can discuss waking activities such as talking with the baby while making eye contact, holding the baby in an upright position (sitting or standing), gently bending the baby back and forth while grasping under the knees and supporting the head and back with the other hand, and gently rubbing the baby's hands and feet. Quieting activities may include swaddling the baby to increase a sense of security; using slow, calming movements; and talking softly, singing, or humming to the baby. The nurse must also be aware of cultural variations in newborn care such as timing of naming of the newborn, giving compliments about the baby, and using good luck charms (see Developing Cultural Competence). The nurse plays a vital role in fostering parent-infant attachment. It is important to be sensitive to the cultural beliefs and values of the family (Figure 30–8 •).

Global Perspectives

In Kenya, the naming of the child is an important event. Names are commonly selected to mirror important or current events. For example, an infant that is born while traveling may be given a name that means "wanderer" or "traveler." Other names may be chosen after a relative who is among the "living-dead" (deceased). It is believed that this results in a partial reincarnation of that relative, especially if the child has characteristics in common with that individual. It is also believed there is a connection between newborns and the spirit world. In some parts of the country, the name is chosen when the child is crying. Different names of the living-dead are called, and when the child quits crying when a particular name is called, that is the given name. In some areas, the name is given on the third day and is marked by a celebration with feasting and rejoicing. On the fourth day, the father of the child commonly hangs an iron necklace on the child's neck. It is at this time that the infant is considered a full human being and the connection with the spirit world is lost.

CLIENT TEACHING ENHANCING ATTACHMENT

Assessment Observe and document the interactions between the parents and their baby immediately after birth to determine the family's needs for teaching, support, or interventions.

Nursing Diagnoses The key nursing diagnoses will probably be ***Altered Family Processes*** related to addition of a new baby to the family or ***Deficient Knowledge*** related to lack of information about emotional needs of newborn.

Nursing Plan and Implementation The teaching plan will include information about the infant's physical status and normal characteristics, comforting techniques, and the baby's emotional needs immediately after birth and during the newborn period. Encourage the parents to maintain continuous contact with the baby through rooming-in, thus providing maximum opportunity for them to interact with their infant.

Client Goals At the completion of teaching, the parents will be able to:

- Demonstrate appropriate nurturing behaviors such as touching, bonding, talking to, kissing, and holding their baby.
- Discuss the normal characteristics and emotional needs of the newborn.
- List at least three comforting techniques.

Teaching Plan

CONTENT	TEACHING METHOD
• Present information on periods of reactivity and expected newborn responses.	Focus on open discussion.
• Describe normal physical characteristics of the newborn.	Present slides showing newborn characteristics.
• Explain the bonding process, its gradual development, and the reciprocal interactive nature of the process.	
• Discuss the infant's capabilities for interaction, such as nonverbal communication abilities. The nonverbal communications include movement, gaze, touch, facial expressions, and vocalizations—including crying. Emphasize that eye contact is considered one of the cardinal factors in developing infant-parent attachment and will be integrated with touching and vocal behaviors.	Show a video on the interactive capabilities of newborns.
• Explain that touching, including stroking, patting, massaging, and kissing, will progress to interactive touch between the parents and their infant; discuss their need to assimilate these behaviors into their daily routine with the baby.	Provide handouts, and use a doll to demonstrate behaviors.
• Describe and demonstrate comforting techniques, including the use of sound, swaddling, rocking, massage, and stroking.	Demonstrate the techniques and ask for a return demonstration.
• Describe the progression of the infant's behaviors as the infant matures, and the importance of the parents' consistent response to their infant's cues and needs.	Allow time for questions and discussion.
• Provide information about available pamphlets, videos, and support groups in the community.	

Evaluation

Evaluate the learning by providing time for discussion, questions, and return demonstrations in the birthing unit, and during the postpartal return visit or home visit. Continue to observe the parents' positive interaction with their baby during the remainder of their stay in the birthing unit.

A Letter From Your Baby

Dear Parents:

I come to you a small, immature being with my own style and personality. I am yours for only a short time; enjoy me.

1. Please take time to find out who I am, how I differ from you, and how much I can bring you joy.
2. Please feed me when I am hungry. I never knew hunger in the womb, and clocks and time mean little to me.
3. Please hold, cuddle, kiss, touch, stroke, and croon to me. I was always held closely in the womb and was never alone before.
4. Please don't be disappointed when I am not the perfect baby that you expected, nor disappointed with yourselves that you are not the perfect parents.
5. Please don't expect too much from me as your newborn baby, or too much from yourself as a parent. Give us both six weeks as a birthday present—six weeks for me to grow, develop, mature, and become more stable and predictable, and six weeks for you to rest and relax and allow your body to get back to normal.
6. Please forgive me if I cry a lot. Bear with me and in a short time, as I mature, I will spend less and less time crying and more time socializing.
7. Please watch me carefully and I can tell you the things that soothe, console and please me. I am not a tyrant who was sent to make your life miserable, but the only way I can tell you that I am not happy is with my cry.
8. Please remember that I am resilient and can withstand the many natural mistakes you will make with me. As long as you make them with love, you cannot ruin me.
9. Please take care of yourself and eat a balanced diet, rest, and exercise so that when we are together, you have the health and strength to take care of me.
10. Please take care of your relationship with others. Relationships that are good for you, support both you and me.

Although I may have turned your life upside down, please realize that things will be back to normal before long.

Thank you,

Your Loving Child

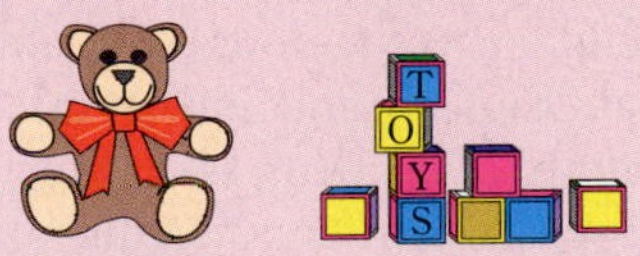

Figure 30–8 • A letter from your baby.

Evaluation

When evaluating the nursing care provided during the newborn period, the nurse may anticipate the following outcomes:

- The baby's physiologic and psychologic integrity is supported.
- The newborn feeding pattern will be satisfactorily established.
- The parents express understanding of the bonding process and display attachment behaviors.

Nursing Care in Preparation for Discharge

Parent Teaching

To meet parent needs for information, the nurse who is responsible for the daily care of the mother and newborn should assume the primary responsibility for parent education. Nearly every contact with the parents presents an opportunity for sharing information that can facilitate their sense of competence in newborn care. The nurse also needs to recognize and respect the fact that there are many good ways to provide safe care. Unless their care methods are harmful to the newborn, the parents' methods of giving care should be reinforced rather than contradicted.

The information that follows is provided to increase the nurse's knowledge of newborn care and is used to meet parents' needs for information. Parents may be familiar with handling and caring for infants, or this may be their first time to interact with a newborn. If they are new parents, the sensitive nurse gently teaches them by example and provides instructions geared to their needs and previous knowledge about the various aspects of newborn care.

The length of stay in the birthing unit for mother and baby after birth is often 48 hours or less. The challenge for the nurse is to use every opportunity to teach, guide, and support parents, fostering the parents' capabilities and confidence in caring for their newborn. Including mother-baby care and home care instruction on the night shift can help meet the teaching needs of early discharge parents.

The nurse observes how parents interact with their infant during feeding and caregiving activities. Even during a short stay, there will be opportunities for the nurse to provide information and evaluate whether the parents are comfortable with changing diapers and wrapping, handling, and feeding their newborn. Do both parents get involved in the infant's care? Is the mother depending on someone else to help her at home? Does the mother give excuses ("I am too tired," "My stitches hurt," or "I will learn later") for not wanting to be involved in her baby's care? As the family provides care, the nurse can enhance parental confidence by giving them

Developing Cultural Competence

Examples of Cultural Beliefs and Practices Regarding Baby Care*

Umbilical Cord

People of Latin American or Filipino cultural background may use an abdominal binder or bellyband to protect against dirt, injury, and umbilical hernia. They may also apply oils to the stump of the cord or tape metal to the umbilicus to ward off evil spirits.

People of northern European ancestry may expect a sterile cutting of the cord at birth. They may allow the stump to air-dry and discard the cord once it falls off.

Some Latin American cultures cauterize the stump with a hot flame, hot coal, or the like (WHO, 1999).

In Kenya, women may express colostrum to the cord stump (WHO, 1999).

In Ecuador, the cord is left long in girls to prevent a small uterus and problems with childbirth (WHO, 1999).

Parent-Infant Contact

People of Asian ancestry may pick up the baby as soon as it cries, or they may carry the baby at all times.

Some Native Americans, notably the Navajos, may use cradle boards.

Korean mothers may be reluctant to pick up or touch their infant, deferring infant care to the paternal grandmother (Schneiderman, 1996).

The Muslim father traditionally calls praise to Allah in the newborn's right ear and cleans the infant after birth (Hutchinson & Baqi-Aziz, 1994).

Feeding

Some people of Asian heritage may breastfeed their babies for the first 1 to 2 years of life. Many Cambodian refugees practice breastfeeding on demand without restriction, or, if formula-feeding, provide a "comfort bottle" in between feedings (Rasbridge & Kulig, 1995).

People of Iranian heritage may breastfeed female babies longer than male babies.

Some people of African ancestry may wean their babies after they begin to walk.

Most Korean mothers resist breastfeeding in the hospital, contending that they do not have "milk," and state that they will begin breastfeeding at home (Schneiderman, 1996).

Some Asians, Hispanics, Eastern Europeans, and Native Americans may delay breastfeeding because they believe colostrum is "bad" (Lipson, Dibble, & Minarik, 1996).

Circumcision

People of Muslim and Jewish ancestry practice circumcision as a religious ritual (Hutchinson & Baqi-Aziz, 1994).

Many natives of Africa and Australia practice circumcision as a puberty rite.

Native Americans and people of Asian and Latin American cultures rarely perform circumcision.

Only 15% of the world's male population is circumcised.

Health and Illness

Some people from Latin American cultural backgrounds may believe that touching the face or head of an infant when admiring it will ward off the "evil eye." They may also neglect to cut the baby's nails to avoid nearsightedness and instead put mittens on the baby's hands to prevent scratching. They also may believe that fat babies are healthy.

Some people of Asian heritage may not allow anyone to touch the baby's head without asking permission.

Some Orthodox Jews believe that saying the baby's name before the formal naming ceremony will harm the baby.

Some Asians and Haitians delay naming their infants (Geissler, 1998).

Some people of Vietnamese ancestry believe that cutting a baby's hair or nails will cause illness.

*Note: The information is meant only to provide examples of some of the behaviors that may be found within certain cultures. Not all members of a culture practice the behaviors described.

positive feedback. If the family encounters problems, the nurse can express confidence in the family's abilities to master the new skill or information, suggest alternatives, and serve as a role model. All these considerations need to be taken into account when evaluating the educational needs of the parents (Ruchala, 2000).

Several methods may be used to teach parents about newborn care. Daily child care classes are a nonthreatening way to convey general information. Individual instruction is helpful to answer specific questions or to clarify an item that may have been confusing in class (Figure 30–9 •). Currently many birthing centers have 24-hour educational video channels or videos to be viewed in the mother's room on a variety of postpartum and newborn care issues. For hearing-impaired clients, videotapes with information in both spoken and signed formats are most helpful. Birthing centers should have handouts available for families who do not speak English and either interpreters or language interpreter phones. With shorter stays, most such teaching tends to focus on infant feeding and immediate physical care needs of the mother, with limited anticipatory guidance in other areas.

One-to-one teaching while the nurse is in the mother's room is shown to be the most effective educational model. Both first-time and experienced postpartum mothers rate individual teaching as the most effective method of instruction.

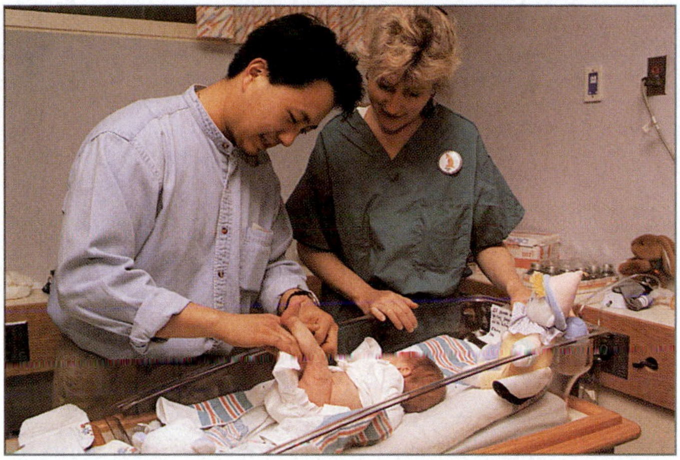

Figure 30–9 • Individualizing parent education. Father returns demonstration of diapering his son.

> *With the new life come new rhythms. Or perhaps I should say no rhythms. The day is divided into phone calls, meals eaten on the run, visitors who've come to see the baby, trips from hospital to home to walk the dog.*
>
> *The new life brings new thoughts, new perceptions of the world. Why don't men take paternity leave? Why is time off, if any, basically reserved for women? Why don't we take a month off? In those first few chaotic days, filled with ecstasy and fear, the family needs to be together. Being together in times of joy and sadness is what a family is. A month's distance from the office grind, from the bottom line, could not help but create a healthier world.*
>
> –Dennis Donziger, *Daddy*–

GENERAL INSTRUCTIONS FOR NEWBORN CARE

How to pick up a newborn is one of the first concerns of anyone who has not had experience. The newborn is easily picked up by sliding one hand under the neck and shoulders and the other hand under the buttocks or between the legs, then gently lifting the newborn. This technique provides security and support for the head (which the baby is unable to consistently support until 3 or 4 months of age).

The baby should never be left alone anywhere but in the crib. The mother is reminded that while she and the newborn are together in the birthing unit, she should never leave the baby alone for security reasons and because newborns spit up frequently the first day or two after birth.

Demonstrating a bath, cord care, and temperature assessment is the best way for the nurse to provide information on these topics to parents (see Chapter 36). Parents should be told to call their healthcare provider if redness, foul odor, bright red bleeding, or greenish yellow drainage occurs at the cord site or if the area remains unhealed 2 to 3 days after the cord stump has sloughed off. Current evidence does not support the routine application of topical antimicrobials to the drying cord (WHO, 1999). See Table 30–3 •: What to Tell Parents about Infant Care.

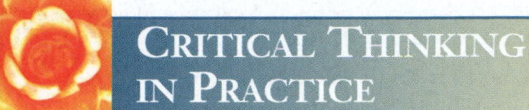

CRITICAL THINKING IN PRACTICE

You are caring for Sarah Feldstein, who had her first child, a daughter, about 4 hours ago. She appears visibly upset when changing her infant's diaper and says she thinks something is wrong because her daughter has tissue protruding from her vagina and some bleeding in her diaper. What would you do?

Answers can be found in Appendix I.

The nurse demonstrates the taking of an axillary temperature and discourages the use of mercury thermometers and ear thermometers for infants. It is important that families understand the differences and know how to select the appropriate device. The newborn's temperature needs to be taken only when signs of illness are present. Parents are advised to call their physician or pediatric nurse practitioner immediately if any signs of illness become apparent.

NASAL AND ORAL SUCTIONING

Most newborns are obligatory nose breathers for the first months of life. They generally maintain air passage patency by coughing or sneezing. During the first few days of life, however, the newborn has increased mucus, and gentle suctioning with a bulb syringe may be indicated. The nurse can demonstrate the use of the bulb syringe in the nose and mouth and have the parents do a return demonstration. The parents should repeat this demonstration before discharge so they will feel more confident and comfortable with the procedure (McCartney, 2000). Care should be taken to apply only gentle suction so nasal bleeding does not occur.

To suction the newborn, the bulb syringe is compressed and the tip is placed in the nostril. The nurse or parent must take care not to occlude the passageway. The bulb is permitted to reexpand slowly by releasing the compression on the bulb (Figure 30–10 •). The bulb syringe is removed from the nostril, and drainage is then compressed out of the bulb onto a tissue. The bulb syringe may also be used in the mouth if the newborn is spitting up and unable to handle the excess secretions. The bulb is compressed, the tip of the bulb syringe is placed about 1 inch to one side of the newborn's mouth, and compression is released. This draws up the excess secretions. The procedure is repeated on the other side of the mouth. The roof of the mouth and back of the throat are avoided because suction in these areas might stimulate the gag reflex. The bulb syringe should be washed in warm, soapy water and rinsed in warm water daily and as needed after use. Rinsing with a half-strength white vinegar solution followed by clear water may help to extend the useful life of the bulb syringe by inhibiting bacterial growth. A bulb syringe should always be kept near the newborn. New parents and nurses who are inexperienced with babies may fear that the baby will choke and may be relieved if they know how to take action if such an event occurs. They

Table 30-3 • WHAT TO TELL PARENTS ABOUT INFANT CARE

Immediate Safety Measures for the Newborn

Watch for excessive mucus: use bulb syringe to remove mucus.

Have baby sleep on his or her back in crib or in someone's arms.

Voiding and Stool Characteristics and Patterns

Urine is straw to amber color without foul smell.

At least 6 to 10 wet diapers a day.

Normal progression of stool changes: (1) meconium (thick, tarry, dark green); (2) transitional stools (thin, brown to green); (3a) breastfed infant: yellow gold, soft or mushy stools; (3b) formula-fed infant: pale yellow, formed and pasty stools.

Only 1 to 2 stools a day for formula-fed baby.

Six to 10 small, loose yellow stools per day or only one stool every few days after breastfeeding is well established (after about 1 month).

Cord Care

Wash hands with clean water and soap before and after care. Keep the cord dry and exposed to air or loosely covered with clean clothes. (If cultural custom demands binding of the abdomen, a sanitary method such as the use of a clean piece of gauze can be recommended.)

Clean cord and skin around base with a cotton swab or cotton ball. Clean 2 to 3 times a day or with each diaper change. Touching the cord, applying unclean substances to it, and applying bandages should be avoided. Do not give tub baths until cord falls off in 7 to 14 days.

Fold diapers below umbilical cord to air-dry the cord (contact with wet or soiled diapers slows the drying process and increases the possibility of infection).

Check cord each day for any odor, oozing of greenish yellow material, or reddened areas around the cord. Expect tenderness around the cord and darkening and shriveling of cord. Report to healthcare provider any signs of infection.

Normal changes in cord: Cord should look dark and dry up before falling off. A small drop of blood may present when cord falls off.

Never pull the cord or attempt to loosen it.

Care Required for Circumcision and Uncircumcised Infants

Circumcision Care

Squeeze soapy water over circumcision site once a day.

Rinse area off with warm water and pat dry.

Apply small amount of petroleum jelly (unless a Plastibell is in place) with each diaper change.

Fasten diaper loosely over penis.

Since the glans is sensitive, avoid placing baby on his stomach.

Check for any foul-smelling drainage or bleeding at least once a day.

Let Plastibell fall off by itself (about 8 days after circumcision).

Plastibell should not be pulled off.

Light, sticky, yellow drainage (part of healing process) may form over head of penis.

Uncircumcised Care

Clean uncircumcised penis with water during diaper changes and with bath.

Do not force foreskin back over the penis; foreskin will retract normally over time (may take 3 to 5 years).

Techniques for Waking and Quieting Newborns

Techniques for Waking Baby

Loosen clothing, change diaper.

Hand-express milk onto baby's lips.

Talk with baby while making eye contact.

Hold baby in upright position (sitting or standing).

Have baby do sit-ups (gently and rhythmically bend baby back and forth while grasping the baby under his or her knees and supporting baby's head and back with your other hand).

Play patty-cake with baby.

Stimulate rooting reflex (brush one cheek with hand or nipple).

Increase skin contact (gently rub hands and feet).

Techniques for Quieting Baby

Check for soiled diaper.

Swaddle or bundle baby (bring arms and legs into midline, which increases sense of security).

Use slow, calming movements with baby.

Softly talk, sing, or hum to baby.

Signs of Illness and Use of Thermometer

See Table 30-4: When Parents Should Call Their Healthcare Provider.

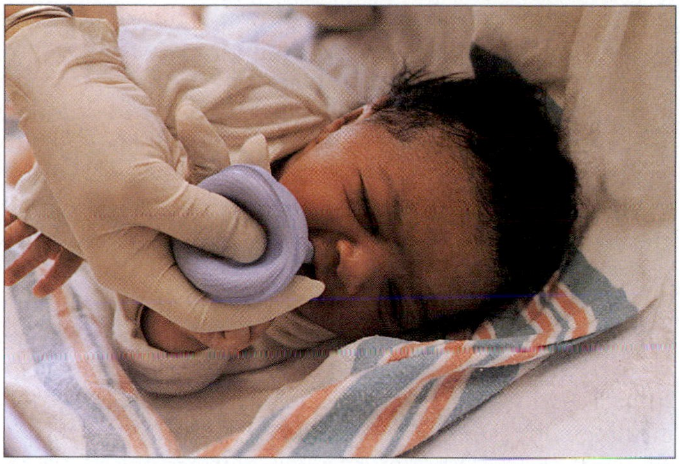

Figure 30–10 • Nasal and oral suctioning. The bulb is compressed, the tip is placed in either the mouth or the nose, and the bulb is released.

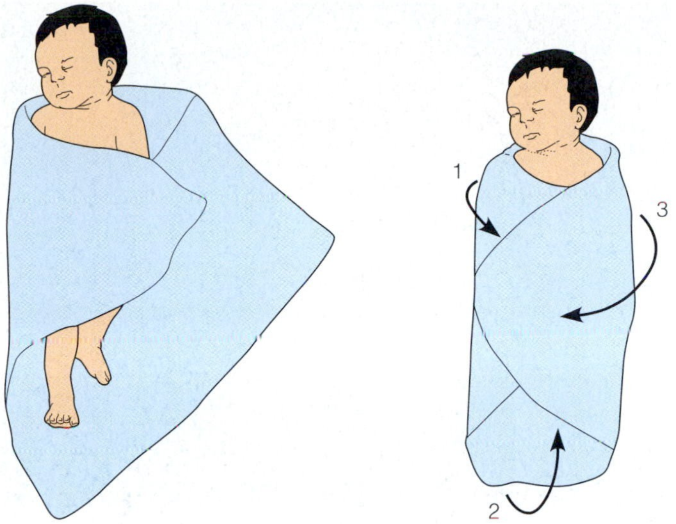

Figure 30–11 • Steps in wrapping a baby.

should be advised to turn the newborn's head to the side or down as soon as there is any indication of gagging or vomiting and to use the bulb syringe as needed.

Some infants may have transient edema of the nasal mucosa following suctioning of the airway after birth. The nurse can demonstrate the use of normal saline to loosen secretions, and instruct parents in the gentle and moderate use of the bulb syringe to avoid further irritation of the mucous membranes. If parents will be using humidifiers at home, they should be instructed to follow the manufacturer's cleaning instructions carefully so that molds, spores, and bacteria from a dirty humidifier do not enter the baby's environment.

Clinical Tip *You'll find that left-handed people tend to hold the baby over their right shoulder, and right-handed people do the opposite. This keeps the dominant hand free. However, most health personnel wear their name tags on the left side. To avoid scratching the baby's face, wear your name tag on the same side as your dominant hand.*

SWADDLING THE NEWBORN

Swaddling (wrapping) helps the newborn maintain body temperature, provides a feeling of closeness and security, and may be effective in quieting a crying baby. A blanket is placed on the crib (or secure surface) in the shape of a diamond. The top corner of the blanket is folded down slightly, and the newborn's body is placed with the head at the upper edge of the blanket. The right corner of the blanket is wrapped around the infant and tucked under the left side (not too tightly—newborns need a little room to move). The bottom corner is then pulled up to the chest, and the left corner is wrapped around the baby's right side (Figure 30–11 •). The nurse can show this wrapping technique to a new mother so she will feel more skilled in handling her baby.

SLEEP AND ACTIVITY

The National Institute of Child Health and Human Development and the American Academy of Pediatrics recommend that healthy term infants be placed on their back to sleep. Parents are taught the importance of following "Back to Sleep Guidelines" to reduce the incidence of sudden infant death syndrome (SIDS). Though infants may need to be placed on their sides initially because of copious or thick secretions, placing them on their backs in the newborn period serves to educate parents regarding infant positioning. Studies indicate that parents position their babies in the same positions they observe in the hospital setting, so nurses must demonstrate this behavior to reduce the risk of SIDS. If exceptions are warranted, these should be explained to families so they do not misinterpret what they observe. The placement of babies in a prone position during wakeful play sessions should be encouraged as well (National Institute of Child Health and Human Development, 2002).

MediaLink: SIDS Resources for Parents

Perhaps nothing is more individual to each baby than the sleep-activity cycle. It is important for the nurse to recognize the individual variations of each newborn and to assist parents as they develop sensitivity to their infant's communication signals and rhythms of activity and sleep. See Chapter 29 for more detailed discussion of the sleep-activity cycle.

CAR SAFETY CONSIDERATIONS

Half the children killed or injured in automobile accidents could have been protected by the use of a federally approved car seat. Newborns should go home from the birthing unit in a car seat adapted to fit newborns (Figure 30–12 •). Babies should never be in the front seat of a car equipped with a passenger-side air bag. The safest spot in any car is the middle of the back seat. The car seat should be positioned to face the rear of the car until the baby is a year old or weighs 20 pounds (9.09 kg) (AAP Committee on Injury and Poison Prevention, 2002). In many states, the use of car seats for

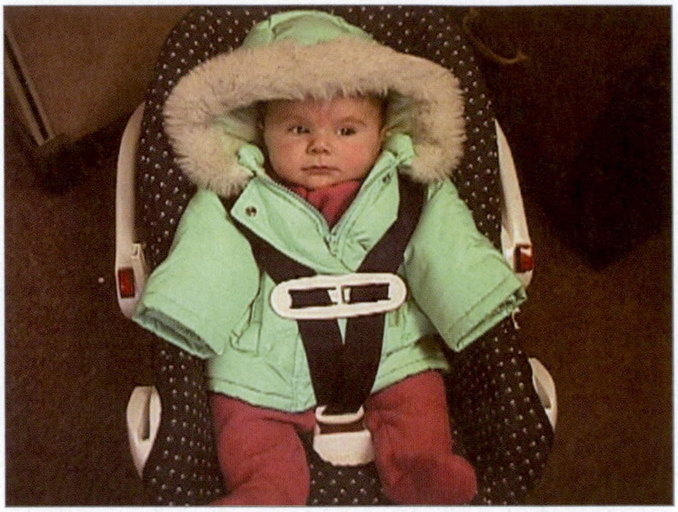

Figure 30–12 • Infant car restraint for use from birth to about 12 months of age.

children up to the age of 4 is mandatory. In some states such as California the age is 6. Nurses need to ensure that all parents are knowledgeable about the benefits of child safety seat use and proper installation.

NEWBORN SCREENING AND IMMUNIZATION PROGRAM

MEDIALINK IMMUNIZATION INITIATIVES

Before the newborn and mother are discharged from the birthing unit, the nurse informs the parents about **newborn screening tests** and tells them when to return to the birthing center or clinic if further tests are needed. The disorders that can be identified from a drop of blood obtained by a heel stick are cystic fibrosis, galactosemia, congenital adrenal hyperplasia, hypothyroidism, biotinidase deficiency, phenylketonuria (PKU), and hemoglobinopathies. Early newborn discharge puts infants at risk for delayed or even missed diagnosis of PKU and congenital hypothyroidism because of decreased sensitivity of screening prior to 24 hours of age. Newborns should be retested by 2 weeks of age if the first test was done prior to 24 hours of age.

Immunization programs against the hepatitis B virus during the newborn period and infancy are in place in many states, at least 20 countries, and high-incidence areas such as Alaska and American Samoa. Universal vaccination of infants is recommended. Infants should receive the first dose of hepatitis B (Hep B) vaccine at birth to 2 months of age. The second dose should be at least one month after the first dose. The third dose should be administered at least 4 months after the first dose and at least 2 months after the second dose, but not before 6 months of age (Centers for Disease Control, 2003). See the Drug Guide: Hepatitis B Vaccine. Parents need to be advised whether their birthing center provides newborn hepatitis vaccination so that an adequate follow-up program can be set in motion.

Early discharge has affected both the timing of newborn metabolic screening tests and the acquisition of subsequent immunization. For example, the accuracy of the test for PKU is directly related to the newborn's age. The likelihood of detecting PKU increases as the infant grows older, and the infant must be at least 24 hours old for a valid test. A second test is required in most states, usually between one week and one month of age, to minimize the chance of a positive child going undetected.

The nurse should teach the family all necessary caregiving methods before discharge. A checklist may be helpful to determine whether the teaching has been completed and to verify the parents' knowledge on leaving the birthing unit (Figure 30–13 •). The nurse needs to review all areas for understanding or any outstanding questions with the mother and father, without rushing, taking time to answer all queries. Any concerns of the parents or nurse are noted.

COMMUNITY-BASED NURSING CARE

The nurse discusses with parents ways to meet their newborn's needs, ensure safety, and appreciate the newborn's unique characteristics and behaviors. By assisting parents in establishing links with their community-based healthcare provider, the nurse can get the new family off to a good start. Parents also need to know the signs of illness, how to reach the pediatrician or after-hours clinic, and the importance of follow-up after discharge. See Table 30–4 •. Parents should also check with their clinician for advice about over-the-counter medications to be kept in the medicine cabinet.

The family should have the care provider's phone number, address, and any specific instructions. Having the birthing unit or nursery phone number is also reassuring to a new-

Table 30–4 • WHEN PARENTS SHOULD CALL THEIR HEALTHCARE PROVIDER

Temperature above 38.4C (101F) rectally or 38C (100.4F) axillary or below 36.1C (97F) rectally or 36.6C (97.8F) axillary
Continual rise in temperature
More than one episode of forceful vomiting or frequent vomiting over a 6-hour period
Refusal of two feedings in a row
Lethargy (listlessness), difficulty in awakening baby
Cyanosis with or without a feeding
Absence of breathing longer than 15 seconds
Inconsolable infant (quieting techniques are not effective) or continuous high-pitched cry
Discharge or bleeding from umbilical cord, circumcision, or any opening (except vaginal mucus or pseudomenstruation)
Two consecutive green, watery stools
No wet diapers for 18 to 24 hours or fewer than six to eight wet diapers per day after 4 days of age
Development of eye drainage

FOR NURSES ONLY

NURSERY TEACHING CHECKLIST

Please read the *Mother/Baby* information booklet given to you after birth. After reading it, please go through the following list and check whether you understand each topic or need to know more.

		I know this already	Doesn't apply to me	I need to know more	Taught/ reviewed/ demonstrated
Baby Care	What to do if baby is choking or gagging				
	Safety				
	How to do skin care/cord care				
	How to take care of the circumcision or genital area				
	How to know if my baby is sick and what to do				
	What is jaundice and how to detect it				
	Use of thermometer				
	Use of bulb syringe				
	How and when to burp baby				
	Newborn behavior: crying/comforting				
	How to position baby after feeding				
	What does demand scheduling mean				
Breastfeeding	I attended breastfeeding class/watched breastfeeding video	YES ☐	NO ☐		
	How to position baby for feeding				
	How to get baby to latch on to my nipple properly				
	When and how long to breastfeed				
	Removal of baby from my nipple				
	What is the supply and demand concept				
	What is the let-down reflex				
	When does breast milk come in				
	Supplementing				
	Proper diet for breastfeeding mothers				
	Prevention and comfort measures for sore nipples				
	Prevention and comfort measures for engorgement				
	When and how to use a breast pump				
	How to express milk by hand				
	How to go back to work and continue to breastfeed				
Bottle-Feeding	How to feed my baby a bottle				
	Reasons for NOT propping bottles				
	How to clean nipple/bottle				
	How to mix formula				
	What formula should my baby drink				
Safety	**Use of infant car seat**				
	Back to Sleep				
	Shaken Baby Syndrome				

Other information: ______________________

I have received and understand the instructions given on the above topics.

______________________ MOTHER'S SIGNATURE ______________ DATE

Videos viewed/ Literature given: ______________________

Language Spoken by Mother:

☐ English ☐ Spanish ☐ Other ______________

Interpreter Used? ☐ Yes ☐ No ☐ Family Interprets

Nurse's Signature(s): ______________________

Figure 30–13 • An infant teaching checklist is completed by the time of discharge.
SOURCE: Adapted from Presbyterian/St. Luke's Medical Center, Denver, CO.

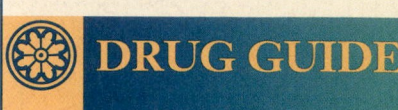

DRUG GUIDE Hepatitis B Vaccine (Engerix-B, Recombivax HB)

• Overview of Neonatal Action

Recombinant hepatitis B vaccine is used as a prophylactic treatment against all subtypes of hepatitis B virus. It provides passive immunization for newborns of HBsAg-negative and HBsAg-positive mothers. Hepatitis B can be transmitted across the placenta, but most newborns are infected during birth.

The vaccine is produced from baker's yeast and plasmid containing the HBsAg gene.

Hepatitis B (thimerosal free) vaccine contains more than 95% HBsAg protein and is an inactivated (noninfective) product. Universal immunization is recommended.

Infants of HBsAg-positive mothers should concurrently receive 0.5 mL of hepatitis B immunoglobulin (HBIG) prophylaxis at separate injection sites (CDC, 2003).

• Route, Dosage, Frequency

The first dose of 0.5 mL (10 mcg) is given intramuscularly into the anterolateral thigh within 12 hours of birth for infants born to HBsAg-positive mothers. The second dose of vaccine is given at 1 month of age and followed by a final dose at 6 months of age.

Infants born to HBsAg-negative mothers receive their first dose of vaccine at birth, the second dose at 1 to 2 months, and the third dose at 6 to 18 months (Zenk et al, 2000).

Infants whose mother's HBsAg status is unknown should receive the same doses of vaccine as infants born to HBsAg-positive mothers.

• Neonatal Side Effects

The only common side effect is soreness at the injection site. Occasionally, there is erythema, swelling, warmth, and induration at the injection site, irritability, or a low-grade fever (37.7 C[99.8F]).

• Nursing Considerations

Delay administration during active infection; the vaccine will not prevent infection during its incubation period.

- The vaccine should be used as supplied. Do not dilute. Shake well.
- Do not inject intravenously or interdermally.
- Monitor for adverse reactions. Monitor temperature closely.
- Have epinephrine available to treat possible allergic reactions.
- Responsiveness to the vaccine is age dependent. Preterm infants weighing less than 1000 g have lower seroconversion rates. Consider delaying the first dose until the infant is term PCA (postconceptual age) or use a four-dose schedule.

Although recent studies show no link between thimerosal-containing immunizations and autism, attention-deficit/hyperactivity disorder, or speech and language delay, the American Academy of Pediatrics and The Public Health Service continue to recommend use of thimerosal-free vaccines whenever available (AAP News Release, 2001).

MediaLink CARE PLAN: INITIAL NEWBORN CARE

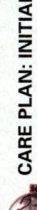

born's family. They are encouraged to call with questions. Follow-up calls lend added support by providing another opportunity for parents to have their questions answered.

To assist parents in caring for their newborn at home, some physicians/healthcare systems encourage prenatal pediatric visits to establish a relationship with caregivers before the birth of the baby. Public health nurses play an important role in this early teaching and preparation in many communities.

Some institutions have initiated postpartum and/or newborn follow-up visits 48 to 72 hours after birth when the family is unable to visit their primary care physician within that time period (Lieu, Braverman, Escobar, et al, 2000). The newborn visit focuses on normal newborn care, assessment for hyperbilirubinemia (jaundice), extreme weight loss, feeding problems, and knowledge deficits related to newborn care and feeding within the family unit.

Routine well-baby visits should be scheduled with the clinic, pediatric nurse practitioner, or physician. Regardless of the type of follow-up services available in the community, the nurse contributes to the newborn's health by stressing the importance of routine care and by helping families who have no follow-up plans to connect to local resources for care.

Evaluation

When evaluating the nursing care provided during the newborn period, the nurse may anticipate the following outcomes:

- The parents demonstrate safe techniques for caring for their newborn.
- The parents verbalize developmentally appropriate behavioral expectations of and community-based follow-up care for their newborn.

CHAPTER REVIEW

EXPLOREMEDIALINK

NCLEX review questions, case studies, and other interactive resources for this chapter can be found on the Web site at http://www.prenhall.com/olds. Click on "Chapter 30" to select the activities for this chapter.

For tutorials including animations and videos, more NCLEX review questions, and an audio glossary, access the accompanying CD-ROM in this book.

Focus Your Study

- The overall goal of newborn nursing care is to provide comprehensive care while promoting the establishment of a well-functioning family unit.
- The period immediately following birth, during which adaptation to extrauterine life occurs, requires close monitoring to identify any deviations from normal.
- Nursing goals during the first 4 hours after birth (admission period) are to maintain a clear airway, maintain a neutral thermal environment, prevent hemorrhage and infection, initiate oral feedings, and facilitate attachment.
- The newborn is routinely given prophylactic vitamin K to prevent possible hemorrhagic disease of the newborn.
- Prophylactic eye treatment for *Neisseria gonorrhoeae* is legally required on all newborns.
- Nursing goals in daily newborn care include maintaining cardiopulmonary function, maintaining a neutral thermal environment, promoting adequate hydration and nutrition, preventing complications, promoting safety, and enhancing attachment and family knowledge of child care.
- Essential daily care includes assessing vital signs, weight, overall color, intake, output, umbilical cord and circumcision, newborn nutrition, parent education, and attachment.
- Following a circumcision, the newborn must be observed closely for signs of bleeding, inability to void, and signs of infection.
- Signs of illness in newborns include temperature above 38C (100.4F) axillary or below 36.6C (97.8F) axillary, more than one episode of forceful vomiting, refusal of two feedings in a row, lethargy, cyanosis with or without a feeding, and absence of breathing for longer than 15 seconds.
- Newborn screening for cystic fibrosis, galactosemia, hypothyroidism, phenylketonuria, congenital adrenal hyperplasia, biotinidase deficiency, and hemoglobinopathies may be done on all newborns in the first 1 to 3 days.

References

American Academy of Pediatrics (AAP) Committee on Fetus and Newborn & American College of Obstetricians and Gynecologists (ACOG) Committee on Obstetrics (2002). *Guidelines for perinatal care* (5th ed.). Evanston, IL: Author.

American Academy of Pediatrics (AAP) Committee on Injury and Poison Prevention. (2002). Selecting and using the most appropriate car safety seats for growing children: Guidelines for counseling parents. *Pediatrics, 109*(3), 550–553.

American Academy of Pediatrics (AAP) News Release. (2001). *IOM report on vaccines should reassure parents that children should be vaccinated.* Retrieved October 1, 2001 from, www.aap.org/advocacy/releases/vaccinesafety

American Academy of Pediatrics (AAP) Task Force on Circumcision. (1999). Circumcision policy statement. *Pediatrics, 103*(3), 686–693.

Andrews, M. M. (1999). Transcultural perspectives in the nursing care of children and adolescents. In M. M. Andrews & J. S. Boyle (Eds.), *Transcultural concepts in nursing care* (3rd ed., pp. 107–159). Philadelphia: Lippincott.

Association of Women's Health Obstetric and Neonatal Nurses (AWHONN). (2001). Evidence-based clinical practice guideline: Neonatal skin care. Washington, DC: Author.

Beers, M., & Berdow, R. (2000). *The Merck manual* (Section 19, p. 2083). Whitehouse Station, NJ: Merck Research Laboratories.

Behring, A., Vezeau, T. M., & Fink, R. (2003). Timing of the newborn first bath: A replication. *Neonatal Network, 22*(1), 39–46.

Blackburn, S. T. (2003). *Maternal, fetal, & neonatal physiology: A clinical perspective.* St. Louis, MO: Saunders.

Carroll, V. (2000). Infant abduction: Lowering the risk. *AWHONN Lifelines, 3*(6), 25–27.

Centers for Disease Control, Advisory Committee on Immunization Practices. (2003). *Recommended childhood and adolescent immunization schedule, United States* 2003. Retrieved Jan 8, 2003 from www.cdc.gov/NLP/acip

Geissler, E. M. (1998). *Pocket guide to cultural assessment* (2nd ed.). St. Louis, MO: Mosby.

Hutchinson, M. K., & Baqi-Aziz, M. (1994). Nursing care of the childbearing Muslim family. *Journal of Obstetric, Gynecologic, and Neonatal Nursing, 23*(9), 767–771.

James, G., & Dinulos, L. (2000). Neonatal skin care. *Pediatric Clinics of North America, 47*(4), 757–782.

Karl, D. J. (1999). The newborn bath: Using infant neurobehavior to connect parents and newborns. *American Journal of Maternal Child Nursing, 24*(6), 280–286.

Kaufman, M. W., Clark, J. Y., & Castro, C. L. (2001). Neonatal circumcision: Benefits, risks, and family teaching. *American Journal of Maternal Child Nursing, 26*(4), 197–201.

Klaus, M., & Klaus, P. (1985). *The amazing newborn.* Menlo Park, CA: Addison-Wesley.

Lieu, T. A., Braverman, P. A., Escobar, G. J., Fischer, A. F., Jensvold, N. G., & Capra, A. M. (2000). A randomized comparison of home and clinic follow-up visits after early postpartum hospital discharge. *Pediatrics, 105* (5), 1058–1065.

Lipson, J. G., Dibble, S. L., & Minarik, P. A. (1996). *Culture and nursing care: A pocket guide.* San Francisco: University of California at San Francisco Nursing Press.

MacMullen, N. J., & Dulski, S. L. (2000). Factors related to sucking ability in healthy newborns. *Journal of Obstetric, Gynecologic, and Neonatal Nursing, 29*(4), 390–396.

McCartney, P. R. (2000). Bulb syringes in newborn care. *American Journal of Maternal Child Nursing, 25*(4), 217.

National Institute of Child Health and Human Development. (2002). Babies sleep best on of their backs: Reduce the risk of sudden infant death syndrome. Retrieved 1/10/2003 from www.NIH.gov

Neonatal Thermoregulation. (1997). *NANN guidelines for practice.* Petaluma, CA: National Association of Neonatal Nurses.

Rasbridge, L. A., & Kulig, J. C. (1995). Infant feeding among Cambodian refugees. *American Journal of Maternal Child Nursing, 20*(4), 213–218.

Reynolds, R. D. (1996). Use of the Mogen clamp for neonatal circumcision. *American Family Physician, 54*(1), 177–182.

Riordan, J., & Auerbach, K. G. (1999). *Breastfeeding and human lactation* (2nd ed.). Boston: Jones & Bartlett.

Ruchala, P. L. (2000). Teaching new mothers: Priorities of nurses and postpartum women. *Journal of Obstetric, Gynecologic, and Neonatal Nursing, 29*(3), 265–273.

Schneiderman, J. U. (1996). Postpartum nursing for Korean mothers. *American Journal of Maternal Child Nursing, 21*(3), 155–158.

Stevens, B., Taddio, A., Ohlsson, A., Einarson, T. (1997). The efficacy of sucrose for relieving procedural pain in neonates—a systematic review and meta-analysis. *Acta Paediatrica, 86*, 837–842.

Taddio, A., Pollock, N., Gilbert-MacLeod, C., Ohlsson, K., & Koren, G. (2000). Combined analgesia and local anesthesia to minimize pain during circumcision. *Archives of Pediatrics & Adolescent Medicine, 154*, 620–622.

Tappero, E. P., & Honeyfield, M. E. (1996). *Physical assessment of the newborn* (2nd ed.). Petaluma, CA: NICU Ink.

World Health Organization (WHO). (1999). *Care of the umbilical cord: A review of the evidence* Retrieved 2/2000 from www.whoint/rht/documents/MSM98-4

Zenk, K. E., Sills, J. H., & Koeppel, R. M. (2000). *Neonatal medications and nutrition: A comprehensive guide* (2nd ed.). Santa Rosa, CA: NICU Ink.

Zupan, J., & Garner, P. (2001). Topical umbilical cord care at birth (Cochrane Review). In *The Cochrane Library*, Issue 2. Oxford: Update Software.

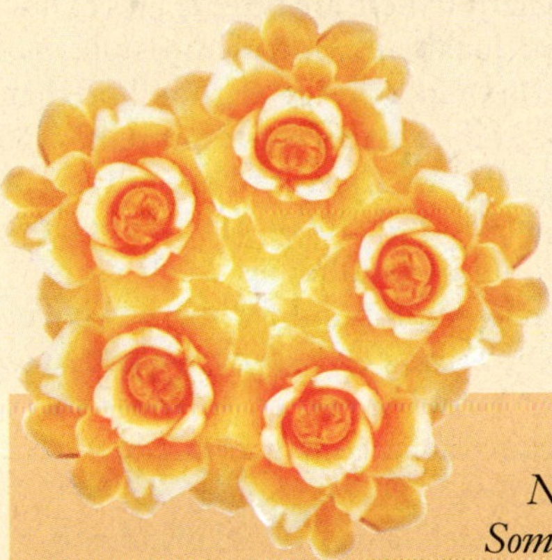

31 Newborn Nutrition

I had been told that most babies ate every three or four hours and slept the rest of the time. Not mine! She wanted to nurse every two hours, and sometimes more often than that. Sometimes she would sleep for an hour, sometimes for fifteen minutes. I loved her, but I also felt consumed by her needs. It was hard to adjust to the fact that I couldn't get anything finished, whether it was an article I was reading or folding the laundry. At the end of the day I would realize I hadn't accomplished anything. Once I accepted the fact that I was not going to function at my old efficient rate (at least for a while) and stopped feeling guilty about what I wasn't getting done, I felt free to enjoy the time I was spending with my baby.

~ The New Our Bodies, Ourselves ~

Objectives

- Compare the nutritional value and composition of breast milk and formula preparations.
- Discuss the advantages and disadvantages of breastfeeding and formula-feeding for both mother and newborn.
- Develop guidelines for helping both breastfeeding and formula-feeding mothers to feed their infants successfully.
- Delineate nursing responsibilities for client teaching about issues the breastfeeding mother may encounter in the birthing center.
- Incorporate knowledge of newborn nutrition and normal growth patterns into parent education and infant assessment.
- Recognize the influence of cultural values on infant care, especially feeding practices.

Key Terms

Colostrum 866
Foremilk 866
Hindmilk 866
La Leche League 868
Let-down reflex 875
Mature milk 866
Milk/plasma ratio 881
Oxytocin 875
Prolactin 875
Transitional milk 866

MediaLink

Additional resources for this content can be found on the Student CD-ROM and on the Companion Website at www.prenhall.com/olds. Click on "Chapter 31" to select the activities for this chapter.

CD-ROM

- Audio Glossary
- NCLEX Review

Companion Website

- Additional NCLEX Review
- Case Study: Breastfeeding Client
- Care Plan Activity: Breastfeeding Concerns

Feeding their newborn is an exciting, satisfying, and often worrisome task for parents. Meeting this essential need of their new child helps parents strengthen their attachment to their baby and fosters their self-images as nurturers and providers. Whether a woman chooses to breastfeed or use infant formula, she can be reassured that she can adequately meet her infant's needs. As questions arise about feeding, the nurse works with the woman to help her develop skill in her chosen method. In every interaction it is the nurse's responsibility to support the parents and promote the family's sense of confidence.

Nutritional Needs of the Newborn

The newborn's diet must supply nutrients to meet the rapid rate of physical and mental growth and development. A neonatal diet should provide adequate calories and include protein, carbohydrate, fat, water, vitamins, and minerals. The recommended dietary allowances (RDAs) for birth through the first 6 months have been established.

The calories (105 to 108 kcal/kg/day or 50 to 55 kcal/lb/day) in the newborn's diet are divided among protein, carbohydrate, and fat. Protein is needed for rapid cellular growth and maintenance. Carbohydrates provide energy. The fat portion of the diet provides calories, regulates fluid and electrolyte balance, and is necessary for the normal development of the neonatal brain and neurologic system.

Fluid requirements are high (140 to 160 mL/kg/day or 64 to 73 mL/lb/day) because of the newborn's inability to concentrate urine. Fluid needs are further increased in illness or hot weather.

The infant's iron needs will be affected by the accumulation of iron stores during fetal life and by the mother's iron and other food intake if she is breastfeeding. Ascorbic acid (usually in the form of fruit or fruit juices) and meat, poultry, and fish are known to enhance absorption of iron. Adequate minerals and vitamins are needed by the newborn to prevent deficiency states such as scurvy, cheilosis, and pellagra.

Formula-fed babies do gain weight faster than breastfed babies because of the higher protein content in commercially prepared formula and the larger volumes of formula that are needed to obtain the necessary nutrients. (Because breast milk is digested more easily than formula, the nutrients are more readily available.) Formula-fed infants tend to regain their birth weight by 10 days after birth and may gain as much as 30 g (1 oz) per day up to 6 months of age. Healthy breastfed babies, however, tend to regain their birth weight about 14 days after birth and gain approximately 15 g (0.5 oz) per day in the first 6 months of life. Formula-fed infants generally double their birth weight in 3.5 to 4 months, whereas breastfeeding infants double their weight at about 5 months of age.

Breast Milk Feeding

The composition of human milk varies with the stage of lactation, the time of day, the time during the feeding, maternal nutrition, and gestational age of the newborn at birth. During the establishment of lactation there are three stages of human milk: colostrum, transitional milk, and mature milk.

Colostrum is a yellowish or creamy-appearing fluid that is thicker than later milk and contains more protein, fat-soluble vitamins, and minerals (American College of Obstetricians and Gynecologists [ACOG], 2000). It also contains high levels of immunoglobulins (antibodies, such as IgA) and can be a source of passive immunity for the newborn. Colostrum production begins early in pregnancy and may last for several days after birth. However, in most cases colostrum is replaced by transitional milk within 2 to 4 days after birth.

Transitional milk is produced from the end of colostrum production until approximately 2 weeks postpartum. This milk contains more fat, lactose, water-soluble vitamins, and calories than colostrum.

The final milk produced, **mature milk,** contains about 10% solids (carbohydrates, proteins, fats) for energy and growth; the rest is water, which is vital for maintaining hydration. The composition of mature milk varies according to the time during the feeding. **Foremilk** is the milk obtained at the beginning of the feeding. It is high in water content and contains vitamins and protein. **Hindmilk** is released after the initial let-down, or release of milk, and has higher fat concentration.

Although mature milk appears similar to skim milk (watery and somewhat bluish in color) and may cause mothers to question whether their milk is "rich enough," mature breast milk provides 20 kcal/oz, as do most prepared formulas. However, the percentage of calories derived from protein is lower in breast milk than in formulas, and a greater proportion of calories is derived from fat. In breastfed babies, protein metabolism produces less nitrogen waste, which has a positive effect on the infant's immature renal system.

ACOG (2000) recommends breast milk as the optimal food for the first 6 to 12 months of life. It is believed that breastfeeding provides newborns and infants with specific immunologic, nutritional, and psychosocial advantages.

IMMUNOLOGIC ADVANTAGES

Immunologic advantages include varying degrees of protection from respiratory and gastrointestinal infections, otitis media, meningitis, sepsis, and allergies (ACOG, 2000). This protection provides coverage for the breastfed baby during the neonatal period until the baby's own immunoglobulins become active by 18 months of age.

Secretory IgA, an immunoglobulin present in colostrum and breast milk, has antiviral, antibacterial, and antigenic-inhibiting properties. Secretory IgA plays a role in decreasing the permeability of the small intestine to antigenic macromolecules. Other properties in colostrum and breast milk that act to inhibit the growth of bacteria or viruses are *Lactobacillus bifidus*, lysozymes, lactoperoxidase, lactoferrin, transferrin, and various immunoglobulins (Biancuzzo, 2003). Immunoglobulins to the poliomyelitis virus are also present in the breast milk of mothers who have immunity to this virus. Because the presence of these immunoglobulins may inhibit the desired intestinal infection and immune response of the infant, some clinics suggest that breastfeedings be withheld for 30 to 60 minutes following the administration of the Sabin oral polio vaccine. In addition to its immunologic properties, breast milk is known to be nonallergenic.

NUTRITIONAL ADVANTAGES

Breast milk is composed of lactose, lipids, polyunsaturated fatty acids, and amino acids, especially taurine, and has a whey:casein protein ratio that facilitates its digestion, absorption, and full use compared to formulas (Biancuzzo, 2003). Some researchers believe that the high concentration of cholesterol and the balance of amino acids in breast milk make it the best food for myelination and neurologic development. High cholesterol levels in breast milk may stimulate the production of enzymes that lead to more efficient metabolism of cholesterol, thereby reducing its harmful long-term effects on the cardiovascular system (Biancuzzo, 2003).

Breast milk is also considered the ideal first food because its composition varies according to gestational age and stage of lactation. For example, the milk of a preterm mother has more long-chain polyunsaturated fatty acids (LC-PUFA) than the milk of a full-term mother. LC-PUFA is essential for brain growth (Blackburn, 2003), and preterm infants are born with very low LC-PUFA reserves.

Breast milk provides newborns with minerals in more appropriate doses than do formulas (Blackburn, 2003). The iron found in breast milk, even though much lower in concentration than that of prepared formulas, is much more readily and fully absorbed and appears sufficient to meet the infant's iron needs for the first 6 months. The American Academy of Pediatrics (AAP) and ACOG (2002) state that breastfed newborns generally do not need supplemental iron before the age of 6 months. Furthermore, supplemental iron may decrease the ability of breast milk to protect the newborn by interfering with lactoferrin, an iron-binding protein that enhances the absorption of iron and has anti-infective properties.

Another advantage of breast milk is that all its components are delivered to the infant in an unchanged form, and vitamins are not lost through processing and heating. Vitamin D supplements may not necessary for the exclusively breastfed infant if the mother is taking daily multivitamins, her diet is adequate, and the baby is exposed to sunlight for 30 minutes a week if wearing only a diaper or 2 hours a week if fully clothed (Shinskie & Lauwers 2002). If the mother's diet or vitamin intake is inadequate or questionable, caregivers may choose to prescribe additional vitamins for the infant.

PSYCHOSOCIAL ADVANTAGES

The psychosocial advantages of breastfeeding are primarily those associated with maternal-infant attachment. The mother's level of oxytocin generally increases with breastfeeding, and studies indicate that this hormonal change coincides with more even mood responses and increased feelings of maternal well-being.

Breastfeeding enhances attachment by providing the opportunity for frequent, direct skin contact between the newborn and the mother. The newborn's sense of touch is highly developed at birth and is a primary means of communication. The tactile stimulation associated with breastfeeding can communicate warmth, closeness, and comfort. The increased closeness provides both newborn and mother with the opportunity to learn each other's behavioral cues and needs. The mother's sense of accomplishment in being able to satisfy her baby's needs for nourishment and comfort is enhanced when the newborn suckles vigorously and is satiated and calmed by the breastfeeding. Some mothers prefer breastfeeding as a means of extending the close, unique, nourishing relationship between mother and baby that existed prior to birth.

In the event of a twin birth, breastfeeding not only is possible but also enhances the mother's individualization and attachment to each newborn. The fantasized single baby is replaced more readily with the reality of two individual babies when the mother has close and frequent contact with each. Fathers can also be actively involved with the feeding experience by offering fresh pumped or thawed (frozen) breast milk to the baby at one or more feedings daily.

CONTRAINDICATIONS AND DISADVANTAGES

There are some medical contraindications to breastfeeding. A mother with a diagnosis of breast cancer should not breastfeed so that she may begin treatment immediately. Women with HIV or AIDS are counseled against breastfeeding except in countries where the risk of neonatal death from diarrhea and other disease (excluding AIDS) is high (Jackson, Chopra, Witten, & Sengwana, 2003).

Maternal medications may preclude breastfeeding, as discussed in Chapters 19 and 32. Medications such as metronidazole (Flagyl) used to treat trichomoniasis pass into breast milk and may be harmful to the breastfeeding infant. Management of jaundice in the newborn may include suspension of breastfeeding (see Chapter 33).

In the dominant Western culture, where women actively pursue activities outside the home, being "tied down" to an infant for 9 to 12 feedings every day may be considered inconvenient and stressful. Another often cited disadvantage of breastfeeding is exclusion of the father from the nurturing involved in feeding the infant. But because nurturing encompasses more than just feeding, the father can comfort and attend to the baby in many other ways (Figure 31–1 •).

Opinion varies as to the advisability of continuing breastfeeding in the event of another pregnancy. Some feel the nutritional demands on the pregnant mother are too great and advocate gradual weaning. Others suggest that with adequate rest, a proper diet, and strong emotional support, continued breastfeeding during pregnancy is a valid choice. The practice of breastfeeding one infant throughout pregnancy and then breastfeeding both infants after birth is called *tandem nursing*. When pregnancy occurs, the decision of how to handle breastfeeding is best made on an individual basis after considering maternal health and motivation and the age of the first child.

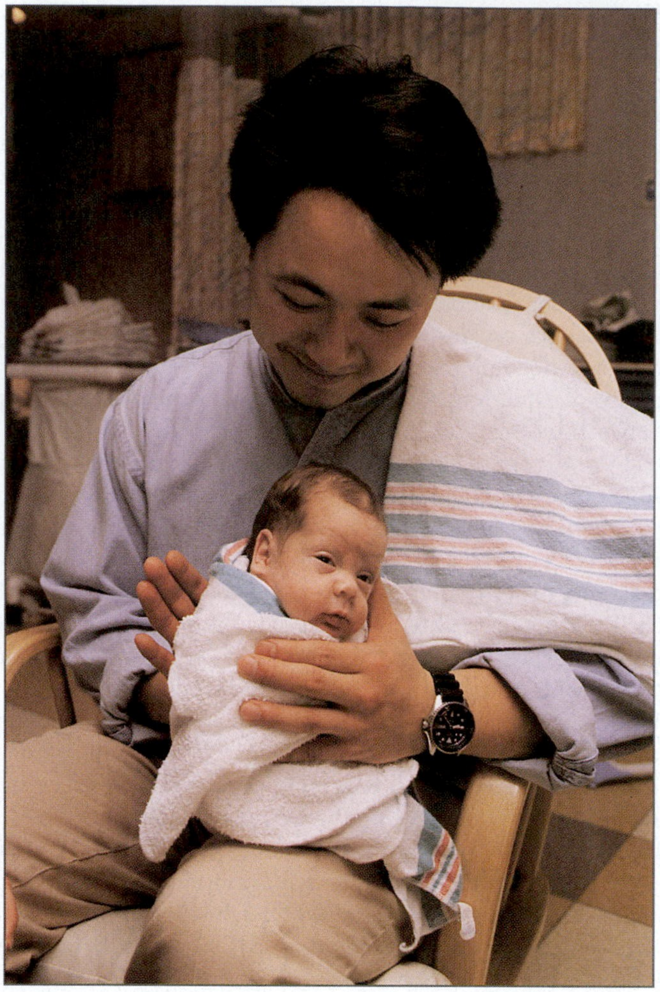

Figure 31–1 • A father can nurture his baby in many ways.

Even though many mothers obtain information about breastfeeding from written sources, family and friends, and the **La Leche League** (an international breastfeeding support and information group), the nurse needs to be a ready source of information, encouragement, and support, as well. The nurse can be helpful when parents are deciding whether to breastfeed, after birth when breastfeedings are just being established, and after the family returns home.

Formula-Feeding

Although breastfeeding is increasing in popularity, formula-feeding continues to be a viable and nurturing choice, particularly in developed countries, and meets the goal of successful growth of the baby. The closeness and warmth that can occur during breastfeeding is also an integral part of formula-feeding. An advantage of formula-feeding is that parents can share equally in this nurturing, caring experience with their baby.

TYPES OF INFANT FORMULAS

Numerous types of commercially prepared formulas meet the nutritional needs of the infant. There are three categories: formulas based on cow's milk protein, soy protein-based formulas, and specialized or therapeutic formulas.

Commercial formulas using a cow's milk base tend to have a higher renal solute load, high protein and casein content, high proportion of saturated fats, low amounts of linoleic acid, poorer mineral bioavailability, and increased risk for allergy to cow's milk proteins (Walker & Creehan, 2001). Some companies have developed cow's milk-based formulas that minimize these harmful components. The formulas have been enriched with tyrosine, phenylalanine, carnitine, and/or taurine; some of them with LC-PUFA; and all of them with vitamins, particularly vitamin D .

Soy protein-based formulas (eg, Isomil, Prosobee, Gerber Soy) substitute soy protein supplemented with methionine for cow's milk protein and are used for infants with primary lactase deficiency or galactosemia, as well as infants of formula-feeding vegan parents. Soy-based infant formulas should not be confused with soy milk, which is not appropriate for infant formula.

The specialized formulas are categorized as casein-hydrolysated or whey-hydrolysated formulas. The AAP recommends casein-hydrolysated formulas (eg, Nutramigen, Pregestimil, Alimentum) for infants with allergy or intolerance to cow's milk protein to avoid risk of concomitant allergy to soy protein (AAP Committee on Nutrition, 2000). Casein-hydrolysate is essentially a "predigested" protein that presents protein fragments too small to be recognized by the infant's immune system as an antigen, thereby decreasing the baby's allergic response. Whey-hydrolysated formulas, such as Carnation Good Start, can also be used with cow's milk allergy but not if the child has an IgE-mediated allergy to cow's milk.

POTENTIAL CONTRAINDICATIONS AND DISADVANTAGES

If formula is prepared with too much powder, the excess salts (ie, sodium) may be detrimental to the newborn's immature kidneys and may lead to thirst, causing overfeeding. If formula is overdiluted, the infant will not receive adequate nutrients.

As discussed earlier, another potential problem with many formulas is an allergic reaction in the newborn. The small intestine of the infant is permeable to macromolecules such as those found in some cow's milk-based and soy-based formulas. The introduction of these foreign proteins in formula may cause an allergic reaction, with signs such as vomiting, colic, diarrhea, colitis, reluctance to feed, and eczema.

Clinicians recommend that parents who are formula-feeding use iron-fortified formulas or supplements because iron deficiency anemia still occurs (AAP & ACOG, 2002). However, parents must be aware that too much iron, such as may be consumed when the infant is started on iron-fortified cereal, may interfere with the infant's natural ability to defend against disease. Parents also need to be informed about the constipation that sometimes results from iron-enriched formulas and about various methods of alleviating it. Many companies make enriched formulas that are similar to breast milk. These formulas have sufficient levels of carbohydrate, protein, fat, vitamins, and minerals to meet the newborn's nutritional needs.

Table 31–1 • COMPARISON OF BREASTFEEDING AND FORMULA-FEEDING

Breast	Bottle (Iron-Enriched Formula)
Nutrition	
Breast milk is species specific (ie, perfect balance of proteins, carbohydrates, fats, vitamins, and minerals for human infants).	Formula is as close to human milk as possible, but nutrients are not as efficiently utilized.
Breast milk contains higher levels of lactose, cystine, and cholesterol, which are necessary for brain and nerve growth.	Nutritional adequacy depends on proper preparation (overdilution results in decreased nutrients delivered to infant).
Proteins are easily digested and fats are well absorbed.	Some babies cannot tolerate the fats or carbohydrates found in regular formula. Companies offer alternative formulas.
Composition varies according to gestational age and stage of lactation, thereby meeting the changing nutritional requirements of individual infants as they grow.	
Infants determine the volume of milk consumed.	Pediatrician or caregiver determines the volume consumed. Overfeeding may occur if caregiver is determined that baby empty bottle.
Frequency of feeding is determined by infant cues.	Feeding is determined by infant's cues.
Anti-Infective and Antiallergic Properties	
Breast milk contains immunoglobulins, enzymes, and leukocytes that protect against pathogens.	Formula is linked to an increased number of gastrointestinal and respiratory infections.
Bacteriostatic properties permit storage at room temperature up to 6 hours, in refrigerator for 24 hours, and freezing for 6 months.	Potential for bacterial contamination exists during preparation and storage.
Breast milk decreases the incidence of allergy by eliminating exposure to potential antigens (cow and soy protein).	Some babies are allergic to cow or soy protein. Formula companies are offering alternative formulas suitable for babies who develop allergies.
Psychosocial Aspects	
Skin-to-skin contact enhances closeness.	Bottle-feeding provides an opportunity for positive parent-infant interaction.
Hormones of lactation promote maternal feelings and sense of well-being.	
The value system of an industrial society can create barriers to successful breastfeeding: Mother may feel ashamed or embarrassed. Breastfeeding after return to work may be difficult.	
Father is not able to breastfeed, but he can feed expressed breast milk from a bottle and nurture the infant in ways other than feeding.	Father can feed the baby.
Cost	
Healthy diet for mother.	Formula is an expense.
Optional, but recommended, items include nursing pads, nursing bras.	Bottles or disposable nursers with plastic liners, nipples, and nipple caps must be purchased.
A breast pump may be needed.	
Refrigeration is necessary for storing expressed milk.	
Convenience	
The milk is always the perfect temperature.	A refrigeration system is necessary if mixing formula for more than one feeding at a time or using large containers of ready-to-feed formula.
No preparation time is needed.	Varying amounts of time are involved in formula preparation.
The mother must be available to feed or provide expressed milk to be given in her absence.	Anyone can feed the baby.
If she misses a feeding, the mother must express milk to maintain lactation.	
The mother may experience slight discomfort in the early days of lactation.	
Maternal medication may interrupt breastfeeding.	

The AAP and ACOG (2002) have recommended that infants be given breast milk or iron-fortified formula rather than whole milk until 1 year of age. Neither whole milk nor skim milk is an acceptable alternative for infant feeding. The levels of protein in cow's milk are much higher (50% to 75% greater) than in human milk. It is poorly digested and may cause bleeding of the gastrointestinal tract. Cow's milk also has higher levels of calcium, phosphorus, sodium, and potassium, which increase the renal solute load and result in greater obligatory water loss. Skim milk lacks adequate calories, fat content, and essential fatty acids necessary for proper development of the newborn's neurologic system. Nutritionists also advise against giving low-fat milk (2% or 1% milk) or skim milk to children under 2 years of age.

Table 31–1 • compares several factors for parents to consider when choosing between breastfeeding and formula-feeding.

Timing of Newborn Feedings

The timing of newborn feedings is determined by physiologic and behavioral cues rather than a set schedule.

Initial Feeding

After birth, the nurse assesses for active bowel sounds, absence of abdominal distention, and a lusty cry that quiets and is replaced with rooting and sucking behaviors when a stimulus is placed near the lips. These signs indicate that the newborn is hungry and physically ready to tolerate the initial feeding. Contraindications to immediate breastfeeding include heavy sedation of the mother and physical compromise of either mother or baby.

Because colostrum is not irritating if aspirated (which may occur because of the newborn's initially uncoordinated sucking and swallowing abilities) and is readily absorbed by the respiratory system, breastfeeding can usually begin immediately after birth. The mother who plans to breastfeed should therefore be encouraged to feed her newborn immediately, allowing the baby to breastfeed to satiety. Early feedings benefit the breastfeeding pair because oxytocin helps expel the placenta and prevent excessive maternal blood loss, lactation is accelerated, and the infant receives the immunologic protection of colostrum.

Throughout the first 2 hours after birth, but especially during the first 20 to 30 minutes, the infant is usually alert and ready to breastfeed. However, newborn suckling patterns vary, and although many babies are eager to suckle at this time, many will simply lick or nuzzle the nipple. This behavior is beneficial because the licking stimulates the release of oxytocin, which aids uterine involution and lactation (let-down). The mother should be encouraged to interpret this as a positive breastfeeding interaction (Biancuzzo, 2003). Within minutes after birth the newborn shows early odor-based recognition of the mother's breasts. Maternal breast odors elicit preferential head orientation, which helps guide the newborn to the nipple.

Formula-feeding newborns are offered the bottle as soon as they show an interest. For both breastfed and formula-fed infants, early feedings stimulate peristalsis, facilitating elimination of the by-products of bilirubin conjugation, which decreases the risk of jaundice and enhances maternal-infant attachment.

The first feeding provides an opportunity for the nurse to assess the effectiveness of the newborn's suck, swallow, and gag reflexes. In addition, assessment of the newborn's physiologic status is of primary and ongoing concern to the nurse throughout the first feeding. Extreme fatigue coupled with rapid respiration, circumoral cyanosis, and diaphoresis of the head and face may indicate cardiovascular complications and should be assessed further. The initial feeding also requires assessment of the infant for rare congenital anomalies such as tracheoesophageal fistula and esophageal atresia (Chapter 32). Findings associated with esophageal anomalies include maternal polyhydramnios and increased oral mucus in the infant. In cases of esophageal atresia, the feeding is taken well initially, but as the esophageal pouch fills, the feeding is quickly regurgitated unchanged by stomach contents. If a fistula is present, the infant gags, chokes, regurgitates mucus, and may become cyanotic as fluid passes through the fistula into the lungs.

It is not unusual for the newborn to regurgitate some mucus, water, or colostrum following a feeding, even if it was taken without difficulty. Consequently, the newborn is observed closely and positioned on the right side after a feeding to aid drainage and facilitate gastric emptying.

Establishing a Feeding Pattern

An "on demand" feeding program facilitates each baby's own rhythm and assists a new mother in establishing lactation. The newborn rapidly digests breast milk and may desire to feed eight to ten times in a 24-hour period. After the initial period of alertness and eagerness to suckle, the infant progresses to light sleep, then deep sleep, followed by increased wakefulness and interest in breastfeeding. As wakefulness and interest increase, the infant will often cluster five to ten feeding episodes over 2 to 3 hours, followed by a 4- to 5-hour deep sleep. After this cluster of minifeeds and deep sleep, the infant will feed frequently, but at more regular intervals. Maternal medications received during labor may affect newborn feeding behavior by delaying these early cluster feedings. Delays in normal feeding patterns depend on the specific drug and its half-life. Newborns whose mothers received epidural analgesia have been noted to be irritable and demonstrate reduced motor organization, poor self-quieting skills, and decreased visual skills and alertness (Biancuzzo, 2003).

Couplet care permits the mother to learn about and respond to her infant's early feeding cues. Early cues that indicate a newborn is interested in feeding include hand-to-mouth or hand-passing-mouth motion, whimpering, sucking, and rooting (Mulford, 1992). Crying is typically a late sign of hunger. Satiety behaviors can include withdrawal of head from nipple, falling asleep, relaxation of hands, and relief of body tension. When couplet care is not available, a supportive nursing staff and flexible nursery policies allow the mother to feed her infant on cue. It is very frustrating to a new mother to attempt to feed a newborn who is sound asleep because he or she is either not hungry or exhausted from crying.

Although people often accept crying as normal and healthy behavior for newborns, it may actually delay the transition to extrauterine life. Crying involves a Valsalva maneuver that results in increased pulmonary vascular pressure, which may cause unoxygenated blood to be shunted into systemic circulation through the foramen ovale and ductus arteriosus. Therefore, it may be advantageous for the baby to be in the room with the mother because she will respond to the baby's needs more quickly than the nursery staff may be able to, resulting in less newborn crying.

Formula-fed newborns may awaken for feedings every 2 to 5 hours but are frequently satisfied with feedings every 3 to 4 hours. Because formula is digested more slowly, the formula-fed infant may go longer between feedings but should not go longer than 4 hours. Babies may begin skipping the night feeding at about 8 to 12 weeks of age (Riordan & Auerbach,

Global Perspectives

In Malaysia, the ingestion of breast milk represents a great deal more than simple nutrition for newborn infants. It is believed that the mother's milk enters the baby's blood. This is thought to cultivate a long life. Breast milk is thought to bind the mother and baby together, creating a sense of respect and closeness. While milk develops the infant's spirit and body, it also develops faith and character. It is thought that the consumption of breast milk formulates a maternal-infant bond that lasts throughout life. This bond cannot be broken by any means. Breastfeeding mothers drink "jamu" (a drink consisting of egg yolk, palm sugar, tamarind, and herbs) to ensure an adequate milk supply.

1999). The need for a night feeding is very individual, depending on the infant's size and development.

Both breastfed and formula-fed infants experience growth spurts at certain times and require increased feeding. The mother of a breastfed infant will meet these increased demands by breastfeeding more frequently to increase her milk supply. It will take about 72 hours for the milk supply to increase adequately to meet the new demand (Biancuzzo, 2003). A slight increase in the amount of formula given at each feeding will meet the needs of the formula-fed infant.

Providing nourishment for her newborn is a major concern for the new mother. Her feelings of success or failure may influence her self-concept as she assumes her maternal role. With proper instruction, support, and encouragement from healthcare providers, feeding becomes a source of pleasure and satisfaction to both parents and infant.

Community-Based Nursing Care

Promotion of Successful Infant Feeding

Parents may see the task of feeding their baby as the center of their relationship with the new family member. Whether the mother has chosen to breastfeed or use formula, the nurse can help the mother have a successful experience while in the birthing center and during the early days at home. Feeding and caring for newborns may be routine tasks for the nurse, but the success or lack of success that a mother achieves the first few times may determine her feelings about herself as an adequate mother.

The newborn's response to caring is an expression of personality but often has great significance for parents. A parent may interpret the newborn's behavior as rejection, which may alter the parent-child relationship. Parents may also interpret the sleepy infant's refusal to suck or inability to retain formula as evidence of their incompetence as parents. The breastfeeding mother may deduce that the newborn does not like her if the baby fails to take her nipple readily. Conversely, infants pick up messages from the muscular tension of those holding them.

A nurse who is sensitive to the needs of the mother can form a relationship with her that permits sharing of knowledge about techniques and emotions connected with feeding. Breastfeeding women frequently express disappointment in the help given to them by birthing unit or hospital nurses, saying they would like more encouragement, support, and practical information about feeding their newborns, especially in the case of early discharge. This need also applies to nonbreastfeeding mothers. Consistency in teaching by nursing personnel is paramount. A new mother becomes very frustrated if she is shown a number of different methods of feeding her newborn. With the technologic advances in formula production and the availability of knowledge about breastfeeding techniques, the mother should be confident that the choice she makes will promote normal growth and development of her newborn.

The decision by the mother about whether or not to breastfeed is usually made by the sixth month of pregnancy and often even before conception. The final decision, however, may not be made until the mother's admission to the birth center. The decision is frequently influenced by relatives, especially the baby's father and maternal grandmother (Chezem, Friesen & Boettcher, 2003), and by friends and social customs, rather than being based on knowledge about the nutritional and psychologic needs of herself and her newborn.

The goals of Healthy People 2010 continue to be that 75% of infants breastfeed at birth and 50% continue to consume at least some human milk until 6 months (Davis, Okuboye, & Ferguson, 2000). It is the healthcare provider's responsibility to provide the parents with accurate information regarding the distinct advantages of breastfeeding to the mother and infant. In times of short stays, the Baby Friendly Hospital Initiative program promotes breastfeeding by designating hospitals as centers for breastfeeding education. Unfortunately, only a few hospitals in the United States have implemented the program (Davis et al, 2000). Parents have a right to hear about the data so they can make an informed choice.

ACOG (2000) supports the following "Ten Hospital Practices to Encourage and Support Breastfeeding" that can increase rates of successful breastfeeding:

- Maintain a written breastfeeding policy that is communicated to all healthcare staff.
- Train all pertinent healthcare staff in skills necessary to implement this policy.
- Inform all pregnant women about the benefits of breastfeeding.
- Offer all mothers the opportunity to initiate breastfeeding within 1 hour of birth.
- Show breastfeeding mothers how to breastfeed and how to maintain lactation even if they are separated from their infants.
- Give breastfeeding infants only breastmilk unless medically indicated.

Evidence-Based Practice

Assisting a New Mother to Establish and Maintain Breastfeeding

Clinical Question

What practices assist a new mother with a healthy term infant to establish and maintain breastfeeding during the first 14 days?

The Evidence

Clinical experts from the International Lactation Consultant Association developed these evidence-based clinical practice guidelines. Evidence to support the guidelines was gathered from research when available and augmented with clinical experience and logical deductions from known scientific facts. The recommendations are supported with evidence ranging from original research to works based on years of clinical experience from a panel of multidisciplinary healthcare providers. Specific references for each intervention are provided in the guideline document.

Best Practice

Twenty-four recommendations are included in this guideline. These include recommendations to:

- Encourage unrestricted breastfeeding 8 to 12 times per 24 hours.
- Provide necessary breastfeeding assistance and monitor closely.
- Encourage parents to avoid the use of pacifiers, artificial nipples, and supplements unless medically indicated, until breastfeeding is well established (4 to 6 weeks).
- Confirm that parents know the signs of ineffective breastfeeding, effective breastfeeding, risk factors that can affect the infant's ability to breastfeed effectively, and common maternal health problems related to breastfeeding.
- Include family members or significant others in breastfeeding education.
- Help parents establish realistic expectations regarding feedings, infant output, and infant weight gain.

For a full list of the recommendations, as well as specific management strategies and references for each, consult the source document.

Reference: International Lactation Consultant Association. (1999). *Evidence-based guidelines for breastfeeding management during the first fourteen days.* Raleigh, NC: Author.

- Facilitate rooming-in; encourage all mothers and infants to remain together during their hospital stay.
- Encourage unrestricted breastfeeding when baby exhibits hunger cues or signals or on request of mother.
- Encourage exclusive suckling at the breast by providing no pacifiers or artificial nipples.
- Refer mothers to established breastfeeding and mother's support groups and services, and foster the establishment of those services when they are not available.

Once an *informed choice* has been made, the nurse's primary responsibility is to support the family's decision and to help the family achieve a positive result. No woman should be made to feel inadequate or superior because of her choice in feeding. There are advantages and disadvantages to breastfeeding and formula-feeding, but positive bonds in parent-child relationships may be developed with either method.

Before feeding, the mother should be made as comfortable as possible. Preparations may include voiding, washing her hands, and assuming a position of comfort. See Figure 31–2 • for a variety of breastfeeding positions.

The woman who has had a cesarean birth needs support so that the newborn does not rest on her abdomen for long periods of time. When she is breastfeeding, she may be more comfortable lying on her side with a pillow behind her back and one between her legs. The nurse can position the newborn next to the woman's breast and place a rolled towel or small pillow behind the infant for support. Initially the mother will need assistance turning from side to side and burping the newborn. She may prefer to breastfeed sitting up with a pillow on her lap and the infant resting on the pillow rather than directly on her abdomen. It may be helpful to place a rolled pillow under the arm supporting the infant's head. An alternative position that avoids pressure on the incision while allowing for maximum visualization of the infant's face is the football hold. Mothers who have undergone cesarean birth frequently use the sitting position to bottle-feed. If incisional pain makes this position difficult, the bottle-feeding mother may also find it helpful to assume the side-lying position. The infant can be positioned in a semi-sitting position against a pillow close to the mother.

Clinical Tip *As you assist new mothers with breastfeeding, it is important to create a relaxed environment and approach to breastfeeding. Encourage mom to get into a comfortable position, well supported with pillows. Remind her to bring the baby to her breast rather than leaning forward to the baby.*

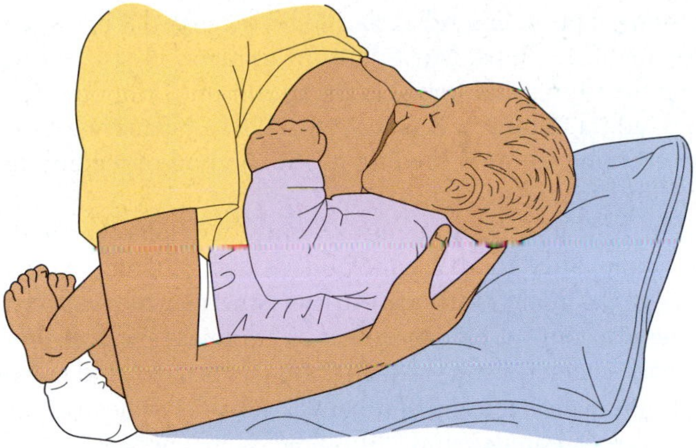

A Football hold

- Hold the baby's back and shoulders in the palm of your hand.
- Tuck the baby up under your arm, lining up the baby's lips with your nipple.
- Support the breast to guide it into the baby's mouth.
- Hold your breast until the baby nurses easily.

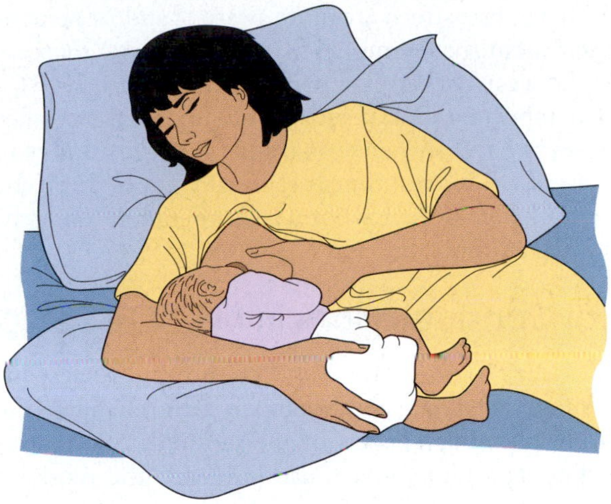

B Lying down

- Lie on your side with a pillow at your back and lay the baby so you are facing each other.
- To start, prop yourself up on your elbow and support your breast with the opposite hand.
- Pull the baby close to you, lining up the baby's mouth with your nipple.
- Lie back down once the baby is nursing well.

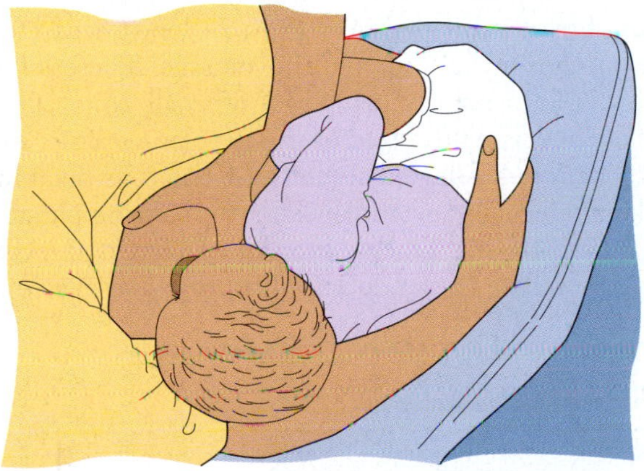

C Cradling

- Cradle the baby in the arm closest to the breast, with the baby's head in the crook of the arm.
- Have the baby's body facing you, tummy-to-tummy.
- Use your opposite hand to support the breast.

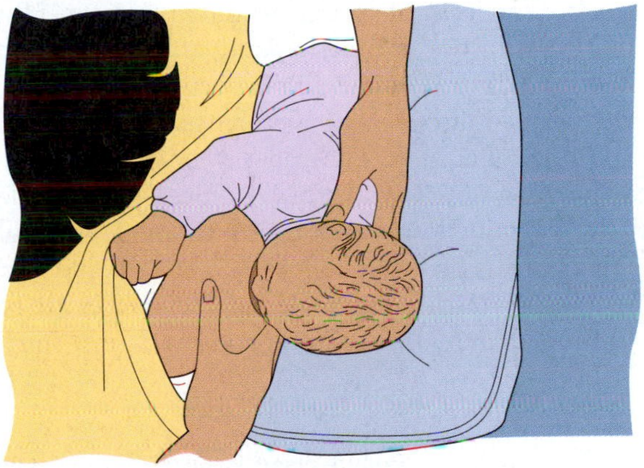

D Across the lap

- Lay your baby on pillows across your lap.
- Turn the baby facing you.
- Reach across your lap to support the baby's back and shoulders with the palm of your hand.
- Support your breast from underneath to guide it into the baby's mouth.

Figure 31–2 • Four common breastfeeding positions. *A,* Football hold. *B,* Lying down. *C,* Cradling. *D,* Across the lap.
SOURCE: *Breastfeeding: A special relationship.* Breastfeeding Education Resources. 1-800-869-7892, Raleigh, NC. Copyright Lactation Consultants of NC.

Depending on the newborn's level of hunger, the parents may want to use the time before feeding to get acquainted with their infant. The presence of the nurse during part of this time to answer questions and provide reinforcement of parenting skills will be helpful for the family. For the sleepy baby, a period of playful activity—such as gently rubbing the feet and hands or adjusting clothing and loosening coverings to expose the infant to room air—may increase alertness so that, when the feeding is initiated, the infant is ready and sucks eagerly. If an infant is overly hungry and upset, talking quietly and rocking gently may provide the baby with an opportunity to calm down so that he or she can find and grasp the nipple effectively. After the feeding, when the infant is satisfied and asleep, parents may explore the characteristics unique to their newborn. Routines must be flexible enough to allow this time for the family. Couplet care offers spontaneous, frequent encounters for the family and provides opportunities to practice handling skills, thereby increasing confidence in care after discharge. It also encourages feeding in response to cues from the baby, rather than feeding by a fixed schedule. Women who continue to breastfeed are more aware of and/or responsive to their infant's cues and state (eg, quiet alert) than are mothers who wean earlier than planned (Biancuzzo, 2003).

It is also important to understand and support the mother who chooses to have her newborn cared for in the nursery so that she can rest. This rest time is especially important if she must care for herself, the newborn, and other children without adult help at home.

Cultural Considerations in Infant Feeding

The nurse needs to understand how culture and society influence infant feeding. Motherhood itself changes the woman's lifestyle. Perceptions of the mother's role and of breastfeeding as a biologic act also influence the mother's comfort with breastfeeding. In one study, some mothers identified shame, modesty, and embarrassment as reasons they chose not to breastfeed. The amount of body contact considered acceptable also influences parental behaviors (Figure 31–3 •). North American and European societies sometimes consider it indecent to expose the breast, believe that too much handling spoils children, and regard weaning as a sign of infant development (Biancuzzo, 2003).

The nurse also needs to understand the impact of the culture on the idiosyncrasies of specific feeding practices. How soon women want to began breastfeeding after birth is culturally determined. For example, in many cultures (Mexican American, Navajo, Filipino, and Vietnamese) and in some countries (Guinea, Pakistan, Bangladesh), colostrum is not offered to the newborn (Geissler, 1998). Breastfeeding begins only after the milk flow is established. In some Asian cultures, the newborn is given boiled water until the mother's milk flows. The newborn is fed on demand, and cries are responded to immediately. If the crying continues, evil spirits may be blamed, and a priest's blessing may be sought. Although many of the Hmong women of Laos combine breastfeeding with some formula-feeding, they find expressing their milk or pumping their breasts unacceptable. Thus other methods of providing relief should be suggested if breast engorgement develops. Most Muslim mothers breastfeed because the Qur'an (Koran) encourages it until the child is 2 years old (Hutchinson & Baqi-Aziz, 1994). Japanese women are returning to breastfeeding as the method of feeding for the baby's first year.

The African American culture tends to emphasize plentiful feeding. Solid foods are introduced early and may even be added to the infant's formula. African American mothers view frequent feeding as an expression of hardiness and a positive behavior characteristic for the future (Biancuzzo, 2003). For the traditional Mexican, a fat baby is considered healthy and infants are fed on demand. "Spoiling" is encouraged.

These are but a few of the cultural practices related to feeding. When faced with an infant care practice different from the ones to which they are accustomed, nurses need to evaluate the effect of the practice. Different practices are not necessarily inferior. The nurse should intervene only if the practice is actually harmful to the mother or baby.

Physiology of the Breasts and Lactation

The female breast is divided into 15 to 24 lobes, separated from one another by fat and connective tissue. These lobes are subdivided into lobules composed of small units called alveoli where milk is synthesized by the alveolar secretory epithelium. The lobules have a system of lactiferous ductules that join larger ducts and eventually open onto the nipple surface (see Figure 10–16). During pregnancy, increased levels of estrogen stimulate breast duct proliferation and develop-

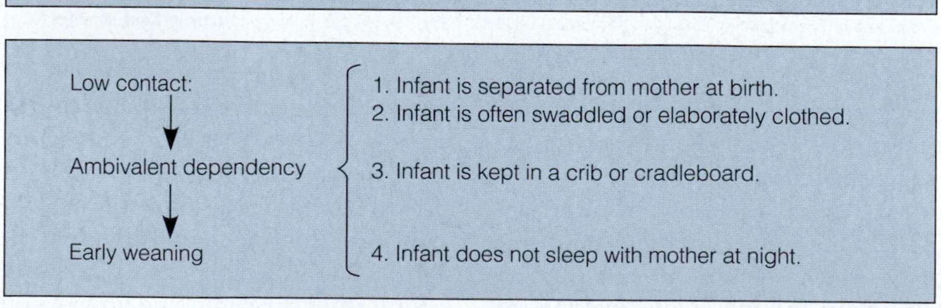

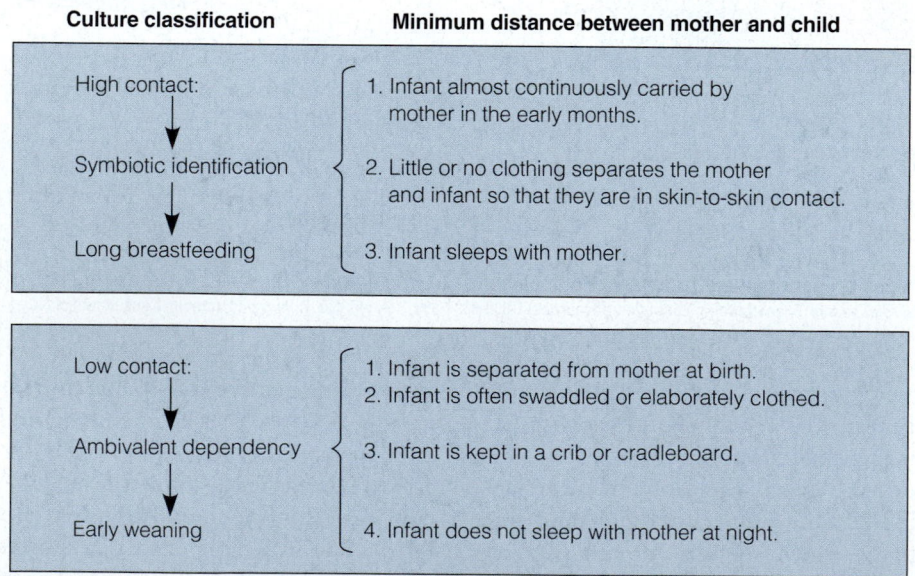

Figure 31–3 • Culturally determined mother-child body interaction and implications for breastfeeding practices. The amount of contact and degree of closeness between mother and infant is often culturally determined and may influence how long the mother will breastfeed.
SOURCE: Lawrence, R. A. (1994). *Breastfeeding: A guide for the medical profession* (4th ed., p. 185). St Louis, MO: Mosby.

ment, and elevated progesterone levels promote the development of lobules and alveoli in preparation for lactation.

Birth results in a rapid drop in estrogen and progesterone with a concomitant increase in the secretion of **prolactin.** This hormone promotes milk production by stimulating the alveolar cells of the breasts. Prolactin levels rise in response to the infant suckling. The newborn's suckling also stimulates the release of **oxytocin** from the pituitary gland. This hormone increases the contractility of the myoepithelial cells lining the walls of the mammary ducts, and a flow of milk results. This is called the **let-down reflex,** or milk ejection. Mothers have described the let-down reflex as a prickling or tingling sensation during which they feel the milk coming down. Other signs of let-down include increased uterine cramps and increased lochia (during the early postpartum period), milk leaking from the other breast, and a feeling of relaxation. It is not unusual for the breasts to leak some milk prior to feeding.

The let-down reflex can be stimulated by the newborn's suckling, presence, or cry, or even by maternal thoughts about her baby. It may also occur during sexual orgasm because oxytocin is released. Conversely, the mother's lack of self-confidence or fear of, embarrassment about, or pain connected with breastfeeding may prevent the milk from being ejected into the duct system.

Milk production is decreased with repeated inhibition of the milk ejection reflex. Failure to empty the breasts frequently and completely also decreases production because as milk accumulates and is not withdrawn, the buildup of pressure in the alveoli suppresses secretion. Once lactation is well established, prolactin production decreases. Oxytocin and suckling continue to be the facilitators of milk production.

Client Education for Breastfeeding

The nurse caring for the breastfeeding mother should help the woman achieve independence and success in her feeding efforts (Figure 31–4 •). Prepared with a knowledge of the anatomy and physiology of the breast and lactation, the components and positive effects of breast milk, and the techniques of breastfeeding, the nurse can help the woman and her family use their own resources to achieve a successful experience. Table 31–2 • summarizes information about breastfeeding.

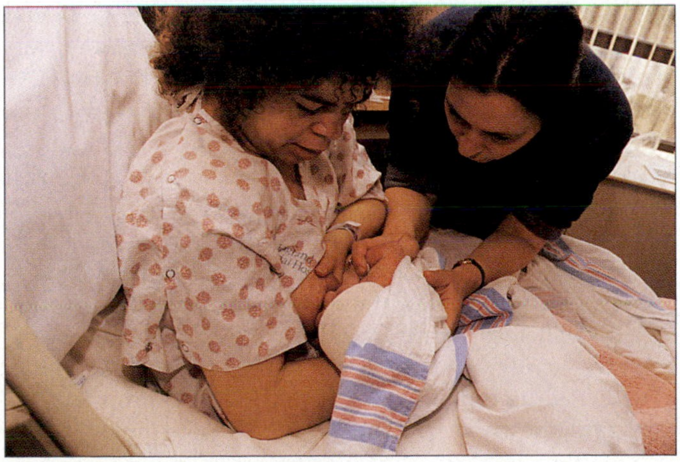

Figure 31–4 • For many mothers, the nurse's support and knowledge are instrumental in establishing successful breastfeeding.

Table 31–2 • INFORMATION HELPFUL TO BREASTFEEDING MOTHERS

Basics of Milk Production
Milk is produced according to demand.
Milk is stored in sinuses under areola.
Adequate maternal fluid intake is required.
Milk supply is established by frequent breastfeeding (every 1 1/2 to 3 hours).
Let-down reflex: Flow of milk is initiated by newborn's sucking, presence, or cry; by mother's thoughts; or during maternal orgasm.
Positioning Baby at the Breast
Turn baby's entire body toward mother with mouth adjacent to nipple and the ear; shoulder and hip are in direct alignment.
Mother should assume a comfortable position with arms supported.
Direct nipple straight into baby's mouth so that during sucking, jaw compresses ducts directly beneath areola.
Lightly brush infant's mouth with breast to stimulate rooting reflex (but avoid touching both cheeks).
Procedure for Feeding
Avoid arbitrary time limits (since let-down reflex may take up to 3 minutes).
Allow baby to nurse at first breast until breast is emptied.
Insert finger in baby's mouth near nipple to break suction.
Burp baby before changing breast.
Burp baby again at end of feeding.
To prevent skin breakdown, wash nipple with warm water and dry thoroughly.
Helpful Hints
Be certain baby is well awake before attempting feeding.
Alternate breast at which baby begins feeding (use safety pin as reminder).
Lift breast slightly or press lightly on breast above nose if mother's breast occludes infant's nares.
Rotate baby's position at breast to avoid undue trauma to nipples and improve emptying of ducts.
Avoid supplementary formula feedings until lactation is established.
Check with caregiver before taking any medication while breastfeeding (because medications may cross into breast milk).

BREASTFEEDING PROCESS

The nurse caring for the breastfeeding mother should help the woman achieve independence and facilitate the woman and her family's use of their own resources to achieve a successful experience. The objectives of breastfeeding are (1) to provide adequate nutrition, (2) to facilitate maternal-infant attachment, and (3) to prevent trauma to the nipples. All information and support are aimed toward these goals. When assisting the mother with breastfeeding, the nurse should use disposable gloves because breast milk and newborn saliva are body substances that call for standard precautions. To facilitate successful breastfeeding, the nurse should arrange for privacy, help the mother find a comfortable position, and help position the baby comfortably close to her. The mother

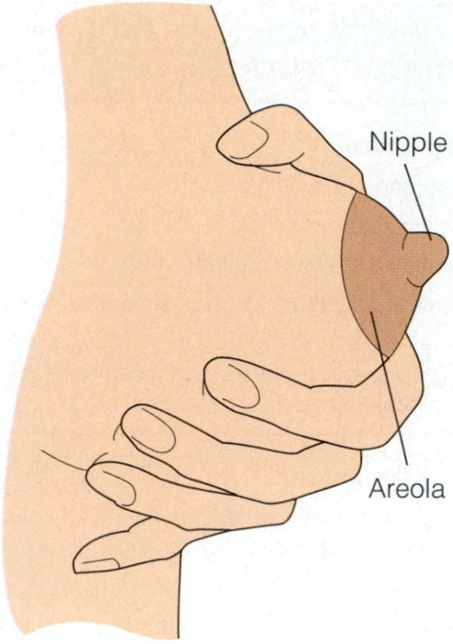

A

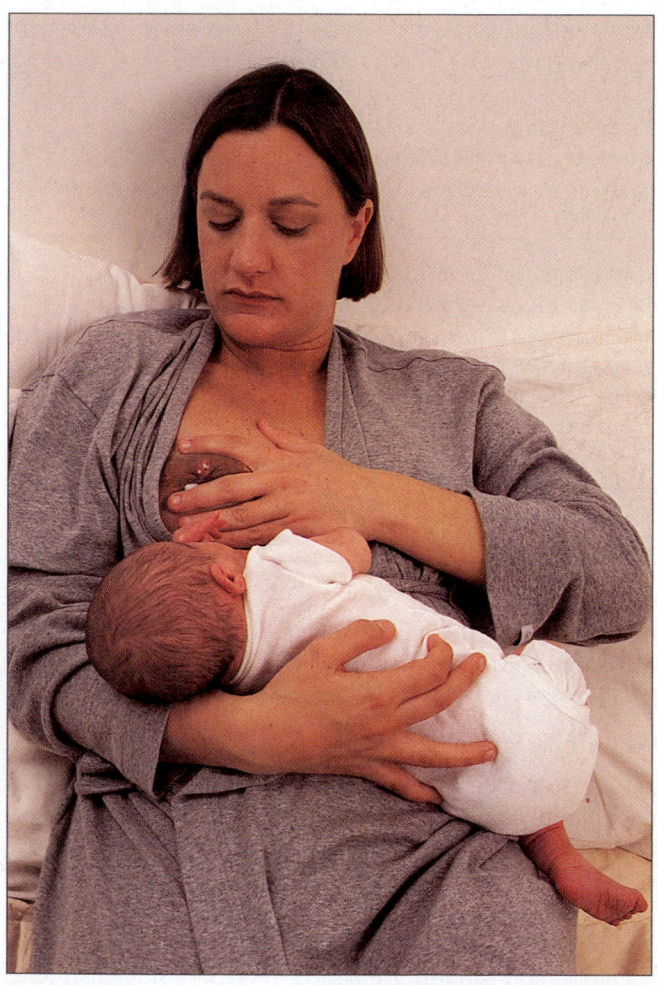

B

Figure 31–5 • *A*, C-hold. *B*, Scissors hold.
SOURCE: Courtesy of Childbirth Graphics Ltd., Rochester, NY.

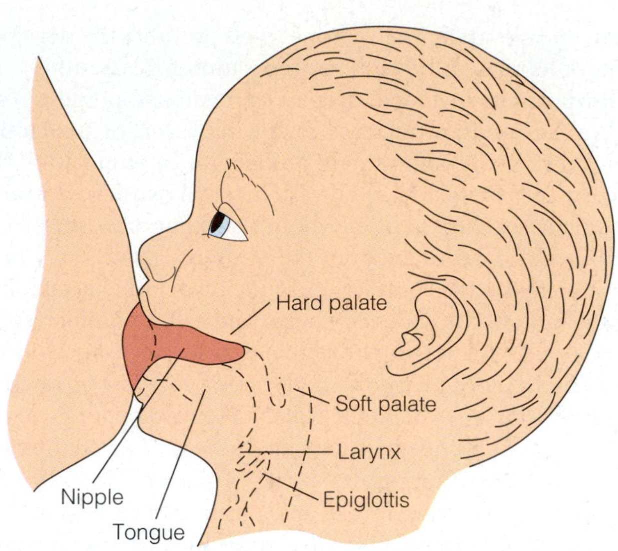

Figure 31–6 • Baby properly positioned at the breast with good latch-on. Nose is near the breast, gums are on the areola, lips are flanged out, tongue is over the bottom gum.
SOURCE: Adapted from Lawrence, R. A. (1994). *Breastfeeding: A guide for the medical profession* (4th ed., p. 219). St. Louis, MO: Mosby.

should support her breast with her hand, using either the C-hold or the scissors hold. For the C-hold, the mother places her thumb well above the areola and the rest of her fingers below the areola and under the breast. The mother may also use the scissors hold, placing her index finger above the areola and her other three fingers below the areola and under the breast. Either method of presenting the breast to the infant is acceptable as long as the hands are well away from the nipple so the baby can "latch on" to the breast (Figure 31–5 •).

The mother should position the baby so that the infant's nose is at the level of the nipple. She then lightly tickles the baby's lower lip with her nipple until the baby opens his or her mouth wide, and then brings the baby to the breast. The baby needs to take the whole nipple into the mouth so that the gums are on the areola. This allows the jaws to compress the milk ducts directly beneath the areola when the baby suckles (Figure 31–6 •). The baby's nose and chin should touch the breast. If the breast occludes the baby's airway, simply lifting up on the breast will usually clear the nares. The baby's lips should be relaxed and flanged outward with the tongue over the lower gum. At this point, the baby should be facing the mother (tummy to tummy or chest to chest), with the ear, shoulder, and hip aligned (Figure 31–7 •).

During these early feedings, the infant should be offered both breasts at each feeding to stimulate the supply-demand response. In some cases, the newborn will suckle only one breast well before falling asleep. As long as each breast is offered frequently (at least every 2 hours), single-breast feeds of whatever duration the baby wishes are an appropriate option until the baby shows a desire for both breasts. The

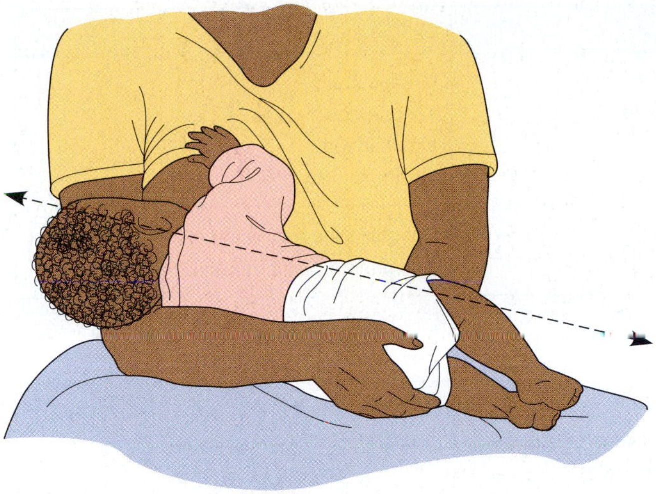

Figure 31–7 • Infant in good breastfeeding position: tummy to tummy; ear, shoulder, and hip aligned.
SOURCE: Riordan, J., & Auerbach, K. (1993). *Breastfeeding and lactation* (p. 248), Jones & Bartlett Publishers, Sudbury, MA. www.jbpub.com. Reprinted with permission.

mother should feed until she becomes relaxed to the point of sleepiness—a delightful side effect of oxytocin secretion—or until she notes cues from the infant suggesting satiety (suckling activity ceases or the baby falls asleep). The length of the feedings is up to the mother; she need not watch a clock. Literature suggests that imposing time limits for breastfeeding does not prevent nipple soreness and in fact interferes with successful feeding. For example, the length of breastfeeding time necessary to stimulate the milk ejection reflex varies with the individual. If the mother feeds according to the clock and disengages the baby prior to let-down too soon, the baby will not get the hindmilk. Because the hindmilk is higher in fat and calories than the foremilk, the baby will be less satisfied, will need to feed again sooner, and will gain less weight. The mother should be encouraged to feed in response to the cues from her baby and her body, not in accordance with an arbitrary time schedule. If the mother wishes to end the feeding before the infant falls asleep or detaches himself or herself, she should break the suction by gently inserting her finger between the baby's gums. Burping between feedings on each breast and at the end of the feeding continues to be necessary. If the infant has been crying, it is also advisable to burp before beginning feeding.

Clinical Tip *Sleepy baby: Unwrap baby, encourage lots of skin-to-skin contact between mom and baby, have mom rest with baby near breast so baby can feel and smell the breast. Encourage mom to watch for feeding cues, such as hand-to-mouth activity, fluttering eyelids, vocalization but not necessarily crying, and mouthing activities.*

BREASTFEEDING ASSESSMENT

During the birthing unit stay, the nurse must carefully monitor the progress of the breastfeeding pair. A systematic assessment of several breastfeeding episodes provides the opportunity to teach the new mother about lactation and the breastfeeding process, provide anticipatory guidance, and evaluate the need for follow-up care after discharge. Criteria for evaluating a breastfeeding session include maternal and infant cues, latch-on, position, let-down, nipple condition, infant response, and maternal response. The literature provides various tools to guide the assessment and documentation of the breastfeeding efforts. The LATCH Scoring Table is one example (Figure 31–8 •).

Clinical Tip *Digital suck training: If baby is pulling tongue back, humping tongue, or thrusting tongue, you can use digital suck training to bring the tongue down and forward. Place a finger in baby's mouth, pad side up. When baby starts sucking well, turn finger so the pad is down. If the baby is sucking correctly, the tongue will come forward and cup the finger, and baby will continue to suckle. Performing this technique prior to feedings encourages the baby to use the tongue correctly.*

LEAKING

Initially, more milk is produced than the infant requires. During the first few weeks, infant needs and maternal responses are not yet well attuned, daily variabilities of feeding frequency and duration are greatest, and most women experience breast leaking. Stimuli that result in let-down or leaking breast milk include hearing a baby cry or even thinking about the baby. The mother should be forewarned of this and use breast pads in her bra to absorb the secretions. She should be cautioned to remove wet pads frequently to avoid irritation of the nipples or infection. (Breast pads with plastic liners interfere with air circulation; the mother should remove the plastic before using them.) Once breastfeeding is well established—usually after the first month—the mother may also be taught to apply direct pressure to the breast with her hand or forearm when leaking occurs.

SUPPLEMENTARY BOTTLE-FEEDINGS

Supplementary bottle-feedings for the breastfeeding infant may weaken or confuse the suckling reflex or decrease the infant's interest in breastfeeding. To grasp the mother's nipple, the newborn has to open her or his mouth wider than needed to grasp a bottle nipple. The shape of the mouth and lips and the sucking mechanism are also different for sucking the breast and the bottle nipple. While suckling at the breast, the infant's tongue moves in a peristaltic manner from front to back, squeezing the milk from the nipple. While sucking on a rubber nipple, the tongue pushes forward against the nipple to

	0	1	2
L Latch	Too sleepy or reluctant No latch achieved	Repeated attempts Hold nipple in mouth Stimulate to suck	Grasps breast Tongue down Lips flanged Rhythmic sucking
A Audible swallowing	None	A few with stimulation	Spontaneous and intermittent <24 hrs old Spontaneous and frequent >24 hrs old
T Type of nipple	Inverted	Flat	Everted (after stimulation)
C Comfort (breast/ nipple)	Engorged Cracked, bleeding, large blisters or bruises Severe discomfort	Filling Reddened/small blisters or bruises Mild/moderate discomfort	Soft Nontender
H Hold (positioning)	Full assist (staff holds infant at breast)	Minimal assist (ie, elevate head of bed, place pillows for support) Teach one side; mother does other Staff holds and then mother takes over	No assist from staff Mother able to position/hold infant

Figure 31–8 ● LATCH: a breastfeeding charting and documentation tool. LATCH was created to provide a systematic method for breastfeeding assessment and charting. It can be used to assist the new mother in establishing breastfeeding and define areas of needed intervention.
SOURCE: AWHONN. (1994). Jensen, D., Wallace, S, & Kelsay, P. A breastfeeding charting system and documentation tool. *Journal of Obstetric, Gynecologic, and Neonatal Nursing, 23*(1): 27–32. (Table 1 Latch Scoring Table and Figure 1 Infant Nursing Care Record, p. 29–30.) Washington, DC: Author. ©1994 by the Association of Women's Health, Obstetric and Neonatal Nurses. All rights reserved.

control the milk flow. Some breastfeeding babies who are given supplementary bottles cannot adjust to these different techniques and push the mother's nipple out of their mouth in subsequent breastfeeding attempts. This can be frustrating for both mother and baby. Breastfeeding mothers should avoid introducing bottles until breastfeeding is well established.

Parents are often concerned because they have no visual assurance of the amount of breast milk consumed. The mother should be taught the signs of milk transfer to the infant (ie, audible swallowing, milk appearing in the baby's mouth, her breasts feeling soft after feeding, milk leaking from the opposite breast) (Mulford, 1992). In addition, if the infant gains weight and has six or more wet diapers a day without supplemental feedings of water or formula, he or she is receiving adequate amounts of milk. Parents should know that because breast milk is more easily digested than formula, the breastfed infant becomes hungry sooner. Thus the frequency of breastfeeding will be greater. The parents may also expect the infant to demand more frequent feeding during growth spurts, such as 10 days to 2 weeks, 5 to 6 weeks, and 2.5 to 3 months.

EXPRESSION OF MILK

If the mother who desires to breastfeed is unable to do so for medical or employment reasons, she needs to know about other means of stimulating milk production and storing the breast milk. The choice of method may depend on the mother's physiologic capabilities to produce the desired amount of milk and her personal preference. During the early postpartum period, if the baby can't feed at the breast (as in the case of some premature or sick infants), the mother needs frequent breast stimulation to establish and increase her milk supply to prepare for later breastfeeding. She should use an electric breast pump at least eight times in each 24-hour period (Shinskie & Lauwers, 2002). Research has shown that a pulsatile electric pump and double setup (allowing both breasts to be stimulated simultaneously) results in higher prolactin levels and a greater volume of milk than does manual expression (Shinskie & Lauwers, 2002) (Figure 31–9 ●). After lactation is established, milk expression may be accomplished by the method that the mother finds most effective and convenient.

To express her milk manually, the woman washes her hands, then massages her breast to stimulate let-down. To massage her breast, the woman grasps the breast with both hands at the base of the breast near the chest wall. Using the palms of her hands, she firmly slides her hands toward her nipple. She repeats this process several times. Then she is ready to begin hand expression. The woman generally uses her left hand for her right breast and right hand for her left breast. However, some women find it preferable to use the hand on the same side as the breast. The nurse should encourage the woman to use the method she finds most effective. The woman grasps the areola with her thumb on the top and her first two fingers on the lower

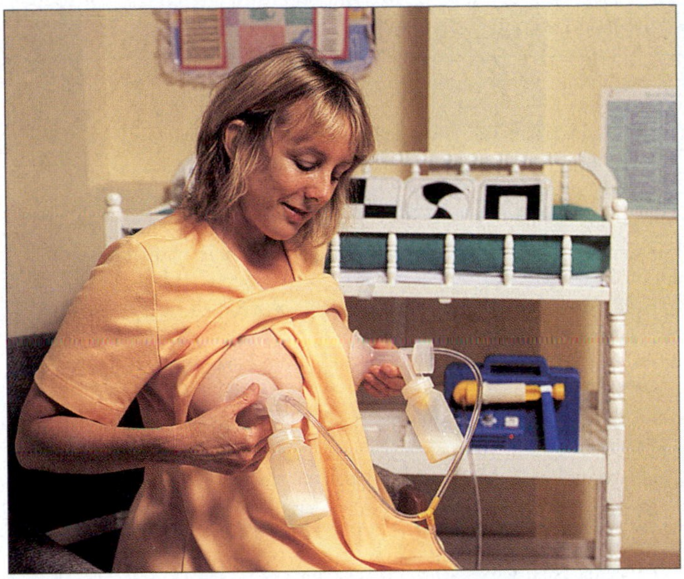

Figure 31–9 ● Mother using electric breast pump and double setup.

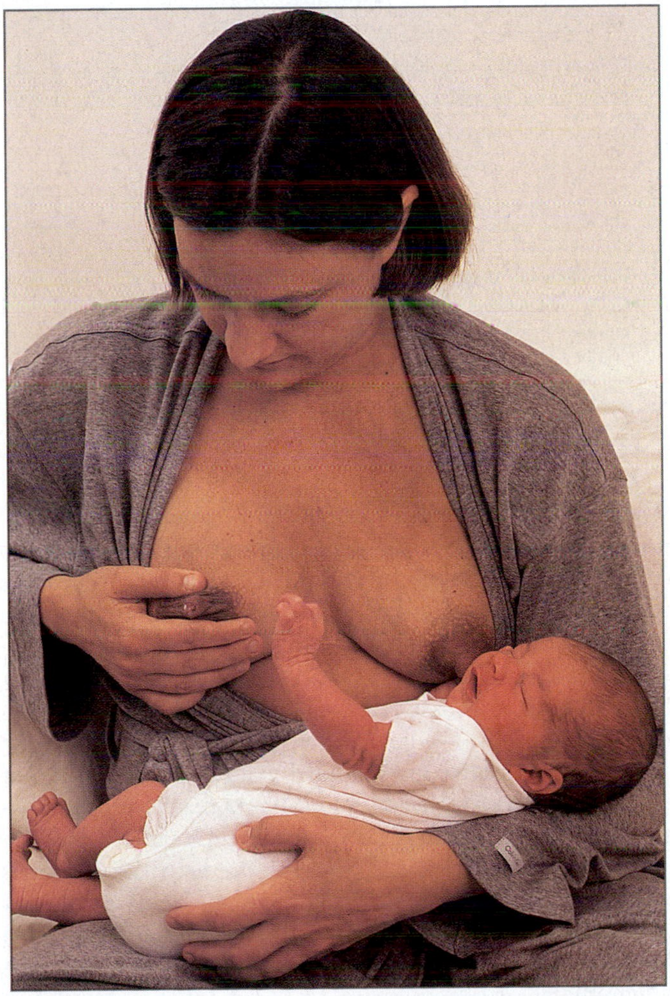

Figure 31–10 ● Hand position for manual expression of milk.

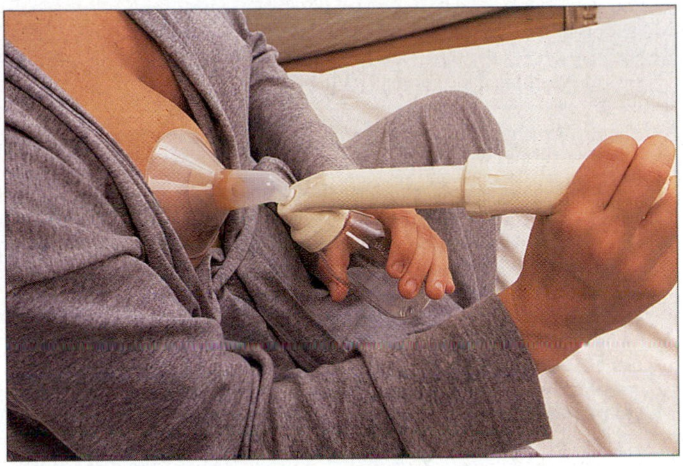

Figure 31–11 ● A mother expresses milk with her Kaneson hand pump.

portion (Figure 31–10 ●). Without allowing her fingers to slide on her skin, she pushes inward toward the chest and then squeezes her fingers together while pulling forward on the areola. She can use a container to catch any fluid that is squeezed out. She then repositions her hand by rotating it slightly so that she can repeat the process. She continues to reposition her hand and repeat the process to empty all the milk sinuses.

Breast pumps use suction to express the milk. Some have collection systems to conveniently store the milk. Hand pumps are portable and inexpensive. Battery-operated pumps are more efficient than hand pumps but are also more expensive. Electric pumps are the most efficient but are bulky and expensive; however, they may be rented in many areas. Many agencies have a variety of pumps available and provide instruction on correct use (Figure 31–11 ●). Videotapes or photographs are also useful in demonstrating the process to new mothers (Table 31–3 ●).

STORING BREAST MILK

Breast milk has bacteriostatic qualities because of the presence of IgA and IgG antibodies, which retard bacterial growth; however, it is recommended that refrigerated milk be used within 3 days (Shinskie & Lauwers, 2002). If breast milk is to be refrigerated and then fed to the infant, it should be stored in clean plastic containers because the white blood cells in the milk will adhere to glass, and their protective effect will be lost. Breast milk may be frozen in either glass or plastic because freezing destroys the white blood cells anyway. Breast milk may be stored in a freezer compartment inside the refrigerator for up to 2 weeks, in a self-contained freezer unit of a refrigerator up to 3 to 4 months, and in a separate deep freeze unit at 0 degrees up to 6 months. Frozen breast milk can be thawed by initially running cool water over the container, then gradually adding warm water until the milk is thawed. The container should be shaken well to

MEDIALINK CASE STUDY: BREASTFEEDING CLIENT

Table 31-3 • RECOMMENDATIONS FOR BREASTFEEDING MOTHER WHO USES A PUMP

General Pumping Recommendations	Recommendations for Specific Types of Pumps
1. Read the instructions on the use and cleaning of a pump before expressing milk with any product. 2. Wash hands before each pumping session. 3. Frequency: For occasional pumping, pump during, after, or between feedings, whichever gives the best results. Most mothers tend to express more milk in the morning. Working mothers should use the pump on a regular basis for the number of feedings that are missed. For premature or ill babies who are not at breast, the number of pumpings should total eight or more in 24 hours. Initiation of pumping should be delayed no longer than 6 hours following birth unless medically indicated. This ensures appropriate development and sensitivity of prolactin receptors. More frequent pumping will avoid the buildup of excessive back pressure of milk during engorgement. 4. Duration: With single-sided pumping, optimal duration is 10 to 15 minutes with an electric pump and 10 to 20 minutes with a manual pump. If double pumping with an electric or two battery-operated pumps, 12 to 15 minutes is optimal. Encourage mothers to tailor these times to their own situation. 5. Technique: • Elicit the milk ejection reflex before using any pump. • Use only as much suction as is needed to maintain milk flow. • Massage the breast in quadrants during pumping to increase intramammary pressure. • Allow enough time for pumping to avoid anxiety. • Use inserts or different flanges if needed to obtain the best fit between pump and breast. • Avoid long periods of uninterrupted vacuum. • Stop pumping when the milk flow is minimal or has ceased.	1. Avoid pumps that use rubber bulbs to generate vacuum; they can cause bruising. 2. Cylinder pumps: • When "O" rings are used, they must be in place for proper suction. • Remove gaskets after each use for cleaning to avoid harboring bacteria in the pump. • Roll the gasket on the inner cylinder back and forth to restore it to its original shape. • The pump stroke may need to be shortened as the outer cylinder fills with milk. • The user may need to empty the outer cylinder once or twice during pumping. • Hand position should be palm up with the elbow held close to the body. 3. Battery-operated pumps: • Use alkaline batteries. • Replace batteries when cycles per minute decrease. • Interrupt vacuum frequently to avoid nipple pain and damage. • Use an AC adapter when possible, especially if the pump generates fewer than six cycles per minute. • Consider renting an electric pump for pumping that will continue for longer than 1 or 2 months. • Use two pumps simultaneously if pumping time is limited or to increase the quantity of milk obtained. • Choose a pump in which the vacuum can be regulated. • Massage the breast by quadrants during pumping. 4. Semiautomatic pumps: • Vacuum may be easier to control if the mother does not lift her finger completely off the hole but rolls it back and forth rhythmically so that the vacuum is efficient but not painful. 5. Automatic electric pumps: • Use the lowest pressure setting that is efficient. • Use a double setup (simultaneous pumping) when time is limited to increase the milk supply and for prematurity, maternal or infant illness, or other special situations.

Source: Adapted from Riordan, J., & Auerbach, K. 1999: *Breastfeeding and human lactation* (2nd ed., p. 397), Boston: Jones & Bartlett Publishers, Sudbury, MA. www.jbpub.com. Reprinted with permission.

return to suspension the fat molecules that separate during freezing. Breast milk should not be defrosted under hot running water or in boiling water. Breast milk should never be microwaved. Uneven heating patterns may alter the composition of the milk and can create hot spots that can burn the baby's mouth.

EXTERNAL SUPPORTS

Childbirth and the beginning of motherhood are a critical time in a woman's life, so physical, psychologic, and social supports are of paramount importance. The father or other partner is the most important support person for her, although the baby can also provide some support in the form of positive feedback. However, extensive family support systems may not be available. Mothers, sisters, and other females who could mentor and care for the new mother may live at a distance or work full-time. As evidenced by the frequent discontinuation of breastfeeding in the early postpartum weeks, there is a need for assistance and follow-up in this area. Nurses, dietitians, childbirth educators, certified nurse-midwives, lactation consultants, mother-to-mother support groups, and physicians must collaborate to provide consistent, timely information and support and to attend to the new mother's special needs. Breastfeeding mothers who work outside the home and who receive support for their decision tend to breastfeed their infants for longer periods of time.

La Leche League International is an organized group of volunteers who provide education about breastfeeding and assistance to women who are breastfeeding. Organized as small, neighborhood-based groups, it sponsors activities, provides printed materials, makes electric breast pumps available for rental, offers one-to-one counseling to mothers with questions or problems, and provides group support to breastfeeding mothers.

Certified lactation consultants are specially trained to offer a wide range of services through private practice and healthcare facilities. A variety of lactation education programs are offered with differing prerequisites and objectives. Numerous books, pamphlets, and educational videos are also available to help the breastfeeding mother. The mother needs the support of all family members, her certified nurse-midwife/physician, her pediatrician or certified nurse practitioner, and all nursing personnel because it is often the attitudes of these people that lead the woman to success or failure.

DRUGS AND BREASTFEEDING

It has long been recognized that certain medications taken by the breastfeeding mother may affect her infant. It should be noted that (1) most drugs pass into breast milk, (2) almost all medications appear in only small amounts in breast milk (usually less than 1% of the maternal dosage), and (3) very few drugs are contraindicated for breastfeeding women.

Characteristics of a drug that influence its passage into breast milk include the following:

1. *Degree of protein binding.* Unbound drugs are most likely to enter the breast milk.
2. *Degree of ionization.* Drugs tend to cross into breast milk in un-ionized form.
3. *Molecular weight.* Drugs with a molecular weight greater than 200 will not cross into breast milk.
4. *Degree of solubility in fat and water.* Alveolar epithelium is a lipid barrier with water-filled pores, but colostrum makes epithelium more permeable to lipid-soluble drugs.
5. *Mechanism of transport.* Drugs enter breast milk by active transport, simple diffusion, or carrier-mediated diffusion.
6. *The pH.* Breast milk, which is acidic, attracts drugs that are weak bases.
7. *Half-life.* Rates of absorption, metabolism, and excretion determine a drug's half-life, or how fast it leaves the body. The longer the half-life, the greater the risk of accumulation in tissues.
8. *Milk/plasma (M/P) ratio.* The higher the **milk/plasma ratio,** the higher the drug concentration in the breast milk compared to the drug concentration in the plasma. An M/P ratio of 1.0 indicates that the milk and plasma contain equal concentrations of the drug. An M/P ratio of less than 1.0 indicates that the concentration of the drug in the milk is lower than its plasma concentration, whereas an M/P ratio greater than 1.0 indicates that the drug's concentration in milk is greater than in plasma.

Other variables that affect the passage of drugs into breast milk include the amount of the drug taken, the frequency and route of administration, and the timing of the dose in relationship to infant feeding. A drug's effects are influenced by the infant's age, the feeding frequency, the volume of milk taken, and the degree of absorption through the gastrointestinal tract.

Five adjustments should be made when administering drugs to a breastfeeding mother to decrease the effects on the infant (Blackburn, 2003):

1. Long-acting forms of drugs should be avoided. The infant may have difficulty metabolizing and excreting them, and accumulation may be a problem.
2. Absorption rates and peak blood levels should be considered in scheduling the administration of the drugs. Less of the drug crosses into the milk if the medication is given immediately after the woman has breastfed her baby.
3. The infant should be closely observed for any signs of drug reaction, including rash, fussiness, lethargy, or changes in sleeping habits or feeding pattern.
4. Whenever alternatives are available, the drug that shows the least tendency to pass into breast milk should be selected.
5. Use single-symptom drugs versus multi-symptom drugs.

The mother should be given information about the potential of most drugs to cross into breast milk. She should also be advised to tell any physician who may prescribe medications for her that she is breastfeeding.

In counseling the breastfeeding mother, the healthcare provider should weigh the benefits of the medication against the possible risk to the infant and its possible effects on the breastfeeding process. The potential risk to the infant must also be weighed against the effect of interrupting breastfeeding.

POTENTIAL PROBLEMS IN BREASTFEEDING

Because mothers are discharged from the hospital before breastfeeding is well established, they are frequently alone when they encounter changes in the breastfeeding process. Many women stop breastfeeding if the situations they encounter seem to pose problems. Nurses can offer anticipatory guidance regarding common breastfeeding phenomena and provide resources for the woman's use after discharge. See Chapter 36 for a complete discussion of self-care measures the nurse can suggest to a woman with a breastfeeding problem after discharge from the birthing unit.

MEDIALINK CARE PLAN: BREASTFEEDING CONCERNS

Client Education for Formula-Feeding

With the great emphasis placed on successful breastfeeding, the teaching needs of the formula-feeding new mother may be overlooked. If she has had only limited experience in feeding infants, she may need some guidelines to feed her newborn successfully. The following information is helpful for parents to facilitate adequate nutrition and foster attachment (see Table 31–4 ●).

The baby is held for all feedings in order to prevent positional otitis media. Positional otitis media may develop when the infant is fed horizontally because milk and nasal mucus may occlude the eustachian tube. Holding the infant provides social and close physical contact for the baby and an

COMPLEMENTARY AND ALTERNATIVE THERAPIES

HERBS, ESSENTIAL OILS, AND HOMEOPATHY FOR BREASTFEEDING

Herbs

Herbs thought to increase milk supply include alfalfa, dandelion, fennel, horsetail, red raspberry, caraway, and anise. The mother may drink caraway tea to reduce colic in the breastfeeding infant. Caraway tea also may be given directly to infants to treat colic (Skidmore-Roth, 2001). Chaste tree (also known as vitex) may also be helpful in cases of insufficient lactation (Blumenthal, 2000). The following herbs may decrease milk supply, so they should be avoided until a woman is no longer breastfeeding: black walnut, sage, parsley, and yarrow (Balch & Balch, 2001; Gladstar, 1993). Black cohosh, blessed thistle, cascara sagrada, horseradish, garlic, cinnamon bark, kava kava, and senna are also contraindicated during lactation (Blumenthal, 2000).

Homeopathy

Pulsatilla, a homeopathic remedy, is used to improve a deficient flow of milk or to dry up the milk if the mother is weaning the child.

Essential Oils

Cracked nipples often respond to calendula cream or ointment, found in health food stores. The breastfeeding mother should wash her nipples off very well before feeding her child. Oil of peppermint, as a cold compress, may relieve breast engorgement or assist in the process of weaning. Four to five drops of peppermint oil are placed in ice cold water. Although essential oils feel like water, chemically they are oils and as such do not mix with the water. A piece of clean fabric is dipped into the water so that the cloth picks up the essential oil on the surface. The fabric is then wrung out and placed on the breasts. Again, the breast should be washed completely before feeding. Women who are allergic to ragweed may find they are also allergic to calendula.

Table 31-4 • INFORMATION HELPFUL TO FORMULA-FEEDING FAMILIES

Types of Formula
Ready-to-feed: Use directly from the can.
Concentrate: Dilute with water before feeding.
Powder: Add water and mix well for proper concentration.
Amount of Formula
Start with 3 oz in each bottle (since a newborn usually takes 1 to 3 oz every 2 1/2 to 4 hours).
Expect increases in baby's appetite with demand feeding (as baby needs more he or she will start finishing each bottle).
Don't feed the baby a partially used bottle after 1 hour at room temperature.
Don't feed the baby a partially used bottle after 4 hours in refrigerator.
Prepare a fresh bottle for each feeding; don't add new formula to old.
Refrigerate bottles made in advance.
Don't feed the baby an opened, refrigerated can of concentrated or ready-to-feed formula after 48 hours.
Temperature of Formula
Mother or family member can try a bottle directly from the refrigerator, but most babies prefer warm formula, close in temperature to breast milk.
Warm bottle under hot tap water, in bottle warmer, or in pan of heated water.
Always test temperature of formula by sprinkling a few drops on wrist.
BE VERY CAREFUL if using a microwave oven to warm formula, as milk is superheated and plastic bottle bags may burst; use "defrost" setting on microwave oven and carefully check temperature of formula before feeding.
Positioning the Baby for Feeding
Hold baby close, establishing eye contact as in breastfeeding.
Hold baby's bottom or foot firmly, keeping his or her back straight to aid digestion and provide a sense of security.
Quiet baby before feeding.
Alternate the side baby is fed from to give baby two-sided stimulation.
Avoid feeding while baby is on his or her back.
Don't prop the bottle.
Procedure for Feeding
Nipple hole should allow only drops of formula to flow.
Keep nipple full with formula to decrease air ingestion.
How to Burp a Baby
Position baby so his or her head rests on mother's shoulder or face down on lap, or sit baby on lap with baby's chin and chest supported.
Gently pat or stroke baby's back.
Burp baby halfway through feeding and at end of feeding.
Learn baby's preferred burping position and whether baby is a slow or quick burper.
Regurgitation of small amounts of formula is common.
Have "burp cloth" available.

opportunity for parent-infant interaction and bonding (Figure 31–12 •).

Nipples should have a hole big enough to allow milk to flow in drops when the bottle is inverted. Too large an opening may cause regurgitation because of rapid feeding. If feeding is too fast, the nipple should be changed, and the infant should be helped to eat more slowly by stopping the feeding frequently for burping and cuddling. The nipple is pointed directly into the mouth, not toward the palate or tongue, and is placed on top of the tongue. The nipple needs to be full of liquid at all times to avoid ingestion of air, which decreases the amount of feeding and increases gastric discomfort. Nipples vary in shape, amount of energy needed to obtain the formula, and rate of formula flow through the nipple unit.

The infant is burped at intervals, preferably at the middle and end of the feeding. The infant who seems to swallow a great deal of air while sucking may need more frequent burping. If the infant has cried before being fed, air may have been swallowed; in such cases, the infant is burped before beginning to feed or after taking just enough to calm down. Burping is done by holding the infant upright on the shoulder or by holding the infant in a sitting position on the

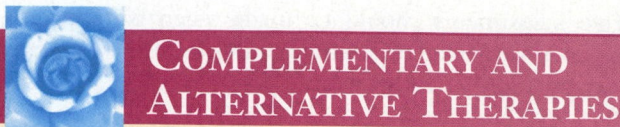

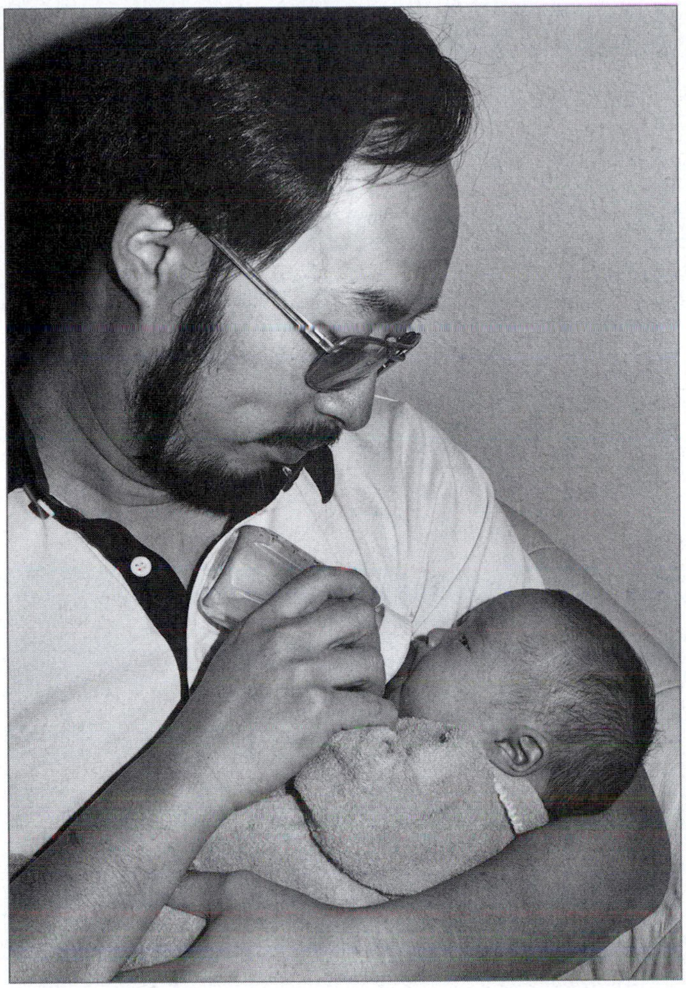

Figure 31–12 ● An infant is supported comfortably during bottle-feeding.

feeder's lap with chin and chest supported on one hand. The back is then gently patted or stroked with the other hand. Too frequent burping may confuse a newborn who is attempting to coordinate sucking, swallowing, and breathing simultaneously.

Newborns frequently regurgitate small amounts of feedings. This may look like a large amount to inexperienced parents, however, and they may require reassurance that this is normal. Initially, regurgitation may be due to excessive mucus and gastric irritation from foreign substances such as aspirated blood in the stomach from birth. Later, regurgitation may result when the infant feeds too rapidly and swallows air. It may also occur when the infant is overfed; the cardiac sphincter allows the excess to be regurgitated. Because this is such a common occurrence, experienced parents and nurses generally keep a "burp cloth" available. Although regurgitation is normal, vomiting or a forceful expulsion of fluid is not. When forceful expulsion occurs, further evaluation may be indicated, especially if other symptoms are present.

Parents should be encouraged to avoid overfeeding or feeding infants every time they cry. Infants should be encouraged to feed and should be allowed to set their own pace once feedings are established. Parents sometimes set artificial goals—"The baby must take all 5 ounces"—and tend to keep feeding the child until those goals are met, even though the infant may not be hungry. During early feedings, however, the infant may need simple tactile stimulation—such as gently rubbing feet and hands, adjusting clothing, and loosening coverings—to maintain adequate sucking for a sufficient time to complete a full feeding.

The desirable amount and frequency of formula-feeding vary with postnatal age of the infant. From birth to 2 months of age, the baby takes six to eight feedings of approximately 2 to 4 ounces of formula at each feeding within a 24-hour period.

There are three forms of formula (Table 31–5 ●). They are ready-to-feed, liquid concentrate, and powdered.

Clinical Tip *When you help a mother bottle-feed her baby for the first time, there are many potential frustrations you can help her avoid. The first is often "flying arms" as the baby waves his or her arms in the air. The second is the "chin plunge" as the baby's head falls forward in the mother's tentative hold. To avoid this, assist the mother with positioning. A third frustration may arise when she tries to get the nipple correctly placed in the mouth. To do this, put your index finger on the baby's chin, and gently pull downward while quickly sliding the nipple in over the tongue.*

The nurse is responsible for discussing formula preparation and sterilization techniques with families. Cleanliness is essential, but sterilization is necessary only if the water source is questionable. Bottles may be effectively prepared in dishwashers or washed thoroughly in warm soapy water and rinsed well. Nipples may be weakened by the temperature of dishwashers and therefore should be washed thoroughly by hand and rinsed well. Tap water, if from an uncontaminated source, may be used for mixing powdered formulas, which are less expensive than the concentrated or ready-to-use prepared formulas. Honey should not be used as a "sugar source" because of the danger of infant botulism.

Bottles may be prepared individually, or up to one day's supply of formula may be prepared at one time. Extra bottles are stored in the refrigerator and should be warmed slightly before feeding. Ready-to-use disposable bottles of formula are very convenient but are also expensive. Formula left in bottles after a feeding should be discarded.

The Special Supplemental Food Program for Women, Infants, and Children (WIC) provides 8 pounds of powdered formula or 403 ounces of concentrated liquid formula per month. Individual states make provisions about when WIC nutritionists may distribute soy formulas and whether prescriptions are needed for special or therapeutic formulas.

Table 31-5 • FORMULA PREPARATION

Ready to Feed	Formula Concentrate	Powdered Formula
(20 kcal/oz; available in 32-oz cans or 4-oz bottles) Use within 30 minutes to 1 hour once opened. Do not dilute. Use directly from can, no mixing required. Just add clean nipple to bottle. Most expensive type of formula preparation.	(available in 13-oz cans) Mix equal amounts of concentrate and water from uncontaminated source. This provides a 20 kcal/30 mL (1 oz) dilution. For example, for a 4-oz feeding mix 2 oz of formula concentrate with 2 oz water. Wash punchtype can opener and top of formula can before opening. Prepare a single feeding by measuring water and liquid directly into nursing bottle. Cover opened concentrate formula cans with foil or plastic wrap and refrigerate until next bottle is made up.	(52 scoops per can) Mix one unpacked level scoop of powdered formula with each 60 mL (2 oz) of warm water. Always pour water into bottle first; then add powder and stir well. Make sure the powder and water are well mixed to ensure the formula composition is 20 kcal/30 mL (1 oz). After opening, keep can tightly covered and use contents within 1 month to ensure freshness. Will keep in refrigerator for up to 24 hours. Least expensive type.

Nutritional Assessment of the Infant

During the early months of life, the food offered to and consumed by infants will be instrumental to their proper growth and development. The infant's nutritional status is assessed at each well-baby visit. Assessment should include four components:

- Nutritional history from the parent
- Weight gain since the last visit
- Growth chart percentiles
- Physical examination

The nutritional history reports the type, amount, and frequency of milk and supplemental foods, vitamins, and minerals being given to the infant on a daily basis. If the baby is taking formula, the history also includes how the formula is mixed (checking for underdilution or overdilution) and stored. The healthy formula-fed infant should generally gain 30 g (1 oz) per day for the first 6 months of life and 15 g (0.5 oz) per day for the second 6 months. Individual charts show the infant's growth with respect to height, weight, and head circumference. The important consideration is that infants continue to grow at their own individual rates.

For a mother who is concerned about whether her infant is getting adequate nutrition, the nurse can recommend looking for an appearance of weight gain and counting the number of wet and soiled diapers in a 24-hour period. Approximately six wet diapers or more and frequent stools in a day indicate adequate nutrition is being attained in the totally breastfed infant. If additional water is ingested, the diaper count should be higher. The presence of urine can most accurately be assessed when the diaper is free of feces. The diaper is most likely to be free of feces prior to feedings because the gastrocolic reflex often stimulates stooling following a feeding. For the anxious parent, another means of reassurance of adequate intake and output is to keep a record of the frequency and duration of feedings, amount of swallowing, and the exact number of wet and/or soiled diapers. Keeping a record tends to give the worried parent a sense of control and a tangible indication on which to rule out or base concern (Table 31–6 •).

Table 31-6 • SUCESSFUL BREASTFEEDING EVALUATION

Babies are probably getting enough milk if

- They are nursing at least eight times in 24 hours.
- In a quiet room, their mothers can hear them swallow while nursing.
- Their mothers' breasts appear to soften after breastfeeding.
- The number of wet diapers increases by the fourth or fifth day after birth, or there are at least six to eight wet diapers every 24 hours after day 5.
- Their stools are yellow or are beginning to lighten in color by the fourth or fifth day after birth.

Offering a supplemental bottle is not a reliable indicator because most babies will take a few ounces even if they are getting enough breast milk.

The physical examination will help identify any nutritional disorders. Iron deficiency should be suspected in an infant who is pale, diaphoretic, and irritable.

By calculating the nutritional needs of infants, the nurse can recommend a diet that supplies appropriate nutrition for infant growth and development. The assessment is especially helpful in counseling mothers of infants under 6 months of age, because there is a tendency to add too many supplemental foods or offer too much formula to infants of this age. Clinicians generally advise that an infant not be given more than 32 oz of formula in 1 day. If additional calories are needed, supplemental foods should be added to the diet. Conversely, if the caloric intake is adequate, formula alone gives the infant enough calories, and introduction of solid foods can be delayed.

Appropriate nutritional intake can be identified by comparing the infant's dietary intake with the desired caloric intake for the infant's weight and age. Most commercial formulas prescribed for the normal healthy newborn contain 20 kcal per 30 mL (1 oz). If the infant is eating solids, the caloric value of those foods must be determined and included in the calculations of nutritional intake. With knowledge of the number of calories needed by the infant according to weight (108 kcal/kg/day [55 kcal/lb/day]), the nurse can counsel the parents about how many ounces per day the infant needs to meet caloric requirements. The following example shows the effectiveness of these assessments and interventions.

Jamie Adams, age 1 week, is visited at home by the nurse associated with her family's health maintenance organization. Jamie is Mrs Adams's first child, and Mrs Adams is concerned about whether Jamie is getting adequate nourishment. Jamie weighed 7 lb at birth and has regained her birth weight after an 11 oz (10%) loss. Mrs Adams reports that Jamie takes 3 oz of formula every 3 hours, does not spit up any formula, and has eight to ten wet diapers a day with one to two soft bowel movements per day. Jamie is a contented baby who sleeps between feedings.

Based on requirements of 108 kcal/kg/day, the nurse calculates 1-week-old Jamie's dietary needs as follows:

- Jamie's weight = 7 lb. Converting weight into kg (2.2 lb/kg), Jamie weighs 3.2 kg.
- Jamie's 24-hour caloric need = 3.2 kg (Jamie's weight) 108 kcal/kg/day = 346 kcal/day.
- Amount of formula (at 20 kcal/oz) needed in 24 hours = 17 oz.
- Jamie's 24-hour intake = 24 oz (3 oz every 3 hours) 20 kcal/oz = 480 kcal.

The nurse makes the following nursing diagnoses:

- ***Deficient Knowledge*** related to lack of information about assessing adequacy of food intake
- ***Altered Nutrition: More than Body Requirements*** related to formula intake that is greater than necessary to meet Jamie's growth needs

The nursing plan outlines the following actions:

- Discuss Jamie's feeding cues with Mrs Adams. How does Mrs Adams decide when to feed Jamie? Is she feeding in response to Jamie or in response to a time schedule? Explain that infants have a need for nonnutritive sucking that can be met with a pacifier.
- Explain normal infant sleep-wake cycles and how babies can self-regulate in phases of light sleep, although they may make stirring noises.
- Explain that Jamie is ingesting more calories than necessary, and point out the need to reduce her intake by approximately 7 oz/day. Mrs Adams can accomplish this by feeding Jamie a little less frequently and feeding slightly less formula (approximately 0.5 oz or less) each feeding. Giving Jamie 75 mL (2.5 oz) at each of seven feedings provides 350 cal/day. Teach Mrs Adams how to feed Jamie in response to feeding cues, such as rooting and hand-to-mouth activity. When Jamie has taken 75 to 90 mL (2.5 to 3 oz) of formula, substitute a pacifier to provide nonnutritive sucking. Explain that if Jamie takes 2.5 to 3 oz and seems to want to eat again before 3 to 4 hours, Mrs Adams should try other comfort measures, such as changing Jamie's diaper, rocking her, giving her a pacifier, or putting her in a swing, before resorting to feeding.
- Discuss with Mrs Adams the behaviors that indicate satiation. These include minimal sucking with release of the nipple and falling asleep with hands and body relaxed. She should not attempt to force the remaining formula, if any, but should discard it because of the potential for bacterial growth even if refrigerated.
- Formula amounts can be increased gradually to meet Jamie's changing caloric needs and growth without excessive caloric intake. Once Jamie is ingesting 32 oz a day, the addition of solid foods can be considered after discussion with the healthcare provider.
- Explore alternative methods for providing comfort to a newborn.

On a follow-up well-baby visit, Jamie is weighed and is gaining 30 g (1 oz) per day. Jamie continues to have approximately eight to ten wet diapers a day and is alert and responsive.

MEDIALINK BREASTFEEDING RESOURCES

CHAPTER REVIEW

EXPLOREMEDIALINK

NCLEX review questions, case studies, and other interactive resources for this chapter can be found on the Web site at http://www.prenhall.com/olds. Click on "Chapter 31" to select the activities for this chapter.

For tutorials including animations and videos, more NCLEX review questions, and an audio glossary, access the accompanying CD-ROM in this book.

Focus Your Study

- The RDA for calories for the newborn is 105 to 108 kcal/kg/day (50 to 55 kcal/lb/day).
- The nurse must monitor the first feeding because this is when the newborn may initially manifest signs of cardiac complications or anomalies of the upper gastrointestinal tract.
- Breast milk has immunologic and nutritional properties that make it the optimal food for the first year of life.
- Mature breast milk and commercially prepared formulas (unless otherwise noted) provide 20 kcal/oz.
- Breastfed infants need supplements of iron after 6 months of age. Infants consuming iron-enriched formula need no other vitamin or mineral supplements.
- Three types of commercial infant formulas are available: those based on cow's milk proteins, soy-based formulas, and specialized or therapeutic hydrolysated formulas.
- Neither cow's milk nor soy milk should be given to infants. The use of skim milk, cow's milk with lowered fat content, or unmodified cow's milk is not recommended for children under 2 years old.
- Signs indicating newborn readiness for the first feeding are active bowel sounds, absence of abdominal distention, and a lusty cry that quiets with rooting and sucking behaviors when a stimulus is placed near the lips.
- Nurses must recognize that cultural values influence infant feeding practices, be sensitive to ethnic backgrounds of minority populations, and understand that the dominant culture in any society defines "normal" maternal-infant feeding interaction.
- Breastfed infants are getting adequate nutrition if they are gaining weight and have at least six wet diapers a day when not receiving additional water supplements.
- Most maternal medications are transmitted through breast milk. The effects on the infant and lactation depend on a variety of factors, including route of administration, timing of the dose with respect to feeding time, and multiple properties of the medication.
- Breastfeeding mothers should be encouraged to ensure that the infant is correctly positioned at the breast, with a large portion of areola in the mouth and not under the tongue. The mother is advised to rotate the baby's position periodically to ensure that all ducts are emptied.
- Formula-fed infants regain their birth weight by 10 days of age and gain 1 oz/day for the first 6 months and 0.5 oz/day for the second 6 months; birth weight is doubled at 3.5 to 4 months of age. Healthy breastfed babies gain approximately 0.5 oz/day in the first 6 months of life, regain their birth weight by about 14 days of age, and double their birth weight at approximately 5 months of age.
- The formula-feeding mother may need help feeding and burping her infant. She will also benefit from information about feeding schedules and types of formula.
- Nutritional assessment of the infant includes nutritional history from the parent, measurement of weight gain, determination of growth chart percentiles, and physical examination.

References

American Academy of Pediatrics (AAP) Committee on Nutrition. (1999). Iron fortification of infant formulas. *Pediatrics, 104*(1), 119–123.

American Academy of Pediatrics (AAP) Committee on Nutrition. (2000). Hypoallergenic infant formulas. *Pediatrics, 106*(2), 346–349.

American Academy of Pediatrics (AAP) and the American College of Obstetricians and Gynecologists (ACOG). (2002). *Guidelines for perinatal care* (5th ed.). Washington, DC: Author.

American College of Obstetricians and Gynecologists (ACOG). (2000). *Breastfeeding: Maternal and infant aspects (ACOG Educational Bulletin No. 258).* Washington, DC: Author.

Balch, J. F., & Balch, P. A. (2001). *Prescription for nutritional healing* (3rd ed.). Garden City, NY: Avery Publishing Group.

Biancuzzo, M., (2003). *Breastfeeding the newborn: Clinical strategies for nurses.* (2nd ed.). St. Louis, MO: Mosby.

Blackburn, S. T. (2003). *Maternal, fetal, & neonatal physiology: Clinical perspective* (2nd ed.). St. Louis, MO: Saunders.

Blumenthal, M. (2000). *Herbal medicine: Expanded commission E monograph.* Austin, TX: American Botanical Council.

Chezem, J., Friesen, C. & Boettcher, J. (2003). Breastfeeding knowledge, breastfeeding confidence, and infant feeding plans: Effects on actual feeding practices. *Journal of Obstetric, Gynecologic, & Neonatal Nursing. 32,* (1). p 40–47.

Davis, L. J., Okuboye, S., & Ferguson, S. L. (2000). Healthy People 2010: Examining a decade of maternal and infant health. *AWHONN Lifelines, 4*(3), 26–33.

Fontaine, K. L. (2000). *Healing practices: Alternative therapies for nursing.* Upper Saddle River, NJ: Prentice Hall.

Geissler, E. M. (1998). *Pocket guide to cultural assessment* (2nd ed.). St. Louis, MO: Mosby.

Gladstar, R. (1993). *Herbal healing for women.* New York: Simon & Schuster.

Hershoff, A. (2000). *Homeopathic remedies.* Garden City Park, NY: Avery Publishing.

Hutchinson, M. K., & Baqi-Aziz, M. (1994). Nursing care of the childbearing Muslim family. *Journal of Obstetric, Gynecologic, and Neonatal Nursing, 23*(9), 767–771.

Jackson, D. J., Chopra, M., Witten, C., & Sengwana, M. J. (2003). HIV and infant feeding: Issues in developed and developing countries. *Journal of Obstetric, Gynecologic, and Neonatal Nursing, 32*(1), 117–127.

Mulford, C. (1992). The mother-baby assessment (MBA): An "Apgar score" for breastfeeding. *Journal of Human Lactation, 8*(2), 79–82.

Riordan, J. M., & Auerbach, K. (1999). *Breastfeeding and Human lactation* (2nd ed.). Boston: Jones & Bartlett.

Riordan, J. M., & Koehn, M. (1997). Reliability and validity testing of three breastfeeding assessment tools. *Journal of Obstetric, Gynecologic, and Neonatal Nursing, 26*(2), 181–187.

Shinskie, D. & Lauwers, J. (2002). *Pocket guide for counseling the nursing mother: A lactation consultant's guide* (1st ed.). Sudbury, MA: Jones & Bartlett.

Skidmore-Roth, L. (2001). *Mosby's handbook of herbs and natural supplements.* St. Louis, MO: Mosby.

Walker, M., & Creehan, P. (2001). Newborn nutrition. In K. R. Simpson & P. A. Creehan (Eds.), *AWHONN perinatal nursing* (2nd ed., pp. 568–571). Philadelphia: Lippincott Williams & Wilkins.

Weil, A. (2000). *Eating well for optimal health.* New York: Alfred A. Knopf.

The Newborn at Risk: Conditions Present at Birth

32

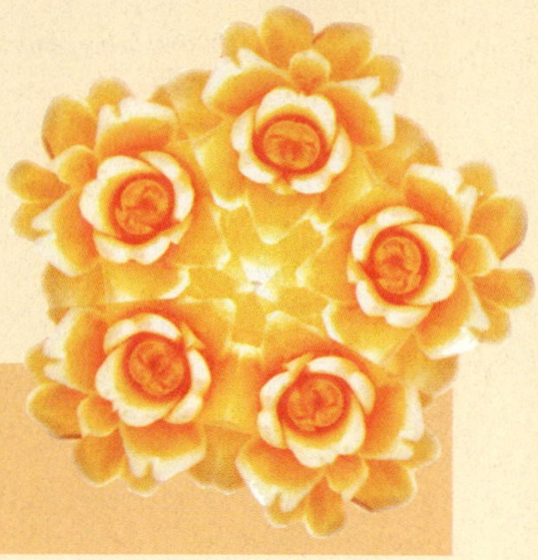

The rhythmic tides of her sleeping and feeding spaciously measured her days and nights.
Her frail absorption was a commanding presence, her helplessness strong as a rock.
~ *Laurie Lee,* Two Women ~

Objectives

- Identify factors present at birth that help identify an at-risk newborn.
- Compare the underlying etiologies of the physiologic complications of small-for-gestational-age (SGA) newborns and preterm appropriate-for-gestational-age (Pr AGA) newborns.
- Describe the impact of maternal diabetes mellitus on the newborn.
- Compare the characteristics and underlying etiologies of potential complications of the postterm newborn and the newborn with postmaturity syndrome.
- Discuss the physiologic characteristics of the preterm newborn that predispose each body system to various complications.
- Identify the data used in developing the nursing diagnoses required to plan interventions for the care of the Pr AGA newborn.
- Discuss the nursing assessments of and initial interventions for a newborn born with congenital anomalies.
- Explain the special care needed by an alcohol- or drug-exposed newborn.
- Relate the consequences of maternal HIV/AIDS to the management of the infant in the neonatal period.
- Identify physical examination findings during the early newborn period that would make the nurse suspect a congenital cardiac defect.
- Explain the special care needed by a newborn with an inborn error of metabolism.

Key Terms

Alcohol-related birth defect (ARBD) 919
Drug-dependent infants 921
Fetal alcohol effects (FAE) 919
Fetal alcohol syndrome (FAS) 919
Inborn errors of metabolism 930
Infant of diabetic mother (IDM) 896
Infant of substance-abusing mother (ISAM) 916
Intrauterine growth restriction (IUGR) 890
Large for gestational age (LGA) 895
Neonatal morbidity 889
Neonatal mortality risk 889
Phenylketonuria (PKU) 930
Postmaturity 899
Postterm newborn 898
Preterm infant 900
Small for gestational age (SGA) 890

MediaLink

Additional resources for this content can be found on the Student CD-ROM and on the Companion Website at www.prenhall.com/olds. Click on "Chapter 32" to select the activities for this chapter.

CD-ROM
- Audio Glossary
- NCLEX Review

Companion Website
- Additional NCLEX Review
- Case Study: Postterm Newborn
- Care Plan Activity: Infant of a Diabetic Mother

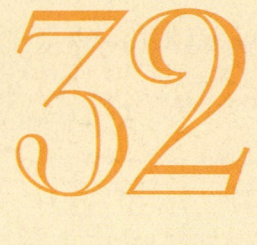

Within the past 30 years, the field of neonatology has expanded greatly. Many levels of nursery care have evolved in response to increasing knowledge about the newborn: special care, intensive care, and convalescent or transitional care. Along with the newborn's parents, the nurse is an important caregiver in all these settings. As a member of the multidisciplinary healthcare team, the nurse provides the holistic care necessary in the often high-tech perinatal environment.

In addition to the availability of excellent intensive care services, a variety of other factors influences the outcomes of at-risk infants, including the following:

- Birth weight
- Gestational age
- Type and length of newborn illness
- Environmental factors
- Maternal factors
- Maternal-infant separation

Identification of At-Risk Newborns

An at-risk newborn is one who is susceptible to illness (morbidity) or even death (mortality) because of dysmaturity, immaturity, physical disorders, or complications during or after birth. In most cases, the infant is the product of pregnancy involving one or more predictable risk factors, including the following:

- Low socioeconomic level of the mother and limited access to healthcare
- Exposure to environmental dangers, such as toxic chemicals and illicit drugs
- Preexisting maternal conditions, such as heart disease, diabetes, hypertension, and renal disease
- Maternal factors, such as age or parity
- Medical conditions related to pregnancy and their associated complications
- Pregnancy complications such as abruptio placentae

Various risk factors and their specific effects on the pregnancy outcome were identified in Table 15–2. Since these factors and the perinatal risks associated with them are known, the birth of at-risk newborns can often be anticipated. The pregnancy can be closely monitored, treatment can be started as necessary, and arrangements can be made for birth to occur at a facility with appropriate resources to care for both mother and baby.

Most at-risk infants can be identified before the onset of labor, so prenatal assessment and care are crucial. However, because the course of labor and birth and the infant's ability to withstand the stress of labor cannot be predicted, the nurse's use of electronic fetal heart monitoring or fetal heart auscultation by Doppler plays a significant role in detecting distress in the fetus. Immediately after birth, the Apgar score is a helpful tool in identifying the at-risk newborn, but it is not the only indicator of possible long-term outcome.

The newborn classification and neonatal mortality risk chart is another useful tool in identifying newborns at risk (Figure 32–1 •). Before this classification tool was developed, birth weight of less than 2500 g was the sole criterion for determination of immaturity. Clinicians then recognized that newborns could weigh more than 2500 g but still be immature. Conversely, an infant weighing less than 2500 g might be functionally mature at term or beyond. Thus birth weight and gestational age together became the criteria used to assess neonatal maturity and mortality risk.

According to the newborn classification and neonatal mortality risk chart, gestation is divided as follows:

- Preterm: less than 37 (completed) weeks
- Term: 38 to 41 (completed) weeks
- Postterm: greater than 42 weeks

As shown in Figure 32–1, large-for-gestational-age (LGA) infants are those that plot above the 90th percentile curve. Appropriate-for-gestational-age (AGA) infants are those that plot between the 10th percentile and 90th percentile curve. Small-for-gestational-age (SGA) infants are those that plot below the 10th percentile curve on the Denver intrauterine growth curves. A newborn is assigned to a category depending on birth weight and gestational age. For example, a newborn classified as Pr SGA is preterm and small for gestational age. The full-term newborn whose weight is appropriate for gestational age is classified F AGA. The assigned newborn classification may vary according to the intrauterine growth curve chart used; therefore, the chart used should correlate with the characteristics of the patient population. It is also important to note that intrauterine growth curve charts are influenced by altitude and the ethnicity of the newborn population used to create the chart.

Neonatal mortality risk is the chance of death within the newborn period, that is, within the first 28 days of life. As indicated in Figure 32–1, the neonatal mortality risk decreases as both gestational age and birth weight increase. Infants who are preterm and SGA have the highest neonatal mortality risk. The previously high mortality rates for LGA infants have decreased at most perinatal centers because of improved management of diabetes in pregnancy and recognition of potential complications of LGA newborns.

Neonatal morbidity can also be anticipated based on birth weight and gestational age. In Figure 32–2 •, the infant's birth weight is located on the vertical axis, and the gestational age in weeks is found along the horizontal axis. The area where the two meet on the graph identifies common problems. This tool assists in determining the needs of particular infants for special observation and care. For example, an infant of 2000 g at 40 weeks' gestation should be carefully

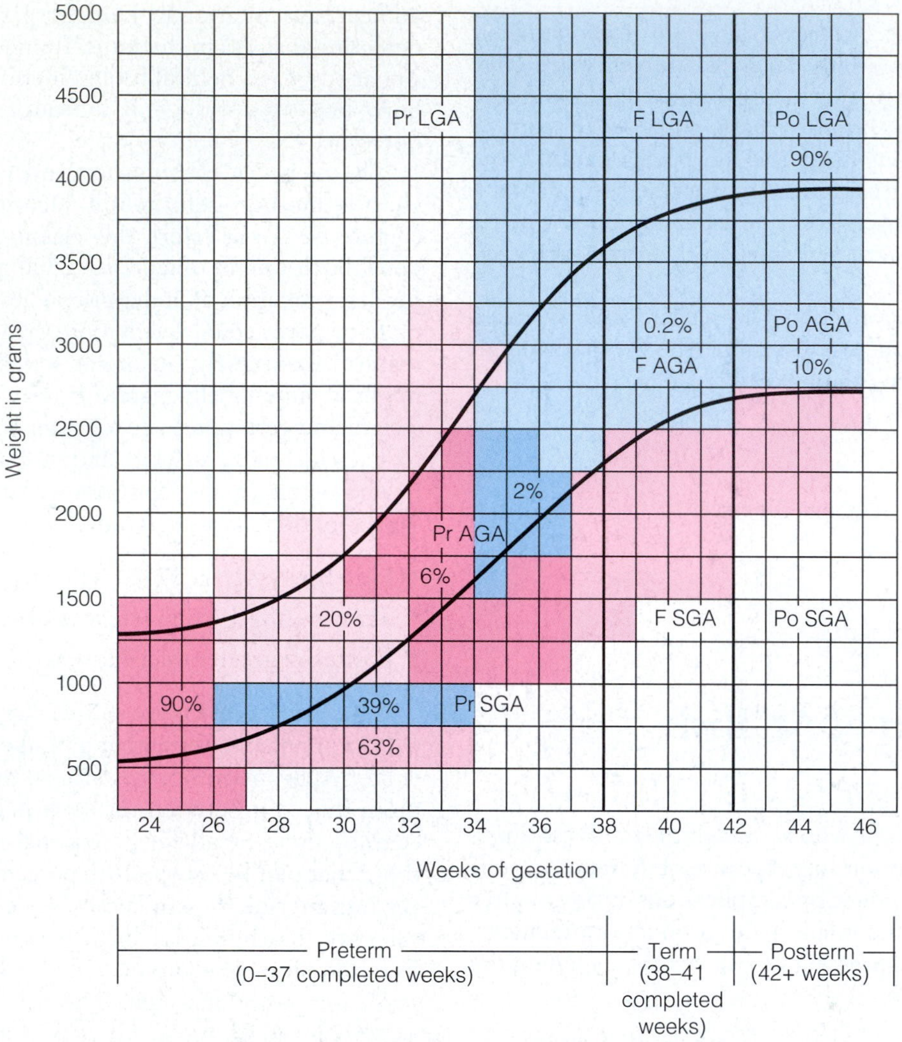

Figure 32–1 • Newborn classification and neonatal mortality risk chart. Infants are classified according to weight as small for gestational age (SGA), appropriate for gestational age (AGA), or large for gestational age (LGA) and by weeks of newborn as preterm (Pr), term (F), or postterm (Po). Corresponding neonatal mortality risks are indicated by the percentages in the various colored regions.

SOURCE: Koops, B. L., Morgan, L. P., & Battaglia, F. C. (1982). Neonatal mortality risk in relationship to birth weight and gestational age. *Journal of Pediatrics, 101*(6), 969.

assessed for evidence of fetal distress, hypoglycemia, congenital anomalies, congenital infection, and polycythemia.

Identifying the nursing care needs of the at-risk newborn depends on minute-to-minute observations of the changes in the newborn's physiologic status. The nursing care management must be directed toward the following:

- Decreasing physiologically stressful situations
- Constantly observing for subtle signs of change in clinical condition
- Interpreting laboratory data and coordinating interventions
- Conserving the infant's energy for healing and growth
- Providing for developmental stimulation and maintenance of sleep cycles
- Assisting the family in developing attachment behaviors
- Involving the family in planning and providing care

Care of the Small-for-Gestational-Age/Intrauterine Growth Restriction Newborn

Infants are considered **small for gestational age (SGA)** when they are less than two standard deviations below the population norm or at less than the third percentile (10th percentile for Denver curves because of the lower birth weight at higher altitudes) (see Figure 32–1). When possible, the birth weight charts used to assign the SGA classification to a newborn should be based on the local population into which the newborn is born (Kliegman & Das, 2002). A SGA newborn may be preterm, term, or postterm. An undergrown newborn may be also said to have **intrauterine growth restriction (IUGR),** which describes the pregnancy circumstance of advanced gestation and limited fetal growth. The terms SGA and IUGR are not necessarily interchangeable.

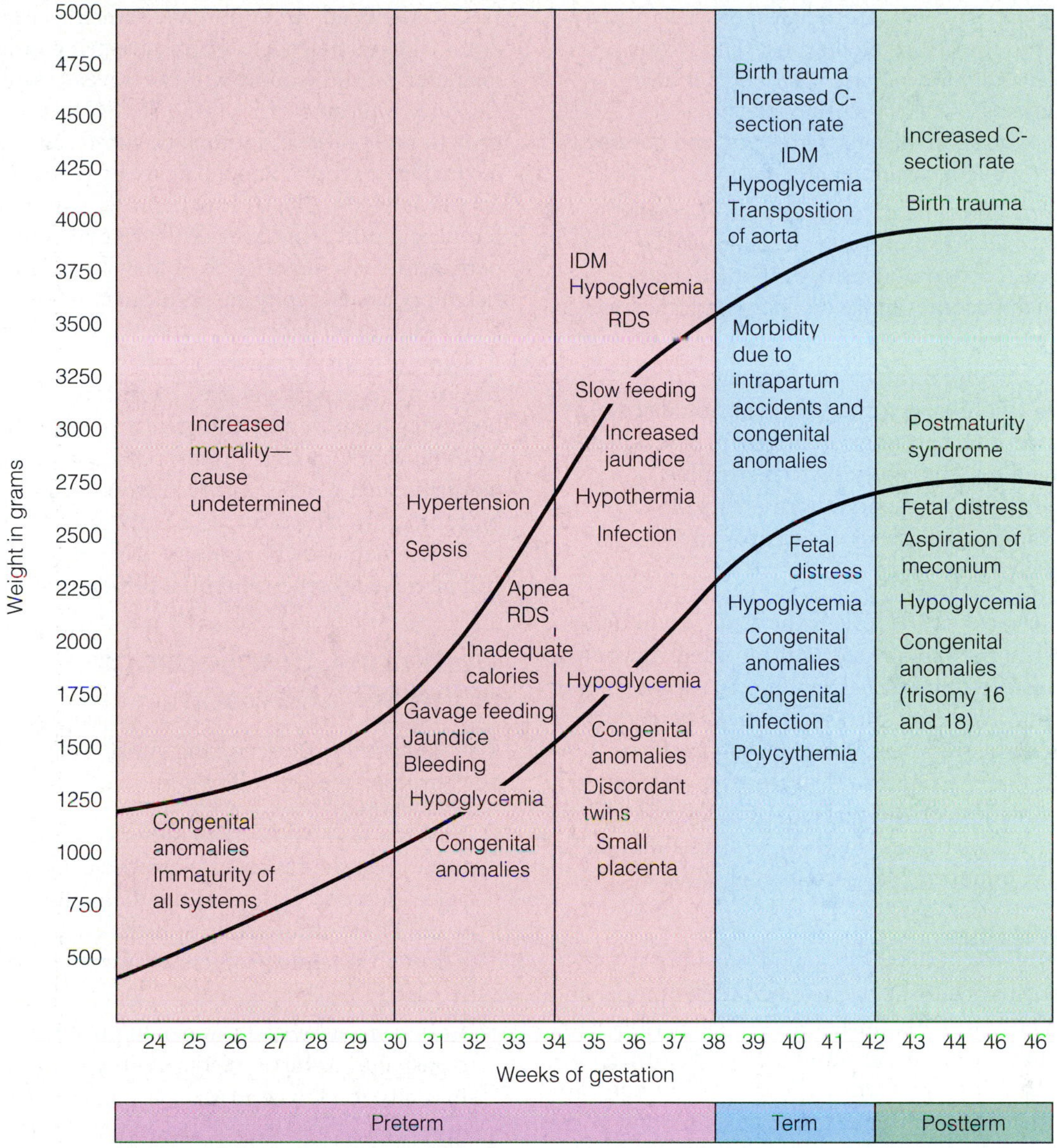

Figure 32–2 • Neonatal morbidity by birth weight and gestational age.
SOURCE: Lubchenco, L. O. (1976). *The high risk infant.* (p. 122) Philadelphia: Saunders.

SGA infants have an increased incidence of perinatal asphyxia and perinatal mortality compared to AGA infants (Bernstein, Gabbe, & Reed, 2002). The incidence of polycythemia and hypoglycemia are also higher in this group of infants.

Factors Contributing to Intrauterine Growth Restriction

IUGR may be caused by maternal, placental, or fetal factors and may not be apparent antenatally. In the normal pregnancy, intrauterine growth is linear from approximately 28 to 38 weeks' gestation. After 38 weeks, growth is variable, depending on the genetic growth potential of the fetus and placental function. The most common factors affecting growth restriction are the following:

- *Maternal factors.* Primiparity, grand multiparity, multiple pregnancy (twins and higher order multiples), lack of prenatal care, age extremes (under 16 or over 40), and low socioeconomic status (which can result in inadequate healthcare, inadequate education, and inadequate living conditions) affect IUGR (Bernstein et al, 2002). Before the third trimester, the nutritional supply to the fetus far exceeds its needs. Only in the third trimester is maternal malnutrition a limiting factor in fetal growth.
- *Maternal disease.* Maternal heart disease, substance abuse (drugs, tobacco, alcohol), sickle cell anemia, phenylketonuria (PKU), and asymptomatic pyelonephritis are associated with SGA. Complications associated with preeclampsia, chronic hypertensive vascular disease, and advanced diabetes mellitus (White's classes D through F) diminish blood flow to the uterus.

- *Environmental factors.* High altitude, exposure to x-rays, excessive exercise, work-related exposure to toxins, hyperthermia, and maternal use of drugs that have teratogenic effects, such as nicotine, alcohol, antimetabolics, anticonvulsants, narcotics, and cocaine, affect fetal growth (Bernstein et al, 2002).
- *Placental factors.* Placental conditions such as small placenta, infarcted areas, abnormal cord insertions, placenta previa, or thrombosis may affect circulation to the fetus, which becomes more deficient with increasing gestational age.
- *Fetal factors.* Congenital infections (rubella, toxoplasmosis, syphilis, cytomegalic inclusion disease), congenital malformations, discordant twins (see Chapter 11), sex of the fetus (females tend to be smaller), chromosomal syndromes, and inborn errors of metabolism can predispose a fetus to growth disturbances.

Identifying fetuses with IUGR is the first step in detecting common disorders associated with affected newborns. The perinatal history of maternal conditions, early dating of pregnancy by first trimester ultrasound measurements, antepartal testing (nonstress test, contraction stress test, biophysical profile—see Chapter 21), Doppler velocimetry, pathology examination of the placenta, gestational age assessment, and the physical and neurologic assessment of the newborn are also important (Bernstein et al, 2002).

Patterns of IUGR

Intrauterine growth occurs by an increase in cell number and cell size. If insult occurs early during the critical period of organ development in the fetus, fewer new cells are formed, organs are small, and organ weight is subnormal. In contrast, growth failure that begins later in pregnancy does not affect the total number of cells, only their size. The organs are normal, but their size is diminished. There are two clinical pictures of IUGR newborns.

Symmetric (proportional) IUGR is caused by long-term maternal conditions (such as chronic hypertension, severe malnutrition, chronic intrauterine infection, substance abuse, and anemia) or fetal genetic abnormalities (Kliegman & Das, 2002). Symmetric IUGR can be noted by ultrasound in the first half of the second trimester. In symmetric IUGR there is chronic prolonged restriction of growth in size of organs, body weight, body length, and, in severe cases, head circumference.

Asymmetric (disproportional) IUGR is associated with an acute compromise of uteroplacental blood flow. Some associated causes are placental infarcts, preeclampsia, and poor weight gain in pregnancy. The growth restriction is usually not evident before the third trimester because although weight is decreased, length and head circumference remain appropriate for that gestational age. After 36 weeks' gestation, the abdominal circumference of a normal fetus becomes larger than the head circumference. In asymmetric IUGR, the head circumference remains larger than the abdominal circumference. Thus measuring only the biparietal diameter on ultrasound will not reveal asymmetric IUGR. An early indicator of asymmetric SGA is a decrease in the growth rate of the abdominal circumference, reflecting subnormal liver growth and a paucity of subcutaneous fat. Birth weight is below the 10th percentile, whereas head circumference, and/or length, may plot between the 10th and 90th percentiles. Asymmetric SGA newborns are particularly at risk for perinatal asphyxia, pulmonary hemorrhage, hypocalcemia, and hypoglycemia in the newborn period.

Despite growth restriction, physiologic maturity develops according to gestational age. Therefore, the term SGA newborn may be more physiologically mature than the preterm AGA newborn and less predisposed to complications of prematurity such as respiratory distress syndrome and hyperbilirubinemia. The term SGA newborn's chances for survival are better because of organ maturity, although this newborn still faces many other potential difficulties.

Common Complications of the SGA Newborn

The complications occurring most frequently in the SGA newborn include the following:

- *Asphyxia.* The SGA infant suffers chronic hypoxia in utero because of placental insufficiency, which leaves little reserve to withstand the demands of labor and birth. Thus intrauterine asphyxia occurs with its potential systemic problems. Cesarean birth may be necessary.
- *Aspiration syndrome.* In utero, hypoxia can cause the fetus to gasp during birth, resulting in aspiration of amniotic fluid into the lower airways. It can also lead to relaxation of the anal sphincter and passage of meconium. This may result in aspiration of the meconium in utero or with the first breaths following birth.
- *Hypothermia.* Diminished subcutaneous fat (used for survival in utero), depletion of brown fat in utero, and a large surface area decrease the IUGR newborn's ability to conserve heat. The effect of surface area is diminished somewhat because of the flexed position assumed by the term SGA newborn.
- *Hypoglycemia.* An increase in metabolic rate in response to heat loss and poor hepatic glycogen stores cause hypoglycemia. In addition, the infant is compromised by inadequate supplies of enzymes to activate gluconeogenesis (conversion of nonglucogen sources, such as fatty acids and proteins, to glucose).
- *Polycythemia.* The number of red blood cells is increased in the SGA newborn. This finding is considered a physiologic response to in utero chronic hypoxic stress. Newborns who have significant IUGR tend to have a poor prognosis, especially when born before 37 weeks' gestation. Factors contributing to poor outcome include:

- *Congenital malformations.* Congenital malformations occur 10 to 20 times more frequently in SGA infants than in AGA infants (Kliegman & Das, 2002). The more severe the IUGR, the greater the chance for malformation as a result of impaired mitotic activity and cellular hypoplasia.
- *Intrauterine infection.* When fetuses are exposed to intrauterine infections such as rubella and cytomegalovirus, they are profoundly affected by direct invasion of the brain and other vital organs by the offending virus, resulting in IUGR.
- *Continued growth difficulties.* SGA newborns tend to be shorter than newborns of the same gestational age. Asymmetric IUGR infants can be expected to catch up in weight and approach their inherited growth potential when given an optimal environment. Symmetric IUGR infants reportedly have varied growth potential but tend not to catch up to their peers (Kliegman & Das, 2002).
- *Cognitive difficulties.* Often SGA newborns can exhibit subsequent learning disabilities. The disabilities are characterized by hyperactivity, short attention span, and poor fine motor coordination (writing and drawing). Some hearing loss and speech defects also occur.

Clinical Therapy

The goal of medical therapy for SGA infants is early recognition and implementation of medical management of the potential problems.

NURSING CARE MANAGEMENT

Nursing Assessment and Diagnosis

The nurse is responsible for assessing gestational age and identifying signs of potential complications associated with SGA infants.

All body parts of the symmetric IUGR infant are in proportion, but they are below normal size for the baby's gestational age. Therefore the head does not appear overly large or the length excessive in relation to the other body parts. These newborns are generally vigorous.

The asymmetric IUGR infant appears long, thin, and emaciated, with loss of subcutaneous fat tissue and muscle mass (Figure 32–3 •). The baby may have loose skin folds; dry, desquamating skin; and a thin and often meconium-stained cord. The head appears relatively large (although it approaches normal size) because the chest size and abdominal girth are decreased. The baby may have a vigorous cry and appear alert and wide eyed.

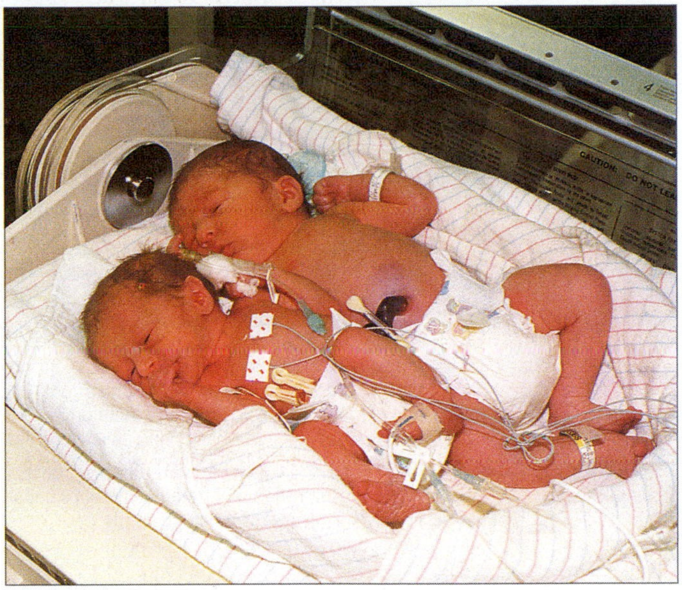

Figure 32–3 • Thirty-five-week gestational age twins. Twin B is SGA and weighs 1260 g. Twin A is AGA and weighs 2605 g.
SOURCE: Courtesy of Carol Harrigan, RNC, MSN, NNP.

Nursing diagnoses that may apply to the SGA newborn include the following:

- ***Impaired Gas Exchange*** related to aspiration of meconium
- ***Hypothermia*** related to decreased subcutaneous fat
- ***Risk for Injury to Tissues*** related to decreased glycogen stores and impaired gluconeogenesis
- ***Altered Nutrition: Less than Body Requirements*** related to SGA's increased metabolic rate
- ***Risk for Altered Tissue Perfusion*** related to polycythemia and increased blood viscosity
- ***Risk for Altered Parenting*** related to prolonged separation of newborn from parents secondary to illness

Nursing Plan and Implementation

Hospital-Based Nursing Care

Hypoglycemia, the most common metabolic complication of IUGR, produces such sequelae as central nervous system abnormalities and mental retardation. Conditions such as asphyxia, hyperviscosity, and cold stress may also affect the baby's outcome. Meticulous attention to physiologic parameters is essential for immediate nursing management and reduction of long-term disorders (see the Clinical Pathway for Small-for-Gestational-Age Newborns on page 894).

Community-Based Nursing Care

The long-term needs of the SGA newborn include careful follow-up evaluation of patterns of growth and possible disabilities that may later interfere with learning or motor functioning. Long-term follow-up care is especially necessary for those infants with congenital malformations, congenital infections, and obvious sequelae from

CLINICAL PATHWAY FOR SMALL-FOR-GESTATIONAL-AGE NEWBORNS

Category	Day of Birth—First 4 Hours	Remaining Day of Birth
Referral	Report from L&D, neonatal nurse practitioner Check ID bands Prn consults: high-risk peds, genetics	Check ID bands q shift As parents desire, obtain circumcision permit after their discussion with MD Lactation consult prn
Assessments	(Refer to Newborn Clinical Pathway, Chapter 30) • Complete set of VS • Admission wt, length, HC • Assess skin color • Gestational age assessment • Assess for s/s hypoglycemia. Chemstrip ASAP after birth, then follow SGA policy and procedure for blood glucose monitoring • Assess for polycythemia: follow policy for treatment prn	Vital signs: T/P/R q4h and prn, BP prn Newborn assessment q shift (See Newborn Clinical Pathway, Chapter 30 Continue hypoglycemia assessments, chemstrips per SGA protocol Assess mother/baby interaction
Teaching/ psychosocial	(See Newborn Clinical Pathway, Chapter 30) Admission activities performed at mother's bedside if possible, orient to nursery, handwashing, assess teaching needs Teach parents rationale for SGA protocol	(See Newborn Clinical Pathway, Chapter 30) Reinforce previous teaching Teach parent/guardian feeding methods, burping, diapering, calming techniques, s/s of stress, elimination norms
Nursing care management and reports	Diagnostic Tests: blood type, Rh, Coombs' on cord blood when applicable, chemstrip within 1 h of birth and q1–2h until feedings initiated per protocol Check chemstrip before at least two feedings or until condition stabilizes (chemstrip $>$ 40 mg/dL x 2)	Femoral pulse or BP all 4 extremities if early DC Hct per policy Hearing screen Cord care per policy Bathe per policy
Activity and comfort	Place under radiant warmer, attach skin probe to maintain NTE Soothe baby as needed with voice, touch, nesting in warmer	Leave in radiant warmer until stable, then swaddle in open crib Incubator if temp instability; adjust incubator for infant size and gestation to maintain NTE
Nutrition	Initiate breast- or formula-feeding as soon as mother and baby condition allows Lavage and gavage prn Supplement breast when medically indicated or ordered by MD per policy Feed SGA infants q3–4h Monitor feeding tolerance, suck	Continue feeding schedule: small frequent feedings, high-calorie formula, nutritional fortifiers
Elimination	Note first void and stool if not at birth	Note all voids, amount and color of stools q4h
Medication	AquaMEPHYTON IM, dosage according to infant wt per MD orders Ilotycin ophth ointment OU	Hep B vaccine as ordered by MD after consent signed by parent
Discharge planning/ home care	Hep B consent reviewed with parents Plan DC with parent/guardian in 1–3 days Evaluate for social services/home care/discharge planning needs	Hep B consent signed by parents Birth certificate instructions/worksheet Car seat for DC
Family Involvement	Evaluate psychosocial needs Evaluate parent teaching Access community resources prn, ie, Teen "Healthy Starts"	Assess parents' knowledge of newborn behavior and reflexes Encourage family involvement in infant's care as possible and as infant tolerates
Date		

Category	Day 1	Day 2/3 (if applicable)
Referral	Check ID bands q shift	Check ID bands q shift ➤ **Expected Outcomes** Mother/baby ID bands correlate at time of discharge. Consults completed prn.
Assessments	Assess thermoregulation Assess for potential complications: perinatal asphyxia, aspiration syndrome, hypoglycemia, hypocalcemia, polycythemia Assess mother/baby interaction	Assess color for jaundice Assess for apnea Assess mother/baby interaction ➤ **Expected Outcomes** Physical assessments, VS WNL; no complications of SGA noted
Teaching/ psychosocial	(See Newborn Clinical Pathway, Chapter 30) Reinforce previous teaching Parent teaching: bathing, cord care, skin/nail care, use of thermometer, activity, sleep patterns, soothing, reflexes, jaundice, growth/feeding patterns	Final Discharge Teaching (See Newborn Clinical Pathway, Chapter 30) Review infant safety, s/s of illness and when to call healthcare provider with parents ➤ **Expected Outcomes** Mother verbalizes comprehension of instructions, demonstrates care capabilities

➤

CLINICAL PATHWAY FOR SMALL-FOR-GESTATIONAL-AGE NEWBORNS *CONTINUED*

Category	Day 1	Day 2/3 (if applicable)
Nursing care management and reports	Scalp treatment BID Daily wt Newborn assessment q shift Check circumcision site q diaper change Unclamp cord clamp Cord care per policy Total bilirubin level prn	Newborn assessment q shift Daily wt Check circumcision site Cord care per policy Note Baer hearing test results Femoral pulse or BP all 4 extremities ➤ **Expected Outcomes** Physical assessments WNL; cord unclamped and dry without s/s of infection; circ site unremarkable; gaining wt or wt stabilized to not > 10% loss, labs WNL
Activity and comfort	Swaddled in open crib Incubator if temp instability; adjust incubator for infant size and gestation to maintain NTE	➤ **Expected Outcomes** Maintains temp WNL swaddled in open crib
Nutrition	Continue enhanced feeding schedule, gavage prn per MD orders Supplement breast only when medically indicated/policy or ordered by MD/NP Encourage on-demand feeds, minimally q3–4h, breast or formula	Continue enhanced feeding schedule, gavage prn per MD/NP orders ➤ **Expected Outcomes** Infant tolerates feedings, feeds on demand, breastfeeds without supplement, nipples without problems; regaining lost wt or wt stabilized
Elimination	Evaluate all voids and stool color q8h ➤ **Expected Outcomes** Voids and stools without difficulty	Note all voids and stool color q shift ➤ **Expected Outcomes** Voids qs, stools without difficulty and WNL
Medication	Hep B vaccine before discharge	➤ **Expected Outcomes** Infant has received ophth ointment OU and AquaMEPHYTON injection; received first Hep B vaccine if ordered and parental consent given
Discharge planning/ home care	Newborn photographs Complete birth certificate packet If vag birth, complete DC teaching	If C/S birth complete DC instructions (See Newborn Clinical Pathway, Chapter 30) ➤ **Expected Outcomes** Infant DC home with mother; mother verbalizes follow-up appointment time/date
Family Involvement	Bath, newborn care and feeding classes Newborn channel as available Assess mother/baby bonding and interaction Incorporate significant others and siblings in care Support positive parenting behaviors Evaluate mother/parent teaching	Assess mother/baby bonding and interaction Identify community referral needs and refer to community agencies ➤ **Expected Outcomes** Demonstrates caring and family incorporation of infant
Date		

ASAP, as soon as possible; C/S birth, cesarean birth; ID, identification; DC, discharge; HC, head circumference; Hct, hematocrit; LD, labor and delivery; NTE, neutral thermal environment; ophth, ophthalmic; OU, both eyes; q, every; SGA, small for gestational age; s/s, signs and symptoms; vag, vaginal; VS, vital signs; wt, weight; WNL, within normal limits.

physiologic problems. In addition, the parents of the IUGR baby need support because a positive atmosphere can enhance the baby's growth potential and the child's ultimate outcome.

Evaluation

Expected outcomes of nursing care include the following:

- The SGA newborn is free from respiratory compromise.
- The SGA newborn maintains a stable temperature and glucose hemostasis.
- The SGA newborn gains weight and takes breast- or formula-feedings without physiologic distress or fatigue.
- The parents verbalize their concerns surrounding their baby's health problems and understand the rationale behind management of their newborn.

Care of the Large-for-Gestational-Age Newborn

A newborn whose birth weight is at or above the 90th percentile on the intrauterine growth curve (at any week of gestation) is considered **large for gestational age (LGA).** Some appropriate-for-gestational-age (AGA) newborns have been incorrectly categorized as LGA because of miscalculation of the date of conception due to postconceptional bleeding. Careful gestational age assessment is essential to identify the potential needs and problems of such infants.

The best known condition associated with excessive fetal growth is maternal diabetes (White's classes A through C; see Table 19–4); however, only a small fraction of LGA newborns are born to diabetic mothers. The cause of the majority of cases of LGA infants is unclear, but certain factors or situations have been found to correlate with their births (Langer, 2000):

- Genetic predisposition is correlated proportionally to the mother's prepregnancy weight and to weight gain during pregnancy. Large parents tend to have large infants.
- Multiparous women have two to three times the number of LGA infants as primigravidas.
- Male infants are typically larger than female infants.
- Infants with erythroblastosis fetalis, Beckwith-Wiedemann syndrome (a genetic condition associated with macroglossia, omphalocele, and newborn hypoglycemia and hyperinsulinemia), or transposition of the great vessels are usually large.

The increase in the LGA infant's body size is characteristically proportional, although head circumference and body length are in the upper limits of intrauterine growth. The exception to this rule is the infant of the diabetic mother, whose body weight is higher but whose length and head circumference may be in the normal range. Macrosomic infants have poor motor skills and have more difficulty in regulating behavioral states. LGA infants tend to be more difficult to arouse and may have problems maintaining a quiet alert state. They may also have feeding difficulties.

Common Complications of the LGA Newborn

Complications of the LGA infant can include the following:

- *Birth trauma due to cephalopelvic disproportion (CPD).* Often LGA newborns have a biparietal diameter greater than 10 cm (4 in) or are associated with a maternal fundal height measurement greater than 42 cm (16 in) without the presence of hydramnios. Because of their excessive size, there are more breech presentations and shoulder dystocia. These complications may result in asphyxia, fractured clavicles, brachial plexus palsy, facial paralysis, phrenic nerve palsy, depressed skull fractures, cephalhematoma, and intracranial hemorrhage due to birth trauma.
- *Increased incidence of cesarean births and oxytocin-induced births due to fetal size.* These births are accompanied by all the risk factors associated with cesarean births (Chatfield, 2001).
- *Hypoglycemia, polycythemia, and hyperviscosity.* These disorders are most often seen in infants of diabetic mothers and infants with erythroblastosis fetalis or Beckwith-Wiedemann syndrome.

NURSING CARE MANAGEMENT

The perinatal history, in conjunction with ultrasonic measurement of fetal skull and gestational age testing, is important in identifying an at-risk LGA newborn. Nursing care is directed toward early identification and immediate treatment of the common disorders. Essential components of the nursing assessment are monitoring vital signs, screening for hypoglycemia and polycythemia, and observing for signs and symptoms related to birth trauma. The nurse should address parental concerns about the visual signs of birth trauma and the potential for continuation of the overweight pattern. The nurse should help parents learn to arouse and console their newborn and facilitate nutritional intake and attachment behaviors. Mothers of LGA infants with bruising of the face or head may be reluctant to interact with their infants because they fear increasing the bruising or causing their infants pain. The nursing care for complications associated with LGA newborns is similar to the care needed by the infant of a diabetic mother and will be discussed in the next section.

Care of the Infant of a Diabetic Mother

Infants of diabetic mothers (IDMs) are considered at risk and require close observation the first few hours to the first few days of life. Mothers with severe diabetes or diabetes of long duration (type 1 or White's classes D through F, associated with vascular complications) may give birth to small-for-gestational-age (SGA) infants. However, the typical IDM (type 1 when the diabetes is poorly controlled, or White's classes A and C) is LGA. The infant is macrosomic, ruddy in color, and has excess adipose fat tissue (Figure 32–4 •). The umbilical cord is thick and the placenta is large. There is a higher incidence of macrosomic infants born to certain ethnic groups (Native Americans, Mexican Americans, African Americans, and Pacific Islanders) (Doshier, 1995; Homko, Sivan, Nyirjesy, et al, 1995).

IDMs have decreased total body water, particularly in the extracellular spaces, and are therefore not edematous. Their excessive weight is due to increased weight of the visceral organs, cardiomegaly (hypertrophy), and increased body fat. The only organ not affected is the brain.

The excessive fetal growth of the IDM is caused by exposure to high levels of maternal glucose, which readily crosses the placenta. The fetus responds to these high glucose levels with increased insulin production and hyperplasia of the pancreatic beta cells. The main action of insulin is to facilitate the entry of glucose into muscle and fat cells.

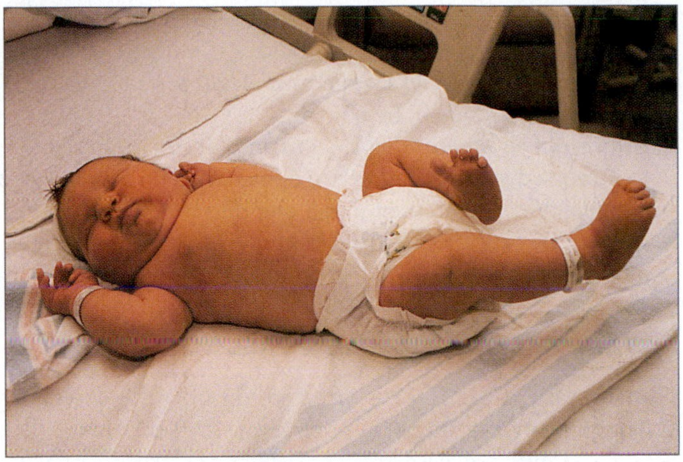

Figure 32–4 • Macrosomic infant of a diabetic mother.

Once in the cells, glucose is converted to glycogen and stored. Insulin also inhibits the breakdown of fat to free fatty acids, thereby maintaining lipid synthesis; increases the uptake of amino acids; and promotes protein synthesis. Insulin is an important regulator of fetal metabolism and has a "growth hormone" effect that results in increased linear growth. IDMs may be obese as children (Landon, Catalano, & Gabbe, 2002).

Common Complications of the IDM

Although IDMs are usually large, they are immature in physiologic functions and exhibit many of the problems of the preterm (premature) infant. The complications most often seen in an IDM are as follows:

- *Hypoglycemia.* Even though the high maternal blood sugar supply is lost, the IDM continues to produce high levels of insulin, which deplete the infant's blood glucose within hours after birth. IDMs also have less ability to release glucagon and catecholamines, which normally stimulate glucagon breakdown and glucose release. The incidence of hypoglycemia in IDMs varies from 30% to 50% (Landon et al, 2002). The incidence varies according to the degree of success in controlling the maternal diabetes, the maternal blood sugar level at the time of birth, the length of labor, the class of maternal diabetes, and early versus late feedings of the newborn. Signs and symptoms of hypoglycemia include tremors, cyanosis, apnea, temperature instability, poor feeding, and hypotonia. Seizures may occur in severe cases.

> **Clinical Tip** *When beginning fluids on an IDM, it is sometimes best to start at a higher concentration of dextrose to avoid hypoglycemia episodes.*

- *Hypocalcemia.* Tremors are the obvious clinical sign of hypocalcemia. This may be due to the IDM's prematurity and to the stresses of difficult pregnancy, labor, and birth. Diabetic women tend to have decreased serum magnesium levels at term secondary to increased urinary calcium excretion, which causes secondary hypoparathyroidism in their infants. Other factors may include vitamin D antagonism, which results from elevated cortisol levels, hypophosphatemia from tissue catabolism, and decreased serum magnesium levels.
- *Hyperbilirubinemia.* This condition may be seen at 48 to 72 hours after birth. It may be caused by slightly decreased extracellular fluid volume, which increases the hematocrit level. This in turn will cause an increase in red blood cell breakdown that will increase bilirubin. The presence of hepatic immaturity may impair bilirubin conjugation. Enclosed hemorrhages resulting from complicated vaginal birth may also cause hyperbilirubinemia.
- *Birth trauma.* Because most IDMs are macrosomic, trauma may occur during labor and birth from shoulder dystocia.
- *Polycythemia.* This condition may be caused by the decreased extracellular fluid volume in IDMs. Fetal hyperglycemia and hyperinsulinism results in increased oxygen consumption, leading to fetal hypoxia (Landon et al, 2002). Hemoglobin A_{1c} binds to oxygen, decreasing the oxygen available to the fetal tissues. This tissue hypoxia stimulates increased erythropoietin production, which increases both the hematocrit level and the potential for hyperbilirubinemia. See Chapter 19 for discussion of hemoglobin A_{1c}.
- *Respiratory distress syndrome (RDS).* This complication occurs more frequently in newborns of White's classes A through C diabetic mothers who are not well controlled (Landon et al, 2002). Insulin antagonizes the cortisol-induced stimulation of lecithin synthesis that is necessary for lung maturation. Therefore, IDMs may have lungs that are less mature than expected for their gestational age. There is also a decrease in the phospholipid phosphatidylglycerol (PG), which stabilizes surfactant. The insufficiency of PG increases the incidence of respiratory distress syndrome (RDS). Therefore, it is important to test for the presence of PG in the amniotic fluid.

  RDS does not appear to be problematic for infants born to diabetic mothers in White's classes D through F; instead, the stresses of poor uterine blood supply may lead to increased production of steroids, which accelerates lung maturation. IDMs may also have a delay in closure of the ductus arteriosus and decreases in postnatal pulmonary artery pressure (Landon et al, 2002).
- *Congenital birth defects.* These may include transposition of the great vessels, ventricular septal defect, left or right ventricular wall hypertrophy, small left colon syndrome, and sacral agenesis (caudal regression) (Landon et al, 2002). Early careful control of maternal glucose before and during pregnancy decreases the risk of birth defects. See Chapter 19.

Clinical Therapy

The goal of clinical therapy is the early detection of and intervention in the problems associated with infants born to diabetic mothers. Prenatal management is directed toward controlling maternal glucose levels, which minimizes the common complications of IDMs.

Because the onset of hypoglycemia occurs between 1 and 3 hours after birth in IDMs (with a spontaneous rise to normal levels by 4 to 6 hours), blood glucose determinations should be performed initially on cord blood then on capillary or venous blood samples hourly during the first 4 hours after birth and at 4-hour intervals until the risk period (about 24 hours) has passed or per agency protocol.

IDMs whose serum glucose falls below 40 mg/dL should have early feedings with formula or breast milk (colostrum). If normal glucose levels cannot be maintained with oral feeding an intravenous infusion of glucose will be necessary. An infusion of D-10-W at a rate of 4 to 6 mg/kg/min usually maintains normoglycemia in the IDM. If higher glucose concentrations are needed to maintain normal serum glucose levels, a central line will be placed to minimize tissue extravasation. Newborns with refractory hypoglycemia may benefit by the administration of intravenous corticosteroids. Once the blood glucose has been stable for 24 hours, the infusion rate can be decreased as oral feedings are increased. The newborn's blood glucose levels must be carefully monitored. Repeated dextrose as a bolus infusion is contraindicated because it may lead to severe rebound hypoglycemia following an initial brief increase in glucose level.

NURSING CARE MANAGEMENT

Nursing Assessment and Diagnosis

The nurse should not be lulled into thinking that a big baby is a mature baby. In almost every case, because of the infant's large size, the IDM will appear older than gestational age scoring indicates. The nurse must consider both the gestational age and whether the baby is AGA or LGA in planning and providing safe care. In caring for the IDM, the nurse assesses for signs of respiratory distress, hyperbilirubinemia, birth trauma, and congenital anomalies.

Nursing diagnoses that may apply to IDMs include the following:

- ***Altered Nutrition: Less than Body Requirements*** related to increased glucose metabolism secondary to hyperinsulinemia
- ***Impaired Gas Exchange*** related to respiratory distress secondary to impaired production of surfactant
- ***Alteration in Calcium Homeostasis*** related to inappropriate parathyroid response
- ***Increased Incidence of Congenital Anomalies*** related to poor maternal metabolic control
- ***Alteration in Hematologic Status: Polycythemia*** related to increased synthesis of erythropoietin secondary to hypoxia due to increased metabolic rate
- ***Ineffective Family Coping: Compromised,*** related to the illness of the baby

Nursing Plan and Implementation

Nursing care of the IDM is directed toward early detection and ongoing monitoring of hypoglycemia (by performing glucose tests) and polycythemia (by obtaining central hematocrits), respiratory distress, and hyperbilirubinemia. For specific nursing interventions for respiratory distress syndrome, hypoglycemia, hyperbilirubinemia, and polycythemia, see Chapter 33. Also assess for signs of birth trauma and congenital anomalies.

Parent teaching is directed toward preventing macrosomia and the resulting fetal-newborn problems and instituting early and ongoing diabetic control. Parents are advised that with early identification and care, most IDMs' complications have no significant sequelae.

Evaluation

Expected outcomes of nursing care include the following:

- The IDM's respiratory and metabolic alteration problems are minimized.
- The parents understand the etiology of the baby's health problems and preventive steps they can initiate to decrease the impact of maternal diabetes on subsequent fetuses.
- The parents verbalize their concerns surrounding their baby's health problems and understand the rationale behind management of their newborn.

Care of the Postterm Newborn

The **postterm newborn** is any newborn born after 42 weeks' gestation. Postterm or prolonged pregnancy occurs in approximately 4% to 14% of all pregnancies (Blackburn, 2003). The cause of most postterm pregnancies is not completely understood, but several factors are known to be associated with it, including primiparity, high multiparity (five or more pregnancies), and a history of prolonged pregnancies. Many pregnancies classified as prolonged are thought to be a result of inaccurate determination of the estimated date of birth (EDB). Postterm pregnancy is more common in Australian, Greek, and Italian ethnic groups.

Most babies born as a result of prolonged pregnancy are of normal size and health; some keep on growing and are over 4000 g at birth, which supports the contention that the postterm fetus can remain well nourished. Potential intrapartal problems for these healthy but large fetuses include cephalopelvic disproportion (CPD) and shoulder dystocia. See Chapter 26 for discussion of the necessary assessments and interventions for CPD and shoulder dystocia.

Common Complications of the Newborn with Postmaturity Syndrome

The term **postmaturity** applies only to the infant who is born after 42 completed weeks of gestation and also demonstrates characteristics of *postmaturity syndrome*. Only about 5% of postterm newborns are also postmature. The truly postmature newborn is at high risk for morbidity and has a mortality rate two to three times higher than that of term infants. Although today the percentages are extremely low, the majority of postmature fetal deaths occur during labor, because by that time the fetus has used up necessary body reserves.

Postmaturity syndrome is characterized by decreased placental function, which impairs nutrition transport and oxygenation, leaving the fetus prone to hypoglycemia and hypoxemia when the stresses of labor begin. The following are common disorders of the postmature newborn:

- Hypoglycemia from nutritional deprivation and resultant depleted glycogen stores.
- Meconium aspiration in response to in utero hypoxia. The presence of oligohydramnios increases the danger of aspirating thick meconium. Severe meconium aspiration syndrome increases the baby's chance of developing persistent pulmonary hypertension, pneumothorax, and pneumonia.
- Polycythemia due to increased production of red blood cells (RBCs) in response to hypoxia.
- Congenital anomalies of unknown cause.
- Seizures due to hypoxic insult.
- Cold stress due to loss or poor development of subcutaneous fat.

The long-term effects of postmaturity syndrome are unclear. At present, studies do not agree on the effect of postmaturity syndrome on weight gain and IQ scores (Divon, 2002).

Prolonged pregnancy by itself is not responsible for the postmaturity syndrome. The characteristics of the postmature newborn are caused primarily by a combination of placental aging and subsequent insufficiency and continued exposure to amniotic fluid.

Clinical Therapy

The aim of antenatal management is to differentiate the fetus who has postmaturity syndrome from the fetus who is large, well nourished, and active and who is tolerating the prolonged (postterm) pregnancy.

Antenatal tests that can be done to evaluate fetal status and determine obstetric management are discussed in more depth in Chapters 21 and 26. If the amniotic fluid is meconium stained, an amnioinfusion may be done during labor. This procedure dilutes the meconium, decreasing the risk of meconium aspiration syndrome. (For detailed discussion of clinical management and care of the newborn at risk for meconium aspiration, see Chapter 33.)

Hypoglycemia is monitored by serial glucose determinations as per agency protocols. The baby may be placed on glucose infusions or given early feedings if respiratory distress is not present, but these measures must be instituted with caution because of the frequency of asphyxia in the first 24 hours. Postmature newborns are often voracious eaters.

As with SGA infants, peripheral and central hematocrits are tested to diagnose polycythemia. Fluid resuscitation can be initiated, and in extreme cases a partial exchange transfusion may be necessary to manage polycythemia and adverse sequelae such as hyperviscosity. Oxygen is provided for respiratory distress. Also, temperature instability and excessive loss of body heat can result from decreased liver glycogen stores. See Chapter 30 for thermoregulation techniques.

NURSING CARE MANAGEMENT

Nursing Assessment and Diagnosis

The newborn with postmaturity syndrome appears alert. This wide-eyed, alert appearance is not necessarily a positive sign because it may indicate chronic intrauterine hypoxia. The infant has dry, cracking, parchmentlike skin without vernix or lanugo (Figure 32–5 ●). Fingernails are long, and scalp hair is profuse. The infant's body appears long and thin. The wasting involves depletion of previously stored subcutaneous tissue, causing the skin to be loose. Fat layers are almost nonexistent.

Postmature newborns frequently have meconium staining, which colors the nails, skin, and umbilical cord. The varying shades (yellow to green) of meconium staining can give some clue about whether the expulsion of meconium was a recent or a chronic problem. Green coloring indicates a more recent event.

Nursing diagnoses that may apply to the postmature newborn include the following:

- ***Hypothermia*** related to decreased liver glycogen and brown fat stores
- ***Altered Nutrition: Less than Body Requirements*** related to increased use of glucose secondary to stress in utero and decreased placental perfusion
- ***Impaired Gas Exchange in the Lungs and at the Cellular Level*** related to airway obstruction from meconium aspiration
- ***Risk for Altered Tissue Perfusion*** related to increased blood viscosity

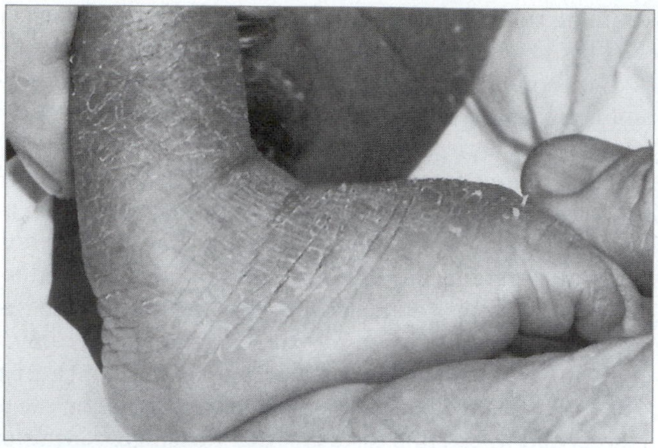

Figure 32–5 • The skin of the postterm infant exhibits deep cracking and peeling.
SOURCE: Dubowitz, L., & Dubowitz, V. (1977). *The gestational age of the newborn.* Menlo Park, CA: Addison-Wesley. Reprinted by permission of V. Dubowitz, MD, Hammersmith Hospital, London, England.

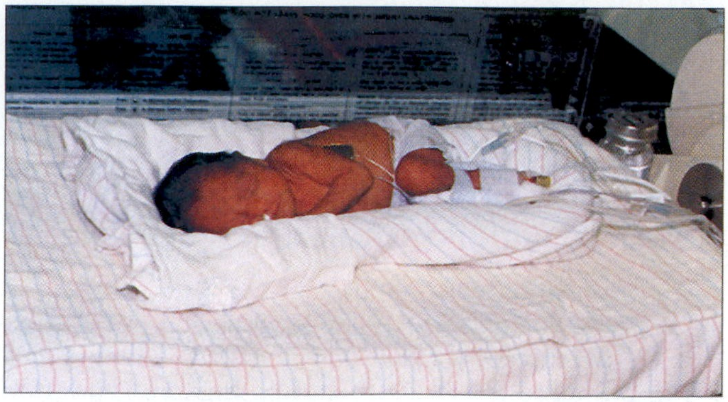

Figure 32–6 • A 6-day-old, 28 weeks' gestational age, 960-g preterm infant.
SOURCE: Courtesy of Carol Harrigan, RNC, MSN, NNP.

MediaLink CASE STUDY: POSTTERM NEWBORN

Nursing Plan and Implementation

Nursing interventions are primarily supportive measures. They include the following:

- Monitor cardiopulmonary status because the stresses of labor are poorly tolerated and can result in hypoxemia in utero and possible asphyxia at birth.
- Provide warmth to counterbalance the infant's poor response to cold stress and decreased liver glycogen and brown fat stores.
- Frequently monitor blood glucose and initiate early feeding (at 1 or 2 hours of age) or intravenous glucose per physician order.
- Obtain a central hematocrit to determine accurately the presence of polycythemia.

The nurse encourages parents to express their feelings and fears regarding the newborn's condition and potential long-term problems. The nurse also gives careful explanations of procedures, includes the parents in developing care plans for their baby, and encourages follow-up care as needed.

Evaluation

Expected outcomes of nursing care include the following:

- The postterm newborn establishes effective respiratory function.
- The postmature baby is free of metabolic alterations (hypoglycemia) and maintains a stable temperature.

Care of the Preterm (Premature) Newborn

A **preterm infant** is an infant born before the completion of 37 weeks' gestation (Figure 32–6 •). With the help of modern technology, infants are surviving at younger gestational ages, but not without significant morbidity. The incidence of preterm births in the United States is approximately 8%. The rise in multiple birth rates has markedly influenced overall rates of low-birth-weight (LBW) infants (Hoyert, Freedman, Strobino, et al, 2001). The rate of LBW infants between 1999 and 2000 has declined slightly among black women (from 13.1% to 12.9%) and was unchanged for non-Hispanic white (6.6%) and Hispanic (6.4%) mothers. A higher incidence is also seen in single women and adolescents. (See Chapter 20 for a discussion of preterm labor.)

The major problem of the preterm newborn is variable immaturity of all systems. The degree of immaturity depends on the length of gestation. The preterm newborn must traverse the same complex, interconnected pathways from intrauterine to extrauterine life as the term newborn; however, the preterm newborn's immature tissues and organs are ill-equipped to make this transition smoothly. Maintenance of the preterm newborn falls within narrow physiologic parameters.

Alteration in Respiratory and Cardiovascular Physiology

The preterm newborn is at risk for respiratory problems because the lungs are not fully mature and not fully ready to take over the process of oxygen and carbon dioxide exchange until 37 to 38 weeks' gestation. Critical factors in the development of respiratory distress include the following:

1. The preterm infant is unable to produce adequate amounts of surfactant. (See Chapter 28 for discussion of respiratory adaptation and development.) Inadequate surfactant lessens compliance (ability of the lungs to fill with air easily), and the inspiratory pressure needed to expand the lungs with air is higher. The collapsed (or atelectatic) alveoli will not facilitate an exchange of oxygen and carbon dioxide. As a result, the infant becomes hypoxic, pulmonary blood flow is inefficient, and the preterm newborn's available energy is depleted.
2. The muscular coat of the pulmonary blood vessels is incompletely developed. Because of this, the

pulmonary arterioles do not constrict as well in response to decreased oxygen levels. This lowered pulmonary vascular resistance leads to increased left-to-right shunting through the ductus arteriosus, which increases the blood flow back into the lungs.

3. The ductus arteriosus usually responds to increasing oxygen levels and prostaglandin E levels by vasoconstriction; in the preterm infant, who has higher susceptibility to hypoxia, the ductus may remain open. A patent ductus increases the blood volume to the lungs, causing pulmonary congestion, increased respiratory effort, carbon dioxide retention, and bounding femoral pulses. The common complications of the cardiopulmonary system in preterm infants are discussed later in the chapter and in Chapter 33.

Alteration in Thermoregulation

Heat loss is a major problem that the nurse can do much to prevent. Two limiting factors in heat production, however, are the availability of glycogen in the liver and the amount of brown fat available for metabolism. Both glycogen and brown fat appear in the third trimester. In the cold-stressed newborn, norepinephrine is released which in turn stimulates the metabolism of brown fat for heat production. As a complicating factor, the hypoxic newborn cannot increase oxygen consumption in response to cold stress because of the already limited reserves and thereby becomes progressively colder. Because the muscle mass is small in preterm infants and voluntary muscular activity is diminished (they are unable to shiver), little heat is produced.

Five physiologic and anatomic factors increase heat loss in the preterm infant:

1. The preterm baby has a high ratio of body surface to body weight. This means that the baby's ability to produce heat (based on body weight) is much less than the potential for losing heat (based on surface area). The loss of heat in a preterm infant weighing 1500 g is five times greater per unit of body weight than in an adult.
2. The preterm baby has very little subcutaneous fat, which is the human body's insulation. Without adequate insulation, heat is easily conducted from the core of the body (warmer temperature) to the surface of the body (cooler temperature). Heat is lost from the body as the blood vessels, which lie close to the skin surface in the preterm infant, transport blood from the body core to the subcutaneous tissues.
3. The preterm baby has thinner, more permeable skin than the term infant. This increased permeability contributes to a greater insensible water loss as well as heat loss.
4. The posture of the preterm baby influences heat loss. Flexion of the extremities decreases the amount of surface area exposed to the environment. Extension increases the surface area exposed to the environment and thus increases heat loss. The gestational age of the infant influences the amount of flexion, from completely hypotonic and extended at 28 weeks to strong flexion displayed by 36 weeks.
5. The preterm baby has a decreased ability to vasoconstrict superficial blood vessels and conserve heat in the body core.

In summary, gestational age is directly proportional to the ability to maintain thermoregulation; thus the more preterm the newborn, the less the infant is able to maintain heat balance. Preventing heat loss by providing a neutral thermal environment is one of the most important considerations in nursing management of the preterm infant. Cold stress, with its accompanying severe complications, can be prevented (see Chapter 33).

Alteration in Gastrointestinal Physiology

The basic structure of the gastrointestinal (GI) tract is formed early in gestation. Maturation of the digestive and absorptive processes is more variable, however, and occurs later in gestation.

As a result of GI immaturity, the preterm newborn has the following ingestion, digestion, and absorption problems:

- A marked danger of aspiration and its associated complications due to the infant's poorly developed gag reflex, incompetent esophageal cardiac sphincter, and poor sucking and swallowing reflexes.
- Difficulty in meeting high caloric and fluid needs for growth due to small stomach capacity.
- Limited ability to convert certain essential amino acids to nonessential amino acids. Certain amino acids, such as histidine, taurine, and cysteine, are essential to the preterm infant but not to the term infant.
- Inability to handle the increased osmolarity of formula protein due to kidney immaturity. The preterm infant requires a higher concentration of whey protein than casein.
- Difficulty absorbing saturated fats due to decreased bile salts and pancreatic lipase. Severe illness of the newborn may also prevent intake of adequate nutrients.
- Difficulty with lactose digestion initially because processes may not be fully functional during the first few days of a preterm infant's life. The preterm newborn can digest and absorb most simple sugars.
- Deficiency of calcium and phosphorus may exist because two thirds of these minerals are deposited in the last trimester. Rickets and significant bone demineralization due to deficiency of calcium and phosphorus are common problems.
- Increased basal metabolic rate and increased oxygen requirements due to fatigue associated with sucking.
- Feeding intolerance and necrotizing enterocolitis (NEC) due to diminished blood flow and tissue perfusion to the intestinal tract due to prolonged hypoxia and hypoxemia at birth.

MEDIALINK RESOURCES FOR FAMILIES OF PREMATURE INFANTS

Alteration in Renal Physiology

The kidneys of the preterm infant are immature in comparison with those of the full-term infant, which poses clinical problems in the management of fluid and electrolyte balance. Specific characteristics of the preterm infant include the following:

- The glomerular filtration rate (GFR) is lower because of decreased renal blood flow. The GFR is directly related to lower gestational age, so the more preterm the newborn, the lower the GFR. The GFR is also decreased in the presence of diseases or conditions that decrease renal blood flow and perfusion, such as severe respiratory distress, hypotension, and perinatal asphyxia. Anuria or oliguria may also be observed.
- The preterm infant's kidneys are limited in their ability to concentrate urine or to excrete excess amounts of fluid. This means that if excess fluid is administered, the infant is at risk for fluid retention and overhydration. If too little is administered, the infant will become dehydrated because of the inability to retain adequate fluid.
- The kidneys of the preterm infant begin excreting glucose at a lower serum glucose level than those of the term infant. Therefore, glycosuria with hyperglycemia is common.
- The buffering capacity of the kidney is reduced, predisposing the infant to metabolic acidosis. Bicarbonate is excreted at a lower serum level, and acid is excreted more slowly. Therefore, after periods of hypoxia or insult, the preterm infant's kidneys require a longer time to excrete the lactic acid that accumulates. Sodium bicarbonate is frequently required to treat the metabolic acidosis.
- The immaturity of the renal system affects the preterm infant's ability to excrete drugs. Because excretion time is longer, many drugs are given over longer intervals (for example, every 24 hours instead of every 12 hours). Urine output must be carefully monitored when the infant is receiving nephrotoxic drugs, such as gentamicin, nafcillin, and vancomycin. In the event of oliguria, drugs can become toxic in the infant much more quickly than in the adult.

Alteration in Hepatic and Hematologic Physiology

Immaturity of the preterm newborn's liver predisposes the infant to several problems. After birth, the glycogen stores in the liver are rapidly used for energy. Glycogen deposits are affected by asphyxia in utero and after birth by both asphyxia and cold stress. The baby born preterm has decreased glycogen stores at birth and frequently experiences stress, which rapidly uses up these limited stores. Therefore, the preterm newborn is at high risk for hypoglycemia and its complications.

Iron is also stored in the liver, especially during the last trimester of pregnancy. Therefore, the preterm newborn is born with low iron stores. If subject to hemorrhage, rapid growth, and excess blood sampling, the preterm infant is likely to become iron depleted more quickly than the term infant. Many preterm babies require transfusions of packed cells to treat symptomatic anemia as a consequence of frequent blood sampling.

Conjugation of bilirubin in the liver is impaired in the preterm infant. Thus bilirubin levels increase more rapidly and to a higher level than in the full-term infant. Early clinical assessment of jaundice associated with indirect hyperbilirubinemia is more difficult in preterm newborns because they lack subcutaneous fat.

The normal cord hemoglobin in an infant of 34 weeks' gestation is approximately 16.8 g/dL, and total blood volume ranges from 80 mL/kg to 100 mL/kg (Blackburn, 2003). Due to the small total blood volume, any blood loss is highly significant to the preterm infant. Therefore, periodic assessments of hemoglobin values are performed during the first weeks of life.

Alteration in Immunologic Physiology

The preterm infant is at a much greater risk for infection than the term infant. This increased susceptibility may be the result of an infection acquired in utero which precipitates preterm labor and birth. However, all preterm infants have immature specific and nonspecific immunity.

In utero the fetus receives passive immunity against a variety of infections from maternal IgG immunoglobulins, which cross the placenta (see Chapter 28). Because most of this immunity is acquired in the last trimester of pregnancy, the preterm infant has few antibodies at birth. These provide less protection and become depleted earlier than in a full-term infant. This may be a contributing factor in the higher incidence of recurrent bacterial infection during the first year of life as well as in the immediate neonatal period.

The other immunoglobulin significant for the preterm infant is secretory IgA, which does not cross the placenta but is found in breast milk in significant concentrations. Breast milk's secretory IgA provides immunity to the mucosal surfaces of the GI tract, protecting the newborn from enteric infections such as those caused by *Escherichia coli* and *Shigella*. Ill preterm infants may be unable to have breast milk and thus are at risk for enteric infection.

Another altered defense against infection in the preterm infant is the skin surface. In very small infants the skin is easily excoriated, and this factor, coupled with many invasive procedures, places the infant at great risk for nosocomial infections. It is vital to use good handwashing techniques in the care of these infants to prevent unnecessary infection.

Alteration in Neurologic Physiology

The general shape of the brain is formed during the first 6 weeks of gestation. Between the second and fourth months of gestation the brain's total complement of neurons proliferate; these neurons migrate to specific sites throughout the central nervous system, and nerve impulse pathways organize. The final step in neurologic development is the covering of these nerves with myelin, which begins in the second trimester of gestation and continues into adult life (Volpe, 2001).

Because the period of most rapid brain growth and development occurs during the third trimester of pregnancy, the closer to term an infant is born, the better the neurologic prognosis. A common interruption of neurologic development in the preterm infant is caused by intraventricular hemorrhage (IVH) and intracranial hemorrhage (ICH). Hydrocephalus may develop as a consequence of an IVH due to the obstruction at the cerebral aqueduct.

Alteration in Reactivity Periods and Behavioral States

The newborn infant's response to extrauterine life is characterized by two periods of reactivity, as discussed in Chapter 31. The preterm infant's periods of reactivity are delayed. In the very ill infant, these periods of reactivity may not be observed at all because the infant may be hypotonic and unreactive for several days after birth.

As the preterm newborn grows and the condition stabilizes, identifying behavioral states and traits unique to each infant becomes increasingly possible. This is a very important part of nursing management of the high-risk infant because it facilitates parental knowledge of their infant's cues for interaction.

In general, stable preterm infants do not demonstrate the same behavioral states as term infants. Preterm infants are more disorganized in their sleep-wake cycles and are unable to attend as well to the human face and objects in the environment. Neurologically, their responses (sucking, muscle tone, states of arousal) are weaker than full-term infants' responses.

By observing each infant's patterns of behavior and responses, especially the sleep-wake states, the nurse can teach parents optimal times for interacting with their infant. The parents and nurse can plan nursing care around the times when the infant is alert and best able to attend. In addition, the more knowledge parents have about the meaning of their infant's responses and behaviors, the better prepared they will be to meet their newborn's needs and to form a positive attachment with their child. See discussion of developmental care for the preterm newborn later in this section.

Management of Nutrition and Fluid Requirements

Early feedings are extremely valuable in maintaining normal metabolism and lowering the possibility of such complications as hypoglycemia, hyperbilirubinemia, hyperkalemia, and azotemia. However, the preterm newborn is at risk for complications that may develop because of the immaturity of the digestive system.

NUTRITIONAL REQUIREMENTS

Oral (enteral) caloric intake necessary for growth in an uncompromised healthy preterm infant is 95 to 130 kcal/kg/day (Blackburn, 2003). In addition to these relatively high caloric needs, the preterm infant requires more protein than full-term infants. To meet these needs, many institutions use fortified breast milk or special preterm formulas.

Whether breast milk or formula is used, feeding regimens are established based on the infant's weight and estimated stomach capacity (Table 32–1 •). Initial formula feedings are gradually increased as the infant tolerates them. It may be necessary to supplement the oral feedings with parenteral fluids to maintain adequate hydration and caloric intake until the baby is on full oral feedings. Those preterm infants who cannot tolerate any oral (enteral) feedings are given nutrition by total parenteral nutrition (TPN).

In addition to a higher calorie and higher protein formula, preterm infants should receive supplemental multivitamins, including vitamin E and trace minerals. A diet high

Table 32–1 • SUGGESTED FEEDING GUIDELINES FOR THE PRETERM INFANT

Weight (g)	Feeding Interval	Beginning Volume (cc/kg/d)	Feeding Increments (cc/kg/d)	Days to Full Feedings†
< 1000	q 3 hour	10–20	10–20	16–13
1000–1500	q 3 hour	10–20	15–20	10–7
1501–1800 sick‡	q 3 hour	10–20	20–30	7–5
1501–1800 healthy‡	q 3 hour	20–40	30–50	5–3
> 1800 sick‡	q 3 hour	20–40	30–75	5–2

†Full feedings are defined as 120 kcal/kg/day of a 24 kcal/oz formula or human milk.

‡ *Sick* refers to infants who have had symptoms of any medical or surgical condition, other than uncomplicated prematurity.

Healthy refers to term or preterm infants who have had no symptomatic medical or surgical conditions.

1. Advancement of feedings should occur only as the infant demonstrates tolerance of enteral feedings. Clinical signs of feeding intolerance or illness dictate discontinuing or holding the advancement of feedings.
2. Infants are started on either full-strength human milk or 24 kcal/oz premature infant formula.
3. At 100–120 mL/kg, fortifier is added to human milk.
4. Iron supplements are added at 2–4 mg/kg/day for the human milk fed infant at full feeds.

Source: *Neonatal nutrition survival guide for the practitioner* by Lisa R. Vanatta, MS, RD, CSP, Clinical Nutrition Services, Phoenix Children's Hospital.

in polyunsaturated fats (which preterm infants tolerate best) increases the requirement for vitamin E. Preterm infants fed iron-fortified formulas have higher red cell hemolysis and lower vitamin E concentrations and thus require additional vitamin E. Preterm formulas also need to contain medium-chain triglycerides (MCT) and additional amino acids such as cysteine, as well as calcium, phosphorus, and vitamin D supplements to increase mineralization of bones. Rickets and significant bone demineralization have been documented in very-low-birth-weight infants and otherwise healthy preterm infants.

Nutritional intake is considered adequate when there is consistent weight gain of 20 to 30 g per day. Initially, no weight gain may be noted for several days, but total weight loss should not exceed 15% of the total birth weight or more than 1% to 2% per day. Some institutions add the criteria of head circumference growth and increase in body length of 1 cm per week once the newborn is stable.

METHODS OF FEEDING

The preterm infant is fed by various methods, depending on the infant's gestational age, health and physical condition, and neurologic status. The three most common oral feeding methods are bottle, breast, and gavage.

Bottle-Feeding

Preterm infants who have a coordinated as well as rhythmic suck-swallow-breathing pattern are usually between 35 and 36 weeks' postconceptual age and may be fed by bottle. Nutritive sucking is a multifaceted process involving the central nervous system and the musculoskeletal system of the mouth, pharynx, esophagus, and face (McGrath & Conliffe-Torres, 2000). To avoid excessive expenditure of energy, a soft, yellow, single-hole nipple is usually used (milk flow is less rapid). The infant is fed in a semisitting position and burped gently after each half ounce or ounce. The feeding should take no longer than 15 to 20 minutes (nippling requires more energy than other methods).

Those preterm infants who are progressing from gavage feedings to bottle-feeding should be started with one session of bottle-feeding a day, and the number of times a day a bottle is given should be increased slowly until the baby tolerates all feedings from a bottle.

The nurse also assesses the infant's ability to suck. Sucking may be affected by postconceptional age, asphyxia, chronic lung disease, intraventricular hemorrhage, or other neurologic insult. Before initiating nipple feeding, the nurse observes the infant for any signs of stress, such as tachypnea (more than 60 respirations per minute), respiratory distress, or hypothermia, which may increase the risk of aspiration. During the feeding, the infant should be observed for signs of difficulty with feeding (tachypnea, a decrease in oxygen saturation levels, bradycardia, lethargy, and uncoordinated suck and swallow). Difficulty in bottle-feeding is often associated with a milk bolus that is too large for the infant's oral cavity which can lead to aspiration (Lemons, 2001).

Breastfeeding

Mothers who wish to breastfeed their preterm infants should be given the opportunity to put the infant to breast as soon as the infant has demonstrated a coordinated suck and swallow reflex, is showing consistent weight gain, and can control body temperature outside of the incubator. Besides breast milk's many benefits for the infant, it allows the mother to contribute actively to the infant's well-being (Figure 32–7 •). The nurse should encourage mothers to breastfeed if they choose to do so. It is important for the nurse to be aware of the advantages of breastfeeding as well as the possible disadvantages if breast milk is the sole source of food for the preterm infant. See Chapter 31 for a detailed discussion of the advantages and disadvantages of breastfeeding. Even if the infant can't be put to the breast, mothers can pump their breasts, and the breast milk can be given via gavage. Use of the double-pumping system produces higher levels of prolactin than sequential pumping of the breasts (see Figure 31–9).

By initiating skin-to-skin holding of low-birth-weight infants in the early intensive care phase, mothers can significantly increase milk volume, thereby overcoming lactation problems (Nyqvist, 2002). Also preterm infants tolerate breastfeeding with higher transcutaneous oxygen pressure and better maintenance of body temperature than during bottle-feeding.

The infant is placed at the mother's breast. It has been suggested that the football hold is a convenient position for preterm babies. Feeding time may take up to 45 minutes, and babies should be burped as they alternate breasts. Length of feeding time must be monitored so that the preterm infant does not burn too many calories.

The nurse should coordinate a flexible feeding schedule so babies can breastfeed during alert times and be allowed to set their own pace. Feedings should be on demand, but a maximum number of hours between feedings should be set. A similar regimen should be used for the baby who is progressing from gavage feeding to breastfeeding. The mother

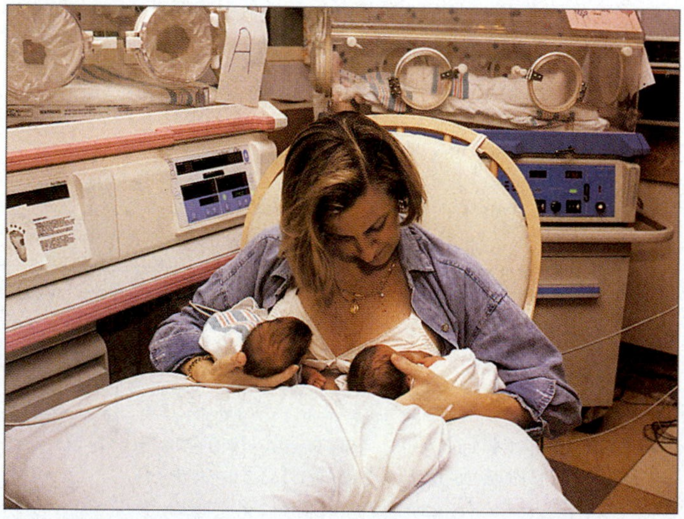

Figure 32–7 • Mother visits neonatal intensive care unit to breastfeed her infants.

RESEARCH IN PRACTICE
Breastfeeding in Preterm Twins

What is this study about? A premature birth presents unique problems for mothers who breastfeed. Because of the newborn's need for specialized care, there is generally a period when the mother and baby are deprived of regular, extended, private contact. This problem is magnified for mothers of preterm twins. However, some mothers do manage successful breastfeeding strategies even with these obstacles. A primary focus of this study was to determine the factors that support or inhibit breastfeeding in preterm twins, and to identify potential improvements in hospital practices so that breastfeeding these at-risk newborns is supported.

How was this study done? This study used a convenience sample of twins born at a Swedish hospital after a gestation of less than 36 weeks. Mothers were included only if they expressed a desire to breastfeed. Infants with serious illness that would affect feeding behavior were also excluded. Thirteen mothers and their twins participated. The majority of the mothers were primiparas. Six of the mothers had a cesarean birth. The newborns' breastfeeding behavior was observed using a structured observation tool at multiple times during the postpartum period. Data were collected from the mothers using a structured interview guide, and responses were categorized into general themes.

What were the results of the study? Eight of the 13 mothers preferred simultaneous breastfeeding, primarily because they found it less time-consuming. The mothers that preferred breastfeeding one infant at a time favored it for their ability to give the infant more guidance and for the facilitation of mother-infant interaction. The majority found the "football hold" the most comfortable and successful. These mothers indicated that their success at breastfeeding was facilitated by information about breast milk production, expression, and positions. The mothers also valued advice about how to interpret and respond to infants' behavioral signals. Mothers appreciated consistent advice from a specific caregiver during the breastfeeding period. Lack of timely information was regarded as an obstacle, and getting conflicting opinions was identified as counterproductive. Mothers' experiences of supportive hospital practices included letting the twins bed together and mother-infant skin-to-skin contact. Delays in initiation of breastfeeding and separate feeding schedules for each twin were perceived as obstacles. Having a noisy, nonprivate environment was also an obstacle.

What additional questions might I have? Sweden's national health system allows mothers to remain in the hospital with their infants. Would these findings be different in the US system, when mothers are sent home before their babies?

How can I use this study? Supporting breastfeeding preterm twins is a complex process requiring consideration of many factors. Nurses are in a key position to provide information that will support this process and enhance the success of mothers who desire to breastfeed. Procedures, the environment, and feeding schedules should be designed to maximize the chance that breastfeeding will be successful for these at-risk newborns.

Source: Nyqvist, K. (2002). Breast-feeding in preterm twins: Development of feeding behavior and milk intake during hospital stay and related caregiving practices. *Journal of Pediatric Nursing, 17*(4), 246–256.

should begin with one feeding at the breast and then gradually increase the number of times during the day that the baby breastfeeds. When breastfeeding is not possible because the infant is too small or too weak to suck at the breast, an option for the mother may be to express her breast milk into a cup. The milk touches the infant's lips and is lapped by the protruding motions of the tongue.

Gavage Feeding

The gavage feeding method is used with preterm infants (less than 34 weeks' gestation) who lack or have a poorly coordinated suck-swallow-breathing pattern or are ill and ventilator dependent. Gavage feeding may be used as an adjunct to nipple feeding if the infant tires easily or as an alternative if an infant is losing weight because of the energy expenditure required for nippling. See Procedure 32–1: Performing Gavage Feeding. Gavage feedings are administered by either the nasogastric or orogastric route and by intermittent bolus or continuous drip method. Early initiation of minimal enteral nutrition (MEN) via gavage is now advocated in the preterm newborn as a supplement to parenteral nutrition. MEN, using formula or human milk in quantities of 10 mL/kg/day, is designed to "prime" the intestinal tract, thereby stimulating many of its hormonal and enzymatic functions (Anderson, 2002). Benefits of early feedings (as early as 24 to 72 hours of life) include the following: no increase in the incidence of NEC; fewer days on TPN, thereby decreasing the incidence of cholestatic jaundice; increased muscle maturation of the gut as well as muscle growth; increase in gut peristalsis; increased gut hormone levels, which can lead to improved feeding tolerance; lower risk of osteopenia; and a possible decrease in the total number of hospital days in the neonatal intensive care unit (NICU) (Anderson, 2002).

Clinical Tip *For an otherwise healthy, growing premature infant who is receiving total enteral intake and has started to experience apnea and bradycardia, one differential diagnosis to think about is reflux rather than sepsis, although sepsis may need to be ruled out.*

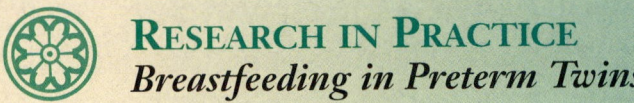

Procedure 32–1 Performing Gavage Feeding

Preparation

1. When choosing the catheter size, consider the size of the infant, the area of insertion (oral or nasal), and the desired rate of flow.
   Rationale: The size of the catheter will influence the rate of flow.
2. Explain the procedure to the parents.
3. Elevate the head of the bed and position the infant on the back or side to allow easy passage of the tube.
4. Measure the distance from the tip of the ear to the nose to the xiphoid process, and mark the point with a small piece of paper tape (Figure 32–8 •) to ensure enough tubing to enter the stomach.

Clinical Tip

The very small infant (less than 1600 g) requires a 5 Fr. feeding tube; an infant greater than 1600 g may tolerate a larger tube.

Orogastric insertion is preferable to nasogastric because most infants are obligatory nose breathers. If nasogastric is used, a 5 Fr. catheter should be used to minimize airway obstruction.

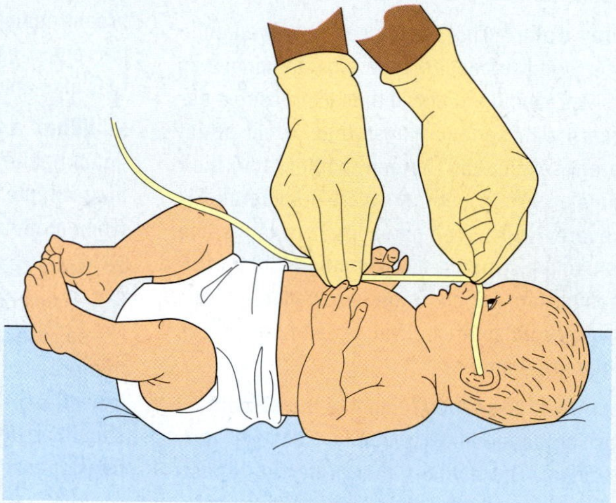

Figure 32–8 • Measuring gavage tube length.

Equipment and Supplies

- No. 5 or no. 8 Fr. feeding tube. See the material below for guidelines for choosing tube size.
- 3- to 5-mL syringe, for aspirating stomach contents
- 1/4-inch paper tape, to mark the tube for insertion depth and to secure the catheter during feeding
- Stethoscope, for auscultating the rush of air into the stomach when testing the tube placement
- Appropriate formula
- Small cup of sterile water to test for tube placement and to act as lubricant

Procedure: Clean Gloves

Inserting and Checking Placement of Tube

1. If inserting the tube nasally, lubricate the tip in a cup of sterile water. Use water instead of an oil-based lubricant, in case the tube is inadvertently passed into a lung. Shake any excess drops to prevent aspiration.
2. If inserting the tube orally, the oral secretions are enough to lubricate the tube adequately.
3. Stabilize the infant's head with one hand and pass the tube via the mouth (or nose) into the stomach to the point previously marked. If the infant begins coughing or choking or becomes cyanotic or phonic, remove the tube immediately as the tube has probably entered the trachea.
4. If no respiratory distress is apparent, lightly tape the tube in position, draw up 0.5 to 1.0 mL of air in the syringe, and connect the syringe to the tubing. Place the

Procedure 32-1 *(continued)*

stethoscope over the epigastrium and briskly inject the air (Figure 32–9 ●). You will hear a sudden rush as the air enters the stomach.

5. Aspirate the stomach contents with the syringe, and note the amount, color, and consistency to evaluate the infant's feeding tolerance. Return the residual to the stomach unless you are asked to discard it. It is usually not discarded because of the potential for electrolyte imbalance.
6. If the aspirated contents contain only a clear fluid or mucus and if it is unclear whether or not the tube is in the stomach, test the aspirate for pH. Stomach aspirate has a pH between 1 and 3.

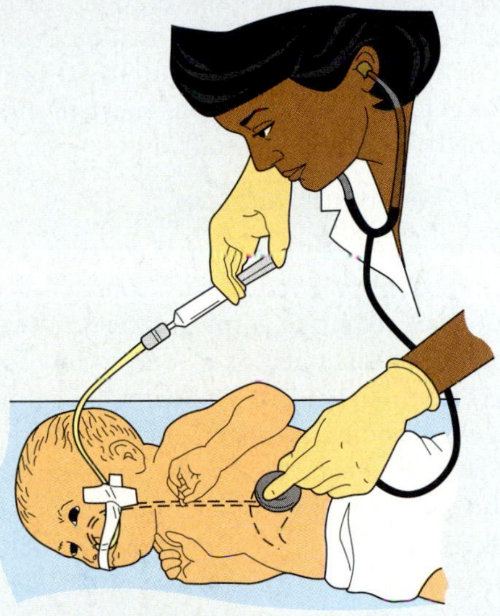

Figure 32–9 ● Auscultation for placement of gavage tube.

Administering the Feeding

1. Hold the infant for feeding, or position the infant on the right side.
   Rationale: This position decreases the risk of aspiration in case of emesis during feeding.
2. Separate the syringe from the tube, remove the plunger from the barrel, reconnect the barrel to the tube, and pour the formula into the syringe.
3. Elevate the syringe 6 to 8 inches over the infant's head, and allow the formula to flow by gravity at a slow, even rate. You may need to initiate the flow of formula by inserting the plunger of the syringe into the barrel just until you see formula enter the feeding tube. Do not use pressure.
4. Regulate the rate to prevent sudden stomach distention leading to vomiting and aspiration. Continue adding formula to the syringe until the infant has absorbed the desired volume.

Clearing and Removing the Tube

1. Clear the tubing with 2 to 3 mL sterile water or with air.
   Rationale: This ensures that the infant has received all of the formula. If the tube is going to be left in place, clearing it will decrease the risk of clogging and bacterial growth in the tube.
2. To remove the tube, loosen the tape, fold the tube over on itself, and quickly withdraw the tube in one smooth motion to minimize the potential for fluid aspiration as the tube passes the epiglottis. If the tube is to be left in, position it so that the infant is unable to remove it. Replace the tube per hospital policy.

Maximize the Feeding Pleasure of the Infant

1. Whenever possible, hold the infant during gavage feeding. If it is too awkward to hold the infant during feeding, be sure to take time for holding after the feeding.
   Rationale: Feeding time is important to the infant's tactile sensory input.
2. Offer a pacifier to the infant during the feeding.
   Rationale: Sucking during feeding comforts and relaxes the infant, making the formula flow more easily. Infants can lose their sucking reflexes when fed by gavage for long periods.

Transpyloric Feeding

An alternative method of feeding, transpyloric feeding (a method in which the stomach is bypassed), is not recommended when beginning enteral feedings. Transpyloric feedings are associated with maldigestion of fat, decreased potassium absorption, and intestinal perforation (Evans & Thureen, 2001). This feeding method should be used only in specially equipped and staffed high-risk nurseries.

Total Parenteral Nutrition

TPN is used in situations that contraindicate feeding the infant through the GI tract. Contraindications include GI anomalies requiring surgical intervention, necrotizing enterocolitis, intolerance of feedings, and asphyxia. TPN may also be used in tandem with enteral feedings, during the early stages of feeding advancement.

The TPN method provides complete nutrition to the infant intravenously. TPN includes use of hyperalimentation and intralipids. Hyperalimentation provides vitamins, minerals, protein, and glucose. Appropriate amino acid intake (1.5 to 3 g/kg/day) is necessary to avoid catabolism and maintain the newborn in a positive-nitrogen balance. A percutaneous central venous catheter (PCVC/PICC) is often used with the low-birth-weight infant to deliver higher concentrations of glucose (greater than D 12.5) as well as to provide an energy substrate. Intralipids are also administered to provide essential fatty acids.

The nurse needs to monitor serum glucose levels and serum chemistries carefully during TPN. Urine is checked for protein, sugar, and specific gravity at least every 12 hours. The intravenous rate is monitored hourly to maintain accurate intake. The rate should not be increased to "catch up" if administration lags behind. The intravenous site should be observed hourly for signs of infiltration—hyperalimentation is extremely caustic and causes severe tissue destruction if it infiltrates. Intake and output are carefully monitored (hyperglycemia causing an osmotic diuresis can lead to dehydration). If hypoglycemia occurs, continuous insulin infusions may be initiated to enhance glucose uptake and utilization (Zylberberg & Pepper, 2001). The nurse needs to be aware of the potential complications associated with intralipid infusions, including increased free bilirubin concentrations, impaired pulmonary functions which can lead to chronic lung disease, and interference with platelet function. Therefore, serum triglyceride levels need to be followed. Daily lipid dose should be spread out over a 24-hour period.

FLUID REQUIREMENTS

Calculation of fluid requirements takes into account the infant's weight and postnatal age. Recommendations for fluid therapy in the preterm infant are approximately 80 to 100 mL/kg/day for day 1, 100 to 120 mL/kg/day for day 2, and 120 to 150 mL/kg/day by day 3 of life. These amounts may be increased up to 200 mL/kg/day if the infant is very small, receiving phototherapy, or under a radiant warmer because of increased insensible water losses. Fluid losses can be minimized through the use of heat shields and humidity, or "swamping."

Common Complications of Preterm Newborns and Their Clinical Management

The goals of clinical therapy are to meet the growth and development needs of the preterm newborn and to anticipate and manage the complications associated with prematurity. Complications associated with prematurity that require clinical intervention are respiratory distress syndrome (RDS), patent ductus arteriosus, apnea, intraventricular hemorrhage, and sepsis. Long-term problems include retinopathy of prematurity, bronchopulmonary dysplasia (BPD) that can lead to chronic lung disease (CLD), pulmonary interstitial emphysema (PIE), and posthemorrhagic hydrocephalus.

An in-depth discussion of RDS, BPD/CLD, and sepsis, including pathophysiology, clinical management, and nursing care, is contained in Chapter 33. Patent ductus arteriosus, apnea, intraventricular hemorrhage, retinopathy of prematurity, and other complications are discussed as follows.

PATENT DUCTUS ARTERIOSUS

The incidence of symptomatic patent ductus arteriosus (PDA) is related to birth weight in preterm infants and has been shown to decrease with increase in birth weight. Symptomatic PDA is often seen around the third day of life, when the premature infant is recovering from RDS. Initially, when the preterm newborn is hypoxic secondary to RDS, the pulmonary vascular resistance (PVR) can be higher than the systemic vascular resistance, and right-to-left shunting through the ductus will occur. However, as the RDS improves and adequate oxygenation is maintained, the pulmonary pressures fall allowing more blood flow into the lungs, leading to ventricular volume overload, pulmonary edema, and congestive failure. Oxygenation is again compromised, and ventilator requirements will increase, leading to the possible difficulty in weaning from the ventilator and long-term pulmonary sequelae. Clinical findings include tachypnea, hyperactive precordium, bounding peripheral pulses, hypotension, widened pulse pressure, tachycardia, and hepatomegaly.

Early identification of symptomatic infants and prompt clinical intervention will minimize long-term complications. There are a multitude of medical management regimens of the PDA. Initial medical management consists of providing adequate respiratory support, restricting fluids, and using diuretics (to decrease pulmonary edema) and perhaps digoxin (to treat congestive heart failure) while waiting for spontaneous closure of the ductus to occur. The administration of prostaglandin synthetase inhibitors, such as indomethacin (Indocin), impairs synthesis of the E series prostaglandins responsible for dilatation of the ductus and can cause ductal closure. Courses of indomethacin therapy vary; the standard, short course consists of three doses of indomethacin, 0.2 mg/kg IV every 12 hours. As an alternative, a long course of indomethacin may be chosen involving dosing over approximately 7 days. A decrease in renal side effects is thought to be the advantage of the longer dosing schedule. Indomethacin is effective, but it is not without side effects and must be used cautiously. Adverse side effects include transient renal dysfunction, oliguria, platelet dysfunction, and GI bleeding.

If medical management is unsuccessful or contraindicated, then the ductus may be surgically ligated. PDA will often prolong the course of illness in a preterm newborn and may lead to chronic pulmonary dysfunction.

APNEA

Apnea of prematurity refers to cessation of breathing for 20 seconds or longer or for less than 20 seconds when associated with cyanosis, pallor, and bradycardia. Apnea is one of the most common problems in the preterm infant presenting between day 2 and day 7 of life. Although the etiology of apnea is multifactorial, it is thought to be primarily a result of neuronal immaturity, a factor that contributes to the preterm infant's irregular breathing patterns (central apnea). Obstructive apnea can occur in the premature infant when there is a cessation of airflow associated with blockage of the upper airway (small airway diameter, increased pharyngeal secretions, improper body alignment and positioning, gastroesophageal reflux).

Differential diagnoses with regard to apnea include sepsis, electrolyte disturbances, hypoglycemia, lung disease (atelectasis, pneumonia), cardiovascular changes (PDA, hypotension), central nervous system disturbances (seizures, intraventricular hemorrhage, meningitis), medication use (narcotics, opioids), thermoregulation problems (hypo- and hyperthermia), and gastrointestinal disturbances (NEC, distention, obstruction, gastroesophageal reflux). Gastroesophageal reflux is defined as a movement of gastric contents into the lower esophagus due to poor lower esophageal sphincter tone, activating the laryngeal chemoreflex causing apnea. Apnea of prematurity is then a diagnosis of exclusion (Theobald, Botwinski, Alabanna, et al, 2000).

Apneic onset is often insidious; cardiorespiratory monitoring allows for early recognition and intervention, thus decreasing the need for resuscitative efforts. Apnea may occur during feeding, suctioning, or stooling. However, there may be no observable activity related to apnea. All episodes of apnea are documented. The documentation includes activity at the time of apnea, length of episode (along with any bradycardia, color change, or desaturation on pulse-oximeter associated with the apneic episode), and treatment required to bring the baby out of the apneic spell. These data are useful in determining etiology and possible treatment.

The nurse makes careful observations, quickly assessing the need for intervention or ascertaining that the infant is having periodic breathing. The intervention required depends on the severity of the apneic episode and the baby's response. Gentle stimulation of the infant may be sufficient. Respiratory support is provided if needed, and methylxanthine drugs (aminophylline, theophylline, or caffeine citrate) are often used to treat apnea of prematurity. Conservative management of apnea associated with gastroesophageal reflux would include dietary modification by adding rice cereal to thicken feedings. Feedings may also be small and frequent to decrease gastric distention. Following feedings, the infant should be placed in a side-lying or prone position with the head of the bed elevated 30 degrees for 20 to 30 minutes to facilitate gastric emptying. Pharmacologic intervention using metoclopramide (Reglan) facilitates gastric emptying and improves GI motility.

INTRAVENTRICULAR HEMORRHAGE

Intraventricular hemorrhage (IVH) is the most common type of intracranial hemorrhage in the small preterm infant, especially those weighing less than 1500 g or of less than 34 weeks' gestation.

The most common site of hemorrhage is the periventricular subependymal germinal matrix in the lateral ventricles of the brain, where there is a rich blood supply and the capillary walls are thin and fragile. The matrix provides little supportive tissue for the fragile blood vessels. Before 32 weeks' gestation, an infant is much more susceptible to hemorrhage of these tiny vessels because they are vulnerable to hypoxic events (such as respiratory distress, birth trauma, birth asphyxia) that damage and rupture vessel walls.

Prenatal interventions include preventing premature birth and transporting the pregnant mother to a tertiary care center. Administration of phenobarbital and vitamin K to the mother is being studied for their preventive effect. Postnatal preventive interventions include careful resuscitation, correction or prevention of major hemodynamic disturbances, and correction of coagulation abnormalities. Potential postnatal preventive pharmacologic interventions include phenobarbital to control seizures, narcotics for sedation, and vitamin E for its antioxidant abilities (Volpe, 2001).

The outcome for the infant depends on the size of the intracerebral bleed and the gestational age of the infant. The most severe hemorrhages may cause motor deficits, posthemorrhagic hydrocephalus, hearing loss, and blindness. Less severe bleeds may have no observable effects. In caring for the infant with an IVH, the nurse provides continuing support for the parents, identifying their level of understanding and facilitating interdisciplinary communication with them.

ANEMIA OF PREMATURITY

The preterm infant is at risk for anemia because of the rapid rate of growth required, shorter red blood cell life, excessive blood sampling, decreased iron stores, and deficiency of vitamin E. The hemoglobin usually reaches its lowest level by 3 to 12 weeks and remains low for 3 to 6 months. Interventions include iron supplementation and administration of recombinant human erythropoietin (rHuEPO). Iron supplementation ensures adequate stores for red blood cell production once erythropoiesis starts. The use of rHuEPO is reported to increase the hematocrit and reticulocyte count and reduce the need for blood transfusions in preterm infants (Blackburn, 2003).

LONG-TERM COMPLICATIONS

The care of the preterm infant and the family does not stop on discharge from the nursery. Follow-up care is extremely important because many developmental problems are not noted until the infant is older and begins to demonstrate motor delays or sensory disability. Within the first year of life, low-birth-weight preterm infants face higher mortality than term infants. Causes of death include sudden infant death syndrome (SIDS)—which occurs about five times more frequently in the preterm infant—respiratory infections, and neurologic defects. Morbidity is also much higher among preterm infants, with those weighing less than 1500 g at highest risk for long-term complications.

The most common long-term problems observed in preterm infants include retinopathy of prematurity, speech defects, neurologic defects, and auditory defects.

Retinopathy of Prematurity

Premature newborns are particularly susceptible to injury of the delicate capillaries of the retina causing characteristic retinal changes known as retinopathy of prematurity (ROP). It is this injury to the developing vascular system of the retina that leads to ischemia resulting in hemorrhage, scarring, and, in extreme cases, retinal detachment. Until recently, ROP was thought to be exclusively the result of excessive use of oxygen in the treatment of premature infants. However, ROP has also occurred in premature infants who never received oxygen, in full-term infants with cyanotic congenital heart disease, and in infants with certain other congenital anomalies. The disease is now viewed as multifactorial in origin. Other risk factors include IVH, CLD, apnea, hypoxia, sepsis, acidosis, multiple gestation, exposure to bright lights, and blood transfusions. Increased survival of very-low-birth-weight infants may be the most important factor in the increased incidence of ROP.

Treatment of the acute stages of ROP with laser photocoagulation and cryotherapy is an option. Because most acute cases of ROP regress spontaneously with no long-term visual impairment, the possibility of regression must be weighed against the risk of an unfavorable outcome from treatment. For infants with bilateral traction and retinal detachment, surgical vitrectomy and scleral buckling are performed. Nursing care for the visually impaired infant must concentrate on parental support and education. When the crisis of premature birth is quickly followed by the devastating news of suspected visual impairment (poor visual acuity, myopia, strabismus, amblyopia, and glaucoma) or blindness, the parents will need extensive support by all members of the interdisciplinary health team. The parents again experience overwhelming anxiety and uncertainty about their infant's future abilities. Premature infants with blindness due to ROP may be at increased risk of cognitive and emotional problems. The evidence suggests that this increased risk may be due to environmental factors rather than to inherent intellectual or neurologic factors.

Speech Defects

The most frequently observed speech defects involve delayed development of receptive and expressive ability that may persist into the school-age years.

Neurologic Defects

The most common neurologic defects include cerebral palsy, hydrocephalus, seizure disorders, lower IQ scores, and learning disabilities. However, the socioeconomic climate and family support systems have been shown to be important factors influencing the child's ultimate school performance in the absence of major neurologic defects. Families can be reminded that risk does not equal injury, injury does not equal damage, and description of damage does not allow a precise prediction about recovery or outcome.

Auditory Defects

Preterm infants have a 1% to 4% incidence of moderate to profound hearing loss and should have a formal audiologic examination prior to discharge and at 3 to 6 months (corrected age). One test currently used to measure hearing functions of the newborn is the evoked otoacoustic emissions (EOAE) test. Earphones are used on each ear and independently measure sounds produced in the inner ear in response to acoustic stimuli. Another test, the automated auditory brain response (AABR), measures electroencephalogram (EEG) waves in response to sound waves generated by the test. The AABR provides information about the auditory pathway to the brainstem. Any infant with repeated abnormal results should be referred to speech-and-language specialists. Infants at increased risk include those with congenital viral infections, hyperbilirubinemia, severe perinatal asphyxia, meningitis, and birth trauma. Damage from ototoxic drugs such as gentamicin and furosemide (Lasix) is variable and related to multiple factors, including renal function, age, duration of treatment, and concomitant administration of other ototoxic agents.

When evaluating an infant's abilities and disabilities, parents must understand that the developmental progress must be evaluated based on chronologic age from the expected date of birth, not from the actual date of birth (corrected age). In addition, the parents need the consistent support of healthcare professionals in the long-term management of their infant. Many new and ongoing concerns arise as the high-risk infant grows and develops; the goal is to promote the highest quality of life possible.

NURSING CARE MANAGEMENT

Nursing Assessment and Diagnosis

Accurate assessment of the physical characteristics and gestational age of the preterm newborn is imperative to anticipate the special needs and problems of this baby. Physical characteristics vary greatly, depending on the gestational age, but the following characteristics are frequently present:

- *Color*: Usually pink or ruddy but may be acrocyanotic (Cyanosis, jaundice, or pallor are abnormal and should be noted.)

- *Skin.* Reddened, translucent, blood vessels readily apparent, lack of subcutaneous fat
- *Lanugo.* Plentiful, widely distributed
- *Head size.* Appears large in relation to body
- *Skull.* Bones pliable, fontanelle smooth and flat
- *Ears.* Minimal cartilage, pliable, folded over
- *Nails.* Soft, short
- *Genitals.* Male: nonrugated, small scrotum; testes may or may not be descended. Female: prominent clitoris and labia minora
- *Resting position.* Flaccid, froglike
- *Cry.* Weak, feeble
- *Reflexes.* Poor suck, swallow, and gag
- *Activity.* Jerky, generalized movements (Seizure activity is abnormal.)

Determining gestational age in preterm newborns requires knowledge and experience in administering gestational assessment tools. The tool used should be specific, reliable, and valid. For a discussion of gestational age assessment tools, see Chapter 29. Nursing diagnoses that may apply to the preterm newborn include:

- ***Impaired Gas Exchange*** related to immature pulmonary vasculature and inadequate surfactant production
- ***Ineffective Breathing Pattern*** related to immature central nervous system
- ***Alteration in Cardiovascular Status*** related to hypotension related to decreased tissue perfusion secondary to PDA
- ***Ineffective Thermoregulation*** related to hypothermia secondary to decreased glycogen and brown fat stores
- ***Altered Nutrition: Less than Body Requirements*** related to weak suck and swallow reflexes and decreased ability to absorb nutrients
- ***Fluid Volume Deficit*** related to high insensible water losses and inability of kidneys to concentrate urine
- ***High Risk for Intraventricular Hemorrhage*** related to fragile capillary network in the germinal matrix
- ***Ineffective Coping*** related to anger/guilt by parents at having given birth to a premature baby
- ***Dysfunctional Grieving*** related to actual or perceived loss of a normal newborn

Nursing Plan and Implementation

Maintenance of Respiratory Function

There is increased danger of respiratory obstruction in preterm newborns because their bronchi and trachea are so narrow that mucus can obstruct the airway. The nurse must maintain patency through judiciously suctioning, but only on an as-needed basis.

Positioning of the newborn can also affect respiratory function. If the baby is in the supine position, the nurse should slightly elevate the infant's head to maintain the airway, being careful not to hyperextend the neck because the trachea will collapse. Also, because the newborn has weak neck muscles and cannot control head movement, the nurse should ensure that this head position is maintained by using a small roll under the shoulders. The prone position splints the chest wall and decreases the amount of respiratory effort used to move the chest wall. The prone position therefore facilitates chest expansion and improves air entry and oxygenation. Weak or absent cough or gag reflexes increase the chance of aspiration in the premature newborn. The nurse should ensure that the infant's position facilitates drainage of mucus or regurgitated formula.

The nurse monitors heart and respiratory rates with cardiorespiratory monitors as well as through physical assessments to identify alterations in the newborn's cardiopulmonary status. Signs of respiratory distress include the following:

- Cyanosis (serious sign when generalized)
- Tachypnea (sustained respiratory rate greater than 60/minute after first 4 hours of life)
- Retractions
- Expiratory grunting
- Nasal flaring
- Apneic episodes
- Presence of rales or rhonchi on auscultation
- Diminished air entry

The nurse who observes any of these alterations records and reports them for further evaluation. If respiratory distress occurs, the nurse administers oxygen per physician/nurse practitioner order to relieve hypoxemia. If hypoxemia is not treated immediately, it may result in patent ductus arteriosus or metabolic acidosis. If oxygen is administered to the newborn, the nurse monitors the oxygen concentration with devices such as the transcutaneous oxygen monitor ($tcPO_2$) or the pulse oximeter. Periodic arterial blood gas sampling to monitor oxygen concentration in the baby's blood is essential because hyperoxemia may lead to ROP.

The nurse also needs to consider respiratory function prior to initiation of feedings as well as during feeding. To prevent aspiration, increased energy expenditure, and increased oxygen consumption, the nurse needs to ensure that the infant's gag and suck reflexes are intact.

Maintenance of Neutral Thermal Environment

Providing a neutral thermal environment minimizes the oxygen consumption required to maintain a normal core temperature; it also prevents cold stress and facilitates growth by decreasing the calories needed to maintain body temperature. The preterm infant's immature central nervous system, as well as small brown fat stores, provides poor temperature control. A small infant (< 1200 g) can lose 80 kcal/kg/day through radiation of body heat. The nurse should implement all the usual thermoregulation measures discussed in Chapter 30. In addition, to minimize heat loss and the effects of temperature instability for preterm and low-birth-weight newborns, the nurse should do the following:

1. Warm and humidify oxygen to minimize evaporative heat loss and decrease oxygen consumption.
2. Place the baby in a double-walled incubator, or use a Plexiglas heat shield over small preterm infants in

single-walled incubators to avoid radiative heat losses. Some institutions use radiant warmers and plastic wrap over the baby and pipe in humidity (swamping). Do not use Plexiglas shields on radiant warmer beds because it blocks the infrared heat.

3. Avoid placing the baby on cold surfaces, such as metal treatment tables and cold x-ray plates (conductive heat loss); pad cold surfaces with diapers and use radiant warmers during procedures; place the preterm infant on prewarmed mattresses; and warm hands before handling the baby to prevent heat transfer via conduction.
4. Use warmed ambient humidity. The use of humidity and its role in decreasing insensible water loss remains controversial (Blackburn, 2003).
5. Keep the skin dry (evaporative heat loss), and place a cap on the baby's head. The head makes up 25% of the total body size.
6. Keep radiant warmers, incubators, and cribs away from windows and cold external walls (radiative heat loss) and out of drafts (conductive heat loss).
7. Open incubator portholes and doors only when necessary, and use plastic sleeves on portholes to decrease convective heat loss.
8. Use a skin probe to monitor the baby's skin temperature. Correlate ambient temperatures with the skin probe in the incubator using the servocontrol rather than the manual mode. The temperature should be 36C to 37C (96.8F to 98.6F). Temperature fluctuations indicate hypothermia or hyperthermia. Be careful not to place skin temperature probes over bony prominences; areas of brown fat; poorly vasoreactive areas, such as extremities; or excoriated areas.
9. Warm formula or stored breast milk before feeding.
10. Use reflector patch over the skin temperature probe when using a radiant warmer bed so that the probe does not sense the higher infrared temperature as the baby's skin temperature and therefore decrease the heater output.

Once preterm infants are medically stable, they should be clothed with a double-thickness cap, cotton shirt, and diaper. If possible, they should be swaddled in a blanket. The nurse begins the process of weaning to a crib when the premature infant is medically stable, doesn't require assisted ventilation, weighs approximately 1500 g, has 5 days of consistent weight gain, and is taking oral feedings, and when apnea and bradycardia episodes have stabilized. The nurse should be familiar with the individual institution's protocol for weaning to crib for preterm infants.

Maintenance of Fluid and Electrolyte Status

Hydration is maintained by providing adequate intake based on the newborn's weight, gestational age, chronologic age, and volume of sensible and insensible water losses. Adequate fluid intake should provide sufficient water to compensate for increased insensible losses and to provide the amount needed for renal excretion of metabolic products. Insensible water losses can be minimized by providing a high-ambient humidity, humidifying oxygen, using heat shields, and placing the infant in a double-walled incubator.

The nurse evaluates the baby's hydration status by assessing and recording signs of dehydration. Signs of dehydration include the following:

- Sunken fontanelles
- Loss of weight
- Poor skin turgor (skin returns to position slowly when tented)
- Dry oral mucous membranes
- Decreased urine output
- Increased urine specific gravity (> 1.013)

The nurse must also identify signs of overhydration by observing the newborn for edema or excessive weight gain and by comparing urine output with fluid intake.

The preterm infant should be weighed at least once daily at the same time each day. *Weight change is the most sensitive indicator of fluid balance.* Weighing diapers is also important for accurate input and output measurement (1 mL = 1 g). A comparison of intake and output measurements over an 8-hour or 24-hour period provides important information about renal function and fluid balance. Assessment of patterns—in particular, whether they show a net gain or loss over several days—is also essential to fluid management. Monitor blood serum levels and pH to evaluate for electrolyte imbalances.

Accurate hourly intake calculations should be maintained when administering intravenous fluids. Because the preterm infant is unable to excrete excess fluid, it is important that the nurse maintain the correct amount of intravenous fluid to prevent fluid overload. This can be accomplished by using neonatal or pediatric infusion pumps. To prevent electrolyte imbalance, overhydration, and dehydration, the nurse must take care to give the correct intravenous solutions and volumes and concentrations of formulas. Urine specific gravity and pH are obtained periodically. Urine osmolality provides an indication of hydration, although this factor must be correlated with other assessments (for example, serum sodium). Hydration is considered adequate when the urine output is 1 to 3 mL/kg/hr.

Provision of Adequate Nutrition and Prevention of Fatigue During Feeding

The feeding method depends on the preterm newborn's feeding abilities and health status. Both nipple and gavage methods are initially supplemented with intravenous therapy until oral intake is sufficient to support growth (110 to 130 kcal/kg/day). Early, small-volume enteral feedings called *minimal enteral nutrition via gavage* have proved to be of benefit to the very-low-birth-weight infant. (See Methods of Feeding, earlier in this chapter). Formula or breast milk (with or without fortifiers to increase caloric content) is incorporated into the feedings slowly; initially, it may be at quarter-strength, then half-strength, and so on. This is done to avoid overtaxing the digestive capacity of the preterm newborn. The nurse should carefully watch for any signs of feeding intolerance, including:

- Increasing gastric residuals
- Abdominal distention (measured routinely before feedings) with visible bowel loops
- Guaiac-positive stools (occult blood in stools)
- Lactose in stools (reducing substance in the stools)
- Vomiting
- Diarrhea

Before each feeding, the nurse measures abdominal girth and auscultates the abdomen to determine the presence and quality of bowel sounds. Such assessments permit early detection of abdominal distention and decreased peristaltic activity, which may indicate NEC or paralytic ileus. The nurse also checks for residual formula in the stomach prior to feeding. This is done when the newborn is fed by gavage method. This procedure also can be performed when the nipple-fed newborn presents with abdominal distention. The presence of residual formula may indicate intolerance to the type or amount of feeding. Residual formula is usually readministered because digestive processes have already been initiated. The residual formula that is obtained is subtracted from the amount to be given at that feeding.

Preterm newborns who are ill or fatigue easily with nipple feedings are usually fed by gavage. The infant is essentially passive with these methods, thus conserving energy and calories. As the baby matures, gavage feedings are replaced with nipple (breast or formula) feedings to assist in strengthening the sucking reflex and meeting oral and emotional needs. Factors used to indicate readiness are a strong gag reflex, presence of nonnutritive sucking, rooting behavior, gestational age of 34 weeks or more, and weight over 1500 g. Both low-birth-weight and preterm infants nipple-feed more effectively in a quiet state (Lemons, 2001). The nurse establishes a gradual nipple-feeding program, such as one nipple feeding per day, then one nipple feeding per shift, and then a nipple feeding every other feeding. Daily weights are monitored because often there is a small weight loss when nipple feedings are started. After feedings, the baby is placed on the right side (with support to maintain this position) or on the abdomen. These positions enhance gastric emptying and decrease the chance of aspiration if regurgitation occurs. Gastroesophageal reflux is not uncommon in preterm newborns.

The nurse involves the parents in feeding their preterm baby. This is essential to the development of attachment between parents and infant. In addition, such involvement increases parental knowledge about the care of their infant and helps them cope with the situation.

Clinical Tip *Residual feeding may indicate early NEC and should be called to the attention of the clinician.*

Prevention of Infection

The nurse is responsible for minimizing the preterm newborn's exposure to pathogenic organisms. The preterm newborn is susceptible to infection because of an immature immune system and thin, permeable skin. Invasive procedures, techniques such as umbilical catheterization and mechanical ventilation, and prolonged hospitalization place the infant at greater risk for infection.

Strict handwashing and the use of separate equipment for each infant help minimize exposure of the preterm newborn to infectious agents. In addition, most nurseries around the country have adopted the Centers for Disease Control and Prevention (CDC) standard precautions whereby every baby is isolated. Staff members are required to scrub 2 to 3 minutes using antibacterial solutions, which inhibit the growth of gram-positive cocci and gram-negative rod organisms. Other nursing interventions include limiting visitors; requiring visitors to wash their hands; and maintaining strict aseptic practices when changing intravenous tubing and solutions (IV solutions should be changed every 24 hours; IV tubing changes vary among institutions), administering parenteral fluids, and assisting with sterile procedures. Incubators and radiant warmers should be changed weekly. Pressure area breakdown is prevented by changing the baby's position, doing range-of-motion exercises, and using a sheepskin (cover sheepskin with blanket, or diaper portion of sheepskin beneath infant's head), a water bed, or an air mattress. To avoid skin tears, a protective transparent covering can be applied over vulnerable joints, but use very sparingly (AWHONN, 2001). Chemical skin preps and tape may cause skin trauma and should be avoided as much as possible.

If infection (sepsis) occurs in the preterm newborn, the nurse may be the first to identify the associated subtle clinical signs. The nurse informs the clinician of the findings immediately and implements the treatment plan per clinician orders in the presence of infection. For specific nursing care required for the newborn with an infection, see Chapter 33.

Promotion of Parent-Infant Attachment

Preterm newborns can be separated from their parents for prolonged periods after illness or complications that are detected in the first few hours or days following birth. The resultant interruption in parent-newborn bonding necessitates intervention to ensure successful attachment of parent and infant.

Nurses should take measures to promote positive parental feelings toward the newborn. Photographs of the baby are given to parents to have at home or to the mother if she is in a different hospital or too ill to come to the nursery and visit. The infant's first name is placed on the incubator as soon as it is known to help the parents feel that their infant is a unique and special person. A weekly card with the baby's footprint, weight, and length is also sent to promote bonding. The nurse provides the parents with the telephone number of the nursery or intensive care unit and names of staff members so that they have access to information about their baby at any time of the day or night. The nurse encourages visits from siblings and grandparents to foster attachment.

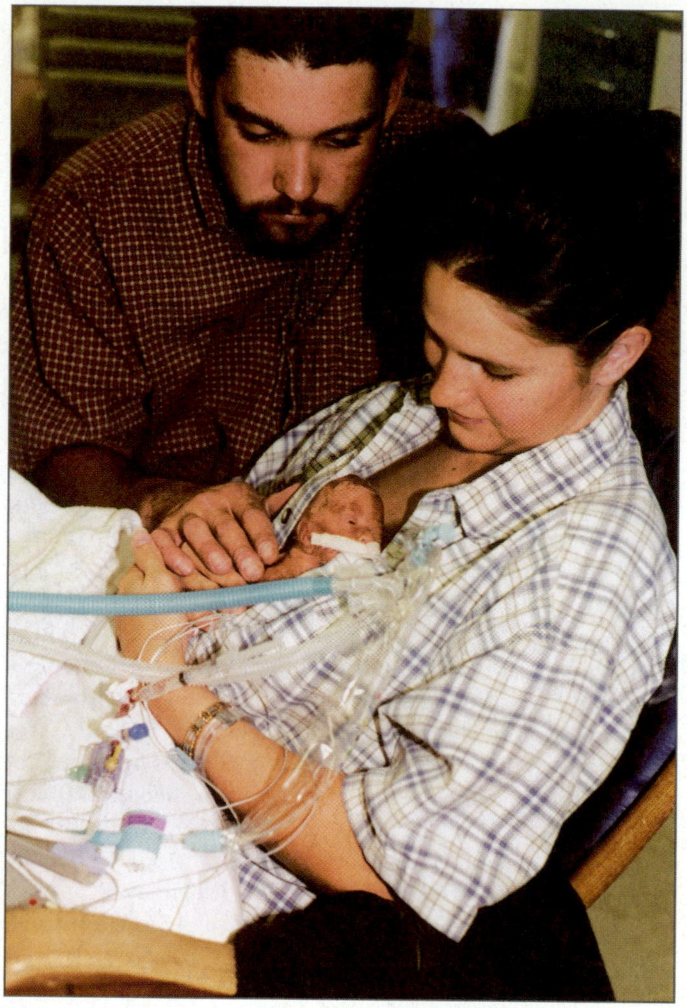

Figure 32–10 • Kangaroo (skin-to-skin) care facilitates a closeness and attachment between parents and their premature infant.
SOURCE: Courtesy of Carol Harrigan, RNC, MSN, NNP.

Early involvement in the care and decisions regarding their baby provides parents with realistic expectations for their baby. The individual personality characteristics of the infant and the parents influence bonding and contribute to the interactive process. Information is another important variable. Parents need education to develop caregiving skills and to understand the premature infant's behavioral characteristics. Their daily participation (if possible) is encouraged, as are early and frequent visits. The nurse provides opportunities for the parents to touch, hold, talk to, and care for the baby. Skin-to-skin holding (*kangaroo care*) helps parents feel close to their small infants. Kangaroo care has been shown to improve sleep periods and parents' perception of their caregiving ability (Feldman, Eidelman, Sirota, et al, 2002) (Figure 32–10 •).

Some parents may progress easily to touching and cuddling their infant; others will not (Figure 32–11 •). Parents need to know that their apprehension is normal and the progression of acquaintanceship is slow. Rooming-in can provide another opportunity for the stable preterm infant and family to get acquainted. Rooming-in is beneficial for both infant and family prior to discharge, as it offers a quiet, private environment where help is readily available.

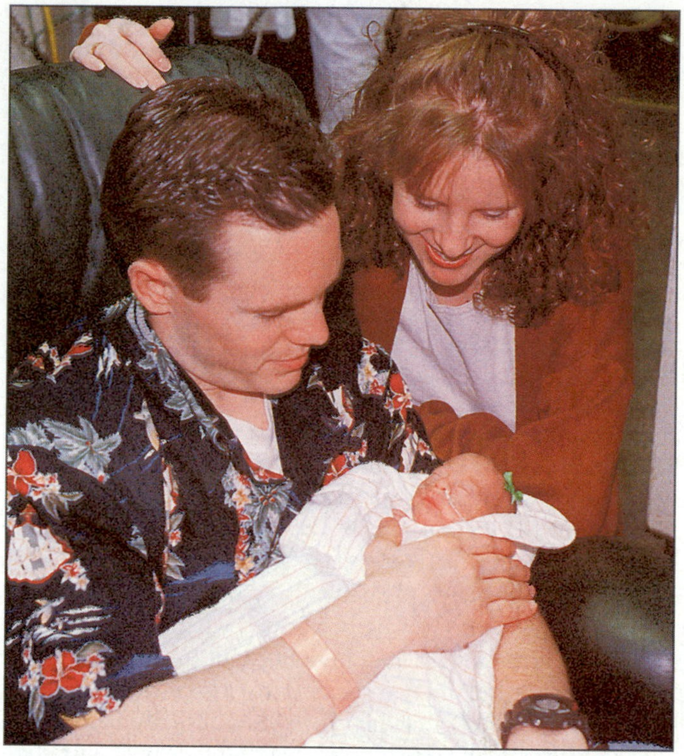

Figure 32–11 • Family bonding occurs when parents have opportunities to spend time with their infant.
SOURCE: Courtesy of Carol Harrigan, RNC, MSN, NNP.

Promotion of Developmentally Supportive Care

Prolonged separation and the NICU environment necessitate individualized sensory stimulation programs for the baby. The nurse plays a key role in determining the appropriate type and amount of visual, tactile, and auditory stimulation.

Research has shown that some preterm infants are not developmentally able to deal with more than one sensory input at a time. The assessment of preterm infant behavior (APIB) scale identifies the individual preterm newborn behaviors according to five areas of development (Als, Lester, Tronick, et al, 1982). The infant's physiologic and behavioral subsystems are autonomic, motor control, state differentiation, attention maintenance and social interaction, and finally overall system regulation or self-regulation. Integration of these subsystems improves with increasing gestational and postconceptual age. If the premature infant's self-regulatory capacity is exceeded and the infant is not able to return to previously integrated subsystem functioning, maladaptive behaviors may result when the infant is confronted with environmental demands. The nurse observes the baby's behavioral reactions to stimulation and then bases developmental interventions on reducing detrimental environmental stimuli to the lowest possible level and providing appropriate opportunities for development (Blackburn, 2003).

COMPLEMENTARY AND ALTERNATIVE THERAPIES

COMPLEMENTARY AND ALTERNATIVE MEDICINE (CAM) IN THE NICU

As NICUs are becoming more and more "developmentally" friendly, complementary and alternative medicine (CAM) has now become an adjunct to that nurturing environment. This holistic approach in caring for the low-birth-weight infant attempts not only to mimic the intrauterine environment, but also to foster parent-infant bonding by simultaneously caring for the body, spirit, and mind.

Aromatherapy is the use of scent to alter mood or behavior to produce a calming and sedating effect. There is an enhanced bonding process between mothers and newborns associated with the natural body odor emitted from the mother (Jones, Kassity, & Duncan, 2001). Aromatherapy is utilized in the NICU by placing an article of clothing belonging to the mother next to the infant to produce a soothing and consoling effect on the infant in her absence. Researchers are also investigating other aromatherapies, including peppermint as a respiratory stimulant, chamomile as a method to regulate sleep-wake cycles, Brazilian guava for its analgesic effects, and lavendar sitz baths for management of diaper rash.

Skin-to-skin (kangaroo) care is becoming more prevalent in NICUs across the United States. It was first practiced in Bogota, Colombia, in the early 1980s because of the fear of the spread of infection from sharing incubators (Eichel, 2001). Skin-to-skin care is defined as the practice of holding infants skin-to-skin next to their parents. The infant is usually naked, except for a diaper, and placed on his/her parent's bare chest. They are then both covered with a blanket. Benefits of skin-to-skin care as a developmental intervention include the following: improved oxygenation as evidenced by an increase in transcutaneous oxygen levels, enhanced temperature regulation, a decline in the episodes of apnea and bradycardia, increased periods of quiet sleep, stabilization of vital signs, positive interaction between parent and infant which enhances attachment and bonding, increased growth parameters, and early discharge (McGrath & Conliffe-Torres 2000). Limitations to skin-to-skin care may be due to staff uneasiness when moving the infant while attached to multiple IV lines, monitor leads, and a ventilator. The limited confines of the nursery may be another limiting factor.

Music therapy as a noninvasive auditory stimulus has been shown to be advantageous for the premature infant (Standley, 2001). The music used in NICUs includes primarily lullabies and soft acoustical pieces which are pleasant, soothing, and calming. Such music has been shown to effect newborn physiologic responses, improving oxygenation and increasing weight gain. It also has behavioral effects, leading to enhanced parental bonding and increased intervals of nonnutritive sucking periods. Language development is also enhanced if the music is live and sung by the mother or another female, which is preferential to the infant (Standley, 2001). The overall noise level in the NICU needs to be considered before including any extra auditory stimulation, including music therapy.

Infant massage and gentle touch have been practiced for many centuries. The types of stimulation include massage with stroking, gentle touch without stroking, and therapeutic touch or "hands on" containment. Practitioners report such physiologic benefits as stimulating blood and lymphatic flow, promoting weight gain in premature infants, and regulating sleep patterns. Many emotional and behavioral benefits are also cited by practitioners. Classes are available to teach parents how to perform massage on their infants. Massage demonstrates compassion while increasing the parent's empathy and understanding of the baby. It helps parents learn to interpret their baby's behavioral cues such as facial expression, various crying patterns, and other body language. At the same time it helps infants learn about their various body parts and boundaries and feel how they integrate into the whole. Therapeutic touch reduces motor activity and energy expenditure by the infant and promotes comfort (Harrison, 2001).

The NICU environment contains many detrimental stimuli that the nurse can help reduce. Noise levels can be lowered by replacing alarms with lights or silencing alarms quickly and keeping conversations away from the baby's bedside. Dimmer switches should be used to shield the baby's eyes from bright lights with blankets over the top portion of the incubator. Dimming the lights may encourage infants to open their eyes and be more responsive to their parents. Nursing care should be planned to decrease the number of times the baby is disturbed. Signs (ie, "Quiet Please") can be placed near the bedside to allow the baby some periods of uninterrupted sleep (Blackburn, 2003). Some other suggested developmentally supportive interventions include:

- Facilitate handling by using containment measures when turning or moving the infant or doing procedures such as suctioning. Use the hands to hold the infant's arms and legs, flexed, close to the midline of the body. This helps stabilize the infant's motor and physiologic subsystems during stressful activities.
- Touch the infant gently, and avoid sudden postural changes.
- Promote self-consoling or soothing activities, such as placing blanket rolls or approved manufactured devices next to the infant's sides and against the feet, to provide "nesting." Swaddle the infant to maintain extremities in a flexed position while ensuring that the hands can reach the face. This permits the infant to do hand-to-mouth activities, which can be consoling (Figure 32–12 ●).
- Simulate the kinesthetic advantages of the intrauterine environment by using sheepskin and approved water beds. Water bed use has been reported to improve sleep

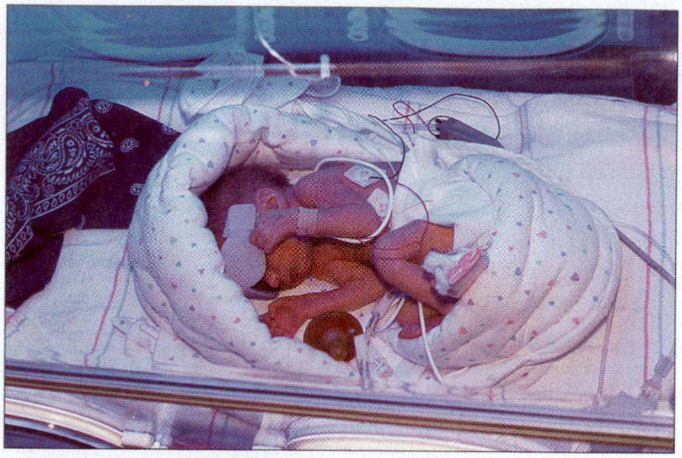

Figure 32–12 • Infant is "nested." Hand-to-face behavior facilitates self-consoling and soothing activities.
SOURCE: Courtesy of Theresa Kledzik, RN, Developmental Nurse, Memorial Hospital, Colorado Springs, Colorado.

and decrease motor activity as well as lead to more mature motor behavior, fewer state changes, and a decreased heart rate.
- Provide opportunities for nonnutritive sucking with a pacifier. This improves transcutaneous oxygen saturation; decreases body movement; improves sleep, especially after feedings; and increases weight gain.
- Provide objects for the infant to grasp (eg, a piece of blanket, oxygen tubing, or a finger) during caregiving. Grasping may comfort the baby.

Teaching the parents to read behavioral cues will help them move at their infant's pace when providing stimulation. Parents are ideally equipped to meet the baby's need for stimulation. Stroking, rocking, cuddling, quiet singing, and talking to the baby can all be an integral part of the baby's care. Visual stimulation in the form of *en face* interaction with the caregivers and mobiles is also important.

Preparation for Home Care

Parents are often anxious when their premature infant is transferred out of the NICU or is discharged home. Parents of preterm babies should receive the same postpartal teaching as any parent taking a new infant home. In preparing for discharge, the nurse encourages the parents to spend time caring directly for their baby. This familiarizes them with their baby's behavior patterns and helps them establish realistic expectations about the infant. Some hospitals have a special room near the nursery where a mother can spend the night with her baby prior to discharge.

Discharge instruction includes breastfeeding and formula-feeding techniques, formula preparation, and vitamin administration. If the mother wishes to breastfeed, the nurse teaches her to pump her breasts to keep the milk flowing and provide milk even before discharge. The nurse gives information on bathing, diapering, hygiene, and normal elimination patterns and prepares the parents to expect changes in the color of the baby's stool, number of bowel movements, and timing of elimination when the infant is switched from formula-feeding to breastfeeding. This information can prevent unnecessary concern by the parents. The nurse also discusses normal growth and development patterns, reflexes, and activity for preterm infants. In these discussions, the nurse should emphasize ways to promote bonding behaviors and deal with newborn crying. Care of the preterm infant with complications, preventing infections, recognizing signs of a sick baby, and the need for continued medical follow-up are other key issues.

Families with preterm infants usually do not need to be referred to community agencies, such as visiting nurse assistance. Referral may be necessary if the infant has severe congenital abnormalities, feeding problems, or complications with infections or respiratory problems or if the parents seem unable to cope with an at-risk baby. Parents of preterm infants can benefit from meeting with others in a similar situation to share common experiences and concerns. Nurses should refer parents to support groups sponsored by the hospital or by others in the community and make connection for parents with early education intervention centers.

Evaluation

Expected outcomes of nursing care include the following:

- The preterm newborn is free of respiratory distress and establishes effective respiratory function.
- The preterm newborn gains weight and shows no signs of fatigue or aspiration during feedings.
- The preterm newborn demonstrates a serial head circumference growth rate of 1 cm per week.
- The parents are able to verbalize their anger, anxieties, and guilt feelings about the birth of a preterm baby and show attachment behavior such as frequent visits and growing confidence in their participatory care activities.

Care of the Newborn with Congenital Anomalies

The birth of a baby with a congenital defect places both newborn and family at risk. Many congenital anomalies can be life threatening if not corrected within hours after birth; others are very visible and cause the families emotional distress. When one congenital anomaly is found, healthcare providers should look for other ones, particularly in body systems that develop at the same time during gestation. Table 32–2 • identifies some of the more common anomalies and their early management and nursing care in the newborn period.

Care of the Infant of a Substance-Abusing Mother

An **infant of a substance-abusing mother (ISAM)** may also be alcohol or drug dependent. After birth, when an infant's connection with the maternal blood supply is severed, the baby

Table 32-2 • CONGENITAL ANOMALIES: IDENTIFICATION AND CARE IN NEWBORN PERIOD

Congenital Anomaly	Nursing Assessments	Nursing Goals and Interventions
Congenital hydrocephalus	Enlarged head Enlarged or full fontanelles Split or widened sutures "Setting sun" eyes Head circumference > 90% on growth chart	Assess presence of hydrocephalus: Measure and plot occipital-frontal baseline measurements; then measure head circumference once a day. Check fontanelles for bulging and sutures for widening. Assist with head ultrasound and transillumination. Maintain skin integrity: Change position frequently. Clean skin creases after feeding or vomiting. Use sheepskin pillow under head. Postoperatively, position head off operative site. Watch for signs of infection.
Choanal atresia	Occlusion of posterior nares Cyanosis and retractions at rest Snorting respirations Difficulty breathing during feeding Obstruction by thick mucus	Assess patency of nares: Listen for breath sounds while holding baby's mouth closed and alternately compressing each nostril. Assist with passing feeding tube to confirm diagnosis. Maintain respiratory function: Assist with taping airway in mouth to prevent respiratory distress. Position with head elevated to improve air exchange.
Cleft lip	Unilateral or bilateral visible defect May involve external nares, nasal cartilage, nasal septum, and alveolar process Flattening or depression of midfacial contour 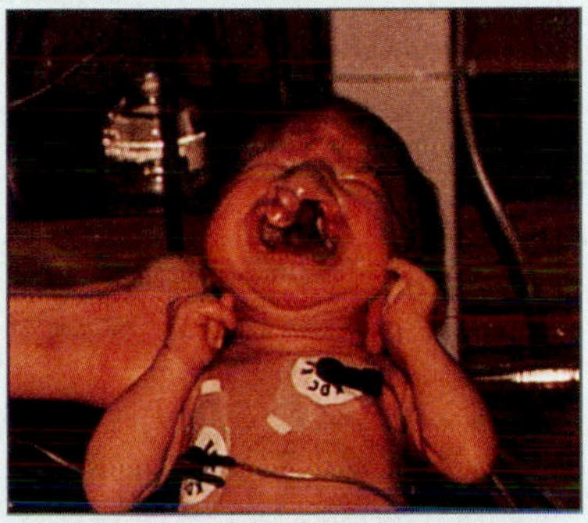	Provide nutrition: Feed with special nipple. Burp frequently (increased tendency to swallow air and reflex vomiting). Clean cleft with sterile water (to prevent crusting on cleft prior to repair). Support parental coping: Assist parents with grief over loss of idealized baby. Encourage verbalization of their feelings about visible defect. Provide role model in interacting with infant. (Parents internalize others' responses to their newborn.) (At left) Unilateral cleft lip with cleft abnormality involving both hard and soft palates.
Cleft palate	Fissure connecting oral and nasal cavity May involve uvula and soft palate May extend forward to nostril involving hard palate and maxillary alveolar ridge Difficulty in sucking Expulsion of formula through nose	Prevent aspiration/infection: Place prone or in side-lying position to facilitate drainage. Suction nasopharyngeal cavity (to prevent aspiration or airway obstruction). During newborn period feed in upright position with head and chest tilted slightly backward (to aid swallowing and discourage aspiration). Provide nutrition: Feed with special nipple that fills cleft and allows sucking. Also decreases chance of aspiration through nasal cavity. Clean mouth with water after feedings. Burp after each ounce (tend to swallow large amounts of air). Thicken formula to provide extra calories. Plot weight gain patterns to assess adequacy of diet. Provide parental support: Refer parents to community agencies and support groups. Encourage verbalization of frustrations because feeding process is long and frustrating. Praise all parental efforts. Encourage parents to seek prompt treatment for upper respiratory infection (URI) and teach them ways to decrease URI.
Tracheoesophageal fistula (type 3)	History of maternal hydramnios Excessive mucous secretions Constant drooling Abdominal distention beginning soon after birth Periodic choking and cyanotic episodes Immediate regurgitation of feeding Clinical symptoms of aspiration pneumonia (tachypnea, retractions, rhonchi, decreased breath sounds, cyanotic spells) Failure to pass nasogastric tube	Maintain respiratory status and prevent aspiration: Withhold feeding until esophageal patency is determined. Quickly assess patency before putting to breast in birth area. Place on low intermittent suction to control saliva and mucus (to prevent aspiration pneumonia). Place in warmed, humidified incubator (liquefies secretions, facilitating removal). Elevate head of bed 20–40 degrees (to prevent reflux of gastric juices). Keep quiet (crying causes air to pass through fistula and to distend intestines, causing respiratory embarrassment). Maintain fluid and electrolyte balance: Give fluids to replace esophageal drainage and maintain hydration. Provide parent education: Explain staged repair—provision of gastrostomy and ligation of fistula, then repair of atresia. Keep parents informed; clarify and reinforce physician's explanations regarding malformation, surgical repair, preoperative and postoperative care, and prognosis (knowledge enhances feelings of self-worth).

(continued on next page)

Table 32–2 • CONTINUED

Congenital Anomaly	Nursing Assessments	Nursing Goals and Interventions
Tracheoesophageal fistula (type 3) continued		Involve parents in care of infant and in planning for future; facilitate touch and eye contact (to dispel feelings of inadequacy, increase self-esteem and self-worth, and promote incorporation of infant into family).
Diaphragmatic hernia	Difficulty initiating respirations Gasping respirations with nasal flaring and chest retraction Barrel chest and scaphoid abdomen Asymmetric chest expansion Breath sounds may be absent (Usually on left side) Heart sounds displaced to right Spasmodic attacks of cyanosis and difficulty in feeding Bowel sounds may be heard in thoracic cavity	Nurse should never ventilate with bag and mask O_2 because the stomach and intestines will become distended with air, further compressing the lungs. Maintain respiratory status: Immediately administer oxygen. May need to be intubated and ventilated. Initiate gastric decompression. Place in high semi-Fowler's position (to use gravity to keep abdominal organs' pressure off diaphragm). Turn to affected side to allow unaffected lung expansion. Carry out interventions to alleviate respiratory and metabolic acidosis. Assess for increased secretions around suction tube (denotes possible obstruction). Aspirate and irrigate tube with air or sterile water.

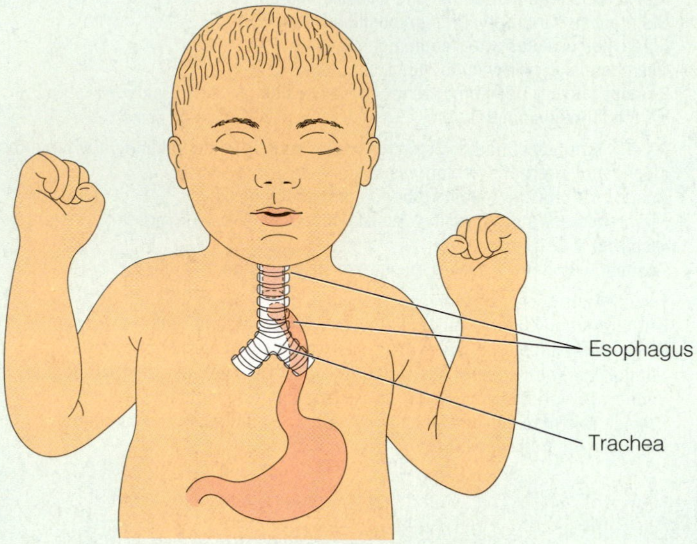

(At left) The most frequently seen type of congenital tracheoesophageal fistula and esophageal atresia.

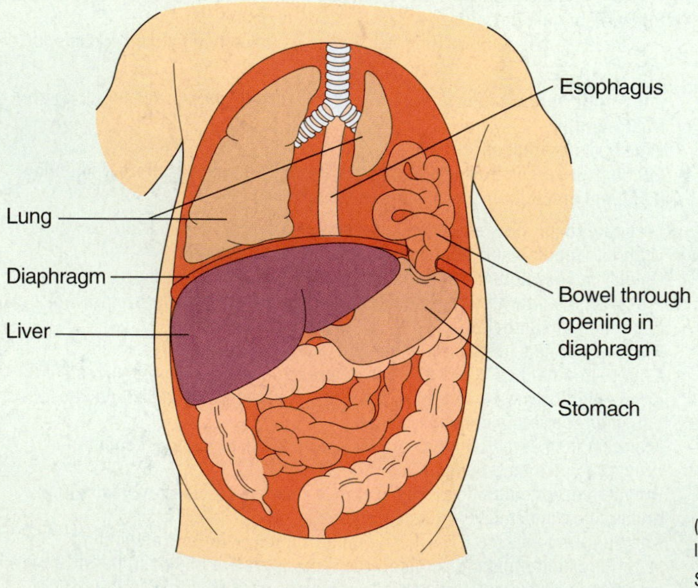

(At left) Diaphragmatic hernia. Note compression of the lung by the intestine on the affected side.

Source: Courtesy of Nancy Houck, RNC, BSN, NNP.

Table 32-2 • CONTINUED

Congenital Anomaly	Nursing Assessments	Nursing Goals and Interventions
Myelomeningocele	Saclike cyst containing meninges, spinal cord, and nerve roots in thoracic and/or lumbar area Myelomeningocele directly connects to subarachnoid space so hydrocephalus often associated No response or varying response to sensation below level of sac May have constant dribbling of urine Incontinence or retention of stool Anal opening may be flaccid	Prevent trauma and infection. Position on abdomen or on side and restrain (to prevent pressure and trauma to sac). Meticulously clean buttocks and genitals after each voiding and defecation (to prevent contamination of sac and decrease possibility of infection). May put protective covering over sac (to prevent rupture and drying). Observe sac for oozing of fluid or pus. Credé bladder (apply downward pressure on bladder with thumbs, moving urine toward the urethra) as ordered to prevent urinary stasis. Assess amount of sensation and movement below defect. Observe for complications. Obtain occipital-frontal circumference baseline measurements; then measure head circumference once a day (to detect hydrocephalus). Check fontanelle for bulging.
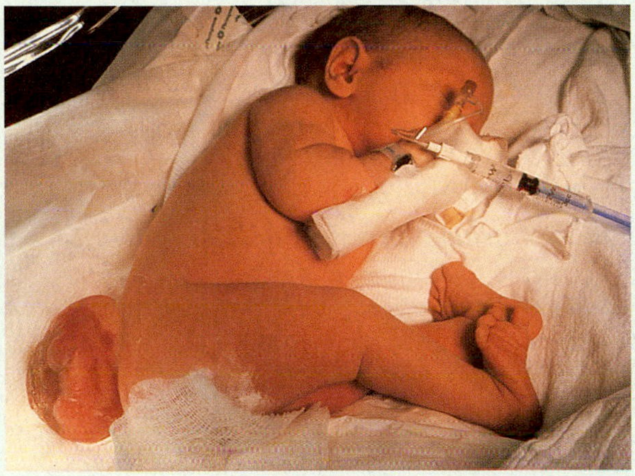		(At left) Newborn with lumbar myelomeningocele. SOURCE: Courtesy Dr Paul Winchester.
Omphalocele	Herniation of abdominal contents into base of umbilical cord May have an enclosed transparent sac covering	Maintain hydration and temperature. Provide D_5LR and albumin for hypovolemia. Place infant in sterile bag up to and covering defect. Cover sac with moistened sterile gauze, and place plastic wrap over dressing (to prevent rupture of sac and infection). Initiate gastric decompression by insertion of nasogastric tube attached to low suction (to prevent distention of lower bowel and impairment of blood flow). Prevent infection and trauma to defect. Position to prevent trauma to defect. Administer broad-spectrum antibiotics.
Gastroschisis	Lateral defect in abdominal wall allowing viscera outside the body to the left of an intact umbilical cord. No sac covering. Associated with intestinal atresia, malrotation	Maintain hydration and temperature. Prevent trauma and infection to defect. Provide D_5LR and albumin for hypovolemia. Place infant in sterile bag up to cord and covering defect. Initiate gastric decompression by insertion of nasogastric tube attached to low suction. Administer broad-spectrum antibiotics.
Imperforate anus, congenital dislocated hip, and clubfoot	See discussion in Chapter 29, Anus and Extremities	Identify defect and initiate appropriate referral early.

Source: Courtesy of Nancy Houck, RNC, BSN, NNP.

may suffer withdrawal. In addition, the drugs the mother ingested may be teratogenic, resulting in congenital anomalies.

Alcohol Dependence

The **fetal alcohol syndrome (FAS)** includes a series of malformations (identified shortly) frequently found in infants exposed to alcohol in utero. It has been estimated that complete FAS occurs in 5.2 live births per 1000 (AAP Committee on Substance Abuse and Committee on Children with Disabilities, 2000). FAS rates are increased among Native Americans and Alaska natives and those of low economic status. **Fetal alcohol effects (FAE),** or **alcohol-related birth defects (ARBD),** are usually determined only by a positive maternal drinking history and cognitive difficulties and usually do not exhibit the classic facial dysmorphology (Rosen & Bateman, 2002). The new diagnostic categories for FAS take into consideration the various clinical manifestations of FAS, the social and family environment, and, if available, the maternal alcohol history.

MediaLink FETAL ALCOHOL SYNDROME RESOURCES

Although it is known that ethanol freely crosses the placenta to the fetus, it is still not known whether the alcohol alone or the breakdown products of alcohol cause the damage. For in-depth discussion of alcohol abuse in pregnancy, see Chapter 19. The effects of other substances that are often combined with alcohol, such as nicotine, marijuana, and caffeine, as well as poor diet, enhance the likelihood of FAS.

LONG-TERM COMPLICATIONS FOR THE INFANT WITH FAS

The long-term prognosis for the FAS newborn is less than favorable. Many FAS infants are evaluated for organic and inorganic failure to thrive. These infants have a delay in the normal progression of oral feeding because of weak suck development. Many FAS infants breastfeed poorly and have persistent vomiting until 6 to 7 months of age. They have difficulty adjusting to solid foods and show little spontaneous interest in food.

Central nervous system (CNS) dysfunctions are the most common and serious problems associated with FAS. Hypotonicity and increased placidity is seen in these infants. They also have a decreased ability to habituate repetitive stimuli. Children exhibiting FAS can be severely mentally retarded or have normal intelligence. The more abnormal the facial features, the lower the IQ scores. Often there is little improvement in intelligence (as measured by IQ) despite positive environmental and educational factors (Rosen & Bateman, 2002). These children show impulsivity, cognitive impairment, speech and language abnormalities, and learning disabilities indicative of CNS involvement (Jacobson, Chiodo, Sokol, et al, 2002).

NURSING CARE MANAGEMENT

Nursing Assessment and Diagnosis

Newborns with FAS show the following characteristics:

- *Abnormal structural development and CNS dysfunction,* including mental retardation, microcephaly, and hyperactivity.
- *Growth deficiencies.* Infants with FAS are often growth retarded with weight, length, and head circumference being affected. These infants continue to show a persistent postnatal growth deficiency with head circumference and linear growth most affected.
- *Distinctive facial abnormalities.* These include short palpebral fissures, epicanthal folds, broad nasal bridge, flattened midfacies, short upturned or beaklike nose, micrognathia (abnormally small lower jaw), hypoplastic maxilla, thin upper lip or vermilion border, and smooth philtrum (groove on upper lip).
- *Associated anomalies.* Abnormalities affecting the heart (primarily septal and valvular defects), eyes, kidneys, and skeletal system (especially those involving joints, such as congenital dislocated hips) are often noted.

Alcohol-exposed infants in the first week of life may show symptoms that include sleeplessness, excessive arousal states, inconsolable crying, abnormal reflexes, hyperactivity with little ability to maintain alertness and attentiveness to environment, jitteriness, abdominal distention, and exaggerated mouthing behaviors such as hyperactive rooting and increased nonnutritive sucking. These symptoms commonly persist throughout the first month of life but may continue longer. Alcohol dependence in the infant is physiologic, not psychologic. Signs and symptoms of withdrawal often appear within 6 to 12 hours and at least within the first 3 days of life. Seizures after the neonatal period are rare.

Nursing diagnoses that may apply to the FAS newborn include the following:

- ***Altered Nutrition: Less than Body Requirements*** related to decreased food intake and hyperirritability
- ***Alteration in Neurodevelopmental Status*** related to central nervous system involvement secondary to maternal alcohol use
- ***Ineffective Coping*** related to dysfunctional family dynamics and substance-dependent mother

Nursing Plan and Implementation

Hospital-Based Nursing Care

The nurse's awareness of the signs and symptoms of FAS is important in structuring and guiding nursing care. Nursing care of the FAS newborn is aimed at avoiding heat loss, providing adequate nutrition, and reducing environmental stimuli. The FAS baby is most comfortable in a quiet, dimly lighted environment. Because of feeding problems, these infants require extra time and patience during feedings. It is important to provide consistency in the staff working with the baby and parents and to keep personnel and visitors to a minimum at any one time.

The nurse should inform the alcohol-dependent mother that breastfeeding is not contraindicated but that excessive alcohol consumption may intoxicate the newborn and inhibit the let-down reflex. The nurse should monitor the newborn's vital signs closely and observe for evidence of seizure activity and respiratory distress.

Community-Based Nursing Care

Infants affected by maternal alcohol abuse are also at risk psychologically. Restlessness, sleeplessness, agitation, resistance to cuddling or holding, and frequent crying can be frustrating to parents as their efforts to relieve the distress are unrewarded. Feeding dysfunction can also result in frustrations for the caregiver and digestive upsets for the infant. Frustration may cause the parents to punish the baby or result in the unconscious desire to stay away from the infant. Either outcome may create an unstable family environment and result in the infant's failure to thrive.

The nurse should focus on providing support for the parents and reinforcing positive parenting activity. Prior to discharge, parents should be given opportunities to provide baby care so that they can feel confident in their interpretations of their baby's cues and their ability to meet the baby's needs. Referring the family to social services and visiting nurse or public health nurse associations is essential for the well-being of the infant. Follow-up care and teaching can strengthen the parents' skills and coping abilities and help them create a stable, healthy environment for their family. The infant with FAS/ARBD should be involved in intervention programs that monitor the child's developmental progress, health, and home environment.

Evaluation

Expected outcomes of nursing care include the following:

- The FAS newborn is able to tolerate feedings and gain weight.
- The FAS infant's hyperirritability is controlled, and the baby has suffered no physical injuries.
- The parents are able to identify and meet the special needs of their newborn and accept outside assistance as needed.

Drug Dependence

Drugs of abuse by the pregnant woman can include the following singularly or in combination: tobacco, cocaine, phencyclidine (PCP), methamphetamines, inhalants, marijuana, heroin, and methadone.

Drug-dependent infants are predisposed to a number of problems. Almost all narcotic drugs cross the placenta and enter the fetal circulation, so the fetus can develop problems in utero or soon after birth. The effects of polydrug use on the newborn must always be taken into consideration.

The greatest risks to the fetus of the drug-dependent mother include the following:

- *Intrauterine asphyxia.* Often a direct result of fetal withdrawal secondary to maternal withdrawal, fetal withdrawal is accompanied by hyperactivity with increased oxygen consumption. If not adequately compensated, this can lead to fetal asphyxia. Moreover, narcotic-addicted women tend to have a higher incidence of preeclampsia, abruptio placentae, and placenta previa, resulting in placental insufficiency and fetal asphyxia.
- *Intrauterine infection.* Sexually transmitted infections, HIV infection, and hepatitis are often connected with the pregnant addict's lifestyle. Such infections can involve the fetus.
- *Alterations in birth weight.* These may depend on the type of drug the mother uses. Women using predominantly heroin or cocaine have infants of lower birth weight who are small for gestational age (SGA). Women maintained on methadone have higher-birth-weight infants, some of whom are large for gestational age (LGA).
- *Low Apgar scores.* These may be related to the intrauterine asphyxia or the medication the woman received during labor. The use of a narcotic antagonist (nalorphine or naloxone) to reverse respiratory depression is contraindicated because it may precipitate acute withdrawal in the infant.

Patterns of abuse of alcohol, marijuana, and heroin in childbearing women have changed very little in the past few years, but the incidence of cocaine (especially "crack") use has recently risen dramatically. (See Chapter 19 for more discussion of maternal substance abuse .) Marijuana, alcohol, and nicotine are often used in conjunction with cocaine.

COMMON COMPLICATIONS OF THE DRUG-DEPENDENT NEWBORN

The newborn of a woman who abused drugs during her pregnancy is predisposed to the following problems:

- *Respiratory distress.* The heroin-addicted newborn frequently suffers respiratory stress, mainly meconium-aspiration pneumonia and transient tachypnea. Meconium aspiration is usually secondary to increased oxygen consumption and activity experienced by the fetus during intrauterine withdrawal. Transient tachypnea may develop secondary to the inhibitory effects of narcotics on the reflex responsible for clearing the lungs. Respiratory distress syndrome, however, occurs less often in heroin-addicted newborns, even in those who are premature, because they have tissue-oxygen unloading capabilities comparable to those of a 6-week-old term infant. In addition, heroin stimulates production of glucocorticoids via the anterior pituitary gland.
- *Jaundice.* Newborns of methadone-addicted women may develop jaundice due to prematurity. By contrast, infants of mothers addicted to heroin or cocaine have a lower incidence of hyperbilirubinemia because these substances contribute to early maturity of the liver.
- *Congenital anomalies and growth restriction.* The incidence of anomalies of the genitourinary and cardiovascular systems is slightly increased in infants of heroin- and cocaine-addicted mothers. Infants of cocaine-addicted mothers exhibit congenital malformations involving bony skull defects, such as microencephaly, and symmetric intrauterine growth restriction, cardiac defects, and genitourinary defects. Congenital anomalies, however, are rare (Weiner & Finnegan, 2002).
- *Behavioral abnormalities.* Babies exposed to cocaine have poor state organization. They exhibit decreased interactive behaviors when tested with the Brazelton Neonatal Behavioral Assessment Scale. These infants also have difficulty moving through the various sleep and awake states and have problems attending to and actively engaging in auditory and visual stimuli.

Table 32–3 • CLINICAL MANIFESTATIONS NEWBORN WITHDRAWAL

Central nervous system signs
- Hyperactivity
- Hyperirritability (persistent shrill cry)
- Increased muscle tone
- Exaggerated reflexes
- Tremors and myoclonic jerks
- Sneezing, hiccups, yawning
- Short, unquiet sleep
- Fever (accompanies the increased neuromuscular activities)

Respiratory signs
- Tachypnea (> 60 breaths per minute when quiet)
- Excessive secretions

Gastrointestinal signs
- Disorganized, vigorous suck
- Vomiting
- Drooling
- Sensitive gag reflex
- Hyperphagia
- Diarrhea
- Abdominal cramping
- Poor feeding (< 15 mL on first day of life; takes longer than 30 minutes per feeding)

Vasomotor signs
- Stuffy nose, yawning, sneezing
- Flushing
- Sweating
- Sudden, circumoral pallor

Cutaneous signs
- Excoriated buttocks, knees, elbows
- Facial scratches
- Pressure-point abrasions

- *Withdrawal.* The most significant postnatal problem of the drug-addicted newborn is narcotic withdrawal (usually from heroin or methadone). The onset of the withdrawal manifestations often occurs after discharge, especially with short birthing unit stays. See Table 32–3 • for a discussion of withdrawal symptoms.

LONG-TERM EFFECTS

During the first 2 years of life, many cocaine-exposed infants demonstrate susceptibility to behavior lability and the inability to express strong feelings such as pleasure, anger, or distress, or even a strong reaction to being separated from their parents. Cocaine-exposed infants are at higher risk for motor development problems, delays in expressive language skills, and feeding difficulties due to swallowing problems (Cambell, 2003).

Infants of drug-addicted mothers often demonstrate a higher incidence of gastrointestinal and respiratory illnesses; it is believed these are related not to drug exposure but to the mothers' lack of education regarding proper infant care, feeding, and hygiene.

Another important long-term complication is the high rate of sudden infant death syndrome (SIDS) for heroin-or methadone-exposed infants and for infants who have a very difficult course of neonatal abstinence syndrome (Weiner & Finnegan, 2002). After birth the infant born to a drug-dependent mother may also be subject to neglect, abuse, or both.

CLINICAL THERAPY

The goal of clinical therapy is to prevent complications through prenatal management (see Chapter 19) and pharmacologic management of newborn narcotic withdrawal. For optimal fetal and newborn outcome, the narcotic-addicted woman should receive complete prenatal care as early as possible. She should be started on a methadone program (Ballard, 2002). The aim of methadone maintenance during pregnancy is to prevent heroin use. The maintenance dose of methadone should be sufficient to ensure this goal. It is not recommended that the woman be withdrawn completely from narcotics while pregnant because this induces fetal withdrawal with poor newborn outcomes.

Newborn treatment may include management of complications; serologic tests for syphilis, HIV, and hepatitis B; urine drug screen and meconium analysis; and social service referral (Weiner & Finnegan, 2002). Drugs used to control withdrawal symptoms vary and may be regionally based. They include phenobarbital, paregoric, oral morphine sulfate solution, and diazepam (Blackburn, 2003; Weiner & Finnegan, 2002). Nutritional support is important in light of the increase in energy expenditure that withdrawal may entail.

NURSING CARE MANAGEMENT

Nursing Assessment and Diagnosis

Early identification of the newborn needing clinical or pharmacologic interventions decreases the incidence of mortality and morbidity. During the newborn period, nursing assessment focuses on the following:

- Discovering the mother's last drug intake and dosage level. This is accomplished through the prenatal history and laboratory tests. Women may be reluctant to disclose this information; therefore, a nonjudgmental interview technique is essential (Lester, ElSohly, Wright, et al, 2001).
- Assessing for congenital malformations and the complications related to intrauterine withdrawal, such

Table 32–4 • NEONATAL ABSTINENCE SCORE SHEET

Neonatal Abstinence Scoring System

System	Signs and Symptoms	Score	AM	PM	Comments
Central Nervous System Disturbances	Excessive high-pitched (or other) cry Continuous high-pitched (or other) cry	2 3			Daily weight:
	Sleeps < 1 hour after feeding Sleeps < 2 hours after feeding Sleeps < 3 hours after feeding	3 2 1			
	Hyperactive Moro reflex Markedly hyperactive Moro reflex	2 3			
	Mild tremors disturbed Moderate-severe tremors disturbed	1 2			
	Mild tremors undisturbed Moderate-severe tremors undisturbed	3 4			
	Increased muscle tone	2			
	Excoriation (specific area)	1			
	Myoclonic jerks	3			
	Generalized convulsions	5			
Metabolic/Vasomotor/ Respiratory Disturbances	Sweating	1			
	Fever < 101 (99–100.8F/37.2–38.2C) Fever > 101 (38.4C and higher)	1 2			
	Frequent yawning (> 3–4 times/interval)	1			
	Mottling	1			
	Nasal stuffiness	1			
	Sneezing (> 3–4 times/interval)	1			
	Nasal flaring	2			
	Respiratory rate > 60/min Respiratory rate > 60/min with retractions	1 2			
Gastrointestinal Disturbances	Excessive sucking	1			
	Poor feeding	2			
	Regurgitation Projectile vomiting	2 3			
	Loose stools Watery stools	2 3			
	Total Score				
	Initials of Scorer				

Source: Finnegan, L. P. (1990). Neonatal abstinence syndrome. In Nelson, N. (Ed.), *Current therapy in neonatal-perinatal medicine* (2nd ed.). Ontario: BC Decker.

as SGA, intrauterine asphyxia, meconium aspiration, and prematurity.

- Identifying the signs and symptoms of newborn withdrawal or neonatal abstinence syndrome (see Table 32–3).

Although many of the signs and symptoms of narcotic withdrawal are similar to those seen with hypoglycemia and hypocalcemia, glucose and calcium values are reported to be within normal limits for this group of infants.

Neonatal abstinence syndrome includes both physiologic and behavioral responses. The severity of withdrawal can be assessed by a scoring system based on observations and measurement of the responses to neonatal abstinence such as the Finnegan scale. It evaluates the infant on potentially life-threatening signs, such as vomiting, diarrhea, weight loss, irritability, tremors, and tachypnea (Table 32–4 •).

Nursing diagnoses that may apply to drug-dependent newborns include the following:

- ***Altered Nutrition: Less than Body Requirements*** related to vomiting and diarrhea, uncoordinated suck and swallow reflex, hypertonia secondary to withdrawal
- ***Impaired Skin Integrity*** related to constant activity
- ***Altered Parenting*** related to hyperirritable behavior of the infant
- ***Ineffective Coping: Disabling*** related to drug abuse, poverty, and lack of education
- ***Sleep Pattern Disturbance*** related to CNS excitation secondary to drug withdrawal

Nursing Plan and Implementation

Hospital-Based Nursing Care

Care of the drug-dependent newborn is based on reducing withdrawal symptoms and promoting adequate respiration, temperature, and nutrition. See the Clinical Pathway for Newborn of a Substance-Abusing Mother for specific nursing care measures. Some general nursing care measures include the following:

- Monitoring temperature for hyperthermia
- Carefully monitoring pulse and respirations every 15 minutes and pulse oximetry until stable; stimulation if apnea occurs
- Small, frequent feedings, especially in the presence of vomiting, regurgitation, and diarrhea
- Intravenous therapy as needed
- Medications as ordered, such as oral morphine, phenobarbital, and paregoric (but not methadone because of possible neonatal addiction to it), use of paregoric is controversial because it contains alcohol and camphor (Weiner & Finnegan, 2002)
- Proper positioning on the right side-lying or semi-Fowler's to avoid possible aspirations of vomitus or secretions
- Monitoring frequency of diarrhea and vomiting, and weighing infant every 8 hours during withdrawal
- Observing for problems of SGA or LGA newborns
- Swaddling with hands near mouth to minimize injury and achieve more organized behavioral state (Offer a pacifier for nonnutritive, excessive sucking. Gentle, vertical rocking can be successful in calming an infant who is out of control.)
- Protecting face and extremities from excoriation by using mittens, and soft sheets or sheepskin
- Placing newborn in quiet, dimly lighted area of nursery

Community-Based Nursing Care

Parents need assistance to prepare for what they can expect for the first few months at home. At the time of discharge, the mother should be instructed to anticipate mild jitteriness and irritability in the newborn, which may persist from 6 days to 8 weeks, depending on the initial severity of the withdrawal (Blackburn, 2003). Infants with neonatal abstinence syndrome are at a significantly higher risk for SIDS when the mother used heroin or cocaine. The infant should sleep supine and home apnea monitoring should be implemented. The nurse should demonstrate and help the mother learn feeding techniques, comforting measures, how to recognize newborn cues, and appropriate parenting responses. Parents are to be counseled regarding available resources, such as support groups, and signs and symptoms that indicate the need for further care. Ongoing evaluation is necessary because of the potential for long-term problems. Follow-up on missed appointments can bring parents back into the healthcare system, thereby improving parent and infant outcomes and promoting a positive, interactive environment after birth.

Evaluation

Expected outcomes of nursing care include the following:

- The newborn tolerates feedings, gains weight, and has a decreased number of stools.
- The parents learn ways to comfort their newborn.
- The parents are able to cope with their frustrations and begin to use outside resources as needed.

Care of the Newborn Exposed to HIV/AIDS

Increasing numbers of newborns are born infected with HIV or at risk for acquiring it in the newborn period or early infancy. Transmission during the perinatal and newborn periods can occur across the placenta or through breast milk or contaminated blood. Maternal-to-newborn vertical transmission rates are about 13% to 40% in the United States (Merenstein, Adams, & Weisman, 2002). The risk of vertical transmission can be decreased in mothers taking zidovudine during gestation. For further discussion of maternal and fetal HIV/AIDS, see Chapter 19. Opportunistic diseases such as gram-negative sepsis and problems associated with prematurity are the primary causes of mortality in HIV-infected babies. Some infants infected by maternal-fetal transmission suffer from severe immunodeficiency, with HIV disease progressing more rapidly during the first year of life.

Early identification of babies with or at risk for HIV/AIDS is essential during the newborn period. However, the currently available HIV serologic tests (ELISA and Western blot test) cannot distinguish between maternal and infant antibodies; therefore, they are inappropriate for infants up to 15 months of age. It may take up to 15 months for infected infants to form their own antibodies to HIV (Merenstein et al, 2002). Testing by HIV DNA polymerase chain reaction (PCR) is the preferred test. Results can be made available within 24 hours. A viral culture may also be performed at birth but it is more expensive and results are not available for 2 weeks (Krist & Crawford-Faucher, 2002). The first DNA PCR test should be performed on the newborn before 48 hours of age. The test is repeated when the infant is 1 to 2 months of age, and again at 4 to 6 months (Krist & Crawford-Faucher, 2002). Umbilical cord blood should not be used for HIV testing. If PCR and viral culture are unavailable, the p24 antigen may be used to assess HIV infection status in infants older than 1 month, but the sensitivity of p24 antigen testing is substantially less than the other tests. For infants who have three negative (at birth and at 1 and 4 months of age) HIV virologic antibody tests, a negative HIV-specific IgG assay (ELISA) at 18 months of age definitively rules out HIV in exposed infants (Krist & Crawford-Faucher, 2002).

CLINICAL PATHWAY FOR NEWBORN OF A SUBSTANCE-ABUSING MOTHER *CONTINUED*

Category	Day of Birth—First 4 Hours	Remainder of Birth Day
Family involvement	Evaluate parent teaching Access community resources prn, ie, Teen "Healthy Starts" Encourage/support positive mothering/parenting behaviors with infant	Evaluate parent teaching Assess parents' knowledge of newborn behavior and reflexes Encourage family involvement in infant's care as soon as possible and as infant tolerates
Date		

Category	Day 1	Day 2/3 (if applicable)
Referral	Check ID bands when baby leaves nursery Lactation consult prn	Check ID bands q shift ➤ **Expected Outcomes** Mother/baby ID bands correlate at time of DC Consults completed prn
Assessments	Assess mother/baby interaction Continue newborn assessments q shift Assess thermoregulation/VS q shift and prn Assess abdominal distention, gastric residuals Assess altered sleep-wake cycle and rhythm at 24–48h Abstinence scoring	Assess mother/baby interaction Assess abdominal distension, gastric residuals, wt gain, s/s drug withdrawal and complications Abstinence scoring ➤ **Expected Outcomes** Physical assessments, VS WNL; no complications of newborn of substance-abusing mother noted
Teaching/ psychosocial	(See Newborn Clinical Pathway, Chapter 30) Reinforce previous teaching Parental teaching: bathing, cord care, skin/nail care, use of thermometer, activity, sleep patterns, calming activities, reflexes, s/s jaundice, growth/feeding patterns, special nutritional needs, report feeding intolerance, circumcision care Evaluate mother/parent teaching; provide information about HIV s/s, group support and community resources for persons with substance abuse issues	Final Discharge Teaching: (See Newborn Clinical Pathway, Chapter 30) Review with parents/guardian infant safety, s/s illness and when to call healthcare provider ➤ **Expected Outcomes** Mother verbalizes comprehension of instructions, demonstrates care capabilities
Nursing care management and reports	Newborn assessment q shift Daily wt Circumcision care q diaper change Femoral pulse or BP all 4 extremities before DC or first 48h Unclamp cord clamp, alcohol to cord q diaper change HSV culture per parental hx of HSV Maintain NTE Newborn screen Continue to monitor for s/s of drug withdrawal, seizure activity Administer meds for withdrawal s/s as ordered; monitor infant response, report to NP/MD prn	Newborn assessment and VS q shift Daily wt Cord care per policy Note OAE or ABR hearing test results Cord care, circumcision care q diaper change ➤ **Expected Outcomes** Physical assessments WNL; cord unclamped and dry without s/s infection; circ site unremarkable; gaining wt or stabilized to not >10% loss; labs WNL; without s/s of substance withdrawal or infection; infant not requiring medication for relief of s/s of drug withdrawal
Activity and Comfort	Note sleep/wake pattern Swaddled in open crib Incubator if temp instability; adjust incubator for infant size, gestation, layers of clothing to maintain NTE	Note sleep/wake pattern Swaddle to allow movement of hands to face Mittens on hands per agency protocol ➤ **Expected Outcomes** Maintains temp WNL, swaddled in open crib, no face or extremity excoriation
Nutrition	• Supplement oral or gavage feedings with intravenous intake per orders; evaluate necessity prn • Give small, frequent feedings q3–4h breast milk or formula as ordered, increasing strength of feeding as tolerated and as ordered (may start with half-strength breast milk/formula) • Feed calorically enhanced breast milk/formula as ordered; monitor infant's tolerance to feedings • Check for gastric residuals before q feeding; adjust volume of feeding prn with high or increasing residuals. Notify NP/MD of increasing residuals • Increase feeding volume as tolerated and as hyperactivity decreases • Supplement breast only when medically indicated and ordered by NP/MD • Feed on demand, minimally q3–4h	Feed on demand, minimally q3–4h Gavage feed prn, as ordered to maintain nutrition Supplement breast only when medically indicated and ordered by NP/MD Encourage frequent feedings during day Monitor infant for s/s of active or residual presence of drugs with breastmilk feedings versus normal satiation after feeding. Consider toxicology screen of breast milk, fresh or frozen, prn ➤ **Expected Outcomes** Infant tolerates feedings, feeds on demand; breastfeeds without supplement, nipples without problems; regaining lost wt or wt stabilized

CLINICAL PATHWAY FOR NEWBORN OF A SUBSTANCE-ABUSING MOTHER

Category	Day of Birth—First 4 Hours	Remainder of Birth Day
Referral	Report from L&D, neonatal nurse practitioner Check ID bands High-risk peds/neonatology consults prn	Check ID bands q shift As parents request, obtain circumcision permit after their discussion with MD
Assessments	Complete set of VS Admission wt, length, HC Assess skin color, skin integrity for rashes, breakdown Gestational age assessment Monitor activity (lethargy, character of cry, exaggerated startle responses) Maternal hx of drugs consumed during each month of pregnancy Obtain prior hx of addiction and treatment Withdrawal s/s: hyperactivity, jitteriness, irritability, shrill high-pitched cry, vomiting, diarrhea, weak suck, stuffy nose, frequent sneezing, yawning, tachycardia, hypertension, apnea, seizure activity Cocaine withdrawal pattern may be unpredictable or may be asymptomatic with only subtle behavioral state organization problems	Vital signs: T/P/R q4h and prn, BP prn Newborn assessment q shift Assess mother/baby interaction Abstinence scoring
Teaching/ psychosocial	(See Newborn Clinical Pathway, Chapter 30) Admission activities performed at mother's bedside if possible; orient parents to NSY, handwashing; assess teaching needs and readiness for learning Evaluate additional psychosocial needs (provide time for verbalizing concerns, determine parental understanding of substance abuse) Provide information including: • s/s of baby's withdrawal, current condition, and rationale of treatment • Newborn capabilities and developmental behaviors, cues • Newborn's need for appropriate stimulation as well as rest, depending on cues • Physical care needs (feeding, bathing, clothing, holding) • Safety-bulb syringe, choking, positioning	Reinforce previous teaching Discuss/teach infant security, identification Discuss/teach temperature maintenance with clothing/blankets Teach parents/guardian feeding methods, burping, diapering, and elimination norms Teach parents calming techniques, s/s of stress and infant cues to stress
Nursing care management and reports	• Serum electrolytes to detect losses from vomiting/diarrhea • Blood type, Rh, Coombs' on cord blood when applicable • Chemstrip prn; BP prn • EOAE/AABR hearing test • Maintain Standard Precautions • Bathe ASAP if-foul-smelling amniotic fluid/cord care per policy • Hep B form reviewed and/or signed by parent, administer if ordered after bath • Peripheral hematocrit per protocol • Toxicology screen to identify drugs and drug levels in infant • CBC and blood cultures to detect sepsis • Intravenous access for meds, hydration, nutritional support	• Check for EOAE or AABR hearing test results • Femoral pulse or BP all 4 extremities if early DC • Vital signs: q4h, T/P/R • Daily wt • Assess color q shift and prn • Cord care per policy • Monitor for s/s of substance withdrawal, seizure activity; notify NP/MD prn, offer supportive care • Maintain intravenous access prn
Activity and comfort	• Adjust and monitor radiant warmer to maintain skin temp until stable • Provide calming techniques: Swaddling infant tightly in side-lying or prone position with blanket roll to back, nest Provide quiet, dim environment for rest Hold, rock, and cuddle infant. Use touching, petting, smiling, talking. Use infant snuggly for closeness, carrying infant. Provide pacifier or swaddle to allow infant's hands to mouth for nonnutritive sucking.	Leave in radiant warmer until stable, then swaddle in open crib Continue calming/soothing techniques prn Cluster care, provide care on infant's schedule Avoid overstimulation Note sleep/waking patterns
Nutrition	Initiate formula feeding Initiate breastfeeding as soon as mother/baby condition allows lavage and gavage prn Supplement breast only when medically indicated or ordered by MD per protocol Assess for increased nutritional needs because of gestational age, weight, uncoordinated suck and swallow, vomiting, diarrhea, and regurgitation	Continue feeding schedule Encourage frequent feedings at least q3–4h during day Feed on demand breast or formula Consider breast milk evaluation to r/o active or residual drug presence
Elimination	Note first void and stool color Urine specific gravity to detect dehydration	Monitor stools for amount, type, consistency, and pattern changes Monitor all voids q shift
Medication	Administer medications for withdrawal as ordered, such as paregoric, chlorpromazine, diazepam, phenobarbital, tincture of opium, observe for effectiveness and side effects AquaMEPHYTON IM, dosage according to infant wt and protocol after bath Ilotycin ophth ointment OU—after bath	Continue medications as ordered and necessary to alleviate s/s substance withdrawal, to allow newborn rest and ability to suck/maintain nutritional status
Discharge planning/ home care	Evaluate for social services, visiting nurses service, and DC planning needs Plan DC with parent/guardian in 1–3 days	Present birth certificate instructions/worksheet Car seat available for DC Newborn photographs

(continued on next page)

CLINICAL PATHWAY FOR NEWBORN OF A SUBSTANCE-ABUSING MOTHER *CONTINUED*

Category	Day 1	Day 2/3 (if applicable)
Elimination	Monitor stools for amount, consistency, pattern changes, occult blood, reducing substances Monitor voids q8h	Continue monitoring of all voids and stools q shift, noting changes ➤ **Expected Outcomes** Voids qs; stools without difficulty qs with stool character WNL; diaper area without s/s breakdown
Medication	Hep B vaccine before DC Administer meds for withdrawal or seizure activity prn as ordered; observe for s/s of effectiveness and side effects	➤ **Expected Outcomes** Infant has received ophth ointment OU and AquaMEPHYTON injection; received first Hep B vaccine if ordered and parental consent received; infant not requiring meds for s/s withdrawal or seizure activity
Discharge planning/ home care	Newborn photographs Complete birth certificate packet If vag birth, complete DC teaching Access community referrals, support groups for mother/family prn, ie, drug rehab, developmental, occupational and physical therapy, WIC, financial resources, public health nursing for home visits	If cesarean birth, complete DC teaching Complete DC summary (See Newborn Clinical Pathway, Chapter 30) ➤ **Expected Outcomes** Infant DC home with mother; mother verbalizes follow-up appointment times, dates, referral sources
Family involvement	Bath, newborn care, and feeding class Newborn channel as available Assess mother/baby bonding/interaction Incorporate significant other/siblings in infant care Support positive parenting behaviors Evaluate mother/parent teaching	Assess mother/baby interaction Identify community referral needs and refer to community agencies Evaluate mother/parent teaching Encourage questions ➤ **Expected Outcomes** Mother/family demonstrates caring and family incorporation of infant
Date		

AABR, automated auditory brain response; ASAP, as soon as possible; DC, discharge; EOAE, evoked otoacustic emissions; HC, head circumference; hx, history; ID, identification; L&D, labor and delivery; NTE, neutral thermal environment; NSY, nursery; OU, both eyes; s/s, signs and symptoms; vag, vaginal; VS, vital signs; WIC, Women, Infants, and Children program; WNL, within normal limits; wt, weight.

NURSING CARE MANAGEMENT

Nursing Assessment and Diagnosis

Many newborns exposed to HIV/AIDS are premature, SGA, or both and show failure to thrive during the newborn and infant periods. They can show signs and symptoms of disease within days of birth. Signs that may be seen in the early infancy period include enlarged spleen and liver, swollen glands, recurrent respiratory infections, rhinorrhea, interstitial pneumonia (rarely seen in adults), recurrent gastrointestinal problems (diarrhea and weight loss), organic failure to thrive, urinary system infections, persistent or recurrent oral and genital candidiasis infections, and loss of developmental milestones (Merenstein et al, 2002). Nursing diagnoses that may apply to the infant exposed to HIV/AIDS include the following:

- ***Altered Nutrition: Less than Body Requirements*** related to formula intolerance and inadequate intake
- ***Risk for Impaired Skin Integrity*** related to chronic diarrhea
- ***Risk for Infection*** related to perinatal exposure and immunoregulation suppression secondary to HIV/AIDS
- ***Impaired Physical Mobility*** related to decreased neuromuscular development
- ***Altered Growth and Development*** related to lack of attachment and stimulation
- ***Altered Parenting*** related to diagnosis of HIV/AIDS and fear of future outcome

Nursing Plan and Implementation

Hospital-Based Nursing Care

Nursing care of the newborn exposed to HIV/AIDS includes all the normal care required for any newborn in a nursery. In addition, the nurse must include care for a newborn suspected of having a blood-borne infection, as with hepatitis B. Standard precautions should be used when caring for the newborn immediately after birth until all maternal blood is removed and when obtaining blood samples via vein puncture or heel stick. (The blood of all newborns must be considered potentially infectious because the status of the infant's blood is often not known until after the infant

Table 32–5 • ISSUES FOR CAREGIVERS OF INFANTS AT RISK FOR HIV/AIDS

Resuscitation	For suctioning use a bulb syringe, mucus extractor, or meconium aspirator with wall suction on low setting. Use masks, goggles, and gloves.	Specimens	Blood and other specimens should be double-bagged and/or sealed in an impervious container and labeled according to agency protocol.
Admission Care	To remove blood from baby's skin, give warm water-mild soap bath using gloves as soon as possible after admission.	Equipment and linen	Articles contaminated with blood or body fluids should be discarded or bagged according to isolation or institution protocol.
Handwashing	Thorough handwashing is indicated before and after caring for infant. Hands must be washed immediately if contaminated with blood or body fluids. Wash hands after removal of gloves.	Body fluid spills	Blood and body fluids should be cleaned promptly with a solution of 5.25% sodium hypochlorite (household bleach) diluted 1:10 with water. Apply for at least 30 seconds then wipe after the minimum contact time.
Gloves	Gloves are indicated with touching blood or other high-risk fluids. Gloves should also be worn when handling newborns before and during their initial baths, cord care, eye prophylactics, and vitamin K administration.	Education and support	Provide education and psychologic support for family and staff. Caregivers who avoid contact with baby at risk or who overdress in unnecessary isolation garb subtly exacerbate an already difficult family situation. Information resources include the National AIDS Hotline (1-800-342-2437) and HIV/AIDS Treatment Enforcement Service Web http://www.hevatis.org
Mask, goggle, and gown	Not routinely needed unless coming in contact with placenta or the blood and amniotic fluid on the skin of the newborn.	Exempted personnel	Immunologically compromised staff (pregnant women may be included in this group) and possibly infectious staff members should not care for these infants.
Needles and syringes	Used needles should not be recapped or bent; they should be disposed of in a puncture-resistant plastic container belonging specifically to that baby. After the newborn is discharged the container is discarded.		

Source: Adapted from American Academy of Pediatrics, Committee on Pediatric AIDS and Committee on Infectious Diseases. (1999). Issues related to human immunodeficiency transmission in schools, child care, medical settings, the home, and community. *Pediatrics, 104*(2), 318–324; Mendez, H., & Jule, J. E. (1990). Care of the infant born exposed to AIDS. *Obstetric and Gynecologic Clinics of North America, 17*(3), 637; Krist, A. H., & Crawford-Faucher, A. (2002). Management of newborns exposed to maternal HIV infection. *American Family Physician, 65*(10), 2049–2056.

is discharged. There is also a window of time before seroconversion occurs, during which the baby is still considered infectious.)

Nursing care involves providing for comfort; keeping the newborn well nourished and protected from opportunistic infections; and facilitating growth, development, and attachment. Most institutions recommend that their caregivers wear gloves during all diaper changes and examination of babies. Disposable gloves are worn when changing diapers or cleaning the diaper area, especially in the presence of diarrhea, because blood may be in the stool (AAP Committee on Pediatric AIDS and Committee on Infectious Diseases, 1999). Good skin care is essential to prevent skin rashes. See Table 32–5 •.

CRITICAL THINKING IN PRACTICE

Mrs Jean Corrigan, a 23-year-old G1P1, positive for HIV, has just given birth to a 7 lb 1 oz baby girl. As she watches you assessing her daughter in the birthing room, she asks why you are wearing gloves and whether her daughter will have to be in isolation. What will your response be?

Answers can be found in Appendix I.

Community-Based Nursing Care

Handwashing is crucial when caring for newborns at risk for AIDS; thus, parents must be taught proper handwashing technique. Nutrition is essential because failure to thrive and weight loss are common. Small, frequent feedings and food supplementation are helpful. The nurse should discuss with the parents sanitary techniques for preparing formula. The nurse should also inform parents that the baby should not be put to bed with juice or formula because of potential bacteria growth. Parents need to be alert to the signs of feeding intolerance, such as increasing regurgitation, abdominal distention, and loose stools. The newborn should be weighed three times a week.

The baby should have his or her own skin care items, towels, and washcloths. Most clothing and linens can be washed with other household laundry. Linen that is visibly soiled with blood or body fluids should be kept separate and washed separately in hot, sudsy water with household bleach. Prompt diaper changing and perineal care can prevent or minimize diaper rash and promote comfort. The diaper-changing area in the home should be separate from the food preparation and serving areas. The diapers are to be placed in plastic bags, sealed, and disposed of daily. Diaper-changing areas should be cleaned with a 1:10 dilution of household bleach after each diaper change. Toys should be kept as clean as possible, and they should not be shared with other children. Toys should be checked for sharp edges to prevent scratches.

The nurse should instruct parents in what signs of infection to be alert for and when to call their healthcare provider. The inability to feed without pain may indicate esophageal yeast infection and may require administration of nystatin (Mycostatin) for oral thrush. Topical Mycostatin or Desitin ointment is used for diaper rashes and oral Mycostatin for oral thrush. If diarrhea occurs, the baby requires frequent perineal care and fluid replacements. Antidiarrheal medications are often ineffective. Taking rectal temperatures should be avoided, as it may stimulate diarrhea. Fluids, antipyretics, and sponging with tepid water are of use in managing fever. Irritability may be the first sign of fever. Preventive care for exposed infants is the same as for other infants and includes routine immunizations, except that the live polio vaccine should be avoided. If the infant is exposed to varicella, the parents should notify their healthcare professional because the baby may need varicella zoster immune globulin [VZIG] within 96 hours of exposure or if exposed to measles (may need vaccination within 72 hours of exposure).

Parents and family members need to be reassured that there are no documented cases of people contracting HIV/AIDS from routine care of infected babies. Emotional support for the family is essential because of the stress and social isolation they may face. Because of these stresses, parents may not bond with the baby or may fail to provide the baby with enough sensory and tactile stimulation. The nurse should instruct the parents to hold the baby during feedings because the infant will benefit from frequent, gentle touch. Auditory stimulation may also be provided using music or tapes of parents' voices. The nurse should offer information to families about support groups, available counseling, and information resources. Current therapeutic information regarding HIV disease is available to both healthcare providers and families through the AIDS Clinical Trials Information Service (1-800-TRIALS-A). The CDC recommends that HIV-infected women in developed countries not breastfeed because HIV can be transmitted via breast milk. Therefore, if there is a viable alternative feeding method, it should be used (Krist & Crawford-Faucher, 2002).

Infants of infected mothers should be given antiretroviral drug therapy such as zidovudine beginning at 8 to 12 hours of life and continuing for 6 weeks (Merenstein et al, 2002). All infants born to HIV-positive mothers require regular clinical, immunologic, and virologic monitoring. At 1 month of age, the baby's physical examination should include a developmental assessment and a complete blood count, including differential blood count, CD4+ count, and platelet count. Prophylaxis for *pneumocystis carinii* pneumonia for all infants born to HIV-infected women should be initiated at 4 to 6 weeks of age, regardless of the infant's CD4+ lymphocyte count (Merenstein et al, 2002). Pediatric HIV disease raises many healthcare issues for the family. The parents, depending on their health status, may or may not be able to care for their infant, and they must deal with many psychosocial and economic issues.

Evaluation

Expected outcomes of nursing care include the following:

- The parents are able to bond with their infant and have realistic expectations about the baby.
- Potential opportunistic infections are identified early and treated promptly.
- The parents verbalize their concerns surrounding their baby's existing and potential health problems and accept outside assistance as needed.

Care of the Newborn with Congenital Heart Defect

The incidence of congenital heart defects is 8 per 1000 live births (Smith, 2001). Because accurate diagnosis and surgical treatment are now available, many deaths can be prevented (American Heart Association, 2003). It is now possible to perform corrective surgery at an earlier age; for example, more than one half of children undergoing surgery are less than 1 year of age, and one fourth are less than 1 month old. It is crucial for the nurse to have comprehensive knowledge of congenital heart disease to detect deviations from normal and to initiate interventions.

Overview of Congenital Heart Defects

In the majority of the cases of congenital heart malformations, the cause is multifactorial with no specific trigger. Other factors that might influence development of congenital heart malformations can be classified as environmental or genetic. Infections of the pregnant woman, such as rubella, cytomegalovirus, coxsackie B, and influenza, have been implicated. Thalidomide, steroids, alcohol, lithium, and some anticonvulsants have been shown to cause malformations of the heart. Seasonal spraying of pesticides has also been linked to an increase in congenital heart defects. Clinicians are also beginning to see cardiac defects in infants of mothers with phenylketonuria who do not follow their diets. Infants with Down syndrome, Turners syndrome, Holt-Oram syndrome, trisomy 13, and trisomy 18 frequently have heart lesions. Increased incidence and risk of recurrence of specific defects occur in families.

It is customary to describe congenital malformations of the heart as either acyanotic (those that do not present with cyanosis) or cyanotic (those that do present with cyanosis). If an opening exists between the right and left sides of the heart, blood will normally flow from the area of greater pressure (left side) to the area of lesser pressure (right side). This process is referred to as left-to-right shunt and does not produce cyanosis because oxygenated blood is being pumped out to the systemic circulation. If pressure in the right side of the heart, due to obstruction of normal flow, exceeds that in the left side, unoxygenated blood will flow from the right side to the left side of the heart and out into the system. This right-to-left shunt causes cyanosis. If the opening is large, there may be a bidirectional shunt with mixing of blood in both sides of the heart, which also produces cyanosis.

The common cardiac defects seen in the first 6 days of life are left ventricular outflow obstructions (mitral stenosis, aortic stenosis, or atresia), hypoplastic left heart, coarctation of the aorta, patent ductus arteriosus (PDA, the most common defect), transposition of the great vessels, tetralogy of Fallot, and large ventricular septal defect or atrial septal defects. Many cardiac defects may not clearly manifest themselves until after discharge from the birthing unit.

NURSING CARE MANAGEMENT

The primary goals of the neonatal nurse are early identification of cardiac defects and initiation of referral to the physician. The three most common manifestations of cardiac defect are cyanosis, detectable heart murmur, and signs of congestive heart failure (tachycardia, tachypnea, diaphoresis, hepatomegaly, and cardiomegaly). Table 32–6 • on page 931–932 presents the clinical manifestations and medical/surgical management of these cardiac defects. Initial repair of heart defects in the newborn period is becoming more commonplace. The NICU staff is now more involved in both the preoperative and postoperative care of cardiac newborns. The benefits for the cardiac infant of being cared for by NICU staff include the staff's knowledge of neonatal anatomy and physiology, experience in supporting the family, and an awareness of the developmental needs of the newborn.

After the baby is stabilized, decisions are made about the special ongoing care needs. The parents need careful and complete explanations and the opportunity to take part in decision making. They also require ongoing emotional support. Families of any baby born with a congenital abnormality need genetic counseling regarding future conception. Parents need to verbalize their concern about their baby's health maintenance and to understand the rationale for follow-up care.

Care of the Newborn with Inborn Errors of Metabolism

Inborn errors of metabolism are a group of hereditary disorders that are transmitted by mutant genes. Each causes an enzyme defect that blocks a metabolic pathway and leads to an accumulation of toxic metabolites. Most of the disorders are transmitted by an autosomal recessive gene, requiring two heterozygous parents to produce a homozygous infant with the disorder. Heterozygous parents carrying some inborn errors of metabolism disorders can be identified by special tests, and some inborn errors of metabolism can be detected and treated in utero.

Many inborn errors of metabolism are now detected neonatally through newborn screening programs. These programs test principally for disorders associated with mental retardation.

Types of Inborn Errors of Metabolism

Phenylketonuria (PKU) is the most common of the group of metabolic errors known as amino acid disorders. Newborn screenings have set its incidence at about 1 in 11,000 live births in the United States; however, the incidence varies considerably among ethnic groups (Kenner & Dreyer, 2000). The highest incidence worldwide is noted in white populations from northern Europe and the United States. It is rarely observed in people of African, Jewish, or Japanese descent.

Phenylalanine is an essential amino acid (found in dietary protein) used by the body for growth, and in the normal individual any excess is converted to tyrosine. The newborn with PKU lacks this converting ability, which results in an accumulation of phenylalanine in the blood. Phenylalanine produces two abnormal metabolites, phenylpyruvic acid and phenylacetic acid, which are eliminated in the urine, producing a musty odor. Excessive accumulation of phenylalanine and its abnormal metabolites in the brain tissue leads to progressive mental retardation.

Maple syrup urine disease (MSUD) is an inborn error of metabolism that, when untreated, is a rapidly progressing and often fatal disease caused by an enzymatic defect in the metabolism of the branched chain amino acids leucine, isoleucine, and valine. Diagnosis of MSUD is made by analyzing blood levels of leucine, isoleucine, and valine. Confirmation of the diagnosis depends on blood assay for the enzyme oxidative decarboxylase.

Homocystinuria is a disorder caused by a deficiency of the enzyme cystathionine β-synthase, which causes an elevated excretion of homocystine and methionine.

Galactosemia is an inborn error of carbohydrate metabolism in which the body is unable to use the sugars galactose and lactose. Enzyme pathways in liver cells normally convert galactose and lactose to glucose. In galactosemia, one step in that conversion pathway is absent, either because of the lack of the enzyme galactose 1-phosphate uridyltransferase or because of the lack of the enzyme galactokinase. High levels of unusable galactose circulate in the blood, causing cataracts, brain damage, and liver damage. There appear to be ethnic differences in age of onset of symptoms and in severity of course. Caucasians have more severe symptoms and earlier onset (3 to 14 days) than people of African descent (14 to 28 days).

Table 32-6 • CARDIAC DEFECTS OF THE EARLY NEWBORN PERIOD

Congenital Heart Defect	Clinical Findings	Medical/Surgical Management
Acyanotic		
Patent ductus arteriosus (PDA) ↑ in females, maternal rubella, RDS, <1500 g preterm newborns, high-altitude births	Harsh grade 2–3 machinery murmur upper left sternal border (LSB) just beneath clavicle ↑ difference between systolic and diastolic pulse pressure Can lead to right heart failure and pulmonary congestion ↑ left atrial (LA) and left ventricular (LV) enlargement, dilated ascending aorta ↑ pulmonary vascularity	Indomethacin—0.2 mg/kg IV (prostaglandin inhibitor) 3 doses q 12 hours Surgical ligation, occlusion coil Use of O_2 therapy and blood transfusion to improve tissue oxygenation and perfusion Fluid restriction and diuretics
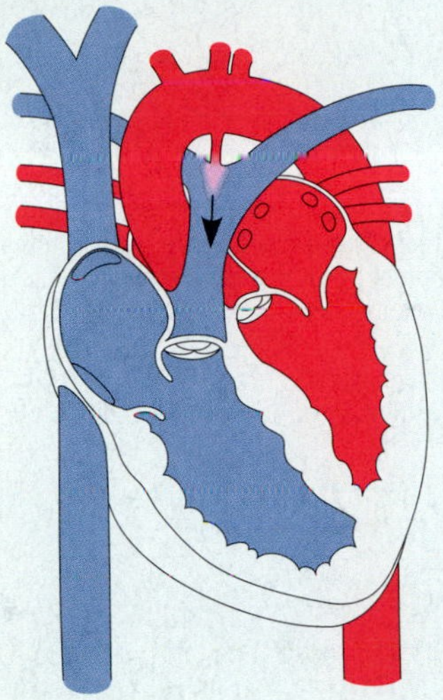	The patent ductus arteriosus is a vascular connection that, during fetal life, short-circuits the pulmonary vascular bed and directs blood from the pulmonary artery to the aorta. Postnatally, blood shunts through the ductus from the aorta to the pulmonary artery.	
Atrial septal defect (ASD) ↑ in females and Down syndrome	Initially frequently asymptomatic Systolic murmur second left intercostal space (LICS) With large ASD, diastolic rumbling murmur lower left sternal (LLS) border Failure to thrive, upper respiratory infection (URI), poor exercise tolerance	Surgical closure with patch or suture Umbrella
Ventricular septal defect (VSD) ↑ in males	Initially asymptomatic until end of first month or large enough to cause pulmonary edema Loud, blowing systolic murmur between the third and fourth intercostal space (ICS) pulmonary blood flow Right ventricular hypertrophy Rapid respirations, growth failure, feeding difficulties Congestive right heart failure at 6 weeks–2 months of age	Follow medically—some spontaneously close Use of Lanoxin and diuretics in congestive heart failure (CHF) Surgical closure with Dacron patch
Coarctation of aorta Can be preductal or postductal	Absent or diminished femoral pulses Increased brachial pulses Late systolic murmur left intrascapular area Systolic BP in lower extremities Enlarged left ventricle Can present in CHF at 7–21 days of life	Surgical resection of narrowed portion of aorta Prostaglandin E, to maintain peripheral perfusion No afterload reducer drugs
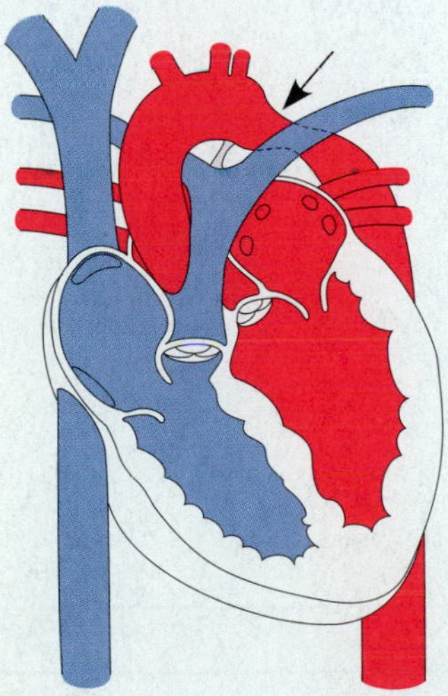	Coarctation of the aorta is characterized by a narrowed aortic lumen. The lesion produces an obstruction to the flow of blood through the aorta, causing an increased left ventricular pressure and workload.	

(continued on next page)

Table 32–6 • CONTINUED

Congenital Heart Defect	Clinical Findings	Medical/Surgical Management
Hypoplastic left heart syndrome	Normal at birth—cyanosis and shocklike congestive heart failure develop within a few hours to days Soft systolic murmur just left of the sternum Diminished pulses Aortic and/or mitral atresia Tiny, thick-walled left ventricle Large, dilated, hypertrophied right ventricle X-ray examination: cardiac enlargement and pulmonary venous congestion	PGE_1 until decision made Norwood procedure Transplant
Cyanotic		
Tetralogy of Fallot (Most common cyanotic heart defect) Pulmonary stenosis Ventricular septal defect (VSD) Overriding aorta Right ventricular hypertrophy 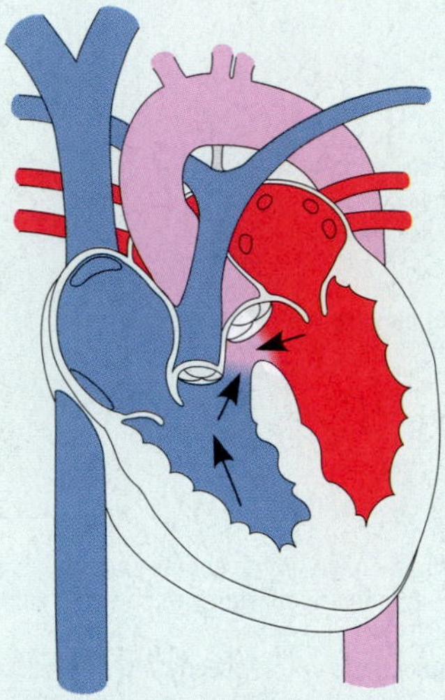 In tetralogy of Fallot, the severity of symptoms depends on the degree of pulmonary stenosis, the size of the ventricular septal defect, and the degree to which the aorta overrides the septal defect.	May be cyanotic at birth or within first few months of life Harsh systolic murmur LSB Crying or feeding increases cyanosis and respiratory distress X-ray: boot-shaped appearance secondary to small pulmonary artery Right ventricular enlargement	Prevention of dehydration, intercurrent infections Alleviation of paroxysmal dyspneic attacks Palliative surgery to increase blood flow to the lungs Corrective surgery—resection of pulmonic stenosis, closure of VSD with Dacron patch
Transposition of great vessels (TGA) (↑ females, IDMs, LGAs) 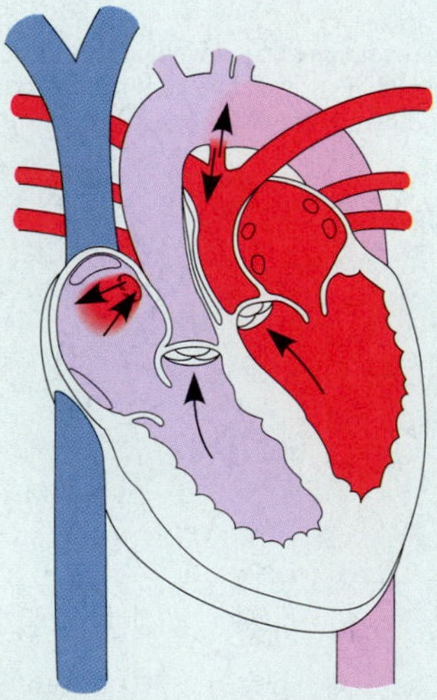 Complete transposition of great vessels is an embryologic defect caused by a straight division of the bulbar trunk without normal spiraling. As a result, the aorta originates from the right ventricle, and the pulmonary artery from the left ventricle. An abnormal communication between the two circulations must be present to sustain life.	Cyanosis at birth or within 3 days Possible pulmonic stenosis murmur Right ventricular hypertrophy Polycythemia "Egg on its side" x-ray finding	Prostaglandin E to vasodilate ductus to keep it open Initial surgery to create opening between right and left side of heart if none exists Total surgical repair—usually the arterial switch procedure—done within first few days of life

Source: All illustrations from *Congenital Heart Abnormalities*. Clinical Education Aid No. 7, Ross Laboratories, Columbus, OH.

Another disorder frequently included in mandatory newborn blood screening tests is *congenital hypothyroidism (CH)*. An inborn enzymatic defect, lack of maternal dietary iodine, or maternal ingestion of drugs that depress or destroy thyroid tissue can cause CH.

The incidence of metabolic errors is relatively low, but for affected infants and their families these disorders pose a threat to survival and frequently require lifelong treatment.

Clinical Therapy

All states have universal screening of newborns for PKU and CH (Matthews & Robin, 2002). Mandatory newborn screening for other inborn errors of metabolism varies among states. Some states simultaneously test all hospitalized newborns for MSUD and homocystinuria. In several states newborn screening includes an enzyme assay for galactose 1-phosphate uridyltransferase; however, this test does not detect galactosemia if it is caused by a deficiency of the enzyme galactokinase.

Identification via newborn screening and early clinical intervention for inborn errors of metabolism becomes more difficult with the advent of early discharge of newborns. If the initial specimen is obtained before 24 hours of age, then a second specimen should be obtained before 5 days of age (Zinn, 2002). Newborns in the NICU who require interhospital transfers and early-discharged healthy newborns are at risk for nonscreening. The first blood specimen test screens for PKU, homocystinuria, MSUD, galactosemia, and sickle cell anemia. A second blood specimen is often required, but the nurse must remember that this second blood specimen tests only for PKU.

NURSING CARE MANAGEMENT

The nurse assesses the newborn for signs of inborn errors of metabolism and carries out state-mandated newborn testing. Parents of affected newborns should be referred to support groups. The nurse should also ensure that parents are informed about centers that can provide them with information about biochemical genetics and dietary management.

Infant with PKU

The clinical picture of a PKU baby involves a normal-appearing newborn, most often with blond hair, blue eyes, and fair complexion. Decreased pigmentation may be related to the competition between phenylalanine and tyrosine for the available enzyme tyrosinase. Tyrosine is needed for the formation of melanin pigment and the hormones epinephrine and thyroxine. Without treatment, the infant fails to thrive and develops vomiting and eczematous rashes. By about 6 months of age, the infant exhibits behavior indicative of mental retardation and other CNS involvement, including seizures and abnormal electroencephalogram (EEG) patterns.

The Guthrie blood test for PKU is required for all newborns before discharge. The Guthrie test uses a drop of blood collected from a heel stick and placed on filter paper. It should be done at least 24 hours after the initiation of feedings containing the usual amounts of breast milk or formula so its metabolites begin to build up in the baby with PKU once milk feedings are initiated. High-risk newborns should be receiving a 60% milk intake, with no more than 40% of their total intake coming from nonprotein intravenous fluids. The PKU testing of high-risk newborns should be deferred for at least 48 hours after hyperalimentation is initiated. It is vital that the parents understand the need for the screening procedure, and a follow-up check is necessary to confirm that the test was done.

The nurse advises parents that once identified, an afflicted PKU infant can be treated by a special diet that limits ingestion of phenylalanine. Special formulas low in phenylalanine, such as Lofenalac, Minafen, and Albumaid XP, are available. Special food lists are helpful for parents of a PKU child (Blackburn, 2003). If treatment is begun before 1 month of age, CNS damage can be minimized. There is an increased risk of producing a child with mental retardation if the mother with PKU is not on a low-phenylalanine diet during pregnancy. It is recommended that the woman reinstate her low-phenylalanine diet a few months before becoming pregnant (Blackburn, 2003).

Infant with MSUD

Newborns with MSUD have feeding problems and neurologic signs (seizures, spasticity, opisthotonos) during the first week of life. A maple syrup odor of the urine is noted, and when ferric chloride is added to the urine, its color changes to gray-green. An ear swab within 6 to 12 hours after birth has a similar smell (Robinson & Drumm, 2001). Diagnosis is confirmed with plasma amino acid analysis.

Newborns with MSUD must be given a formula that is low in the branched-chain amino acids leucine, isoleucine, and valine. This diet must be continued indefinitely. Dietary treatment prior to 12 days of life has been reported to result in normal intelligence.

Infant with Homocystinuria

Homocystinuria varies in its presentation, but the more common characteristics are skeletal abnormalities, dislocation of ocular lenses, intravascular thromboses, and mental retardation. Abnormalities occur because of the toxic effects of the accumulation of methionine and the metabolite homocystine in the blood.

Infants with homocystinuria are managed on a diet that is low in methionine but supplemented with cystine and pyridoxine (vitamin B_6). Early diagnosis and careful management may prevent mental retardation.

Infant with Galactosemia

Clinical manifestations of galactosemia include vomiting soon after ingestion of milk-based formula or breast milk, diarrhea, poor weight gain, hepatosplenomegaly, jaundice, and mental retardation. The condition is frequently associated with anemia, sepsis, and cataracts in the newborn period (Zinn, 2002). Except for cataracts and mental retardation, those findings are reversible when galactose is excluded from the diet. Mental retardation can be prevented by early diagnosis and careful dietary management.

A baby with galactosemia is placed on a galactose-free diet. Galactose-free formulas include Nutramigen (a protein hydrolysate process formula), meat-based formulas, or soybean formulas. As the infant grows, parents must be educated not only to avoid giving their child milk and milk products but also to read all labels carefully and avoid any foods containing dry milk products. Even with early treatment, children may have learning disabilities, speech problems, and female ovarian failure (Zinn, 2002).

Infant with CH

A large tongue, umbilical hernia, cool and mottled skin, low hairline, hypotonia, and large fontanelles (especially the posterior fontanelle in term infants) are frequently associated with congenital hypothyroidism. Early symptoms include prolonged newborn jaundice, poor feeding, constipation, low-pitched cry, poor weight gain, inactivity, and delayed motor development. In addition, premature infants of less than 30 weeks' gestation frequently have lower T_4 and thyroid-stimulating hormone (TSH) values than those of term infants. This difference may reflect the premature infant's inability to bind thyroid and a risk for hypothyroidism.

Babies with CH need frequent laboratory monitoring and adjustment of thyroid medication to accommodate their growth and development. With adequate treatment, children remain free of symptoms, but if the condition is untreated, stunted growth and mental retardation occur.

Evaluation

Expected outcomes of nursing care include the following:

- The risk of inborn errors of metabolism is promptly identified, and early intervention is initiated.
- The parents verbalize their concerns about their baby's nutritional status, health problems, long-term care needs, and potential outcomes.
- The parents are aware of available community health resources and use them as indicated.

CHAPTER REVIEW

EXPLOREMEDIALINK

NCLEX review questions, case studies, and other interactive resources for this chapter can be found on the Web site at http://www.prenhall.com/olds. Click on "Chapter 32" to select the activities for this chapter.

For tutorials including animations and videos, more NCLEX review questions, and an audio glossary, access the accompanying CD-ROM in this book.

Focus Your Study

- Early identification of potential high-risk fetuses through assessment of preconception, prenatal, and intrapartal factors facilitates strategically timed nursing observations and interventions.
- High-risk newborns, whether they are premature, SGA, LGA, postterm, or infants of a diabetic or substance-abusing mother, have many similar problems, although their problems are based on different physiologic processes.
- Small-for-gestational-age newborns are associated with perinatal asphyxia and resulting aspiration syndrome, hypothermia, hypoglycemia, hypocalcemia, polycythemia, congenital anomalies, and intrauterine infections. Long-term problems include continued difficulties with growth and learning.
- Large-for-gestational-age newborns are at risk for birth trauma as a result of cephalopelvic

disproportion, hypoglycemia, polycythemia, and hyperviscosity.

- Infants of diabetic mothers are at risk for hypoglycemia, hypocalcemia, hyperbilirubinemia, polycythemia, and respiratory distress due to delayed maturation of their lungs.
- Postterm newborns often encounter intrapartal problems such as CPD, shoulder dystocia, and birth traumas, hypoglycemia, polycythemia, meconium aspiration, cold stress, and possible seizure activity. Long-term complications may involve poor weight gain and low IQ scores.
- The common problems of the preterm newborn are results of the baby's immature body systems. Potential problem areas include respiratory distress (respiratory distress syndrome), patent ductus arteriosus, hypothermia and cold stress, feeding difficulties and necrotizing enterocolitis, marked insensible water loss and loss of buffering agents through the kidneys, infection, anemia of prematurity, apnea and intraventricular hemorrhage, retinopathy of prematurity, and behavioral state disorganization. Long-term needs and problems include bronchopulmonary dysplasia, speech defects, sensorineural hearing loss, and neurologic defects.
- Newborns of alcohol-dependent mothers are at risk for alterations in physical characteristics and the long-term complications of feeding problems; CNS dysfunction, including lower IQ, hyperactivity, and language abnormalities; and congenital anomalies.
- Newborns of drug-dependent mothers experience drug withdrawal as well as respiratory distress, jaundice, congenital anomalies, and behavioral abnormalities. With early recognition and intervention, the potential long-term physiologic and emotional consequences of these difficulties can be avoided or at least lessened in severity.
- Newborns of mothers with AIDS require early recognition and treatment so that the physiologic and emotional consequences may be lessened in severity and CDC guidelines implemented.
- Cardiac defects are a significant cause of morbidity and mortality in the newborn period. Early identification and nursing and medical care of newborns with cardiac defects are essential to the improved outcome of these infants. Care is directed toward lessening the workload of the heart and decreasing oxygen and energy consumption.
- Inborn errors of metabolism such as galactosemia, PKU, homocystinuria, and maple syrup urine disease are usually included in a newborn screening program designed to prevent mental retardation through dietary management and medication.
- The nursing care of the newborn with special problems involves understanding normal physiology, the pathophysiology of the disease process, clinical manifestations, and supportive or corrective therapies. Only with this theoretical background can the nurse make appropriate observations concerning responses to therapy and development of complications.

References

Als, H., Lester, B. M., Tronick, E., & Brazelton, T. B. (1982). Assessment of preterm infant behavior (APIB). In B. M. Fitzgerald Lester & M. W. Yogman (Eds.), *Theory and research in behavioral pediatrics* (Vol. 1). New York: Plenum.

American Academy of Pediatrics (AAP) Committee on Pediatric AIDS. (2000). Identification and care of HIV-exposed and HIV-infected infants, children, and adolescents in foster care. *Pediatrics, 102*(1), 149–153.

American Academy of Pediatrics (AAP) Committee on Pediatric AIDS and Committee on Infectious Diseases. (1999). Issues related to human immunodeficiency virus transmission in schools, child care, medical settings, the home, and community. *Pediatrics, 104*(2), 318–324.

American Academy of Pediatrics (AAP) Committee on Substance Abuse and Committee on Children with Disabilities. (2000). Fetal alcohol syndrome and alcohol-related neurodevelopmental disorders. *Pediatrics, 106*(2), 358–361.

American Heart Association. (2003). *Congenital cardiovascular disease statistics.* Retrieved 2/28/2003 from http://www.americanheart.org/children

Anderson, D. M. (2002). Feeding the ill or preterm infant. *Neonatal Network, 21*(7), 7–14.

Association of Women's Health, Obstetric and Neonatal Nurses (AWHONN). (2001). Evidence-based clinical practice guidelines. Neonatal skin care. Washington, DC: Author.

Ballard, J. L. (2002). Treatment of neonatal abstinence syndrome with breast milk containing methadone. *Journal of Perinatal and Neonatal Nursing, 15*(4), 76–85.

Bernstein, I., Gabbe, S. G., & Reed, K. L. (2002). Intrauterine growth restriction. In S. G. Gabbe, J. R. Niebyl, & J. L. Simpson (Eds.), *Obstetrics: Normal and problem pregnancies* (4th ed., pp. 869–891). Philadelphia: Churchill Livingstone.

Blackburn, S. (2003). *Maternal-fetal-neonatal physiology: A clinical perspective* (2nd ed.). Philadelphia: Saunders.

Cambell, S. (2003). Prenatal cocaine exposure and neonatal/infant outcomes. *Neonatal Network, 22*(1), 19–21.

Chatfield, J. (2001). ACOG issues guidelines on fetal macrosomia. *American Family Physician, 64*(1), 169–170.

Divon, M. Y. (2002). Prolonged pregnancy. In S. G. Gabbe, J. R. Niebyl, & J. L. Simpson (Eds.), *Obstetrics: Normal and problem pregnancies* (4th ed., pp. 931–942). Philadelphia: Churchill Livingstone.

Doshier, S. (1995). What happens to the offspring of diabetic pregnancies? *American Journal of Maternal Child Nursing, 20*(1), 25–28.

Eichel, P. (2001). Kangaroo care: Expanding our practice to critically ill neonates. *Newborn and Infant Nursing Reviews, 1*(4), 224–228.

Evans, R., & Thureen, P. J. (2001). Early feeding strategies in preterm and critically ill neonates. *Neonatal Network, 20*(7), 7–16.

Feldman, R., Eidelman, A. I., Sirota, L., & Weller, A. (2002). Comparison of skin-to-skin (kangaroo) and traditional care: Parenting outcomes and preterm infant development. *Pediatrics, 110*(1), 16–26.

Harrison, L. (2001). The use of comforting touch and massage to reduce stress for preterm infants in the neonatal intensive care unit. *Newborn and Infant Nursing Reviews, 1*(4), 235–241.

Homko, C. J., Sivan, E., Nyirjesy, P., & Reece, E. A. (1995). The interrelationship between ethnicity and gestational diabetes in fetal macrosomia. *Diabetes Care, 18*(11), 1442–1445.

Hoyert, D. L., Freedman, M. A., Strobino, D. M., & Guyer, B. (2001). Annual summary of vital statistics: 2000. *Pediatrics, 108*(6), 1241–1255.

Jacobson, S. W., Chiodo, L. M., Sokol, R. J., & Jacobson, J. L. (2002). Validity of maternal report of prenatal alcohol, cocaine, and smoking in relation to neurobehavioral outcome. *Pediatrics, 109*(5), 815–825.

Jones, J., Kassity, N., & Duncan, K. (2001). Complementary care: Alternatives for the neonatal intensive care unit. *Newborn and Infant Nursing Reviews, 1*(4), 207–210.

Kenner, C., & Dreyer, L. A. (2000). Prenatal and neonatal testing and screening: A double-edged sword. *Nursing Clinics of North America, 35*(3), 627–641.

Kliegman, R. M., & Das, U. G. (2002). Intrauterine growth restriction. In A. A. Fanaroff & R. J. Martin (Eds.), *Neonatal-perinatal medicine: Diseases of the fetus and infant* (7th ed., pp. 228–262). St. Louis, MO: Mosby.

Krist, A. H., & Crawford-Faucher, A. (2002). Management of newborns exposed to maternal HIV infection. *American Family Physician, 65*(10), 2049–2056.

Landon, M. B., Catalano, P. M., & Gabbe, S. G. (2002). Diabetes mellitus. In S. G. Gabbe, J. R. Niebyl, & J. L. Simpson (Eds.), *Obstetrics: Normal and problem pregnancies* (4th ed., pp. 1081–1116). Philadelphia: Churchill Livingstone.

Langer, O. (2000). Fetal macrosomia: Etiologic factors. *Clinical Obstetrics and Gynecology, 43*(2), 283–297.

Lemons, P. K. (2001). From gavage to oral feedings: Just a matter of time. *Neonatal Network, 20*, 7–13.

Lester, B. M., ElSohly, M., Wright, L. L., Smeriglio, V. L., Verter, J., Bauer, C. R., et al. (2001). The maternal lifestyle study: Drug use by meconium toxicology and maternal self-report. *Pediatrics, 107*(2), 309–317.

Lutes, L. M., & Altimier, L. (2001). Co-bedding multiples. *Newborn and Infant Nursing Reviews, 1*(4), 242–246.

Matthews, A. L., & Robin, N. H. (2002). Genetic disorders, malformations, and inborn errors of metabolism. In G. B. Merenstein & S. L. Gardner, *Handbook of neonatal intensive care* (5th ed., pp. 679–701). St. Louis, MO: Mosby.

McGrath, J. M., & Conliffe-Torres, S. (2000). *Feeding the preterm infant. Self-study guide.* Glenview, IL: National Association of Neonatal Nurses.

Merenstein, G. B., Adams, K., & Weisman, L. E. (2002). Infection in the neonate. In G. B. Merenstein & S. L. Gardner, *Handbook of neonatal intensive care* (5th ed., pp. 462–484). St. Louis, MO: Mosby.

Newell, S. J. (2000). Enteral feeding of the micropremie. *Clinics in Perinatology, 27*(1), 221–234.

Nyqvist, K. H. (2002). Breast-feeding in preterm twins: Development of feeding behavior and milk intake during hospital stay and related caregiving practices. *Journal of Pediatric Nursing, 17*(4), 246–256.

Robinson, D., & Drumm, L. (2001). Maple syrup disease: A standard of nursing care. *Pediatric Nursing, 27*(3), 255–264, 270.

Rosen, T. S., & Bateman, D. A. (2002). Infants of addicted mothers. In A. A. Fanaroff & R. J. Martin (Eds.), *Neonatal-perinatal medicine: Diseases of the fetus and infant* (7th ed., pp. 661–673). St. Louis, MO: Mosby.

Smith, P. (2001). Primary care in children with congenital heart disease. *Journal of Pediatric Nursing, 16*(5), 308–319.

Standley, J. M. (2001). Music therapy for the neonate. *Newborn and Infant Nursing Reviews, 1*(4), 211–216.

Strodtbeck, F. (2003). Assessment and management of the opthalmic system. In C. Kenner & J. Wright Lott, *Comprehensive neonatal care: A physiologic perspective.* (3rd ed., pp. 742–753). St. Louis, MO: Saunders.

Theobald, K., Botwinski, C., Alabanna, S., & McWilliam, P. (2000). Apnea of prematurity: Diagnosis, implications for care and pharmacologic management. *Neonatal Network, 19*(16), 17–24.

Volpe, J. J. (2001). *Neurology of the newborn.* Philadelphia: Saunders.

Weiner, S. M., & Finnegan, L. P. (2002). Drug withdrawal in the neonate. In G. B. Merenstein & S. L. Gardner, *Handbook of neonatal intensive care* (5th ed., pp. 163–178). St. Louis, MO: Mosby.

Zinn, A. B. (2002). Inborn errors of metabolism. In A. A. Fanaroff & R. J. Martin (Eds.), *Neonatal-perinatal medicine: Diseases of the fetus and infant* (7th ed., pp. 1468–1516). St. Louis, MO: Mosby.

Zylberberg, R., & Pepper, M. (2001). Continuous insulin infusion: Promoting growth in low birth weight infants. *Neonatal Network, 20*(1), 17–24.

33 The Newborn at Risk: Birth-Related Stressors

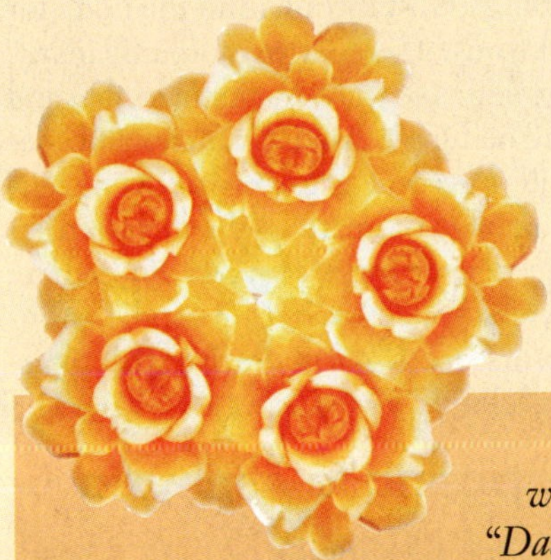

I watched her breathe every precious breath on the respirator. I saw her covered with wires and tubes. I kept watch. She was special to me and I would tell her over and over, "Daddy is here. Daddy loves you." The three days she lived were hell—not knowing if she would make it, uncertain about what plans we should make. Somehow I thought she would live; I was hopeful. When she died, at least I was there with her. The grief was unbearable. But there was also a sense of relief. The uncertainty, the waiting were finally over.

~ *When Pregnancy Fails* ~

Objectives

- Discuss how to identify infants in need of resuscitation and the appropriate method of resuscitation based on the labor record and observable physiologic indicators.
- Based on clinical manifestation, differentiate among the various types of respiratory distress (respiratory distress syndrome, transient tachypnea of the newborn, meconium aspiration syndrome, and persistent pulmonary hypertension).
- Identify the components of nursing care for a newborn with respiratory distress syndrome.
- Identify nursing interventions appropriate for preventing complications of respiratory therapy in newborns.
- Discuss selected metabolic abnormalities (including cold stress and hypoglycemia), their effects on the newborn, and their nursing implications.
- Differentiate between physiologic and pathologic jaundice according to onset, cause, possible sequelae, and specific management.
- Explain the circumstances that must be present for the development of erythroblastosis and ABO incompatibility.
- Identify the nurse's role in the care of an infant with hemolytic disease.
- Identify the nursing responsibilities in caring for the newborn receiving phototherapy.
- Discuss selected hematologic problems such as anemia and polycythemia and the nursing implications associated with each one.
- Describe the nursing assessment that would lead the nurse to suspect newborn sepsis.
- Relate the consequences of selected maternally transmitted infections, such as maternal syphilis, gonorrhea, herpesvirus, or chlamydia, to the management of the infant in the neonatal period.
- Describe interventions to facilitate parental attachment with the at-risk newborn.
- Identify the special initial and long-term needs of parents of at-risk infants.

Key Terms

Bronchopulmonary dysplasia (BPD)/chronic lung disease of prematurity (CLD) 956
Cold stress 958
Erythroblastosis fetalis 963
Hemolytic disease of the newborn 963
Hydrops fetalis 963
Hyperbilirubinemia 963
Hypoglycemia 959
Jaundice 963
Meconium aspiration syndrome (MAS) 951

MediaLink

Additional resources for this content can be found on the Student CD-ROM and on the Companion Website at www.prenhall.com/olds. Click on "Chapter 33" to select the activities for this chapter.

CD-ROM
- Audio Glossary
- NCLEX Review

Companion Website
- Additional NCLEX Review
- Case Study: Newborn with Jaundice
- Care Plan Activity: Infection in a Newborn

Key Terms

Persistent pulmonary hypertension of the newborn (PPHN) 954
Phototherapy 965
Physiologic anemia 971
Polycythemia 972
Respiratory distress syndrome (RDS) 943
Sepsis neonatorum 973

Marked homeostatic changes occur during the transition from fetal to newborn life. The most rapid anatomic and physiologic changes of this period occur in the cardiopulmonary system. Thus the major problems of the newborn are usually related to this system. These problems include asphyxia, respiratory distress syndrome, cold stress, jaundice, hemolytic disease, and anemia. Ideally, most problems are anticipated and identified prenatally, and appropriate intervention measures are begun at or immediately after birth.

Care of the Newborn at Risk Due to Asphyxia

Newborn asphyxia results from circulatory, respiratory, and biochemical factors. Circulatory patterns that accompany asphyxia indicate an inability to make the transition to extrauterine circulation—in effect, a return to fetal circulatory patterns. Failure of lung expansion and establishment of respiration rapidly produces hypoxia (decreased PaO_2), acidosis (decreased pH), and hypercarbia (increased PCO_2). These biochemical changes result in pulmonary vasoconstriction and high pulmonary vascular resistance in relation to the lower systemic vascular resistance (following birth the pulmonary vascular resistance should be markedly lower than the systemic vascular resistance), hypoperfusion of the lungs, and a large right-to-left shunt through the ductus arteriosus. As right atrial pressure exceeds left atrial pressure, the foramen ovale reopens, and blood flows from right to left. See Chapter 28 for review of normal newborn cardiopulmonary adaptation.

Biochemical changes that occur in asphyxia contribute to these circulatory and respiratory factors. The most serious biochemical abnormality is a change from aerobic to anaerobic metabolism due to hypoxia. This change results in the accumulation of lactate and the development of metabolic acidosis. Simultaneously, respiratory acidosis may also occur in response to a rapid increase in PCO_2 during asphyxia. In response to hypoxia and anaerobic metabolism, the amounts of free fatty acids (FFA) and glycerol in the blood increase. Glycogen stores are mobilized to provide a continuous glucose source for the brain. Hepatic and cardiac stores of glycogen may be used up rapidly during an asphyxial attack.

The newborn is supplied with protective mechanisms against hypoxic insults. These include a relatively immature brain and a resting metabolic rate lower than that observed in the adult, an ability to mobilize substances within the body for anaerobic metabolism and to use the energy more efficiently, and an intact circulatory system able to redistribute lactate and hydrogen ions in tissues still being perfused. Unfortunately, severe prolonged hypoxia will overcome these protective mechanisms, resulting in brain damage or death of the newborn.

The newborn who is apneic at birth requires immediate resuscitative efforts. The need for resuscitation can be anticipated if specific risk factors are present during the pregnancy or labor and birth period.

Risk Factors Predisposing to Asphyxia

The need for resuscitation may be anticipated if the mother demonstrates the antepartal and intrapartal risk factors described in Tables 15–1 and 23–1. Neonatal risk factors are as follows (Heinonen & Saarikoski, 2001):

- Nonreassuring fetal heart rate pattern
- Difficult birth
- Fetal scalp/capillary blood sample-acidosis
- History of meconium in amniotic fluid
- Apneic episode unresponsive to tactile stimulation
- Inadequate ventilation
- Prematurity
- Male infant
- Low birth weight
- Small for gestational age
- Multiple births
- Structural lung abnormality (congenital diaphragmatic hernia, lung hypoplasia)
- Congenital heart disease
- Sepsis with cardiovascular collapse

At times, no risk factors may be apparent prenatally. Particular attention must be paid to all at-risk pregnancies during the intrapartal period. Certain aspects of labor and birth challenge the oxygen supply to the fetus, and often the at-risk fetus has less tolerance to the stress of labor and birth.

Clinical Therapy

The initial goal of clinical management is to identify the fetus at risk for asphyxia so that resuscitative efforts can begin at birth.

Fetal biophysical assessment (see Chapter 21) combined with monitoring of fetal pH, fetal heart rates, and fetal oximetry if available during the intrapartal period may help identify fetal distress. If fetal distress is present, appropriate measures can be taken to deliver the fetus immediately, before major damage occurs, and to treat the asphyxiated newborn.

The fetal biophysical profile enhances the ability to predict an abnormal perinatal outcome. In addition, fetal scalp blood sampling may indicate asphyxic insult and the degree of fetal acidosis, when considered in relation to the stage of labor, uterine contractions, and nonreassuring fetal heart rate (FHR) patterns. During labor, a fetal pH of 7.25 or higher is considered normal (nonacidemia). A pH value of 7.20 or less is considered an ominous sign of intrauterine asphyxia (acidemia). However, low fetal pH without associated hypoxia can be caused by maternal acidosis resulting from prolonged labor, dehydration, and maternal lactate production.

The treatment of fetal or newborn asphyxia is resuscitation. The goal of resuscitation is to provide an adequate airway with expansion of the lungs, to decrease the PCO_2 and increase the PO_2, to support adequate cardiac output, and to minimize oxygen consumption by reducing heat loss.

Initial resuscitative management of a compromised newborn is extremely important. Caregivers should keep the newborn in a head-down position before the first gasp to avoid aspiration of the oropharynx secretions and must suction the oropharynx and nasopharynx immediately. Clearing the nasal and oral passages of fluid that may obstruct the airway establishes a patent airway. Suction of the mouth first and then the nose is always performed before resuscitation so that mucus, blood, or meconium is not aspirated into the lungs.

After the first few breaths, the nurse places the newborn in a level position under a radiant heat source and dries the baby quickly with warm blankets to maintain skin temperature at about 36.5C (97.7F). The newborn may be placed on the mother's chest or abdomen "skin to skin" as another heat source (American Academy of Pediatrics [AAP] & American College of Obstetrics and Gynecologists [ACOG] 2002). Drying is also a good stimulation to breathing. Heat loss through evaporation is tremendous during the first few minutes of life. The temperature of a wet 1500-g baby in a cold room (16C [62F]) drops 1C every 3 minutes. Hypothermia increases oxygen consumption. In an asphyxiated infant, it increases the hypoxic insult and may lead to severe acidosis and development of respiratory distress.

Assessment of the newborn's need for resuscitation begins at the time of birth. The time of the first gasp, first cry, and onset of sustained respirations should be noted in order of occurrence. The Apgar score (see Chapter 24) may be helpful in determining the severity of neonatal depression and may be predictive of neonatal survival (Casey, McIntire, & Leveno, 2001; Patel, Piotrowski, Nelson, et al, 2001).

Breathing is established by employing the simplest form of resuscitative measures initially, with progression to more complicated methods as required, for example:

1. Simple stimulation is provided by rubbing the back.
2. If respirations have not been initiated or are inadequate (gasping or occasional respirations), the lungs must be inflated with positive pressure. The mask is positioned securely on the face (over nose and mouth, avoiding the eyes) with the head in "sniffing" or neutral position (Figure 33–1 •). Hyperextension of the infant's neck will obstruct the trachea. An airtight connection is made between the baby's face and the mask (thus allowing the bag to inflate). The lungs are inflated rhythmically by squeezing the bag. Oxygen can be delivered at 100% with an anesthesia or modified self-inflating bag and adequate liter flow of at least 5L/min. The self-inflating bag delivers only 40% oxygen unless it has been adapted with an attached oxygen reservoir (AAP & ACOG, 2002). In addition, it may not be possible to maintain adequate inspiratory pressure with Ambu or Hope bags. In a crisis situation, it is crucial that 100% O_2 be delivered with adequate pressure.

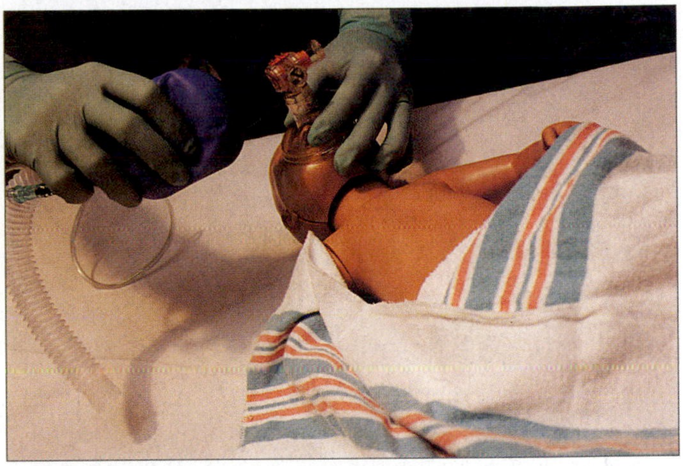

Figure 33–1 • Demonstration of resuscitation of an infant with bag and mask. Note that the mask covers the nose and mouth and that the head is in a neutral position. The resuscitation bag is placed to the side of the baby so that chest movement can be seen.

3. The rise and fall of the chest are observed for proper ventilation. Air entry and heart rate are checked by auscultation. Manual resuscitation is coordinated with any voluntary efforts. The rate of ventilation should be between 40 and 60 breaths per minute. Pressure should be adequate to move the chest wall. The pressure gauge (manometer) must be in place to avoid overdistention of the newborn's lungs and other problems such as pneumothorax or abdominal distention. In newborns with normal lungs, 15 to 25 cm H_2O may be adequate. If the newborn has lung disease, 20 to 40 cm H_2O may be necessary. If the newborn has not taken a first breath after birth, pressures of greater than 30 cm H_2O may be transiently required to expand collapsed alveoli. If ventilation is adequate, the chest moves with each inspiration, bilateral breath sounds are audible, and the lips and mucous membranes become pink. Distention of the stomach is controlled by inserting a nasogastric tube for decompression.
4. Endotracheal intubation (Figure 33–2 •) may be needed. However, most newborns, except for very-low-birth-weight (VLBW) (<1500 g) infants, can be resuscitated by bag and mask ventilation. With preterm newborns, positive end-expiratory pressure (PEEP) is required to help prevent alveolar collapse (Wong & Stenson, 2001). If color and heart rate fail to respond to ventilatory efforts, poor or improper

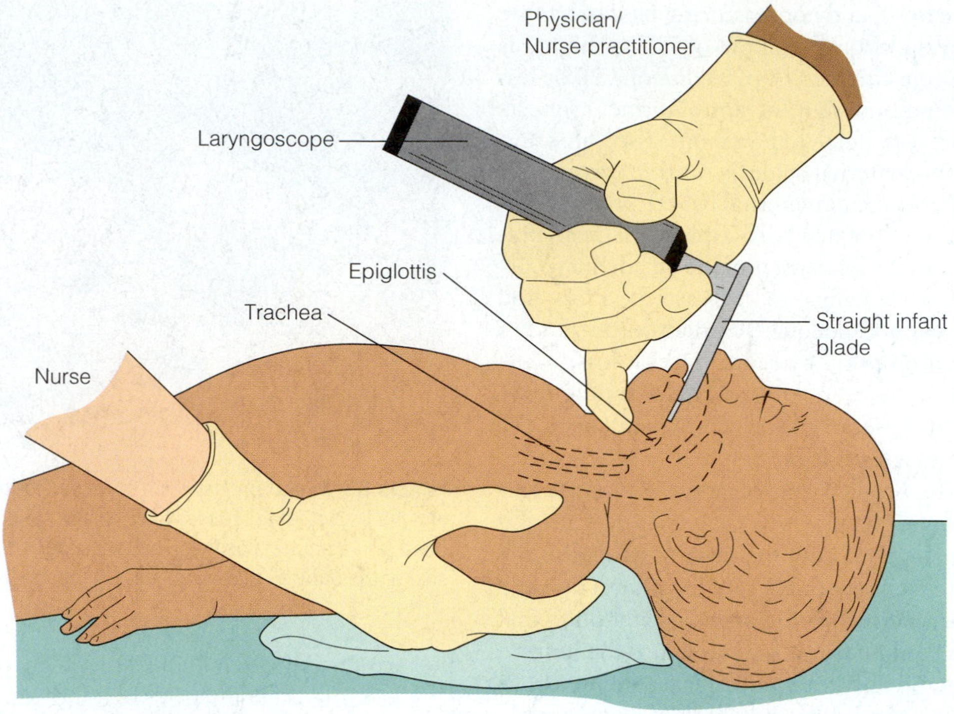

Figure 33–2 ● Endotracheal intubation is accomplished with the infant's head in the "sniffing" position. The clinician places the fifth finger under the chin to hold the tongue forward and inserts the laryngoscope blade. Once the blade is in position as shown, an endotracheal tube is inserted through the groove in the laryngoscope blade. The endotracheal tube is not seen in this illustration.

placement of an endotracheal tube may be the cause. If the baby is intubated properly, pneumothorax, diaphragmatic hernia, or hypoplastic lungs (Potter's association) may exist.

Once breathing has been established, the heart rate should increase to over 100 beats per minute. If the heart rate is absent or the heart rate remains less than 60 beats per minute after 30 seconds of effective positive pressure with 100% oxygen, external cardiac massage (chest compression) is begun. Chest compressions are started immediately if there is no detectable heartbeat. Following is the procedure for performing chest compression:

1. The infant is positioned properly on a firm surface.
2. The resuscitator may stand at the foot of the infant and place both thumbs over the lower third of the sternum (just below an imaginary line drawn between the nipples) with the fingers wrapped around and supporting the back (Figure 33–3, *A* ●). Alternatively, the examiner can use two fingers instead of the thumbs (Figure 33–3, *B*). The two-thumb method is preferred because it may provide better coronary perfusion pressure; however, it makes access to the umbilical cord for medication administration more difficult (Klaus & Fanaroff, 2001).
3. The sternum is depressed to sufficient depth to generate a palpable pulse or approximately one third of the anterior-posterior depth of the chest at a rate of 90 beats per minute (AAP & ACOG, 2002). Use a 3:1 ratio of heartbeat to assisted ventilation.

Drugs that should be available in the birthing area include those needed in the treatment of shock, cardiac arrest, and narcosis.

If after 30 seconds of ventilation and cardiac compression, the newborn has not responded with spontaneous respirations and a heart rate above 60 beats per minute, it is necessary to administer resuscitative medications (AAP & ACOG, 2002). The most accessible route for administering medications is the umbilical vein. If bradycardia is present, epinephrine (0.1 to 0.3 mL/kg of a 1:10,000 solution or 0.01 to 0.03 mg/kg) is given through the umbilical vein catheter or the peripheral IV setup. When epinephrine is administered by endotracheal tube, two to three times the IV dose of epinephrine is given followed immediately by 1 mL of normal saline. Sodium bicarbonate is rarely given in the delivery room. It is given only in the case of a severely asphyxiated newborn to correct metabolic acidosis and only after adequate ventilation is established. Dextrose is given to prevent progression of hypoglycemia. A 10% dextrose in water intravenous solution is usually sufficient to prevent or treat hypoglycemia in the birthing area. Naloxone hydrochloride (0.1 mg/kg), a narcotic antagonist, is used to reverse narcotic depression (Young & Mangum, 2001). See Drug Guide: Naloxone Hydrochloride (Narcan).

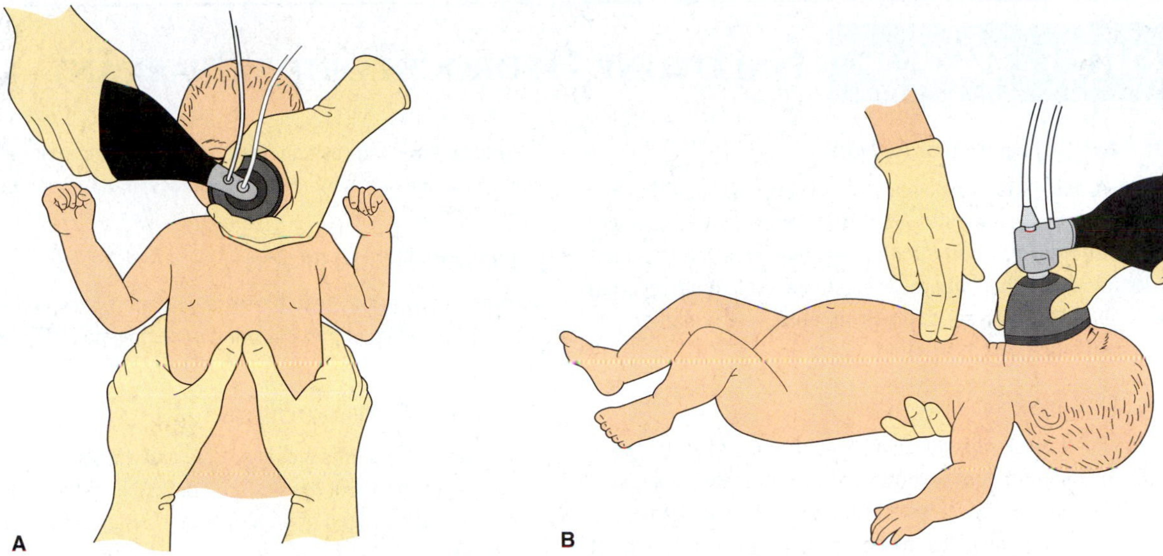

Figure 33–3 • External cardiac massage. The lower third of the sternum is compressed with two fingertips or thumbs at a rate of 90 beats per minute. *A,* In the thumb method, the fingers support the infant's back, and both thumbs compress the sternum. *B,* In the two-fingers method, the tips of two fingers of one hand compress the sternum, and the other hand or a firm surface supports the infant's back.

If shock develops (eg, low blood pressure or poor peripheral perfusion), the baby may be given a volume expander such as 5% albumin, lactated Ringer's, or normal saline in a dose of 10 mL/kg. Whole blood (O negative cross-matched against the mother's blood), fresh-frozen plasma, plasmanate, and packed red blood cells can also be used for volume expansion and treatment of shock. In some instances of prolonged resuscitation associated with shock and poor response to resuscitation, dopamine (5 mg/kg/min) may be necessary.

NURSING CARE MANAGEMENT

Nursing Assessment and Diagnosis

Communication between the obstetric office or clinic and the birthing area nurse facilitates the identification of newborns who may be in need of resuscitation. When the woman arrives in the birthing area, the nurse should have the antepartal record and should note any contributory prenatal history factors and assess present fetal status. As labor progresses, nursing assessments include ongoing monitoring of fetal heartbeat and its response to contractions, assisting with fetal scalp blood sampling, and observing the presence of meconium in the amniotic fluid to identify fetal asphyxia. In addition, the nurse should alert the resuscitation team and the practitioner responsible for the care of the newborn of any potential high-risk laboring woman.

Nursing diagnoses that may apply to the newborn with asphyxia and the newborn's parents include:

- ***Ineffective Breathing Pattern*** related to lack of spontaneous respirations at birth secondary to in utero asphyxia
- ***Decreased Cardiac Output*** related to impaired oxygenation
- ***Ineffective Family Coping: Compromised*** related to baby's lack of spontaneous respirations at birth and fear of losing their newborn

Nursing Plan and Implementation

Hospital-Based Nursing Care

Following identification of possible high-risk situations, the next step in effective resuscitation is assembling the necessary equipment and ensuring proper functioning. It is desirable to provide for pH and blood gas determinations as well. Necessary equipment includes a radiant warmer that provides an overhead radiant heat source (a thermostatic mechanism that is secured to the infant's abdomen, over a solid organ like the liver triggers the radiant warmer to turn on or off in order to maintain a level of thermoneutrality) and an open bed for easy access to the newborn. It is essential that the nurse keep the infant warm. To do so, the nurse dries the newborn quickly with warmed towels or blankets to prevent evaporative heat loss and places the baby under a prewarmed radiant warmer with servocontrol set at 36.5C (97.7F).

Resuscitative equipment in the birthing room must be sterilized after each use. In the high-risk nursery, the need for resuscitation may occur at any time. The reliability of the equipment must be maintained before an emergency arises,

DRUG GUIDE Naloxone Hydrochloride (Narcan)

Overview of Neonatal Action

Naloxone hydrochloride (Narcan) is used to reverse respiratory depression due to acute narcotic toxicity. It displaces morphinelike drugs from receptor sites on the neurons; therefore the narcotics can no longer exert their depressive effects. Naloxone reverses narcotic-induced respiratory depression, analgesia, sedation, hypotension, and pupillary constriction.

Route, Dosage, Frequency

Intravenous dose is 0.1 mg/kg (0.25 mL/kg of 0.4 mg/mL preparation or 0.1 cc/kg of 1 mg/cc) concentration at birth, including premature infants. This drug is usually given through the umbilical vein or endotracheal tube, although naloxone can be given intramuscularly or subcutaneously if adequate perfusion.

Reversal of drug depression occurs within 1 to 2 minutes after IV administration and within 15 minutes of IM administration. The duration of action is variable (minutes to hours) and depends on the amount of the drug present and the rate of excretion. Dose may be repeated in 3–5 minutes. If there is no improvement after two or three doses, discontinue naloxone administration. If initial reversal occurs, repeat dose as needed (Young & Mangum, 2001).

Neonatal Contraindications

Naloxone should not be administered to infants of narcotic-addicted mothers because it may precipitate acute withdrawal syndrome (increased HR and BP, vomiting, seizures, tremors).

Respiratory depression may result from nonmorphine drugs, such as sedatives, hypnotics, anesthetics, or other nonnarcotic CNS depressants.

Neonatal Side Effects

Excessive doses may result in irritability, increased crying, and possible prolongation of partial thromboplastin time (PTT). Tachycardia may occur.

Nursing Considerations

- Monitor respirations closely—rate and depth.
- Assess for return of respiratory depression when naloxone effects wear off and effects of longer acting narcotics reappear.
- Have resuscitative equipment, O_2, and ventilatory equipment available.
- Monitor bleeding studies.
- Note that naloxone is incompatible with alkaline solutions.
- Store at room temperature and protect from light.
- Compatible with heparin.

and the equipment must be restocked immediately after use. The nurse inspects all equipment—bag and mask, pressure manometer, oxygen and flow meter, laryngoscope, and suction machine—for damaged or nonfunctioning parts before a birth or when setting up an admission bed. A systematic check of the emergency cart and equipment is a routine responsibility of each shift.

Training and knowledge about resuscitation are vital to personnel in the birth setting for both normal and high-risk births. Resuscitation is at least a two-person effort, and the nurse should call for additional support as needed. The resuscitative efforts are recorded on the newborn's chart so that all members of the healthcare team will have access to this information.

Parent Teaching

Birthing room resuscitation is particularly distressing for the parents. If the need for resuscitation is anticipated, the parents should be assured that a team will be present at the birth to care specifically for their newborn. As soon as stabilization is accomplished, a member of the interdisciplinary team needs to discuss the baby's condition with the parents. The parents may have many fears about the reasons for resuscitation and the condition of their baby following the resuscitation.

Evaluation

Expected outcomes of nursing care include the following:

- The risk of asphyxia is promptly identified, and intervention is started early.
- The newborn's metabolic and physiologic processes are stabilized, and recovery proceeds without complications.
- The parents can describe the reason for resuscitation and what was done to resuscitate their newborn.
- The parents can verbalize their fears about the resuscitation process and potential implications for their baby's future.

Care of the Newborn with Respiratory Distress

One of the severest conditions to which the newborn may fall victim is respiratory distress—an inappropriate respiratory adaptation to extrauterine life. The nursing care of a baby with respiratory distress requires understanding of the normal pulmonary and circulatory physiology (Chapter 28), the pathophysiology of the disease process, clinical manifestations, and supportive and corrective therapies . Only with this knowledge can the nurse make appropriate observations concerning responses to therapy and development of complications. Unlike the verbalizing adult client, the newborn communicates needs only by exhibiting behaviors or physiologic parameters that must be interpreted by the neonatal intensive care unit (NICU) nurse. The neonatal nurse interprets this behavior as clues about the individual baby's condition. In this section, we discuss respiratory distress syndrome, transient tachypnea of the newborn, meconium aspiration syndrome, and persistent pulmonary hypertension.

Respiratory Distress Syndrome

Respiratory distress syndrome (RDS), also referred to as *hyaline membrane disease (HMD)*, is the result of a primary absence, deficiency, or alteration in the production of pulmonary surfactant. It is a complex disease that affects approximately 20,000 to 30,000 infants a year in the United States, most of whom are preterm. RDS is a complication of about 1% of pregnancies. The syndrome occurs more frequently in premature Caucasian infants than in infants of African descent and almost twice as often in males as in females.

All the factors precipitating the pathologic changes of RDS have not been determined, but the main factors associated with its development are as follows:

1. *Prematurity.* All preterm newborns—whether appropriate for gestational age (AGA), small for gestational age (SGA), or large for gestational age (LGA)—and especially infants of diabetic mothers are at risk for RDS. The incidence of RDS increases with the degree of prematurity, with most deaths occurring in newborns weighing less than 1500 g. The maternal and fetal factors resulting in preterm labor and birth, complications of pregnancy, indications for cesarean birth, and familial tendency are all associated with RDS.
2. *Surfactant deficiency disease.* Normal pulmonary adaptation requires adequate surfactant, a lipoprotein that coats the inner surface of the alveoli. Surfactant provides alveolar stability by decreasing the alveoli's surface tension and tendency for collapse. Surfactant is produced by type II alveolar cells starting at about 24 weeks' gestation. In the normal or mature newborn lung, it is continuously synthesized, oxidized during breathing, and replenished. Adequate surfactant levels lead to better lung compliance and permit breathing with less work. RDS is due to alterations in surfactant quantity, composition, function, or production.

Clinical Tip *An alveolus can be thought of as a small balloon filled with water and no air. When the balloon is emptied, the water droplets which remain inside the balloon increase the surface tension. As a result, the sides of the balloon stick together. The increased surface tension makes reinflation very difficult.*

Development of RDS indicates a failure to synthesize surfactant, which is required to maintain alveolar stability (see Chapter 28). Upon expiration, the instability increases atelectasis, which causes hypoxia and acidosis because of the lack of gas exchange. These conditions further inhibit surfactant production and cause pulmonary vasoconstriction. The resulting lung instability causes the biochemical problems of hypoxemia (decreased PO_2), hypercarbia (increased PCO_2), and acidemia (decreased pH), which further increases pulmonary vasoconstriction and hypoperfusion. The cycle of events of RDS leading to eventual respiratory failure is diagrammed in Figure 33–4 •.

Because of these pathophysiologic conditions, the newborn must expend increasing amounts of energy to reopen the collapsed alveoli with every breath, so that each breath becomes more difficult than the last. The progressive expiratory atelectasis upsets the physiologic homeostasis of the pulmonary and cardiovascular systems and prevents adequate gas exchange. Lung compliance decreases, which accounts for the difficulty of inflation, labored respirations, and the increased work of breathing.

The physiologic alterations of RDS produce the following complications:

1. *Hypoxia.* As a result of hypoxia, the pulmonary vasculature constricts, pulmonary vascular resistance increases, and pulmonary blood flow is reduced. Increased pulmonary vascular resistance may precipitate a return to fetal circulation as the ductus arteriosus opens and blood flow is shunted around the lungs. This increases the hypoxia and further decreases pulmonary perfusion. Hypoxia also causes impairment or absence of metabolic response to cold; reversion to anaerobic metabolism, resulting in lactate accumulation (acidosis); and impaired cardiac output, which decreases perfusion to vital organs.
2. *Respiratory acidosis.* Increased PCO_2 and decreased pH are results of alveolar hypoventilation. A persistent rise in PCO_2 is a poor prognostic sign of pulmonary function and adequacy.
3. *Metabolic acidosis.* Because of the lack of oxygen at the cellular level, the newborn begins an anaerobic pathway of metabolism, with a resultant base deficit (loss of bicarbonate) and an increase in acidemia (decrease in pH).

The classic radiologic picture of RDS is diffuse reticulogranular density that occurs bilaterally, with portions of the air-filled tracheobronchial tree (air bronchogram) outlined by the opaque ("white-out") lungs with widespread atelectasis (Blackburn, 2003) (Figure 33–5 •). Opacification of the lungs on x-ray image may be due to massive atelectasis, diffuse alveolar infiltrate, or pulmonary edema. The progression of x-ray findings parallels the pattern of resolution, which usually occurs in 7 to 10 days, and the time of surfactant reappearance, unless surfactant replacement therapy and mechanical ventilation has been used (Blackburn, 2003).

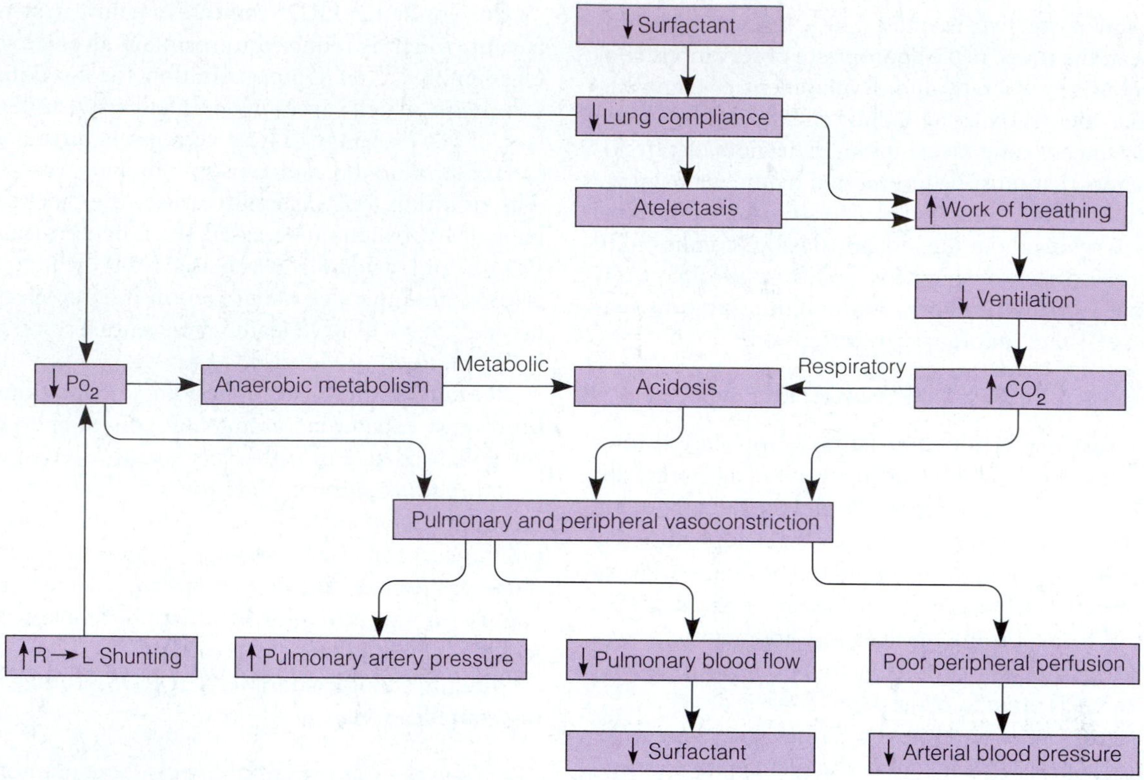

Figure 33–4 • Cycle of events of RDS leading to eventual respiratory failure.
SOURCE: Modified from Gluck, L., & Kulovich, M. V. (1973). Fetal lung development. *Pediatric Clinics of North America, 20,* 375.

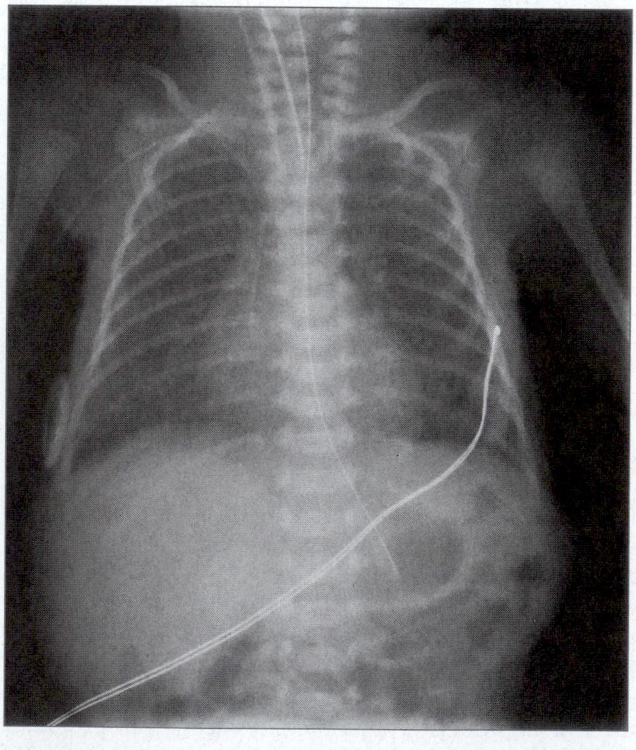

Figure 33–5 • RDS chest x-ray. Chest radiograph of respiratory distress syndrome characterized by a reticulogranular pattern with areas of microatelectasis of uniform opacity and air bronchograms.
SOURCE: Courtesy of Carol Harrigan, RNC, MSN, NNP.

Echocardiography is a valuable tool in diagnosing vascular shunts that shunt blood either away from or toward the lungs.

CLINICAL THERAPY

The primary goal of prenatal management is to prevent preterm birth through aggressive treatment of preterm labor and administration of glucocorticoids to enhance fetal lung development (see Chapter 20). Clinical trials have shown that multiple courses of antenatal steroids reduce the incidence of RDS in singleton premature newborns born within 1 week of the last dose; however, there is a decrease in head circumference (Abbasi, Hirsch, Davis, et al, 2000). The goals of postnatal therapy are to maintain adequate oxygenation and ventilation, to correct acid-base abnormalities, and to provide the supportive care required to maintain homeostasis.

Supportive medical management consists of oxygenation, ventilatory therapy, transcutaneous oxygen and carbon dioxide monitoring, blood gas monitoring, correction of acid-base imbalance, environmental temperature regulation, adequate nutrition, and protection from infection. Ventilatory therapy is directed toward preventing hypoventilation and hypoxia. Mild cases of RDS may require only increased humidified oxygen concentrations. Use of continuous positive airway pressure (CPAP) may be required in moderately afflicted infants. Babies with severe cases of RDS require mechanical ventilatory assistance from a respirator (Figure 33–6 •). Surfactant replacement therapy is now available for infants to de-

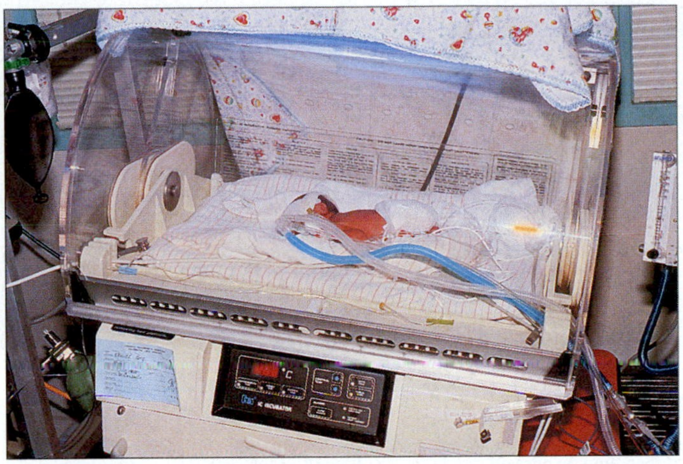

Figure 33–6 • One-day-old, 29 weeks' gestational age, 1450-g baby on respirator and in isolette.
SOURCE: Carol Harrigan, RNC, MSN, NNP.

crease the severity of RDS in low-birth-weight newborns. Surfactant replacement therapy is delivered through an endotracheal tube, and it may be given either in the delivery room or in the nursery after hospitalization and as indicated by the severity of RDS. Repeat doses are often required. The most generally reported response to treatment is rapidly improved oxygenation and decreased need of ventilatory support.

High-frequency ventilation and extracorporeal membrane oxygenation (ECMO), a form of heart-lung bypass, have been tried when conventional ventilator therapy has not been successful. Both of these have specific protocols for eligibility for use and require specially trained nurses and respiratory therapists. Nitric oxide inhalation therapy may also be a useful adjunctive therapy for infants with RDS (Lemons, Blackmon, Kanto, et al, 2000). According to a study by Rimensberger, Beghetti, Hanquinet, et al (2000), very-low-birth-weight newborns with RDS benefited from early placement on high-frequency ventilation by decreasing long-term lung problems. However, according to Moriette, Brunhes, and Jarreau (2000) there is an increased incidence of severe intraventricular hemorrhage with early use. In some institutions, morphine or fentanyl is used for its analgesic and sedative effects. Sedation may be indicated for infants most likely to have air leak respiratory problems. Use of pancuronium for muscle relaxation in infants with RDS is controversial.

Clinical Tip *In babies with respiratory distress syndrome who are on ventilators, increased urination (determined by weighing diapers) may be an early clue that the baby's condition is improving. As fluid moves out of the lungs into the bloodstream, alveoli open, and kidney perfusion increases, which results in increased voiding. At this point, the nurse must monitor chest expansion closely. If chest expansion is increasing, ventilator settings may have to be decreased. Too high a ventilator setting may "blow the lungs," resulting in pneumothorax.*

NURSING CARE MANAGEMENT

Nursing Assessment and Diagnosis

Characteristics of RDS the nurse should look for are increasing cyanosis, tachypnea (> 60 respirations per minute), grunting respirations, nasal flaring, significant retractions, and apnea. Table 33–1 • reviews clinical findings associated with respiratory distress in general. The Silverman-Andersen index (Figure 33–7 •) may be helpful in evaluating the signs of respiratory distress and can be done in the birthing area.

Nursing diagnoses that may apply to the newborn with respiratory distress syndrome include the following:

- ***Impaired Gas Exchange*** related to inadequate lung surfactant
- ***Altered Nutrition: Less than Body Requirements*** related to increased metabolic needs of stressed infants
- ***Risk for Infection*** related to invasive procedures

Nursing Plan and Implementation

Hospital-Based Nursing Care

Based on clinical parameters, the neonatal nurse implements therapeutic approaches to maintain physiologic homeostasis and provides supportive care to the newborn with RDS. See Clinical Pathway for Care of a Newborn with Respiratory Distress on pages 948 to 951.

Nursing interventions and criteria for instituting mechanical ventilatory assistance are done per institutional protocol. Methods of noninvasive oxygen monitoring and nursing interventions are described in Table 33–2 •. (The nursing care of infants on ventilators or with umbilical artery catheters is not discussed here. These infants have severe respiratory distress and are cared for in intensive care nurseries by nurses with advanced knowledge and training.) Ventilatory assistance with high-frequency ventilators has shown positive results. The parents of a baby born having respiratory distress should be provided with a very supportive environment.

Evaluation

Expected outcomes of nursing care include the following:

- The risk of RDS is promptly identified, and early intervention is initiated.
- The newborn is free of respiratory distress and metabolic alterations.
- The parents verbalize their concerns about their baby's health problem and survival and understand the rationale behind management of their newborn.

Table 33–1 • CLINICAL ASSESSMENTS ASSOCIATED WITH RESPIRATORY DISTRESS

Clinical Picture	Significance
Skin Color	
Pallor or mottling	These represent poor peripheral circulation due to systemic hypotension and vasoconstriction and pooling of independent areas (usually in conjunction with severe hypoxia).
Cyanosis (bluish tint)	Depending on hemoglobin concentration, peripheral circulation, intensity and quality of viewing light, and acuity of observer's color vision, this is frankly visible in advanced hypoxia. Central cyanosis is most easily detected by examination of mucous membranes and tongue.
Jaundice (yellow discoloration of skin and mucous membranes due to presence of unconjugated [indirect] bilirubin)	Metabolic alterations (acidosis, hypercarbia, asphyxia) of respiratory distress predispose to dissociation of bilirubin from albumin-binding sites and deposition in the skin and central nervous system.
Edema (presents as slick, shiny skin)	This is characteristic of preterm infants because of low total protein concentration with decrease in colloidal osmotic pressure and transudation of fluid. Edema of hands and feet is frequently seen within first 24 hours and resolved by fifth day in infants with severe RDS.
Respiratory System	
Tachypnea (normal respiratory rate 30–60/min, elevated respiratory rate 60+/min)	Increased respiratory rate is the most frequent and easily detectable sign of respiratory distress after birth. This compensatory mechanism attempts to increase respiratory dead space to maintain alveolar ventilation and gas exchange in the face of an increase in mechanical resistance. As a decompensatory mechanism it increases workload and energy output by increasing respiratory rate, which causes increased metabolic demand for oxygen and thus increases alveolar ventilation of an already overstressed system. During shallow, rapid respirations, there is an increase in dead space ventilation, thus decreasing alveolar ventilation.
Apnea (episode of nonbreathing for more than 20 seconds; periodic breathing, a common "normal" occurrence in preterm infants, is defined as apnea of 5–10 seconds alternating with 10–15 seconds of ventilation)	This poor prognostic sign indicates cardiorespiratory disease, CNS disease, metabolic alterations, intracranial hemorrhage, sepsis, or immaturity. Physiologic alterations include decreased oxygen saturation, respiratory acidosis, and bradycardia.
Chest	Inspection of the thoracic cage includes shape, size, and symmetry of movement. Respiratory movements should be symmetrical and diaphragmatic; asymmetry reflects pathology (pneumothorax, diaphragmatic hernia). Increased anteroposterior diameter indicates air trapping (meconium aspiration syndrome).
Labored respirations (Silverman-Andersen chart in Figure 33–7 indicates severity of retractions, grunting, and nasal flaring, which are signs of labored respirations)	Indicates marked increase in the work of breathing.
Retractions (inward pulling of soft parts of the chest cage—suprasternal, substernal, intercostal, subcostal—at inspiration)	These reflect the significant increase in negative intrathoracic pressure necessary to inflate stiff, noncompliant lungs. Infants attempt to increase lung compliance by using accessory muscles. Lung expansion markedly decreases. Seesaw respirations are seen when the chest flattens with inspiration and the abdomen bulges. Retractions increase the work of breathing and O_2 need so that assisted ventilation may be necessary due to exhaustion.
Flaring nares (inspiratory dilation of nostrils)	This compensatory mechanism attempts to lessen the resistance of the narrow nasal passage.
Expiratory grunt (Valsalva maneuver in which the infant exhales against a closed glottis, thus producing an audible moan)	This increases transpulmonary pressure, which decreases or prevents atelectasis, thus improving oxygenation and alveolar ventilation. Intubation should not be attempted unless the infant's condition is rapidly deteriorating, because it prevents this maneuver and allows the alveoli to collapse.
Rhythmic body movement with labored respirations (chin tug, head bobbing, retractions of anal area)	This is a result of using abdominal and other respiratory accessory muscles during prolonged forced respirations.
Auscultation of chest reveals decreased air exchange with harsh breath sounds or fine inspiratory rales; rhonchi may be present	Decrease in breath sounds and distant quality may indicate interstitial or intrapleural air or fluid.
Cardiovascular System	
Continuous systolic murmur may be audible	Patent ductus arteriosus is a common occurrence with hypoxia, pulmonary vasoconstriction, right-to-left shunting, and congestive heart failure.
Heart rate usually within normal limits (fixed heart rate may occur with a rate of 110–120/min)	A fixed heart rate indicates a decrease in vagal control.
Point of maximal impulse usually located at fourth to fifth intercostal space, left sternal border	Displacement may reflect dextrocardia, pneumothorax, or diaphragmatic hernia.
Hypothermia	This is inadequate functioning of metabolic processes that require oxygen to produce necessary body heat.
Muscle Tone	
Flaccid, hypotonic, unresponsive to stimuli Hypertonia and/or seizure activity	These may indicate deterioration in the newborn's condition and possible CNS damage due to hypoxia, acidemia, or hemorrhage.

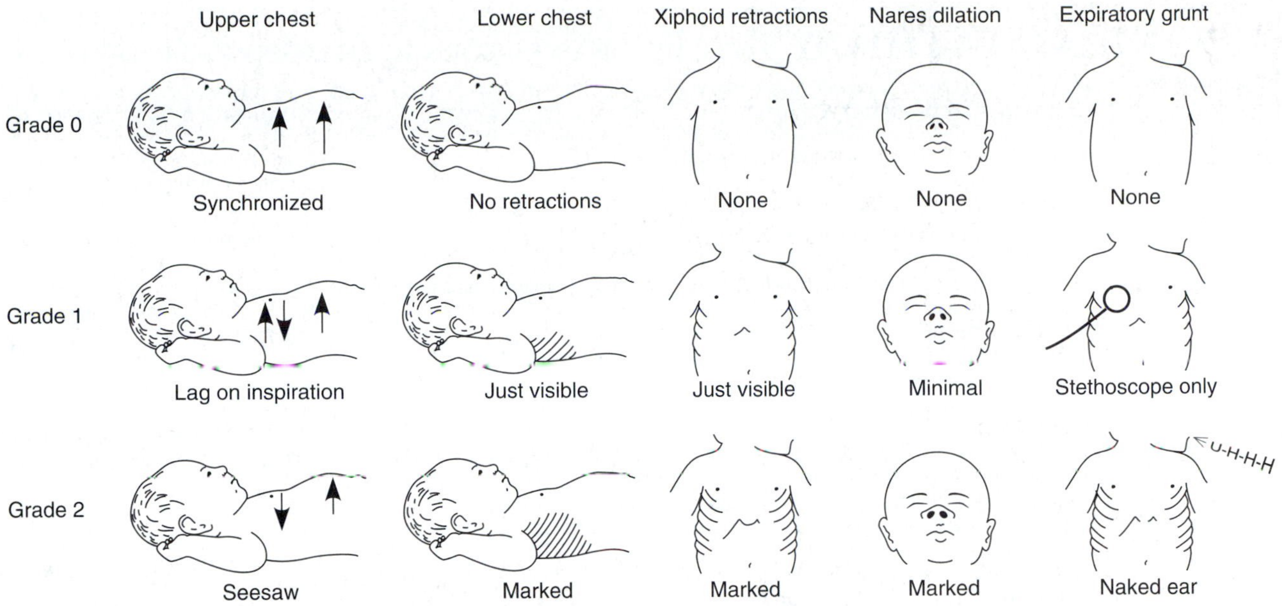

Figure 33–7 • Evaluating respiratory status using the Silverman-Andersen index. The baby's respiratory status is assessed. A grade of 0, 1, or 2 is determined for each area, and a total score is charted in the baby's record or on a copy of this tool and placed in the chart.
SOURCES: Ross Laboratories, Nursing Inservice Aid No. 2, Columbus, OH; Silverman, W. A., & Andersen, D. H. (1956). *Pediatrics, 17*, 1. Copyright 1956, American Academy of Pediatrics.

CRITICAL THINKING IN PRACTICE

You are caring for baby girl Linn, who is a 39-week, AGA female born by repeat cesarean birth to a 34-year-old G3 now P3 mother. Baby Linn's Apgar scores were 7 and 9 at 1 and 5 minutes. At 2 hours of age, an elevated respiratory rate of 70 to 80 and mild cyanosis were noted. She is now receiving 30% oxygen and has a respiratory rate of 100 to 120. The baby's clinical course, chest x-ray examination, and lab work are all consistent with transient tachypnea of the newborn. Her mother calls you to ask about her baby. She tells you that her last child was born at 30 weeks' gestation, had respiratory distress syndrome requiring ventilator support, and was hospitalized for 6 weeks. She asks you, "Is this the same respiratory distress?" What will you tell her?

Answers can be found in Appendix I .

Transient Tachypnea of the Newborn

Some newborns, primarily AGA and near-term infants, may develop progressive respiratory distress that clinically can resemble RDS. They may have had intrauterine or intrapartal asphyxia due to maternal oversedation, maternal bleeding, prolapsed cord, breech birth, or maternal diabetes. The resultant effect on the newborn is failure to clear the airway of lung fluid, mucus, and other debris, or an excess of fluid in the lungs due to aspiration of amniotic or tracheal fluid. Transient tachypnea of the newborn occurs in 11 per 1000 live births. It is more prevalent in cesarean-born newborns who have not had the thoracic squeeze that occurs during vaginal birth and removes some of the lung fluid (Blackburn, 2003).

Usually the newborn experiences little or no difficulty at the onset of breathing. However, shortly after birth, expiratory grunting, flaring of the nares, and mild cyanosis may be noted in the newborn breathing room air. Tachypnea is usually present by 6 hours of age, with respiratory rates as high as 100 to 140 breaths per minute. Mild respiratory and metabolic acidosis may be present at 2 to 6 hours.

CLINICAL THERAPY

Initial x-ray findings may be identical to those showing RDS within the first 3 hours. However, radiographs of infants with transient tachypnea usually reveal a generalized overexpansion of the lungs (hyperaeration of alveoli), which is identifiable principally by flattened contours of the diaphragm. Dense streaks (increased vascularity) radiate from the hilar region and represent engorgement of the lymphatic vessels, which clear alveolar fluid on initiation of air breathing. Within 72 hours, the chest x-ray examination is normal (Hagedorn, Gardner, & Abman, 2002).

Ambient oxygen concentrations of 30% to 50%, usually under an oxyhood, may be required to correct the mild

CLINICAL PATHWAY FOR CARE OF A NEWBORN WITH RESPIRATORY DISTRESS

Category	Day of Birth—First 4 Hours	Remainder of Birth Day
Referral	Report from L&D, Neonatal Nurse Practitioner Check ID bands Consults prn: High-risk peds, neonatology	Check ID bands q shift Lactation consult prn
Assessments	Assess development of s/s respiratory distress: • Tachypnea (>60 respirations/min) • Expiratory grunting (audible), subcostal/intercostal/suprasternal retractions, nasal flaring on inspiration • Cyanosis and pallor • Signs of increased air hunger (apnea, hypotonus), labored respirations • Arterial blood gases (indicating respiratory failure): Pao_2 less than 50 mm Hg, and Pco_2 above 60 mm Hg Auscultation: • Initially breath sounds may be normal, then decreased air exchange occurs with harsh breath sounds and, upon deep inspiration, rales • Later, a low-pitched systolic murmur indicates patent ductus arteriosus Determine baseline of respiratory effort and ventilatory adequacy: • Observe chest wall movement • Assess skin, mucous membranes color, capillary refill • Auscultate quality of air entry bilaterally • Assess arterial blood gases and pH Increasing oxygen concentration requirements to maintain adequate Po_2 levels VS: temp (ax), pulse, respirations, BP Admission wt, length, HC, peripheral pulses × 4 Monitor pulse oximeter Gestational age assessment (only as tolerated without increasing infant's work of breathing, or defer) Gestational history: recent episodes of fetal or intrapartal stress (maternal hypotension, bleeding, maternal and resultant fetal oversedation), fetal lung circulation compromise Lung maturity assessment: amniotic, tracheal and/or gastric aspirates as available for PG Newborn Hx: birth asphyxia resulting in acute hypoxia, hypothermia, low Apgar scores, bag/mask resuscitation Monitor activity (increasing lethargy, s/s seizure activity)	Continue previous assessments q2–4h and prn Assess color, respiratory status Assess mother/baby interaction as appropriate Observe infant for temperature instability, signs of increased oxygen consumption and metabolic acidosis Observe infant for s/s sepsis: apnea, lethargy, cyanosis, temp instability
Teaching/ psychosocial	Admission activities performed at mother's bedside as possible; orient parents to nursery, handwashing; assess teaching needs and readiness for learning Provide parents information on infant's condition, minimal handling rationale, equipment and monitoring devices prn	Reinforce previous teaching; keep parents apprised of infant's status Discuss/teach infant security, identification Teach parents s/s respiratory distress, calming techniques, bulb syringe, positioning, when to call for assistance
Nursing care management and reports	Admit directly to special care nursery prn Labs as ordered: blood type, Rh, Coombs' on cord blood prn, tracheal or gastric aspirate for PG, chemstrip, peripheral hct, blood cultures, CBC, electrolytes, arterial or capillary blood gas Administer IV antibiotics as ordered Intravenous access for meds, hydration, nutritional support Assist MD/NP with placement of umbilical or arterial lines prn Attach servo probe to infant's skin, radiant warmer bed on servo control Attach 3-lead EKG for continuous cardiac, resp monitoring prn Attach pulse oximeter to infant extremity Set up, monitor oxygen administration prn (or assist respiratory therapist prn), nasal cannula, oxygen hood	Vital signs: q4h and prn, use monitoring devices to decrease infant stimulation; daily wt using bedscale as necessary Monitor antibiotic drug levels Continue assessments q4h and prn Cord care per policy (alcohol to cord q diaper change after infant stable and possibility of placing umbilical lines remote) Rotate pulse oximetry sites q8h and prn; TCOM sites q4h and prn depending on infant's skin integrity
Activity and comfort	Adjust and monitor radiant warmer to maintain skin temp and NTE Provide calming techniques Cluster cares (allow recovery time between procedures), nest Minimal stimulation, quiet and dim environment Provide pacifier for nonnutritive sucking	Leave in radiant warmer until stable, then swaddle and move to isolette or open crib as condition allows Encourage parent interaction/holding as soon as infant tolerates Avoid overstimulation, cluster cares, assess on infant's schedule Reposition for comfort q4h, prn; position on surfboard while prone

CLINICAL PATHWAY FOR CARE OF A NEWBORN WITH RESPIRATORY DISTRESS *CONTINUED*

Category	Day of Birth—First 4 Hours	Remainder of Birth Day
Nutrition	Provide total parenteral nutrition (TPN) as ordered and indicated Provide adequate caloric intake: consider amount of intake, route of administration, need for supplementation of intake by other routes, type of feeding breast/formula Gavage feeding prn Maintain IV rate via infusion pump (usually 60–80 mL/kg/day dependent on gestational age, and organ efficiency) • Record intake hourly (oral, parenteral type and amount) • Monitor vital signs, lung auscultation, heart sounds for s/s fluid overload	Advance intake as tolerated from parenteral to gastrointestinal Gavage or nipple feed, supplementing with IV prn, discontinue IV when oral intake sufficient Initiate breastfeeding as soon as mother/baby condition allows Supplement breastfeeding only when medically indicated and ordered by MD/NP Initiate formula feeding as applicable
Elimination	Note first void and stool Record hourly output Monitor urine specific gravity	Continue accurate hourly output monitoring (1–3 mL/kg/h) Monitor stools for amt, type, pattern changes Continue specific gravity monitoring
Medication	AquaMEPHYTON IM, dosage according to infant wt per MD order Ilotycin ophth ointment OU after retinal assessment by MD/NP Antibiotic therapy as ordered	Continue antibiotic therapy as ordered
Discharge planning/ home care	Plan DC with parent/guardian Evaluate for Social Services/home care/DC planning needs	Birth certificate instructions/worksheet Car seat available for DC
Family involvement	Evaluate psychosocial needs: provide time for expressions of concerns, determine parents' understanding of respiratory distress syndrome (RDS) Evaluate parent teaching	Encourage family involvement in infant's care as possible and as infant tolerates Keep family apprised of infant's progress and current status Evaluate parent teaching
Category	**Day 1 after Birth**	**Day 2/3 (as applicable) after birth**
Referral	Check ID bands q shift	Check ID bands q shift ➤ **Expected Outcomes** Mother/baby ID bands correlate at time of DC Consults completed prn
Assessments	Continue high-risk assessment for RDS q4h Assess respiratory effort and ventilatory adequacy Assess mother/baby interaction Assess thermoregulation Assess abdominal distention, gastric residuals Monitor blood gases, capillary refill, O_2 saturation, pulses all 4 extremities	Assess respiratory effort and level of distress Continue high-risk assessment for resp distress q4h as needed Assess mother/baby interaction Continue monitoring blood gases, capillary refill, O_2 saturation, pulses all 4 extremities q4h prn, wean to q8h as infant recovers ➤ **Expected Outcomes** Physical assessments, VS WNL; no complications or residual respiratory distress noted
Teaching/ psychosocial	(See Newborn Clinical Pathway, Chapter 30) Reinforce previous teaching Parental teaching: bathing, cord care, skin/nail care, use of thermometer, activity, sleep patterns, calming methods, reflexes, jaundice, growth/feeding patterns, burping, diapering, elimination norms Provide information including: • Newborn capabilities and developmental behaviors, cues • Temperature maintenance with clothing and blankets • Safety (choking, positioning, use of bulb syringe)	Final discharge teaching: (See Newborn Clinical Pathway, Chapter 30) Review infant safety, s/s illness and when to call healthcare provider with parents ➤ **Expected Outcomes** Mother verbalizes comprehension of instructions, demonstrates care capabilities

(continued on next page)

CLINICAL PATHWAY FOR CARE OF A NEWBORN WITH RESPIRATORY DISTRESS *CONTINUED*

Category	Day 1 after Birth	Day 2/3 (as applicable) after Birth
Nursing care management and reports	Maintain on respiratory and cardiac monitors: • Check and calibrate all monitoring and measuring devices q8h • Calibrate oxygen devices to 21% and 100% O_2 concentrations Provide warmed air and humidified oxygen Monitor oxygen concentrations at least q1h Femoral pulses or BPs all 4 extremities before DC or at 48h VS q4h Daily wt Continue high-risk assessments for resp distress q4h, wean to q8h as infant stabilizes and recovers Isolette if temp instability • Adjust and monitor to maintain skin temp and NTE Use servo control to maintain constant temp regulation Monitor activity Administer meds as ordered Newborn screen, monitor therapeutic drug levels, blood gases prn	Newborn/high-risk assessment q8h if resp status WNL and stable Baer hearing test Daily wt VS q8h and prn Continue oxygen administration as warranted (oxyhood, nasal cannula) Monitor O_2 concentrations q1–2h Prepare infant for/assist with circumcision as applicable Cord care per policy (alcohol to cord q diaper change) Administer antibiotics/monitor levels as ordered Continue Standard Precautions HSV culture per parental hx of HSV Wean from radiant warmer or isolette to open crib if VS WNL, stable ➤ **Expected Outcomes** Physical assessments WNL; cord unclamped and dry without s/s infection; circ site unremarkable; no s/s respiratory distress; labs WNL; wt stabilized to not >10% loss
Activity and comfort	Change position q4h and prn Swaddled in open crib as condition permits Isolette if temp instability; adjust temp for infant size, gestation layers of clothing to maintain NTE	Swaddled in open crib as condition permits Allow movement of hands to face ➤ **Expected Outcomes** Maintains temp WNL swaddled in open crib
Nutrition	Supplement breast only when medically indicated/ordered Gavage feed prn Encourage on-demand feedings as tolerated, minimally q3–4h Breast feeding on demand Decrease parenteral support as oral feedings increase	Continue feeding schedule Feed on demand breast or formula Supplement breast only when medically indicated/ordered ➤ **Expected Outcomes** Infant tolerates feedings, feeds on demand; breastfeeds without supplement, nipples without problems or s/s increased WOB; regaining lost wt or wt stabilized after birth
Elimination	Monitor stools for amount, consistency, pattern changes, occult blood, reducing substances Monitor voids q8h Continue accurate intake and output as warranted	Continue monitoring of all voids and stools q shift, noting changes. Accurate intake and output as warranted ➤ **Expected Outcomes** Voids qs, stools without difficulty qs, stool character WNL
Medication	Hep B vaccine as ordered by MD/NP after consent signed by parent	Hep B vaccine before DC ➤ **Expected Outcomes** Infant has received ophthalmic ointment OU and AquaMEPHYTON injection; received first Hep B vaccine if ordered and parental consent given; antibiotics regimen completed with resolution RDS
Discharge planning/ home care	Newborn photographs Complete birth certificate packet Continue DC teaching Access community referrals, support groups for mother/family prn, ie, WIC, financial resources, public health nursing	Complete DC teaching Complete DC summary, give written copy DC instructions (See Newborn Clinical Pathway, Chapter 30) Set up appointment for follow-up newborn screening blood test All discharge referrals made, follow-up appointments scheduled ➤ **Expected Outcomes** Infant discharged home with family; mother verbalizes f/u appointments times and dates; mother verbalizes comprehension of DC instructions and available resources, ie, lactation, new parents support groups

➤

CLINICAL PATHWAY FOR CARE OF A NEWBORN WITH RESPIRATORY DISTRESS *CONTINUED*

Category	Day 1 after Birth	Day 2/3 (as applicable) after Birth
Family Involvement	Bath and feeding class Newborn channel as available Assess mother/baby bonding/interaction Incorporate significant other/siblings in care Support positive parenting behaviors Evaluate mother/parent teaching Encourage significant other's presence during MD visits with mother on infant's progress, current status, and plan formation	Assess mother/baby bonding/interaction Identify community referral needs and refer to community agencies ➤ **Expected Outcomes** Demonstrates caring and family incorporation of infant
Date		

BP, blood pressure; DC, discharge; EKG, electrocardiograph; f/s, follow-up; HC, head circumference; Hx, history; ID, identification; IM, intramuscular; IV, intravenous; L&D, labor and delivery; Meds, medications; MD, medical doctor; MD/NP, medical doctor/nurse practitioner; NTE, neutral thermal environment; OU, both eyes; O_2, oxygen; Peds, pediatrics; PG, phosphatidylglycerol; prn, as needed; RDS, respiratory distress syndrome; Resp, respiratory, respiratoy, s/s, signs and symptoms; Temp, temperature; TCOM, transcutaneous oxygen monitor; TPN, total parenteral nutrition; Via, by way of; VS, vital signs; WIC, Women, Infants, and Children; WNL, within normal limits; WOB, work of breathing.

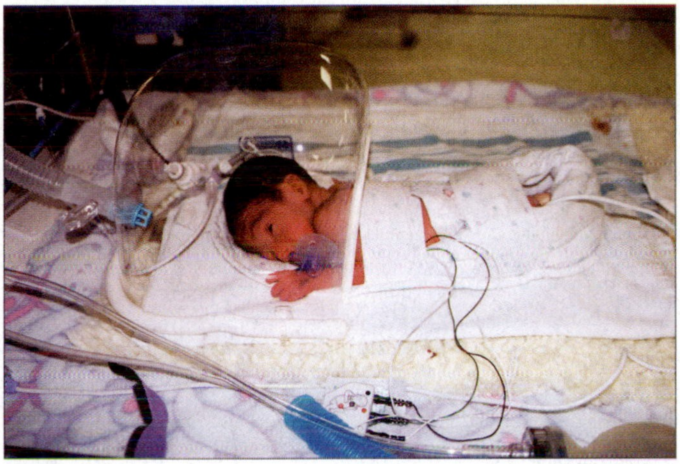

Figure 33–8 • Premature infant under oxygen hood. Infant is nested and has a nonnutritive sucking pacifier.
SOURCE: Courtesy of Lisa Smith-Pedersen, RNC, MSN, NNP.

hypoxemia (Figure 33–8 •). Fluid and electrolyte requirements should be met with intravenous fluids during the acute phase of the disease. Oral feedings are contraindicated because of rapid respiratory rates. The infant should be improving by 8 to 24 hours. The duration of the clinical course of transient tachypnea is approximately 72 hours (Hagedorn et al, 2002).

When hypoxemia is severe and tachypnea continues, persistent pulmonary hypertension must be considered and treatment measures initiated. If pneumonia is suspected initially, antibiotics may be administered prophylactically.

NURSING CARE MANAGEMENT

For nursing actions, see the Clinical Pathway for Care of the Newborn with Respiratory Distress on pages 948 to 951.

Meconium Aspiration Syndrome

The presence of meconium in amniotic fluid indicates an asphyxial insult to the fetus before or during labor unless the baby is in breech position. The physiologic response to asphyxia is increased intestinal peristalsis, relaxation of the anal sphincter, and passage of meconium into the amniotic fluid. However, passage of meconium in a breech position does not necessarily indicate asphyxia.

Among all pregnancies, 13% of live born infants are born through meconium-stained amniotic fluid (MSAF). Of the newborns born through MSAF, 4% to 11% develop **meconium aspiration syndrome (MAS)** (Blackburn, 2003). This fluid may be aspirated into the tracheobronchial tree by the fetus in utero or during the first few breaths taken by the newborn. This syndrome primarily affects term, SGA, and postterm newborns and those who have experienced a long labor.

Presence of meconium in the lungs produces a ball-valve action (air is allowed in but not exhaled), so that alveoli overdistend; rupture with pneumomediastinum or pneumothorax is a common occurrence. The meconium also initiates a chemical pneumonitis in the lung with oxygen and carbon dioxide trapping and hyperinflation. Secondary bacterial pneumonias can occur.

Clinical manifestations of MAS include (1) fetal hypoxia in utero a few days or a few minutes prior to birth, indicated by a sudden increase in fetal activity followed by diminished activity, slowing of fetal heart rate or weak and irregular heartbeat, loss of beat-to-beat variability, and meconium staining of amniotic fluid; and (2) presence of signs of distress at birth, such as pallor, cyanosis, apnea, slow heartbeat, and low Apgar scores (below 6) at 1 and 5 minutes. As victims of intrauterine asphyxia, meconium-stained newborns or newborns who have aspirated meconium often have respiratory depression at birth and require resuscitation to establish adequate respiratory effort.

After the initial resuscitation, the severity of clinical symptoms correlates with the extent of aspiration. Many infants require mechanical ventilation at birth due to immediate signs

Table 33-2 • OXYGEN MONITORS

Type	Function and Rationale	Nursing Interventions
Pulse Oximetry—Spo_2		
Estimates beat-to-beat arterial oxygen saturation. Microprocessor measures saturation by the absorption of red and infrared light as it passes through tissue. Changes in absorption related to blood pulsation through vessel determine saturation and pulse rate.	Calibration is automatic. Less dependent on perfusion than $TcPo_2$ and $TcPco_2$; however, functions poorly if peripheral perfusion is decreased due to low cardiac output. Much more rapid response time than $TcPo_2$—offers "real-time" readings. Can be located on extremity, digit, or palm of hand, leaving chest free; not affected by skin characteristics. Requires understanding of oxyhemoglobin dissociation curve. Pulse oximeter reading of 85% to 95% reflects clinically safe range of saturation. Extreme sensitivity to movement; decreases if average of 7th or 14th beat is selected rather than beat to beat. Poor correlation with extreme hyperoxia.	Understand and use oxyhemoglobin dissociation curve. Monitor trends over time and correlate with arterial blood gases. Check disposable sensor at least q8h. Use disposable cuffs (reusable cuffs allow too much ambient light to enter, and readings may be inaccurate).
Transcutaneous Oxygen Monitor—$TcPo_2$		
Measures oxygen diffusion across the skin. Clark electrode is heated to 43C (preterm) or 44C (term) to warm the skin beneath the electrode and promote diffusion of oxygen across the skin surface. Po_2 is measured when oxygen diffuses across the capillary membrane, skin, and electrode membrane.	When transcutaneous monitors are properly calibrated and electrodes are appropriately positioned, they will provide reliable, continuous, noninvasive measurements of Po_2, Pco_2, and oxygen saturation. Readings vary when skin perfusion is decreased. Reliable as trend monitor. Frequent calibration necessary to overcome mechanical drift. Following membrane change, machine must "warm up" 1 hour prior to initial calibration; otherwise, after turning it on, it must equilibrate for 30 minutes prior to calibration. When placed on infant, values will be low until skin is heated; approximately 15 minutes required to stabilize.	Use $TcPo_2$ to monitor trends of oxygenation with routine nursing care procedures. Clean electrode surface to remove electrolyte deposits; change solution and membrane once a week. Allow machine to stabilize before drawing arterial gases; note reading when gases are drawn, and use values to correlate. Ensure airtight seal between skin surface and electrode; place electrodes on clean, dry skin on upper chest, abdomen, or inner aspect of thigh; avoid bony prominences.
	Second-degree burns are rare but can occur if electrodes remain in place too long. Decreased correlations noted with older infants (related to skin thickness); with infants with low cardiac output (decreased skin perfusion); and with hyperoxic infants.	Change skin site and recalibrate at least every 4 hours; inspect skin for burns; if burns occur, use lowest temperature setting and change position of electrode more frequently.
	The adhesive that attaches the electrode may abrade the fragile skin of the preterm infant. May be used for both preductal and postductal monitoring of oxygenation for observations of shunting.	Adhesive disks may be cut to a smaller size, or skin prep may be used under the adhesive circle only; allow membrane to touch skin surface at center.

of distress (generalized cyanosis, tachypnea, and severe retractions). An overdistended, barrel-shaped chest with increased anteroposterior diameter is common. Auscultation reveals diminished air movement with prominent rales and rhonchi. Abdominal palpation may reveal a displaced liver caused by diaphragmatic depression resulting from the overexpansion of the lungs. Yellowish/pale green staining of the skin, nails, and umbilical cord is usually present.

The chest x-ray film for newborns with MAS reveals nonuniform, coarse, patchy densities and hyperinflation (9- to 11-rib expansion) (Carey & Trotter, 2000). Evidence of pulmonary air leak is frequently present. These infants have serious biochemical alterations, which include (1) extreme metabolic acidosis resulting from the cardiopulmonary shunting and hypoperfusion; (2) extreme respiratory acidosis due to shunting and alveolar hypoventilation; and (3) extreme hypoxia, even in 100% O_2 concentrations and with ventilatory assistance. The extreme hypoxia is also caused by the cardiopulmonary shunting and resultant failure to oxygenate and can lead to *persistent pulmonary hypertension of the newborn (PPHN)*, discussed shortly.

CLINICAL THERAPY

The combined efforts of the maternity and pediatric teams are needed to prevent MAS. The most effective form of preventive management is outlined as follows:

1. After the head of the newborn is born and the shoulders and chest are still in the birth canal, the baby's oropharynx and then the nasopharynx are suctioned by the birth attendant with use of a DeLee attached to wall suction. (The same procedure is followed with a cesarean birth.) To decrease the possibility of HIV transmission, low-pressure wall suction is used.
2. If the infant is vigorous even if there is thick or thin meconium in the amniotic fluid, no subsequent special resuscitation is indicated (Wiswell, Gannon, Jacob, et al, 2000).
3. If the infant has absent or depressed respirations, heart rate less than 100 beats per minute, or poor muscle tone, direct tracheal suctioning is recommended. The glottis is visualized with a laryngoscope and the trachea suctioned (Weber, 2000; Wiswell et al, 2000).

If the newborn's head is not adequately suctioned on the perineum (at the time the head is born but the shoulder and chest are still in the vagina), respiratory or resuscitative efforts will push meconium into the airway and into the lungs. Stimulation of the newborn should be avoided to minimize respiratory movements. Further resuscitative efforts are undertaken as indicated, following the same principles mentioned in clinical/medical therapy for asphyxia earlier in this chapter. Resuscitated newborns should be immediately transferred to the nursery for closer observation. An umbilical arterial line may be used for direct monitoring of arterial blood pressures; blood sampling for pH and blood gases; and infusion of intravenous fluids, blood, or medications.

Treatment usually involves delivery of high oxygen concentrations and high-pressure ventilation. Low positive end-expiratory pressures (PEEP) are preferred to avoid air leaks such as pneumothorax. Unfortunately, high pressures may be needed to cause sufficient expiratory expansion of the obstructed terminal airways or to stabilize airways that are weakened by inflammation so that the most distal atelectatic alveoli are ventilated.

Surfactant replacement therapy is most effective when given as a prophylactic measure. It improves oxygenation and decreases the incidence of air leaks (Dargaville, South, & McDougall, 2001). Systemic blood pressure and pulmonary blood flow must be maintained. Dopamine or dobutamine and/or volume expanders may be used to maintain systemic blood pressure.

Newborns over 2 kg with respiratory failure who are not responding to conventional ventilator therapy may require treatment with high-frequency ventilation and/or nitric oxide therapy or ECMO (Blackburn, 2003). ECMO has proven successful for newborns with meconium aspiration, pneumonia, and PPHN who are not responding to traditional treatment modalities.

Treatment also includes chest physiotherapy (chest percussion, vibration, and drainage) to remove the debris. Prophylactic antibiotics are frequently given. Bicarbonate to correct metabolic acidosis may be necessary for several days for severely ill newborns. Mortality in term or postterm infants is very high because the cycle of hypoxemia and acidemia is difficult to break.

NURSING CARE MANAGEMENT

Nursing Assessment and Diagnosis

During the intrapartal period, the nurse should observe for signs of fetal hypoxia and meconium staining of amniotic fluid. At birth, the nurse assesses the newborn for signs of distress. During the ongoing assessment of the newborn, the nurse carefully observes for complications such as pulmonary air leaks; anoxic cerebral injury manifested by convulsions; myocardial injury evidenced by congestive heart failure or cardiomegaly; disseminated intravascular coagulation (DIC) resulting from hypoxic hepatic damage with depression of liver-dependent clotting factors; anoxic renal damage demonstrated by hematuria, oliguria, or anuria; fluid overload; sepsis secondary to bacterial pneumonia; and any signs of intestinal necrosis from ischemia, including gastrointestinal obstruction or hemorrhage.

Nursing diagnoses that may apply to the newborn with meconium aspiration syndrome and the infants' parents include the following:

- ***Ineffective Gas Exchange*** related to aspiration of meconium and amniotic fluid during birth
- ***Altered Nutrition: Less than Body Requirements*** related to respiratory distress and increased energy requirements
- ***Ineffective Family Coping: Compromised*** related to life-threatening illness in a term newborn

Nursing Plan and Implementation

Hospital-Based Nursing Care

Initial interventions are aimed primarily at preventing the aspiration by assisting with the removal of the meconium from the infant's oropharynx and nasopharynx prior to the first extrauterine breath.

When significant aspiration occurs, therapy is supportive with the primary goals of maintaining appropriate gas exchange and minimizing complications. Nursing interventions after resuscitation should include maintaining adequate oxygenation and ventilation, regulating temperature, performing glucose testing by glucometer at 2 hours of age to check for hypoglycemia, observing intravenous fluids, calculating necessary fluids (which may be restricted in the first 48 to 72 hours because of cerebral edema), providing caloric requirements, and monitoring intravenous antibiotic administration.

Evaluation

Expected outcomes of nursing care include the following:

- The risk of MAS is promptly identified, and early intervention is initiated.
- The newborn is free of respiratory distress and metabolic alterations.
- The parents verbalize their concerns about their baby's health problem and survival and understand the rationale behind management of their newborn.

Persistent Pulmonary Hypertension of the Newborn

Persistent pulmonary hypertension of the newborn (PPHN) is a serious disorder that may affect 10,000 near-term, term, or postterm newborns in the United States annually. There is a fivefold increase in the incidence of PPHN in infants born by elective cesarean over those born vaginally (Levine, Ghai, Barton, et al, 2001). PPHN has also been called *persistent fetal circulation (PFC)* because the problems that occur are a result of right-to-left (R-L) shunting of blood away from the lungs and through the fetal ductus arteriosus and patent foramen ovale (Clark, Kueser, Walker, et al, 2000).

PPHN has been associated with several events causing hypoxemia and acidosis: postmaturity syndrome, RDS, MAS, intrapartal asphyxia, pneumonia, group B streptococcal sepsis, and diaphragmatic hernia. Many fetuses have problems that compromise fetal oxygenation prior to the onset of labor.

Depending on the cause, PPHN is classified as primary or secondary. Primary disease results from pulmonary vascular changes prior to birth, which cause abnormally high pulmonary vascular resistance (PVR). Secondary PPHN occurs when the initial sequences of respiration and change in circulation after birth are interrupted by events that increase the PVR. Hypoxemia and acidosis are the most potent stimulants of pulmonary vasoconstriction. The increased vascular resistance increases pulmonary artery pressure, hypoxemia, and R-L shunting of pulmonary blood across fetal shunts. Once this process has begun, it is self-perpetuating and difficult to interrupt. Clinical deterioration is rapid.

CLINICAL THERAPY

The first goal of medical management is early diagnosis of this disorder to halt the progressive worsening of the R-L shunt. Certain diagnostic tests are often used to evaluate the increased PVR and shunting. Simultaneous preductal and postductal blood gases or pulse oximetry and/or transcutaneous monitoring can be used to demonstrate ductal shunting. The hyperoxia-hyperventilation test is the most definitive test for PPHN. A positive indication of PPHN is when the prehypertension PaO_2 is less than 50 mm Hg and rises to greater than 100 mm Hg with hyperoxia and hyperventilation. The improved oxygenation can be noted clinically if the infant's mucous membranes turn pink. Echocardiography (bubble echo) can demonstrate R-L shunting and a prolonged ratio of right ventricular ejection period to right ventricular ejection time in infants with PPHN.

The goal of therapeutic intervention is to lower the PVR and reverse the process of shunting. This can be accomplished with the use of nitric oxide, which is a selective pulmonary vasodilator, when other methods fail (Clark et al, 2000). Maintaining tissue oxygenation in the presence of R-L shunting presents the greatest therapeutic challenge but is essential to minimize complications. With PPHN, oxygen acts as a potent vasodilator and these babies are very labile so it is important to be careful in weaning them from oxygen.

Ventilatory management is undertaken to decrease the PVR and increase oxygenation. Hyperventilation to achieve respiratory alkalosis (pH 7.55) will cause pulmonary vasodilatation, which increases oxygenation. Sodium bicarbonate infusions may be required to induce alkalosis. To prevent respiratory interference and achieve hypocarbia, most infants require paralysis with a neuromuscular blocking agent such as fentanyl. Either respiratory or metabolic alkalosis may decrease pulmonary vascular resistance.

If alkalosis alone does not lead to a decrease in the PVR, pharmacologic vasodilators may be given to decrease pulmonary vascular resistance. In the presence of systemic hypotension, volume expanders such as isotonic crystalloids, albumin, plasma, or packed red cells should be administered. Infusion of vasopressors (such as dopamine, dobutamine, or isoproterenol) and/or afterload reducers (nitroprusside) are also advocated. Vasopressors increase the systemic vascular resistance, thereby decreasing the amount of R-L shunting, which increases cardiac output.

Oxygenation, ventilation, and drug therapy efforts continue until the PaO_2 can be consistently maintained greater than 100 mm Hg. Alkalosis and hyperoxia may have to be maintained for several days to avoid a sudden return of hypoxemia and increased PVR. Inhaled nitric oxide and high frequency or oscillatory jet ventilation are also used.

NURSING CARE MANAGEMENT

The nurse assesses for the onset of symptoms, which usually occur in the first 12 to 24 hours of life. Affected newborns exhibit signs of respiratory distress (grunting, nasal flaring, tachypnea), with increased anteroposterior diameter and cyanosis. They typically fail to respond to conventional methods of oxygenation and ventilation. Significant unexplained hypoxemia exists in the absence of congenital heart disease. The chest radiograph might show no evidence of pulmonary parenchymal disease (depending on the underlying disease). The hypoxemia and cyanosis associated with PPHN are characteristic of extreme changeability. Marked, rapid changes in PaO_2 and color are seen with agitation, stimulation, therapeutic intervention (suctioning), or rapid changes in ambient oxygen.

Infants with PPHN are critically ill and require experienced, highly skilled nurses to provide optimal care with minimal manipulation. Any disturbance may cause agitation, which leads to hypoxemia. If a paralyzing agent is used, nursing care includes monitoring the newborn's response to artificial oxygenation and mechanical ventilation. The nurse ensures that the oxygen is delivered in correct amounts and route and records the percentage of oxygen flow. The ventilator settings are checked frequently and recorded every 1 to 2 hours. The nurse carefully suctions the endotracheal tube only as necessary while assessing the effect of the procedure on the baby's oxygenation and perfusion. The amount and type of secretions are noted. The nurse carefully assesses arterial blood gases and notifies the clinician if the results are out of the acceptable range. Oxygen monitoring is essential for identifying activities that may compromise the infant's status. (Nursing interventions required for noninvasive oxygen monitoring are discussed in Table 33–2.) Continuous monitoring of vital signs and blood pressure is required, and careful inspection of the skin during positioning is necessary to avoid pressure necrosis.

Pharmacologic vasodilation may lead to precipitous central hypotension, which must be quickly identified and corrected. If tolazoline therapy is used, the infant is monitored for other side effects, such as increased gastric secretion, gastrointestinal bleeding, and oliguria.

Aggressive ventilation poses a potential risk for pneumothorax. The nurse can best prevent complications by advanced preparation and close monitoring for signs of compromise. (See Pneumothorax later in this chapter for appropriate nursing interventions.)

Many infants suffering PPHN are born at or near term at a time when parents least expect problems—especially life-threatening problems—to occur. The magnitude of the infant's illness and the rapid deterioration may be overwhelming to parents. The nurse should assess their level of understanding and assist them by providing information about their baby's condition and therapies in easily understandable terms.

Attachment becomes difficult when the infant responds poorly to touching (as seen by decreased PaO_2). Instead, the nurse can encourage parents to talk very softly to their infant because this will usually not compromise the baby's condition. Continuity of nursing care is helpful because it will be less threatening for the parents to relate to a smaller group of nurses.

Expected outcomes of nursing care include the following:

- The risks for development of persistent pulmonary hypertension of the newborn (PPHN) are identified early, and immediate action is taken to minimize the development of sudden, severe illness.
- The newborn is free of respiratory distress and establishes effective respiratory function.
- The parents verbalize their concerns about their baby's illness and understand the rationale behind the management of their newborn.

Care of the Newborn with Complications Due to Respiratory Therapy

Oxygen and mechanical ventilation, although required as therapeutic interventions to reduce hypoxia, hypercarbia, ischemia, and infarction to vital organs, may also have harmful effects. The concentrations of ambient oxygen administered to the newborn must be titrated according to oxygen tension within arterial blood to avoid development of retinopathy of prematurity or bronchopulmonary dysplasia/chronic lung disease. In addition, pulmonary air leaks occur in approximately 15% of mechanically ventilated newborns; however, air leaks can be a consequence of injury due to the disease rather than the mechanical ventilation.

Pulmonary Interstitial Emphysema

Pulmonary interstitial emphysema (PIE) is the accumulation of air in lung tissues. It may be unilateral or bilateral. Extra-alveolar air collections are most common with use of positive pressure ventilation. Air collections outside the lung are a function of lung compliance and use of increased pressures to ventilate. Overdistention of alveoli may progress to PIE when rupture occurs and air escapes into the interstitial spaces. Air moves along perivascular spaces but not into the pleural space or mediastinum. As the air collections increase, blood vessels are constricted, and blood gas exchange is impaired. The air does not decrease on expiration. This condition is highly associated with subsequent bronchopulmonary dysplasia (BPD). It may also precede pneumothorax or pneumomediastinum.

Pneumothorax

Pneumothorax, a common complication of respiratory therapy, is an accumulation of air in the thoracic cavity between the parietal and visceral pleura. Pneumothorax occurs when alveoli are overdistended, usually by excessive intra-alveolar pressure and rupture; air then leaks into the thoracic cavity.

Pneumothorax in the newborn causes several physiologic changes: collapse of the lung, compression of the heart and lungs, compromise of venous return to the right heart with mediastinal air, and development of tension in the pleural space. Symptoms of pneumothorax include a sudden, unexplained deterioration in the newborn's condition; decreased breath sounds; apnea; bradycardia; cyanosis; increased oxygen requirements; higher PCO_2; decrease in pH; mottled, asymmetric chest expansion; decreased arterial blood pressure; shocklike appearance; and a shift in the apical cardiac impulses to the side opposite the pneumothorax.

Transillumination of the chest is used for rapid evaluation of pneumothorax. Transillumination is the visualization of light through the air in the affected side (or sides, for bilateral pneumothorax) of the baby's chest. However, x-ray examination is the main method of diagnosing this complication (Figure 33–9 •).

Pneumothorax is a life-threatening situation for the newborn and demands immediate removal of the accumulated air. The thoracentesis procedure is done only as an emergency measure and carries a risk of damaging the lung pleura with needle tracks as the air is evacuated and the collapsed lung reexpands. Only skilled and specifically trained personnel should perform this procedure. For complete resolution of the pneumothorax, a chest tube may be inserted.

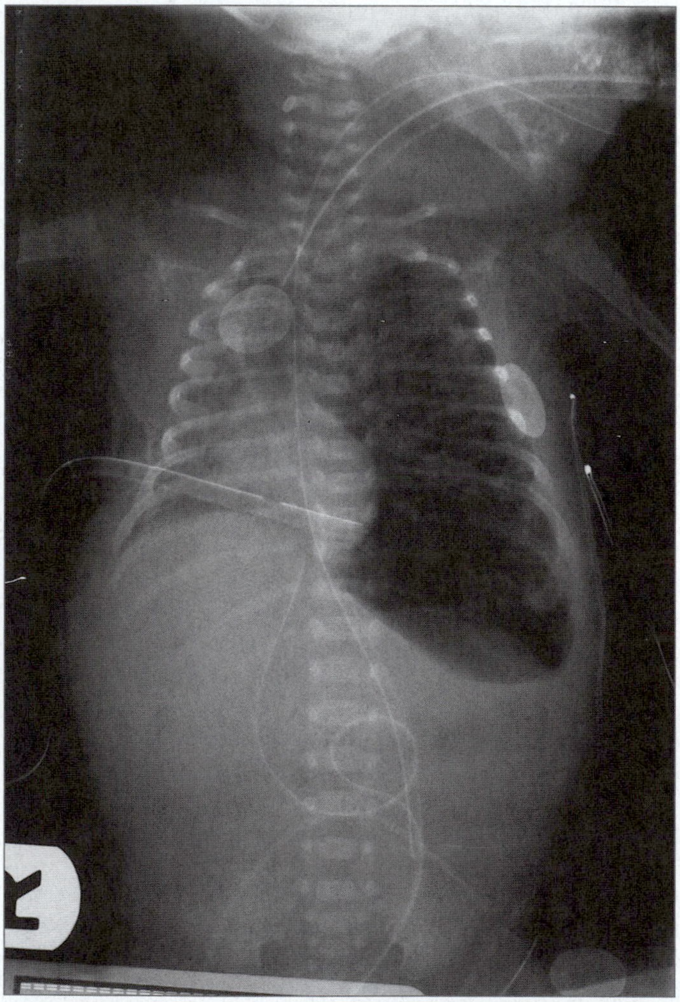

Figure 33–9 • Chest x-ray of a left-sided pneumothorax. A rupture of the alveolic sacs allows air to leak through the pleura forming collections of air outside the lung (air shows on x-ray as dark area over lung).
SOURCE: Courtesy of Carol Harrigan, RNC, MSN, NNP.

Bronchopulmonary Dysplasia/Chronic Lung Disease

Bronchopulmonary dysplasia (BPD), also known as **chronic lung disease of prematurity (CLD),** most commonly occurs in very compromised low-birth-weight (LBW) infants who require oxygen therapy and assisted mechanical ventilation for the treatment of respiratory distress syndrome. It has also been associated with neonatal pneumonia, MAS, PPHN, congenital heart disease (patent ductus arteriosus), other congenital anomalies requiring high levels of ventilatory support, and low-grade or asymptomatic pulmonary infection with *Ureaplasma urealyticum*. The cause is multifactorial. The process of BPD is one of continuous lung tissue injury and repair, delaying both lung and body growth.

CLINICAL THERAPY

The goals of therapeutic intervention for the newborn with BPD are to provide adequate oxygenation and ventilation, prevent further lung damage, promote optimal nutrition, and give supportive care to ensure adequate rates of growth and development. New therapies, such as exogenous surfactant administration, high-frequency ventilation, and steroids (prenatal and postnatal) have altered the severity of BPD, but chronic lung disease remains a major clinical problem. A low vitamin A level in infants weighing less than 750 g is postulated to increase the risk for development of chronic lung disease (Atkinson, 2001; Shenai, Mellen, & Chytil, 2000). Because of the chronic nature of BPD, therapeutic intervention must be individualized to meet the specific needs of the infant. Diuretics and fluid restriction are frequently used to control pulmonary fluid retention and to improve lung function; electrolyte supplements are necessary to offset the results of chronic diuretic therapy (Hagedorn et al, 2002). In addition, bronchodilators are indicated to decrease airway resistance and to control bronchospasm. The infant with chronic lung disease is often on long-term steroids. Serial echocardiography is used to monitor cardiac response to the chronic pulmonary disease.

NURSING CARE MANAGEMENT

Hospital-Based Nursing Care

The nurse observes carefully any changes in the newborn's oxygenation, giving special attention to maintaining the prescribed oxygen concentration during all activities, especially during periods of stress, such as when the infant is crying; when blood is drawn; while starting an IV infusion; and during a lumbar puncture (LP), suctioning, chest physiotherapy (CPT), and feeding (Figure 33–10 •).

The current goal is to adjust the level of supplemental oxygen to consistently keep O_2 saturations between 90% and 95%, depending on the presence of associated clinical problems such as poor growth, recurrent bradycardia, and pulmonary hypertension. The nurse obtains blood gases based on the institution's chronic blood gas protocol—for example, every 3 days, 20 minutes after a permanent change in ambient oxygen concentration (FiO_2), or more frequently if the infant experiences increasing respiratory distress or increasing lethargy.

Postural drainage, CPT, and vibration followed by suctioning are carried out with close attention to the baby's tolerance. It is essential to time the care activities with rest periods to avoid fatiguing the infant. The nurse maintains the infant's body temperature because hypothermia or hyperthermia will increase oxygen consumption and may increase oxygen requirements. Positioning on the abdomen helps the baby maintain higher transcutaneous oxygen saturation ($TcPO_2$) and improved ventilation.

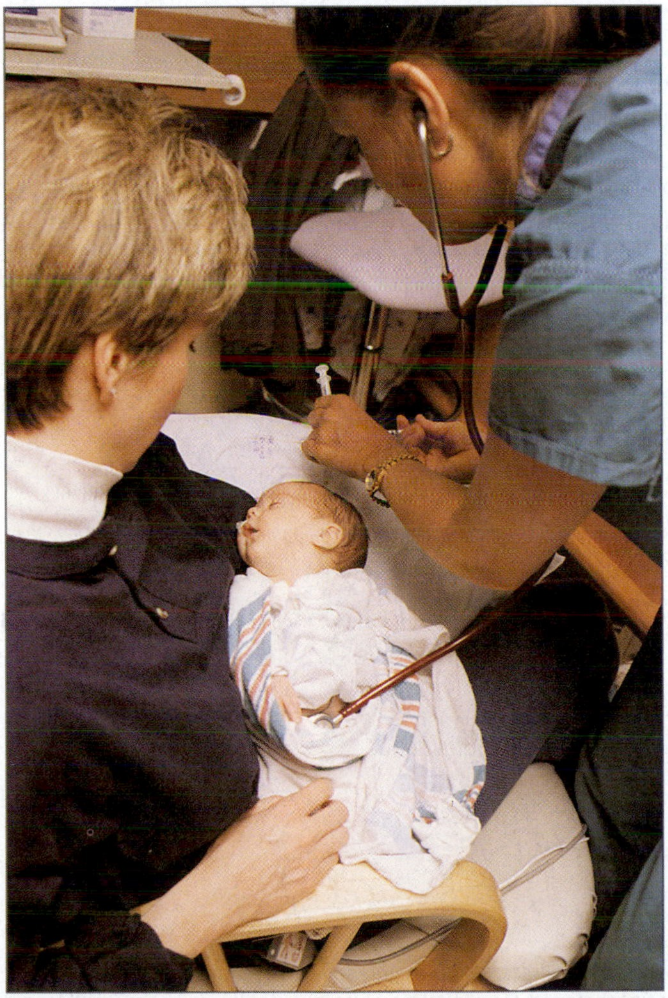

Figure 33–10 • The baby with BPD has ongoing oxygen and nutritional needs as well as the need for gentle individualized care.

Bronchodilators such as theophylline, albuterol, and terbutaline; diuretics; steroids; and electrolyte supplements may be used in the clinical management of the BPD infant (American Academy of Pediatrics & Canadian Pediatric Society, 2002). Appropriate timing of administration is essential to maintain adequate blood levels. Many of the side effects of these drugs, such as hypokalemia and mineral losses (fractures), can be avoided by giving the diuretics every other day.

Providing for adequate nutrition enhances formation of new alveoli and enlargement of the airway diameter. The nurse helps provide adequate nutrition and monitors the newborn's caloric intake and the energy expended during the feeding process. The more severely ill the baby, the higher the caloric need to meet the greater expenditure of energy for survival and healing. As soon as tolerated, a 24 kcal/oz formula for preterm infants is started, especially if the baby is on fluid restriction. More oxygen may be required during feeding, and the least energy-consuming feeding method should be used. If the feeding schedule is too stressful, smaller, more frequent feedings may be initiated (Hagedorn et al, 2002).

Infants with BPD frequently experience negative oral sensations due to suctioning and intubation. These can adversely affect their transition to nipple or spoon feeding. Positioning is often the key to adequate intake and decreasing gastroesophageal reflux (GER). In addition, most infants receive numerous, possibly unpalatable, medications with meals. Attempts must be made to include pleasurable activities such as cuddling at mealtime to develop positive associations with appropriate feeding behaviors. Premature infants with BPD frequently require some type of feeding therapy to help them eat successfully.

Infants with BPD are very susceptible to infection, especially if they are on long-term steroids; therefore, it is important to discourage anyone with early signs of infectious disease from having contact with them. The infant's behavior and vital signs should be monitored for changes that might indicate early developing infection. Changes in color, quantity, or quality of pulmonary secretions are noted and reported. The frequency of CPT and suctioning may need to be increased.

Because BPD infants require prolonged hospitalization and/or home care, the nurse should give special attention to formulating a program of early stimulation activities. Psychomotor delays are seen frequently in these infants and are most likely due in part to prolonged exposure to the hospital environment. Because the illness limits these infants' tolerance level for activity, the nurse must individualize activities for each baby. Families need to be included in the plans for their baby.

Community-Based Nursing Care

When the infant develops BPD and the family becomes aware of the implications of chronic illness and prolonged hospitalization, they may experience despair and find it difficult to cope with this added burden. The nurse can help the family cope by encouraging them to take an active role in their infant's daily activities. Their involvement will help dispel feelings of inadequacy and prepare them to perform the unique tasks necessary to meet their infant's needs.

Parents need to demonstrate their ability to provide all the care their child will require at home before leaving the hospital. This may include feeding, adjusting O_2 support, O_2 saturation monitoring, suctioning and airway management, CPT, bathing, and giving medications. They also need to know when to call the home health nurse who is providing care. Parents should be taught how to assess the infant's respiratory condition and understand the BPD baseline respiratory pattern (frequency of respiration, rhythm, degree of retractions, and color of skin and mucous membranes) (Vaucher, 2001). Finally, parents must be taught to evaluate their infant's tolerance of activities and to recognize signs of distress due to poor oxygenation, inadequate ventilation, infection, fluid retention, and bronchospasm.

Care of the Newborn with Cold Stress

Cold stress is excessive heat loss resulting in the use of compensatory mechanisms (such as increased respirations and nonshivering thermogenesis) to maintain core body temperature. Heat loss that results in cold stress occurs in the newborn through the mechanisms of evaporation, convection, conduction, and radiation. (See Chapter 28 for a detailed discussion of thermoregulation.) Heat loss at birth that leads to cold stress can play a significant role in the severity of respiratory distress syndrome (RDS) and the ultimate outcome for the infant. Both preterm and small-for-agestational-age (SGA) newborns are at increased risk for cold stress because they have decreased adipose tissue, brown fat stores, and glycogen available for metabolism.

The amount of heat lost by an infant depends to a large extent on the actions of the nurse or caregiver. Following the transfer of a neonatal intensive care unit (NICU) newborn from one bed to another, a transient, although not significant, decrease in temperature for up to one hour may be noted.

As discussed in Chapter 28, the newborn's major source of heat production in nonshivering thermogenesis (NST) is brown fat metabolism. The ability of an infant to respond to cold stress by NST is impaired in the presence of several conditions:

- Hypoxemia (PO_2 less than 50 torr)
- Intracranial hemorrhage or any central nervous system (CNS) abnormality
- Hypoglycemia (blood glucose < 40 mg/dL)

When these conditions occur, the infant's temperature should be monitored more closely and the neutral thermal environment conscientiously maintained. It is important for the nurse to recognize these conditions and treat them as soon as possible. The metabolic consequences of cold stress can be devastating and potentially fatal to an infant. Oxygen requirements increase; even prior to noting a change in temperature, glucose use increases; acids are released into the bloodstream; and surfactant production decreases. The effects are graphically depicted in Figure 33–11.

Prevention is especially critical in the very-low-birth-weight (VLBW) infant. Placing the VLBW newborn in a polyethylene wrapping immediately following birth can decrease the postnatal fall in temperature that normally occurs. Both convective and evaporative heat loss can be reduced (Blackburn, 2003).

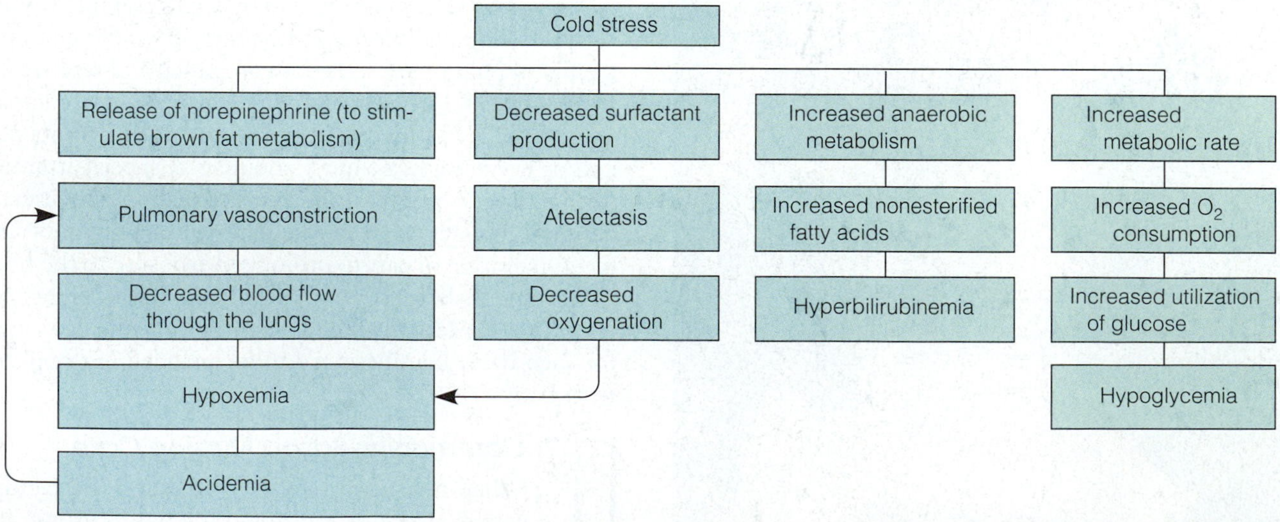

Figure 33–11 • Cold stress chain of events. The hypothermic, or cold-stressed, newborn attempts to compensate by conserving heat and increasing heat production. These physiologic compensatory mechanisms initiate a series of metabolic events that result in hypoxemia and altered surfactant production, metabolic acidosis, hypoglycemia, and hyperbilirubinemia.

NURSING CARE MANAGEMENT

The nurse observes the baby for signs of cold stress. These include increased movements and respirations, decreased skin temperature and peripheral perfusion, development of hypoglycemia, and possibly development of metabolic acidosis.

Skin temperature assessments are used because initial response to cold stress is vasoconstriction, resulting in a decrease in skin temperature. Therefore, monitoring rectal temperature is not satisfactory. A decrease in rectal temperature means that the infant has long-standing cold stress with decompensation in the ability to maintain core body temperature.

If a decrease in skin temperature is noted, the nurse determines whether hypoglycemia is present. Hypoglycemia is a result of the metabolic effects of cold stress and is suggested by glucose strip values below 45 mg/mL, tremors, irritability or lethargy, apnea, or seizure activity.

If hypothermia occurs, the following nursing interventions should be initiated (Blackburn, 2003):

- Keep the ambient air temperature 1C to 1.5C higher than the infant's temperature.
- Warm the newborn slowly, because rapid temperature elevation may cause hypotension and apnea.
- Increase the air temperature in hourly increments of 1C until infant's temperature is stable.
- Monitor skin temperature every 15 to 30 minutes to determine whether the newborn's temperature is increasing.
- Remove plastic wrap, caps, and heat shields while rewarming the infant so that cool air as well as warm air is not trapped.
- Warm intravenous fluids prior to infusion.
- Initiate efforts to block heat loss by evaporation, radiation, convection, and conduction. Maintain the newborn in a neutral thermal environment.

The nurse assesses the presence of anaerobic metabolism and initiates interventions for the resulting metabolic acidosis. Attempts to burn brown fat increase oxygen consumption, lactic acid levels, and metabolic acidosis. Hypoglycemia may be reversed by adequate glucose intake, as described in the following section.

Care of the Newborn with Hypoglycemia

A widely used cutoff point or threshold for intervention in newborn hypoglycemia is a plasma blood glucose concentration of 40 mg/dL (45 mg/dL if symptomatic) (Cowett & Loughead, 2002). Plasma glucose values less than 20 to 25 mg/dL should be treated with parenteral glucose, regardless of the age or gestation. **Hypoglycemia** is the most common metabolic disorder occurring in infants of diabetic mothers (IDM) SGA infants, the smaller of twins, infants born to mothers with preeclampsia, male infants, and preterm AGA infants (Cowett & Loughead, 2002). The pathophysiology of hypoglycemia differs for each classification.

AGA preterm infants have not been in utero a sufficient time to store glycogen and fat. As a result, they have a decreased ability to carry out gluconeogenesis. This situation is further aggravated by increased use of glucose by the tissues (especially the brain and heart) during stress and illness (chilling, asphyxia, sepsis, and respiratory distress syndrome).

Infants of White's classes A through C or type 1 diabetic mothers (women with diagnosed or gestational diabetes) have increased stores of glycogen and fat (see Chapters 19 and 32). Circulating insulin and insulin responsiveness are also higher when compared with other newborns. Because the high glucose loads present in utero stop at birth, the newborn experiences rapid and profound hypoglycemia (Cornblath & Ichord, 2000). The SGA infant has used up glycogen and fat stores because of intrauterine malnutrition and has a blunted hepatic enzymatic response with which to produce and use glucose. Any newborn stressed at birth from asphyxia or cold also quickly uses up available glucose stores and becomes hypoglycemic. Also epidural anesthesia may alter maternal-fetal glucose homeostasis, resulting in hypoglycemia (Kalhan & Parimi, 2002).

Clinical Therapy

The goal of medical management includes early identification of hypoglycemia through observation and screening of newborns at risk (Cornblath & Ichord, 2000). The baby may be asymptomatic, or any of the following may occur:

- Lethargy, jitteriness
- Poor feeding, poor sucking
- Vomiting
- Hypothermia
- Pallor
- Apnea, irregular respirations, respiratory distress, cyanosis
- Hypotonia, possible loss of swallowing reflex
- Tremors, jerkiness, seizure activity
- High-pitched cry
- Exaggerated Moro reflex, coma

Differential diagnosis of a newborn with nonspecific hypoglycemic symptoms includes determining whether the newborn has any of the following:

- CNS disease
- Sepsis

- Metabolic aberrations
- Polycythemia
- Congenital heart disease
- Drug withdrawal
- Temperature instability
- Hypocalcemia

Aggressive treatment is recommended after a single low blood glucose value if the infant shows any of these symptoms. In at-risk infants, routine screening should be done frequently during the first 4 hours of life and then whenever any of the noted clinical manifestations appear or at 4-hour intervals until the risk period has passed.

Hypoglycemia may also be defined as a glucose oxidase reagent strip below 45 mg/dL, but only when corroborated with laboratory blood glucose (see Procedure 33–1: Performing a Heel Stick on a Newborn). Bedside glucose oxidase strip tests can screen for hypoglycemia, but laboratory determinations must confirm the results before a diagnosis of hypoglycemia can be made. Glucose reagent strips should not be used by themselves to screen and diagnose hypoglycemia because their results depend on the baby's hematocrit (they react to the glucose in the plasma, not the red blood cells), and there is a wide variance (5 to 15 mg/dL) when compared to laboratory determinations.

Clinical Tip *Wrapping the foot in a warm washcloth or disposable diaper is a simple way to create adequate vasodilation for taking a blood specimen.*

Blood glucose sampling techniques can significantly affect the accuracy of the blood glucose value. Common bedside methods use whole blood, an enzymatic reagent strip, and a reflectance meter or color chart. It is important to note that whole blood glucose concentrations are 10% to 15% lower than plasma glucose concentration (Kalhan & Parimi, 2002). The higher the hematocrit, the greater the difference between whole blood and plasma values. Also, venous blood glucose concentrations are approximately 15% to 19% lower than arterial blood glucose concentrations because the tissues extract some glucose before the blood enters the venous system ("Neonatal Hypoglycemia," 2000). Newer techniques, such as using a glucose oxidase analyzer or an optical bedside glucose analyzer, are more reliable for bedside screening but must also be validated with laboratory chemical analysis.

Clinical Tip *Blood samples for the laboratory should be placed on ice and analyzed within 30 minutes of drawing to prevent the red blood cells from continuing to metabolize glucose.*

Adequate caloric intake is important. Early breastfeeding or formula-feeding is one of the major preventive approaches. If early feeding or intravenous glucose is started to meet the recommended fluid and caloric needs, the blood glucose is likely to remain above the hypoglycemic level. During the first hours after birth, asymptomatic newborns may be given oral glucose, and then another plasma glucose measurement is obtained within 30 to 60 minutes after feeding. Intravenous infusions of a dextrose solution (5% to 10%) begun immediately after birth should prevent hypoglycemia. Plasma glucose levels are obtained when the parenteral infusion is started. However, in the very small AGA infant, infusions of 10% dextrose solution may cause hyperglycemia to develop, requiring an alteration in the glucose concentration (Cornblath & Ichord, 2000). Infants require 6 to 8 mg/kg/min of glucose to maintain normal glucose concentrations. Therefore an intravenous glucose solution should be calculated based on body weight of the infant and fluid requirements and correlated with blood glucose tests to determine adequacy of the infusion treatment.

A rapid infusion of 25% to 50% dextrose is contraindicated because it may lead to profound rebound hypoglycemia following an initial brief increase. In more severe cases of hypoglycemia, corticosteroids may be administered. It is thought that steroids enhance gluconeogenesis from noncarbohydrate protein sources (Kalhan & Parimi, 2002).

CT and MRI scans reveal generalized occipital lobe cortical thinning in the newborn suffering from hypoglycemia (Kinnala, Korvenranta, & Parkkola, 2000). The prognosis for untreated hypoglycemia is therefore poor. The untreated hypoglycemia may result in permanent, untreatable, CNS damage or death.

NURSING CARE MANAGEMENT

Nursing Assessment and Diagnosis

The objective of nursing assessment is to identify newborns at risk and to screen symptomatic infants. For newborns who are diagnosed with hypoglycemia, assessment is ongoing with careful monitoring of glucose values. Glucose strips, urine dipsticks, and urine volume (monitor only if above 1 to 3 mL/kg/hr) are evaluated frequently for osmotic diuresis and glycosuria.

Nursing diagnoses that may apply to the newborn with hypoglycemia include the following:

- ***Altered Nutrition: Less than Body Requirements*** related to increased glucose use secondary to physiologic stress
- ***Ineffective Breathing Pattern*** related to tachypnea and apnea
- ***Acute Pain*** related to frequent heel sticks for glucose monitoring

Procedure 33-1 Performing a Heel Stick on a Newborn

Preparation

1. Explain to parents what will be done.
2. Select a clear, previously unpunctured site.
   Rationale: The selection of a previously unpunctured site minimizes the risk of infection and excessive scar formation.
3. The infant's lateral heel is the site of choice because it precludes damaging the posterior tibial nerve and artery, plantar artery, and the important longitudinally oriented fat pad of the heel, which in later years could impede walking (Figure 33–12 •). This is especially important for infants undergoing multiple heel stick procedures. Toes are acceptable sites if necessary.

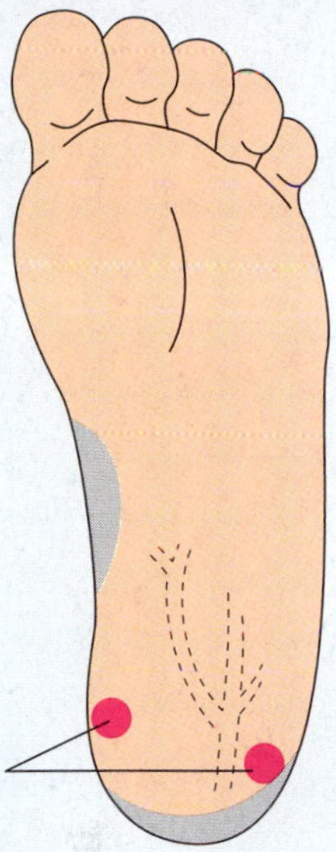

Figure 33–12 • Potential sites for heel sticks. Avoid shaded areas in order to avoid injury to arteries and nerves in the foot.

Equipment and Supplies

- Microlancet (do not use a needle)
- Alcohol swabs
- 2 × 2 sterile gauze squares
- Small bandage
- Transfer pipette or capillary tubes
- Glucose reagent strips or reflectance meters
- Gloves

Rationale: A needle may nick the periosteum. Gloves are used to implement standard precautions and prevent nosocomial infections.

Procedure: Clean Gloves

1. Apply gloves.
2. Use a warm wet wrap or specially designed chemical heat pad to warm the infant's heel for 5 to 10 seconds to facilitate blood flow.

Performing the Heel Stick

1. Grasp the infant's lower leg and foot so as to impede venous return slightly. This will facilitate extraction of the blood sample (Figure 33–13 •).
2. Clean the site by rubbing vigorously with 70% isopropyl alcohol swab.
   Rationale: Friction produces local heat, which aids vasodilation.

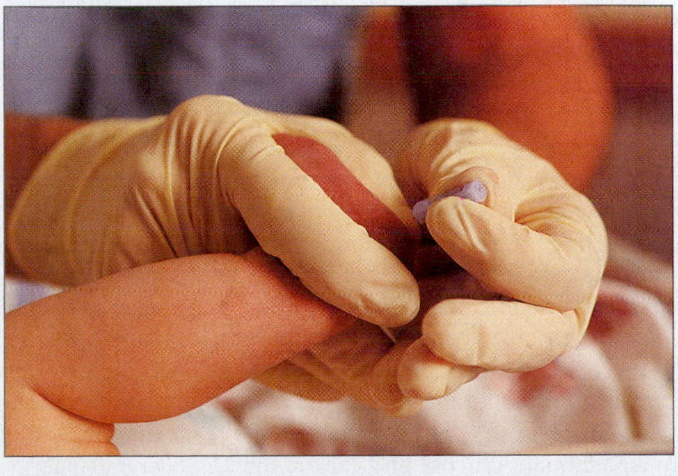

Figure 33–13 • Heel stick.

(continued on next page)

Procedure 33–1 Performing a Heel Stick on a Newborn *(continued)*

3. Blot the site dry completely with dry gauze square before lancing.
   Rationale: Alcohol is irritating to injured tissue and it may also produce hemolysis.
4. With a quick, piercing motion, puncture the lateral heel with a microlancet. Be careful not to puncture too deeply. Optimal penetration is 4 mm.
5. Wipe the first drop of blood away with the gauze.
   Rationale: The first drop may be contaminated by skin contact and the blood cells may have been traumatized during the stick.

Collecting the Blood Sample

1. Use transfer pipette to place drop of blood on glucose reflectance meter.
2. Use capillary tube for hematocrit testing.

Prevent Excessive Bleeding

1. Apply a folded gauze square to the puncture site and secure it firmly with a bandage.
2. Check the puncture site frequently for the first hour after sampling.

Record the Findings on the Infant's Chart.

Nursing Plan and Implementation

The nurse should monitor blood glucose levels in at-risk groups no later than 2 hours after birth and before feedings or whenever there are abnormal signs (Cornblath & Ichord, 2000). Monitor the IDM within 30 minutes of birth. Once an at-risk infant's blood sugar level is stable, glucose testing every 2 to 4 hours (or per agency protocol), or prior to feedings, adequately monitors glucose levels (Cornblath & Ichord, 2000). See Procedure 33–1: Performing a Heel Stick on a Newborn. The infant's lateral heel is the preferred site for the glucose sample, so that the posterior tibial nerve and artery and the important longitudinally oriented fat pad of the heel will not be damaged.

Calculating glucose requirements and maintaining intravenous glucose will be necessary for any symptomatic infant with low serum glucose levels. Careful attention to glucose monitoring is again required when the transition from intravenous to oral feedings is attempted. Titration of intravenous glucose may be required until the infant is able to take adequate amounts of formula or breast milk to maintain a normal blood sugar level. This titration is accomplished by decreasing the concentration of parenteral glucose gradually to 5%, then reducing the rate of infusion to 6 mg/kg/min, then to 4 mg/kg/min, and slowly discontinuing it over 4 to 6 hours. Enteral feeds are increased to maintain an adequate glucose and caloric intake (Cornblath & Ichord, 2000).

Complementary and Alternative Therapies

Pain Relief in the NICU

Oral administration of *sucrose for pain management* from procedural pain (heel sticks, venipuncture, IM injections, oral suctioning, etc.) has been introduced in the NICU. The sweetness of the sucrose, a disaccharide, elevates the pain threshold through endogenous opioid release in the central nervous system (Noerr, 2001). A range of 0.5 to 2 mL of 24% sucrose is administered on the anterior part of the tongue via a syringe or nipple approximately 2 minutes prior to the procedure (Noerr, 2001). Care must be taken, however, with repeated doses of sucrose, as the concern for hyperglycemia may arise.

The method of feeding greatly influences glucose and energy requirements. In addition, the therapeutic nursing measure of nonnutritive sucking during gavage feedings has been reported to increase the baby's daily weight gain and lead to earlier formula-feeding or breastfeeding and discharge. Nonnutritive sucking may also lower activity levels, which allows newborns to conserve their energy stores. Activity can increase energy requirements; crying alone can double the baby's metabolic rate. Establishment and maintenance of a neutral thermal environment has a potent influence on the newborn's metabolism. The nurse pays careful attention to environmental conditions, physical activity, and organization of care and integrates these factors into nursing care. The nurse identifies any discrepancies between the baby's caloric requirements and received calories and weighs the newborn daily at consistent times, preferably before a feeding. Only then can findings of unusual weight losses or gains, as well as the pattern of weight gain, be considered reliable.

Evaluation

Expected outcomes of nursing care include the following:

- The risk of hypoglycemia is promptly identified, and intervention is started early.
- The newborn's metabolic and physiologic processes are stabilized; recovery proceeds without sequelae.

Care of the Newborn with Jaundice

The most common abnormal physical finding in newborns is **jaundice** (*icterus neonatorum*). Jaundice develops from the deposit of yellow pigment bilirubin in lipid tissues, as described in Chapter 28. Fetal unconjugated bilirubin is normally cleared by the placenta in utero, so total bilirubin at birth is usually less than 3 mg/dL unless an abnormal hemolytic process has been present. Postnatally, the infant must conjugate bilirubin (convert a lipid-soluble pigment into a water-soluble pigment) in the liver.

The rate and amount of conjugation of bilirubin depend on the rate of hemolysis, the bilirubin load, the maturity of the liver, and the presence of albumin-binding sites. See Chapter 28 for discussion of conjugation of bilirubin. A normal, healthy, full-term infant's liver is usually mature enough and produces enough glucuronyl transferase that the total serum bilirubin concentration does not reach a pathologic level. However, physiologic jaundice remains a common problem for the term newborn and may require treatment with phototherapy. It is typically due to the newborn's increased red cell mass, shorter red cell lifespan, slower uptake by the liver, lack of intestinal bacteria, and/or poorly established hydration.

Pathophysiology

Serum albumin-binding sites are usually sufficient to meet the normal demands. However, certain conditions tend to decrease the number or quality of available binding sites. Fetal or neonatal asphyxia decreases the binding affinity of bilirubin to albumin, as acidosis impairs the capacity of albumin to hold bilirubin. Hypothermia and hypoglycemia release free fatty acids that dislocate bilirubin from albumin. Neonatal medications such as indomethacin also decrease albumin binding. Maternal medications such as sulfa drugs and salicylates compete with bilirubin for these sites. Finally, premature infants have less albumin available for binding with bilirubin.

Neurotoxicity is possible because unconjugated bilirubin has a high affinity for extravascular tissue, including subcutaneous fatty tissue and the tissues of the brain. Bilirubin not bound to albumin is free to cross the blood-brain barrier, damage cells of the CNS, and produce kernicterus or bilirubin encephalopathy (Porter & Dennis, 2002). *Kernicterus* (meaning "yellow nucleus") usually refers to the deposition of unconjugated bilirubin in the basal ganglia of the brain and to permanent neurologic sequelae of untreated hyperbilirubinemia. The classic bilirubin encephalopathy of kernicterus most commonly found with Rh and ABO blood group incompatibility is less common today because of aggressive treatment with phototherapy and exchange transfusions. But cases of kernicterus are reappearing as a result of early discharge and the increased incidence of dehydration (a result of discharge before mother's milk is established). Current therapy can reduce the incidence of kernicterus encephalopathy but cannot distinguish all infants who are at risk.

Causes of Hyperbilirubinemia

A primary cause of pathologic **hyperbilirubinemia** is **hemolytic disease of the newborn** secondary to Rh incompatibility. All pregnant women who are Rh negative or who have blood type O (possible ABO incompatibility) should be asked about outcomes of any previous pregnancies, including abortions, and their history of blood transfusion. Prenatal amniocentesis with spectrophotographic examination may be indicated in some cases. Cord blood from newborns is evaluated for bilirubin level, which normally does not exceed 5 mg/dL. Newborns of Rh-negative and O blood type mothers are carefully assessed for blood type status, appearance of jaundice, and levels of serum bilirubin.

Isoimmune hemolytic disease, also known as **erythroblastosis fetalis,** occurs when an Rh-negative mother is pregnant with an Rh-positive fetus and transplacental passage of maternal antibodies takes place. Maternal antibodies enter the fetal circulation, then attach to and destroy the fetal red blood cells. The fetal system responds by increasing red blood cell production. Jaundice, anemia, and compensatory erythropoiesis result. A marked increase in immature red blood cells (erythroblasts) also occurs, hence the designation erythroblastosis fetalis. Because of the widespread use of Rh immune globulin (Rho GAM), the incidence of erythroblastosis fetalis has dropped dramatically.

Hydrops fetalis, the most severe form of erythroblastosis fetalis, causes multiple organ system failure. Cardiomegaly with severe cardiac decompensation and hepatosplenomegaly occur. Severe generalized massive edema (anasarca) and generalized fluid effusion into the pleural cavity (hydrothorax), pericardial sac, and peritoneal cavity (ascites) develop. Jaundice is not present until the newborn period because the bilirubin pigments for the fetus are being excreted through the placenta into the maternal circulation. The hydropic hemolytic disease process is also characterized by hyperplasia of the adrenal cortex and pancreatic islets, which predisposes the infant to neonatal hypoglycemia similar to that of IDMs. These infants also have increased bleeding tendencies due to associated thrombocytopenia and hypoxic damage to the capillaries. Hydrops is a frequent cause of intrauterine death among infants with Rh disease.

ABO incompatibility (the mother is blood type O and the baby is blood type A or B) may result in jaundice, although it rarely results in hemolytic disease severe enough to be clinically diagnosed and treated. Hepatosplenomegaly may be found occasionally in newborns with ABO incompatibility, but hydrops fetalis and stillbirth are rare.

Certain prenatal and perinatal factors predispose the newborn to hyperbilirubinemia. During pregnancy, maternal conditions that predispose to neonatal hyperbilirubinemia include hereditary spherocytosis, diabetes, intrauterine infections, gram-negative bacilli infections that stimulate production of maternal isoimmune antibodies, drug ingestion (such as sulfas, salicylates, novobiocin, and diazepam), and oxytocin.

In addition to Rh or ABO incompatibility, other newborn conditions predispose to hyperbilirubinemia: polycythemia (central hematocrit 65% or more), pyloric stenosis, obstruction or atresia of the biliary duct or of the lower bowel, low-grade urinary tract infection, sepsis, hypothyroidism, enclosed hemorrhage (cephalhematoma, extensive bruising), asphyxia neonatorum, hypothermia, acidemia, and hypoglycemia. Neonatal hepatitis, atresia of the bile ducts, and gastrointestinal atresia all can alter bilirubin metabolism and excretion.

The prognosis for a newborn with hyperbilirubinemia depends on the extent of the hemolytic process and the underlying cause. Severe hemolytic disease may result in fetal or early neonatal death from the effects of anemia—cardiac decompensation, edema, ascites, and hydrothorax. The neurologic damage of kernicterus may be responsible for cerebral palsy, mental retardation, sensory difficulties, or, to a lesser degree, perceptual impairment, delayed speech development, hyperactivity, muscle incoordination, or learning difficulties.

Clinical Therapy

The best treatment for hemolytic disease is prevention. Prenatal identification of the fetus at risk for Rh or ABO incompatibility will allow prompt treatment. See Chapter 20 for discussion of in utero management of this condition.

When one or more of the predisposing factors are present, the maternal and neonatal blood types should be tested in the laboratory for Rh or ABO incompatibility. Other necessary laboratory evaluations include Coombs' test, serum bilirubin levels (direct and total), hemoglobin, reticulocyte percentage, white blood cell count, and positive smear for cellular morphology.

Neonatal hyperbilirubinemia must be considered pathologic if any of the following criteria are met (Porter & Dennis, 2002):

1. Clinically evident jaundice in the first 24 hours of life
2. Serum bilirubin concentration rising by more than 5 mg/dL per day
3. Total serum bilirubin concentrations exceeding 15 mg/dL in term infants
4. Conjugated bilirubin concentrations greater than 2 mg/dL or more than 20% of the total serum bilirubin concentration

Initial diagnostic procedures are aimed at differentiating jaundice resulting from increased bilirubin production, impaired conjugation or excretion, increased intestinal reabsorption, or a combination of these factors. Coombs' test is performed to determine whether jaundice is due to Rh or ABO incompatibility.

If the hemolytic process is due to Rh sensitization, laboratory findings reveal the following: (1) an Rh-positive newborn with a positive Coombs' test, (2) increased erythropoiesis with many immature circulating red blood cells (nucleated blastocysts), (3) anemia, in most cases, (4) elevated levels (5 mg/dL or more) of bilirubin in cord blood, and (5) a reduction in albumin-binding capacity. Maternal data may include an elevated anti-Rh titer and spectrophotometric evidence of fetal hemolytic process.

The indirect Coombs' test measures the amount of Rh-positive antibodies in the mother's blood. Rh-positive red blood cells are added to the maternal blood sample. If the mother's serum contains antibodies, the Rh-positive red blood cells will agglutinate (clump) when rabbit immune antiglobulin is added, and the test results are labeled positive.

The direct Coombs' test reveals the presence of antibody-coated (sensitized) Rh-positive red blood cells in the newborn. Rabbit immune antiglobulin is added to the specimen of neonatal blood cells. If the neonatal red blood cells agglutinate, they have been coated with maternal antibodies, a positive result.

If the hemolytic process is due to ABO incompatibility, laboratory findings reveal an increase in reticulocytes. The resulting anemia is usually not significant during the newborn period and is rare later on. The direct Coombs' test may be negative or mildly positive; the indirect Coombs' test may be strongly positive. Infants with a positive direct Coombs' test have increased incidence of jaundice with bilirubin levels in excess of 10 mg/dL. Increased numbers of spherocytes (spherical, plump, mature erythrocytes) are seen on a peripheral blood smear. Increased numbers of spherocytes are not seen on smears from Rh disease infants.

Because of the shorter lifespan of red blood cells in the newborn, a significant bilirubin load is produced. When bilirubin breaks down, carbon monoxide (CO) is released. This production of carbon monoxide is being investigated as a marker in the study of bilirubin production. Measuring end-tidal CO (ETCO) has been shown to provide results similar to laboratory measures of bilirubin (Gilbert Frank, Cooper, & Merenstein, 2002; Halamek & Stevenson, 2002).

Regardless of the cause of hyperbilirubinemia, management of these infants is directed toward alleviating anemia, removing maternal antibodies and sensitized erythrocytes, increasing serum albumin levels, reducing serum bilirubin levels, and minimizing the consequences of hyperbilirubinemia. Early discharge of newborns from birthing centers has significantly influenced the diagnosis and management of neonatal jaundice, increasing the emphasis on outpatient and home care management.

Therapeutic methods of management of hyperbilirubinemia include phototherapy, exchange transfusion, infusion of albumin, and drug therapy. If hemolytic disease is present, it may be treated by phototherapy, exchange transfusion, and drug therapy. When determining the appropriate management of hyperbilirubinemia due to hemolytic disease, the three variables that must be taken into account are the newborn's (1) serum bilirubin level, (2) birth weight, and (3) age in hours. If a newborn has hemolysis with an unconjugated bilirubin level of 14 mg/dL, weighs less than 2500 g (birth weight), and is 24 hours old or less, an exchange transfusion may be the best management. However, if that same newborn is over 24 hours old, which is past the time where an increase in bilirubin would occur due to pathologic causes, phototherapy may be the treatment of choice to prevent the possible complications of kernicterus.

PHOTOTHERAPY

Phototherapy is the exposure of the newborn to high-intensity light. It may be used alone or in conjunction with exchange transfusion to reduce serum bilirubin levels. Exposure of the newborn to high-intensity light (fluorescent light bulbs or bulbs in the blue-light spectrum) decreases serum bilirubin levels in the skin by facilitating biliary excretion of unconjugated bilirubin. This occurs when light absorbed by the tissue converts unconjugated bilirubin into two isomers called photobilirubin. The photobilirubin moves from the tissues to the blood by a diffusion mechanism. In the blood it is bound to albumin and transported to the liver. It moves into the bile and is excreted into the duodenum for removal with feces without requiring conjugation by the liver. In addition, the photodegradation products formed when light oxidizes bilirubin can be excreted in the urine.

Phototherapy plays an important role in preventing a rise in bilirubin levels but does not alter the underlying cause of jaundice, and hemolysis may continue to produce anemia. It is generally accepted that phototherapy should be started at 4 to 5 mg/dL below the calculated exchange level for each infant. Sick newborns of less than 1000 g should have phototherapy instituted at a bilirubin concentration of 5 mg/dL. Many authors have recommended initiating phototherapy "prophylactically" in the first 24 hours of life in high-risk, very-low-birth-weight infants (Cashore, 2000). Sick preterm infants who are at least 1500 g should have phototherapy instituted when the bilirubin level is 10 mg/dL. Any term newborn with a bilirubin level of 20 mg/dL or above at 24 to 48 hours of age may need an exchange transfusion if illness or associated conditions are present (Table 33–3 •).

Phototherapy can be provided through conventional banks of phototherapy lights or by a fiberoptic blanket attached to a halogen light source around the trunk of the newborn or a combination of both delivery methods. With the fiberoptic blanket, the light stays on at all times, and the newborn is accessible for care, feeding, and diaper changes. The eyes are not covered. Fluid and weight loss are not complications of this system. Furthermore, it makes the infant accessible to the parents and is less alarming to parents than standard phototherapy (Hannon, Willis, & Scrimshaw, 2001). A combination of a fiberoptic light source in the mattress under the baby and a standard light source above may also be used (Porter & Dennis, 2002). Many institutions and pediatricians use fiberoptic blankets for home care.

EXCHANGE TRANSFUSION

Exchange transfusion is the withdrawal and replacement of the newborn's blood with donor blood. It is used to treat anemia with red blood cells that are not susceptible to maternal antibodies, remove sensitized red blood cells that would be

Table 33–3 • AMERICAN ACADEMY OF PEDIATRICS GUIDELINES FOR THE MANAGEMENT OF HYPERBILIRUBINEMIA IN THE HEALTHY TERM NEWBORN

	Total Serum Bilirubin Level, mg/dL (μmol/L)			
Age (hours)	Consider Phototherapy°	Phototherapy	Exchange Transfusion if Intensive Phototherapy Fails†	Exchange Transfusion and Intensive Phototherapy
25–48‡	≥12 (170)	≥15 (260)	≥20 (340)	≥25 (430)
49–72	≥15 (260)	≥18 (310)	≥25 (430)	≥30 (510)
>72	≥17 (290)	≥20 (340)	≥25 (430)	≥30 (510)

°Phototherapy at these total serum bilirubin (TSB) levels is a clinical option, meaning that the intervention is available and may be used on the basis of individual clinical judgment.

†Intensive phototherapy should produce a decline of TSB of 1 to 2 mg/dL within 4 to 6 hours, and the TSB level should continue to decline and remain below the threshold level for exchange transfusion. If this does not occur, phototherapy has failed. Intensive phototherapy includes the use of more than one bank of lamps containing "special blue" bulbs, maximizing the surface area illuminated by using a phototherapy blanket or other means, and providing phototherapy on a continuous, noninterrupted schedule.

‡Term infants who are clinically jaundiced at ≤24 hours old are not considered healthy and require further evaluation.

Source: Used with permission of the American Academy of Pediatrics (1994). Practice parameter: Management of hyperbilirubinemia in the healthy term newborn. *Pediatrics, 94,* 560.

lysed soon, remove serum bilirubin, and provide bilirubin-free albumin and increase the binding sites for bilirubin. Concerns over doing an exchange transfusion are related to the use of blood products and associated potential for HIV infection and hepatitis.

NURSING CARE MANAGEMENT

Nursing Assessment and Diagnosis

Assessment is aimed at identifying prenatal and perinatal factors that predispose to development of jaundice and identifying jaundice as soon as it is apparent. Clinically, ABO incompatibility presents as jaundice and occasionally as hepatosplenomegaly. Fetal hydrops or erythroblastosis fetalis is rare (see Chapter 20). Hemolytic disease of the newborn is suspected if the placenta is enlarged, if the newborn is edematous with pleural and pericardial effusion plus ascites, if pallor or jaundice is noted during the first 24 to 36 hours, if hemolytic anemia is diagnosed, or if the spleen and liver are enlarged. The nurse carefully notes changes in behavior and observes for evidence of bleeding. If laboratory tests indicate elevated bilirubin levels, the nurse checks the newborn for jaundice about every 2 hours and records observations.

To check for jaundice in lighter skinned babies, the nurse should blanch the skin over a bony prominence (forehead, nose, or sternum) by pressing firmly with the thumb. After pressure is released, if jaundice is present, the area appears yellow before normal color returns. The nurse should check oral mucosa and the posterior portion of the hard palate and conjunctival sacs for yellow pigmentation in darker skinned babies. Assessment in daylight gives best results, because pink walls and surroundings may mask yellowish tints and yellow light makes differentiation of jaundice difficult. The time of onset of jaundice is recorded and reported. If jaundice appears, careful observation of the increase in depth of color and the infant's behavior is mandatory.

In addition to visual inspection, reflectance photometers that measure transcutaneous bilirubin should be used to screen and monitor neonatal jaundice (Halamek & Stevenson, 2002). Another portable screening tool is the analysis for end-tidal carbon monoxide. This analysis allows for rapid identification of newborns with significant hemolytic disease who may be at risk for the sequelae of unconjugated hyperbilirubinemia (Halamek & Stevenson, 2002).

The newborn's behavior is assessed for neurologic signs associated with hyperbilirubinemia, which are rare but may include hypotonia, diminished reflexes, lethargy, or seizures.

Nursing diagnoses that may apply to a newborn with jaundice include the following:

- ***Fluid Volume Deficit*** related to increased insensible water loss and frequent loose stools
- ***Risk for Injury*** related to use of phototherapy
- ***Sensory/Perceptual Alterations*** related to neurologic damage secondary to kernicterus
- ***Risk for Altered Parenting*** related to parenting a newborn with jaundice

Nursing Plan and Implementation

Hospital-Based Nursing Care

Hospital-based care is described in the Clinical Pathway for Care of a Newborn with Hyperbilirubinemia on page 967. Ideally, the entire skin surface of the newborn is exposed to the light. Minimal covering may be applied over the genitals and buttocks to expose maximum skin surface while still protecting the bedding from soiling. Phototherapy success is measured every 12 hours or daily by serum bilirubin levels. The lights must be turned off while drawing blood for serum bilirubin levels. Because it is not known whether phototherapy injures the delicate eye structures, particularly the retina, the nurse applies eye patches over the newborn's closed eyes during exposure to banks of phototherapy lights (Figure 33–14 •). Phototherapy is discontinued and the eye patches are removed at least once per shift to assess the eyes for the presence of conjunctivitis. Patches are also removed to allow eye contact during feeding (for social stimulation) or when parents are visiting (to promote parental attachment).

Most phototherapy units will provide this level of irradiance 45 to 50 cm below the lamps. The nurse can use a photometer to measure and maintain desired irradiance levels. Disadvantages of lights are that they create a difficult work environment and can distort an infant's color.

The newborn's temperature is monitored to prevent hyperthermia or hypothermia. The newborn will require additional fluids to compensate for the increased water loss through the skin and loose stools. Loose stools and increased urine output are the results of increased bilirubin excretion. The infant is observed for signs of dehydration and perianal excoriation.

A benign transient bronze discoloration of the skin may occur with phototherapy when the infant has elevated direct serum bilirubin levels or liver disease. As a side effect of phototherapy, some newborns develop a maculopapular rash. In addition to assessing the newborn's skin color for jaundice and bronzing, the nurse examines the skin for developing pressure areas. The newborn should be repositioned at least every 2 hours to permit the light to reach all skin surfaces, to prevent pressure areas, and to vary the stimulation to the infant. The nurse keeps track of the number of hours each lamp is used so that each can be replaced before its effectiveness is lost. The nurse must be careful about using ointment under bilirubin lights because they may cause burns.

The terms *jaundice*, *hyperbilirubinemia*, *exchange transfusion*, and *phototherapy* may sound frightening and threatening. Some

CLINICAL PATHWAY FOR CARE OF A NEWBORN WITH HYPERBILIRUBINEMIA

Category	Day 1	Day 2/Discharge
Referral	Refer to lactation consultant	➤ **Expected Outcomes** Consults completed
Assessments	Lab work (CBC, Rh, Coombs'-direct, retic count, bilirubin level, both direct and indirect) Baer hearing test if bilirubin >18 Obtain maternal/paternal history Obtain birth and newborn history Assess sclera and skin color for jaundice; assess mucous membranes for jaundice with dark pigmented skin Continue routine newborn assessments (See Newborn Clinical Pathway in Chapter 30)	Bilirubin levels as ordered BID Assess for s/s of dehydration Assess sclera and skin color for progression of jaundice ➤ **Expected Outcomes** Physical assessments, VS WNL; skin/mucous membranes pink, sclera clear of jaundice color; laboratory work WNL, total bilirubin level stabilized or decreasing
Teaching/ psychosocial	Evaluate additional psychosocial needs of parents/family Orient family to nursery, equipment, client room if rooming-in Instruct parents on s/s of hyperbilirubinemia (slight lethargy, irritability) Discuss possible side effects of phototherapy (stool character changes, increased fluid loss, temp changes, rash, altered sleep/wake patterns) Instruct parents on care and treatment of hyperbilirubinemia: • Phototherapy rationale, indications and precautions • Placement of bili mask over closed eyes • Lab draws; rationale, frequency • Accurate intake and output to monitor for s/s dehydration Review cord care, skin care, care of genitalia (circumcision care as applicable) Review role of pumping breasts if necessary and offering formula for limited period of time	Teach/encourage parents to provide cuddling, tactile stimulation and eye contact during diaper changes and feedings, talk to baby frequently Reinforce previous teaching; evaluate parental comprehension Provide opportunities for parents to express concerns/feelings ➤ **Expected Outcomes** Parents verbalize comprehension of care of infant with hyperbilirubinemia and potential sequelae of no treatment; parents verbalize comprehension of the risks/benefits of phototherapy as treatment; parents demonstrate developmentally appropriate care for infant during diaper changes and feedings; parents verbalize concerns, ask appropriate questions prn
Nursing care management and reports	Vital signs q4h with axillary temps Monitor thermoregulation Daily wt Initiate phototherapy as indicated and ordered • Maintain bili mask over eyes • Keep genitalia covered per policy • Check eyes for discharge, excessive pressure, corneal abrasions • Expose as much skin surface as possible to bili lights • Bilimeter reading q shift • No lotion or ointment on infant skin • Turn bili lights off during lab draws Continue infant assessments including: • Note and document skin color q shift • Thorough skin care with diaper changes; note s/s breakdown, rash • Assess neuro status for s/s abnormality q interaction (hypotonia, lethargy, poor sucking reflex)	VS q4h with axillary temps Monitor thermoregulation, maintain NTE Daily wt Continue phototherapy as indicated • Maintain bili mask over eyes • Cover genitalia per policy • Check eyes for discharge, conjunctivitis, corneal abrasions • Expose as much skin surface as possible to bili lights • Bilimeter reading q shift • No lotion or ointment on infant skin • Turn bili lights off during lab draws Continue infant assessments as per Day 1 ➤ **Expected Outcomes** VS WNL; wt stabilized or gaining wt; no s/s kernicterus; skin integrity intact; skin and mucous membranes pink; eyes without drainage, sclera clear; labs WNL with stabilized or decreasing bilirubin level
Activity and comfort	Nest in open crib if infant able to maintain temp beneath bili lights Isolette if infant unable to maintain temp beneath bili lights Reposition q2–4h Remove bili mask, swaddle and cuddle during feedings Cluster cares, remove from lights for feedings	Nest in open crib if infant's temp stable beneath bili lights Isolette if infant unable to maintain temp beneath bili lights ➤ **Expected Outcomes** Infant's temp WNL; infant able to rest with nested boundaries; infant cuddled, has eye contact with caregiver during cares and feedings
Nutrition	Breast- or formula-feed q2–4h Monitor for dehydration, supplement with oral/IV fluid as indicated Remove newborn from bili lights, remove mask for feedings	Continue to feed q2–4h, monitor for dehydration, cuddle for feeding ➤ **Expected Outcomes** Infant tolerating feedings q2–4h without sequelae
Elimination	Record urine color and frequency Specific gravity each void Record quantity and characteristics each stool Strict intake and output (weigh diapers before discarding)	Continue noting urine and stool quantity and characteristics ➤ **Expected Outcomes** Voids qs, stools qs without difficulty, stool characteristics WNL for resolving hyperbilirubinemia; specific gravity WNL, no s/s dehydration

Bili, bilirubin; CPR, cardiopulmonary resuscitation; DC, discharge; info, information; IV, intravenous; lab draws, laboratory blood withdrawal; MD/NP, medical doctor/nurse practitioner; NSY, nursery; NTE, neutral thermal environment; PRN, as needed; s/s, signs and symptoms; VS, vital signs; WNL, within normal limits; wt, weight.

(continued on next page)

CLINICAL PATHWAY FOR CARE OF A NEWBORN WITH HYPERBILIRUBINEMIA *CONTINUED*

Category	Day 1 after Birth	Day 2/Discharge
Medication	Evaluate routine meds Evaluate need for IV fluids	➤ **Expected Outcomes** Routine meds given; IV fluids administered prn, IV fluids tapered as oral intake adequate to prevent dehydration
Discharge planning/ home care	Evaluate social services/visiting nurse/DC planning needs Possible home phototherapy Schedule follow-up bili levels as outpatient; follow-up with MD/NP	Offer info on CPR classes and/or film, give CPR booklet ➤ **Expected Outcomes** Infant DC home with parent(s); mother verbalizes follow-up appointments
Family involvement	Evaluate additional psychosocial needs Orient family to NSY, equipment, room Discuss rationale for treatment and possible side effects of phototherapy with family (stool changes, increased fluid loss, possible temp instability, slight lethargy, rash, altered sleep/wake patterns) Instruct family on infant's care while undergoing phototherapy: • Safety precautions—bili mask, isolette door closed and latched, covering genitalia per policy • Skin care, cord care, circ care as appropriate • Lab draws, rationale for intake and output As necessary, review role of pumping breasts and offering formula for limited time Encourage parents/significant others/sibling involvement in infant care as possible Evaluate family's understanding of information	Encourage parents to provide tactile stimulation during feeding and diaper changes Encourage cuddling and eye contact during feedings Offer suggestions to comfort restless infant: • Nesting beneath bili lights • Talking softly/singing quietly to infant • Taped music or tape recording of evening activities from home • Rhythmic patting of infant's buttocks • Firm, nonstroking touch, assisting with control of extremities • Pacifier for nonnutritive sucking Encourage family/friend support of mother/parents, ie, meals, rest, child care for siblings, allow expression of concerns/feelings ➤ **Expected Outcomes** Parents verbalize understanding of rationale and possible side effects of phototherapy; parents/family demonstrate safety precautions when caring for infant; parents getting meals, rest, verbalize support given
Date		

parents may feel guilty about their baby's condition and think they have caused the problem. Under stress, parents may not be able to understand the physician/nurse practitioner's first explanations. The nurse must expect that the parents will need explanations repeated and clarified and that they may need help voicing their questions and fears. Eye and tactile contact with the infant is encouraged. The nurse can coach parents when they visit with the baby. After the mother's discharge, parents are kept informed of their infant's condition and are encouraged to return to the hospital or telephone at any time so that they can be fully involved in the care of their infant. Tell parents that they can expect a rebound of 1 to 2 mg/dL after discontinuation of phototherapy and a follow-up bilirubin test may be done (Porter & Dennis, 2002).

While the mother is still hospitalized, phototherapy can also be carried out in the mother's room if the only problem is hyperbilirubinemia. The mother must be willing to keep the baby in the room for 24 hours a day, be able to take emergency action, as for choking, if necessary, and complete instruction checklists. Some institutions require that parents sign a consent form. The nurse gives the instructions to the parents but also continues to monitor the infant's temperature, activity, intake and output, and positioning of eye patches (if conventional light banks are used) at regular intervals (Table 33–4 •).

Table 33–4 • INSTRUCTIONAL CHECKLIST FOR IN-ROOM PHOTOTHERAPY

Explain and demonstrate the placement of eye patches and explain that they must be in place when the infant is under the lights.

Explain the clothing to be worn (diaper under lights, dress and wrap when away from the lights).

Explain the importance of taking the infant's temperature regularly.

Explain the importance of adequate fluid intake.

Explain the charting flow sheet (intake, output, eyes covered).

Explain how to position the lights at a proper distance.

Explain the need to keep the infant under phototherapy except during feeding and diaper changes.

Community-Based Nursing Care

The Fetus and Newborn Committee of the American Academy of Pediatrics has not endorsed home phototherapy but has issued strict guidelines for its use (Halamek & Stevenson, 2002). Some studies have shown that with early discharge of newborns and their mothers comes an increase in hospital readmission and elevated risk of pathological hyperbilirubinemia. There is an increased need for close follow-up of all newborns in the first days and weeks of life.

Procedure 33–2 Infant Receiving Phototherapy

Preparation

1. Explain the purpose of phototherapy, the procedure itself (including the need to use eye patches), and possible side effects such as dehydration.
2. Note evidence of jaundice in skin, sclera, and mucous membranes (in infants with darkly pigmented skin). Be sure that recent serum bilirubin levels are available.
   Rationale: The decision to use phototherapy is based on a careful assessment of the newborn's condition over a period of time. The most recent results prior to starting therapy serve as a baseline to evaluate the effectiveness of therapy.

Equipment and Supplies

- Bank of phototherapy lights
- Eye patches
- Small scale to weigh diapers

Procedure

1. Obtain vital signs including axillary temperature.
   Rationale: Provides baseline data.
2. Remove all of the infant's clothing except the diaper.
   Rational: Exposure of the newborn to high-intensity light (a bank of fluorescent lightbulbs or bulbs in the blue-white spectrum) decreases serum bilirubin levels in the skin by aiding biliary excretion of unconjugated bilirubin. Because the tissue absorbs the light, best results are obtained when there is maximum skin surface exposure.
3. Apply eye coverings (eye patches or a bili mask) to the infant according to agency policy. (See Figure 33–14 •.)
   Rationale: Eye coverings are used because it is not known if phototherapy injures delicate eye structures, particularly the retina.
4. Place the infant in an open crib or isolette (more commonly used in preterm infants and infants who are sicker) about 45 to 50 cm below the bank of phototherapy lights. Reposition every 2 hours.
   Rationale: The isolette helps the infant maintain his or her temperature while undressed. Repositioning exposes different areas of skin to the lights, prevents the development of pressure areas on the skin, and varies the stimulation the infant receives.
5. Monitor vital signs every 4 hours with axillary temperatures.
   Rationale: Temperature assessment is indicated to detect hypothermia or hyperthermia. Deviation in pulse and respirations may indicate developing complications.
6. Cluster care activities.
7. Discontinue phototherapy and remove eye patches at least once per 8-hour shift. Also discontinue phototherapy and remove patches when feeding the infant and when the parents visit.
   Rationale: Care activities are clustered to help ensure that the newborn has maximum time under the lights. Eye patches are removed to assess for signs of complications such as excessive pressure, discharge, or conjunctivitis. Patches are also removed to provide some social stimulation and to promote parental attachment.

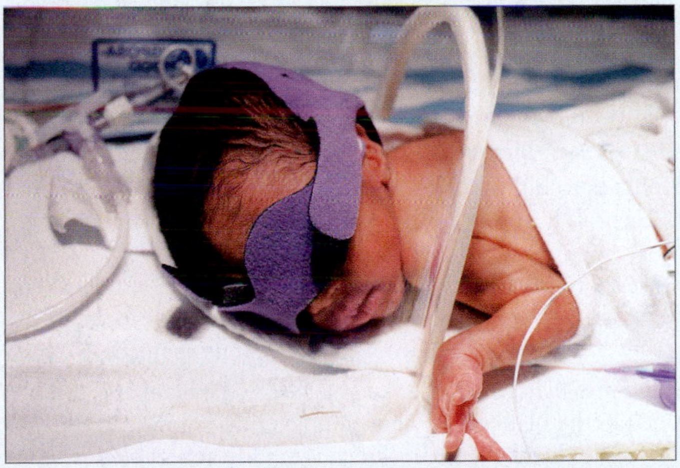

Figure 33–14 • Infant receiving phototherapy. The phototherapy light is positioned over the incubator. Bilateral eye patches are always used during photo light therapy to protect the baby's eyes.
SOURCE: Courtesy of Lisa Smith-Pedersen, RNC, MSN, NNP.

(continued on next page)

Procedure 33–2 Infant Receiving Phototherapy *(continued)*

8. Maintain adequate fluid intake. Evaluate need for IV fluids.
9. Monitor intake and output carefully. Weigh diapers before discarding. Record quantity and characteristics of each stool.
   Rationale: Infants undergoing phototherapy treatment have increased water loss and loose stools as a result of bilirubin excretion. This increase their risk of dehydration.
10. Assess specific gravity with each voiding. Weigh newborn daily.
    Rationale: Specific gravity provides one measure of urine concentration. Highly concentrated urine is associated with a dehydrated state. Weight loss is also a sign of developing dehydration in the newborn.
11. Observe the infant for signs of perianal excoriation and institute therapy if it develops.
    Rationale: Perianal excoriation may develop because of the irritating effect of diarrhea stools.
12. Ensure that serum bilirubin levels are drawn regularly according to orders or agency policy. Turn the phototherapy lights off while the blood is drawn.
    Rationale: Serum bilirubin levels provide the most accurate indication of the effectiveness of phototherapy. They are generally drawn every 12 hours, but at least once daily. The phototherapy lights are turned off to ensure accurate serum bilirubin levels.
13. Examine the newborn's skin regularly for signs of developing pressure areas, bronzing, maculopapular rash, and changes in degree of jaundice.
    Rationale: Pressure areas may develop if the infant lies in one position for an extended period. A benign, transient bronze discoloration of the skin may occur with phototherapy when the infant has elevated direct serum bilirubin levels or liver disease. A maculopapular rash is another transient side effect of phototherapy that develops occasionally.
14. Avoid using lotion or ointment on the exposed skin.
    Rationale: Lotion and ointments on a newborn receiving phototherapy may cause skin burns.
15. Provide parents with opportunities to hold the newborn and assist in the infant's care. Answer their questions accurately and keep them informed of developments or changes.
    Rationale: A sick infant is a source of great anxiety for parents. Information helps them deal with their anxiety. Moreover, they have a right to be kept well informed of their baby's status so that they are able to make informed decisions as needed.

    Note: Phototherapy may also be provided using lightweight, fiberoptic blankets ("bili blankets"). The baby is wrapped in the blanket, which is plugged into an outlet. The eyes are not covered. With fiberoptic blankets the newborn is readily accessible for care, feedings, and diaper changes. The baby does not get overheated, and fluid and weight loss are not complications of this system. The infant is accessible to the parents and the procedure seems less alarming to parents than standard phototherapy. A combination of a fiberoptic light source in the mattress under the baby and a standard phototherapy light source above is also used by some agencies. In addition, many agencies and pediatricians use fiberoptic blankets for home care.

Clinical Tip *If the area of jaundice about the eyes begins to disappear, it is probable that the eye patches are allowing light to enter and better eye protection is needed.*

If the baby is to receive phototherapy at home, parents are taught to record the infant's temperature, weight, fluid intake and output, stools, and feedings and to use the phototherapy equipment. In addition, if phototherapy lights are being used, parents must agree that the baby will be exposed to the lights for long periods of time; that they will hold the baby for only short periods for feedings, comforting, and cleansing of the perineal area; and that the room temperature will be regulated to minimize heat loss. Fiberoptic phototherapy blankets eliminate the need for eye patches, decrease heat loss because the baby is clothed, and provide more opportunities for interaction between the baby and parents. The best method of home phototherapy depends on the cause of the hyperbilirubinemia and the rate of progression of the jaundice. Ongoing monitoring of bilirubin levels is essential with home phototherapy and can be carried out in the home, in the follow-up clinic, or in the clinician's office (Madlon-Kay, 2001).

Jaundice and its treatment can be very disturbing to parents and may generate feelings of guilt and fear. Reassurance and support are vital especially for the breastfeeding mother, who may question her ability to adequately nourish her newborn. The parents' perception of and/or misconceptions about jaundice can affect parent-infant interactions (Hannon et al, 2001). The nurse should explain the causes of jaundice and emphasize that it is usually a transient problem and one to which all infants must adapt after birth. It is essential that the impact of cultural beliefs be considered. Some Latina women believe that showing strong maternal emotions during pregnancy and during breastfeeding can be detrimental. "Bilis" associated with anger may be blamed by some Latina women for jaundice. Cultural beliefs lead mothers to interpret illness within their cultural framework, especially when left without clear and understood explanations (Hannon et al, 2001). Maternal reactions can be lessened by careful explanations to the mothers about the diagnosis, prognosis, duration, management options for jaundice, and possibility of recurrence.

Evaluation

Expected outcomes of nursing care include the following:

- The risks for development of hyperbilirubinemia are identified, and action is taken to minimize the potential impact of hyperbilirubinemia.
- The baby will not have any corneal irritation or drainage, skin breakdown, or major fluctuations in temperature.
- Parents will understand the rationale for, goal of, and expected outcome of therapy. Parents verbalize their concerns about their baby's condition and identify how they can facilitate their baby's improvement.

Care of the Newborn with Anemia

Neonatal anemia is often difficult to recognize by clinical evaluation alone. The hemoglobin concentration in a full-term newborn is 15 to 20 g/dL, slightly higher than in premature infants, in whom the mean hemoglobin is 14 to 18 g/dL. According to a study by Lubetzky, Ben-Shachar, Mimouni, et al (2000), the hematocrit is lower if an infant is born by cesarean. Infants with hemoglobin values of less than 14 mg/dL (term) and 13 g/dL (preterm) are usually considered anemic. The most common causes of neonatal anemia are blood loss, hemolysis, and impaired red blood cell production.

Blood loss (hypovolemia) occurs in utero from placental bleeding (placenta previa or abruptio placentae). Intrapartal blood loss may be fetomaternal, fetofetal, or the result of umbilical cord bleeding. Birth trauma to abdominal organs or the cranium may produce significant blood loss, and cerebral bleeding may occur because of hypoxia.

Excessive hemolysis of red cells is usually a result of blood group incompatibilities but may be due to infections. The most common cause of impaired red cell production is a deficiency in G-6-PD, which is genetically transmitted. Anemia and jaundice are the presenting signs.

A condition known as **physiologic anemia** exists as a result of the normal gradual drop in hemoglobin for the first 6 to 12 weeks of life and corresponds with the decline in fetal hemoglobin. Theoretically, the bone marrow stops production of red blood cells in response to the elevated oxygenation of extrauterine respirations. When the amount of hemoglobin decreases, reaching levels of 10 to 11 g/dL at about 6 to 12 weeks of age, the bone marrow begins production of red blood cells again, and the anemia disappears.

Anemia in preterm newborns occurs earlier, and reversal by bone marrow is initiated at lower levels of hemoglobin (7 to 9 g/dL). The preterm baby's hemoglobin reaches a low sooner (4 to 8 weeks after birth) than does a term newborn's (6 to 12 weeks) because preterm red blood cell survival time is shorter than in the term newborn (Manco-Johnson, Rodden, & Collins, 2002). This difference is due to several factors: the preterm infant's rapid growth rate, decreased iron stores, and an inadequate production of erythropoietin (Blackburn, 2003).

Clinical Therapy

Hematologic problems can be anticipated based on the pregnancy history and clinical manifestations. The age at which anemia is first noted is also of diagnostic value.

Clinically, light-skinned anemic infants are very pale in the absence of other symptoms of shock and usually have abnormally low red blood cell counts. In acute blood loss, symptoms of shock may be present, such as pallor, low arterial blood pressure, and a decreasing hematocrit value. The initial laboratory work-up should include hemoglobin and hematocrit measurements, reticulocyte count, examination of peripheral blood smear, bilirubin determinations, direct Coombs' test of infant's blood, and examination of maternal blood smear for fetal erythrocytes (Kleihauer-Betke test). Clinical management depends on the severity of the anemia and whether blood loss is acute or chronic. The baby should be placed on constant cardiac and respiratory monitoring. Mild or chronic anemia in an infant may be treated adequately with iron supplements alone or with iron-fortified formulas. Frequent determinations of hemoglobin, hematocrit, and bilirubin levels (in hemolytic disease) are essential. In severe cases of anemia, transfusions are the preferred method of treatment. Management of anemia of prematurity includes recombinant human erythropoietin and supplemental iron. Blood transfusions (dedicated units of blood) are kept to a minimum.

NURSING CARE MANAGEMENT

The nurse assesses the newborn for symptoms of anemia (pallor). If the blood loss is acute, the baby may exhibit signs of shock (a capillary filling time greater than 3 seconds, decreased pulses, tachycardia, and low blood pressure). Continued observations will be necessary to identify physiologic anemia as the preterm newborn grows. Signs of compromise include poor weight gain, tachycardia, tachypnea, and apneic episodes. The nurse promptly reports any symptoms indicating anemia or shock. The amount of blood drawn for all laboratory tests is recorded in tenths of a milliliter, so that total blood removed can be assessed and replaced by transfusion when necessary. If the newborn exhibits signs of shock, the nurse may need to initiate interventions.

Care of the Newborn with Polycythemia

Polycythemia, a condition in which blood volume and hematocrit values are increased, is observed more commonly in small-for-gestational-age (SGA) and full-term infants with delayed cord clamping, infants receiving maternal-fetal or twin-to-twin transfusions, infants of diabetic mothers (IDM), babies of mothers who smoke, and infants who experience chronic intrauterine hypoxia (Al-Alawi & Jenkins, 2000). An infant is considered polycythemic when the central venous hematocrit value is greater than 65% to 70% or the venous hemoglobin level is greater than 20 to 22 g/dL during the first week of life. Other conditions that present with polycythemia are chromosomal anomalies such as trisomy 21, 18, and 13; endocrine disorders such as hypoglycemia and hypocalcemia; and births at altitudes over 5000 feet.

Many infants are asymptomatic, but as symptoms develop, they are related to the increased blood volume, hyperviscosity (thickness) of the blood, and decreased deformability of red blood cells, all of which result in poor perfusion of tissues. The infants have a characteristic plethoric (ruddy) appearance. The most common symptoms observed include the following:

- Tachycardia and congestive heart failure due to the increased blood volume
- Respiratory distress with grunting, tachypnea, and cyanosis; increased oxygen need; or hemorrhage in respiratory system due to pulmonary venous congestion, edema, and hypoxemia
- Hyperbilirubinemia due to increased numbers of red blood cells breaking down
- Decrease in peripheral pulses, discoloration of extremities, renal vein thrombosis with decreased urine output, hematuria, or proteinuria due to thromboembolism
- Jitteriness, decreased activity and tone, seizures due to decreased perfusion of the brain, and increased vascular resistance secondary to sluggish blood flow (This can result in neurologic or developmental problems.)

Clinical Therapy

The goal of therapy is to reduce the central venous hematocrit to a range of 55% to 60% in symptomatic infants. To decrease the red cell mass, the symptomatic infant receives a partial exchange transfusion in which blood is removed from the infant and replaced milliliter for milliliter with fresh plasma, Plasmanate, or 5% albumin. Supportive treatment of presenting symptoms is required until resolution, which usually occurs spontaneously following the partial exchange transfusion.

NURSING CARE MANAGEMENT

The nurse assesses, records, and reports symptoms of polycythemia. The nurse also does an initial screening of the newborn's hematocrit on admission to the nursery. If a capillary hematocrit is done, warming the heel prior to obtaining the blood helps to decrease falsely high values (Procedure 33–1: Performing Heel Stick on a Newborn). Peripheral free-flowing venous hematocrit samples are usually obtained from the antecubital fossa.

The nurse observes closely for signs of distress or change in vital signs during the partial exchange. The nurse assesses carefully for potential complications resulting from the exchange such as transfusion overload (which can result in congestive heart failure), irregular cardiac rhythm, bacterial infection, hypovolemia (because of decreased plasma volume), and anemia. Parents need specific explanations about polycythemia and its treatment. The newborn needs to be reunited with the parents as soon after the exchange as the baby's status permits.

Care of the Newborn with Infection

Newborns up to 1 month of age are particularly susceptible to infection, referred to as **sepsis neonatorum,** caused by organisms that do not cause significant disease in older children. Once any infection occurs in the newborn, it can spread rapidly through the bloodstream, regardless of its primary site. The incidence of primary neonatal sepsis is 1 to 5 per 1000 live births (0.1% to 0.5%) (Edwards, 2002). Nosocomial infection frequency is less in normal newborn infants and increases for infants in the neonatal intensive care unit (NICU).

One factor predisposing the newborn to infection is prematurity. Prematurity and low birth weight are associated with nosocomial infection rates up to 5% higher than average. The general debilitation and underlying illness often associated with prematurity necessitates invasive procedures such as umbilical catheterization, intubation, resuscitation, ventilatory support, monitoring, and parenteral alimentation (especially lipid emulsions); and prior broad-spectrum antibiotic therapy. However, even full-term infants are susceptible because their immunologic systems are immature. They lack the complex factors involved in effective phagocytosis and the ability to localize infection or to respond with a well-defined recognizable inflammatory response. In addition, newborns lack IgM immunoglobulin, which is necessary to protect against bacteria, because it does not cross the placenta (refer to Chapter 28 for immunologic adaptations in the newborn period).

Most nosocomial infections in the NICU present as bacteremia/sepsis, urinary tract infections, meningitis, or pneumonia. Maternal antepartal infections such as rubella, toxoplasmosis, cytomegalic inclusion disease, and herpes may cause congenital infections and resulting disorders in the newborn. Intrapartal maternal infections, such as amnionitis and those resulting from premature rupture of membranes (PROM) and precipitous birth, are sources of neonatal infection. (See Chapter 20 for more detailed information). Passage through the birth canal and contact with microorganisms in the vaginal flora (β-hemolytic streptococci, herpes, *Listeria*, and gonococci) expose the infant to infection (Table 33–5 •). With infection anywhere in the fetus or newborn, the adjacent tissues or organs are very easily penetrated, and the blood-brain barrier is ineffective. Septicemia is more common in males, except for those infections caused by group B β-hemolytic streptococcus.

At present gram-negative organisms (especially *E coli*, *Enterobacter*, *Proteus*, and *Klebsiella*) and the gram-positive organism β-hemolytic streptococcus are the most common causative agents. *Pseudomonas* is a common fomite contaminant of ventilatory support and oxygen therapy equipment. Gram-positive bacteria, especially coagulase-negative staphylococci, are common pathogens in nosocomial bacteremias, pneumonias, and urinary tract infections. Other gram-positive bacteria frequently isolated are enterococci and *Staphylococcus aureus* (Edwards, 2002).

Protection of the newborn from infections starts prenatally and continues throughout pregnancy and birth. Prenatal prevention should include maternal screening for sexually transmitted infection and monitoring of rubella titers in women who test negative. Intrapartally, sterile technique is essential. Smears from genital lesions are taken, and placenta and amniotic fluid cultures are obtained if amnionitis is suspected. If genital herpes is present toward term, cesarean birth may be indicated. Local eye treatment with silver nitrate or an antibiotic ophthalmic ointment is given to all newborns to prevent damage from gonococcal infections. Prophylactic antibiotic therapy, for asymptomatic GBS-culture-positive women during the intrapartum period, has been shown to be beneficial in preventing early-onset sepsis.

Clinical Therapy

Infants with a history of possible exposure to infection in utero (for example, PROM more than 24 hours before birth or questionable maternal history of infection) should have cultures taken as soon after birth as possible. Cultures are obtained before antibiotic therapy is begun.

1. Two blood cultures are obtained from different peripheral sites. They are taken from a peripheral rather than an umbilical vessel because catheters have yielded false-positive results due to contamination. The skin is prepared by cleaning with an antiseptic solution, such as one containing iodine, and allowed to dry; the specimen is obtained with a sterile needle/syringe.
2. Spinal fluid culture is done following a spinal tap/lumbar puncture.
3. The specimen for urine culture is best obtained by a suprapubic bladder aspiration.
4. Skin cultures are taken of any lesions or drainage from lesions or reddened areas.
5. Nasopharyngeal, rectal, ear canal, and gastric aspirate cultures may be obtained.

Other laboratory investigations include a complete blood count, chest x-ray examination, serology, and Gram stains of cerebrospinal fluid, urine, skin exudate, and umbilicus. White blood cell (WBC) count with differential may indicate the presence or absence of sepsis. A level of 30,000 WBC may be normal in the first 24 hours of life, whereas low WBC may be indicative of sepsis. A low neutrophil count and high band (immature white cells) count indicate that an infection is present. Stomach aspirate should be sent for culture and smear if a gonococcal infection or amnionitis is suspected. C-reactive protein may or may not be elevated. Serum IgM levels are elevated (normal level less than 20 mg/dL) in response to transplacental infections. If available, counterimmunoelectrophoresis tests for specific bacterial antigens are performed.

Evidence of congenital infections may be seen on skull x-rays or CT scan for cerebral calcifications (cytomegalovirus, toxoplasmosis), on bone x-rays (syphilis, cytomegalovirus),

Table 33–5 • MATERNITY TRANSMITTED NEWBORN INFECTIONS

Infection	Nursing Assessment	Nursing Plan and Implementation
Group B Streptococcus 1% to 2% colonized with one in ten developing disease. Early onset—usually within hours of birth or within first week. Late onset—1 week to 3 months.	Severe respiratory distress (grunting and cyanosis). May become apneic or demonstrate symptoms of shock. Meconium-stained amniotic fluid seen at birth.	Early assessment of clinical signs necessary. Assist with x-ray examination—shows aspiration pneumonia or hyaline membrane disease. Immediately obtain blood, gastric aspirate, external ear canal and nasopharynx cultures. Administer antibiotics, usually aqueous penicillin or ampicillin combined with gentamicin, as soon as cultures are obtained. Early assessment and intervention are essential to survival. Initiate referral to evaluate for blindness, deafness, learning or behavioral problems.
Syphilis Spirochetes cross placenta after 16th–18th week of gestation.	Check perinatal history for positive maternal serology. Assess infant for Elevated cord serum IgM and FTA-ABS IgM Rhinitis (snuffles) Fissures on mouth corners and excoriated upper lip Red rash around mouth and anus Copper-colored rash over face, palms, and soles Irritability Generalized edema, particularly over joints; bone lesions; painful extremities Hepatosplenomegaly, jaundice Congenital cataracts SGA and failure to thrive	Initiate isolation techniques until infants have been on antibiotics for 48 hours. Administer penicillin. Provide emotional support for parents because of their feelings about mode of transmission and potential long-term sequelae.
Gonorrhea Approximately 30%–35% of newborns born vaginally to infected mothers acquire the infection.	Assess for Ophthalmia neonatorum (conjunctivitis) Purulent discharge and corneal ulcerations Neonatal sepsis with temperature instability, poor feeding response, and/or hypotonia, jaundice	Administer ophthalmic antibiotic ointment (see Drug Guide: Erythromycin [Ilotycin] Ophthalmic Ointment in Chapter 30) or penicillin . Initiate follow-up referral to evaluate any loss of vision.
Herpes Type 2 1 in 7500 births. Usually transmitted during vaginal birth; a few cases of in utero transmission have been reported.	Small cluster vesicular skin lesions over all the body. Check perinatal history for active herpes genital lesions. Disseminated form—DIC, pneumonia, hepatitis with jaundice, hepatosplenomegaly, and neurologic abnormalities. Without skin lesions, assess for fever or subnormal temperature, respiratory congestion, tachypnea, and tachycardia.	Carry out careful handwashing and gown and glove isolation with linen precautions. Administer intravenous vidarabine (Vira A) or acyclovir (Zovirax). Initiate follow-up referral to evaluate potential sequelae of microcephaly, spasticity, seizures, deafness, or blindness. Encourage parental rooming-in and touching of their newborn. Show parents appropriate handwashing procedures and precautions to be used at home if mother's lesions are active. Obtain throat, conjunctiva, cerebral spinal fluid (CSF), blood, urine, and lesion cultures to identify herpesvirus type 2 antibiotics in serum IgM fraction. Cultures positive in 24–48 hours.
Oral Candidal Infection (Thrush) Acquired during passage through birth canal.	Assess newborn's buccal mucosa, tongue, gums, and inside the cheeks for white plaques (seen 5 to 7 days of age). Check diaper area for bright red, well-demarcated eruptions. Assess for thrush periodically when newborn is on long-term antibiotic therapy.	Differentiate white plaque areas from milk curds by using cotton tip applicator (if it is thrush, removal of white areas causes raw, bleeding areas). Maintain cleanliness of hands, linen, clothing, diapers, and feeding apparatus. Instruct breastfeeding mothers on treating their nipples with nystatin. Administer gentian violet (1% to 2%) swabbed on oral lesions 1 hour after feeding or nystatin instilled in baby's oral cavity and on mucosa. Swab skin lesions with topical nystatin. Discuss with parents that gentian violet stains mouth and clothing. Avoid placing gentian violet on normal mucosa; it causes irritation.
Chlamydia Trachomatis Acquired during passage through birth canal.	Assess for perinatal history of preterm birth. Symptomatic newborns present with pneumonia—conjunctivitis after 3–4 days. Chronic follicular conjunctivitis (corneal neovascularization and conjunctival scarring).	Instill ophthalmic erythromycin (see Drug Guide: Erythromycin [Ilotycin] Ophthalmic Ointment in Chapter 30) . Initiate follow-up referral for eye complications and late development of pneumonia at 4–11 weeks postnatally.

and in serum-specific IgM levels (rubella). Cytomegalovirus infection is best diagnosed by urine culture.

Because neonatal infection causes high mortality, therapy is instituted before results of the sepsis work-up are obtained. A combination of two broad-spectrum antibiotics, such as ampicillin and gentamicin, is given in large doses until a culture with sensitivities results is obtained.

After the pathogen and its sensitivities are determined, appropriate specific antibiotic therapy is begun. Combinations of penicillin or ampicillin and kanamycin have been used in the past, but new kanamycin-resistant enterobacteria and penicillin-resistant staphylococcus necessitate increasing use of gentamicin.

Rotating aminoglycosides has been suggested to prevent development of resistance. Use of cephalosporins and, in particular, cefotaxime has emerged as an alternative to aminoglycoside therapy in the treatment of neonatal infections. Duration of therapy varies from 7 to 14 days (Table 33–6 •). However, if cultures are negative and symptoms subside, antibiotics may be discontinued after 3 days. Supportive physiologic care may be required to maintain respiratory, hemodynamic, nutritional, and metabolic homeostasis.

NURSING CARE MANAGEMENT

Nursing Assessment and Diagnosis

Symptoms of infection are most often noticed by the nurse during daily care of the newborn. The infant may deteriorate rapidly in the first 12 to 24 hours after birth if β-hemolytic streptococcal infection is present, with signs and symptoms mimicking respiratory distress syndrome. In other cases, the onset of sepsis may be gradual, with more subtle signs and symptoms (Hashim & Guillet, 2002). The most common symptoms include the following:

- Subtle behavioral changes—the infant "isn't doing well" and is often lethargic or irritable (especially after first 24 hours), hypotonic, and hypotensive. Color changes may include pallor, duskiness, cyanosis, or a "shocky" appearance. Skin is cool and clammy.
- Temperature instability, manifested most commonly by hypothermia (recognized by a decrease in skin temperature) or, rarely in newborns, hyperthermia (elevation of skin temperature) necessitates a corresponding increase or decrease in incubator temperature to maintain a neutral thermal environment.
- Feeding intolerance is evidenced by a decrease in total intake, abdominal distention, vomiting, poor sucking, lack of interest in feeding, and diarrhea.
- Hyperbilirubinemia.
- Tachycardia initially, followed by spells of apnea/bradycardia.

Signs and symptoms may suggest central nervous system disease (jitteriness, tremors, seizure activity), respiratory system disease (tachypnea, labored respirations, apnea, cyanosis), hematologic disease (jaundice, petechial hemorrhages, hepatosplenomegaly), or gastrointestinal disease (diarrhea, vomiting, bile-stained aspirate, hepatomegaly). A differential diagnosis is necessary because of the similarity of symptoms to other more specific conditions.

Nursing diagnoses that may apply to the infant with suspected sepsis neonatorum and the family include the following:

- ***Risk for Infection*** related to immature immunologic system
- ***Fluid Volume Deficit*** related to feeding intolerance
- ***Ineffective Family Coping: Compromised*** related to present illness resulting in prolonged hospital stay for the newborn

Nursing Plan and Implementation

In the nursery, controlling the environment and preventing acquired infection are the responsibilities of the neonatal nurse. The nurse must promote strict handwashing technique for all who enter the nursery, including nursing colleagues; physicians; laboratory, x-ray, and inhalation technicians; and parents. The nurse must be prepared to assist in the aseptic collection of specimens for laboratory investigations. Scrupulous care of equipment—changing and cleaning incubators at least every 7 days, removing and sterilizing wet equipment every 24 hours, preventing cross-use of linen and other equipment, cleaning sinkside equipment such as soap containers periodically, and taking special care with the open radiant warmers (access without prior handwashing is much more likely than with the closed incubator)—will prevent fomite contamination or contamination through improper hand washing. An infected newborn can be effectively isolated in an incubator and receive close observation. Visits to the nursery area by unnecessary personnel should be discouraged.

MEDIALINK CARE PLAN: INFECTION IN A NEWBORN

Antibiotic Therapy Provision

The nurse administers antibiotics as ordered by the nurse practitioner/physician. It is the nurse's responsibility to be knowledgeable about the following:

- The proper dose to be administered, based on the weight of the newborn and desired peak and trough levels
- The appropriate route of administration, because some antibiotics cannot be given intravenously
- The appropriate rate of administration
- Admixture incompatibilities because some antibiotics are precipitated by intravenous solutions or by other antibiotics
- Side effects and toxicity

In the case of term infants who are being treated for infections, neonatal home infusion of antibiotics should be considered as a viable alternative to continued hospitalization.

Table 33-6 • NEONATAL SEPSIS ANTIBIOTIC THERAPY

Drug	Dose (mg/kg) Total Daily Dose	Schedule for Divided Doses	Route	Comments
Ampicillin	50–100 mg/kg	Every 12 hours–* Every 8 hours†	IM or IV	Effective against gram-positive microorganisms, *Haemophilus influenzae*, and most *Escherichia coli* strains. Higher doses indicated for meningitis. Used with aminoglycoside for synergy.
Cefotaxime	50 mg/kg 100–150 mg/kg/day	Every 12 hours* Every 8 hours†	IM or IV	Active against most major pathogens in infants; effective against aminoglycoside-resistant organisms; achieves CSF bactericidal activity; lack of ototoxicity and nephrotoxicity; wide therapeutic index (levels not required); resistant organisms can develop rapidly if used extensively; ineffective against *Pseudomonas, Listeria*.
Gentamicin	2.5–3 mg/kg 5–7.5 mg/kg/day 4–5 mg/kg/dose (first week of life)	Every 12–24 hours*‡ Every 8–24 hours† Every 24–48 hours	IM or IV	Effective against gram-negative rods and staphylococci; may be used instead of kanamycin against penicillin-resistant staphylococci and *E. coli* strains and *Pseudomonas aeruginosa*. May cause ototoxicity and nephrotoxicity. Need to follow serum levels. Must never be given as IV push. Must be given over at least 30–60 minutes. In presence of oliguria or anuria, dose must be decreased or discontinued. In infants less than 1000 g or 29 weeks, lower dosage 2.5–3 mg/kg/day. Monitor serum levels before administration of second dose. Peak 5–12 μg/mL Trough 0.5–1 μg/mL
Methicillin	25–50 mg/dose 50–100 mg/kg/day	Every 12 hours* Every 6–8 hours†	IM or IV	Effective against penicillinase-resistant staphylococci. Monitor CBC and UA. Slow IV push.
Nafcillin	25–50 mg/kg 50–100 mg/kg/day	Every 8–12 hours* Every 6–8 hours†	IM or IV	Effective against penicillinase-resistant staphylococci. Caution in presence of jaundice.
Penicillin G (aqueous crystalline)	25,000–50,000 IU/kg 50,000–125,000, up to 400,000 IU/kg/day for group B strep meningitis IU/kg/da	Every 12 hours* Every 8 hours†	IM or IV	Initial sepsis therapy effective against most gram-positive microorganisms except resistant staphylococci; can cause heart block in infants.
Vancomycin	10–20 mg/kg 30 mg/kg/day	Every 12–24 hours*† Every 8 hours†	IV	Effective for methicillin-resistant strains (*Staphylococcus epidermis*); must be administered by slow intravenous infusion to avoid prolonged cutaneous eruption. For smaller infants, < 1200 g, < 29 weeks, smaller dosages and longer intervals between doses. Nephrotoxic, especially in combination with aminoglycosides. Slow IV infusion over at least 60 minutes. Peak 25–40 μg/mL Trough 5–10 μg/mL

*Up to 7 days of age. †Greater than 7 days of age. ‡Dependent on GA.

The infusion of antibiotics at home by skilled RNs facilitates parent-infant bonding while meeting the ongoing healthcare needs of the infant.

Provision of Supportive Care

In addition to antibiotic therapy, physiologic supportive care is essential in caring for a septic infant. The nurse should carry out the following:

- Observe for resolution of symptoms or development of other symptoms of sepsis.
- Maintain a neutral thermal environment with accurate regulation of humidity and oxygen administration.
- Provide respiratory support: Administer oxygen and observe and monitor respiratory effort.
- Provide cardiovascular support: Observe and monitor pulse and blood pressure; observe for hyperbilirubinemia, anemia, and hemorrhagic symptoms.
- Provide adequate calories, because oral feedings may be discontinued due to increased mucus, abdominal distention, vomiting, or aspiration.
- Provide fluids and electrolytes to maintain homeostasis. Monitor weight changes, urine output, and urine specific gravity.
- Observe for the development of hypoglycemia, hyperglycemia, acidosis, hyponatremia, and hypocalcemia.

Restricting parental visits has not been shown to have any effect on the rate of infection and may be harmful to the newborn's psychologic development. With instruction and guidance from the nurse, both parents should be allowed to handle the baby and participate in daily care. Support to the parents is crucial. They need to be informed of the newborn's prognosis as treatment continues and to be involved in care as much as possible. They also need to understand how infection is transmitted.

Evaluation

Expected outcomes of nursing care include the following:

- The risks for development of sepsis are identified early, and immediate action is taken to minimize the development of the illness.
- Appropriate use of aseptic technique protects the newborn from further exposure to illness.
- The baby's symptoms are relieved, and the infection is treated.
- The parents verbalize their concerns about their baby's illness and understand the rationale behind the management of their newborn.

Care of the Family with Birth of an At-Risk Newborn

The birth of a preterm or ill infant or an infant with a congenital anomaly is a serious crisis situation for a family. Throughout the pregnancy, both parents, together and separately, have felt excitement, experienced thoughts of acceptance, and pictured what their baby would look like. Both parents have wished for a perfect baby and feared a damaged, unhealthy one. Each parent and family member must accept and adjust when the fantasized fears become reality.

Parental Responses

Acute *grief reactions* follow the loss of the perfect baby the parents have fantasized. In the case of a preterm birth, the mother is denied the last few weeks of pregnancy that seem to prepare her psychologically for the stress of birth and the attachment process. Attachment at this time is fragile, and interruption of the process by separation can affect the future mother-child relationship. Parents express grief as shock and disbelief, denial of reality, anger toward self and others, guilt, blame, and concern for the future. Self-esteem and feelings of self-worth are jeopardized.

Feelings of guilt and failure often plague mothers of preterm newborns. They may ask themselves, "Why did labor start? What did I do (or not do)?" A woman may have guilt fantasies and wonder what she may have done to cause the early labor: "Was it because I carried three loads of wash up from the basement?" "Am I being punished for something I did in the past—even in childhood?"

Honest, simple, and positive facts can be shared: "Your baby is alive"; "Your baby is a girl"; "Your baby has a strong heartbeat but needs some help with breathing"; "Your baby is alive but needs some special care right now"; "The pediatrician/nurse practitioner is helping your baby now and will talk with you soon." The information that nurses share with parents must always be honest data that nurses can observe and document. Nurses should not make promises that they cannot fulfill and should refrain from offering empty reassurances that everything will be all right.

The period of waiting between suspicion and confirmation of abnormality or dysfunction is a very anxious one for parents because it is difficult, if not impossible, to begin attachment to the infant if the newborn's future is questionable. During the "not knowing period," parents need support and acknowledgment that this is an anxious time and must be kept informed about efforts to gather additional data and maintain the infant's livelihood. It is helpful to tell both parents about the problem at the same time with the baby present. An honest discussion of the problem and anticipatory management at the earliest possible time by health professionals help the parents (1) maintain trust in the physician and nurse, (2) appreciate the reality of the situation by dispelling fantasy and misconception, (3) begin the grieving process, and (4) mobilize internal and external support.

Nurses need to be aware that anger is a universal response and that it is best directed outward because holding it in check requires great energy, which is diverted away from grieving and physical recovery from pregnancy and giving birth. Anger may be directed unjustifiably at the physician and/or nurse, at the food, at nursing care, or at hospital regulations and routines. Parents rarely show anger with the baby and such responses can precipitate guilt feelings.

Although reactions and steps of attachment are altered by the birth of these infants, a healthy parent-child relationship can occur. Kaplan and Mason (1974) identified four psychologic tasks as essential for coping with the stress of an at-risk newborn and for providing a basis for the maternal-infant relationship:

1. Anticipatory grief as a psychologic preparation for possible loss of the child while still hoping for his or her survival.
2. Acknowledgment of maternal failure to produce a term or perfect newborn expressed as anticipatory grief and depression and lasting until the chances of survival seem secure.
3. Resumption of the process of relating to the infant, which was interrupted by the threat of nonsurvival. This task may be impaired by a continuous threat of death or abnormality, and the mother may be slow in her response of hope for the infant's survival.
4. Understanding of the special needs and growth patterns of the at-risk newborn, which are temporary and yield to normal patterns.

Solnit and Stark (1961) postulated that grief and mourning of the loss of the loved object—the idealized child—mark parental reactions to an infant with abnormalities. Grief work, the emotional reaction to significant loss, must occur before adequate attachment to the actual baby is possible. Parental detachment precedes parental attachment. The parents must first grieve the loss of the wished-for perfect child, and then must adopt the imperfect child as the new love object.

Parental responses to an infant with health problems may also be viewed as a five-stage process (Klaus & Kennell, 1982):

1. Shock is felt at the reality of the birth of this baby. This stage may be characterized by forgetfulness, amnesia of the situation, and a feeling of desperation.
2. There is denial (disbelief) of the reality that the child is defective. This stage is exemplified by assertions such as, "It didn't really happen!" "There has been a mistake; it's someone else's baby."
3. Depression over the reality of the situation and a corresponding grief reaction follows acceptance of the situation. This stage is characterized by much crying and sadness. Anger about the reality of the situation may also occur at this stage. A projection of blame on others or on self and feelings of "why me?" are characteristic of this stage.
4. Equilibrium and acceptance are characteristic of a decrease in the emotional reactions of the parents. This stage is variable and may be prolonged because of continuing threat to the infant's survival. Some parents experience chronic sorrow in relation to their child.
5. Reorganization of the family is necessary to deal with the child's problems. Mutual support of the parents facilitates this process, but the crisis of the situation may precipitate alienation between the mother and father.

Developmental Consequences

The baby who is born prematurely, is ill, or has a malformation or disorder is at risk in emotional and intellectual, as well as physical, development. The risk is directly proportional to the seriousness of the problem and the length of treatment.

Medical, surgical, and technical advances in recent years have been responsible for salvaging increasing numbers of preterm and ill newborns. However, the necessary physical separation of family and infant and the tremendous emotional and financial burdens adversely affect the parent-child relationship. A considerable percentage of these children have been rescued only to be emotionally or physically battered by the parents. The most recent trend in many hospitals is to involve the parents with the newborn early, repeatedly, and over protracted periods of time. Early and continued involvement may only mean opportunities to look at or stroke the baby (Figure 33–15 •). Later, when the mother's and baby's conditions warrant it, the mother should participate in her baby's care (to the extent she is willing) and in planning for the future. This type of involvement facilitates early bonding, attachment, and emotional investment. The parents need a sense of personal success, self-worth, self-esteem, and confidence from the knowledge that they can cope with the situation. This atmosphere aids the baby, as well—the child may escape abuse and may instead be assisted toward self-actualization.

The parents must have a clear picture of the reality of the handicap and the types of developmental hurdles ahead. Unexpected behaviors and responses from the baby due to his or her defect or disorder can be upsetting and frightening. For example, parents may find it difficult to cope with a baby's lack of motor or social responsiveness, interpreting this as rejection. The parents may in return respond with rejection, and an unfortunate cycle is begun.

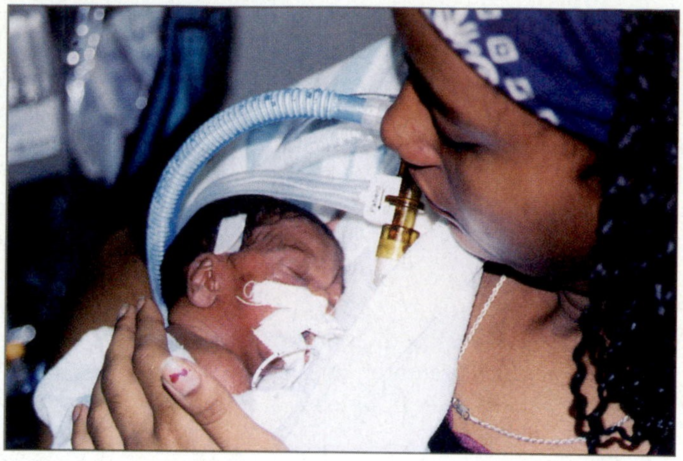

Figure 33–15 • Mother of a 26 weeks' gestational age infant with respiratory distress syndrome on a ventilator is getting acquainted with her baby. Physical contact is vital to the bonding process and should be encouraged whenever possible.
SOURCE: Courtesy of Lisa Smith-Pedersen, RNC, MSN, NNP.

The demands of care of the child and disputes regarding management or behavior stress family relationships. A variety of behavioral patterns may occur. For example, one or more members of the family may make a scapegoat of the child. Another may become the youngster's champion to the exclusion of others. One or the other spouse may feel pushed aside or denied attention and thus may withdraw or leave the family unit. Parents or siblings may feel that their own needs (schooling, material goods, freedom of movement) are being set aside while all assets (financial and other) go to support the one child's needs.

The entire multidisciplinary team may need to pool their resources and expertise to help parents of children born with problems or disorders so that both parents and children can thrive.

NURSING CARE MANAGEMENT

Nursing Assessment and Diagnosis

Development of a nurse-family relationship facilitates information gathering in areas of concern. A concurrent illness of the mother or other family members or other concurrent stress (lack of hospitalization insurance, loss of job, age of parents) may alter the family response to the baby. Feelings of apprehension, guilt, failure, and grief that are verbally or nonverbally expressed are important aspects of the nursing history. These observations enable all professionals to be aware of the parental state, coping behaviors, and readiness for attachment, bonding, and caretaking. Appropriate nursing observations while interviewing and relating to the family may include:

1. *Level of understanding.* Observations concerning the family's ability to assimilate information given and to ask appropriate questions; the need for constant repetition of "the same" information
2. *Behavioral responses.* Appropriateness of behavior in relation to information given; lack of response; "flat" affect
3. *Difficulties with communication.* Deafness (reads lips only); blindness; dysphasia; unable to understand English
4. *Paternal and maternal education level.* For example: parents unable to read or write; only eighth grade completed; mother an MD, RN, or PhD; and so on

Documentation of such information, obtained by the nurse through continuing contact and development of a therapeutic family relationship, enables all professionals to understand and use the nursing history in providing continuous individual care.

Visiting and caregiving patterns indicate the level or lack of parental attachment. A record of visits, caretaking procedures, affect (in relating to the newborn), and telephone calls from parents is essential. Serial observations, rather than just isolated instances of concern, must be obtained. Grant (1978) developed a conceptual framework depicting adaptive and maladaptive responses to parenting of a preterm or less-than-perfect infant (Figure 33–16 ●). If a pattern of distancing behaviors evolves, the nurse should institute appropriate

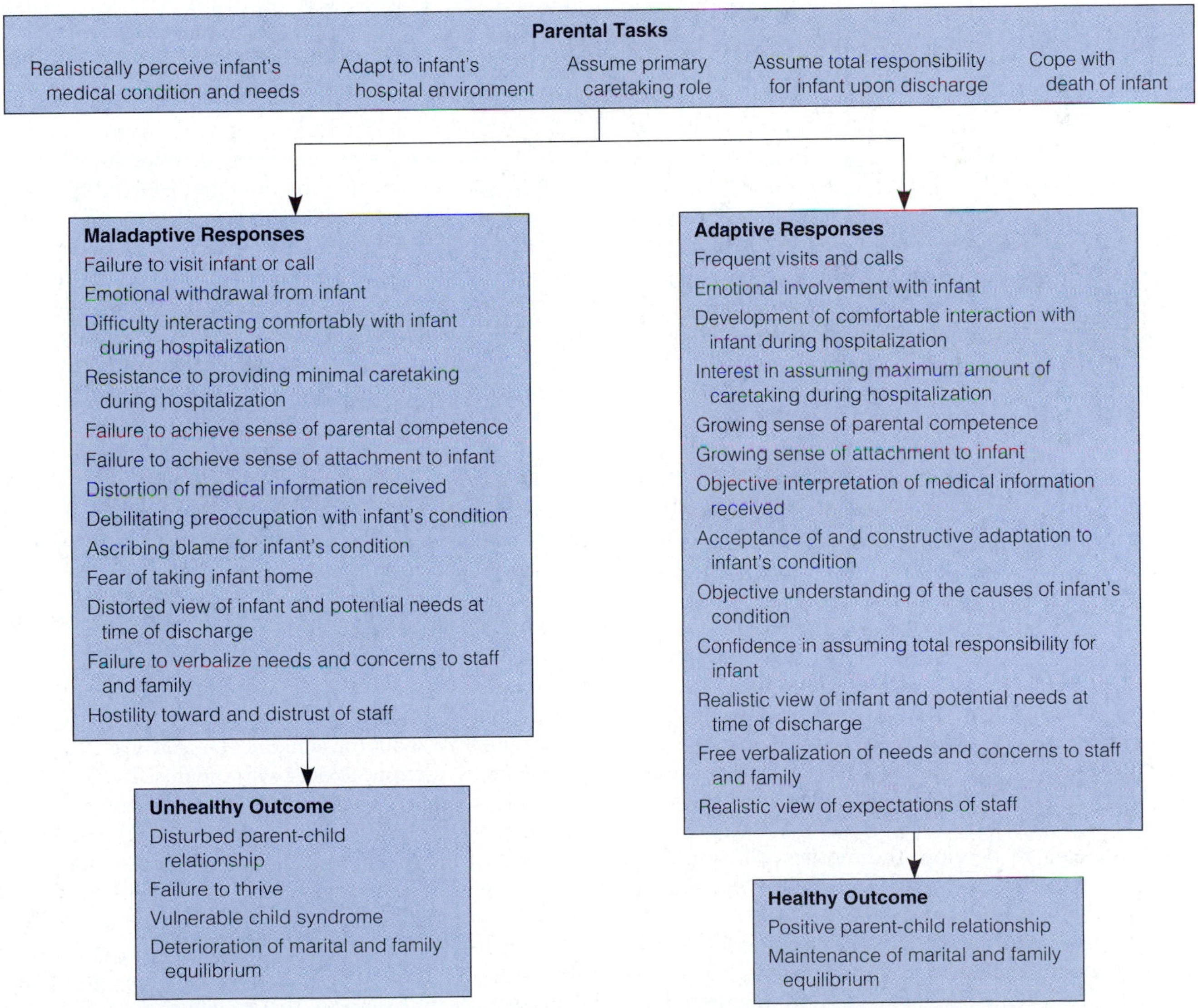

Figure 33–16 ● Maladaptive and adaptive parental responses during crisis period, showing unhealthy and healthy outcomes.
SOURCE: Grant, P. (1978). Psychological needs of families of high-risk infants. *Family & Community Health,* 11, Fig. 1. Philadelphia: Lippincott Williams & Wilkins.

intervention. Follow-up studies have found that a statistically significant number of preterm, sick, and congenitally defective infants suffer from failure to thrive, battering, or other disorders of parenting. Early detection and intervention may prevent these aberrations in parenting behaviors from leading to irreparable damage or death.

Nursing diagnoses that may apply to the family of a newborn at risk include the following:

- ***Dysfunctional Grieving*** related to loss of idealized newborn
- ***Fear*** related to emotional involvement with an at-risk newborn
- ***Altered Parenting*** related to impaired bonding secondary to feelings of inadequacy about caretaking activities

Nursing Plan and Implementation

Hospital-Based Nursing Care

In their sensitive and vulnerable state, parents are acutely perceptive about others' responses and reactions (particularly nonverbal) to the child. Parents can be expected to identify with the responses of others. Therefore, it is imperative that medical and nursing staff be fully aware of their feelings and come to terms with those feelings so that they are comfortable and at ease with the baby and the grieving family.

Nurses may feel uncomfortable not knowing what to say to parents or may fear confronting their own feelings as well as those of the parents. Each nurse must work out personal reactions with instructors, peers, clergy, parents, or significant others. It is helpful to have a stockpile of therapeutic questions and statements to initiate meaningful dialog with parents. Opening statements can be as follows: "You must be wondering what could have caused this"; "Are you thinking that you (or someone else) may have done something?"; "How can I help?"; "Go ahead and cry. It's worth crying about"; or "Are you wondering how you are going to manage?" Avoid statements such as, "It could have been worse"; "It's God's will"; "You have other children"; "You are still young and can have more"; and "I understand how you feel." This child is important now.

Support of Parents in Initial Viewing of the Newborn

Before parents see their child, the nurse must prepare them for the visit. It is important that a positive, realistic attitude regarding the infant, rather than a pessimistic one, be presented to the parents. An overly negative, fatalistic attitude further alienates the parents from their infant and retards attachment behaviors. In this case, instead of allowing attachment and bonding to develop, the mother will begin the process of grieving for the loss of her infant. Once started, this process is very difficult to reverse.

In preparing parents for the first view of their infant, the professional should have already looked at the baby. The nurse should prepare the parents to see both the deviations and the normal aspects of their infant. All infants exhibit strengths as well as deficiencies. The nurse may say, "Your baby is small, about the length of my two hands. She weighs 2 lb 3 oz but is very active and cries when we disturb her. She is having some difficulty breathing but is breathing without assistance and on only 35% oxygen and room air is 21%."

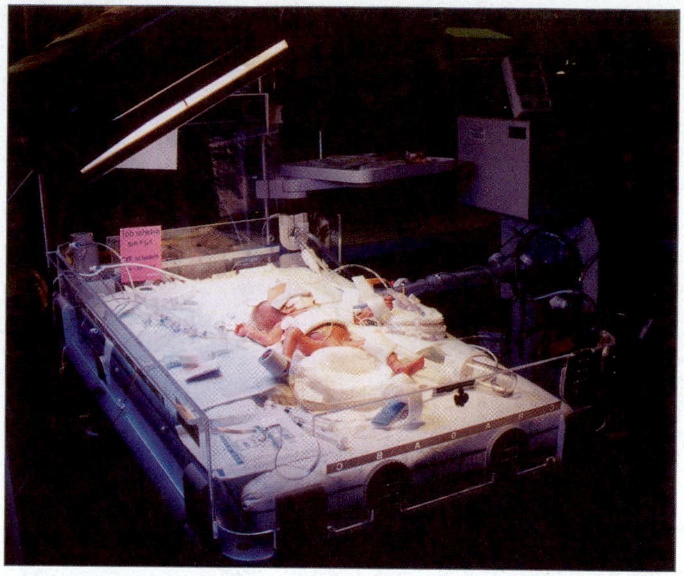

Figure 33–17 • This 25 weeks' gestational age infant with respiratory distress syndrome may be frightening for her parents to see for the first time due to the technology that is attached to her.
SOURCE: Courtesy of Lisa Smith-Pedersen, RNC, MSN, NNP.

The equipment being used for the at-risk newborn and its purpose should be described before the parents enter the intensive care unit. Many NICUs have booklets for parents to read before entering the unit. Through explanations and pictures, the parents can be better prepared to deal with the feelings they may experience when they see their infant for the first time (Figure 33-17 •).

On entering the unit, parents may be overwhelmed by the sounds of monitors, alarms, and respirators, as well as by the unfamiliar language and "foreign" atmosphere. Preparing the parents by having the same healthcare professional(s) accompany them to the unit can be reassuring. The primary nurse and physician caring for the newborn should be with the parents when they first visit the baby. Parental reactions vary, but there is usually an element of initial shock. Providing them with chairs and time to regain composure will assist the parents. Slow, complete, and simple explanations—first about the infant and then about the equipment—allay fear and anxiety.

As parents attempt to deal with the initial stages of shock and grief, they may fail to grasp new information. The parents may need repeated explanations about the procedures, equipment, and the infant's condition on subsequent visits.

Many physicians show parents "before" and "after" photographs of conditions requiring surgical intervention. Parents also may benefit from meeting other parents who have faced the same problem through a parental support group or organization that is specific to that problem. Specialists (plastic surgeons, perinatal clinic nurse specialists, neurosurgeons, orthopedists, oral surgeons, dentists, and rehabilitation therapists) can be reassuring and supportive of parents in their short- and long-term goals. However, these types of interventions must be carefully timed to the readiness of the parents.

Concern about the infant's physical appearance is common, yet may remain unvoiced. Parents may express such concerns as, "He looks so small and red—like a drowned rat." "Why do her genitals look so abnormal?" "Will that awful looking mouth [cleft lip and palate] ever be normal?" Such questions need to be anticipated by the nurse and addressed. Use of pictures, such as of an infant after cleft lip repair, may be reassuring to doubting parents. Knowledge of the development of a "normal" preterm infant will allow the nurse to make reassuring statements such as "The baby's skin may look very red and transparent with lots of visible veins, but it is normal for her maturity. As she grows, subcutaneous fat will be laid down, and these superficial veins will begin to disappear."

The tone of the NICU is set by the nursing staff. Development of a safe, trusting environment depends on viewing the parents as essential caregivers, not as visitors or nuisances in the unit. It is important to provide parents privacy when needed and easy access to staff and facilities. An uncrowded and welcoming atmosphere lets parents know, "You are welcome here." However, even in crowded physical surroundings an attitude of openness and trust can be conveyed by the nursing staff.

A trusting relationship is essential for collaborative efforts in caring for the infant. Nurses must therapeutically use their own responses to relate on a one-to-one basis with the parents. Each individual has different needs, different ways of adapting to crisis, and different means of support. Professionals must use techniques that are real and spontaneous to them and avoid adopting words or actions that are foreign to them. Nurses must also gauge their interventions to match the parents' pace and needs.

Nurses show concern and support by planning time to spend with the parents, by being psychologically as well as physically present, by encouraging open discussion and grieving, by repetitious explanations (as necessary), by providing privacy as needed, and by encouraging contact with the newborn. Identifying and clarifying feelings and fears decrease distortions in perception, thinking, and feeling. Nurses invest the baby with value in the eyes of the parents when they provide meticulous care to the newborn, talk and coo (especially in the face-to-face position) while holding or providing care to the newborn, refer to the child by gender or name, and relate the newborn's activities ("He took a whole ounce of formula"; "She took hold of the blanket and just wouldn't let go"). Nurses should note the "normal" characteristics and capabilities of each newborn as well as the newborn's needs. The nurse should also learn the baby's name and refer to him or her by name.

Facilitation of Attachment if Neonatal Transport Occurs

In the event that a small hospital may not be able to care for a sick infant, transport to a regional referral center may be necessary. These centers may be as far as 500 miles from the parents' community; it is therefore essential that the mother see and touch her infant before the infant is transported.

Bringing the mother to the nursery or taking the infant in a warmed transport incubator to the mother's bedside will allow her to see the infant before transportation to the center. When the infant reaches the referral center, a staff member should call the parents with information about the infant's condition during transport, safe arrival at the center, and present condition.

Support of parents, with explanations from the professional staff, is crucial. Occasionally, the mother may be unable to see the infant prior to transport, for example, if she is still under general anesthesia or experiencing postpartum complications. In these cases, the infant should be photographed before transport. The picture should be given to the mother, along with an explanation of the infant's condition, present problems, and a detailed description of the infant's characteristics, to facilitate the attachment process until the mother can visit. An additional photograph is also helpful for the father to share with siblings or the extended family. With the increased attention to improved fetal outcome, prenatal maternal transports, rather than neonatal transports, are occurring more frequently. This practice gives the mother of an at-risk infant the opportunity to visit and care for her infant during the early postpartal period.

Promotion of Touching and Parental Caretaking

Parents visiting a small or sick infant may need several visits to become comfortable and confident in their abilities to touch the infant without injuring her or him. Barriers such as incubators, incisions, monitor electrodes, and tubes may delay the mother's confidence. Knowledge of this "normal" delay in touching behavior will enable the nurse to understand parental behavior.

Klaus and Kennell (1982) found a significant difference in the amount of eye contact and touching behaviors of mothers of normal newborns and mothers of preterm infants. Whereas mothers of normal newborns progress within minutes to palm contact of the infant's trunk, the mother of a preterm infant is slower to progress from fingertip to palm contact and from the extremities to the trunk. The progression to palm contact with the infant's trunk may take several visits to the nursery.

Through support, reassurance, and encouragement, the nurse can facilitate the mother's positive feelings about her ability and her importance to her infant. Touching facilitates "getting to know" the infant and thus establishes a bond with the infant. Touching as well as seeing the infant helps the mother to realize the "normals" and potentials of her baby (Figure 33–18 •).

The nurse can also encourage parents to meet their newborn's need for stimulation. Stroking, rocking, cuddling, singing, and talking should be an integral part of the parents' caretaking responsibilities. Bonding can be facilitated by encouraging parents to visit and become involved in their baby's care (Figure 33–19 •). When visiting is impossible, the parents should feel free to phone whenever they wish to receive information about their baby. A warm receptive

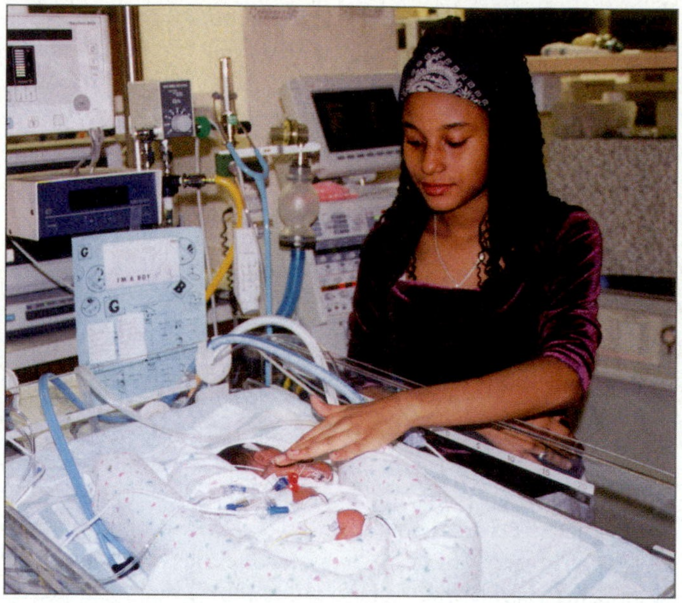

Figure 33–18 • Mother of this 26 weeks' gestational age 600-g baby begins attachment through fingertip touch.
SOURCE: Courtesy of Lisa Smith-Pedersen, RNC, MSN, NNP.

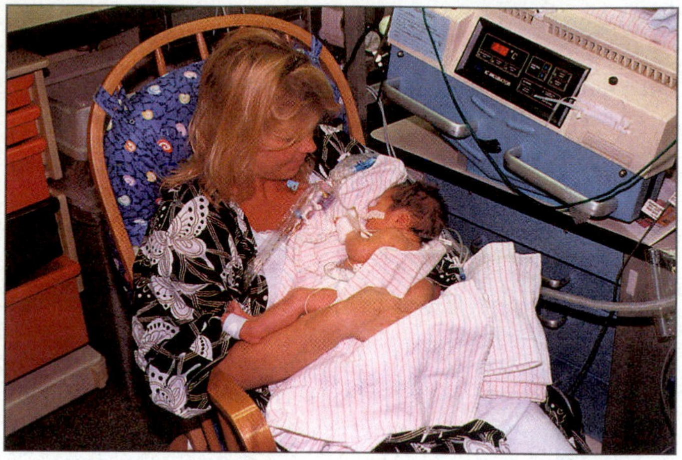

Figure 33–19 • This mother of a 35 weeks' gestational age infant with respiratory distress syndrome is spending time with her newborn and meeting the baby's need for cuddling.
SOURCE: Courtesy of Carol Harrigan, RNC, MSN, NNP.

attitude on the part of the nurse is very supportive. A study by Riper (2001) that examined and described the relationship between healthcare providers and the mothers of preterm newborns in the NICU reached the conclusion that the mothers who were able to develop a positive rapport with the staff viewed the hospital experience as positive. The mothers experienced a level of comfort with the staff and were more likely to enlist the staff for help.

The variety of equipment needed for life support is hardly conducive to anxiety-free caretaking by the parents. However, even the sickest infant may be cared for, if only in a small way, by the parents. As a facilitator of parental caretaking, the nurse should promote the parents' success. Demonstration and explanation, followed by support of the parents in initial caretaking behaviors, positively reinforce this behavior. Changing the infant's diaper, giving their infant skin care or oral care, or helping the nurse turn the infant may at first be anxiety provoking for the parents, but they will become more comfortable and confident in caretaking and receive satisfaction from the baby's reactions and their ability "to do something." Complimenting the parent's competence in caretaking also increases their self-esteem, which has received recent "blows" of guilt and failure. It is vitally important that the parents never be given a task if there is any possibility they will not be able to accomplish it. Cues that the parents are ready to become involved with the child's care include their reference to the baby by name and their questioning as to amount of feeding taken, sleeping patterns, appearance today, and the like (Loo, Espinosa, Tyler & Howard, 2003).

Parents may feel inadequate or guilty when they do not feel love for their baby. For example, a mother of a girl born with a severe cleft lip and palate said, "God help me. I can't stand looking at her. I wish she weren't mine. What a horrid thing to say, but I just can't." She could not bring herself to hold or touch the infant prior to cleft lip repair. She needed considerable reassurance in a nonjudgmental and accepting atmosphere before she could admit her feelings and—after surgery—hold her infant.

Occasionally, parents may become overprotective and overoptimistic shortly after the baby's birth. The nurse should accept this behavior but continue to remind the parents that it is okay and natural to feel disappointment, a sense of failure, helplessness, or anger. The overprotectiveness and overoptimism are defense mechanisms. To deny the negative feelings only entrenches them further, delays their resolution, and delays realistic planning.

Often mothers of high-risk infants have ambivalent feelings toward the nurse. As the mother watches the nurse competently perform the caretaking tasks, she feels both grateful for the nurse's abilities and expertise and jealous of the nurse's ability to care for her infant (Bruns & McCollum, 2002). These feelings may be acted out in criticism of the care being received by the infant, manipulation of staff, or personal guilt. Instead of fostering (by silence) these inferiority feelings within mothers, nurses should recognize such feelings and intervene appropriately to enhance mother-infant attachment. The nurse needs to deal with ambivalent feelings that contribute to a competitive atmosphere. For example, the nurse should avoid making unfavorable comparisons between the baby's response to parental caretaking and the child's responses to the nurses. During a quiet time, it may help for the nurse to encourage the parents to talk about their hopes and fears and to facilitate their involvement in parent groups.

Verbalizations by the nurse that improve parental self-esteem are essential and easily shared. The nurse can point out that, in addition to physiologic use, breast milk is important because of the emotional investment of the mother. Pumping, storing, labeling, and delivering quantities of breast milk is time-consuming and a "labor of love" for mothers. Positive remarks regarding breast milk reinforce the ma-

RESEARCH IN PRACTICE
Maternal Needs and Priorities in the NICU

What is this study about? It is important to involve parents in the care of a premature infant, but this is often difficult to accomplish in the neonatal intensive care unit (NICU) environment. The birth of an ill child is stressful for the parents. Past studies have shown that there are often barriers to effective nurse-parent interactions when a child is in the NICU. This study investigated the priorities mothers report about their needs during this stressful period.

How was this study done? A structured self-reporting data collection procedure was used to gather data from 209 mothers who had infants in an NICU. Data were collected for 2 years. A self-assessment called the "Critical Care Maternal Needs Inventory" was used to collect data about needs. Factor analysis was used to group the needs into meaningful categories. After classifying the needs, the researchers then used a second sample of mothers to rank them in order of importance.

What were the results of the study? Clear priorities emerged during analysis. Ninety-three percent of the mothers placed a high priority on the need for accurate infant-related information. Communication with professionals was the second most frequent priority. Maternal needs, although altruistically rated lower than infant-related needs, reflected a desire for social and emotional support.

What additional questions might I have? How did the staff nurses in the NICU rate these needs? Would nurse ratings be different than parental ratings? Were the nurses able to accurately predict the kinds of needs the parents have? What are the obstacles that prevent the NICU staff nurse from meeting these needs?

How can I use this study? Providing infant-related information to parents of babies in the NICU should be a priority. Families are in crisis during this stressful time, and an appropriate focus on the infant's needs should include efforts to communicate clearly and listen carefully. Opportunities for social and emotional support are also ways to address the needs of the mother.

Source: Bialoskurski, M., Cox, D., & Wiggins, R. (2002). The relationship between maternal needs and priorities in a neonatal intensive care environment. *Journal of Advanced Nursing, 37*(1), 62–69.

ternal behavior of caretaking and providing for her infant: "Breast milk is something that only you can give your baby" or "You really have brought a lot of milk today" or "Even small amounts of milk are important, and look how rich it is."

If the infant begins to gain weight while being fed breast milk, it is important to point this out to the mother. Parents should also be advised that initial weight loss with beginning nipple feedings is common because of the increased energy expended when the infant begins active rather than passive nutritional intake.

Provision of care by the parents is appropriate even for a very sick infant who is likely to die. It has been found that detachment is easier after attachment because the parents are comforted by the knowledge that they did all they could for their child while he or she was alive.

Facilitation of Family Adjustment

During crisis, maintaining interpersonal relationships is difficult. Yet in a newborn intensive care area, the parents are expected to relate to many different care providers. It is important that parents have as few professionals as possible relaying information to them. A primary nurse should coordinate and provide continuity in the information given to parents. Care providers are individuals and thus will use different terms, inflections, and attitudes. These subtle differences are monumental to parents and only confuse, confound, and produce anxiety. The transfer of the baby from the NICU to a step-down unit or transport back to the home hospital is very anxiety producing for the parents because they must now deal with new healthcare professionals. The nurse not only functions as a liaison between the parents and the wide variety of professionals interacting with the infant and parents, but also offers clarification, explanation, interpretation of information, and support to the parents.

The nurse should encourage the parents to deal with the crisis with help from their support system. The support system attempts to meet the emotional needs and provide support for the family members in crisis and stress situations. Biologic kinship is not the only valid criterion for a support system; an emotional kinship is the most important factor. In our mobile society of isolated nuclear families, the support system may be a next-door neighbor, a best friend, or perhaps a schoolmate. The nurse must search out the significant others in the lives of the parents and help them understand the problems so that they can be a constant parental support.

The impact of the crisis on the family is individual and varied. The nurse obtains information about the family's ability to adapt to the situation through the relationship with the family. To institute appropriate interventions, the nurse should view the birth of the infant (normal newborn, preterm infant, infant with illness or congenital anomaly) as defined by the family.

Because the family is a unit composed of individuals who must deal with the situation, it is important to encourage open intrafamily communication. The nurse should discourage the family from keeping secrets from one another, especially between spouses, because secrets undermine the trust of their relationship. Well-meaning rationales such as, "I want to protect her," "I don't want him to worry about it," and so on, can be destructive to open communication and to the basic element of a relationship—trust.

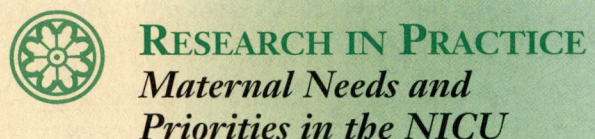

The nurse should encourage open communication among family members, particularly between spouses. Open communication is especially important when the mother is hospitalized apart from the infant. The first person to visit the infant relays information regarding the infant's care and condition to the mother and family. In this situation, the mother has had minimal contact, if any, with her infant. Because of her anxiety and isolation, she may mistrust all those who provide information (the nurse, physician, or extended family) until she can see the infant for herself. This can put tremendous stress on the relationship between family members. The parents (and family) should be given information together. This practice helps overcome misunderstandings and misinterpretations and promotes mutual "working through" of problems.

The nurse should encourage the entire family—siblings as well as extended relatives—to visit and receive information about the baby. Methods of intervention in assisting the family to cope with the situation include providing support, confronting the crisis, and helping the family understand the reality. Support, explanations, and the helping role must extend to the kin network, as well as to the nuclear family, to aid them in communication and support ties with the nuclear family.

The needs of siblings should not be overlooked. They have been looking forward to the new baby, and they too suffer a degree of loss. Young children may react with hostility and older ones with shame at the birth of an infant with an anomaly. Both reactions make them feel guilty. Parents, preoccupied with working through their own feelings, often cannot give the other children the attention and support they need. Sometimes another child becomes the focus of family tension. Anxiety thus directed can take the form of finding fault or of overconcern. This is a form of denial; the parents cannot face the real worry—the infant at risk. After assessing the situation, the observant nurse could see to it that another family member or friend step in and give the needed support to the siblings of the affected baby.

The nurse must respect and facilitate the desires and needs of the individuals involved; differences are tolerable and should be able to exist side by side. The nurse can easily elicit the parents' feelings and the meaning of this experience to them by asking, "How are you doing?" The emphasis is on "you," and the interest must be sincere. Parents from minority cultures must deal with language barriers and cultural differences that can make feelings of isolation and uncertainly more acute (Bracht, Kandankery, Nodwell, & Stade, 2002). Feelings of isolation and uncertainty influence not only the parent's emotional responses to the ill newborn, but also the utilization of services and their interaction with health professionals. Hospital cultural interpreters programs can assist families with interactions with staff, provide translation during family meetings and multidisciplinary family conferences, and in parent support groups (Bracht et al., 2002).

Families with children in the NICU become friends and support one another. To encourage the development of these friendships and to provide support, many units have established parent groups. The core of the groups consists of parents who previously have had an infant in the intensive care unit. Most groups make contact with families within a day or two of the infant's admission to the unit, either through phone calls or visits to the hospital. Early one-on-one parent contacts help families work through their feelings better than discussion groups. This personalized method gives the grieving parents an opportunity to share personal feelings about the pregnancy, labor, and birth and their "different from expected" infant with others who have experienced the same feelings and with whom they can identify.

Community-Based Nursing Care

Predischarge planning begins once the infant's condition becomes stable and indications suggest the newborn will survive (AAP Committee on Fetus and Newborn and American College of Obstetricians and Gynecologists, ACOG) (2002). NICU nursing staff is the fulcrum for aiding in the transition of high-risk infants from the intensive care unit to the home. Effective open communication with the families during the entire discharge-planning phase of care empowers the families to assume the role of primary caregiver for their children (Allen, Donohue, & Porter, 2002). Adequate predischarge teaching will help the parents transform their feelings of inadequacy and competition with the nurse into feelings of self-assurance and attachment. Cobedding of twins allows for clustering of care and facilitates parents' ability to spend time with both of their children (Figure 33–20 •). From the beginning, the

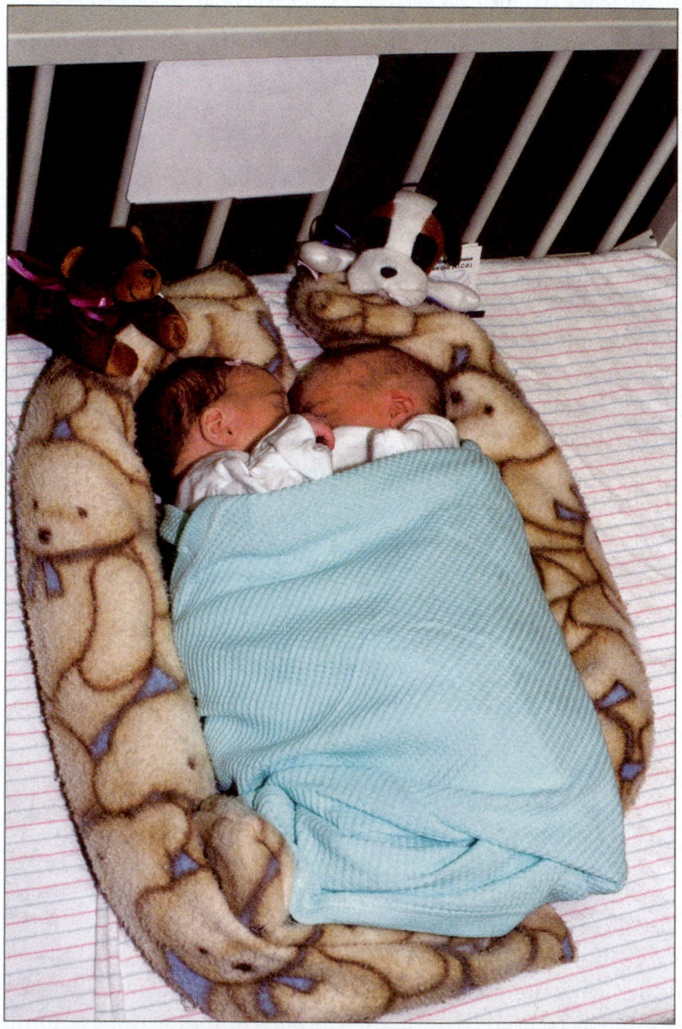

Figure 33–20 • Cobedding of twins facilitates delivery of care and parent interaction with healthcare members.
SOURCE: Courtesy of Carol Harrigan, RNC, MSN, NNP.

COMPLEMENTARY AND ALTERNATIVE THERAPIES

COMPLEMENTARY AND ALTERNATIVE THERAPIES IN THE NICU

As NICUs have become more and more "developmentally" friendly, complementary and alternative therapies have become an adjunct to that nurturing environment.

Cobedding of stable twins and higher order multiples replicates the closeness of the in utero environment whereby the siblings are placed together in the same incubator or crib to maintain physical contact (see Figure 33–20). Clustering of care provided by the bedside nurse is a true advantage to cobedding. This in turn proves beneficial to the parents because they have interactions with fewer nurses and other members of the health-care team. In addition, the parents can care for and visit with all the infants at one time (Lutes & Altimier 2001). Discharge teaching, therefore, is easily facilitated. Cobedding is also a strategy to maximize the synchronization of sleep-wake cycles (Lutes & Altimier 2001).

parents should be taught about their infant's special needs and growth patterns (Sydnor-Greenberg & Dokken, 2000). This teaching and involvement are best facilitated by a nurse who has been familiar with the infant and family over a period of time and who has developed a comfortable and supportive relationship with them.

The nurse's responsibility is to provide home care instructions in an optimal environment for parental learning. Learning should take place over time, to avoid the necessity of bombarding the parents with instructions in the day or hour before discharge. Parents often enjoy doing minimal caretaking tasks with gradual expansion of their role.

Many intensive care units provide facilities for parents to room-in with their infants for a few days before discharge. This allows parents a degree of independence in the care of their infant with the security of nursing help nearby. This practice is particularly helpful for anxious parents, parents who have not had the opportunity to spend extended time with their infant, or parents who will be giving complex physical care at home, such as tracheostomy care.

Alternatively, use of a *transitional care center (TCC)* also allows the parents to master caring for their at-risk newborn prior to discharge. TCCs shorten the length of hospitalization and decrease readmission rates (Allen, Donohue, & Porter, 2002). The families are able to interact with the staff while preparing for discharge and gradually transition to sole caretakers of their medically complex high-risk infant.

The basic elements of discharge and home care instruction are as follows:

1. Teach parents routine well-baby care, such as bathing, temperature taking, formula preparation, and breastfeeding.
2. Train parents to do special procedures as needed by the newborn, such as gavage or gastrostomy feedings, tracheostomy or enterostomy care, medication administration, cardiopulmonary resuscitation (CPR), and operation of an apnea monitor. Before discharge, the parents should be as comfortable as possible with these tasks and should demonstrate independence. Written tools and instructions are useful for parents to refer to once they are home with the infant, but these should not replace participation in the infant's care.
3. Make sure that all applicable screening (metabolic, vision, hearing) tests, immunizations, and respiratory syncytial virus (RSV) prophylaxis are done prior to discharge and that all records are given to the primary care provider and parents.
4. Refer parents to community health and support organizations. The visiting nurses association, public health nurses, or social services can assist the parents in the stressful transition from hospital to home by providing the necessary home teaching and support. Some intensive care nurseries have their own parent support groups to help bridge the gap between hospital and home care. Parents can also find support from a variety of community support organizations, such as mothers of twins groups, March of Dimes Birth Defects Foundation, handicapped children services, and teen mother and child programs. Each community has numerous agencies capable of assisting the family in adapting emotionally, physically, and financially to the chronically ill infant. The nurse should be familiar with community resources and help the parents identify which agencies may benefit them.
5. Help parents recognize the growth and development needs of their infant. A developmental care program begun in the hospital can be continued at home, or parents may be referred to an infant development program in the community.
6. Arrange medical follow-up care before discharge. The infant will need to be followed up by a family pediatrician, a well-baby clinic, or a specialty clinic. The first appointment should be made before the infant is discharged from the hospital.
7. Evaluate the need for durable medical equipment for infant care (such as a respirator, oxygen, apnea monitor, feeding pump) in the home. Any extra equipment or supplies should be placed in the home before the infant's discharge.
8. Arrange for neonatal hospice for parents of the medically fragile infant as needed.

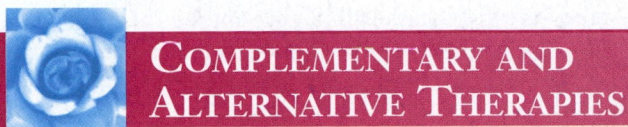

Further evaluation after the infant has gone home is useful in determining whether the crisis has been resolved satisfactorily. The parents are usually given the intensive care nursery's telephone number to call for support and advice. The staff can follow up each family with visits or telephone calls at intervals for several weeks to assess and evaluate the infant's (and parents') progress. Taylor, Klein, Minich, et al (2001) examined the families of children who were born with birth weight less than 750 g and found that the sequelae related to both health and behavioral problems of these children continue to impact on the families for years following discharge from the NICU.

Evaluation

Expected outcomes of nursing care include the following:

- The parents are able to verbalize their feelings of grief and loss.
- The parents verbalize their concerns about their baby's health problems, care needs, and potential outcome.
- The parents are able to participate in their infant's care and show attachment behaviors.

Considerations for the Nurse Who Works with At-Risk Newborns

Support cannot be given unless it can be received. Working in an emotional environment of "lots of living and lots of dying" takes its toll on staff. NICUs are among the most stressful areas in healthcare for clients, families, and nurses. Nurses bear most of the stress and largely determine the atmosphere of the NICU. The nurse's ability to cope with stress is the key to creating an emotionally healthy environment and a positive working atmosphere. The emotional needs and feelings of the staff must be recognized and dealt with to enable them to support the parents. An environment of openness to feelings and support in dealing with their own human needs and emotions is essential for staff. As caregivers, nurses may be unaware of their need to grieve for their own losses in the NICU. Nurses must also go through the grief work that parents experience. Techniques such as group meetings, individual support, and primary care nursing may assist in maintaining staff mental health.

The NICU nurses may never see the long-term results of the specialized, sensitive care they give to parents and their newborns. Their only immediate evidence of effective care may be the beginning of resolution of parental grief, discharge of a recovered thriving infant to the care of happy parents, and the beginning of reintegration of family life.

CHAPTER REVIEW

EXPLOREMEDIALINK

NCLEX review questions, case studies, and other interactive resources for this chapter can be found on the Web site at http://www.prenhall.com/olds. Click on "Chapter 33" to select the activities for this chapter.

For tutorials including animations and videos, more NCLEX review questions, and an audio glossary, access the accompanying CD-ROM in this book.

Focus Your Study

- The sick newborn—whether preterm, term, or postterm—must be managed within narrow physiologic parameters.
- These parameters (respiratory, cardiovascular, and thermal regulation) will maintain physiologic homeostasis and prevent introduction of iatrogenic stress to the already stressed infant.
- The nursing care of the newborn with special problems involves understanding normal physiology, the pathophysiology of the disease process, clinical manifestations, and supportive or corrective therapies. Only with this theoretic background can the nurse make appropriate observations concerning responses to therapy and development of complications.
- Asphyxia results in significant circulatory, respiratory, and biochemical changes in the newborn that make the successful transition to extrauterine life difficult. Asphyxia requires early identification and resuscitative management.
- Newborn conditions that commonly present with respiratory distress and require oxygen and ventilatory assistance are respiratory distress syndrome, transient tachypnea of the newborn, meconium aspiration syndrome, and persistent pulmonary hypertension.
- Management of respiratory problems can result in further respiratory compromising conditions such as pulmonary interstitial emphysema, pneumothorax, and bronchopulmonary dysplasia/chronic lung disease.

- Cold stress sets up the chain of physiologic events of hypoglycemia, pulmonary vasoconstriction, hyperbilirubinemia, respiratory distress, and metabolic acidosis.
- Nurses are responsible for early detection and initiation of treatment for hypoglycemia.
- Differentiation between pathologic and physiologic jaundice is key to early and successful intervention.
- Anemia (decreased amount of red blood cell volume) or polycythemia (excess amount) place the newborn at risk for alterations in blood flow and the oxygen-carrying capacity of the blood.
- Nursing assessment of the septic newborn involves identifying very subtle clinical signs that are also seen in other clinical disease states.
- The nurse is the facilitator for interdisciplinary communication with the parents, identifying their understanding of their infant's care and their needs for emotional support.
- Parents of at-risk newborns need support from nurses and healthcare providers to understand the special needs of their baby and to feel comfortable in an overwhelming and often unfamiliar environment.

References

Abbasi, S., Hirsch, D., Davis, J., Tolosa, J., Stouffer, N., Debbs, R., et al. (2000). Effect of single versus multiple courses of antenatal corticosteroids on maternal and neonatal outcome. *American Journal of Obstetrics and Gynecology, 182*(5), 1243–1249.

Al-Alawi, E., & Jenkins, D. (2000). Does maternal smoking increase the risk of neonatal polycythemia? *Irish Medical Journal, 93*(6), 175–176.

Allen, M. C., Donohue, P. K., & Porter, M. (2002). Follow-up of the NICU infant. In G. B. Merenstein & S. L. Gardner, *Handbook of intensive care* (5th ed., pp. 787–800). St. Louis, MO: Mosby.

American Academy of Pediatrics (AAP) Committee on Fetus and Newborn & American College of Obstetricians and Gynecologists (ACOG) committee on Obstetrics (2002). *Guidelines for perinatal care* (5th ed.). Evanston, Ill: Author.

American Academy of Pediatrics & Canadian Pediatric Society. (2002). Postnatal corticosteroids to treat or prevent chronic lung disease in preterm infants. *Pediatrics, 109*(2), 330–338.

Atkinson, S. A. (2001). Special nutritional needs for prevention of and recovery from bronchopulmonary dysplasia. *Journal of Nutrition, 131*, 942S–946S.

Blackburn, S. T. (2003). *Maternal, fetal, & neonatal physiology: A clinical perspective* (2nd ed.). St. Louis, MO: Saunders.

Bracht, M., Kandankery, A., Nodwell, S., & Stade, B. (2002). Cultural differences and parental responses to the preterm infant at risk: Strategies for supporting families. *Neonatal Network, 21*(6), 31–38.

Bruns, D. A., & Mc Collum, J. A. (2002). Partnerships between mothers and professionals in the NICU: Caregiving, information exchange, and relationships. *Neonatal Network, 21*(7), 15–23.

Carey, B., & Trotter, C. (2000). Radiology basics, Part III: TTN, MAS and neonatal pneumonia. *Neonatal Network, 19* (4), 37.

Casey, B. M., McIntire, D. D., & Leveno, K. J. (2001). The continuing value of the Apgar score for the assessment of newborn infants. *New England Journal of Medicine, 344*(7), 467–471.

Cashore, W. J. (2000). Bilirubin and jaundice in the micropremie. *Clinics in Perinatology, 27*(1), 171–178.

Clark, R. H., Kueser, T. J., Walker, M. W., Southgate, W. M., Huckaby, J. L., Perez, J. A., et al., (2000). Low-dose nitric oxide therapy for persistent pulmonary hypertension of the newborn. *Massachusetts Medical Society, 342*(7), 469–474.

Cornblath, M., & Ichord, R. (2000). Hypoglycemia in the neonate. *Seminars in Perinatology, 24*(2), 136–149.

Cowett, R. M., & Loughead, J. L. (2002). Neonatal glucose metabolism: Differential diagnoses, evaluation, and treatment of hypoglycemia, *Neonatal Network, 21*(4), 9–19.

Dargaville, P. A., South, M., & McDougall, P. N. (2001). Surfactant and surfactant inhibitors in meconium aspiration syndrome. *Journal of Pediatrics, 138*(1), 113–115.

Edwards, M. S. (2002). Postnatal bacterial infections. In A. A. Fanaroff & R. J. Martin (Eds.), *Neonatal-perinatal medicine. Diseases of the fetus and infant* (7th ed, Vol. 2, pp. 706–745). St. Louis, MO: Mosby.

Gilbert, Frank C., Cooper, S. C., & Merenstein, G. B. (2002). Jaundice. In G. B. Merenstein & S. L. Gardner, *Handbook of intensive care* (5th ed., pp. 443–461). St. Louis, MO: Mosby.

Grant, P. (1978). Psychological needs of families of high risk infants. *Family and Community Health, 1*(3), 91–102.

Hagedorn, M. E., Gardner, S. L., & Abman, S. H. (2002). Respiratory disease. In G. B. Merenstein & S. L. Gardner, *Handbook of intensive care* (5th ed., pp. 485–575). St. Louis, MO: Mosby.

Halamek, L. P., & Stevenson, D. K. (2002). Neonatal jaundice and liver disease. In A. A. Fanaroff & R. J. Martin (Eds.), *Neonatal-perinatal medicine: Diseases of the fetus and infant* (7th ed., Vol. 2, pp. 1309–1350). St. Louis, MO: Mosby.

Hannon, P. R., Willis, S. K., & Scrimshaw, S. C. (2001). Persistence of maternal concerns surrounding neonatal jaundice: An exploratory study. *Archives of Pediatrics & Adolescent Medicine 155*, 1357–1363.

Hashim, M. J., & Guillett, R. (2002). Common issues in the care of sick neonates. *American Family Physician, 66*(9) 1685–1692.

Heinonen, S., & Saarikoski, S. (2001). Reproductive risk factors of fetal asphyxia at delivery: A population based analysis. *Journal of Clinical Epidemiology, 54*, 407–410.

Kalhan, S. C., & Parimi, P. S. (2002). Metabolic and endrocrine disorders. In A. A. Fanaroff & R. J. Martin (Eds.), *Neonatal-perinatal medicine: Diseases of the fetus and infant* (7th ed., Vol. 2, pp. 1351–1376). St. Louis, MO: Mosby.

Kaplan, D. M., & Mason, E. A. (1974). Maternal reactions to premature birth viewed as an acute emotional disorder. In H. J. Parad (Ed.), *Crisis intervention.* New York: Family Services Association of America.

Kinnala, A., Korvenranta, H., & Parkkola, R. (2000). Newer techniques to study neonatal hypoglycemia. *Seminars in Perinatology, 24*(2), 116–119.

Klaus, M. H., & Fanaroff, A. A. (2001). *Care of the high-risk neonate* (5th ed.). Philadelphia: Saunders.

Klaus, M. H., & Kennell, J. H. (1982). *Maternal-infant bonding* (2nd ed.). St. Louis, MO: Mosby.

Lemons, J. A., Blackmon, L. R., Kanto, W. P., MacDonald, H. M., Miller, C. A., Rosenfeld, W., et al. (2000). Use of inhaled nitric oxide. *Pediatrics, 106*(2), 344–345.

Levine, E. M., Ghai, V., Barton, J. J., & Strom, C. M. (2001). Mode of delivery and risk of respiratory diseases in newborns. *Obstetrics & Gynecology, 97*(3), 439–442.

Loo, K. K., Espinosa, M., Tyler, R., & Howard, J. (2003). Using knowledge to cope with stress in the NICU: How parents integrate learning to read the physiologic and behavioral cues of the infant. *Neonatal Networks, 22*(1), 31–37.

Lubetzky, R., Ben-Shachar, S., Mimouni, F. B., & Dollberg, S. (2000). Mode of delivery and neonatal hematocrit. *American Journal of Perinatology, 17*(3), 163–165.

Lutes, L. M., & Altimier, L. (2001). Co-bedding multiples. *Newborn and Infant Nursing Reviews, 1*, 242–246.

Madlon-Kay, D. J. (2001). Home health nurse clinical assessment of neonatal jaundice: Comparison of 3 methods. *Archives of Pediatrics & Adolescent Medicine, 155*, 583–585.

Manco-Johnson, M., Rodden, D. J., & Collins, S. (2002). Newborn hematology. In G. B. Merenstein & S. L. Gardner, *Handbook of intensive care.* (5th ed., pp. 419–442). St. Louis, MO: Mosby.

Moriette, G., Brunhes, A., & Jarreau, P. (2000). High-frequency oscillatory ventilation in the management of respiratory distress syndrome. *Biology of the Neonate, 77*, 14–16.

Neonatal hypoglycemia. (2000). *In NANN guidelines for practice* (pp. 1–16). Des Plaines, IL: National Association of Neonatal Nurses.

Noerr, B. (2001). Sucrose for neonatal procedural pain. *Neonatal Network, 20*(7), 63–67.

Patel, D., Piotrowski, Z. H., Nelson, M. R., & Sabich, R. (2001). Effects of statewide neonatal resuscitation training program on Apgar scores among high-risk neonates in Illinois. *Pediatrics, 107* (4), 648–655.

Porter, M. L., & Dennis, B. L. (2002). Hyperbilirubinemia in the term newborn. *American Family Physician, 65*(4), 599–606.

Rimensberger, P. C., Beghetti, M., Hanquinet, S., & Berner, M. (2000). First intention high-frequency oscillation with early lung volume optimization improves pulmonary outcome in very low birth weight infants with respiratory distress syndrome. *Pediatrics, 105*(6), 1202–1208.

Riper, M. V. (2001). Family-provider relationships and well-being in families with preterm infants in the NICU. *Heart and Lung, 30* (1), 74–84.

Shenai, J. P., Mellen, B. G., & Chytil, F. (2000). Vitamin A status and postnatal dexamethasone treatment in bronchopulmonary dysplasia. *Pediatrics, 106*(3), 547–553.

Solnit, A., & Stark, M. (1961). Mourning and the birth of a defective child. *Psychoanalytic Study of the Child, 16*, 505.

Sydnor-Greenberg, N., & Dokken, D. (2000). Coping and caring in different ways: Understanding and meaningful involvement. *Pediatric Nursing, 26*(2), 185–190.

Taylor, H. G., Klein, N., Minich, N. M., & Hack, M. (2001). Long-term family outcomes for children with very low birth weights. *Archives of Pediatrics & Adolescent Medicine, 155*, 155–161.

Vaucher, Y. (2001). "What can I do to enhance the development of a premature infant with chronic lung disease?" *Pediatrics, 107*(4), 966–970.

Weber, T. S. (2000). Intubation ineffective in vigorous meconium-stained infants. *Journal of Family Practice, 49*(4), 301.

Wiswell, T. E., Gannon, C. M., Jacob, J., Goldsmith, L., Szyld, E., Weiss, K., et al. (2000). Delivery room management of the apparently vigorous meconium-stained neonate: Results of the multicenter, international collaborative trial. *Pediatrics, 105*(1), 1–7.

Wong, C. M., & Stenson, B. J. (2001). Resuscitation of the preterm neonate. *Current Paediatrics, 11*, 172–176.

Young, T. E., & Mangum, B. (2001). *Neofax* (14th ed.). Raleigh, NC: Acorn.

SEVEN

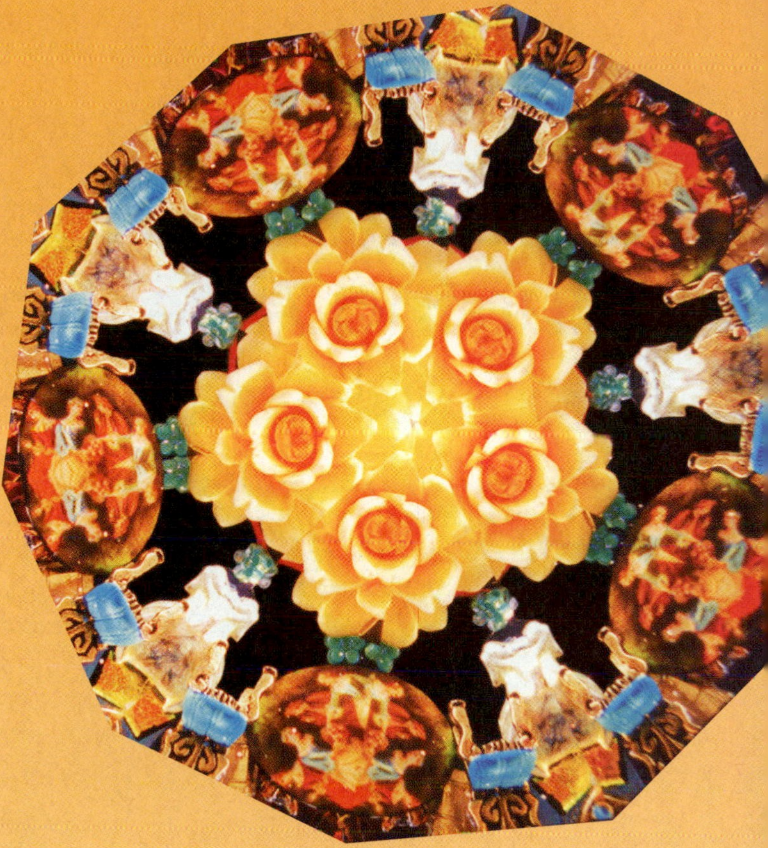

Postpartum

Postpartal Adaptation and Nursing Assessment

34

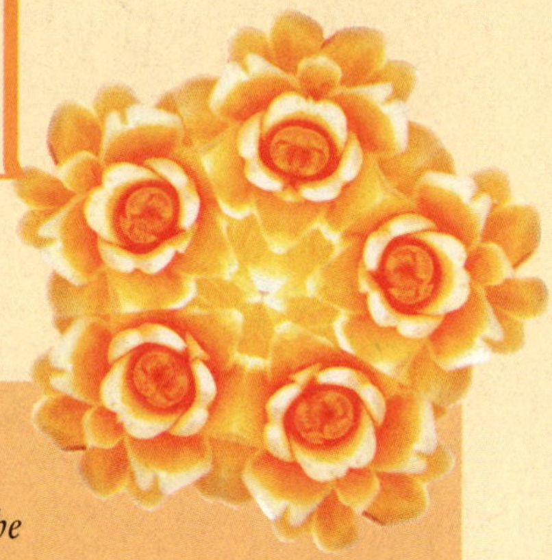

I had heard about the negatives—the fatigue, the loneliness, loss of self. But nobody told me about the wonderful parts: holding my baby close to me, seeing her first smile, watching her grow and become more responsive day by day. How can I describe the way I felt when she stroked my breast while nursing, or looked into my eyes or arched her eyebrows like an opera singer? This was the deepest connection I'd felt to anybody. Sometimes the intensity almost frightened me. For the first time I cared about somebody else more than myself, and I would do anything to nurture and protect her.
~ *The New Our Bodies, Ourselves* ~

Objectives

- Describe the basic physiologic changes that occur in the postpartal period as a woman's body returns to its prepregnant state.
- Identify those organs that will not return completely to a prepregnant state following childbirth.
- Discuss the psychologic adjustments that normally occur during the postpartal period.
- Delineate the physiologic and psychosocial components of a normal postpartal assessment.
- Summarize the physical and developmental tasks that the mother must accomplish during the postpartal period.

Key Terms

Afterpains 995
Boggy uterus 992
Diastasis recti abdominis 993
En face 998
Engrossment 999
Fundus 991
Involution 991
Lochia 992
Lochia alba 992
Lochia rubra 992
Lochia serosa 992
Maternal role attainment 996
Newborns' and Mothers' Health Protection Act (NMHPA) 1014
Postpartum blues 997
Puerperium 991
Reciprocity 998
Subinvolution 992

MediaLink

Additional resources for this content can be found on the Student CD-ROM and on the Companion Website at www.prenhall.com/olds. Click on "Chapter 34" to select the activities for this chapter.

CD-ROM
- Audio Glossary
- NCLEX Review
- Video: Postpartum Assessment

Companion Website
- Additional NCLEX Review
- Case Study: Mother-Infant Bonding

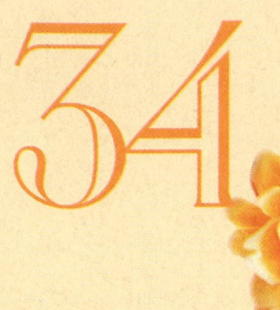

The **puerperium,** or postpartal period, is the period during which the woman adjusts, physically and psychologically, to pregnancy and birth. It begins immediately after birth and continues for approximately 6 weeks or until the body has returned to a near prepregnant state.

This chapter describes the physiologic and psychologic changes and adaptations that occur postpartally and the basic aspects of a thorough postpartal assessment.

Postpartal Physical Adaptations

Comprehensive nursing assessment is based on a sound understanding of the normal anatomic and physiologic processes of the puerperium. These processes involve the reproductive organs and other major body systems.

Reproductive System

INVOLUTION OF THE UTERUS

The term **involution** is used to describe the rapid reduction in size of the uterus and its return to a condition similar to its prepregnant state, although it remains slightly larger than it was before the first pregnancy. Specifically, the weight of the uterus decreases from 1000 g in the immediate postpartal period to 500 g at the end of the first week. It reaches 300 g by the end of the second week, finally terminating the involution process with a weight of 100 g or less (Cunningham, Gant, Leveno, et al, 2001).

The mechanisms of involution are as follows. Immediately after separation of the placenta, the decidua of the uterus is irregular, jagged, and varied in thickness. With the dramatic decrease in the levels of circulating estrogen and progesterone following placental separation, the uterine cells atrophy, and the hyperplasia of pregnancy begins to reverse. The process is one in which the size of the cells decreases markedly; the number of cells does not decrease. Proteolytic enzymes are released, and macrophages migrate to the uterus to promote autolysis (self-digestion). Protein material in the uterine wall is broken down and absorbed. The spongy layer of the decidua is cast off as lochia, and the basal layer of the decidua remains in the uterus to become differentiated into two layers within the first 48 to 72 hours after birth. The outermost layer becomes necrotic and is sloughed off in the lochia. The layer closest to the myometrium contains the fundi of the uterine endometrial glands, and these glands lay the foundation for the new endometrium. Except at the placental site, this process is completed in approximately 3 weeks.

Involution of the placental site is a similar process but takes up to 6 to 7 weeks for completion. Following separation, the placental site contracts to an area about 8 to 10 cm in diameter that appears raised, irregular, and 4 to 10 cm above the surface of the uterus. Following the completion of the second week the healing placental site is 3 to 4 cm in diameter (Blackburn, 2003). Bleeding from the larger uterine vessels of the placental site is controlled by compression of the retracted uterine muscle fibers. The clotted blood is gradually absorbed by the body. Some of these vessels are eventually obliterated and replaced by new vessels with smaller lumens.

Rather than forming a fibrous scar in the decidua, the placental site heals by a process of exfoliation. The placental site is undermined by the growth of the endometrial tissue, both from the margins of the site and from the fundi of the endometrial glands left in the basal layer of the site. The infarcted superficial tissue then becomes necrotic and is sloughed off. *Exfoliation* is one of the most important aspects of involution. If the healing of the placental site left a fibrous scar, the area available for further implantation would be limited, as would the number of possible pregnancies.

Factors that enhance involution include an uncomplicated labor and birth, complete expulsion of the amniotic membranes and the placenta, breastfeeding, manual removal of the placenta during a cesarean birth, and early ambulation. Factors that slow uterine involution and the rationale for each factor are listed in Table 34–1 •.

CHANGES IN FUNDAL POSITION

Immediately following the expulsion of the placenta, the uterus contracts firmly to the size of a large grapefruit. The **fundus** (top portion of the uterus) is situated in the midline of the abdomen, one half to two thirds of the way between the symphysis pubis and the umbilicus (Figure 34–1 •). The walls of the contracted uterus, each about 4 to 5 cm thick, are close together, and the uterine blood vessels are firmly compressed by the myometrium. Within 6 to 12 hours after

Table 34–1 • FACTORS THAT RETARD UTERINE INVOLUTION

Factor	Rationale
Prolonged labor	Muscles relax because of prolonged time of contraction during labor.
Anesthesia	Muscles relax.
Difficult birth	The uterus is manipulated excessively.
Grandmultiparity	Repeated distention of uterus during pregnancy and labor leads to muscle stretching, diminished tone, and muscle relaxation.
Full bladder	As the uterus is pushed up and usually to the right, pressure on it interferes with effective uterine contraction.
Incomplete expulsion of placenta or membranes	The presence of even small amounts of tissue interferes with ability of uterus to remain firmly contracted.
Infection	Inflammation interferes with uterine muscle's ability to contract effectively.
Overdistention of uterus	Overstretching of uterine muscles with conditions such as multiple gestation, hydramnios, or a very large baby may set the stage for slower uterine involution.

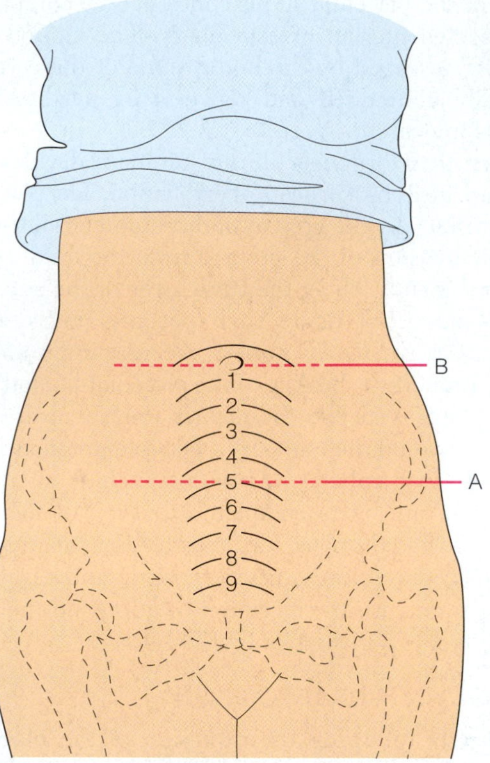

Figure 34–1 • Involution of the uterus. Immediately after delivery of the placenta, the top of the fundus is in the midline and approximately halfway between the symphysis pubis and the umbilicus (*A*). About 6 to 12 hours after birth, the fundus is at the level of the umbilicus (*B*). The height of the fundus then decreases about one fingerbreadth (approximately 1 cm) each day.

birth, the fundus of the uterus rises to the level of the umbilicus because of blood and clots that remain within the uterus and changes in support of the uterus by the ligaments. A fundus that is above the umbilicus and boggy (feels soft and spongy rather than firm and well contracted) is associated with excessive uterine bleeding. As blood collects and forms clots within the uterus, the fundus rises; firm contractions of the uterine muscle are interrupted, causing a **boggy uterus.** When the fundus is higher than expected and deviated from the midline (usually to the right), bladder distention should be suspected. Because the uterine ligaments are still stretched, a full bladder can move the uterus.

After birth, the top of the fundus remains at the level of the umbilicus for about half a day. On the first postpartum day (first day following birth), the top of the fundus is located about 1 cm below the umbilicus. The top of the fundus descends approximately one fingerbreadth (width of index, second, or third finger), or 1 cm, per day until it descends into the pelvis within 2 weeks on average (Cunningham et al, 2001). According to a study by Cluett, Alexander, and Pickering, (1997) the average time that the uterine fundus was no longer palpable was 13.57 days, with a range in healthy women of 11 to 22 days.

If the mother is breastfeeding, the release of endogenous oxytocin from the posterior pituitary in response to suckling may hasten this process. Barring complications, such as infection or retained placental fragments, the uterus approaches its prepregnant size and location by 4 weeks (Cunningham et al, 2001). In women who had an oversized uterus during the pregnancy (hydramnios, birth of a large-for-gestational-age [LGA] infant, or multiple gestation), the time frame for immediate uterine involution process is lengthened. If intrauterine infection is present, the uterine fundus descends much more slowly. When infection is suspected, other clinical signs such as fever and tachycardia in addition to delay in involution must be assessed. Any slowing of descent is called **subinvolution** (for further discussion of subinvolution, see Chapter 37).

LOCHIA

One of the unique capabilities of the uterus is its ability to rid itself of the debris remaining after birth. This discharge, termed **lochia,** is classified according to its appearance and contents. **Lochia rubra,** named for the Latin word for *red,* is dark red in color. It is present for the first 3 to 4 days postpartum and contains epithelial cells, erythrocytes, leukocytes, bacteria, shreds of the decidua, and occasionally fetal meconium, lanugo, and vernix caseosa. Lochia should not contain large clots; if it does, the cause should be investigated without delay. A few small clots (no larger than a nickel) are considered normal. **Lochia serosa** is a pinkish to brownish color. It follows from about the fourth to the tenth day. Lochia serosa is composed of serous exudate (hence the name), shreds of degenerating decidua, erythrocytes, leukocytes, cervical mucus, and numerous microorganisms (Blackburn, 2003).

The red blood cell component decreases gradually, and a creamy or yellowish discharge persists for an additional week or two. This final discharge, termed **lochia alba** from the Latin word for *white,* is composed primarily of leukocytes, decidual cells, epithelial cells, fat, cervical mucus, cholesterol crystals, and bacteria. According to a study by Marchant, Alexander, Garcia, et al (1999), lochia alba may continue for 2 to 86 days, with an average of 24 days. In breastfeeding women, lochia may continue beyond 6 weeks postpartum. It is believed that the flow is associated with the exfoliation process of the placental site, which does not terminate until after this time (Marchant et al, 1999). When the lochia stops the cervix is considered closed, and chances of infection ascending from the vagina to the uterus decrease.

Like menstrual discharge, lochia has a musty, stale odor that is not offensive. Microorganisms are always present in the vaginal lochia, and by the second day following birth the uterus is contaminated with the vaginal bacteria. Researchers speculate that infection does not develop because the organisms involved are relatively nonvirulent. In addition, by the time the bacteria reach the raw, exposed surface of the uterus, the process of granulation has begun, forming a protective barrier. Any foul smell to the lochia or used peripad suggests infection and the need for prompt additional assessment, such as white blood cell count and differential and assessment for uterine tenderness and fever.

The total volume of lochia is approximately 240 to 270 mL (8 to 9 oz), and the daily volume decreases gradually (Blackburn, 2003). Discharge is greater in the morning because of pooling in the vagina and uterus while the mother lies sleeping. The amount of lochia may also be increased by exertion or breastfeeding.

Evaluation of lochia is necessary not only to determine the presence of hemorrhage but also to assess uterine involution. The type, amount, and consistency of lochia determine the state of healing of the placental site, and a progressive color change from bright red at birth to dark red to pink to white or clear should be observed. Persistent discharge of lochia rubra or a return to lochia rubra indicates subinvolution or late postpartal hemorrhage (see Chapter 37).

The nurse should exercise caution in evaluating bleeding immediately after birth. The continuous seepage of blood is more consistent with cervical or vaginal lacerations and may be effectively diagnosed when the bleeding is evaluated in conjunction with the consistency of the uterus. Lacerations should be suspected if the uterus is firm and of expected size and if no clots can be expressed.

CERVICAL CHANGES

Following birth, the cervix is spongy, flabby, and formless and may appear bruised. The lateral aspects of the external os are frequently lacerated during the birth process (Cunningham et al, 2001). However, the original form of the cervix is regained within the first week (Harrison, 2000). The external os is markedly irregular and closes slowly. It admits two fingers for a few days following birth, but by the end of the first week it will admit only a fingertip.

The shape of the external os is permanently changed by the first childbearing. The characteristic dimplelike os of the nullipara changes to the lateral slit (fish-mouth) os of the multipara. After significant cervical laceration or several lacerations, the cervix may appear lopsided. Because of the slight change in the size of the cervix, a diaphragm or cervical cap will need to be refitted if the woman is using one of these methods of contraception.

VAGINAL CHANGES

Following birth, the vagina appears edematous and may be bruised. Small superficial lacerations may be evident, and the rugae have been obliterated. The apparent bruising of the vagina is due to pelvic congestion and will quickly disappear. The hymen, torn and jagged, heals irregularly, leaving small tags called the *carunculae myrtiformes.*

The size of the vagina decreases and rugae return within 3–4 weeks (Blackburn, 2003). This facilitates the gradual return to smaller, although not to nulliparous, dimensions. By 6 weeks, the nonlactating woman's vagina usually appears normal. The lactating woman is in a hypoestrogenic state because of ovarian suppression, and her vaginal mucosa may be pale and without rugae. This may lead to dyspareunia (painful intercourse). Tone and contractibility of the vaginal opening may be improved by perineal tightening exercises (Kegel exercises, discussed in Chapter 16), which may begin soon after birth. The labia majora and labia minora are looser in the woman who has borne a child than in the nullipara.

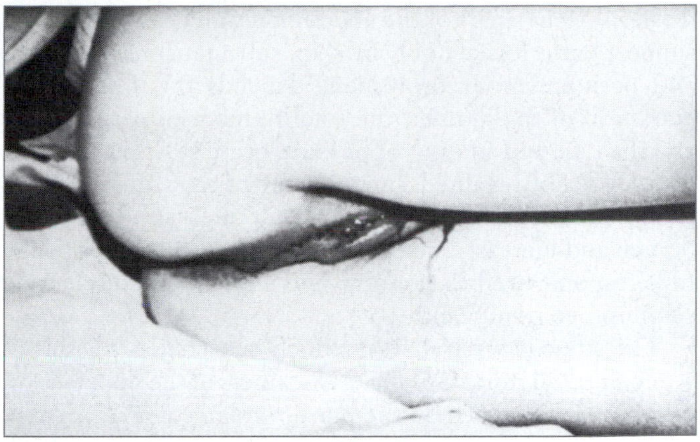

Figure 34–2 ● Bruising and edema of the vulva and perineum in a primipara 3 days after a forceps delivery.
SOURCE: Bennett, V. R., & Brown, L. K. (1989). *Myles textbook for midwives* (11th ed., p. 235). Edinburgh, Scotland: Churchill Livingstone.

PERINEAL CHANGES

During the early postpartal period, the soft tissue in and around the perineum may appear edematous with some bruising (Figure 34–2 ●). If an episiotomy or laceration is present, the edges should be approximated. Occasionally, ecchymosis occurs, and this may delay healing.

RECURRENCE OF OVULATION AND MENSTRUATION

The return of menstruation and ovulation varies for each postpartal woman. Menstruation generally returns in nonbreastfeeding mothers between 6 and 8 weeks after birth, and the first cycle is anovulatory (Cunningham et al, 2001). Overall, 90% of nonbreastfeeding mothers resume menstruation by 12 weeks after birth (Scroggins, 2000).

The return of menstruation and ovulation in breastfeeding mothers is usually prolonged and is associated with the length of time the woman breastfeeds and whether formula supplements are used. If a mother breastfeeds for less than 1 month, the return of menstruation and ovulation is similar to the nonbreastfeeding mother. In women who exclusively breastfeed, menstruation is usually delayed for at least 3 months. However, since ovulation precedes menstruation, breastfeeding is not a reliable means of contraception, especially after the first 3 weeks postpartum (American College of Obstetricians and Gynecologists [ACOG], 2000).

Abdomen

The uterine ligaments (notably the round and broad ligaments) are stretched and require time to recover. The stretched abdominal wall appears loose and flabby, but it will respond to exercise within 2 to 3 months. In the grand-multipara, in the woman whose abdomen is overdistended, or in the woman whose muscle tone was poor before pregnancy, the abdomen may fail to regain good tone and will remain flabby. **Diastasis recti abdominis,** a separation of the rectus abdominis muscles, may occur with pregnancy, especially in women with poor abdominal muscle tone. If diastasis occurs, part of the abdominal wall has no muscular support but is formed only by skin, subcutaneous fat, fascia, and peritoneum. Improvement depends on the physical condition of the mother, the total number of pregnancies, and the type and amount of physical exercise. If rectus muscle tone is not regained, support may be inadequate during future pregnancies. This may result in a pendulous abdomen and increased maternal backache. Fortunately, diastasis responds well to exercise, and abdominal muscle tone can improve significantly.

The striae (stretch marks), which occurred as a result of stretching and rupture of the elastic fibers of the skin, take on different colors based on the mother's skin color. The striae of Caucasian mothers are red to purple at the time of birth and gradually fade to silver or white. The striae of mothers with darker skin are darker than the surrounding skin and remain darker. The appearance of striae (stretch marks) can be improved with the use of prescription topical agents.

Lactation

During pregnancy, the breasts develop in preparation for lactation as a result of the influence of both estrogen and progesterone. After birth, the interplay of maternal hormones leads to the establishment of milk production (see Chapter 31).

Gastrointestinal System

Hunger following birth is common, and the mother may enjoy a light meal. Frequently, she is quite thirsty and will drink large amounts of fluid. Drinking fluids helps replace fluid lost during labor, in the urine, and through perspiration.

The bowels tend to be sluggish after birth because of the lingering effects of progesterone and decreased abdominal muscle tone. Women who have had an episiotomy may tend to delay elimination for fear of increasing their pain or in the belief that their stitches will be torn if they bear down. In most instances the initial bowel movement is not uncomfortable. However, refusing or delaying the bowel movement may cause constipation and more discomfort when elimination finally occurs.

The woman with a cesarean birth may receive clear liquids shortly after surgery. Once bowel sounds are present, the diet is quickly advanced to solid food. The woman may experience some initial discomfort from flatulence. This is relieved by early ambulation and use of antiflatulent medications. It may take a few days for the bowel to regain its tone. The woman who has had a cesarean or a difficult birth may benefit from stool softeners. In some cases it may be necessary to administer an enema or suppository to promote elimination.

Urinary Tract

The postpartal woman has an increased bladder capacity, swelling and bruising of the tissues around the urethra, decreased sensitivity to fluid pressure, and decreased sensation of bladder filling. Consequently, she is at risk for overdistention, incomplete emptying, and buildup of residual urine. Women who have had an anesthetic block have inhibited neural functioning of the bladder and are more susceptible to bladder distention, difficulty voiding, and bladder retention. In addition, immediate postpartal use of oxytocin to facilitate uterine contractions following expulsion of the placenta has an antidiuretic effect. Following cessation of the oxytocin the woman will experience rapid bladder filling (Cunningham et al, 2001).

Urinary output increases during the early postpartal period (first 12 to 24 hours) due to *puerperal diuresis.* The kidneys must eliminate an estimated 2000 to 3000 mL of extracellular fluid with a normal pregnancy, which causes rapid filling of the bladder. Thus adequate bladder elimination is an immediate concern. Women with preeclampsia, chronic hypertension, and diabetes experience even greater fluid retention, and postpartal diuresis is increased accordingly.

Bladder elimination presents an immediate problem. If stasis exists, chances increase for urinary tract infection because of bacteriuria and the presence of dilated ureters and renal pelves, which persist for about 6 weeks after birth. A full bladder may also increase the tendency of the uterus to relax by displacing the uterus and interfering with its contractility, leading to hemorrhage.

Hematuria, resulting from bladder trauma, may occasionally occur after birth, but the presence of lochia may mask this sign. If hematuria occurs in the second or third postpartal week, there may be a bladder infection. Acetone may be present in the urine of women with diabetes or of women with prolonged labor and dehydration. Slight (1+) proteinuria may occur during the first week following birth. However, proteinuria may be associated with an infectious process (cystitis, pyelitis), so it should be evaluated further. A urine specimen contaminated with lochia may falsely indicate proteinuria, so any specimen should be obtained as a midstream or a catheterized specimen.

Vital Signs

During the postpartal period, with the exception of the first 24 hours, the woman should be afebrile. A temperature of up to 38C (100.4F) may normally occur up to 24 hours after birth as a result of the exertion and dehydration of labor. An increase in temperature to between 37.8C and 39C may also occur during the first 24 hours after the mother's milk comes in (Cunningham et al, 2001). However, in women not meeting these criteria, infection must be considered in the presence of an increased temperature (see Chapter 37).

Blood pressure readings should remain stable and within normal range following the birth. A decrease may indicate physiologic readjustment to decreased intrapelvic pressure, or it may be related to uterine hemorrhage. Blood pressure elevations, especially when they are accompanied by headache (nondependent edema or proteinuria) suggest preeclampsia, and the woman should be evaluated further.

Puerperal bradycardia with rates of 50 to 70 beats per minute commonly occurs during the first 6 to 10 days of the postpartal period. It may be related to decreased cardiac strain, the decreased blood volume following placental separation, contraction of the uterus, and increased stroke volume. Tachycardia occurs less frequently and is related to increased blood loss or difficult, prolonged labor and birth.

Blood Values

Blood values should return to the prepregnant state by 6 to 9 weeks after birth. Pregnancy-associated activation of coagulation factors may continue for variable amounts of time. This condition, in conjunction with trauma, immobility, or sepsis, predisposes the woman to development of thromboembolism. The incidence of thromboembolism is reduced by early mobilization (Harrison, 2000). Plasma fibrinogen is maintained at pregnancy levels for a week following childbirth, accounting for the higher sedimentation rate observed in the early postpartum period.

Leukocytosis with white blood cell (WBC) counts up to 30,000 per mL persists in the early postpartal days (Cunningham et al, 2001). The leukocytosis does not necessarily indicate infection. An increase of greater than 30% in 6 hours is an indication of pathology. Other clinical signs of infection (elevation of temperature, redness, swelling, and pain) must be evaluated.

Blood loss averages 200 to 500 mL with a vaginal birth and 700 to 1000 mL with a cesarean birth. Hemoglobin and erythrocyte values vary during the early puerperium, but they should approximate or exceed prelabor values within 2 to 6 weeks. As extracellular fluid is excreted, hemoconcentration occurs, with a concomitant rise in hematocrit. A drop in values indicates an abnormal blood loss. The following is a convenient rule to remember: a 2-point drop in hematocrit equals a blood loss of 500 mL. Anemia is a common postpartal complication with an incidence of greater than 50%. The majority of these cases are related to decreased iron levels (Milasinovic, Kapamadzija, Dobric, et al, 2000).

Weight Loss

An initial weight loss of 10 to 12 lb occurs as a result of the birth of infant, placenta, and amniotic fluid. Puerperal diuresis accounts for the loss of an additional 5 lb during the early puerperium. By the sixth to eighth week after birth, many women have returned to approximately prepregnant weight if they gained the average 25 to 30 lb. For others, a return to prepregnant weight takes longer or does not occur. A woman who is physically active prior to, during, and after pregnancy completion retains less weight (8.6 lb) than a comparable, but less active counterpart (11.3 lb). Younger women, married women, and women who experience lower weight gain during pregnancy are more likely to obtain their prepregnancy weights.

Postpartal Chill

Most mothers experience a shaking chill immediately after birth, which may be related to a neurologic response or to vasomotor changes. Covering the woman with warmed blankets will help alleviate the chill and increase her comfort. The mother may also find a warm beverage helpful. Chills and fever later in the puerperium indicate infection and require further evaluation.

Postpartal Diaphoresis

The elimination of excess fluid and waste products via the skin during the puerperium greatly increases perspiration. Diaphoretic episodes frequently occur at night, and the woman may awaken drenched with perspiration. This perspiration is not significant clinically, but the mother should be protected from chilling.

Afterpains

Afterpains occur more commonly in multiparas than in primiparas and are caused by intermittent uterine contractions. Although the uterus of the primipara usually remains consistently contracted, the lost tone of the uterus of the multipara results in alternate contraction and relaxation. This phenomenon also occurs if the uterus has been markedly distended, as with multiple pregnancies or hydramnios, or if clots or placental fragments were retained. These afterpains may cause the mother severe discomfort for 2 to 3 days following birth. The administration of oxytocic agents (intravenous infusion with Pitocin or oral administration of Methergine) stimulates uterine contraction and increases the discomfort of the afterpains. Because oxytocin is released naturally when the infant suckles, breastfeeding also increases the severity of the afterpains. The breastfeeding mother may find it helpful to take a mild analgesic agent approximately 1 hour before feeding her infant. The nurse can assure the mother that the prescribed analgesic agents are not harmful to the newborn and help improve the quality of the breastfeeding experience. An analgesic agent is also helpful at bedtime if the afterpains interfere with the mother's rest.

Postpartal Psychologic Adaptations

The postpartal period is a time of readjustment and adaptation for the entire childbearing family, but especially for the mother. The woman experiences a variety of responses as she adjusts to a new family member, postpartal discomforts, changes in her body image, and the reality that she is no longer pregnant. One young mother described her responses well:

> *I feel like it's the day after Christmas. I'm relieved that everything went well and I have a fine baby, but I feel so let down. I had an image of what childbirth would be like, but everything was a little different. I figured that as soon as I gave birth, I would feel fine. Why didn't someone tell me I would still be sore? The pain didn't magically disappear! When I was pregnant, everyone treated me as though I was a little fragile. Now when people call or visit, all they*

talk about is the baby. I don't think I'm really jealous, but I do miss the attention. During this past day I've started to realize that my life will never, ever be the same again. I've always wanted to be a mother, but I'm not really sure how to do it. Isn't that strange?"

Taking-In and Taking-Hold

Over 40 years ago, research on maternal postpartal adaptation suggested the existence of two distinct periods of adjustment to motherhood. During the first day or two following birth, the woman was said to be in the *taking-in* period (Rubin, 1961), which was characterized by passivity and dependence on others. The new mother follows suggestions, is hesitant about making decisions, and is still rather preoccupied with her needs. She may have a great need to talk about her perceptions of her labor and birth. This helps her work through the process, sort out the reality from her fantasized experience, and clarify anything that she did not understand. Food and sleep are major focuses.

By the second or third day after birth, the new mother was observed to be ready to resume control of her body, her mothering, and her life in general. Rubin (1961) labeled this phase as *taking-hold.* If she is breastfeeding, the mother may worry about her technique or the quality of her milk. If her baby spits up following feeding, she may view it as a personal failure. She may also feel demoralized by the fact that the nurse or an older family member handles her baby proficiently while she feels unsure and tentative. She requires assurance that she is doing well as a mother.

Today's birthing care has changed drastically from the time of Rubin's research. More important, mothers are more independent and adjust more rapidly. Thus, the paradigm first described by Rubin (1961) is no longer relevant as originally stated. Ament (1990) found that women did exhibit behavior characteristics of taking-in and taking-hold, but found that the time frames were shorter than those cited by Rubin. Martell (1996) discovered that aspects of taking-in and taking-hold both surfaced during the first 12 hours postpartally. Examples cited by study participants of taking-in were inactivity, tiredness, and a desire to converse regarding the labor and birth process. Plans for discharge, proactive personal control, and requests for needs were aspects of the taking-hold phase recounted by participants. These behaviors were found to be elements of the original concepts described by Rubin; however, a new theory directed at contemporary postpartal clients is needed.

Maternal Role Attainment

A prime focus of research in recent years has been maternal role attainment. **Maternal role attainment** is the process by which a woman learns mothering behaviors and becomes comfortable with her identity as a mother. The formation of a maternal identity indicates that the woman has attained the maternal role. This process occurs with each child a woman bears. As the mother grows to know this child and forms a relationship with her or him, the mother's maternal identity gradually and systematically evolves, and she "binds in" to the infant (Rubin, 1984).

Maternal role attainment occurs in four stages (Mercer, 1995):

1. The *anticipatory stage* occurs during pregnancy. The woman looks to role models, especially her own mother, for examples of how to mother.
2. The *formal stage* begins when the child is born. The woman is still influenced by the guidance of others and tries to act as she believes others expect her to act.
3. The *informal stage* begins when the mother begins to make her own choices about mothering. The woman begins to develop her own style of mothering and finds ways of functioning that work well for her.
4. The *personal stage* is the final stage of maternal role attainment. When the woman reaches this stage, she is comfortable with the notion of herself as "mother."

The formal and informal stages of maternal role attainment correspond with the taking-in and taking-hold stages previously identified by Rubin (1961).

In most cases, maternal role attainment occurs within 3 to 10 months following birth. A study by Fowles (1998) revealed that most women experience comfort in their role as a mother within 4 months of childbirth. Social support, the woman's age and personality traits, the temperament of her infant, and the family's socioeconomic status all influence the woman's success in attaining the maternal role, as does the woman's culture. For example, attaining the role of "mother" is typically viewed as a major and joyous accomplishment for African American women (Gichia, 2000). In contrast, new mothers whose birth experience did not go as envisioned because of premature birth, unplanned cesarean birth, or lack of expected support system may perceive themselves to be less competent in infant care (Fowles, 1998).

Following the birth, the woman initially experiences sensations that are profoundly opposite in meaning, such as devotion/sacrifice or happiness/frustration. The woman gives unselfishly of herself while establishing a new role. Following that phase, the woman goes through a metamorphosis in which she finally evolves as a mother of a young infant. This changes other facets of her life, such as professional goals or personal relationships (McVeigh, 2000a).

The postpartal woman faces a number of challenges as she adjusts to her new role (Mercer, 1995):

- For many women, finding time for themselves is one of the greatest challenges. It is often difficult for the new mother to find time to read a book, talk to her partner, or even eat a meal without interruption.
- Women also report feelings of incompetence because they have not mastered all aspects of the mothering role. Often they are unsure of what to do in a given situation.
- The next greatest challenge involves fatigue resulting from sleep deprivation. The demands of nighttime care

are tremendously draining, especially if the woman has other children.

- One challenge the new mother faces involves the feeling of responsibility that having a child brings. Women experience a sense of lost freedom, an awareness that they will never again be quite as carefree as they were before becoming mothers.
- Mothers sometimes cite the infant's behavior as a problem, especially when the child is about 8 months old. Stranger anxiety develops, the infant begins crawling and getting into things, teething may cause fussiness, and the baby's tendency to put everything in his or her mouth requires constant vigilance by the parent.

Adjustment to Altered Body Image

Postpartally, the woman must adjust to a changed body image. Often women, especially primiparas, are surprised and rather dismayed to discover that they do not return to their prepregnant weight and shape as soon as the baby is born. Women often express dissatisfaction about their appearance and concern about the return of their weight and figure to normal. Multiparas tend to be more positive about their appearance postpartally than primiparas. This may be because the multipara's previous experience has prepared her for the fact that the body does not immediately return to a prepregnant state. A recent study by Morin, Brogan, and Flavin (2002) studied African American mothers' perception of their body image in the postpartum period. African American women, in general, tend to have a positive body image irrespective of their body size. In the postpartum period they often continue this slightly more positive attitude toward their body, and increased body weight is less of a concern.

Postpartum Blues

The term **postpartum blues** describes a transient period of depression that occurs in most women during the first week or two after birth. It may be manifested by mood swings, anger, weepiness, anorexia, difficulty sleeping, and a feeling of letdown. Because most new mothers are discharged within 2 to 3 days, the depression often occurs at home. Psychologic adjustments and hormonal changes are thought to be the main causes, although fatigue, discomfort, and overstimulation may play a part. The postpartum blues usually resolve naturally, especially if the woman receives understanding and support. If symptoms persist or intensify, the woman may need evaluation for postpartum depression (see Chapter 37).

Importance of Social Support

The psychologic outcomes of the postpartal period are far more positive when the parents have access to a support network. Women and their partners may find that family relationships become increasingly important, and the attention that their infant receives from family members is a source of satisfaction to the new parents. In many cases, the ties to the

GLOBAL PERSPECTIVES

In many patriarchal countries in the Middle East, the new mother and her infant stay with the husband's family following the birth of the infant. Frequent visits from the woman's family are discouraged and may even be viewed as burdensome by the husband's family. Typically, only women visit the new mother during the postpartum period. For the birth of the first baby, the wife's parents are expected to purchase all of the supplies and clothing for the baby.

woman's family become especially good. Fathers may report that their relationships with their in-laws become far more positive and supportive. But the increased family interaction can be a source of stress, especially for the new mother, who tends to have more contact with the families.

Childbearing couples often change their social network somewhat following the birth of their child. Once the new parents have made the transition to parenthood, they both tend to have more contact with other parents of small children. For the woman, interaction with coworkers often declines postpartally, but contact with friends increases. Thus the woman maintains the size of her support group but alters it to meet the changes that have occurred in her lifestyle.

Perhaps the greatest concern involves women and their partners who have no family available and no friends to form a social network. Isolation during a time in which the woman feels an increased need for support can result in tremendous stress and is often a contributing factor in situations of child neglect or abuse.

Development of Parent-Infant Attachment

A mother's first interaction with her infant is influenced by many factors, including her family of origin, her relationships, the stability of her home environment, the communication patterns she has developed, and the degree of nurturing she received as a child. Certain characteristics of the mother are also important:

- *Level of trust.* What level of trust has this mother developed in response to her life experiences? What is her philosophy of childrearing? Will she be able to treat her infant as a unique individual with changing needs that should be met as much as possible?
- *Level of self-esteem.* How much does she value herself as a woman and as a mother? Does she feel generally able to cope with the adjustments of life?
- *Capacity for enjoying herself.* Is the mother able to find pleasure in everyday activities and human relationships?
- *Interest in and adequacy of knowledge about childbearing and childrearing.* What beliefs about the course of pregnancy,

MEDIALINK POSTPARTUM DEPRESSION RESOURCES

MEDIALINK CASE STUDY: MOTHER-INFANT BONDING

the capacities of newborns, and the nature of her emotions may influence her behavior at first contact with her infant and later?

- *Her prevailing mood or usual feeling tone.* Is the woman predominantly content, angry, depressed, or anxious? Is she sensitive to her own feelings and those of others? Will she be able to accept her own needs and to obtain support in meeting them?
- *Reactions to the present pregnancy.* Was the pregnancy planned? Did it go smoothly? Were there ongoing life events that enhanced her pregnancy or depleted her reserves of energy?

By the time of birth, each mother has developed an emotional orientation of some kind to the baby based on these factors, as well as a physical awareness of the fetus within her and her fantasy images and perceptions.

INITIAL ATTACHMENT BEHAVIOR

New mothers demonstrate a fairly regular pattern of maternal behaviors at first contact with a normal newborn. In a progression of touching activities, the mother proceeds from fingertip exploration of the newborn's extremities toward palmar contact with larger body areas and finally to enfolding the infant with the whole hand and arms. The time taken to accomplish these steps varies from minutes to days, depending, it appears, on the timing of the first contact, the clothing barriers present, and the physical condition of the baby. Maternal excitement and elation tend to increase during the time of the initial meeting. The mother also increases the proportion of time spent in the **en face** position (Figure 34–3 •). She arranges herself or the newborn so that she has direct face-to-face and eye-to-eye contact. There is an intense interest in having the infant's eyes open. When the eyes are open, the mother characteristically greets the newborn and talks in high-pitched tones to him or her.

In most instances the mother relies heavily on her senses of sight, touch, and hearing in getting to know what her baby is really like. She tends also to respond verbally to any sounds emitted by the newborn, such as cries, coughs, sneezes, and grunts. The sense of smell may also be involved, although this possibility has not yet been adequately studied.

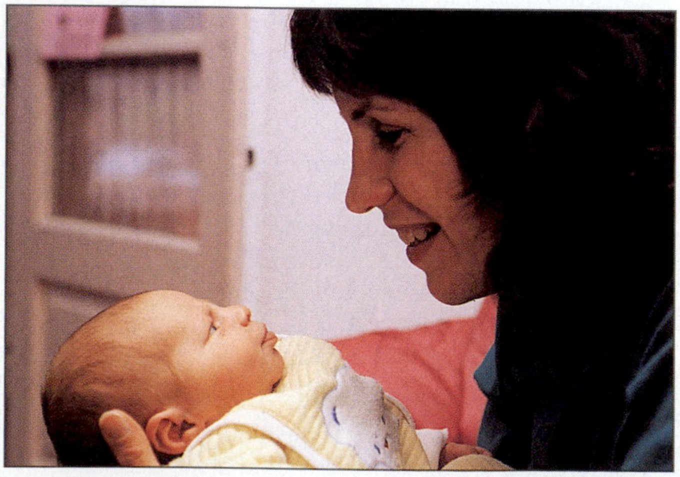

Figure 34–3 • The mother has direct face-to-face and eye-to-eye contact in the *en face* position.

In addition to interacting with the newborn, the mother is undergoing her own emotional reactions to the birth and, more specifically, to the baby as she perceives him or her. The frequency of the "I can't believe" reaction leads to speculation that human beings meet gains as well as losses with a degree of shock, disbelief, and denial. Among mothers, a feeling of emotional distance from the newborn is quite common: "I felt he was a stranger." However, the mother may express feelings of connectedness between the newborn and the rest of the family, either in positive or in negative terms: "She's got your cute nose, Daddy,"or "Oh, no! He looks just like the first one, and he was an impossible baby." A mother's facial expression or the frequency and content of her questions may demonstrate concerns about the infant's general condition or normality, especially if her pregnancy was complicated or if a previously born baby was not normal.

During the first few days after her child's birth, the new mother applies herself to the task of getting to know her baby. This is termed the *acquaintance phase.* If the infant gives clear behavioral cues about needs, the infant's responses to mothering will be predictable, which will make the mother feel effective and competent. Other behaviors that make an infant more attractive to caretakers are smiling, grasping a finger, breastfeeding eagerly, cuddling, and being easy to console.

During this time the newborn is also becoming acquainted. Within a few days after birth, infants show signs of recognizing recurrent situations and responding to changes in routine. To the extent that their mother is their world, it can be said that they are actively acquainting themselves with her.

During the *phase of mutual regulation,* mother and infant seek to deal with the degree of control to be exerted by each in their relationship. In this phase of adjustment, a balance is sought between the needs of the mother and the needs of the infant. The most important consideration is that each should obtain a good measure of enjoyment from the interaction. During the mutual adjustment phase, negative maternal feelings are likely to surface or intensify. Because they feel that they are expected to love their babies, mothers often fail to express these negative feelings, which often then build up. If the mother does express these feelings, friends, relatives, or healthcare personnel often respond by denying them: "You don't mean that." Some negative feelings are normal in the first few days after birth, and the nurse should be supportive when the mother vocalizes these feelings.

When mutual regulation arrives at the point where both mother and infant primarily enjoy each other's company, reciprocity has been achieved. **Reciprocity** is an interactional cycle that occurs simultaneously between mother and infant. It involves mutual cuing behaviors, expectancy, rhythmicity, and synchrony. The mother develops a new relationship with an individual who has a unique character and evokes a response entirely different from the fantasy response of pregnancy. When reciprocity is synchronous, the interaction between mother and infant is mutually gratifying and is sought and initiated by both partners. They find pleasure and delight in each other's company and grow in mutual love. A new mother who experiences comfort and competence in her role provides an environment that is stimulating and nurturing, which in turn facilitates her infant's development (Fowles, 1998).

FATHER-INFANT INTERACTIONS

Traditionally in Western cultures, the primary role of the expectant father has been one of support for the pregnant woman. Commitment to family-centered maternity care, however, has fostered interest in understanding the feelings and experiences of the new father. Evidence suggests that the father has a strong attraction to his newborn and that the feelings he experiences are similar to the mother's feelings of attachment (Figure 34–4 •). The characteristic sense of absorption, preoccupation, and interest in the infant demonstrated by fathers during early contact has been termed **engrossment.**

SIBLINGS AND OTHERS

Infants are capable of maintaining a number of strong attachments without loss of quality. These attachments may include siblings, grandparents, aunts, and uncles. The social setting and personality of the individual seem to be significant factors in the development of multiple attachments. The advent of open visiting hours and rooming-in permits siblings and grandparents to participate in the attachment process.

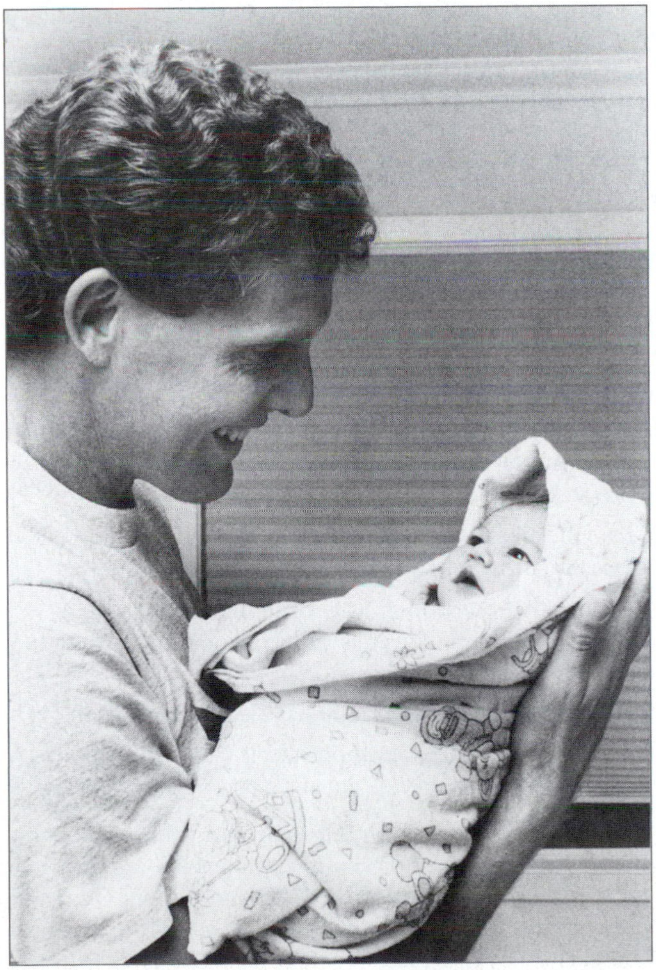

Figure 34–4 • The father experiences strong feelings of attraction during engrossment.

Cultural Influences in the Postpartal Period

Whereas Western culture places primary emphasis on the events of birth, many other cultures place greater emphasis on the postpartum period. Some cultures may proscribe contact with others, contact with food or objects, and sexual relationships. These practices may serve to reduce the risks of infection; and promote healing, lactation, and attachment (Andrews & Boyle, 1999). The new mother's culture and personal values also influence her beliefs about her postpartal care. Her expectations regarding food, fluids, rest, hygiene, medications, relief measures, support, and counsel—as well as other aspects of her life—will be influenced by the beliefs and values of her family and cultural group. Sometimes a new mother's wishes will differ from the expectations of the certified nurse-midwife/physician or nurse. (See Chapter 2 for in-depth discussion.)

As a part of the healthcare cultural group, nurses implement practices that support their general beliefs, such as offering food in the recovery period following birth, providing iced fluids, expecting the woman to ambulate as soon as possible, and assuming the woman will want to shower and perhaps wash her hair soon after birth. However, these practices may be in opposition to the woman's beliefs and expectations. To individualize care for each mother, the nurse needs to assess the woman's preferences, have her exercise her choices when possible, and support those choices, with the help of cultural awareness and a sound knowledge base.

Although describing the practices of different cultural groups always involves some generalization, it is helpful for nurses to understand some of the possible differences in beliefs and practices (Mayberry, Affonso, Shibuya, et al, 1999). For example, a woman of European heritage may expect to eat a full meal and have a large amount of iced fluids following the birth, in the belief that the food restores energy and the fluids help replace fluid lost during the labor. She may want to ambulate shortly after the birth, shower, wash her hair, and put on a fresh gown. She may expect a relatively short stay in the hospital and may or may not be interested in educational classes. Women of the Islamic faith may have specific modesty requirements; the woman must be completely covered, with only her feet and hands exposed. A man, other than the husband or family member, may not be alone with the woman (Al-Oballi Kridli, 2002).

Many cultures emphasize postpartal rituals for mother and baby which are designed to restore the hot-cold balance of the body (Howard & Berbiglia, 1997). For example, some women of Indian, Mexican, African, and Asian cultures may avoid cold after birth. This prohibition includes cold air, wind, and all water (even if heated). Dietary changes also reflect the need to avoid cold foods and restore the balance between hot and cold (Andrews & Boyle, 1999; Al-Oballi Kridli, 2002). For instance, a traditional Mexican woman may avoid eating "hot" foods, such as pork, just after the birth of her baby. It is important to note that each individual or cultural group may define hot and cold conditions as well as hot and cold foods differently. Therefore, the nurse should ask each woman what she can eat and what foods she thinks would be helpful for healing (Choudhry, 1997). The nurse may encourage family members to bring preferred food and drink for the mother.

In many cultures, the extended family plays an essential role during the puerperium. The grandmother is often the primary helper to the mother and newborn. She brings wisdom and experience, allowing the new mother time to rest as well as giving her ready access to someone who can help with problems and concerns as they arise. It is important to ensure access of all family members during the postpartal period. Visiting rules may be waived to allow family members or authority figures access to the mother and newborn. These practices show respect and foster a blending of old and new behaviors to meet the goals of all concerned (Cesario, 2001). African American mothers model their mothering skills after their older female relatives. In addition, these same older female relatives usually provide child care as needed (Gichia, 2000). People of Jewish faith observe a Sabbath from sundown Friday to sundown Saturday. During this time, conservative Jews do not perform any manual labor; for the postpartal woman, this includes turning on or off the lights, pressing the call bell, or raising/lowering the head of the bed (DeSovo, 1997). Jewish clients may also request a kosher diet. Some traditional Jewish couples avoid physical contact while the woman is experiencing any vaginal discharge; thus, the man may be viewed as unsupportive by the staff during the postpartal period.

MediaLink VIDEO: POSTPARTUM ASSESSMENT

Postpartal Nursing Assessment

Comprehensive care is based on a thorough assessment, with identification of individual needs or potential problems. (See the accompanying Assessment Guide: Postpartal—First 24 Hours After Birth.)

Risk Factors

The emphasis on ongoing assessment and education during the puerperium is designed to meet the needs of the childbearing family and to detect and treat possible complications. Table 34–2 • identifies factors that may place the new mother at risk during the postpartal period. The nurse uses this knowledge during the assessment and is particularly alert for possible complications that may occur in an individual because of identified risk factors.

Table 34–2 • POSTPARTAL HIGH-RISK FACTORS

Factor	Maternal Implication
Preeclampsia	↑ Blood pressure ↑ CNS irritability ↑ Need for bed rest → ↑ risk thrombophlebitis
Diabetes	Need for insulin regulation Episodes of hypoglycemia or hyperglycemia ↓ Healing
Cardiac disease	↑ Maternal exhaustion
Cesarean birth	↑ Healing needs ↑ Pain from incision ↑ Risk of infection ↑ Length of hospitalization
Overdistention of uterus (multiple gestation, hydramnios)	↑ Risk of hemorrhage ↑ Risk of anemia ↑ Stretching of abdominal muscles ↑ Incidence and severity of afterpains
Abruptio placentae, placenta previa	Hemorrhage → anemia ↓ Uterine contractility after birth → ↑ infection risk
Precipitous labor (<3 hours)	↑ Risk of lacerations to birth canal → hemorrhage
Prolonged labor (>24 hours)	Exhaustion ↑ Risk of hemorrhage Nutritional and fluid depletion ↑ Bladder atony and/or trauma
Difficult birth	Exhaustion ↑ Risk of perineal lacerations ↑ Risk of hematomas ↑ Risk of hemorrhage → anemia
Extended period of time in stirrups at birth	↑ Risk of thrombophlebitis
Retained placenta	↑ Risk of hemorrhage ↑ Risk of infection

Physical Assessment

The nurse should use the following principles in preparing for and completing an assessment of the postpartal woman:

- Select the time that will provide the most accurate data. Palpating the fundus when the woman has a full bladder, for example, may give false information about the progress of involution.
- Provide an explanation of the purposes of regular assessment to the woman.
- Ensure that the woman is relaxed before starting; perform the procedures as gently as possible to avoid unnecessary discomfort.
- Record and report the results as clearly as possible.
- Take appropriate precautions to prevent exposure to body fluids.

While completing the physical assessment, the nurse should also teach the woman. For example, when assessing the breasts of a breastfeeding woman, the nurse can discuss breast milk production, the let-down reflex, and breast self-examination. Mothers may be very receptive to instruction on postpartal abdominal tightening exercises when the nurse assesses the woman's fundal height and diastasis. The assessment also

Assessment Guide: Postpartal—First 24 Hours After Birth

PHYSICAL ASSESSMENT/ NORMAL FINDINGS	ALTERATIONS AND POSSIBLE CAUSES*	NURSING RESPONSES TO DATA†
➤ VITAL SIGNS		
➤ ***Blood pressure (BP):*** Should remain consistent with baseline BP during pregnancy.	High BP (preeclampsia, essential hypertension, renal disease, anxiety). Drop in BP (may be normal; uterine hemorrhage).	Evaluate history of preexisting disorders and check for other signs of preeclampsia (edema, proteinuria). Assess for other signs of hemorrhage (↑pulse, cool clammy skin).
➤ ***Pulse:*** 50–90 beats/minute. May be bradycardia of 50–70 beats/minute.	Tachycardia (difficult labor and birth, hemorrhage).	Evaluate for other signs of hemorrhage (↓BP, cool clammy skin).
➤ ***Respirations:*** 16–24/minute.	Marked tachypnea (respiratory disease).	Assess for other signs of respiratory disease.
➤ ***Temperature:*** 36.6–38C (98–100.4F).	After first 24 hours temperature of 38C (100.4F) or above suggests infection.	Assess for other signs of infection; notify physician/certified nurse-midwife.
➤ BREASTS		
➤ ***General appearance:*** Smooth, even pigmentation, changes of pregnancy still apparent; one may appear larger.	Reddened area (mastitis).	Assess further for signs of infection.
➤ ***Palpation:*** Depending on postpartal day, may be soft, filling, full, or engorged.	Palpable mass (caked breast, mastitis). Engorgement (venous stasis). Tenderness, heat, edema (engorgement, caked breast, mastitis).	Assess for other sign of infection: If blocked duct, consider heat, massage, position change for breastfeeding. Assess for further signs. Report mastitis to physician/certified nurse-midwife.
➤ ***Nipples:*** Supple, pigmented, intact; become erect when stimulated.	Fissures, cracks, soreness (problems with breastfeeding), not erectile with stimulation (inverted nipples).	Reassess technique; recommend appropriate interventions.
➤ ABDOMEN		
➤ ***Musculature:*** Abdomen may be soft, have a "doughy" texture; rectus muscle intact.	Separation in musculature (diastasis recti abdominis).	Evaluate size of diastasis; teach appropriate exercises for decreasing the separation.
➤ ***Fundus:*** Firm, midline; following expected process of involution.	Boggy (full bladder, uterine bleeding).	Massage until firm; assess bladder and have woman void if needed; attempt to express clots when firm. If bogginess remains or recurs, report to physician/certified nurse-midwife.
May be tender when palpated.	Constant tenderness (infection).	Assess for evidence of endometritis.
➤ LOCHIA		
Scant to moderate amount, earthy odor; no clots.	Large amount, clots (hemorrhage). Foul-smelling lochia (infection).	Assess for firmness, express additional clots; begin peripad count. Assess for other signs of infection; report to physician/certified nurse-midwife.
	*Possible causes of alterations are placed in parentheses.	† This column provides guidelines for further assessment and initial nursing actions.

(continued on next page)

Assessment Guide: Postpartal—First 24 Hours After Birth *continued*

PHYSICAL ASSESSMENT/ NORMAL FINDINGS	ALTERATIONS AND POSSIBLE CAUSES*	NURSING RESPONSES TO DATA†
➤ LOCHIA *(continued)*		
Normal progression: First 1–3 days: rubra. Following rubra: Days 3–10: serosa (alba seldom seen in hospital).	Failure to progress normally or return to rubra from serosa (subinvolution).	Report to physician/certified nurse-midwife.
➤ PERINEUM		
Slight edema and bruising in intact perineum.	Marked fullness, bruising, pain (vulvar hematoma).	Assess size; apply ice glove or ice pack; report to physician/certified nurse-midwife.
➤ ***Episiotomy:*** No redness, edema, ecchymosis, or discharge; edges well approximated.	Redness, edema, ecchymosis, discharge, or gaping stitches (infection).	Encourage sitz baths; review perineal care, appropriate wiping techniques.
➤ ***Hemorrhoids:*** None present; if present, should be small and nontender.	Full, tender, inflamed hemorrhoids.	Encourage sitz baths, side-lying position; Tucks pads, anesthetic ointments, manual replacement of hemorrhoids, stool softeners, increased fluid intake.
➤ COSTOVERTEBRAL ANGLE (CVA) TENDERNESS		
None	Present (kidney infection).	Assess for other symptoms of urinary tract infection (UTI); obtain clean-catch urine; report to physician/certified nurse-midwife.
➤ LOWER EXTREMITIES		
No pain with palpation; negative Homans' sign.	Positive findings (thrombophlebitis).	Report to physician/certified nurse-midwife.
➤ ELIMINATION		
➤ ***Urinary output:*** Voiding in sufficient quantities at least every 4–6 hours; bladder not palpable.	Inability to void (urinary retention). Symptoms of urgency, frequency, dysuria (UTI).	Employ nursing interventions to promote voiding; if not successful, obtain order for catheterization. Report symptoms of UTI to physician/certified nurse-midwife.
➤ ***Bowel elimination:*** Should have normal bowel movement by second or third day after birth.	Inability to pass feces (constipation due to fear of pain from episiotomy, hemorrhoids, perineal trauma).	Encourage fluids, ambulation, roughage in diet; sitz baths to promote healing of perineum; obtain order for stool softener.

CULTURAL ASSESSMENT‡	VARIATIONS TO CONSIDER	NURSING RESPONSES TO DATA†
Determine customs and practices regarding postpartum care. Ask the mother whether she would like fluids, and ask what temperature she prefers.	Individual preference may include • Room-temperature or warmed fluids rather than iced drinks.	Provide for specific request if possible. If woman is unable to provide specific information, the nurse may draw from general information regarding cultural variation.

‡ These are only a few suggestions. It is not our intent to imply this is a comprehensive cultural assessment.

*Possible causes of alterations are placed in parentheses.

† This column provides guidelines for further assessment and initial nursing actions.

➤

Assessment Guide: Postpartal—First 24 Hours After Birth *continued*

CULTURAL ASSESSMENT‡	VARIATIONS TO CONSIDER	NURSING RESPONSES TO DATA†
Ask the mother what foods or fluids she would like.	Special foods or fluids to hasten healing after childbirth.	Mexican women may want food and fluids that restore hot-cold balance to the body. Women of European background may ask for iced fluids.
Ask the mother whether she would prefer to be alone during breastfeeding.	Some women may be hesitant to have someone with them when their breast is exposed.	Provide privacy as desired by mother.

PSYCHOSOCIAL ASSESSMENT/ NORMAL FINDINGS	VARIATIONS TO CONSIDER	NURSING RESPONSES TO DATA†
➤ PSYCHOLOGIC ADAPTATION		
➤ ***During first 24 hours:*** Passive; preoccupied with own needs; may talk about her labor and birth experience; may be talkative, elated, or very quiet.	Very quiet and passive; sleeps frequently (fatigue from long labor; feelings of disappointment about some aspect of the experience; may be following cultural expectation).	Provide opportunities for adequate rest; provide nutritious meals and snacks that are consistent with what the woman desires to eat and drink; provide opportunities to discuss birth experience in nonjudgmental atmosphere if the woman desires to do so.
➤ ***By 12 hours:*** Beginning to assume responsibility; some women eager to learn; easily feels overwhelmed.	Excessive weepiness, mood swings, pronounced irritability (postpartum blues; feelings of inadequacy; culturally proscribed behavior).	Explain postpartum blues; provide supportive atmosphere; determine support available for mother; consider referral for evidence of profound depression.
➤ ATTACHMENT		
En face position; holds baby close; cuddles and soothes; calls by name; identities characteristics of family members in infant; may be awkward in providing care.	Continued expressions of disappointment in sex, appearance of infant; refusal to care for infant; derogatory comments; lack of bonding behaviors (difficulty in attachment, following expectations of cultural/ethnic group).	Provide reinforcement and support for infant caretaking behaviors; maintain nonjudgmental approach and gather more information if caretaking behaviors are not evident.
Initially may express disappointment over sex or appearance of infant but within 1–2 days demonstrates attachment behaviors.		
➤ CLIENT EDUCATION		
Has basic understanding of self-care activities and infant care needs; can identify signs of complications that should be reported.	Unable to demonstrate basic self-care and infant care activities (knowledge deficit; postpartum blues; following prescribed cultural behavior and will be cared for by grandmother or other family member).	Determine whether woman understands English and provide interpreter if needed; provide reinforcement of information through conversation and through written material (remember that some women and their families may not be able to understand written materials because of language difficulties or inability to read);

‡ These are only a few suggestions. It is not our intent to imply this is a comprehensive cultural assessment.

† This column provides guidelines for further assessment and initial nursing actions.

(continued on next page)

Assessment Guide: POSTPARTAL—FIRST 24 HOURS AFTER BIRTH *continued*

PSYCHOSOCIAL ASSESSMENT/ NORMAL FINDINGS	VARIATIONS TO CONSIDER	NURSING RESPONSES TO DATA†
➤ **CLIENT EDUCATION** *(continued)*		
		provide information regarding infant care skills that are culturally consistent; give woman opportunity to express her feelings; consider social service home referral for women who have no family or other support, are unable to take in information about self-care and infant care, and demonstrate no caretaking activities.
‡ These are only a few suggestions. It is not our intent to imply this is a comprehensive cultural assessment.		† This column provides guidelines for further assessment and initial nursing actions.

provides an excellent time to provide information about the body's postpartal physical and anatomic changes as well as common postpartal concerns (Table 34-3 •). Because the time the woman spends in the postpartum unit is limited, nurses should use every available opportunity for client teaching regarding self-care. To assist nurses in recognizing these opportunities, examples of client teaching during the assessment have been provided throughout the following discussion.

VITAL SIGNS

The nurse may organize the physical assessment in a variety of ways. Many nurses choose to begin by assessing vital signs because the findings are more accurate when they are obtained with the woman at rest. In addition, establishing whether the vital signs are within the expected normal range will assist the nurse in determining other assessments that might be needed. For instance, if the temperature is elevated, the nurse considers the time since birth and begins to gather information to determine whether the woman is dehydrated or whether an infection is developing.

Alterations in vital signs may indicate complications, so they are assessed at regular intervals. The blood pressure should remain stable. The pulse often shows a characteristic slowness that is no cause for alarm. Pulse rates return to prepregnant norms very quickly unless complications arise. The nurse should evaluate any temperature elevation in light of other signs and symptoms and should carefully review the woman's history to identify other factors, such as premature rupture of membranes (PROM) or prolonged labor, that might increase the incidence of infection in the genital tract.

The nurse informs the woman of the results of the vital signs assessment, providing information regarding the normal changes in blood pressure and pulse. This may also be an opportunity to assess whether the mother knows how to take her own and her infant's temperatures, how to read a thermometer, and how to select a thermometer from the wide variety now available.

Table 34–3 • COMMON POSTPARTAL CONCERNS

Several postpartal occurrences cause special concern for mothers. The nurse will frequently be asked about the following events:

Source of Concern	Explanation
Gush of blood that sometimes occurs when she first arises	Due to normal pooling of blood in vagina when the woman lies down to rest or sleep. Gravity causes blood to flow out when she stands.
Night sweats	Normal physiologic occurrence that results as body attempts to eliminate excess fluids that were present during pregnancy. May be aggravated by plastic mattress pad.
Afterpains	More common in multiparas. Due to contraction and relaxation of uterus. Increased by oxytocin, breastfeeding. Relieved with mild analgesics and time.
"Large stomach" after birth and failure to lose all weight gained during pregnancy	The baby, amniotic fluid, and placenta account for only a portion of the weight gained during pregnancy. The remainder takes approximately 6 weeks to lose. Abdomen also appears large due to ↓ muscle tone. Postpartal exercises will help.

Clinical Tip *During the first few hours after birth, the woman may have some orthostatic hypotension. This will cause her to have a lower blood pressure reading in a sitting position. For the most accurate reading, measure her blood pressure with her in the same position each time, preferably lying on her back with her arm at her side.*

AUSCULTATION OF LUNGS

The breath sounds should be clear. Women who have been treated for preterm labor or preeclampsia are especially at risk for pulmonary edema (see Chapter 19).

BREASTS

A properly fitting bra provides support to the breasts and helps maintain breast shape by limiting stretching of supporting ligaments and connective tissue. The nurse can first assess the fit and support provided by the woman's bra. The nurse provides information about how to select a bra. If the mother is breastfeeding, the straps of the bra should be cloth, not elastic (because cloth has less stretch and provides more support) and easily adjustable. The back should be wide and have at least three rows of hooks to adjust for fit. Traditional nursing bras have a fixed inner cup and a separate half-cup that can be unhooked for breastfeeding while continuing to support the breast. Purchasing a nursing bra one size too large during pregnancy will usually result in a good fit because the breasts increase in size with milk production.

The bra is then removed so the breasts can be examined. The nurse notes the size and shape of the breasts and any abnormalities, reddened areas, or engorgement. The nurse also palpates the breasts lightly for softness, slight firmness associated with filling, or firmness associated with engorgement, warmth, or tenderness. The nipples are assessed for fissures, cracks, soreness, or inversion. The nurse teaches the woman the characteristics of the breast and explains how to recognize problems such as fissures or cracks in the nipples.

The nurse assesses the nonbreastfeeding mother for evidence of breast discomfort and provides relief measures if necessary. (See discussion of lactation suppression in the nonbreastfeeding mother in Chapter 35.) Breast assessment findings for a nonbreastfeeding woman may be recorded as follows: "Breasts soft, filling, no evidence of nipple tenderness or cracking."

ABDOMEN AND FUNDUS

The woman should void before her abdomen is examined. This practice ensures that a full bladder is not causing displacement of the uterus or any uterine atony; if atony is present, other causes (such as uterine relaxation associated with a regional block, overstretched uterus, or distended bladder) must be investigated.

The nurse determines the relationship of the fundus to the umbilicus and also assesses the firmness of the fundus. The nurse notes whether the fundus is in the midline or displaced to either side of the abdomen. The most common cause of displacement is a full bladder; thus this finding requires further assessment. If the fundus is in the midline but higher than expected, it is usually associated with clots within the uterus. The results of the assessment should then be recorded. (See Procedure 34–1 on page 1006.)

While completing the assessment, the nurse teaches the woman about fundal position and how to determine firmness. The mother can be taught to massage her fundus gently if it is not firm.

Clinical Tip *During postpartal assessment, a firm uterus typically feels like a grapefruit because the muscles are well contracted. If the uterus loses its ability to contract and begins to relax, it is called boggy. A boggy uterus feels softer, like a sponge, or may become so relaxed that you can't feel it at all. If the uterus is boggy but you can still feel it, massage it until it becomes firm. If you can't feel it at all, place the side of one hand just above the woman's symphysis pubis to provide stability. Then place the other hand at the level of the umbilicus. (The fundus may have risen to this level because it is relaxed and filling with blood.) Press deeply into the abdomen and massage in a circular motion. You will usually feel the uterus begin to firm up under your hand. If you don't, move your hand slightly lower on the abdomen, and repeat the process.*

A well-contracted uterus feels as firm as the uterus does during a strong labor contraction. If handled gently, the uterus should not be overly tender. Excessive pain in the uterus during postpartal examination should alert the nurse to possible uterine infection. If the uterus is not firm, the nurse should gently massage the fundus with the fingertips of the examining hand, and then assess the results. If the uterus becomes firm, the chart should read: "Uterus: boggy → firm with light massage." A good habit for the nurse to develop during the postpartal examination is to have the woman lie flat on her back with her head on a pillow and legs flexed. Then the nurse can release the perineal pad to observe the results of uterine massage based on the amount of expelled blood. Occasionally, oxytocic agents, such as an intravenous Pitocin infusion or methylergonovine maleate (Methergine), need to be administered postpartally to maintain uterine contraction and prevent or treat hemorrhage (see Drug Guide: Methylergonovine Maleate [Methergine] in Chapter 35).

A boggy uterus that does not contract with light, gentle massage may need more vigorous massage. The nurse assesses the amount and character of any expelled blood obtained while massaging the fundus. When a woman has postpartal uterine atony (the uterus does not remain firm), the nurse should do the following:

1. Reevaluate for full bladder; if the bladder is full, have the woman void.
2. Question the woman on her bleeding history since the birth or last examination. How heavy does her flow seem? Has she passed any clots? How frequently has she changed pads? Were the pads saturated? Look at the discarded pads.
3. For the breastfeeding mother, put the newborn to the mother's breast for feeding to stimulate oxytocin production.
4. Assess maternal blood pressure and pulse to identify hypotension.

Procedure 34–1 Assessing the Status of the Uterine Fundus After Birth

Preparation

1. Explain the procedure, the information it provides, and what it might feel like.
2. Ask the woman to void.
   Rationale: A full bladder can cause uterine atony.
3. Have the woman lie flat in bed with her head on a pillow. If the procedure is uncomfortable, she may find that it helps to flex her legs.
   Rationale: The supine position prevents falsely high assessment of fundal height. Flexing the legs relaxes the abdominal muscles.

Equipment and Supplies

- A clean perineal pad (see Procedure 34–2)

Procedure

1. Gently place one hand on the lower segment of the uterus. Using the side of the other hand, palpate the abdomen until you locate the top of the fundus.
   Rationale: One hand stabilizes the uterus while the other hand locates the top of the fundus.
2. Determine whether the fundus is firm. If it is, it will feel like a hard round object in the abdomen. If it is not firm, massage the abdomen lightly until the fundus is firm.
   Rationale: A firm fundus indicates that the uterine muscles are contracted and bleeding will not occur.
3. Measure the top of the fundus in fingerbreadths above, below, or at the fundus. See Figure 34–5 •.
   Rationale: Fundal height gives information about the progress of involution.

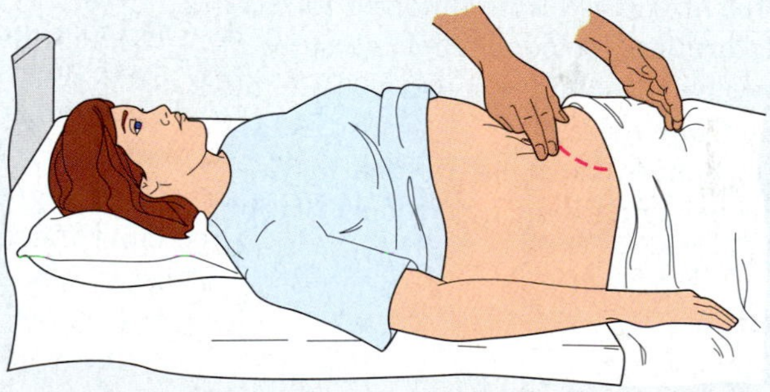

Figure 34–5 • Measuring the descent of the fundus. The fundus is located two fingerbreadths below the umbilicus.

4. Determine the position of the fundus in relation to the midline of the body. If it is not in the midline, locate it and then evaluate the bladder for distention.
   Rationale: The fundus may deviate from the midline when the bladder is full because the enlarged bladder pushes the uterus aside.
5. If the bladder is distended, use nursing measures to help the woman void. If she is not able to void after a specified period of time, catheterization may be necessary.
6. Measure urine output for the next few hours until normal elimination is established.
   Rationale: During the postpartum as diuresis occurs; the bladder may fill far more rapidly than normal, putting the woman at risk for uterine atony and hemorrhage.
7. Assess the lochia (see Procedure 34–2).

Procedure 34–1 *(continued)*

8. During the first few hours postpartum, if the fundus becomes boggy frequently or is located high above the umbilicus and the woman's bladder is empty, the uterine cavity may be filled with clots of blood. In this case, do the following:
   - Release the front of the perineal pad and lay it back so that you can see the perineum and the pad laying between the woman's legs.
   - Massage the uterine fundus until it is firm.
   - Keep one hand in position stabilizing the lower portion of the uterus. With the hand you used to massage the fundus, put steady pressure on the top of the now-firm fundus and see if you are able to express any clots. (Watch the pad between her legs for clots to pass from the vagina.)

   Rationale: If the woman's uterus is filled with blood, it acts as an irritant and the uterus will not remain contracted. When the muscle fibers relax, bleeding results, further aggravating the problem. Pushing on a uterus that is not firm is dangerous because it is possible to cause the uterus to invert, a true emergency.
9. Provide the woman with a clean perineal pad.
10. Record findings. Fundal height is recorded in fingerbreadths (eg "2 FB ↓ U" or "1 FB ↑ U").
11. If fundal massage was necessary, note that fact: "Uterus boggy → firm with light massage."

5. Reassess the fundus; if the fundus is still boggy, alert the certified nurse-midwife or physician immediately, because further intervention, such as intravenous fluids and an oxytocic medication, are needed.

In the woman who has had a cesarean birth, the nurse should inspect the abdominal incision for signs of healing, such as approximation and minimal redness, and for any signs of infection, including drainage, foul odor, or redness. During the assessment, the nurse teaches the woman about her incision. The nurse can also review characteristics of normal healing and discuss signs of infection.

LOCHIA

Lochia is then assessed for character, amount, odor, and the presence of clots. The nurse must wear disposable gloves when assessing the perineum and lochia. Nurses may put on the gloves before beginning the assessment, just before assessing the abdomen and fundus, or when they are ready to assess the perineum and lochia. During the first 1 to 3 days, the lochia should be rubra. A few small clots are normal and occur as a result of blood pooling in the vagina. However, the passage of numerous or large clots is abnormal, and the cause should be investigated immediately. After 3 to 4 days, the lochia becomes serosa.

Lochia should never exceed a moderate amount, such as that needed to partially saturate four to eight peri-pads daily, with an average of six. However, the number of pads alone is not the sole indicator; the nurse must also consider two other factors. First, some birth facilities use peri-pads that are super absorbent; a saturated pad of this type would contain a greater amount of lochia than a regular pad. The nurse needs to assess the volume absorbed in the pad. The other factor is the individual woman's pad-changing practices. The nurse should ask the mother how long the current pad has been in use, and whether any clots were passed prior to this examination, such as during voiding. If heavy bleeding is reported but not seen, the nurse asks the woman to put on a clean perineal pad and reassesses the discharge in 1 hour (see Procedure 34-2 and Figure 34–6 •).

Research suggests that visual estimations of blood loss are influenced by the brand of peri-pad used (Luegenbiehl, 1997). Consequently, the clinical facility's standards for estimating blood loss should be brand specific and need to be reassessed whenever brands are changed. When a more accurate

CRITICAL THINKING IN PRACTICE

You have completed your assessment of Patty Clark, a 24-year-old G2P2 woman who is 24 hours past birth. The fundus is just above the umbilicus and slightly to the right. Lochia rubra is present, and a pad is soaked every 2 hours. What would you do?

Answers can be found in Appendix I.

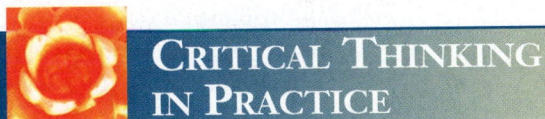

Procedure 34–2 Evaluating Lochia

Preparation

1. Explain why lochia occurs, why it is assessed, how it is assessed, and how it changes during the postpartum.
2. Ask the woman to void.
   Rationale: A full bladder can cause uterine atony and increase the amount of lochia.
3. Complete the assessment of uterine fundal height and firmness.
   Rationale: *In almost all cases, fundal height and firmness are evaluated with an assessment of lochia. This practice provides a more thorough assessment.*
4. If she has not already done so for the fundal assessment, ask the woman to flex her legs. Then ask her to spread her legs apart. Use the bed sheet as a drape to preserve her modesty.
   Rationale: *This position allows you to see the perineum and the perineal pad more effectively.*

Equipment and Supplies

Note: Gloves are put on before assessing the perineum and lochia.

- Gloves
- Clean perineal pad

Procedure: *Clean Gloves*

1. Don gloves.
2. Lower the perineal pad and observe the amount of lochia on the pad. Because women's pad-changing practices vary, ask her about the length of time the current pad has been in use, whether the amount is normal, and whether any clots were passed before this examination, such as during voiding.
   Rationale: During the first 1 to 3 days the woman's lochia should be rubra, which is dark red in color. A few small clots are normal and occur as a result of pooling of blood in the vagina when the woman is lying down. The passage of large clots is abnormal and the cause should be investigated immediately.
3. If the woman reports heavy bleeding or clots, ask her to put on a clean perineal pad and then reassess the pad in 1 hour. Also ask her to call you before flushing any clots she passes into the toilet during voiding.
4. When the uterine fundus is firm and stabilized with the nondominant hand, press down on it with the dominant hand while watching to see if any clots are expelled. (See procedure 34–1, step 8.)
5. Determine the amount of lochia, using the following guide (see Figure 34–6):
   - Heavy amount—Perineal pad has a stain larger than 6 inches in length within 1 hour; 30 to 80 mL lochia.

Clinical Tip

If blood loss exceeds the guidelines given in this chapter, weigh the perineal pads and the chux pads to estimate the blood loss more accurately. Typically, 1 g = 1 mL blood. Because blood can pool below the woman on the chux pad, the pads are included in your assessment.

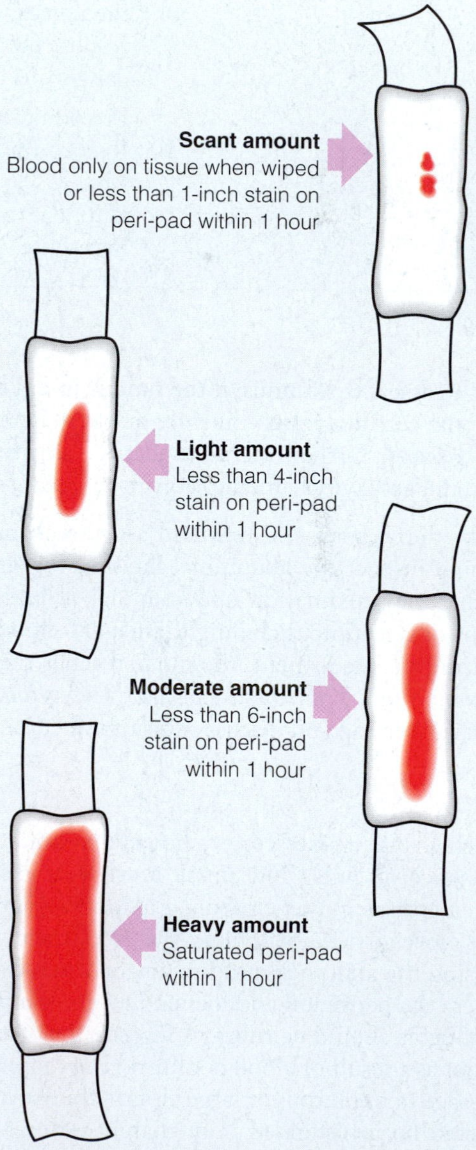

Figure 34–6 • Suggested guidelines for assessing lochia volume.
SOURCE: Jacobson, H. (1985, May-June). A standard for assessing lochia volume. *American Journal of Maternal Child Nursing, 10,* 175.

Procedure 34–2 *(continued)*

- Moderate amount—Perineal pad has a stain less than 6 inches in length within 1 hour; 25 to 50 mL lochia.
- Small (light) amount—Perineal pad has a stain less than 4 inches in length after 1 hour; 10 to 25 mL lochia.
- Scant amount—Perineal pad has a stain less than 1 inch in length after 1 hour or lochia is only on tissue when the woman wipes.

Rationale: Lochia should never exceed a moderate amount such as 4 to 8 partially saturated perineal pads daily. Using a consistent standard for measuring lochia improves the accuracy of the information charted and conveyed to others.

6. In most cases, a woman is discharged while her lochia is still rubra. Provide her with information about lochia serosa and lochia alba.
   Rationale: Accurate discharge information enables the woman to assess herself more accurately and enables her to judge better when to contact her caregiver.
7. Record the findings specifically. For example, "Lochia moderate rubra, no clots passed."

assessment of blood loss is needed, the perineal pads can be weighed, with 1 g considered equivalent to 1 mL blood.

Clots and heavy bleeding may be caused by uterine relaxation (atony) or retained placental fragments, and they require further assessment. Because of the evacuation of the uterine cavity during cesarean birth, women with such surgery usually have less lochia after the first 24 hours than mothers who give birth vaginally. Therefore, amounts of lochia that would be normal in women who had vaginal births are suspect in women who have undergone cesarean birth.

If the woman is at increased risk for bleeding or is actually experiencing heavy flow of lochia rubra, her blood pressure, pulse, and uterus need to be assessed frequently, and the physician may prescribe methylergonovine maleate (Methergine). The odor of the lochia is nonoffensive and never foul. If foul odor is present, so is an infection. When using narrative nursing notes, the amount of lochia is charted first, followed by character, for example, "Lochia: moderate rubra" or "Lochia: small rubra/serosa."

Client teaching that the nurse may address during assessment of the lochia may center on normal changes that can be expected in the amount and color of the flow. Hygienic measures, such as wiping the perineum from front to back and washing her hands after toileting and changing pads, may be reviewed if appropriate. The nurse should approach the timing of teaching hygienic practices delicately, along with the content to be included. By establishing positive goals for the teaching—promoting comfort, enhancing tissue healing, and preventing infection—the nurse can avoid value-laden statements regarding personal beliefs about the need for cleanliness or control of body odor.

PERINEUM

The perineum is inspected with the woman lying in Sims' position. The buttock is lifted to expose the perineum and anus.

If an episiotomy was performed or a laceration required suturing, the nurse assesses the wound. To evaluate the state of healing, the nurse inspects the wound for redness, edema, ecchymosis, discharge, and approximation. After 24 hours, some edema may still be present, but the skin edges should be "glued" together (well approximated) so that gentle pressure does not separate them. Gentle palpation should elicit minimal tenderness, and there should be no hardened areas suggesting infection. Ecchymosis interferes with normal healing, as does infection. Foul odors associated with drainage indicate infection.

The nurse next assesses whether hemorrhoids are present around the anus. If present, they are assessed for size, number, and pain or tenderness (Procedure 34–3 and Figure 34–7 •).

During the assessment, the nurse talks with the woman to determine the effectiveness of comfort measures that have been used. The nurse provides teaching about the episiotomy. Some women do not thoroughly understand what an episiotomy is and where it is and may believe that the stitches must be removed, as with other types of surgery. Frequently, when women fear that the stitches must be removed manually, they are afraid to ask about them. While explaining the findings of the assessment, the nurse can provide information about the episiotomy, its location, and signs that are being assessed. In addition, the nurse can casually add that the sutures dissolve slowly over the next few weeks as the tissues heal. By the time the sutures are dissolved, the tissues are strong, and the incision edges will not separate. This is also an opportunity to teach comfort measures that may be used (see Chapter 35).

An example of charting a perineal assessment might read: "Midline episiotomy; no edema, tenderness, or ecchymosis present. Skin edges well approximated. Woman reports sitz bath and pain relief measures are controlling discomfort."

Procedure 34-3 Postpartum Perineal Assessment

Preparation

1. Explain the purpose and the procedure for assessing the perineum during the postpartum period.
2. Complete the assessment of fundal height and lochia as described in Procedures 34–1 and 34–2.
   Rationale: Typically, perineal assessment is the final step of the postpartum assessment.
3. At this point in a postpartal assessment, the woman is lying on her back with her knees flexed. Her perineal pad has already been lifted away from her perineum to permit inspection of the lochia. If an episiotomy was performed or if the birth was difficult, the woman may be using an ice pack on her perineum to reduce swelling. The ice pack would also have been removed for inspection of the lochia.
4. Ask her to turn onto her side with her upper knee drawn forward and resting on the bed (Sims' position).
   Rationale: When the woman is supine, even with her knees flexed, it is very difficult to expose the posterior portion of the perineum. Thus, Sims' position makes it easiest to inspect the perineum and anal area.

Equipment and Supplies

- Clean perineal pad
- Small light source such as a penlight may be necessary

Procedure: *Clean Gloves*

1. Use a systematic approach to assessment.
   Rationale: A systematic approach helps ensure that you don't overlook a significant finding.
2. In evaluating the perineum, begin by asking the woman's perceptions. How does she describe her discomfort? Does it seem excessive to her? Has it become worse since the birth? Does it seem more severe than you would expect? (Note: Pain that seems disproportionately severe may indicate that the woman is developing a vulvar hematoma.)
   Rationale: Information from the client herself often helps identify developing problems.
3. After talking with the woman, assess the condition of the tissue. To allow for full visualization, it may be helpful to ask the woman to life the knee of her upper leg to expose her perineum more fully. In some cases it may help to use the nondominant hand to lift the buttocks and tissue. Note any swelling (edema) and bruising (ecchymosis).
   Rationale: The tissue is often traumatized by the birth and mild bruising is not unusual. However, excessive bruising may indicate that a hematoma is developing.
4. Evaluate the episiotomy, if there is one, or any repaired laceration for its state of healing. Is it reddened? Note the edges of the incision. Are they well approximated? Tell the woman that you are going to palpate the incision gently, then do so. Note any areas of hardness. Note whether the incision is warmer to the touch than the surrounding tissue.
   Rationale: Gentle palpation should elicit minimal tenderness and there should be no redness, warmth, or areas of hardness, which suggest infection. Both bruising and infection interfere with normal healing. Typically, within 24 hours the edges of the incision should be "glued" together (well approximated).
5. During the assessment be alert for odors. Typically the lochia has an earthy, but not unpleasant, smell that is easily identifiable.
   Rationale: A foul odor associated with drainage often indicates infection.

> **Clinical Tip**
>
> *In evaluating the perineum, use the REEDA scale as a quick reminder of what to assess. Specifically:*
>
> *R = redness*
>
> *E = edema or swelling*
>
> *E = ecchymosis or bruising*
>
> *D = drainage*
>
> *A = approximation (how well the edges of an incision—the episiotomy—or a repaired laceration seem to be holding together)*

Procedure 34–3 Postpartum Perineal Assessment *(continued)*

6. Finally, assess for hemorrhoids. To visualize the anal area, lift the upper buttocks to fully expose the anal area. (See Figure 34–7 •.) If hemorrhoids are present, note the size, number, and pain or tenderness.
   Rationale: Hemorrhoids often develop during pregnancy or labor and can cause considerable discomfort. If hemorrhoids are present, the woman may benefit from available comfort measures.

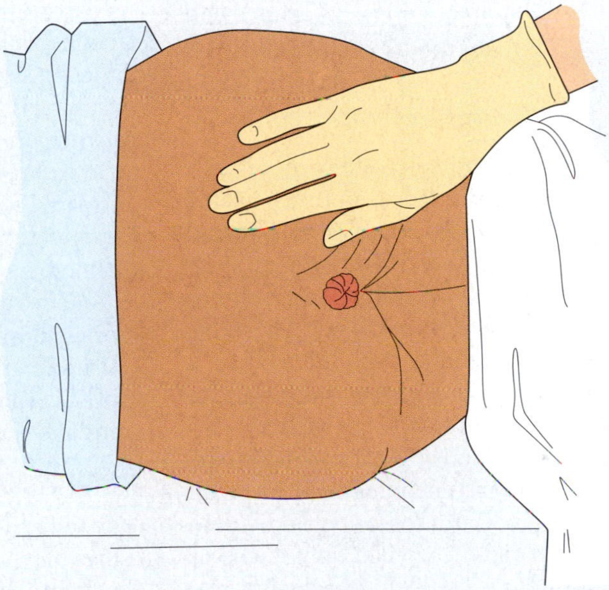

Figure 34–7 • Intact perineum with hemorrhoids.

7. During the assessment, talk to the woman about the effectiveness of comfort measures being used. Provide teaching about care of the episiotomy, hemorrhoids, and the like.
   Rationale: Health teaching is an important part of nursing care. Many women have concerns about the episiotomy and may not know, for example, that the suture used is dissolvable. This is an excellent time to provide information about good healthcare practices in both the short and long term.
8. Provide the woman with a clean perineal pad. Replenish the ice pack if necessary.
9. Record findings. For example: "Midline episiotomy; no edema, ecchymosis, or tenderness. Skin edges well approximated. Woman reports pain relief measures are controlling discomfort."

LOWER EXTREMITIES

If thrombophlebitis occurs, the most likely site will be the woman's legs. To assess for this condition, the nurse should have the woman stretch her legs out, with the knees slightly flexed and the legs relaxed. The nurse then grasps the foot and dorsiflexes it sharply. No discomfort or pain should be present. If pain is elicited, the nurse notifies the certified nurse-midwife or physician that the woman has a positive Homans' sign (see Figure 37–3). The pain is caused by inflammation of a vessel. The nurse also evaluates the legs for edema, noting any areas of redness, tenderness, and increased skin temperature.

Early ambulation is an important aspect of preventing thrombophlebitis. Most women are able to get up shortly after birth or once they have fully recovered from the effects of the regional anesthetic agent, if one has been used. The cesarean birth client requires passive range-of-motion exercises until she is ambulating more freely.

Client teaching associated with assessment of the lower extremities focuses on the signs and symptoms of thrombophlebitis. In addition, the nurse may review self-care measures to promote circulation and prevent thrombophlebitis, such as leg exercises that may be performed in bed, dorsiflexion on an hourly basis while on bed rest, ambulation, avoiding pressure behind the knees, avoiding use of the knee gatch on the bed, and avoiding crossing the legs.

Usually, the nurse records the results of the assessment on a flowsheet or a summary nursing note. If tenderness and warmth have been noted, they might be recorded as follows: "Tenderness, warmth, slight edema, and slight redness noted on posterior aspect of left calf—positive Homans'. Woman advised to avoid pressure to this area; lower leg elevated and moist heat applied per agency protocol. Call placed to Dr Garcia to report findings."

ELIMINATION

During the hours after birth, the nurse carefully monitors a new mother's bladder status. A displaced uterus, palpable bladder, or boggy uterus is a sign of bladder distention and requires nursing intervention.

Following birth, the postpartal woman should void within 4 hours, and at least every 4 to 6 hours thereafter. The nurse should assess the bladder for distention until the woman is able to completely empty her bladder with each voiding. The nurse may employ techniques to assist voiding, such as helping the woman out of bed to void, pouring warm water on the vulva, running water in the sink, and encouraging the woman to relax and take deep breaths. Catheterization is required when the bladder is distended and the woman cannot void or when she is voiding small amounts (<100 mL) frequently. Although many physicians/CNMs write orders stating that the woman can be catheterized in 8 hours if she has not voided, the nurse needs to assess the bladder and any voiding pattern frequently prior to the end of the 8-hour period. Some women may require catheterization sooner. The cesarean birth mother may have an indwelling catheter inserted prophylactically. The nurse should perform the same assessments in evaluating bladder emptying once the catheter is removed.

During the physical assessment, the nurse elicits information from the woman regarding the adequacy of her fluid intake, whether she feels she is emptying her bladder completely when she voids, and any signs of urinary tract infection (UTI) she may be experiencing.

In the same way, the nurse obtains information about the new mother's intestinal elimination and any concerns she may have about it. Many mothers fear that the first bowel movement will be painful and possibly even damaging if an episiotomy has been performed. Stool softeners may be ordered to increase bulk and moisture in the fecal material and to allow more comfortable and complete evacuation. Constipation may cause pressure on sutures and increase discomfort and therefore should be prevented. Encouraging ambulation, forcing fluids (up to 2000 mL/day or more), and providing fresh fruits and roughage in the diet enhance bowel elimination and help the woman reestablish her normal bowel pattern.

During the assessment, the nurse may provide information regarding postpartum diuresis, explaining why the woman may be emptying her bladder so frequently. Information about the need for additional fluid intake, with suggestions of specific amounts, may be helpful. The woman should drink at least eight 8-oz glasses of water or juice in addition to other fluids. The nurse discusses signs of retention and overflow voiding and reviews symptoms of UTI with the mother at this time if it seems an appropriate moment for teaching. The nurse can also review methods of assisting bowel elimination and provide opportunities for the woman to ask questions.

REST AND SLEEP STATUS

As part of the postpartal assessment, the nurse evaluates the amount of rest the new mother is getting. If the woman reports difficulty sleeping at night, the nurse should try to determine the cause. If it is simply the strange environment, a warm drink, backrub, or mild sedative may prove helpful. Appropriate nursing measures are indicated if the woman is bothered by normal postpartal discomforts such as afterpains, diaphoresis, or episiotomy or hemorrhoidal pain. The impact of rooming-in on the mother's ability to rest should be assessed.

A daily rest period should be encouraged, and hospital activities should be scheduled to allow time for napping. The nurse can also provide information about the fatigue a new mother experiences and the impact it can have on her emotions and sense of well-being.

NUTRITIONAL STATUS

The nurse determines postpartal nutritional status by evaluating information provided by the mother and by direct assessment. During pregnancy, the daily recommended dietary allowances call for increases in calories, proteins, and most vitamins and minerals. After birth, the nonbreastfeeding mother's dietary requirements return to prepregnancy levels.

Visiting mothers during mealtime provides an opportunity for unobtrusive nutritional assessment and counseling. The nonbreastfeeding mother should be advised about the need to reduce her caloric intake by about 300 kcal and to return to prepregnancy levels for other nutrients. The breastfeeding mother should increase her caloric intake by about 200 kcal over the pregnancy requirements, or a total of 500 kcal over the nonpregnant requirement. Basic discussion will usually prove helpful, followed by referral as needed. In all cases, the nurse should provide literature on nutrition so that the woman will have a source of information following discharge.

The dietitian should be informed of any mother who is a vegetarian or whose cultural or religious beliefs require specific foods. Appropriate meals can then be prepared for her. Many women, especially those who gained more than the recommended number of pounds, are interested in losing weight after birth. The dietitian can design weight-reduction diets to meet nutritional needs and food preferences. The nurse may also refer women with unusual eating habits or numerous questions about good nutrition to the dietitian.

New mothers are also advised that it is common practice to prescribe iron supplements for 3 months after birth. Hemoglobin and hematocrit values are assessed at a postpartal visit to detect any anemia.

Table 34–4 • DAILY EATING TO ENCOURAGE HEALTHFUL NUTRITION DURING THE POSTPARTAL PERIOD

2–3 servings of milk, yogurt, and cheese group
2–3 servings of meat or protein group
3–5 servings of vegetable group
4 servings of whole grain
2–4 servings of fruit group
6–11 servings of bread, cereal, rice, and pasta group
Fats, oils, and sweets sparingly

As a part of the nutritional assessment, the nurse can provide teaching about the nutritional needs of the woman during the postpartal period. See Table 34–4 • as well as the discussion in Chapter 18.

Psychologic Assessment

Adequate assessment of the mother's psychologic adjustment is an integral part of postpartal evaluation. This assessment focuses on the mother's general attitude, feelings of competence, available support systems, and caregiving skills. It also evaluates her fatigue level, sense of satisfaction, and ability to accomplish her developmental tasks.

The concepts of postpartal/childbearing fatigue and tiredness are not synonymous. During the initial hospitalization following childbirth, the woman typically suffers from tiredness, which is less severe and more easily relieved; fatigue, by contrast, tends to be more severe and lasts longer, with both physiologic and psychologic aspects (Bozoky & Corwin, 2002). Women are more fatigued at 14 to 19 months postpartum than they were at 6 weeks postpartum. This fatigue level is the same or higher than at the time of birth. There was no correlation between quality of sleep and energy or level of fatigue. Frequently, the woman is so tired from a long labor and birth that everything seems to be an effort. To avoid inadvertently classifying a very tired mother as one with a potential attachment problem, the nurse should perform the psychologic assessment on more than one occasion. After a nap, the new mother is often far more receptive to her baby and her surroundings (Bozoky & Corwin, 2002).

Some new mothers have little or no experience with newborns and may feel totally overwhelmed. They may show these feelings by asking questions and reading all available material or by becoming passive and quiet because they simply cannot deal with their feelings of inadequacy. Unless a nurse questions the woman about her plans and previous experience in a supportive, nonjudgmental way, the nurse might conclude that the woman is uninterested, withdrawn, or depressed. Clues that may indicate a problem include excessive, continued fatigue; marked depression; excessive preoccupation with physical status or discomfort; evidence of low self-esteem; lack of support systems; marital problems; inability to care for or nurture the newborn; and current family crises (such as illness or unemployment). These characteristics frequently indicate a potential for maladaptive parenting, which may lead to child abuse or neglect (physical, emotional, intellectual) and cannot be ignored. Referrals to public health nurses or other available community resources may provide greatly needed assistance and alleviate potentially dangerous situations.

Assessment of Early Attachment

Attachment is a desired outcome of maternal-newborn interactions during the postpartal period. The nurse in the postpartum setting can periodically observe and note the mother's progress toward attachment. The following questions can be addressed in the course of nurse-client interaction:

1. Is the mother attracted to her newborn? To what extent does she seek face-to-face contact and eye contact? Has she progressed from fingertip touch to palmar contact, to enfolding the infant close to her own body? Is attraction increasing or decreasing? If the mother does not exhibit increasing attraction, why not? Do the reasons lie primarily within her, in the baby, or in the environment?
2. Is the mother inclined to nurture her infant? Is she progressing in her interactions with her infant?
3. Does the mother act consistently? If not, is the source of unpredictability within her or her infant?
4. Is her mothering consistently carried out? Does she seek information and evaluate it objectively? Does she develop solutions based on adequate knowledge of valid data? Does she evaluate the effectiveness of her maternal care and make appropriate adjustments?
5. Is she sensitive to the newborn's needs as they arise? How quickly does she interpret her infant's behavior and react to cues? Does she seem happy and satisfied with the infant's responses to her efforts? Is she pleased with feeding behaviors? How much of this ability and willingness to respond is related to the baby's nature, and how much to her own?
6. Does she seem pleased with her baby's appearance and sex? Is she experiencing pleasure in interaction with her infant? What interferes with the enjoyment? Does she speak to the baby frequently and affectionately? Does she call him or her by name? Does she point out family traits or characteristics she sees in the newborn?
7. Are there any cultural factors that might modify the mother's response? For instance, is it customary for the grandmother to assume most of the child care responsibilities while the mother recovers from childbirth?

When the nurse has addressed these questions and assembled the facts, the nurse's intuition and formal background of knowledge combine to answer three more questions: Is there a problem in attachment? What is the problem? What is its source? The nurse can then devise a creative approach to the problem as it presents itself in the context of a unique, developing mother-infant relationship.

Discharge Assessment and Follow-up

Goals of postpartal nursing care include promoting physical stability for both mother and baby, ensuring the mother's ability to care for the infant, and providing follow-up care (Ruchala, 2000).

Newborns' and Mothers' Health Protection Act

The **Newborns' and Mothers' Health Protection Act** of 1996 **(NMHPA)** went into effect January 1, 1998. This law states that a woman who has given birth vaginally in a health-care setting cannot be forcibly discharged within 48 hours of the time of birth for insurance reasons. A woman who had a cesarean birth is covered by her insurance until 96 hours following the time of giving birth. If a mother with an uncomplicated birth and her physician/caregiver mutually decide that discharge prior to this time frame is required this can be accomplished. When this occurs it is recommended that the newborn be seen in a follow-up setting within 48 hours (Lieu, Braveman, Escobar, et al, 2000). According to a study by Dato, Saraiya, & Ziskin. (2000) the mean length of a hospital stay following an uncomplicated vaginal birth was 1.9 days with 62% of the women feeling this was an adequate length of time. Older married women working outside of the home felt their length of stay was shorter than needed due to concerns of physical well-being of the baby and perceived need of rest.

Maternal Concerns Questionnaire

Mothers may have a variety of concerns related to their own physiologic changes, newborn care, and methods to manage their recovery. The Maternal Concerns Questionnaire developed by Sheil, Bull, Moxon, et al (1995) is a useful tool for nurses. It helps the mother identify the degree of concern she has regarding her own and the baby's needs, concerns related to her partner and family, and concerns related to the community. For each area, the mother can note specific needs and rate each as of no concern, little concern, moderate concern, or much concern. After the mother completes the questionnaire, the nurse can identify the woman's concerns and informational needs and address each one. Postpartum nurses must be aware of the long-term adjustments and stresses that the childbearing family faces as its members adjust to new and different roles. Nurses can help by providing anticipatory guidance about the realities of being a mother. Agencies should have literature available for reference at home. Ongoing parenting groups give parents an opportunity to discuss problems and become comfortable in new roles.

Critical Thinking in Practice

You walk in and find Dana Sullivan, a 29-year-old G2P2 at 48 hours post repeat cesarean, crying. She states, "I'm not ready to go home. With my first baby they made me go home after 2 days. Can they make me again?"

Answers can be found in Appendix I.

Assessment of Physical and Developmental Tasks

During the first several weeks postpartum, the woman must accomplish several physical and developmental tasks critical to her own and her newborn's health and well-being. Assessment of her progress toward accomplishing these tasks is usually carried out both in the community—in ambulatory clinics—as well as in the home.

Postpartum physical and developmental tasks include the following:

- Restoring physical condition
- Developing competence in caring for and meeting the needs of her infant
- Establishing a relationship with her new child
- Adapting to altered lifestyles and family structure resulting from the addition of a new member

The new mother and her family may have an inadequate or incorrect understanding of what to expect during the early postpartal weeks. She may be concerned with restoring her figure and surprised because of continuing physical discomfort from sore breasts, episiotomy, or hemorrhoids. Fatigue is perhaps her greatest, yet most underestimated, problem during the early weeks. This may be aggravated if she has no extended family support or if there are other young children at home.

Developing skill and confidence in caring for an infant may provoke extreme anxiety in a new mother. As she struggles to establish a mutually acceptable pattern with her baby, small unanticipated concerns may seem monumental. The woman may begin to feel inadequate and, if she lacks support systems, isolated. Gjerdingen (2000) studied first-time parents' predictions about the change in their workload. Eighty-five percent of mothers expected a greater change in their workloads in comparison to 53% of fathers following the birth of their child. These increases tended to fall along stereotypical gender lines, with women planning to do more child care and housework, and men expecting to spend more time in their employment or doing odd jobs around the house. A study by McVeigh, Baafi, and Williamson (2002) found that even though most fathers maintained their level of participation in household and family activities during the postpartum period, few increased their involvement when a new family member was added.

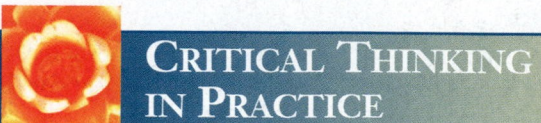

Postpartal Assessment in the Community

Nurses have been in the forefront of healthcare providers attempting to improve the care given during the postpartal period. Many obstetricians, certified nurse-midwives, and nurse practitioners now routinely see all postpartal women 1 to 2 weeks after birth in addition to the routine 6-week checkup. These visits provide opportunities for physical assessment as well as assessment of the mother's psychologic and informational needs and needs of the family. Glazener, Abdalla, Stroud, et al (1995) discovered that 87% of the women they studied suffered from self-described health problems during the first 8 weeks postpartum. Seventy-six percent of the study population continued to suffer from at least one health problem at 18 months following birth.

Women may readily discuss physical problems postpartally, but they may be reluctant to divulge their emotional needs. Developing skill and confidence in caring for an infant may provoke extreme anxiety in a new mother. As she struggles to establish a mutually acceptable pattern with her baby, small unanticipated concerns may seem monumental. The woman may begin to feel inadequate and, if she lacks support systems, isolated. According to Fowles (1998), a woman who experiences marked difficulty in maternal role attainment will exhibit depressive symptoms within 2 to 3 months of giving birth. During this time, contact with her obstetrician, certified nurse-midwife, or nurse practitioner is essential. In addition, the study author recommends that pediatricians and pediatric nurse practitioners also assess the mother's physical, mental, and emotional health during "well baby" visits.

In summary, the results of all of these studies indicate that healthcare professionals across the spectrum need to have a greater awareness of the physical and psychologic needs and potential problems the postpartal woman may experience.

Postpartal Assessment in the Home

Nurses may provide postdischarge care for the postpartal woman by home visits, follow-up phone calls, or both. A home visit 1 to 3 days after discharge provides opportunities for further assessment and teaching. The follow-up phone call is usually initiated by a nurse from the postpartal unit of the agency where the mother gave birth. It is made soon after discharge (within 24 to 48 hours) and is designed to provide assessment and, if necessary, care; to reinforce knowledge and provide additional teaching; and to make referrals if indicated.

The routine physical assessment, which can be made rapidly, focuses on the woman's general appearance, breasts, reproductive tract, bladder and bowel elimination, and any specific problems or complaints. (See the Assessment Guide: Postpartal—First Home Visit and Anticipated Progress at 6 Weeks, in Chapter 36.) In addition, the nurse should talk with the mother about her diet, fatigue level, family adjustment, and psychologic status. The nurse explores any problems with child care and refers the mother to a pediatric nurse practitioner or pediatrician if needed. Available community resources, including public health department follow-up visits, are mentioned when appropriate. If not already discussed, teaching about family planning is appropriate at this time, and the nurse provides information regarding birth control methods. Women who gave birth vaginally tend to abstain from resuming sexual intercourse for a longer period of time than the women who had a cesarean birth. Couples who breastfed resumed sexual relations later than couples who did not breastfeed.

In ideal situations, a family approach involving the father, newborn, and other siblings permits a total evaluation and provides an opportunity for all family members to ask questions and express concerns. In addition, a family approach can sometimes enable the nurse to identify disturbed family patterns more readily and suggest, or even institute, therapeutic measures to prevent future problems of neglect or abuse.

CHAPTER REVIEW

EXPLOREMEDIALINK

NCLEX review questions, case studies, and other interactive resources for this chapter can be found on the Web site at http://www.prenhall.com/olds. Click on "Chapter 34" to select the activities for this chapter.

For tutorials including animations and videos, more NCLEX review questions, and an audio glossary, access the accompanying CD-ROM in this book.

Focus Your Study

- The uterus involutes rapidly, primarily through a reduction in cell size.
- Involution is assessed by measuring fundal height. The fundus is at the level of the umbilicus within a

few hours after birth and should decrease by approximately one fingerbreadth per day.

- The placental site heals by a process of exfoliation, so no scar formation occurs.
- Lochia progresses from rubra to serosa to alba and is assessed in terms of type, quantity, and characteristics.
- The abdomen may have decreased muscle tone (flabby consistency) initially. The nurse should assess for diastasis recti abdominis, separation of the rectus abdominis muscles.
- Constipation may develop postpartally because of decreased tone in the abdominal muscles, limited diet, and denial of the urge to defecate due to fear of pain.
- Decreased bladder sensitivity, increased capacity, and postpartal diuresis may lead to problems with bladder elimination. Frequent assessment and prompt intervention are indicated. A fundus that is boggy but does not respond to massage, is higher than expected, or deviates to the side usually indicates a full bladder.
- Postpartally, a healthy woman should be normotensive and afebrile. Bradycardia is common.
- Postpartally the WBC count is often elevated. Activation of clotting factors predisposes the woman to thrombus formation.
- Psychologic adaptations of the postpartal woman are traditionally described as "taking-in" and "taking-hold."
- In consideration of the client's background, the nurse should recognize and respect cultural variations and individual preferences.
- Postpartal assessment should be completed in a systematic way, usually head to toe, and should include assessment of rest and sleep, nutrition, and attachment. The assessment provides opportunities for informal client teaching.
- In the weeks following birth, the woman's physical condition returns to a nonpregnant state, and she gains competence in caregiving and confidence in herself as a parent.

References

Al-Oballi Kridil, S. (2002). Health beliefs and practices among Arab women. *American Journal of Maternal Child Nursing, 27*(3), 178–182.

Ament, L. A. (1990). Maternal tasks of the puerperium reidentified. *Journal of Obstetric, Gynecologic, and Neonatal Nursing, 19*(4), 330–335.

American College of Obstetricians and Gynecologists (ACOG). (2000). Breast feeding: Maternal and infant aspects (*Education Bulletin* No. 258). Washington, DC: Author.

Andrews, M. M., & Boyle, J. S. (1999). *Transcultural concepts in nursing care* (3rd ed.). Philadelphia: J. B. Lippincott.

Blackburn, S. T. (2003). *Maternal, fetal, & neonatal physiology: A clinical perspective.* (2nd ed.). St. Louis, MO: Saunders.

Bozoky, I., & Corwin, E. J. (2002). Fatigue as a predictor of postpartum depression. *Journal of Obstetric, Gynecologic, and Neonatal Nursing, 31*(4), 436–443.

Cesario, S. K. (2001). Care of the Native American woman: Strategies for practice, education, and research. *Journal of Obstetric, Gynecologic, and Neonatal Nursing, 30*(1), 13–18.

Choudhry, U. K. (1997). Traditional practices of women from India: Pregnancy, childbirth, and newborn care. *Journal of Obstetric, Gynecologic, and Neonatal Nursing, 26*(5), 533–539.

Cluett, E. R., Alexander, J., & Pickering, R. M. (1997). What is the normal pattern of uterine involution? *Midwifery, 13*(1), 9–16.

Cunningham, F. G., Gant, N. F., Leveno, K. J., Gilstrap, L. C., III, Hauth, J. C., & Wenstrom, K. D. (2001). *Williams obstetrics* (21st ed.). New York: Lippincott Williams & Wilkins.

Dato, V. M., Saraiya, M., & Ziskin, L. (2000). Use of a comprehensive state birth data system to assess mother's satisfaction with length of stay. *Maternal and Child Health Journal, 4*(4), 223–231.

De Sovo, M. R. (1997, August). Keeping the faith: Jewish traditions in pregnancy and childbirth. *Lifelines, 1*(4), 46–49.

Fowles, E. R. (1998). The relationship between maternal role attainment and postpartum depression. *Health Care for Women International, 19*, 83–94.

Gichia, J. E. U. (2000). Mothers and others: African-American women's preparation for motherhood. *American Journal of Maternal Child Nursing, 25*(2), 86–91.

Gjerdingen, D. (2000). Expectant parents' anticipated changes in workload after the birth of their first child. *Journal of Family Practice, 49*(11), 993–997.

Glazener, C. M., Abdalla, M., Stroud, P., Naji, S., Templeton, A., & Russell, I. T. (1995). Postnatal maternal morbidity: Extent, causes, prevention and treatment. *British Journal of Obstetrics and Gynaecology, 102*(4), 282–287.

Harrison, J. M. (2000). Physiological changes of the puerperium. *British Journal of Midwifery, 8*(8), 483–488.

Howard, J. Y., & Berbiglia, V. A. (1997). Caring for childbearing Korean women. *Journal of Obstetric, Gynecologic, and Neonatal Nursing, 26*(6), 665–671.

Jacobson, H. (1985). A standard for assessing lochia volume. *American Journal of Maternal Child Nursing, 10*(3), 174–175.

Lieu, T. A., Braveman, P. A., Escobar, G. J., Fischer, A. F., Jensvold, N. G., & Capra, A. M. (2000). A randomized comparison of home and clinic follow-up visits after early postpartum hospital discharge. *Pediatrics, 105*(5), 1058–1065.

Luegenbiehl, D. L. (1997). Improving visual estimation of blood volume on peripads. *American Journal of Maternal Child Nursing, 22*(6), 294–298.

Marchant, S., Alexander, J., Garcia, J., Ashurst, H., Alderdice, F., & Keene, J. (1999). A survey of women's experiences of vaginal loss from 24 hours to three months after childbirth (the BliPP study). *Midwifery, 15*(2), 72–81.

Martell, L. K. (1996). Is Rubin's "taking-in" and "taking-hold" a useful paradigm? *Health Care for Women International, 17*(1), 1–13.

Mayberry, L. J., Affonso, D. D., Shibuya, J., & Clemmens, D. (1999). Integrating cultural values, beliefs, and customs into pregnancy and postpartum care: Lessons learned from a Hawaiian public health nursing project. *Journal of Perinatal and Neonatal Nursing, 13*(1), 15–26.

McVeigh, C. A. (2000a). Anxiety and functional status after childbirth. *Australian College of Midwives Journal, 13*(1), 14–18.

McVeigh, C. A. (2000b). Satisfaction with social support and functional status after childbirth. *Maternal Child Nursing Journal, 25*(1), 25–30.

McVeigh, C. A., Baafi, M., & Williamson, M. (2002). Functional status after fatherhood: An Australian study. *Journal of Obstetric, Gynecologic, and Neonatal Nursing, 31*(2), 165–171.

Mercer, R. T. (1995). *Becoming a mother.* New York: Springer.

Milasinovic, L., Kapamadzija, A., Dobric, L., & Petrovic, D. (2000). Postpartal anemia: Incidence and etiology. *Medicinski Pregled, 53*(7–8), 394–399.

Morin, K. H., Brogan, S., & Flavin, S. K. (2002). Attitudes and perceptions of body image in postpartum African American women. *American Journal of Maternal Child Nursing, 27*(1), 20–25.

Rubin, R. (1961). Puerperal change. *Nursing Outlook, 9*, 753.

Rubin, R. (1984). *Maternal identity and the maternal experience.* New York: Springer.

Ruchala, P. L. (2000). Teaching new mothers: Priorities of nurses and postpartum women. *Journal of Obstetric, Gynecologic, and Neonatal Nursing, 29*(3), 265–273.

Scroggins, J. (2000). Physical and psychological changes. In S. Mattson & J. Smith (Eds.), *AWHONN: Core curriculium for maternal-newborn nursing* (2nd ed., pp. 302–316). Philadelphia: Saunders.

Sheil, E. P., Bull, M. J., Moxon, B. E., Muehl, P. A., Kroening, K. L., Peterson-Palmberg, G., & Kelber, S. (1995). Concerns of childbearing women: A Maternal Concerns Questionnaire as an assessment tool. *Journal of Obstetric, Gynecologic, and Neonatal Nursing, 24*(2), 149–155.

Stark, M. A. (2000). Is it difficult to concentrate during the third trimester and postpartum? *Journal of Obstetric, Gynecologic, and Neonatal Nursing, 29*(4), 378–389.

Troy, N. W. (1999). A comparison of fatigue and energy levels at 6 weeks and 14 to 19 months postpartum. *Clinical Nursing Research, 8*(2), 135–152.

The Postpartal Family: Needs and Care

35

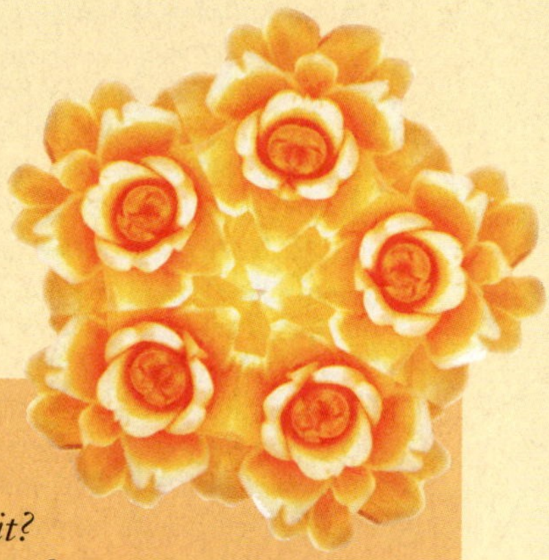

I have always associated the word "family" with positive thoughts and experiences. I vividly remember growing up as the oldest of six children, and yet receiving constant love, support, and affection from my parents. I have often wondered, "How did they do it? How did they nurture and raise so many kids and still make every one of us feel special and important?" I truly believed that I would never be able to match their success in parenting, and I was scared to begin a family of my own. When I shared these thoughts with my husband before we married, it turned out that he had anxieties of his own, but we decided that, if we supported each other every step of the way, we could do it. Seven years later, our family continues to grow quite rapidly. Trying to raise a 4-year-old, 2-year-old, and 10-week-old is extremely challenging, but it is the most rewarding experience of our lives.

In addition to parenting three very small children, we balance full-time jobs. I manage a postpartal nursing unit, and I completed my master's degree this spring. All of this has demanded an enormous amount of energy and self-control, but it has increased my confidence in myself and my empathy for my clients. I realize now that, when new parents confess their uncertainty about being able to provide enough love and care for their infant, their concern itself shows that they are going to be just fine.

Objectives

- Delineate nursing responsibilities for client teaching during the early postpartal period.
- Discuss appropriate nursing interventions to promote maternal comfort and well-being.
- Describe the nurse's role in promoting maternal rest and helping the mother to resume gradually an appropriate level of activity.
- Identify client teaching topics for promoting postpartal family wellness.
- Compare the nursing needs of a woman who experienced a cesarean birth with the needs of a woman who gave birth vaginally.
- Summarize the nursing needs of the childbearing adolescent during the postpartal period.
- Describe possible approaches to sensitive, holistic nursing care for the woman who relinquishes her newborn.
- Determine the nurse's responsibilities related to early postpartum discharge.

Key Terms

Bogginess 1023
Couplet care 1033
Mother-baby care 1033
Patient-controlled analgesia (PCA) 1038

MediaLink

Additional resources for this content can be found on the Student CD-ROM and on the Companion Website at www.prenhall.com/olds. Click on "Chapter 35" to select the activities for this chapter.

CD-ROM

- Audio Glossary
- NCLEX Review

Companion Website

- Additional NCLEX Review
- Case Study: Postpartum Client
- Care Plan Activity: Postpartal Care Following Vaginal Birth
- Care Plan Activity: Postpartal Care Following Cesarean Birth

Certain premises form the basis of effective nursing care during the postpartal period.

- The best postpartal care is family centered and disrupts the family unit as little as possible. This approach uses the family's resources to support an early and smooth adjustment to the newborn by all family members.
- Knowledge of the range of normal physiologic and psychologic adaptations occurring during the postpartal period allows the nurse to recognize alterations and initiate interventions early. Communicating information about postpartal adaptations to the family facilitates their adjustment to their situation.
- Nursing care is aimed at accomplishing specific goals that ultimately meet individual needs. These goals are formulated after careful assessment and consideration of factors that could influence the outcome of care.

Chapter 34 provides a thorough discussion of postpartal assessment ∞. This chapter describes nursing care during the immediate postpartal period. Specific nursing responses to the mother's physical needs and the family's psychosociocultural needs are described at length, and are summarized in the Clinical Pathway for the Postpartal Period on pages 1020–1021.

Nursing Care During the Early Postpartal Period

For most postpartal women, physical recovery proceeds smoothly and is considered a healthy process. Because of this perception, it is all too common for caregivers to think that the woman and her family have no "real" needs and thus no care plan is needed. Nothing can be further from the truth. Every member of the family has needs, although they may not be obvious, especially if educational or emotional.

Nursing Diagnosis

The postpartal family's needs, which should be identified during assessment, are the basis for developing nursing diagnoses. Once a nursing diagnosis is made and recorded, systematic action, as delineated in a nursing care plan, can be taken to meet the identified need.

Often agencies prefer to use only the North American Nursing Diagnosis Association (NANDA) list. Consequently, physiologic alterations form the basis of many postpartal diagnoses. Examples of such diagnoses include the following:

- ***Altered Patterns of Urinary Elimination*** related to dysuria or urinary retention
- ***Constipation*** related to fear of tearing stitches or pain
- ***Pain*** related to perineal edema from birth, episiotomy, and generalized muscular discomfort
- ***Sleep Pattern Disturbance*** related to frequent interruption of rest for newborn care

Diagnoses related to family coping or instructional needs are also used frequently. Examples of these diagnoses include the following:

- ***Health-Seeking Behavior:*** Information about infant care related to an expressed desire to understand an infant's needs.
- ***Family Coping: Potential for Growth*** related to successful adjustment to new baby

After completing the assessment and diagnosis steps of the nursing process, the nurse identifies expected outcomes and selects nursing interventions that will effect the expected outcomes.

Nursing Plan and Implementation

Nursing care management is individualized to meet the needs of each postpartal woman, her newborn, and her family. The plan of care needs to consider the newborn's schedule of activities during the day, such as feeding times, because they frequently determine the mother's schedule. Flexibility is crucial since most breastfeeding infants feed on demand at frequent intervals.

An important component of nursing care is client teaching, which is designed to help the woman and her family learn how to perform self-care and provide effective newborn care. Sophisticated, detailed forms and guidelines are often available to assist in health teaching. Such tools are a useful adjunct but cannot take the place of the nurse's client-specific plan. As part of client teaching, the nurse should discuss cultural beliefs, desired outcomes, and goals with the mother as soon as possible on her arrival in the postpartum unit. Examples of these desired client outcomes (adapted from the Rose Women's Center, Denver, Colorado) include the following:

- Maintains health for self and baby
- Reviews educational resources for self and baby care
- Demonstrates care for self and baby
- Displays appropriate interaction between parent and baby
- Practices principles of infant safety
- Demonstrates proper breastfeeding and breast care or describes formula preparation for formula-feeding, feeding techniques, and breast care
- Identifies the symptoms of postpartum depression and available resources

Additional outcomes for the cesarean birth mother include the following:

- States in own words the reason for the cesarean birth
- Maintains desired pain control
- Maintains moderate mobility level

In summary, all components of nursing care management are designed to achieve the desired outcomes identified for the woman and her family.

CLINICAL PATHWAY FOR THE POSTPARTAL PERIOD

Category	First 4 Hours	4–8 Hours Past Birth	8–24 Hours Past Birth
Referral	Report from labor nurse if not continuing in an LDR room	Lactation consultation as needed	Home nursing, WIC referral if indicated ➤ **Expected Outcomes** Referrals made
Assessments	Postpartum assessments q30min × 2, q1h × 2, then q4h. Includes: • Fundus firm, midline, at or below umbilicus • Lochia rubra < 1 pad/h; no free flow or passage of clots with massage • Bladder: voids large amounts of urine spontaneously; bladder not palpable following voiding • Perineum: sutures intact; no bulging or marked swelling; no c/o severe pain. Minimal bruising may be present. If hemorrhoids present, no tenseness or marked engorgement; < 2 cm diameter • Breasts: soft, colostrum present Vital Signs: • BP WNL; no hypotension; not >30 mm systolic or 15 mm diastolic over baseline • Temperature: < 38C (100.4F) • Pulse: bradycardia normal, consistent with baseline • Respirations: 12–20/min; quiet, easy Comfort level: < 3 on scale of 1–10	Continue postpartum assessment q4h × 2, then q8h Breast: evaluate nipple status; should be no evidence of cracks or bruising Observe feeding technique with newborn Vital signs assessment q8h; all WNL; report temperature > 38C (100.4F) Assess Homan's sign q8h Continue assessment of comfort level	Continue postpartum assessment q8h Breasts: nipples should remain free of cracks, fissures, bruising Feeding technique with newborn: should be good or improving Vital signs assessment q8h; all WNL; report temperature > 38C (100.4F) Continue assessment of comfort level ➤ **Expected Outcomes** Vital signs medically acceptable, voids qs, postpartum assessment WNL; comfort level: < 3 on 1–10 scale, involution of uterus in process, demonstrates and verbalizes appropriate newborn feeding techniques
Teaching/ psychosocial	Explain postpartum assessments Teach self-massage of fundus and expected findings; rationale for fundal massage Instruct to call for assistance first time OOB and PRN Demonstrate peri-care, surgigator, sitz bath PRN Explain comfort measures Begin newborn teaching; bulb suctioning, positioning, feeding, diaper change, cord care Orient to room if transferred from LDR room Provide information on early postpartal period Assess mother/infant attachment	Discuss psychologic changes of postpartum period; facilitate transition through tasks of taking on maternal role Discuss peri-care/hygiene; encourage use of supportive brassiere for breast- or formula-feeding Stress need for frequent rest periods Continue newborn teaching: soothing/comforting techniques, swaddling; return demonstrations indicate woman's understanding Provide opportunities for questions and review; reinforce previous teaching Breastfeeding: nipple care: air-drying, lanolin; proper latch-on technique; tea bags Formula-feeding: supportive bra, ice bags, breast binder Assess mother/infant attachment	Reinforce previous teaching, complete teaching evaluation Discuss involution; anticipated physical changes in first 2 weeks postpartum; postpartal exercises; need to limit visitors Discuss postpartal nutrition; balanced diet Breastfeeding: • Increase calories by 500 kcal over nonpregnant state (200 kcal over pregnant intake) • Explain milk production, let-down reflex, use of supplements, breast pumping, and milk storage Formula-feeding: • Return to nonpregnant caloric intake • Explain formula preparation and storage Discuss birth control options, sexuality Discuss sibling rivalry and plan for supporting siblings at home Discuss pets; suggestions for improving acceptance of infant by pets ➤ **Expected Outcomes** Mother verbalizes teaching comprehension. Positive bonding and emotional behaviors observed.
Nursing care management and reports	Ice pack to perineum to decrease swelling and increase comfort Straight catheter prn × 1 if distended or voiding small amounts If continues unable to void or voiding small amounts, insert Foley catheter and notify CNM/physician	Sitz baths prn If woman Rh− and infant Rh+, RhoGAM work-up; obtain consent; complete teaching Determine rubella status Obtain consent for rubella vaccine if indicated; explain purpose, procedure, implications of vaccine Obtain hematocrit	Continue sitz baths PRN May shower if ambulating without difficulty DC heparin lock if present Administer rubella vaccine as indicated ➤ **Expected Outcomes** Using sitz bath; voids qs; lab work WNL; performs ADL without sequelae

➤

CLINICAL PATHWAY FOR THE POSTPARTAL PERIOD *CONTINUED*

Category	First 4 Hours	4–8 Hours Past Birth	8–24 Hours Past Birth
Activity	Assistance when OOB first time, then PRN Ambulate ad lib Rests comfortably between assessments	Encourage rest periods Ambulate ad lib; may leave birthing unit after notifying staff of plan to ambulate off unit	Up ad lib ➤ **Expected Outcomes** Ambulates ad lib
Comfort	Institute comfort measures: • Perineal discomfort: peri-care; sitz baths, topical analgesics • Hemorrhoids: sitz baths, topical analgesics, digital replacement of external hemorrhoids; side-lying or prone position • Afterpains: prone with small pillow under abdomen; warm shower or sitz baths; ambulation • Administer pain medication ________	Continue with pain management techniques Offer alternative pain management options: distraction with music, television, visitors; massage; warmed blankets or towels to affected area; using breathing techniques when infant latches on to breast and/or during cramping until medication's action is felt	Continue with pain management techniques ➤ **Expected Outcomes** Comfort level < 3 on 1–10 scale Verbalizes alternative pain management options
Nutrition	Regular diet Fluid $\geqq$ 2000 mL/day	Continue diet and fluids	Continue diet and fluids ➤ **Expected Outcomes** Regular diet/fluids tolerated
Elimination	Voiding large amounts straw-colored urine	Voiding large quantities May have bowel movement	Same ➤ **Expected Outcomes** Voiding qs; passing flatus or bowel movement
Medications	Pain medications as ordered Methergine 0.2 mg q4h po if ordered Stool softener ________________ Tucks pad prn, perineal analgesic spray	Continue meds Lanolin to nipples PRN; tea bags to nipples if tender; heparin flush to heparin lock (if present) q8h or as ordered May take own prenatal vitamins	Continue medications RhoGAM and rubella vaccine administered if indicated ➤ **Expected Outcomes** Vaccines administered; pain controlled
Discharge planning/home care	Evaluate knowledge of normal postpartum and newborn care Evaluate support systems	Discuss typical newborn schedule; plan for periods of rest Birth certificate paperwork completed Evaluate plans for transporting newborn; car seat available	Review discharge instruction sheet/checklist Describe postpartum warning signs and when to call CNM/physician Provide prescriptions. Gift packs given appropriate for formula- or breastfeeding Arrangements for baby pictures as per agency protocol. Postpartum and newborn visits scheduled ➤ **Expected Outcomes** Discharged home; mother verbalizes postpartum warning s/s, follow-up appointment times/dates
Family involvement	Identify available support persons Assess family perceptions of birth experience Parenting: demonstrates culturally expected early parenting behaviors	Involve support persons in care, teaching; answer questions Evidence of parental bonding behaviors present	Continue to involve support persons in teaching, involve siblings as appropriate. Plans made for providing support to mother following discharge ➤ **Expected Outcomes** Evidence of parental bonding behavior; support persons verbalize understanding of woman's need for rest, good nutrition, fluids, and emotional support
Date			

Information is included for both vaginal birth (VB) and cesarean birth (CB). However, since many of the nursing care interventions are the same for either, specific interventions or suggestions related to vaginal birth are designated VB, and those specific to cecesarean birth are designated CB.

ADL, activities of daily living; BP, blood pressure; CB, cesarean birth; CNM, certified nurse-midwife; DC, discontinue; LDR, labor, delivery, and recovery; OOB, out of bed; OR, operating room; PCA patient controlled analgesia, PRN, as needed; VB, vaginal birth; WNL within normal limits; PP, postpartum, qs, quantity sufficient; VS, vital signs; c/o, complaints of; LOS, level of sensation; LOC, level of conscienceness; TC & DB, turn-cough and deep breathe; D/C, discharge; s/s, signs and symptoms.

COMMUNITY-BASED NURSING CARE

Various services are available to meet the needs of the childbearing family during the immediate postpartal period and beyond. These services range from educational opportunities, such as classes on nutrition, breastfeeding, exercise, infant care and development, and parenting, to specific healthcare programs, such as well-baby checkups, immunization clinics, and family-planning services. Some are offered by private caregivers, some are provided by volunteer and charitable organizations, and some are the domain of city, state, or federal agencies. In all cases, the goal is consistent: to help ensure that the mother, the father (if he is involved), siblings, and the newborn have the opportunity to meet specific healthcare needs regardless of their personal resources.

Home healthcare is one of the most important forms of community-based nursing care offered to postpartal families. Home care visits and phone contacts (telephone follow-up) help ensure that families have the necessary skills and resources to care for an infant and to meet their own health needs. Because of its importance today in caring for childbearing families, home care is discussed in depth in Chapter 36.

Promotion of Effective Parent Learning

Meeting the educational needs of the new mother and her family is one of the primary challenges facing the postpartum nurse. Each woman's educational needs vary according to age, background, culture, experience, and expectations. However, because the mother spends only a brief period of time in the postpartal area, identifying and addressing individual instructional needs can be difficult. Effective education provides the childbearing family with sufficient knowledge to meet many of their own health needs and to seek assistance if necessary.

The nurse assesses the learning needs of the new mother through observation, sensitivity to nonverbal clues, and tactfully phrased questions. For example, "What plans have you made for handling things when you get home?" will elicit a more detailed response than, "Will someone be available to help you at home?" To assess learning needs, some agencies provide a client handout listing the most frequently identified areas of concern for new mothers. The mother checks those that apply to her or writes in concerns not included.

The nurse should plan and implement learning experiences in a logical, nonthreatening way based on knowledge of and respect for the family's cultural values and beliefs. For example, many Hmong and Southeast Asian women learn and seek advice from their elders and view folk traditions as important (Mayberry, Affonso, Shibuya, et al, 1999). The nurse needs to recognize this and honor the role the elders play in the family. Unless there is a culturally related activity the nurse believes would be harmful, most cultural customs can be supported and encouraged.

Methods and Timing of Teaching

The educational method the nurse chooses varies. Agencies with many clients and limited staff may rely heavily on structured classes. Smaller units may provide individualized instruction through the use of one-on-one teaching or prepared videotapes. Some agencies use a television channel to show instructional videotapes at scheduled times during the day. Women should have a pencil and paper to jot down questions that arise as they view the material. Afterward, nurses need to be available to clarify material or answer any questions about the content. Because more effective learning occurs when there is sensory involvement and active participation, videotapes (sight and hearing) are more helpful than lecture (hearing only). Demonstration-return demonstration (sight, touch, hearing, and possibly smell and taste) is even more effective.

Timing is important in implementing educational activities. The new mother is more receptive to teaching after the first 24 to 48 hours, when she is ready to assume responsibility for her own care and that of her newborn (Lamp & Howard, 1999). However, many women are discharged in the early, dependent phase. Because of this, the nurse needs to provide whatever teaching the woman is ready for, with written handouts for future reference.

Timing is also important for new fathers, who are more likely to attend sessions planned for them if they are scheduled in the evening after visiting hours. If material is planned for siblings, late afternoon teaching after school or naps might be more effective.

Content of Teaching

Research suggests that after new mothers return home, they want additional information on self-care topics such as postpartum complications, exercise and activity, emotions/mood changes, and breast care. They also desire more information on infant care topics such as signs of infant illness, infant feeding, circumcision care, and cord care (Ruchala, 2000). These needs may be addressed through home visits, in postpartum educational programs, and by nurses in obstetric and pediatric offices.

Teaching should not be limited to "how to" activities, however. Anticipatory guidance is essential in assisting the family to cope with role changes and the realities of a new baby. Small-group discussions provide a chance for the new parents to talk about fears and expectations. Questions may arise about sexuality, contraception, child care, and even the grief associated with giving up the fantasized infant in order to accept the actual one.

Content must be individualized for families with special education needs—the mother who had a cesarean birth, the adolescent mother, the parents of an infant with congenital anomalies, and so on (Koniak-Griffin, Mathenge, Anderson, et al, 1999). They may feel overwhelmed, have difficult feelings to work through, and not even realize what it is they need to know. Nurses who are attuned to these individual problems can begin providing guidance as soon as possible.

Table 35–1 • identifies important topic areas to be included in postpartal client teaching.

Evaluating Learning

Methods for evaluating learning vary according to the objectives and teaching methods. Return demonstrations, question-and-answer sessions, and even programmed instruction are opportunities for evaluating learning, as are formal evaluation tools.

Evaluation of attitudinal or less concrete learning is more difficult. For example, a mother's ability to express her frustrations over an unanticipated cesarean birth or a decision to delay for several weeks a family dinner originally scheduled for the first weekend after the birth may be the nurse's only clues that learning has occurred. Follow-up phone calls and home visits after discharge may provide additional evaluative information and continue the helping process as the nurse assesses the family's current educational needs and begins planning accordingly.

Promotion of Maternal Comfort and Well-Being

The nurse promotes and restores maternal physical well-being by monitoring the woman's vital signs, cardiovascular status, and elimination. These assessments were discussed in the previous chapter. The nurse also monitors the status of the woman's uterus, and performs nursing activities aimed at relieving specific discomforts, such as an edematous perineum or a distended bladder. In addition, medications may be needed to promote comfort, treat anemia, provide immunity to rubella, and prevent development of antibodies in the nonsensitized Rh-negative woman. Finally, the woman may be experiencing alterations in her emotional well-being. Interventions for these conditions are discussed in this section.

Monitoring Uterine Status

The nurse completes an assessment of the uterus as discussed in Chapter 34. The assessment interval is every 15 minutes for the first hour after childbirth, every 30 minutes for the next hour, and then hourly for approximately 2 hours. Thereafter, the nurse monitors uterine status every 8 hours or more frequently if problems arise, such as **bogginess** (softening of the uterus due to inadequate contraction of the muscle tissue), positioning out of midline, heavy lochia flow, or the presence of clots (Table 35–2 •).

The amount, consistency, color, and odor of the lochia are monitored on an ongoing basis. Changes in lochia that need to be assessed further, documented, and reported to the physician/certified nurse-midwife are presented in Table 35–3 •.

Occasionally a medication such as methylergonovine maleate (Methergine) is prescribed to promote uterine contractions. In some cases an intravenous infusion of oxytocin (Pitocin) may be necessary if the uterus does not remain firm and uterine bleeding is excessive. See Drug Guide: Methylergonovine Maleate (Methergine) in this chapter and Drug Guide: Pitocin in Chapter 27.

Nipple stimulation can also be utilized to promote contraction of the uterus. The release of oxytoxin can also be facilitated by breastfeeding.

TEACHING FOR SELF-CARE

The nurse teaches the woman to assess her fundus for firmness and position and to massage the fundus gently to promote uterine contraction. In addition, the nurse instructs her to monitor the amount and color of the lochia. Being aware of normal involutional changes will help the woman identify problems. Discharge instructions should specify that women should call their healthcare provider if their bleeding is equal to or more than two sanitary pads per hour.

Relief of Perineal Discomfort

Many nursing interventions are available for relieving perineal discomfort. Before selecting a method, the nurse needs to have assessed the perineum to determine the degree of edema and other problems. It is also important to ask the woman whether there are special measures that she feels will be particularly effective and to offer her choices when possible. Some cultures believe the use of "cold" versus "hot" may alter the recovery or spirit of the new mother. These beliefs will affect the choices made by the new mother. The nurse uses disposable gloves while applying all relief measures and washes hands before and after using the gloves.

It is important to use good hygienic practices, such as moving from the front (area of the symphysis pubis) to the back (area around the anus) of the perineum. The nurse should follow this principle when placing ice packs, placing perineal pads, and applying topical anesthetic agents or pain relief products. Avoiding contamination between the anal area and the urethral-vaginal area is essential to prevent infection.

Clinical Tip *You may be surprised by how quickly the postpartal woman shows signs of bladder distention, possibly as soon as 1 to 2 hours after childbirth. This is because of normal postpartal diuresis. You can help prevent overdistention by palpating the woman's bladder frequently and encouraging her to void. When urinating the first time after vaginal birth, some mothers may feel the urge to urinate but are unable to begin the flow of urine. Possible interventions include letting her hear running water by turning water on in the sink; running warm water in the sink and having her place one hand in the water; having her place one foot in a basin of warm water; squirting warm water over her perineum using a peri-bottle; and placing a few drops of peppermint oil in the urine collection device ("hat"). Be sure to measure the first few voidings. The amount should be at least 150/mL. If she is still unable to void and catheterization becomes necessary, be prepared for difficulty in visualizing the urethra because of localized swelling and discomfort and tenderness in the area.*

Table 35–1 • AREAS TO INCLUDE IN POSTPARTAL TEACHING

Knowledge and Skills To Be Taught	Teaching Method: Video	Verbal Only	Verbally Reinforced	Demonstration
Care of the Mother				
Breast care				
Breastfeeding or lactation suppression				
Possible problems and care				
Involutional changes				
Position of fundus				
Afterpains				
Changes in lochia				
Signs of possible problems				
Bladder function				
Fluid needs				
Signs of possible problems				
Bowel function				
Normal patterns				
Dietary assistance				
Perineal care				
Expected healing changes in episiotomy				
Comfort measures (rinsing with warm water, use of icepacks, use of analgesic/anesthetic spray, sitz bath), home care				
Signs of possible problems				
Rest and activity				
Scheduling rest periods, handling fatigue				
Ambulation				
Watching for circulatory problems in legs				
Emotional changes				
Changes in mood, crying, depression				
Care of the Father/Partner				
Emotional changes				
Emotional changes and challenges that may occur				
Encouragement to seek support as needed				
Physiologic and psychologic changes that may occur in the mother and newborn				
Infant care concerns				
Possible supportive measures for the new family				
Care of the Baby				
Observing the baby				
General appearance				
Senses				
Visual				
Hearing				
Touch				
Smell				
Taste				
Vital signs				
Normal parameters				
How to take a temperature				
Skin				
Coloring				
Normal rashes				
Diaper care				
Elimination cycles of stool/urine				
Normal characteristics				
Signs of diarrhea and treatment				
Signs of constipation and treatment				

Table 35–1 • CONTINUED

Knowledge and Skills To Be Taught	Teaching Method: Video	Verbal Only	Verbally Reinforced	Demonstration
Emotional and comforting needs				
Protective reflexes				
Blinking				
Sneezing				
Swallowing				
Normal reflexes				
Moro				
Fencing				
Head lag				
Stepping				
Feeding the baby				
Schedule				
Breastfeeding				
Positioning, initiating and ending feeding				
Infant cues for feeding				
Identifying problem areas and possible solutions				
Signs of dehydration				
Formula-feeding				
Positioning				
Preparation of bottles and formula				
Burping or bubbling the baby				
Holding, wrapping, and diapering the baby				
Various holds (cradle, football)				
Securing baby in blanket to provide warmth				
Diapering				
Comparison of reusable (cloth) and single use (paper)				
Methods of diapering and care of soiled diapers				
Perineal skin care				
Positioning the baby for sleep				
Bathing the baby				
Supplies				
Method				
Safety				
Use of bulb syringe and care if choking				
Positioning				
Car seat				
Health promotion				
When to call healthcare provider				
Temp				
Diarrhea				
Eating problems				
Malaise				
Protecting baby from infections				
Immunization schedule				
Aspects of Parenting				
Interaction with newborn				
Newborn cues and capacity for interaction				
Parenting needs				
Acquaintance with individual characteristics of their newborn and possible techniques to use				
Resources available				

Table 35–2 • KEY FACTS TO REMEMBER ABOUT MONITORING POSTPARTAL UTERINE STATUS

Position of the Uterine Fundus Following Birth

Immediately after birth: The top of the fundus is in the midline about midway between the symphysis pubis and umbilicus.

Six to 12 hours after birth: The top of the fundus is in the midline and at the level of the umbilicus.

One day after birth: The top of the fundus is in the midline and one finger breadth below the umbilicus.

Second day after birth and thereafter: The top of the fundus remains in the midline and descends about one fingerbreadth per day.

Normal Characteristics of Lochia

Lochia rubra is red and is present for the first 2–3 days.

Lochia serosa is pinkish red and is present from day 3 to day 10.

Lochia alba is creamy white and is present from day 11 to about day 21.

MediaLink CASE STUDY: POSTPARTUM CLIENT

PERINEAL CARE

Perineal care after each elimination (urination or defecation) cleanses the perineum and helps promote comfort. Many agencies provide "peri-bottles" that the woman can use to squirt warm tap water over her perineum following elimination. To cleanse her perineum, the woman may use a Surgigator, moist antiseptic towelettes, or toilet paper in a blotting (patting) motion. She should be taught to start at the front (area just under the symphysis pubis) and proceed toward the back (area around the anus) to prevent contamination from the anal area. In addition, to prevent contamination, the perineal pad should be applied from front to back, placing the front portion against the perineum first. Perineal pads should be changed regularly to prevent infection.

Teaching for Self-Care

The nurse demonstrates how to cleanse the perineum and assists the woman as necessary, for example, by offering additional information regarding the use of perineal pads. Many women have never used a perineal pad or belt and will need instruction in using them during the postpartal period. (See Client Teaching: Episiotomy Care.) Some women may prefer to use the pads designed for urinary incontinence. The pads are also highly absorbent and are usually self-adherent.

ICE PACK

If an episiotomy is performed at the time of birth or a laceration occurs, an ice pack is generally applied to reduce edema and numb the tissues, which promotes comfort. In some agencies, chemical ice bags are used. These are usually activated by folding both ends toward the middle. Prior to applying the ice pack the nurse should ask the woman for permission and consider cultural norms when appropriate. Inexpensive ice bags can be made by filling a disposable glove with ice chips or crushed ice and then tying the top of the glove closed, like a balloon. The gloves should always be wrapped in either a cotton or disposable washcloth to prevent damage to the tissue from excessively cold temperatures. To protect the perineum from burns caused by contact with the ice pack, the disposable glove is first rinsed under running water to remove any powder that may be present and then wrapped in an absorbent towel or washcloth before it is placed against the perineum. To attain the maximum effect of this cold treatment, the ice pack should remain in place approximately 20 minutes and then be removed for about 10 minutes before it is replaced. Ice packs may be continued for as long as necessary. Usually, they are needed for the first 24 hours.

Teaching for Self-Care

The nurse provides information about the purpose of the ice pack, anticipated effects, benefits, possible problems, and ways of preparing an ice pack for home use if edema is present and early discharge is planned.

SITZ BATH

The warmth of the water in the sitz bath provides comfort, decreases pain, and increases circulation to the tissues, which promotes healing and reduces the incidence of infection. Sitz baths may be ordered three times daily (TID) or as needed (PRN). The nurse cleanses the portable sitz bath and then fills it with water at 102F to 105F. The nurse instructs the woman to remain in the sitz bath for 20 minutes. It is important for the woman to have a clean towel to pat dry her perineum after the sitz bath and to have a clean perineal pad ready to apply. The woman should be advised to pat her perineal area dry rather than use a more rigorous rubbing technique.

Recently, cool sitz baths have gained popularity because they are effective in reducing perineal edema. Until definite research supports one temperature (warm or cold) as more effective, it may be best to offer the woman a choice.

Table 35–3 • CHANGES IN LOCHIA THAT CAUSE CONCERN

Change	Possible Problem	Nursing Action
Presence of clots	Inadequate uterine contractions that allow bleeding from vessels at the placental site.	Assess location and firmness of fundus. Assess voiding pattern. Record and report findings.
Persistent lochia rubra	Inadequate uterine contractions; retained placental fragments; infection	Assess location and firmness of fundus. Assess activity pattern. Assess for signs of infection. Record and report findings.

DRUG GUIDE Methylergonovine Maleate (Methergine)

• Overview of Action

Methylergonovine maleate (Methergine) is an ergot alkaloid that stimulates smooth muscle tissue. Because the smooth muscle of the uterus is especially sensitive to this drug, it is used postpartally to stimulate the uterus to contract in order to decrease blood loss by clamping off uterine blood vessels and to promote the involution process. In addition, the drug has a vasoconstrictive effect on all blood vessels, especially the larger arteries. This may result in hypertension, particularly in a woman whose blood pressure is already elevated.

• Route, Dosage, and Frequency

Methergine has a rapid onset of action and may be given orally or intramuscularly.

Usual IM dose: 0.2 mg following expulsion of the placenta. The dose may be repeated every 2–4 hours if necessary.

Usual oral dose: 0.2 mg every 4 hours (six doses).

• Maternal Contraindications

Pregnancy, hepatic or renal disease, cardiac disease, hypertension or preeclampsia contraindicate this drug's use. Methylergonovine maleate must be used with caution during lactation (PDR Nurse's Handbook, 1999).

• Maternal Side Effects

Hypertension, nausea, vomiting, headache, bradycardia, dizziness, tinnitus, abdominal cramps, palpitations, dyspnea, chest pain, and allergic reactions may be noted.

• Effects on Fetus or Newborn

Because Methergine has a long duration (3 hours [Karch, 1999]) and action and can thus produce tetanic contractions, it **should never be used during pregnancy or in labor,** when it may result in a sustained uterine contraction that may cause amniotic fluid embolism (increased pressure in uterus may allow entry of amniotic fluid under the edge of the placenta and thus entry into the maternal venous system), uterine rupture, cervical and perineal lacerations (resulting from tetanic contractions and rapid birth of the baby), and hypoxia and intracranial hemorrhage in the baby (because of tetanic contractions, which severely decrease the maternal-placental-fetal blood flow, or uterine rupture, which causes cessation of blood flow to the unborn baby) (PDR Nurse's Handbook, 1999).

• Nursing Considerations

- Monitor fundal height and consistency and the amount and character of the lochia.
- Assess the blood pressure before and routinely throughout drug administration.
- Observe for adverse effects or symptoms of ergot toxicity (ergotism) such as nausea and vomiting, headache, muscle pain, cold or numb fingers and toes, chest pain, and general weakness (PDR Nurse's Handbook, 1999).
- Provide client/family teaching regarding importance of not smoking during methergine administration (nicotine from cigarettes leads to constricted vessels and may lead to hypertension), signs of toxicity.

Teaching for Self-Care

The nurse provides information about the purpose and use of the sitz bath, anticipated effects, benefits, possible problems, and safety measures to prevent injury from possible slipping or excessive water temperature. Home use of sitz baths may be recommended for the woman with an extensive episiotomy or laceration; the woman may use a portable sitz bath or her bathtub. It is important for the nurse to emphasize that in using a bathtub, the woman should draw only 4 to 6 inches of water, assess the temperature of the water, and use the water only for the sitz, not for bathing. If the woman takes a tub bath, she should release the water, clean the tub, and draw new water prior to the sitz to prevent infection.

TOPICAL AGENTS

Topical anesthetic agents may be used to relieve perineal discomfort. The woman is advised to apply the anesthetic agent after a sitz bath or perineal care.

Witch hazel compresses may be used to relieve perineal discomfort and edema. Nupercainal ointment or Tucks pads may be ordered for relief of both perineal and hemorrhoidal pain. It is important for the nurse to emphasize that the woman should wash her hands before and after using the topical treatments.

Teaching for Self-Care

The nurse provides information about the anesthetic spray or topical agent. The woman needs to understand the purpose, use, anticipated effects, benefits, and possible problems associated with the product. The nurse can combine an explanation with a demonstration of correct application. A return demonstration is a useful method of evaluating the woman's understanding.

Relief of Hemorrhoidal Discomfort

Some mothers experience hemorrhoidal pain after giving birth. Relief measures include the use of sitz baths, anesthetic ointments, rectal suppositories, or witch hazel pads applied directly to the anal area. Rectal suppositories should

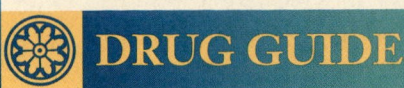

CLIENT TEACHING — EPISIOTOMY CARE

Assessment During the time following labor and birth, assess the woman's understanding of the purpose of the episiotomy, the factors that contribute to wound healing, and the comfort measures available if needed. The woman's level of knowledge may be influenced by several factors, including, for example, childbirth preparation activities and previous childbirth experience.

Nursing Diagnosis The key nursing diagnosis will probably be ***Health-seeking behavior:*** Information about self-care measures to promote episiotomy healing and personal comfort.

Nursing Plan and Implementation The teaching will focus on the process of healing, factors that increase the risk of infection, and steps the woman can take to promote healing and increase her personal comfort.

Client Goals At the completion of teaching, the woman will be able to:

- Identify the factors that both promote and interfere with wound healing.
- Summarize self-care activities to promote healing and increase personal comfort.
- Demonstrate the correct procedure for taking a sitz bath.
- Discuss the judicious use of prescribed analgesics as needed.

Teaching Plan

CONTENT	TEACHING METHOD
• Describe the process of wound healing, including the value of healing by first intention as opposed to a jagged tear. Discuss the risk of contamination of the episiotomy by bacteria from the anal area.	Many women do not consider the episiotomy a surgical incision. Discussion helps them understand the importance of good wound care.
• Explain techniques that are used to keep the episiotomy clean and promote healing such as: • Sitz bath • Use of peri-bottle following each voiding or defecation • Pad change following each elimination and at regular intervals	Focus on open discussion. Demonstrate correct use of the peri-bottle or sitz bath if necessary.
• Describe comfort measures: • Ice pack or glove immediately following birth • Sitz bath • Judicious use of analgesics or topical anesthetics • Tightening buttocks before sitting	Focus on discussion and provide an opportunity for questions.
• Identify signs of episiotomy infection. Advise the woman to contact her caregiver if infection develops.	Encourage discussion and provide printed handouts. Some of this content may also be covered during a small postpartum class.

Evaluation

At the end of the teaching session the woman will be able to verbalize the principles of wound healing and episiotomy care. She will also be able to demonstrate self-care measures such as peri-care and taking a sitz bath.

not be used by women who have had a fourth-degree laceration during birth.

TEACHING FOR SELF-CARE

The woman can be taught to digitally replace external hemorrhoids in her rectum. She may also find it helpful to maintain a side-lying position when possible or to tighten her buttocks when sitting down to reduce contact of the perineum with the seat and to avoid prolonged sitting. The mother is encouraged to maintain an adequate fluid intake, and is given stool softeners to ensure greater comfort with bowel movements. The hemorrhoids usually disappear a few weeks after birth if the woman did not have them prior to her pregnancy.

Relief of Afterpains

Afterpains are the result of intermittent uterine contractions. A primipara may not notice afterpains because her uterus is able to maintain a contracted state. Multiparous women and those who have had an overdistended uterus (due to multiple gestation or hydramnios) frequently experience discomfort from afterpains as the uterus intermittently contracts more vigorously. Breastfeeding women are also more likely to experience afterpains than formula-feeding women because of the release of oxytocin when the infant suckles. The nurse can suggest the woman lie prone with a small pillow under the lower abdomen, explaining that the discomfort may be intensified for about 5 minutes but then will diminish greatly, if not completely. The prone position applies pressure to the uterus and therefore stimulates contractions. When the uterus maintains a constant contraction, the afterpains cease. Additional nursing interventions include positioning, ambulation, or administration of an analgesic agent, such as Motrin, Tylenol, or Percocet. The mother's description of the type and severity of her pain is usually the most reliable method of determining which analgesic agent would provide her the comfort she desires. Many women who are breastfeeding have concerns about the effects of medications on the infant. For breastfeeding mothers, a mild analgesic agent administered an hour before feeding will promote comfort and enhance maternal-infant interactions.

TEACHING FOR SELF-CARE

The nurse provides information about the cause of afterpains and methods to decrease discomfort. The nurse also explains any medications that are ordered, expected effect, benefits, possible side effects, and any special considerations such as the possibility of dizziness or sleepiness with particular medications.

Relief of Discomfort from Immobility and Muscle Strain

Discomfort may also be caused by immobility and muscle strain. The woman who pushed for a long time during labor may experience muscular aches. It is not unusual for women to experience joint pains and discomfort in both arms and legs, depending on the effort they exerted during the second stage of labor. Early ambulation is encouraged to help reduce the incidence of complications such as constipation and thrombophlebitis. It also helps promote a general feeling of well-being.

The nurse assists the woman the first few times she gets up during the postpartal period. Fatigue, effects of medications, loss of blood, and possibly even lack of food may cause feelings of dizziness or faintness when the woman stands up. Because this may be a problem during the woman's first shower, the nurse should remain in the room, check the woman frequently, and have a chair close by in case she becomes faint. Dizziness may be aggravated by standing still and by the warmth of the water, so it is best to wait until the woman has shown stability when ambulating and has eaten. The first shower should be somewhat brief. On many postpartal units, ammonia inhalants (referred to as "smelling salts") are taped to the bathroom door for use in case of fainting. During this first shower the nurse instructs the woman in the use of the emergency call button in the bathroom; if she becomes faint during a future shower, she can call for assistance.

TEACHING FOR SELF-CARE

The nurse provides information about ambulation and the importance of monitoring any signs of dizziness or weakness. If she becomes dizzy, the woman should sit down and call for assistance.

Postpartal Diaphoresis

Postpartal diaphoresis (excessive perspiration) may cause discomfort for new mothers. The nurse can offer a fresh dry gown and bed linens to enhance comfort.

Some women may feel refreshed by a shower. It is important to consider cultural practices and realize that some women may prefer not to shower in the first few days following birth. For example, some Hispanic and Asian women prefer to delay showering. Nurses can offer these women a warm washcloth to increase maternal comfort. Because diaphoresis also may lead to increased thirst, the nurse can offer fluids as the woman desires. Again, cultural practices are important to consider. Women of western European background may prefer iced water; Asian women may prefer water at room temperature. The nurse should ascertain the woman's wishes rather than operate solely from the nurse's own values or cultural belief system.

TEACHING FOR SELF-CARE

The nurse provides information about the normal physiologic changes that cause diaphoresis and methods to increase comfort.

Suppression of Lactation in the Non-breastfeeding Mother

For the woman who chooses not to breastfeed, lactation may be suppressed by mechanical inhibition. Previously, medications were administered to mothers who were not planning on breastfeeding; however, use of these medications has been discontinued due to adverse side effects. Although signs of engorgement do not usually occur until the third or fourth day postpartum, engorgement is best prevented by beginning mechanical methods of lactation suppression as soon as possible after birth. Ideally, this involves having the woman begin wearing a supportive, well-fitting bra within 6 hours after birth. The bra is worn continuously until lactation is suppressed (usually about 5 to 10 days) and is removed only for showers. The bra provides support and eases the discomfort that can occur with tension on the breasts because of fullness. A snug breast binder may be used if the woman does not have a bra available or if she finds the binder more comfortable. Ice packs should be applied over the axillary area of each breast for 20 minutes four times daily. This, too, should begin soon after birth. Ice is also useful in relieving discomfort if engorgement occurs. Research has shown that cabbage leaves can be effective in decreasing lactation and relieving engorgement. Women are advised to boil the cabbage slightly until the leaves are softened. The leaves are then peeled from the head and placed in the refrigerator. The woman can apply the cabbage leaves to her breast by placing them within her bra. The leaves should be changed as they "wilt." A chemical excreted by the cabbage is effective in suppressing milk production and promotes maternal comfort.

TEACHING FOR SELF-CARE

The mother is advised to avoid any stimulation of her breasts by her baby, herself, breast pumps, or her sexual partner until the sensation of fullness has passed (usually about 5 to 10 days). Such stimulation will increase milk production and delay the suppression process. Heat is avoided for the same reason, and the mother is encouraged to let shower water flow over her back rather than her breasts. Suppression takes only a few days in most cases, but small amounts of milk may be produced up to a month after birth.

Pharmacologic Interventions

Pharmacologic preparations, including pain medications, vaccinations, and Rh immune globulin, are frequently administered in the postpartal period. (See Table 35–4 •.)

RUBELLA VACCINE

Women who have a rubella titer of less than 1:10 or are ELISA antibody negative are usually given rubella vaccine in the postpartal period (Technical Working Group, 1999). Administering the injection just after childbirth is advantageous because the woman is definitely not pregnant and typically does not want another pregnancy within 3 months.

Teaching for Self-Care

The nurse needs to ensure that the woman understands the purpose of the vaccine and that she must avoid becoming pregnant in the next 3 months. To ensure that the woman understands, an informed consent is usually signed prior to administration. Because avoiding pregnancy is so important, counseling regarding contraception is suggested.

RH IMMUNE GLOBULIN (RHOGAM)

All Rh-negative women with Rh-positive babies should receive Rh immune globulin (RhoGAM) within 72 hours after childbirth to prevent sensitization from a fetomaternal transfusion of Rh-positive fetal red blood cells. See discussion of criteria in Procedure 20-2.

Teaching for Self-Care

The Rh-negative woman needs to understand the implications of her Rh-negative status in future pregnancies. (See Chapter 20 for a detailed discussion.) The nurse provides opportunities for questions during teaching.

Relief of Emotional Stress

The birth of a child, with the role changes and increased responsibilities it produces, is a time of emotional stress for the new mother. This stress is increased by the tremendous physiologic changes that occur as her body adjusts to a nonpregnant state. During the early postpartal days, mood swings and tearfulness are common.

At first the mother may repeatedly discuss her experiences in labor and birth and how it compared with her fantasized picture. This storytelling allows her to relive and integrate her experiences (Banks-Wallace, 1999). If she feels that she did not cope well with labor, she may have feelings of inadequacy and may benefit from reassurance that she did well. Open discussion of feelings is possible only if the postpartum nurse has established a warm, supportive relationship with the woman. Follow-up visits from the nurse who assisted her in labor and birth provide additional opportunities for the mother to relive her experiences and come to terms with them.

During the postpartal period, the mother must also adjust to the loss of her fantasized child and accept the child she has borne. This may be more difficult if the child is not of the desired sex or has birth defects.

Immediately following the birth (the taking-in period), the mother is dependent and focused inward on bodily concerns. During this time, teaching other than for self-care may not be totally effective. Because early discharge has become so common, however, the nurse should offer classes and information and provide printed handouts for reference as questions arise at home.

Once the woman's self-care needs have been met, her focus will shift to the care of her newborn and her ability as a parent (the taking-hold period). Skillful intervention by the nurse, with continual reassurance that the woman is a successful mother, is vital. During this time the mother is most receptive to teaching, and tactful instruction and demonstration assist her in developing mothering skills. The nurse must carefully avoid "taking over" the infant. By functioning as an adviser and allowing the mother to perform the actual care, the nurse demonstrates confidence in the mother's skill and ability, which in turn increases the mother's self-confidence about her effectiveness as a parent. Recognition and praise of her success help the mother develop feelings of competence in caring for her baby.

Usually the mother is discharged before the onset of mood disturbances and disorders associated with the postpartal period. These include postpartum "baby blues," true postpartum depression, and postpartum psychosis, and are described in detail in Chapter 37.

TEACHING FOR SELF-CARE

The nurse should advise the mother that physical, psychologic, and hormonal factors all influence an individual's response to childbirth. Normal responses include a brief

Table 35-4 • ESSENTIAL INFORMATION FOR COMMON POSTPARTUM DRUGS

TYLENOL No. 3 (300 mg Acetaminophen and 30 mg codeine)

Drug Class: Narcotic analgesic.

Dose/Route: Usual adult dose: 1–2 tablets PO every 4 hours PRN.

Indication: For relief of mild to moderate pain.

Adverse Effects: Respiratory depression, apnea, light-headedness, dizziness, nausea, sweating, dry mouth, constipation, facial flushing, suppression of cough reflex, ureteral spasm, urinary retention, pruritus, hepatotoxicity (overdose).

Nursing Implications: Determine whether woman is sensitive to acetaminophen or codeine; has history of impaired hepatic or renal function. Monitor bowel sounds, respirations, urine output.

Administer with food or after meals if GI upset occurs; encourage woman to drink one full glass (240 mL) with the tablet to reduce the risk of the tablet lodging in the esophagus.

Client Teaching: Inform client about name of drug, expected action, possible side effects, that it is secreted in breast milk (Note: Some physicians/certified nurse-midwives may avoid ordering this medication for breastfeeding mothers), and review safety measures (assess for dizziness, use side rails, call for assistance when getting out of bed and ambulating, report to nurse any signs of adverse effects); ask if she has any questions.

Nursing Diagnoses Related to Drug Therapy: ***Health-Seeking Behavior:*** Information regarding drug therapy.
Risk for injury related to dizziness secondary to effect of drug.
Constipation related to slowed gastrointestinal activity secondary to effects of medications.

PERCOCET (325 mg acetaminophen and 5 mg oxycodone)

Drug Class: Narcotic analgesic.

Dose/Route: 1–2 tablets PO every 4 hours PRN.

Indication: For moderate to moderately severe pain. Can be used in aspirin-sensitive women.

Adverse Effects: Acetaminophen: Hepatotoxicity, headache, rash, hypoglycemia.

Oxycodone: Respiratory depression, apnea, circulatory depression, euphoria, facial flushing, constipation, suppression of cough reflex, ureteral spasm, urinary retention.

Nursing Implications: Determine whether woman is sensitive to acetaminophen or codeine; has bronchial asthma, respiratory depression, convulsive disorder.

Observe woman carefully for respiratory depression if given with barbiturates or sedative/hypnotics. Consider that postcesarean-birth woman may have depressed cough reflex, so teaching and encouragement to deep breathe and cough are needed.

Monitor bowel sounds, urine and bowel elimination.

Client Teaching: Teaching should include name of drug, expected effect, possible adverse effects, that drug is secreted in the breast milk, encouragement to report any signs of adverse effects immediately.

Nursing Diagnoses Related to Drug Therapy: ***Ineffective Breathing Pattern*** related to respiratory depression.
Constipation related to slowed gastrointestinal activity secondary to the effects of medications.

RUBELLA VIRUS VACCINE, LIVE (Meruvax 2)

Dose/Route: Single-dose vial, inject subcutaneously in outer aspect of the upper arm.

Indication: Stimulate active immunity against rubella virus.

Adverse Effects: Burning or stinging at the injection site; about 2–4 weeks later may have rash, malaise, sore throat, or headache.

Nursing Implications: Determine whether woman has sensitivity to neomycin (vaccine contains neomycin); is immunosuppressed, or has received blood transfusions (not to be administered within 3 months of blood transfusion, plasma transfusion, or serum immune globulin). To be given at discharge.

Client Teaching: Name of drug, expected effect, possible adverse effects, possible comfort measures to use if adverse effects occur; rubella titer will be assessed in about 3 months. Instruct woman to AVOID PREGNANCY FOR 3 MONTHS following vaccination. Provide information regarding contraceptives and their use.

Nursing Diagnoses Related to Drug Therapy: ***Knowledge Deficit*** regarding drug therapy. ***Health-Seeking Behavior:*** Information about postpartum contraception related to an expressed desire to avoid pregnancy following rubella vaccination.
Pain related to rash and malaise.

RhoGAM (Rh immune globulin specific for D antigen)

Dose/Route: Postpartum: One vial IM within 72 hours of birth. Antepartal: One vial microdose RhoGAM IM at 28 weeks in Rh-negative women; after amniocentesis, spontaneous or therapeutic abortion, or ectopic pregnancy.

Indication: Prevention of sensitization to the Rh factor in Rh-negative women and to prevent hemolytic disease in the newborn in subsequent pregnancies. Mother must be Rh negative, not previously sensitized to Rh factor. Infant must be Rh positive, direct antiglobulin negative.

Adverse Effects: Soreness at injection site.

Nursing Implications: Confirm criteria for administration are present. Ensure correct vial is used for the client (each vial is cross-matched to the specific woman and must be carefully checked).

Inject entire contents of vial.

Client Teaching: Name of drug, expected action, possible side effects; report soreness at injection site to nurse; woman should carry information regarding Rh status and dates of RhoGAM injections with her at all times; explain use of RhoGAM with subsequent pregnancies.

Nursing Diagnoses Related to Drug Therapy: ***Health-Seeking Behavior:*** Information about future need for Rh immune globulin related to an expressed desire to understand the long-term implications of her Rh-negative status.
Pain related to soreness at injection site.

(continued on next page)

Table 35–4 • ESSENTIAL INFORMATION FOR COMMON POSTPARTUM DRUGS (CONTINUED)

AMBIEN (Zolpidem tartrate)

Drug Class: Hypnotic, sedative.

Dose/Route: 5–10 mg PO at bedtime.

Indication: Promote sleep.

Adverse Effects: Dizziness, daytime drowsiness, diarrhea, drugged feelings, amnesia.

Nursing Implications: Determine if woman has compromised respiratory function. Monitor respirations, blood pressure, pulse. Modify environment to increase relaxation and promote sleep. Monitor for drug interaction if woman is taking other CNS depressants.

Client Teaching: Name of drug, expected effect, possible adverse effects, safety measures (siderails, use call bell, ask for assistance when out of bed); medication is secreted in breast milk.

Nursing Diagnoses Related to Drug Therapy: ***Risk for Injury*** related to possible ataxia or vertigo.
Altered Thought Processes related to drug-induced confusion.
Health-Seeking Behavior: Information regarding drug therapy.

period of irritability, mood swings, crying spells, and other mood-related symptoms. Generally, this period lasts from several days to a week. Women who experience a longer duration of symptoms should be advised to contact their physician/certified nurse-midwife. It is often helpful to discuss normal adaptations in the postpartum period with both the mother and her partner. This ensures that her partner will be aware of the normal patterns of psychologic responses in the early postpartum period. The nurse should review symptoms of postpartum depression and indicate when these symptoms warrant medical intervention. When women are so disabled from feelings of sadness or depression, or are unable to care for themselves or the baby, postpartum depression is suspected. Women should be counseled that feeling overwhelmed by their new or changing role, sleep deprivation, and a feeling of social isolation are all common for new mothers.

Promotion of Maternal Rest and Activity

Following birth, some women feel exhausted and in need of rest. Other women are euphoric and full of psychic energy, ready to retell their experience of birth repeatedly. The nurse evaluates individual needs, always with the goal of providing opportunities for rest. The nurse can provide time for the excited, euphoric woman to air her feelings and then can encourage a period of rest. The nurse may also help the family limit visitors and provide a comfortable sleep chair or bed for the partner.

Relief of Fatigue

Physical fatigue often affects other adjustments and functions of the new mother. For example, fatigue may reduce milk flow, thereby increasing problems with establishing breastfeeding. The mother requires energy to make the psychologic adjustments to a new infant and to assume new roles. She makes these adjustments more smoothly when she gets adequate rest. The nurse can encourage rest by organizing activities to avoid frequent interruptions for the woman. If the new mother chooses, rest times may be arranged by having the newborn remain in the holding nursery for a period of time, or the mother can rest or sleep when the baby is sleeping in her room. It is important for the new mother to know that physical fatigue may persist for a number of months. Persistent fatigue is affected by physiologic, psychologic, situational, and environmental factors (Parks, Lenz, Milligan, et al, 1999).

Although most mothers feel fatigued, they tend to view themselves as healthy and well if they perceive pregnancy and birth as natural processes. Some mothers, however, view the postpartal period as a time of rest. For instance, new West Indian mothers recuperate for up to a week in bed and are cared for by female family members. Middle Eastern mothers often stay home and recuperate for 40 days, during which time they rest and are cared for by their families (Mayberry et al, 1999). They are expected to eat special foods with their meals. These foods are believed to help restore the energy lost by the mother during childbirth.

TEACHING FOR SELF-CARE

Nearly all new mothers experience some degree of fatigue or sleep deprivation during the postpartum period. Women who have had a cesarean birth are coping with both the constant demands of the baby and their own recovery needs. The nurse should advise the mother to take frequent rest periods, to nap when the baby is napping, and to avoid performing unnecessary chores and activities. It is not uncommon for new mothers to attempt to "do it all" and end up feeling exhausted and irritable. Many women feel self-induced pressure to take care of household chores while the infant is napping. Once a woman becomes sleep deprived, it is difficult to "catch up." The nurse should advise the new mother to take naps and allow others to assist with household tasks. Well-wishing friends who call and ask if anything is needed can be encouraged to prepare a meal or pick up items at the grocery store. The woman will discover that friends and family are usually anxious to provide assistance. Her energy can then be concentrated on caring for herself and the baby.

Resumption of Activity

Ambulation and activity may gradually increase after discharge. The new mother should avoid heavy lifting, excessive stair climbing, and strenuous activity. One or two daily naps are essential and are most easily achieved if the mother sleeps when her baby does.

By the second week at home, the new mother may begin some light housekeeping activities. Although it is customary to delay returning to work for 6 weeks, most women are physically able to resume practically all activities by 4 to 5 weeks when the lochia flow has stopped. Delaying returning to work until after the final postpartal examination will minimize the possibility of problems.

TEACHING FOR SELF-CARE

The nurse can provide the new mother with suggestions for resuming her normal level of activity. Women should be encouraged to limit the number of activities to prevent excessive fatigue, increase in lochia, and negative psychologic reactions, such as feeling overwhelmed. The nurse can encourage the new mother to avoid the temptation to catch up on housework during infant naps, but instead use the time to rest herself. If excessive fatigue or an increase in lochia occurs, the woman should increase rest periods and decrease extra activities.

Postpartal Exercises

The nurse should encourage the woman to begin simple exercises while in the birthing unit and continue them at home, advising her that increased lochia or pain means she should reevaluate her activity and make necessary reductions. Most agencies provide a booklet describing suggested postpartal activities. (Exercise routines vary for women undergoing tubal ligation following birth and for cesarean birth clients.) See Figure 35–1 • on page 1034 for a description of some commonly used exercises. According to Sampselle, Seng, Yeo, et al (1999), exercise during the prenatal period is associated with positive views of the childbirth experience. The postpartal woman is more likely to have positive views of her own well-being and less fatigue if she continues to do stretching and/or her own programmed pattern of exercise.

TEACHING FOR SELF-CARE

The nurse should advise the woman to begin Kegel exercises immediately after birth. The nurse can explain that these exercises will assist in returning vaginal tone and preventing urinary leakage. If no complications exist, normal exercise can be initiated at 2 weeks after birth. Women should be advised to take short walks outside if the weather is appropriate. Abdominal exercises can be suggested to retone the abdominal muscles. A regular exercise program can be initiated after her 6 week postpartum examination.

Promotion of Family Wellness

A satisfactory maternity experience may have a positive impact on the entire family. The new or expanding family that receives appropriate information and has adequate time to interact with its newest member in a supportive environment will feel more comfortable and secure at home.

In the past, newborns were typically separated from their parents immediately after birth. Today most facilities support family-centered care, which is focused on keeping the mother and baby together as much as the mother desires. **Mother-baby care**, or **couplet care** (care of both the mother and her baby), is an important part of the family-centered approach, in which the infant remains at the mother's bedside and both are cared for by the same nurse. Couplet care allows the nurse to teach and role-model and to integrate the entire family into the care of the woman and her infant. It also enables the mother to have time to bond with her baby and learn to care for him or her in a supportive environment.

In a mother-baby unit, the newborn's crib is placed near the mother's bed, where she can see her baby easily. The crib should be a self-contained unit stocked with items the mother might require in providing care. A bulb syringe for suctioning the mouth or nares should always be accessible, and the mother and father/partner should be familiar with its use. The mother-baby unit is conducive to a self-demand feeding schedule for both breastfeeding and formula-feeding infants.

Mothers are frequently very tired after birth, so the responsibility for providing total infant care could be overwhelming. The mother-baby policy must be flexible enough to permit the mother to return the baby to the nursery if she finds it necessary because of fatigue or physical discomfort. Some mother-baby units also return the newborns to a central nursery at night so the mothers can get more rest.

Many agencies have unlimited visiting hours for the father or significant others of the mother's choice. These opportunities to hold and care for the child promote paternal self-confidence and foster paternal attachment.

Reactions of Siblings

Sibling visitation helps meet the needs of both the siblings and their mother. A visit to the hospital reassures children that their mother is well and still loves them. It also provides an opportunity for the children to become familiar with the new baby. For the mother, the pangs of separation are lessened as she interacts with her children and introduces them to the newest family member.

Most agencies now recognize the importance of providing siblings with opportunities to see their mother and meet the infant during the early postpartal period (Figure 35–2 •). Approaches to this issue vary from specified visiting hours for siblings to unlimited visiting privileges.

TEACHING FOR SELF-CARE

Although the parents have prepared the child for the presence of a new brother or sister, the actual arrival of the infant requires some adjustments. Some children may be present for the birth and have an opportunity to spend time with their new sibling and their parents immediately following

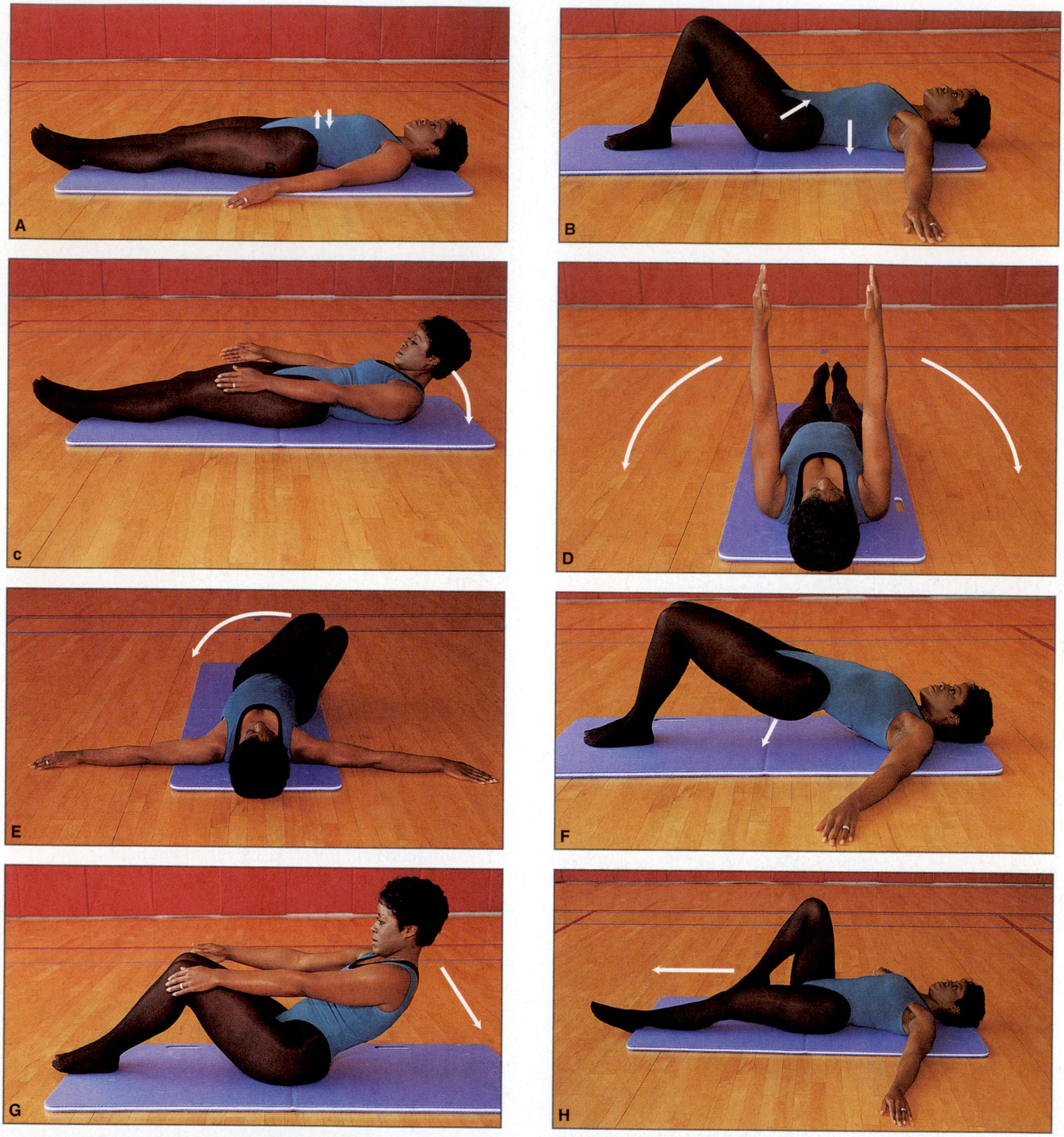

Figure 35–1 • Postpartal exercises. Begin with five repetitions two or three times daily, and gradually increase to ten repetitions. First day: *A,* Abdominal breathing. Lying supine, inhale deeply, using the abdominal muscles. The abdomen should expand. Then exhale slowly through pursed lips, tightening the abdominal muscles. *B,* Pelvic rocking. Lying supine with arms at sides, knees bent, and feet flat, tighten abdomen and buttocks, and attempt to flatten back on floor. Hold for a count of ten; then arch the back, causing the pelvis to "rock." On the second day, add *C,* Chin to chest. Lying supine with legs straight, raise head and attempt to touch chin to chest. Slowly lower head. *D,* Arm raises. Lying supine, arms extended at a 90-degree angle from body, raise arms so that they are perpendicular and hands touch. Lower slowly. On fourth day, add *E,* Knee rolls. Lying supine with knees bent, feet flat, arms extended to the side, roll knees slowly to one side, keeping shoulders flat. Return to original position, and roll to opposite side. *F,* Buttocks lift. Lying supine, arms at sides, knees bent, feet flat, slowly raise the buttocks, and arch the back. Return slowly to starting position. On sixth day, add *G,* Abdominal tighteners. Lying supine, knees bent, feet flat, slowly raise head toward knees. Arms should extend along either side of legs. Return slowly to original position. *H,* Knee to abdomen. Lying supine, arms at sides, bend one knee and thigh until foot touches buttocks. Straighten leg and lower it slowly. Repeat with other leg. After 2 to 3 weeks, more strenuous exercises, such as sit-ups and side leg raises, may be added as tolerated. Kegel exercises, begun antepartally, should be done many times daily during postpartum to restore vaginal and perineal tone.

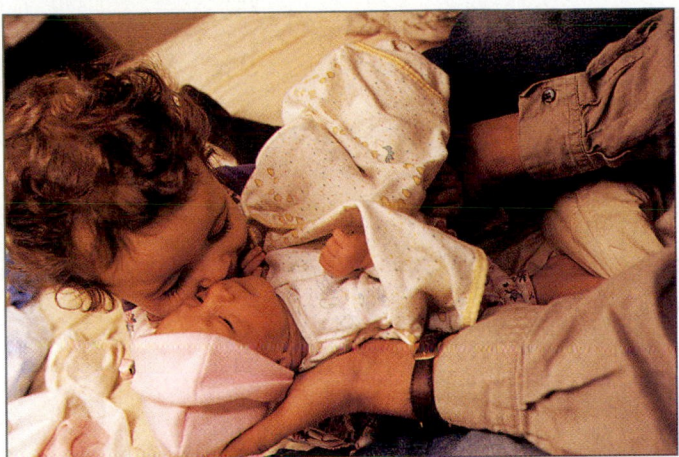

Figure 35–2 • The sister of this newborn becomes acquainted with the new family member.

the birth. They may even remain throughout the woman's hospitalization, especially if it is brief, and all go home as a family.

For the mother who is returning home to small children, it is often helpful to have the father carry the new baby inside. This practice keeps the mother's arms free to hug and hold her older children. She thereby reaffirms her love for them before introducing them to their new sibling. Many mothers have found that bringing a doll home with them for the older child is helpful. The child cares for the doll alongside his or her parents, thereby identifying with the parent. This identification helps decrease anger and the need to regress to get attention.

Often older children enjoy working with the parents to care for the newborn. Involvement in care helps the older child develop a sense of closeness to the baby. It also helps the child learn acceptable behavior toward the newborn, feel a sense of accomplishment, and develop tenderness and caring. With constant supervision and assistance as necessary, even very young children can hold the baby or a bottle during feeding.

Regression is a common occurrence even when siblings have been well prepared. The nurse can provide anticipatory guidance so that parents do not become overly upset if their previously toilet-trained child begins to have accidents or requests a bottle.

Regardless of age, an older sibling needs reassurance that he or she is still special to the parents, a truly loved and valued family member. Words of love and praise coupled with hugs and kisses are very important. So, too, is special parent-child time. Both parents should spend quality time in a one-to-one experience with each of their older children. This may require some careful planning, but its worth cannot be overestimated. It confirms the parents' love for the child and often helps the child accept the new baby.

The child, especially one of the opposite sex from the newborn, may raise queries about the appearance of the genitals as compared to his or her own. A simple explanation, such as, "That's what little girls (boys) look like," is often sufficient.

Resumption of Sexual Activity

Nursing interventions in the postpartal period acknowledge that the parent is also a sexual being. Couples were formerly discouraged from engaging in sexual intercourse until 6 weeks postpartum. Currently, the couple is advised to abstain from intercourse until the episiotomy is healed and the lochial flow has stopped (usually by the third to sixth week postpartum). During this period, couples can be encouraged to express their affection and love through kissing, holding, and talking. Because the vaginal vault is still "dry" (hormone-poor), some form of lubrication, such as K Y jelly, may be necessary initially during intercourse. The female-superior or side-by-side positions for coitus may be preferable because they enable the woman to control the depth of penile penetration.

Breastfeeding couples should be forewarned that during orgasm, milk may spout from the nipples because of the release of oxytocin. Some couples find this pleasurable or amusing; other couples choose to have the woman wear a bra during sexual activity. Breastfeeding the baby prior to lovemaking may reduce the chance of milk release.

Other factors may inhibit satisfactory sexual experience. The baby's crying may "spoil the mood," the woman's changed body may be unattractive to her or to her partner, and maternal sleep deprivation may interfere with a mutually satisfying experience. Couples may also be frustrated if there is decreased libido or other changes in the woman's physiologic response to sexual stimulation. These changes are due to hormonal changes and may persist for several months.

Maternal fatigue is often a significant factor limiting the resumption of sexual intercourse. Consequently, couples should be encouraged to find a time for lovemaking when both are interested and awake. By 3 months postpartum, sexual interest and activity are generally regular in frequency.

Anticipatory guidance during the prenatal and postnatal periods can forewarn the couple of these eventualities and of their temporary nature. See Client Teaching: Resuming Sexual Activity after Childbirth.

TEACHING FOR SELF-CARE

The nurse should discuss normal sexual changes that frequently occur in the postpartum period. A discussion that includes both partners can facilitate an open dialog between them and can provide an opportunity for questions and answers.

Contraception

Because many couples resume sexual activity before the postpartal examination, family-planning information should be made available before discharge. A couple's decision to use a contraceptive is often motivated by a desire to gain control over the number of children they will conceive or to determine the spacing of future children. In choosing a specific method, consistency of use outweighs the absolute reliability of a given method. The nurse must identify risk factors and

Client Teaching: Resuming Sexual Activity After Childbirth

Assessment Recognize that couples, especially if they have become parents for the first time, may have questions about resuming sexual activity. Although the woman may initiate this discussion, you can often best assess the woman's (and her partner's) understanding by providing general information followed by some tactful questions.

Nursing Diagnosis The key nursing diagnosis will probably be ***Health-Seeking Behavior:*** Information about changes in sexual activity that commonly occur postpartally.

Nursing Plan and Implementation First establish rapport with the couple and promote an environment that is conducive to teaching and discussion. It is helpful to provide privacy during the session so that the couple feels free to ask questions without fear of interruption. The format is generally a question-and-answer or discussion approach.

Client Goals At the completion of teaching, the couple will be able to:

- Discuss the changes in the woman's body that affect sexual activity.
- Formulate alternative approaches to sexual activity based on an understanding of these changes.
- Identify the length of time it is advisable to wait before resuming sexual activity.
- Discuss information needed to make contraceptive choices.

Teaching Plan

CONTENT

- Present information about changes that may affect sexual activity, including the following:
  - Tenderness of the vagina and perineum
  - Presence of lochia and the healing process
  - Dryness of the vagina
  - Breast engorgement and tenderness
  - Escape of milk during sexual activity
- Discuss healing at the placental site and stress that the presence of lochia indicates that healing is not yet complete. Point out that because the vagina is "hormone-poor" postpartally, vaginal dryness may pose a problem. This can be avoided by using a water-soluble lubricant. Explain that escape of milk during sexual activity can be minimized by breastfeeding the baby immediately beforehand.
- Discuss the importance of contraception during the early postpartal period. Provide information on the advantages and disadvantages of different methods. The woman's body needs adequate time to heal and recover from the stress of pregnancy and childbirth. Couples who are opposed to contraception may choose abstinence at this time.
- Discuss the impact of fatigue and the new baby's schedule on the woman's feelings of desire. Refer the couple to a physician or certified nurse-midwife for additional information if needed.

TEACHING METHOD

Discussion is a logical approach. It may be useful to make a universal statement and link it with a question to determine a couple's initial level of knowledge. For example, "Many women experience vaginal dryness when they resume intercourse for the first several weeks after childbirth. Are you familiar with this change and the cause for it?" Use the information gained during this discussion to determine the depth to which to cover the material.

Provide printed information to clarify content and serve as a resource for the couple following discharge.

Provide samples of different types of contraceptives.

Provide literature on specific contraceptive methods.

Many couples are unprepared for the impact of fatigue and the baby's schedule on lovemaking. Information enables the couple to anticipate this impact.

Evaluation

Determine the couple's learning by providing time for discussion and questions. If the couple indicates that they plan to use a particular contraceptive method, you may ask them about aspects of the method to ascertain that they have correct and complete information.

Table 35–5 • PARENT ATTACHMENT BEHAVIORS

Assessment Area	Attachment	Behavior Requiring Assessment and Information
Caretaking	Talks with baby. Demonstrates and seeks eye-to-eye contact. Touches and holds baby. Changes diapers when needed. Baby is clean. Clothing is appropriate for room temperature. Feeds baby as needed and baby is gaining weight. Positions baby comfortably and checks on baby.	Does not refer to baby. Completes activities without addressing the baby or looking at the baby. Lack of interaction. Does not recognize need for or demonstrate concern for baby's comfort or needs. Feeding occurs intermittently. Baby does not gain weight. Waits for baby to cry and then hesitates to respond.
Perception of the baby	Has knowledge of expected child development. Understands that the baby is dependent and cannot meet parent's needs. Accepts sex of child and characteristics.	Has unrealistic expectations of the baby's abilities and behaviors. Expects love and interaction from the baby. Believes that the baby will fulfill parent's needs. Is strongly distressed over sex of baby or feels that some aspect of the baby is unacceptable.
Support	Has friends who are available for support. Seems to be comfortable with being a parent. Has realistic beliefs of parenting role.	Is alone or isolated. Is on edge, tense, anxious, and hesitant with the baby. Demonstrates difficulty incorporating parenting with own wants and needs.

Please note: These are a few of the behaviors that may be associated with attachment. It is vitally important for the nurse to observe the parents on more than one occasion and to take into consideration individual characteristics, values, beliefs, and customs.

contraindications of the various methods to help the couple select a contraceptive method that has practical application and is compatible with the couple's health and physical needs.

Often different methods of contraception are appropriate at different times in the couple's life. Thus they should have a clear understanding of all of the methods available to them so that they can make an appropriate choice. The currently available contraceptive methods are discussed in detail in Chapter 5 .

TEACHING FOR SELF-CARE

The nurse should discuss available contraceptive methods with both partners prior to discharge. Written information should also be provided for the couple to refer to at a later time. The nurse should stress the fact that pregnancy can occur before the first menstrual period returns and that contraception before that time is imperative. The nurse should be frank and open with the couple, answering questions as needed.

Parent-Infant Attachment

Nursing interventions to enhance the quality of parent-infant attachment should be designed to promote feelings of well-being, comfort, and satisfaction. Table 35–5 • describes parental attachment behaviors and those that require further assessment. Following are some suggestions for ways of achieving this.

- Determine the childbearing and childrearing goals of the infant's mother and father, and adapt them wherever possible in planning nursing care for the family. This includes considering cultural preferences, and giving the parents choices about their labor and birth experience and their initial time with their new infant.
- Postpone eye prophylaxis for 1 hour after birth to facilitate eye contact between parents and their newborn (eye ointment further clouds the newborn's vision and makes eye contact difficult for the baby).
- Provide time in the first hour after birth for the new family to become acquainted, with as much privacy as possible.
- Arrange the healthcare setting so that the individual nurse-client relationship can be developed and maintained. A primary nurse can develop rapport and assess the mother's strengths and needs.
- Encourage the parents to involve the siblings in integrating the infant into the family by bringing them to the birthing center for sibling visits.
- Use anticipatory guidance from conception through the postpartal period to prepare the parents for expected problems of adjustment.
- Include parents in any nursing intervention, planning, and evaluation. Give choices whenever possible.
- Initiate and support measures to alleviate fatigue in the parents.
- Help parents identify, understand, and accept both positive and negative feelings related to the overall parenting experience.
- Support and assist parents in determining the personality and unique needs of their infant.

Whenever possible and culturally acceptable, the mother should be allowed to care for her baby. This practice gives the mother a chance to learn her newborn's normal patterns and develop confidence in caring for him or her. It also allows the father more uninterrupted time with his infant in the first days of life. Early discharge may be advantageous if mother and baby are doing well, help is available for the mother at home, and the family and certified nurse-midwife/physician agree.

The nurse may observe beginnings of parent-newborn attachment in the first few hours after birth, and when continuing assessments in home visits after discharge. As the nurse assesses attachment, it is important to remember that cultural values, beliefs, and practices will direct child care activities and self-care practices. For example, some Arabic women wrap the infant's abdomen in a firm binder as a means of preventing the umbilical stump from protruding. Nurses should incorporate cultural norms into the care of the newborn whenever possible.

TEACHING FOR SELF-CARE

Some new parents may feel awkward in their new role as parents. The nurse should provide reassurance and advise new parents of normal infant behavior and activity. The nurse assesses attachment prior to discharge. If the nurse identifies a possible alteration in attachment, the parents can be referred to a new parent support group, parenting classes, or counseling to assist them with their transition into their new roles. The nurse can explain that new attachments are being formed, and like all new relationships, both the infant and the parents are discovering each other. The nurse should discuss possible risk factors of altered attachment such as inability or lack of desire to care for the infant.

Nursing Care Following Cesarean Birth

After a cesarean birth, the new mother has postpartal needs similar to those of women who gave birth vaginally. Because she has undergone major abdominal surgery, however, the woman also has nursing care needs similar to those of other surgical clients.

Promotion of Maternal Physical Well-Being after Cesarean Birth

Immobility after the use of narcotic and sedative agents and alterations in the immune response of postoperative clients increase the chances of pulmonary infection. For this reason, the woman is encouraged to cough and deep breathe and to use incentive spirometry every 2 to 4 hours while awake for the first few days following cesarean birth.

Immobility increases the risk of abdominal distention and discomfort, blood clots, deep vein thrombosis, and pulmonary embolisms. Within the first 12 to 24 hours postoperatively, unless medically contraindicated, the woman should be assisted to dangle her legs on the side of the bed. The woman should be assisted out of bed in the next 24 to 36 hours.

The nurse continues to assess the woman's pain level and provide relief measures as needed. Sources of pain include incisional pain, gas pain, referred shoulder pain, periodic uterine contractions (afterbirth pains), and pain from voiding, defecation, or constipation.

Nursing interventions are oriented toward preventing or alleviating pain or helping the woman cope with pain. The nurse should undertake the following measures:

- Administer analgesic medications as needed, especially during the first 24 to 72 hours. Their use will relieve the woman's pain and enable her to be more mobile and active.
- Promote comfort through proper positioning, backrubs, oral care, and the reduction of noxious stimuli, such as noise and unpleasant odors.
- Encourage the presence of significant others, including other children, and the newborn. This provides distraction from the painful sensations and helps reduce the woman's fear and anxiety.
- Encourage the use of breathing, relaxation, and distraction techniques (for example, stimulation of cutaneous tissue) taught in childbirth preparation class.
- Encourage adequate rest periods. This may include limiting excessive visitors and phone calls.
- Encourage early ambulation to prevent abdominal distention that can occur with excess accumulation of gas in the intestines.

Epidural analgesia administered just after the cesarean birth is an effective method of pain relief for most women in the first 24 hours following birth (see Drug Guide: Postpartum Epidural Morphine).

The physician may prescribe **patient-controlled analgesia (PCA).** With this approach, the woman is given a bolus of analgesia, usually morphine or meperidine, at the beginning of therapy. Using a special IV pump system, the woman presses a button to self-administer small doses of the medication as needed. For safety, the pump is preset with a time lockout so that the pump cannot deliver another dose until a specified time has elapsed. Women using PCA feel less anxious and have a greater sense of control with less dependence on the nursing staff. The frequent smaller doses help the woman experience rapid pain relief without grogginess and also eliminate the discomfort of injections.

If general anesthesia was used, abdominal distention from the accumulation of gas in the intestines may produce discomfort for the woman during the first postpartal days. Additional measures to prevent or minimize gas pains include leg exercises, abdominal tightening, avoiding carbonated or very hot or cold beverages, avoiding the use of straws, and providing a high-protein liquid diet for the first 24 to 48 hours until bowel sounds return. The woman may find it helpful to lie prone or on her left side. Lying on the left side allows gas to rise from the descending colon to the sigmoid colon so that it can be expelled more readily. Other women report that a rocking chair helps them obtain relief. Medical interventions for gas pain include the use of antiflatulents (such as Mylicon), suppositories, and enemas.

The nurse can minimize discomfort and promote satisfaction as the mother assumes the activities of her new role. In-

DRUG GUIDE POSTPARTUM EPIDURAL MORPHINE

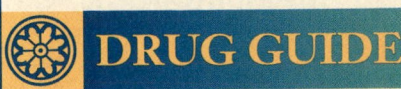

• Overview of Obstetric Action

Epidural morphine is used to provide relief of pain associated with cesarean birth, extensive episiotomies (mediolaterals), or third- and fourth-degree lacerations. Epidural morphine pain relief results directly from its effect on the opiate receptors in the spinal cord (it depresses pain impulse transmission). Morphine binds opiate receptors, thereby altering both the perception of and emotional response to pain. Women experience little or no discomfort or pain during recovery and for up to 24 hours afterward. There is no motor or sympathetic block or associated hypotension. Onset of analgesia is slower, but duration is longer.

• Route, Dosage, and Frequency

Five to seven and one-half mg of morphine is injected through a catheter into the epidural space, providing pain relief for about 24 hours (Datta, 1995).

• Maternal Contraindications

Allergy to morphine, narcotic addiction, chronic debilitating respiratory disease, infection at the injection site, or administration of parenteral corticosteroids in past 14 days (PDR Nurse's Handbook, 1999).

• Maternal Side Effects

Late-onset respiratory depression (rare but may occur 8–12 hours after administration), nausea and vomiting (occurring between 4 and 7 hours after injection), itching (begins within 3 hours and lasts up to 10 hours), urinary retention, and, rarely, somnolence. Side effects can be managed with naloxone.

• Neonatal Effects

No adverse effects since medication is injected after birth of baby.

• Nursing Considerations

- Obtain history: sensitivity (allergy) to morphine, presence of any contraindications (PDR Nurse's Handbook, 1999).
- Assess orientation, reflexes, skin color, texture, breath sounds, presence of lesions or infection over area of lumbar spine, voiding pattern, urinary output within normal limits (Karch, 1999).
- Monitor and evaluate analgesic effect. Ask client about comfort level and notify anesthesiologist of inadequate pain relief.
- Check catheter for obvious knots, breaks, and leakage at insertion site and catheter hub.
- Assess for pruritus (scratching and rubbing, especially around face and neck).
- Administer comfort measures for narcotic-induced pruritus, such as lotion, backrubs, cool/warm packs, or diversional activities. If the itching can be tolerated, naloxone should be avoided, especially since it counteracts the pain relief.
- If allergic reaction (urticaria, edema, or respiratory difficulties) occurs, administer naloxone or diphenhydramine per physician order.
- Provide comfort measures for nausea/vomiting, such as frequent oral hygiene or gradual increase of activity; administer naloxone, trimethobenzamide (Tigan), or metoclopramide HCl per physician order.
- Assess postural blood pressure and heart rate before ambulation.
- Assist client with her first ambulation and then as needed.
- Assess respiratory function every hour for 24 hours, then q2–8 hr as needed. Also assess level of consciousness and mucous membrane color. May need to monitor client via apnea monitor for 24 hours.
- Monitor urinary output and assess bladder for distention. Assist client to void.

struction and assistance in assuming comfortable positions when holding or breastfeeding the infant will do much to increase the mother's sense of competence and comfort. Sitting in a chair or tailor fashion in bed, leaning slightly forward with the infant propped on a pillow in her lap, will prevent irritation to the incision. Another preferred position for breastfeeding during the first postoperative days is lying on the side with the newborn positioned along the mother's body.

By the first or second day after the cesarean birth, the mother is usually receptive to learning how to care for herself and her infant. Demonstration of proper body mechanics in getting out of bed without the use of a side rail and ways of caring for the infant that prevent strain and torsion on the incision are also indicated. The nurse needs to place special emphasis on home management, encouraging the woman to let others assume responsibility for housekeeping and cooking. Fatigue not only prolongs recovery but also interferes with breastfeeding and mother-infant interaction.

The woman usually does extremely well postoperatively. If spinal anesthesia was used, the side effects of general anesthesia are absent. Even after general anesthesia, however, most women are ambulating by the day after the surgery. Usually by the second postpartal day, the incision can be covered with plastic wrap so the woman can shower, which seems to provide a mental as well as physical lift. If staples have been used, the incision is sometimes left open to the air, and showering is permitted without covering it. Most women are discharged on the third postoperative day.

Research suggests that women with cesarean births have several special needs following discharge: increased need for rest and sleep; incisional care; assistance with household chores, infant care, and self-care; and relief of pain and discomfort. Nurses need to address these areas during hospitalization and discharge planning. Perhaps one of the most important considerations for cesarean birth mothers is the need to plan for additional assistance at home to enable the new mother to rest and heal.

TEACHING FOR SELF-CARE

The nurse can assist the woman in identifying interventions to relieve discomfort or pain. The woman should be encouraged to take pain medication regularly, engage in frequent rest periods, avoid prolonged activity, and observe for signs of "overdoing it" (such as discomfort and fatigue). The nurse should advise the woman that recovery after a surgical procedure involves healing time and that fatigue and soreness are common symptoms of too much activity too quickly. The nurse can assist the family in identifying resources for assisting the new mother at home, such as assistance from friends and family, cleaning services, or food delivery services.

Promotion of Parent-Infant Interaction after Cesarean Birth

Many factors associated with cesarean birth may hinder successful and frequent maternal-infant interaction. These include the physical condition of the mother and newborn and maternal reactions to stress, anesthesia, and medications. The mother and her infant may be separated after birth because of hospital routines, prematurity, or neonatal complications. A healthy infant born by an uncomplicated cesarean birth is no more fragile than an infant born vaginally. Many agencies are beginning to provide time for the family together in the operating room if the mother's and infant's conditions permit, but some agencies still automatically place cesarean birth newborns in a high-risk nursery for a time.

Signs of depression, anger, or withdrawal in the cesarean birth mother may indicate a grief response to the loss of the fantasized vaginal birth experience. Fathers as well as mothers may experience feelings of "missing out," guilt that the

RESEARCH IN PRACTICE
Risk Factors for Surgical Site Infections Following Cesarean Section

What is this study about? Mothers who have cesarean births are at higher risk for maternal morbidity and mortality and have nearly ten times the number of infectious complications than their counterparts with vaginal births. These complications include postpartum endometritis and surgical wound infections. While clinical trials have demonstrated the efficacy of prophylactic antibiotics in the prevention of infections associated with cesarean birth, controversy exists as to the timing of antibiotic administration and the best subjects for prophylaxis. This study had at its objective the identification of risk factors associated with the development of surgical site infections after a cesarean and the evaluation of antibiotic prophylaxis in these women.

How was this study done? This study was a prospective cohort study conducted in an academic tertiary-care center using methodology recommended by the National Nosocomial Infections Surveillance System. For a six-month period during each of three sequential years, women were followed for incisional infections and endometritis for 30 days following cesarean birth. Data were collected for 765 subjects. Infections were identified by readmission to the hospital or by a post-discharge survey. The presence or absence of prophylactic antibiotics was documented for each subject. Risk factors were determined using logistic regression techniques.

What were the results of the study? Of these subjects, 7.7% had a surgical site infection, of which 5.1% developed endometritis, and 2.6% developed incisional infections. Analysis indicted four factors that were independently associated with an increased risk of infection: absence of antibiotic prophylaxis; surgery time; fewer than seven prenatal visits; and hours of ruptured membranes. Lack of prophylactic antibiotics was associated with both types of infections, and women who had received antibiotic prophylaxis had a lower overall infection rate (5.9%) than those who did not receive prophylaxis (12.7%). In addition, ruptured membranes were associated with an increased risk of endometritis, while multiple procedures were more common in women with incisional infection. Women with surgical site infections had a longer mean postoperative length of stay than those without infections, with the increased length of stay associated primarily with endometritis. There was no significant difference in length of stay for women with incisional infections.

What additional questions might I have? The post-discharge survey had a low physician response rate; did the researchers account for those women whose physician did not complete the post-discharge survey? What complications may have been caused by the prophylactic antibiotics? What is the increased cost of using prophylactic antibiotics?

How can I use this study? Multiple factors were determined to be associated with surgical site infections after cesarean birth. Of these–limited prenatal care and prophylactic antibiotics–can be changed in an effort to prevent infections. Birthing units need to conduct an evaluation to determine if their post-cesarean infection rate warrants consideration of antibiotic prophylaxis for all cesarean birth clients.

Source: Killian, C.A., Raffunder, E.M., Vinciguerra, T.J., & Venezia, R.A. (2001). Risk factors for surgical-site infections following cesarean section. *Infection Control & Hospital Epidemiology, 22*(10): 613-7.

surgery was the result of something they did "wrong," and even jealousy toward another couple who had a vaginal birth. The cesarean birth couple may also feel guilty that they are considering their personal needs and not simply the welfare of the infant.

The nurse can support the parents in a variety of ways. Initially, nurses must work through their own feelings about cesarean birth. The nurse who considers a vaginal birth "normal" and refers to it as such indicates that a cesarean birth is "abnormal," rather than simply an alternative method. Thus language and terminology, though seemingly insignificant, can convey to the couple negative messages about their cesarean birth experience.

The nurse should offer positive support to the couple. The cesarean birth couple may need the opportunity to tell their story repeatedly to work through their feelings. The nurse can provide factual information about their situation and support the couple's effective coping behaviors. The nurse should provide the parents with choices by allowing them to participate in decision making about the options available to them.

The presence of the father or significant other during the birth process positively influences the woman's perception of the birth event. His or her presence not only reduces the woman's fears but also enhances her sense of control and enables the couple to share feelings and respond to one another with touch and eye contact. Later they have the opportunity to relive the experience and fill in any gaps or missing pieces. This is especially valuable if the mother has had general anesthesia. The father or significant other can take pictures, hold the baby, and foster the discovery process by directing the mother's attention to details about her newborn.

The perception of and reactions to a cesarean birth experience depend on how the woman defines that experience. Her reality is what she perceives it to be. If the woman's attitude is more positive than negative, successful resolution of subsequent stressful events is more likely. Because the definition of events is transitory in nature, the possibility of change and growth is present. Often the mothering role is perceived as an extension of the childbearing role, and inability to fulfill expected childbearing behavior (vaginal birth) may lead to parental feelings of role failure and frustration. The nurse can help families alter their negative definitions of cesarean birth and bolster and encourage positive perceptions.

TEACHING FOR SELF-CARE

The nurse should advise the mother that she is able to hold, cuddle, lift, and feed her infant despite her surgical incision. The nurse can assist the woman in finding positions that are comfortable for holding and feeding the baby. Upon discharge, the woman should be encouraged to care for the infant and allow family members or friends to assist with household duties rather than infant care practices.

Nursing Care of the Postpartal Adolescent

Over half the teens who become pregnant give birth and keep their babies (Ventura, Mathews, & Hamilton, 2001). The adolescent mother's ability to relate to her infant is important. Earlier studies demonstrated that teenage mothers interact less positively with their babies than older mothers do. However, recent research suggests that this is related more to self-esteem, perceived social support (McVeigh & Smith, 2000), and the amount of support an adolescent receives in the prenatal period (Koniak-Griffin et al, 1999).

During the postpartal period, the adolescent may have special needs, depending on her level of maturity, support systems, and cultural background. The nurse should assess maternal-infant interaction, roles of support people, plans for discharge, knowledge of childrearing, and plans for follow-up care. It is imperative to have a community health service be in touch with the young woman shortly after discharge.

Contraception counseling is an important part of teaching. Often the young woman tells the nurse that she does not plan on engaging in sex again. This denial mechanism is unrealistic, and the nurse must help the young woman realize this. The nurse should make sure that the woman has some method of birth control available to her and that she understands ovulation and fertility in relation to her menstrual cycle. This is an excellent opportunity for sex education.

The nurse has many opportunities for teaching the adolescent about the newborn in the postpartal unit. Because the nurse serves as a role model, the manner in which she handles the baby greatly influences the young mother. The father, if involved, should be included in as much of the teaching as possible.

A newborn physical examination performed at the bedside gives the adolescent immediate feedback about the newborn's health and shows her methods of handling an infant. The nurse can teach as the examination progresses, giving the new mother information about the fontanelles, cradle cap, shampooing the newborn's hair, and so on. The nurse might also use this time to teach the young mother about infant stimulation techniques. Because adolescent mothers tend to concentrate their interactions in the physical domain, they need to comprehend the importance of verbal, visual, and auditory stimulation for newborns as well.

Performing an examination at the bedside also gives the adolescent permission to explore her baby, which she may have been hesitant to do. A Brazelton neonatal assessment (Chapter 29) will help the mother understand the newborn's response to stimuli, a key factor in the adolescent's response to the individuality of her newborn once she goes home. Parents who have some idea of what to expect from their infants will be less frustrated with the newborn's behavior.

The adolescent mother appreciates positive feedback about her fine newborn and her developing maternal responses. This praise and encouragement will increase her confidence and self-esteem.

Group classes for adolescent mothers should include infant care skills, information about growth and development, infant feeding, well-baby care, and danger signals in the ill newborn. If classes are offered in the hospital during the postpartum stay, the adolescent mother should be strongly encouraged to attend. If the child's father is involved, he should also be encouraged to attend and participate. The nurse can correct misconceptions and unrealistic expectations about growth and development. The nurse should also make a thorough assessment of the support systems and resources already in place for the mother and additional resources from the hospital or the community that may be appropriate for the situation.

Ideally, teenage mothers should visit adolescent clinics where mother and baby are assessed for several years after birth. In this way, classes on parenting, vocational guidance, and school attendance can be followed closely. School systems' classes for young mothers are an excellent way of helping adolescents finish school and learn how to parent at the same time.

In the event that a woman decides to keep an unwanted child, the nurse should be aware of the potential for parenting problems. Families with unwanted children are more prone to crisis than others, although in many cases, parents grow to love their child after attachment occurs. The nurse should be ready to initiate crisis management strategies or make appropriate referrals as the need arises.

Nursing Care of the Woman Who Relinquishes Her Infant

Mothers who choose to give their infants up for adoption typically are young, unmarried, or both. Some relinquishing mothers are living in poverty, or their pregnancy may have resulted from incest or rape. Other women may dislike children or the idea of being a mother, and still others are not emotionally ready for parenthood. At times a woman may desperately want to keep her child but her partner disapproves; he may even have threatened to leave her if she brings the baby home. These and many other reasons may cause the woman to relinquish her baby.

The mother who chooses to let her child be adopted often experiences intense ambivalence about her decision. Several factors contribute to this ambivalence. First, there are social pressures against giving up one's child even when relinquishment appears to be in the baby's best interest. Additionally, the woman usually has made considerable adjustments in her lifestyle to carry and give birth to this child. She may be unaware of her growing bond with her child until she actually gives birth, at which point all her sensible plans may suddenly be thrown into doubt by the intensity of her feelings of protectiveness and attachment to the newborn. At the same time, she may not have told friends and relatives about the pregnancy and so may lack an extended support system to help her cope with the grief, anxiety, doubt, guilt, and shame that may arise at the thought of relinquishing her child.

Throughout the perinatal period, the nurse can help the relinquishing mother by encouraging her to express her grief, loneliness, guilt, and other feelings. When the relinquishing mother is admitted to the birthing unit, the staff should be informed about the mother's decision to relinquish the infant. Any special requests regarding the birth should be respected, and the woman should be encouraged to express her emotions. Her feelings of ambivalence may heighten just before birth. If the woman is accompanied by family members or a significant other, the nurse provides support to them throughout the labor and birth. If no support person is present, the nurse acts as the primary support person and ensures that the woman has a clear understanding of all that occurs.

After the birth, the mother should be able to decide whether she wants to see the newborn. Seeing the newborn often facilitates the grieving process. When the mother sees her baby, she may feel strong attachment and love, and her ambivalence may be especially pronounced. The nurse needs to assure the woman that these feelings do not mean that her decision to relinquish the child is a wrong one; relinquishment is often a painful act of love (Arms, 1990).

> “*I have had the pleasure of working with several mothers who have decided to relinquish their infants. Their selfless act of love is one of the greatest acts of mothering I have ever seen, as was the case with Lashonda, the mother of a 3-year-old boy and 18-month-old twin girls. As I entered the room, she was profoundly quiet with tears in her eyes. I asked her how she was doing. She responded, "It's so hard." I asked her if she was having second thoughts and she said, "No, I want her to have all the things I can't give her, all the love and time she deserves." She said that as a single mother, she was having difficulty financially supporting and caring for three children. I then asked her if she wanted to see her infant. She hesitated, said no, and asked me if she was doing "okay." I told her the baby was fine. After several moments of silence, she asked me for a favor. "Would you go and hold her for a minute, give her a kiss, and tell her I really did love her?" With that, I left the room and entered the nursery. The tiny girl with dark black curly hair was truly beautiful. I rocked her for a long time. As I placed her in her crib, I kissed her tiny forehead and whispered, "Your mama loves you so much." It may have been my imagination but I swear that the faintest smile emerged as I laid her down. Then it was my turn to cry.*”

Society views relinquishing as a voluntary choice and does not acknowledge that a loss has occurred; therefore, there is no expectation of the birth mother to grieve. Research has indicated that birth mothers have not received acknowledgment of their loss from healthcare providers. Simple recognition of loss and its significance to the woman will go a long way toward assisting with resolution of grief (Askern & Brown, 1999).

After the birth, the nurse can ask the mother if she wishes to remain on the postpartum unit or if she would prefer to be cared for on another unit. The mother's choice should be supported. Many mothers who relinquish their infants may opt for a shortened hospital stay. Nurses should facilitate discharge instructions in the immediate postpartum period.

Discharge Information

The postpartum stay allowed by most third-party payers has decreased dramatically in recent years. Hospital stays that were measured in weeks in the 1940s are now measured in hours. Postpartum nursing care that has traditionally included a strong focus on the adjustments of the mother, newborn, and family is very difficult to accomplish because of the brief length of stay. Mothers and newborns are being discharged before many of their important postbirth healthcare needs can be addressed. These include establishing breastfeeding, ruling out infections, supporting infant-family bonding, and client teaching. Home health services are increasingly being recognized as a cost-effective means of meeting the postbirth needs of mothers and newborns. Home care of the postpartal family is the subject of the next chapter.

Ideally, preparation for discharge begins the moment a woman enters the birthing unit to give birth. Nursing efforts should be directed toward assessing the couple's knowledge, expectations, and beliefs and then providing anticipatory guidance and teaching accordingly (see Table 35–1). Because teaching is one of the primary responsibilities of the postpartum nurse, many agencies have elaborate teaching programs and classes. Before the actual discharge, however, the nurse should spend time with the couple to determine whether they have any last-minute questions. In general, discharge teaching should include at least the following.

1. The woman should contact her caregiver if she develops any of the signs of possible complications:
    a. Sudden persistent or spiking fever or chills
    b. Change in the character of the lochia—foul smell, return to bright red bleeding, excessive amount (more than two pads in 1 hour)
    c. Evidence of mastitis, such as breast tenderness, reddened areas, malaise, fever, chills
    d. Evidence of thrombophlebitis, such as calf pain, tenderness, redness
    e. Evidence of urinary tract infection, such as urgency, frequency, burning on urination
    f. Evidence of infection in an incision (either episiotomy or cesarean), such as redness, edema, pain or discomfort, discharge, or lack of approximation
    g. Continued severe or incapacitating postpartal depression, inability to care for self or baby, feelings of self-harm
2. The woman should review the literature she has received that explains recommended postpartum exercises, the need for adequate rest, the need to avoid overexertion initially, and the recommendation to abstain from sexual intercourse until lochia has ceased. The woman may take a shower and may continue sitz baths at home if she desires.
3. The woman should be given the phone numbers of the postpartum unit, lactation consultant, and nursery and be encouraged to call if she has any questions, no matter how simple.
4. The woman should receive information on local agencies or support groups, such as La Leche League and Mothers of Twins, that might be of particular assistance to her.
5. Both breastfeeding and formula-feeding mothers should receive information geared to their specific nutritional needs. They should also be told to continue their vitamin and iron supplements until their postpartal examination.
6. The woman should have a scheduled appointment for her postpartal examination and for her infant's first well-baby examination before they are discharged.
7. The mother should clearly understand the correct procedure for obtaining copies of her infant's birth certificate.
8. The new parents should be able to provide home care for their infant and should know when to anticipate that the cord will fall off, when the infant can have a tub bath, when the infant will need his or her first immunizations, and so on. They should also be comfortable feeding and handling the baby and should be aware of basic safety considerations, including the need to use a car seat whenever the infant is in a car. These topics are covered in Chapter 36.
9. The parents should be aware of signs and symptoms in the infant that indicate possible problems and whom they should contact about them.

The nurse can also use this final period to reassure the couple of their ability to be successful parents, stressing the infant's need to feel loved and secure. The nurse can also urge parents to talk to each other and work together to solve any problems that may arise.

The nurse addresses follow-up visits when appropriate. If not already discussed, teaching about family planning is appropriate at this time, and the nurse can provide information regarding birth control methods.

In ideal situations, a family approach involving the father, infant, and possibly other siblings would permit a total evaluation and provide an opportunity for all family members to ask questions and express concerns. In addition, a family approach can enable the nurse to identify disturbed family patterns more readily and initiate interventions to prevent future problems of neglect or abuse.

Evaluation

Anticipated outcomes of comprehensive nursing care of the postpartal family include the following:

- The mother demonstrates effective pain control and verbalizes understanding of self-comfort measures.

- The mother is rested and verbalizes understanding of the importance of gradual return to activities.
- The mother verbalizes understanding of the nature and prevalence of postpartum "baby blues" and identifies the symptoms of postpartum depression.
- The new parents demonstrate safe and effective care of their baby.
- The new parents display appropriate attachment to their baby.
- The cesarean birth mother states in her own words the reason for the cesarean birth.
- The cesarean birth mother demonstrates effective pain control and maintains moderate mobility level.
- The adolescent mother has been supported physically and emotionally.
- The woman relinquishing her newborn verbalizes rationale for her decision and demonstrates acceptance of her decision.
- In summary, all components of nursing care are designed to achieve the desired outcomes identified for the woman and her family.

Chapter Review

ExploreMediaLink

NCLEX review questions, case studies, and other interactive resources for this chapter can be found on the Web site at http://www.prenhall.com/olds. Click on "Chapter 35" to select the activities for this chapter.

For tutorials including animations and videos, more NCLEX review questions, and an audio glossary, access the accompanying CD-ROM in this book.

Focus Your Study

- Effective parent learning requires precise timing of teaching, as well as choice of a teaching method that is effective for the family, such as videotapes, return-demonstration, and so on. Content on self-care, infant care, and anticipatory guidance is important.
- Postpartum discomfort may be due to a variety of factors, including an edematous perineum, an episiotomy or extension, engorged hemorrhoids, hematoma formation, afterpains, immobility, diaphoresis, or engorged breasts. Various self-care approaches are helpful in promoting comfort. Cultural values are incorporated in providing care to the new family.
- Lactation may be suppressed by mechanical techniques or by administering medication.
- The first day or two following birth are marked by maternal behaviors that are more dependent and oriented to the woman's comfort. Thereafter the woman becomes more independent and ready to assume responsibility.
- The new mother requires opportunities to discuss her childbirth experience with an empathetic listener.
- Maternal rest is promoted by advising the woman to take frequent rest periods, nap when the baby is napping, avoid unnecessary activities, and use her social support system. Ambulation and activity should be resumed gradually.
- Rooming-in provides the childbearing family with opportunities to interact with their new member during the first hours and days of life. This enables the family to develop some confidence and skill in a "safe" environment.
- Sexual intercourse may resume once the episiotomy has healed and lochia has stopped. Couples should be forewarned of possible changes; for example, the vagina may be "dry," fatigue may inhibit the level of desire, or the woman's breasts may leak milk during orgasm.
- Following cesarean birth, a woman has the nursing care needs of a surgical client in addition to her needs as a postpartum client. She may also require assistance in working through her feelings if the cesarean birth was unexpected.
- Postpartally, the nurse evaluates the adolescent mother in terms of her level of maturity, available support systems, cultural background, and existing knowledge and then plans care accordingly.
- The mother who decides to relinquish her baby needs emotional support. She should be able to decide whether to see and hold her baby and should

have any special requests regarding the birth honored.

- Prior to discharge, the nurse should give the couple any information necessary for the woman to provide appropriate self-care. They should have a beginning skill in caring for their newborn and should be familiar with warning signs of possible complications for mother or baby. Printed information is valuable in helping couples deal with questions that may arise at home.
- Because of the trend toward early discharge, follow-up care is more important than ever. Many approaches are used, especially home visits.

References

Arms, S. (1990). *Adoption: A handful of hope.* Berkeley, CA: Celestial Arts.

Askren, H. A., & Brown, K. C. (1999). Postadoptive reactions of the relinquishing mother: A review. *Journal of Obstetric, Gynecologic, and Neonatal Nursing, 28*(4), 395–400.

Banks-Wallace, J. (1999). Storytelling as a tool for providing holistic care to women. *American Journal of Maternal Child Nursing, 24*, 20–24.

Beckerman, C. R. B., & Dystart, D. (2000). The challenge of multicultural medical care. *Contemporary OB/GYN, 45*(12), 12–33.

Callister, L. C. (2001). Culturally competent care of women and newborns: Knowledge, attitude, and skills. *Journal of Obstetric, Gynecologic, and Neonatal Nursing, 30*, 209–215.

Calvert, S., & Fleming, V. (2000). Minimizing postpartum pain: A review of research pertaining to perineal care in childbearing women. *Journal of Advanced Nursing, 32*(2), 407–415.

Datta, S. (1995). *The obstetric anesthesia handbook.* St. Louis: Mosby.

DeJonge, A. (2001). Support for teenage mothers: A qualitative study into the views of women about the support they received as teenage mothers. *Journal of Advanced Nursing, 36*(1), 49–57.

Karch, A. M. (1999). *Lippincott's nursing drug guide.* Philadelphia: Lippincott.

Koniak-Griffin, D., Mathenge, C., Anderson, N. L. R., & Verzemnieks, I. (1999). An early intervention program for adolescent mothers: A nursing demonstration project. *Journal of Obstetric, Gynecologic, and Neonatal Nursing, 28*, 51–59.

Lamp, J. M., & Howard, P. A. (1999). Guiding parents' use of the internet for newborn education. *American Journal of Maternal Child Nursing, 24*, 33–36.

Mayberry, L. J., Affonso, D. D., Shibuya, J. & Clemmens, D. (1999). Integrating cultural values, beliefs, and customs into pregnancy and postpartum care: Lessons learned from a Hawaiian public health nursing project. *Journal of Perinatal and Neonatal Nursing, 13*(1), 15–26.

McVeigh, C., & Smith, M. (2000). A comparison of adult and teenage mother's self esteem and satisfaction with social support. *Midwifery, 16*(4), 269–276.

Montgomery, A. M. (2000). Breastfeeding and postpartum maternal care. *Primary Care, 27*(1), 237–249.

Parks, P. L., Lenz, E. R., Milligan, R. A., & Han, H.R. (1999). What happens when fatigue lingers for 18 months after delivery? *Journal of Obstetric, Gynecologic, and Neonatal Nursing, 28*, 87–93.

PDR Nurse's Handbook. (1999). Montvale, NJ: Medical Economics.

Ruchala, P. L. (2000). Teaching new mothers: Priorities of nurses and postpartum women. *Journal of Obstetric, Gynecologic, and Neonatal Nursing, 29*(3), 265–273.

Sampselle, C. M., Seng, J., Yeo, S., Killion, C., & Oakley, D. (1999). Physical activity and postpartum well-being. *Journal of Obstetric, Gynecologic, and Neonatal Nursing, 28*, 41–49.

Schwarts, M. A., Wang, C. C., Eckert, L. O., & Critchlow, C. W. (1999). Risk factors for urinary tract infection in the postpartum period. *American Journal of Obstetrics and Gynecology, 181*(3), 547–553.

Technical Working Group, World Health Organization. (1999). Postpartum care of the mother and newborn: A practical guide. *Birth, 26*(4), 255–258.

Thoyre, S. M. (2000). Mothers' ideas about their role in feeding their high-risk infants. *Journal of Obstetric, Gynecologic, and Neonatal Nursing, 29*(6), 613–624.

Ventura, S. J., Mathews, T. J., & Hamilton, B. E. (2001). Births to teenagers in the United States, 1940–2000. *National Vital Statistics Report, 49*(10), 1–23.

Home Care of the Postpartal Family

36

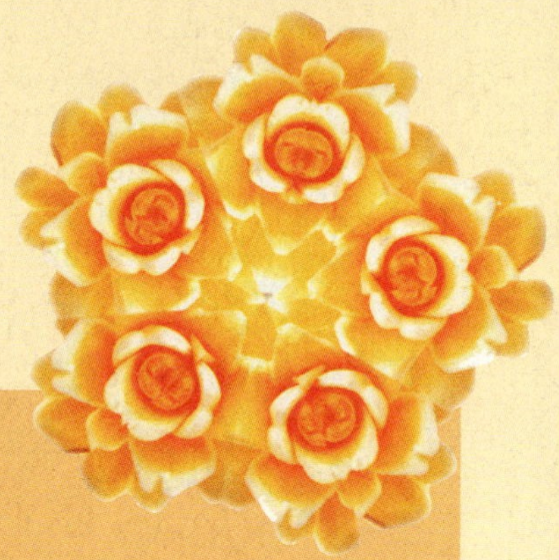

I am amazed by the fact that I love making home visits. I always thought that nothing could be more enjoyable than hospital nursing, but when I go into a home and help a family with a teaching need or work out a problem using my knowledge, common sense, and the resources available in the community, I know I am making an incredible difference in the lives of a new family.

Objectives

- Explain the current controversy surrounding length of stay.
- Discuss the components of postpartal home care.
- Identify the main purposes of home visits during the postpartum period.
- Summarize actions the nurse should take to ensure personal safety during a home visit.
- Delineate aspects of fostering a caring relationship in the home.
- Describe assessment, care of the newborn, and reinforcement of parent teaching in the home.
- Discuss maternal and family assessment and anticipated progress after birth.
- Identify appropriate nursing interventions for women who are experiencing breastfeeding difficulties.
- Provide client teaching regarding resumption of sexual activity.
- Identify postpartum resources that are available to new families.

Key Terms

Active alert state 1057
Cosleeping 1057
Crying state 1057
Deep sleep 1057
Drowsy state 1057
Light sleep 1057
Quiet alert state 1057
Postpartal home care 1047
Sudden infant death syndrome (SIDS) 1056

MediaLink

Additional resources for this content can be found on the Student CD-ROM and on the Companion Website at www.prenhall.com/olds. Click on "Chapter 36" to select the activities for this chapter.

CD-ROM
- Audio Glossary
- NCLEX Review

Companion Website
- Additional NCLEX Review
- Case Study: Follow-Up With the Client at Home
- Care Plan Activity: Breastfeeding Pain

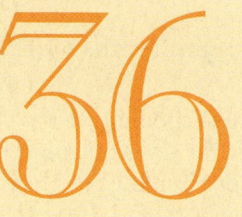

Home care is an essential component of perinatal nursing care, particularly as caregivers struggle to find an appropriate balance between providing quality client care and managing escalating healthcare costs. The hospital length of stay (LOS) following childbirth dominated this controversy during the last years of the 20th century. The average LOS decreased during the early 1990s in an effort to contain healthcare costs. Discharge occurring less than 24 hours after vaginal birth was not uncommon (Brumfield, 1998), with 24 hours being the average LOS following a vaginal birth in 1997 (Thilo & Rosenberg, 2001). The public protested, and changes in legislation followed (Dahlberg, 2001).

Role of Length of Stay in Postpartum Home Care

The Newborns' and Mothers' Health Protection Act (NMHPA) of 1996 was signed into law in 1997 and took effect in January 1998. The bill provides for a guaranteed minimum stay of up to 48 hours following an uncomplicated vaginal birth and 96 hours following an uncomplicated cesarean birth at the discretion of the new mother and her healthcare provider (Carpenter, 1998). Although the bill did not require follow-up visits for women discharged earlier than the mandated time, more than half the states passed legislation requiring coverage for home care follow-up. Since these changes were implemented, a number of studies have been done that illustrate the benefits of home care and support the use of perinatal home care programs in conjunction with relatively early discharge in providing quality care, promoting client satisfaction, and managing costs (Lieu, Braveman, Escobar, et al, 2000; Ortenstrand, Winbladh, Nordstrom, et al, 2001).

The American Academy of Pediatrics (AAP) and the American College of Obstetricians and Gynecologists (ACOG) have developed guidelines for LOS and follow-up care for mothers and newborns. A home visit or follow-up telephone call by a healthcare provider such as a lactation nurse within 48 hours of discharge is recommended for mothers with a shortened hospital stay. An examination by a healthcare provider is recommended within 48 hours of discharge for newborns who go home before 48 hours of age. The exam may be completed in the home by personnel competent in newborn assessment, provided that the results are reported to the physician that day (AAP & ACOG, 2002; Dahlberg, 2001). Optimal timing of discharge needs to be determined by considering the medical, social, and financial factors in each case. Suggested discharge criteria are found in Table 36–1 •.

Controversy still exists as to whether an increase in LOS from 1 to 2 days decreases the risk of neonatal readmission and negative outcomes (Simpson, Thorman, & Ropp, 2001). According to Eaton (2001, p. 401), "Current scientific knowledge does not provide conclusive evidence about ideal delivery length of stay, in-hospital services, or post-discharge services for the general population of infants and mothers."

Table 36–1 • MINIMAL CRITERIA FOR DISCHARGE OF NEWBORNS

1. Uncomplicated prenatal, intrapartal, and postpartal course and vaginal birth.
2. A single baby who is term, 38–42 weeks, and AGA (average weight for gestational age).
3. The newborn's vital signs are within normal limits and have been stable for the 12 hours preceding discharge. (Respirations < 60/min; apical pulse 120–160 beats/min; axillary temperature of 36.1C–37C in an open crib with appropriate clothing)
4. The newborn has passed at least one stool and has urinated.
5. At least two feedings have been successfully completed, and the baby's ability to coordinate sucking, swallowing, and breathing has been observed and documented.
6. No physical abnormalities have been found that require continued hospitalization.
7. If a circumcision has been done, no excessive bleeding has been evident for at least 2 hours before discharge.
8. There has been no significant jaundice in the first 24 hours of life.
9. The mother has received education about breastfeeding or formula-feeding; the newborn's expected stool and urinary patterns; care of circumcision; cord, skin, and genital care; ways to recognize signs of illness or distress and common infant problems; signs of jaundice and who to contact if it develops; infant safety, including positioning of baby after feeding and for sleep; and use of a car seat.
10. Review of pertinent laboratory data including maternal syphilis and hepatitis B surface antigen status; cord or infant blood type.
11. Completion of screening tests (eg, phenylketonuria [PKU]).
12. First hepatitis B vaccine has been administered or appointment for administration has been scheduled within the first week.
13. Method and schedule for continuing care has been ascertained and planned, and the family is aware of the plan.
14. Family assessment has been completed for social and environmental risk factors such as history of previous child abuse or neglect; spousal or partner abuse either preceding or beginning during the pregnancy; parental substance abuse; lack of support within the family or community; lack of funds, shelter, or food; mental illness of one of the parents that impairs ability to care for self and newborn; single first-time mother without social support.

Source: Adapted from the Committee on Fetus and Newborn (1995). Hospital stay for healthy term newborns. *Pediatrics, 96*(4), 788.

Regardless of the exact time of discharge, the LOS remains "relatively short" for mothers to recover and to assimilate the knowledge they need to care appropriately for themselves and their newborns. In addition, a growing shortage of hospital nurses increases the number of clients cared for by each nurse (Martell, 2000). The greater ratio of mother-infant couplets to one nurse affects the level of nursing services possible, particularly in regard to time available for teaching. Although many educated, well-prepared women with strong support systems are eager to return home and often press for early discharge, the shorter stay has implications for new mothers who are less prepared. Mothers who lack family and other social supports, first-time mothers, breastfeeding mothers, and single mothers are priority candidates for follow-up home care.

Home care for the postpartal family is focused more on assessment, teaching, and counseling than on physical care. **Postpartal home care** provides opportunities for expanding information and reinforcing self- and infant care techniques initially presented in the birth setting. In addition, the home setting provides an opportunity for the nurse and family to interact in a more relaxed environment, one in which the family has control of the setting. It also provides an invaluable opportunity for the nurse to assess home safety in the setting where the family will grow together. In some instances, a home provides unique challenges in assessing and enhancing the woman's self-care and infant care, and the nurse has many opportunities to exercise critical thinking and develop creative options with the family.

Considerations for the Home Visit

In planning a home visit, the nurse should clearly understand the purpose of the visit and identify the maximum amount of content to be addressed. Other important considerations include ways of creating and fostering relationships with families, techniques for preplanning and executing the visit while maintaining safety, documenting the visit, and ensuring telephone follow-up.

The postpartal home visit differs from community health visits in that only one or two postpartal visits are typically planned, and long-term follow-up by the postpartal nurse is not anticipated. Although the postpartal home visit is comprehensive, it is more specifically focused on a postpartal family's needs and care.

Because of the established guidelines for early discharge of the mother and baby (refer to Table 36–1), the nurse can logically expect to find certain levels of health and wellness. However, because the status of the mother and newborn can change, the nurse should stay alert for deviations from the norm.

Purpose and Timing of the Home Visit

The Association of Women's Health, Obstetric, and Neonatal Nurses (AWHONN) provides guidelines for the home care of women and newborns. Care in the home setting can provide the family with both physical and psychologic support. According to AWHONN (1998), "The importance of considering the mother of newborns as a whole person is underscored in the home care environment. Care is often provided by a multidisciplinary team, with the nurse coordinating the components." The postpartal home visit usually occurs within 24 to 48 hours of discharge and is conducted by a registered nurse who is experienced in postpartal maternal and newborn care. This timing is designed to provide assistance to the family as they deal with questions or concerns that may arise as they begin caring for their new infant. The visit typically occurs on about the infant's third day of life, when the breastfeeding mother's milk volume has increased significantly. This provides an opportunity for her to ask questions about infant feeding, nipple care, and the like. At this point, too, the infant's bilirubin levels are peaking and the nurse can assess for jaundice.

MediaLink POSTPARTUM HOME VISITS

Fostering a Caring Relationship with the Family

Although the nurse in the birthing center strives to enhance family autonomy and control, the inherent atmosphere of the institutional environment may cause the new mother and family to feel unempowered. It is important for the professional nurse to recognize that the parameters of the home visit are different in many ways from those of the hospital or birthing center environment. In the home, the family has control of their environment and the nurse is an invited visitor. The nurse can rely on the same characteristics of a caring relationship that have been integral to hospital-based practice—regard for clients, genuineness, empathy, and establishment of trust and rapport—but the relationship may take on new elements as the nurse moves into the home setting for the first time (Table 36–2 •).

Clinical Tip *When visiting a culturally diverse family the nurse may be invited to take part in specific rituals or customs. Whenever possible, the nurse should accept the invitation and join the mother and other family members. Willingness to accept the family's customs will assist the care provider in establishing a positive relationship with the family and signifies acceptance of cultural diversity.*

Table 36–2 • FOSTERING A CARING RELATIONSHIP

Demonstrated Goal	Approaches to Achieve Goal
Regard	Introduce yourself to the family. Call the family members by their surnames until you have been invited to use the given or a less formal name. Ask to be introduced to other members of the family who are present. Allow the mother or spokesperson to assume this role. Use active listening. Maintain objectiveness. Ask permission before sitting.
Genuineness	Mean what you say. Make sure that your verbal and nonverbal messages are congruent. Be nonjudgmental. Don't make assumptions about individuals or settings. Always strive to demonstrate caring behaviors. Be prepared for the visit, honestly answer questions and provide information, and be truthful. If you don't know the answer to a question, tell the client you will find the information and report back.
Empathy	Listen to the mother and family without judgment, trying to view events and circumstances from their point of view. Be attentive to what the birthing experience means to them so that you will understand their concerns from their perspective. Remember empathy denotes understanding, not sympathy.
Trust and rapport	Do what you say you will do. Be prepared for the visit and be on time. Follow up on any areas that are needed.

GLOBAL PERSPECTIVES

In Pakistan, it is customary for the woman to drink a ceremonial drink made from soaking cinnamon in water overnight. The extract is thought to prevent postpartum hemorrhage and provide good health after giving birth. It is also customary for visiting female companions to consume the drink during a celebration several days after the infant is born.

Planning the Home Visit

Prior to the home visit, the nurse prepares by identifying the purpose of the home visit and gathering anticipated materials and equipment. A personal contact while the woman is still in the birth setting or a previsit telephone call is used to arrange the appointment with the woman and her family. During the previsit contact, it is important for the nurse to identify clearly the purpose and goals of the visit and to begin establishing a rapport.

Maintaining Safety

In the past, nurses were viewed as a mainstay of communities and could move in most settings without fear or concern for safety. However, in current times some communities are not safe for visiting nurses. Thus it is important for the nurse to follow some basic safety rules when conducting a home visit. Specifically, the nurse should:

- Know the exact address, and ask for directions during the previsit contact.
- Trace out the route to the client's home on a map before leaving for the visit and take the map along.
- Notify an instructor or supervisor when leaving for a visit and check in as soon as the visit is completed.
- Carry a cellular phone or another method of communication, or carry a phone card or enough change to make a call from a pay phone if needed.
- Ensure that the vehicle used for the visit is well maintained and has sufficient fuel.
- Wear a name tag.
- Carry a flashlight, particularly for night visits.
- Avoid wearing expensive jewelry.

Many agencies that provide home care services have established violence prevention programs to help ensure safety. Nurses in the community need to be aware of their environment and alert to environmental cues, whether overt or subtle. In addition, the following recommendations are important (Durkin & Wilson, 1999):

- Invest time in personal safety by driving around a neighborhood before making an initial visit to identify potential cues to violence.
- Before starting out (or prior to arriving at the home) lock personal belongings in the trunk of the car, out of sight.
- Pay attention to the body language of anyone present during the visit, not just the client.
- Be alert for signs that a person is becoming enraged (reddened neck and/or face, clenched fists, pacing).
- Be aware of personal body language and how it might be interpreted (for example, avoid crossing arms or shoving hands in pockets; remain calm and convey a sense of respect at all times).
- Leave the home immediately if a gun is visible and the client or family member refuses requests to put it away.
- If a situation arises that feels unsafe, terminate the visit.

If the visit is in an area that seems very unsafe, it may be wise for two nurses to go together. Nurses should avoid entering areas where violence is in progress. In such cases, they should return to the car and contact the appropriate facility, such as 911.

Most people are more comfortable in familiar settings and have some hesitation in entering other residential areas. It is always important for nurses to be aware of their surroundings and the people who are nearby. First home visits may feel uncomfortable because they are unfamiliar, but with experience comfort increases (Figure 36–1 ●).

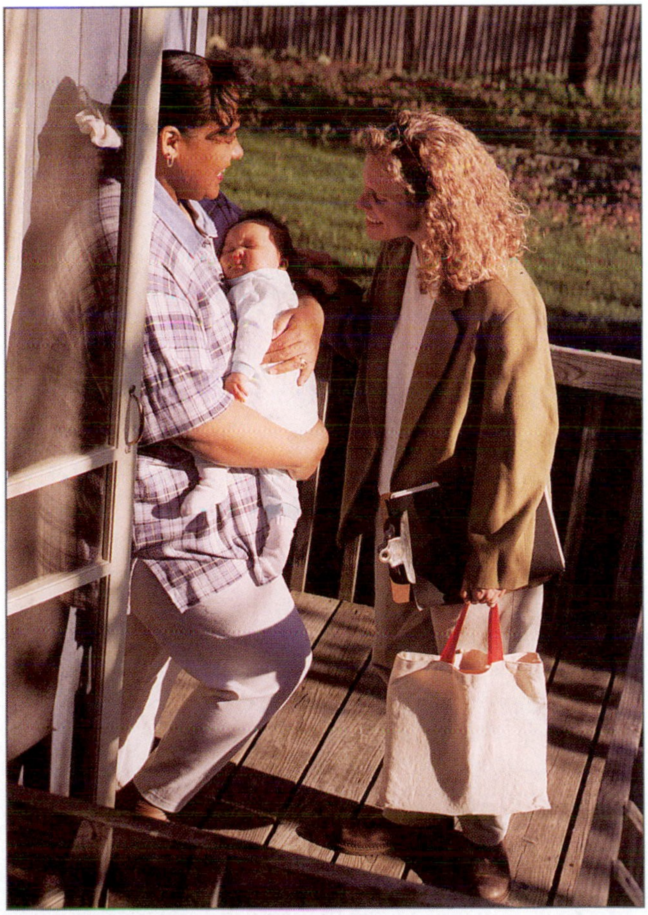

Figure 36–1 ● Nurse arriving for a home visit.

RESEARCH IN PRACTICE
Home Care of a Compromised Infant

What is this study about? While the incidence of premature and low birth weight births has remained stable for the past 30 years, neonatal mortality has declined. As a result, many medically fragile infants are discharged to the home care of their families. Unfortunately, the decline in morbidity for these compromised newborns has not kept pace with the decline in mortality. Health problems, some severe, are common. The home care of a compromised infant presents considerable challenge to the family, particularly the mother, who is generally the primary caregiver. This study examined the effects of a low birth weight infant's medical vulnerability on the mental health of the mothers who care for these infants, and on the functioning of their families. The goal was to devise nursing interventions that can support these families in providing home care for their at-risk babies.

How was this study done? The subjects in this sample were 125 low birth weight infants and their mothers. The ethnically diverse sample of newborns had an average gestational age of 32 weeks at birth. A clinical nurse specialist (CNS) made a baseline assessment of the mother's mental health. The infant's vulnerability was measured relative to four characteristics: birth weight; perinatal risk status; interactive capacity, and severity of physical health problems. In subsequent home visits, the CNS videotaped a typical feeding episode and administered four questionnaires to the mother. These questionnaires measured the mother's symptoms of mental illness and three aspects of family functioning: family cohesion, family coping, and family interaction. The videotape of the feeding was analyzed using a formal scale to measure the infant's interactive capacity. Two additional mental health assessments of the mother were made in the home when the infant was six months and one year of age. Information about the infant's physical condition was recorded every 2 to 3 months throughout the year.

What were the results of the study? Infant responsiveness and the presence of a partner were related to better maternal mental health; increased severity of physical health problems was related to worse maternal mental health. All family functioning characteristics were related to some aspect of maternal mental health except the family's use of external coping strategies. The strongest correlation relationships were between maternal mental health and perceived emotional support, family adaptability, and cohesion. Infant responsiveness was related to the family's adaptability and cohesion as well. These findings support the conclusion that infant vulnerability, particularly how it is manifested in responsiveness and physical problems, is indeed related to both maternal mental health and family functioning.

What additional questions might I have? Were these relationships significant over all time periods, or did they become less severe as the child got older? What were some of the strategies that helped families successfully deal with these pressures?

How can I use this study? Families of compromised newborns need substantial support following discharge if mothers are to stay mentally healthy and supported by a functioning family. In particular, families of newborns who are less responsive and who demonstrate significant health problems are at risk. The home care nurse is in a position to identify these risk factors and plan interventions to reduce their impact on both the mother and her family. The nurse may strengthen a family's functioning by teaching them ways to engage the infant and support his or her development. Particularly for the mother, ongoing support and education are needed to deal with the health problems that will arise for the at risk infant.

Source: Weiss, S. & Jyu-Lin, C. (2002). Factors influencing maternal mental health and family functioning during the low birthweight infant's first year of life. *Journal of Pediatric Nursing, 17*(2), 114–123.

Carrying Out the Home Visit

When the door is answered, the nurse should introduce herself or himself and confirm that the location is correct. If a place to sit is not indicated, the nurse may inquire, "Where is the best place to sit so that we can talk for a while?" In some homes, the mother or family may offer refreshments, and this may be an important aspect of welcoming a visitor. In this case, it is beneficial to the relationship to accept the refreshment graciously. Other culturally appropriate customs should be respected in the home setting whenever possible.

Many agencies have developed a uniform assessment tool to be used during postpartum home visits. This ensures that the nurse completes a physical assessment of both the mother and the newborn; assesses infant feeding and weight gain; evaluates maternal psychosocial adjustment, parental bonding, parenting behaviors, family adaptation, and coping skills; and determines environmental strengths and risk factors. Based on these assessments the nurse may do any of the following:

- Provide direct physical care (assessments, interventions, consultation, and referrals).
- Carry out client and family teaching.
- Consult with the physician or a specialist, such as a lactation consultant.
- Refer the woman or family to appropriate community agencies.
- Schedule additional home visits or telephone follow-up.

The unique aspect of home care is that the nurse is practicing alone. Critical thinking and appropriate communication skills are essential. The nurse needs to recognize any findings outside of normal limits, inform the family, contact the primary healthcare provider, and coordinate appropriate follow-up care (Dahlberg, 2001).

The remainder of the chapter focuses on specific aspects of newborn and maternal care that are assessed, addressed, and evaluated during the home visit.

Home Care: The Newborn

When the family provides care for their newborn, the nurse can instill confidence by giving them positive feedback. If the family encounters problems, the nurse can suggest alternatives and serve as a role model. Each newborn has variations in normal physiologic responses and in growth and development patterns. Parents need to learn to interpret these changes in their child. To help parents care for their newborn at home, some physicians encourage prenatal pediatric visits to establish contact before the birth. Public health nurses have long been involved as guides in newborn care and parent education. Many birthing units are now expanding their primary care functions to the new family to include one home visit by the nurse who cared for the family in the birthing unit. The birthing unit nursery staff may also make themselves available as a 24-hour telephone resource for the new family that needs additional support and consultation during the first few days at home with their newborn.

Routine well-baby visits should be scheduled with the clinic, pediatric nurse practitioner, or physician.

The family should have been taught all necessary caregiving methods before discharge. However, during the home visit the nurse may use a checklist to determine that the family clearly understands the material. If not, the nurse should complete pertinent teaching. The nurse needs to review with the couple all areas for understanding and answer any questions they may have, making sure that the mother has the phone number and address of, and any specific instructions from, the certified nurse-midwife/nurse practitioner/physician and lactation consultant. Having the nursery phone number is also reassuring to a new family. The nurse encourages them to call with questions.

Physical Assessment of the Newborn at Home

In the home, a newborn physical exam is performed to assess vital signs, fontanelles, color, evidence of jaundice, skin condition, the umbilical cord, circumcision if done, reflexes (suck, grasp, and Moro), nutritional status and feeding, elimination, activity, sleep-wake cycles, and weight (Dahlberg, 2001). The nurse will also assess and reinforce knowledge related to infant care as detailed in the following paragraphs.

Positioning and Handling

The nurse demonstrates methods of positioning and handling the newborn as needed. When the newborn is out of the crib, one of the following holds can be used (Figure 36–2 ●). The cradle hold is frequently used during feeding. It provides a sense of warmth and closeness, permits eye contact, frees one of the adult's hands, and provides security because the cradling protects the newborn's body. Extra security is provided by gripping the thigh with the hand while the arm supports the newborn's body. The upright position provides security and a sense of closeness and is ideal for burping. One hand should support the neck and shoulders while the other hand holds the buttocks or is placed between the newborn's legs. The

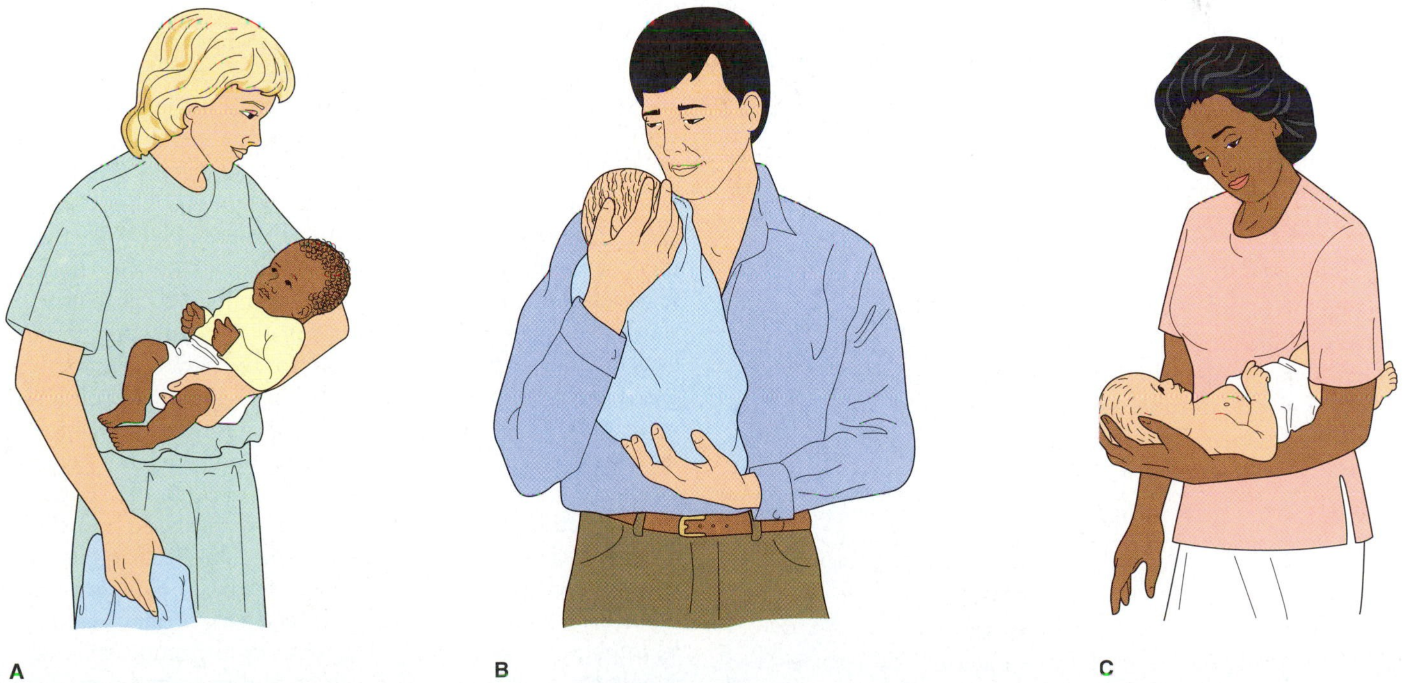

A B C

Figure 36–2 ● Various positions for holding an infant. *A,* Cradle hold. *B,* Upright position. *C,* Football hold.

newborn may also be held upright in a cloth sling carrier that gently holds the baby against the mother's or father's chest and frees the hands for other tasks. The football hold frees one of the caregiver's hands and permits eye contact. This hold is ideal for shampooing, carrying, or breastfeeding. It frees the caregiver to talk on the telephone, answer the door, or do the myriad tasks that await attention at this busy time.

The awake newborn is frequently positioned on her or his side with the dependent arm forward to provide support and to prevent rolling. The side-lying position aids drainage of mucus and allows air to circulate around the cord. It is also comfortable for the newly circumcised male. After feeding, the newborn may be placed on the right side to aid digestion and to prevent aspiration of regurgitated feedings; this position also makes it easier to expel air bubbles from the stomach. Although this position is appropriate when the infant is awake and under observation, infants should sleep on their backs.

Bathing

An actual bath demonstration is the best way for the nurse to provide information to parents. Because excess bathing and use of soap removes natural skin oils and dries out the newborn's sensitive skin, bathing should be done two to three times per week. Cleansing agents with a neutral pH and minimal dyes and perfumes should be used (Mendenhall & Eichenfield, 2000). Sponge baths are recommended for the first 2 weeks or until the umbilical cord completely falls off and the umbilicus has healed. Some agencies use a tub bath for the bath demonstration. See Client Teaching: Newborn Bathing.

Supplies can be kept in a plastic bag or some type of container to eliminate the necessity of hunting for them each time (Table 36–3 •). At home, the family may want to use a small plastic dishpan, a clean kitchen or bathroom sink, or a large bowl as the baby's tub. Plastic baby tubs are not necessary, but some prefer to purchase them.

Before starting, if no one else is at home, the parent may want to take the phone off the hook and put a sign on the door to avoid being disturbed. Having someone home during the first few baths is helpful, because that person can get forgotten items, attend to interruptions, and provide moral support. The room should be warm and free of drafts.

SPONGE BATH

After the supplies are gathered, the tub (or any of the containers mentioned) is filled with water that is warm to the touch. Even though the newborn won't be placed in the tub, the bath giver carefully tests the water temperature with an elbow or forearm. Families may also choose to purchase a thermometer to help them determine when the bath water is at approximately 37.8C (100F) and safe to use. Soap should not be added to the water. The newborn should be wrapped in a blanket, with a T-shirt and diaper on, to keep him or her warm and secure.

Table 36–3 • BATH SUPPLIES

Washcloths (2)	Petrolatum product if indicated
Towels (2)	Cotton balls
Blankets (2)	Diapers
Unperfumed mild soap	Clean clothes
Shampoo	

To start the bath, the adult wraps a washcloth around the index finger once. Each eye is gently wiped from inner to outer canthus. This direction prevents the potential for clogging the tear duct at the inner canthus, where the eye naturally drains. A different portion of the washcloth is used for each eye to prevent cross-contamination. Cotton balls can also be used for this purpose, using a new one for each eye. Some eye swelling and drainage may be present the first few days after birth as a result of the eye prophylaxis.

The bath giver washes the ears next by wrapping the washcloth once around an index finger and gently cleaning the external ear and behind the ear. Cotton swabs are never used in the ear canal because it is possible to put the swab too far into the ear and damage the eardrum. In addition, the swab may back any discharge farther down into the ear canal.

The caregiver then wipes the remainder of the baby's face with the soap-free washcloth. Many babies start to cry at this point. The face should be washed every day and the mouth and chin wiped off after each feeding.

The neck is washed carefully but thoroughly with the washcloth. A mild soap may now be used. Formula or breast milk and lint collect in the skinfolds of the neck, so it may be helpful to sit the newborn up, supporting the neck and shoulders with one hand while washing the neck with the other hand.

The bath giver now unwraps the blanket, removes the T-shirt, and wets the chest, back, and arms with the washcloth. The bath giver may then lather the hands with soap and wash the baby's chest, back, and arms. Wetting the cord is avoided, if possible, because it delays drying. Soap is rinsed off with the wet washcloth, and the upper part of the body is dried with a towel or blanket. The newborn's upper body is then wrapped with a clean, dry blanket to prevent chill.

Next the bath giver unwraps the newborn's legs, wets them with the washcloth, and lathers, rinses, and dries them well. If the newborn has dry skin, a small amount of an emollient such as petroleum may be used. Products without perfumes or dyes are recommended (Mendenhall & Eichenfield, 2000). Ointments are thought to be better than lotions for dry, cracked feet and hands. Baby oil is not recommended because it clogs skin pores. Families should be warned that baby powder can cause serious respiratory problems for the baby if it is inhaled, and therefore should not be used. The genital area is cleansed after each wet or dirty diaper. Females are washed from the front of the genital area toward the rectum to avoid fecal contamination of the urethra and thus the bladder. Newborn females often have a thick, white mucous discharge or a slight bloody discharge from the vaginal area. This discharge is normal for the first 1 to 2 weeks after birth. The mucous may come off if wiped gently after diaper changes but should not be intentionally scrubbed off. Parents of uncircumcised males should cleanse the penis daily. Even minimal retraction of the foreskin is not advised (see in-depth discussion of care of un-

CLIENT TEACHING NEWBORN BATHING

Assessment During the postpartum home visit, the nurse can observe the mother giving the newborn a sponge bath. The nurse should observe for safety issues, proper technique, and use of appropriate bathing supplies and products.

Nursing Diagnosis The key nursing diagnosis will probably be ***Health-seeking behavior:*** Information or experience in performing newborn bathing.

Nursing Plan and Implementation The teaching will focus on safety issues for the newborn related to bathing, providing comfort for the infant during the bath, and proper instruction on appropriate supplies and bathing technique.

Client Goals At the completion of the teaching, the family will be able to:

1. Identify appropriate timing of sponge and tub baths for newborns.
2. List appropriate supplies for bathing.
3. Demonstrate proper bathing procedures for both sponge and tub baths.
4. Discuss the use of appropriate skin care agents for newborn use.

Teaching Plan

CONTENT	TEACHING METHOD
Describe the proper timing and environment (including safety factors) for sponge and tub bathing for newborns.	Clarify information related to sponge bathing and the proper timing of tub baths for safe newborn bathing. Explain that the proper environment is needed for newborn safety and comfort.
Identify proper bathing supplies that are needed for both sponge and tub baths.	Encourage mother to assemble supplies prior to beginning the newborn bath to avoid cold exposure and ensure that proper supplies are being used.
Demonstrate sponge bathing.	Demonstrate proper technique and encourage the family to ask questions as they arise. Help instill confidence in new parents.
Discuss and demonstrate tub bathing using an infant model.	
Explain the need for neutral pH, fragrance-free, and dye-free cleansing products for newborn use.	Clarify the need for appropriate cleansing agents for newborns.

Evaluation At the end of the teaching session the woman or family will be able to verbalize the principles of proper bathing for the newborn. They will be able to demonstrate the proper techniques to ensure safety during both sponge and tub baths.

circumcised male babies in Chapter 30 (link)). Males who have been circumcised also need their penis cleansed daily. A very wet washcloth is squeezed above the baby's penis, allowing clear water to run over the circumcision site. The area is gently patted dry. A mild soap may be used and then rinsed off beginning several days after the circumcision. A small amount of an emollient such as petrolatum, petrolatum-impregnated gauze, or Aquaphor may be applied during each diaper change for the first 24 to 48 hours. Emollients promote comfort and healing and prevent adherence of the diaper to the site. Antimicrobial ointments are not recommended (Lund, Osborne, Kuller, et al, 2001). It is important to avoid using ointments if a Plastibell is in place because ointments may cause the Plastibell ring to slip off the penis too early. The Plastibell usually falls off within 5 to 8 days. If it doesn't, the family needs to call the healthcare provider.

The diaper area should be cleansed and well dried with each diaper change to prevent diaper rash. Even when this cleansing is done regularly, a diaper rash may occasionally occur. Baby powder (or cornstarch) is not recommended for diaper rash. Baby powder may cake with urine and irritate the perineal area. Cornstarch may promote fungal infection.

Moisturizers such as petrolatum provide protection from wetness and promote healing of mildly irritated skin. Generous application of a protective skin barrier containing zinc oxide is recommended to prevent further injury if diaper rash occurs. Fecal material should be removed with each diaper change, but the skin barrier should be maintained if possible and reapplied.

If the ointment does not help the rash, families using single-use (disposable) diapers should try another brand. Superabsorbent gelled diapers help to keep the skin dry (Mendenhall & Eichenfield, 2000). If the family uses cloth diapers, a different mild detergent, more thorough rinsing, and hanging them in the sun to dry may alleviate the problem. If the rash persists, parents should discuss the problem with their nurse practitioner or physician, because it may be due to a yeast or fungal infection. In this case, the provider may recommend an antifungal ointment or cream.

The umbilical cord should be kept clean and dry (Lund et al, 2001). The close proximity of the umbilical vessels makes the cord a potential entry area for serious infection. The cord stump generally falls off in 7 to 14 days. The diaper should be folded down to allow air to circulate around the cord. The parents should consult their healthcare provider if redness, bright red bleeding, or puslike drainage with foul odor appears around the umbilicus, or if the area remains unhealed 2 to 3 days after the cord stump has sloughed off.

Although many facilities continue to clean the umbilical cord with alcohol after each diaper change, research does not support this practice (Mendenhall & Eichenfield, 2000). Parents should be instructed to simply keep the area clean and dry unless directed to do otherwise by their healthcare provider. While natural drying may occasionally result in a cord that is smelly or appears "mucky," this is a natural process. Studies have found no statistically significant difference in infection rates or in time until separation in naturally drying cords versus alcohol-treated cords (Mendenhall & Eichenfield, 2000).

The last step in bathing is washing the hair (some prefer to do this step first). The newborn is swaddled in a dry blanket, leaving only the head exposed, and held in the football hold with the head tilted slightly downward to prevent water from running in the eyes. Water should be brought to the head by a cupped hand. Parents should avoid placing the infant's head directly under running water as changes in water temperature could cause burns or discomfort. The hair is moistened and lathered with a small amount of shampoo. A very soft brush may be used to massage the shampoo over the entire head, including the fontanelles, which families often call the "soft spots." The hair is then rinsed and toweled dry. The fingers can be placed over the infant's ears to prevent water from entering the ear canal, although this usually does not cause any medical complications. Oils or lotions are not used on the newborn's head unless there is evidence of cradle cap. Moistening the scaly area with lotion or mineral oil a half an hour or more before shampooing softens the crusts or scales and makes it easier to remove them with a soft brush during the shampoo.

TUB BATHS

The baby may be put in a small tub after the cord has fallen off and the circumcision site is healed (approximately 2 weeks) (Figure 36–3 •). Newborns usually enjoy a tub bath more than a sponge bath, although some cry during either one.

The tub is filled with 3 to 4 inches of water. To prevent slipping, a washcloth is placed in the bottom of the tub or sink. Some parents choose to bring the newborn into the tub with them. Since all clothes will be removed for the duration of a tub bath, it is particularly important to keep the room warm and draft-free and to limit the time young infants spend in the tub. Parents should be instructed never to turn their back on a baby or young child in a tub because of the potential for drowning, even in small amounts of water.

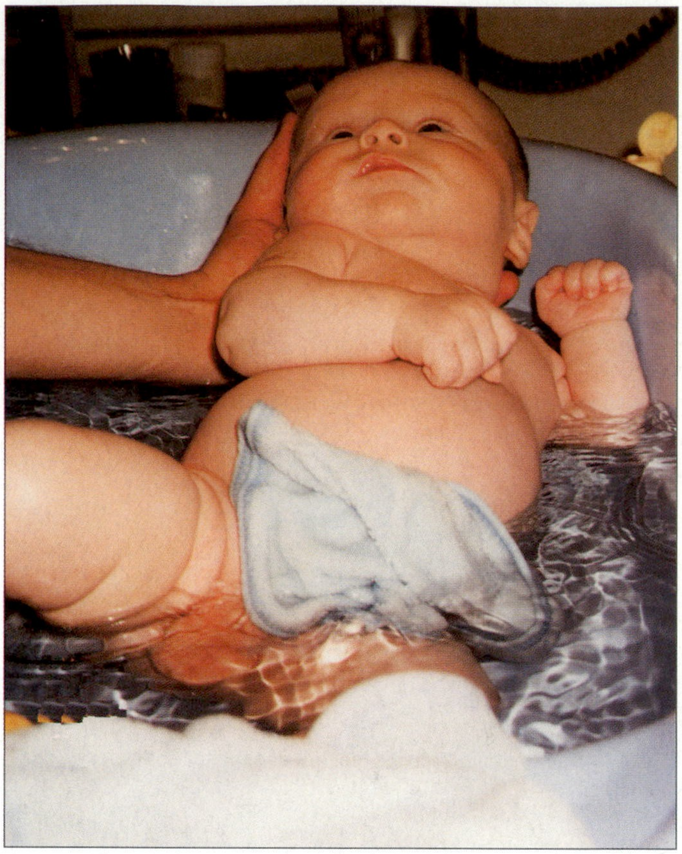

Figure 36–3 • When bathing the newborn, the caregiver must support the head. Wet babies are very slippery.

The baby's face is washed in the same manner as for a sponge bath. The parent then places the newborn in the tub using the cradle hold and grasping the distal thigh. The neck is supported by the parent's elbow in the cradle position. An alternative hold is to support the newborn's head and neck with the forearm while grasping the distal shoulder and arm.

Because wet newborns are slippery, some parents pull a cotton sock (with holes cut out for the fingers) over the supporting arm to provide a "nonskid" surface. The newborn's body is washed with a soapy washcloth or hand. To wash the back, the bath giver places the noncradling hand on the newborn's chest with the thumb under the newborn's arm closest to the adult. Gently tipping the newborn forward onto the supporting hand frees the cradling arm to wash the back. After the bath, the newborn is lifted out of the tub in the cradle position, dried well, and wrapped in a dry blanket. The hair is then washed in the same way as for a sponge bath.

Nail Care

The nails of the newborn are seldom cut in the birthing center. During the first days of life, the nails may adhere to the skin of the fingers, and cutting is contraindicated. Within a week the nails separate from the skin and frequently break off. If the nails are long or if the newborn is scratching his or her face, the nails may be gently filed using a newborn file. This is most easily done while the infant is asleep.

Dressing the Newborn

Newborns need to wear a T-shirt, diaper (diaper cover if using cloth diapers), and a sleeper. At home, the amount of clothing the newborn wears is determined by the temperature. Families who maintain their home at 60F to 65F should dress the infant more warmly than those who maintain a temperature of 70F to 75F.

Newborns should wear a head covering outdoors to protect their sensitive ears from drafts and to prevent heat loss. A blanket can also be wrapped around the baby, leaving one corner free to place over the head for added protection while outdoors or in crowds. The nurse must advise families about the ease with which a newborn's skin can burn when exposed to the sun. To prevent sunburn, the newborn should remain shaded, wear a light layer of clothing, or be protected with sunscreen specifically formulated for infants. Many healthcare professionals recommend avoiding sunscreen until the infant is at least 6 months old.

Diaper shapes vary and are subject to personal preference (Figure 36–4 •). Prefolded and disposable diapers are usually rectangular. Cloth diapers may also be triangular or kite-folded. Extra material is placed in front for males and toward the back for females to increase absorbency.

Baby clothing should be laundered separately with a mild soap or detergent. Diapers are generally presoaked before washing. All clothing should be rinsed twice to remove soap and residue and to decrease the possibility of rash. Some newborns may not tolerate clothing treated with fabric softeners added to the washer or dryer.

Temperature Assessment

As the nurse prepares to teach parents about taking their baby's temperature, it is important to provide opportunities for discussion and demonstration. Families often need a review of how to take their infant's temperature and when to call their primary healthcare provider.

Clinical Tip *Dressing a newborn baby with a T-shirt may be quite a challenge. The T-shirt is first pulled over the baby's head. The next challenge is getting the arms in the sleeves, because the newborn grasps at the fabric of the T-shirt as you try to pull it over the hands and arms. It helps to put your hand through the right sleeve of the T-shirt and hold the baby's right hand. Then pull the sleeve over your hand. Repeat the same movements for the left sleeve.*

When taken properly, the axillary method is an accurate way to measure an infant's temperature (Fallis & Christiani, 1999). The nurse shows the family how to take an axillary temperature and discusses the different types of thermometers. It is important that parents understand the differences and how to select an appropriate one.

Digital and electronic thermometers are appropriate for healthy newborns (Sganga, Wallace, Kiehl, et al, 2000), but there are many varieties available on the market today. The parents may want to discuss their choice with their primary healthcare provider. It is also helpful for nurses to periodically check thermometer availability at local retailers and review current literature and manufacturer's literature.

Although mercury-containing glass thermometers are a very reliable method of measuring core temperature in infants, the risks outweigh the benefits. Breakage of mercury thermometers has caused symptomatic mercury poisoning in children and adults. **Mercury thermometers should not be used or kept in homes** and should be disposed of at a hazardous waste collection site. Many organizations have initiated programs where mercury thermometers can be turned in for nonmercury substitutes, and many retailers have phased out their sales of mercury thermometers (Shannon, 2001). The nurse should ask about this during the safety assessment and inform parents of local programs or hazardous waste facilities where the thermometers may be turned in.

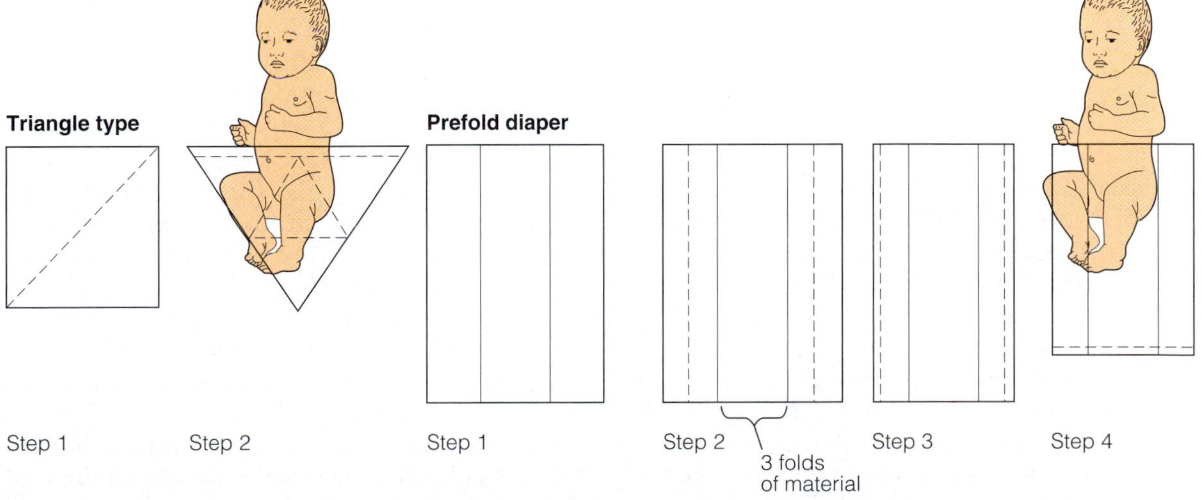

Figure 36–4 • Two basic cloth diaper shapes. Dotted lines indicate folds.

Parents need to take the newborn's temperature only when signs of illness are present. Most physicians agree that a septic work-up is indicated in febrile infants less than 3 months of age, because their immunologic immaturity makes newborns susceptible to severe infections and infections caused by unusual organisms (McCarthy, 2000). Additionally, infected newborns may not be febrile but may exhibit more subtle manifestations such as inability to tolerate feedings, irritability, or lethargy (Gotoff, 2000). Therefore, parents of young infants should call their primary care provider immediately for any signs of illness and/or fever, rather than treating the infant at home.

Parents of older babies will want to discuss the management of colds, flu, teething, constipation, diarrhea, and other common ailments with their clinician before they occur. The healthcare provider can make recommendations regarding over-the-counter analgesics and antipyretic medications, such as acetaminophen and ibuprofen. Aspirin use for viral illness has been linked to Reye syndrome in children and therefore should not be used.

Stools and Urine

The appearance and frequency of a newborn's stools can cause concern for parents. The nurse prepares them by discussing and showing pictures of meconium stools and transitional stools and by describing the difference between breast milk and formula stools. Although each baby develops his or her own stooling patterns, parents can get an idea of what to expect (see Figure 28–12).

- Breastfed newborns may have 6 to 10 small, semiliquid, yellow stools per day by the third or fourth day after milk production is established, unless the mother is having problems with her milk supply. Once breastfeeding is well established, usually by 1 month, the newborn may have only 1 stool every few days because of the increased digestibility of breast milk, or the newborn may still have several daily. Constipation is unlikely to occur in newborns receiving only breast milk. Infrequent stooling in the first few weeks may indicate inadequate milk intake.
- Formula-fed babies may have only 1 or 2 stools a day; they are more formed and yellow or yellow-brown.

The parents may also be shown pictures of a constipated stool (small, pelletlike) and diarrhea (loose, green, or perhaps blood-tinged). Families should understand that a green color is common in transitional stools so that they do not mistake transitional stools for diarrhea during the first week of a newborn's life. Constipation may indicate that the newborn needs additional fluid intake.

Babies normally void (urinate) five to eight times per day. Fewer than six to eight wet diapers a day may indicate the newborn needs more fluids. Frequency of voiding is easy to assess with cloth diapers. Parents who use superabsorbent single-use disposable diapers may have difficulty determining voiding patterns because the surface of the diaper feels dry. The liquid pools inside the filling of the diaper.

Sleeping

When, where, and for how long their baby sleeps are common concerns of parents. The following sections address SIDS prevention, cribs, and cosleeping. The newborn's sleep/wake states are then described.

SIDS PREVENTION

Sudden infant death syndrome (SIDS) is the primary cause of infant death beyond the neonatal period in the United States. African Americans and Native Americans experience rates two to three times higher than the national average. The risk factors with the greatest potential for modification include prone sleeping position, sleeping on soft surfaces, maternal smoking (especially during pregnancy), and overheating (AAP, 2000). Nurses have the opportunity to assess for risk factors in the home environment and to educate families, particularly clients in groups at high risk for SIDS.

The AAP has recommended sleeping in non-prone positions since 1992 to reduce the risk of SIDS. The "Back to Sleep" campaign was initiated in 1994 to educate the public on recommendations. Since then, the frequency of prone sleeping has decreased from more than more than 70% to about 20% of US infants, and the SIDS rate has decreased by over 40%. There is no evidence of an increase in aspiration or vomiting with the increased use of the supine positioning (AAP, 2000). However, a newborn should not be left unattended in the supine position after feedings for the first few days of life.

The infant's position should be changed periodically during the early months of life, because skull bones are soft, and permanently flattened areas may develop if the infant consistently lies in one position. The AAP (2000) recommends placing infants to sleep with the supine head to one side for a week or so and then changing to the other. Changing the infant's orientation to outside activity is helpful as well. Infants should also spend some time in the prone position each day when awake and observed to promote development and muscle strength.

As mentioned, another SIDS risk factor is sleeping on soft surfaces. Therefore, a firm flat mattress should be provided for the newborn who should sleep directly on the mattress and sheet, without blankets or other soft materials under his or her body. Parents who are concerned their infant will "catch cold" may dress the infant in one-piece sleepwear not requiring additional blankets. If parents insist on blankets, the infant's feet should be able to reach the foot of the crib, with the blankets tucked in around the crib mattress and reaching only to the level of the infant's chest. The nurse also cautions about overheating the infant, since this has been noted as a SIDS risk factor as well.

These recommendations are for healthy infants, and parents should follow them unless otherwise directed by their healthcare provider in response to a particular medical condition (AAP, 2000). Parents can be encouraged to attend infant cardiopulmonary resuscitation (CPR) classes, especially if there is a family history of SIDS, prematurity, or another health problem.

CRIB SAFETY

During the home visit, the nurse discusses with the family their newborn's sleeping arrangements, and observes the crib, bassinet, cradle, mat, or other device. Infants should not have pillows, loose bedding, or stuffed animals near them while they sleep; these items could cause suffocation. Crib bumpers can be used to keep the infant's head from hitting the crib bars; however, they should be securely tied using all the strings, and removed as soon as the infant is able to stand so they are not used for climbing out of the crib.

The crib headboard and footboard should be solid, with no large designs cut out of the wood, as the infant's head could become entrapped in them. Crib slats should be no more than 2 3/8 inches apart. If the crib is older and painted, ensure that the paint is non-lead based. If there is any doubt, the crib should not be used unless it is stripped and painted with new enamel. Mattresses should fit snugly to prevent entrapment and suffocation, and should always be lowered to a level at which the infant cannot fall out. Parents should always leave the side rails up when the baby is in the crib, even if they are in the room. Parents should inspect the crib regularly to determine whether it is in safe working order, with no splinters, sharp edges, or loose parts.

COSLEEPING

In recent years, much debate has ensued over the parental issue of cosleeping. **Cosleeping** is the practice whereby an infant or child regularly sleeps in an adult bed with the parents. Also known as the *family bed,* this practice has for centuries been the norm in many cultures. It is estimated that 25% to 30% of Americans engage in this practice.

In 1999, the Consumer Product Safety Commission (CPSC) issued a warning that cosleeping with infants may put them at risk for suffocation or strangulation (Centuori, Burmax, Ronfani, et al, 1999). The recommendation was based on a 7-year review of injury data that linked adult beds to 515 infant deaths. The deaths resulted from suffocation associated with cosleeping with an adult, entrapment between the mattress or other object, airway obstruction on waterbed mattresses, and strangulation due to entrapment of the head in rails or bed openings (Centuori et al, 1999).

This CPSC warning raised a huge debate between detractors and supporters of cosleeping. La Leche League International (1999) issued a statement supporting cosleeping for its role in promotion of breastfeeding, regulation of maternal and infant sleep patterns, effectiveness in promoting development of maternal responses to infant cues, and promotion of sleep for both mothers and infants. Some opponents even raised issues on the appropriateness of the CPSC issuing a statement on this topic.

Conflicting research has further clouded the issue of cosleeping. For example, while some studies have shown an increase in the incidence of SIDS with cosleeping, others have cited a decline. Although much of the debate continues, certain recommendations have been agreed upon. Families should be counseled to follow these guidelines:

- Place the infant on a firm mattress, never on comforters, pillows, or a waterbed.
- Never sleep with your infant if you have been using drugs or have become intoxicated.
- Ensure that the infant is protected from rolling off the bed, or becoming entrapped in bed rails or a space between the frame and the mattress.
- As with crib sleeping, remove all decorative pillows, stuffed animals or toys, or blankets that could impair the baby's breathing. Do not cover the baby with blankets or sheets.
- Avoid down comforters.
- Make sure the baby is sleeping on his or her back.
- Ensure plenty of ventilation to the infant.
- Avoid overdressing the infant since the parents' body heat will reduce the infant's need for excess clothing.
- Never smoke in bed with an infant.
- If additional children are also in the bed, make sure they are not sleeping directly next to the infant.

The nurse's role in counseling new parents on the issue of cosleeping should support the family's personal and cultural beliefs. The nurse should review safety information with parents to ensure safe sleeping practices.

Sleep-Wake States

The newborn demonstrates several different sleep-wake states after the initial periods of reactivity. It is not uncommon for a newborn to sleep almost continuously for the first 2 to 3 days following birth, awakening only for feedings every 3 to 4 hours. Some newborns bypass this stage of deep sleep and require only 12 to 16 hours of sleep. The parents need to know that this is normal.

Pearson (1999) discussed the six sleep-wake states and caregiving implications related to each state. Sleep states include **deep sleep** and **light sleep.** During *deep sleep* the infant will be nearly still except for occasional startles, twitches, and sucking. The infant will arouse to intense stimuli, and care and feeding at this time will be frustrating. *Light sleep* makes up the highest proportion of newborn sleep and usually precedes awakening. It is characterized by some body movements, rapid eye movements (REM), and brief fussing or crying. The infant may arouse, remain in light sleep, or return to deep sleep in response to stimuli. Infants are not usually ready to feed in this state.

Awake states include **drowsy, quiet alert, active alert,** and **crying** states. *Drowsy* infants open and close their eyes, but the eyes appear glazed and face is often still. They may return to sleep or awaken further in response to stimuli. The *quiet alert state* is characterized by a brightening of the eyes and face. Infants are most attentive to their environment in this state and provide positive feedback to caregivers. It is usually easiest to initiate feeds during this state (AWHONN, 2000; International Lactation Consultant Association [ILCA], 1999). The *active alert state* brings about an increase in facial and body movement, with periods of fussiness occurring. The infant in this state has increased sensitivity to disturbing stimuli, and intervention to console the infant at this point is beneficial.

Crying is evidenced by increased motor activity, grimaces, eyes tightly closed or open, and extreme responsiveness to stimuli. Infants may be able to console themselves, or they may require consoling from a caregiver.

For newborns, crying is a spontaneous response to unpleasant stimuli, and their only means of expressing their needs vocally. After 2 or 3 days, newborns settle into individual patterns and families learn to distinguish different tones and qualities of this newborn's cry. The amount of crying is also highly individual. Some newborns cry as little as 15 to 30 minutes in 24 hours, or as long as 2 or more hours. When crying continues after such causes as discomfort or hunger are eliminated, the newborn may be comforted by swaddling, rocking, or other reassuring activities. There is some indication that newborns who are held more tend to be calmer and cry less when not being held. Some parents may be afraid that holding will "spoil" the newborn, and need reassurance that is not the case. On the contrary, picking babies up when they cry teaches them that adults are responsive to them. This helps build a sense of trust in humankind. Of course, the nurse documents and assesses any crying, and provides teaching and referrals as necessary. See Table 36–4 • for the characteristics and caregiving implication of each state.

> *It was so exciting to go home with our new baby. That first day went quite well and Joe and I felt that we were on our way as new parents. Our son had been fed and diapered a number of times and it was now time for bed. When we snuggled him in his bassinet, he lay quietly and didn't cry. Then we looked at each other, and at the same time said, "What if we don't hear him in the middle of the night?" We went on to bed but with much trepidation. Our baby's first cry in the night woke us immediately. We both sat up and simultaneously said, "There he is!"*
>
> *After a few weeks, we could laugh at the anxiety we had during those first few days. I'm sure all new parents must have had similar experiences.*

Injury Prevention

Injuries are the leading cause of death in children and account for significant healthcare costs. During the home visit, the nurse observes the environment and identifies changes that need to be made in order to childproof the home. For example, accessible electrical outlets can cause severe injury or death. Childproof covers should be installed to decrease the risk of electrocution. Unattended pots and pans on stoves

Evidence-Based Practice

Interventions in Infantile Colic

Clinical Question

Which behavioral interventions, drugs, and dietary changes reduce infantile colic?

The Evidence

Following a systematic review, results from 27 published studies on the treatment of infantile colic were combined. Reduction in crying or colic was the main outcome measured in these 27 studies.

The following interventions were effective for reducing excessive crying:

- In formula-feeding infants, elimination of cows' milk protein
- In breastfeeding mothers, maternal consumption of herbal tea containing chamomile, vervain, licorice, fennel, and balm mint
- Treatment of infant with anticholinergic drugs
- Increase in parental responsiveness with prompt reduction in stimulation and advice to leave the infant when the caregiver finds the crying intolerable

Replacing cows' milk with hypoallergenic formula milk reduced crying, whereas using soy formula milk did not. However, increasing parental responsiveness was more effective than replacing cows' milk protein with hypoallergenic formula milk. Dicyclomine and dicycloverine produced adverse events in a small proportion of the infants.

Interventions that were not effective for reducing crying were lowering the lactose content in formula milk, adding fiber to formula milk, using simethicone treatment, and increased carrying of infants.

Best Practice

Advice to parents of colicky infants should include elimination of cows' milk protein, drinking herbal tea, and use of anticholinergic drugs (specifically dicyclomine). Parents should be guided in being responsive to the infant and quickly decreasing stimulation. Recommendations should not include low-lactose or fiber-enriched formula milk, simethicone, or increased carrying of infants.

Reference: Lucassen, P. L., Assendelft, W. J., & Gubbels, J. W., et al. (1998). Effectiveness of treatments for infantile colic: A systematic review. *British Medical Journal, 316,* 1563–1569.

Table 36–4 • INFANT STATE* CHART (SLEEP AND AWAKE STATES)

Infant States	Characteristics of State: Body Activity	Eye Movements	Facial Movements	Breathing Pattern	Level of Response	Implications for Caregiving
Sleep States						
Deep sleep	Nearly still, except for occasional startle or twitch	None	Without facial movements, except for occasional sucking at regular intervals	Smooth and regular	Threshold to stimuli very high so that only very intense or disturbing stimuli will arouse infants	Caregivers trying to feed infants in deep sleep will probably find the experience frustrating. Infants will be unresponsive, even if caregivers use disturbing stimuli (flicking feet) to arouse infants. Infants may arouse only briefly and then become unresponsive as they return to deep sleep. If care givers wait until infants move to a higher, more responsive state, feeding or caregiving will be much more pleasant.
Light sleep	Some body movements	Rapid eye movements (REM) Fluttering of eyes beneath closed eyelids	May smile and make brief fussy or crying sounds	Irregular	Infants are more responsive to internal and external stimuli (When these stimuli occur, infants may remain in light sleep, return to deepsleep, or arouse to drowsy.)	Light sleep makes up the highest proportion of newborn sleep and usually precedes wakening. The brief fussy or crying sounds made during this state may make caregivers who are not aware that these sounds occur normally think it is time for feeding, and they may try to feed infants before they are ready to eat.
Awake States						
Drowsy	Activity level variable, with mild startles interspersed from time to time; movement usually smooth	Eyes open and close occasionally, are heavy lidded with dull, glazed appearance	Some facial movements possible (Often there are none, and the face appears still.)	Irregular	Infants react to sensory stimuli, although responses are delayed (State change after stimulation is frequently noted.)	From the drowsy state, infants *may* return to sleep or awaken further. To facilitate waking, caregivers can provide something for infants to see, hear, or suck. This may arouse them to a quiet alert state, a more responsive state. Infants left alone without stimuli may return to a sleep state.
Quiet alert	Minimal	Brightening and widening of eyes	Face bright, shining, sparkling	Regular	Infants attend most to environment, focusing attention on any stimuli that are present	Infants in quiet alert state provide much pleasure and positive feedback for caregivers. Providing something for infants to see, hear, or suck will often maintain this state. In the first few hours after birth, most newborns commonly experience a period of intense alertness before going into a long sleeping period.
Active alert	Much body activity; periods of fussiness possible	Eyes open with less brightening	Much facial movement; face not as bright as quiet alert state	Irregular	Infants are increasingly sensitive to disturbing stimuli (hunger, fatigue, noise, excessive handling)	Caregivers may intervene at this stage to console and to bring infants to a lower state.
Crying	Increased motor activity, with color changes	Eyes tightly closed or open	Grimaces	More irregular	Infants are extremely responsive to unpleasant external or internal stimuli	Crying is the infants' communication signal. It is a response to unpleasant stimuli from the environment or from within infants (fatigue, hunger, discomfort). Crying tells us infants' limits have been reached. Sometimes infants can console themselves and return to lower states. At other times, they need help from caregivers.

**State* is a group of characteristics that regularly occur together: body activity, eye movements, facial movements, breathing pattern, and level of response to external stimuli (eg, handling) and internal stimuli (eg, hunger).

Source: Blackburn S., Kang B. Early Parent-Infant Relationships, 2nd edition, module 3, series 1. *The First Six Hours after Birth.* White Plains, NY: March of Dimes Birth Defects Foundation, 1991. Reprinted with permission of the copyright holder.

can easily be pulled over, scalding or seriously burning young children. The nurse can advise the family to install a stove guard (a plastic partition that prevents small children from touching hot stoves or pulling down pots or pans). Handles should also be turned inward and should not protrude over the edge of the stove.

It is important for nurses to be aware of the impact they can have on the safety of families through the use of home visits. A study of one-time home visits by trained research assistants to families of toddlers (median age of 2) found that the visits significantly decreased injuries in the intervention group (King, Klassen, LeBlanc, et al, 2001). Although these findings may not be generalizable to the postpartum population, they indicate what a home visit by a nurse has the potential to accomplish in relation to safety. The AAP (1998) has recommended that home visits be used to improve the safety of children in high-risk families. The AAP (2001) has also made a number of recommendations to address and prevent shaken baby injuries, including home visitation programs and any other child abuse prevention efforts that prove efficacious. Home visits provide an ideal opportunity to educate parents and provide appropriate resources and referrals.

Newborn Screening and Immunization Program

Before the newborn and mother are discharged from the hospital, the nurse informs parents about the normal screening tests for newborns and tells them when to return for further tests if needed. Newborn screening tests detect disorders that cause mental retardation, physical handicaps, or death if left undiscovered. Disorders that can usually be detected from a drop of blood obtained by a heel stick on the second or third day include: galactosemia, cystic fibrosis, congenital adrenal hyperplasia, hypothyroidism, phenylketonuria (PKU), and sickle cell anemia. Parents should be instructed that a second blood specimen will be required from the newborn after 7 to 14 days. In some states, the second blood specimen is not recommended if the first specimen is obtained prior to 24 hours of age. However, it must be clarified that an abnormal test result is not diagnostic. More definitive tests must be performed to verify the results. It is important to follow protocols that incorporate state laws about newborn testing.

If additional tests are positive, treatment is initiated. These conditions may be treated by dietary means or by administering missing hormones. The inborn conditions cannot be cured, but they can be treated. They are not contagious, but they may be inherited (Chapter 32).

The nurse should ensure that the family has information regarding the current childhood immunization schedule and has plans to begin or continue immunizations. The nurse should be familiar with current recommendations and should share information about immunizations with the family as necessary.

Home Care: The Mother and Family

Assessment of the Mother and Family at Home

During the home visit, the nurse can complete ongoing postpartum assessment following discharge. The initial goal is to assess the woman's perceptions of her current circumstances, her recovery from childbirth, her adjustment and that of her partner to parenthood, the newborn's condition, family-newborn bonding, and any problems or concerns the woman may have. The nurse asks specifically about the following areas: (1) progression of lochia (color, amount of flow, presence of foul odor or clots); (2) fever or malaise; (3) dysuria or difficulty voiding; (4) pain in the pelvis or perineum; (5) painful, reddened hot spots or shooting pains in the breasts during or between feedings; and (6) areas of redness, edema, tenderness, or warmth in the legs.

The nurse should also talk with the mother about her diet, fatigue level, ability to rest and sleep, pain management, signs of postpartal complications, activity level, sexuality issues, self-care ability, social support system, and any pertinent cultural or religious practices related to postpartum or newborn care (Dahlberg, 2001).

Low energy and fatigue are frequent problems during the first 3 months postpartum. Lee and Zaffke (1999) found fatigue to be related to fragmented sleep and low ferritin and hemoglobin levels. Younger women were more fatigued than older women. The nurse can inform new mothers that fatigue may be a problem and stress the need for good nutrition and periods of uninterrupted sleep if possible. The nurse can also discuss continued use of prenatal vitamins and iron, particularly if the client is breastfeeding.

Before performing the physical assessment, the nurse ensures privacy. The physical assessment focuses on maternal physical adaptation, which is assessed by evaluating vital signs, breasts, abdominal musculature, elimination patterns, fundal height and location, the perineum, lochia, edema, and laboratory values.

The psychologic assessment focuses on attachment, adjustment to the parental role, sibling adjustment, and educational needs. When appropriate, the nurse mentions available community resources, including the public health department, which can be used for follow-up visits. In ideal situations, a family approach involving the presence of the father and any siblings provides an opportunity to observe family interactions and opportunities for all family members to ask questions and express concerns. In addition, this approach may surface any questionable family interaction pattern, such as one suggestive of abuse or neglect; the nurse can consider further referral if needed. See the Assessment Guide: Postpartal—First Home Visit and Anticipated Progress at Six Weeks.

If not addressed previously, the nurse provides information about family-planning options at this time (see

ASSESSMENT GUIDE POSTPARTAL—FIRST HOME VISIT AND ANTICIPATED PROGRESS AT SIX WEEKS

PHYSICAL ASSESSMENT/ NORMAL FINDINGS	ALTERATIONS AND POSSIBLE CAUSES*	NURSING RESPONSES TO DATA†
➤ VITAL SIGNS		
➤ ***Blood pressure:*** Return to normal prepregnant level.	Elevated blood pressure (anxiety, essential hypertension, renal disease) preeclampsia (can occur postpartum).	Review history, evaluate normal baseline; refer to physician/CNM if necessary.
➤ ***Pulse:*** 60–90 beats/min (or prepregnant normal rate).	Increased pulse rate, tachycardia, chest pain (excitement, anxiety cardiac disorders).	Count pulse for full minute, note irregularities; marked tachycardia or beat irregularities require additional assessment and possible physician/CNM referral.
➤ ***Respirations:*** 16–24/min.	Marked tachypnea or abnormal patterns (respiratory disorders).	Evaluate for respiratory disease; refer to physician/CNM if necessary.
➤ ***Temperature:*** 36.6C–37.6C (98F–99.6F)	Increased temperature (infection).	Assess for signs and symptoms of infection or disease state.
➤ WEIGHT		
2 days: Possible weight loss of 12–20+ lb.	Minimal weight loss (fluid retention, preeclampsia).	Evaluate for fluid retention, edema, deep tendon reflexes, and blood pressure elevation.
6 weeks: Returning to normal prepregnant weight.	Retained weight (excessive caloric intake).	Determine amount of daily exercise. Provide dietary teaching. Refer to dietitian if necessary for additional dietary counseling.
	Extreme weight loss (excessive dieting, inadequate caloric intake).	Discuss appropriate diets, refer to dietitian for additional counseling if necessary.
➤ BREASTS		
➤ ***Nonbreastfeeding*** 2 days: May have mild tenderness; small amount of milk may be expressed. 6 weeks: Soft, with no tenderness; return to prepregnant size.	Some engorgement (incomplete suppression of lactation). Redness; marked tenderness (mastitis). Palpable mass (tumor).	Engorgement may be seen in nonbreastfeeding mothers. Advise client to wear a supportive, well-fitted bra, avoid very warm showers, avoid pumping or any stimulation of breasts, use ice packs for comfort, evaluate for signs and symptoms of mastitis (rare in nonbreastfeeding mothers).
➤ ***Breastfeeding*** Full, with prominent nipples; lactation established.	Cracked, fissured nipples (feeding problems). Redness, marked tenderness, or even abscess formation (mastitis). Palpable mass (full milk duct, tumor).	Counsel about nipple care. Observe infant feeding. Evaluate client condition, evidence of fever; refer to physician/ certified nurse-midwife for initiation of antibiotic therapy, if indicated. Opinion varies as to value of breast examination for breastfeeding mothers; some feel a breastfeeding mother should examine her breasts monthly, after feeding, when breasts are empty; if palpable mass is felt, refer to physician for further evaluation.

*Possible causes of alterations are placed in parentheses.

†This column provides guidelines for further assessment and initial nursing intervention.

(continued on next page)

Assessment Guide: Postpartal—First Home Visit and Anticipated Progress at Six Weeks *continued*

PHYSICAL ASSESSMENT/ NORMAL FINDINGS	ALTERATIONS AND POSSIBLE CAUSES*	NURSING RESPONSES TO DATA†
➤ **BREASTS** *(continued)*		For breast inflammation instruct the mother to **1.** Keep breast empty by frequent feeding. **2.** Rest when possible. **3.** Take prescribed pain relief med. **4.** Force fluids. **5.** Take antibiotics if ordered. If symptoms persist for more than 24 hours, or if accompanied by fever, or flu-like symptoms, redness, instruct her to call her physician/CNM.
➤ **ABDOMINAL MUSCULATURE**		
2 days: Improved firmness, although "bread dough" consistency is not unusual, especially in multipara. Striae pink and obvious.	Marked relaxation of muscles.	Evaluate exercise level; provide information on appropriate exercise program.
Cesarean incision healing.	Drainage, redness, tenderness, pain, edema (infection).	Evaluate for infection; refer to physician/CNM if necessary.
6 weeks: Muscle tone continues to improve; striae may be beginning to fade, may not achieve a silvery appearance for several more weeks; linea nigra fading.		
➤ **ELIMINATION PATTERN**		
➤ ***Urinary Tract*** Return to prepregnant urinary elimination routine.	Urinary incontinence, especially when lifting, coughing, laughing, and so on (urethral trauma, cystocele).	Assess for cystocele; instruct in appropriate muscle tightening exercises; refer to physician/CNM.
	Pain or burning when voiding, urgency and/or frequency, pus or white blood cells (WBC) in urine, pathogenic organisms in culture (urinary tract infection).	Evaluate for urinary tract infection; obtain clean-catch urine; refer to physician/CNM for treatment if indicated.
Routine urinalysis within normal limits (proteinuria disappeared).	Sugar or ketone in urine—may be some lactose present in urine of breastfeeding mothers (diabetes).	Evaluate diet; assess for signs and symptoms of diabetes; refer to physician/CNM.
➤ ***Bowel Habits*** 2 days: May be some discomfort with defecation, especially if client had severe hemorrhoids or third- or fourth-degree extension.	Severe constipation or pain when defecating (trauma or hemorrhoids).	Discuss dietary patterns; encourage fluid, adequate roughage. Continue use of stool softener if necessary to prevent pain associated with straining; continue sitz baths, periods of rest for severe hemorrhoids; assess healing of episiotomy and/or lacerations; severe constipation may require administration of laxatives, stool softeners, and an enema if not contraindicated (check with physician/CNM).

*Possible causes of alterations are placed in parentheses.

†This column provides guidelines for further assessment and initial nursing intervention.

➤

ASSESSMENT GUIDE: POSTPARTAL—FIRST HOME VISIT AND ANTICIPATED PROGRESS AT SIX WEEKS *continued*

PHYSICAL ASSESSMENT/ NORMAL FINDINGS	ALTERATIONS AND POSSIBLE CAUSES*	NURSING RESPONSES TO DATA†
➤ ELIMINATION PATTERN *(continued)*		
6 weeks: Return to normal prepregnancy bowel elimination.	Marked constipation (inadequate fluid/fiber intake).	See previous discussed interventions.
	Fecal incontinence or constipation (rectocele).	Assess for evidence of rectocele, instruct in muscle tightening exercises; refer to physician/CNM.
➤ REPRODUCTIVE TRACT		
➤ ***Lochia*** 2 days: Lochia rubra or lochia serosa, scant amounts, fleshy odor.	Excessive amounts and/or large clots (nonfirm uterus), foul odor (infection), passing tissue (possible retained placenta).	Assess for evidence of infection and/or failure of the uterus to decrease in size; refer to physician/CNM.
6 weeks: No lochia, or return to normal menstruation pattern.	See above.	See above.
➤ ***Fundus and Perineum*** 2 days: Fundus is at least two fingerbreadths below the umbilicus; uterine muscles still somewhat lax; introitus of vagina lacks tone—gapes when intra-abdominal pressure is increased by coughing or straining.	Uterus not decreasing in size appropriately (infection).	Assess fundus for firmness and/or signs of infection; refer to physician/CNM if indicated.
Episiotomy and/or lacerations healing; no signs of infection; may have some bruising and tenderness.	Evidence of redness, severe pain, poor tissue approximation in episiotomy and/or laceration (wound infection).	
6 weeks: Uterus almost returned to prepregnant size with almost completely restored muscle tone.	Continued flow of lochia, failure to decrease appropriately in size (subinvolution).	Assess for evidence of subinvolution and/or infection; refer to physician for further evaluation and treatment if necessary.
➤ HEMOGLOBIN AND HEMATOCRIT LEVELS		
6 weeks: Hb 12 g/dL. Hct 37% ±5%	Hb < 12 g/dL. Hct 32% (anemia).	Assess nutritional status, assess for signs or symptoms of anemia, begin (or continue) supplemental iron; for marked anemia (Hb ≤ 9 g/dL) additional assessment and/or physician/CNM referral may be necessary.
➤ ATTACHMENT		
Bonding process demonstrated by soothing, cuddling, and talking to infant; appropriate feeding techniques; eye-to-eye contact; calling infant by name.	Failure to bond demonstrated by lack of behaviors associated with bonding process, calling infant by nickname that promotes ridicule, inadequate infant weight gain, infant is dirty, hygienic measures are not being maintained, severe diaper rash, failure to obtain adequate supplies to provide infant care (malattachment).	Provide counseling; talk with the woman about her feelings regarding the infant; provide support for the caretaking activities that are being performed; refer to public health nurse for continued home visits; refer if abuse or neglect is suspected.

*Possible causes of alterations are placed in parentheses.

†This column provides guidelines for further assessment and initial nursing intervention.

(Continued on next page)

Assessment Guide: IPostpartal—First Home Visit and Anticipated Progress at Six Weeks *continued*

PHYSICAL ASSESSMENT/ NORMAL FINDINGS	ALTERATIONS AND POSSIBLE CAUSES*	NURSING RESPONSES TO DATA†
➤ ATTACHMENT *(continued)*		
Parent interacts with infant and provides soothing, caretaking activities.	Parent is unable to respond to infant needs (inability to recognize needs, inadequate education and support, fear, family stress).	Provide support for caretaking activities observed; provide information regarding caretaking activities, such as responding to infant cry; methods of wrapping infant; methods of soothing the infant such as swaddling, rocking, increasing stimuli by singing to the infant or decreasing stimuli by putting infant to rest in quiet room; methods of holding the infant; differences in the cry. Identify support system such as friends, neighbors; provide information regarding community resources and support groups.
Parents express feelings of comfort and success with the parent role.	Evidence of stress and anxiety (difficulty moving into or dealing with the parent role).	Provide support and encouragement; provide information regarding progression into parent role and assist parents in talking through their feelings; refer to community resources and support groups.
Woman is in the informal or personal stage of maternal role attainment.	Woman is still greatly influenced by others, has not developed an image or style of her own (woman remains in the anticipatory stage).	Provide role modeling for the woman in working through problem solving with the infant, provide encouragement as she thinks through decisions and develops her sense of problem solving; encourage her to make decisions regarding infant care.
➤ ADJUSTMENT TO PARENTAL ROLE		
Parents are coping with new roles in terms of division of labor, financial status, communication, readjustment of sexual relations, and adjusting to new daily tasks.	Inability to adjust to new roles (immaturity, inadequate education and preparation, ineffective communication patterns, inadequate support, current family crisis).	Provide counseling, refer to parent groups.
➤ EDUCATION		
Mother understands self-care measures.	Inadequate knowledge of self-care (inadequate education).	Provide education and counseling.
Parents are knowledgeable regarding infant care.	Inadequate knowledge of infant care (inadequate education).	
Siblings are adjusting to new baby.	Excessive sibling rivalry.	
Parents have a method of contraception.	Birth control method not chosen.	
	*Possible causes of alterations are placed in parentheses.	†This column provides guidelines for further assessment and initial nursing intervention.

Chapter 5) and answers any questions the woman or her partner may have about methods of birth control.

During the home visit, the nurse continues to provide teaching to the mother and her family and describes self-care measures as needed. The nurse also reviews the signs of developing illness with the woman and her partner. If signs of potential complications are present, the nurse completes a more in-depth evaluation and determines whether it is necessary for the woman to see her primary care provider.

Breastfeeding Concerns Following Discharge

The *Healthy People 2010 Breastfeeding Goals* state that by 2010, 75% of women will initiate breastfeeding, 50% will continue breastfeeding for at least 6 months, and 24% will continue until the infant is at least one year of age (US Department of Health and Human Services [USDHHS], 2000). Breastfeeding benefits maternal as well as newborn health, and results in cost savings for parents, insurers, and employers. Therefore, it has a high economic as well as medical value for society (Ball & Bennett, 2001). However, most mothers are discharged before breastfeeding is well established and many require anticipatory guidance and support in order to continue once they go home.

Gill (2001) found that breastfeeding mothers expected nurses to support them by providing information, encouragement, and interpersonal support, and to remain with them during initial feeding attempts. Many of the nurses felt that providing verbal and written information was helpful, but they did not remain with clients. The mothers in this study found the lack of support to be frustrating, which is consistent with previous research findings.

A home visit a few days after discharge can identify at-risk infants before they lose excessive weight and at a time when intervention can correct most breastfeeding problems before they become complicated by insufficient milk. A home visit program developed to provide breastfeeding support to families discharged within 24 hours of birth resulted in fewer infant readmissions and a decreased number of unnecessary phone calls and visits to physicians (Johnson, Brennan, & Flynn-Tymkow, 1999). The home health nurse can assess the infant and the breastfeeding process, provide appropriate education to promote breastfeeding, and initiate referrals to a lactation consultant or primary healthcare provider as needed. Additionally, the nurse can provide individualized support and encouragement as desired by the client.

BREASTFEEDING ASSESSMENT

Breastfeeding infants discharged before 48 hours of age should be assessed within 48 to 72 hours after discharge by a physician or nurse, who should observe a feeding episode if indicated, to ensure correct position, maternal and infant feeding cues, latch-on, position, let-down, nipple condition, infant response, and maternal response. The nurse can assess the parents' ability to identify infant feeding cues such as rooting, hand-to-mouth movements, sucking, opening of mouth in response to stimulation, and infant transition from sleep to drowsy to quiet alert states. Various tools are available to assess the breastfeeding session including the LATCH Scoring Table provided in Chapter 31 . Assessment of the mother's ability to perceive infant satiety cues such as a gradual decrease in sucking, pulling away and releasing the nipple, relaxation, sleep, contentment, and a small amount of milk visible in the mouth can be accomplished at this time as well (AWHONN, 2000; ILCA, 1999).

The assessment should also include the infant's weight, number of feedings per 24 hours, elimination over 24 hours, and presence of jaundice (AWHONN, 2000). According to AAP criteria, the infant's weight should remain within 10% of his or her birth weight and the infant should feed at least eight to ten times per day by the fourth day of life. The infant should have at least three voids and one to two stools per 24 hours by the third day of life and at least six voids and three stools per 24 hours by the fourth day. Parents should awaken the infant to feed at least eight times in 24 hours until the infant begins to awaken on his or her own (AWHONN, 2000).

Infant signs of ineffective breastfeeding include failure to meet the AAP criteria, or weight loss of more than 7%, continued weight loss after day 3, passing meconium after day 4, an infant who does not begin to gain weight by day 5, and an infant who has not returned to birth weight by day 14. The infant may be irritable or sleepy and refusing to feed (ILCA, 1999). Both home and early clinic visits have been found to decrease the incidence of neonatal dehydration and malnutrition in breastfeeding infants (Gagnon, Dougherty, Jiminez, et al, 2002).

Many new mothers have breastfeeding difficulties including leaking, nipple soreness, cracked nipples, breast engorgement, and plugged ducts. The nurse can assess for these complications at the home visit and provide interventions to decrease maternal discomfort.

MEDIALINK BREASTFEEDING ISSUES

NIPPLE SORENESS

Nipple soreness is a common complaint and frequent reason for early discontinuation of breastfeeding (Adams, Berger, Conning, et al, 2001). Primary causes of sore nipples are poor positioning and improper latch. Therefore, assistance with proper position and latching technique is essential to the prevention of soreness (AWHONN, 2000; Biancuzzo, 2003; Brent, Rudy, Redd, et al, 1998; Lauwers & Shinskie, 2000). Observation of feeding and assistance with positioning and latch during the home visit can promote nipple comfort and prevent problems.

Some discomfort often occurs initially; it peaks between the third and sixth days and then recedes. Discomfort that lasts throughout the feeding or past the first week demands attention (Riordan & Auerbach, 1999).

The baby's position at the breast is a critical factor in nipple soreness. The mother's hand should be off the areola, and the baby should be facing the mother's chest, with ear, shoulder, and hip aligned (see Figure 31–6). Because the area of greatest stress to the nipple is in line with the

Critical Thinking in Practice

Ann calls you from home in tears on her third postpartum day. She states that, although breastfeeding was going well in the hospital, her breasts are now swollen, hard, and very painful, and her baby is refusing to suckle. Ann expresses extreme disappointment that "the breastfeeding didn't work" because she truly believes that breast milk is best for babies and she had enjoyed her breastfeeding experience in the hospital, especially feeding the baby immediately after birth. But she also states she has not been able to stop crying all day and can no longer tolerate her painful breasts. In addition she says that the baby "seems happier" with the bottle. What would you do?

Refer to Appendix I.

newborn's chin and nose, nipple soreness may be decreased by encouraging the mother to rotate positions when feeding the infant. Changing positions alters the focus of greatest stress and promotes more complete breast emptying.

Nipple soreness may also develop if the infant has faulty sucking habits. Nipples may have injured tips that are bruised, scabbed, or blistered from the nipple entering the baby's mouth at an upward angle and rubbing against the roof of the mouth (Riordan & Auerbach, 1999).

A study of sore nipples found significant associations between the early use of pacifiers and/or supplemental feedings and sore nipples (Centuori, et al, 1999). Therefore, use of artificial nipples should be discouraged if possible. Soreness may also result from continuous negative pressure related to improper use of breast pumps, prolonged nonnutritive sucking, or delayed let-down. Attempting to remove the infant from the breast prior to breaking suction may result in soreness as well (Biancuzzo, 2003).

Chewed nipples, which result from improper positioning, are cracked or tender at or near the base. In these cases, the baby's jaw is closed only on the nipple instead of on the areola, the baby's mouth is not opened wide enough, or the infant's mouth has slipped down to the nipple from the areola as a result of engorgement. Soreness on the underside of the nipple is caused by the infant suckling with the bottom lip tucked in rather than out, causing a friction burn. In such cases, even vigorous sucking produces little milk because the milk sinuses under the areola are not compressed. The situation results in a frustrated infant and marked soreness for the mother. The problem is overcome by positioning the infant with as much areola as possible in his or her mouth with bottom lip out, and rotating the baby's positions at the breast.

Nipple soreness is especially pronounced during the first few minutes of a feeding. If the mother is not expecting this discomfort, she may become discouraged and quickly stop. The let-down reflex may take a few minutes to activate, and it may not occur if the mother stops breastfeeding too quickly. The infant is unsatisfied, and the possibility of breast engorgement increases.

Nipple soreness can also result from the vigorous feeding of the overeager infant. Thus the mother may find it helpful to feed the baby more frequently. She can massage the breast prior to breastfeeding to soften the breast and stimulate the milk ejection reflex. Alternatively, the woman can apply ice to her nipples and areola for a few minutes before feeding to promote nipple erectness and to numb the painful tissue (Riordan & Auerbach, 1999).

The nurse can instruct the mother in a number of measures to promote comfort and healing to prevent skin breakdown. The application of warm water compresses followed by air-drying with the bra flaps down after feedings is helpful. Expressing some breast milk and applying it to the nipples and areola followed by air-drying after feedings promotes healing and prevents infection (Riordan & Auerbach, 1999). Drying the nipples with a hair dryer on low heat held 6 to 8 inches from the body facilitates drying when the mother is unable to air-dry (Biancuzzo, 2003). If a woman finds that her bra or clothing rubs against her nipples and adds to her discomfort, she may find it helpful to use breast shells between feedings. Breast shells are hard plastic molded devices that are worn inside the woman's bra. While they are commonly used for women with flat nipples to aid in nipple protrusion, they can also be worn by mothers with sore nipples to prevent further irritation to the nipples.

A number of research studies spanning the last 40 years have found warm water to be the most effective treatment for sore nipples (Riordan & Auerbach, 1999). A recent randomized trial found warm moist compresses to be more beneficial than ointment in the treatment of sore nipples as well (Centuori et al, 1999). Table 36–5 • lists helpful interventions for sore nipples and other breastfeeding problems.

Many lactation consultants recommend 100% anhydrous modified lanolin for nipple soreness resistant to more natural treatment (Lansinoh, Purelan, Marcalan). This has been studied and found to reduce soreness. Other forms of lanolin should not be used because of potential problems related to allergens or pesticides (Riordan & Auerbach, 1999). A study comparing the use of Lansinoh along with breast shells to the use of hydrogel wound dressings in the treatment of damaged nipples found the combined use of shells and Lansinoh to be more beneficial than the more expensive dressings. Additionally, the hydrogel dressings were associated with higher rates of infection than expected, and the study was terminated early (Hagen, 1999).

Although a number of other products have been marketed for or tried by breastfeeding mothers over the years for the prevention and cure of sore nipples, they have not been clinically proven to be effective. Additionally, a number of them can cause irritation, delay healing, or be harmful to the infant (Lauwers & Shinskie, 2000). Massé cream, Mammol ointment, Eucerin cream, Bag Balm, A and

Table 36-5 • BREASTFEEDING PROBLEMS AND REMEDIES

Nipples Not Graspable

Flat or inverted nipples

- Use Hoffman technique to break adhesions.
- Wear milk cups to encourage nipples to protrude.
- Use nipple tug and roll to increase protractility.
- Form the nipple prior to breastfeeding by hand shaping, ice, wearing milk cups a half-hour before feeding.
- As a last resort, use nipple shield for first few minutes of feeding to draw out nipple; then place baby on breast.

Engorged breasts

Treat engorgement by relieving fullness with hand expression of milk prior to breastfeeding and instituting frequent feedings so nipple is more prominent.

Large breasts

- Support breast with opposite hand, or use rolled towel under breast to bring nipple to the level of baby's mouth.
- Use C-hold to make nipple accessible to baby.

Engorgement

Missed or infrequent feedings

- Breastfeed frequently (every $1\frac{1}{2}$ hours).
- Massage and hand express or pump to empty breasts completely when feedings are missed or when a full feeling develops in breasts and baby is not available or willing to feed.

Breasts not emptied at feedings

- Breastfeed long enough to empty breasts (10–15 minutes on each side at each feeding).
- If baby will not feed long enough to empty breasts, hand express or pump after feeding.

Inadequate let-down

- Use relaxation techniques, massage, and warm or cool compresses before breastfeeding.
- Relax in warm shower with water running from back over shoulders and breasts, hand expressing to relieve fullness.
- If due to anxiety, try to eliminate the source of tension.

Baby sleepy or not eager to feed

- Use rousing techniques (eg, hold baby upright, unwrap blanket, change diaper).
- Pre-express milk onto nipple or baby's lips to entice baby.
- Avoid use of bottles of water or formula; these will decrease baby's willingness to suckle.

Inadequate Let-Down

Let-down not well established

- Give the baby ample time at the breast (at least 15 minutes per side) to allow for let-down and complete emptying.
- Breastfeed in a quiet spot away from distractions.
- Massage breasts before breastfeeding.
- Drink juice, water, tea (no caffeine) before and during breastfeeding.
- Condition let-down by setting up a routine for beginning feedings.
- Use relaxation and breathing techniques.
- Stimulate the nipple manually before breastfeeding.
- Concentrate thought on the baby and milk flow; turn on a faucet so that the sound of running water helps stimulate let-down.
- Use synthetic oxytocin nasal spray several times during a feeding. (This should condition let-down within 24 hours. Then it is no longer needed. Spray must be prescribed by a doctor.)

Mother overtired or overextended

- Nap or rest when the baby rests.
- Lie down to breastfeed.
- Breastfeed the baby in bed at night.
- Simplify daily chores; set priorities.

Mother tense, pressured

- Identify the causes of tensions and eliminate or minimize them.
- Decrease fatigue.

Mother caught in cycle of little milk, worry, less milk

- Try all the actions above.
- Develop confidence in mothering skills. (A home visit by a counselor may help.)

Cracked Nipples

All causes of sore nipples carried to extreme

- Refer to all actions for sore nipples.
- Consult doctor about using aspirin, acetaminophen (Tylenol), or other painkiller.
- Improve nutritional status, increasing protein, vitamin C, zinc.

Local infection (baby with staph or other organism may have infected mother's nipples)

Refer to physician.

Plugged Ducts

Poor positioning

Try a variety of positions for complete emptying.

Incomplete emptying of breast

- Breastfeed at least 10 minutes per side after let-down.
- Alternate breastfeeding positions.
- If baby does not empty breasts, pump or express milk after feedings.

External pressure on breast

- Use larger size bras, insert bra extender, or go braless.
- Use nursing bra instead of pulling up conventional bra to breastfeed to avoid pressure on ducts.
- Avoid bunching up sweater or nightgown under arm during breastfeeding.

Sore Nipples

Poor positioning

- Alternate breastfeeding positions throughout the day.
- Bring the baby close to feed so the baby does not pull on the breast.
- Place the nipple and some of the areola in the baby's mouth.
- Check to ensure the baby is put on and off the breast properly.
- Check to ensure the nipple is back far enough in the baby's mouth.
- Hold the baby closely during feeding so the nipple is not constantly being pulled.

Baby chewing or nuzzling onto nipple

- Form the nipple for the baby.
- Set up a pattern of getting the baby onto the breast using the rooting reflex.

Baby sucking on end of nipple

- Ensure the nipple is way back in the baby's mouth by getting the baby properly onto the breast.
- Check for an inverted nipple.
- Check for engorgement.

Baby chewing his or her way off the nipple (nipple being pulled out of baby's mouth at end of feeding)

- Remove the baby from the breast by placing a finger between the baby's gums to ensure suction is broken.
- End feeding when the baby's suckling slows, before he or she has a chance to chew on the nipple.

Table 36–5 • BREASTFEEDING PROBLEMS AND REMEDIES (CONTINUED)

Sore Nipples ***continued***

Baby overly eager to nurse

- Breastfeed more often.
- Pre-express milk to hasten let-down, avoiding vigorous suckling.

Dry colostrum or milk causing nipple to stick to bra or breast pads

Moisten bra or pads before taking off so as not to remove keratin.

Nipples not allowed to dry

- Remove plastic liners from milk pads.
- Air dry breast completely after nursing.
- Change milk pads frequently.

Improper use of breast shield

- Use shield only to draw out nipple; then have the baby breastfeed.
- Cut tip of shield back bit by bit and eventually discard.

Nipple skin not resistant to stress

- Improve diet, especially adding fresh fruits and vegetables and vitamin supplements.
- Eliminate or decrease use of sugary foods, alcohol, caffeine, cigarettes.
- Check use of cleansing or drying agents.

Natural oils removed or keratin layers broken down by drying agents (soap, alcohol, shampoo, deodorant)

- Eliminate irritants.
- Wash breasts with water only.

Source: Adapted from Lauwers J., Woessner C. *Counseling the Nursing Mother: A Reference Handbook for Health Care Providers and Lay Counselors,* 2nd ed. Garden City Park, NY: Avery, 1990, pp 385–397.

D ointment, Vaseline, and vitamin E are examples of products that could potentially be harmful to breastfeeding infants (Riordan & Auerbach, 1999).

The home care nurse should discourage the use of such products. Since sore nipples may also indicate the presence of infection, the home care nurse should refer clients to a lactation consultant or to their primary care provider if sore nipples are not readily improved by the use of proper positioning, breast milk or warm water compress application, and air-drying.

Burning pain or itching of the nipple or burning and shooting pains deep in the breast may be caused by a fungal infection (thrush). The nipples may be bright pink with a pale or shiny spot on the areola. The newborn may present with white or gray patches on the buccal mucosa, gums, or tongue. The infant may exhibit diaper rash related to *Candida albicans* in the intestines and stools as well (Walker & Creenhan, 2001). The client should see her primary care provider for simultaneous treatment of herself and her infant with an antifungal agent.

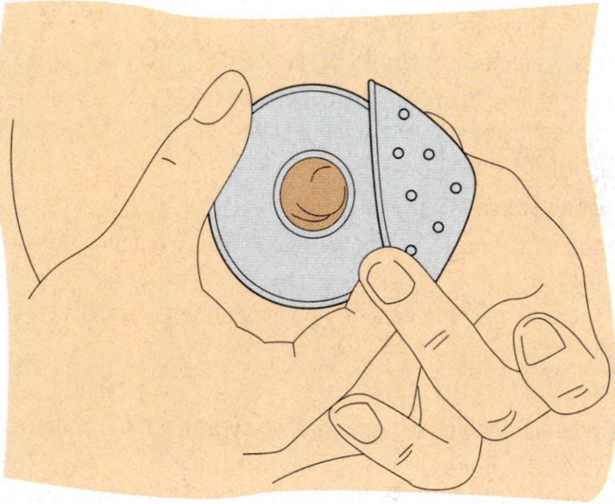

Figure 36–5 • Breast shells can help correct flat or inverted nipples.
SOURCE: Courtesy of Medula Breastfeeding information guide (p. 5). McHenry, IL.

CRACKED NIPPLES

Nipple soreness is often coupled with cracked nipples. When a breastfeeding mother complains of soreness, the nurse carefully examines the nipples for fissures or cracks and observes the mother during breastfeeding to see whether the infant is correctly positioned at the breast. If cracks exist, interventions are necessary. All the interventions described for sore nipples may be used. It may also help the mother to begin breastfeeding on the breast that is less sore for a couple of feedings. This approach allows the let-down reflex to occur in the affected breast and permits the infant to do more vigorous sucking on the less tender breast, which decreases trauma to the cracked nipple.

MediaLink CARE PLAN: BREASTFEEDING PAIN

FLAT OR INVERTED NIPPLES

Many women with flat or inverted nipples who had difficulty with breastfeeding in the immediate postpartum period will continue to have difficulties at home. The home health nurse can assess the nipples for protrusion characteristics. Women with flat or inverted nipples may benefit from wearing breast shells (Figure 36–5 •). These hard plastic cups are placed in the woman's bra between feedings to encourage nipple protrusion. The nurse can also teach the woman to roll her nipple between her thumb and forefinger or to stretch the nipple by pulling it inward and outward prior to infant feedings (Hoffman's technique). Nurse can also recommend use of an electric breast pump to pull the nipple into a prominent position prior to latching the baby onto the breast. Nipple shields are another device that may aid breastfeeding women. Shields are made of latex or rubber and cover the nipple in a tight-fitting manner. The infant then sucks the shield instead of the mother's nipple. The use of all rubber or latex shields is typically not recommended since they correct nipple position by having the baby suck the plastic instead of the mother's nipple. These devices have been shown to decrease milk transfer by up to 58% and increase the infant's suck effort and rate. This can result in infant fatigue and nipple confusion. Newer latex shields are available that do not alter sucking patterns, but still result in a reduction in milk transfer. These devices should only be used as a last resort, typically under the continued direction of a lactation consultant.

BREAST ENGORGEMENT

A distinction exists between breast fullness and engorgement. All lactating women experience a transition fullness at first, initially due to venous congestion and later due to accumulating milk. However, this fullness generally lasts only 24 hours, the breasts remain soft enough for the newborn to suckle, and there is no pain. Engorged breasts are hard, painful, and warm and appear taut and shiny.

The infant should suckle for an average of 15 minutes per feeding and should feed at least eight times in 24 hours (Riordan & Auerbach, 1999). If the baby is unable to feed more frequently, the mother may express some milk manually or with a pump, taking care to avoid traumatizing the breast tissue. Warm compresses, breast massage, and manual expression of milk before breastfeeding stimulate let-down and soften the breast so that the infant can grasp the areola more easily. The mother should wear a well-fitting nursing bra 24 hours a day to support the breasts and prevent discomfort from tension.

The use of fresh green cabbage leaves placed inside the bra to treat engorgement is a long-recognized home remedy that has sparked renewed interest. Although the exact action of the cabbage is not understood, it appears to reduce the edema of engorgement. The amount of relief women experience varies. Some women report relief in as little as 30 minutes, whereas other women require more continuous use to perceive an effect. It should be noted that prolonged use of cabbage can cause the milk to dry up, which may be helpful if sudden weaning is necessary (Lauwers & Shinskie, 2000).

Analgesics may be appropriate as directed by a primary healthcare provider. It is best to avoid breastfeeding when drug levels are peaking in maternal plasma. This is usually best accomplished by taking the drug right after a feeding. However, if relief is needed for the mother to tolerate feedings, she may want to take the drug shortly before a feeding (usually 30 minutes or less), so the drug's onset coincides with the feeding (AWHONN, 2000; Biancuzzo, 2003; Hale, 2002).

PLUGGED DUCTS

Some mothers experience plugging of one or more ducts, especially in conjunction with or following engorgement. Manifested as an area of tenderness or lumpiness in an otherwise well woman, plugging may be relieved by the use of heat and massage. The nurse can encourage the mother to massage her breasts from her chest wall forward to the nipple while standing in a warm shower or following the application of moist heat to the breast. The mother should then breastfeed her infant, starting on the affected breast to promote drainage. Frequent breastfeeding and the use of a variety of positions to ensure complete emptying help prevent the problem (Riordan & Auerbach, 1999). If these interventions do not relieve the tenderness or if lumpiness remains, a breast pump may be effective in unplugging the duct.

Continued milk stasis and plugged ducts increase the risk for mastitis, an inflammatory condition of the breast. Symptoms of mastitis include fever (> 100.4F), a hot red tender area on the breast, and flulike symptoms. The mastitis may also involve a bacterial infection, in which case the client will require antibiotic therapy from her primary care provider (Walker & Creehan, 2001).

EFFECT OF ALCOHOL AND MEDICATIONS

Mothers may ask the home care nurse about use of alcohol and prescription medications and social alcohol use while breastfeeding. Although alcohol use was considered acceptable in the past, it is no longer recommended for breastfeeding women. Alcohol levels in breast milk parallel those found in maternal plasma, peaking 30 to 60 minutes after consumption. Mothers who do occasionally drink while lactating should be advised to consume the alcohol after breastfeeding rather than shortly before a feeding in order to minimize the amount the infant receives (Menella, 2002).

As discussed in Chapter 31, most medications do pass into the breast milk. ACOG (2000) recommends that women consult with their primary care providers prior to taking any medications, vitamins, or herbal supplements. Helpful references are listed in Table 36–6 •.

BREASTFEEDING AND THE WORKING MOTHER

Mothers frequently cite returning to work as a reason for discontinuing breastfeeding (Adams et al, 2001). The home care nurse can help the woman to explore options and solve problems related to breastfeeding in the workplace to promote continuation (AWHONN, 2000). The earlier the breastfeeding mother returns to work, the more often she will need to pump her breasts to express the breast milk. Recommendations for mothers who are using a breast pump can be found in Table 31–3. Because milk production follows the principle of supply and demand, if breasts are not pumped, the milk supply will decrease. The nurse can review pumping and storage of breast milk with the mother. An electric pump and double collection system is optimal for the working mother. Working mothers can also obtain printed materials on pumping, storage, working while breastfeeding, and related issues from breastfeeding support groups, such as La Leche League.

The nurse can also discuss methods of maintaining breast milk supply such as relaxation, stress reduction, proper nutrition, adequate fluid intake, and frequent nursing during the evenings, in the mornings, and on days off. The nurse

Table 36–6 • BOOKS ON MEDICATIONS AND THEIR EFFECTS ON BREAST MILK

Briggs, G. G., Freeman, R. K., & Yaffe, S. J. (2001). *Drugs in pregnancy and lactation* (6th ed.). Baltimore, MD: Williams & Wilkins.

Hale, T. D. (2002). *Medications and mothers' milk* (10th ed.). Amarillo, TX: Pharmasoft Medical.

Newman, J., & Pitman, T. (2000). *The ultimate breastfeeding book of answers.* Westminster, MD: Crown Publishing Group.

and client can explore options such as pumping at work, visiting the infant or having the infant brought to work during the mother's lunch, and having the child care provider give expressed breast milk (AWHONN, 2000; Zinn, 2000).

Night breastfeeding presents a dilemma. It may help a working mother maintain her milk supply, but it may also contribute to fatigue. For the mother who works long hours or has a rigid work schedule, the best alternative may be to limit breastfeeding to morning and evening feeds, with supplemental feedings at other times. This choice allows her to maintain a close relationship with the infant and provides some of the unique benefits of breast milk.

WEANING

The decision to *wean* the baby from the breast may be made for a variety of reasons, including family or cultural pressures, changes in the home situation, pressure from the woman's partner, or a personal opinion about when weaning should occur. For the woman who is comfortable with breastfeeding and well informed about the process, the appropriate time to wean her infant will become evident if she is sensitive to the child's cues. Often weaning falls between periods of great developmental activity for the child. Thus weaning commonly occurs at 8 to 9 months, 12 to 14 months, 18 months, 2 years, and 3 years of age. The infant who is weaned before 12 months should be given formula, not cows' milk (ACOG, 2000).

If weaning is timed to respond to the child's cues, and if the mother is comfortable with the timing, it can be accomplished with less difficulty than if the process begins before mother and child are ready emotionally. Nevertheless, weaning is a time of emotional separation for mother and baby; it may be difficult for them to give up the closeness of their breastfeeding sessions. The nurse who is understanding about this possibility can help the mother see that her infant or toddler is growing up and plan other comforting, consoling, and play activities to replace breastfeeding.

A gradual approach is the easiest and most comforting way to wean the child from breastfeedings. During weaning, the mother should substitute one cup feeding or bottle-feeding for one breastfeeding session over 4 to 7 days so that her breasts gradually produce less milk. Eliminating the breastfeedings associated with meals first facilitates the mother's ability to wean the infant, because satiation with food lessens the desire for milk. Over a period of several weeks she can substitute more cup feedings or bottle-feedings for breastfeedings. The slow method of weaning prevents breast engorgement, allows infants to alter their eating methods at their own rates, and provides time for psychologic adjustments.

CULTURAL CONSIDERATIONS RELATED TO BREASTFEEDING

Despite increases in breastfeeding in the United States during the 1990s, minority women still breastfeed at lower rates than white women. Many immigrants breastfeed less than family members from their native countries after moving to the United States.; lack of family support decreases the likelihood that the woman will continue breastfeeding once she goes home (Riordan & Gill-Hopple, 2001).

Although cultural considerations related to each group are beyond the scope of this chapter, it is important for the home care nurse to individualize care for minority women by incorporating their cultural beliefs and practices related to breastfeeding. For further discussion regarding cultural influences on infant feeding practices, see Chapter 2.

BREASTFEEDING REFERRALS AND SOCIAL SUPPORT

Support from the woman's family and social contacts is very important with regard to the initiation and continuation of breastfeeding. Weissinger (2002) highly recommends referral to local support groups where women can learn over time and observe role models to enhance their breastfeeding experience. The home care nurse should be familiar with local lay support groups and encourage breastfeeding mothers to contact them.

Other Types of Follow-Up Care

Other types of follow-up care may include return home visits, telephone follow-up, and postpartal classes or support groups.

Return Visits

If the mother and family and physician/certified nurse-midwife have chosen discharge earlier than 48 hours after vaginal birth, the mother may, in some states, request a total of three visits. In such cases, the nurse would schedule the first visit about 24 hours after discharge and then space out the other two visits over the next week. In other instances, the nurse may schedule additional home visits based on the findings of the first home visit and the follow-up phone call.

Telephone Follow-Up

The postpartum home care nurse usually makes a follow-up phone call a few days after the home visit. During the call, the nurse may provide additional information, address questions or areas of confusion, and make referrals.

Some families may be offered or may request a telephone follow-up at the time of discharge. A mutually agreeable time is set for the call, typically within 3 days of discharge, or earlier if desired. Calls typically last about 20 minutes, and are preplanned and goal directed.

To perform an effective telephone assessment, the nurse must be able to listen skillfully, use open-ended questions, and wait for answers. The nurse projects a warm, caring attitude so that the mother feels comfortable talking to a faceless caller. When assessment reveals signs of an initial or recurring postpartum complication, the nurse refers the woman to her primary care provider for further evaluation.

The plan of care developed and implemented during a telephone conversation is limited to supportive counseling, teaching, and referral. The new mother may have many questions, especially about newborn care, and is generally at a high level of learning readiness. The nurse can answer the woman's questions and use the questions as a "stepping stone" for further teaching.

In addition to these scheduled follow-up telephone calls, nurses on birthing, newborn, and postpartum units as well as nurses in clinic settings often receive phone calls from postpartal families seeking advice or care. These calls must be triaged—that is, sorted according to urgency—so that clients with potentially life-threatening needs are not left on hold. Nurses engaged in telephone triage must consider several important strategies to provide optimum care and avoid legal pitfalls. These strategies include the following (Cady, 1999):

- Develop and follow triage protocols for calls with the most commonly occurring themes.
- Document all triage calls carefully and accurately.
- Initiate timely follow-up contacts. This may include instructions to the client to call back after a specific period or if the condition does not improve. It also involves calls from the nurse to the client for follow-up.

Finally, many communities have established 24-hour help lines for new parents to call when they have questions or need support. In areas where help lines are not available, parents may be directed to call the birthing center. In either case, the nurse provides the number so that it is readily accessible for the family.

Postpartal Classes and Support Groups

Postpartal classes are becoming more common as caregivers recognize the continuing needs of the childbearing family. In many instances, classes are prepared to meet the specific needs of a variety of families so that, for example, single mothers and adolescent mothers can attend class with peers. A series of structured classes may focus on topics such as parenting, postpartal exercise, or nutrition, or there may be loosely structured group sessions that address mothers' concerns as they arise. Such classes offer chances for the new mother to socialize, share her concerns, and receive encouragement. Because baby-sitting arrangements may be difficult or expensive, it is desirable to provide child care for newborns and siblings. In some instances, infants may remain with mothers in the class.

Some cities offer support groups through birthing centers or hospitals or as a community effort. Once again, the support group provides an opportunity for parents to interact with one another and to share information and experiences.

Many parents look to Internet resources for additional information on parenting and newborn care. Internet sites can be devised by anyone, so the quality, usefulness, and accuracy of the information may vary. Nurses have an opportunity to assist parents in evaluating the reliability of the information they find. Criteria that suggest Internet information is reliable and high in quality include affiliation with a university medical or nursing school; inclusion of the authors' credentials, education, board certification, and affiliations; referencing of information; currency of information; similarity of information when compared with other sources; and easy accessibility (Beyea, 2002).

MEDIALINK CASE STUDY: FOLLOW-UP WITH THE CLIENT AT HOME

CHAPTER REVIEW

EXPLOREMEDIALINK

NCLEX review questions, case studies, and other interactive resources for this chapter can be found on the Web site at http://www.prenhall.com/olds. Click on "Chapter 36" to select the activities for this chapter.

For tutorials including animations and videos, more NCLEX review questions, and an audio glossary, access the accompanying CD-ROM in this book.

Focus Your Study

- The Newborns' and Mothers' Health Protection Act took effect in January 1998, and provides for a guaranteed minimum stay of up to 48 hours following an uncomplicated vaginal birth and 96 hours following an uncomplicated cesarean birth. For women discharged earlier than the mandated time, more than half of all states in the United States require coverage for home care follow-up.
- The overall goal of postpartal home visits is to enhance opportunities for smooth transition of the new family. The home visit provides opportunities for assessment, teaching, breastfeeding support, and fostering a caring relationship with new families.
- In planning the home visit, the nurse needs to take precautions to maintain safety, such as carrying a cellular phone, notifying supervisors of location of

visit, keeping personal belongings out of sight, assessing the neighborhood and home for signs of danger, and if present, terminating the visit.

- Physical assessment of the newborn during a home visit includes assessments of vital signs, weight, overall color, intake/output, umbilical cord and circumcision, newborn nutrition, newborn safety, parent education, and attachment.
- Teaching goals during home visits include reinforcing daily newborn care, including demonstrations of positioning and handling, sponge and tub bathing, nail care, and dressing; discussing temperature assessment and maintenance of a neutral thermal environment; discussing assessment of the newborn's stools; promoting safe and appropriate newborn sleeping, including SIDS prevention; promoting crib safety; encouraging childproofing of the home environment; and encouraging newborn screening and immunization.
- The physician or pediatric nurse practitioner should be notified if there is evidence of redness around the newborn's umbilicus, if there is bright red bleeding or puslike drainage near the cord stump, or if the umbilicus remains unhealed.
- A primary risk factor for sudden infant death syndrome is sleeping in the prone position.
- Newborn screening for galactosemia, hemocystinuria, hypothyroidism, maple syrup urine disease, phenylketonuria, and sickle cell anemia is performed on all newborns in the first 1 to 3 days, with a second blood specimen drawn after 7 to 14 days.
- Signs of illness in mothers include pain or burning with urination, passage of clots or placental tissue, excessive perineal pain, chest pain, difficulty breathing, excessive or foul-smelling lochia, failure of fundus to descend at anticipated rate, temperature of 101.4F or above, elevation of blood pressure, and tenderness, redness, or pain in the legs or breasts.
- Difficulties with breastfeeding include sore, cracked, flat, or inverted nipples, breast engorgement, and plugged ducts.
- Breastfeeding mothers require information on effect of alcohol and various medications on breast milk; pumping; weaning; and breastfeeding referrals and social support.
- Return visits, telephone follow-up, classes, and support groups can provide valuable information and support to new mothers and their families.

References

Adams, C., Berger, R., Conning, P., Cruikshank, L., & Dore, K. (2001). Breastfeeding trends at a community breastfeeding center: An evaluative survey. *Journal of Obstetric, Gynecologic, and Neonatal Nursing, 30*(4), 392–400.

Agency for Healthcare Policy and Research. (1999). *Hospital inpatient statistics.* Silver Spring, MD: AHCPR Publications Clearinghouse.

American Academy of Pediatrics (AAP) and American College of Obstetricians and Gynecologists (ACOG). (2002). *Guidelines for perinatal care* (5th ed.). Elk Grove Village, IL: Author.

American Academy of Pediatrics (AAP) Committee on Child Abuse and Neglect. (2001). Shaken baby syndrome: Rotational cranial injuries—technical report. *Pediatrics, 108,* 206–209.

American Academy of Pediatrics (AAP) Council on Child and Adolescent Health. (1998). The role of home-visitation programs in improving health outcomes for children and families. *Pediatrics, 101,* 486–489.

American Academy of Pediatrics (AAP) Task Force on Infant Sleep Position and Sudden Infant Death Syndrome. (2000). Changing concepts of sudden infant death syndrome: Implications for infant sleeping environment and sleep position. *Pediatrics, 105*(3), 650–656.

American College of Obstetricians and Gynecologists (ACOG). (2000). *Breastfeeding: Maternal and infant aspects* (ACOG Educational Bulletin No. 258). Washington, DC. Author.

Association of Women's Health, Obstetric, and Neonatal Nurses (AWHONN). (1998). *Standards and guidelines for professional nursing practice in the care of women and newborns* (5th ed.). Washington, DC: Author.

Association of Women's Health, Obstetric, and Neonatal Nurses (AWHONN). (2000). *Evidenced based clinical practice guideline. Breastfeeding support: Prenatal care through the first year* (Practice Guideline). Washington, DC: Author.

Avery, M. C., Duckett, L., & Frantzich, C. R. (2000). The experience of sexuality during breastfeeding among primiparous women. *Journal of Midwifery and Women's Health, 45*(3), 227–237.

Ball, T. M., & Bennett, D. M. (2001). The economic impact of breastfeeding. *Pediatric Clinics of North America, 48*(1), 253–262.

Bennett, R. L., & Tandy, L. J. (1998). Postpartum home visits: Extending the continuum of care from hospital to home. *Home Healthcare Nurse, 16*(5), 294–303.

Beyea, S. C. (2002). Finding patient safety Internet resources. *Association of Perioperative Registered Nurses Journal, 75*(6), 1171–1173.

Biancuzzo, M. (2003). *Breastfeeding the newborn: Clinical strategies for nurses.* (2nd ed.). St. Louis, MO: Mosby.

Brent, N., Rudy, S. J., Redd, B., Rudy, T. E., & Roth, L. A. (1998). Sore nipples in breast-feeding women: A clinical trial of wound dressings vs conventional care. *Archives of Pediatrics & Adolescent Medicine, 152*(11), 1077–1082.

Brumfield, C. G. (1998). Early postpartum discharge. *Clinical Obstetrics and Gynecology, 41*(3), 611–625.

Byrd, J. E., Hyde, J. S., DeLamater, J. D., & Plant, E. A. (1998). Sexuality during pregnancy and the year postpartum. *Journal of Family Practice, 47*(4), 305–308.

Cady, R. (1999). Telephone triage: Avoiding the pitfalls. *American Journal of Maternal-Child Nursing, 24*(4), 209.

Carpenter, J. A. (1998). Shortening the short stay. *AWHONN Lifelines, 2*(1), 29–34.

Centuori, S., Burmax, T., Ronfani, L., Fragiacomo, M., Quintero, S. & Pavan, C., (1999). CPSC warns against placing babies in adult beds (CPSC Document No. 5091). Washington, DC: Consumer Product Safety Commission.

Dahlberg, N. F. (2001). Postpartum home care. In K. R. Simpson & P. A. Creehan (Eds.), *AWHONN perinatal nursing* (2nd ed.) (pp. 643–655). Philadelphia: Lippincott.

Davanzo, R., & Cattaneo, A. (1999). Nipple care, sore nipples, and breastfeeding: A randomized trial. *Journal of Human Lactation, 15*(2), 125–130.

Dore, S., Buchan, D., Coulas, S., Hamber, L., Stewart, M., Cowan, D., et al. (1998). Alcohol versus natural drying for newborn cord care. *Journal of Obstetric, Gynecologic, and Neonatal Nursing, 27*(6), 621–627.

Durkin, N., & Wilson, C. (1999). Simple steps to keep yourself safe. *Home Healthcare Nurse, 17*(7), 430–435.

Eaton, A. P. (2001). Commentary. Early postpartum discharge: Recommendations from a preliminary report to Congress. *Pediatrics, 107*(2), 400–403.

Fallis, W. M., & Christiani, P. (1999). Neonatal axillary temperature measurements: A comparison of electronic thermometer predictive and monitor modes. *Journal of Obstetric, Gynecologic, and Neonatal Nursing, 28*(4), 389–394.

Gagnon, A. J., Dougherty, G., Jiminez, V., & Leduc, N. (2002). Randomized trial of postpartum care after hospital discharge. *Pediatrics, 109*(6), 1074–1080.

Gill, S. L. (2001). The little things: Perceptions of breastfeeding support. *Journal of Obstetric, Gynecologic, and Neonatal Nursing, 30*(4), 401–409.

Gotoff, S. P. (2000). Infections of the neonatal infant: Clinical syndromes. In R. E. Behrman, R. M. Kliegman, & H. B. Jenson, (Eds.), *Nelson textbook of pediatrics* (16th ed.) (pp. 544–552). Philadelphia: W.B. Saunders.

Hagen, R. L. (1999). Lanolin for sore nipples. *Archives of Pediatrics & Adolescent Medicine, 153*(6), 658.

Hale, T. (2002). *Medications and mothers' milk* (10th ed.). Amarillo, TX: Pharmasoft Medical.

International Lactation Consultant Association (ILCA). (1999). *Evidence-based guidelines for breastfeeding management during the first fourteen days.* Raleigh, NC: Author.

James, D. C. (2001). Postpartum care. In K. R. Simpson & P. A. Creehan, (Eds.), *AWHONN perinatal nursing* (2nd ed.) (pp. 446–472). Philadelphia: Lippincott.

Johnson, T. S., Brennan, R. A., & Flynn-Tymkow, C. D. (1999). A home visit program for breastfeeding education and support. *Journal of Obstetric, Gynecologic, and Neonatal Nursing, 28*(5), 480–485.

King, W. J., Klassen, T. P., LeBlanc, J., Bernard-Bonnin, A. C., Robitaille, Y., Pham, B., et al. (2001). The effectiveness of a home visit to prevent childhood injury. *Pediatrics, 108*, 382–388.

La Leche League International. (1999, September 30). *La Leche League International and co-sleeping expert find study to be inaccurate* (La Leche League Press Release). Schaumburg, IL: Author.

Lauwers, J., & Shinskie, D. (2000). *Counseling the nursing mother: A lactation consultant's guide* (3rd ed.). Boston: Jones & Bartlett.

Lee, K. A., & Zaffke, M. (1999). Longitudinal changes in fatigue and energy during pregnancy and the postpartum period. *Journal of Obstetric, Gynecologic, and Neonatal Nursing, 28*(2), 183–191.

Lieu, T. A., Braveman, P. A., Escobar, G. J., Fischer, A. F., Jensvold, N. G., & Capra, A. M., (2000). A randomized comparison of home and clinic follow-up visits after early postpartum hospital discharge. *Pediatrics, 105*(5), 1058–1065.

Locklin, M. P., & Jansson, M. J. (1999). Home visits: Strategies to protect the breastfeeding newborn at risk. *Journal of Obstetric, Gynecologic, and Neonatal Nursing, 28*(1), 33–40.

Lund, C. H., Osborne, J. W., Kuller, J., Lane, A. T., Lott, J. W., & Raines, D. A. (2001). Neonatal skin care: Clinical outcomes of the AWHONN/NANN evidence-based clinical practice guideline. *Journal of Obstetric, Gynecologic, and Neonatal Nursing, 30*(1), 41–45.

Martell, L. K. (2000). The hospital and the postpartum experience: A historical analysis. *Journal of Obstetric, Gynecologic, and Neonatal Nursing, 29*(1), 65–72.

McCarthy, P. L. (2000). Evaluation of the sick child in the office and clinic. In R. E. Behrman, R. M. Kliegman, & H. B. Jenson. (Eds.), *Nelson textbook of pediatrics* (16th ed.) (pp. 228–231). Philadelphia: W. B. Saunders.

Mendenhall, A. K., & Eichenfield, L. F. (2000). Back to basics: Caring for the newborn's skin. *Contemporary Pediatrics, 17*(8), 98–100, 103–104, 107–108.

Menella, J. A. (2002). Alcohol use during lactation: The folklore versus the science. In K. Auerbach (Ed.), *Current issues in clinical lactation: 2002* (pp. 3–9). Boston: Jones & Bartlett.

Neifert, M. R. (2001). Prevention of breastfeeding tragedies. *Pediatric Clinics of North America, 48*(2), 273–297.

Ortenstrand, A., Winbladh, B., Nordstrom, G., & Waldenstrom, U. (2001, October). Early discharge of preterm infants followed by domiciliary nursing care: Parents' anxiety, assessment of infant health and breastfeeding. *Acta Paediatrica, 90*(10), 1190–1195.

Pearson, J. (1999). Crying and calming: Important information and effective techniques to teach parents of full-term newborns. *Mother-Baby Journal, 4*, 39–42.

Riordan, J., & Auerbach, K. (1999). *Breastfeeding and human lactation* (2nd ed.). Boston: Jones & Bartlett.

Riordan, J., & Gill-Hopple, K. (2001). Breastfeeding care in multicultural populations. *Journal of Obstetric, Gynecologic, and Neonatal Nursing, 30*(2), 216–223.

Sganga, A., Wallace, R., Kiehl, E., Irving, T., & Witter, L. (2000). A comparison of four methods of normal newborn temperature measurement. *American Journal of Maternal Child Nursing, 25*(2), 76–79.

Shannon, M. (2001). Pediatricians, parents urged to stop using mercury thermometers. *AAP News, 19*(1), 21.

Simpson, K. R., Thorman, K. E., & Ropp, A. (2001). Managing the quality of care. In K. R. Simpson & P. A. Creehan (Eds.), *AWHONN perinatal nursing* (2nd ed.) (pp. 2–20). Philadelphia: Lippincott.

Thilo, E. H., & Rosenberg, A. A. (2001). The newborn infant. In W. W. Hay, A. R. Hayward, M. J. Levin, & J. M. Sondheimer, (Eds.), *Current pediatric diagnosis and treatment* (15th ed.) (pp. 1–59). New York: McGraw-Hill.

US Department of Health and Human Services. (2000). *Healthy people 2010* (conference edition, in two volumes). Washington, DC: Author.

Walker, M., & Creehan, P. (2001). Newborn nutrition. In K. R. Simpson, & P. Creehan, (Eds.), *AWHONN perinatal nursing* (2nd ed.) (pp. 550–574). Philadelphia: Lippincott.

Weissinger, D. (2002). Last step first. In K. Auerbach (Ed.), *Current issues in clinical lactation* (pp. 69–73). Boston: Jones & Bartlett.

Zinn, B. (2000). Supporting the employed breastfeeding mother. *Journal of Midwifery & Women's Health, 45*(3), 216–225.

The Postpartal Family at Risk 37

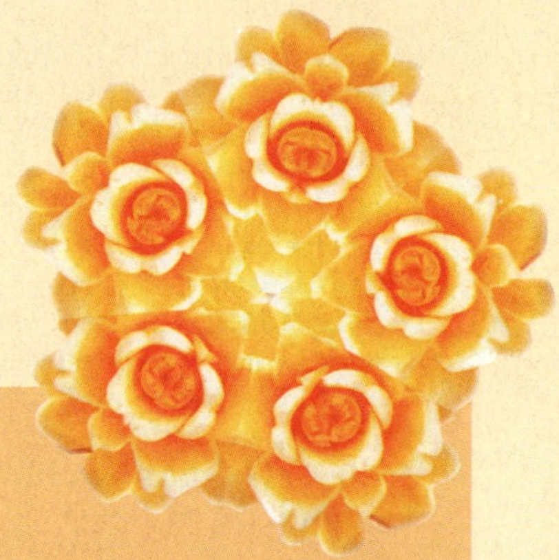

We are surviving. Just. Why don't they give the Croix de Guerre to people who can go without more than two hours total daily sleep for five weeks? I thought babies ate at six-ten-two-six-ten-two—mine does. He also eats at five-seven-nine-eleven and four-eight-twelve. I am getting rather used to going around with my breasts hanging out. They are either drying from the last feed or getting ready for the next one. But the love—I never knew, never imagined that I would love him like this. This incredible feeling of boundless, endless love—a wish to protect his innocence from ever being hurt or wounded or scratched. And that awful, horrible, mad feeling in the first week that you'll never be able to keep anything so precious and so vulnerable alive.

~ THE NEW OUR BODIES, OURSELVES ~

Objectives

- Describe assessment of the woman for predisposing factors, signs, and symptoms of various postpartum complications to facilitate early and effective management of complications.
- Incorporate preventive measures for various complications of the postpartal period into nursing care of the postpartum woman.
- List the causes of and appropriate nursing interventions for hemorrhage during the postpartal period.
- Develop a nursing care plan that reflects a knowledge of etiology, pathophysiology, and current clinical management for the woman experiencing postpartal hemorrhage, reproductive tract infection, urinary tract infection, mastitis, thromboembolic disease, or a postpartal psychiatric disorder.
- Evaluate the mother's knowledge of self-care measures, signs of complications to be reported to the primary care provider, and measures to prevent recurrence of complications.
- Describe the role of telephone follow-up and home care in the extended care of postpartal families at risk.

Key Terms

Early postpartal hemorrhage 1075
Late postpartal hemorrhage 1075
Mastitis 1090
Metritis (endometritis) 1082
Pelvic cellulitis (parametritis) 1083
Peritonitis 1083
Postpartum blues (adjustment reaction with depressed mood) 1100
Postpartum depression (postpartum major mood disorder) 1101
Postpartum psychosis 1100
Puerperal infection 1082
Puerperal morbidity 1082
Subinvolution 1079
Thrombophlebitis 1093
Uterine atony 1075

MEDIALINK

Additional resources for this content can be found on the Student CD-ROM and on the Companion Website at www.prenhall.com/olds. Click on "Chapter 37" to select the activities for this chapter.

CD-ROM
- Audio Glossary
- NCLEX Review

Companion Website
- Additional NCLEX Review
- Case Study: Postpartal Thromboembolic Disease
- Care Plan Activity: Postpartal Perineal Pain

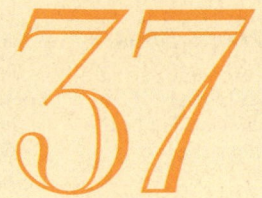

The postpartal period is typically seen as a smooth, uneventful time that follows the anticipation of pregnancy and the excitement and work of labor and birth—and often it is. However, it is important for the nurse to be aware of problems that may develop postpartally, and to teach the family the signs of postpartal complications; findings to report to the physician or certified nurse-midwife; and preventive measures, if available. Written instructions to supplement any discussion will be of great value in the early weeks at home with a newborn, when life can be chaotic and verbal instructions may be forgotten. The family should have telephone numbers for postpartum follow-up services and other resources for getting answers to questions. By communicating an attitude of willingness to answer questions and listen to concerns, the nurse enhances the family's comfort in making calls later for what they might otherwise perceive as "too trivial to bother someone about."

When a telephone follow-up or an examination at the home visit provides evidence of a developing complication, the nurse shares these findings or impressions with the woman, and they mutually plan an appropriate next step. In the case of telephone follow-up, the nurse usually counsels the woman to notify her physician or certified nurse-midwife, being prepared to schedule an appointment immediately if risk assessment indicates. The nurse who identifies a complication at the home visit will need to communicate the clinical findings to the physician or certified nurse-midwife and document them and any interventions for the permanent record. Complications, by their very nature, suggest the need for immediate collaborative management.

The most common complications of the postpartal period are hemorrhage, infection, thromboembolic disease, and postpartum psychiatric disorders. These are the focus of this chapter.

Care of the Woman with Postpartal Hemorrhage

Hemorrhage in the postpartum period is described as either early (immediate) or late (delayed) postpartal hemorrhage. **Early postpartal hemorrhage** occurs in the first 24 hours after childbirth. **Late postpartal hemorrhage** occurs from 24 hours to 6 weeks after birth. Postpartal hemorrhage continues to be a cause of significant maternal mortality and morbidity and accounts for 10.5% of maternal deaths attributable to pregnancy-related hemorrhage in the United States (Andersen & Hopkins, 2002).

The traditional definition of postpartal hemorrhage has been a blood loss of greater than 500 mL following childbirth. This definition is being questioned, because careful quantification indicates that the average blood loss in a vaginal birth is actually greater than 500 mL, and the average blood loss after cesarean childbirth exceeds 1000 mL (Benedetti, 2002). Clinical estimates of blood loss tend to underestimate actual loss by up to 50%. Some clinicians believe that postpartal hemorrhage can be objectively and reliably defined as a decrease in the hematocrit of 10 points between the time of admission and the time postbirth, or the need for blood transfusion following childbirth. Clinical estimation of blood loss at childbirth may be difficult because blood mixes with amniotic fluid and is obscured as it oozes onto sterile drapes or is sponged away; without vigilance, it may be difficult over the next hours to appreciate the significance of slow, steady blood loss. As the amount of blood loss increases, as in the case of hemorrhage, estimates are likely to be even less accurate. Moreover, postpartal hemorrhage may occur intra-abdominally, into the broad ligament, or into hematomas arising from genital tract trauma, wherein the blood loss is concealed. Given the increased blood volume of pregnancy, the clinical signs of hemorrhage—such as decreased blood pressure, increasing pulse, and decreasing urinary output—do not appear until as much as 1800 to 2100 mL has been lost, shortly before the woman becomes hemodynamically unstable (Gilbert & Harmon, 2003).

Clinical Tip *Women who are natural redheads tend to experience heavier bleeding after childbirth.*

Early Postpartal Hemorrhage

At term, blood volume and cardiac output have increased so that 20% of cardiac output, or 600 mL per minute, perfuses the pregnant uterus, supporting the developing fetus. When the placenta separates from the uterine wall, the many uterine vessels that have carried blood to and from the placenta are severed abruptly. The normal mechanism for hemostasis after birth of the placenta is contraction of the interlacing uterine muscles to occlude the open sinuses that previously brought blood into the placenta. Absence of prompt and sustained uterine contraction (uterine atony) can cause significant blood loss. Other causes of postpartal hemorrhage include laceration of the genital tract; episiotomy; retained placental fragments; vulvar, vaginal, or subperitoneal hematomas; uterine inversion; uterine rupture; problems of placental implantation; and coagulation disorders.

UTERINE ATONY

Uterine atony (relaxation of the uterus) is a common cause of early postpartum hemorrhage (Cunningham, Gant, Leveno, et al, 2001). Although uterine atony can occur after any childbirth, its contributing factors include the following:

- Overdistention of the uterus due to multiple gestation, hydramnios, or a large infant (macrosomia)
- Dysfunctional or prolonged labor, which indicates that the uterus is contracting abnormally
- Oxytocin augmentation or induction of labor
- Grandmultiparity, because stretched uterine musculature contracts less vigorously

- Use of anesthesia (especially halothane) or other drugs such as magnesium sulfate or terbutaline (Brethine), which cause the uterus to relax
- Prolonged third stage of labor—more than 30 minutes
- Preeclampsia
- Asian or Hispanic heritage
- Operative birth
- Retained placental fragments
- Placenta previa

Hemorrhage from uterine atony may be slow and steady or sudden and massive. The blood may escape vaginally or collect in the uterus, evident as large clots. The uterine cavity may distend with up to 1000 mL or more of blood while the perineal pad and linen protectors remain suspiciously dry. A treacherous feature of postpartal hemorrhage is that maternal blood pressure and pulse may not change until significant blood loss has occurred because of the increased blood volume associated with pregnancy. The woman with preeclampsia is an exception to this finding because she does not have the normal hypervolemia of pregnancy and cannot tolerate even normal postchildbirth blood loss (Cunningham et al, 2001).

Ideally, postpartal hemorrhage is prevented, beginning with adequate prenatal care, good nutrition, avoidance of traumatic procedures, risk assessment, early recognition, and management of complications as they arise. Any woman at risk should be typed and cross-matched for blood and have intravenous lines in place with needles suitable for blood transfusion (18-gauge minimum). Excellent labor management and childbirth techniques are imperative.

After expulsion of the placenta, the fundus is palpated to ensure that it is firmly contracted. If it is not firm, fundal massage is performed until the uterus contracts. Fundal massage is painful for the woman who has not received regional anesthesia; she will need explanations for why this uncomfortable procedure is necessary and support as massage is initiated. If bleeding is excessive, the clinician will likely order intravenous oxytocin at a rapid infusion rate and may elect to do a bimanual massage (Figure 37–1 ●). Other uterine stimulants may be necessary to manage postpartal uterine atony. Table 37–1 ● summarizes critical nursing information about the use of uterine stimulants. The need for intravenous fluid replacement and blood transfusion is determined on the basis of hemoglobin and hematocrit results.

In addition to the previously described measures, severe uncontrolled hemorrhage may require radiographic-guided embolization of the pelvic vessels (Benedetti, 2002). Ligation of the uterine vessel may be used to slow blood loss and allow normal clotting mechanisms to occur (Benedetti, 2002). Hysterectomy may be necessary to control hemorrhage but is usually reserved as a last resort for women of high parity when other measures have failed and excessive bleeding has become life threatening. Uterine packing, common in the past in cases of postpartum hemorrhage, is no longer advocated because it dilates the uterine cavity and may actually increase bleeding.

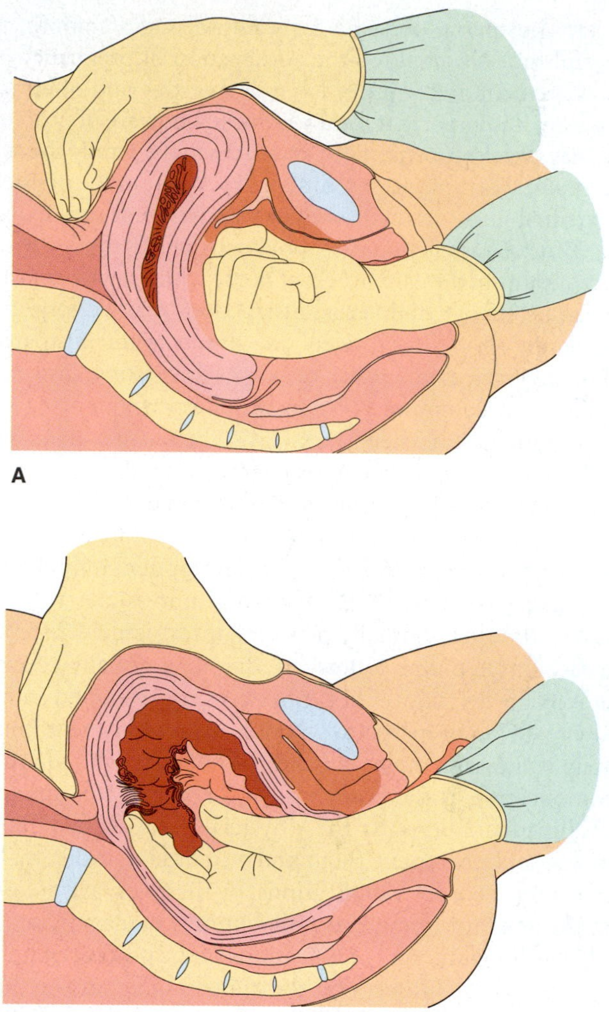

A

B

Figure 37–1 ● *A,* Manual compression of the uterus and massage with the abdominal hand usually will effectively control hemorrhage from uterine atony. *B,* Manual removal of placenta. The fingers are alternately abducted, adducted, and advanced until the placenta is completely detached. Both procedures are performed only by the medical clinician.

SOURCE: Adapted from Cunningham, F. G., MacDonald, P. C., & Gant, N. F. (Eds.). (1989). *Williams obstetrics* (18th ed., pp. 417–418). Norwalk, CT: Appleton & Lange.

LACERATIONS OF THE GENITAL TRACT

Early postpartum hemorrhage is associated with lacerations of the perineum, vagina, or cervix. Several factors predispose women to higher risk of reproductive tract lacerations:

- Nulliparity
- Epidural anesthesia
- Precipitous childbirth
- Macrosomia
- Forceps- or vacuum-assisted birth

Thorough inspection of the genital tract by the birth attendant allows recognition and timely repair of most lacerations. Genital tract lacerations should be suspected

Table 37-1 • UTERINE STIMULANTS USED TO PREVENT AND MANAGE UTERINE ATONY

Drug	Dosing Information	Contraindications	Expected Effects	Side Effects
Oxytocin (Pitocin, Syntocinon)	IV use: 10–40 units in 500–1000 mL crystalloid fluid @ 50 m U/min administration rate. Onset: immediate. Duration: 1 h. **IV bolus administration not recommended.** IM use: 10–20 units. Onset: 3–5 min. Duration: 2–3 h.		Rhythmic uterine contractions that help to prevent or reverse postpartal hemorrhage caused by uterine atony.	Uterine hyperstimulation, mild transient hypertension, water intoxication rare in postpartum use.
Methylergonovine maleate (Methergine)	IM use: 0.2 mg q2–4h. Onset: 2–5 min. Duration: 3 h (× 5 dose maximum). PO use: 0.2 mg q6–12h. Onset: 7–15 min. Duration: 3 h (× 1 week). **IV administration not recommended.**	Women with labile or high blood pressure or known sensitivity to drug.	Sustained uterine contractions that help to prevent or reverse postpartal hemorrhage caused by uterine atony; management of postpartal subinvolution.	Hypertension, dizziness, headache, flushing/hot flashes, tinnitus, nausea and vomiting, palpitations, chest pain. Overdose or hypersensitivity is recognized by seizures; tingling and numbness of fingers and toes from vasoconstrictive effect, leading rarely to gangrene; hypertension; weak pulse; chest pain.
Ergonovine maleate (Ergotrate Maleate)	IM use: 0.2 mg q2–4h. Onset 7 min. Duration: 3 h (5 dose maximum). PO use: 0.2 mg q6–12h. Onset: 15 min. Duration: 3 h (× 2–7 days). **IV administration not recommended.**	Women with labile or high blood pressure or known sensitivity to drug.	Sustained uterine contractions that help to prevent or reverse postpartal hemorrhage caused by uterine atony; management of postpartal subinvolution.	Hypertension, dizziness, headache, nausea and vomiting, chest pain. Hypersensitivity is noted by systemic vasoconstrictive effects: seizure, chest pain, and tingling and numbness of fingers and toes that leads rarely to gangrene.
Prostaglandin ($PGF_{2\alpha}$, Hemabate, Prostin/15M)	IM use: 0.25 mg repeated up to maximum 5 doses; may be repeated q15–90min. Physician may elect to administer by direct intramyometrial injection.	Women with active cardiovascular, renal, liver disease, or asthma or with known hypersensitivity to drug.	Control of refractory cases of postpartal hemorrhage caused by uterine atony; generally used after failed attempts at control of hemorrhage with oxytocic agents.	Nausea, vomiting, diarrhea, headache, flushing, bradycardia, bronchospasm, wheezing, cough, chills, fever.

Implications for Nursing Management of the Postpartal Woman Receiving Uterine Stimulants

- Assess fundus for evidence of contraction and amount of uterine bleeding at least q10–15min × 1–2 h after administration, then q30–60min until stable. **More frequent assessments are determined by the woman's condition or by orders of the physician or certified nurse-midwife.**
- Weigh pads to estimate blood loss.
- Monitor blood pressure and pulse q15min for at least 1 h after administration, then q30–60min until stable.
- Note expected duration of action of drug being administered, and take care to recheck fundus at that time.
- When the drug is ineffective, the fundus remains atonic (boggy or uncontracted) and bleeding continues, massage the fundus. If massage fails to cause sustained contraction, notify the physician or certified nurse-midwife immediately.
- Monitor woman for signs of known side effects of the drug; report to physician or certified nurse-midwife if side effects occur.
- Remind the woman and her support person that uterine cramping is an expected result of these drugs and that medication is available for discomfort. Administer analgesic medications as needed for pain relief. Provide nonpharmacologic comfort measures. If analgesic medication ordered is insufficient for pain relief, notify the physician or certified nurse-midwife.

When Prostaglandin Is Used

- Check temperature q1–2h and/or after chill. Administer antipyretic medication as ordered for prostaglandin-induced fever.
- Auscultate breath sounds frequently for signs of adverse respiratory effects.
- Assess for nausea, vomiting, and diarrhea. Administer antiemetic and antidiarrheal medications as ordered. (In some settings, women are premedicated with these drugs.)

when vaginal bleeding persists in the presence of a firmly contracted uterus. The nurse who suspects a laceration should notify the clinician so that the laceration can be immediately sutured to control hemorrhage and repair the integrity of the reproductive tract (Andersen & Hopkins, 2002).

Episiotomies can be a source of postpartal blood loss. Episiotomy is an underappreciated source because of slow, steady bleeding. The risk for bleeding is increased with mediolateral episiotomies.

Nurses who care for postpartum clients are wise to appreciate that most deaths from postpartum hemorrhage are not due to gross bleeding but to ineffective management of slow, steady blood loss.

RETAINED PLACENTAL FRAGMENTS

Retained placental fragments may be a cause of early postpartal hemorrhage and are also the most common cause of late hemorrhage. Retention of fragments is usually attributable to partial separation of the placenta during massage of the fundus prior to spontaneous placental separation, so this practice should be avoided.

Following birth, the placenta should always be inspected for intactness and evidence of missing fragments or cotyledons on the maternal side and for vessels that traverse to the edge of the placenta outward along the membranes of the fetal side, which may indicate succenturiate placenta and a retained lobe. Uterine exploration may be required at that time to remove missing fragments. (Figure 37–1B.) This cause should be immediately suspected if bleeding persists and no lacerations are noted. Sonography may be used to diagnose retained placental fragments. Curettage, formerly standard treatment, is now thought by some to traumatize the implantation site, thereby increasing bleeding and the potential for uterine adhesions. It may be necessitated by the degree of hemorrhage, however (Cunningham et al, 2001).

VULVAR, VAGINAL, AND PELVIC HEMATOMAS

Hematomas occur as a result of injury to a blood vessel from birth trauma, often without noticeable trauma to the superficial tissue, or from inadequate hemostasis at the site of repair of an incision or laceration. The soft tissue in the area offers little resistance, and hematomas containing 250 to 500 mL of blood may develop rapidly. Hematomas may be vulvar (involving branches of the pudendal artery), vaginal (especially in the area of the ischial spines), vulvovaginal, or subperitoneal. The latter are rare but most dangerous because of the large amount of blood loss that can occur without clinical symptoms until the woman becomes hemodynamically unstable. Subperitoneal hematomas involve the uterine artery branches or vessels in the broad ligaments.

Risk factors for hematomas include the following: preeclampsia, use of pudendal anesthesia, first full-term birth, precipitous labor, prolonged second stage of labor, macrosomia, forceps- or vacuum-assisted births, and history of vulvar varicosities. Frequent assessment of the perineum of the woman under the effects of regional anesthesia is important. Once the effects of anesthesia have subsided, vaginal and vulvar hematomas are generally associated with perineal pain, often intense and out of proportion to what seems apparent in the area. If the hematoma is localized in the posterior vaginal area, rectal pressure may also be a presenting complaint. Hematomas that develop in the upper vagina may cause difficulty voiding because of pressure against the urinary meatus or urethra. Rather than automatically attributing complaints of perineal pain to the presence of an episiotomy, the nurse should examine the perineal area for signs of hematomas: ecchymosis, edema, tenseness of tissue overlying the hematoma, a fluctuant mass bulging at the introitus, and extreme tenderness to palpation. Estimating the size on first assessment of the perineum enables the nurse to better identify increases in size and the potential blood loss. The nurse notifies the physician or certified nurse-midwife if a hematoma is suspected.

Hematomas less than 5 cm in size and nonexpanding are managed expectantly with ice packs and analgesia. They usually resolve over several days. For larger hematomas and those that expand, surgical management is usually required: the hematoma is evacuated, the bleeding vessel ligated, and the wound closed, with or without a vaginal packing. An indwelling urinary catheter may be necessary for 24 to 36 hours because voiding may be impossible with a vaginal pack in place (Benedetti, 2002).

The initial sign of subperitoneal hematoma may be hypovolemic shock; however, the woman may also complain of severe pelvic pain, flank pain, or abdominal distention. A parametrial mass may be identified on bimanual examination. Expectant management with serial ultrasonography and hematocrit may be possible. In rare cases, angiographic embolization or ligation of the hypogastric vessels may be required to manage the hemorrhage associated with postpartal hematomas.

The hematoma site is an ideal medium for proliferation of flora normally present in the genital tract. Consequently, broad-spectrum antibiotics are usually ordered to prevent infection or abscess.

The nurse can decrease the risk of vulvar or vaginal hematoma by applying an ice pack to the woman's perineum during the first hour after birth and intermittently thereafter for the next 8 to 12 hours. If a hematoma develops despite preventive measures, a sitz bath after the first 12 hours will aid fluid absorption once bleeding has stopped and will promote comfort, as will the judicious use of analgesic agents.

UTERINE INVERSION

Uterine inversion, a prolapse of the uterine fundus to or through the cervix so that the uterus is, in effect, turned inside out after birth, is a rare (the incidence is 1 in 2000 or more) but life-threatening cause of postpartal hemorrhage (Benedetti, 2002). Although not always preventable, uterine inversion is often associated with these factors: fundal implantation or abnormal adherence of the placenta, weakness of the uterine musculature or other uterine abnormalities, protracted labor, uterine relaxation secondary to anesthesia or drugs such as magnesium sulfate, and excess traction on the umbilical cord or vigorous manual removal of the placenta.

UTERINE RUPTURE

Spontaneous rupture of the uterus is rare in the United States but continues to be seen in developing countries where emergency surgery for obstructed labors may be less immediately accessible. The woman with a ruptured uterus will have acute, severe abdominal pain, with minimal to diffuse external bleeding. Concealed hemorrhage may occur in the abdominal cavity or broad ligaments, undetected until the woman becomes symptomatic from hypovolemic shock. Risk factors for uterine rupture include prior uterine surgery, including cesarean birth; fetal malpresentation; grandmultiparity; operative vaginal birth; and oxytocic induction of labor. With uterine rupture, immediate surgery is required with fluid and blood replacement as needed (Toppenberg & Block, 2002).

ABNORMAL PLACENTAL IMPLANTATION

Normally, a layer of decidual tissue separates the proliferating placental villi from the myometrium at the site of placental implantation. A defect in the formation of this decidual layer, possibly related to a poor blood supply, can contribute to a placenta that directly adheres to the myometrium (placenta accreta) or penetrates deeply into the myometrium (placenta increta). See Chapter 27. Abnormally adherent placentas are rare in normal pregnancies but occur in 5% of women with placenta previa, especially those with cesarean births. Placenta accreta accounts for 80% of retained placental fragments (Alexander & Schneider, 2000). Even if successfully removed, uncontrollable hemorrhage is possible; as a result, this complication is often associated with emergency hysterectomy (Alexander & Schneider, 2000).

COAGULATION DISORDERS (COAGULOPATHIES)

Coagulopathies should be suspected when postpartal bleeding persists with no identifiable cause (Benedetti, 2002). Preexisting coagulation defects, such as von Willebrand disease and idiopathic thrombocytopenic purpura, should have been identified prenatally and managed in consultation with a hematologist. A consumptive coagulopathy such as disseminated intravascular coagulation (DIC) may occur during pregnancy as a result of preeclampsia, amniotic fluid embolism, sepsis, abruptio placentae, or prolonged intrauterine fetal demise syndrome. Coagulopathy can also result from excessive blood loss (Gilbert & Harmon, 2003). Oozing from a puncture site or development of petechiae may be initial clues of coagulopathy. Coagulation studies (prothrombin time, partial thromboplastin time, platelet count, fibrinogen level, and fibrin split products) should be assessed immediately (Gilbert & Harmon, 2003).

Late Postpartal Hemorrhage

Although early postpartal hemorrhage most often occurs within hours of birth, delayed hemorrhage occurs most often within 1 to 2 weeks after childbirth, most frequently as a result of subinvolution of the placental site or retention of placental tissue. Blood loss at this time may be excessive but rarely poses the same risk as that from immediate postpartal hemorrhage. The incidence of late postpartum hemorrhage is 0.7% (Cash & Glass, 2000).

The site of placental implantation is always the last area of the uterus to regenerate after childbirth. In the case of subinvolution, adjacent endometrium and the decidua basalis fail to regenerate to cover the placental site. Deficiency of immunologic factors has been implicated as a cause. Faulty implantation in the less vascular lower uterine segment, retention of placental tissue, or infection may contribute to subinvolution. With **subinvolution,** the postpartum fundal height is greater than expected. In addition, lochia often fails to progress from rubra to serosa to alba normally. Lochia rubra that persists longer than 2 weeks postpartum is highly suggestive of subinvolution (Cunningham et al, 2001). Some women report scant brown lochia or irregular heavy bleeding. Leukorrhea, backache, and foul lochia may occur if infection is a cause. There may be a history of heavy early postpartal bleeding or difficulty in expulsion of the placenta.

When portions of the placenta have been retained in the uterus, bleeding continues because normal uterine contraction that constricts the bleeding site is prohibited. Presence of placental tissue within the uterus can be confirmed by pelvic ultrasonography. Occasionally the placental fragment becomes necrotic over time and, when it separates from the uterus, hemorrhage occurs suddenly.

Subinvolution is most commonly diagnosed during the routine postpartal examination at 4 to 6 weeks. The woman may relate a history of irregular or excessive bleeding or describe the symptoms listed previously. An enlarged, softer than normal uterus, palpated bimanually, is an objective indication of subinvolution. Treatment includes oral administration of methylergonovine maleate (Methergine) 0.2 mg orally every 3 to 4 hours for 24 to 48 hours (see Drug Guide: Methergine, in Chapter 35). When uterine infection is present, antibiotics are also administered. The woman is reevaluated in 2 weeks. If retained placenta is suspected or other treatment is ineffective, curettage may be indicated (Cunningham et al, 2001).

NURSING CARE MANAGEMENT

Nursing Assessment and Diagnosis

Careful and ongoing assessment of the woman during labor and birth and evaluation of her prenatal history will help identify factors that put her at risk for postpartal hemorrhage. Following birth, periodic assessment for evidence of bleeding is a major nursing responsibility. Regular and frequent assessment of fundal height and evidence of uterine tone or contractility will alert the nurse to the possible development or recurrence of hemorrhage. Careful observation and documentation of vaginal bleeding are important to determine whether further medical intervention is needed. This assessment can be done visually, by pad counts, or by weighing the perineal pads. Nursing diagnoses that may apply when a woman experiences postpartal hemorrhage include the following:

- ***Health Seeking Behaviors*** related to lack of information about signs of delayed postpartal hemorrhage
- ***Fluid Volume Deficit*** related to blood loss secondary to uterine atony, lacerations, hematomas, coagulation disorders, or retained placental fragments

MediaLink
CARE PLAN: POSTPARTAL PERINEAL PAIN

Nursing Plan and Implementation

If the nurse detects a soft, boggy uterus, it is massaged until firm. If the uterus is not contracting well and appears larger than anticipated, the nurse may express clots during fundal massage. Once clots are removed, the uterus tends to contract more effectively.

If the woman seems to have a slow, steady, free flow of blood, the nurse begins weighing the perineal pads (1mL = 1g) and monitors the woman's vital signs at least every 15 minutes—more frequently if indicated. If the fundus is displaced upward or to one side because of a full bladder, the nurse encourages the woman to empty her bladder—or catheterizes her if she is unable to void—to allow for efficient uterine contractions.

When there are risk factors for postpartal hemorrhage or frequent fundal massage has been necessary to sustain uterine contractions, the nurse should maintain the vascular access (IV) initiated during labor in case additional fluid or blood becomes necessary. Sometimes physicians and certified nurse-midwives write orders that specify "discontinue IV after present bottle." The astute postpartum nurse will assess the consistency of the fundus and the presence of normal versus excessive lochia prior to discontinuing the infusion. If the assessments are not reassuring, the nurse continues the IV and notifies the physician or certified nurse-midwife.

> **Clinical Tip** *As you know, bogginess indicates that the uterus is not contracting well, which results in increased uterine bleeding. This blood may remain in the uterus and form clots or may result in increased flow. In assessing the amount of blood loss, you must first massage the uterus until it is firm and then express clots. Don't be misled by the fact that a woman has a firm uterus. Significant bleeding can occur from causes other than uterine atony. To accurately determine the amount of blood loss, it is not sufficient to assess only the peri-pad. You should also ask the woman to turn on her side so you can assess underneath her for pooling of blood.*

In most settings, postpartum collection of blood for hemoglobin and hematocrit determination is routine. The nurse reviews these findings when available, compares them to the admission baseline, and notifies the physician or certified nurse-midwife if the hematocrit has decreased by 10 points or more. In cases where there is risk of postpartal hemorrhage and blood has been cross-matched earlier, the nurse checks that blood is available in the blood bank.

The nurse evaluates the woman for signs of anemia, such as fatigue, pallor, headache, thirst, and orthostatic changes in pulse or blood pressure, and reviews the results of all hematocrit determinations. All medical interventions, intravenous infusions, blood transfusions, oxygen therapy, and medications such as uterine stimulants are monitored as necessary and evaluated for effectiveness. Urinary output should be monitored to determine adequacy of fluid replacement and renal perfusion, with amounts less than 30 mL per hour reported to the physician. The nurse also helps the woman plan activities so that adequate rest is possible.

The woman who is experiencing anemia and fatigue related to hemorrhage may need assistance with self-care and progressive ambulation for several days. When she is able to be out of bed to shower, use of a shower chair permits independence while providing a measure of safety should the woman experience weakness or dizziness. The emergency call light should be easily accessible.

The mother may find it difficult to care for her baby because of the fatigue associated with blood loss. The nurse can often find ways to promote attachment while still recognizing the health needs of the mother. The mother may require additional assistance in caring for her infant. If she has intravenous lines in place, even carrying the newborn may be awkward. For the mother who feels compelled to do as much as possible, the nurse may also need to "give permission" to the mother to return her infant to the nursery so she can have adequate periods of uninterrupted rest.

If the father of the child is involved in the birth experience, including him in the plan of care is a productive strategy. He supports the mother's recovery by helping to meet her physical needs while encouraging her to rest. The mother is likely to feel less concern over her limited opportunities for newborn care if she can witness the father's interactions with and care for the newborn. The couple may wish for arrangements to be made for the father to stay in the hospital room, sleeping on a cot and eating with the mother so that limited rooming-in with the newborn is still an option. In that way, even if the mother is too fatigued to care for the infant, she can enjoy the infant's presence and initiate bonding. The extent to which the father becomes involved with the care of the mother and baby must be carefully balanced with his need to be rested for the extra responsibilities he will assume when his partner and newborn child are discharged from the hospital.

Teaching for Self-Care

The woman and her family or other support persons should receive clear, preferably written, explanations of the normal postpartal course, including changes in the lochia and fundus and signs of abnormal bleeding. Instructions for the prevention of bleeding should include fundal massage, ways to assess the fundal height and consistency, and inspection of the episiotomy and lacerations, if present. The woman should receive instruction in perineal care. The woman and her family are advised to contact their caregiver if any of the following occur: excessive or bright red bleeding (saturation of more than one pad per hour), a boggy fundus that does not respond to massage, abnormal clots, leukorrhea, high temperature, or any unusual pelvic or rectal discomfort or backache. See Table 37–2 •. If iron supplementation is ordered, instructions for proper dosage should be provided in order to enhance absorption and avoid constipation and nausea.

Table 37-2 • SIGNS OF POSTPARTAL HEMORRHAGE
Excessive or bright red bleeding
A boggy fundus that does not respond to massage
Abnormal clots
Any unusual pelvic discomfort or backache
Persistent bleeding in the presence of a firmly contracted uterus
Rise in the level of the fundus of the uterus
Increased pulse or decreased BP
Hematoma formation or bulging/shiny skin in the perineal area
Decreased level of consciousness

Community-Based Nursing Care

For most postpartal women, routine discharge instructions include advice such as: "You take care of the baby, and let someone else care for you, the family, and the household." Because of her fatigue and weakened condition, the woman who experienced postpartal hemorrhage may be unable even to care for her newborn unassisted. The caregivers at home need clear, concise explanations of her condition and needs for recovery. For example, all should understand the woman's need to rest and to be given extra time to rest after any necessary activity.

To ensure her safety, the woman should be advised to rise slowly to minimize the likelihood of orthostatic hypotension. Until she regains strength, the mother should be seated when holding the newborn.

The person who assumes responsibility for grocery shopping and meal preparation will need advice about the importance of including foods high in iron in the daily menus. Having the woman indicate her preferences from a list of such foods will promote cooperation with the diet. The nurse also explains the rationale for continuing medications containing iron.

The woman should continue to count perineal pads for several days so she can recognize any recurring problem with excessive blood loss. The debilitated condition and anemia associated with hemorrhage increase the woman's risk of puerperal infection. She and her caregivers should use good handwashing technique and minimize exposure to infection in the home. They should be given a list of signs of infection and should understand the importance of alerting the physician immediately should signs occur.

A sense of emergency often exists in the event of late postpartal hemorrhage. Because it commonly occurs 1 to 2 weeks after birth, the couple is generally at home, involved in the day-to-day activities demanded by their new roles, when the unexpected, excessive bleeding begins. Quick decisions about child care arrangements must often be made so that the mother can return to the hospital. Both mother and father are likely to be alarmed by the excessive bleeding and concerned about her prognosis. There will be additional worries about separation from the newborn, especially when the mother is breastfeeding. The father may find himself torn between the needs of the mother and those of the newborn. Ideally, arrangements can be made to minimize separation of the family members.

In addition to meeting the woman's physical needs, the nurse will assess the couple for impending crisis by addressing these factors: (1) What is their perception of the current situation? Is the perception realistic? (2) What coping strategies have been helpful in previous difficult circumstances? Are they in use at this time, and are they effective? (3) What degree of support do they have from significant others? Do they have necessary resources? Providing realistic information, offering to call those in their support network, and exploring effective coping strategies can be of immeasurable value as they try to maintain a sense of balance in this difficult situation.

Evaluation

Expected outcomes of nursing care include:

- Signs of postpartal hemorrhage are detected quickly and managed effectively.
- Maternal-infant attachment is maintained successfully.
- The woman is able to identify abnormal changes that might occur following discharge and understands the importance of notifying her caregiver if they develop.

Care of the Woman with a Reproductive Tract Infection or Wound Infection

Because shortened inpatient stays are the norm in maternity care, women will be discharged following childbirth before clinical signs of puerperal infection are evident. Consequently, hospital-based nurses are challenged to analyze the woman's history and clinical course for risk assessment and to recognize the sometimes early subtle signs of infection so that discharge may be delayed as needed. Prior to discharge, the nurse advises the postpartal woman about preventive measures and signs of infection. Community and home care nurses review the prenatal and birth record for continuity of risk assessment, conduct physical assessment for objective findings of infection, collect specimens as ordered for diagnosing infection, and collaborate with the primary caregiver in managing infection.

Obviously, postpartal women are at risk for both genital and other sources of infection. A thorough history, including antepartal and intrapartal risk assessments, helps differentiate the site of infection, including the possibility of exposure to illness prior to admission in labor. When fever occurs, the physical examination should include the pharynx, neck, lungs, costovertebral angle (CVA) region, breasts, abdomen, extremities, IV sites, and incisions. The timing of fever also helps in differentiating the source of infection: atelectasis generally occurs within the first 48 hours; pneumonia or urinary tract infection usually occurs within 72 hours after childbirth; and wound infections and septic thrombophlebitis are likely to occur at 3 to 7 days postpartum, with wound abscess formation at 7 to 14 days. Postpartum infections develop in

1% to 7% of women, accounting for more than 200,000 infections annually in the United States (Gravett, 2002).

Puerperal infection is an infection of the reproductive tract associated with childbirth that occurs at any time up to 6 weeks postpartum. The most common postpartal infection is metritis (endometritis), which is limited to the uterus. Indeed, the cause of postpartal fever is presumed to be metritis until proven otherwise. However, infection can spread by way of the lymphatic system and circulatory system to become a progressive disease resulting in parametrial cellulitis and peritonitis. The woman's prognosis is directly related to the stage of the disease at the time of diagnosis, the causative organism, and the state of her health and immune system.

The standard definition of **puerperal morbidity** established in the 1930s by the Joint Committee on Maternal Welfare is a temperature of 38C (100.4F) or higher, with the temperature occurring on any 2 of the first 10 days postpartum, exclusive of the first 24 hours, and when taken by mouth by a standard technique at least four times a day. However, serious infections can occur in the first 24 hours or may cause only persistent low-grade temperatures. Therefore, careful assessment of all postpartal women with elevated temperatures is essential.

Antibiotic therapy alone has not caused the decrease in postpartal morbidity and mortality that is seen today. Aseptic technique, fewer traumatic operative births, a better understanding of labor dystocia, improved surgical intervention, and a population that is generally at less risk from malnutrition and chronic debilitative disease have also contributed to this reduction.

The vagina and cervix of approximately 70% of all healthy pregnant women contain pathogenic bacteria that, alone or in combination, are sufficiently virulent to cause extensive infections. Why the organisms do not cause infection during pregnancy is not altogether clear; possibly the acidic vaginal pH of pregnancy prevents overgrowth of vaginal flora. In the postpartum, the vaginal pH becomes alkaline, favoring growth of aerobes; however, recent studies indicate that more than the presence of a pathogen in the woman's reproductive tract is necessary for infection to begin.

Although the uterus is considered a sterile cavity prior to rupture of the fetal membranes, bacterial contamination of amniotic fluid with the membranes still intact at term is more common than previously believed and may contribute to premature labor. Following rupture of the membranes and during labor, contamination of the uterine cavity by vaginal or cervical bacteria can easily occur. Despite that finding, uterine infections are relatively uncommon following uncomplicated vaginal births. They continue to be a major source of morbidity for women who give birth by cesarean.

Postpartal Uterine Infection

Postpartal uterine infection is known variously as metritis, endometritis, endomyometritis, and endoparametritis. Because the infection involves the decidual lining of the uterus, the myometrium, and parametrial tissue, some authorities are proposing the terminology *metritis with parametrial cellulitis* (Cunningham et al, 2001). Risk factors for postpartal uterine infection include the following:

- Cesarean birth is the single most significant risk (20 times greater than in vaginal births) (Baxley, 2001)
- Prolonged premature rupture of the amniotic membranes (PROM)
- Prolonged labor preceding cesarean birth
- Multiple vaginal examinations during labor
- Compromised health status (low socioeconomic status, anemia, obesity, smoking, use of illicit drugs or alcohol)
- Use of fetal scalp electrode or intrauterine pressure catheter for internal monitoring during labor
- Obstetric trauma—episiotomy, laceration of perineum, vagina, or cervix
- Chorioamnionitis
- Preexisting bacterial vaginosis or *Chlamydia trachomatis* infection
- Instrument-assisted childbirth—vacuum or forceps
- Manual removal of the placenta
- Lapses in aseptic technique by surgical staff or prolonged duration of surgery

METRITIS

Metritis, or **endometritis,** an inflammation of the endometrium, may occur postpartally in 2% to 5% of women who give birth vaginally and 15% to 20% of those who give birth by cesarean (Quilligan & Zuspan, 2000). After expulsion of the placenta, the placental site provides an excellent culture medium for bacterial growth. The site in the contracted uterus is a round, dark red, elevated area of 4 cm, with a nodular surface composed of numerous veins, many of which may become occluded because of clot formation. The remaining portion of the decidua is also susceptible to infection because of its thinness (approximately 2 mm) and its large blood supply. The cervix presents a bacterial breeding ground because of multiple small lacerations attending normal labor and spontaneous birth. Pathogenic bacteria deposited at the cervix during vaginal examinations and those that are already present infect the decidua and eventually involve the entire mucosa. If the infection is confined to this region, the area will be necrotic and will be sloughed off within 3 to 5 days. With the extra surgical trauma associated with cesarean birth, more tissue is devitalized and there are more foreign bodies (eg, sutures) and blood, which can act as a medium for bacterial proliferation, making infection more probable. Both aerobic and anaerobic organisms cause metritis, which is often polymicrobial (Quilligan & Zuspan, 2000). See Table 37–3 • for a list of common causative organisms.

Clinical findings of metritis in the initial 24 to 36 hours postpartum tend to be related to group B streptococcus (GBS) (Quilligan & Zuspan, 2000). Late-onset postpartal endometritis/metritis is most commonly associated with genital mycoplasmas and *Chlamydia trachomatis. Chlamydia trachomatis* has a longer replication time and latency period

Table 37–3 • COMMON CAUSATIVE ORGANISMS IN METRITIS

Aerobes	Anaerobes
• Group A, B, D streptococcus	• *Peptostreptococcus*
• Enterococcus	• *Clostridium* species
• *Staphylococcus* species	• *Bacteroides* species
• *Escherichia coli*	• *Chlamydia trachomatis*
• *Klebsiella pneumoniae*	• Genital *mycoplasma*
• *Proteus mirabilis*	

Source: Compiled from Baxley, E. G. (2001). Postpartum biomedical concerns. Section B postpartum endometritis. In S. D. Ratcliffe, E. G. Baxley, J. E. Byrd, & E. L. Sakornbut (Eds.), *Family practice obstetrics* (2nd ed., pp. 602–607). Philadelphia: Hanley & Belfus; Cash, J. C., & Glass, C. A. (2000). *Family practice guidelines*. Philadelphia: Lippincott; Scarr, E. M., & Sammone, L. N. (1999). Endometritis. In W. L. Star, M. T. Shannon, L. L. Lommel, & Y. M. Gutierres (Eds.), *Ambulatory obstetrics* (3rd ed., pp. 379–383). San Francisco: UCSF Nursing Press.

than other bacteria and is not consistently eradicated by antibiotics used for early postpartal infections.

In mild cases of metritis, the woman generally has vaginal discharge that may be scant or profuse, bloody, and foul smelling. In more severe cases, she also has uterine tenderness; sawtooth temperature spikes, usually between 38.3C (101F) and 40C (104F); tachycardia; and chills. Foul-smelling lochia is cited as a classic sign of endometritis, but in the case of infection with β-hemolytic streptococcus, the lochia may be scant, serosanguineous, and odorless (Cunningham et al, 2001).

PELVIC CELLULITIS (PARAMETRITIS)

Pelvic cellulitis (parametritis) is infection involving the connective tissue of the broad ligament or, in more severe forms, the connective tissue of all the pelvic structures. The infection generally ascends upward in the pelvis by way of the lymphatic vessels in the uterine wall but may also occur if pathogenic organisms invade a cervical laceration that extends upward into the connective tissue of the broad ligament—a direct pathway into the pelvis. Infection involving the peritoneal cavity is **peritonitis.**

A pelvic abscess may form in the case of postpartal peritonitis and most commonly is found in the uterine ligaments, the cul-de-sac of Douglas, and the subdiaphragmatic space. Pelvic cellulitis may be a secondary result of pelvic vein thrombophlebitis. This condition occurs when the clot, usually in the right ovarian vein, becomes infected, and the wall of the vein breaks down from necrosis, spilling the infection into the connective tissues of the pelvis.

As the course of pelvic cellulitis advances, a mass of exudate develops along the base of the broad ligament that may push the uterus toward the opposite wall (if the infection is unilateral), where it will become fixed. If the exudate spreads into the rectocervical septum, a firm mass develops behind the cervix instead. The abscess that results should be drained or resolved through appropriate antibiotic therapy to avoid rupture of the abscess into the peritoneal cavity and development of a possibly fatal peritonitis.

A woman suffering from parametritis may demonstrate a variety of symptoms, including marked high temperature (38.9C to 40C or 102F to 104F), chills, malaise, lethargy, abdominal pain, subinvolution of the uterus, tachycardia, and local and referred rebound tenderness. If peritonitis develops, the woman will be acutely ill with severe pain; marked anxiety; high fever; rapid, shallow respirations; pronounced tachycardia; excessive thirst; abdominal distention; nausea; and vomiting.

Perineal Wound Infections

Given the degree of bacterial contamination that occurs with normal vaginal birth, it is surprising that more women do not have infections of the episiotomy or repaired lacerations of perineum, vagina, or vulva. When perineal wound infection does occur, it is recognized by the classic signs: redness, warmth, edema, purulent drainage, and later, gaping of the wound that has previously been well approximated. Local pain may be severe. Infected perineal wounds, like other infected wounds, are treated by draining purulent material. Sutures are removed, and the wound is left open. A regimen of broad-spectrum antibiotics is used. When the surface of the wound is free of infectious exudate and tissue granulation is evident, the mother returns for secondary closure of the wound under regional anesthesia (Cunningham et al, 2001).

Cesarean Wound Infections

The infection rate following cesarean births is 3% to 5%, with the highest rate occurring after emergency cesarean births because there is more traumatization of the tissue (Duff, 2002). Predisposing factors include obesity, diabetes mellitus, prolonged postpartal hospitalization, PROM, metritis, prolonged labor, anemia, steroid therapy, and immunosuppression (Duff, 2002). Signs of an abdominal wound infection, which may not be evident until after discharge, include erythema; warmth; skin discoloration; edema; tenderness; purulent drainage, sometimes mixed with serosanguineous fluid; or gaping of the wound edges. Fever, pain, malodorous lochia, and other systemic signs of infection are also common. Abdominal distention and decreased bowel sounds may be noted. Culture of wound drainage commonly reveals mixed pathogens.

Postpartal wound dehiscence (opening of wound edges) is uncommon because pregnant women are usually a healthy population and because lower uterine skin incisions (called *Pfannenstiel* incisions) rarely dehisce. An infected open wound may be left open for delayed closure after the debridement.

Clinical Therapy

The infection site and causative organism are diagnosed by careful history and complete physical examination, blood tests, aerobic and anaerobic endometrial cultures (although this may be of limited value, because multiple organisms are usually present), and urinalysis to rule out urinary tract infection. When a localized infection develops, it is treated with antibiotics, sitz baths, and analgesics as necessary for pain relief. If an abscess has developed or a stitch site is infected, the suture is removed, and the area is allowed to drain. Packing the wound with saline gauze twice to three times daily, using aseptic technique, allows removal of necrotic debris when packing is removed. Broad-spectrum antibiotic coverage is used to treat postpartal wound infections. Cephalosporins, penicillinase-resistant penicillin, and vancomycin are commonly used with anaerobic coverage by clindamycin or ampicillin/sulbactam (Gravett, 2002).

The incidence of metritis has been reduced by prophylactic administration of antibiotics to women undergoing cesarean childbirth. Metritis, once diagnosed, is treated by the administration of intravenous antibiotics. With appropriate antibiotic coverage, improvement should occur within a few days. Antibiotics are generally continued until the woman is afebrile for 24 to 48 hours. If the clinical manifestations show no response to the drugs, the clinician should consider the possibility of nonpelvic causes of infection, septic thrombophlebitis, or pelvic abscess. The route and dosage are determined by the severity of the infection. Careful monitoring is also necessary to prevent the development of a more serious infection.

Parametritis and peritonitis are treated with intravenous antibiotics. Broad-spectrum antibiotics effective against the most common causative organisms are chosen initially until the results of culture and sensitivity reports are available. If multiple organisms are present, the approach to antibiotic therapy is continued unless no improvement is observed; then the antibiotic is changed.

An abscess is frequently manifested by the development of a palpable mass and may be confirmed with ultrasound. An abscess usually requires incision and drainage to avoid rupture into the peritoneal cavity and the possible development of peritonitis. After drainage of the abscess, the cavity may be packed with iodoform gauze to promote drainage and facilitate healing.

The woman with a severe systemic infection is acutely ill and may require care in an intensive care unit. Supportive therapy includes maintenance of adequate hydration with intravenous fluids, analgesic medications, ongoing assessment of the infection, and possibly continuous nasogastric suctioning if paralytic ileus develops.

Standard antibiotic coverage for metritis has been provided by clindamycin and gentamicin, broad-spectrum antibiotics with nearly 90% effectiveness. Single-agent therapy with effectiveness against aerobic and anaerobic organisms is slightly less effective. Cephalosporins, such as cefoxitin or cefotetan, are used as are expanded penicillins (mezlocillin, piperacillin, ticarcillin) and beta-lactam/beta-lactamase inhibitor combinations, like ticarcillin-clavulanate or ampicillin-sulbactam. The occasional resistant organism requires adjustment of antibiotics. Antibiotics are generally continued until the woman has been afebrile for 48 hours. Oral antibiotics are rarely needed on discharge.

NURSING CARE MANAGEMENT

Nursing Assessment and Diagnosis

The nurse should inspect the woman's perineum every 8 to 12 hours for signs of early infection. The REEDA scale helps the nurse remember to consider *r*edness, *e*dema, *e*cchymosis, *d*ischarge, and *a*pproximation. Any degree of induration (hardening) should be immediately reported to the clinician.

Fever, malaise, abdominal pain, foul-smelling lochia, larger than expected uterus, tachycardia, and other signs of infection should be noted and reported immediately so that treatment can begin. The white blood cell (WBC) count, a usual objective measure of infection, cannot be used reliably because of the normal increase in WBCs during the postpartum period; a WBC count of 14,000 to 16,000 mm^3 is not an unusual finding. Some clinicians believe that WBC counts of even 20,000 plus are not abnormal at this time, but likely result from the physiologic stress response of labor. The initial increase may only be seen in the neutrophils. An increase in WBC level of more than 30% in a 6-hour period, however, is indicative of infection.

Nursing diagnoses that may apply to the women with a puerperal infection include the following:

- ***Risk for Injury*** related to the spread of infection
- ***Pain*** related to the presence of infection
- ***Deficient Knowledge*** related to lack of information about condition and its treatment
- ***Risk for Altered Parenting*** related to delayed parent-infant attachment secondary to woman's malaise and other symptoms of infection

Nursing Plan and Implementation

Hospital-Based Nursing Care

Careful attention to aseptic technique during labor, birth, and postpartum is essential.

The nurse caring for a woman during the postpartal period is responsible for teaching the woman self-care measures that are helpful in preventing infection. The woman should understand the importance of good perineal care, hygiene practices to prevent contamination of the perineum (such as wiping from front to back, changing the perineal pad after voiding), and thorough handwashing. Once edema and perineal pain are under control, the nurse can also encourage sitz baths, which are cleansing and promote healing. Adequate fluid intake, coupled with a diet high in protein and vitamin C, which are necessary to promote wound healing, also helps prevent infection.

If the woman has a draining wound or purulent lochia, it is especially important that those in contact with soiled items and linens practice good handwashing. Clear, concise instructions about wound care and how to discard of soiled dressings appropriately must be provided to safeguard the woman and her caregivers.

If the woman is seriously ill, ongoing assessment of urine specific gravity and intake and output is necessary. The nurse also carefully administers antibiotics as ordered and regulates the intravenous fluids. Ongoing assessment of the woman's condition is vital to detect subtle changes in her health status. The nurse also recognizes the woman's comfort needs related to hygiene, positioning, oral hygiene, and pain relief.

Promoting maternal-infant attachment can be difficult with the acutely ill woman. The nurse may provide pictures of the infant and keep the mother informed of the infant's well-being. Mementos, such as a footprint, a note written by the father "from the baby," or a videotape of the baby can be comforting to the mother during their separation. If she feels up to it, the new mother will also benefit from brief visits with her newborn.

The woman who wishes to breastfeed when her condition allows can maintain lactation by pumping her breasts regularly. Understanding that the opportunity to breastfeed is simply delayed, not eliminated, by the infectious process may improve the woman's morale.

The partner of a seriously ill woman will be concerned about her condition and torn about spending time with her and with their newborn. Because maternal-infant bonding may be compromised, father-newborn bonding can be especially important.

See the Clinical Pathway for the Woman with a Puerperal Infection on pages 1086 to 1088 for specific nursing measures.

Community-Based Nursing Care

The woman with a puerperal infection needs assistance when she is discharged from the hospital. If the family cannot provide this home assistance, a referral to home care services is needed. Home care services should be contacted as soon as puerperal infection is diagnosed so that the nurse can meet with the woman for a family and home assessment and development of a home care plan.

The family needs instruction in the care of a newborn, including feeding, bathing, cord care, immunizations, and significant observations that should be reported. A well-baby appointment should be scheduled. Breastfeeding mothers receiving antibiotics should be instructed to inspect the infant's mouth for signs of thrush and to report the finding to their physician.

The mother should be instructed regarding activity, rest, medications, diet, and signs and symptoms of complications, and she should be scheduled for a return medical visit. She needs to know the importance of taking the entire course of prescribed antibiotics even though she may begin to feel better before the bottle is empty. She also needs to be informed about the importance of pelvic rest; that is, she should not use tampons or douches nor have intercourse until she has been examined by the physician and told it is safe to resume those activities.

Evaluation

Expected outcomes of nursing care include:

- The infection is quickly assessed, and treatment is instituted successfully without further complications.
- The woman understands the nature of the infection and the purpose of therapy; she carries out any ongoing antibiotic therapy necessary after discharge.
- Maternal-infant attachment is maintained.

Care of the Woman with a Urinary Tract Infection

Urinary tract infection (UTI) is a common postpartal infection. The postpartal woman is at increased risk of developing urinary tract problems because of the normal postpartal diuresis, increased bladder capacity, decreased bladder sensitivity from stretching or trauma, and possible inhibited neural control of the bladder following the use of general or regional anesthesia and contamination from catheterization.

Overdistention of the Bladder

Overdistention occurs postpartally when the woman is unable to empty her bladder, usually because of trauma or the effects of anesthesia. Women who have not sufficiently recovered from the effects of anesthesia cannot void spontaneously, and catheterization is often necessary. After the effects of anesthesia have worn off and the woman should therefore be able to void spontaneously and completely, urinary retention is highly indicative of UTI.

CLINICAL THERAPY

Overdistention in the early postpartal period is often managed by draining the bladder with a straight catheter as a one-time measure. If the overdistention recurs or is diagnosed later in the postpartal period, an indwelling catheter is generally ordered for 24 hours.

NURSING CARE MANAGEMENT

Nursing Assessment and Diagnosis

The overdistended bladder appears as a large mass, reaching sometimes to the umbilicus and displacing the uterine fundus upward. There is increased vaginal bleeding, the fundus is boggy, and the woman may complain of cramping as the uterus attempts to contract. Some women also experience backache and restlessness.

CLINICAL PATHWAY FOR THE WOMAN WITH A PUERPERAL INFECTION

Category	1–4 Hours Postpartum	4–8 Hours Postpartum	8–24 Hours Postpartum
Referral	Report from labor nurse if not continuing in an LDR room	Lactation consultation if needed	Home nursing referral if indicated ➤ **Expected Outcomes** Appropriate resources identified and utilized
Assessment	Postpartum assessments q½ h ×2, q1h ×2, then q4h. Includes: • Fundus firm, in midline, at or below umbilicus • Lochia rubra <1 pad/h; no free flow or passage of clots with massage • Bladder: voids large amounts of urine spontaneously; bladder not palpable following voiding • Perineum: sutures intact; no bulging or marked swelling; no c/o severe pain. Minimal bruising may be present. If hemorrhoids present, no tenseness or marked engorgement; <2 cm diameter • Breasts: soft, colostrum present Vital signs: • BP WNL; no hypotension; not >30 mm systolic or 15 mm diastolic over baseline • Temperature: <38C (100.4F) • Pulse: Bradycardia normal; consistent with baseline • Respirations: 12–20/min; quiet; easy Comfort level: <3 on scale of 1 to 10	Continue postpartum assessment q4h ×2, then q8h • Assess for bowel sounds • Assess lochia for color, odor, amount Breasts: evaluate nipple status; should be no evidence of cracks or bruising Observe feeding technique with newborn Assess VS q8h; all WNL; report temp >38C (100.4F) Continue assessment of comfort level q3–4h	Continue postpartum assessment q8h Breasts: nipples should remain free of cracks, fissures, bruising Feeding technique with newborn should be good or improving Assess VS q4h; report temp >38C (100.4F) Continue assessment of comfort level q3–4h Continue s/s of infection (ie, episiotomy, endometritis, pelvic cellulitis, or puerperal peritonitis) Inspect incision/episiotomy for redness, approximation, and drainage Assess for signs of progressive infection (ie, uterine subinvolution, foul-smelling lochia, uterine tenderness, severe lower abdominal pain, fever, elevated WBC, malaise, chills, lethargy, tachycardia, nausea and vomiting, abdominal rigidity) ➤ **Expected Outcomes** Findings indicate infection identified, treated and reduced or eliminated in timely manner No additional complications found
Comfort	Institute comfort measures: • Perineal discomfort: peri-care, sitz baths, topical analgesics • Hemorrhoids: sitz baths, topical analgesics, digital replacement of external hemorrhoids, side-lying or prone position • Afterpains: prone with small pillow under abdomen; warm shower or sitz baths; ambulation Administer pain medication as needed	Continue with pain management techniques	Continue with pain management techniques Promote comfort by: • Ensuring adequate periods of rest • Minimizing disturbing environmental stimuli • Judicious use of analgesics and antipyretics • Providing emotional support • Using supportive nursing measures (ie, backrubs, instruction in relaxation techniques, maintenance of cleanliness, provision of diversional activities)
Teaching/ psychosocial	Explain postpartum assessments Teach self-massage of fundus and expected findings Instruct to call for assistance first time OOB and prn Demonstrate peri-care, surgigator, sitz baths prn Explain comfort measures Begin newborn teaching (bulb suctioning, positioning, feeding, diaper change, cord care) Orient to room if transferred from LDR room Provide information on early postpartum period If mother is unable to breastfeed, assist her in pumping her breasts to maintain adequate milk supply	Discuss psychologic changes of postpartum period Stress need for frequent rest periods Continue newborn teaching: soothing/comforting techniques, swaddling; return demonstrations indicate woman's understanding Provide opportunities for questions and review; reinforce previous teaching Breastfeeding: nipple care; air-drying, lanolin; tea bags; proper latch-on technique Formula-feeding: supportive bra; ice bags, breast binder ➤ **Expected Outcomes** Client verbalizes/demonstrates understanding of teaching and related plan of care Client incorporates teaching into self-care	Reinforce previous teaching: answer questions Discuss need to take antibiotics until course completed Discuss involution; anticipated physical changes in first 2 weeks postpartum; postpartum exercises; need to limit visitors Breastfeeding/formula-feeding: • Explain milk production, let-down reflex, use of supplements, breast pumping, and milk storage • If cannot breastfeed, assist mother with pumping her breasts • Explain formula preparation and storage Discuss sibling rivalry; mother should have plan for supporting siblings at home Teaching evaluation completed

➤

CLINICAL PATHWAY FOR THE WOMAN WITH A PUERPERAL INFECTION *CONTINUED*

Category	1–4 Hours Postpartum	4–8 Hours Postpartum	8–24 Hours Postpartum
Therapeutic nursing interventions and reports	Ice pack to perineum to decrease swelling and increase comfort Straight cath prn × 1 if distended or voiding small amounts If continues unable to void or voiding small amounts, insert Foley catheter and notify CNM/physician	Sitz baths prn If woman Rh− and infant Rh+, RhoGAM work-up; obtain consent; complete teaching Obtain consent for rubella vaccine if indicated; explain purpose, procedure, implications Obtain hematocrit Determine rubella status ➤ **Expected Outcomes** Labs and cultures indicate infection reduced/resolved Complications have been minimized	Continue sitz baths 2–3 times/day or surgigator May shower if ambulating without difficulty Obtain blood cultures per dr order if temp elevated Obtain wound culture and assist with wound drainage and packing Use principles of medical asepsis in handwashing and disposal of contaminated material by client and caregiver Promote normal wound healing by peri-care, wiping front to back after each voiding, frequent changing of pads
Activity	Assistance when OOB first time, then prn Ambulate ad lib Rests comfortably between checks	Encourage rest periods Ambulate ad lib; may leave birthing unit	Up ad lib ➤ **Expected Outcomes** Optimal comfort and activity maintained
Nutrition	Regular diet, high in vit C and protein Fluid intake ≥2000 mL/day	Continue diet and fluids ➤ **Expected Outcomes** Nutritional needs met with emphasis on calories needed for healing	Continue diet and fluids Increase calories by 500 kcal over nonpregnant state (200 kcal over pregnant intake) if breastfeeding Return to normal caloric intake for nonpregnant state if formula-feeding
Elimination	Voiding large amounts straw-colored urine	Voiding large quantities May have bowel movement, assess bowel sounds	Monitor I/O, urine specific gravity, and level of hydration ➤ **Expected Outcomes** Intake and output WNL
Medications	Methergine 0.2 mg q4h prn if ordered Stool softener as ordered Tucks pads prn	Continue meds Lanolin to nipples prn; tea bags to nipples if tender; heparin flush to buffalo cap (if present) q8h or as ordered	IV antibiotics Continue meds May take own prenatal vitamins RhoGAM administered if indicated Rubella vaccine administered if indicated ➤ **Expected Outcomes** Infection successfully treated Medications utilized to further support health
Discharge planning/ home care	Evaluate knowledge of normal postpartum, newborn care Evaluate support systems	Discuss typical newborn schedule; plan for periods of rest Birth certificate paperwork completed Evaluate plans for transporting newborn; car seat used	Provide information regarding predisposing factors, s/s, and treatment Discuss the value of a nutritious diet in promoting healing Review hygiene practice (ie, correct wiping after voiding, and handwashing, to prevent the spread of infection) Discuss home care routines to be used following postpartal infection Review discharge instruction sheet and checklist Describe postpartum and infection warning signs and when to call CNM/physician Provide prescriptions; gift pack given to woman Arrangements made for baby pictures if desired Postpartum visit scheduled Newborn check scheduled ➤ **Expected Outcomes** Woman participates in self-care and continued medication therapy Discharge teaching complete with emphasis on follow-up care, adequate rest, and infant attachment

(continued on next page)

CLINICAL PATHWAY FOR THE WOMAN WITH A PUERPERAL INFECTION *CONTINUED*

Category	1–4 Hours Postpartum	4–8 Hours Postpartum	8–24 Hours Postpartum
Family involvement	Identify available support persons Assess family perceptions of birth experience Parenting: demonstrates culturally expected early parenting behaviors	Involve support persons in care, teaching; answer questions Evidence of parental bonding behaviors apparent Provide and maintain mother-infant interaction: • Provide opportunities for the mother to see and hold her infant • Encourage partner or support person to discuss infant with woman and to become involved in infant's care if the woman is not able to do so	Continue to involve support persons in teaching Evidence of parental bonding behaviors continued Plans made for providing support to mother following discharge. Support persons verbalize understanding of need for woman to rest, eat nutritionally, recover ➤ **Expected Outcomes** Family demonstrates understanding of resources Support network identified Family development unimpaired
Date			

ad lib, as desired; BSI, body substance isolation: CNM, certified nurse-midwife; dr, doctor; hep-lock, intravenous catheter that allows intermittent access, I/O, intake and output; IV, intravenous; LDR, labor, delivery, and recovery; meds, medications; OOB, out of bed; peri-care, perineal care; prn, as desired; s/s, signs and symptoms; vit C, vitamin C; VS, vital signs; WBC, white blood count; WNL, within normal limits.

Nursing diagnoses that may apply when a woman has difficulties due to overdistention include the following:

- ***Risk for Infection*** related to urinary stasis secondary to overdistention
- ***Urinary Retention*** related to decreased bladder sensitivity and normal postpartal diuresis

Nursing Plan and Implementation

Diligent monitoring of the bladder during the recovery period and preventive health measures greatly reduce the chance for overdistention of the bladder. Encouraging the mother to void spontaneously and helping her use the toilet, if possible, or the bedpan if she has received conductive anesthesia, prevents overdistention in most cases. The nurse assists the woman to a normal position for voiding (ie, sitting with the legs and feet lower than the trunk) and provides privacy to encourage voiding. The woman should be medicated for whatever pain she may be having before attempting to void because pain may cause a reflex spasm of the urethra. Perineal ice packs applied after birth will minimize any edema, which may interfere with voiding. Pouring warm water over the perineum or having the woman void in a sitz bath may also be effective.

If catheterization becomes necessary, careful, meticulous, aseptic technique should be employed during catheter insertion. The vagina and vulva are traumatized to some degree by vaginal birth, and edema is common. This edema may obscure the urinary meatus; therefore, the nurse needs to be extremely careful in cleansing the vulva and inserting the catheter. It is imperative to discard a catheter that has inadvertently been introduced into the vagina and thus contaminated. Because catheterization is an uncomfortable procedure due to the postpartal trauma and edema of the tissue, the nurse should be careful and gentle not only in inserting the catheter but also in handling and cleaning the perineal area.

If the amount of urine drained from the bladder reaches 900 to 1000 mL, the catheter should be clamped and taped firmly to the woman's leg. The nurse should carefully document the procedure, including taking the woman's vital signs before and after the procedure and noting her responses. After an hour, the catheter may be unclamped and removed or, in the case of an indwelling catheter, placed on gravity drainage. This technique protects the bladder and avoids rapid intra-abdominal decompression. When the indwelling catheter is removed, a urine specimen is often sent to the laboratory. The tip of the catheter may also be removed and sent for culture.

Evaluation

Expected outcomes of nursing care include:

- The woman voids adequately to meet the demands of the increased fluid shifts during the postpartal period.
- The woman doesn't develop infection due to stasis of urine.
- The woman actively incorporates self-care measures to decrease bladder overdistention.

Cystitis (Lower Urinary Tract Infection)

Retention of residual urine, bacteria introduced at the time of catheterization, and a bladder traumatized by childbirth combine to provide an excellent environment for the development of cystitis. As many as 5% of women who have one catheterization, and 50% of those with intermittent catheterization develop cystitis. *Escherichia coli* has been demonstrated to be the causative agent in most cases of postpartal cystitis and pyelonephritis (in both lower and upper UTI). In most cases, the infection ascends the urinary tract from the urethra to the bladder. If cystitis is not treated, the infection can spread to the kidneys (pyelonephritis) because vesiculoureteral reflux forces contaminated urine into the renal pelvis.

CLINICAL THERAPY

When cystitis is suspected, a clean-catch midstream urine sample is obtained for microscopic examination, culture, and sensitivity tests. The specimen may require collection by the nurse with the woman on a bedpan because few postpartal women can collect a true midstream, clean-catch specimen without contaminating the specimen with lochia. A catheterized specimen is avoided when possible because of the increased risk of infection. When the bacterial concentration is greater than 100,000 colonies of the same organism per milliliter of fresh urine, infection is generally present. Counts between 10,000 and 100,000 may also suggest infection, particularly if clinical symptoms are noted.

Treatment is theoretically delayed until urine culture and sensitivity reports are available. In the clinical setting, however, antibiotic therapy is often initiated using trimethoprim-sulfamethoxazole–double strength (Bactrim DS, Septra DS), one of the short-acting sulfonamides, nitrofurantoin (Macrobid), or, in the case of sulfa allergy, ampicillin or amoxicillin. The antibiotic is begun immediately and then can be changed if indicated by the results of the sensitivity report (Duff, 2002). Antispasmodic or urinary analgesic agents, such as Pyridium, may be given to relieve discomfort.

Pyelonephritis (Upper Urinary Tract Infection)

Pyelonephritis is an infection of the upper urinary tract. In most cases, the infection has ascended from the lower urinary tract. It occurs more commonly on the right, although both kidneys may be affected. If untreated, the renal cortex may be damaged and kidney function impaired.

CLINICAL THERAPY

When pyelonephritis is diagnosed, intravenous antibiotic therapy is begun immediately. If sensitivity reports so indicate, the antibiotic can be changed later. Bed rest and careful monitoring of intake and output are necessary to detect the development of bacterial shock. Fluids are encouraged. Antispasmodic, analgesic, and antipyretic medications are given to relieve discomfort. The woman usually continues to take antibiotics for 2 to 4 weeks after clinical and bacteriologic response. A clean-catch urine culture should be obtained 2 weeks after completion of therapy and then periodically for the next 2 years. An intravenous pyelogram may be ordered in 2 to 4 months to identify any residual renal damage.

Continuation of breastfeeding during therapy is limited only by the degree of the mother's malaise and clinical discomfort. For the breastfeeding mother, the antibiotic should be selected carefully to avoid problems for the infant via the milk.

NURSING CARE MANAGEMENT

Nursing Assessment and Diagnosis

Symptoms of cystitis often appear 2 to 3 days after birth. The initial symptoms of cystitis may include frequency, urgency, dysuria, and nocturia. Hematuria and suprapubic pain may also be present. A slightly elevated temperature may occur, but systemic symptoms are often absent.

When a urinary tract infection progresses to pyelonephritis, systemic symptoms usually occur, and the woman becomes acutely ill. Symptoms include chills, high fever, flank pain (unilateral or bilateral), nausea, and vomiting, in addition to all the signs of lower UTI. Costovertebral angle tenderness on palpation and pain also may or may not be present. The nurse obtains a urine culture so that sensitivity tests can identify the causative organism.

Nursing diagnoses that may apply if a woman develops a UTI postpartally include the following:

- ***Pain*** with voiding related to dysuria secondary to infection
- ***Deficient Knowledge*** related to lack of information about self-care measures to prevent UTI

Nursing Plan and Implementation

Screening for asymptomatic bacteriuria in pregnancy should be routine. Frequent emptying of the bladder during labor and postpartum should be encouraged to prevent overdistention and trauma to the bladder. Catheterization technique and nursing actions to prevent overdistention (previously discussed) also apply. The woman with pyelonephritis must understand the importance of follow-up care after discharge to prevent recurrence or further complications.

Teaching for Self-Care

The nurse should advise the postpartal woman to continue good perineal hygiene following discharge. The nurse also advises her to maintain a good fluid intake, especially of water, and to empty her bladder whenever she feels the urge to void, but at least every 2 to 4 hours while awake. Once sexual intercourse is resumed, the new mother should void before (to prevent bladder trauma) and following intercourse (to wash contaminants from the vicinity of the urinary meatus). Wearing cotton-crotch underwear to facilitate air circulation also reduces the risk of UTI.

Acidification of the urine is thought to aid in preventing and managing UTI. The nurse thus advises the woman to avoid carbonated beverages, which increase alkalinity of urine, and to drink cranberry, plum, apricot, and prune juices and take vitamin C, which increase the acidity of urine (Gilbert & Harmon, 2003).

Evaluation

Expected outcomes of nursing care include:

- Signs of urinary tract infection are detected quickly, and the condition is treated successfully.
- The woman incorporates self-care measures to prevent the recurrence of UTI as part of her personal hygiene routine.
- The woman continues with any long-term therapy or follow-up.
- Maternal-infant attachment is maintained; the woman is able to care for her newborn effectively.

Care of the Woman with Mastitis

Mastitis is an infection of the breast connective tissue, primarily occurring in women who are lactating; the incidence is 2% to 5% of breastfeeding women (Baxley, 2001). The usual causative organisms are *Staphylococcus aureus*, *Haemophilus parainfluenzae*, *H influenzae*, *Escherichia coli*, and *Streptococcus* species. Infectious mastitis is characterized by either rapid or insidious onset of fever (38.5C [101F] or higher), chills, headache, flulike muscle aches and malaise, and a warm, reddened, painful area of the breast that is often wedge-shaped because of septal distribution of connective tissue (Figure 37–2 •). Because symptoms rarely occur before the second to fourth week postpartum, hospital-based nurses often are not fully aware of how uncomfortable and acutely ill the woman may be. No definitive data exist to allow caregivers to predict which women will experience mastitis, so all breastfeeding women need to be taught preventive techniques, ways of recognizing it, and the appropriate response of immediate notification of their physician or certified nurse-midwife.

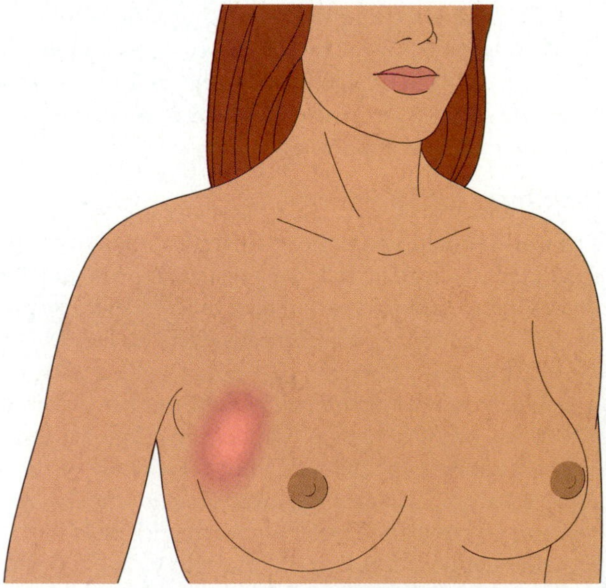

Figure 37–2 • Mastitis. Erythema and swelling are present in the upper outer quadrant of the breast. Axillary lymph nodes are often enlarged and tender. The segmental anatomy of the breast accounts for the demarcated, often V-shaped wedge of inflammation.

Table 37–4 • FACTORS ASSOCIATED WITH DEVELOPMENT OF MASTITIS

Milk stasis
Failure to change infant position to allow emptying all lobes
Failure to alternate breasts at feedings
Poor suck
Poor let-down
Actions that promote access / multiplication of bacteria
Poor handwashing technique
Improper breast hygiene
Failure to air-dry breasts after breastfeeding
Use of plastic-lined breast pads that trap moisture against nipple
Breast/nipple trauma
Incorrect positioning for breastfeeding
Poor latch-on
Failure to rotate position on nipple
Incorrect or aggressive pumping technique
Obstruction of ducts
Restrictive clothing
Constricting bra
Underwire bra
Change in number of feedings / failure to empty breasts
Attempted weaning
Missed feeding
Prolonged sleeping, including sleeping through night
Favoring side of nipple soreness
Lowered maternal defenses
Fatigue
Stress

The infection usually begins when bacteria invade the breast tissue after it has been traumatized in some way (see the factors commonly associated with mastitis in Table 37–4 •). Milk serves as a favorable medium for the invasive bacteria to multiply; thus, milk stasis is another risk factor (Shinskie & Lauwers, 2002). The most common source of the causative organism is the infant's nasopharynx, although other sources include the hands of the mother or nursing staff or the woman's circulating blood. Infants of women with mastitis generally remain well.

In some cases, *Candida albicans* is the causative organism of mastitis, entering the breast through a small fissure or abrasion on the nipple; the baby will often have thrush, a candidal infection of the mouth. There may be a history of a recent course of antibiotics in the woman. Signs include nipple pain, itching, and burning followed by a shooting pain throughout or between feedings. The affected nipple(s) may be bright pink or red. Eventually, the skin of the affected breast may become pink, flaking, and pruritic. Women may notice a yeasty odor to their milk.

Complementary and Alternative Therapies

Probiotics

Probiotics are a category of dietary supplements consisting of beneficial microorganisms (*pro* means "for" and *biotic* means "life" versus *antibiotic,* which literally means "against life"). Probiotics compete with disease-causing microorganisms in the gastrointestinal tract. When antibiotics are taken, they kill many of the beneficial bacteria that exist naturally in the digestive tract. Supplementing with probiotics after a course of antibiotics is frequently prescribed by nutritionists and complementary practitioners. Commonly used probiotics include *Lactobacillus acidophilus* and *Bifidobacterium bifidum;* there are other species of *Lactobacillus* and *Bifidobacterium* that have been shown to be effective in such conditions as diarrhea and vaginal infections (Elmer, 2001). Bifidobacterium also competes against *Candida albicans.* Probiotics can be taken in the form of powder, capsules, and suppositories, or in fermented milk products such as yogurt or *kefir.*

Clinical Therapy

Diagnosis is usually based on history and physical examination but culture and sensitivity testing of breast milk may be done. Some clinicians question the worth of milk culture since it is not ductal tissue that is infected and recommend antibiotic coverage empirically based on the most common etiologic organisms. If a culture of the breast milk is ordered either for initial diagnosis or with recurrence or failed treatment of mastitis, it is more reliable with a mid stream-type collection process. The nipple is washed first; then, the first 3 mL of breast milk are manually expressed and discarded, after which the actual specimen is collected. Normally, breast milk contains 1000 to 4000 leukocytes per mL. A leukocyte count greater than 10^6 and a bacterial count greater than 10^3 suggests infectious mastitis (Newton, 2002).

Treatment of mastitis involves bed rest for at least 24 hours, increased fluid intake (at least 2 to 3 liters per day), a supportive bra, frequent breastfeeding, local application of moist heat, and analgesics that are compatible with breastfeeding. Additionally, a 10-day course of antibiotics is appropriate, usually a penicillinase-resistant penicillin or cephalosporin (Gravett, 2002).

Candidal infections can be stubborn. If initial antifungal therapy fails, a second course may be necessary. Initial treatment generally involves antifungal creams or ointments once or twice daily. Oral Diflucan is excreted in breast milk but is not considered toxic to the infant and can be used if other agents fail. Women should be instructed to cleanse their nipples with warm water and allow air-drying before application of the antifungal medication. For the woman who prefers to avoid medication, an alternative treatment is cleansing of the nipples with a solution of one tablespoon of vinegar in one cup of water or one teaspoon of baking soda in one cup of water, followed by air-drying.

Improved outcome, a decreased duration of symptoms, and decreased incidence of a breast abscess result if the breasts continue to be emptied by either breastfeeding or pumping. The plan of care should include contacting the woman within 24 hours of initiation of treatment to ensure that symptoms are subsiding.

Ten percent of cases will progress to abscess formation if mastitis remains untreated, treatment fails, or the infant is abruptly weaned. Abscess is more common when there is a lag of 24 hours or more between onset of symptoms and when the woman seeks care (Baxley, 2001). Abscess is suspected when symptoms of mastitis fail to respond to antibiotics. When a breast abscess forms, the affected breast is likely to remain erythematous and painful; there is a distinct palpable mass or area of fullness, usually in the periphery of the breast; and fever and other systemic symptoms persist. Ultrasonography may be used to confirm the diagnosis of abscess. Contaminated fluid may be aspirated with a fine-needle technique and sent for culture and sensitivity. Antibiotics and comfort measures are continued; a surgical incision and drainage may be necessary. The breast should be kept emptied to promote healing. If the wound is too close to the nipple for comfortable breastfeeding, gentle pumping can be used. The woman should be advised to begin each breastfeeding session on the unaffected side; this enables her to capitalize on the let-down reflex for breastfeeding more comfortably on the affected breast. On occasion with breast abscess, the infant may refuse to breastfeed because of the increase in sodium chloride in the milk; lactation can be continued with pumping in conjunction with the let-down reflex of the other breast.

Nursing Care Management

Nursing Assessment and Diagnosis

Daily assessment of breast consistency, skin color, surface temperature, nipple condition, and presence of pain is essential to detect early signs of problems that may predispose to mastitis. The mother should be observed breastfeeding her baby to ensure use of proper technique.

If an infection has developed, the nurse should assess for contributing factors such as cracked nipples, poor hygiene, engorgement, supplemental feedings, change in routine or infant feeding pattern, abrupt weaning, or lack of proper breast support so that these factors may be corrected as part of the treatment plan.

Nursing diagnoses that may apply to the woman with mastitis include the following:

- ***Health Seeking Behaviors*** related to lack of information about appropriate breastfeeding practices
- ***Ineffective Breastfeeding*** related to pain secondary to development of mastitis

Nursing Plan and Implementation

Preventing mastitis is far simpler than treating it. Ideally, mothers should be instructed in proper breastfeeding technique prenatally. The nurse should help the mother breastfeed soon after birth and should review correct technique. Comanagement of breastfeeding between the nurse and a certified lactation specialist is often possible. All women, even those not breastfeeding, are encouraged to wear a good supportive bra at all times to avoid milk stasis, especially in the lower lobes.

Meticulous handwashing by the breastfeeding mother and all personnel is the primary measure for preventing epidemic nursery infections and subsequent maternal mastitis. Prompt attention to mothers who have blocked milk ducts eliminates stagnant milk as a growth medium for bacteria. If the mother finds that one area of her breast feels distended, she can rotate the position of her infant for breastfeeding, manually express milk remaining in the breast after feeding (usually only necessary if the infant is not sucking well), or massage the caked area toward the nipple as the infant suckles. Mothers who have developed mastitis can apply warm, moist compresses to the affected area before breastfeeding. The nurse encourages the mother to breastfeed frequently, starting with the unaffected breast until let-down occurs in the affected breast, then encourages feeding from the affected breast until it is emptied completely (Shinskie & Lauwers, 2002). After breastfeeding, the mother can leave a small amount of milk on each nipple to prevent cracking and allow nipples to air dry. Early identification of and intervention for sore nipples are also essential, as is prompt assessment of the breastfeeding mother's breasts when thrush is discovered in her newborn's mouth.

Teaching for Self-Care

The nurse stresses to the breastfeeding woman the importance of adequate breast and nipple care to prevent the development of cracks and fissures, a common portal for bacterial entry. For a detailed discussion of breastfeeding, see Chapter 31.

The woman should be aware of the importance of regular, complete emptying of the breasts to prevent engorgement and stasis. She should also understand the role of let-down in successful breastfeeding, correct positioning of the infant on the nipple, proper latch-on, and the principles of supply and demand. Breastfeeding mothers who will be returning to work outside the home need information on how to do so successfully. Because mastitis tends to develop following discharge, it is important to include information about signs and symptoms in the discharge teaching (Table 37–5 •). All flulike symptoms should be considered a sign of mastitis until proved otherwise. If symptoms develop, the woman should contact her caregiver immediately, because prompt treatment helps to avoid abscess formation. The woman with symptoms will benefit from a skilled assessment by an experienced professional nurse or lactation consultant.

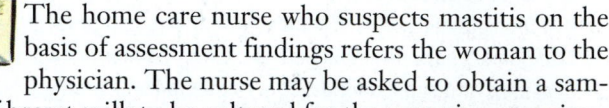

Community-Based Nursing Care

The home care nurse who suspects mastitis on the basis of assessment findings refers the woman to the physician. The nurse may be asked to obtain a sample of breast milk to be cultured for the causative organism.

If the mother feels too ill to breastfeed or develops an abscess that prevents breastfeeding, the home care nurse can help the mother obtain an appropriate breast pump to help her maintain lactation and can provide opportunities for demonstration and return demonstration of pumping. The nurse can assist the mother to deal with her feelings about temporarily being unable to breastfeed. Referral to a lactation consultant or to La Leche League can be invaluable to the woman's physical and emotional adjustment to mastitis.

Evaluation

Expected outcomes of nursing care include:

- The woman is aware of the signs and symptoms of mastitis.
- The woman's mastitis is detected early and treated successfully.
- The woman continues breastfeeding if she chooses.
- The woman understands self-care measures she can use to prevent recurrence of mastitis.

Table 37–5 • COMPARISON OF FINDINGS OF ENGORGEMENT, PLUGGED DUCT, AND MASTITIS

Characteristics	Engorgement	Plugged Duct	Mastitis
Onset	Gradual, immediately postpartum	Gradual, after feedings	Sudden, after 10 days
Site	Bilateral	Unilateral	Usually unilateral
Swelling and heat	Generalized	May shift, little or no heat	Localized, red, hot, and swollen
Pain	Generalized	Mild but localized	Intense but localized
Body temperature	<38.4C (101.1F)	<38.4C (101.1F)	>38.4C (101.1F)
Systemic symptoms	Feels well	Feels well	Flulike symptoms

Source: Lawrence, R. A. & Lawrence, R. M., *Breastfeeding: A guide for the medical profession.* (5th ed., p.276). Copyright 1999, Mosby Inc., with permission from Elsevier Science.

Table 37-6 • FACTORS ASSOCIATED WITH INCREASED RISK OF THROMBOEMBOLIC DISEASE
• Cesarean birth
• Inactivity
• Obesity
• Cigarette smoking
• Previous thromboembolic disease
• Trauma to extremity (can include injury from incorrect positioning or prolonged interval in stirrups during labor)
• Varicose veins
• Diabetes mellitus
• Advanced maternal age
• Inherited coagulation disorders
• Multiparity
• Anemia

Care of the Woman with Postpartal Thromboembolic Disease

Thromboembolic disease may occur antepartally, but it is generally considered a postpartal complication. Venous thrombosis refers to formation of a blood clot at an area of impeded blood flow in a superficial or deep vein. Inflammatory changes in the vessel wall generally accompany thrombus formation, hence the name **thrombophlebitis.** Thrombophlebitis may occur in either superficial or deep veins, usually in the legs. Pulmonary embolism, a rare, life-threatening condition, occurs when thrombi formed in the deep leg veins are carried to the pulmonary artery, obstructing pulmonary blood flow to one or both lungs. Together, these conditions are known as thromboembolic disease.

Three major causes of thromboembolic disease are hypercoagulability of blood, venous stasis, and injury to the epithelium of the blood vessel. Changes in the woman's coagulation system in pregnancy contribute to hypercoagulability, and compression of the common iliac vein by the gravid uterus leads to venous stasis. These factors increase the risk of this phenomenon in pregnant and postpartum women approximately fivefold (Walling, 2001). Superficial thrombophlebitis complicates the childbearing period for 1 in 500 to 750 women. Deep vein thrombosis (DVT), which is more serious, occurs most commonly in postpartum women between postpartum days 10 to 20 (Matteson, 2001).

Factors associated with increased risk of thromboembolic disease are identified in Table 37–6 •. Factors contributing directly to the development of thromboembolic disease postpartally include (1) increased amounts of certain blood clotting factors; (2) postpartal thrombocytosis (increased quantity of circulating platelets and their increased adhesiveness); (3) release of thromboplastin substances from the tissue of the decidua, placenta, and fetal membranes; and (4) increased amounts of fibrinolysis inhibitors. Because women are at risk for thromboembolic disease during the childbearing period, attention should be given to measures that might prevent this complication (Table 37–7 •).

Superficial Leg Vein Disease

Superficial thrombophlebitis is far more common postpartally than during pregnancy. Often the clot involves the saphenous veins. This disorder is more common in women with preexisting varicose veins, although it is not limited to these women. Symptoms usually become apparent about the third or fourth postpartal day and include tenderness in a portion of the vein, some local heat, swelling and redness, absent or low-grade fever, and occasionally slight elevation of the pulse. A tender palpable cord may be noted along a portion of the vein. Treatment involves application of local, moist heat, elevation of the affected limb, bed rest and analgesic agents, and the use of elastic support hose. Anticoagulants are usually not necessary unless complications develop. Pulmonary embolism is extremely rare. There is generally little risk beyond discomfort.

Table 37–7 • MEASURES TO DECREASE RISK OF THROMBOEMBOLIC DISEASE IN CHILDBEARING WOMEN

Antepartum Measures	Intrapartum Measures	Postpartum Measures
Advise woman to avoid sedentary lifestyle and to exercise as possible (walking is ideal).	Encourage ambulation unless contraindicated in early labor. Later, encourage leg exercises.	Encourage early ambulation.
Recommend plenty of fluids to avoid dehydration.	Do not gatch bed or use pillows under knees.	For clients on bed rest, advise or assist with turning and leg exercises every 2 hours (woman may be encouraged to rotate ankles and to "write baby's name in air with toes").
Advise to quit smoking.	Pad stirrups.	Encourage fluids to avoid dehydration.
Teach to avoid prolonged standing or sitting in one position or sitting with legs crossed.	Ensure correct positioning in stirrups that minimizes pressure on the popliteal area.	Advise no smoking.
Encourage elevation of legs when sitting.	Limit time in stirrups as possible.	Use antiembolism stockings with those at risk, including after cesarean birth.
Teach to avoid tight knee-high hose or other constrictive garments.	After cesarean birth, initiate leg/foot exercises as soon as possible (in recovery).	Advise against prolonged sitting and crossing legs.
Encourage to take frequent breaks during long car trips to walk around, thereby preventing prolonged venous stasis.	Use antiembolism stockings for women at risk of DVT.	Encourage elevation of legs while sitting.

Deep Vein Thrombosis

Deep venous thrombosis or thrombophlebitis is more frequently seen in women with a history of thrombosis. Certain obstetric complications such as hydramnios, preeclampsia, and operative birth are associated with an increased incidence. After a clinical diagnosis of DVT, a woman's risk in a subsequent pregnancy is as high as 20% (Clarke-Pearson, 2000).

Clinical manifestations may include edema of the ankle and leg and an initial low-grade fever often followed by high temperature and chills. Depending on the vein involved, the woman may complain of pain in the popliteal and lateral tibial areas (popliteal vein), entire lower leg and foot (anterior and posterior tibial veins), inguinal tenderness (femoral vein), or pain in the lower abdomen (iliofemoral vein). Homans' sign (Figure 37–3 •) may or may not be positive, but pain often results from calf pressure. Because of reflex arterial spasm, sometimes the limb is cool to the touch—the so-called milk leg or phlegmasia alba dolens—and peripheral pulses may be decreased.

Septic Pelvic Thrombophlebitis

Septic pelvic thrombophlebitis is a complication that develops in conjunction with infections of the reproductive tract and is more common in women who have had a cesarean birth. Infection ascends upward along the venous system, and thrombophlebitis develops in the uterine, ovarian, or hypogastric veins (Cunningham et al, 2001). This diagnosis is suspected with clinical findings resembling metritis that fail to respond to antibiotics. Abdominal or flank pain, or both, sometimes accompanied by guarding, occurs on the second or third day postpartum with fever and tachycardia. Bimanual exam may or may not reveal a parametrial mass; the uterus is generally exquisitely tender. On occasion, paralytic ileus develops. A complete blood count (CBC), blood chemistry, coagulation profile, chest x-ray examination, pelvic ultrasonography, computed tomography (CT), and magnetic resonance imaging (MRI) are useful for diagnosis. Treatment consists of anticoagulation and antibiotic therapy. Although most women show significant clinical improvement with antibiotics, a sawtooth fever spike and chills may persist (Laros, 1999).

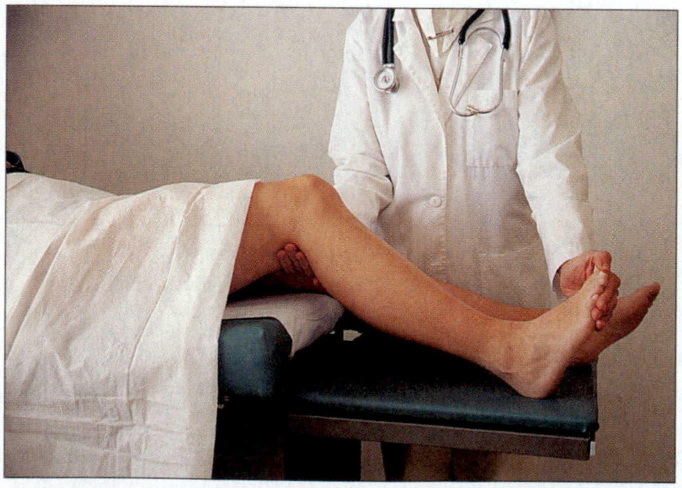

Figure 37–3 • Homans' sign. With the client's knee flexed to decrease the risk of embolization, the nurse dorsiflexes the client's foot. Pain in the foot or leg is a positive Homans' sign.

CRITICAL THINKING IN PRACTICE

Lei Chang, G1P1, had a cesarean birth after a prolonged labor and failure to progress. As she is walking in the hallway with her husband, you notice that Lei is limping slightly, and you comment on that observation. Lei responds that she is having pain in her right lower leg. She says, "Maybe I pulled a muscle during labor." What would you do?

Answers can be found in Appendix I.

Pulmonary Embolism

Pulmonary embolism (PE) is a particularly catastrophic event with a high mortality rate; most fatalities occur within 30 minutes; however, early recognition and prompt action can decrease the mortality rate to between 2% and 8% (Wells & Salyer, 2001). Although the incidence of DVT in pregnancy is now believed to be almost comparable to that of postpartum DVT, pulmonary embolism develops most commonly in postpartal women (Walling, 2001). The most common risk factors are proximal DVT and recurrent thromboembolic disease. Diagnosis may be difficult because the most common clinical findings include nonspecific signs and symptoms such as dyspnea, chest pain, cough with hemoptysis, cyanosis, tachypnea and tachycardia, syncope, or sudden hypotension. The nurse who recognizes these findings, especially in a woman at risk, should alert the woman's physician immediately, as time can be critical. Elevating the head of the woman's bed may facilitate ease of breathing; oxygen by face mask at 8 to 10 L per minute is often used. Narcotics may be ordered for pain and to decrease anxiety, thereby decreasing the respiratory effort. Chest x-ray, arterial blood gases, and electrocardiogram (ECG) may be ordered to rule out other diagnoses; if the initial tests do not diagnose some other cause for symptomalogy, ventilation-perfusion (V/Q) lung scanning may be ordered. If the results are not diagnostic and the woman is clinically stable, an ultrasound or MRI may be done of the lower extremities to assess for DVT. In some cases, a CT scan or pulmonary angiography, an invasive procedure, may be used to diagnose pulmonary embolus. The primary treatment is anticoagulation with standard or low molecular weight heparins (LMWH)(Hull, Kane, & Tapson, 2000). In some cases, thrombolytics (streptokinase or urokinase) or embolectomy may be used.

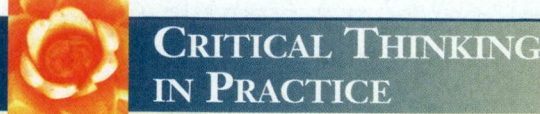

Clinical Therapy

Because cases of thromboembolic disease are seldom clear-cut, diagnosis involves a variety of approaches, such as client history and physical examination, occlusive cuff impedance plethysmography (IPG), Doppler ultrasonography, and contrast venography. In questionable cases, contrast venography provides the most accurate diagnosis of deep vein thrombosis. Unfortunately, venography is not practical for multiple examinations or prospective screening and may itself induce phlebitis.

Treatment involves the administration of intravenous heparin, using an infusion pump to permit continuous, accurate infusion of medication. Strict bed rest and elevation of the affected leg are required, and analgesics are given as necessary to relieve discomfort. If fever is present, deep thrombophlebitis is suspected, and the woman is also given antibiotic therapy. In most cases thrombectomy is not necessary.

Once the symptoms have subsided (usually in several days), the woman may begin walking while wearing elastic support stockings. Intravenous heparin is continued, and treatment with sodium warfarin (Coumadin) is begun. When prothrombin time reaches 1.5 to 1.7, the heparin is discontinued. The woman will continue on Coumadin for 2 to 6 months at home. While the woman is on warfarin, prothrombin times are assessed periodically to maintain correct dosage levels.

NURSING CARE MANAGEMENT

Nursing Assessment and Diagnosis

The nurse carefully assesses the woman's history for factors predisposing to development of thrombosis or thrombophlebitis. In addition, as part of regular postpartal assessment, the nurse is alert to any client complaints of pain in the leg, inguinal area, or lower abdomen because such pain may indicate deep venous thrombosis. The nurse also assesses the woman's legs for evidence of edema, temperature change, or pain with palpation.

Nursing diagnoses that may apply to a postpartal woman with thromboembolic disease include the following:

- ***Altered Tissue Perfusion*** in periphery related to obstructed venous return
- ***Pain*** related to tissue hypoxia and edema secondary to vascular obstruction
- ***Risk for Altered Parenting*** related to decreased maternal-infant interaction secondary to bed rest and intravenous lines
- ***Altered Family Processes*** related to illness of family member
- ***Deficient Knowledge*** related to lack of information about the DVT/thrombophlebitis, its treatment, preventive measures, and the medication (warfarin)

Nursing Plan and Implementation

Women with varicosities should be evaluated for the need for support hose during labor and postpartum. Adequate fluid intake is necessary during labor to avoid dehydration. Because trauma is often a factor in the development of thrombophlebitis, the nurse avoids keeping the woman's legs elevated in stirrups for prolonged periods. If stirrups are used, they should be comfortably padded and adjusted to provide correct support and prevent pressure on popliteal vessels. In addition, early ambulation is encouraged following birth, and the use of the knee gatch on the bed should be avoided. Women confined to bed following a cesarean birth are encouraged to perform regular leg exercises to promote venous return.

Once the diagnosis of deep venous thrombosis is made, the nurse maintains the heparin therapy, provides for appropriate comfort measures, and monitors the woman closely for signs of pulmonary embolism. The nurse also assesses for evidence of bleeding related to heparin and keeps the antagonist for heparin, protamine sulfate, readily available.

The nurse instructs the woman to avoid prolonged standing or sitting, because these positions contribute to venous stasis. She is also instructed to avoid crossing her legs because of the pressure it causes. The nurse also advises her to take frequent breaks, such as when taking car trips or at a job where she sits most of the day. Walking is acceptable because it promotes venous return. The woman is reminded to identify her history of thrombosis or thrombophlebitis to her physician during subsequent pregnancies so that preventive measures may be instituted early.

Women discharged on warfarin sodium should be taught about the drug and safety factors associated with its use. Clients need to be educated about foods high in vitamin K (Table 37–8 •) and the need to strive for consistent daily intake. In moderation, these foods can remain a part of the daily diet. When the dietary intake of such foods decreases significantly, there is a risk of bleeding. Binge alcohol use inhibits warfarin metabolism; an occasional alcoholic beverage does not affect coagulation adversely. Many multivitamins contain vitamin K; clients on warfarin may take them but should do so consistently. Vitamin C doses up to 500 mg per day and vitamin E doses up to 400 IU per day are considered safe; higher doses can affect coagulation. While taking anticoagulants, the woman will be asked to undergo frequent coagulant tests to guide dosing. Point-of-care testing is now available to decrease the inconvenience of going into a laboratory environment for testing. Home self-testing involves a single capillary finger stick (Coaguchek, ProTime, Avocet) to test thromboplastin-mediated clotting expressed as prothrombin time (PT) or international normalized ratio (INR). The risk of bleeding increases significantly when the INR is greater than 5. (Nadeau, Alpert, Costantino, et al, 2000). Bleeding should be reported if it fails to stop within 10 minutes.

Table 37-8 • FOODS HIGH IN VITAMIN K

- Basil
- Broccoli
- Brussels sprouts
- Cabbage
- Cauliflower
- Chives
- Collard greens
- Coriander
- Kale
- Lettuce
- Mint
- Mustard greens
- Parsley
- Peppers
- Spinach
- Turnips
- Watercress
- Green and black tea
- Canola oil, soybean oil, mayonnaise

Source: Used with permission: *Patient Care for the Nurse Practitioner* 2002, *3*(12). Copyright Medical Economics Company, Thomson Healthcare, 2002.

MediaLink CASE STUDY: POSTPARTAL THROMBOEMBOLIC DISEASE

Although warfarin sodium (Coumadin) cannot be used in pregnancy, it is commonly used to anticoagulate women who experience postpartum DVT. Warfarin is excreted in breast milk but is not considered hazardous to breastfeeding infants (Nadeau et al, 2000).

Women who are discharged on warfarin must understand the purpose of the medication and be alert to signs of hemorrhage, such as bleeding gums, epistaxis, petechiae or ecchymosis, or evidence of blood in the urine or stool. Because careful monitoring is important, the woman should clearly understand the need to keep scheduled appointments for prothrombin time assessment. Certain medications, such as aspirin and other nonsteroidal anti-inflammatory drugs, increase anticoagulant activity, so they should be avoided. In fact, while she is taking warfarin the woman should check for possible medication interaction before taking *any* other medication. Many herbals affect the efficacy of warfarin; for example, garlic, ginger, and ginkgo prolong prothrombin time and should be avoided. The nurse should encourage the woman to carry a MedicAlert card in case of emergency and to inform all medical care providers, including dentists, that she is taking anticoagulants. She should also have vitamin K available in case bleeding occurs. See the Clinical Pathway for the Woman with Thromboembolic Disease for specific nursing care measures.

Community-Based Nursing Care

Because the mother with postpartal thromboembolic disease will depend on others for much of her initial home care, it is helpful for the father to be involved in preparations for discharge. The nurse should provide ample opportunities to answer questions and clarify instructions, verbally and in writing. The nurse will evaluate the extent to which both mother and father have understood instructions regarding the plan of care. It is especially important before discharge to assess the couple's plans in order to ensure complete bed rest for the mother. They might explore ways for her to maintain bed rest and still spend quality time with her newborn and any other children. For example, young children can sit on the bed for storytelling or play quiet games, and the newborn's crib can be placed adjacent to the mother's bed.

The father may be assuming multiple roles in the circumstances—household manager, parent, worker, and caregiver. Fatigue is inevitable. There may be financial concerns as a result of prolonged healthcare or his extended time away from work to care for the family. Referral to social services and assessment of the presence and use of a support system and coping strategies are necessary to avert potential crises. The nurse should plan telephone or home visit follow-up care.

Signs of postpartum thrombophlebitis may not occur until after discharge from the hospital. Consequently, all couples must be taught about the signs and symptoms and to appreciate the importance of reporting them immediately and of not massaging the affected leg. Should signs and symptoms occur after discharge from the postpartum unit, a short readmission might be required. Every effort is made in that case to allow mother, father, and newborn to remain together.

Evaluation

Expected outcomes of nursing care include:

- If thrombosis or thrombophlebitis develops, it is detected quickly and managed successfully without further complications.
- At discharge, the woman is able to explain the purpose, dosage regimen, and necessary precautions associated with any prescribed medications, such as anticoagulants.
- The woman can discuss self-care measures and ongoing therapies (such as the use of elastic stockings) that are indicated.
- The woman has bonded successfully with her newborn and is able to care for the baby effectively.

Care of the Woman with a Postpartum Psychiatric Disorder

The relationship of affective disorders to childbirth is reflected in the fact that the rate of admission to a psychiatric hospital is greater during the year after childbirth than at any other time in a woman's life (Gjerdinger & Byrd, 2001).

Types of Postpartum Psychiatric Disorders

Many types of psychiatric problems may occur in the postpartum. Their classification is a subject of some controversy. The *Diagnostic and Statistical Manual of Mental Disorders*, 5th

CLINICAL PATHWAY FOR THE WOMAN WITH THROMBOEMBOLIC DISEASE*

Category	Antepartal Management	Intrapartal Management	Postpartal Management
Referral	Perinatologist Internist Social worker Psychiatric clinical nurse practitioner Dietary/nutritionist Infectious disease consult	Obtain prenatal record	Home nursing referral if indicated ➤ **Expected Outcomes** Appropriate resources identified and utilized
Assessment	Obtain hx of present pregnancy Assess estimated gestational age Assess any sensitivity to medications Obtain complete physical examination to include: • Fetal size, fetal status (FHR), and fetal maturity • Signs of fatigue, weakness, recurrent diarrhea, pallor, night sweats • Present weight and amount of weight gain or weight loss Obtain diagnostics studies: • Ultrasound • Fetal maturity studies (L/S ratio, PG, creatinine) • Hemoglobin, hematocrit, platelet count • WBC and differential • HIV-I • CD4+ T lymphocyte count • ESR		Monitor daily Hct Continue normal postpartum assessment q8h Feeding technique with newborn: should be good or improving TPR assessment: q8h; all WNL; report temperature >38C (100.4F) Continue assessment of comfort level Assess for superficial thrombophlebitis: • Tenderness along involved vein • Areas of palpable thrombosis • Warmth and redness in the involved area Deep venous thrombosis (DVT): • Positive Homans' sign (pain occurs when foot is dorsiflexed with knee slightly flexed) • Tenderness and pain in affected area • Fever (initially low, followed by high fever and chills) • Edema in affected extremity • Pallor and coolness in affected limb • Diminished peripheral pulses • Increased potential for pulmonary embolus Immediately report the development of any signs of pulmonary embolism, including the following: • Sudden onset of severe chest pain, often located substernally • Apprehension and sense of impending catastrophe • Cough (may be accompanied by hemoptysis) • Tachycardia • Fever • Hypotension • Diaphoresis, pallor, weakness • Shortness of breath • Neck engorgement • Friction rub and evidence of atelectasis upon auscultation ➤ **Expected Outcomes** Findings indicate complications of thrombosis minimized, and condition stable/improved
Comfort			Continue with pain management techniques. No aspirin or ibuprofen. Acetaminophen may be ordered. Provide supportive nursing comfort measures such as backrubs, provision of quiet time for sleep, diversional activities Maintain warm moist soaks as ordered with legs elevated Advise not to rub leg

(continued on next page)

CLINICAL PATHWAY FOR THE WOMAN WITH THROMBOEMBOLIC DISEASE *CONTINUED*

Category	Antepartal Management	Intrapartal Management	Postpartal Management
Teaching/ psychosocial	Room orientation Explain s/s of labor Increase client awareness of fetal monitoring Evaluation of client teaching	Tour of ICN Discuss with woman: • Mode of childbirth • Postpartum expectation	Implement normal postpartum teaching and psychosocial support (see Chapter 35) Maintain mother/infant attachment; when mother is on bed rest provide frequent contacts for mother and infant; modified rooming-in is possible if the crib is placed close to the mother's bed and nurse checks often to help mother lift or move infant ➤ **Expected Outcomes** Woman demonstrates/verbalizes understanding of plan of care and teaching Infant/maternal bonding unimpaired
Nursing care management and reports	Assess emotional response so that support and teaching can be planned accordingly Weigh woman Obtain food history Establish rapport Provide opportunities to talk without interruption Monitor for signs of infection Maintain appropriate isolation precautions	Ongoing monitoring of blood pressure Electronic fetal monitoring in place Try to have same nurses caring for woman during her hospitalization Monitor for signs of infection ➤ **Expected Outcomes** Maternal/fetal circulation optimized	Continue sitz baths prn May shower if ambulating without difficulty (DC heparin lock if present or cover with plastic) Monitor for signs of infection For DVT obtain prothrombin time (PT), INR, and review prior to beginning warfarin. Repeat periodically per physician order ➤ **Expected Outcomes** Thromboembolic disease treated successfully, without related complications
Activity and comfort	Decreased stimulation in room including visitors		Maintain bed rest and limb in elevated position Initiate progressive ambulation following the acute phase; provide properly fitting elastic stockings prior to ambulation for management of superficial thrombophlebitis and DVT ➤ **Expected Outcomes** Activity initiated as appropriate Optimal comfort maintained
Nutrition	Plan high-protein, high-calorie diet		Continue diet and fluids Continue consistent intake of food sources of vitamin K ➤ **Expected Outcomes** Nutritional needs met
Elimination			
Medications		Continuous IV infusion	May take own prenatal vitamins RhoGAM administered if indicated Rubella vaccine administered if indicated For DVT administer intravenous heparin as ordered by continuous intravenous drip, heparin lock, or subcutaneously, including: • Monitor IV or heparin lock site for signs of infiltration • Obtain Lee-White clotting times or partial thromboplastin time (PTT) per physician order, and review prior to administering heparin • Observe for signs of anticoagulant overdose with resultant bleeding, including the following: hematuria, epistaxis, ecchymosis, and bleeding gums • Provide protamine sulfate per physician order to combat bleeding problems related to heparin overdosage ➤ **Expected Outcomes** Thrombosis resolved and control of related bleeding problems achieved Minimized complications and side effects

➤

CLINICAL PATHWAY FOR THE WOMAN WITH THROMBOEMBOLIC DISEASE *CONTINUED*

Category	Antepartal Management	Intrapartal Management	Postpartal Management
Discharge planning/ home care	Assess home care needs Provide support and counseling		Discuss ways of avoiding circulatory stasis such as avoiding prolonged standing, sitting, and crossing legs Review need to wear support stockings and to plan for rest periods with legs elevated In the presence of DVT, discuss the following: • The use of warfarin, its side effects, possible interactions with other medications, and need to have dosage assessed through periodic checks of the prothrombin time • Signs of bleeding, which may be associated with warfarin sodium and which need to be reported immediately, including the following: hematuria, epistaxis, ecchymosis, bleeding gums, and rectal bleeding • Monitor menstrual flow: bleeding may be heavier • Review need for woman to eat a consistent amount of leafy green vegetables (lettuce, cabbage, brussels sprouts, broccoli) every day (high in vit K so affects dose of warfarin and PT balance) • Instruct the woman to report any bleeding that continues more than 10 minutes Instruct the woman to do the following: • Routinely inspect the body for bruising • Carry MedicAlert card indicating she is on anticoagulant therapy • Use electric razor to avoid scratching skin and take care with other sharps • Use soft bristle toothbrush and floss gently • Avoid alcohol intake or keep intake at minimum • Avoid taking any other drugs without checking with the physician • Note that stools may change color to pink, red, or black as a result of anticoagulant use • Advise all health providers, including dentists, that she is taking anticoagulants • Review follow-up agenda and expectations Review discharge instructions and checklist Provide list or make appropriate referrals to available community resources Describe postpartum warning signs and when to call CNM/physician Provide prescriptions: Gift pack given to woman Arrangements made for baby pictures if desired Postpartum visit scheduled Newborn check scheduled ➤ **Expected Outcomes** Client discharge teaching done with emphasis on follow-up care, continued therapy needs and precautions Support network identified

(continued on next page)

CLINICAL PATHWAY FOR THE WOMAN WITH THROMBOEMBOLIC DISEASE *CONTINUED*

Category	Antepartal Management	Intrapartal Management	Postpartal Management
Family involvement	Assess support systems	Encourage family member to stay with the woman as long as possible throughout labor and childbirth	Involve support persons in teaching Plans made for providing support to mother following discharge. Support persons verbalize understanding of need for woman to rest, eat nutritionally, recover Encourage woman to express her concerns to her partner. Assist couple in planning ways to manage while woman is hospitalized and after her discharge Encourage partner or support person to bring other children to hospital to visit mother and meet new sibling Encourage partner or support person to bring in family pictures. Encourage phone calls Contact social services if indicated to obtain additional assistance for family if needed ➤ **Expected Outcomes** Family demonstrates resource availability and utilization Family bonding and development unimpaired
Date			

*All of the interventions for a normal labor and birth and postpartal client may be found in those appropriate clinical pathways.

CNM, certified nurse-midwife; DC, discharge; Hct, hematocrit; NICU, neonatal intensive care unit; IV, intravenous; heparin lock, intravenous catheter that allows intermittent access; hx, history; prn, as needed; s/s, signs and symptoms; TPR, temperature, pulse, and respiration; WNL, within normal limits; INR, international normalized ratio.

edition, has added a postpartum-onset specifier to the mood disorder diagnostic category of psychiatric disorders. It is proposed that postpartum psychiatric disorders be considered one diagnosable syndrome with three subclasses: (1) adjustment reaction with depressed mood, (2) postpartum psychosis, and (3) postpartum major mood disorder. The incidence, etiology, symptoms, treatment, and prognosis vary with each subclass.

ADJUSTMENT REACTION WITH DEPRESSED MOOD

Adjustment reaction with depressed mood is commonly known as **postpartum blues,** or as *maternal* or *"baby" blues.* It occurs in as many as 50% to 70% of mothers and is characterized by mild depression interspersed with happier feelings (Bowes & Katz, 2002). Postpartum blues typically occur within a few days after the baby's birth and are self-limiting, lasting from a few hours to 10 days or longer. It is more severe in primiparas and seems related to the rapid alteration of estrogen, progesterone, and prolactin levels after birth. New mothers experiencing postpartum blues commonly report feeling overwhelmed, unable to cope, fatigued, anxious, irritable, and oversensitive. A key feature is episodic tearfulness, often without an identifiable reason.

Validating the existence of this phenomenon, labeling it as a real but normal adjustment reaction, and providing reassurance can offer a measure of relief. Assistance with self and infant care, information, and family support is helpful to recovery. The partner should be encouraged to watch for and report signs that the new mother is not returning to a more normal mood but is instead slipping into a deeper depression.

POSTPARTUM PSYCHOSIS

Postpartum psychosis, which has an incidence of 0.14% to 0.26%, usually becomes evident within the first 3 months postpartum (Bowes & Katz, 2002). Symptoms include agitation, hyperactivity, insomnia, mood lability, confusion, irrational thoughts and behaviors, difficulty remembering or concentrating, poor judgment, delusions, and hallucinations. With appropriate treatment, improvement is seen in 95% of women in 2 to 3 months (Meighan, Davis, Thomas, et al, 2000). There is a 10% to 25% recurrence rate in subsequent pregnancies.

Risk factors include (1) previous puerperal psychosis; (2) history of bipolar (manic-depressive) disorder; (3) prenatal stressors, such as lack of social support, lack of a partner, and low socioeconomic status; (4) obsessive personality; and (5) a family history of a mood disorder. Treatment may include hospitalization, antipsychotic medications, sedatives, electroconvulsive therapy, removal of the infant, social support, and psychotherapy.

Postpartum psychosis is considered an emergency because of the risk of suicide and/or infanticide. The psychotic woman may experience delusions or hallucinations that support her perceptions that the infant should not be allowed to live. For example, she may believe that her newborn is evil and will harm her other children, or she may believe that her newborn would be "better off dead" than living in such an evil world. She may contemplate suicide because she believes that her child would be better off without a mother than with her as such a "terrible, crazy mother." Illogical thinking or evidence of bonding difficulties may serve as cues to infanticide and suicide risk; however, this assessment is often challenging because of the lucidity seen in some psychotic clients (Mills, 2001).

POSTPARTUM MAJOR MOOD DISORDER

Postpartum major mood disorder, also known as **postpartum depression,** develops in about 8% to 20% of all postpartal women (Bowes & Katz, 2002). Although it may occur at any time during the first year postpartum, the greatest risks occur around the fourth week, just prior to the initiation of menses, and upon weaning. Surprisingly, it is not associated with depression during pregnancy.

Many of the symptoms of this major depression are indistinguishable from serious depression at other times: sadness, frequent crying, insomnia or excessive sleeping, appetite change, difficulty concentrating and making decisions, feelings of worthlessness, obsessive thoughts of inadequacy as a person and parent, lack of interest in usual activities (including sexual relations), and lack of concern about personal appearance. Persistent anxiety further contributes to the woman's feeling of being out of control. Irritability and hostility toward others, including the newborn, may be evident. Beck (1993) described these debilitating symptoms as "teetering on the edge" between sanity and insanity. Women participating in Beck's qualitative research on postpartum depression described a sense of living their daily life in a sort of fog, from which they believed they would never emerge. Once they improved, they often grieved over the time lost with their newborns while in this "fog." The duration of symptoms varies but as many as half continue to be symptomatic at 6 months (Gjerdinger & Byrd, 2001).

Risk factors for postpartum depression include the following:

- Primiparity
- Ambivalence about maintaining the pregnancy
- History of depression or bipolar illness
- Previous postpartum depression (most significant risk)
- Family history of psychiatric disorders
- Lack of social support
- Lack of a stable relationship with parents or partner
- The woman's dissatisfaction with herself, including body image problems and eating disorders
- Lack of a supportive relationship with her parents, especially her father, as a child

Alcohol has depressive effects as can "coming down from" illicit drugs such as amphetamines and cocaine. Some prescription medications widely used by postpartum women can also cause depression. These include certain contraceptives, drugs used to treat gastroesophageal reflux and peptic ulcer disease, and several others. Women with postpartum depression are at risk of suicide, most prominently as they enter or exit the deeply depressed state. In a deep depression, the woman is unlikely to be able to plan and carry out suicide. For that reason, signs of improvement in depression should be celebrated with some caution.

Whereas the woman with postpartal psychosis may attempt suicide because of illogical thought processes, the woman with major depression attempts suicide because her suffering is so great that dying seems a more favorable option than continuing to live in such pain. She may also attempt suicide in order to save her newborn from some perceived or real threat—including the threat that she herself might harm the baby. The risk of suicide is greater in those who have attempted suicide previously, have a specific plan, and can access the means or weapon identified within the plan. The more specific the plan, the greater is the probability of an attempt.

Clinical Therapy

Medication, individual or group psychotherapy, and practical assistance with child care and other demands of daily life are common treatment measures. Treatment of postpartum depression is not unlike treatment of any significant depression: psychotherapy and antidepression medications, usually the selective serotonin reuptake inhibitors such as sertraline (Zoloft), paroxetine (Paxil), and fluoxetine (Prozac) or tricyclic agents, such as amitriptyline (Elavil) or imipramine (Tofranil). Support groups have proved to be successful adjuncts to such treatment. Within a support group of postpartal women and their partners, a couple may feel consolation that they are not alone in their experience. Moreover, the support group provides a forum for gaining information about postpartum depression, learning stress reduction measures, and experiencing renewed self-esteem and support. If a support group is not available locally, the woman and her family may be encouraged to contact Depression After Delivery (DAD), a national support network that provides literature and volunteers, at PO Box 1282, Morrisville, PA 19067, or 800-944-4773.

Women with a history of depression or postpartum psychosis should be referred to a mental health professional for counseling and biweekly visits between the second and sixth week postpartum for evaluation of depression.

Treatment of postpartum psychosis is directed at the specific type of psychotic symptoms displayed. Emergency hospitalization in an inpatient psychiatric unit is usually indicated. Treatment may include lithium; antipsychotic medications, such as chlorpromazine (Thorazine) or haloperidol (Haldol); or electroconvulsive therapy in combination with psychotherapy. It is important for the nurse to realize that many of the drugs used in treating postpartum psychiatric conditions are contraindicated in breastfeeding women.

NURSING CARE MANAGEMENT

Nursing Assessment and Diagnosis

Assessment for factors predisposing a client to postpartum depression or psychosis should begin prenatally (Beck, 2002). Questions designed to detect problems can be included as part of the routine prenatal history interview or questionnaire. Women with a personal or family history of psychiatric disease, particularly postpartum depression or psychosis, need prenatal instructions on the signs and symptoms of depression and may need additional emotional support. Ideally the assessment should be completed each trimester to update a pregnant woman's risk status (Beck, 2002). If not done previously, the nurse assesses the woman for predisposing factors during her labor and postpartum stay.

Becoming a mother is idealized by most societies as a joyful event. Consequently, the woman who experiences depression, instead of joy, often suffers silently because she feels guilty and hesitant to disclose her honest feelings with family and caregivers. Some women believe that admission of emotional difficulty and mothering inadequacy will be used against them and that their children will be taken away. Prior to assessment for evidence of depression, the nurse can give voice to this societal myth of joyful motherhood, giving the woman permission to share negative feelings and thoughts she might be having. Several depression scales are available for assessing postpartum depression. The Edinburgh Postnatal Depression Scale (Table 37–9 •) is likely the most widely used screening tool for postpartum depression in large populations of women. The tool has been validated, computerized, and used as a telephone screening. No matter what approach the nurse uses to assess for postpartum depression, enabling the woman's voice to be heard about her feelings of maternal role transition and how she is adjusting in this vulnerable time is of inestimable value. Listening to her story provides a critical emic (insider's) view of her circumstances as opposed to an etic (outsider's) view.

Mothers who score above 12 on the Edinburgh Postnatal Depression Scale, are likely to be suffering from postpartum depression.

Beck (2001) revised her practical and simple screening checklist for use during routine care with all postpartal women to identify those who might be experiencing postpartum depression so that early management might be initiated. There are 13 symptoms on the Postpartum Depression Predictors Inventory (PDPI-Revised). Questions are asked to elicit yes/no answers about each symptom; when a "yes" answer is elicited, the nurse provides opportunities for additional exploration, using open-ended questions (Table 37–10 •). Willingness to listen as the mother

Table 37–9 • EDINBURGH POSTNATAL DEPRESSION SCALE

In the past 7 days:

1. I have been able to laugh and see the funny side of things
   As much as I always could
   Not quite so much now
   Definitely not so much now
   Not at all
2. I have looked forward with enjoyment of things
   As much as I ever did
   Rather less than I used to
   Definitely less than I used to
   Hardly at all

*3. I have blamed myself unnecessarily when things went wrong
   Yes, most of the time
   Yes, some of the time
   Not very often
   No, never

4. I have been anxious or worried for no good reason
   No, not at all
   Hardly ever
   Yes, sometimes
   Yes, very often

*5. I have felt scared or panicky for no very good reason
   Yes, quite a lot
   Yes, sometimes
   No, not much
   No, not at all

*6. Things have been getting on top of me
   Yes, most of the time I haven't been able to cope at all
   Yes, sometimes I haven't been coping as well as usual
   No, I have been coping quite well
   No, I have been coping as well as ever

*7. I have been so unhappy that I have had difficulty sleeping
   Yes, most of the time
   Yes, sometimes
   Not very often
   No, not at all

*8. I have felt sad or miserable
   Yes, most of the time
   Yes, quite often
   Not very often
   No, not at all

*9. I have been so unhappy that I have been crying
   Yes, most of the time
   Yes, quite often
   Only occasionally
   No, never

*10. The thought of harming myself has occurred to me
   Yes, quite often
   Sometimes
   Hardly ever
   Never

Note: Response categories are scored 0,1,2, and 3 according to increased severity of the symptoms. Items marked with an asterisk are reversed scored (3,2,1,0). The total score is calculated by adding together the scores for each of the 10 items. A score above the threshold of 12–13 out of 30 indicates with 86% sensitivity, that the woman is suffering from postpartum depression.

Source: Cox, J.L., Holden, J.M., & Sagovsky, R. (1987). Detection of postnatal depression: Development of the 10-item Edinburgh Postnatal Depression Scale. *British Journal of Psychiatry, 150,* 782–786. Users may reproduce the scale without further permission provided they respect copyright by quoting the names of the authors, the title, and the source of the paper in all reproduced copies.

Table 37-10 • POSTPARTUM DEPRESSION PREDICTORS INVENTORY (PDPI)—REVISED AND GUIDE QUESTIONS FOR ITS USE

During Pregnancy		
Marital Status	*Check One*	
1. Single	O	
2. Married/cohabitating	O	
3. Separated	O	
4. Divorced	O	
5. Widowed	O	
6. Partnered	O	
Socioeconomic status		
Low	O	
Middle	O	
High	O	
Self-esteem	*Yes*	*No*
Do you feel good about yourself as a person?	O	O
Do you feel worthwhile?	O	O
Do you feel you have a number of good qualities as a person?	O	O
Prenatal depression		
1. Have you felt depressed during your pregnancy?	O	O
If yes, when and how long have you been feeling this way?		
If yes, how mild or severe would you consider your depression?		
Prenatal anxiety		
Have you been feeling anxious during your pregnancy?	O	O
If yes, how long have you been feeling this way?		
Unplanned/unwanted pregnancy		
Was the pregnancy planned?	O	O
Is the pregnancy unwanted?	O	O
History of previous depression		
1. Before this pregnancy, have you ever been depressed?	O	O
If yes, when did you experience this depression?		
If yes, have you been under a physician's care for this past depression?	O	O
If yes, did the physician prescribe any medication for your depression?	O	O
Social support		
1. Do you feel you receive adequate emotional support from your partner?	O	O
2. Do you feel you receive adequate instrumental support from your partner (eg, help with household chores or baby-sitting)?	O	O
3. Do you feel you can rely on your partner when you need help?	O	O
4. Do you feel you can confide in your partner? (repeat same questions for family and again for friends)	O	O
Marital satisfaction		
1. Are you satisfied with your marriage (or living arrangement)?	O	O
2. Are you currently experiencing any marital problems?	O	O
3. Are things going well between you and your partner?	O	O
Life stress		
1. Are you currently experiencing any stressful events in your life such as:		
financial problems	O	O
marital problems	O	O
death in the family	O	O
serious illness in the family	O	O
moving	O	O
unemployment	O	O
job change	O	O

Table 37-10 • POSTPARTUM DEPRESSION PREDICTORS INVENTORY (PDPI)—REVISED AND GUIDE QUESTIONS FOR ITS USE (CONTINUED)

	Yes	No
After delivery, add the following items		
Child care stress		
1. Is your infant experiencing any health problems?	O	O
2. Are you having problems with your baby feeding?	O	O
3. Are you having problems with your baby sleeping?	O	O
Infant temperament		
1. Would you consider your baby irritable or fussy?	O	O
2. Does your baby cry a lot?	O	O
3. Is your baby difficult to console or soothe?	O	O
Maternity blues		
1. Did you experience a brief period of tearfulness and mood swings during the 1st week after delivery?	O	O

COMMENTS:

____

____

____

Source: AWHONN. (2002). Beck, C. T. Revision of the postpartum predictors inventory. *Journal of Obstetric, Gynecologic, and Neonatal Nursing, 31*(4): 394–402. (Table 2 and Table 3 on PDPI, p. 399–401). Washington, DC Author.

shares her experience of postpartum depression not only enables the nurse to recognize symptoms and initiate timely management, but also is commonly perceived by the mother as caring (Beck, 2002).

In providing daily care, the nurse observes the woman for objective signs of depression—anxiety, irritability, poor concentration, forgetfulness, sleeping difficulties, appetite change, fatigue, and tearfulness—and listens for statements indicating feelings of failure and self-accusation. Severity and duration of symptoms should be noted. Behavior and verbalization that are bizarre or seem to indicate a potential for violence against herself or others, including the infant, are reported as soon as possible for further evaluation.

The nurse needs to be aware that many normal physiologic changes of the puerperium are similar to symptoms of depression (lack of sexual interest, indecisiveness, appetite change, sleep disturbance, and fatigue). It is essential that observations be as specific and as objective as possible and that they be carefully documented.

A central challenge for nursing is identifying women at risk of suicide. Like others with psychologic disorders, the postpartum woman is likely ambivalent about suicide, and may be "rescuable" if suicide ideation is assessed and timely action follows. Assessment of suicide risk reflects the standard of care; contrary to myth, asking a depressed woman about suicidal thoughts does not increase her risk, but it may save her life. Introducing the issue of suicide can be as simple as saying something like, "I'm concerned about the amount of emotional pain you're feeling, and I'm wondering whether you've ever thought of hurting yourself." Ambivalence about suicide is likely to make the woman answer candidly. A suicide prevention contract may be established with the woman to exact an agreement that she will seek help immediately if she begins to consider self-harm. For example, the nurse might say, "Promise me that should you begin to feel as if you are going to hurt yourself, you will telephone me or the hot line immediately—that you will not act without talking to someone." Because of the hope this offers, the woman is likely to respond by seeking help; she does not want to renege on a promise she made to a nurse who has shown such caring for her.

If a woman admits that she has thought of hurting herself, assessment of the risk that she will follow through is imperative. The mnemonic **SAL** is useful for risk assessment: Is there a **S**pecific plan with a designated time? Is there an **A**ccessible weapon or other means? How **L**ethal is the method identified in the plan? A specific plan that identifies a highly lethal method that is immediately accessible is evidence of very high risk of suicide. Immediate intervention is critical; emergency psychiatric hospitalization is likely necessary. Those considered a threat to themselves or others may be admitted to involuntary hospitalization for a minimum of 48 hours until further evaluation is complete.

Family members of the depressed woman should also be alert to signals that she may be intent on self-harm; they must be advised that threats should always be taken seriously. Cues to suicide that might be noted by family are comments such as " I don't deserve to live," "Life is no longer worth living," or "You won't have to worry about me for long." Someone who is considering suicide may also telephone or write family or friends to say good-bye or give away prized possessions. Family members should be told to be especially vigilant for suicide when the woman seems to be feeling better.

Possible nursing diagnoses that may apply to a woman with a postpartum psychiatric disorder include the following:

- ***Ineffective Individual Coping*** related to postpartum depression
- ***Risk for Altered Parenting*** related to postpartal mental illness

Nursing Plan and Implementation

Nurses working in antepartal settings or teaching childbirth classes play indispensable roles in helping prospective parents appreciate the lifestyle changes and role demands associated with parenthood. Offering realistic information and anticipatory guidance and debunking myths about the perfect mother or perfect newborn may help prevent postpartum depression.

The nurse should alert the mother, partner, and other family members to the possibility of postpartum blues in the early days after birth and reassure them of the short-term nature of the condition. Symptoms of postpartum depression should be described and the mother encouraged to call her healthcare provider if symptoms become severe, if they fail to subside quickly, or if at any time she feels she is unable to function. Encouraging the mother to plan how she will manage at home and providing concrete suggestions on how to cope will aid in her adjustment to motherhood. Table 37–11 • indicates suggestions that serve as primary prevention for postpartum depression.

Table 37–11 • PRIMARY PREVENTION STRATEGIES FOR POSTPARTUM DEPRESSION

1. Celebrate childbirth but appreciate that it is a life-changing transition that can be stressful—at times it can seem overwhelming. Share your feelings with each other and/or others.
2. Consider keeping a journal where you write down feelings. Not only is it emotionally cathartic, it provides a great memory book.
3. Appreciate that you do not have to know everything to be a good parent—it is okay to seek advice during this transition.
4. Connect to others who are parents—use them as a support and information network.
5. Set a daily schedule and follow it even if you do not feel like it. Structuring activity helps counteract inertia that comes with feeling sad or unsettled.
6. Prioritize daily tasks. Decide what must be done and what can wait. Try to get one major thing done every day. Remember, you do not always have to look like a magazine fashion model.
7. Remember that you do not have to entertain or care for everyone who drops by. Doing something for someone else, however, often tends to make you feel better.
8. If someone volunteers to help you with tasks or baby care, take them up on it. While your volunteer is in action, do something pleasurable or get some rest.
9. Maintain outside interests. Plan some time every day—even if it's just 15 minutes—to do something exclusively for "you" that is pleasurable.
10. Eat a healthful diet. Limit alcohol. Quit smoking. Get some exercise. (All of these can positively affect the immune system.)
11. Get as much sleep as possible. Rest whenever you can, such as when the baby is napping. If you have other young children, bring them onto your bed to read or play quietly while you lie down.
12. Limit major changes (moves, job changes, etc) the first year insofar as possible.
13. Spend time with others.
14. If things get overwhelming, and you feel yourself slipping into depression, reach out to someone for help.
15. Attend a postpartum support group if one is available. Consider also an international program:

Postpartum Support International
927 North Kellogg Avenue
Santa Barbara, CA 93111
1-805-967-7636 or online at http://www.postpartum.net

Community-Based Nursing Care

Home visits, especially for early discharge families, are invaluable to fostering positive adjustments for the new family constellation. Telephone follow-up at 3 weeks postpartum to ask whether the mother is experiencing difficulties is also helpful.

In all women, the presence of three symptoms (identified earlier) on one day or one symptom for 3 days may signal serious postpartum depression and requires immediate referral to a mental health professional. Immediate referral should also be made if rejection of the infant or threatened or actual aggression against the infant has occurred. In such cases, the newborn is never left unattended with the mother.

Depression does appear to interfere with optimal mothering; there is less interaction between mother and child, more mood and cognitive development problems, and more visits to the doctor in these children (Beck, 2002).

A diagnosis of postpartum depression or other psychiatric disorder will pose major problems for the family, especially the father. The symptoms of these disorders are difficult to witness and may be harder to understand than physical problems such as hemorrhage or infection. The father may feel hurt by his partner's hostility and may worry that she is becoming insane, or be baffled by her mood swings and lack of concern about herself, the newborn, or household responsibilities. He may be troubled by their lack of intimacy or deteriorating communication. Certainly, he has cause for concern about how the newborn and any other children are being affected. There may be very real practical matters to handle—running the household; managing the children, including the totally dependent newborn; and caring for the mother—added to his usual routines and work responsibilities. It is not surprising that even in the most supportive families relationships may suffer in response to these circumstances. It is often a family member who in desperation makes contact with the healthcare agency. This is especially difficult when the mother is reluctant to admit she is suffering emotional difficulty or is too ill to recognize her own needs.

MEDIALINK POSTPARTUM SUPPORT

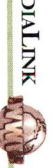

Information, emotional support, and assistance in providing or obtaining care for the infant may be needed. The nurse can assist family members by identifying community resources and making referrals to public health nursing services and social services. Postpartum follow-up is especially important, as well as visits from a psychiatric home health nurse.

Evaluation

Expected outcomes of nursing care include:

- Signs of potential postpartal psychiatric disorders are detected quickly, and therapy is implemented.
- The newborn is cared for effectively by the father or another support person until the mother is able to do so.

Chapter Review

ExploreMediaLink

NCLEX review questions, case studies, and other interactive resources for this chapter can be found on the Web site at http://www.prenhall.com/olds. Click on "Chapter 37" and select the activities for this chapter.

For tutorials including animations and videos, more NCLEX review questions, and an audio glossary, access the accompanying CD-ROM in this book.

Focus Your Study

- Nursing assessment and intervention play a large role in preventing postpartum complications.
- The main causes of early postpartal hemorrhage are uterine atony, lacerations of the vagina and cervix, and retained placental fragments.
- The most common postpartal infection is metritis, which is limited to the uterine cavity.
- A postpartal woman is at increased risk for developing urinary tract problems because of normal postpartal diuresis, increased bladder capacity, decreased bladder sensitivity from stretching or trauma, and, possibly, inhibited neural control of the bladder following the use of anesthetic agents.
- Mastitis is an inflammation of the breast often caused by *Staphylococcus aureus*, *Escherichia coli*, and *Streptococcus* species. Mastitis is seen primarily in breastfeeding women. Symptoms seldom occur before the second to fourth postpartal week.
- Thromboembolic disease originating in the veins of the leg, thigh, or pelvis may occur antepartally or postpartally and carries with it the potential for creating a pulmonary embolus.
- Although many different types of psychiatric problems may be encountered in the postpartal period, postpartum blues is the most common. Postpartum blues episodes occur frequently in the week after birth and are typically transient.
- Postpartum depression risk factors should be screened for each trimester during pregnancy and during the immediate postpartum period.
- Telephone calls and home visits are effective measures for extending comprehensive care into the home setting of the postpartal family at risk.

References

Alexander, J. D., & Schneider, F. D. (2000). Vaginal bleeding associated with pregnancy. *Primary Care, 27*(1), 137–145.

American Psychiatric Association (APA). (2000). *Diagnostic and statistical manual of mental disorders* (5th ed.). Washington, DC: Author.

Andersen, H. F., & Hopkins, M. P. (2002). Postpartum hemorrhage. In J. J. Sciarri (Ed.), *Gynecology and obstetrics* (Vol. 2, pp.1–10). Philadelphia: Lippincott Williams & Wilkins.

Baxley, E. G. (2001). Postpartum biomedical concerns. Section B postpartum endometritis. In S. D. Ratcliffe, E. G. Baxley,

J. E. Byrd, & E. L. Sakornbut (Eds.), *Family practice obstetrics* (2nd ed., pp. 602–607). Philadelphia: Hanley & Belfus.

Beck, C. T. (1993). Teetering on the edge: A substantive theory of postpartum depression. *Nursing Research, 42*(1), 42–48.

Beck, C. T. (2001). Predictors of postpartum depression: An update. *Nursing Research, 50*, 275–285.

Beck, C. T. (2002). Revision of the postpartum depression predictors inventory. *Journal of Obstetric, Gynecologic, and Neonatal Nursing, 31*(4), 394–402.

Beck, C. T., & Gable, R. (2000). Postpartum depression screening scale: Development and psychometric testing. *Nursing Research, 49*(5), 272–282.

Benedetti, T. J. (2002). Obstetric hemorrhage. In S. G. Gabbe, J. R. Niebyl, & J. L. Simpson (Eds.), *Obstetrics: Normal and problem pregnancies* (4th ed., pp. 503–538). New York: Churchill Livingstone.

Bowes, W. A., & Katz, V. L. (2002). Postpartum care. In S. G. Gabbe, J. R. Niebyl, & J. L. Simpson (Eds.), *Obstetrics: Normal and problem pregnancies* (4th ed., pp. 701–726). New York: Churchill Livingstone.

Cash, J. C., & Glass, C. A. (2000). *Family practice guidelines.* Philadelphia: Lippincott.

Clarke-Pearson, D. L. (2000). Venous thromboembolic disease in pregnancy. In E. J. Quilligan & F. P. Zuspan (Eds.), *Current therapy in obstetrics and gynecology* (5th ed., pp. 368–371). Philadelphia: W.B. Saunders.

Cox, J. L., Holden, J. M., & Sagovsky, R. (1987). Detection of postnatal depression: Development of the 10-item Edinburgh Postnatal Depression Scale. *British Journal of Psychiatry, 150*, 782–786.

Cunningham, F. G., Gant, N. F., Leveno, K. J., Gilstrap, L. C., III, Hauth, J. C., & Wenstrom, K. D. (2001). *Williams obstetrics* (21st ed.). New York: McGraw-Hill.

Duff, P. (2002). Maternal and perinatal infection. In S. G. Gabbe, J. R. Niebyl, & J. L. Simpson (Eds.), *Obstetrics: Normal and problem pregnancies* (4th ed., pp. 1293–1345). New York: Churchill Livingstone.

Elmer, G. W. (2001). Probiotics: "Living drugs." *American Journal of Health System Pharmacy, 58*(12), 1101–1109.

Gilbert, E. S., & Harmon, J. S. (2003). *Manual of high risk pregnancy and delivery* (3rd ed.). St.Louis, MO: Mosby.

Gjerdinger, D., & Byrd, J. E. (2001). Postpartum psychosocial concerns. In S. D. Ratcliff, E. G. Baxley, J. E. Byrd, & E. L. Sakornbut (Eds.), *Family practice obstetrics* (2nd ed., pp. 625–638). Philadelphia: Hanley & Belfus.

Gravett, M. G. (2002). Intra-amniotic and postpartum infections. In J. J. Sciarri (Ed.), *Gynecology and obstetrics* (Vol. 3, pp.1–18). Philadelphia: Lippincott Williams & Wilkins.

Hull, R. D., Kane, G. C., & Tapson, V. F. (2000, August). Improving survival in pulmonary embolism. *Patient Care, 30*(8), 50–63.

Laros, R. K. (1999). Thromboembolic disease. In R. K. Creasy & R. Resnik (Eds.), *Maternal-fetal medicine* (4th ed., pp. 821–832). Philadelphia: Saunders.

Lawrence, R. A., & Lawrence, R. M. (1999). *Breastfeeding: A guide for the medical profession.* St. Louis, MO: C.V. Mosby.

Matteson, P. S. (2001). *Women's health during the childbearing years: A community-based approach.* St. Louis, MO: C.V. Mosby.

Meighan, M., Davis, M. W., Thomas, S. P., & Droppleman, P. G. (2000). Living with postpartum depression: The father's perspective. *American Journal of Maternal Child Nursing, 24*(4), 202–208.

Mills, M. (2001, April). *The moody blues mood disorders in pregnancy.* Presented at Obstetrical Challenges of the New Millennium, Phoenix, AZ.

Nadeau, C., Alpert, B., Costantino, T., McGinn, R., Coyne, M., Ahern, K., et al. (2000). The challenges of oral anticoagulation. *Patient Care for the Nurse Practitioner, 3*(12), 12–25.

Newton, E. R. (2002). Physiology of lactation and breast-feeding. In S. G. Gabbe, J. R. Niebyl, & J. L. Simpson (Eds.), *Obstetrics: Normal and problem pregnancies* (4th ed., pp. 105–138). New York: Churchill Livingstone.

Quilligan, E. J., & Zuspan, F. P. (2000). *Current therapy in obstetrics and gynecology* (5th ed.). Philadelphia: W.B. Saunders.

Scarr, E. M., & Sammone, L. N. (1999). Endometritis. In W. L. Star, M. T. Shannon, L. L. Lommel, Y. M. Gutierres, (Eds.), *Ambulatory obstetrics* (3rd ed., pp. 379–383). San Francisco: UCSF Nursing Press.

Shinskie, D., & Lauwers, J. (2002). *Pocket Guide: Counseling the nursing mother.* Boston: Jones & Bartlett.

Toppenberg, K. S., & Block, W. A. (2002). Uterine rupture: What family physicians need to know. *American Family Physician, 66*(3), 823–828.

Walling, A. D. (2001). Thromboembolism in pregnancy: Clinical guidelines. *American Family Physician.* Retrieved 2/1/2001 from www.aafp.org/afp20011020/tips/7.html

Wells, J. L., & Salyer, S. W. (2001). Diagnosing pulmonary embolism. *Clinician Reviews, 11*(2), 67–79.

Appendices

APPENDIX A

Common Abbreviations in Maternal-Newborn and Women's Health Nursing

AC Abdominal circumference
accel Acceleration of fetal heart rate
AFAFP Amniotic fluid alpha-fetoprotein
AFI Amniotic fluid index
AFP Alpha-fetoprotein
AFV Amniotic fluid volume
AGA Average for gestational age
AI Amnioinfusion
AMOL Active management of labor
AOP Apnea of prematurity *or* Anemia of prematurity
ARBOW Artificial rupture of bag of waters
AROM Artificial rupture of membranes
ART Artificial reproductive technology
BAT Brown adipose tissue (brown fat)
BBT Basal body temperature
BBOW Bulging bag of water
BL Baseline (fetal heart rate baseline)
BOW Bag of waters
βCG Beta-human chorionic gonadotropin
BPD Biparietal diameter *or* Bronchopulmonary dysplasia
BPP Biophysical profile
BRB Bright red bleeding *or* Breakthrough bleeding
BR CA Breast cancer
BSE Breast self-examination
BSST Breast self-stimulation test
CC Chest circumference *or* Cord compression
C-H Crown-to-heel length
CID Cytomegalic inclusion disease
CLD Chronic lung disease
CM Certified midwife
CMV Cytomegalovirus
CNM Certified nurse-midwife
CNP Certified nurse practitioner
CNS Clinical nurse specialist
CP Chest pain
CPAP Continuous positive airway pressure
CPD Cephalopelvic disproportion *or* Citrate-phosphate-dextrose
CRL Crown-rump length
CRNP Certified registered nurse practitioner
C/S Cesarean section (or C-section)
CST Contraction stress test
CT Chlamydia
CVA Costovertebral angle
CVS Chorionic villus sampling
D&C Dilatation and curettage
D&E Dilatation and evacuation
decels Deceleration of fetal heart rate
DFMR Daily fetal movement response
dil Dilatation
DTR Deep tendon reflexes
DV Domestic violence
EAB Elective abortion
ECMO Extracorporal membrane oxygenator
EDB Estimated date of birth
EDC Estimated date of confinement
EDD Estimated date of delivery
EFM Electronic fetal monitoring
EFW Estimated fetal weight
EIA Enzyme immunoassay
ELF Elective low forceps
ELISA Enzyme-linked immunosorbent assay
EP Ectopic pregnancy
epis Episiotomy
FAD Fetal activity diary
FAE Fetal alcohol effects
FAS Fetal alcohol syndrome
FBD Fibrocystic breast disease
FBM Fetal breathing movements
FBS Fetal blood sample *or* Fasting blood sugar test
FECG Fetal electrocardiogram
FeSO4 Iron supplement
FHR Fetal heart rate
FHT Fetal heart tones
Fhx Family history
FL Femur length
FMC Fetal movement count
FMR Fetal movement record
FPG Fasting plasma glucose test
FSE Fetal scalp electrode
FSH Follicle-stimulating hormone

FSHRH	Follicle-stimulating hormone–releasing hormone
G or grav	Gravida
GC	Gonorrhea
GDM	Gestational diabetes mellitus
GIFT	Gamete intrafallopian transfer
GnRF	Gonadotropin-releasing factor
GnRH	Gonadotropin-releasing hormone
GTD	Gestational trophoblastic disease
GTPAL	Gravida, term, preterm, abortion, living children; a system of recording maternity history
HA	Head-abdominal ratio, headache
HAI	Hemagglutination-inhibition test
HC	Head compression
hCG	Human chorionic gonadotropin
hCS	Human chorionic somatomammotropin (same as hPL)
HIV	Human immunodeficiency virus
HMD	Hyaline membrane disease
hMG	Human menopausal gonadotropin
hPL	Human placental lactogen
HPV	Human papilloma virus
HRT	Hormone replacement therapy
HSV	Herpes simplex virus
ICSI	Intracytoplasmic sperm injection
IDM	Infant of a diabetic mother
IPG	Impedance phlebography
ISAM	Infant of a substance-abusing mother
IU	International units
IUD	Intrauterine device
IUFD	Intrauterine fetal death
IUGR	Intrauterine growth restriction
IUPC	Intrauterine pressure catheter
IUS	Intrauterine system
IVF	In vitro fertilization
LADA	Left-acromion-dorsal-anterior
LADP	Left-acromion-dorsal-posterior
LBW	Low birth weight
LDR	Labor, delivery, and recovery room
LGA	Large for gestational age
LH	Luteinizing hormone
LHRH	Luteinizing hormone–releasing hormone
LMA	Left-mentum-anterior
LML	Left mediolateral (episiotomy)
LMP	Last menstrual period *or* Left-mentum-posterior
LMT	Left-mentum-transverse
LOA	Left-occiput-anterior
LOF	Low outlet forceps
LOP	Left-occiput-posterior
LOS	Length of stay
LOT	Left-occiput-transverse
L/S	Lecithin/sphingomyelin ratio
LSA	Left-sacrum-anterior
LSP	Left-sacrum-posterior
LST	Left-sacrum-transverse
MAS	Meconium aspiration syndrome
mec	Meconium
mec st	Meconium stain
MLE	Midline episiotomy
MSAFP	Maternal serum alpha-fetoprotein
MUGB	4-methylumbelliferyl quanidinobenzoate
multip	Multipara
NEC	Necrotizing enterocolitis
NGU	Nongonococcal urethritis
NP	Nurse practitioner
NSCST	Nipple stimulation contraction stress test
NST	Nonstress test *or* Nonshivering thermogenesis
NSVD	Normal sterile vaginal delivery
NTD	Neural tube defects
NTE	Neutral thermal environment
OA	Occiput anterior
OCPs	Oral contraceptive pills
OCT	Oxytocin challenge test
OF	Occipitofrontal diameter of fetal head
OFC	Occipitofrontal circumference
OGTT	Oral glucose tolerance test
OM	Occipitomental (diameter)
OP	Occiput posterior
p	Para
Pap smear	Papanicolaou smear
PDA	Patent ductus arteriosus
PEEP	Positive end-expiratory pressure
PG	Phosphatidylglycerol *or* Prostaglandin
PID	Pelvic inflammatory disease
Pit	Pitocin
PKU	Phenylketonuria
PMS	Premenstrual syndrome
PNV	Prenatal vitamins
PPHN	Persistent pulmonary hypertension
Premie	Premature infant
primip	Primipara
PROM	Premature rupture of membranes
PSI	Prostaglandin synthesis inhibitor
PUBS	Percutaneous umbilical blood sampling
RADA	Right-acromion-dorsal-anterior

RADP	Right-acromion-dorsal-posterior
RDS	Respiratory distress syndrome
REM	Rapid eye movements
RIA	Radioimmunoassay
RLF	Retrolental fibroplasia
RMA	Right-mentum-anterior
RMP	Right-mentum-posterior
RMT	Right-mentum-transverse
ROA	Right-occiput-anterior
ROM	Rupture of membranes
ROP	Right-occiput-posterior *or* Retinopathy of prematurity
ROT	Right-occiput-transverse
RRA	Radioreceptor assay
RSA	Right-sacrum-anterior
RSP	Right-sacrum-posterior
RST	Right-sacrum-transverse
SAB	Spontaneous abortion
SET	Surrogate embryo transfer
SGA	Small for gestational age
SIDS	Sudden infant death syndrome
SMB	Submentobregmatic diameter
SOB	Suboccipitobregmatic diameter
SPA	Sperm penetration assay
SRBOW	Spontaneous rupture of bag of waters
SROM	Spontaneous rupture of membranes
STD	Sexually transmitted disease
STI	Sexually transmitted infection
STS	Serologic test for syphilis
SVE	Sterile vaginal exam
TAB	Therapeutic abortion
TC	Thoracic circumference
TCM	Transcutaneous monitoring
TDI or THI	Therapeutic donor insemination (*H* designates mate is donor)
TET	Tubal embryo transfer
TOL	Trial of labor
TORCH	Toxoplasmosis, rubella, cytomegalovirus, herpesvirus hominis type 2
TSS	Toxic shock syndrome
ū	Umbilicus
UA	Uterine activity
UAC	Umbilical artery catheter
UAU	Uterine activity units
UC	Uterine contraction
UPI	Uteroplacental insufficiency
US	Ultrasound
VBAC	Vaginal birth after cesarean
VDRL	Venereal Disease Research Laboratories
VIP	Voluntary interruption of pregnancy
VLBW	Very low birth weight
WIC	Supplemental food program for Women, Infants, and Children
ZIFT	Zygote intrafallopian transfer

APPENDIX B

Conversions and Equivalents

TEMPERATURE CONVERSION

(Fahrenheit temperature − 32) × 5/9 = Centigrade temperature

(Centigrade temperature × 9/5) + 32 = Fahrenheit temperature

SELECTED CONVERSION TO METRIC MEASURES

Known Value	Multiply by	To find
inches	2.54	centimeters
ounces	28	grams
pounds	454	grams
pounds	0.45	kilogram

SELECTED CONVERSION FROM METRIC MEASURES

Known Value	Multiply by	To find
centimeters	0.4	inches
grams	0.035	ounces
grams	0.0022	pounds
kilograms	2.2	pounds

CONVERSION OF POUNDS AND OUNCES TO GRAMS

	Ounces															
S (Pounds)	0	1	2	3	4	5	6	7	8	9	10	11	12	13	14	15
0	—	28	57	85	113	142	170	198	227	255	283	312	340	369	397	425
1	454	482	510	539	567	595	624	652	680	709	737	765	794	822	850	879
2	907	936	964	992	1021	1049	1077	1106	1134	1162	1191	1219	1247	1276	1304	1332
3	1361	1389	1417	1446	1474	1503	1531	1559	1588	1616	1644	1673	1701	1729	1758	1786
4	1814	1843	1871	1899	1928	1956	1984	2013	2041	2070	2098	2126	2155	2183	2211	2240
5	2268	2296	2325	2353	2381	2410	2438	2466	2495	2523	2551	2580	2608	2637	2665	2693
6	2722	2750	2778	2807	2835	2863	2892	2920	2948	2977	3005	3033	3062	3090	3118	3147
7	3175	3203	3232	3260	3289	3317	3345	3374	3402	3430	3459	3487	3515	3544	3572	3600
8	3629	3657	3685	3714	3742	3770	3799	3827	3856	3884	3912	3941	3969	3997	4026	4054
9	4082	4111	4139	4167	4196	4224	4252	4281	4309	4337	4366	4394	4423	4451	4479	4508
10	4536	4564	4593	4621	4649	4678	4706	4734	4763	4791	4819	4848	4876	4904	4933	4961
11	4990	5018	5046	5075	5103	5131	5160	5188	5216	5245	5273	5301	5330	5358	5386	5415
12	5443	5471	5500	5528	5557	5585	5613	5642	5670	5698	5727	5755	5783	5812	5840	5868
13	5897	5925	5953	5982	6010	6038	6067	6095	6123	6152	6180	6209	6237	6265	6294	6322
14	6350	6379	6407	6435	6464	6492	6520	6549	6577	6605	6634	6662	6690	6719	6747	6776
15	6804	6832	6860	6889	6917	6945	6973	7002	7030	7059	7087	7115	7144	7172	7201	7228
16	7257	7286	7313	7342	7371	7399	7427	7456	7484	7512	7541	7569	7597	7626	7654	7682
17	7711	7739	7768	7796	7824	7853	7881	7909	7938	7966	7994	8023	8051	8079	8108	8136
18	8165	8192	8221	8249	8278	8306	8335	8363	8391	8420	8448	8476	8504	8533	8561	8590
19	8618	8646	8675	8703	8731	8760	8788	8816	8845	8873	8902	8930	8958	8987	9015	9043
20	9072	9100	9128	9157	9185	9213	9242	9270	9298	9327	9355	9383	9412	9440	9469	9497
21	9525	9554	9582	9610	9639	9667	9695	9724	9752	9780	9809	9837	9865	9894	9922	9950
22	9979	10007	10036	10064	10092	10120	10149	10177	10206	10234	10262	10291	10319	10347	10376	10404

APPENDIX C

Spanish Translations of English Phrases[*]

This appendix includes phrases you might find helpful in working with families during pregnancy, labor, and birth, and after the birth. There are many ways to phrase questions. We have chosen some statements we consider essential and have tried to phrase them in a straightforward way. The phrases are designed to help you in situations in which translation is not possible at the moment.

This list begins with introductory statements, which are presented in a logical conversational flow. The remaining phrases are arranged according to the phases of pregnancy and birth during which they are most applicable.

Essential Introductory Phrases	Frases Introductoras Esenciales
Hello	Hola
I am a nurse.	Soy enfermera (enfermero).[†]
I am a student nurse.	Soy estudiante de enfermería.
My name is ____________________.	Mi nombre es ____________________.
	Me llamo ____________________.
What is your name?	¿Cuál es su nombre?
	¿Cómo se llama?
What name should I call you?	¿Cómo quiere que la llamemos?
	¿Cómo quiere ser llamada?
Thank you	Gracias
Please	Por favor
Is someone here with you?	¿Hay alquien aquí con usted?
Does he (she) speak English?	¿Habla él (ella) inglés?
Goodbye	Adiós.

Phrases for the Antepartal Period	Frases para el Periodo Prenatal
Are you taking any medications now?	¿Está tomando algunas medicinas ahora?
Show me the medicine bottles please.	Por favor, muéstreme los frascos.
Have you ever had trouble with your blood pressure?	¿Ha tenido problemas alguna vez con la presión arterial?
When was the first day of your last period?	¿Cuál fue el primer día de su última regla?
	¿Cuál fue el primer día de su última menstruación?
Have you had any spotting or bleeding since your last period?	¿Ha sangrado o ha tenido manchas de sangre desde su última regla?
Have you been on birth control pills?	¿Ha estado tomando píldoras anticonceptivas?
When did you stop taking them?	¿Cuándo dejó de tomarlas?
Do you have an intrauterine device (IUD)?	¿Usa un aparato intrauterino?
How many times have you been pregnant?	¿Cuántas veces ha estado usted embarazada?
Are you having any problems with your pregnancy?	¿Tiene problemas con su embarazo?
Is there anything that is worrying you?	¿Hay algo o alguna cosa que la preocupe?
I would like to take your blood pressure.	Quisiera tomarle la presió arterial.
I would like to take your pulse.	Quisiera tomarle el pulso.
I would like to take your temperature.	Quisiera tomarle la temperatura.
I would like to listen to your heart and lungs.	Quisiera escucharle el corazon y los pulmones.

I would like to check your uterus.	Quisiera examinarle el útero.
Please urinate in this cup and leave it in the bathroom.	Puede orinar en este vaso y dejarlo en el baño.
Please stand up.	Por favor, levántese.
Please sit down.	Por favor, siéntese.
Please lie down.	Por favor, acuéstese.

Phrases Related to Client Safety / Frases Relacionadas con la Seguridad del Cliente

I would like to talk to you alone.	Quisiera hablar a solas con usted.
Are you safe at home?	¿Sufre de peligros en casa?
Are you afraid of your partner?	¿Le tiene miedo a su compañero?
During your pregnancy has your partner hit, slapped, kicked, or punched you?	Durante su embarazo, ¿la ha golpeado? ¿la ha abofeteado? ¿la ha pateado? o ¿le ha dado puñetazos?
How many times?	¿Cuántas veces?
Do you have someone for support?	¿Cuénta con alguien que la pueda ayudar?

Questions the Mother or Father May Ask / Posibles Preguntas que Madres o Padres Hacen

How big is my baby?	¿De qué tamaño es el (la) bebé?
How much does the baby weigh now?	¿Cuánto pesa el bebé ahora?
When will I feel my baby move?	¿Cuándo lo (la) voy a sentir moverse?

Phrases for the Intrapartal Period / Frases Durante el Parto

Note: Review the essential introductory phrases for beginning a conversation.	*Nota:* Repase las frases introductoras para comenzar una conversación.
Are you having labor pains?	¿Tiene dolores de parto?
Are you having contractions?	¿Tiene contracciones?
Are you having pain?	¿Tiene dolores?
Do you need medicine for pain?	¿Necesita medicina para el dolor?
Do you need to urinate?	¿Necesita orinar?
This is a bedpan to urinate in.	Aquí tiene el bacín (la chata) (el pato) para orinar.
Can I help you to the bathroom?	¿La ayudo a ir al baño?
Do you need to have a bowel movement?	¿Necesita mover el vientre (obrar)? Necesita "Hacer caca"— coloquial
Has your bag of water broken?	¿Se le ha roto la bolsa de agua(s)?
Have you had any bright-red bleeding during your pregnancy?	¿Ha tenido algún sangramiento de color rojo durante su embarazo?
How many births have you had?	¿Cuántos niños le han nacido?
I need to do a vaginal examination.	Necesito hacerle un examen vaginal.
I will help you.	La voy a ayudar.
I will stay with you.	Me quedaré con usted.
Please pant. I will show you how.	Por favor, jadee. Le voy a mostrar cómo.
Do not push now.	No puje ahora.
Push now.	Puje ahora.
Stop pushing.	Pare de pujar. No puje más.
The doctor needs to do a cesarean birth.	El doctor le va a hacer una operación cesárea.

This is medicine for your pain. You will feel better soon.	Esta medicina es para el dolor. Va a sentirse mejor pronto.
When is your baby supposed to be born?	¿Cuando está supuesto a nacer el bebé?
January	enero
February	febrero
March	marzo
April	abril
May	mayo
June	junio
July	julio
August	agosto
September	septiembre
October	octubre
November	noviembre
December	diciembre
What is your doctor's name?	¿Cuál es el nombre de su doctor?
What is your midwife's name?	¿Cuál es el nombre de su comadrona (partera)?
Your baby is having some trouble now.	El bebé está pasando por algunos problemas. El bebé está sufriendo algunas dificultades.
I need to put this oxygen mask on you. It will help your baby. It may smell funny, but it is OK.	Le voy a poner esta máscara de oxígeno. Va a ayudar al bebé. Huele extraño, pero no hay problemas.
Please turn on your left side.	Por favor voltéese al lado izquierdo.
Please turn on your right side.	Por favor voltéese al lado derecho.
Your baby is OK.	El bebé está bien.

Phrases for the Postpartal Period and the Newborn Area / Frases para el Periodo Despues del Parto y el Area del Recien Nacido

Note: Review the essential introductory phrases for beginning a conversation.	*Nota:* Repase las frases introductoras para comenzar una conversación.
Are you hungry?	¿Tiene hambre?
Are you thirsty?	¿Tiene sed?
Are you cold?	¿Tiene frío?
Are you tired?	¿Está cansada?
I am going to put antibiotic ointment in the baby's eyes.	Le voy a poner al bebé un ungüento antibiótico alrededor de los ojos.
It will help protect your baby from some infections.	Lo (la) va a proteger contra algunos infecciones.
I am going to take some blood from your baby's foot to check the blood sugar and hemocrit.	Le voy a sacar sangre del pie al bebé para determinar el azúcar de la sangre y el hematocrítico.
If your baby begins to spit up, please turn him (her) on his (her) side.	Si el bebé comienza a vomitar, colóquelo (colóquela) de costado.
It may help to position your baby like this.	Lo (la) ayudará— si lo coloca así. Lo (la) ayudaría—si lo colocara así.
I would like to suggest that you clean your nipples this way before you breastfeed your baby.	Es bueno que se lave los pezones de esta manera antes de darle el pecho al bebé.
It is better that you clean your baby's cord this way.	Es mejor para el bebé que le lave el ombligo de esta manera.
It is better that you bathe your baby this way.	Es mejor que lo (la) bañe de esta manera.
It is better that you clean your baby's penis this way.	Es mejor que le limpie el pene así.

I would like to suggest that you fold the diaper this way.	Le sugiero que doble el pañal así.
I would like to suggest that you fasten the diaper this way.	Le sugiero que asegure el pañal así.
Take the baby's temperature this way.	Tómele la temperatura así.
I need to check (your breasts, your uterus, your flow, your stitches, your legs and feet).	Necesito examinarle (los pechos, el útero, el flujo, los puntos, las piernas y los pies).
I need to feel your uterus.	Necesito examinarle el útero.
I need to massage your uterus.	Necesito darle un masaje en la región del útero.
Place your baby on its side.	Coloque al bebé de costado.
Place the baby's used diapers here.	Coloque aquí los pañales usados.
Please rub your uterus every half hour to keep it firm. I will show you how.	Necesita darse un masaje en la región del útero cada media hora para mantenerlo firme. Le voy a mostrar cómo.
Would you like to see your baby now?	¿Quiere ver a su bebé ahora?
Would you like me to help you feed your baby?	¿Quiere que le ayude a alimentarlo (la)?
Your baby needs a car seat to go home in.	El (la) bebé necesita un asiento para bebé en el automóvil.

Special Neonatal Needs / Necesidades del Recien Nacido

We are giving your baby oxygen.	Le vamos a dar oxígeno al (a la) bebé.
Your baby is having problems breathing.	El (la) bebé tiene problemas al respirar.
Your baby needs extra help.	El (la) bebé necesita ayuda especial.
Your baby needs to go to a special care nursery.	El (la) bebé necesita ir a la sala de cuidados especiales para bebés.

*Prepared by Elizabeth Medina, Ph.D. Associate Professor of Spanish, Regis University, Denver, Colorado.

†In Spanish, nouns that end in *a* indicate female gender; nouns that end in *o* indicate male gender.

APPENDIX D

Guidelines for Working with Deaf Clients and Interpreters

1. First, remember that it requires trust on the part of the client to allow nonsigning caregivers and an interpreter into her life.
2. It is important to use a registered interpreter. Medical interpreters are registered with the Registry of Interpreters for the Deaf. Although family members and friends may offer to interpret, it is best to use registered medical interpreters because they are required to translate the clients' and nurses' words accurately without adding in any other opinion.
3. Greet the client and family with a handshake and body posture that indicates welcome. You may point to your name tag and use the American Sign Language (ASL) alphabet cards to spell out your name. The client may wish to select cards to indicate her name. It is especially important as you work together to make the effort to provide a greeting as you would with speaking clients; greetings help develop rapport.
4. Once the interpreter is present, continue to look at the client and speak directly to her. There will be a temptation to look at the interpreter, and it will help to remember that you are speaking to the client.
5. Avoid phrasing your words as if you are talking to the interpreter (eg, "Can you tell her . . . ?"). Instead, phrase your questions as you do with speaking clients (eg, "I'm going to ask you some questions now.").
6. Depend on the deaf client to ask questions.
7. Look at the client's face for signs of difficulty in understanding. Deaf clients have a behavior of "gesturing" that involves shaking their heads as if to indicate "yes" even when they do not understand. If the client is nodding "yes," ask her to repeat the directions you have just given.
8. Be as direct as possible. Keep to what you want to know or what you want to convey. Speak in short sentences, using nontechnical words. Avoid colloquial or slang words. Be sure to explain what you want to do before you do it. For instance, tell her you want to start an IV and explain the equipment. Then, with her permission, start the IV.
9. Be aware that deaf clients may have difficulty understanding when to take medications. It will be helpful to associate taking medications or completing some treatment or activity with meals. (For instance, while showing her the two capsules she is to take when she goes home, tell her to take the two capsules at breakfast and another two capsules at bedtime.) Avoid saying "take two capsules at 8:00 A.M., 2:00 P.M., and 12:00 A.M."
10. The difference in interpreting time may also affect obtaining a history. It is best to begin with a specific event in the past and work forward.

What to Do Until the Interpreter Arrives

1. Role-play as much as possible.
2. Demonstrate what you want the client to do or what you want to do.
3. Be resourceful.
4. Remember that some deaf clients can read lips. Some may read written language, but use care in assuming the client understands.

What to Do to Prepare for Working with a Deaf Client

1. Contact local agencies that work with deaf clients to see what resources are available. Ask about classes in ASL. Being able to use some basic signs will be very helpful while waiting for an interpreter to arrive.
2. Read to learn more about the deaf culture. Contact your local agency or the National Information Center on Deafness, Silver Springs, Maryland, to get suggestions on books you might read.
3. Investigate your health facility. What is available to assist you? Look for videos used for teaching in the maternal-child unit and note if they have captions. Remember that many deaf clients do not read written language, so it will be important to review the content of the video with an interpreter present.

Prepared with the kind assistance of Mr. Gerald Dement, Interpreter Coordinator, Pikes Peak Center on Deafness, Colorado Springs, Colorado.

Appendix E

Sign Language for Healthcare Professionals

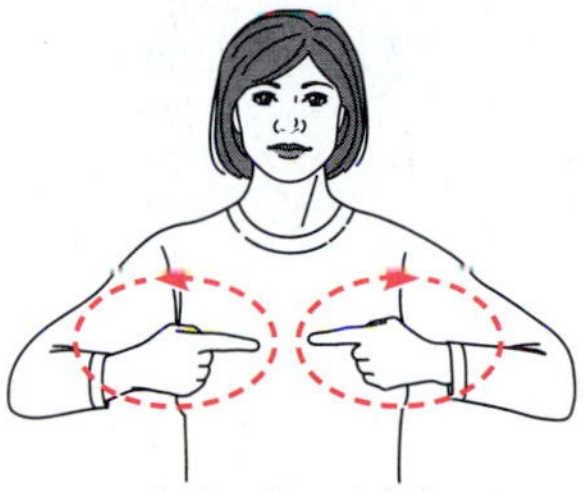
Ache (or pain)

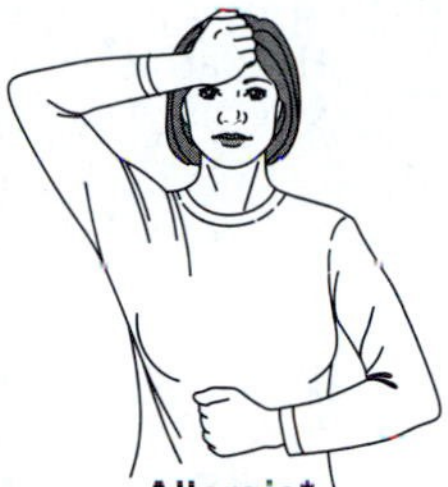
Allergic*

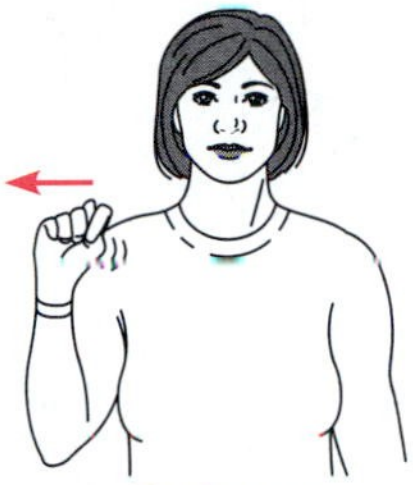
Bathroom

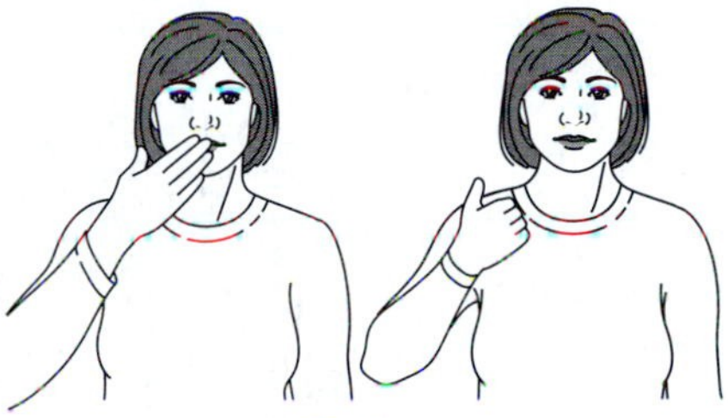
Better

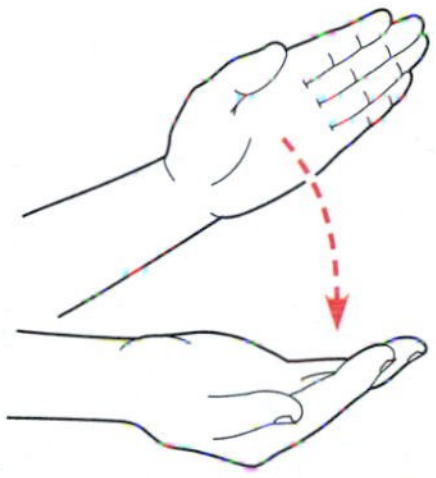
Congratulate (or praise)

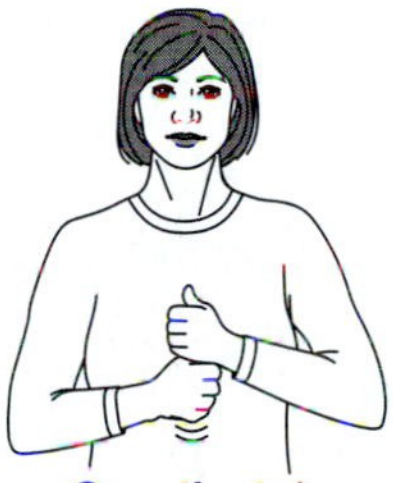
Constipate*

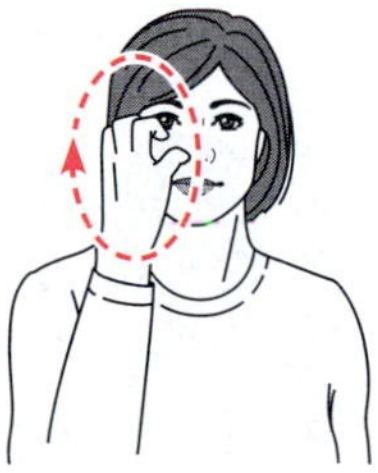
Dizzy

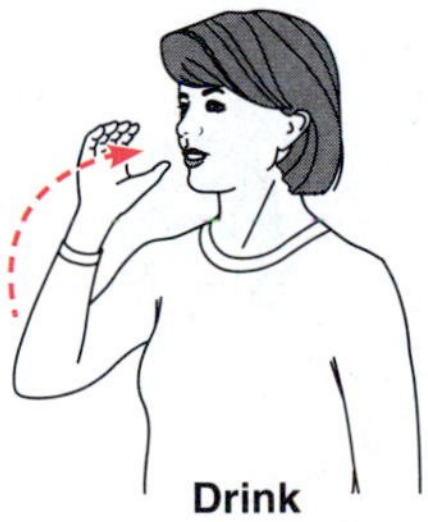
Drink

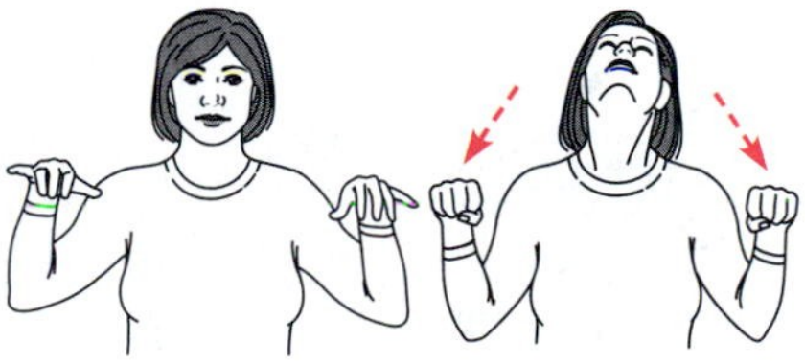
Faint

*Indicates signs that are in manually signed English. Those without an asterisk are in American Sign Language.

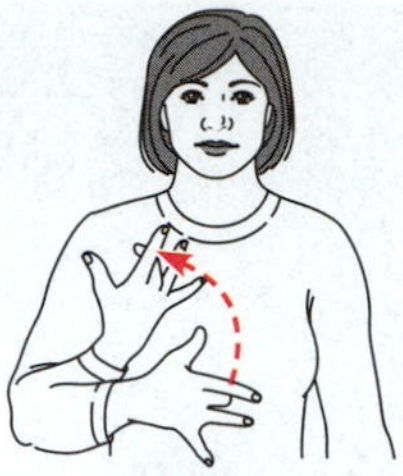
Feel

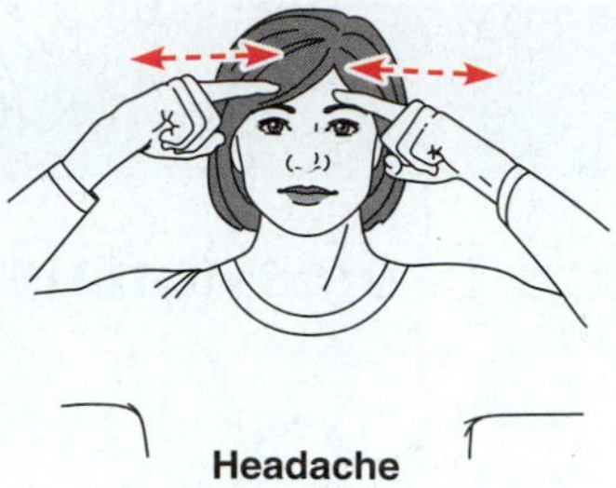
Headache

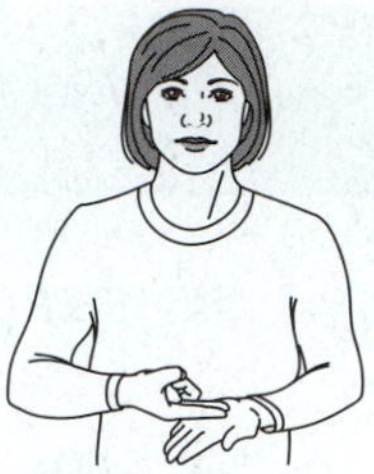
Lie down

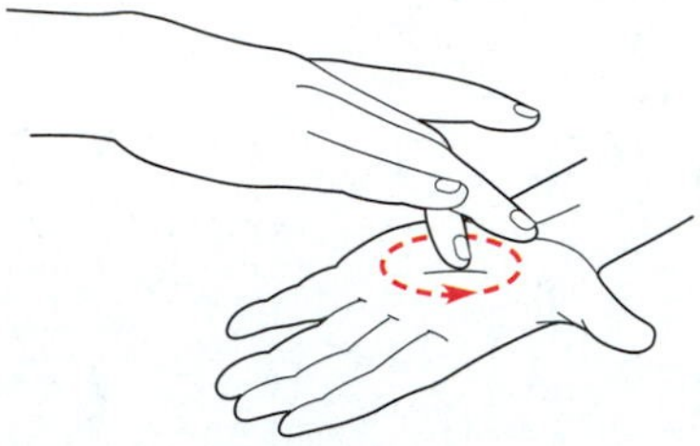
Medicine

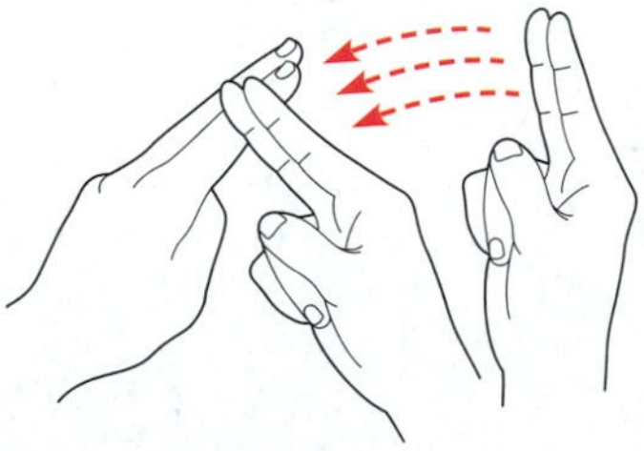
Name

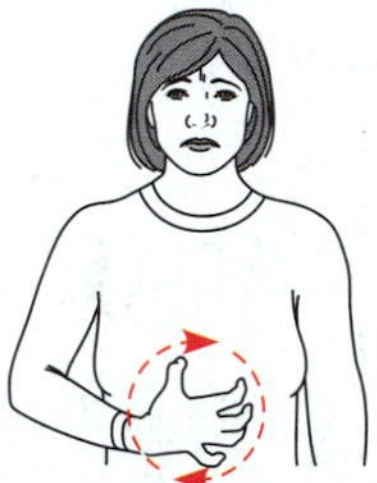
Nauseous

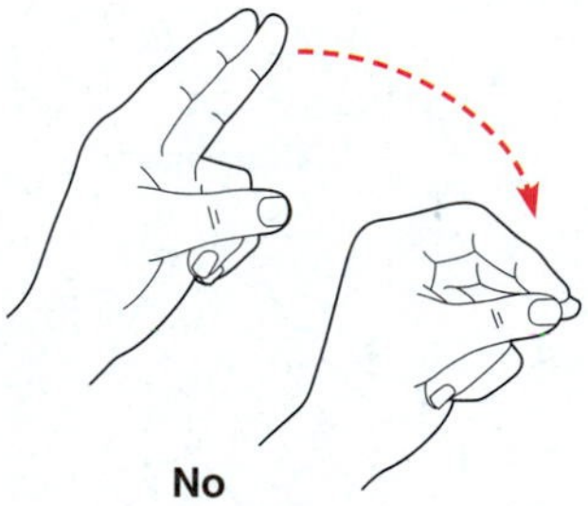
No

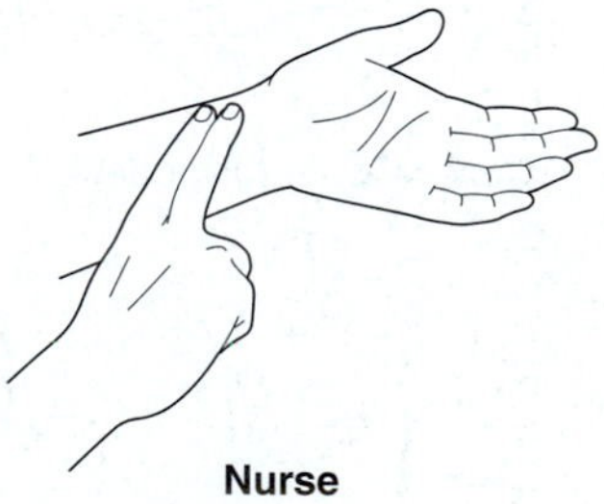
Nurse

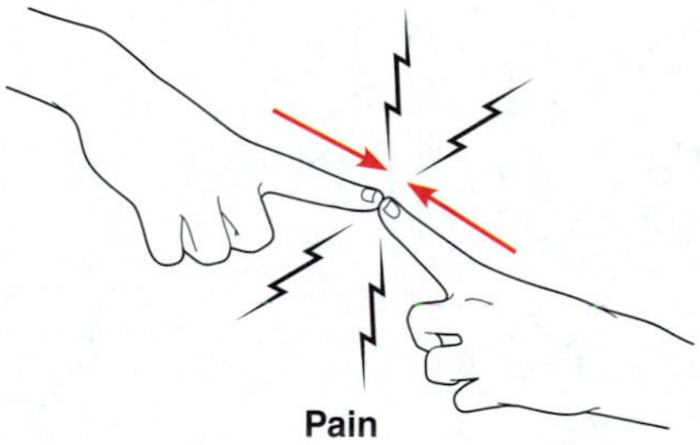
Pain

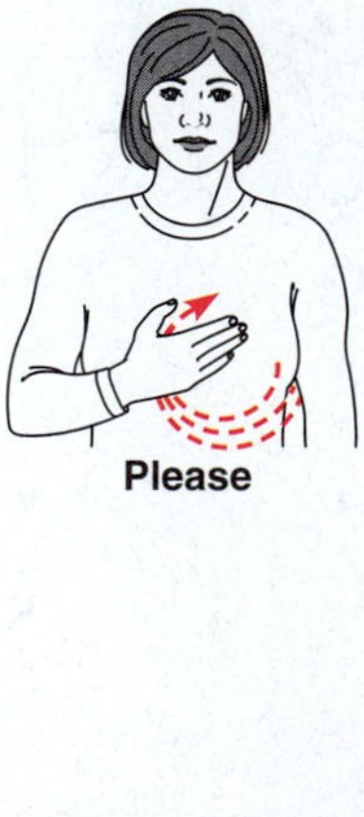
Please

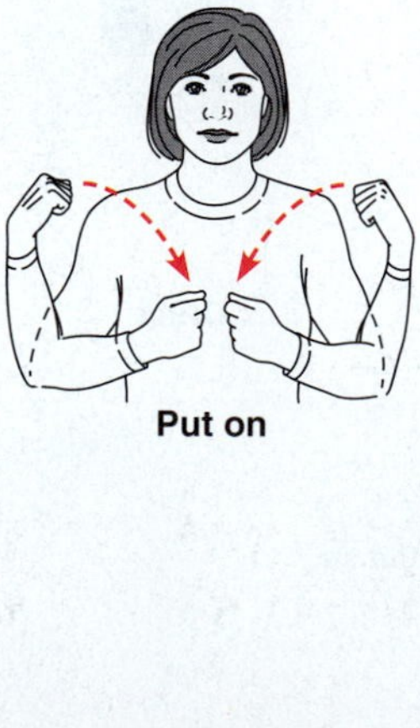
Put on

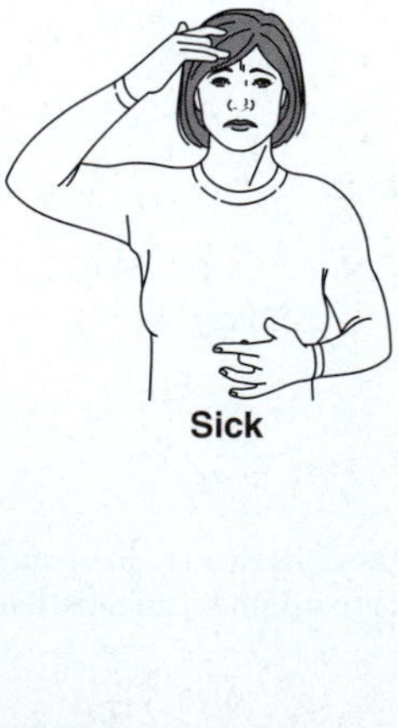
Sick

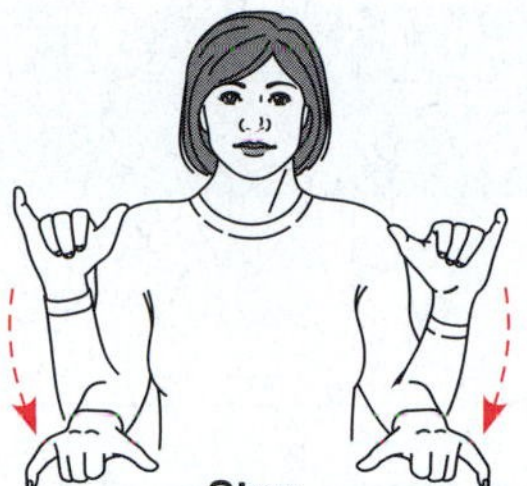
Stay

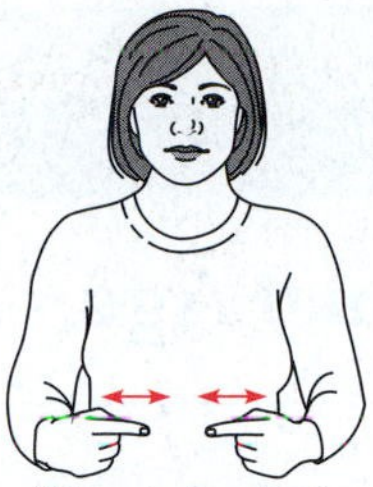
Stomachache*

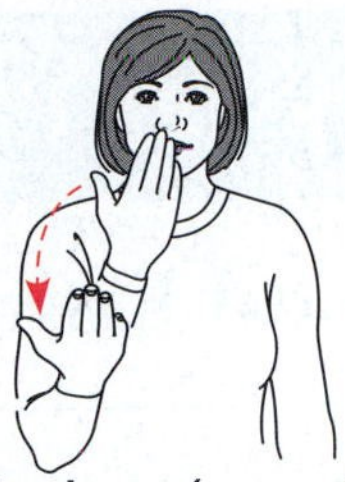
Thank you (or good)

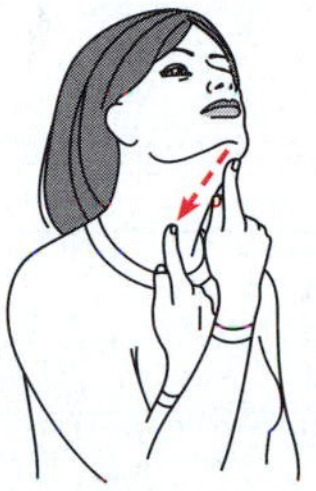
Thirsty

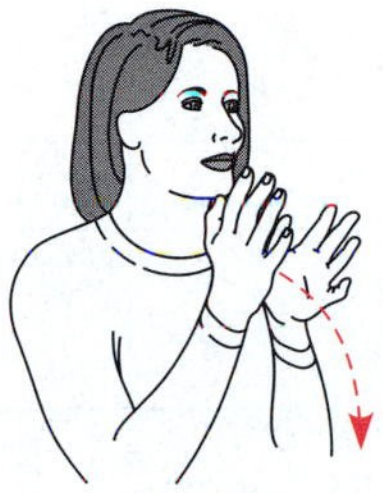
Vomit

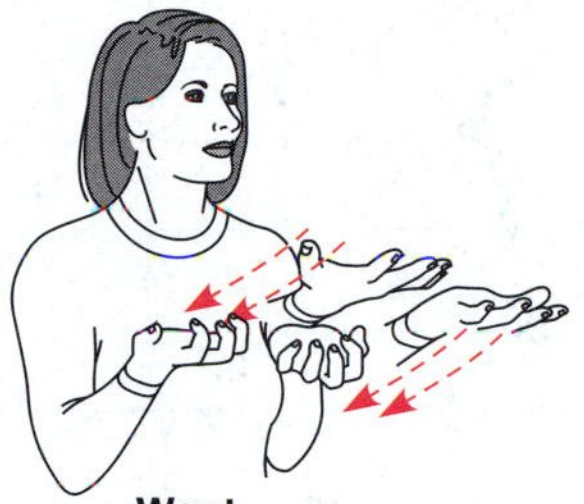
Want

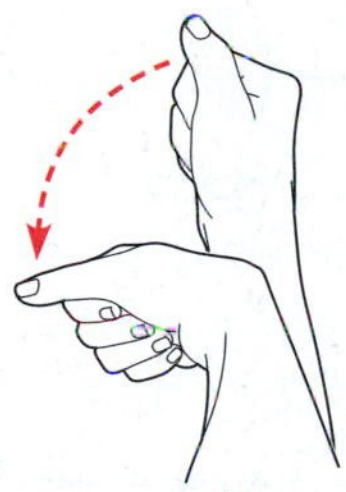
Yes

APPENDIX F

Clinical Estimation of Gestational Age

Examination First Hours

CLINICAL ESTIMATION OF GESTATIONAL AGE

An Approximation Based on Published Data*

Weeks gestation: 20 21 22 23 24 25 26 27 28 29 30 31 32 33 34 35 36 37 38 39 40 41 42 43 44 45 46 47 48

Physical Findings		Stage 1	Stage 2	Stage 3	Stage 4	Stage 5	Stage 6	Stage 7	Stage 8
VERNIX		APPEARS	COVERS BODY, THICK LAYER	ON BACK, SCALP, IN CREASES	SCANT, IN CREASES	NO VERNIX			
BREAST TISSUE AND AREOLA		AREOLA & NIPPLE BARELY VISIBLE NO PALPABLE BREAST TISSUE	AREOLA RAISED	1-2 MM NODULE	3-5 MM	5-6 MM	7-10 MM	?12 MM	
EAR	FORM	FLAT, SHAPELESS	BEGINNING INCURVING SUPERIOR	INCURVING UPPER 2/3 PINNAE	WELL-DEFINED INCURVING TO LOBE				
	CARTILAGE	PINNA SOFT, STAYS FOLDED	CARTILAGE SCANT RETURNS SLOWLY FROM FOLDING	THIN CARTILAGE SPRINGS BACK FROM FOLDING	PINNA FIRM, REMAINS ERECT FROM HEAD				
SOLE CREASES		SMOOTH SOLES $\bar{s}$ CREASES	1-2 ANTERIOR CREASES	2-3 ANTERIOR CREASES	CREASES ANTERIOR 2/3 SOLE	CREASES INVOLVING HEEL	DEEPER CREASES OVER ENTIRE SOLE		
SKIN	THICKNESS & APPEARANCE	THIN, TRANSLUCENT SKIN, PLETHORIC, VENULES OVER ABDOMEN EDEMA	SMOOTH THICKER NO EDEMA	PINK	FEW VESSELS	SOME DESQUAMATION PALE PINK	THICK, PALE, DESQUAMATION OVER ENTIRE BODY		
	NAIL PLATES	APPEAR	NAILS TO FINGER TIPS	NAILS EXTEND WELL BEYOND FINGER TIPS					
HAIR		APPEARS ON HEAD	EYE BROWS & LASHES	FINE, WOOLLY, BUNCHES OUT FROM HEAD	SILKY, SINGLE STRANDS LAYS FLAT	?RECEDING HAIRLINE OR LOSS OF BABY HAIR SHORT, FINE UNDERNEATH			
LANUGO		APPEARS	COVERS ENTIRE BODY	VANISHES FROM FACE	PRESENT ON SHOULDERS	NO LANUGO			
GENITALIA	TESTES	TESTES PALPABLE IN INGUINAL CANAL	IN UPPER SCROTUM	IN LOWER SCROTUM					
	SCROTUM	FEW RUGAE	RUGAE, ANTERIOR PORTION	RUGAE COVER	PENDULOUS				
	LABIA & CLITORIS	PROMINENT CLITORIS LABIA MAJORA SMALL WIDELY SEPARATED	LABIA MAJORA LARGER NEARLY COVERED CLITORIS	LABIA MINORA & CLITORIS COVERED					
SKULL FIRMNESS		BONES ARE SOFT	SOFT TO 1" FROM ANTERIOR FONTANELLE	SPONGY AT EDGES OF FONTANELLE CENTER FIRM	BONES HARD SUTURES EASILY DISPLACED	BONES HARD, CANNOT BE DISPLACED			
POSTURE	RESTING	HYPOTONIC LATERAL DECUBITUS	HYPOTONIC	BEGINNING FLEXION THIGH	STRONGER HIP FLEXION	FROG-LIKE	FLEXION ALL LIMBS	HYPERTONIC	VERY HYPERTONIC
	RECOIL - LEG	NO RECOIL	PARTIAL RECOIL	PROMPT RECOIL					
	ARM	NO RECOIL	BEGIN FLEXION NO RECOIL	PROMPT RECOIL MAY BE INHIBITED	PROMPT RECOIL AFTER 30" INHIBITION				

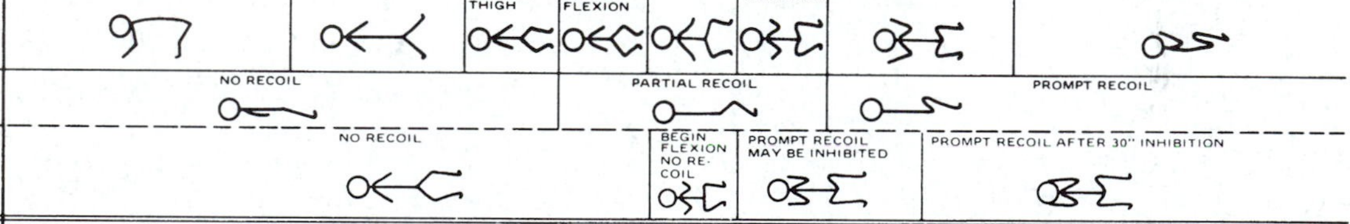

*Brazie, J. V., & Lubchenco, L. O. (1974). The estimation of gestational age chart. In Kempe, C. H., Silver, H. K., & O'Brien, D. (Eds.), *Current pediatric diagnosis and treatment* (3rd ed., chap. 4). Los Altos, CA: Lange Medical Publications. Form courtesy of Mead Johnson Laboratories, Evansville, IN.

Appendix G

Actions and Effects of Selected Drugs During Breastfeeding*

Anticoagulants

Coumarin derivatives (warfarin, dicumarol): Relatively safe to use; only small amount in breast milk; check PTT

Heparin: Does not cross into breast milk; check PTT

Anticonvulsants

Phenytoin (Dilantin), phenobarbital: Generally considered safe; if high doses of phenobarbital are ingested, may cause drowsiness; short-acting phenobarbiturates (secobarbital) preferred, because they appear in lower concentration in milk

Magnesium sulfate: Lactogenesis may be delayed

Antidepressants

SSRI class (fluoxetine, fluvoxamine): Effect on newborn unknown current concern

Antihistamines

Diphenhydramine (Benadryl), pheniramine (Dimetane), Claritin, Allegra: May cause decreased milk supply; infant may become drowsy or irritable

Antimetabolites

Unknown, probably long-term anti-DNA effect on the infant; potentially very toxic

Antimicrobials

Aminoglycosides: May cause ototoxicity or nephrotoxicity if given for more than 2 weeks

Ampicillin: Skin rash, candidiasis; diarrhea

Azithromycin: No risk to newborn

Chloramphenicol: Possible bone marrow suppression; too low a dose for Gray syndrome; refusal of breast

Methacycline: Possible inhibition of bone growth; may cause discoloration of the teeth; use should be avoided

Metronidazole (Flagyl): Possible neurologic disorders or blood dyscrasias; delay breastfeeding for 12 hours after dose

Penicillin: Possible allergic response; candidiasis

Quinolones (synthetic antibiotics): Can cause arthropathies

Sulfonamides: May cause hyperbilirubinemia; use contraindicated until infant over 1 week old

Tetracycline: Long-term use and large doses should be avoided; may cause tooth staining or inhibition of bone growth

Antithyroids

Thiouracil: Contraindicated during lactation; may cause goiter or agranulocytosis

Barbiturates

Propylthiouracil: Safe; monitor infant thyroid function

Phenothiazines: May produce sedation

Bronchodilators

Aminophylline: May cause insomnia or irritability in the infant

Ephedrine, cromolyn (Intal): Relatively safe

Caffeine

Excessive consumption may cause jitteriness or wakefulness

Cardiovascular

Methyldopa: Increase in milk volume

Propranolol (Inderal): May cause hypoglycemia; possibility of other blocking effects, especially if infant has renal or liver dysfunction

Quinidine: May cause arrhythmias in infant

Reserpine (Serpasil): Nasal stuffiness, lethargy, or diarrhea in infant

Corticosteroids

Adrenal suppression may occur with long-term administration of doses greater than 10 mg/day

Diuretics

Furosemide (Lasix): Not excreted in breast milk

Thiazide diuretics (Esidrix, HydroDIURIL, Oretic): Safe but can cause dehydration, reduce milk production

Heavy Metals

Gold: Potentially toxic; gold salts—compatible with breastfeeding

Lead: Excreted in breast milk; high maternal levels can affect neuropsychologic development

Mercury: Excreted in the milk and hazardous to infant

Hormones

Androgens: Suppress lactation

Thyroid hormones: May mask hypothyroidism

Laxatives

Peri-Colace, Dulcolax: Relatively safe

Milk of magnesia, Metamucil: Relatively safe

Narcotic analgesics

Codeine: Accumulation may lead to neonatal depression

Meperidine: May lead to neonatal depression

Morphine: Long-term use may cause newborn addiction

Nonnarcoti analgesics, nsaids

Acetaminophen (Tylenol): Relatively safe for short-term analgesia

Ibuprofen (Motrin): Safe

Propoxyphene (Darvon): May cause sleepiness and poor breastfeeding in infant

Salicylates (aspirin): Safe after first week of life; monitor protime

Oral Contraceptives

Combined estrogen/progestin pills: Significantly decrease milk supply; may alter milk composition; may cause gynecomastia in male infants

Progestin only (DMPA, Norplant): Safe if started after lactation is established

Radioactive Materials for Testing

Gallium citrate (^{67}G): Insignificant amount excreted in breast milk; no breastfeeding for 2 weeks

Iodine: Contraindicated; may affect infant's thyroid gland

^{125}I: Discontinue breastfeeding for 48 hours

^{131}I: Breastfeeding should be discontinued until excretion is no longer significant; may be resumed after 10 days

Technetium-99m: Discontinue breastfeeding for 3 days (half-life = 6 hours)

Sedatives/tranquilizers

Diazepam (Valium): May accumulate to high levels; may increase neonatal jaundice; may cause lethargy and weight loss

Lithium: Contraindicated; may cause neonatal flaccidity and hypotonia

Substance abuse

Alcohol: Potential motor developmental delay; mild sedative effect

Amphetamines: Controversial; may cause irritability, poor sleeping pattern

Cocaine, crack: Extreme irritability, tachycardia, vomiting, apnea

Marijuana: Drowsiness

Heroin: Tremors, restlessness, vomiting, poor feeding

Nicotine (smoking): Shock, vomiting, diarrhea, decreased milk production

*Based on data from Riordan, J., & Auerbach, K. J. (1999). *Breastfeeding and human lactation* (2nd ed., pp. 163–220). Boston: Jones & Bartlett; Briggs, G. G., Freeman, R. K., & Yaffe, S. J. (2002). *Drugs in pregnancy and lactation* (6th ed.). Baltimore: Williams & Wilkins; Hale, T. (2000). *Medications and mothers' milk.* (9th ed.). Amarillo, TX: Pharmasoft Publishing; Committee on Drugs, American Academy of Pediatrics. (1994). The transfer of drugs and other chemicals into human milk. *Pediatrics, 93,* 137–150.

APPENDIX H

Selected Maternal-Newborn Laboratory Values

NORMAL MATERNAL LABORATORY VALUES

Test	Nonpregnant Values	Pregnant Values
Hematocrit	37%–47%	32%–42%
Hemoglobin	12–16 g/dL**	10–14 g/dL**
Platelets	150,000–350,000/mm^3	Significant increase 3–5 days after birth (predisposes to thrombosis)
Partial thromboplastin time (PTT)	12–14 seconds	Slight decrease in pregnancy and again in labor (placental site clotting)
Fibrinogen	250 mg/dL	400 mg/dL
Serum glucose		
..Fasting	70–80 mg/dL	65 mg/dL
..2-hour postprandial	60–110 mg/dL	Less than 140 mg/dL
Total protein	6.7–8.3 g/dL	5.5–7.5 g/dL
White blood cell total	4500–10,000/mm^3	5000–15,000/mm^3
Polymorphonuclear cells	54%–62%	60%–85%
Lymphocytes	38%–46%	15%–40%

**At sea level

NORMAL TERM NEONATAL CORD BLOOD LABORATORY VALUES

Test	Normal Values
Hematocrit	43%–63%*
Hemoglobin	14–20 g/dL
Platelets	150,000–350,000/mm^3
Reticulocyte	3%–7%
White blood cell total	10,000–30,000/mm^3
White blood cell differential	
..Polymorphonuclear (segs)	40%–80%
..Lymphocytes	20%–40%
..Monocytes	3%–10%
Serum glucose	45–96 mg/dL*
Serum electrolytes	
..Sodium	126–166 mEq/L*
..Potassium	5.6–12.0 mEq/L*
..Chloride	98–110 mEq/L*
..Carbon dioxide	13–29 mmol/L
..Bicarbonate	18–23 mEq/L
..Calcium	8.2–11.1 mg/dL
Total protein	4.8–7.3 g/dL

Note: From Fanaroff, A. A., & Martin, R. J. (Eds.). (2002). *Neonatal-perinatal medicine* (7th ed.). St. Louis, MO: Mosby. Adapted.

* All laboratory values are approximate. Consult your local laboratory for guidelines as to normal values.

APPENDIX I

Suggested Answers to Critical Thinking in Practice Questions

Chapter 4

Rita has described a normal menstrual cycle. Although it is variable in frequency, it is not outside the range of what is acceptable in a teenager. The flow that she thinks is heavy is really quite normal, and her cramps indicate that she is having ovulatory cycles.

It is important to reassure Rita that there is nothing wrong with her menstrual cycle. It would be appropriate to suggest an antiprostaglandin such as ibuprofen for the relief of dysmenorrhea. Of utmost importance is to follow up on her request for birth control pills. She may be considering becoming sexually active and may need contraception. Sometimes teenagers have a difficult time asking for what they really want, and this is an ideal situation in which to bring up issues of sexuality with a young woman.

Chapter 5

Monique's concern about taking action beforehand eliminates the diaphragm, cervical cap, female condom, contraceptive sponge, and spermicides as options. Because she is interested in two men and little is known about their sexual histories, the IUD would not be a good choice even though it is very reliable and its use is removed from the act of intercourse. Combined oral contraceptives (COCs) would be an excellent choice because Monique is a nonsmoker with no known contraindications. COCs remove contraception from coitus and are extremely reliable. Similarly, Monique might consider Lunelle or Depo-Provera, if she doesn't mind the injections.

Regardless of the method she chooses, it is important that you talk to Monique about requiring that any sexual partners use condoms. Condoms offer protection for both parties and are an important element in safe sex.

Chapter 6

The use of feminine hygiene products can result in vaginitis and actually promote sexually transmitted diseases, especially PID. Feminine hygiene products, especially douches, alter the acid-base balance of the vagina, allowing opportunistic organisms to replicate. Also, douching washes out the protective normal flora of the vagina, and the altered acid-base vaginal environment prevents the protective bacteria from growing. The action of douching can propel pathogenic organisms upward and promote an ascending infection such as PID. Ella should be told that douching is seldom necessary, and that cleansing daily with soap and water is an adequate hygienic measure. Ella should be told that she is at increased risk for PID because she has multiple sexual partners, uses an IUD, and douches. She should be counseled to consider other forms of contraceptives that are more protective against STIs and to consider limiting her sexual activity to a monogamous relationship.

Chapter 9

Marsha's story of how she got her injury is not consistent with the type of injury she has. Injuries that are accidental are usually to the extremities and not to the trunk. Also, the bruising and edema suggest that the injury happened several hours ago. You should suspect that Marsha received her injuries from physical abuse, probably by Fred. The type of injury and the delay in coming for treatment are possible indicators of abuse. Also the fact that she looks to Fred to agree with her statements is suspicious. You should make every attempt to separate Marsha from Fred so that she can speak more openly if she chooses. It is likely that if Fred is in the room she will deny the abuse for fear of further abuse. You do not want to put her in danger. You may need to be creative in separating Fred from Marsha, since often the abuser does not want to leave.

Chapter 11

She is correct that drugs may be teratogenic. But severe hyperthermia such as this (T 104F) is known to cause neural tube defects (spina bifida and anencephaly at this stage gestation). Therefore, the healthcare provider must weigh the risk of teratogenicity of an antipyretic with a teratogenic potential, such as low-dose aspirin, against the risk of hyperthermia.

Chapter 14

Elena's height and prepregnancy weight are normal. Her weight gain during pregnancy has been appropriate but not excessive. Research indicates that assessment of fundal height is more accurate between 22–24 and 34 weeks' gestation. At 33 weeks Elena's baby was growing normally. Thus this finding is not abnormal by itself and may simply be a reflection of decreased accuracy of the procedure late in pregnancy. It may also reflect variations in growth of the baby. To make your best assessment you need further information about the results of this week's examination. If during her examination there are no indicators of problems, such as decreased fetal activity, maternal urinary tract infection, maternal hypertension, and so forth, you can reassure Elena that this finding is probably a normal variation.

Chapter 15

Karen should be encouraged to continue with her exercising program. Benefits of exercise for pregnant women include reduced weight gain, increase in weight loss after birth, improved mood, improved sleep patterns, lower use of epidural anesthesia in labor, less need for Pitocin in labor, shorter labors, and fewer operative births. The following guidelines should be followed in pregnancy: do not exercise to the point of exhaustion or breathlessness; wear comfortable footwear;

drink large quantities of water during the exercise session; take frequent breaks; avoid exercising outdoors in hot weather; avoid heavy weight lifting (especially weights over the head or exercises that put stress on the back); avoid lying flat on the back; and avoid large increases in heart rate (a pulse of over 150 can raise the core maternal body temperature). Karen should be advised that swimming and the use of heated pools is safe in pregnancy. High water temperatures (> 100F) are not advised. If Karen wishes to use a hot tub where she can control the temperature (such as at her own home), that is safe in pregnancy. In most commercial hot tubs in gyms or resorts, however, temperatures average 110F to 120F. If she does not know the temperature of the hot tub she intends to use, she should be advised not to use it. Since the chlorine in the water can cause excessive skin dryness, she should be encouraged to rinse off after using a chlorinated hot tub or pool and to apply a moisturizing cream or lotion.

Chapter 16

Competing in the marathon is not recommended. Even though Constance is in excellent shape, we do not know what impact prolonged participation in such a strenuous event might have on her fetus. The normal fetus seems able to withstand decreased uterine blood flow during exercise as blood is shunted to the muscles. We do not know, however, whether this decreased blood flow to the fetus interferes with the fetus's ability to dissipate heat, especially since the fetus is not able to decrease temperature via perspiration or respiration. With this in mind, during pregnancy, competitive athletes avoid competition, and all women should avoid reaching their maximal physical effort by maintaining their pulse at 140 beats per minute or less.

Chapter 17

Begin by gathering information. Discuss with Rachel her reasons for considering this option. Don't be opinionated about what option might be best but rather determine what factors are making Rachel feel that adoption is the right choice for her. Then help Rachel find appropriate resources. Refer her to a social worker to discuss the issue of infant relinquishment. If possible, participate in the discussion and be a support person for Rachel if she desires it. Help Rachel come to terms with issues related to sharing this information with significant others. If Rachel continues with this decision, the social worker will assist with the decision of open versus closed adoption and will link Rachel with adoption agencies and resources.

It is important to support Rachel in her decision. Recognize that most women who relinquish their infants do this because they believe it is the best option for the baby. The positive support of healthcare providers during the entire perinatal period is very important.

Chapter 18

Although Jaya's intake is supporting an appropriate weight gain, her diet is not nutritionally adequate. Comparing her diet to the Food Guide Pyramid shows that she lacks servings from the grain and dairy groups and that she has a high intake from the meat group.

Grain group Jaya should not restrict her intake from this group. Breads, pasta, and other grain products will not cause weight gain unless they are prepared with large amounts of fat or eaten in excessive quantities.

Meat group The number of servings from this group exceeds the recommended intake. This contributes to Jaya's fat and calorie intake even though she may be selecting lean cuts of meat. The number of servings should be decreased and each portion size should be about 2 to 3 ounces.

Dairy group A restricted dairy intake has decreased Jaya's calcium intake. The items she consumes from this group tend to have a high fat content. She could use dairy products that have a reduced fat content in order to limit her calorie intake but maintain the calcium level in her diet.

Vegetable group Broccoli and green leafy vegetables such as beet greens, collards, and kale will provide calcium to the diet but must be consumed in amounts greater than usual serving sizes for Jaya to obtain adequate calcium. Most salad greens contain very little calcium.

Beverages The total amount of fluid consumed is adequate. The consumption of soda should be limited because it would increase the calorie intake without contributing to the nutrient content of the diet.

Chapter 19

It is not unusual for women to be upset and frustrated with news that they may have newly diagnosed glucose intolerance during pregnancy. It has been described that women with gestational diabetes approach the new diagnosis as a crisis or anxiety-provoking situation. These women may experience more difficulty with coping and learning than do women with chronic diabetes who become pregnant.

It is important for the nurse to first assess the woman's knowledge about gestational diabetes before attempting to provide any teaching. The woman will benefit most from discussions that build on her current knowledge level. It will usually take several sessions to ensure that the new information is accurately understood and retained.

The nurse can reassure Patti that the baby should be fine and can stress the importance of keeping her glucose levels in a normal range. Women with gestational diabetes may require treatment with diet therapy alone, or they may need insulin administration to control hyperglycemia.

It is believed that gestational diabetes does not cause birth defects because it occurs later in pregnancy, after the baby's organs are formed. The two most common risks to the baby are macrosomia, potentially causing a problem in labor and birth, and hypoglycemia.

Chapter 20

This approach is not appropriate for Jena. Although it is unusual for a nonpregnant woman to develop pyelonephritis from a bladder infection, a significant number of pregnant women with bacteriuria develop cystitis or pyelonephritis unless their bladder infection is treated. This is related to the anatomic and physiologic changes of pregnancy, including decreased ureteral peristalsis, ureteral dilation, and increased bladder capacity. Since Jena is 6 months pregnant, she is probably being seen monthly for prenatal care. Because prompt treatment is essential, you should urge her to call her caregiver and discuss her symptoms.

Chapter 25

We hope you would encourage her to take medication if she felt she needed it. There are many types of analgesic agents and many types of regional blocks that can help her if she decides she needs them. Sometimes, giving permission for someone to ask relieves her anxiety and decreases the need for intervention.

Chapter 26

The pattern described is within normal limits. No further action is needed because the pattern is reassuring.

Chapter 27

Once uterine contractions reach the desired characteristics (frequency of every 2 to 3 minutes, duration of 40 to 60 seconds, and moderate to strong intensity), and cervical dilatation is 5 to 6 cm, the infusion rate can be decreased by increments similar to those by which it was increased. In this case you should decrease the rate to the step it was just prior to 6 mU/min (36 mL/hr). If the frequency, duration, or intensity decreases after reducing the oxytocin infusion rate, the infusion can be increased and maintained at the rate at which desired characteristics (described above) reoccur.

Chapter 28

The twin at greatest risk of developing tissue hypoxia is David. Hypoxia develops when there is inadequate delivery of oxygen to the tissues. This occurs when there is inadequate circulation to the tissues or, as in this case, the blood delivered to the tissues has a decreased oxygen-carrying capacity. The oxygen-carrying capacity of blood is calculated as: 1.26 mL O_2/gram of hemoglobin (the O_2-carrying capacity of fetal hemoglobin) multiplied by the grams of hemoglobin in the sample. Thus, the oxygen vols% and the oxygen-carrying capacity of David's blood is $1.26 \times 11 = 13.86$ vols%. Therefore, David is at greater risk of developing tissue hypoxia than is his brother.

Caution should be exercised when using oxygen saturation monitors to assess hypoxia. The monitors determine the amount of oxygenated versus deoxygenated hemoglobin in the blood and report this value as a percentage; for example, "94% saturated" means 94% of the hemoglobin has bound to oxygen molecules. The monitors do not evaluate the amount of hemoglobin present in the blood, nor the actual oxygen-carrying capacity. In this case, David is at greater risk of developing tissue hypoxia despite his oxygen saturation of 100% because he has a lower oxygen-carrying capacity and his tissues are receiving less oxygen per volume of blood.

Chapter 29

The unique behavioral and temperamental characteristics of newborn infants should be discussed. Additionally, aspects of the Brazelton exam may be helpful to show Mrs Reyes how her infant changes state with different stimuli and intervention. Teaching her how to console her newborn may also be helpful.

Chapter 30

Although babies may make occasional cooing sounds, brand new babies tend to either cry or be silent. The nurse needs to immediately assess the situation as the "cute little noises" may be early signs of respiratory distress such as grunting.

Chapter 30

Reassure Aisha that you will help her baby as you carry out the following activities:

Position the infant with her head lowered and to the side.

Bulb suction the nares and mouth repeatedly until the airway is cleared.

Hold and comfort the infant when normal respirations are restored.

Reassure Aisha and review this procedure with her.

Note: If bulb suctioning alone does not clear the airway, use DeLee wall suction and administer oxygen as needed to restore normal respirations.

Chapter 30

We hope you would first examine the infant's genitalia and wipe between the labia to verify the source of bleeding. If there were no external lacerations, you would explain to the mother that a small amount of bleeding, called pseudomenstruation, sometimes occurs in newborn girls because of maternal hormone levels. This is considered normal and generally resolves in a few days. The tissue she observes is a vaginal skin tag, also a normal finding. It usually disappears in a few weeks.

Chapter 32

We hope that you would tell her that nurses always wear gloves during the initial assessment of a newborn, during all admission procedures until the newborn has its first bath, and sometimes during diaper changes. You should also tell her that her baby will not be isolated from the other babies when in the nursery and that her baby can remain with her if she wishes. It is important to recognize the concern that Mrs Corrigan may have about people knowing that her baby may have HIV and to assess her own feelings of social isolation.

Chapter 33

It is important to give this mother clear, factual information regarding the type, cause, and usual course of the baby's respiratory problem. You see that Linn's laboratory tests, chest x-ray, and clinical course so far are indicative of transient tachypnea of the newborn. Respiratory distress syndrome is probably not the problem since Linn is not premature and did not have any asphyxia at birth. You recognize that prior experience with a premature newborn with respiratory distress and prolonged hospitalization will add to this mother's fear and anxiety regarding her new baby. Therefore, in addition to giving factual information regarding the baby's condition, it is important for you to see whether the mother can be brought to the nursery to see her baby or to have the mother receive a picture of the baby for reassurance. Before the mother visits the baby, clearly describe the oxygen and monitoring equipment that is helping Linn so that the mother will not be alarmed upon seeing her daughter.

Chapter 34

These findings are not within the normal range. At 24 hours past birth the fundus should be approximately one finger breadth below the umbilicus and located in the midline. A uterus that is deviated to the right may indicate that the bladder is full and the woman needs to urinate. You should determine whether she is having difficulty urinating and emptying her bladder; if so, you can try some nursing measures to help her void. The lochia will still be rubra, but the amount is excessive and may be related to a boggy uterus.

Chapter 34

Your best response would be, "You can only be discharged if both you and your physician feel you are ready. Federal law now states that you can stay in the hospital for up to 4 days (96 hours) when you have had a cesarean birth."

Chapter 36

Acknowledge Ann's frustration and pain. Tell her you are glad she called and ask how you may be of help. Let her ventilate about how she feels. Explain that her breasts are engorged, which is a problem that many women encounter. It is not unusual for infants to refuse to breastfeed when the breast is hard and the nipple difficult to grasp.

Identify methods to relieve the engorgement.

1. Try warm or cool soaks, whichever she prefers, for comfort and to stimulate let-down.
2. Express a small amount of milk.
3. Put the baby to breast after stimulating let-down and expressing a little milk. (The breast will be softer and it will be easier to grasp the nipple.)
4. Use analgesics. (If taken immediately before breastfeeding, less medication will go to the baby.)

Explain to Ann that her emotional upheaval is probably the "baby blues" or "postpartum blues" and that they usually subside in 24 to 72 hours. Instruct her to call her physician if the blues do not subside, or if she develops symptoms of depression.

Ask why she started supplemental feedings. Upon questioning, Ann tells you that she had started supplementing her baby with formula after each feeding because her mother-in-law told her that the baby was breastfeeding too frequently (every 1 to 3 hours, sometimes clustering 3 to 4 feedings in one 2- to 3-hour period). She told Ann that the baby was obviously not getting enough breast milk. After receiving supplemental feedings, the baby began feeding once every 3 to 5 hours.

Tactfully explain that although Ann's mother-in-law meant well, her comments indicate a lack of information about breastfeeding; that is,

1. Breast milk digests faster than formula, so breastfeeding babies feed more frequently.
2. On average, babies breastfeed 8 to 12 times in 24 hours.
3. After lactation is well established, the baby will breastfeed less frequently. During growth spurts, however, all babies breastfeed more frequently for a few days.

Explain that Ann may still breastfeed successfully, and if she desires to continue breastfeeding, she should stop supplementing with formula.

Chapter 37

You should have Lei return to her room via wheelchair. Assess her leg for warmth, edema, redness, tenderness, and Homans' sign. Discuss with Lei that she should not massage her leg or get out of bed until you consult with the primary provider concerning your findings. Notify her primary healthcare provider and document your assessment findings.

Glossary

Abdominal effleurage Gentle stroking used in massage.

Abortion Loss of pregnancy before the fetus is viable outside the uterus; miscarriage.

Abruptio placentae (ab-rŭp´shē-ō pla-sen´tē) Partial or total premature separation of a normally implanted placenta.

Abstinence Refraining voluntarily, especially from indulgence in food, alcoholic beverages, or sexual intercourse.

Acceleration Periodic increase in the baseline fetal heart rate.

Acculturation The process by which people adapt to a new cultural norm.

Acini cells Secretory cells in the human breast that create milk from nutrients in the bloodstream.

Acme Peak or highest point; time of greatest intensity (of a uterine contraction).

Acrocyanosis Cyanosis of the extremities.

Acrosomal reaction Breakdown of the hyaluronic acid in the corona radiata by enzymes from the heads of sperm; allows one spermatozoon to penetrate the ovum zona pellucida.

Active acquired immunity Formation of antibodies by the pregnant woman in response to illness or immunization.

Active alert state Alert state marked by an increase in facial and body movement, with periods of fussiness occurring. The infant in this state has increased sensitivity to disturbing stimuli.

Active management of labor Medical protocol for augmentation of labor that includes (1) a strict criterion for labor admission, (2) early amniotomy, (3) high-dose oxytocin infusion for inefficient labor contractions, and (4) a commitment to provision of continuous nursing care.

Acupressure (sometimes called *Chinese massage*) Therapy using pressure from the fingers and thumbs to stimulate pressure points.

Acupuncture Therapy using very fine (hairlike) stainless steel needles to stimulate specific acupuncture points depending on the client's medical assessment and condition.

Adequate intake (AI) A value cited for a nutrient when there are not sufficient data to calculate an estimated average requirement.

Adnexa Adjoining or accessory parts of a structure, such as the uterine adnexa: the ovaries and fallopian tubes.

Adolescence Period of human development initiated by puberty and ending with the attainment of young adulthood.

Afterbirth Placenta and membranes expelled after the birth of the infant, during the third stage of labor. Also called *secundines*.

Afterpains Cramplike pains due to contractions of the uterus that occur after childbirth. They are more common in multiparas, tend to be most severe during breastfeeding, and last 2 to 3 days.

AIDS (acquired immune deficiency syndrome) An immunologic disorder caused by infection with the human immunodeficiency virus (HIV) and characterized by increasing susceptibility to opportunistic infections and rare cancers.

Alcohol-related birth defect (ARBD) Birth defects and cognitive difficulties occurring in infants born to mothers who drink.

Alpha fetoprotein (AFP) A fetal protein produced in the yolk sac for the first 6 weeks of gestation and then by the fetal liver.

Alternative therapy A substance or procedure used as a therapy that has not undergone rigorous scientific testing in this country, although it might have been thoroughly tested in other countries.

Alveoli Small units of the breast tissue in which milk is synthesized by the alveolar secretory epithelium.

Amenorrhea Suppression or absence of menstruation.

Amniocentesis Removal of amniotic fluid by insertion of a needle into the amniotic sac; amniotic fluid is used to assess fetal health or maturity.

Amnioinfusion Procedure used to infuse a sterile fluid (such as normal saline) through an intrauterine catheter into the uterus in an attempt to increase the fluid around the umbilical cord to decrease or prevent cord compression during labor contractions; also used to dilute thick meconium-stained amniotic fluid.

Amnion The inner of the two membranes that form the sac containing the fetus and the amniotic fluid.

Amnionitis Infection of the amniotic fluid.

Amniotic fluid The liquid surrounding the fetus in utero. It absorbs shocks, permits fetal movement, and prevents heat loss.

Amniotic fluid embolism Amniotic fluid that has leaked into the chorionic plate and entered the maternal circulation.

Amniotic fluid index (AFI) A method of reporting fluid volume. The AFI is calculated by dividing the maternal abdomen into four quadrants with the umbilicus as the reference point. Then, the deepest vertical pocket is measured. These measurements are summed to calculate the AFI.

Amniotomy (am-nē-ot´ō-mē) The artificial rupturing of the amniotic membrane.

Ampulla The outer two-thirds of the fallopian tube; fertilization of the ovum by a spermatozoon usually occurs here.

Androgen Substance producing male characteristics, such as the male hormone testosterone.

Android pelvis Male-type pelvis.

Antepartum Time between conception and the onset of labor; usually used to describe the period during which a woman is pregnant.

Anterior fontanelle Diamond-shaped area between the two frontal and two parietal bones just above the newborn's forehead.

Anthropoid pelvis Pelvis in which the anteroposterior diameter is equal to or greater than the transverse diameter.

Apgar score A scoring system used to evaluate newborns at 1 minute and 5 minutes after birth. The total score is achieved by assessing five signs: heart rate, respiratory effort, muscle tone, reflex irritability, and color. Each of the signs is assigned a score of 0, 1, or 2. The highest possible score is 10.

Apnea A condition that occurs when respirations cease for more than 20 seconds, with generalized cyanosis.

Areola Pigmented ring surrounding the nipple of the breast.

Aromatherapy The use of certain essential oils, derived from plants, whose odor or aroma is believed to have a therapeutic effect.

Artificial rupture of membranes (AROM) Use of a device such as an amnihook or allis forceps to rupture the amniotic membranes.

Assimilation Phenomenon in which a minority group completely changes its cultural identity to become part of the majority culture.

Assisted reproductive technology (ART) Term used to describe the highly technologic approaches used to produce pregnancy.

Attachment Enduring bonds or relationship of affection between persons.

Attitude In perinatal care, the relationship of the fetal parts to each other.

Autosome A chromosome that is not a sex chromosome.

Ayurveda The classical system of Hindu medicine. The term *ayurveda* means the knowledge of how to live a vital, healthful life.

Babinski reflex Reflex found normally in infants under 6 months of age in which the great toe dorsiflexes when the sole of the foot is stimulated.

Bacterial vaginosis A bacterial infection of the vagina, formerly called *Gardnerella vaginalis* or *Hemophilus vaginalis,* characterized by a foul-smelling, grayish vaginal discharge that exhibits a characteristic fishy odor when 10% potassium hydroxide (KOH) is added. Microscopic examination of a vaginal wet prep reveals the presence of "clue cells" (vaginal epithelial cells coated with gram-negative organisms).

Bag of waters (BOW) The membrane containing the amniotic fluid and the fetus.

Ballottement (bal-ot-maw´) A technique of palpation to detect or examine a floating object in the body. In obstetrics, the fetus, when pushed, floats away and then returns to touch the examiner's fingers.

Barlow maneuver A test designed to detect subluxation or dislocation of the hip. A dysplastic joint will be felt to be dislocated as the femur leaves the actabulum.

Barr body Deeply staining chromatin mass located against the inner surface of the cell nucleus. It is found only in normal females. Also called *sex chromatin.*

Basal body temperature (BBT) The lowest waking temperature.

Baseline rate The average fetal heart rate observed during a 10-minute period of monitoring.

Baseline variability Changes in the fetal heart rate that result from the interplay between the sympathetic and the parasympathetic nervous systems.

Battledore placenta Placenta in which the umbilical cord is inserted on the periphery rather than centrally.

Beta hCG (Beta human chorionic gonadotropin) A product of the trophoblast or placenta that is detected through serum testing and is a very accurate marker of the presence of pregnancy and placental health.

Bimanual palpation Examination of the pelvic organs by placing one hand on the abdomen and one or two fingers of the other hand into the vagina.

Biofeedback The use of monitoring devices to help individuals learn to control their autonomic responses.

Biophysical profile (BPP) Assessment of five variables in the fetus that help to evaluate fetal risk: breathing movement, body movement, tone, amniotic fluid volume, and fetal heart rate reactivity.

Birth center A setting for labor and birth that emphasizes a family-centered approach rather than obstetric technology and treatment.

Birth plan A written document prepared by the expectant parents that is used to identify available options in the birth setting.

Birthing room A room for labor and birth with a relaxed atmosphere.

Birth preference plan Decisions made by the expectant couple about aspects of the childbearing experience that are most important to them.

Birth rate Number of live births per 1000 population.

Bishop score A prelabor scoring system to assist in predicting whether an induction of labor may be successful. The total score is achieved by assessing five components: cervical dilatation, cervical effacement, cervical consistency, cervical position, and fetal station. Each of the components is assigned a score of 0 to 3, and the highest possible score is 13.

Blastocyst The inner solid mass of cells within the morula.

Bloody show Pink-tinged mucous secretions resulting from rupture of small capillaries as the cervix effaces and dilates.

Body stalk Future umbilical cord; structure that attaches the embryo to the yolk sac and contains blood vessels that extend into the chorionic villi.

Bogginess The softening of the uterus due to inadequate contraction of the muscle tissue.

Boggy uterus A term used to describe the uterine fundus when it is not firmly contracted after the birth of the baby and in the early postpartum period; excessive bleeding occurs from the placental site, and maternal hemorrhage may occur.

Bonding Process of parent-infant attachment occurring at or soon after birth.

Brachial palsy Partial or complete paralysis of portions of the arm resulting from trauma to the brachial plexus during a difficult birth.

Braxton Hicks contractions Intermittent painless contractions of the uterus that may occur every 10 to 20 minutes. They occur more frequently toward the end of pregnancy and are sometimes mistaken for true labor signs.

Brazleton's neonatal behavioral assessment A brief examination used to identify the infant's behavioral states and responses.

Breasts Mammary glands.

Breast self-examination (BSE) A manual examination conducted monthly by a woman to evaluate her own breasts for signs of masses, changes, nipple discharge, or evidence of abnormalities.

Breech presentation A birth in which the buttocks and/or feet are presented instead of the head.

Broad ligament The ligament extending from the lateral margins of the uterus to the pelvic wall; keeps the uterus centrally placed and provides stability within the pelvic cavity.

Bronchopulmonary dysplasia (BPD) Chronic pulmonary disease of multifactorial etiology characterized initially by alveolar and bronchial necrosis, which results in bronchial metaplasia and interstitial fibrosis. Appears in x-ray films as generalized small, radiolucent cysts within the lungs.

Brown adipose tissue (BAT) Fat deposits in newborns that provide greater heat-generating activity than ordinary fat. Found around the kidneys, adrenals, and neck; between the scapulas; and behind the sternum. Also called *brown fat.*

Calorie Amount of heat required to raise the temperature of 1 kg of water 1 degree centigrade.

Capacitation Removal of the plasma membrane overlying the spermatozoa's acrosomal area with the loss of seminal plasma proteins and the glycoprotein coat. If the glycoprotein coat is not removed, the sperm will not be able to penetrate the ovum.

Caput succedaneum (kap´ut suk_s″ē -dáne-um) Swelling or edema occurring in or under the fetal scalp during labor.

Cardinal ligaments The chief uterine supports, suspending the uterus from the side walls of the true pelvis.

Cardinal movements of labor The positional changes of the fetus as it moves through the birth canal during labor and birth. The positional changes are descent, flexion, internal rotation, extension, restitution, and external rotation.

Cardiopulmonary adaptation Adaptation of the newborn's cardiovascular and respiratory systems to life outside the womb.

Cephalhematoma (sef´ăl-hé-mă-tōmă) Subcutaneous swelling containing blood found on the head of an infant several days after birth; it usually disappears within a few weeks to 2 months.

Cephalic presentation Birth in which the fetal head is presenting against the cervix.

Cephalopelvic disproportion (CPD) A condition in which the fetal head is of such a shape or size, or in such a position, that it cannot pass through the maternal pelvis.

Certified nurse-midwife (CNM) An RN who has received special training and education in the care of the family during childbearing and the prenatal, labor and birth, and postpartal periods. After a period of formal education, the nurse-midwife takes a certification test to become a CNM.

Certified registered nurse (RNC) A registered nurse who has shown expertise in a specific field by passing a national certification examination.

Cervical cap A cup-shaped device placed over the cervix to prevent pregnancy.

Cervical dilatation Process in which the cervical os and the cervical canal widen from less than 1 cm to approximately 10 cm, allowing birth of the fetus.

Cervical funneling A cone-shaped indentation in the cervical os which is common in cases of cervical incompetence.

Cervical ripening Softening of the cervix; occurs normally as a physiologic process prior to labor or is stimulated to occur through the process of induction of labor.

Cervix The "neck" between the external os and the body of the uterus. The lower end of the cervix extends into the vagina.

Cesarean birth Birth of fetus accomplished by performing a surgical incision through the maternal abdomen and uterus.

Chadwick's sign Violet bluish color of the vaginal mucous membrane caused by increased vascularity; visible from about the fourth week of pregnancy.

Chemical conjunctivitis Irritation of the mucous membrane lining of the eyelid; may be due to instillation of silver nitrate ophthalmic drops.

Child abuse Nonaccidental physical or threatened harm, including mental or emotional injury, sexual abuse, and sexual exploitation.

Child neglect Failure by parents or other custodians to meet the medical, emotional, physical, or supervisory needs of a child.

Chiropractic Third largest independent health profession found in the United States. Uses spinal manipulation to address abnormal nerve transmission (subluxation) caused by misalignment of the spine.

Chlamydial infection Caused by Chlamydia trachomatis, this infection is the most common bacterial sexually transmitted infection in the United States.

Chloasma (klō-az´mă) Brownish pigmentation over the bridge of the nose and the cheeks during pregnancy and in some women who are taking oral contraceptives. Also called *mask of pregnancy.*

Chorioamnionitis (kō'rē -ō-am´nē -ō-ī´tis) An inflammation of the amniotic membranes stimulated by organisms in the amniotic fluid, which then becomes infiltrated with polymorphonuclear leukocytes.

Chorion The fetal membrane closest to the intrauterine wall that gives rise to the placenta and continues as the outer membrane surrounding the amnion.

Chorionic villus sampling Procedure in which a specimen of the chorionic villi is obtained from the edge of the developing placenta at about 8 weeks' gestation. The sample can be used for chromosomal, enzyme, and DNA tests.

Chromosomes The threadlike structures within the nucleus of a cell that carry the genes.

Circumcision Surgical removal of the prepuce (foreskin) of the penis.

Circumoral cyanosis Bluish appearance around the mouth.

Circumvallate (ser-kŭm-val´āt) **placenta** A placenta with a thick, white fibrous ring around the edge.

Cleavage Rapid mitotic division of the zygote; cells produced are called *blastomeres.*

Client Person seeking assistance from professionals that have the special skills and knowledge the individual lacks.

Client advocacy An approach to client care in which the nurse educates and supports the client and protects the client's rights.

Climacteric The period of time that marks the cessation of a woman's reproductive function; the "change of life," or menopause.

Clinical nurse specialist (CNS) A nurse possessing a master's degree and specialized knowledge and competence in a specific clinical area.

Clitoris Female organ homologous to the male penis; a small oval body of erectile tissue situated at the anterior junction of the vulva.

Coitus interruptus Method of contraception in which the male withdraws his penis from the vagina prior to ejaculation.

Cold stress Excessive heat loss resulting in compensatory mechanisms (increased respirations and nonshivering thermogenesis) to maintain core body temperature.

Colostrum (kō -los´trŭm) Secretion from the breast before the onset of true lactation; contains mainly serum and white blood corpuscles. It has a high protein content, provides some immune properties, and cleanses the newborn's intestinal tract of mucus and meconium.

Colposcopy The use of an instrument inserted into the vagina to examine the cervical and vaginal tissues by means of a magnifying lens.

Combined decelerations The occurrence of two different types of deceleration patterns occurring at the same time (for example, early/late, early/variable, or variable/late).

Combined oral contraceptives (COCs) Commonly called birth control pills or "the pill" cocs are a form of contraception that uses a combination of a synthetic estrogen and a progestin.

Comparable worth The standard that the same wages should be paid for different types of work that require comparable skills, responsibility, education, and experience.

Complementary therapy An adjunct to conventional medical treatment that has been through rigorous scientific testing which shows that it has some reliability.

Conception Union of male sperm and female ovum; fertilization.

Conceptional age The number of complete weeks since the moment of conception. Because the moment of conception is almost impossible to determine, conceptional age is estimated at 2 weeks less than gestational age.

Condom A rubber sheath that covers the penis to prevent conception or disease.

Conduction Loss of heat to a cooler surface by direct skin contact.

Condyloma (kon-di-lō'mă) Wartlike growth of skin, usually seen on the external genitals or anus. There are two types, a pointed variety and a broad, flat form usually found with syphilis.

Condylomata acuminata Known also as genital or venereal warts, they are a common sexually transmitted infection caused by the human papilloma virus (HPV).

Conjugate Important diameter of the pelvis, measured from the center of the promontory of the sacrum to the back of the symphysis pubis. The diagonal conjugate is measured and the true conjugate is estimated.

Conjugate vera The true conjugate, which extends from the middle of the sacral promontory to the middle of the pubic crest.

Contraception The prevention of conception or impregnation.

Contraction Tightening and shortening of the uterine muscles during labor, causing effacement and dilatation of the cervix; contributes to the downward and outward descent of the fetus.

Contraction stress test A method of assessing the reaction of the fetus to the stress of uterine contractions. This test may be utilized when contractions are occurring spontaneously or when contractions are artificially induced by oxytocin challenge test (OCT) or breast self-stimulation test (BSST).

Convection Loss of heat from the warm body surface to cooler air currents.

Coombs' (kōōmz) **test** A test for antiglobulins in the red cells. The indirect test determines the presence of Rh-positive antibodies in maternal blood; the direct test determines the presence of maternal Rh-positive antibodies in fetal cord blood.

Cornua The elongated portions of the uterus where the fallopian tubes open.

Corpus The upper two thirds of the uterus.

Corpus luteum A small yellow body that develops within a ruptured ovarian follicle; it secretes progesterone in the second half of the menstrual cycle and atrophies about 3 days before the beginning of menstrual flow. If pregnancy occurs, the corpus luteum continues to produce progesterone until the placenta takes over this function.

Cosleeping (family bed) Practice whereby children and parents regularly sleep together in an adult bed.

Cotyledon (kot-i-lē´don) One of the rounded portions into which the placenta's uterine surface is divided, consisting of a mass of villi, fetal vessels, and an intervillous space.

Couplet care A family-centered approach for maternal-child nursing where both the mother and her baby are cared for by the same nurse, with the baby remaining at the mothers' bedside.

Couvade (kū-vahd´) In some cultures, the male's observance of certain rituals and taboos to signify the transition to fatherhood.

Crack A form of freebase cocaine that is smoked.

Crisis intervention Actions taken by the nurse to help the client deal with an impending, potentially overwhelming crisis; regain his or her equilibrium; grow from the experience; and improve coping skills.

Critical thinking Intellectual processes that include separating fact from opinion, identifying prejudices and stereotypes that may influence interpretation of information, exploring differing ideas and views, and arriving at conclusions or insights.

Crowning Appearance of the presenting fetal part at the vaginal orifice during labor.

Crying state A state in the infant sleep/awake cycle in which the infant exhibits increased motor activity, grimaces, eyes tightly closed or open, and extreme responsiveness to stimuli.

Cultural beliefs Those beliefs that reflect the predominating values, attitudes, and practices accepted by a population, community, or ethnic group.

Cultural competency Referring to the skills and knowledge necessary to appreciate, understand, and work with individuals from different cultures.

Culture The beliefs, values, attitudes, and practices that are accepted by a population, community, or an individual.

Cycle of violence A theory that postulates that battering takes place in a cyclic fashion through three phases: the tension-building phase, the acute battering incident, and the tranquil phase (honeymoon period).

Cystocele The downward displacement of the bladder, which appears as a bulge in the anterior vaginal wall.

Date rape A form of acquaintance rape that occurs between a dating couple.

Deceleration Periodic decrease in the baseline fetal heart rate.

Decidua (dē-sid´ yū ă) Endometrium or mucous membrane lining of the uterus in pregnancy that is shed after childbirth.

Decidua basalis The part of the decidua that unites with the chorion to form the placenta. It is shed in lochial discharge after childbirth.

Decidua capsularis The part of the decidua surrounding the chorionic sac.

Decidua vera (parietalis) Nonplacental decidua lining the uterus.

Decrement Decrease or stage of decline, as of a contraction.

Deep sleep State of sleep in which the infant will be nearly still except for occasional startles, twitches, and sucking.

Depo-Provera A long-acting, injectable progestin contraceptive.

Descriptive statistics Statistics that describe or summarize a set of data.

Desquamation (des-kwă-mā´ shŭn) Shedding of the epithelial cells of the epidermis.

Diagonal conjugate Distance from the lower posterior border of the symphysis pubis to the sacral promontory; may be obtained by manual measurement.

Diaphragm A flexible disk that covers the cervix to prevent pregnancy.

Diastasis (dī-as´tă-sis) **recti** (rek´ti) **abdominis** Separation of the recti abdominis muscles along the median line. In women, it is seen with repeated childbirths or multiple gestations. In the newborn, it is usually caused by incomplete development.

Dilatation and curettage (D&C) Stretching of the cervical canal to permit passage of a curette, which is used to scrape the endometrium to empty the uterine contents or to obtain tissue for examination.

Dilatation of the cervix Expansion of the external os from an opening a few millimeters in size to an opening large enough to allow the passage of the infant.

Diploid number of chromosomes Containing a set of maternal and a set of paternal chromosomes; in humans, the diploid number of chromosomes is 46.

Disability Impairment in one or more of five function categories: cognition, communication, motor abilities, social abilities, or patterns of interactions.

Dissociation relaxation A pattern of active relaxation in which the woman learns to tighten one area of the body and then relax other areas simultaneously. This relaxation pattern is very effective for some women during labor.

Domestic violence Defined as the collective methods used to exert power and control by one individual over another in an adult intimate relationship. Forms of abuse typically fall into three categories: psychological abuse, physical abuse, and sexual abuse.

Doula A supportive companion who accompanies a laboring woman to provide emotional, physical, and informational support and acts as an advocate for the woman and her family.

Down syndrome An abnormality resulting from the presence of an extra chromosome number 21 (trisomy 21); characteristics include mental retardation and altered physical appearance. Formerly called *mongolism.*

Drowsy awake state Awake state in which infants open and close their eyes although the eyes appear glazed and the face is often still. They may return to sleep or awaken further in response to stimuli.

Drowsy state A state in the infant sleep/awake cycle that occurs between light sleep and the quiet alert state. It is marked by the infant opening and closing their eyes, but the eyes appear glazed and face is often still. They may return to sleep or awaken further in response to stimuli.

Drug-dependent infant The newborn of an alcoholic or drug-addicted woman.

Ductus arteriosus A communication channel between the main pulmonary artery and the aorta of the fetus. It is obliterated after birth by rising Po_2 and changes in intravascular pressure in the presence of normal pulmonary functioning. It normally becomes a ligament after birth but sometimes remains patent (patent ductus arteriosus, a treatable condition).

Ductus venosus A fetal blood vessel that carries oxygenated blood between the umbilical vein and the inferior vena cava, bypassing the liver; it becomes a ligament after birth.

Duncan's mechanism Occurs when the maternal surface of the placenta rather than the shiny fetal surface presents upon birth.

Duration The time length of each contraction, measured from the beginning of the increment to the completion of the decrement.

Dysfunctional uterine bleeding (DUB) A condition characterized by anovulatory cycles with abnormal uterine bleeding that does not have a demonstrable organic cause.

Dysmenorrhea Painful menstruation.

Dyspareunia Painful intercourse.

Dystocia (dis-tō´sē-ă) Difficult labor due to mechanical factors produced by the fetus or the maternal pelvis or due to inadequate uterine or other muscular activity.

Early adolescence Referring to adolescents who are age 14 and under.

Early decelerations Periodic change in fetal heart rate pattern caused by head compression; deceleration has a uniform appearance and early onset in relation to maternal contraction.

Early postpartal hemorrhage See *Postpartal hemorrhage.*

Eclampsia (ek-lamp´sē-ă) A major complication of pregnancy. Its cause is unknown; it occurs more often in the primigravida and is accompanied by elevated blood pressure, albuminuria, oliguria, tonic and clonic convulsions, and coma. It may occur during pregnancy (usually after the 20th week of gestation) or within 48 hours after childbirth.

Ectoderm Outer layer of cells in the developing embryo that gives rise to the skin, nails, and hair.

Ectopic pregnancy Implantation of the fertilized ovum outside the uterine cavity; common sites are the abdomen, fallopian tubes, and ovaries. Also called *oocyesis.*

Effacement Thinning and shortening of the cervix that occurs late in pregnancy or during labor.

Effleurage (e-fler-ahz´) A light stroking movement of the fingertips over the abdominal area during labor; used to provide distraction during labor contractions.

Ejaculation Expulsion of the seminal fluids from the penis.

Elder abuse Any deliberate action or lack of action that causes harm to an elderly person.

Electronic fetal monitoring (EFM) A method of placing a fetal monitor on the fetus in order to obtain a continuous tracing of the FHR, which allows many characteristics of the fetal heart rate to be observed and evaluated.

Emancipated minors Minors who are legally considered to have assumed the rights of an adult. An adolescent may be considered emancipated if he or she is self-supporting and living away from home, married, pregnant, a parent, or in the military.

Embryo The early stage of development of the young of any organism. In humans the embryonic period is from about 2 to 8 weeks' gestation and is characterized by cellular differentiation and predominantly hyperplastic growth.

Embryonic membranes The amnion and chorion.

Endoderm The inner layer of cells in the developing embryo that give rise to internal organs such as the intestines.

Endometrial biopsy Procedure providing information about the effects of progesterone produced by the corpus luteum after ovulation and endometrial receptivity.

Endometriosis Ectopic endometrium located outside the uterus in the pelvic cavity. Symptoms may include pelvic pain or pressure, dysmenorrhea, dispareunia, abnormal bleeding from the uterus or rectum, and sterility.

Endometritis Infection of the endometrium.

Endometrium (en´dō-mē´trē-ŭm) The mucous membrane that lines the inner surface of the uterus.

En face An assumed position in which one person looks at another and maintains his or her face in the same vertical plane as that of the other.

Engagement The entrance of the fetal presenting part into the superior pelvic strait and the beginning of the descent through the pelvic canal.

Engorgement Vascular congestion or distention. In obstetrics, the swelling of breast tissue brought about by an increase in blood and lymph supply to the breast, preceding true lactation.

Engrossment Characteristic sense of absorption, preoccupation, and interest in the infant demonstrated by fathers during early contact with their infants.

Entrainment Phenomenon in which a newborn moves in rhythm to adult speech.

Epidural block Regional anesthesia effective through the first and second stages of labor.

Episiotomy (ĕ-piz-ē-ot´o-mē) Incision of the perineum to facilitate birth and to avoid laceration of the perineum.

Epstein's (ep´stīnz) **pearls** Small, white blebs found along the gum margins and at the junction of the hard and soft palates; commonly seen in the newborn as a normal manifestation.

Erb-Duchenne palsy Paralysis of the arm and chest wall as a result of a birth injury to the brachial plexus or a subsequent injury to the fifth and sixth cervical nerves.

Erythema toxicum Innocuous pink papular rash of unknown cause with superimposed vesicles; it appears within 24 to 48 hours after birth and resolves spontaneously within a few days.

Erythroblastosis fetalis Hemolytic disease of the newborn characterized by anemia, jaundice, enlargement of the liver and spleen, and generalized edema. Caused by isoimmunization due to Rh incompatibility or ABO incompatibility.

Estimated date of birth (EDB) During a pregnancy, the approximate date when childbirth will occur; the "due date."

Estrogens The hormones estradiol and estrone, produced by the ovary.

Ethnicity A social identity that is associated with shared beliefs, behaviors, and patterns.

Ethnocentrism An individual's belief that the values and practices of his or her own culture are the best ones.

Evaporation Loss of heat incurred when water on the skin surface is converted to a vapor.

Evidence-based practice An approach to problem-solving and decision-making based on the consideration of data from research, statistical analysis, quality measures, risk management measurements, and other sources of reliable information.

Exchange transfusion The replacement of 70% to 80% of circulating blood by withdrawing the recipient's blood and injecting a donor's blood in equal amounts, for the purpose of preventing the accumulation of bilirubin or other by-products of hemolysis in the blood.

External (cephalic) version (ECV) Procedure involving external manipulation of the maternal abdomen to change the presentation of the fetus from breech to cephalic.

External os The opening between the cervix and the vagina.

Fallopian tubes Tubes that extend from the lateral angle of the uterus and terminate near the ovary; they serve as a passageway for the ovum from the ovary to the uterus and for the spermatozoa from the uterus toward the ovary. Also called *oviducts* and *uterine tubes*.

False labor Contractions of the uterus, regular or irregular, that may be strong enough to be interpreted as true labor but that do not dilate the cervix.

False pelvis The portion of the pelvis above the linea terminalis; its primary function is to support the weight of the enlarged pregnant uterus.

Family Two or more persons who are joined together by bonds of sharing and emotional closeness and who identify themselves as being part of a family.

Family assessment The process by which a nurse collects data regarding a family's current level of functioning, support systems, sociocultural influences, home and work environment, type of family, family structure, and needs.

Family-centered care An approach to healthcare based on the concept that a hospital can provide professional services to mothers, fathers, and infants in a homelike environment that would enhance the integrity of the family unit.

Family development The changes that families experience over time, including changes in relationships, communication patterns, roles, and interactions.

Family planning Actions an individual or a couple takes to avoid a pregnancy, to space future pregnancies for a specific reason, or to gain control over the number of children conceived.

Family power The individual who has either the potential or actual ability to change the behavior of other family members.

Family roles The specific roles of individuals within a family unit. Examples of roles include breadwinner, homemaker, mother, father, social planner, and family peacemaker.

Family values A system of ideas, attitudes, and beliefs about the worth of an entity or a concept that consciously or unconsciously bind together the members of the family in a common culture.

Female condom A thin, disposable polyurethane sheath with a flexible ring at each end that is placed inside the vagina and serves to prevent sperm from entering the cervix, thus preventing conception.

Female reproductive cycle (FRC) The monthly rhythmic changes in sexually mature women.

Feminization of later life Worldwide trend for women to comprise a majority of the elderly population.

Feminization of poverty Term used to describe the fact that, in the United States, women comprise a majority of the adult poor.

Ferning Formation of a palm-leaf pattern by the crystallization of cervical mucus as it dries at mid-menstrual cycle. Helpful in determining time of ovulation. Observed via microscopic examination of a thin layer of cervical mucus on a glass slide. This pattern is also observed when amniotic fluid is allowed to air dry on a slide and is a useful and quick test to determine whether amniotic membranes have ruptured.

Ferning capacity Formation of a palm-leaf pattern by the crystallization of cervical mucus as it dries at mid-menstrual cycle. The formation can be helpful in determining time of ovulation. Observed via microscopic examination of a thin layer of cervical mucus on a glass slide. This pattern is also observed when amniotic fluid is allowed to air dry on a slide and is a useful and quick test to determine whether amniotic membranes have ruptured.

Fertility awareness methods Also known as natural family planning, fertility awareness methods are based on an understanding of the changes that occur throughout a woman's ovulatory cycle. All these methods require periods of abstinence and recording of certain events throughout the cycle; cooperation of the partner is important.

Fertility rate Number of births per 1000 women aged 15 to 44 in a given population per year.

Fertilization Impregnation of an ovum by a spermatozoon; conception.

Fetal acoustic stimulation test (FAST) A fetal assessment test that uses sound from a speaker, bell, or artificial larynx to stimulate acceleration of the fetal heart; may be used in conjunction with the nonstress test.

Fetal activity diary (FAD) A method for tracking fetal activity taught to pregnant women.

Fetal alcohol effects (FAE) The less severe fetal manifestations of maternal alcohol ingestion, including mild to moderate cognitive problems and physical growth retardation.

Fetal alcohol syndrome (FAS) Syndrome caused by maternal alcohol ingestion and characterized by microcephaly, intrauterine growth restriction, short palpebral fissures, and maxillary hypoplasia.

Fetal attitude Relationship of the fetal parts to one another. Normal fetal attitude is one of moderate flexion of the arms onto the chest and flexion of the legs onto the abdomen.

Fetal blood sampling Blood sample drawn from the fetal scalp (or from the fetus in breech position) to evaluate the acid-base status of the fetus.

Fetal bradycardia A fetal heart rate less than 120 beats per minute during a 10-minute period of continuous monitoring.

Fetal death Death of the developing fetus after 20 weeks' gestation. Also called *fetal demise.*

Fetal distress Evidence that the fetus is in jeopardy, such as a change in fetal activity or heart rate.

Fetal fibronectin (fFN) A glycoprotein that is produced by the trophoblast and fetal tissues whose presence between 20 and 34 weeks gestation is a strong predictor of pre-term birth associated with pre-term spontaneous rupture of membranes.

Fetal heart rate (FHR) The number of times the fetal heart beats per minute; normal range is 120 to 160.

Fetal lie Relationship of the cephalocaudal axis (spinal column) of the fetus to the cephalocaudal axis (spinal column) of the woman. The fetus may be in a longitudinal or transverse lie.

Fetal movement record See *Fetal activity diary (FAD).*

Fetal position Relationship of the landmark on the presenting fetal part to the front, sides, or back of the maternal pelvis.

Fetal presentation The fetal body part that enters the maternal pelvis first. The three possible presentations are cephalic, shoulder, and breech.

Fetal scalp blood sample A collection of fetal blood collected via the vagina from the fetal head by making a small nick with a scalpel and collecting a blood sample which is used to identify the fetal acid-base status and determine if hypoxia is occurring during labor.

Fetal tachycardia A fetal heart rate of 160 beats per minute or more during a 10-minute period of continuous monitoring.

Fetoscope An adaptation of a stethoscope that facilitates auscultation of the fetal heart rate.

Fetoscopy A technique for directly observing the fetus and obtaining a sample of fetal blood or skin.

Fetus The child in utero from about the seventh to ninth week of gestation until birth.

Fibrocystic breast changes Benign breast changes characterized by bilateral, cyclic breast pain and breast nodularities that may be unilateral or bilateral, and often in the upper outer quadrants of the breasts.

Fibrocystic breast disease Benign breast disorder characterized by a thickening of normal breast tissue and the formation of cysts.

Fimbria Any structure resembling a fringe; the fringelike extremity of the fallopian tubes.

Folic acid An important vitamin directly related to the outcome of pregnancy and to maternal and fetal health.

Follicle-stimulating hormone (FSH) Hormone produced by the anterior pituitary during the first half of the menstrual cycle, stimulating development of the graafian follicle.

Fontanelle (fon´tănel´) In the fetus, an unossified space, or soft spot, consisting of a strong band of connective tissue lying between the cranial bones of the skull.

Foramen ovale Special opening between the atria of the fetal heart. Normally, the opening closes shortly after birth; if it remains open, it can be repaired surgically.

Forceps Obstetric instrument occasionally used to aid in childbirth.

Forceps-assisted birth A birth in which a set of instruments, known as forceps, are applied to the presenting part of the fetus to provide traction or to enable the fetal head to be rotated to an occiput-anterior position. Forceps-assisted birth is also known as *instrumental delivery, operative delivery, or operative vaginal delivery.*

Forceps marks Reddened areas over the cheeks and jaws caused by the application of forceps. The red areas usually disappear within 1 to 2 days.

Foremilk Breast milk obtained at the beginning of the breastfeeding episode.

Fourth trimester First several postpartal weeks during which the woman returns to an essentially prepregnant state and becomes competent in caring for her newborn.

Frequency The time between the beginning of one contraction and the beginning of the next contraction.

Fundus The upper portion of the uterus between the fallopian tubes.

Galactorrhea Nipple discharge.

Gamete (gam´ēt) Female or male germ cell; contains a haploid number of chromosomes.

Gamete intrafallopian transfer (GIFT) Retrieval of oocytes by laparoscopy; immediately combining oocytes with washed, motile sperm in a catheter; and placement of the gametes into the fimbriated end of the fallopian tube.

Gametogenesis The process by which germ cells are produced.

General anesthesia A state of induced unconsciousness that may be achieved through intravenous injection, inhalation of anesthetic agents, or a combination of both methods.

Genotype The genetic composition of an individual.

Gestation (jes-tā´shŭn) Period of intrauterine development from conception through birth; pregnancy.

Gestational age The number of complete weeks of fetal development, calculated from the first day of the last normal menstrual cycle.

Gestational age assessment tools Systems used to evaluate the newborn's external physical characteristics and neurologic and/or neuromuscular development to accurately determine gestational age. These replace or supplement the traditional calculation from the woman's last menstrual period.

Gestational diabetes mellitus A form of diabetes of variable severity with onset or first recognition during pregnancy.

Gestational trophoblastic disease (GTD) Disorder classified into two types: benign (hydatidiform mole) and malignant.

Gonadotropin-releasing hormone (GnRH) A hormone secreted by the hypothalamus that stimulates the anterior pituitary to secrete FSH and LH.

Gonorrhea A sexually transmitted infection caused by the bacterium *Neisseria gonorrhoeae*.

Goodell's sign Softening of the cervix that occurs during the second month of pregnancy.

Graafian follicle The ovarian cyst containing the ripe ovum; it secretes estrogens.

Grasping reflex Normal newborn reflex elicited by stimulating the palm with a finger or object, resulting in newborn firmly holding on to the finger or object.

Gravida (grav´i-dă) A pregnant woman.

Grief work The inner process of working through or managing the bereavement.

Guided imagery A state of intense, focused concentration used to create compelling mental images. It is sometimes considered a form of hypnosis.

Gynecoid pelvis Typical female pelvis in which the inlet is round instead of oval.

Habituation (ha-bit-chū-ā´shŭn) Infant's ability to diminish innate responses to specific repeated stimuli.

Haploid number of chromosomes Half the diploid number of chromosomes. In humans there are 23 chromosomes, the haploid number, in each germ cell.

Harlequin sign A rare color change that occurs between the longitudinal halves of the newborn's body, such that the dependent half is noticeably pinker than the superior half when the newborn is placed on one side; it is of no pathologic significance.

Hatha yoga The physical branch of yoga; in the United States, it is commonly practiced for wellness, illness prevention, and healing.

Hegar's sign A softening of the lower uterine segment found upon palpation in the second or third month of pregnancy.

HELLP syndrome A cluster of changes including *h*emolysis, *e*levated *l*iver enzymes, and *l*ow *p*latelet count; sometimes associated with severe preeclampsia.

Hemolytic disease of the newborn *Hyperbilirubinemia* secondary to Rh incompatibility.

Herpes genitalis A life-long, recurrent sexually transmitted infection caused by the herpes simplex virus (HSV).

Heterozygous A genotypic situation in which two different alleles occur at a given locus on a pair of homologous chromosomes.

Hindmilk Breast milk released after initial let-down reflex; high in fat content.

Homeopathy Term derived from the Greek word *homos* meaning the same, and describing a healing system that uses as remedies minute dilutions of substances that, if ingested in larger amounts, would produce effects *similar* to the symptoms of the disorder being treated.

Homozygous A genotypic situation in which two similar genes occur at a given locus on homologous chromosomes.

Hormone replacement therapy (HRT) Administration of hormones, usually estrogen and a progestin, to alleviate the symptoms of menopause.

Huhner test Postcoital examination to evaluate sperm and cervical mucus.

Human chorionic gonadotropin (hCG) A hormone produced by the chorionic villi and found in the urine of pregnant women. Also called *prolan*.

Human immunodeficiency virus (HIV) A virus that causes a progressive disease that ultimately results in the development of acquired immunodeficiency syndrome (AIDS).

Human placental lactogen (hPL) A hormone synthesized by the syncytiotrophoblast that functions as an insulin antagonist and promotes lipolysis to increase the amounts of circulating free fatty acids available for maternal metabolic use.

Hydatidiform (hī-da-tid´i-form) **mole** Degenerative process in chorionic villi, giving rise to multiple cysts and rapid growth of the uterus, with hemorrhage.

Hydramnios (hī-dram´nē-os) An excess of amniotic fluid, leading to overdistention of the uterus. Frequently seen in diabetic pregnant women, even if there is no coexisting fetal anomaly. Also called *polyhydramnios*.

Hydrops fetalis See *Erythroblastosis fetalis*.

Hydrotherapy Type of therapy that makes use of hot or cold moisture in any form. Hydrotherapy is used to relax muscles, promote rest, decrease pain, reduce swelling, promote healing, cleanse wounds and burns, reduce fever, lessen cramps, and improve well-being.

Hyperbilirubinemia (hī-per-bil´i-rū-bi-nē´mē-ă) Excessive amount of bilirubin in the blood; indicative of hemolytic processes due to blood incompatibility, intrauterine infection, septicemia, neonatal renal infection, and other disorders.

Hyperemesis gravidarum Excessive vomiting during pregnancy, leading to dehydration and starvation.

Hyperventilation Rapid breathing that occurs over a prolonged period of time resulting in an imbalance of oxygen and carbon dioxide that can result in tingling or numbness in the tip of nose, lips, fingers, or toes; dizziness; spots before the eyes; or spasms of the hands or feet (carpal-pedal spasms).

Hypnosis Whether guided by a trained hypnotherapist or self-induced, a state of great mental and physical relaxation during which a person is very open to suggestions.

Hypoglycemia Abnormally low level of sugar in the blood.

Hysterectomy Surgical removal of the uterus.

Hysterosalpingogram Result of testing by instillation of radiopaque substance into the uterine cavity to visualize the uterus and fallopian tubes.

Hysterosalpingography (HSG) Testing by instillation of radiopaque substance into the uterine cavity to visualize the uterus and fallopian tubes.

Hysteroscopy Use of a special endoscope to examine the uterus.

Inborn error of metabolism A hereditary deficiency of a specific enzyme needed for normal metabolism of specific chemicals.

Incompetent cervix The premature dilatation of the cervix, usually in the second trimester of pregnancy.

Increment Increase or addition; to build up, as of a contraction.

Induction of labor The process of causing or initiating labor by use of medication or surgical rupture of membranes.

Infant A child under 1 year of age.

Infant mortality rate Number of deaths of infants under 1 year of age per 1000 live births in a given population per year.

Infant of a diabetic mother (IDM) At-risk infant born to a woman previously diagnosed as diabetic or who develops symptoms of diabetes during pregnancy.

Infant of substance-abusing mother (ISAM) Formerly called infant of an addicted mother, an infant born to a mother who abuses or is addicted to drugs or alcohol.

Inferential statistics Statistics that allow an investigator to draw conclusions about what is happening between two or more variables in a population and to suggest or refute causal relationships between them.

Infertility Diminished ability to conceive.

Informed consent A legal concept that protects a person's rights to autonomy and self-determination by specifying that no action may be taken without that person's prior understanding and freely given consent.

Infundibulopelvic ligament Ligament that suspends and supports the ovaries.

Intensity The strength of a uterine contraction during acme.

Internal os An inside mouth or opening; the opening between the cervix and the uterus.

Internal version Procedure used for the vaginal birth of a second twin. The obstetrician inserts a hand into the uterus, grasps the feet of the fetus, and changes the fetus from a transverse to a breech presentation.

Intrapartum The time from the onset of true labor until the birth of the infant and expulsion of the placenta.

Intrauterine device (IUD) Small metal or plastic form that is placed in the uterus to prevent implantation of a fertilized ovum.

Intrauterine fetal surgery Surgery performed on a fetus to correct anatomic lesions that are not compatible with life if left untreated.

Intrauterine growth restriction (IUGR) Fetal undergrowth due to any etiology, such as intrauterine infection, deficient nutrient supply, or congenital malformation. A term used to describe fetuses falling below the 10th percentile in ultrasonic estimation of weight at a given gestational age.

Intrauterine pressure catheter (IUPC) A catheter that can be placed through the cervix into the uterus to measure uterine pressure during labor. Some types of catheters may be inserted for the purpose of infusing warmed saline to add additional intrauterine fluid when oligohydramnios is present.

Intrauterine resuscitation Interventions initiated when nonreassuring fetal heart rate patterns are noted; they are directed at improving intrauterine blood flow.

Introitus Opening or entrance into a cavity or canal such as the vagina.

In vitro fertilization (IVF) Procedure during which oocytes are removed from the ovary, mixed with spermatozoa, fertilized, and incubated in a glass petri dish; then up to four viable embryos are placed in the woman's uterus.

Involution Rolling or turning inward; the reduction in size of the uterus following childbirth.

Ischial spines Prominences that arise near the junction of the ilium and ischium and jut into the pelvic cavity; used as a reference point during labor to evaluate the descent of the fetal head into the birth canal.

Isthmus The straight, narrow part of the fallopian tube with a thick muscular wall and an opening (lumen) 2 to 3 mm in diameter; the site of tubal ligation. Also, a constriction in the uterus that is located above the cervix and below the corpus.

Jaundice Yellow pigmentation of body tissues caused by the presence of bile pigments. See also *Physiologic jaundice*.

Karyotype The set of chromosomes arranged in a standard order.

Kegel exercises Perineal muscle tightening that strengthens the pubococcygeus muscle and increases its tone.

Kernicterus (ker-nik´ter-ŭs) An encephalopathy caused by deposition of unconjugated bilirubin in brain cells; may result in impaired brain function or death.

Kilocalorie (kcal) Equivalent to 1000 calories, it is the unit used to express the energy value of food.

Klinefelter syndrome A chromosomal abnormality caused by the presence of an extra X chromosome in the male. Characteristics include tall stature; sparse pubic and facial hair; gynecomastia; small, firm testes; and absence of spermatogenesis.

Labor The process by which the fetus is expelled from the maternal uterus. Also called *childbirth, confinement,* or *parturition.*

Labor induction The stimulation of uterine contractions before the spontaneous onset of labor, with or without ruptured fetal membranes, for the purpose of accomplishing birth.

Lactase deficiency (lactose intolerance) A condition characterized by difficulty digesting milk and dairy products. Results from an inadequate amount of the enzyme lactase, which breaks down the milk sugar lactose into smaller digestible substances.

Lactation The process of producing and supplying breast milk.

Lacto-ovovegetarians Vegetarians who include milk, dairy products, and eggs in their diets and occasionally fish, poultry, and liver.

Lactose intolerance A condition in which an individual has difficulty digesting milk and milk products.

Lactovegetarians Vegetarians who include dairy products but no eggs in their diets.

La Leche League Organization that provides information on and assistance with breastfeeding.

Lamaze method A method of childbirth preparation.

Lanugo (lă-nū´ gō) Fine, downy hair found on all body parts of the fetus, with the exception of the palms of the hands and the soles of the feet, after 20 weeks' gestation.

Laparoscopy Procedure that enables direct visualization of pelvic organs.

Large for gestational age (LGA) Excessive growth of a fetus in relation to the gestational time period.

Last menstrual period (LMP) The last normal menstrual period experienced by the woman prior to pregnancy; sometimes used to calculate the infant's gestational age.

Late adolescence A term referring to adolescents who are ages 18 to 19 years.

Late decelerations Symmetrical decrease in fetal heart rate beginning at or after the peak of the contraction and returning to baseline only after the contraction has ended, indicating possible uteroplacental insufficiency and potential that the fetus is not receiving adequate oxygenation.

Late postpartal hemorrhage See *Postpartal hemorrhage.*

Lecithin-sphingomyelin (les´i-thin sfing´gō-mī´ē-lin) **(L/S) ratio** Lecithin and sphingomyelin are phospholipid components of surfactant; their ratio changes during gestation. When the L/S ratio reaches 2:1, the fetal lungs are thought to be mature and the fetus will have a low risk of respiratory distress syndrome (RDS) if born at that time.

Leiomyoma A benign tumor of the uterus, composed primarily of smooth muscle and connective tissue. Also referred to as a myoma or a fibroid.

Leopold's maneuvers A series of four maneuvers designed to provide a systematic approach whereby the examiner may determine fetal presentation and position.

Let-down reflex Pattern of stimulation, hormone release, and resulting muscle contraction that forces milk into the lactiferous ducts, making it available to the infant. Also called *milk ejection reflex.*

Leukorrhea Mucous discharge from the vagina or cervical canal that may be normal or pathologic, as in the presence of infection.

Lie Relationship of the long axis of the fetus and the long axis of the pregnant woman. The fetal lie may be longitudinal, transverse, or oblique.

Light sleep State that makes up the highest proportion of newborn sleep and precedes awakening; characterized by some body movements, rapid eye movements (REM), and brief fussing or crying.

Lightening Moving of the fetus and uterus downward into the pelvic cavity.

Linea nigra (lin´ē-ă ni´gră) The line of darker pigmentation extending from the umbilicus to the pubis noted in some women during the later months of pregnancy.

Local anesthesia Injection of an anesthetic agent into the subcutaneous tissue in a fanlike pattern.

Lochia (lō´kē-ă) Maternal discharge of blood, mucus, and tissue from the uterus; may last for several weeks after birth.

Lochia alba White vaginal discharge that follows lochia serosa and that lasts from about the 10th to the 21st day after birth.

Lochia rubra Red, blood-tinged vaginal discharge that occurs following birth and lasts 2 to 4 days.

Lochia serosa Pink, serous, and blood-tinged vaginal discharge that follows lochia rubra and lasts until the 7th to 10th day after birth.

Long-term variability (LTV) Large rhythmic fluctuations of the FHR that occur from two to six times per minute.

Luteinizing hormone (LH) Anterior pituitary hormone responsible for stimulating ovulation and for development of the corpus luteum.

Macrosomia (mak-rō-sō´mē-ă) A condition seen in newborns of large body size and high birth weight (more than 4000 to 4500 g (8 lb, 13 oz to 9 lb, 14 oz)), such as those born of prediabetic and diabetic mothers.

Malposition An abnormal position of the fetus in the birth canal.

Malpresentation A presentation of the fetus into the birth canal that is not "normal"— that is, brow, face, shoulder, or breech presentation.

Mammogram A soft-tissue radiograph of the breast without the injection of a contrast medium.

Massage therapy Manipulation of the soft tissues of the body to reduce stress and tension, increase circulation, diminish pain, and promote a sense of well-being.

Mastitis Inflammation of the breast.

Maternal mortality rate The number of maternal deaths from any cause during the pregnancy cycle per 100,000 live births.

Maternal role attainment Process by which a woman learns mothering behaviors and becomes comfortable with her identity as a mother.

Maternal serum alpha-fetoprotein (MSAFP) Screening test performed between 16 and 22 gestational weeks that utilizes the multiple markers (the "triple screen") of alpha-fetoprotein (AFP), human chorionic growth hormone (hCG), and urine estriol (uE3) to screen pregnancies for NTD, Down syndrome, and trisomy 18.

Mature milk Breast milk that contains 10% solids for energy and growth.

McDonald's sign A probable sign of pregnancy characterized by an ease in flexing the body of the uterus against the cervix.

Meconium Dark green or black material present in the large intestine of a full-term infant; the first stools passed by the newborn.

Meconium aspiration syndrome (MAS) Respiratory disease of term, postterm, and SGA newborns caused by inhalation of meconium or meconium-stained amniotic fluid into the lungs; characterized by mild to severe respiratory distress, hyperexpansion of the chest, hyperinflated alveoli, and secondary atelectasis.

Meiosis The process of cell division that occurs in the maturation of sperm and ova that decreases their number of chromosomes by one-half.

Menarche (me-nar´kē) Beginning of menstrual and reproductive function in the female.

Mendelian inheritance A major category of inheritance whereby a trait is determined by a pair of genes on homologous chromosomes. Also called *single gene inheritance.*

Menopause The permanent cessation of menses.

Menorrhagia Excessive or profuse menstrual flow.

Menstrual cycle Cyclic buildup of the uterine lining, ovulation, and sloughing of the lining occurring approximately every 28 days in nonpregnant females.

Mentum The chin.

Mesoderm The intermediate layer of germ cells in the embryo that gives rise to connective tissue, bone marrow, muscles, blood, lymphoid tissue, and epithelial tissue.

Metrorrhagia Abnormal uterine bleeding occurring at irregular intervals.

Middle adolescence A term referring to adolescents who are ages 15 to 17 years.

Milia (mil´ē -ă) Tiny white papules appearing on the face of a newborn as a result of unopened sebaceous glands; they disappear spontaneously within a few weeks.

Milk/plasma ratio The comparison of the concentration of substances in the breast milk and the maternal blood serum.

Miscarriage See *Spontaneous abortion.*

Mitosis Process of cell division whereby both daughter cells have the same number and pattern of chromosomes as the original cell.

Molding Shaping of the fetal head by overlapping of the cranial bones to facilitate movement through the birth canal during labor.

Mongolian spot Dark, flat pigmentation of the lower back and buttocks noted at birth in some infants; usually disappears by the time the child reaches school age.

Moniliasis Yeastlike fungal infection caused by *Candida albicans.*

Monosomies A genetic condition that occurs when a normal gamete unites with a gamete that is missing a chromosome.

Mons pubis (monz pu´bis) Mound of subcutaneous fatty tissue covering the anterior portion of the symphysis pubis.

Morning sickness A term that refers to the nausea and vomiting that a woman may experience in early pregnancy. This lay term is sometimes used because these symptoms frequently occur in the early part of the day and disappear within a few hours.

Moro reflex Flexion of the newborn's thighs and knees accompanied by fingers that fan, then clench, as the arms are simultaneously thrown out and then brought together, as though embracing something. This reflex can be elicited by startling the newborn with a sudden noise or movement. Also called the *startle reflex.*

Morula Developmental stage of the fertilized ovum in which there is a solid mass of cells.

Mosaicism Condition of an individual who has at least two cell lines with differing karyotypes.

Mottling (mot´ling) Discoloration of the skin in irregular areas; may be seen with chilling, poor perfusion, or hypoxia.

Mucous plug A collection of thick mucus that blocks the cervical canal during pregnancy. Also called *operculum.*

Multigravida (mŭl-tē-grav´i-dă) Woman who has been pregnant more than once.

Multipara (mŭl-tip´ă-ră) Woman who has had more than one pregnancy in which the fetus was viable.

Multiple pregnancy More than one fetus in the uterus at the same time.

Music therapy Form of sound therapy using one or more musical instruments and improvisations or musical compositions. *Sound therapy* is based on the premise that when the body is exposed to the correct sound frequency (including some very low and very high frequencies that humans cannot normally hear) the body restores itself.

Myometrium Uterine muscular structure.

Nägele's rule A method of determining the estimated date of birth (EDB): after obtaining the first day of the last menstrual period, subtract 3 months and add 7 days.

Naturopathy A healing system that employs various natural means of preventing and treating human disease, such as foods, herbs, rest, etc. (Also called *natural medicine.*)

Neonatal morbidity The risk of death during the newborn period—the first 28 days of life.

Neonatal mortality rate Number of deaths of infants in the first 28 days of life per 1000 live births.

Neonatal mortality risk The chance of death within the newborn period.

Neonatal transition The first few hours of life, in which the newborn stabilizes its respiratory and circulatory functions.

Neonate Infant from birth through the first 28 days of life.

Neonatology The specialty that focuses on the management of at-risk conditions of the newborn.

Neutral thermal environment (NTE) An environment that provides for minimal heat loss or expenditure.

Nevus (nē´vŭs) **flammeus** (flaem´iŭs) Large port-wine stain.

Nevus vasculosus "Strawberry mark": raised, clearly delineated, dark-red, rough-surfaced birthmark commonly found in the head region.

Newborn screening tests Tests that detect inborn errors of metabolism that, if left untreated, cause mental retardation and physical handicaps.

Newborns' and mothers' health protection act (NMHPA) Legislation which states that women who have given birth vaginally cannot be forcibly discharged from the hospital within 48 hours of the time of birth for insurance reasons. Cesarean birth mothers are covered by their insurance for 96 hours following the time of birth.

Nidation Implantation of a fertilized ovum in the endometrium.

Nipple A protrusion about 0.5 to 1.3 cm in diameter in the center of each mature breast.

Nipple preparation Prenatal activities designed to toughen the nipple in preparation for breastfeeding.

Nonmendelian (multifactorial) inheritance The occurrence of congenital disorders that result from an interaction of multiple genetic and environmental factors.

Nonstress test (NST) An assessment method by which the reaction (or response) of the fetal heart rate to fetal movement is evaluated.

Norplant A subdermal progestin contraceptive that is implanted in a woman's arm and provides contraceptive protection for up to 5 years.

Nuchal cord Term used to describe the umbilical cord when it is wrapped around the neck of the fetus.

Nulligravida (nŭl-i-grav´i-dă) A woman who has never been pregnant.

Nullipara A woman who has not given birth to a viable fetus.

Obstetric conjugate Distance from the middle of the sacral promontory to an area approximately 1 cm below the pubic crest.

Oligohydramnios (ol´i-gō-hī-dram´nē-os) Decreased amount of amniotic fluid, which may indicate a fetal urinary tract defect.

Oocyte Early primitive ovum before it has completely developed.

Oogenesis Process during fetal life whereby the ovary produces oogonia, cells that become primitive ovarian eggs.

Oophoritis Infection of the ovaries.

Ophthalmia (of-thal´mē-ă) **neonatorum** Purulent infection of the eyes or conjunctiva of the newborn, usually caused by gonococci.

Oral contraceptives Birth control pills that work by inhibiting the release of an ovum and by maintaining a type of mucus that is hostile to sperm.

Orientation Infant's ability to respond to auditory and visual stimuli in the environment.

Ortolani maneuver A manual procedure performed to rule out the possibility of developmental dysplastic hip.

Osteoporosis A condition most common in postmenopausal women that is characterized by decreased bone strength related to diminished bone density and bone quality. It is thought to be associated with lowered estrogen and androgen levels. Osteoporosis puts an individual at increased risk for fractures of the hip, forearm, and vertebrae.

Ovarian ligaments Ligaments that anchor the lower pole of the ovary to the cornua of the uterus.

Ovary Female sex gland in which the ova are formed and in which estrogen and progesterone are produced. Normally there are two ovaries, located in the lower abdomen on each side of the uterus.

Ovulation Normal process of discharging a mature ovum from an ovary approximately 14 days prior to the onset of menses.

Ovum Female reproductive cell; egg.

Oxygen toxicity Excessive levels of oxygen therapy that result in pathologic changes in tissue.

Oxytocin Hormone normally produced by the posterior pituitary, responsible for stimulation of uterine contractions and the release of milk into the lactiferous ducts.

Oxytocin challenge test (OCT) See *Contraction stress test.*

Papanicolaou (Pap) smear Procedure to detect the presence of cancer of the uterus by microscopic examination of cells gently scraped from the cervix.

Para (par´ă) A woman who has borne offspring who reached the age of viability.

Parametritis Inflammation of the parametrial layer of the uterus.

Parent-newborn attachment Close affectional ties that develop between parent and child. See also *Attachment.*

Passive acquired immunity Transfer of antibodies (IgG) from the mother to the fetus in utero.

Patient-controlled analgesia (PCA) A method of pain control where anesthesia, usually morphine or meperidine, is initially administered by the anesthesiologist and subsequent doses are self-administered by pushing a button controlled by a special IV pump system.

Pedigree Graphic representation of a family tree.

Pelvic cavity Bony portion of the birth passages; a curved canal with a longer posterior than anterior wall.

Pelvic cellulitis Infection involving the connective tissue of the broad ligament or, in severe cases, the connective tissue of all the pelvic structures.

Pelvic diaphragm Part of the pelvic floor composed of deep fascia and the levator ani and the coccygeal muscles.

Pelvic floor Muscles and tissue that act as a buttress to the pelvic outlet.

Pelvic inflammatory disease (PID) An infection of the fallopian tubes that may or may not be accompanied by a pelvic abscess; may cause infertility secondary to tubal damage.

Pelvic inlet Upper border of the true pelvis.

Pelvic outlet Lower border of the true pelvis.

Pelvic tilt Also called *pelvic rocking;* exercise designed to reduce back strain and strengthen abdominal muscle tone.

Penis The male organ of copulation and reproduction.

Percutaneous umbilical blood sampling (PUBS) A technique used to obtain pure fetal blood from the umbilical cord while the fetus is in utero. Also called *cordocentesis.*

Perimenopause A term referring to the period of time prior to menopause during which the woman moves from normal ovulatory cycles to cessation of menses.

Perimetrium The outermost layer of the corpus of the uterus. Also known as the serosal layer.

Perinatal mortality rate The number of neonatal and fetal deaths per 1000 live births.

Perinatology The medical specialty concerned with the diagnosis and treatment of high-risk conditions of the pregnant woman and her fetus.

Perineal (per´i-nē-ăl) **body** Wedge-shaped mass of fibromuscular tissue found between the lower part of the vagina and the anal canal.

Perineum (per´i-nē´ŭm) The area of tissue between the anus and scrotum in a man or between the anus and vagina in a woman.

Periodic breathing Sporadic episodes of apnea, not associated with cyanosis, that last for about 10 seconds and commonly occur in preterm infants.

Periods of reactivity Predictable patterns of newborn behavior during the first several hours after birth.

Peritonitis Infection involving the peritoneal cavity.

Persistent occiput posterior position Malposition of the fetus in which the fetal occiput is posterior in the maternal pelvis.

Persistent pulmonary hypertension of the newborn (PPHN) Respiratory disease resulting from right-to-left shunting of blood away from the lungs and through the ductus arteriosus and patent foramen ovale.

Phenotype The whole physical, biochemical, and physiologic makeup of an individual as determined both genetically and environmentally.

Phenylketonuria (fen´il-kē´tō-nū´ rē-ă) A common metabolic disease caused by an inborn error in the metabolism of the amino acid phenylalanine.

Phosphatidylglycerol (PG) (fos-fă-tī´dĭl-glis´er-ol) A phospholipid present in fetal surfactant after about 35 weeks' gestation.

Phototherapy The treatment of jaundice by exposure to light.

Physiologic anemia A condition resulting from a normal, gradual drop in hemoglobin for the first 6 to 12 weeks of life.

Physiologic anemia of infancy A harmless condition in which the hemoglobin level drops in the first 6 to 12 weeks after birth, then reverts to normal levels.

Physiologic anemia of pregnancy Apparent anemia that results because during pregnancy the plasma volume increases more than the erythrocytes increase.

Physiologic jaundice A harmless condition caused by the normal reduction of red blood cells, occurring 48 or more hours after birth, peaking at the 5th to 7th day, and disappearing between the 7th and 10th day.

Pica The eating of substances not ordinarily considered edible or to have nutritive value.

Placenta (plă-sen´tă) Specialized disk-shaped organ that connects the fetus to the uterine wall for gas and nutrient exchange. Also called *afterbirth.*

Placenta accreta Partial or complete absence of the decidua basalis and abnormal adherence of the placenta to the uterine wall.

Placenta increta A high risk condition that occurs when the placenta attaches to the uterine wall and invades or attaches itself within the myometrium.

Placenta percreta A high risk condition that occurs when the placenta penetrates the myometrium, sometimes attaching to peritoneal structures within the abdominal cavity, where the removal of the uterus (hysterectomy) is sometimes necessary.

Placenta previa Abnormal implantation of the placenta in the lower uterine segment. Classification of type is based on proximity to the cervical os: *total*—completely covers the os; *partial*—covers a portion of the os; *marginal*—is in close proximity to the os.

Platypelloid pelvis An unusually wide pelvis, having a flattened oval transverse shape and a shortened anteroposterior diameter.

Podalic version Type of version used to turn a second twin during a vaginal birth.

Polar body A small cell resulting from the meiotic division of the mature oocyte.

Polycythemia An abnormal increase in the number of total red blood cells in the body's circulation.

Polydactyly (pol-ē-dak´ti-lē) A developmental anomaly characterized by more than five digits on the hands or feet.

Polypharmacy The act of taking multiple drugs to treat symptoms, when the etiology of the symptoms is actually a side effect from one or more prescribed medications.

Positive signs of pregnancy Indications that confirm the presence of pregnancy.

Postcoital contraception A form of combined hormonal contraception that is used when a woman is worried about pregnancy because of unprotected intercourse, rape, or possible contraceptive failure (eg, broken condom, slipped diaphragm, missed oral contraceptives, or too long a time between DMPA injections).

Postconception age periods Period of time in embryonic/fetal development calculated from the time of fertilization of the ovum.

Postmature newborn See *Postterm newborn.*

Postmaturity See *Postterm newborn.*

Postpartal hemorrhage A loss of blood of greater than 500 mL following birth. The hemorrhage is classified as *early* if it occurs within the first 24 hours and *late* if it occurs after the first 24 hours.

Postpartal home care Home visits for postpartal families occurring in the home setting. This provides opportunities for expanding information and reinforcing self- and infant care techniques initially presented in the birth setting.

Postpartum After childbirth.

Postpartum blues A maternal adjustment reaction occurring in the first few postpartal days, characterized by mild depression, tearfulness, anxiety, headache, and irritability.

Postpartum depression (postpartum major mood disorder) Severe depression that occurs within the first year after giving birth with increase incidence at about the fourth week postpartum, just prior to resumption of menses, and upon weaning.

Postpartum psychosis Psychosis occurring within the first 3 months after birth.

Postterm labor Labor that occurs after 42 weeks' gestation.

Postterm newborn Any infant born after 42 weeks' gestation.

Postterm pregnancy Pregnancy that lasts beyond 42 weeks' gestation.

Precipitous birth (1) Unduly rapid progression of labor. (2) A birth in which no physician is in attendance.

Precipitous labor Labor lasting less than 3 hours.

Preeclampsia (prē-ē-klamp´sē-ă) Toxemia of pregnancy, characterized by hypertension, albuminuria, and edema. See also *Eclampsia.*

Premature infant See *Preterm infant.*

Premature rupture of the membranes (PROM) See *Rupture of membranes (ROM).*

Premenstrual syndrome (PMS) Cluster of symptoms experienced by some women, typically occurring from a few days up to 2 weeks prior to the onset of menses.

Prenatal education Programs offered to expectant families, adolescents, women, or partners to provide education regarding the pregnancy, labor, and birth experience.

Prep Shaving of the pubic area.

Presentation The fetal body part that enters the maternal pelvis first. The three possible presentations are cephalic, shoulder, and breech.

Presenting part The fetal part present in or on the cervical os.

Presumptive signs of pregnancy Symptoms that suggest but do not confirm pregnancy, such as cessation of menses, quickening, Chadwick's sign, and morning sickness.

Preterm infant Any infant born before 38 weeks' gestation.

Preterm labor Labor occurring between 20 and 38 weeks of pregnancy. Also called *premature labor.*

Primigravida (prī-mi-grav´i-dă) A woman who is pregnant for the first time.

Primipara (prī-mip´ă-ră) A woman who has given birth to her first child (past the point of viability), whether or not that child is living or was alive at birth.

Probable signs of pregnancy Manifestations that strongly suggest the likelihood of pregnancy, such as a positive pregnancy test, enlarging abdomen, and positive Goodell's, Hegar's, and Braxton Hicks signs.

Professional nurse A person who has graduated from an accredited basic program in nursing, has successfully completed the nursing licensure examination (NCLEX), and is currently licensed as a registered nurse (RN).

Progesterone A hormone produced by the corpus luteum, adrenal cortex, and placenta whose function is to stimulate proliferation of the endometrium to facilitate growth of the embryo.

Progressive relaxation A relaxation technique that involves relaxing first one portion of the body and then another portion, until total body relaxation is achieved; may be used during labor.

Prolactin A hormone secreted by the anterior pituitary that stimulates and sustains lactation in mammals.

Prolapsed cord Umbilical cord that becomes trapped in the vagina before the fetus is born.

Prolonged decelerations Decelerations in which the FHR decreases from the baseline for 2 to 10 minutes.

Prolonged labor Labor lasting more than 24 hours.

Prostaglandins Complex lipid compounds synthesized by many cells in the body.

Pseudomenstruation Blood-tinged mucus from the vagina in the newborn female infant; caused by withdrawal of maternal hormones that were present during pregnancy.

Psychological disorders Abnormal mental or emotional conditions characterized by alterations in thinking, mood or behavior.

Ptyalism Excessive salivation.

Puberty The developmental period between childhood and the attainment of adult sexual characteristics and functioning.

Pubic Pertaining to the pubes or pubis.

Pubis Pertaining to the pubes or pubic area.

Pudendal (pyū-den´dăl) **block** Injection of an anesthetizing agent at the pudendal nerve to produce numbness of the external genitals and the lower one-third of the vagina, to facilitate childbirth and permit episiotomy if necessary.

Puerperal infection Infection of the reproductive tract associated with childbirth and occurring any time up to 6 weeks postpartum.

Puerperal morbidity A maternal temperature of 38C (100.4F) or higher on any 2 of the first 10 postpartal days, excluding the first 24 hours. The temperature is to be taken by mouth at least four times per day.

Puerperium (pyū-er-pēr´ē-ŭm) The period after completion of the third stage of labor until involution of the uterus is complete, usually 6 weeks.

Quickening The first fetal movements felt by the pregnant woman, usually between 16 and 18 weeks' gestation.

Quiet alert state Alert state characterized by a brightening of the eyes and face. Infants are most attentive to their environment in this state and provide positive feedback to caregivers.

Radiation Heat loss incurred when heat transfers to cooler surfaces and objects not in direct contact with the body.

Rape Sexual activity, often intercourse, against the will of the victim.

Rape trauma syndrome A term which refers to a variety of symptoms, clustered in phases, that a rape survivor experiences following an assault.

Reciprocal inhibition The principle that it is impossible to feel relaxed and tense at the same time; the basis for relaxation techniques.

Reciprocity An interactional cycle that occurs simultaneously between mother and infant. It involves mutual cuing behaviors, expectancy, rhythmicity, and synchrony.

Recommended dietary allowances (RDA) Government recommended allowances of various vitamins, minerals, and other nutrients.

Reflexology Form of massage involving the application of pressure to designated points or reflexes on the client's feet, hands, or ears using the thumb and fingers.

Regional analgesia The temporary and reversible loss of sensation produced by injecting an anesthetic agent (called a local anesthetic) into an area that will bring the agent into direct contact with nervous tissue.

Regional anesthesia Injection of local anesthetic agents so that they come into direct contact with nervous tissue.

Reiki Tibetan-Japanese hand-mediated therapy designed to promote healing, reduce stress, and encourage relaxation. During Reiki sessions, practitioners place their hands on or above specific problem areas and transfer energy from themselves to their clients in order to restore the balance of the client's energy fields.

Relaxin A water-soluble protein secreted by the corpus luteum that causes relaxation of the symphysis and cervical dilatation.

Religion An institutionalized system that shares a common set of beliefs and practices.

Respiratory distress syndrome (RDS) Respiratory disease of the newborn characterized by interference with ventilation at the alveolar level, thought to be caused by the presence of fibrinoid deposits lining the alveolar ducts. Formerly called *hyaline membrane disease.*

Retained placenta Retention of the placenta beyond 30 minutes after birth.

Retinopathy (ret-i-nop´ă-thē) **of prematurity (ROP)** Formation of fibrotic tissue behind the lens; associated with retinal detachment and arrested eye growth, seen with hypoxemia in preterm infants.

Rh factor Antigens present on the surface of blood cells that make the blood cell incompatible with blood cells that do not have the antigen.

RhoGAM An anti-Rh (*D*) gamma globulin given after birth to an Rh-negative mother of an Rh-positive fetus or child. Prevents the development of permanent active immunity to the Rh antigen.

Rhythm method The timing of sexual intercourse to avoid the fertile time associated with ovulation.

Risk factors Any findings that suggest the pregnancy may have a negative outcome, for either the woman or her unborn child.

Roles Patterns of behavior normatively defined and expected of an occupant of a given social position.

Rooting reflex An infant's tendency to turn the head and open the lips to suck when one side of the mouth or cheek is touched.

Round ligaments Ligaments that arise from the side of the uterus near the fallopian tube insertion to help the broad ligament keep the uterus in place.

Rugae (rū´ gē) Transverse ridges of mucous membranes lining the vagina that allow the vagina to stretch during the descent of the fetal head.

Rupture of membranes (ROM) Rupture may be PROM (premature), SROM (spontaneous), or AROM (artificial). Some clinicians may use the abbreviation RBOW (rupture of bag of waters).

Sacral promontory A projection into the pelvic cavity on the anterior upper portion of the sacrum; serves as an obstetric guide in determining pelvic measurements.

Salpingitis Infection of the fallopian tubes.

Saltatory pattern A fetal heart rate pattern of marked or excessive variability.

Scalp stimulation test (SST) A test used during labor to assess fetal well-being by pressing a fingertip on the fetal scalp. A fetus not under excessive stress will respond to the digital stimulation with heart rate accelerations.

Scarf sign The position of the elbow when the hand of a supine infant is drawn across to the other shoulder until it meets resistance.

Schultze's mechanism Expulsion of the placenta with the shiny, or fetal, surface presenting first.

Self-quieting activity Infant's ability to use personal resources to quiet and console him- or herself.

Semen Thick whitish fluid ejaculated by the male during orgasm and containing the spermatozoa and their nutrients.

Sepsis neonatorum Infections experienced by a newborn during the first month of life.

Sex chromosomes The X and Y chromosomes, which are responsible for sex determination.

Sexually transmitted infection (STI) Refers to infections ordinarily transmitted by direct sexual contact with an infected individual. Also called *sexually transmitted disease*.

Short-term variability (STV) Refers to the differences between successive heart beats as measured by the R–R wave interval of the QRS cardiac cycle. Measured only by internal electronic fetal monitoring.

Show A pinkish mucous discharge from the vagina that may occur a few hours to a few days prior to the onset of labor.

Simian line A single palmar crease frequently found in children with Down syndrome.

Sinusoidal pattern A waveform of fetal heart rate in which long-term variability is present but there is no short-term variability.

Situational contraceptives Contraceptive methods that involve no prior preparation (eg, abstinence or coitus interruptus).

Skin turgor Elasticity of skin; provides information on hydration status.

Small for gestational age (SGA) Inadequate weight or growth for gestational age; birth weight below the 10th percentile.

Spermatogenesis The process by which mature spermatozoa are formed, during which the number of chromosomes is halved.

Spermatozoa Mature sperm cells of the male animal, produced by the testes.

Spermicides A variety of creams, foams, jellies, and suppositories that, when inserted into the vagina prior to intercourse, destroy sperm or neutralize any vaginal secretions and thereby immobilize sperm.

Spinal block Injection of a local anesthetic agent directly into the spinal fluid in the spinal canal to provide anesthesia for vaginal and cesarean births.

Spinnbarkheit The elasticity of the cervical mucus that is present at ovulation.

Spirituality A belief in a transcendent power pertaining to the spirit or soul.

Spontaneous abortion Abortion that occurs naturally. Also called *miscarriage*.

Spontaneous rupture of membranes (SROM) The breaking of the "water" or membranes marked by the expulsion of amniotic fluid from the vagina.

Station Relationship of the presenting fetal part to an imaginary line drawn between the pelvic ischial spines.

Sterilization An inclusive term that refers to surgical procedures that permanently prevent pregnancy. In the male, sterilization is achieved through a procedure called a vasectomy. In the female, sterilization is done by tubal ligation.

Stillbirth The birth of a dead infant.

Striae (strī´ā) **gravidarum** Stretch marks; shiny reddish lines that appear on the abdomen, breasts, thighs, and buttocks of pregnant women as a result of stretching the skin.

Subconjunctival hemorrhage (sŭb´kon-jŭnk-tī´văl hem´ō rij) Hemorrhage on the sclera of a newborn's eye, usually caused by changes in vascular tension during birth.

Subdermal implants See *Norplant*.

Subfertility A couple who has difficulty conceiving because both partners have reduced fertility.

Subinvolution (sŭb-in-vō-lū´ shŭn) Failure of a part to return to its normal size after functional enlargement, such as failure of the uterus to return to normal size after pregnancy.

Sucking reflex Normal newborn reflex elicited by inserting a finger or nipple in the newborn's mouth, resulting in forceful, rhythmic sucking.

Sudden infant death syndrome (SIDS) The sudden death of an infant; the primary cause of infant death beyond the neonatal period in the United States.

Supine hypotensive syndrome (also called **vena caval syndrome** or **aortocaval compression)** Referring to a condition that can develop during pregnancy when the enlarging uterus puts pressure on the vena cava when the woman is supine. This pressure interferes with returning blood flow and produces a marked decrease in blood pressure with accompanying dizziness, pallor, and clamminess, which can be corrected by having the woman lie on her left side.

Surfactant (ser-fak´tănt) A substance composed of phospholipid, which stabilizes and lowers the surface tension of the alveoli during extrauterine respiratory exhalation, allowing a certain amount of air to remain in the alveoli during expiration.

Suture Fibrous connection of opposed joint surfaces, as in the skull.

Symphysis pubis Fibrocartilaginous joint between the pelvic bones in the midline.

Syndactyly (sin-dak´ti-lē) Malformation of the fingers or toes in which there may be webbing or complete fusion of two or more digits.

Syphilis A chronic, sexually transmitted infection caused by the spirochete *Treponema pallidum*.

Taboos Behaviors or objects that are avoided by individuals or groups.

Telangiectatic nevi (tel-an´jē-ek-tat´ik nē´vī) **(stork bites)** Small clusters of pink-red spots appearing on the nape of the neck and around the eyes of infants; localized areas of capillary dilatation.

Teratogens Nongenetic factors that can produce malformations of the fetus.

Term The normal duration of pregnancy.

Testes The male gonads, in which sperm and testosterone are produced.

Testosterone The male hormone; responsible for the development of secondary male characteristics.

Therapeutic abortion Medically induced termination of pregnancy when a malformed fetus is suspected or when the woman's health is in jeopardy.

Therapeutic insemination Procedure to produce a pregnancy in which sperm obtained from a woman's husband or from a donor is desposited in the woman's vagina.

Therapeutic touch Complementary therapy grounded in the belief that people are a system of energy with a self-healing potential. The therapeutic touch practitioner, often a nurse, unites his or her energy field with that of the client, directing it in a specific way to promote well-being and healing.

Thrombophlebitis Inflammation of a vein wall, resulting in thrombus.

Thrush A fungal infection of the oral mucous membranes caused by *Candida albicans*. Most often seen in infants; characterized by white plaques in the mouth.

Tocolysis Use of medications to arrest preterm labor.

Tonic neck reflex Postural reflex seen in the newborn. When the supine infant's head is turned to one side, the arm and leg on that side extend while the extremities on the opposite side flex. Also called the *fencing position*.

TORCH An acronym used to describe a group of infections that represent potentially severe problems during pregnancy. TO, toxoplasmosis; R, rubella; C, cytomegalovirus; H, herpesvirus.

Total serum bilirubin Sum of conjugated (direct) and unconjugated (indirect) bilirubin.

Touch relaxation A relaxation technique that involves relaxing an area of one's body as another person provides a "touch" cue to that specific area. Touch relaxation is very effective during labor contractions.

Toxic shock syndrome Infection caused by *Staphylococcus aureus*, found primarily in women of reproductive age.

Traditional Chinese medicine (TCM) System of medicine developed more than 3000 years ago in China that seeks to ensure the balance of energy, which is called *chi* or *qi* (pronounced "chee"). Chi is thought to maintain health and vitality and enable the body to carry out its physiologic functions.

Transitional milk Breast milk produced from the end of colostrum production until about 2 weeks postpartum.

Transvaginal ultrasound A follicular monitoring test that is used in women undergoing induction cycles, for timing ovulation for insemination and intercourse, for retrieving oocytes for in vitro fertilization, and for monitoring early pregnancy.

Transverse diameter The largest diameter of the pelvic inlet; helps determine the shape of the inlet.

Transverse lie A lie in which the fetus is positioned crosswise in the uterus.

Trichomonas vaginalis A parasitic protozoan that may cause inflammation of the vagina, characterized by itching and burning of vulvar tissue and by white, frothy discharge.

Trichomoniasis A sexually transmitted infection caused by *Trichomonas vaginalis*, a microscopic motile protozoan that thrives in an alkaline environment.

Trimester Three months, or one third of the gestational time for pregnancy.

Trisomy The presence of three homologous chromosomes rather than the normal two.

Trophoblast The outer layer of the blastoderm that will eventually establish the nutrient relationship with the uterine endometrium.

True pelvis The portion that lies below the linea terminalis, made up of the inlet, cavity, and outlet.

Trunk incurvation (galant reflex) Reflex resulting from the stroking of the spine which causes the pelvis to turn to the stimulated side.

Tubal embryo transfer (TET) Procedure in which eggs are retrieved and incubated with the man's sperm then transferred back into the women's body at the embryo stage.

Tubal ligation Sterilization of a woman accomplished by transecting or occluding the fallopian tubes.

Turner syndrome A number of anomalies that occur when a woman has only one X chromosome. Characteristics include short stature; little sexual differentiation; webbing of the neck, with a low posterior hairline; and congenital cardiac anomalies.

Ultrasound High-frequency sound waves that may be directed, through the use of a transducer, into the maternal abdomen. The ultrasonic sound waves reflected by the underlying structures of varying densities allow identification of various maternal and fetal tissues, bones, and fluids.

Umbilical cord (ŭm-bil´i-kăl kōrd) The structure connecting the placenta to the umbilicus of the fetus and through which nutrients from the woman are exchanged for wastes from the fetus.

Urinary tract infection (UTI) Significant *bacteriuria* in the presence of symptoms.

Uterine atony Relaxation of uterine muscle tone following birth.

Uterine inversion Prolapse of the uterine fundus through the cervix into the vagina; may occur just prior to or during expulsion of the placenta; associated with massive hemorrhage, requiring emergency treatment.

Uterosacral ligaments Ligaments that provide support for the uterus and cervix at the level of the ischial spines.

Uterus The hollow muscular organ in which the fertilized ovum is implanted and in which the developing fetus is nourished until birth.

Vacuum extraction An obstetric procedure used to assist in the birth of a fetus by applying suction to the fetal head with a soft suction cup attached to a suction bottle (pump) by tubing and placing the device against the occiput of the fetal head.

Vagina The musculomembranous tube or passageway located between the external genitals and the uterus of a woman.

Vaginal birth after cesarean (VBAC) Practice of permitting a trial of labor and possible vaginal birth for women following a previous cesarean birth for nonrecurring causes such as fetal distress or placenta previa.

Variable deceleration Periodic change in fetal heart rate caused by umbilical cord compression; decelerations vary in onset, occurrence, and waveform.

Vasa previa Condition occurring when the fetal vessels course through membranes and are present at the cervical os. Although this is a rare cause of antepartum bleeding, it has a high rate of fetal death.

Vasectomy Surgical removal of a portion of the vas deferens (ductus deferens) to produce infertility.

Vegan A "pure" vegetarian; one who consumes no food from animal sources.

Vena caval syndrome Symptoms of dizziness, pallor, and clamminess that result from lowered blood pressure when a pregnant woman lies supine and the enlarged uterus presses on the vena cava. Also known as supine hypotensive syndrome.

Vernix caseosa (ver´niks kā´sē-ō-sā) A protective, cheeselike, whitish substance made up of sebum and desquamated epithelial cells that is present on the fetal skin.

Version Turning of the fetus in utero.

Vertex The top or crown of the head.

Vibroacoustic stimulation Application of device delivering 90 dB of sound and vibration for 1 to 3 seconds to the mother's abdomen to stimulate movement in the fetus, thereby accelerating the fetal heart rate. (Also called FAST for fetal acoustic stimulation test or VST for vibroacoustic stimulation test.)

Vicarious trauma (also called secondary trauma effect) A condition that can occur as a result of working with people who are trauma victims.

Visualization Complementary therapy in which a person goes into a relaxed state and focuses on or "visualizes" soothing or positive scenes such as a beach or a mountain glade. Visualization helps reduce stress and encourage relaxation.

Vulva The external structure of the female genitals, lying below the mons veneris.

Vulvovaginal candidiasis (VVC) Also called moniliasis or yeast infection, VVC is a genital infection most often caused by *Candida albicans*.

Weaning The process of discontinuing breastfeeding and accustoming an infant to another feeding method.

Wharton's *(hwar'tunz)* **jelly** Yellow-white gelatinous material surrounding the vessels of the umbilical cord.

Zona pellucida Transparent inner layer surrounding an ovum.

Zygote A fertilized egg.

Zygote intrafallopian transfer (ZIFT) Retrieval of oocytes under ultrasound guidance, followed by in vitro fertilization and laparoscopic replacement of fertilized eggs into the fimbriated end of the fallopian tube.

Index

D

SINGLE PC LICENSE AGREEMENT AND LIMITED WARRANTY

READ THIS LICENSE CAREFULLY BEFORE OPENING THIS PACKAGE. BY OPENING THIS PACKAGE, YOU ARE AGREEING TO THE TERMS AND CONDITIONS OF THIS LICENSE. IF YOU DO NOT AGREE, DO NOT OPEN THE PACKAGE. PROMPTLY RETURN THE UNOPENED PACKAGE AND ALL ACCOMPANYING ITEMS TO THE PLACE YOU OBTAINED THEM. ***THESE TERMS APPLY TO ALL LICENSED SOFTWARE ON THE DISK EXCEPT THAT THE TERMS FOR USE OF ANY SHAREWARE OR FREEWARE ON THE DISKETTES ARE AS SET FORTH IN THE ELECTRONIC LICENSE LOCATED ON THE DISK:***

1. GRANT OF LICENSE and OWNERSHIP: The enclosed computer programs and data ("Software") are licensed, not sold, to you by Pearson Education, Inc. ("We" or the "Company") and in consideration of your purchase or adoption of the accompanying Company textbooks and/or other materials, and your agreement to these terms. We reserve any rights not granted to you. You own only the disk(s) but we and/or our licensors own the Software itself. This license allows you to use and display your copy of the Software on a single computer (i.e., with a single CPU) at a single location for academic use only, so long as you comply with the terms of this Agreement. You may make one copy for back up, or transfer your copy to another CPU, provided that the Software is usable on only one computer.

2. RESTRICTIONS: You may not transfer or distribute the Software or documentation to anyone else. Except for backup, you may not copy the documentation or the Software. You may not network the Software or otherwise use it on more than one computer or computer terminal at the same time. You may not reverse engineer, disassemble, decompile, modify, adapt, translate, or create derivative works based on the Software or the Documentation. You may be held legally responsible for any copying or copyright infringement which is caused by your failure to abide by the terms of these restrictions.

3. TERMINATION: This license is effective until terminated. This license will terminate automatically without notice from the Company if you fail to comply with any provisions or limitations of this license. Upon termination, you shall destroy the Documentation and all copies of the Software. All provisions of this Agreement as to limitation and disclaimer of warranties, limitation of liability, remedies or damages, and our ownership rights shall survive termination.

4. LIMITED WARRANTY AND DISCLAIMER OF WARRANTY: Company warrants that for a period of 60 days from the date you purchase this SOFTWARE (or purchase or adopt the accompanying textbook), the Software, when properly installed and used in accordance with the Documentation, will operate in substantial conformity with the description of the Software set forth in the Documentation, and that for a period of 30 days the disk(s) on which the Software is delivered shall be free from defects in materials and workmanship under normal use. The Company does not warrant that the Software will meet your requirements or that the operation of the Software will be uninterrupted or error-free. Your only remedy and the Company's only obligation under these limited warranties is, at the Company's option, return of the disk for a refund of any amounts paid for it by you or replacement of the disk. THIS LIMITED WARRANTY IS THE ONLY WARRANTY PROVIDED BY THE COMPANY AND ITS LICENSORS, AND THE COMPANY AND ITS LICENSORS DISCLAIM ALL OTHER WARRANTIES, EXPRESS OR IMPLIED, INCLUDING WITHOUT LIMITATION, THE IMPLIED WARRANTIES OF MERCHANTABILITY AND FITNESS FOR A PARTICULAR PURPOSE. THE COMPANY DOES NOT WARRANT, GUARANTEE OR MAKE ANY REPRESENTATION REGARDING THE ACCURACY, RELIABILITY, CURRENTNESS, USE, OR RESULTS OF USE, OF THE SOFTWARE.

5. LIMITATION OF REMEDIES AND DAMAGES: IN NO EVENT, SHALL THE COMPANY OR ITS EMPLOYEES, AGENTS, LICENSORS, OR CONTRACTORS BE LIABLE FOR ANY INCIDENTAL, INDIRECT, SPECIAL, OR CONSEQUENTIAL DAMAGES ARISING OUT OF OR IN CONNECTION WITH THIS LICENSE OR THE SOFTWARE, INCLUDING FOR LOSS OF USE, LOSS OF DATA, LOSS OF INCOME OR PROFIT, OR OTHER LOSSES, SUSTAINED AS A RESULT OF INJURY TO ANY PERSON, OR LOSS OF OR DAMAGE TO PROPERTY, OR CLAIMS OF THIRD PARTIES, EVEN IF THE COMPANY OR AN AUTHORIZED REPRESENTATIVE OF THE COMPANY HAS BEEN ADVISED OF THE POSSIBILITY OF SUCH DAMAGES. IN NO EVENT SHALL THE LIABILITY OF THE COMPANY FOR DAMAGES WITH RESPECT TO THE SOFTWARE EXCEED THE AMOUNTS ACTUALLY PAID BY YOU, IF ANY, FOR THE SOFTWARE OR THE ACCOMPANYING TEXTBOOK. BECAUSE SOME JURISDICTIONS DO NOT ALLOW THE LIMITATION OF LIABILITY IN CERTAIN CIRCUMSTANCES, THE ABOVE LIMITATIONS MAY NOT ALWAYS APPLY TO YOU.

6. GENERAL: THIS AGREEMENT SHALL BE CONSTRUED IN ACCORDANCE WITH THE LAWS OF THE UNITED STATES OF AMERICA AND THE STATE OF NEW YORK, APPLICABLE TO CONTRACTS MADE IN NEW YORK, AND SHALL BENEFIT THE COMPANY, ITS AFFILIATES AND ASSIGNEES. HIS AGREEMENT IS THE COMPLETE AND EXCLUSIVE STATEMENT OF THE AGREEMENT BETWEEN YOU AND THE COMPANY AND SUPERSEDES ALL PROPOSALS OR PRIOR AGREEMENTS, ORAL, OR WRITTEN, AND ANY OTHER COMMUNICATIONS BETWEEN YOU AND THE COMPANY OR ANY REPRESENTATIVE OF THE COMPANY RELATING TO THE SUBJECT MATTER OF THIS AGREEMENT. If you are a U.S. Government user, this Software is licensed with "restricted rights" as set forth in subparagraphs (a)-(d) of the Commercial Computer-Restricted Rights clause at FAR 52.227-19 or in subparagraphs (c)(1)(ii) of the Rights in Technical Data and Computer Software clause at DFARS 252.227-7013, and similar clauses, as applicable.

Should you have any questions concerning this agreement or if you wish to contact the Company for any reason, please contact in writing: Prentice-Hall, New Media Department, One Lake Street, Upper Saddle River, NJ 07458.